ROOK / WILKINSON / EBLING

Textbook of Dermatology

ROOK/WILKINSON/EBLING

Textbook of Dermatology

EDITED BY

R.H.CHAMPION
MA, MB, BChir, FRCP
Emeritus Consultant Dermatologist, Department of Dermatology,
Addenbrooke's Hospital, Cambridge

J.L.BURTON
BSc, MD, FRCP
Professor of Dermatology
University of Bristol, Bristol

D.A.BURNS
MB BS, FRCP, FRCP(Edin)
Consultant Dermatologist and Honorary Senior Lecturer in Dermatology,
Department of Dermatology, Leicester Royal Infirmary, Leicester

S.M.BREATHNACH
MA, MB, BChir, MD, PhD, FRCP
Consultant Dermatologist and Senior Lecturer,
St John's Institute of Dermatology, St Thomas's Hospital, London
Consultant Dermatologist,
Epsom Healthcare NHS Trust, Epsom, Surrey

IN FOUR VOLUMES
VOLUME 4

SIXTH EDITION

b
Blackwell
Science

© 1968, 1972, 1979, 1986, 1992, 1998 by
Blackwell Science Ltd
Editorial Offices:
Osney Mead, Oxford OX2 0EL
25 John Street, London WC1N 2BL
23 Ainslie Place, Edinburgh EH3 6AJ
350 Main Street, Malden
  MA 02148 5018, USA
54 University Street, Carlton
  Victoria 3053, Australia
10, rue Casimir Delavigne
  75006 Paris, France

Other Editorial Offices:
Blackwell Wissenschafts-Verlag GmbH
Kurfürstendamm 57
10707 Berlin, Germany

Blackwell Science KK
MG Kodenmacho Building
7–10 Kodenmacho Nihombashi
Chuo-ku, Tokyo 104, Japan

The right of the Authors to be
identified as the Authors of this Work
has been asserted in accordance
with the Copyright, Designs and
Patents Act 1988.

Set by Setrite Typesetters, Hong Kong
Printed and bound in Italy by
Rotolito Lombarda S.p.A., Milan

First published 1968
Reprinted 1969
Second edition 1972
Reprinted 1975
Third edition 1979
Reprinted 1982, 1984
Fourth edition 1986
Reprinted 1988, 1990
Fifth edition 1992
Reprinted 1993, 1994
Sixth edition 1998

The Blackwell Science logo is a
trade mark of Blackwell Science Ltd,
registered at the United Kingdom
Trade Marks Registry

DISTRIBUTORS
Marston Book Services Ltd
PO Box 269
Abingdon, Oxon OX14 4YN
(*Orders*: Tel: 01235 465500
          Fax: 01235 465555)
USA
Blackwell Science, Inc.
Commerce Place
350 Main Street
Malden, MA 02148 5018
(*Orders*: Tel: 800 759 6102
          781 388 8250
          Fax: 781 388 8255)
Canada
Login Brothers Book Company
324 Saulteaux Crescent
Winnipeg, Manitoba R3J 3TZ
(*Orders*: Tel: 204 224-4068)

Australia
Blackwell Science Pty Ltd
54 University Street
Carlton, Victoria 3053
(*Orders*: Tel: 3 9347 0300
          Fax: 3 9347 5001)

A catalogue record for this title
is available from the British Library

ISBN 0-632-03796-2 (BSL)
    0-632-04904-9 (CD-ROM)

Library of Congress
Cataloging-in-publication data

Rook/Wilkinson/Ebling textbook of
  dermatology.—6th ed./edited by R.H.
  Champion . . . [et al.]
      p.   cm.
    Rev. ed. of: Textbook of dermatology/
  edited by Arthur Rook, D.S. Wilkinson,
  F.J.G. Ebling. 2nd ed. 1972.
  Includes bibliographical references and
  index.
  ISBN 0-632-03796-2. —
  ISBN 0-632-04904-9 (CD-ROM)
    1 Skin—Diseases. 2 Dermatology.
  I Rook, Arthur. II Wilkinson, D.S.
  (Darrell Sheldon) III Ebling, F.J.G.
  (Francis John Govier), 1918–   . IV
  Champion, Robert H.V. Rook, Arthur.
  Textbook of dermatology.
    [DNLM: 1 Skin Diseases. WR 140
  R7771 1998]
  RL71.R744 1998
  616.5—dc21
  DNLM/DLC
  for Library of Congress   97-51464
                                       CIP

Contents

Contributors

ADRIAANS, Beverley
MD, FRCP
Consultant Dermatologist, Greenwich District Hospital,
    Vanbrugh Hill, Greenwich, London SE10 9HE
Co-author of
    Chapter 27: Bacterial Infections

ARCHER, Clive B
BSc, MB BS, MD, PhD(Lond), FRCP(Lond & Edin)
Consultant Dermatologist and Clinical Senior Lecturer,
    Department of Dermatology, Bristol Royal Infirmary
    (UBHT), Bristol BS2 8HW
Author of
    Chapter 4: Functions of the Skin
    Chapter 63: The Skin and the Nervous System

ATHERTON, David John
MA, MB, BChir, FRCP
Consultant Dermatologist and Senior Lecturer, Department of
    Dermatology, Great Ormond Street Hospital for Children,
    London WC1N 3JH
Author of
    Chapter 14: The Neonate
    Chapter 15: Naevi and other Developmental Defects

BARAN, Robert
MD
Head of Nail Disease Centre, 42 rue des Serbes,
    06400 Cannes, France
Co-author of
    Chapter 65: Disorders of Nails

BLACK, Martin Munro
MD, FRCP, FRCPath
Consultant Dermatologist and Chairman, Department of
    Dermatology, St John's Institute of Dermatology, St
    Thomas's Hospital, Lambeth Palace Road, London SE1 7EH
Author of
    Chapter 41: Lichen Planus and Lichenoid Disorders
Co-author of
    Chapter 57: Subcutaneous Fat
    Chapter 59: Metabolic and Nutritional Disorders

BLEEHEN, Stanley Sholom
BA, MB, BChir, FRCP
Emeritus Professor of Dermatology, Department of Medicine,
    University of Sheffield
Honorary Consultant Dermatologist, St John's Institute of
    Dermatology, St Thomas's Hospital, Lambeth Palace Road,
    London SE1 7EH
Author of
    Chapter 39: Disorders of Skin Colour

BREATHNACH, Stephen Michael
MA, MB, BChir, MD, PhD, FRCP
Consultant Dermatologist and Senior Lecturer, St John's
    Institute of Dermatology, St Thomas's Hospital, Lambeth
    Palace Road, London SE1 7EH
Consultant Dermatologist, Epsom Healthcare NHS Trust,
    Dorking Road, Epsom, Surrey KTI8 7EG
Editor
Author of
    Chapter 77: Drug Reactions
Co-author of
    Chapter 10: Clinical Immunology and Allergy

BRYCESON, Anthony David Malcolm
MD, FRCPE, FRCP, DTM&H
Consultant Physician, Hospital for Tropical Diseases, 4 St
    Pancras Way, London NW1 0PE
Professor of Tropical Medicine, London School of Hygiene and
    Tropical Medicine, Keppel Street, London WC1E 7HT
Co-author of
    Chapter 29: Leprosy
    Chapter 32: Parasitic Worms and Protozoa

BURD, Andrew
MD, FRCS(Edin)
Consultant Plastic Surgeon, Department of Plastic Surgery,
    Frenchay Hospital, Bristol BS16 1LE
Contributor to
    Chapter 23: Mechanical and Thermal Injury

BURGE, Susan M
BSc, DM, FRCP

Consultant Dermatologist, Department of Dermatology, The
Oxford Radcliffe Hospital, Headington, Oxford OX3 7LJ
Co-author of
Chapter 40: Bullous Eruptions

BURNAND, Kevin Guiver
MB BS, FRCS
Professor of Surgery and Chairman, Department of Surgery,
UMDS, St Thomas's Hospital, Lambeth Palace Road,
London SE1 7EH
Co-author of
Chapter 50: Diseases of the Veins and Arteries: Leg Ulcers

BURNS, David Anthony
MB BS, FRCP, FRCP(Edin)
Consultant Dermatologist and Honorary Senior Lecturer in
Dermatology, Department of Dermatology, Leicester Royal
Infirmary, Leicester LE1 5WW
Editor
Author of
Chapter 33: Diseases caused by Arthropods and other
Noxious Animals
Co-author of
Chapter 2: Comparative Dermatology

BURTON, John Lloyd
BSc, MD, FRCP
Professor of Dermatology, Department of Dermatology, Bristol
Royal Infirmary (UBHT), Bristol BS2 8HW
Address for correspondence: Norland House, 33 Canynge Road,
Bristol BS8 3LD
Editor
Author of
Chapter 71: The Breast
Co-author of
Chapter 1: Introduction and Historical Bibliography
Chapter 5: Diagnosis of Skin Disease
Chapter 17: Eczema, Lichenification and Prurigo
Chapter 44: Disorders of Connective Tissue
Chapter 67: The Skin and the Eyes
Chapter 70: The Lips

CAMP, Richard Doyle Reginal
PhD, FRCP, FFDerm(SA)
Professor of Dermatology, Division of Dermatology, University
of Leicester, Maurice Shock Medical Sciences Building,
University Road, Leicester LE1 9HN
Author of
Chapter 35: Psoriasis

CERIO, Rino
BSc, MB BS, FRCP(Edin & Lond), DipRCPath
Consultant Dermatologist and Clinical Director, Department of
Dermatology, Royal London Hospital, Whitechapel Road,
London E1 1BB

Senior Lecturer in Dermatopathology, Institute of Pathology,
St Bartholomew's and Royal London School of Medicine
and Dentistry, London E1 1BD
Author of
Chapter 7: Histopathology of the Skin: General Principles

CHAMPION, Robert Harold
MA, MB, BChir, FRCP
Emeritus Consultant Dermatologist, Department of
Dermatology, Addenbrooke's Hospital, Cambridge
CB2 2QQ
Address for correspondence: 7 Dogget Lane, Fulbourn, Cambridge
CB1 5BT
Editor
Author of
Chapter 43: Disorders of Sweat Glands
Co-author of
Chapter 1: Introduction and Historical Bibliography
Chapter 5: Diagnosis of Skin Disease
Chapter 45: Disorders of Blood Vessels
Chapter 47: Urticaria
Chapter 48: Purpura

CHU, Anthony C
MB, BSc, FRCP
Senior Lecturer and Honorary Consultant Dermatologist,
Imperial College of Science, Technology and Medicine,
Hammersmith Hospital, Du Cane Road, London W12 0HS
Author of
Chapter 53: Histiocytoses

COTTERILL, John Anthony
BSc, MD, FRCP
Consultant Dermatologist, Department of Dermatology, BUPA
Hospital, Leeds LS8 1NT
Co-author of
Chapter 64: Psychocutaneous Disorders
Chapter 75: General Aspects of Treatment

CUNLIFFE, William James
MD, FRCP
Professor of Dermatology, Department of Dermatology,
General Infirmary at Leeds, Great George Street, Leeds
LS1 3EX
Author of
Chapter 52: Necrobiotic Disorders
Co-author of
Chapter 42: Disorders of the Sebaceous Glands
Chapter 57: Subcutaneous Fat

DAWBER, Rodney Peter Richard
MA, MB, ChB, FRCP
Consultant Dermatologist, Department of Dermatology, The
Oxford Radcliffe Hospital, Headington, Oxford OX3 7LJ

Co-author of
    Chapter 65: Disorders of Nails
    Chapter 66: Disorders of Hair
    Chapter 80: Physical and Laser Therapies
    Chapter 81: Dermatological Surgery

de BERKER, David
BA, MRCP
Consultant Dermatologist and Clinical Senior Lecturer,
    Department of Dermatology, Bristol Royal Infirmary
    (UBHT), Bristol BS2 8HW
Co-author of
    Chapter 65: Disorders of Nails
    Chapter 66: Disorders of Hair

DOWD, Pauline M
MD, FRCP
Professor of Dermatology and Consultant Dermatologist,
    Department of Dermatology, Middlesex Hospital, Mortimer
    Street, London W1N 8AA
Author of
    Chapter 24: Reactions to Cold
Co-author of
    Chapter 45: Disorders of Blood Vessels
    Chapter 48: Purpura

EADY, Robin Anthony Jeffrey
MB BS, FRCP, DSc (Med)
Professor of Experimental Dermatopathology and Consultant
    Dermatologist, St John's Institute of Dermatology, Lambeth
    Palace Road, St Thomas's Hospital, London SE1 7EH
Author of
    Chapter 13: Prenatal Diagnosis of Genetic Skin Disease
Co-author of
    Chapter 3: Anatomy and Organization of Human Skin
    Chapter 40: Bullous Eruptions

EBLING, Francis John Govier [Deceased]
DSc, PhD, CBiol
Emeritus Professor of Zoology, Independent Research Worker
    in Dermatology, Academic Division of Medicine, Royal
    Hallamshire Hospital, Sheffield S10 2JF
Co-author of
    Chapter 2: Comparative Dermatology

FERGUSON, Mark William James
BSc, BDS, PhD, FFD, FDS
Professor of Cell and Structural Biology, The School of
    Biological Sciences, 3.239 Stopford Building, University of
    Manchester, Oxford Road, Manchester M13 9PT
Co-author of
    Chapter 11: Wound Healing

GAWKRODGER, David John
MD, FRCP, FRCPE
Consultant Dermatologist and Honorary Clinical Lecturer in

Dermatology, University of Sheffield, Royal Hallamshire
    Hospital, Sheffield S10 2JF
Author of
    Chapter 28: Mycobacterial Infections
    Chapter 60: Sarcoidosis
    Chapter 73: Racial Influences on Skin Disease
Co-author of
    Chapter 59: Metabolic and Nutritional Disorders

GOODFIELD, Mark Jeremy David
MA, MB, BChir, MRCP
Consultant Dermatologist, Department of Dermatology, Leeds
    General Infirmary, Great George Street, Leeds LS1 3EX
Co-author of
    Chapter 58: The 'Connective Tissue Diseases'

GRAHAM, Robert Martin
MB, FRCP
Consultant Dermatologist, Dermatology Department, James
    Paget Healthcare NHS Trust, Gorleston, Great Yarmouth
    and Waveney District, Norfolk NR31 6LA
Author of
    Chapter 62: Reiter's Disease
Co-author of
    Chapter 61: Systemic Disease and the Skin

GRAHAM-BROWN, Robin Alan Charles
BSc, MB BS, FRCP
Consultant and Honorary Senior Lecturer in Dermatology,
    Department of Dermatology, Leicester Royal Infirmary,
    Leicester LE1 5WW
Author of
    Chapter 74: The Ages of Man and their Dermatoses

GREAVES, Malcolm Watson
MD, PhD, FRCP
Professor of Clinical Dermatology and Consultant
    Dermatologist, St John's Institute of Dermatology,
    St Thomas's Hospital, Lambeth Palace Road, London
    SE1 7EH
Author of
    Chapter 16: Pruritus
    Chapter 46: Flushing and Flushing Syndromes, Rosacea and
        Perioral Dermatitis
    Chapter 54: Mastocytoses
Co-author of
    Chapter 76: Systemic Therapy

GRIFFITHS, William Andrew David
MA, MD, FRCP
Consultant Dermatologist, St John's Institute of Dermatology,
    St Thomas's Hospital, Lambeth Palace Road, London
    SE1 7EH
Co-author of
    Chapter 34: Disorders of Keratinization
    Chapter 78: Topical Therapy

HARPER, John Irwin
MD, FRCP, FRCPCH
Consultant in Paediatric Dermatology, Great Ormond Street
  Hospital for Children, London WC1N 3JH
Author of
  Chapter 12: Genetics and Genodermatoses

HARRAD, Richard A
MA, MRCP, FRCOphth
Consultant Ophthalmic Surgeon, Bristol Eye Hospital, Lower
  Maudlin Street, Bristol BS1 2LX
Co-author of
  Chapter 67: The Skin and the Eyes

HAWK, John LM
BSc, MD, FRACP, FRCP
Consultant Dermatologist and Head of Photobiology
  Department, St John's Institute of Dermatology, St Thomas's
  Hospital, Lambeth Palace Road, London SE1 7EH
Author of
  Chapter 25: Cutaneous Photobiology

HAY, Roderick James
MA, DM, FRCP, FRCPath
Mary Dunhill Professor of Cutaneous Medicine, St John's
  Institute of Dermatology, Guy's Hospital, London SE1 9RT
Co-author of
  Chapter 27: Bacterial Infections
  Chapter 31: Mycology
  Chapter 32: Parasitic Worms and Protozoa
  Chapter 76: Systemic Therapy

HOLDEN, Colin Arthur
BSc, MD, FRCP
Consultant Dermatologist, Department of Dermatology,
  St Helier Hospital, Carshalton, Surrey SM5 1AA
Co-author of
  Chapter 17: Eczema, Lichenification and Prurigo
  Chapter 18: Atopic Dermatitis

IVE, Francis Adrian
MB BS, FRCP
Consultant Dermatologist, Department of Dermatology,
  Dryburn Hospital, North Road, Durham DH1 5TW
Author of
  Chapter 72: The Umbilical, Perianal and Genital Regions

JUDGE, Mary R
MD, MRCP(Ireland & Lond), DCH
Consultant Dermatologist, Royal Bolton Hospital, Farnworth,
  Bolton BL4 0JR
Consultant Paediatric Dermatologist, Hope Hospital, Salford
  M6 8HD
Co-author of
  Chapter 34: Disorders of Keratinization

KENNEDY, Cameron Thomas Campbell
MA, MB, BChir, FRCP
Consultant Paediatric Dermatologist, Bristol Royal Hospital for
  Sick Children, St Michael's Hill, Bristol BS2 8BJ
Consultant Dermatologist and Clinical Senior Lecturer,
  Department of Dermatology, Bristol Royal Infirmary
  (UBHT), Bristol BS2 8HW
Author of
  Chapter 23: Mechanical and Thermal Injury
  Chapter 68: The External Ear

KERDEL-VEGAS, Francisco
CBE, MD, MSc, FACP
Former Professor of Dermatology, Central University of
  Venezuela
Ambassador of Venezuela to France, 11 rue Copernic, 75116
  Paris, France
Contributor to
  Chapter 30: The Treponematoses
  Chapter 32: Parasitic Worms and Protozoa

KOBZA BLACK, Anne
MD, FRCP
Consultant Dermatologist and Senior Lecturer, St John's
  Institute of Dermatology, St Thomas's Hospital, Lambeth
  Palace Road, London SE1 7EH
Co-author of
  Chapter 47: Urticaria

KURTZ, John Bellair
MA, MB, BChir, MRCP, FRCPath
Consultant Virologist, John Radcliffe Hospital, Oxford
  OX3 9DU
Co-author of
  Chapter 26: Viral Infections

LAWRENCE, Clifford M
MD, FRCP
Consultant Dermatologist, Department of Dermatology, Royal
  Victoria Infirmary, Queen Victoria Road, Newcastle upon
  Tyne NE1 4LP
Co-author of
  Chapter 80: Physical and Laser Therapies
  Chapter 81: Dermatological Surgery

LEIGH, Irene May
MD, FRCP
Professor of Dermatology, Centre for Cutaneous Research, St
  Bartholomew's and Royal London School of Medicine and
  Dentistry, Queen Mary and Westfield College, 2 Newark
  Street, London E1 2AT
Co-author of
  Chapter 3: Anatomy and Organization of Human Skin
  Chapter 11: Wound Healing
  Chapter 34: Disorders of Keratinization

LOCKWOOD, Diana NJ
BSc, MD, MRCP
Consultant Leprologist, Hospital for Tropical Diseases,
    4 St Pancras Way, London NW1 0PE
London School of Hygiene and Tropical Medicine, Keppel
    Street, London, WC1E 7HT
Co-author of
    Chapter 29: Leprosy

LOVELL, Christopher R
MD, FRCP
Consultant Dermatologist, Kinghorn Dermatology Unit, Royal
    United Hospital, Combe Park, Bath BA1 3NG
Co-author of
    Chapter 44: Disorders of Connective Tissue

MACKIE, Rona McLeod
MD, DSc, FRCP, FRCPath, FRSE
Professor of Dermatology, Department of Dermatology,
    Robertson Building, University of Glasgow, Glasgow
    G12 8QQ
Author of
    Chapter 36: Epidermal Skin Tumours
    Chapter 37: Tumours of the Skin Appendages
    Chapter 38: Melanocytic Naevi and Malignant Melanoma
    Chapter 55: Soft-Tissue Tumours
    Chapter 56: Cutaneous Lymphomas and Lymphocytic
        Infiltrates

MILLARD, Leslie Graham
MD, FRCP(Lond & Edin)
Consultant Dermatologist, Skin Surgery Suite, Department of
    Dermatology, C Floor South Block, Queen's Medical Centre,
    Nottingham NG7 2UH
Co-author of
    Chapter 64: Psychocutaneous Disorders

MOORE, Mary
MA, PhD
Lecturer, Mycology Department, UMDS, St John's Institute of
    Dermatology, St Thomas's Hospital, Lambeth Palace Road,
    London SE1 7EH
Co-author of
    Chapter 31: Mycology

MORTIMER, Peter S
MD, FRCP
Consultant Skin Physician, Department of Dermatology,
    St George's Hospital, London SW17 0QT
Reader in Dermatology, University of London, St George's
    Hospital Medical School, London SW17 0RE
Author of
    Chapter 51: Disorders of Lymphatic Vessels

MORTON, Robert Steel
MBE, MD, FRCP(Edin), DHMSA

Honorary Lecturer in History of Medicine, University of
    Sheffield
Address for correspondence: 9 Cotworth Road, Sheffield S11 9LN
Author of
    Chapter 30: The Treponematoses

PARISH, William Everett
MA, PhD, BVSc, MRCVS, FRCPath
Principal Scientist, Unilever Research, Colworth Laboratory,
    Colworth House, Sharnbrook, Bedford MK44 1LQ
Author of
    Chapter 9: Inflammation
Co-author of
    Chapter 10: Clinical Immunology and Allergy
    Chapter 18: Atopic Dermatitis
Contributor to
    Chapter 7: Histopathology of the Skin: General Principles

POPE, F Michael
MB BCh, MD, FRCP (Lond, Edin & Glas)
Honorary Head of MRC Connective Tissue Genetics Group,
    Institute of Medical Genetics, University Hospital, Heath
    Park, Cardiff, CF4 4XN
Consultant Dermatologist, Department of Dermatology,
    Princess of Wales Hospital, Bridgend and District NHS
    Trust, Bridgend CF31 1YE
Co-author of
    Chapter 3: Anatomy and Organization of Human Skin

REES, Jonathan L
MB BS, B Med Sci, FRCP
Professor of Dermatology, Medical School, University of
    Newcastle, Framlington Place, Newcastle upon Tyne
    NE2 4HH
Author of
    Chapter 8: Molecular Biology

ROWELL, Neville Robinson
MD, FRCP, DCH
Emeritus Professor of Dermatology, University of Leeds
Address for Correspondence
    15 Radlyn Oval, 20 Park Avenue, Harrogate, North
    Yorkshire HG2 9BG
Co-author of
    Chapter 58: The 'Connective Tissue Diseases'

RYAN, Terence John
DM(Oxon), FRCP
President of the International Society of Dermatology and
    Emeritus Professor of Dermatology, Oxford University and
    Oxford Brookes University
Address for correspondence: Hill House, Abberbury Avenue,
    Iffley, Oxford, OX4 4EU
Author of
    Chapter 49: Cutaneous Vasculitis

Co-author of
    Chapter 50: Diseases of the Veins and Arteries: Leg Ulcers

RYCROFT, Richard John Graham
MD, FRCP, FFOM, DIH
Consultant Dermatologist, St John's Institute of Dermatology, St Thomas's Hospital, Lambeth Palace Road, London SE1 7EH
Author of
    Chapter 21: Principal Irritants and Sensitizers
    Chapter 22: Occupational Dermatoses

SCULLY, Crispian
MD, PhD, MDS, FDS, FFD, FRCPath
Dean and Director, Eastman Dental Institute, University of London, 256 Gray's Inn Road, London WC1X 8LD
Author of
    Chapter 69: The Oral Cavity
Co-author of
    Chapter 70: The Lips

SEYMOUR, Carol Anne
BM, BCh, MA(Oxon), MA(Cantab), MSc, PhD, MRCPath FRCP
Professor of Clinical Biochemistry and Metabolic Medicine, Division of Cardiological Sciences, St George's Hospital Medical School, London SW17 0RE
Co-author of
    Chapter 59: Metabolic and Nutritional Disorders

SHAW, Stephanie
MB, ChB, FRCP
Honorary Consultant Dermatologist, Department of Dermatology, Amersham General Hospital, Whielden Street, Amersham, Bucks HP7 0JD
Co-author of
    Chapter 20: Contact Dermatitis: Allergic

SIMPSON, Nicholas B
MD, FRCP(Lond & Glas)
Consultant Dermatologist, Department of Dermatology, Royal Victoria Infirmary, Queen Victoria Road, Newcastle upon Tyne NE1 4LP
Co-author of
    Chapter 42: Disorders of the Sebaceous Glands

SPITTLE, Margaret Flora
MSc, FRCP, FRCR
Consultant Clinical Oncologist, Meyerstein Institute of Oncology, The Middlesex Hospital, Mortimer Street, London W1N 8AA
St John's Institute of Dermatology, St Thomas's Hospital, Lambeth Palace Road, London SE1 7EH
Author of
    Chapter 79: Radiotherapy and Reactions to Ionizing Radiation

STERLING, Jane Carolyn
MA, MB, BChir, PhD, FRCP
Consultant Dermatologist and Clinical Lecturer Department of Dermatology, Addenbrooke's Hospital, Hills Road, Cambridge CB2 2QQ
Co-author of
    Chapter 26: Viral Infections

WALKER, Neil Patrick John
BSc, MB BS, FRCP
Department of Dermatology, The Oxford Radcliffe Hospital, Headington, Oxford OX3 7LJ
Co-author of
    Chapter 80: Physical and Laser Therapies
    Chapter 81: Dermatological Surgery

WARIN, Andrew Peter
MB, FRCP
Consultant Dermatologist, Royal Devon and Exeter Hospital, Exeter, Devon EX2 5DW
Co-author of
    Chapter 75: General Aspects of Treatment
    Chapter 76: Systemic Therapy

WEISMANN, Kaare
MD, PhD
Consultant Dermatologist, Department of Dermatology, Bispebjerg Hospital, DK-2400 Copenhagen NV, Denmark
Co-author of
    Chapter 59: Metabolic and Nutritional Disorders
    Chapter 61: Systemic Disease and the Skin

WILKINSON, Darrell Sheldon
MD, FRCP
Retired Consultant Dermatologist, Whitecroft, Hervines Road, Amersham, Bucks HP6 5HT
Author of
    Chapter 83: Glossary of Dermatological Terms

WILKINSON, John Darrell
MB BS, MRCS, FRCP
Consultant Dermatologist, Department of Dermatology, Amersham General Hospital, Whielden Street, Amersham, Bucks HP7 0JD
Author of
    Chapter 82: Formulary of Topical Applications
Co-author of
    Chapter 19: Contact Dermatitis: Irritant
    Chapter 20: Contact Dermatitis: Allergic
    Chapter 78: Topical Therapy

WILLIAMS, Hywel C
MSc, PhD, FRCP
Senior Lecturer in Dermato-Epidemiology, Department of Dermatology, Queen's Medical Centre, Nottingham NG7 2UH

Author of
    Chapter 6: Epidemiology of Skin Disease

WILLIS, Carolyn M
BSc, PhD
Research Director, Department of Dermatology, Amersham
    General Hospital, Whielden Street, Amersham, Bucks
    HP7 0JD
Co-author of
    Chapter 19: Contact Dermatitis: Irritant

WOJNAROWSKA, Fenella
MA, MSc, BM, BChir, DM, FRCP
Reader in Dermatology, University of Oxford Consultant
    Dermatologist, Department of Dermatology, The Oxford
    Radcliffe Hospital, Headington, Oxford OX3 7LJ
Co-author of
    Chapter 40: Bullous Eruptions
    Chapter 66: Disorders of Hair

Preface to the Sixth Edition

Thirty years have passed since the first edition of *Textbook of Dermatology* was published under the leadership of Arthur Rook, Darrell Wilkinson and John Ebling.

Arthur Rook, a wise clinician with an encyclopaedic knowledge of medical literature, and a man of great linguistic talent and enormous energy, died in 1991 (see Preface to the fifth edition).

John Ebling, who continued as an editor right up to the fifth edition, died on 29th May 1992. He too occupied a unique position in British dermatology, as a full-time Professor of Zoology, a distinguished research worker and a man of enormous erudition and editorial skills. He made great contributions to British dermatology research, particularly in the field of pilo-sebaceous biology. His breadth of knowledge covered the whole of biology and we owe him a great debt for his tremendous and untiring work over 25 years on this textbook. His obituaries may be read in *The Times* dated 13th June 1992 and in the *Journal of Investigative Dermatology* 1993, **101**, 2S–3S.

The fifth edition, published in 1992, was edited by Champion, Burton and Ebling, with invaluable advice and the very useful 'Glossary of Dermatological Terms' from Darrell Wilkinson.

For this sixth edition, Bob Champion and John Burton have been joined by two new editors, Tony Burns and Stephen Breathnach. We would all like to express our great respect and gratitude to the three original editors whose influence still shines through the whole book.

The text has grown from the original 1964 pages in two volumes to 3683 pages in four volumes, despite careful pruning of out-dated material. However, it remains true to its original aim to compile a comprehensive guide to all recognized dermatological diseases, and to encourage understanding and development of scientific aspects of dermatology, although not intended to provide a comprehensive guide to research in the basic sciences.

For this edition every chapter has been updated, many have been completely rewritten and about 25–30% of the references are new. There are 21 new contributors, mostly clinical dermatologists practising in the United Kingdom, three new chapters and well over 100 new clinical entities. There are many new illustrations and all the clinical pictures are now in colour. The reference system has been slightly changed and is now Vancouver style.

As in previous editions, we have been helped by several colleagues, in addition to the contributors, who have given helpful advice at the manuscript stage to give us the benefit of their special expertise. We are most grateful to these colleagues, some of whom are acknowledged in the relevant chapters. We would also like to acknowledge our indebtedness to contributors to earlier editions, who have generously allowed some of their original material to be retained for the present edition.

We are very grateful also to all those colleagues who have donated colour photographs. Their help is acknowledged under each figure. Where no acknowledgment is given the figures have been provided by the authors of that chapter.

Our wives and families deserve our thanks for their forbearance and support over many years.

Last, but not least, we should like to thank the staff of Blackwell Science for their great efforts throughout the production of this edition. Edward Wates, Julie Elliott and Jonathan Rowley from the Book Production Department have been most closely involved. We are also grateful to Caroline Sheard for the excellent index. We hope that readers will agree with us that the quality of the production remains a great credit to the Blackwell team.

R.H. Champion
J.L. Burton
D.A. Burns
S.M. Breathnach

Preface to the First Edition

No comprehensive reference book on dermatology has been published in the English language for ten years and none in England for over a quarter of a century. The recent literature of dermatology is rich in shorter texts and in specialist monographs but the English-speaking dermatologist has long felt the need for a substantial text for regular reference and as a guide to the immense monographic and periodical literature. The editors have therefore planned the present volume primarily for the dermatologist in practice or in training, but have also considered the requirements of the specialist in other fields of medicine and of the many research workers interested in the skin in relation to toxicology or cosmetic science.

An attempt has been made throughout the book to integrate our growing knowledge of the biology of skin and of fundamental pathological processes with practical clinical problems. Often the gap is still very wide but the trends of basic research at least indicate how it may eventually be bridged. In a clinical textbook the space devoted to the basic sciences must necessarily be restricted but a special effort has been made to ensure that the short accounts which open many chapters are easily understood by the physician whose interests and experience are exclusively clinical.

For the benefit of the student we have encouraged our contributors to make each chapter readable as an independent entity, and have accepted that this must involve the repetition of some material.

The classification employed is conventional and pragmatic. Until our knowledge of the mechanisms of disease is more profound no truly scientific classification is possible. In so many clinical syndromes multiple aetiological factors are implicated. To emphasize one at the expense of others is often misleading. Most diseases are to some extent influenced by genetic factors and a large proportion of common skin reactions are modified by the emotional state of the patient. Our knowledge is in no way advanced by classifying hundreds of diseases as genodermatoses and dozens as psychosomatic.

The true prevalence of a disease may throw light on its aetiology but reported incidence figures are often unreliable and incorrectly interpreted. The scientific approach to the evaluation of racial and environmental factors has therefore been considered in some detail.

The effectiveness of any physician in practice must ultimately depend on his ability to make an accurate clinical diagnosis. Clinical descriptions are detailed and differential diagnosis is fully discussed. Histopathology is here considered mainly as an aid to diagnosis but references to fuller accounts are provided.

The approach to treatment is critical but practical. Many empirical measures are of proven value and should not be abandoned merely because their efficacy cannot yet be scientifically explained. However, many familiar remedies old and new have been omitted either because properly controlled clinical trials have shown them to be of no value or because they have been supplanted by more effective and safer preparations.

There are over nine hundred photographs but no attempt has been made to provide an illustration of every disease. To have done so would have increased the bulk and price of the book without increasing proportionately its practical value. The conditions selected for illustrations are those in which a photograph significantly enhances the verbal description. There are a few conditions we wished to illustrate, but of which we could not obtain unpublished photographs of satisfactory quality.

The lists of references have been selected to provide a guide to the literature. Important articles now of largely historical interest have usually been omitted, except where a knowledge of the history of a disease simplifies the understanding of present concepts and terminology. Books and articles provided with a substantial bibliography are marked with an asterisk.

Many of the chapters have been read and criticized by several members of the team and by other colleagues. Professor Wilson Jones, Dr R.S. Wells and Dr W.E. Parish have given valuable assistance with histopathological, genetic and immunological problems respectively. Many advisers, whose services are acknowledged in the following pages, have helped us with individual chapters. Any errors which have not been eliminated are, however, the responsibility of the editors and authors.

The editors hope that this book will prove of value to all those who are interested in the skin either as physicians or as research workers. They will welcome readers' criticisms and suggestions which may help them to make the second edition the book they hope to produce.

Chapter 62
Reiter's Disease

R.M.GRAHAM

Reiter's disease

SYN. FIESSINGER–LEROY SYNDROME, DYSENTERIC ARTHRITIS

Definition

A disease in which a non-suppurative polyarthritis lasting more than 1 month follows closely a lower urogenital or enteric infection, particularly in young men carrying the human leukocyte antigen (HLA) B27. Inflammatory eye disease and mucocutaneous manifestations are common.

History [1]

The disease was first recognized in 1818 [2] and fully established during World War I by Reiter [3], Fiessinger and Leroy [4] and others [1]. The observations of Paronen [5] during a massive outbreak accompanying epidemic dysentry in Finland significantly added to our knowledge of the disease. The discovery of the strong association with HLA-B27 [6,7] provided an invaluable genetic marker allowing recognition of incomplete and even mono-symptomatic forms [8,9]. The association with acquired immune deficiency syndrome (AIDS) [10] retaining a link with HLA-B27 supports the theory of a genetically orchestrated host response to various infective agents and indicates that immunoregulatory factors are relevant to the pathogenesis.

Incidence

In the UK the incidence following urethritis is about 0.8%

[11], but about 2% of Finnish males develop the disease after non-gonococcal urethritis (NGU) [12], a difference attributable to the higher prevalence (14%) of the B27 antigen in the Finnish compared with the British population (5%) [13]. It has been calculated that the relative risk of a B27-positive person developing the disease is 25-fold as compared with a B27-negative individual in Finland [14]. Reiter's disease develops in about 20% of B27-positive people following an appropriate infection [13], implying that in a population in which 5% of individuals are B27 positive, approximately 1% are at risk. The prevalence of Reiter's syndrome in AIDS appears to be 4.6%; if 71% of AIDS cases of Reiter's are B27 positive then around three-quarters of the HLA-B27-positive AIDS cases will develop Reiter's syndrome [15].

Epidemiology [16,17]

Reliable data depend on acceptable and uniform diagnostic criteria. The suggestions of the American Rheumatism Association (ARA) include peripheral arthritis occurring in association with urethritis and/or cervicitis. The characteristic episode is of more than 1 month's duration [18,19].

Another proposed definition suggests 'seronegative asymmetrical arthropathy lasting more than a month plus one or more of urethritis or cervicitis, dysentery, inflammatory eye disease or mucocutaneous disease' [20]. These criteria were fulfilled by more than 80% of patients considered by experienced investigators to have Reiter's disease while 98% of 'control' patients with seronegative arthropathy did not do so [21].

The disease is worldwide. In the UK and North America the postdysenteric form is rare [22]. In the form preceded by urogenital infection, the evidence strongly implicates venereal origin since most cases follow promiscuous sexual intercourse [11]. It appears that the urethritis of the dysenteric form is not venereal, since sexual exposure has usually been lacking, associated gonorrhoea is rare and the disease has developed in children [1]. With an increasing incidence of AIDS and an approximate association with Reiter's syndrome of 5%, AIDS may eventually become the commonest clinical scenario in which it occurs. Consequently, and somewhat speculatively, the more common use of contraceptive sheaths may reduce the proportion of venereally precipitated Reiter's syndrome in the non-AIDS population at risk.

REFERENCES

1 Keat A. Reiter's syndrome and reactive arthritis in perspective. *N Engl J Med* 1983; **309**: 1606–15.
2 Brodie BC. *Pathological and Surgical Observations on Diseases of the Joints*. London: Longman, 1818: 49–53.
3 Reiter H. Ueber eine bisher unekannte Spirochäteninfektion (Spirochaetosis arthritica). *Dtsche Med Wochenschr* 1916; **42**: 1535–6.
4 Fiessinger N, Leroy ME. Contribution a l'étude d'une épidémie de dysenterie dans la Somme. *Bull Mem Soc Med Hop* 1916; **40**: 2030–70.
5 Paronen I. Reiter's disease, a study of 344 cases observed in Finland. *Acta Med Scand* 1948; **131** (Suppl. 212): 1–112.
6 Aho K, Ahvonen P, Lassus A *et al.* HL-A antigen 27 and reactive arthritis. *Lancet* 1973; **ii**: 157.
7 Brewerton DA, Nicholls A, Oates JK *et al.* Reiter's disease and HL-A 27. *Lancet* 1973; **ii**: 996–8.
8 Arnett FC. Incomplete Reiter's syndrome: clinical comparisons with classical triad. *Ann Rheum Dis* 1979; **38** (Suppl.): 73–8.
9 Arnett FC, McClusky E, Schacter BZ *et al.* Incomplete Reiter's syndrome: discriminating features and HL-A B27 in diagnosis. *Ann Intern Med* 1976; **84**: 8–12.
10 Winchester R, Bernstein DH, Fischer HD *et al.* The occurrence of Reiter's syndrome and acquired immunodeficiency. *Ann Intern Med* 1987; **106**: 19–26.
11 Csonka GW. Workshop I. Features and prognosis of Reiter's syndrome. Clinical aspects of Reiter's syndrome. *Ann Rheum Dis* 1979; **38** (Suppl.): 4–7.
12 Paavonen J, Kousa M, Saikku P *et al.* Examination of men with nongonococcal urethritis and their sexual partners for *Chlamydia trachomatis* and *urealyticum*. *Sex Transm Dis* 1978; **5**: 93–6.
13 Lassus A, Kousa M. Reiter's disease. In: Harris JR, ed. *Recent Advances in Sexually Transmitted Disease*, No. 2. Edinburgh: Churchill Livingstone, 1981: 187–99.
14 Kousa M. Clinical observations on Reiter's disease with special reference to the venereal and non-venereal aetiology. *Acta Derm Venereol (Stockh)* 1978; **58** (Suppl. 81): 1–36.
15 Brancato L, Hesau S, Skovron ML *et al.* Aspects of the spectrum, prevalence and disease susceptibility determinants of Reiter's syndrome and related disorders associated with HIV infection. *Rheumatol Int* 1989; **9**: 137–41.
16 Masi AT. Epidemiology of B27-associated diseases. *Ann Rheum Dis* 1979; **38** (Suppl.): 131–4.
17 Michet CT, Machado EB, Ballard DJ *et al.* Epidemiology of Reiter's syndrome in Rochester, Minnesota 1950–1980. *Arthritis Rheum* 1988; **31**: 428–31.
18 Wilkens RF, Arnett FC, Butler T. Reiter's syndrome, evaluation of preliminary criteria for definite disease. *Arthritis Rheum* 1981; **24**: 844–9.
19 Wilkens RF, Arnett FC, Butler T *et al.* Reiter's syndrome: evaluation of proposed criteria. *Ann Rheum Dis* 1979; **38** (Suppl.): 8–11.
20 Calin A. Workshop III. Management of Reiter's syndrome. *Ann Rheum Dis* 1979; **38** (Suppl.): 96–7.
21 Fisk P. Reiter's Disease. *Br Med J* 1982; **284**: 3–4.
22 Tozzi MA, Stamm R, Bigelli AJ *et al.* Reiter's syndrome, a review and case report. *J Am Pediatr Assoc* 1981; **71**: 418–22.

Pathogenesis

Two problems are central: to determine if and why certain individuals are especially prone, and to recognize the presumed infective triggering agents. Clinical genetic data, supported by HLA studies, point clearly to a constitutional predisposition and demonstrate familial aggregation of the disease [1]. Molecular mimicry between HLA-B27 and bacterially encoded epitopes may, in some situations, be an explanation for this reactive process [2]. Susceptibility to Reiter's syndrome also appears to be associated with alleles of *TAP* (transporters associated with antigen processing) genes, independent of HLA-B27 [3].

Genetic aspects [4–6]

The disease has been described in several pairs of brothers, including twins [7,8], and in several members of a family, sometimes living hundreds of miles apart [9]. A family history of chronic rheumatism was found in 15% of patients with post-urethritic Reiter's disease, but only in 2% of patients with uncomplicated urethritis [7].

Similar figures have been obtained in the postdysenteric disease [10] where, in one family, five of seven children with dysentery developed Reiter's disease. In a thorough family survey in the UK, the frequency of ankylosing spondylitis and sacroiliitis in relatives of patients with Reiter's disease was much higher than normal and comparable to that found in relatives of patients with ankylosing spondylitis itself [11]. B27-related symptoms are common in B27-positive parents of patients with Reiter's disease [12]. In a clinical and epidemiological study of Reiter's syndrome in Greenland 34% of sufferers had a close relative with the disease [13]. Thus, familial clustering of Reiter's disease is undisputed.

Usually there is a highly significant (70–90%) association of HLA-B27 with Reiter's disease [5,14], although some data suggest that in the Israeli population Reiter's syndrome is less often associated with HLA-B27 and that B7-CREG antigens may be an additional marker [15]. As with ankylosing spondylitis, psoriatic spondylitis, reactive arthritis following certain infections and arthropathies associated with chronic bowel disease [16], the association with B27 normally holds true in both urogenital and enteric forms of the disease [17,18]. HLA studies have also shed light on the extra-articular manifestations of the disease, in which conjunctivitis and uveitis are common. In patients presenting with anterior uveitis alone, 42% are B27 positive [19] and over 70% have evidence of chronic prostatitis [20], suggesting that uveitis may be regarded as a monosymptomatic form of the disease. Similarly B27 positivity is common in patients with circinate balanitis without other clinical evidence of Reiter's disease [14].

The association between B27 and Reiter's disease is complex. B27-negative individuals occasionally develop the disease, so the single gene cannot be essential. Cross-reactive HLA antigens have been reported in B27-negative patients with Reiter's disease [21]. The possibility that B27 is only a marker for another pathogenic gene on the same haplotype of the short arm of chromosome 6 has been raised, but seems unlikely [22]. The pathogenic role of HLA-B27 remains unclear, but T-cell receptor variability warrants further investigation [22]. Reiter's syndrome and ankylosing spondylitis are the main spondyloarthropathies linked with HLA-B27 and while the mechanism of development is uncertain a process of molecular mimicry has been postulated between HLA-B27 and *Klebsiella*, which may predispose patients to these spondyloarthropathies. A sequence of six consecutive amino acids appears to be shared [23]. *Yersinia* may also cross-react and a similar sequence has been found in a plasmid of *Shigella flexneri* [2], but whether these similarities are of pathogenic importance needs further substantiation. As HLA-B27 appears to have a preferential approach to β_2-microglobulin, and cytomegalovirus has a propensity to coat itself with this microglobulin, this may result in alternative views on mechanisms [22] and have possible implications in human immunodeficiency virus (HIV) associations. The *TAP* genes are genetically separate but functionally linked to class I genes [3] and provide another pathway to Reiter's syndrome susceptibility.

Triggering infections

No single infective agent is responsible for provoking Reiter's disease. The most important urogenital infective agent is *Chlamydia trachomatis* [24], but T-strain mycoplasma (*Ureaplasma*) and other unidentified organisms may be important [16]; coexistent *Chlamydia* and *Ureaplasma* infection is documented [25]. The most common stool isolate in the enteric form is *Shigella* (*flexneri* and *dysenteriae*) [26], but also *Salmonella* [27], *Yersinia enterocolitica* [28,29] and *Campylobacter fetus* [30,31]. *Klebsiella pneumoniae* and *Escherichia coli* seem more implicated in ankylosing spondylitis than Reiter's disease [32]. Evidence exists that colonic infection with *Clostridium difficile* may trigger Reiter's disease [33]. *Mycobacterium phlei* has been reported as the only infective agent in septic arthritis presenting as infantile Reiter's disease [34]. Ocular, genital and articular manifestations compatible with Reiter's syndrome have been reported after intravesical immunotherapy with bacillus Calmette–Guérin (BCG) [35]. A further tie-up with *Borrelia burgdorferi* [36] takes one full circle back to Reiter's original postulate of spirochaetosis arthritica [37]. Some HIV-positive patients may have increased exposure to many opportunistic organisms, and, if the HIV infection is acquired secondary to permissive sexual activities, exposure to many urethritic and enteric organisms may put particularly HLA-B27/HIV-positive individuals at increased risk of the conventional trigger mechanisms.

Brancato *et al.* [5] have emphasized the epidemiological similarity of Reiter's disease developing in a background of HIV infection with its occurrence in non-HIV infected patients. Whether the heightened risk of Reiter's disease in the HIV positive is principally a result of immune dysfunction, primary or secondary viral effects or enhanced exposure to trigger mechanisms, remains to be seen. A combination effect seems likely, although a direct link is disputed by some studies [38]. Hypozincaemia has also been implicated as an exacerbating factor [39].

Chlamydia trachomatis is regarded as a major aetiological factor in non-gonococcal urethritis. Fifteen serotypes have been identified of which eight (D, E, F, G, H, I, J, K) cause lower urogenital tract infection [24]. Since the original reports [40] linking chlamydiae with Reiter's disease many confirmatory studies have been published [41,1]. Serological data [41–43] lend support to the results of *Chlamydia* cultures [44], although a Reiter's specific antigen in *C. trachomatis* has not been identified [45].

Although the association with *Chlamydia* is established it is still debatable whether *Chlamydia* is a trigger mechanism or an epiphenomenon with the patient rendered liable to persistent chlamydial infection. There does not appear to be a specific pattern of humoral immune response to *Chlamydia* for Reiter's disease or HLA-B27 positivity; nor are there differentiating factors between B27 positive or negative Reiter's disease with chlamydial infection [45]. There is no increased prevalence of *Chlamydia* in the urethra of healthy B27-positive individuals [46]. A fatal endocarditis due to *C. trachomatis* in a pregnant woman is documented [47], and *C. trachomatis* has been isolated from joint material culture in Reiter's disease [48]. There is increasing evidence which suggests that all or part of the *Chlamydia* organism is present in the synovium of some Reiter's disease cases; this is supported by immunocytochemical and immunoelectron microscopic studies where chlamydial particles and antigens have been demonstrated in the synovium [49].

The role of T-strain mycoplasma (*Ureaplasma urealyticum*) in Reiter's disease remains controversial. There is evidence that it can cause experimental [50] and naturally occurring non-gonococcal urethritis [17,51], supported by clinical [52] and epidemiological evidence [53]. Serological evidence of involvement exists [25,54], but its significance in causation is difficult to assess. It has been demonstrated that synovial mononuclear cells obtained from knee effusions in patients with sexually transmitted Reiter's disease respond characteristically to ureaplasmal (and chlamydial) antigens [55]. Isolation of the organism from a patient with Reiter's disease adds further support [56].

Shigella dysentery was the first enteric infection demonstrated to be associated with Reiter's disease [10]. Extensive outbreaks were reported in the 1950s among French troops in Algeria [26]. Cases after 'non-specific' diarrhoea may have been due to *Campylobacter fetus* [30].

Although arthritis is a common complication of *Yersinia enterocolitica* [29] and *Salmonella* [27] infections, the full triad of Reiter's disease is rare [27,57]. Post-*Salmonella* reactive arthropathy can complicate ankylosing spondylitis some considerable time after onset of the ankylosing spondylitis, without modifying the course of the underlying disease [58], although confusion may arise as to which aspect is responsible for any subsequent sacroiliitis. The Chinese may be at particular risk of *Yersinia* arthritis [57].

In view of the possible albeit indirect association of HIV positivity with Reiter's disease [5,38,59] and the exponential increase of HIV-positive patients, together with the relative rarity of Reiter's disease in the population in general, its development in an 'at-risk' person may be an indication for HIV testing, as well as conventional urological and gastrointestinal bacterial screening.

REFERENCES

1 Kousa M, Lassus A, Karvonen J et al. Family study of Reiter's disease and HLA-B27 distribution. *J Rheumatol* 1977; **4**: 95–102.

2 Stieglitz H, Fosmire S, Lipsky PE. Bacterial epitopes involved in the induction of reactive arthritis. *Am J Med* 1988; **85** (Suppl. 6A): 56–8.

3 Barron KS, Reveille JD, Carrington M et al. Susceptibility to Reiter's syndrome is associated with alleles of TAP genes. *Arthritis Rheum* 1995; **38**: 684–9.

4 Albert ED, Scholz S, Christ U. Genetics of B27-associated diseases—2. *Ann Rheum Dis* 1979; **38** (Suppl.): 142–4.

5 Brancato L, Hesu S, Skovron ML et al. Aspects of the spectrum, prevalence and disease susceptibility determinants of Reiter's syndrome and related disorders associated with HIV infection. *Rheumatol Int* 1989; **9**: 137–41.

6 Woodrow JC. Genetics of B27-associated diseases—1. *Ann Rheum Dis* 1979; **38** (Suppl.): 135–41.

7 Csonka G. Multiple cases in Reiter's syndrome. *Br J Vener Dis* 1969; **45**: 157–60.

8 Mowat AG, Nicols CS. Reiter's disease in two brothers. *Br J Vener Dis* 1968; **44**: 334–6.

9 Gough KR. Reiter's syndrome in a father and son. *Ann Rheum Dis* 1962; **21**: 292–4.

10 Paronen I. Reiter's disease, a study of 344 cases observed in Finland. *Acta Med Scand* 1948; **131** (Suppl. 212): 1–112.

11 Lawrence JS. Family survey of Reiter's disease. *Br J Vener Dis* 1974; **50**: 140–5.

12 McCarthy MK, Gibbons RB, Jennings PB et al. Familial studies in HLA-B27 positive Reiter's syndrome. *Milit Med* 1977; **142**: 674–7.

13 Bardin T, Enel C, Lathrop MG. Fiessinger–Leroy–Reiter syndrome in Greenland: clinical and epidemiological aspects. *Rev Rhum Mal Osteoartic* 1987; **54**: 37–43.

14 Lassus A, Tiilikainen A, Stubb J et al. Circinate erosive balanitis and HLA 27. *Acta Derm Venereol (Stockh)* 1975; **55**: 199–207.

15 Ben-Chetrit E, Brantbar T, Rubinow A. HLA-antigens in Reiter's syndrome in Israeli patients. *Ther Umsch* 1985; **42**: 652–8.

16 Lassus A, Kousa M. Reiter's disease. In: Harris JR, ed. *Recent Advances in Sexually Transmitted Diseases*, No 2. Edinburgh: Churchill Livingstone, 1981: 187–99.

17 Aho K, Ahvonen P, Lassus A et al. HLA-A27 in reactive arthritis: a study of *Yersinia* arthritis and Reiter's disease. *Arthritis Rheum* 1974; **17**: 521–6.

18 Sairanen E, Tiilikainen A. HL-A27 in Reiter's disease following Shigellosis. *Abstr Scand J Rheumatol* 1975; **4** (Suppl. 8): 30–11.

19 Brewerton DA. Many genes, many clinical features. *Ann Rheum Dis* 1979; **38** (Suppl.): 145–8.

20 Perkins ES. Uveitis in B27-related disease. *Ann Rheum Dis* 1979; **38** (Suppl.): 92–5.

21 Arnett FC, Jr, Hochberg MC, Bias WB. Cross reactive HLA antigens in B27-negative Reiter's syndrome and sacroiliitis. *Johns Hopkins Med J* 1977; **141**: 193–7.

22 Feltkamp TE. New views on B27 associated disease. *Netherlands J Med* 1989; **35**: 119–22.

23 Schwimmbeck PL, Oldstone MB. Molecular mimicry between human leukocyte antigen B27 and *Klebsiella*: consequences for spondyloarthropathies. *Am J Med* 1988; **85**: 51–3.

24 Dunlop EM. Venereal disease: *Chlamydia trachomatis* and *Ureaplasma urealyticum* in a patient with Reiter's disease. *Br J Hosp Med* 1983; **29**: 6–11.

25 Smith RJ. Evidence for chlamydial genital infection and its complications. *Br J Hosp Med* 1983; **29**: 5–11.

26 Roumagnac H. Le syndrome de Fiessinger–Leroy–Reiter en Algerie. *Rev Practicien* 1960; **10**: 2516–24.

27 Jones RA. Reiter's disease after *Salmonella typhimurium* enteritis. *Br Med J* 1977; **i**: 1391.

28 Ahvonen P. Human yersinosis in Finland ii: clinical features. *Ann Clin Res* 1972; **4**: 39–48.

29 Laitinen O, Leirisala M, Skylv G. Relation between HLA-B27 and clinical features in patients with *Yersinia* arthritis. *Arthritis Rheum* 1977; **20**: 1121–4.

30 Ponka A, Martio J, Kosunen TU. Reiter's syndrome in association with enteritis due to *Campylobacter fetus* ssp. *jejuni*. *Ann Rheum Dis* 1981; **40**: 414–15.

31 Urman JD, Zurier RB, Rothfield NF. Reiter's syndrome associated with *Campylobacter fetus* infection. *Ann Intern Med* 1977; **86**: 444–5.

32 Bunning VK, Raybourne RB, Archer DL. Foodborne enterobacterial pathogens and rheumatoid disease. *J Appl Bact* 1988; (Symposium Suppl.): 87s–107s.

33 Hayward KS, Wensel RH, Kibsey P. Relapsing *Clostridium difficile* colitis and Reiter's syndrome. *Am J Gastroenterol* 1980; **85**: 752–6.

34 Aguilar JL, Sanchez EE, Carillo C et al. Septic arthritis due to *Mycobacterium phlei* presenting as infantile Reiter's syndrome. *J Rheumatol* 1989; **16**: 1377–8.

35 Pancaldi P, Van Linthoudt D, Alborino D et al. Reiter's syndrome after intravesical bacillus Calmette–Guerin treatment for superficial bladder carcinoma. *Br J Rheumatol* 1993; **32**: 1096–8.

36 Weyland CM, Goronzy JJ. Immune responses to *Borrelia burgdorferi* in patients with reactive arthritis. *Arthritis Rheum* 1989; **32**: 1057–64.

37 Reiter H. Ueber eine bisher unerkannte Spirochäteninfektion (Spirochaetosis arthritica). *Dtsch Med Wochenschr* 1916; **42**: 1535–6.

38 Clark MR, Solinger AM, Hochberg MC. Human immunodeficiency virus is not associated with Reiter's syndrome. *Rheum Dis Clin North Am* 1992; **18**: 267–76.

39 Hausmann G, Castel T, Iranzo P et al. Reiter's syndrome associated with hypozincemia in a HIV-positive patient. *Int J Dermatol* 1988; **27**: 342–3.

40 Siboulet A, Galistin P. Arguments in favour of a virus aetiology of non-gonococcal urethritis illustrated by three cases of Reiter's disease. *Br J Vener Dis* 1962; **38**: 209–11.

41 Schachter J. Chlamydial infection. *N Engl J Med* 1978; **298**: 490–5.

42 Amor B, Kahan A, Orfila J et al. Immunological evidence of chlamydial infection in Reiter's syndrome. *Ann Rheum Dis* 1979; **38** (Suppl.): 116–17.

43 Grandal H, Nordhorst CH. Chlamydia infection and arthritis. *Scand J Rheumatol* 1975; **4** (Suppl. 8): Abstr 05–06.

44 Kousa M. Clinical observations on Reiter's disease with special reference to the venereal and non-venereal aetiology. *Acta Derm Venereol (Stockh)* 1978; **58** (Suppl.): 1–36.

45 Inman RD, Johnston ME, Chiu B et al. Immunochemical analysis of immune response to *Chlamydia trachomatis* in Reiter's syndrome and non-specific urethritis. *Clin Exp Immunol* 1987; **69**: 246–54.

46 Keat AC, Maini RN, Nkwazi GC et al. Role of *Chlamydia trachomatis* and HLA B27 in sexually acquired reactive arthritis. *Br Med J* 1978; **i**: 605–7.

47 Van der Bel-Kahn JM, Watanakunakom C, Menefee MG et al. *Chlamydia trachomatis* endocarditis. *Am Heart J* 1978; **95**: 627–36.

48 Vilppula AH, Yli-Kertulla UL, Ahlroos AK et al. Chlamydial isolations and serology in Reiter's syndrome. *Scand J Rheumatol* 1981; **10**: 181–5.

49 Rahman MU, Hudson AP, Schumacher HR. Chlamydia and Reiter's syndrome (Reactive Arthritis). *Rheum Dis Clin North Am* 1992; **18**: 67–79.

50 Taylor-Robinson D, Csonka GW, Prentice MJ. Human intra-urethral inoculation of ureaplasmas. *Q J Med* 1977; **46**: 309–26.

51 McCormack WM, Braun P, Lee YH et al. The genital Mycoplasmas. *N Engl J Med* 1973; **288**: 78–89.

52 Bowie WR, Floyd JF, Miller Y et al. Differential response of chlamydial and ureaplasma-associated urethritis and ureaplasma-associated urethritis to sulphafurazole (sulfisoxazole) and aminocyclitols. *Lancet* 1976; **ii**: 1276–8.

53 Ford DK, Henderson E. Non-gonococcal urethritis due to T-Mycoplasma (*Ureaplasma urealyticum*) serotype 2 in a conjugal sexual partnership. *Br J Vener Dis* 1976; **52**: 341–2.

54 Ford DK, Da Roza DM, Shah P *et al*. Cell mediated immune response of synovial mononuclear cells in Reiter's syndrome against Ureaplasma and Chlamydial antigens. *J Rheumatol* 1980; **7**: 751–5.

55 Ford DK, Da Roza DM, Shah P. Cell-mediated immune responses of synovial mononuclear cells to sexually transmitted enteric and mumps antigen in patients with Reiter's syndrome, rheumatoid arthritis and ankylosing spondylitis. *J Rheumatol* 1981; **8**: 220–32.

56 Kossman JE, Floret D, Renaud H *et al*. Reiter's syndrome in children associated with Ureaplasma urealyticum. *Pediatrie* 1980; **35**: 237–42.

57 Ford DK. *Yersinia*-induced arthritis and Reiter's syndrome. *Ann Rheum Dis* 1979; **38** (Suppl.): 127–8.

58 Herrero-Beaumont G, Elswood J, Will R *et al*. Postsalmonella reactive phenomena in 2 patients with ankylosing spondylitis. No modification of the underlying disease. *J Rheumatol* 1990; **17**: 250–1.

59 Winchester R, Bernstein DH, Fischer HD *et al*. The co-occurrence of Reiter's syndrome and acquired immunodeficiency. *Ann Intern Med* 1987; **106**: 19–26.

General features and mode of onset [1–3]

The disease occurs predominantly in men, mostly young. The reason for the male predominance is unclear; the prostate gland serving as a focus for persistent infection is a possibility. In various series only 2–10% of cases were in women [4,5]. However, the disease was often overlooked in females [6] and a high index of suspicion is required [7]. When women are affected, the incomplete form of the disease seems more common. They are more frequently HLA-B27 negative and generally have a lower erythrocyte sedimentation rate (ESR) than males; urological and arthritic changes and triggering factors appear the same [8]. Female HIV-positive cases have been described [9], although the current preponderance of male HIV-positive cases makes it difficult to interpret whether an increased proportion of HIV-positive females will develop the condition compared with HIV-negative women, but this seems likely.

Reiter's disease is not common in children. Understandably they have a higher incidence of enteric trigger factors [10–12] compared with adults. The incidence and frequency of urethritis appear to increase with adolescence [13] and presumably with sexual activity. It has been reported as a sequel to traveller's diarrhoea [14] in children and following Yersinia infection [15].

Septic arthritis due to *Mycobacterium phlei* presenting as infantile Reiter's disease has also been described [16]. An adolescent female who was HLA-B27 positive with serological evidence of both *Chlamydia* and *Ureaplasma* has also been reported [17]. In general, the presentation of Reiter's disease in children is similar to the adult form, but appears shorter lived, more benign in behaviour, with a lower incidence of ophthalmic involvement [15,17] and more remittent joint involvement [12].

Urethritis, often unnoticed or denied, occurs 4–20 days after sexual exposure. Arthritis appears most commonly 10–14 days later, usually accompanied by conjunctivitis, followed shortly by circinate balanitis, but the latter can precede the arthritis or be delayed for several weeks [2]. In enteric cases, the diarrhoea is followed generally after 10–30 days by urethritis, arthritis and conjunctivitis, usually developing within 10 days of each other. In both types urethritis and conjunctivitis are often fleeting and inconspicuous and may be missed if the physician faced with unexplained arthritis is not alert to the possibility of this disease. Moderate fever often accompanies the arthritis for 1–4 weeks.

Urethritis [2]

The features are those of non-gonococcal urethritis. When mild, the inflammation is symptomless or accompanied only by slight dysuria.

Mucoid material containing numerous polymorphs can be expressed and shreds are present in the first flow of urine. In the average case, a mucopurulent discharge is noticed, especially on waking. When more severe, the urethritis is associated with constant purulent discharge, severe dysuria and sometimes meatal inflammation. Acute abacterial cystitis with severe frequency and sometimes haematuria may supervene. Acute prostatitis is uncommon, but low-grade chronic prostatitis is almost inevitable: the latter is generally symptomless, but may occasionally be accompanied by aching in the perineum. Acute epididymitis can occur. In women the most prominent and persistent urogenital involvement causes cervicitis, salpingitis, pyuria and dysuria [7,8]; urethritis, vaginitis, bartholinitis and cystitis also occur [18]. Chlamydial proctitis can occur in both sexes [19,20]. Urethritis occurs in most enteric cases, but is usually mild and transient.

Eye lesions

Approximately half the venereal cases have early eye involvement, usually conjunctivitis, and the proportion in dysenteric cases is similar [21–23]. Iritis is more characteristic of late recurrent attacks, but occurs in 3–8% of first episodes [2]. The conjunctivitis is usually bilateral, transient and often, being subtarsal, may be missed.

Anterior uveitis is particularly associated with chronic prostatitis [24], sacroiliitis [22] and B27 positivity [25]. *Yersinia* infection may have a more particular association with anterior uveitis than other trigger factors [26]. Typically, anterior uveitis presents as a sudden attack of redness, pain and blurred vision. Slit-lamp microscopy reveals exudation of cells and protein into the aqueous humour, often with hypopyon formation. The pupil contracts and may adhere to the lens to form posterior synechiae [24]. Recurrent uveitis may lead to glaucoma. Keratitis occurs less commonly, characterized by epithelial erosions and pleomorphic infiltrates in the anterior stroma [27].

Herpetiform corneal lesions may be the ocular equivalent of circinate balanitis. A report on the ocular manifestations in eight patients with Reiter's disease following *Salmonella* enteritis demonstrates that conjunctivitis occurred in all cases, but was mild and cleared in 10 days [28].

Transient keratitis and corneal erosions occurred in one of these cases. Several developed unilateral acute anterior uveitis 3–4 years after the onset [28]. An association reported with retinal detachment and Reiter's disease is likely to be fortuitous [29].

Arthritis

It has now been reasonably established that bacteria, bacterial fragments, DNA, RNA and bacterial lipopolysaccharides can be detected in the joints of patients with Reiter's disease and reactive arthritis. The mode of transportation of these bacterial components to the joint is uncertain, but it is unlikely that they are viable [30].

Joint involvement is characteristically non-suppurative, polyarticular and affecting predominantly the joints of the lower limbs and sacroiliac joints. Attacks tend to be self-limiting but are liable to recur over years or decades leading to chronic disability. In a first or early attack, four or five joints are generally involved, especially knees, ankles, tarsal or metatarsophalangeal joints [2]. The joint involvement spreads rapidly, reaching its height within 10–14 days. Infrequently, the arthritis is monoarticular and occasionally only soft tissue pain and swelling are found. During the evolution of the arthritis, its activity tends to wax and wane and spontaneous pain is usual, sometimes of great severity albeit short lived. Paediatric arthritis often is more remittent and less recurrent than adult forms [12]. Dusky erythema is seen over affected joints in a minority of cases. It is usually mild and transient, but when severe can simulate cellulitis. Rarely it leaves petechial haemorrhages as it retreats [31]. As the attack progresses, fresh joints are involved as inflammation in others regresses, involvement of the feet and knees being the most persistent. Reiter's disease differs from psoriatic arthritis in its predominant involvement of the lower limbs, particularly the feet with relative sparing of the hands and wrists [32]. Eventually arthritis of the lower limb joints occurs in over 50% of cases, but at any one time is seldom symmetrical.

Soft-tissue inflammation is usual and may be limited to one section of the periarticular tissues or adjacent tendon sheaths or bursae. Rheumatoid nodules do not occur. Symptoms of soft-tissue involvement may include fleeting sometimes vague pains in the back, feet, heels or calves. In the feet, calcaneal spurs, plantar fasciitis and relapsing Achilles tendonitis may all be a source of pain apart from arthritis of the tarsal and metatarsophalangeal joints. Hip joint disease is very uncommon and pain in the region of the hips is more likely to signify sacroiliitis. Most first attacks last 1–4 months.

Recurrent attacks are the rule and may occur within months or be delayed for decades. Recovery after each is complete in a diminishing proportion of patients as a chronic erosive arthritis of the lower limbs and sacroiliac joints supervenes. Recurrent attacks of iritis may occur. The mechanism of recurrent attacks is uncertain. Early in the disorder, episodes were originally attributed to a fresh exposure to the respective trigger factor; clearly in some situations this may be relevant, but later the correlation becomes more tenuous. Features of rheumatoid arthritis, ankylosing spondylitis and Reiter's disease have rarely been described in the same patient [33].

Involvement with an erosive arthritis of the temporomandibular joint (TMJ) has been reported as an uncommon finding in Reiter's disease [34] although a Finnish study showed a quarter of men with subjective TMJ symptoms [35]. An association with relapsing polychondritis has been described [36]. Features at onset appear unrelated to HLA type. Sacroiliitis, osteitis pubis, pelvic whiskering, and vertebral squaring appear at least in part to be associated with B27 positivity, but syndesmophyte formation does not [3].

Spinal involvement

The incidence and degree of spinal involvement increase with time, more than half the patients eventually developing spinal disease, radiologically if not clinically [37]. The likelihood of developing sacroiliitis is also related to the severity and extent of the first attack and to the number of subsequent relapses [21]. However, sacroiliitis is commonly asymptomatic [38] and self-limiting, unobtrusive signs such as low backache or early morning stiffness the only findings [21]. Involvement of the remainder of the spine is uncommon and severe functional impairment seldom found [39]. A chronic spondylitis may supervene, but it is difficult to distinguish this from ankylosing spondylitis and psoriatic spondylitis. Sacroiliac arthritis may be asymmetrical or even unilateral in both Reiter's disease and psoriatic arthritis. Sclerotic patches of bone just above the sacroiliac joints were reported in a modest proportion of patients with Reiter's disease, but not with psoriatic arthritis; the numbers involved were, however, small [40]. In the vertebrae, radiological changes indistinguishable from those of ankylosing spondylitis or psoriatic arthritis may be seen, but often the changes are atypical for ankylosing spondylitis with large asymmetrical syndesmophytes and 'skipped segments'. However, these features may be seen in psoriatic arthritis [39]. Paravertebral ossification occurred in five out of 35 cases, in one report of Reiter's disease [41]. Cervical involvement is comparatively rare [42], but atlantoaxial subluxation is occasionally reported [43].

Radiological features [37,44]

Although overlap with other arthropathies is common, certain combinations of features are characteristic of Reiter's disease. They can be summarized as: severe involvement of the feet with relative sparing of the hands; predilection for the calcaneus, the interphalangeal joints of the halluces and the metatarsophalangeal joints; periosteal bone deposition near affected joints; sacroiliitis, especially asymmetrical, often large bridging syndesmophytes involving mainly the lateral aspects of the vertebral bodies with relative sparing of their anterior surfaces [37].

REFERENCES

1 DHSS, Chief Medical Officer. Sexually transmitted diseases. *Br J Vener Dis* 1980; **56**: 178–81.
2 King A. *Recent Advances in Venereology*. Churchill: London, 1964.
3 Marks JS, Holt PJ. The natural history of Reiter's disease: 21 years of observations. *Q J Med* 1986; **60**: 685–97.
4 Willkens RF, Arnett FC, Bittner T *et al.* Reiter's syndrome: evaluation of preliminary criteria for definite disease. *Arthritis Rheum* 1981; **24**: 844–9.
5 Wright V. Seronegative polyarthritis: a unified concept. *Arthritis Rheum* 1978; **21**: 619–33.
6 Calin A. Reiter's syndrome. *Med Clin North Am* 1977; **61**: 365–76.
7 Edwards L, Hansen RC. Reiter's syndrome of the vulva. *Arch Dermatol* 1992; **128**: 811–14.
8 Yli-Kerttula UI. Clinical characteristics in male and female Reiter's syndrome. *Clin Rheumatol* 1984; **3**: 351–60.
9 Winchester R, Berstein DH, Fischer HD *et al.* The co-occurrence of Reiter's syndrome and acquired immunodeficiency. *Ann Intern Med* 1987; **106**: 19–26.
10 Iveson JM, Nanda BS, Hancock JA *et al.* Reiter's disease in three boys. *Ann Rheum Dis* 1975; **34**: 364–8.
11 Singssen BH, Bernstein BH, Koster-King KG *et al.* Reiter's syndrome in childhood. *Arthritis Rheum* 1977; **20** (Suppl.): 402–7.
12 Cuttica RJ, Scheines EJ, Garay M *et al.* Juvenile onset Reiter's syndrome. A retrospective study of 26 patients. *Clin Exp Rheumatol* 1992; **10**: 285–8.
13 Lopez-Lango FJ, Monteaguido-Saez I, Cobeta-Garcia JC. Sindrome de Reiter: consideraciones sobre la frecuencia y la evolucions a medio plazo de su forma juvenil. *Ann Esp Pediatr* 1988; **29**: 298–301.
14 Ravin JG. Reiter's syndrome in childhood, a sequel to travellers diarrhea. *J Pediatr Ophthalmol* 1972; **9**: 87–9.
15 Russell AS. Reiter's syndrome in children following infection with *Yersinia enterocolitica* and *Shigella*. *Arthritis Rheum* 1977; **20**: 471–2.
16 Aguilar JL, Sanchez EE, Carillo C *et al.* Septic arthritis due to *Mycobacterium phlei* presenting as infantile Reiter's syndrome. *J Rheumatol* 1989; **16**: 1377–8.
17 Smith RT. Evidence for *Chlamydia trachomatis* and *Ureaplasma urealyticum* in a patient with Reiter's disease. *J Adolesc Health Care* 1989; **10**: 155–9.
18 Dunlop EM. Chlamydial genital infection and its complications. *Br J Hosp Med* 1983; **29**: 6–11.
19 Quinn TC, Goodell SE, Mkrtichian E *et al.* Chlamydia trachomatis proctitis. *N Engl J Med* 1981; **305**: 195–200.
20 Schachter J. Confirmatory serodiagnosis of lymphogranuloma venereum proctitis may yield false positive results due to other chlamydial infections of the rectum. *Sex Transm Dis* 1981; **8**: 26–8.
21 Csonka GW. Workshop I. Features and prognosis of Reiter's syndrome. *Ann Rheum Dis* 1979; **38** (Suppl.): 4–7.
22 Lee DA, Barker SM, Su WP *et al.* The clinical diagnosis of Reiter's syndrome. Ophthalmic and non-ophthalmic aspects. *Ophthalmology* 1986; **93**: 350–6.
23 Willkens RF, Arnett FC, Bitter T *et al.* Reiter's syndrome: evaluation of proposed criteria. *Ann Rheum Dis* 1979; **38** (Suppl.): 8–11.
24 Perkins ES. Uveitis in B27-related disease. *Ann Rheum Dis* 1979; **38** (Suppl.): 92–5.
25 Mapstone R, Woodrow JC. HL-A27 and acute anterior uveitis. *Br J Ophthalmol* 1975; **59**: 270–5.
26 Wakefield D, Stahlberg TH, Toivanen A *et al.* Serological evidence of Yersinia infection in patients with anterior uveitis. *Arch Ophthalmol* 1990; **108**: 219–21.
27 Wiggins RE, Steinkuller PG, Bowes Hamill M. Reiter's keratoconjunctivitis. *Arch Ophthalmol* 1990; **108**: 280–1.
28 Saari KM, Vilppula A, Lassus A *et al.* Ocular inflammation in Reiter's disease after Salmonella enteritis. *Am J Ophthalmol* 1980; **90**: 63–8.
29 Belcon MC, Bensen WG, Zahoruk RM. Bilateral retinal detachment in a case of Reiter's disease. *Postgrad Med J* 1984; **60**: 47–8.
30 Hughes RA, Keat AC. Reiter's syndrome and reactive arthritis: a current view. *Semin Arthritis Rheum* 1994; **24**: 190–210.
31 Oates JK, Hancock JA. Neurological symptoms and lesions occurring in the course of Reiter's disease. *Am J Med Sci* 1959; **238**: 79–84.
32 Gold RH, Bassett LW, Seeger LL. The other arthritides: roentgenologic features of osteoarthritis, erosive osteoarthritis, ankylosing spondylitis, psoriatic arthritis, Reiter's disease, multicentric reticulohistiocytosis and progressive systemic sclerosis. *Radiol Clin North Am* 1988; **26**: 1195–212.
33 Lavery H, Honer T, Roberts SD. Rheumatoid arthritis, ankylosing spondylitis and Reiter's syndrome occurring simultaneously. Case report. *Br J Vener Dis* 1982; **58**: 196–9.
34 Bomalaski JS, Jiemenez SA. Erosive arthritis of the temporomandibular joint in Reiter's syndrome. *J Rheumatol* 1984; **11**: 400–2.
35 Koononen M. Signs and symptoms of craniomandibular disorders in men with Reiter's disease. *J Craniomandib Disord Facial Oral Pain* 1992; **6**: 247–253.
36 Pazirandeh M, Ziram BH, Khandelwal BK *et al.* Relapsing polychondritis and spondylarthropathies. *J Rheumatol* 1988; **60**: 630–2.
37 Martel W. Radiological manifestations of Reiter's syndrome. *Ann Rheum Dis* 1979; **38** (Suppl.): 12–23.
38 McGuigan LE, Hart HH, Gow PJ *et al.* The functional significance of sacroiliitis and ankylosing spondylitis in Reiter's syndrome. *Clin Exp Rheumatol* 1985; **3**: 311–15.
39 Prohaska E, Obererlacher J, Hawel R *et al.* Achsenskelettbefall bei chronischem Reitersyndrom. *Z Rheumatol* 1986; **45**: 155–60.
40 Wright V. Psoriatic arthropathy and seronegative rheumatoid arthritis with psoriasis; distinguishing features from Reiter's syndrome. *Ann Rheum Dis* 1979; **38** (Suppl.): 59–67.
41 Sundaram M, Patton JT. Paravertebral ossification in psoriasis and Reiter's disease. *Br J Radiol* 1975; **48**: 628–33.
42 Moilanen A, Yli-Kertula U, Vilppula A. Cervical spine involvement in Reiter's syndrome. *Fortschr Rontgenstr* 1984; **141**: 84–7.
43 Melson RD, Benjamin JC, Barnes CG. Spontaneous atlantoaxial subluxation, an unusual presenting manifestation of Reiter's syndrome. *Ann Rheum Dis* 1989; **48**: 170–2.
44 Jensen PR, Ringsdal VS. Radiologisk päviste ossøse forandringer ved morbus Reiter. *Ugeskr Laeger* 1988; **150**: 1621–3.

Skin and mucosal lesions [1]

The incidence of mucocutaneous lesions is variably reported between 8 and 31% of all cases [1]. However, a much lower incidence of about 1% has been attributed to postdysenteric cases [2,3].

Keratoderma blenorrhagicum usually appears 1–2 months after the onset of arthritis and conjunctivitis, but may accompany or rarely precede the initial manifestations. The soles of the feet are almost always involved (Fig. 62.1), but the extensor surfaces of the legs, the dorsal aspects of toes (Fig. 62.2), feet, hands, fingers (Fig. 62.3), nails and scalp are common sites. Occasionally the eruption is very widespread and it may evolve into generalized exfoliative dermatitis (erythroderma). The initial lesion is a dull red macule which rapidly becomes papular and pseudovesicular. Its colour changes from yellow to orange–red as the roof thickens to form a hyperkeratotic plaque. A scaly collarette is sometimes present (Fig. 62.4). The

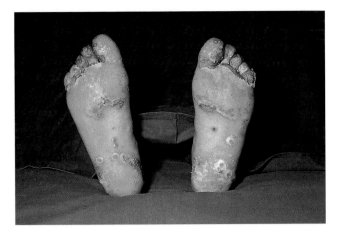

Fig. 62.1 Involvement of the feet with circinate lesions showing early hyperkeratosis. (Courtesy of Dr P. Forster, The James Paget Hospital, Great Yarmouth, UK.)

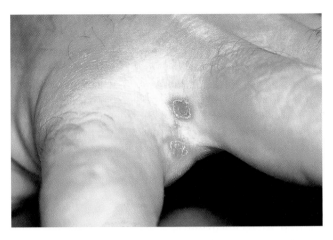

Fig. 62.4 Close up of web space lesion showing an orange red macule with adjacent pseudovesicular lesion. Note peripheral scaling. (Courtesy of Dr P. Forster, The James Paget Hospital, Great Yarmouth, UK.)

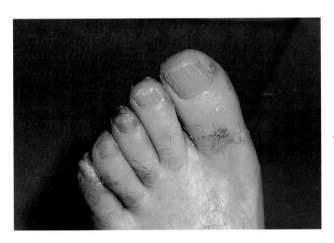

Fig. 62.2 Lesions involving the dorsal surface of toes. Note hyperkeratosis and pustule formation. (Courtesy of Dr P. Forster, The James Paget Hospital, Great Yarmouth, UK.)

mature lesion has a limpet-like appearance and may stand out a centimetre or so from the skin surface. New lesions may emerge together forming an irregular heaped-up dull yellow mass with a 'relief map' appearance and feel. Sometimes the parakeratosis is more diffuse or the lesions are frankly pustular from the outset and may extend into a flaccid bulla with yellowish-brown, cheesy contents covering much of the foot (see Fig. 62.1). On moist skin, for example flexural areas, confluent circinate erosions (Fig. 62.4) or greasy brown maculopapules occur. Conversely, involvement of the palms and soles may be grossly hyperkeratotic.

Nail and perionychial involvement is common and often severe. Painless red swelling at the base of the nailfold (Fig. 62.5) evolves into parakeratotic scaling along the length of the nailfold followed by thickening, opacity or ridging of the nailplate. Subungual pustules may be seen and eventually much friable subungual parakeratosis

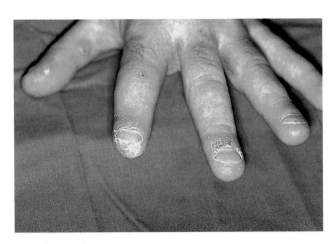

Fig. 62.3 Dorsal surface of the fingers and web space involvement. Note the tendency to peripheral scaling. (Courtesy of Dr P. Forster, The James Paget Hospital, Great Yarmouth, UK.)

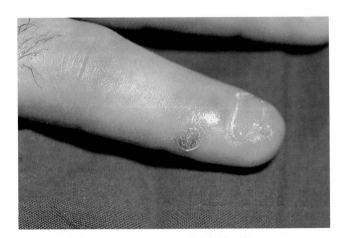

Fig. 62.5 Painless red swelling at the base of the nail. (Courtesy of Dr P. Forster, The James Paget Hospital, Great Yarmouth, UK.)

causes the nailplate to be shed. Onycholysis alone is very unusual [4]. Circinate vulvitis has been described [5] as has ulcerative vulvitis [6,7]. Reiter's disease is uncommon in females, frequently takes incomplete forms and may be difficult to distinguish from genital candidiasis and psoriasis. A high index of suspicion is therefore required to link cutaneous, mucosal and systemic manifestations [8].

Penile lesions

These occur in about 25% of patients, their morphology on the glans depending on the presence or absence of a foreskin. In the uncircumcised male a shallow, red, moist erosion develops with some marginal erythema (Fig. 62.6). The coalescence of multiple lesions leads to so-called circinate balanitis (Fig. 62.7). A more diffuse balano-posthitis may be precipitated by secondary infection. Involvement may occur down the shaft of the penis and including the scrotum (Fig. 62.8). On the circumcised penis, the erosions quickly become covered by a mixture of crust and scale and may evolve into typical keratoderma as seen elsewhere.

Both clinically and histologically all the features of Reiter's disease are psoriasiform and fall within a spectrum of changes seen in idiopathic psoriasis [9]. Typical mild keratoderma corresponds to 'rupioid' psoriasis and the acral changes may also be seen in the absence of arthritis or other involvement. In view of the morphological similarities, evolution into banal psoriasis [10], psoriatic arthritis [4], HLA and family studies [11], it seems possible that keratoderma represents the provocation of a psoriatic diathesis by the disease. Nevertheless, the overall pattern, course and distribution of the eruption in Reiter's disease are usually distinctive [12].

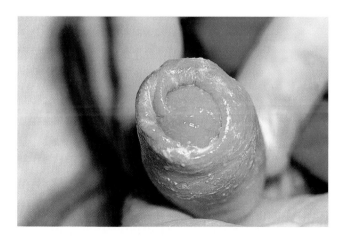

Fig. 62.6 Moist red eroded lesions of the uncircumcised penis. (Courtesy of Dr P. Forster, The James Paget Hospital, Great Yarmouth, UK.)

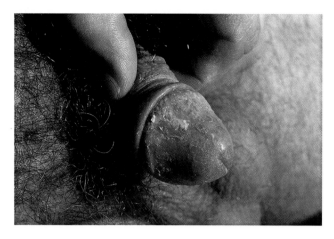

Fig. 62.7 Delicate lesions of circinate balanitis on the glans penis.

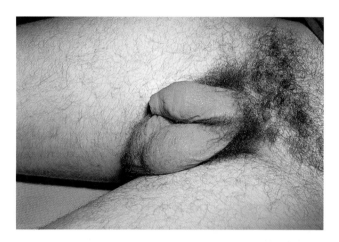

Fig. 62.8 Involvement of the foreskin, shaft of the penis and scrotum. (Courtesy of Dr P. Forster, The James Paget Hospital, Great Yarmouth, UK.)

Keratoderma is often self-limiting, lasting weeks or months. Evolution into universal psoriatic erythroderma occasionally ensues, usually with severe arthritis and constitutional illness; if left untreated, this severe form may lead to chronic incapacity and death. Circinate balanitis may precede other manifestations of the disease by months or years as a *forme fruste* of the disease [1,13].

Oral lesions

In order of frequency, the palate, uvula, tongue, buccal mucosa and lips are involved. The pharynx may also be affected. Such lesions tend to be transient and painless and are seen in about 10–15% of patients, although the published rates of incidence have varied between 3 and 33% [1]. Small vesicles rapidly evolve into erosions with marginal erythema. Larger granular circinate erosions are seen rarely covered with a whitish epithelium simulating leukoplakia. Patchy erythema without erosions may involve the soft palate, uvula or faucial areas. On the tongue, areas of reddened papillae or frank erosions may be seen; these may mimic geographical tongue.

REFERENCES

1 Calin A. Keratoderma blenorrhagicum and mucocutaneous manifestations of Reiter's syndrome. *Ann Rheum Dis* 1979; **38** (Suppl.): 68–72.
2 Paronen I. Reiter's disease a study of 344 cases observed in Finland. *Acta Med Scand* 1948; **131** (Suppl. 212): 1–112.
3 Roumagnac H, Ferreand M, Pernod J *et al*. Etude statisque sur le syndrome de Fiessinger–Leroy. *Rev Corps Milit* 1958; **14**: 502–22.
4 Wright V. Psoriatic arthropathy and seronegative rheumatoid arthritis with psoriasis: distinguishing features from Reiter's syndrome. *Ann Rheum Dis* 1979; **38** (Suppl.): 59–67.
5 Thambar IV, Dunlop R, Thin RN. Circinate vulvitis in Reiter's syndrome. *Br J Vener Dis* 1977; **53**: 260–2.
6 Daunt SO, Kotowsk KE, O'Reilly AP. Ulcerative vulvitis in Reiter's syndrome: a case report. *Br J Vener Dis* 1982; **58**: 405–7.
7 Kanerva L, Kousa M, Niemi KM *et al*. Ultrahistopathology of balanitis circinata. *Br J Vener Dis* 1982; **58**: 188–95.
8 Edwards L, Hansen RC. Reiter's syndrome of the vulva. *Arch Dermatol* 1992; **128**: 811–14.
9 Zachariae H. Significance of the pustular reaction in psoriasis. In: Farber EM, Cox AJ, Jacobs PH *et al*., eds. *Psoriasis; Proceedings of the Second International Symposium*. New York: Yorke Medical Books, 1977: 163–70.
10 Wright V, Reed WB. The link between Reiter's syndrome and psoriatic arthritis. *Ann Rheum Dis* 1964; **23**: 12–21.
11 Lawrence J. Family survey of Reiter's disease. *Br J Vener Dis* 1974; **50**: 140–5.
12 Lassus A, Kousa M. Reiter's disease. In: Harris JR, ed. *Recent Advances in Sexually Transmitted Disease*, No 2. Edinburgh: Churchill Livingstone, 1981: 187–99.
13 Lassus A, Tiilikainen A, Stubb J *et al*. Circinate erosive balanitis and HLA-27. *Acta Derm Venereol (Stockh)* 1975; **55**: 199–201.

Complications

The disease may involve the heart and central nervous system [1]. The heart was involved in 7% of a Finnish series [2] and in 6% of a British series. Kousa [3] found electrocardiogram (ECG) changes in 9% of patients in an acute attack, particularly flattened inverted T waves and prolonged Q–R intervals. More important are the late and chronic cardiac sequelae which can include: complete or incomplete atrioventricular heart block, which may or may not respond to corticosteroids [4,5]; aortic incompetence, which like the conduction defects may be more broadly linked with the seronegative spondyloarthropathies [6]; myocarditis and pericarditis [7]. Transient, incomplete heart block was reported in 4% of one series [8]. Coronary artery stenosis secondary to aortitis has been documented [9].

Neurological manifestations occur in about 1% of patients [8,10]. These have included peripheral neuritis, optic neuritis and various cranial nerve palsies; meningoencephalitis [8], neuralgic amyotrophy [11] and polyradiculitis [3] have been described. An unusual case of reversible ascending motor neuropathy linked with quiescent Reiter's disease appears to be an isolated finding [12].

Lymphadenopathy [13], salivary gland enlargement [14] and erythema nodosum [3] have been reported, but it may be difficult to distinguish direct associations from other mechanisms. Gut involvement of course is linked via a genetic predisposition with the histocompatibility antigen HLA-B27 and inflammatory bowel disease; this association complicates the clinical picture [15]. A case of incomplete Reiter's disease has been reported with ischaemic colitis [16]. Although amyloidosis is infrequently associated [17,18], involvement of the colon has been documented [19]. Ulceration of the middle and distal oesophagus has been described with Reiter's disease [20].

Thyroiditis has been associated [3]. Unusual genito-urinary sequelae include urethral stricture [8] and pyelonephritis [5]. Thrombophlebitis of the deep calf veins was recorded in 4% of patients [8]. Pulmonary involvement with pleurisy and pneumonitis is rare [3]. A report with writer's cramp cryptically infers more than a phonetic link [21].

Complications from the concurrence of Reiter's disease and acquired immune deficiency syndrome appear related to the degree of immunosuppression and whether or not immunosuppressive therapy has been administered for Reiter's disease prior to the recognition of AIDS [22]. Certainly both Kaposi's sarcoma, fulminant AIDS and profound immunosuppression have resulted from methotrexate therapy in AIDS-related complex linked with Reiter's disease [23,24]. An incomplete form of Reiter's disease has been reportedly induced by systemic interferon-α treatment [25], although the role of the patient's chronic active hepatitis C is uncertain. Reiter's disease in an HIV-positive patient has been associated with hypozincaemia, and whilst this is unlikely to be aetiological, it could exacerbate the cutaneous manifestations [26].

REFERENCES

1 Good AE. Reiter's disease; a review with special attention to cardiovascular and neurologic sequelae. *Semin Arthritis Rheum* 1974; **3**: 253–86.
2 Paronen I. Reiter's disease: a study of 344 cases observed in Finland. *Acta Med Scand* 1948; **131** (Suppl. 212): 1–112.
3 Kousa M. Clinical observations on Reiter's disease with special reference to the venereal and non-venereal aetiology. *Acta Derm Venereol (Stockh)* 1978; **58** (Suppl.): 1–36.
4 Nielsen H. Complete heart block in Reiter's syndrome. *Acta Cardiol* 1986; **41**: 451–5.
5 Thomsen NH, Horslev-Petersen K, Simonsen EE. Complete heart block in Reiter's syndrome. *Dan Med Bull* 1985; **32**: 272–3.
6 Qaiyami S, Hassau ZU, Toone E. Seronegative spondyloarthropathies in lone aortic insufficiency. *Arch Intern Med* 1985; **145**: 822–4.
7 Csonka GW, Litchfield JW, Oates JK *et al*. Cardiac lesions in Reiter's disease. *Br Med J* 1961; **i**: 243–7.
8 Csonka GW. Workshop I. Features and prognosis of Reiter's syndrome. Clinical aspects of Reiter's syndrome. *Ann Rheum Dis* 1979; **38** (Suppl.): 4–7.
9 Hoogland YT, Pendelton Alexander E, Patterson RH *et al*. Coronary artery stenosis in Reiter's syndrome: a complication of aortitis. *J Rheumatol* 1994; **21**: 757–9.
10 Weinberger HJ, Ropes MW, Kulka JP *et al*. Reiter's syndrome: clinical and pathologic observations. *Medicine* 1962; **41**: 35–91.
11 Catterall RD, Rooney KJ, Kirby B. Neurologic amyotrophy in Reiter's disease. *Br J Vener Dis* 1965; **41**: 62–4.
12 Taurog JD, Moore PM. An unusual motor neuropathy occurring during quiescent Reiter's disease. A case report. *Clin Exp Rheumatol* 1986; **4**: 147–9.

13 Reich H. Lymphknotenbeteiligung bei Reiterscher Krankheit. *Hautarzt* 1966; **17**: 406–11.

14 Reckless JP. Reiter's syndrome with parotitis in the female. *Br J Vener Dis* 1972; **48**: 207–8.

15 McNiesch LM, Bora JG. Reiter's disease complicated by ulcerative colitis: a case report. *Milit Med* 1986; **151**: 550–2.

16 Lempp F, Butzow GH, Wassilew S *et al.* Ischäimische Kolitis bei Reiter's-syndrome. *Z Gastroenterol* 1985; **23**: 52–9.

17 Caughey DE, Wakem CJ, Auckland NL. A fatal case of Reiter's disease, complicated by amyloidosis. *Arthritis Rheum* 1973; **16**: 695–700.

18 Stone G, Wolfe F. Collateral ligament calcification complicating amyloidosis and Reiter's syndrome. *J Rheumatol* 1984; **11**: 248–50.

19 Bleehen SS, Everall JD, Tighe JR. Amyloidosis complicating Reiter's syndrome. *Br J Vener Dis* 1966; **42**: 88–92.

20 Nakamura S, Iida M, Kohrogi N *et al.* Esophageal ulcer complicated by Reiter's syndrome. *J Clin Gastroenterol* 1992; **14**: 148–51.

21 Hughes RA, Keat AC. Reiter's cramp. *Ann Rheum Dis* 1990; **49**: 47.

22 Winchester R, Bernstein DH, Fischer HD. The co-occurrence of Reiter's syndrome and acquired immunodeficiency. *Ann Intern Med* 1987; **106**: 19–26.

23 Brancato L, Hescu S, Skovron ML *et al.* Aspects of the spectrum, prevalence and disease susceptibility determinants of Reiter's syndrome and related disorders associated with HIV infection. *Rheumatol Int* 1989; **9**: 137–41.

24 Wilkens RF, Arnett FC, Bitter T *et al.* Reiter's syndrome: evaluation of preliminary criteria for definite disease. *Arthritis Rheum* 1981; **24**: 844–9.

25 Cleveland MG, Mallory SB. Incomplete Reiter's syndrome induced by systemic interferon alpha treatment. *J Am Acad Dermatol* 1993; **29**: 788–9.

26 Hausmann G, Castel T, Iranzo P *et al.* Reiter's syndrome associated with hypozincemia in an HIV-positive patient. *Int J Dermatol* 1988; **27**: 342–3.

Differential diagnosis

Other forms of arthritis should be considered [1]. The differentiation between joint involvement associated with Reiter's disease, psoriasis and ankylosing spondylitis is probably not worthwhile as the development and pattern have a common link via the HLA-B27 haplotype. If the joint involvement is monoarticular and painful, pyogenic arthritis should be excluded and has been reported following a dysenteric illness [2]; septic arthritis can mimic Reiter's disease [3]. Gonococcal arthritis and septicaemia may be more common in women especially in pregnancy; the characteristic pustulosis is clearly different from the expected cutaneous changes in Reiter's disease. The arthritides may be difficult to differentiate, but gonoccocal arthritis does not affect the spine [4]. In the female atypical vulval changes may be difficult to distinguish from candidiasis associated with flexural psoriasis [5]. Scabies, erythema multiforme and lichen planus need to be differentiated from the penile, buccal and other skin lesions; taken in the clinical context this is seldom difficult.

In the eye the severe uveitis of Behçet's disease is distinguished by signs of a retinal vasculitis [6]. Posterior uveitis usually points to toxoplasmosis.

In HIV-positive patients distinction needs to be made between AIDS-associated psoriasis, other linked papulo-squamous eruptions and Reiter's disease [7].

Investigations

No specific laboratory test exists to confirm the diagnosis of Reiter's disease. In an unexplained arthritis, clinical evidence of mucocutaneous changes, anterior uveitis and occult urethritis should be sought. An important investigation is the examination of the overnight urethral secretion by smear and culture. Examination of the urine should be carried out, but is less helpful. Stool samples should be sent for culture and examination for cysts. Aspirated joint fluid may be turbid and yellow, but usually sterile. Serology and complement fixation tests should be sent for the relevant infectious triggering agents. The ESR, C-reactive protein, α_2-globulin and gammaglobulin are usually raised. Leukocytosis is variable. Serum complement levels are often normal, but may be raised. Immune complexes may be detectable in the serum [8].

After appropriate counselling the HIV status should be established for all patients in whom it is reasonable to do so. This is particularly important if immunosuppressive therapy is to be entertained [9]. Depending on geographical location, history of travel and clinical circumstances, *Borrelia burgdorferi* antibodies should be looked for [10].

The detection of HLA-B27 positivity helps to support the diagnosis and is a useful epidemiological detail. Tests for rheumatoid factor should be negative. Radiological changes in bones and joints may not be helpful, but in recurrent arthritis the detection of articular erosions, periostitis and plantar spurs aids diagnosis. In suspected cases, formal ophthalmological assessment is justified even in the absence of eye symptoms.

The presence of unexplained iritis in young men requires the exclusion of urogenital infection, radiography of the sacroiliac joints and testing for HLA-B27.

Skin biopsy is of little discriminatory value once a diagnosis of Reiter's disease is considered. Early pustular lesions from the palms or feet may show a spongiform macropustule in the upper epidermis. There is parakeratosis and elongation of the rete ridges. Older lesions may show just non-specific acanthosis, hyperkeratosis and parakeratosis with a pattern resembling psoriasis [11].

Prognosis

Calin *et al.* [12,13] evaluated 104 patients after a mean of 6.4 years. Only 16% were free of symptoms; 22% had annoying symptoms and in another 35% symptoms interfered with work. A further 15% had been forced to change jobs and the residual 12% were unemployable. In this series polyarthritis, back and heel pain, painful calcaneal spurs, tendonitis and eye disease were the chief sources of discomfort or disability. Similar findings were obtained in another American study of 48 patients [14,15]. One hundred postdysenteric cases in Finland were assessed after 20 years [16]. Only 20% were symptom free; 18% had active peripheral arthritis and another 32% had clinical or radiographic evidence of sacroiliitis. The remaining 30% had evidence of inactive chronic arthritis. Other authors have studied the evolution of sacroiliitis in detail [17].

A recurrence rate of 15% per patient per year has been calculated [18]; in total 40% of this series had a second or subsequent attack. Serious systemic lesions (cardiac or neurological) occurred in 3% and mortality was 1%. In general the longer and more stormy the initial attack, the greater the chance of serious long-term disease [18]. HLA-B27-negative individuals with limited joint involvement, without systemic involvement and disease involving children may have a milder, less protracted course. Fatal cases of Reiter's disease are rare, sometimes related to the side-effects of therapy rather than to the disease itself, but do occur [19]. The association with HIV positivity clearly alters the prognosis and within the guarded prognosis of the HIV-positive population, the appearance of severe psoriasis and particularly Reiter's disease is regarded as a poor prognostic indicator [7]. Chronic disability is unlikely to be a problem in this group, but in general it is usually attributable to the arthropathy and associated deformities. Rarely, neurological sequelae, aortic incompetence, glaucoma due to repeated iritis, urethral stricture or chronic erythroderma can condemn the patient to chronic illness. Reiter's disease is unpredictable in its outcome and a severe, debilitating, relapsing chronic disorder may result; patients need to have the nature and potential of the complaint explained, particularly so that the link with re-exposure to infection and reactivation or exacerbation of the disease is taken on board in the hope of modifying behaviour.

Treatment [20]

There is no cure for Reiter's disease. However, around two-thirds of patients will have complete disease resolution within 6 months. Within this group the aim of management is to maintain mobility and reassurance based on a confident diagnosis [20]. This may include rest in the early stages with careful attention to correct posture; heel supports; gentle, non-weight-bearing, passive movements; and simple analgesia. Aspiration of painful effusions may be necessary and local intraarticular steroid injections can benefit. With increasing involvement of the joints non-steroidal antiinflammatory agents are the next line of treatment with aspirin and in particular indomethacin being the drugs of choice. Indomethacin suppositories at night may assist in preventing morning stiffness.

It is sensible to treat infectious triggering agents when present with appropriate therapy. Non-gonococcal urethritis and concomitant gonorrhoea should be treated, but there is no evidence that this modifies the course of the disease [21]. For chlamydial infection and as a first-line measure when sexually transmitted triggers are suspected, tetracycline 500 mg four times a day for 14 days (longer if complications) or until signs of urethritis or cervicitis have cleared, is the treatment of choice [22]. Alternatives include doxycycline, 100 mg twice daily after meals and taken with fluid for 14–21 days [22]. Minocycline and erythromycin are other possible agents. Lymecycline, a water-soluble tetracycline active against *Chlamydia* and many dysenteric Gram-negative organisms, is another alternative. As with any genital infection the sexual partner should be examined and treated. With enteric triggers specific antimicrobial therapies are not always indicated and these must be treated on their own specific merits. Some evidence exists to suggest that long-term antibiotic treatment may be of value [23].

With aggressive and chronic, potentially destructive disease more toxic therapies may have to be used. However, before contemplating immunosuppressive therapy it is important to establish the HIV status of the patient, as Kaposi's sarcoma and fulminant AIDS have been precipitated by immunosuppressive treatment in the HIV-positive individual [9]. An alternative, in general, for the skin and joint manifestations is etretinate or acitretin [24], and specifically in AIDS patients where skin disease tends to be severe and recalcitrant [25–27]. HIV-positive patients with Reiter's who have lowered CD4 lymphocytes may require zidovudine therapy. In non-HIV-positive cases systemic corticosteroids may rarely be needed to control fulminating polyarthritis; up to 60 mg daily of oral prednisolone can be required in the early stages to prevent irreversible joint damage. Azathioprine (1.5–2.5 mg/kg body weight daily) appears to be a potentially successful therapy for relentlessly progressive disease [28]. Methotrexate (0.2–0.5 mg/kg body weight once weekly) has its supporters, for similarly severe involvement [29,30]. Most of these interventions will suppress cutaneous manifestations of the disorder. Gold salts, d-penicillamine and antimalarials do not appear to be effective [20]. Levamisole may be of benefit, but a high incidence of side-effects has prevented more widespread adoption as a treatment [20]. Remission has been described in four patients with Reiter's disease of enteropathic aetiology with the use of bromocriptine [31]. If conjunctivitis is trivial, simple eye toilet suffices; severe conjunctivitis responds to topical steroids, often combined with antibiotic eye-drops or chloretetracyline eye ointment. Anterior uveitis calls for intensive corticosteroid treatment and specialist ophthalmic advice. Rarely, generalized erythroderma will call for systemic treatment. There is increasing evidence that etretinate or acitretin may be the first choice, in such circumstances and particularly in the HIV-positive patients [26,27], but corticosteroids or methotrexate have been employed and may be acceptable in the HIV-negative patients.

Promiscuity will increase the exposure to many infectious trigger factors and the human immunodeficiency viruses. Clearly the use of a condom sheath during sexual activities would help reduce this risk. Those who are knowingly HLA-B27 positive could be forewarned of the risk; however, heightened anxiety may result and general advice in the light of recognized AIDS risks for the public at large may be the best approach. The routine adoption of contraceptive sheaths by the 'at-risk groups' for Reiter's disease could change the epidemiology of the disease; this may already have occurred as a result of the anti-AIDS campaigns from 1984–85 onwards [32].

REFERENCES

1 Wright V. Psoriatic arthropathy and seronegative rheumatoid arthritis with psoriasis: distinguishing features from Reiter's syndrome. *Ann Rheum Dis* 1979; **38** (Suppl.): 59–67.

2 Vartiainen J, Huni L. Arthritis due to *Salmonella typhimurium*. Report of 12 cases of migratory arthritis in association with *Salmonella typhimurium* infection. *Acta Med Scand* 1964; **175**: 771–6.

3 Aguilar JL, Sanchez EE, Carillo C *et al*. Septic arthritis due to *Mycobacterium phlei*. *J Rheumatol* 1989; **16**: 1377–8.

4 Hurd FR, Johns J, Chubick A. Comparative study of gonococcal arthritis and Reiter's syndrome. *Ann Rheum Dis* 1979; **38** (Suppl.): 55–8.

5 Edwards L, Hansen RC. Reiter's syndrome of the vulva. *Arch Dermatol* 1992; **128**: 811–14.

6 Perkins ES. Uveitis in B-27 related disease. *Ann Rheum Dis* 1979; **38** (Suppl.): 92–5.

7 Duvic M, Johnson TM, Rapin RP *et al*. Acquired immunodeficiency syndrome, associated psoriasis and Reiter's syndrome. *Arch Dermatol* 1987; **123**: 1622–32.

8 Rosenbaum JT, Theofilopoulos AN, McDevitt HO *et al*. Presence of circulating immune complexes in Reiter's syndrome and ankylosing spondylitis. *Clin Immunol Immunopathol* 1981; **18**: 291–7.

9 Winchester R, Bernstein DH, Fisher HD. The co-occurrence of Reiter's syndrome and acquired immunodeficiency. *Ann Intern Med* 1987; **106**: 19–26.

10 Arnett FC. The Lyme spirochaete: another cause of Reiter's syndrome. *Arthritis Rheum* 1989; **32**: 1182–4.

11 Lever WF, Schaumberg-Lever G. *Histopathology of the Skin*, 7th edn. Philadelphia: Lippincott Co, 1990: 164–5.

12 Calin A, Fox R, Gerber RC. Prognosis and natural history of Reiter's syndrome. *Ann Rheum Dis* 1979; **38** (Suppl.): 29–31.

13 Calin A, Fox R, Gerber RC *et al*. The natural history of Reiter's syndrome (RS) in academic and community settings. *Arthritis Rheum* 1978; **21**: 548–9.

14 Butler MJ, Russell AS, Percy JS *et al*. A follow-up study of 48 patients with Reiter's syndrome. *Am J Med* 1979; **67**: 808–10.

15 Russell AS, Butler MJ. Scintigraphic evaluation and prognosis of patients with Reiter's syndrome. *Ann Rheum Dis* 1979; **38** (Suppl.): 34–7.

16 Sairanen E, Paronen I, Mahonen H. Reiter's syndrome: a follow up study. *Acta Med Scand* 1969; **185**: 57–63.

17 Good AE. Reiter's syndrome: long term follow up in relation to development of ankylosing spondylitis. *Ann Rheum Dis* 1979; **38** (Suppl.): 39–45.

18 Csonka GW. Workshop I. Features and prognosis of Reiter's syndrome. *Ann Rheum Dis* 1979; **38** (Suppl.): 4–7.

19 Wattiaux MJ, Bourgeois P, Picard O *et al*. Two familial cases of malignant Reiter's syndrome. *Clin Exp Rheumatol* 1989; **7**: 541–5.

20 Anonymous. Treating Reiter's syndrome. *Lancet* 1987; **ii**: 1125–6.

21 Popert AJ, Gill AJ, Laird SM. A prospective study of Reiter's syndrome. An interim report on the first 82 cases. *Br J Vener Dis* 1964; **40**: 160–5.

22 Dunlop EM. Venereal disease: chlamydial genital infection and its complications. *Br J Hosp Med* 1983; **29**: 6–11.

23 Hughes RA, Keat AC. Reiter's syndrome and reactive arthritis: a current view. *Semin Arthritis Rheum* 1994; **24**: 190–210.

24 Benoldi D, Almori A, Bianchi G *et al*. Reiter's disease: successful treatment of the skin manifestations with oral etretinate. *Acta Derm Venereol (Stockh)* 1984; **64**: 352–4.

25 Belz J, Breneman DL, Nordulund JJ *et al*. Successful treatment of a patient with Reiter's syndrome and acquired immunodeficiency syndrome using etretinate. *J Am Acad Dermatol* 1989; **20**: 898–903.

26 Louthrenoo W. Successful treatment of severe Reiter's syndrome associated with human immunodeficiency virus infection with etretinate. Report of 2 cases. *J Rheumatol* 1993; **20**: 1243–46.

27 Williams HC, Du Vivier AW. Etretinate and AIDS-related Reiter's disease. *Br J Dermatol* 1991; **124**: 389–92.

28 Calin A. A placebo controlled crossover study of azothioprine. *Ann Rheum Dis* 1986; **45**: 653–5.

29 Chu SM. Reiter's syndrome: treatment with methotrexate. *Singapore Med J* 1976; **17**: 101–3.

30 Owen ET, Cohen ML. Methotrexate in Reiter's disease. *Ann Rheum Dis* 1979; **38**: 48–50.

31 Bravo G, Zazueta B, Lavalle C. An acute remission of Reiter's syndrome in male patients treated with bromocriptine. *J Rheumatol* 1992; **19**: 747–50.

32 Iliopoulos A, Karras D, Ioakimidis D *et al*. Changes in the epidemiology of Reiter's syndrome in the post-AIDS era? An analysis of cases appearing in the Greek army. *J Rheumatol* 1995; **22**: 252–4.

Chapter 63
The Skin and the Nervous System

C.B. ARCHER

Introduction

The sensory innervation of the skin allows the detection of a number of stimuli from the surrounding environment and the transmission of this information to the central nervous system (CNS) (see Chapter 4). The relationship between the nervous system and the skin is complex, and many neurocutaneous diseases have been described. For those who prefer to consider disease mechanisms, the idea of committing to memory the plethora of neurocutaneous syndromes, often accompanied by offputting eponymous titles, may seem a rather daunting prospect. It is!

The neurocutaneous diseases have been considered in terms of: (i) those in which an embryonic or developmental defect affects cells in the skin and nervous system; (ii) those in which a pathological event simultaneously affects vulnerable cells of both the skin and nervous system; and (iii) those in which there is a primary abnormality of the nervous system, which subsequently gives rise to symptoms and signs in the skin [1]. Embryonic abnormalities in the nervous system and skin may progress in parallel without having any direct interaction, as one sees in neurofibromatosis and tuberous sclerosis (see Chapter 16). Pathogenic events affecting the skin and nervous system simultaneously might include a metabolic abnormality (e.g. the mucopolysaccharidoses, Refsum's syndrome and Tangier disease, see Chapter 59), a deficiency state (e.g. pellagra, see Chapter 59), and exposure to a toxin (e.g. arsenic poisoning) or an infective agent (e.g. *Meningococcus*).

The aim of this chapter is to consider skin diseases arising as a result of a primary abnormality or abnormalities in the nervous system. These may be divided broadly into disorders associated with sensory abnormalities and those associated with autonomic abnormalities, although there is some overlap between these two groups. Skin manifestations may occur when the pathology is predominantly located either in the CNS, such as the spinal cord, or in the peripheral nervous system. Post-herpetic neuralgia is relatively common and will be considered first.

REFERENCE

1 Short PM, Adams RD. Neurocutaneous diseases. In: Fitzpatrick TB, Eisen AZ, Wolff K *et al.*, eds. *Dermatology in General Medicine*. New York: McGraw-Hill, 1993: 2249–90.

Post-herpetic neuralgia [1,2]

Herpes zoster (Chapter 26) is itself painful, and is sometimes followed by neuralgia. The risk of developing post-herpetic neuralgia rises with age, which influences both the duration and the severity of the neuralgia once it appears [1]. Post-herpetic neuralgia, defined as pain persisting beyond 4 weeks, occurred in 16% of patients younger than 60 years but in 47% of those older than 60 years [3]. Only about one-quarter of those with pain 4 weeks after the vesicles have healed still have pain a year later [4], but this pain can be so severe that it interferes with sleep and causes depression or even suicidal tendencies. The pain is a combination of burning, aching or itching, with paroxysms of stabbing or burning pain, sometimes provoked by stimuli which are normally non-noxious, such as contact with clothing or changes in temperature.

Why some patients develop post-herpetic neuralgia is incompletely understood. There is, for example, no consistent relationship between this type of pain and a loss of large fibres in the damaged nerves, but *in vitro* studies [5] suggest that the virus itself may cause normally silent neurones to produce spontaneous action potentials.

Two controlled studies [6,7] suggested that the use of systemic steroids during the acute episode of herpes zoster might reduce the risk of developing post-herpetic neuralgia, and in neither was generalized herpes zoster a problem. However, given its immunosuppressive effects, and potential for serious complications, this treatment is not recommended by all authorities: indeed some of the evidence in its favour is flawed or conflicting [8,9].

In older adults with localized herpes zoster, oral aciclovir (800 mg five times daily for 7 days) reduces acute pain and healing times if treatment is initiated within 72 h of the onset of the eruption [10]. A reduction in ocular complications, particularly keratitis and anterior uveitis, occurs with treatment of herpes zoster ophthalmicus [11]. However, no reproducible effect on post-herpetic neuralgia has been found [12–15]. Valaciclovir (1000 mg three times daily for 7 days) may provide more prompt relief of zoster-associated pain than aciclovir in acute herpes zoster in older adults (over 50 years of age) [16].

In immunocompromised patients with herpes zoster, intravenous aciclovir (500 mg/m^2/8h for 7 days) reduces viral shedding, healing times, the risks of cutaneous dissemination and visceral complications, as well as the length of hospital stay in disseminated zoster [17].

Famciclovir is the prodrug of penciclovir, and lacks intrinsic antiviral activity. Penciclovir is similar to aciclovir in its spectrum of activity and potency against varicella–zoster virus [18]. Oral famciclovir is approved currently for the treatment of localized herpes zoster of less than 3 days' duration in immunocompetent adults. Famciclovir (500 mg three times daily for 7 days) is as effective as conventional acyclovir treatment in treating acute herpes zoster [19,20]. In addition, it seems that famciclovir does not decrease the frequency, but may reduce the duration, of post-herpetic neuralgia, particularly in patients older than 50 years of age.

In mild and moderate cases of established post-herpetic neuralgia, simple analgesics help, but in severe cases they may have little effect, and a variety of medical and surgical treatments have been tried [21,22], including division of the dorsal root or tractotomy. Injection of the ganglion or sensory root is considered unreliable in trigeminal herpes zoster. Amitryptiline, sometimes in combination with a phenothiazine derivative, may prove helpful [22,23]. Shooting pains may be helped by carbamazepine (200 mg three or four times daily) but therapy may have to continue for many months.

Other treatments reported to benefit some patients include baclofen [24], epidural injections of steroids and local injections of triamcinolone with or without procaine. In one patient, the local application of a lignocaine–prilocaine cream proved effective [25]. Acupuncture, transcutaneous stimulation and topical capsaicin applications [26] may also be worth considering, although their efficacy is unpredictable.

REFERENCES

1 Russell K, Portenoy RK, Duma C *et al.* Acute herpetic and postherpetic neuralgia: clinical review and current management. *Ann Neurol* 1986; **20**: 651–64.

2 Watson PN, Evans RJ. Post-herpetic neuralgia. *Arch Neurol* 1986; **43**: 836–46.

3 Rogers RS, Tindall JP. Geriatric herpes zoster. *J Am Geriatr Soc* 1971; **19**: 495–503.

4 Ragozzino MW, Melton LJ, Kurland LT *et al.* Population based study of herpes zoster and its sequelae. *Medicine* 1982; **61**: 310–16.

5 Schon F, Mayer ML, Kelly JS. Pathogenesis of post-herpetic neuralgia. *Lancet* 1987; **ii**: 366–8.

6 Eaglestein WH, Katz R, Brown JA. The effects of early corticosteroid therapy on the skin eruptions of herpes zoster. *JAMA* 1970; **211**: 1681–3.

7 Keczkes K, Basheer AM. Do corticosteroids prevent post-herpectic neuralgia? *Br J Dermatol* 1980; **102**: 511–15.

8 Esmann Y, Geil JP, Kroon S *et al.* Prednisolone does not prevent post-herpetic neuralgia. *Lancet* 1987; **ii**: 126–9.

9 Post BT, Philbrick J. Do corticosteroids prevent post-herpetic neuralgia? *J Am Acad Dermatol* 1988; **18**: 605–10.

10 Wood MJ, Ogan PH, McKendrick MW *et al.* Efficacy of oral acyclovir treatment of acute herpes zoster. *Am J Med* 1988; **85** (Suppl. 2A): 79–83.

11 Cobo LM, Foulks GN, Liesegang T *et al.* Oral acyclovir in the treatment of acute herpes zoster ophthalmicus. *Ophthalmology* 1986; **93**: 763–70.

12 Crooks RJ, Bell AR, Fiddian FP. Treatment of shingles and postherpetic neuralgia. *Br Med J* 1989; **299**: 392–3.

13 Flowers FP, Araujo OE, Turner LA. Recent advances in anti-herpetic drugs. *Int J Dermatol* 1988; **27**: 612–16.

14 Jolleys JV. Treatment of shingles and post-herpetic neuralgia. *Br Med J* 1989; **299**: 393.

15 McKendrick MW, McGill JI, Wood MJ. Lack of effect of acyclovir on post herpetic neuralgia. *Br Med J* 1989; **298**: 431.

16 Beutner KR, Friedman DJ, Forszpaniack C *et al.* Valaciclovir compared with acyclovir for improved therapy for herpes zoster in immunocompetent adults. *Antimicrob Agents Chemother* 1995; **39**: 1546–53.

17 Whitley RJ, Gnann JW, Jr, Hinthorn D *et al.* Disseminated herpes zoster in the immunocompromised host: a comparative trial of acyclovir and vidarabine. *J Infect Dis* 1992; **165**: 450–5.

18 Boyd MR, Kern ER, Safrin S. Penciclovir: a review of its spectrum of activity, selectivity and cross-resistance pattern. *Antiviral Chem Chemother* 1993; **4** (Suppl. 1): 3–11.

19 Degreef H and the Famciclovir Herpes Zoster Clinical Study Group. Famciclovir, a new oral antiherpes drug: results of the first controlled clinical study demonstrating its efficacy and safety in the treatment of uncomplicated herpes zoster in immunocompetent patients. *Int J Antimicrob Agents* 1994; **4**: 241–6.

20 Tyring S, Barbarash RA, Nahlik JE *et al.* Famciclovir for the treatment of acute herpes zoster: effects on acute disease and postherpetic neuralgia. A randomised, double-blind, placebo-controlled trial. *Ann Intern Med* 1995; **123**: 89–96.

21 Jolleys JV. Treatment of shingles and post-herpetic neuralgia. *Br Med J* 1989; **298**: 1537–8.

22 Watson CP, Evans RJ, Reed K *et al.* Amitryptiline versus placebo in post-herpetic neuralgia. *Neurology* 1982; **32**: 670–3.

23 Merskey H, Hester RA. Treatment of chronic pain with psychotropic drugs. *Postgrad Med J* 1982; **48**: 594–8.

24 Steordo L, Leo A, Marano E. Efficacy of baclofen in trigeminal neuralgia and other painful conditions: a clinical trial. *Eur Neurol* 1984; **23**: 51–5.

25 Milligan KA, Atkinson RE, Schofield PA. Lignocaine–prilocaine cream in post-herpetic neuralgia. *Br Med J* 1989; **298**: 253.

26 Bernstein JE. Bickers DR, Dahl MV *et al.* Treatment of post-herpetic neuralgia with topical capsaicin: a preliminary study. *J Am Acad Dermatol* 1987; **17**: 93–6.

Neurotrophic ulcer

This is a form of chronic ulceration, also known as 'perforating ulcer', that develops in anaesthetic skin. Characteristically, it is painless, persistent and uninflamed, appearing on areas subject to trauma or pressure.

Aetiology. The essential factors are loss of pain sensation, and trauma. Other influences such as interference with the triple response (Chapter 45), with autonomic function, and with presumed neurotrophic impulses may be of importance.

A number of neurological disorders may underlie the development of trophic ulcers, including peripheral neuropathy, syringomyelia, tabes dorsalis, spinal dysraphism, spinal cord injury, and hereditary sensory and autonomic neuropathies. In one series of 47 patients [1], diabetes complicated by peripheral neuropathy was the most frequent cause of neurotrophic ulcers of the foot. Friction and abrasion from badly fitting shoes, and from the ill-advised treatment of corns, are important precipitating factors.

Clinical features. Neurotrophic ulcers on the feet are seen, particularly on the pressure-bearing areas—under the heads of the metatarsals and on the heel (Fig. 63.1). The denervated skin is often hyperkeratotic, usually diffusely so, but occasionally localized in the form of callosities, and is anhidrotic.

All injuries heal slowly. A neurotrophic ulcer often begins as a hyperkeratotic and fissured area, which becomes infected. A sinus may then develop. Within the ulcer, necrotic material is seen, and when the underlying bone if affected, small sequestra may be present. The location of the ulcer is determined by trauma, the local topography and the nature of the underlying neurological disorder. Osteoporosis is frequently associated with sensory impairment. On the foot, a sinogram may be required to show communication of the sinus with a joint or a subfascial plantar abscess. Although usually painless, deep sensation may remain intact and referred pain can be present in an anaesthetic ulcer.

Treatment. This is often unsatisfactory, but, particularly in younger patients, considerable benefits can be obtained. Efforts should be made to relieve pressure, to control infection, and to assist, if possible, the return of normal sensation. Education about, and protection from, unperceived trauma are essential. Individually made shoes can be of considerable help, as can occlusive dressings provided that the ulcer is clean. When ischaemia is present, improvement of the circulation will sometimes initiate healing in elderly patients.

REFERENCE

1 Kelly PJ, Coventry MB. Neurotrophic ulcers of the feet. Review of 47 cases. *JAMA* 1958; **168**: 388–93.

Peripheral neuropathy

Peripheral neuropathy may be sensory, motor or mixed. In most types of peripheral neuropathy, the involvement is symmetrical and symptoms begin in the extremities with sensory loss in a glove and stocking distribution. In contrast to this is the patchy involvement of peripheral nerves of mononeuritis multiplex seen, for example, in polyarteritis nodosa, or sarcoidosis (Chapter 60). The causes of peripheral neuropathy are numerous and include diabetes mellitus, carcinomatous neuropathy, vitamin B group deficiency, and drugs or chemicals (Table 63.1).

The clinical picture includes recurrent acral skin ulcers and a history of repeated injuries that may progress to a substantial deformity. Patients with peripheral neuropathy may complain that their extremities feel 'numb', 'lifeless' or 'dead', or of a vague discomfort specified as 'burning', 'aching', 'pins and needles' or 'tenderness'. Lightning pains may be a feature of tabes dorsalis and angiokeratoma corporis diffusum (Fabry's disease). Some neuropathies also affect the autonomic nervous system and, in addition to postural hypotension, blurred vision and sphincter problems, patients may notice areas of hypohidrosis. The inherited sensory neuropathies are discussed in more detail below.

Trigeminal trophic syndrome

This is an uncommon disorder in which trophic ulceration follows minor, repetitive trauma to anaesthetic skin within the trigeminal area. Ulceration often begins on the ala nasi

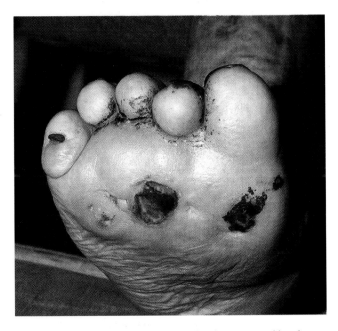

Fig. 63.1 Neurotrophic ulcers lying under the metatarsal heads.

Table 63.1 List of causes of peripheral neuropathy.

Metabolic	Diabetes mellitus, porphyria, myxoedema, acromegaly, uraemia, POEMS syndrome
Neoplastic	Carcinomatous neuropathy
Nutritional	Deficiencies of vitamins B_1, B_{12} or E
Toxic	Alcohol, heavy metals (lead, mercury, gold), drugs (e.g. isoniazid, dapsone, nitrofurantoin, disulfiram, phenytoin, vincristine, metronidazole), other toxic agents (e.g. organophosphates, acrylamide)
Infective	Diphtheria, leprosy, Guillain–Barré syndrome
Inflammatory	Rheumatoid arthritis, polyarteritis nodosa, sarcoidosis, systemic lupus erythematosus
Genetic	Hereditary neuropathies

POEMS, polyneuropathy, organomegaly, endocrinopathy, M-protein, skin changes.

and patients are often unaware of the tendency to scratch the skin.

Aetiology. Neurotrophic changes in the trigeminal area may follow the destruction of fibres conveying pain and temperature sensation. Many cases are due to attempts to relieve intractable trigeminal neuralgia by surgery or by alcohol injections into the Gasserian ganglion: the proportion of patients who have undergone these procedures and then develop the trigeminal trophic syndrome varies from 0 to 18% [1]. Other causes of the same clinical picture include occlusion of the posterior inferior cerebellar artery [2,3], syringobulbia, leprous trigeminal neuritis and, perhaps more commonly than widely appreciated, herpes zoster.

Trauma is an important contributory factor. Pronounced paraesthesiae may cause the patient to keep touching the area. These sensations include burning, itching, crawling and tickling. The nose and face may be repeatedly picked, rubbed or scratched. Elderly patients sometimes have a compulsion to pick at the skin.

Clinical features. A small, crusted area appears, followed by a crescentic ulcer, which may extend to destroy the nasal cartilage. The ulcer slowly spreads towards the cheek and the upper lip, which may be drawn up by a band of scarring. Bleeding may be troublesome and can lead to iron-deficiency anaemia. Characteristically, the tip of the nose is spared. Sites involved less frequently include the forehead, scalp and cheeks.

Ulceration is particularly intractable and, although painless, often causes considerable distress (especially to those who care for elderly patients). The clinical similarity to a basal cell carcinoma may be striking, since neurotrophic ulcers show little inflammatory reaction. The pattern of ulceration may be sufficiently bizarre to suggest dermatitis artefacta.

Treatment. The aim of therapy is to prevent the repeated trauma and to control secondary infection. A plastic prosthesis may be useful as protection. Surgical approaches in the past have included cervical sympathectomy [4]. More recently, good results have followed plastic surgery, in which innervated flaps from the unaffected side of the midline were used to cover the defect [5]. One patient responded well to transcutaneous electrical stimulation [6]. Often, however, the treatment of elderly and sometimes demented patients remains rather unsatisfactory. If necessary, oral iron supplements should be given.

REFERENCES

1 Finlay AY. Trigeminal trophic syndrome. *Arch Dermatol* 1979; **115**: 1118.
2 Freeman AG. Neurotrophic ulceration of the face with erosion of the ala nasi in vascular disorders of the brain. *Br J Dermatol* 1966; **78**: 322–31.
3 Walton, SL, Keczkes K. Trigeminal neurotrophic ulceration—a report of four patients. *Clin Exp Dermatol* 1985; **10**: 485–90.
4 McKenzie KG. Observations on the operative treatment of trigeminal neuralgia. *Can Med Assoc J* 1933; **29**: 492–6.
5 Tatnall FM, Stearns N, Sarkany I. Trigeminal trophic syndrome. *Br J Dermatol* 1985; **113** (Suppl. 29): 86–7.
6 Westerhof W, Bos JD. Trigeminal trophic syndrome: a successful treatment with transcutaneous electrical stimulation. *Br J Dermatol* 1983; **108**: 601–4.

Peripheral nerve injury

Section or severe contusion of a peripheral nerve has been held responsible for a variety of cutaneous changes. Skin manifestations are found in some 20% of patients with the carpal tunnel syndrome [1], and include a reddish discoloration of the fingers with bullae, small foci of necrosis, and nail dystrophy [2]. Nail dystrophy and other trophic changes are also sometimes caused by a cervical rib [3]. In one report, injury to the lateral femoral cutaneous nerve during appendicectomy [4] was followed 6 days later by the development of bullae on the outer aspect of the right lower leg, with subsequent ulceration and scarring.

Cooling also affects conduction in peripheral nerves. Loss of sensation in the feet has been reported after prolonged immersion in cold seawater [5]. Areas of skin looking like partial thickness burns, and blistering, were found on the feet of 25 out of 160 participants in a barefoot run: a temporary cold-induced neuropathy of the feet had allowed them to continue running despite these injuries [6]. Neuropathy may be induced by cryotherapy, and in one series of 183 lesions treated in this way, some subsequent sensory loss was demonstrated in 28%. This was usually mild and transient, although rarely long lasting [7].

REFERENCES

1 Aratari E, Regesta G, Rebora A. Carpal tunnel syndrome appearing with prominent skin symptoms. *Arch Dermatol* 1984; **120**: 517–19.
2 Pfister PR: Zur Klinik der Haut- und Nagelveränderungen beim Carpal-Tunnel syndrom. *Hautarzt* 1954; **5**: 440.
3 Rubin LC, Cipollaro AC. Onychodystrophy caused by cervical rib. *Arch Dermatol* 1939; **39**: 430–3.
4 Wagner W. Skin changes caused by damage of the lateral femoral cutaneous nerve. *Dermatol Wochenschr* 1957; **136**: 971–3.
5 Ungley CC, Channell GD, Richards RL. Immersion foot syndrome. *Br J Surg* 1945; **33**: 17–31.
6 Reichl M. Neuropathy of the feet due to running on cold surfaces. *Br Med J* 1987; **294**: 348–9.
7 Faber WR, Naafs B, Smitt JHS. Sensory loss following cryosurgery of skin lesions. *Br J Dermatol* 1987; **117**: 343–7.

Syringomyelia [1,2]

This is a rare disorder in which a longitudinal cyst in the cervical cord and/or brain stem (syringobulbia) occurs immediately anterior to the central canal and spreads, usually asymmetrically, to each side. It may be due to outflow obstruction of the fourth ventricle. An association with other abnormalities, such as a short neck and a low hairline, suggests a developmental origin. Symptoms usually appear in young adults and the disease is generally slowly progressive over 20–30 years.

Early involvement of pain and temperature fibres, where they cross the midline anteriorly, leads to a characteristic dissociated sensory loss, in which pain and temperature sensation is lost early in the upper limbs, while other sensory modalities carried in the posterior columns (e.g. touch, vibration and position sense) may remain relatively intact. These changes are responsible for the earliest manifestation of the disease, a tendency to sustain painless burns and cuts on the hands and forearms. Later, weakness, wasting and loss of reflexes in the arms may be accompanied by upper motor neurone signs in the legs.

Extension of cavitation into the medulla may disrupt the vestibular pathways, the descending root of the trigeminal nerve, the sympathetic and taste pathways, and the hypoglossal nerve. The symptoms and signs may then include vertigo with nystagmus, dissociated sensory loss over the face, loss of taste, a wasted tongue, Horner's syndrome and sometimes paralysis of the vocal cords. Facial oedema confined to areas of sensory loss has been described [3].

Many of the skin changes accompanying syringomyelia are the result of repeated burns or other injuries, particularly of the hands, where the skin over the fingers and knuckles may become thickened, swollen, cyanotic and keratotic. Analgesia renders the patient liable to minor injuries which heal slowly. Gangrene rarely occurs but damage to, or loss of, terminal phalanges or nails is not uncommon. The French term 'la main succulente' refers to the swollen and oedematous hands of syringomyelia sufferers. Other changes include loss of sweating, or ex-

cessive sweating, usually over the face and upper arms, which may be spontaneous or excited reflexly when the patient consumes hot or highly seasoned food.

Also seen occasionally is a combination of progressive pain loss, perforating ulcers, loss of soft tissue and resorption of the phalanges with muscular atrophy (Morvan's syndrome). Such changes may also occur in leprosy and hereditary sensory neuropathy.

REFERENCES

1 Anderson NE. The natural history of syringomyelia. *Clin Exp Neurol* 1986; **22**: 71–80.
2 Tashiro K, Fukazawa T, Moriwaka F *et al.* Syringomyelia syndrome: clinical features in 31 cases confirmed by CT myelography or magnetic resonance imaging. *J Neurol* 1987; **235**: 26–30.
3 McFadden JP, Handfield-Jones SE, Harman RRM. Hemi-facial oedema complicating a case of syringomyelia. *Clin Exp Dermatol* 1988; **13**: 42–5.

Tabes dorsalis [1]

This is still the most common form of neurosyphilis, and the one with the longest incubation period (usually 10–20 years: range 5–50 years), affecting men more often than women. The main symptoms are due to degeneration of the afferent fibres of the dorsal roots. It is characterized by a triad of symptoms (lightning pains, dysuria and ataxia) and a triad of signs (Argyll Robertson pupils, areflexia and loss of proprioceptive sense).

Usually, sensory symptoms precede ataxia by months or years. Lightning pains are the most characteristic early symptom and occur in 90% of cases at some stage, most often affecting the legs. Pain sensibility is also impaired early, the deep tissues becoming insensitive before the skin does. This may be demonstrated by squeezing the Achilles tendon. True Argyll Robertson pupils, which respond to accommodation but do not react to light, are found in about half of the patients.

Later features may include ataxia, with a wide-based gait, made worse by the elimination of visual clues, dribbling overflow incontinence, visceral crises, optic atrophy and a painless distortion of the hips, knees or ankles (Charcot's joints).

The commonest trophic change in the skin is the perforating ulcer, usually seen beneath the pad of the great toe or at other pressure points on the sole. The first stage is an epidermal thickening resembling a corn. Later, either spontaneously or as a result of attempted excision, an indolent ulcer develops. Sometimes a sinus will extend deeply as far as the underlying bone, leading to bony disorganization and deformity. Symptomatic herpes zoster may occur, as in other conditions affecting dorsal roots.

The clinical features and laboratory findings may be modified by the widespread use of antibiotics and corticosteroids for treating unrelated diseases [2]. This sometimes leads to difficulty in deciding whether tabes dorsalis is active or 'burned-out', with a neurological deficit due to fixed structural damage. Penicillin treatment will arrest the course of the disease, but residual lightning pains, gastric crises and urinary incontinence are likely to persist.

REFERENCES

1 Simon R. Neurosyphilis. *Arch Neurol* 1985; **42**: 606–13.
2 Kolar OJ, Burkhart JE. Neurosyphilis. *Br J Vener Dis* 1977; **53**: 221–5.

Spinal dysraphism [1]

A raphe is a line of junction between symmetrical embryological structures: dysraphism is a failure of this type of fusion. Spinal dysraphism leads to malformations of midline dorsal structures [2]. The term therefore includes spina bifida (defective closure of the neural tube and associated abnormalities of the vertebral column), but is broader, and embraces other abnormalities such as those in which cutaneous ectoderm is carried deeply, causing dermoid cysts or dermal sinuses to form.

A review of 200 published cases of spinal dysraphism [3] included 102 with cutaneous abnormalities, often in combination. A dermatologist may be the first physician to see such patients, and should be aware of possible associations with underlying neurological abnormalities.

Spina bifida

Several varieties of spina bifida are described, differing in the nature and severity of the spinal defect. In the severe form, a sac protrudes through the vertebral opening and transmits an impulse on crying or coughing. In the least severe cases (spina bifida occulta) there is no such protrusion, but a defect in the vertebral lamina may be felt as a depression, and is sometimes covered by a tuft of hair or a dimple (Fig. 63.2). Spina bifida occulta may give rise to no symptoms, and be a chance finding in the course of a routine examination. However, lesions preventing the ascent of the spinal cord, which occurs during normal growth, can lead to undue traction on the lower end of the cord and cauda equina.

The neurological changes will then be those of a chronic lesion of the cauda equina. Such patients may have been slow to learn to walk. Sensation may be impaired over the areas innervated by the lowest sacral segments, leading to a characteristic saddle-shaped area of analgesia over the buttocks and dorsa of the thighs. Trophic changes are conspicuous in some cases, and are rarely lacking altogether. In milder cases, the feet are usually cold and cyanosed: cutaneous injuries are slow to heal and tend to ulcerate, not only on the feet but also in the analgesic skin of the buttocks and thighs. The most severe neurological abnormality is a flaccid paraparesis with sphincter paralysis.

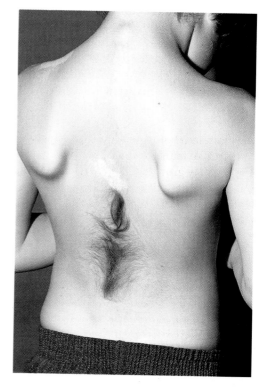

Fig. 63.2 An obvious tuft of hair in association with spina bifida.

The diagnosis is confirmed by radiography, showing defective fusion of the laminae in the affected region, usually the first sacral and fifth lumbar vertebrae. A magnetic resonance imaging (MRI) scan or myelography may be helpful. Estimation of α-fetoprotein in the amniotic fluid or in the maternal serum may successfully identify a fetus with a severe malformation of the CNS such as spina bifida cystica or anencephaly.

The treatment of spina bifida lies in the domain of the paediatrician or neurologist, but the dermatologist may be asked for advice on the trophic ulcers.

Congenital dermal sinuses [1,4]

These lie close to the midline, and may be no more than a millimetre or two in diameter. Hairs may protrude from the opening, but these sinuses differ from pilonidal sinuses in that they connect directly to the contents of the spinal canal and so serve as a portal of entry for infection. Probing is therefore unwise. Such sinuses may expand into cysts deeply, and these may press on the spinal cord.

Subcutaneous lipomas

These were found in 41 of 200 published cases of spinal dysraphism [3], often in association with spina bifida and usually in the midline of the lumbosacral area. The overlying skin is usually normal.

Vascular naevi

These were seen in 7 of the 200 patients in the same series. Capillary haemangiomas in the midline of the back should be suspected as being part of spinal dysraphism.

Hairy patches

These occurred in 30 of the 200 patients [3], and may be present at birth. A 'faun's tail' is an area where coarse hair in the midline may grow to several inches in length: more than 40% of patients with diastematomyelia have such patches of long hair [5]. Pigmented macules may also be found.

REFERENCES

1 Storer JS, Hawk RJ. Cutaneous signs of spinal dysraphism. In: Schachner LA, Hansen RC, eds. *Paediatric Dermatology*, Vol. I. New York: Churchill Livingstone, 1988: 275–7.
2 Lichtenstein BW. Spinal dysraphism: spina bifida and myelodysplasia. *Arch Neurosurg Psychiatry* 1940; **44**: 792–809.
3 Tavafoghi V, Ghandchi A, Hambrick GW *et al*. Cutaneous signs of spinal dysraphism. *Arch Dermatol* 1978; **114**: 573–7.
4 Harris HW, Miller OF. Midline cutaneous and spinal defects. *Arch Dermatol* 1976; **112**: 1724–8.
5 Keim HA, Greene AF. Diastematomyelia and scoliosis. *J Bone Joint Surg* 1973; **55**: 1425–35.

Spinal cord injury [1]

The spinal cord may be injured directly by penetrating wounds. More frequently, it suffers indirectly as a result of dislocations or fracture dislocations of the vertebral column. The commonest sites for spinal injuries are the lower cervical region and the thoracolumbar junction.

Seborrhoea and seborrhoeic dermatitis have been reported in quadriplegia patients. In one study [2] of 20 patients with spinal injury but no seborrhoeic dermatitis on admission, 13 developed the condition on the face and trunk within a few weeks. Nummular eczema may also occur below the level of the lesion [1]. Twenty-one patients with complete paralysis below levels varying from C5 to T12 were investigated for sebum excretion rate, skin temperature and the presence of acne [3]. An increased incidence of acne was found on the back and buttocks, often occurring for the first time after the onset of paralysis. Sebum excretion on the forehead did not differ from that of normals, but was significantly increased below the neurological lesion. This could not be explained by changes in skin temperature.

The changes in eccrine sweating after spinal cord injuries are complex [4]. Episodes of profuse sweating on the face, neck and upper trunk, in patients with lesions at or above T6, may occur as an exaggerated response to stimuli such as bowel or bladder distension (autonomic dysreflexia). Facial flushing and headache may be associated with these episodes. Other patients develop sweating of the face and arms after dizziness due to postural hypotension. Finally, post-traumatic syringomyelia can lead to hyperhidrosis [5]. Dryness of the skin, particularly noticeable on the soles, is an effect of anhidrosis.

Chronic decubitus ulceration can be a problem, and local osteomyelitis rarely leads to secondary amyloidosis. Excellent nursing, prevention of pressure and attention to the patient's general health are essential. Patient aids such as ripple mattresses help to reduce localized pressure.

REFERENCES

1 Reed WB, Pidgeon J, Becker SW. Patients with spinal cord injury: clinical cutaneous studies. *Arch Dermatol* 1961; **83**: 379–85.
2 Wilson CL, Walshe M. Incidence of seborrhoeic dermatitis in spinal injury patients. *Br J Dermatol* 1988; **119** (Suppl. 33): 48.
3 Thomas SE, Conway J, Ebling FJG *et al*. Measurement of sebum excretion rate and skin temperature above and below the neurological lesion in paraplegic patients. *Br J Dermatol* 1985; **112**: 569–73.
4 Sato K, Kang WH, Saga K *et al*. Biology of sweat glands and their disorders. II. Disorders of sweat gland function. *J Am Acad Dermatol* 1989; **20**: 713–26.
5 Stanworth PA. The significance of hyperhidrosis in patients with post-traumatic syringomyelia. *Paraplegia* 1982; **20**: 282–7.

Disorders associated with autonomic abnormalities

Hereditary sensory and autonomic neuropathies [1,2]

Hereditary sensory and autonomic neuropathies (HSAN) are rare. Three main types have been distinguished.

HSAN type I is inherited as an autosomal dominant with variable manifestations. Symptoms start during the second or later decades. Callosities develop on the plantar surfaces of the toes and under the metatarsal heads. These may blister or turn black and ulcerate. Such ulcers may heal but usually reopen with the discharge of pus or serosanguinous material. Episodes of cellulitis or lymphangitis may follow, and later osteomyelitis may lead to loss of bone and acral mutilation. Sensory loss may also occur in the fingers but hand infections are less common than in HSAN type II.

Other features include recurring lancinating pains, and an association in some families with peroneal muscular atrophy, and in others with a disabling sensorineural deafness.

Dissociated sensory loss, with loss of pain and temperature sensation but retained tactile sensibility, brings syringomyelia into the differential diagnosis. Leprosy and neuritic amyloidosis (Chapter 59) should also be considered. Treatment revolves around the prevention of foot ulcers. Shoes must be roomy and comfortable. Ulcers should be cleaned and debrided as necessary, and antibiotics may be needed. The need for amputation implies a failure of treatment, and conservative measures are to be preferred [3].

HSAN type II. The inheritance here is recessive. Symptoms occur in infancy or childhood, and include painless paronychia, whitlows and ulcers of the fingers and feet leading to a mutilating acropathy. All modalities of sensation are lost distally, and acral sweating may be reduced. The lips and tongue are also at risk of damage. Unrecognized fractures and Charcot joints may occur. Preventive treatment is less successful than in HSAN type I.

HSAN type III (syn. familial dysautonomia; Riley–Day syndrome) [4–6]. There is some overlap between this disorder and other types of HSAN, but here autonomic symptoms predominate. The disorder is recessively inherited and seen most often in Ashkenazi Jews originating from eastern Europe.

The condition starts in early infancy. Impaired pharyngeal and oesophageal motility leads to feeding difficulties. Recurrent fevers occur, with or without pneumonia, and affected children may sweat heavily and develop blotchy erythema when overheated. Erythematous macules 2–5 cm in diameter may occur on the trunk and limbs in response to emotional upsets [7].

A diagnosis is sometimes made in infancy because the child cries without producing tears. Absent fungiform papillae on the tongue, absent tendon and corneal reflexes, and an absence of the flare normally induced as an axon reflex after intradermal histamine, complete the picture. Later, the child may show delayed growth and episodes of hypertension and postural hypotension. Abnormalities of cutaneous temperature discrimination and nociception are found in most patients [8]. This tends to worsen with age. Charcot joints have been described [9]. The mortality rate is high. Death may follow inhalation during attacks of vomiting, and hypotension and cardiac arrest are risks with a general anaesthetic. There is no satisfactory treatment. When pulmonary infection is a problem, antibiotics should be used.

REFERENCES

1 Axelrod FB, Iver K, Fish I *et al*. Progressive density loss in dysautonomia. *Paediatrics* 1981; **67**: 517–22.
2 Dyck PG. In: Dyck PJ, Thomas PK, Lambert EH, Bunge R, eds. *Peripheral Neuropathy*, 2nd edn. Philadelphia: WB Saunders, 1984: 1557–641.
3 Berginer V, Baruchin A, Ben-Yakar *et al*. Plantar ulcers in hereditary sensory neuropathy: a plea for conservative treatment. *Int J Dermatol* 1984; **23**: 664–8.
4 Brunt PW, McKusick VA. Familial dysautonomia: a report of genetic and clinical studies with a review of the literature. *Medicine* 1970; **49**: 343–74.
5 Mahloudji M, Brunt PW, McKusick VA. Clinical neurological aspects of familial dysautonomia. *J Neurol Sci* 1970; **11**: 383–95.
6 Riley CM, Day RL, Greeley DM *et al*. Central autonomic dysfunction with defective lacrimation: report of five cases. *Paediatrics* 1949; **3**: 468–78.
7 Fellner MJ. Manifestations of familial autonomic dysfunction: report of a case with an analysis of 125 cases in the literature. *Arch Dermatol* 1964; **89**: 190–5.
8 Bundey S. *Genetics and Neurology*. Edinburgh: Churchill Livingstone, 1985: 194–223.
9 Brunt PW. Unusual case of Charcot joints in early adolescence (Riley Day syndrome). *Br Med J* 1967; **iv**: 277–8.

Congenital insensitivity to pain [1]

In some individuals, the threshold to pain may be high, and they are therefore insensitive to pain. This is a prominent feature of certain HSAN. Other patients with congenital insensitivity to pain have been described, who seemed to have no neuropathic abnormalities. However, they were examined when current techniques for the investigation of sensory neuropathies were not available. Three such children have now been investigated in this way [1]: one, without other apparent neurological deficit was found to have a rare type of HSAN (type V); another had HSAN type II; and a third had congenital pansensory neuropathy with retinitis pigmentosa. It is likely that the many cases described earlier had neuropathic changes that would now be detected by modern methods.

Patients with generalized analgesia of the types mentioned above should, strictly speaking, not be labelled as indifferent to pain. In pain indifference, the subjective threshold to pain may be within normal limits, and yet there may be a high tolerance so that the subject is truly indifferent to stimulation which a normal person would regard as painful. It is difficult to re-evaluate earlier published cases of congenital indifference to pain [2].

Asymbolia for pain [3] may follow localized lesions of the parietal lobe—in five of the original 10 cases it was transient. The brain lesion makes it impossible to build up a full perception of pain—a phenomenon akin to apraxia.

REFERENCES

1 Dyck PJ, Mellinger JF, Reagan TJ *et al*. Not 'indifference to pain' but varieties of hereditary sensory and autonomic neuropathy. *Brain* 1983; **106**: 373–90.
2 Winkelmann RK, Lambert EH, Hayles AB. Congenital absence of pain. *Arch Dermatol* 1962; **85**: 325–39.
3 Schilder P, Stengel E. Asymbolia for pain. *Arch Neurol Psychiatry* 1931; **25**: 598–600.

Sympathetic nerve injury [1]

When the sympathetic supply of the skin is interrupted, loss of vasoconstrictor impulses leads to erythema. There is passive vasodilatation and the denervated area is anhidrotic. The skin may become noticeably dry with scaliness and fine fissures. The affected area heals only slowly following minor trauma, and some patients complain that it is hyperaesthetic. It has been shown that after sympathetic ganglionectomy, there can be dissociation of sudomotor and pilomotor activity [2]. In the denervated areas, there is no loss of cutaneous sensation, and the phenomenon may be due to the regeneration of post-ganglionic cholinergic fibres. In general, the areas of vasodilatation correspond to the areas of anhidrosis, suggesting a close correspondence of sudomotor and vasoconstrictor fibres [3]. Measurements of sweating and vasomotor responses can help to determine the extent of autonomic denervation.

As discussed earlier in this chapter, when sympathetic denervation is combined with a loss of somatic sensation, as, for instance, in peripheral nerve injury or severe peripheral neuropathy, neurotrophic ulcers may be encountered. These result from local minor trauma and are characteristically painless and slow to heal. Sympathetic denervation may also slow or prevent the normal greying of hair that takes place with increasing age [4,5], and in one case it seemed to cause hyperpigmentation of the skin in the affected area [6].

REFERENCES

1 Munro PAG. *Sympathectomy: an Anatomical and Physiological Study with Clinical Applications.* Oxford: Oxford University Press, 1959.
2 Brown GE, Adson AW. Physiologic effects of thoracic and of lumbar sympathetic ganglionectomy or section of the trunk. *Arch Neurol Psychiatry* 1929; **22**: 322–57.
3 Silver A, Versaci A, Montagna W. Studies of sweating and sensory function in cases of peripheral nerve injuries of the hand. *J Invest Dermatol* 1963; **40**: 243–58.
4 Lerner AB. Grey hair and sympathectomy: report of a case. *Arch Dermatol* 1966; **93**: 235–6.
5 Ortonne J-P, Thivolet J, Guillet R. Greying of hair with age and sympathectomy. *Arch Dermatol* 1982; **118**: 876–7.
6 Samuel C, Bird DR, Burton JL. Hyperpigmentation after sympathectomy. *Clin Exp Dermatol* 1980; **5**: 349–50.

Reflex sympathetic dystrophy [1]

Reflex sympathetic dystrophy is a broad term that encompasses a group of disorders characterized by sympathetic hyperactivity, associated with persistent pain and responding to sympathetic denervation. It includes, for example, causalgia (occurring after peripheral nerve injury), mimocausalgia (after an insult to the CNS) and the shoulder–hand syndrome (associated with 'frozen shoulder' and occurring after myocardial infarction).

Aetiology. Causalgia follows damage to a peripheral nerve, either its incomplete division or involvement in scar tissue. Most commonly it follows injury to the median or sciatic nerves or arises in the divided fibres in an amputation stump; the pain is then referred distally into the phantom limb. Iatrogenic cases have followed nerve damage from improperly placed injections, and operations [2], including nail biopsy [3]. The unique factor responsible for the burning pain of causalgia may be a sudden stretching or deformation of the nerve without complete severance. Some damage to the sympathetic nervous system is also essential, but it is still not clear how the condition can be provoked by factors as disparate as those recorded in one series of 125 cases [4].

Clinical features. The pain begins at the time of the injury in about 50% of cases. It is hot and burning in character, and may worsen with dependency, physical contact or emotional upset. At first, oedema and increased nail and hair growth occur in the affected area. Later, the tissues may become indurated, the skin cool and sweaty, and livedo or cyanosis may be seen. Hair loss may then occur and the nails may become ridged and brittle. At this stage pain is constant and made worst by any stimulus. As a result, the patient protects the limb and uses it less. This leads to further trophic changes with a thin, shiny skin, muscle wasting and sometimes contractures. Demineralization of bone may be marked (Sudek's atrophy). The disorder may last for months or even years.

Diagnosis. This is clinical, assisted by the use of differential neural blockage to relieve the pain.

Treatment. Treatment is successful only when the focus of therapy is the sympathetic nervous system. Many patients obtain symptomatic relief from interruption of the sympathetic fibres by surgical ganglionectomy, local anaesthetic blocking of the paravertebral ganglia by direct infiltration [1], or by pharmacological interruption with adrenergic blocking agents. Exercises should be directed towards improving mobility of the affected extremity, but are only effective if undertaken after adequate pain relief has been obtained. A few patients benefit from transcutaneous nerve stimulation [5]. Oral guanethidine has been helpful [6]. The use of systemic corticosteroids, in high or moderate dosage, has led to good or excellent responses in more than half of the patients [7], and should be considered for those who cannot tolerate treatments that directly block sympathetic activity.

REFERENCES

1 Schwartzman RJ, McLellan TL. Reflex sympathetic dystrophy: a review. *Arch Neurol* 1987; **44**: 555–61.
2 Horowitz SH. Iatrogenic causalgia, classification, clinical findings and legal ramifications. *Arch Neurol* 1984; **41**: 821–4.
3 Ingram GJ, Scher RK, Lally EV. Reflex sympathetic dystrophy following nail biopsy. *J Am Acad Dermatol* 1987; **16**: 253–6.
4 Subbarao J, Stillwell GK. Reflex sympathetic dystrophy of the upper extremity: analysis of total outcome of management of 125 cases. *Arch Phys Med Rehabil* 1981; **62**: 549–54.
5 Mayer GA, Fields HL. Causalgia treated by selective large fibre stimulation of peripheral nerves. *Brain* 1972; **95**: 163–8.
6 Tabira T, Shibasaki H, Kuroiwa Y. Reflex sympathetic dystrophy (causalgia); treatment with guanethidine. *Arch Neurol* 1983; **40**: 430–2.
7 Kozin F. Ryan LM, Carrera GF *et al.* The reflex sympathetic dystrophy syndrome III. *Am J Med* 1981; **70**: 23–30.

Horner's syndrome [1]

This follows partial or complete interruption of the sympathetic pathways of the face. It is characterized by ptosis, miosis and anhidrosis.

Aetiology. The fibres responsible for the sympathetic nerve supply to the skin of the face travel from the hypothalamus via the spinal cord to relay at the level of the first and second thoracic segments in the lateral column of the spinal grey matter. The preganglionic fibres emerge from the cord in the anterior rami of the first and second thoracic spinal nerves, and pass up the cervical sympathetic chain to relay in the superior cervical ganglion. From here, postganglionic fibres pass to supply the eye and the skin of a small central area of the face via the internal carotid sympathetic plexus. Other fibres pass along the external carotid artery and its branches to innervate the greater part of the facial skin with vasomotor and sudomotor fibres.

This pathway can be interrupted centrally in the spinal cord, for example by medullary infarction, syringomyelia, multiple sclerosis or intraspinal tumours. The more peripheral fibres can be damaged by an aortic aneurysm, cervical lymphadenopathy, surgery, regional anaesthetic procedures or tumours.

Clinical features. An irritative phase is described but rarely seen, in which there is transient unilateral hyperhidrosis and vasoconstriction. The paralytic phase is characterized by a drooping of the eyelid (ptosis) with narrowing of the palpebral fissure. The pupil is small, but will show normal reflex constriction to light and accommodation. There may be a slight retraction of the globe of the eye into the orbit (enophthalmos). Sweating is absent on that side of the face; Horner's syndrome with normal sweating on the affected side is seen in Raeder's paratrigeminal syndrome. Cases of bilateral Horner's syndrome are rarely encountered.

Treatment. This should be directed to the underlying cause; usually, however, this is not amenable to therapy.

REFERENCE

1 Smith SA. Pupillary function in autonomic failure. In: Bannister R, ed. *Autonomic Failure*, 2nd edn. Oxford: Oxford Medical Publications, 1988: 393–412.

Gustatory hyperhidrosis

The autonomic nervous system has a propensity for regrowth [1]. Damage to adjacent preganglionic parasympathetic fibres and postganglionic sympathetic fibres may be followed by parasympathetic fibres regrowing into the sympathetic nerves, and thereby directly controlling sweat-gland function. In the neck, for example, following damage to the sympathetic cervical trunk and the vagus (parasympathetic) at the time of thyroidectomy or after trauma, such reinnervation may result in gustatory hyperhidrosis even after eating bland foods [2]. A similar event may occur on the cheeks or chin following surgery to the parotid or submandibular glands—the so-called auriculotemporal syndrome (Frey's syndrome) [3]. Fortunately, topical preparations such as those containing aluminium chloride hexahydrate often control these symptoms well, but may themselves produce an irritant dermatitis.

Other disorders

The following probably result from an abnormal and paroxysmal discharge of nerve impulses via the autonomic nervous system.

Ciliary neuralgia or 'cluster headaches'

A unilateral and periorbital headache is accompanied by lacrimation with conjunctival injection, nasal congestion and unilateral flushing of the face. The attacks are paroxysmal and sometimes Horner's syndrome is found on the affected side. Ergotamine may prove effective in treating these attacks.

Hypertensive diencephalic syndrome

This paroxysmal disorder is characterized by excessive sweating and blotchiness of the skin of the face and neck, with salivation, tachycardia and sustained hypertension. These cases require careful assessment and screening for a possible phaeochromocytoma.

Sphenopalatine syndrome

In this disorder, there is chronic and intermittent oedema of the face associated with lacrimation on the affected side. In addition, unilateral rhinitis and paroxysms of swelling alternating with erythema affecting the side of the bridge of the nose are sometimes seen.

REFERENCES

1 Murray JG, Thompson JW. The occurrence and function of collateral sprouting in the sympathetic nervous system of the cat. *J Physiol* 1957; **135**: 133–62.
2 Cunliffe WJ, Johnson CE. Gustatory hyperhidrosis: a complication of thyroidectomy. *Br J Dermatol* 1967; **79**: 519–26.
3 Bloor K. Post-parotidectomy gustatory sweating. *Br Med J* 1958; **ii**: 1295.

Chronic skin pain

The diagnosis of dysmorphophobia or dermatological non-disease [1,2] should always be considered when patients present with chronic skin pain, especially when areas important to body image are involved. These include burning vulva syndrome (vulvodynia) and burning scrotum syndrome discussed further in Chapter 72, as well as orodynia (Chapter 69). However, one should keep an open mind about other entities including notalgia paraesthetica [3–5] and skin-ache syndrome [6]. Postherpetic neuralgia is discussed earlier in this chapter.

Notalgia paraesthetica

This is characterized by episodes of localized itch or skin pain, usually close to the medial border of the scapula. It was first described and named in 1934 [3]. Pigmentation within the symptomatic patch has been reported, apparently resulting from the trauma-induced presence of melanin within macrophages [4]. Other features in lesional skin include necrotic keratinocytes in the epidermis [5], and proliferation of substance P-immunoreactive nerve endings [7]. In one study [8], 70% of patients treated with topical capsaicin and 30% of patients receiving vehicle reported some degree of improvement, but it was difficult to maintain the double-blind design of the study because of the symptoms produced by capsaicin itself. An association with macular localized cutaneous amyloidosis has been recorded.

Skin-ache syndrome

Bassoe [6] has suggested the term 'skin-ache syndrome' for a situation in which patients experience pain of unknown aetiology, characterized by cutaneous trigger points. Relief of symptoms was reported after injection of lidocaine or surgical removal of the skin trigger point.

REFERENCES

1 Cotterill JA. Dermatological non-disease: a common and potentially fatal disturbance of cutaneous body image. *Br J Dermatol* 1981; **104**: 611–18.
2 Cotterill JA. Clinical features of patients with dermatological non-disease. *Semin Dermatol* 1983; **2**: 203–5.
3 Astwazaturow M. Uber paresthetishe Neuralgien und eine bezondere Form derselben-Notalgias paresthetica. Nervenarzt 1934; **133**: 88–96.
4 Leibson I, Honecke H, Mas P. Puzzling posterior pigmented pruritic patches. *Cutis* 1973; **23**: 471–3.
5 Weber PJ, Poullos EG. Notalgia paresthetica. *J Am Acad Dermatol* 1988; **18**: 25–30.
6 Bassoe C-F. Skin-ache syndrome. *J R Soc Med* 1995; **88**: 565–9.
7 Springall DR, Kranth SS, Kirkham N *et al.* Symptoms of notalgia paresthetica may be explained by increased dermal innervation. *J Invest Dermatol* 1991; **97**: 555–61.
8 Wallengren J, Klinker M. Successful treatment of notalgia paresthetica with topical capsaicin: vehicle-controlled, double-blind, crossover study. *J Am Acad Dermatol* 1995; **32**: 287–9.

Chapter 64
Psychocutaneous Disorders

J.A.COTTERILL & L.G.MILLARD

The psychological importance of the skin [1,2]

Some cutaneous stimulation is a basic need. Newborn mammals require the stimulus of licking and stroking, and caressing favours emotional development. Experimental work with rats has shown that those which are caressed learn faster and grow faster [3]. As an organ of touch, temperature and pain sensation, and as an erogenous zone, the skin has great psychological importance at all ages. It is an organ of emotional expression and a site for the discharge of anxiety. Its texture and colour have meaning socially and politically, and its disorders carry with them a disproportionately heavy psychological punishment.

REFERENCES

1 Messeri P, Montagna W. Ethologic implications of the skin and its disturbances. In: Panconesi E, ed. *Clinics in Dermatology*, Vol. 2. *Psychosomatic Dermatology*. 1984: 27–36.
2 Montagu A. The skin, touch and human development. In: Panconesi E, ed. *Clinics in Dermatology*, Vol. 2. *Psychosomatic Dermatology*. 1984: 17–26.
3 Ruegamer WR, Bernstein L, Benjamin JD. Growth, food utilization and thyroid activity in the albino rat as a function of extra handling. *Science* 1954: **120**: 184–5.

Emotional factors in diseases of the skin [1–4]

It has been estimated that the effective management of at least one-third of patients attending skin departments depends to some extent upon the recognition of emotional factors [5]. Yet in only a few instances, such as dermatitis artefacta, do these play a primary and pathogenic role. The relationships between the mind and the skin are usually more complex than this.

One important aspect of the subject is the way in which emotional reactions or psychiatric disorders may trigger or exacerbate skin diseases or affect the outcome of treatment. The mechanisms involved may be obvious or less obvious. An example of the former is the hand dermatitis brought on by the hand-washing rituals of those with obsessive compulsive disorders [6]. Less obvious examples are the role of the impaired parent–child relationships in intractable atopic eczema [7], the triggering of pemphigus by stress [8] and the way in which the successful treatment of warts depends upon the personality traits of the patient [9].

It has to be admitted that, despite intensive research devoted to these problems, our knowledge of the psycho-dynamic and peripheral mechanisms involved is still rudimentary. The new subject of 'psychoneuroimmunology' [4,10,11] (see below) may have much to add by extending Selye's concept of stress to include changes in susceptibility to infections, in immune responsiveness and even in the pathogenesis of neoplastic disorders. Similarly, work on the relationship between mental activity and peripheral blood flow [12] may shed light on the exacerbation of some inflammatory dermatoses by stress, and perhaps on the effect of stress on itching. Neuropeptides (e.g. substance P(SP)) may also be involved [10,13].

Nevertheless, many of the conditions mentioned in this chapter form obvious groups, shading from one into another. One such spectrum ranges from natural anxiety over disfiguring skin lesions, through disproportionate worry over minor blemishes, to disturbances of body image that lead patients to become obsessed with their skin in the absence of any abnormality, and, finally, to psychotic delusions about their skin, for example of parasitosis, which may occasionally be due to organic brain damage [14]. These are dealt with in more detail on page 2790.

Another important concept is that of somatization. In general practice, an emotionally distressed patient is more likely to consult with physical symptoms than to complain about psychological or social problems [15]. Many studies confirm that this type of patient, with unrecognized psychiatric morbidity, is often passed on to medical and surgical clinics [16], and clearly to dermatological clinics also. Indeed, dermatology inpatients are known to have a higher prevalence of psychiatric disorders than general medical inpatients and dermatology outpatients a higher prevalence than the general population [17].

Somatizing patients are not without psychological symptoms, but these are overshadowed by physical complaints that allow those reluctant to accept the stigma of mental illness still to occupy the 'sick role' [18]. Depression and anxiety are the commonest underlying psychological disorders but their mood disturbance and characteristic patterns of thinking are not volunteered. Some somatic symptoms are amplifications of normal physiological sensations, for example itching, which tend to worsen under stress [19]; others relate to the physiological accompaniments of anxiety, such as excessive

sweating. This type of behaviour merges imperceptibly with hypochondriasis. In some patients, this amplification of physical symptoms is an enduring personality trait [20]. Others seem to be reacting to transient life stresses [21].

Those areas of overlap between psychiatry and dermatology are important, and a competent dermatologist should be able to pick up any emotional and psychological clues and cues that may be advanced by the patient during consultation. For example, a polysymptomatic patient is often neurotic, as are patients who describe symptoms in a highly exaggerated manner. Their rashes tend to be 'painful' or 'burning'. The anxious patient sits on the edge of the seat, or in an uncomfortable position, and on the couch writhes in every direction but the one that the examining doctor requires. Folded arms may indicate a defensive posture. The slow gait and dropping shoulders of a depressed patient contrast markedly with the gallop and expansive gestures of the hypomanic. A dermatology–psychiatry liaison clinic has proved to be a useful way of introducing dermatologists to the psychological dimension of their subject [22].

REFERENCES

1 Koblenzer CS. Psychosomatic concepts in dermatology. *Arch Dermatol* 1983; **119**: 501–12.
2 Koo JYM. Psychodermatology. In: *Current Concepts*. Kalamazoo: Upjohn, 1989: 1–45.
3 Panconesi E, ed. Stress and skin disease. In: *Clinics in Dermatology*, Vol. 2. *Psychosomatic Dermatology*. 1984: 1–276.
4 Panconesi E, Hautmann G. Psychophysiology of stress in dermatology: the psychologic pattern of psychosomatics. In: *Dermatologic Clinics* no. 3. 1996: 399–421.
5 Sneddon J, Sneddon I. Acne excoriée: a protective device. *Clin Exp Dermatol* 1983; **8**: 65–8.
6 Rasmussen SA. Obsessive compulsive disorder in dermatologic practice. *J Am Acad Dermatol* 1985; **13**: 965–7.
7 Koblenzer CS, Koblenzer PJ. Chronic intractable atopic eczema. Its occurrence as a physical sign of impaired parent–child relationships and psychologic developmental arrest: improvement through parent insight and education. *Arch Dermatol* 1988; **124**: 1673–7.
8 Brenner S, Bar-Nathan EA. Pemphigus vulgaris triggered by emotional stress. *J Am Acad Dermatol* 1984; **11**: 524–5.
9 Kalivas L, Penick E, Kalivas J. Personality factors as predictors of therapeutic response to cryosurgery in patients with warts. *J Am Acad Dermatol* 1989; **20**: 429–32.
10 Farber EM, Nickoloff BJ, Recht B *et al*. Stress, symmetry and psoriasis: possible role of neuropeptides. *J Am Acad Dermatol* 1986; **14**: 305–11.
11 Panconesi E, Petrini N. The future is here: cutaneous psychoneuro-immunology as a premise. *Clin Dermatol* 1984; **2**: 78–93.
12 Wilkin JK, Trotter K. Cognitive activity and cutaneous blood flow. *Arch Dermatol* 1987; **123**: 1503–6.
13 Matis WL, Larker RM, Murphy GF. Substance P induces the expression of an endothelial-leukocyte adhesion molecule by micro-vascular endothelium. *J Invest Dermatol* 1990; **94**: 492–5.
14 Shelley WB, Shelley ED. Delusions of parasitosis associated with coronary bypass surgery. *Br J Dermatol* 1988; **118**: 309–10.
15 Murphy M. Somatization: embodying the problem. *Br Med J* 1989; **298**: 1311–12.
16 Lloyd G. Medicine without signs. *Br Med J* 1983; **287**: 539–42.
17 Hughes JE, Barraclough BM, Hamblin LG, White JE. Psychiatric symptoms in dermatology patients. *Br J Psychiatry* 1983; **143**: 51–4.
18 Goldberg DP, Bridges K. Somatic presentation of psychiatric illness in a primary case setting. *J Psychosom Res* 1988; **32**: 137–44.

19 Fjellner B, Arnetz BB. Psychological predictors of pruritus during mental stress. *Acta Derm Venereol (Stock)* 1985; **65**: 504–8.
20 Barsky AJ. Patients who amplify bodily symptoms. *Ann Intern Med* 1979; **91**: 63–70.
21 Mechanic D. Social psychologic factors affecting the presentation of bodily symptoms. *N Engl J Med* 1972; **286**: 1331–9.
22 Gould WM, Gragg TM. A dermatology–psychiatry liaison clinic. *J Am Acad Dermatol* 1983; **9**: 73–7.

Psychoneuroimmunology

The immune system can no longer be regarded as autonomous because immunoregulatory processes are part of an integrated system of defence [1]. Psychoneuroimmunology is the study of this integrated system and of behavioural–neuroendocrine–immune system interactions in particular.

The brain and immune system are linked by the autonomic nervous system and the neuroendocrine outflow via the pituitary gland. Communication between the immune system and the brain is bidirectional and probably largely mediated by neuropeptides [2]. More than 50 neuropeptides have now been identified, the smallest ones containing only two amino acids while the larger peptides contain 40 or more amino acids. The neuropeptides act, not only as neurotransmitters, but also as neuromodulators.

Lymphoid tissue is innervated by noradrenergic postganglionic sympathetic nerve fibres, and peptidergic nerve fibres have also been identified in lymph nodes, thymus, spleen and bone marrow [3]. These nerve fibres form close neuroeffective junctions with lymphocytes and macrophages, which also possess receptors for neuropeptides [1].

The neuropeptides of particular interest to dermatologists include SP, calcitonin gene-related peptide (CGRP), vasoactive intestinal polypeptide (VIP) and neuropeptide Y (NPY). Moreover, lymphocytes have receptors for corticotropin-releasing hormone (CRH), adrenocorticotrophic hormone (ACTH) and endogenous opioids, and both endorphins and enkephalins are known to directly influence antigen-specific and non-specific *in vivo* and *in vitro* responses [1].

The most clinically evident beneficial effect on the immune system is achieved by either the administration of glucocorticoids or through endogenous ACTH-induced release of glucocorticoids, leading to a reduction in inflammatory response, and physiological amounts of cortisol are essential for a normal immune response.

Each neuropeptide has a wide range of functions [2]. SP facilitates lymphocyte migration to the site of inflammation, stimulates phagocytosis and is a potent vasodilator. *In vitro* SP has been shown to stimulate IgA production and is a potent mediator of both pain and pruritus.

Farber [4,5] has proposed a psychoneuroimmunological basis for psoriasis, and the evidence for this proposition has been reviewed recently [2]. Thus, psoriatic skin has been shown to have a significant increase in SP-containing nerves. Psoriatic lesions are rich in neuropeptides such as SP and VIP. Proliferation of keratinocytes, a central feature of psoriasis, could be triggered by release of both SP and VIP, while SP could also induce localized lymphocytic proliferation. Moreover, the initiation and maintenance of the lymphocytic infiltrate characteristic of psoriasis could be induced by SP, CGRP and VIP, which all induce the production of endothelial leucocyte adhesion molecule-I (ELAM-I) on endothelium. Further evidence is provided by the fact that capsaicin, an SP depletor, will improve psoriasis to some extent [2].

With regard to atopic eczema, both SP and VIP have been demonstrated in lesional skin. Moreover, NPY, a very potent vasoconstrictor, has been detected in the Langerhans' cells of six of 11 patients with atopic eczema, but not in normal control subjects. Other neuropeptides possibly involved in atopic eczema include somatostatin and endorphins [2].

Behavioural–immune interactions

Changes in both humoral and cell-mediated immunity have been found as a result of exposure to either naturally occurring or experimentally induced stress. Bereavement is often associated with depression and many changes in immune function have been shown in depressed patients. Depression is associated with an increased number of circulating neutrophils, a decreased number of natural killer (NK) cells, T and B lymphocytes, and helper and suppressor cytotoxic T cells. There are also alterations in B-cell function, manifest by increased antibody titres to herpes simplex and cytomegalovirus [1]. Changes in both humoral and cell-mediated immunity have been found following marital separation and divorce [6] and alterations in immune function may occur during examinations [7]. Slowing of human wound healing has also been shown to be associated with stress, possibly mediated by depression of local production of the cytokine interleukin 1B [8].

The bidirectional communication between the central nervous system (CNS) and the immune system provides the basis, not only for behaviourally induced alterations in immune function, but also for immunologically based changes in behaviour [1]. These pathways may explain how emotional stress influences a wide range of disorders.

REFERENCES

1 Ader R, Cohen N, Felten D. Psychoimmunology: interactions between the nervous system and the immune system. *Lancet* 1995; **345**: 99–103.
2 Panconesi E, Hautmann G. Pathophysiology of stress in dermatology: the psychobiologic pattern of psychosomatics. *Dermatol Clin* 1996; **14**: 399–421.
3 Felten SY, Felten DL. The innervation of lymphoid tissue. In: Ader R, Cohen N, Felten DL, eds. *Psychoneuroimmunology*, 2nd edn. New York: Academic Press, 1991: 27–70.

4 Farber EM, Nickoloff BJ, Recht B *et al*. Stress, symmetry and psoriasis: possible role of neuropeptides. *J Am Acad Dermatol* 1986; **14**: 305–11.

5 Farber EM, Rein G, Lanigan SW. Stress in psoriasis: psychoneuroimmunologic mechanisms. *Int J Dermatol* 1991; **30**: 8–12.

6 Glaser R, Rice J, Sheridan J *et al*. Stress-related immune suppression: health implications. *Brain Behav Immun* 1987; **1**: 7–20.

7 Lycke E, Norrby R, Roos BE. A serological study on mentally ill patients with particular reference to the problems of herpes virus infections. *Br J Psychiatry* 1974; **124**: 273–9.

8 Kielcote-Glaser JK, Marucha PT, Malarkey WB *et al*. Slowing of wound healing by psychological stress. *Lancet* 1995; **346**: 1194–6.

Emotional reactions to skin disease [1]

Disorders of the skin lead to emotional as well as physical damage. An extreme example of this occurs in genital herpes when the initial shock and emotional numbing may be followed by a frantic search for a cause, and later by a sense of loneliness and isolation. Some 10–15% of patients with genital herpes never adjust satisfactorily and continue to experience difficulties in all areas of their lives, which become increasingly reclusive and monastic [2]. The special emotional and psychological problems faced by a patient who learns he or she is human immunodeficiency virus (HIV) positive is another example [3].

Other skin disorders carry their own unique but usually less dramatic sets of emotional problems. Common to most are shame and embarrassment [4] and a poor self-image and low self-esteem, easily demonstrated by appropriate questionnaires. Patients with psoriasis, in addition, often feel that others stare at them, and experience much social distress [1]. A related phenomenon may be heavy drinking, which in male psoriatics correlates with the severity of their skin trouble and with its duration [5]. Ten per cent of patients with psoriasis reported a death wish and 6% reported active suicidal ideation in one study [6]. Sufferers from vitiligo adjust better to their disorder than do those with psoriasis, but also tend to have low self-esteem [7], and the disease may have a negative impact on sexual relations [8]. The impaired self-image and psychological distress of patients with acne improve with successful treatment of the skin lesions [9], but acne patients of both sexes have a higher rate of unemployment than controls [10]. Acne scarring can lead to profound depression and suicide [11].

The concept of stigmatization is important in this context. It can be defined as a biological or social mark that sets a person apart from others, is discrediting and disrupts interactions with others [12]. In a study of 100 adults with psoriasis, those who were older at the onset of the disease seemed less likely to anticipate rejection, and to be less sensitive to the opinions of others and to feelings of guilt, shame and secretiveness [12]. Episodes of bleeding from the psoriatic lesions proved to be the strongest predictor of feelings of stigmatization and despair [12].

Atopic dermatitis in children is associated with high levels of psychological morbidity [13]. The disturbance was best predicted by the distribution of the eczema rather than its extent, and children with eczema on the face had high levels of psychological distress.

Disfiguring skin lesions may profoundly influence the emotional development of a child, which is also affected by the attitude of the parents and, later, the teachers. The dermatologist's main function at this stage is to explain, to reassure as far as possible and often to protect the child from ill-advised interference.

With the approach of puberty, a disfiguring skin disease becomes an increasing anxiety to many children and may handicap them in developing easy relationships with the opposite sex. Some children become increasingly introspective and solitary, while others become aggressive and uncooperative. The dermatologist should interpret such changes with empathy. However, it is impossible to generalize about the effect of such lesions; the number of variable factors is too great. With sensible and affectionate parents and intelligent teachers, children with disfiguring skin lesions will often adjust extremely well, form satisfactory sexual relationships and establish themselves in successful careers. On the surface they seem to be blessed with the reverse of dysmorphophobia; but a study of the psychological difficulties of 71 patients with port-wine stains shows that many suffer psychological distress that is not apparent in their social interactions, and that does not lessen with increasing age [14].

REFERENCES

1 Ginsburg IH. The psychosocial impact of skin disease: an overview. *Dermatol Clin* 1996; **14**: 473–84.

2 Luby EB, Klinge V. Genital herpes—a pervasive psychosocial disorder. *Arch Dermatol* 1985; **121**: 494–7.

3 King MB. *Aids, HIV and Mental Health*. Cambridge: Cambridge University Press, 1993: 15.

4 Jowett S, Ryan T. Skin disease and handicap: an analysis of the impact of skin conditions. *Soc Sci Med* 1985; **20**: 425–9.

5 Melotti E, Herpeisen SM, Polenghi MM. Alcohol consumption in psoriasis. *Ann Ital Dermatol Clin Sper* 1987; **41**: 343–8.

6 Gupta MA, Schork NJ, Gupta AK *et al*. Suicidal ideation in psoriasis. *Int J Dermatol* 1993; **32**: 188–90.

7 Porter JR, Beuf AH, Lerner A *et al*. Psychosocial effect of vitiligo. *J Am Acad Dermatol* 1986; **15**: 220–4.

8 Porter JR, Beuf AH, Lerner AB, Nordlund JJ. The effect of vitiligo on sexual relationships. *J Am Acad Dermatol* 1990; **22**: 221–2.

9 Rubinov PR, Peck GL, Squillace KM *et al*. Reduced anxiety and depression in cystic acne patients after successful treatment with oral isotretinoin. *J Am Acad Dermatol* 1987; **17**: 25–32.

10 Cunliffe WJ. Acne and unemployment. *Br J Dermatol* 1986; **115**: 386.

11 Cotterill JA, Cunliffe WJ. Suicide in dermatological patients. *Br J Dermatol* 1997; **137**: 246–50.

12 Ginsburg IH, Link BG. Feelings of stigmatization in patients with psoriasis. *J Am Acad Dermatol* 1989; **20**: 53–63.

13 Jacobs B, Green J, David TJ. A self-concept of children with atopic dermatitis. *Br J Dermatol* 1995; **133**: 1004.

14 Lanigan SW, Cotterill JA. Psychological disabilities amongst patients with port-wine stains. *Br J Dermatol* 1989; **121**: 209–15.

Disability

This aspect of dermatology is covered in more detail in Chapter 75.

Conventional dermatological teaching in medicine describes skin disorders in relatively complicated diagnostic terminology, which takes little account of the effect of a particular skin disease on the individual patient. From the patient's point of view, however, it is much more important to try and determine the degree of disability that a particular skin disease confers [1].

The concept of skin failure is just as valid as that of renal, heart or respiratory failure [2]. The effect on the quality of life induced by psoriasis, eczema and acne have been assessed using disability indices [3–5], which can also be used to quantify reduction in disability before and after treatment [6]. In patients with psoriasis, the area of involvement with the skin disease is often not a reliable guide to disability. For instance, the most trivial psoriasis affecting the fingertips in a blind patient may completely devastate that person's life by making it impossible to read braille, and the presence of relatively trivial amounts of psoriasis on an individual's face may induce disparate depression. The anxiety and anger induced by severe acne are recognized [7].

The language of disability is understood, not only by patients, but also by potential fund-distributing administrators. Management around the basis of handicap and disability forms a basis of a caring consultation [1]. Moreover, the language of disability and the concept of skin failure encourage compliance and may be much more relevant to the training of medical personnel in the developing world than the rather more paternalistic diagnosis-based medicine currently taught in most so-called 'advanced' countries.

REFERENCES

1 Ryan TJ. The confident nude—or—whither dermatology? *Dermatol Pract* 1987; **5**: 8–18.
2 Ryan TJ. Disability in dermatology. *Br J Hosp Med* 1991; **46**: 33–6.
3 Eun HC, Finlay AY. Measurement of atopic dermatitis disability. *Ann Dermatol* 1990; **2**: 9–12.
4 Finlay AY, Kelly SE. Psoriasis—an index of disability. *Clin Exp Dermatol* 1987; **12**: 8–11.
5 Motley RJ, Finlay AJ. How much disability is caused by acne? *Clin Exp Dermatol* 1989; **14**: 194–8.
6 Salek MS, Finlay AY, Luscombe DK *et al.* Cyclosporin greatly improves the quality of life of adults with severe atopic dermatitis. A randomized double-blind placebo controlled trial. *Br J Dermatol* 1993; **129**: 422–30.
7 Wu SF, Kinder BN, Trunnell TN *et al.* Role of anxiety and anger in acne patients: a relationship with severity of the disorder. *J Am Acad Dermatol* 1988; **18**: 325–33.

Body image

Body image can be conceptualized by individuals in many different ways. There are a multiplicity of definitions, but the simplest is that of Critchley [1] who defined body image as 'the physical properties of a person carried into the imagery of himself'. It is important to remember that body image is completely abstract in conceptualization depending on many factors, including memory, intellect, perception and early life experiences.

Body image may be conceptualized as largely cutaneous, and the most important areas include the face, scalp, hair, breasts in females and genital areas. The nose, which is the central part of the face, is also central to body-image conceptualization and it is not surprising, therefore, that skin disease manifesting itself, even as a tiny spot on the nose, may produce disparate cosmetic distress, while a much larger lesion on an adjacent cheek may be completely ignored. As the face is both visible and in a very important body-image area, skin disease in this area may produce major distress and lowering of self-esteem.

Thus, Shuster *et al.* [2] first demonstrated that individuals with severe acne, particularly female, had a significant depression of their body image and self-esteem, which was reversible with successful antibiotic treatment. As mentioned earlier, individuals with acne are less successful at gaining employment [3]. It may be that potential employers perceive individuals with acne as unattractive, but also the interviewees themselves may reflect their lower self-esteem and confidence at interviews. Eczema and psoriasis are both likely to produce the same sort of effects, particularly at times of life when the individual would normally be beginning to socialize. Adolescence can be particularly difficult for the teenager with acne, facial psoriasis or eczema. The stigmatization induced by a port-wine stain may also deter individuals, particularly males, from making any sort of contact with the opposite sex [4].

It is important to recognize that individuals with skin problems in important body-image areas may be manifestly depressed. These individuals will be helped by effective treatment and also helped by an empathetic medical practitioner. In some instances, a clinical psychologist may help a person to come to terms with his or her problems while, in a minority, the depression is severe enough to merit treatment with antidepressants and the help of a psychiatrist. A liaison clinic is particularly helpful in managing this type of patient, where at times there may be a definite risk of suicide or parasuicide.

REFERENCES

1 Critchley M. Corporeal awareness: body image; body scheme. In: *The Divine Banquet of the Brain and other Essays.* New York: Raven Press, 1980: 92–105.
2 Shuster S, Fisher G, Harris E *et al.* The effect of skin disease on self-image. *Br J Dermatol* 1978; **99** (Suppl. 16): 18–19.
3 Cunliffe WJ. Acne and unemployment. *Br J Dermatol* 1986; **115**: 386.
4 Lanigan S, Cotterill JA. Psychological disabilities amongst patients with port-wine stains. *Br J Dermatol* 1989; **121**: 209–15.

Classification

No entirely satisfactory classification has yet been devised. The psychodynamic mechanisms involved remain largely unknown, and individual variability is too complex to be assigned easily to compartments.

Many of the proposed classifications have much merit [1–3] but, as their authors admit, all include inconsistencies and overlaps. This led van der Schaar [4] to suggest a classification based on the patients' behaviour as a consequence of the dermatosis rather than on the dermatological diagnosis *per se*. However, this may be side-stepping the main problem.

The following clinical groupings may serve as a general guide.

Conditions that are primarily psychiatric but that commonly present to dermatologists

Delusions of parasitosis (Ekbom's disease).
Delusions of body image (e.g. dysmorphophobia, body dysmorphic disorder, dermatological non-disease, including atypical pain disorders such as glossodynia and essential vulvodynia).
Phobic states (e.g. syphilophobia, acquired immune deficiency syndrome (AIDS) phobia, venereophobia, wart and mole phobia).
Compulsive hand washing.

Dermatoses primarily factitious in origin

Dermatitis artefacta.
Artefact by proxy.
Witchcraft syndrome.
Dermatological pathomimicry.
Malingering.
Munchausen's syndrome.
Munchausen's syndrome by proxy.
Deliberate self-cutting.
Self mutilation.
Religious stigmata and psychogenic purpura.

Dermatoses aggravated by harmful habits and compulsions

Lichen simplex.
Neurotic excoriations.
Prurigo nodularis.
Acne excoriée.
Hair plucking.
Trichotillomania.
Trichophagia.
Nail destruction.
Onychotillomania.
Lip-licking cheilitis.

Dermatoses due to accentuated physiological responses

Hyperhidrosis.
Blushing.

Dermatoses in which emotional precipitating or perpetuating factors may be important

Vesicular eczema of the palms and soles.
Atopic dermatitis in the adult.
Seborrhoeic dermatitis.
Psoriasis.
Some cases of localized or generalized pruritus.
Alopecia areata.
Aphthosis.
Rosacea.
Chronic urticaria.

It is over the last group that most of the debate rages. Different views are held by dermatologists who assess differently the importance of the role of stress, for example, in psoriasis [5–7] or urticaria.

REFERENCES

1 Koblenzer CS. Psychosomatic concepts in dermatology. *Arch Dermatol* 1983; **119**: 501–12.
2 Medansky RS, Handler RM. Dermatopsychosomatics: classification, physiology and therapeutic approaches. *J Am Acad Dermatol* 1981; **5**: 125–36.
3 Whitlock FA. *Psychophysiological Aspects of Skin Disease*. London: WB Saunders, 1976.
4 Van Der Schaar WW. Relationship between skin disease and behaviour variables. *Br J Dermatol* 1986; **115**: 586.
5 Gaston L, Lassone M, Bernier-Buzzanga J *et al.* Psoriasis and stress: a prospective study. *J Am Acad Dermatol* 1987; **17**: 82–6.
6 Paljan D, Kansky A, Cividini-Stranic E. Psychosomatic factors influencing the course of psoriasis. *Acta Derm Venereol (Stockh)* 1984; **113** (Suppl. 1): 121–2.
7 Seville RH. Stress and psoriasis: the importance of insight and empathy in prognosis. *J Am Acad Dermatol* 1989; **20**: 97–100.

Dermatological delusional disease

Although patients with delusions of parasitosis are relatively easily recognized, they are also rare and dermatologists will see more patients with other types of dermatological delusional disease. Indeed, as Lyell [1] has stated, it is possible to spend a lifetime as a dermatologist and never see a patient with delusions of parasitosis.

The broad spectrum of dermatological delusional disease may be divided into three main types, depending on which sensory system is predominantly involved. First, there are patients with delusional parasitosis who build up delusions around their skin sensations, in particular, around touch. Second, is a group of patients who present with visual delusions centred on their body image. This is the commonest type of patient seen in practice. Third, and much more rare, are those patients whose delusions or overvalued ideas revolve around the sensation of smell. They may present with the delusion that they smell excessively badly to everyone around them.

Delusions of parasitosis [1–4]

Definition. The patient with delusions of parasitosis has an unshakeable conviction that his or her skin is infested by parasites: this must be differentiated from parasitophobia—the fear of becoming infested.

Aetiology. Delusions of parasitosis in a young adult suggest illicit exposure to drugs such as amphetamine or cocaine, or are part of a delusion shared with another member of the family (folie à deux). The term monosymptomatic hypochondriacal psychosis may be applied to patients with a single, fixed hypochondriacal delusion that is apparently not secondary to another psychiatric disorder [5]. Most patients with delusions of parasitosis fit into this category. Such patients are often intelligent, and the professions are well represented, including doctors and even psychiatrists, but they are often rather solitary people and sometimes thought to be eccentric individuals. Indeed, Lyell has commented that it is hard to know where eccentricity ends and madness begins [3]. Moreover, some patients have a rather obsessional premorbid personality. Those seen by psychiatrists are more likely to be labelled schizophrenic or depressed or both. Delusions of perception may follow disease in the non-dominant hemisphere, and so delusions of parasitosis are sometimes seen in patients after a cerebrovascular accident involving that side of the brain [3]. Delusions of parasitosis have also been described in pellagra [6], vitamin B_{12} deficiency [7], following coronary bypass surgery [8], as a side-effect of phenelzine [9] and in severe renal disease [3]. It is particularly important to exclude the possibility of a real infestation, and 6% of Lyell's series developed delusions of parasitosis following real infestation.

Incidence. Patients with delusions of parasitosis are extremely rare. The condition affects both sexes equally below the age of 50 years, but after that age three times as many women are affected as men [1,3].

Clinical features. Like all patients with dermatological delusional disease, those with delusions of parasitosis are often 'doctor shoppers' and complain bitterly about the incompetence of their medical advisers. They see their problems in clear dermatological terms, whereas their medical advisers see them in strictly psychiatric terms. It is sometimes impossible to bridge this gap in communication.

The presenting symptoms are often ill-defined. Some speak of a sensation in their skin as though an insect is crawling around, and may describe and draw the insect or insects concerned. No obvious skin disease may be present, but excoriations are common and follow attempts by the patient to extract the 'parasites'. Usually, the patient will bring a small container to the clinic, such as a matchbox, which, the doctor is told, contains their insects. On microscopy these offerings are usually found to be fragments of skin and hair, but may include living organisms such as ants or flies. Purification rituals rapidly become established and patients will go to great lengths to cleanse the skin and their environment. Indeed, environmental health officers and private pest control organizations are likely to meet more of these patients than do dermatologists. Specimens are also sent for examination to local university zoology departments and to institutions such as the British Museum.

It is not uncommon for delusions to be shared, more often by a husband and wife, but sometimes by a whole family, which becomes isolated as the affected patient forbids the others to meet outsiders.

Diagnosis. The diagnosis is usually obvious, but often the referring family physician has been persuaded by the patient to collude with the delusion. True infestation should be ruled out and the specimens brought by the patient should be carefully examined. It is also important to rule out underlying organic disease, although this is rare.

Management. The management of patients with delusional parasitosis is always difficult. It is important not to collude with the patient and it is better to say 'I can't see any of the parasites today', than to tell the patient that he or she has a mental problem. Sometimes, patients can be persuaded to accept the medication if told that it has helped previous patients with similar problems. Initially, it is often best to admit the patient to hospital. This reduces pressure at home on other family members and ensures compliance with medication. A psychiatric colleague can more easily be asked to see the patient in the dermatology ward.

The response to pimozide is often good in these patients and the initial dose, 2 mg, is increased weekly by 2-mg increments as necessary to a maximum of 12 mg daily [1,3]. On higher doses, patients develop extrapyramidal symptoms. On doses of pimozide of 20 mg or greater per day there is a definite risk of ventricular arrhythmias and other electrocardiogram (ECG) abnormalities such as prolongation of the Q–T interval and T-wave changes. Doses of this magnitude are rarely required in patients with delusions of parasitosis, and if response to pimozide is poor an alternative drug such as sulpiride 200 mg twice daily initially could be tried.

However, an ECG should be performed before pimozide therapy, and the drug should not be given to patients with a prolonged Q–T interval or to patients with a history of cardiac arrhythmia. Patients taking long-term pimozide should have a regular ECG at least once a year and if the Q–T interval is prolonged, treatment should be reviewed or withdrawn [10]. Moreover, concurrent treatment with other antipsychotics, tricyclic antidepressants and other drugs that prolong the Q–T interval, such as the antihistamines terfenadine and astemizole, antimalarials or drugs such as diuretics that alter the electrolyte status, should be avoided [10]. Hypokalaemia may predispose to the cardiotoxic effects of pimozide and care should be taken in patients with hepatic or renal dysfunction [11].

For most patients, pimozide is slightly stimulant so is best given in the morning. However, some find it hypnotic and this minority should take the drug in the evening.

Some patients with delusions of parasitosis are depressed, and have been treated with conventional tricyclic antidepressants, often with pimozide as well [4]. It may be that a selective serotonin reuptake inhibitor (see below) would be a safer option for combined therapy with pimozide.

It should be remembered that suicide is an ever-attendant risk in these patients [1,4].

The main problem is poor patient compliance. Patients frequently defect from follow-up clinics. When compliance is a problem, depot neuroleptics may be used [2].

REFERENCES

1 Lyell A. Delusions of parasitosis. *Semin Dermatol* 1983; **2**: 189–95.
2 Frithz A. Delusions of infestation: treatment by depot injections of neuroleptics. *Clin Exp Dermatol* 1979; **4**: 485–8.
3 Lyell A. Delusions of parasitosis. *Br J Dermatol* 1983; **108**: 485–99.
4 Monk BE, Rao YJ. Delusions of parasitosis with fatal outcome. *Clin Exp Dermatol* 1994; **19**: 341–2.
5 Munro A. Delusional parasitosis: a form of monosymptomatic hypochondriacal psychosis. *Semin Dermatol* 1983; **2**: 197–202.
6 Aleshire I. Delusions of parasitosis: report of a successful cure with antipellagrous treatment. *JAMA* 1954; **155**: 15–17.
7 Pope FM. Parasitophobia as a presenting symptom of Vit. B12 deficiency. *Practitioner* 1970; **204**: 421–2.
8 Shelley WB, Shelley ED. Delusions of parasitosis associated with coronary bypass surgery. *Br J Dermatol* 1988; **118**: 309–10.
9 Aixenberg D, Schwartx B, Zemishlany Z. Delusional parasitosis associated with phenelzine. *Br J Psych* 1991; **159**: 716–17.
10 Committee of Safety of Medicines. *Current Problems in Pharmacovigilance. Cardiac Arrhythmias with Pimozide (Orap)*. London: Medical Control Agency, 1995; **21**: 2.
11 Committee on Safety of Medicines. *Current Problems*. London: Medical Control Agency, 1990: 29.

Dermatological non-disease [1–3]

SYN. DYSMORPHOPHOBIA; BODY DYSMORPHIC DISORDER [4–6]

The term 'dermatological non-disease' was introduced to describe patients who are rich in symptoms (especially in areas important in the body image) but poor in signs of organic skin disease [1]. Nevertheless, these patients *are* ill, the commonest psychiatric disease present being depression [7]. Dermatological non-disease presents with symptoms in three main areas: the face, including the mouth; the scalp; and the genital area. Facial symptoms include complaints of excessive redness, blushing, a burning feeling, scarring, large pores, excessive facial hair and facial greasiness. Patients with orodynia or glossodynia fit into this group with their defect in pain perception involving the mouth. Scalp symptoms include a feeling of intense burning, unremitting by day or night, and excessive hair loss. Perineal symptoms in males include complaints of an excessively red scrotum, discomfort in the genital area, often spreading on to the anterior thighs and making the wearing of clothes uncomfortable, urethral discharge, herpes and acquired immune deficiency syndrome (AIDS). The female equivalent, vulvodynia (the burning vulva syndrome) consists of several different clinical entities, including vulval dermatosis, cyclic vulvitis, vulval papillomatosis, the vulva vestibular syndrome and essential vulvodynia [8]. In essential vulvodynia, the discomfort may be so severe that the patient will neither sit down nor go to bed, and this drives every other member of the family to distraction. Women with essential vulvodynia are more distressed than patients with an identified physical cause of vulval pain [9].

Those patients with facial and scalp problems are more often female than male, but those with perineal symptoms are more likely to be male than female. There is a definite risk of suicide in patients with dermatological non-disease [1,6] and 29% had made a suicide attempt in a large series of 130 patients with body dysmorphic disorder [5].

Aetiology. The aetiology is unknown. Some patients may be examples of monosymptomatic hypochondriacal psychosis [10] in that they have an isolated delusion. Like patients with delusions of parasitosis, affected individuals are often solitary, unmarried or divorced. As a whole they socialize poorly and do not like contact with other people. Their symptoms may appear after severe emotional, especially marital, problems and perineal symptoms in men may follow imagined or real sexual exposure. An obsessional premorbid personality is not unusual. The commonest associated psychiatric illness is depression [3,7] but patients seldom admit to this. Many, however, do wake early. Dysmorphophobic symptoms in a teenager or adult may be the presentation of schizophrenia, while in an elderly patient dementia should be considered. As with delusions of parasitosis, there is usually no evidence of any underlying organic disease.

Other clinical features. In one study, the average age of onset was 15 years and the average duration of symptoms was 18 years [11]. Patients with dermatological non-disease are 'doctor shoppers' and will have often seen many doctors over the years about their many problems. They never respond to placebos. Indeed, they often develop symptoms that they attribute to it. A consultation with a patient with dermatological non-disease always takes much longer than one with a patient with organic disease. The same ground has to be gone over repeatedly and the patient never appreciates normal non-verbal communication emanating from the doctor. An individual patient is likely to return to the clinic within a few minutes of being seen and may repeatedly telephone the doctor asking questions that have already been answered many times in the immediate past. The extreme preoccupation with a perceived dermatological problem is reflected by excessive mirror checking, which is a clinical feature in over 70% of patients [11].

Management. The management of patients with dermatological delusional disease is always difficult, although latterly the introduction of specific serotonin reuptake inhibitors (SSRIs) such as fluoxetine, fluvoxamine and paroxetine has enabled some progress to be made in treatment. Unfortunately, there are no clinical trials to date.

Treatment with SSRIs. It has been claimed that nearly 50% of patients may respond completely or partially to fluoxetine or clomipramine, whereas there was only a 5% response to all other medications [5]. A subsequent larger study yielded similar results, but only 20% of patients reported decreased distress and time preoccupied on their perceived problems. Also, in many patients there is a significant improvement in the social prognosis evidenced by an ability to return to school or work, and this is accompanied by a reduction in ritualistic behaviour, such as mirror checking and skin picking. Phillips [5] observed that only a small proportion of patients responding to SSRI drugs experience any change in insight.

It is important to note that the effective dosage of SSRI drugs is usually higher than the dosage conventionally used to treat depression. Thus, the average dose for a reasonable response to clomipramine was found to be 175 mg/day, for fluoxetine 50 mg/day and for fluvoxamine 260 mg/day. In short, the dose of SSRI needs to be high and the duration of treatment is long term, with response taking, on average, 2 months, and sometimes as long as 3.5 months.

There are several pharmacological options for patients who fail to respond to this type of regimen, and resistant patients have been defined as those who failed to respond to fluoxetine 60 mg/day, or clomipramine 150–200 mg/day, given for 3 months [5].

The initial question to pose in patients not responding to therapy is about compliance, which is a common problem in patients with body dysmorphic disorder. However, in resistant cases it has been recommended to try the addition of buspirone to the SSRI medication in a dose of 30–60 mg/day. This is helpful in about one-third of treated patients. If the patient has a truly delusional body dysmorphic disorder, sometimes the addition of the antipsychotic agent pimozide may be helpful. It is important, however, not to combine pimozide with clomipramine because both drugs prolong the Q–T interval. Occasionally, patients respond to a combination of clomipramine with an SSRI, but in this situation it is important to monitor blood clomipramine concentrations because SSRIs potentiate clomipramine concentration in blood. If all else fails, a monoamine oxidase inhibitor can be tried [5].

Fourteen of 16 patients with minimal acne but gross cosmetic distress responded well to treatment with isotretinoin given for 16 weeks [12].

Dermatological and plastic-surgical treatment. Most patients with dysmorphophobia perceive the solution to their problems in dermatological or plastic-surgical terms and so come to haunt dermatologists and plastic surgeons rather than psychiatrists. It is interesting that a significant proportion of patients presenting with dysmorphophobia have previously received plastic surgery, most commonly to change the shape of their nose. However, occasionally plastic surgery in carefully selected cases may be helpful, but there is always a risk that the patients themselves may then move to a preoccupation with another part of the body. In a series of 130 patients, it was found that 30% of patients had received previous cosmetic surgery, with a mean of 2.0 ± 1.3 procedures [5] and as many as six procedures had occurred in individual patients. Furthermore, 81% of patients with body dysmorphic disorder were either dissatisfied or very dissatisfied with their consultation and results of surgery [6]; therefore, if plastic surgery is planned in this group of patients it is very important to have careful preoperative psychiatric assessment. Those contemplating surgery should remember that some patients with body dysmorphic disorder are angry and go to litigation relatively easily. A perfect cosmetic result may be perceived by a depressed, dysmorphophobic patient as worse than the situation before surgery. Photography before and after surgery is important to refute such claims objectively.

Other non-pharmacological psychiatric treatment [5]. Simple behavioural treatment, such as encouraging patients to avoid ritualistic behaviour and mirror checking, and urging the patient to give up unnecessary cosmetic camouflage, while gradually exposing the patient to the most feared social situations, can be helpful, especially if combined with a cognitive approach involving self-esteem building and modification of distorted thinking, coupled with coping strategies. All these techniques are more likely to be effective when combined with SSRI treatment, and initially some patients may be too ill to benefit from a cognitive behavioural approach.

Supportive psychotherapy can be helpful in patients with overvalued ideas and who are not truly deluded, but it is very time consuming and emotionally demanding. As a generalization, patients with body dysmorphic disorder are poor communicators and difficulty with interpersonal relationships may be one of the central crucial and earliest features of this disorder. The physician, therefore, undertaking supportive psychotherapy has to be patient and very tolerant. Dysmorphophobic patients are poor attenders at clinics, but the consultation may, in some cases, be the only opportunity that a patient has to talk to another human being, a reflection of the isolated life these patients often lead.

Olfactory delusions

Patients with olfactory delusions should be treated with some care as their delusions can drive them to homicide. Those with delusions that they are passing excessively smelly flatus are usually referred to gastroenterologists, who then exclude steatorrhoea. Dermatologists are more likely to see patients who complain that their axillae, genitals or feet smell excessively badly. Like other patients with dermatological delusional disease, they are usually eccentric and often socially isolated. They may go to extraordinary lengths to try and rid themselves of their imagined odour, perhaps changing their shoes and socks several times a day. These patients are best managed by a competent psychiatrist.

REFERENCES

1 Cotterill JA. Dermatological non-disease: a common and potentially fatal disturbance of cutaneous body image. *Br J Dermatol* 1981; **104**: 611–18.
2 Cotterill JA. Clinical features of patients with dermatological non-disease. *Semin Dermatol* 1983; **2**: 203–5.
3 Cotterill JA. Dermatologic non-disease. *Dermatol Clin* 1996; **14**: 439–45.
4 Cotterill JA. Body dysmorphic disorder. *Dermatol Clin* 1996; **14**: 457–63.
5 Phillips KA. Body dysmorphic disorder: clinical features and drug treatment. *CNS Drugs* 1995; **3**: 30–40.
6 Veale D, Boocock A, Gournay K *et al*. Body dysmorphic disorder: a survey of fifty cases. *Br J Psychiatry* 1996; **169**: 169–201.
7 Hardy GE, Cotterill JA. A study of depression and obsessionality in dysmorphophobic and psoriatic patients. *Br J Psychol* 1982; **140**: 19–20.
8 McKay M. Vulvodynia. A multifactorial clinical problem. *Arch Dermatol* 1989; **125**: 256–62.
9 Stewart DE, Reicher AE, Gerulath AH, Boydell KM. Vulvodynia and psychological distress. *Obstet Gynecol* 1994; **84**: 587–90.
10 Munro A. Delusional parasitosis: a form of monosymptomatic hypochondriacal psychosis. *Semin Dermatol* 1983; **2**: 197–202.
11 Phillips KA, McElroy SL, Keck PE *et al*. Body dysmorphic disorder: 30 cases of imagined ugliness. *Am J Psychiatry* 1993; **150**: 302–8.
12 Hull SM, Cunliffe WJ, Hughes BR. Treatment of the depressed and dysmorphophobic acne patient. *Clin Exp Dermatol* 1991; **16**: 210–11.

Phobic states

Obsessive–compulsive disorder [1,2]

While relatively few patients with obsessive–compulsive disorder present directly to psychiatrists, it has been claimed that up to 14% of anxious, itchy dermatological patients have this psychiatric disorder [1]. Thus, psy-chiatrists will rarely have the opportunity to diagnose this condition, while dermatologists often fail to recognize it in their patients. Obsessions involve anxious ideas about contamination by germs, dirt or bodily secretions. The typical patient realizes that these persistent ideas are inappropriate, but they continue to engender much distress and anxiety. Attempts are made to ameliorate the anxiety resulting from the obsession by compulsive acts and rituals which vary, from rubbing, lip licking or touching the skin, to more complex rituals involving washing, cleaning, hair pulling, skin excoriation and other cutaneous damaging behaviour.

Patients' phobias about dirt and bacteria may present to dermatologists with hand eczema induced by repeated hand washing and the final psychiatric diagnosis is usually of an obsessional neurosis. Indeed, this psychiatric diagnosis should be considered in all patients with refractory hand eczema. A similar presentation may be seen in patients with anorexia nervosa (see below).

Patients who are phobic about warts and afraid to touch anything in the consulting room, and indeed in the hospital, are encountered. Such patients will wear gloves when shopping or filling their car with petrol, and even the sight of a wart in another individual can induce acute panic. Wart-phobic patients will bring other family members to dermatologists, and attempts will be made to make the dermatologist collude with the phobia and treat a wide variety of minute skin lesions in both the patient and their immediate relatives. A sterile pack may be produced so that there is no question of the patient's bare feet coming in contact with anything in the consulting room. Tights and socks are abandoned on the consulting room floor because they are regarded as contaminated by the patient. The obsessive concern about warts may reach such proportions that patients become exhausted and even suicidal. The obsessional ideas become heightened during periods of emotional stress.

Mole phobia has also become more common since the recent publicity campaigns about the early diagnosis of malignant melanoma. Affected individuals consult dermatologists repeatedly, along with their unwilling family members. A clinical psychologist is often helpful in supporting these obsessional patients through their phobic crises and a total mole clearance, using the Q-switched frequency doubled Nd:YAG laser, may provide the only relief for the exhausted patient and the rest of his or her family.

Patients with overvalued ideas

Patients with an overvalued idea about the possibility of venereal disease, including AIDS and herpes simplex, may be anxious or depressed and a rather obsessional personality trait is also not unusual in this group of patients [3].

Anorexia nervosa

Anorexia nervosa can be looked upon as a phobia about body weight, and many dermatological sequelae have been described, including pseudojaundice due to raised blood-carotene levels, increased lanugo body hair, diffuse non-scarring alopecia involving scalp hair, brittle nails, dry skin and calluses on the fingers produced by repetitive self-induced vomiting. In the mouth, there may be dental enamel erosion and gingivitis and some patients develop a Sjögren-like syndrome. Other cutaneous features may result from the use of laxatives, such as phenolphthalein, producing a fixed drug reaction, and thiazide diuretics, producing photosensitivity, while the use of the emetic ipecac can be associated with a dermatomyositis-like syndrome [4]. Compulsive hand washing and trichotillomania may result from accompanying psychiatric illness [5]. Severe perniosis is also seen in individuals with anorexia nervosa [6]. Drenching night sweats during weight recovery, possibly due to secondary changes in thermoregulation, which occur with rapid refeeding, have also recently been described in patients with eating disorders [7] as has acne [8].

The management of obsessive–compulsive disorder may be difficult. Behavioural, cognitive and joint behavioural and cognitive techniques have been used with some success [9]. If this approach fails, SSRIs, such as fluoxetine and fluvoxamine, are usually effective, but no more so than clomipramine, which is much cheaper [10]. The dose required is usually much higher than the dose required to treat depression. An initial dose of clomipramine 25 mg daily increasing over 2 weeks to 100–150 mg daily is usually recommended. For fluoxetine an initial dose of 20 mg daily, rising after several weeks to a maximum of 60 mg daily, is recommended, compared with a fixed dose of 20 mg daily for depression [10].

REFERENCES

1 Hatch ML, Paradis C, Friedman S *et al.* Obsessive-compulsive disorder in patients with chronic pruritic conditions: case studies and discussion. *J Am Acad Dermatol* 1992; **26**: 549–51.
2 Warnock JK, Kestenbaum T. Obsessive-compulsive disorder. *Dermatol Clin* 1996; **14**: 465–72.
3 Oates JK, Gomaz J. Venereophobia. *Br J Hosp Med* 1984; **31**: 435–6.
4 Gupta MA, Gupta AK. Psychodermatology: an update. *J Am Acad Dermatol* 1996; **34**: 1030–46.
5 Gupta MA, Gupta AK. Dermatologic signs in anorexia nervosa and bulimia nervosa. *Arch Derm* 1987; **123**: 1386–90.
6 Luck P, Wakerling A. Increased cutaneous vasoreactivity to cold in anorexia nervosa. *Clin Sci* 1981; **61**: 559–67.
7 Anderson AE. Drenching nocturnal sweats during weight recovery in eating disordered patients: a new syndrome. Paper presented at the 6th International Conference on Eating Disorders, New York, April 1994.
8 Marshman GM, Hanna MJ, Ben-Tovin DI, Walker MK. Cutaneous abnormalities in anorexia nervosa. *Australas J Dermatol* 1990; **31**: 9–12.
9 Veale D. Friday the 13th and obsessive compulsive disorder: better understanding has brought some success in treatment. *Br Med J* 1995; **311**: 963–4.
10 Editorial. Selective serotonin reuptake inhibitors in obsessive/compulsive disorder. *Drugs Ther Bull* 1995; **33**: 47–8.

Blushing and erythrophobia

Although blushing itself is normal under certain circumstances, blushing that is grossly excessive in both frequency and extent is sometimes seen in women and may be the cause of considerable embarrassment and give rise to erythrophobia, a compulsive state related to fear of blushing [1]. Occasionally, erythrophobia may represent a hysterical conversion symptom. These patients frequently suffer from emotional difficulties and inhibitions and can sometimes be helped by a sympathetic clinical psychologist. Fairly frequent flushing can be a manifestation of hyperthyroidism and the distinctive flushing of the carcinoid syndrome must also be excluded (Chapter 46).

REFERENCE

1 Parkes-Weber F. *Rare Diseases*, 2nd edn. London: Staples, 1947: 61.

Self-inflicted and simulated skin disease

There are normal behaviour habits associated with the skin that appear particularly at times of stress and anxiety. Picking, plucking, sucking, rubbing, biting and pulling behaviour on skin, nails and hair are stress-relieving activities seen particularly in children, in many adolescents, but less often in adults [1].

Each of these behaviours is physically transient and on most occasions a conscious activity that does not intrude on normal skin function. However, when these habits become entrenched as part of a daily routine, or progress beyond the stage where they are an incidental stress-relieving activity, then they are recognizable as a number of dermatological disorders. Nail biting has been recorded from the age of 15 months [1] but is commoner after the age of 3 years and is present in over one-third of children between the ages of 7 and 10 years [2]. Up to half of adolescents continue to bite their nails, but there is no information about adults, although obsessive onychophagia is well recorded [3]. Studies of college students [4,5] showed 1.5% of males and 3.4% of females continued hair pulling but only 0.5% satisfied the *Diagnostic and Statistical Manual of Mental Disorders* (DSM)-III-R criteria for trichotillomania.

Scratching behaviour may progress to lichen simplex or nodular prurigo. Destructive picking activity may progress to neurotic excoriations, acne excoriée, persistent nose picking and in extreme cases trigeminal trophic syndrome (Chapter 63). Persistent pluckers most commonly abuse their hair and can present as trichotillomania. Perioral dermatitis can be a consequence of chronic licking behaviour and chronic cheilitis the result of lip biting (Chapter 70). Chronic nail disease such as paronychia follows from nail biting and onychophagia (Chapter 65).

REFERENCES

1 Illingworth RS. *Body Manipulations in The Normal Child* 5th edn. Edinburgh: Churchill Livingstone, 1972: 318.
2 Leung AK, Robson WL. Nailbiting. *Clin Paediatr* 1990; **29**: 690–2.
3 Leonard HL, Lenane MC, Swedo SE *et al*. Treatment of severe onychophagia. *Arch Gen Psychiatry* 1991; **48**: 821–7.
4 Christenson GA, Pyle RL, Mitchell JE. Estimated lifetime prevalence of trichotillomania in college students. *J Clin Psychiatry* 1991; **52**: 415–17.
5 Tynes LL, Winsted DK. Behavioural aspects of trichotillomania. *J Louis Med Soc* 1992; **144**: 459–63.

Lichen simplex and neurodermatitis
(see also Chapter 17)

Lichenification describes the pattern of response of the predisposed skin to repeated rubbing. In some instances, a minor initiating event, such as trauma, infection or other itchy lesion, precipitates continuous scratching. Itching is the major complaint, scratching the chronic accompaniment. This behaviour takes the form of rubbing with either the hands or knuckles and in extreme cases sometimes with the use of an instrument such as a hairbrush, a pen or some other domestic implement. The actions may not be conscious ones and may proceed without continuous conscious control. However, in some cases patients subject themselves to frenetic, prolonged spasms of uncontrollable self-damage. Lichen simplex and neurodermatitis are much less common in the elderly.

Regular rubbing and pressure on the skin produces the characteristic thickened, coarsely grained nodules on the skin with hyperpigmentation. The classic sites of involvement are within easy reach, particularly on the nape and sides of the neck, elbows, thighs, knees and ankles. These areas may be in varying stages of evolution, from early papules with surface excoriations to chronic areas that present as plaques with pigment changes, described as 'dermatological worry beads'. Localized patches of lichen simplex presenting as pruritis ani and vulvae are described in Chapters 17 & 72.

These lesions are most often found in females and occur predominantly after puberty. They are found, very rarely, as isolated phenomena in children, even in atopics. Most authors have commented on the relationship of emotional tension to bouts of scratching [1]. Patients are usually described as stable but anxious individuals, whose reactions to stress are relieved by ritualized behaviour such as rubbing [2]. Aggression and hostility related to anxiety [3] caused by emotional disturbance may lead to itching. This maladaptive response has been treated successfully with behaviour therapy [4] to break the itch–scratch cycle.

Treatment with antihistamines is helpful, but antidepressants, particularly tricyclic compounds such as doxepin in doses as low as 25–50 mg/day, have been shown to be more effective [5].

REFERENCES

1 Allerhand ME, Gough HG, Grais ML. Personality factors in neurodermatitis. *Psychosom Med* 1950; **12**: 386–9.
2 Freid RG. Evaluation and treatment of psychogenic pruritis and self excoriation. *J Am Acad Dermatol* 1994; **30**: 993–9.
3 Jordan JM, Whitlock FA. Atopic dermatitis—anxiety and conditioned response. *J Psychosom Res* 1974; **18**: 297–9.
4 Jordan JM, Whitlock FA. Emotions and the skin. *Br J Dermatol* 1972; **86**: 574–7.
5 Melin L, Noren P. Behavioural treatment of scratching in patients with atopic dermatitis. *Br J Dermatol* 1986; **115**: 467–74.

Destructive excoriations

The commonest of the self-inflicted dermatoses are neurotic excoriations and acne excoriée. They differ from other artefactual disorders as those who suffer readily admit to an urge to pick and gouge at their skin. Both of these clinical syndromes are characterized by the preponderance of females, the destructive scarring nature of the lesions and the relationship to psychological stress. Some patients show features of both conditions and one condition may merge into the other.

Neurotic excoriations [1,2]

This is seen most frequently in middle-aged women [1,2]. The average age of onset is between 30 and 50 years of age [1,3], but significantly the average duration of disease before presentation can be up to 10 years [1]. This group make up the most severe cases, where the problem tends to be persistent and unremitting. These patients are described as rather rigid and obsessional individuals with repressed emotions [4]. They have difficulty in verbalizing their problems and are aggressive but also insecure [3]. Depression was a very common feature in one series [5]. The picking and excoriation proceeds in bouts that exceed the bounds of simple habit, and patients describe picking, scratching, gouging and using implements on their skin, to produce bleeding and pain. There is a compulsive quality about the need to continue until pain is produced. The duration of these bouts may last for some hours and can be ritualized to a set time and place. Psychosocial stresses have been reported to precede exacerbations of excoriations in 30–90% of patients [1,3]. Immediately following such behaviour, patients are characteristically unhappy and guilty about the disfigurement.

Clinical features. Lesions can be seen in all stages of development. The acute lesions are usually less than 1 cm in diameter with an erythematous edge and covered with a serosanguinous crust. They may be quite deep, extending into dermis, and are distributed symmetrically within reach

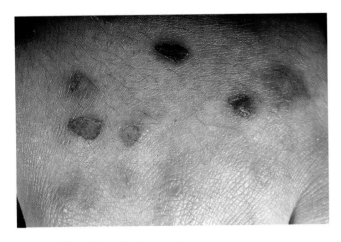

Fig. 64.1 Neurotic exoriations.

of the hands. The lesions may be around the hair margins, on the face, sides of the neck and appear most particularly on the shoulders and anterior chest. Older lesions show pink or red scars, some of which may be hypertrophic and surrounded by an area of hypopigmentation (Fig. 64.1). Very chronic lesions may also show atrophic scars, which coalesce and are eventually seen as linear, coalescent areas. Lesions appear at all stages of development and may number from a few to several hundred.

Differential diagnosis. It is important to exclude excoriations caused by generalized pruritus, bullous disorders, such as pemphigus, and linear excoriated lesions, which may be the presenting signs of lichen planus or lupus erythematosus.

Treatment. The compulsive nature of this disorder responds well to antidepressants and in particular to serotonin re-uptake inhibitor drugs, such as fluoxetine [6]. Clomipramine [7] and doxepin [8] have been reported to work well. Simple, empathic, supportive psychotherapy can produce significant improvement, whereas insight-orientated analysis may exacerbate symptoms [9]. Cognitive behaviour therapy has improved some patients [10], although the management of underlying personality difficulties may require the specific skills of a psychotherapist. Whilst these cases eventually resolve, the most difficult cases are middle-aged women with established patterns of excoriation, which may have been continuing for decades. It may be necessary to continue antidepressants in these patients for some years.

REFERENCES

1 Gupta M, Gupta A, Haberman H. Neurotic excoriations: a review and some new perspectives. *Compr Psychiatry* 1986; **27**: 381–6.
2 Nielsen H, Fruensgaard K, Hjorshoj A. Controlled neuropsychological investigations of patients with neurotic excoriations. *Psychother Psychosom* 1980; **34**: 52–61.

3 Fruensgaard K. Neurotic excoriations. *Int J Dermatol* 1987; **17**: 761–7.
4 Musaph H. Psychodermatology. In: Hill O, ed. *Modern Trends in Psychosomatic Medicine*. London: Butterworths, 1974: 216–19.
5 Koo JVM, Wintraub B, Odom R. Chronic psychogenic excoriations a manifestation of major depression. *Abstracts of the First Congress of European Academy of Dermatology and Venereology*. Florence: Tipographia, 1989: 132 .
6 Primeau F, Fontaine R. Obsessive disorder with self mutilation: a subgroup responsive to pharmacotherapy. *Can J Psychiatry* 1987; **32**: 699–702.
7 DeVeaugh-Geiss J, Landau P, Katz R. Preliminary results from a multicenter trial of clomipramine in obsessive compulsive disorder. *Pharmacol Bull* 1989; **25**: 36–40.
8 Harris BA, Sheretz EF, Flowers FP. Improvement of chronic neurotic excoriations with oral doxepin therapy. *Int J Dermatol* 1983; **26**: 541–3.
9 Seitz PFD. Psychocutaneous aspects of persistent pruritus and excessive excoriation. *Arch Dermatol Syphiligr* 1951; **64**: 136–41.
10 Welkowitz LA, Held JL, Held AL. Management of neurotic scratching with behavioural therapy. *J Am Acad Dermatol* 1989; **21**: 802–4.

Acne excoriée (see Chapter 42) [1,2]

Squeezing and pinching of acne lesions is almost universal. Brocq in 1898 described acne excoriée particularly in adolescent girls under emotional stress who picked and squeezed acne spots. Excoriation that produced mutilating scars persisting into adult life, or even beginning without pre-existing acne, caused Wrong [2] to consider the condition a variant of neurotic excoriation with the lesions largely confined to the face. Acne excoriée is commoner in women [1–4] and seen in an older age group than acne vulgaris, with a mean age of about 30 years [3,4]. Psychological studies have shown no diagnosable DSM-III-R disorder [4,5], although associated phobic states [1] and depressive and delusional disorders [6] have been described.

The clinical lesions resemble those of neurotic excoriation. They are found predominantly around the forehead, hairline, preauricular, cheek and chin areas. Extension to the neck and occipital hairline is often seen. Chronic lesions characteristically show white, atrophic scarring with peripheral hyperpigmentation. One study showed a strong association with atopy [3], suggesting an overlap with prurigo mitis.

Patients with acne excoriée rarely respond to simple acne therapy, and most require in addition systemic antibiotics, and isotretinoin. Whilst this may arrest the development of new lesions and scarring, the physical course of the disease is poor without psychological support [1]. In all cases, the benefit of simple supportive consultation and psychotherapy should not be underestimated [7]. Compulsive behaviour that leads to further scarring may respond to habit-reversal therapy [8].

REFERENCES

1 Sneddon J, Sneddon I. Acne excoriée; a protective device. *Clin Exp Dermatol* 1983; **8**: 65–8.
2 Wrong NM. Excoriated acne of young females. *Arch Dermatol Syphiligr* 1954; **70**: 574–82.
3 Gebhart W, Brosner C, Jurecka W, Schmidt J. Acne excoriée: the dermatologist's view. *Abstracts of the First International Congress on Dermatology and Psychiatry*.

Florence: Tipographia, 1989: 50–1.
4 Zadro-Jaeger S, Musalek M. Acne excoriée psychiatric studies. *Abstracts of the Third International Congress on Dermatology and Psychiatry.* Florence: Tipographia, 1991.
5 Bach M, Bach D. Psychiatric and psychometric issues in acne excoriée. *Psychother Psychosom* 1993; **60**: 207–8.
6 Koo JM, Smith LL. Psychologic aspects of acne. *Pediatr Dermatol* 1991; **8**: 185–9.
7 Ginsburg IH. The psychosocial impact of skin disease. *Dermatol Clin* 1996; **14**: 473–84.
8 Kent A, Drummond LM. Acne excoriée: a case report using habit reversal. *Clin Exp Dermatol* 1989; **14**: 163–4.

Trichotillomania [1,2]

Definition. Trichotillomania is defined as the irresistable urge to pull out the hair, and a sense of relief after the hair has been plucked. The term was originally used by Hallopeau in 1889 and literally means a morbid craving to pull out hair. DSM-IV [3] lists trichotillomania under impulse-control disorders in company with compulsive gambling and kleptomania.

Aetiology and pathogenesis [1,2,4]. The epidemiology of this complaint is not absolutely clear. However, there appear to be two distinct populations: those who present in childhood [2,5] and who probably represent the bulk of cases, and fewer but more chronic cases who present as adults who have continued hair-pulling activity from adolescence or developed the disorder in early adult life [1]. The number of affected children may be seven times that of adults [4]. This early-onset group, usually between the ages of 2 and 6 years, show benign, self-limiting behaviour [2] with equal sex distribution [2,5] or male predominance [6]. The adult age groups are associated with greater psychopathology and show distinct female preponderance [1,2,5,6], usually 4:1, but 15:1 being most evident in the oldest group [1]. This remains true for different racial groups [7–9]. The association with nail biting and thumb sucking is common in children [2,5,10,11]. In children, there is an association with anxiety and dysthymia [12], learning disability and iron deficiency [13]. Emotional problems in the pre-adolescent group tend to be less severe, more a reflection of a stressful life event rather than serious psychopathology [14]. The adult patients show more diverse psychopathology with depression, anxiety disorder, obsessive–compulsive disorder and panic attacks prominent [1,2,11]. Substance abuse and eating disorders may also be evident [1,2]. Whilst it has been proposed that adult chronic trichotillomania is a variant of obsessive–compulsive disorder, with positive correlation in family studies [15], this definition is too narrow for many patients [1], and has not been supported by psychometric testing [16].

Clinical features [1]. All patients describe an increased sense of tension before hair pulling or a sense of relief after the act. This is usually a deliberate conscious act but some patients may have incomplete awareness until the pattern has been established [17].

Hair pulling and plucking is commonest from the scalp, but only 5% do so in response to scalp symptoms. Most pull hair from the vertex, but temporal, occipital and frontal hair loss in children may be more obvious on the side of manual dominance. The hair loss may be minimal, but visible hair thinning may progress to virtual total depilation. Typically, the hairs are short, irregular, broken and distorted. In extreme cases, this shows as a 'tonsure pattern' [18] or 'Friar Tuck' [10] distribution. The eyelashes, eyebrows, facial and pubic hair may also be primarily affected. Two-thirds of adults pulled hair from two or more sites and one-third from three areas [2].

Licking, chewing and eating the hair has been reported in over 10% of adults, who usually report no abdominal symptoms. However, the accumulation of ingested hair in the stomach and small intestine eventually forms a trichobezoar. Anorexia, abdominal pain, weight loss and eventual obstructive ileus have been recorded in children [7,19,20] and the mentally retarded [21].

Investigations. Scalp biopsy has been shown to be most useful [5]. The most important findings include multiple catagen hairs, pigment casts and traumatized hair bulbs.

Differential diagnosis. See Chapter 66.

Treatment. For pre-adolescent children, identification of stressful episodes with accompanying support, and parent education is usually all that is necessary. Behaviour therapy was effective in children [22] and reduced symptoms by 90% in 19 adults [23]. Swedo *et al.* [24] demonstrated that clomipramine was more effective than desipramine, although relapse may be common [25]. In two further studies [26,27], fluoxetine in doses up to 80mg/day decreased severity by 60%. Low-dose pimozide has been shown to augment this response [28].

REFERENCES

1 Christenson GA, Mackenzie TB, Mitchell JE. Characteristics of 60 adult chronic hair pullers. *Am J Psychiatry* 1991; **148**: 365–70.
2 Swedo SE, Rapoport JL. Trichotillomania. *J Clin Psychol Psychiatry* 1991; **32**: 401–9.
3 American Psychiatric Association. *Diagnostic and Statistical Manual of Mental Disorders; DSM-IV*, 4th edn. Washington DC, 1994.
4 Mehregan AH. Trichotillomania: a clinicopathologic study. *Arch Dermatol* 1970; **102**: 129–33.
5 Muller SA. Trichotillomania: a histopathologic study in sixty six patients. *J Am Acad Dermatol* 1990; **23**: 56–62.
6 Dawber R. Self induced hair loss. *Semin Dermatol* 1985; **4**: 53–7.
7 Bhatia MS, Singhal PK, Rastogi V, Dhar NK. Clinical profile of trichotillomania. *J Ind Med Assoc* 1991; **89**: 137–9.
8 Chang CH, Lee MB, Chiang YC, Lu YC. Trichotillomania: a clinical study of 36 patients. *J Formosan Med Assoc* 1991; **90**: 176–80.
9 Hussein SH. Trichotillomania. *Psychopathology* 1992; **25**: 289–93.
10 Dimino-Emme L, Camisa C. Trichotillomania associated with the 'Friar Tuck' sign and nail biting. *Cutis* 1991; **47**: 107–10.

11 Mannino FV, Delgado RA. Trichotillomania in children. *Am J Psychiatry* 1969; **126**: 505–11.

12 Reeve EA, Bernstein GA, Christenson GA. Clinical characteristics and psychiatric comorbidity in children with trichotillomania. *J Am Acad Child Adolesc Psychiatry* 1992; **31**: 132–8.

13 Oranje AP, Peereboom-Wynia JD, DeRaeymacker DM. Trichotillomania in childhood. *J Am Acad Dermatol* 1986; **15**: 614–19.

14 Krishnan RRK, Davidson JRT, Guajardo C. Trichotillomania: a review. *Compr Psychiatry* 1985; **26**: 123–8.

15 Lenane MC, Swedo SE, Rapoport JL *et al*. Rates of obsessive compulsive disorder in first degree relatives of patients with trichotillomania. *J Clin Psychiatry* 1992; **33**: 925–33.

16 Stanley MA, Prather RC, Wagner AL *et al*. Can the Yale–Brown Obsessive Compulsive Scale be used to assess trichotillomania? *Behav Res Ther* 1993; **31**: 171–7.

17 Demaret A. Onychophagia, trichotillomania and grooming. *Ann Med Psychol (Paris)* 1973; **1**: 235–42.

18 Sanderson KV, Hall-Smith P. Tonsure trichotillomania. *Br J Dermatol* 1970; **82**: 343–50.

19 Delsmann BM, Nikolaidis N, Schomacher PH. Trichobezoar as a rare cause of ileus. *Deutsche Med Wochen* 1993; **118**: 1361–4.

20 Minerva. *Br Med J* 1994; **309**: 282.

21 Wadlington WB, Rose M, Holcomb GW. Complications of trichobezoars: a 30-year experience. *South Med J* 1992; **85**: 1020–2.

22 Vitulano LA, King RA, Scahill L, Cohen DJ. Behavioural treatment of children and adolescents with trichotillomania. *J Am Acad Child Adolesc Psychiatry* 1992; **31**: 139–46.

23 Azrin NH. Treatment of hair-pulling. A comparative study of habit reversal and negative practice training. *J Behav Ther Exp Psychiatry* 1980; **11**: 80–5.

24 Swedo S, Leonard HL, Rapoport JL. A double blind comparison of clomipramine and desipramine in the treatment of trichotillomania. *N Engl J Med* 1989; **321**: 497–501.

25 Pollard CA, Ibe I, Krojanker DN *et al*. Clomipramine treatment of trichotillomania: a follow-up report on four cases. *J Clin Psychiatry* 1991; **52**: 128–30.

26 Koran LM, Ringold A, Hewlett W. Fluoxetine for trichotillomania. *Psychopharmacol Bull* 1992; **28**: 145–9.

27 Winchel RM, Jones JS, Stanley B *et al*. Clinical characteristics of trichotillomania and its response to fluoxetine. *J Clin Psychiatry* 1992; **53**: 304–8.

28 Stein DJ, Hollander E. Low dose pimozide augmentation of SSR blockers in trichotillomania. *J Clin Psychiatry* 1992; **53**: 123–6.

Onychotillomania and onychophagia [1,2]
(see also Chapter 65)

The compulsive habits of nail picking and nail biting have been shown to be common in children and adolescents [2,3]. The aetiologies suggested include stress, imitation of family members and a transference from the thumb sucking habit. Nail biting is usually confined to the fingernails, but nail picking, especially in adults may involve all digits. Damage to cuticles and nails causes paronychia, nail dystrophy and longitudinal melanonychia [4]. In chronic cases, there is an association with trichotillomania [1]. Compulsive biting, tearing or picking with instruments such as scissors, knives or razorblades may lead to permanent destruction [5].

Onychotillomania is often denied by the patient but some do admit to the habit. Of these the commonest problem is a compulsive action, not always at times of stress. Self-induced anonychia of the toenails was produced by one man who plucked out the nails with pliers rather than suffer recurrent paronychia of previously crushed toes [6]. Delusions of parasitosis may provoke self-destruction of the nails [7] as can a folie à deux in the confused elderly [8]. Successful response to treatment has been shown with clomipramine [9] and pimozide [8].

REFERENCES

1 Demaret A. Onychophagia, trichotillomania and grooming. *Ann Med Psychol (Paris)* 1973; **1**: 235–42.

2 Leung AK, Robson WL. Nailbiting. *Clin Paediatr* 1990; **29**: 690–2.

3 Odenrick B, Fattstrom V. Nailbiting: frequency and association with root resorption during orthodontic treatment. *Br J Orthod* 1985; **12**: 78–81.

4 Baran R. Nail biting and picking as a cause of longitudinal melanonychia. *Dermatologica* 1990; **181**: 126–8.

5 Sait MA, Reddy BSN, Garg BR. Onychotillomania. *Dermatologica* 1985; **171**: 200–2.

6 Hurley PT, Balu V. Self inflicted anonychia. *Arch Dermatol* 1982; **118**: 956–7.

7 Alkiewicz J. Uber Onychotillomanie. *Dermatol Wochenschr* 1934; **98**: 519–21.

8 Hamman K. Onychotillomania treated with pimozide. *Acta Derm Venereol (Stockh)* 1982; **62**: 346–8.

9 Leonard HL, Lenane MC, Swedo SE *et al*. A Double blind comparison of clomipramine and desipramine in severe onychophagia. *Arch Gen Psychiatry* 1991; **48**: 821–7.

Psychogenic purpuras [1]

This group of disorders is incompletely understood. The common features are the presence of purpura, bruising or frank bleeding in patients who show severe emotional disturbance. The patients are predominantly female. For clarification it is helpful to consider the following separate categories, although some overlap is apparent:

1 autoerythrocyte sensitization syndrome (Gardner–Diamond syndrome) [2];

2 psychogenic purpura without autoerythrocyte sensitization but with other abnormalities [3,4];

3 psychogenic purpura with no measurable abnormality [5,6];

4 purpura factitia [7–9];

5 religious stigmata.

Autoerythrocyte sensitization syndrome [2]
SYN. GARDNER–DIAMOND SYNDROME

In this rare but well recognized condition (Chapter 48), exquisitely tender bruises arise after minimal trauma or emotional stress. In the original cases, it was noted there was a preceding history of an injury involving extensive bruising or major surgery. These bizarre tender lesions are most commonly located on the arms and legs [10]. The bruising is heralded by a burning or stinging sensation followed after a few hours by oedema and erythema. The bruising appears a day or so later [11]. Abdominal pain, bleeding from internal organs and neurological symptoms may occur [1]. Psychiatric symptoms were present in 21 of 30 cases reported [12]. Severe emotional disturbances are a constant feature and the relationship to religious stigmatization has been discussed by Ratnoff [1] and Whitlock [13].

Typical ecchymoses can be reproduced by the intra-dermal injection of the patient's own erythrocytes and in some cases red-cell phosphotidyl-L-serine [14]. Gomi and Miura [15] described a case with associated thrombocytosis where busulphan therapy induced a reduction in attacks. Increased fibrinolytic activity has also been noted at the appearance of fresh lesions in some patients [4,16]. One case seemed to have been made worse by a copper-containing intrauterine contraceptive [17]. This condition is so bizarre that emergency departments should be aware of its features and differential diagnosis [18].

Psychiatric treatment using psychotherapy [1,10,13] or psychotropics [14] has been reported.

Psychogenic purpura without autoerythrocyte sensitization but with other abnormalities [3,4]

A very similar clinical syndrome has been reported but with a negative reaction to intradermal red cells. Rowell [4] described two women with painful bleeding and bruises in association with increased fibrinolytic activity and with mental stress. A further condition in this group consists of autosensitivity to DNA [3] described as painful, itchy eccymoses, which recurred over a number of years.

Psychogenic purpura with no measurable abnormality [5,6]

Sorensen *et al.* [6] considered that patients with psychogenic purpura with no abnormal tests shared the same emotional background and other clinical features and should be regarded as part of the same syndrome. The lesions may be less tender and dramatic [5].

Purpura factitia [7–9]

Bleeding, bruising and purpura have all been reported as artefactual disease. Agle [7] described malingerers who misuse anticoagulants, whilst aspirin has also been taken to similar effect. Mechanical purpuras are ingenious and well reported [8,9].

REFERENCES

1 Ratnoff OD. The psychogenic purpuras: a review of autoerythrocyte sensitization, autosensitization to DNA, 'hysterical' and factitious bleeding, and the religious stigmata. *Semin Hematol* 1980; **17**: 192–213.
2 Gardner FH, Diamond LK. Autoerythrocyte sensitization: a form of purpura producing painful bruising following autosensitization to red blood cells in certain women. *Blood* 1955; **10**: 675–90.
3 Chandler D, Nalbandian RN. DNA autosensitivity. *Am J Med Sci* 1966; **251**: 145–7.
4 Rowell NR. A painful bleeding syndrome with increased fibrinolytic activity. *Br J Dermatol* 1974; **91**: 591–3.
5 Ogston D, Ogston WD, Bennett NB. Psychogenic purpura. *Br Med J* 1971; i: 30.
6 Sorenson RU, Newman AJ, Gordon EM. Psychogenic purpura in adolescent patients. *Clin Paediatr* 1985; **21**: 700–4.
7 Agle D, Ratnoff OD, Spring GK. The anticoagulant malingerer. *Ann Intern Med* 1970; **73**: 67–72.
8 Sneddon IB. Simulated disease: problems in diagnosis and management. *J R Coll Physicians Lond* 1983; **17**: 199–205.
9 Yates VM. Factitious purpura. *Clin Exp Dermatol* 1992; **17**: 238–9.
10 Berman DA, Roenigk HH, Green D. Autoerythrocyte sensitization syndrome (psychogenic purpura). *J Am Acad Dermatol* 1992; **27**: 829–32.
11 Verstraete M. Psychogenic haemorrhages. *Verhandelingen* 1991; **53**: 5–28.
12 Hersle K, Mobacken H. Autoerythrocyte sensitization syndrome (psychogenic purpura): report of two cases and review of the literature. *Br J Dermatol* 1969; **81**: 574–87.
13 Whitlock FA. Self inflicted and related dermatoses. In: Whitlock FA, ed. *Psychophysiological Aspects of Skin Disease.* London: WB Saunders, 1976: 98–107.
14 Strunecka A, Krpejsova L, Palecek J *et al.* Transbilayer redistribution of phosphatidylserine in erythrocytes of a patient with autoerythrocyte sensitization syndrome (psychogenic purpura). *Folia Haematol* 1990; **117**: 829–41.
15 Gomi H, Miura T. Autoerythrocyte sensitization syndrome with thrombocytosis. *Dermatology* 1994; **188**: 160–2.
16 Lotti T, Benci M, Sarti MG *et al.* Psychogenic purpura with abnormally increased tPA dependent cutaneous fibrinolytic activity. *Int J Dermatol* 1993; **32**: 521–3.
17 Grossman RA. Autoerythrocyte sensitization worsened by a copper containing IUD. *Obstet Gynecol* 1987; **70**: 526–8.
18 Tomec RJ, Waugh M, Garcia JC. Diagnosis of autoerythrocyte sensitization syndrome in the emergency department. *Ann Emerg Med* 1989; **18**: 780–2.

Factitious skin disease

There are a series of recognized skin diseases characterized by the essential features that, firstly they are caused by the fully aware patient and secondly, the desire to hide the cause from their doctors. This definition includes dermatitis artefacta, dermatological pathomimicry, dermatitis simulata and dermatitis passivata. These syndromes are additionally distinguishable from others where there is a secondary gain, such as Munchausen's syndrome and malingering.

Dermatitis artefacta

Definition. Dermatitis artefacta is an artefactual skin disease caused entirely by the actions of the fully aware patient on the skin, hair, nails or mucosae. These patients hide the responsibility for their actions from their doctors. There is no rational motive for this behaviour [1].

Epidemiology and aetiology. All studies have shown the preponderance of females, the ratio of female to male varying from 8:1 to 4:1 [2–6]. Lesions have been found in children from the age of 8 years [5]. Whilst these series confirm that the majority of cases commence in adolescence and in adults under 30 years of age, there is an important subgroup whose age of onset is significantly older. This subgroup is distinguished by being more likely to be male (male to female ratio 1:2) to produce more subtle skin lesions [4,5] and to have a past history of somatizing illness [7,8]. Previous work has suggested that dermatitis artefacta is more common in health-care workers and their families [4,9,10] because this environment provides a ready 'model to copy'. However, this bias may now be less obvious [5] perhaps because medical information is more available via the media.

Much has been written about the psychopathology of artefact [1,3,11,12]. In many cases, the psychosocial stress of a major life event may be apparent. Children and adolescents commonly show anxiety and immaturity of coping styles in response to these stresses, possibly in response to a dysfunctional parent–child relationship [12]. Childhood dermatitis artefacta has also been precipitated by child abuse. Adults may be neurotic and react to adverse situations in an immature, impulsive manner [3,12]. However, there may also be significant depression [3,5]. The more chronic patients tend to have a demonstrable personality disorder more particularly borderline or hysterical in females and paranoid in males [1,5,10,12].

Clinical features. The first distinct feature of dermatitis artefacta is the 'hollow history' [13]. This describes the sudden appearance of complete lesions with little or no prodrome. The signs invariably appear overnight, or in a lunch break, or on the way home from school or work. Lesions appear at the same identical stage in development in crops or groups either symmetrically or scattered apparently at random. There is a significant lack of a history of a progression of lesions from an initial lesion to its fully developed state, in contrast to the prolonged and elaborate descriptions of complications and failure to heal once it has appeared. Characteristically, established lesions may undergo sudden deterioration at the same time as new areas appear. It has been suggested that the patients show a 'belle indifference' to their predicament as part of a dissociative state [4] and that, in the presence of visible disease, manifest a nonchalance and innocence transmitted through an enigmatic 'Mona Lisa' smile. However, this is not always the case and considerable anger may be shown by the patient, but more particularly by parents, carers, husbands or partners, at the incompetence of the medical profession [1,14]. This may extend further to recruiting other doctors, university academics, nurses and social workers to support their case [5]. More than one person may be involved, as in the 'folie à deux' of two patients with factitious ulcers [15].

Clinical signs [4,10,14]. The commonest sites involved are exposed areas such as the face, particularly cheeks, the hands, arms and legs. The genitalia and breasts may show considerable mutilation. Involvement of the back, axillae and external ear is uncommon.

The cutaneous lesions represent every known means of damaging the skin. Crude, destructive processes are commonest; less commonly dermal lesions from blunt trauma or injections are found. Oedema from constricting bands and hysterical dependent posture have been described [6] (Secretan's syndrome).

Excoriations may be made with nail files, sanding boards, wood or wire to produce raw, crusty, linear or arciform lesions with characteristic angulated edges (Fig. 64.2). Punched out, necrotic areas, initially with blisters developing into indurated necrotic scars are typical of thermal burns from cigarettes, soldering irons or ovens. These are usually uniform in size and scattered haphazardly. Urticarial lesions that progress subsequently to crusting and scarring may be produced by chemical damage.

Characteristically, these areas may show the 'drip-sign', where corrosive liquids have been allowed to run over the skin (Fig. 64.3). Bleaches, soaps and household cleaners are most commonly employed by women; industrial acids and automotive fluids by men. Purpuras and bruising are seen after suction, friction or blunt trauma. Children produce purpura on the chin by sucking on cups and on limbs by direct mouth suction or with the use of a toy or tool. Shearing stress also produces purpura, tending to show as linear limb lesions.

Subtle artefact [4,5,10] is seen as fixed urticaria, vasculitis (Fig. 64.4) dermal nodules, panniculitis-type lesions and boggy fluctuant swellings. Considerable atrophy and

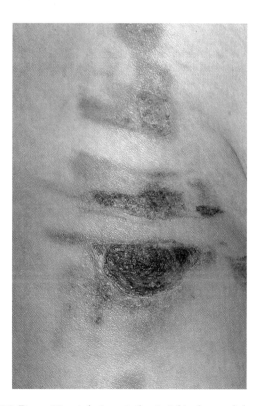

Fig. 64.2 Dermatitis artefacta: note the straight edges and sharp angulation of some of the lesions.

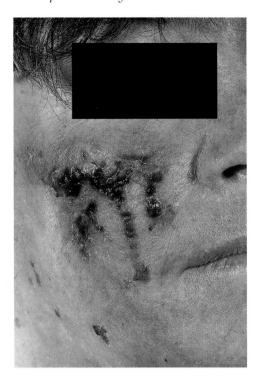

Fig. 64.3 Dermatitis artefacta showing the drip sign.

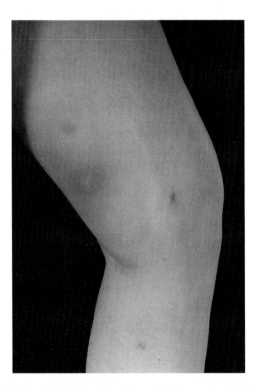

Fig. 64.4 Vasculitic lesions showing acute inflammatory lesions and old monomorphic atrophic scars.

pigment change occur with resolution. Careful examination may reveal the presence of a needle track where milk, air, faeces or urine has been injected [16].

Differential diagnosis. The physical signs of the crude artefact are diagnostic. However, blistering, crusty lesions may simulate ecthyma, herpes simplex, bullous disorders or porphyria cutanea tarda. The collagen–vascular diseases including vasculitis and pyoderma gangrenosum must be excluded as must the curious linear dermatoses such as Nékam's syndrome and linear drug eruptions [17]. The diverse hereditary sensory neuropathies can show chronic non-healing ulcers and be mistaken for artefact [18] as can the cutaneous changes of reflex sympathetic dystrophy. The haematological purpuras and tissue purpuric reactions such as cutaneous amyloid should be excluded in addition to autoerythrocyte sensitization (see Chapter 48).

REFERENCES

1 Consoli S. Dermatitis artefacta: a general review. *Eur J Dermatol* 1995; **5**: 5–11.
2 Campbell R, Donovan O, Rogers S. Dermatitis artefacta. A clinical review of 42 cases. *Proceedings of the Sixth International Congress on Dermatology and Psychiatry.* Amsterdam: ESDaP, 1995: 7.
3 Fabisch W. Psychiatric aspects of dermatitis artefacta. *Br J Dermatol* 1980; **102**: 29–34.
4 Lyell A. Dermatitis artefacta in relation to the syndrome of contrived disease. *Clin Exp Dermatol* 1976; **1**: 109–26.
5 Millard L. Dermatitis artefacta in the 1990s. *Br J Dermatol* 1996; **135** (Suppl. 47): 27.
6 Smith RJ. Factitious lymphoedema of the hand. *J Bone Joint Surg* 1975; **57**: 89–94.
7 Millard LG. Factitious dermatological disorders in the somatising patient. *Abstracts of the Fifth International Meeting European Society for Dermatology and Psychiatry.* Bordeaux: ESDaP, 1993.
8 Sneddon IB. Simulated disease: problems in diagnosis and management. *J R Coll Physicians Lond* 1983; **17**: 199–205.
9 Fras I. Factitial Disease. An Update. *Psychosomatics* 1978; **19**: 119–22.
10 Sneddon I, Sneddon J. Self inflicted injury: a follow-up study of 43 patients. *Br Med J* 1975; **3**; 527–30.
11 Cotterill J. Self-stigmatization: artefact dermatitis. *Br J Hosp Med* 1992; **47**: 115–19.
12 Koblenzer C. Psychologic aspects of skin disease. In: Fitzpatrick TB, Eisen AZ, Wolff K *et al.,* eds. *Dermatology in General Medicine.* New York: McGraw-Hill, 1993: 14–26.
13 Gandy DT. The concept and clinical aspects of factitial dermatitis. *South Med J* 1953; **46**: 551–5.
14 Lyell A. Cutaneous artefactual disease. *J Am Acad Dermatol* 1979; **1**: 391–407.
15 Hubler WR, Hubler WR, Sr. Folie à deux factitious ulcers. *Arch Dermatol* 1980; **116**: 1303–4.
16 Aduan RP, Fauci AS, Dale DC *et al.* Factitious fever and self-induced infection. *Ann Intern Med* 1979; **90**; 230–42.
17 Miori L, Vignini M, Rabbiosi G. Flagellate dermatitis after bleomycin. *Am J Dermatopathol* 1990; **12**; 598–602.
18 Mahood JM. Familial amyloid neuropathy. *Postgrad Med J* 1980; **56**: 658–9.

Factitious cheilitis (Fig. 64.5)

SYN. LE TIC DES LEVRES

Artefactual lesions of the lips are not common, but are seen equally in males and females [1,2]. Persistent inflammation of the lips with crusting and variable haemorrhage has been recorded, caused by picking, biting, rubbing and licking [3]. Differential diagnosis includes contact dermatitis, actinic damage, chronic lip-licking habit and causes of granulomatous cheilitis.

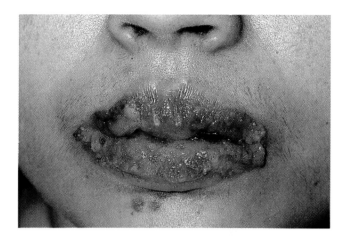

Fig. 64.5 Factitial cheilitis—a type of dermatitis artefacta of the lips.

REFERENCES

1 Crotty CP, Dicken CH. Factitious lip crusting. *Arch Dermatol* 1981; **117**: 338–40.
2 Thomas JR, Greene SL, Dicken CH. Factitious Cheilitis. *J Am Acad Dermatol* 1983; **3**: 368–72.
3 Kuffer R. Cheilitis and lip lesions artificially induced. *Ann Dermatol Vénéréol* 1990; **117**: 477–86.

Nail artefact

Chronic paronychia caused by the insertion of nails, pins or splinters has been recorded in soldiers avoiding duty but also in children [1]. Characteristic lesions show purpura and haemorrhage. Similarly, Lyell [2] described a patient who induced haemorrhagic nail loss using a nail file. Traumatic nail loss may occur singly or on one hand only. The differential diagnosis is described in Chapter 65.

REFERENCES

1 Sneddon IB. Simulated disease: problems in diagnosis and management. *J R Coll Physicians Lond* 1983; **17**: 199–205.
2 Lyell A. Dermatitis artefacta and self-inflicted disease. *Scot Med* 1972; **17**; 187–95.

Hair artefact

A bizarre pattern of hair loss may occur after cutting or shaving. It differs from the plucked appearance of trichotillomania and usually appears acutely either as rough, cropped areas of hair loss or unnatural patterned alopecia of scalp or eyebrows (Fig. 64.6).

Differential diagnosis. See Chapter 66.

Artefact by proxy [1]
WITCHCRAFT SYNDROME

Artefact dermatitis can be provoked on an unknowing and unsuspecting victim by proxy. As an act of revenge, the

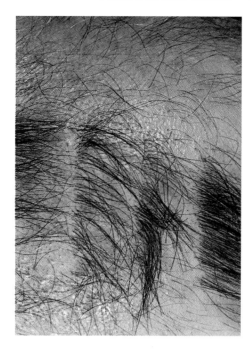

Fig. 64.6 Bizarre pattern of alopecia on the scalp with regimented rows of surviving hairs.

daughter of a hairdresser applied benzyl ether of nicotinic acid to the customers' skin. This induced hyperaemia with some oedema within 10 m but not on the perpetrator since absorption of the agent is very low on the palm of the hand so she could easily apply it to the customer's skin without harm to herself.

REFERENCE

1 Bandmann, Wahl B. Contact urticaria artefacta (witchcraft syndrome). *Contact Dermatitis* 1982; **8**: 145–6.

Dermatitis artefacta with artefact of patch tests [1]

Bullous dermatitis artefacta in a female veterinary assistant healed with occlusive dressings. New bullae on the other arm prompted the parents to demand 'allergy' tests. Ten patch tests to yellow petrolatum were applied to the back, which provoked a non-inflammatory bulla on one of the sites 2 days later. Two other cases are cited.

REFERENCE

1 Maurice PDL, Rivers JK, Jones C, Cronin E. Dermatitis artefacta with artefact of patch tests. *Clin Exp Dermatol* 1987; **12**: 204–6.

Investigations

Whilst the diagnosis is based clinically upon a high index of suspicion, litmus paper has been reported as a valuable aid to diagnosis, since it detects strong alkali or acid, particularly in new lesions [1]. Ordinary histopathology will confirm the nature of skin damage in crude artefact, whilst deeper lesions of vasculitis and panniculitis may show injection tracks and foreign material [2,3]. It has also been shown that serial biopsy may be diagnostically helpful in sophisticated artefact [4].

REFERENCES

1 Sneddon IB. Simulated disease: problems in diagnosis and management. *J R Coll Physicians Lond* 1983; **17**: 199–205.
2 Ackerman BA, Mosher DT, Schwamm HA. Factitial Weber–Christian Syndrome. *JAMA* 1966; **198**: 155–60.
3 Winkelmann RK, Barker SM. Factitial traumatic panniculitis. *J Am Acad Dermatol* 1985; **13**: 988–94.
4 Speight EL, Stevens A, Millard LG. The kaleidoscope of cutaneous artefact: histological clues. *J Am Acad Dermatol* (in press).

Treatment

There are three therapeutic aims. The first is to treat the cutaneous damage, then to identify the nature and extent of the psychological problem and finally to effect a transference to psychiatric care if necessary. Efficient occlusive bandaging will allow most lesions to heal except for those of the most devious and determined [1,2]. The psychological problems should be approached in a non-confrontational manner [1–5] allowing the patient to express their difficulties in a passive, confidential environment. Children usually respond well to this approach particularly if a cause of psychosocial pressure is identifiable. However, chronic persistent self-damage is predictive of long-term emotional illness and referral to a child psychiatrist is imperative [5]. The management and prognosis in adults is that of the primary psychological disorder [3]. Acute stress reaction can be addressed in a series of short consultations at the time when the dressings are changed. Depression responded well in two series [4,6] to tricyclics, or SSRI antidepressants, even when no precipitating event was identifiable. Tacit acceptance that the cause of the rash has been identified, without further challenge, helps to make the transfer to formal psychiatric care easier if needed [5]. Between one-third and a half of patients continue to develop chronic lesions [2,6]. Such cases usually have a personality disorder, commonly hysterical, paranoid or borderline [3,5,6] and need psychiatric assessment [7]. Unfortunately, this is frequently unacceptable to the patient.

REFERENCES

1 Lyell A. Dermatitis artefacta in relation to the syndrome of contrived disease. *Clin Exp Dermatol* 1976; **1**: 109–26.
2 Sneddon I, Sneddon J. Self inflicted injury: a follow-up study of 43 patients. *Br Med J* 1975; **3**: 527–30.
3 Consoli S. Dermatitis artefacta: a general review. *Eur J Dermatol* 1995; **5**: 5–11.

4 Fabisch W. Psychiatric aspects of dermatitis artefacta. *Br J Dermatol* 1980; **102**: 29–34.
5 Koblenzer C. Psychologic aspects of skin disease. In: Fitzpatrick TB, Eisen AZ, Wolff K *et al.* eds. *Dermatology in General Medicine*. New York: McGraw-Hill, 1993: 14–26.
6 Millard L. Dermatitis artefacta in the 1990s. *Br J Dermatol* 1996; **135** (Suppl. 47): 27.
7 van Moffaert MM. Integration of medical and psychiatric management in self-mutilation. *Gen Hosp Psychiatry* 1991; **13**: 59–67.

Dermatological pathomimicry [1]

Intentional aggravation of an existing dermatosis is distinguishable from dermatitis artefacta. Self-inflicted delayed healing of surgical and traumatic wounds is common. However, a group of 13 patients who had deliberately caused recurrence of their existing skin disease by reintroducing the precipitating factor have also recently been described [1,2]. The commonest provocative agents were atopic allergens, contact allergens, drug sensitivities and irritants applied to chronic leg disorders. Other reports have described irritant contact dermatitis [3] and artificial oedema of an arm or leg [4]. Most patients were young women who had lost support from within their family group. More direct confrontational discussion without recrimination proved helpful and follow-up showed only minor recurrence in two patients 5 years later [2].

REFERENCES

1 Millard LG. Dermatological pathomimicry: a form of patient maladjustment. *Lancet* 1984; **2**: 969–71.
2 Millard LG. Dermatological pathomimicry—a follow up study. *Proceedings of the First International Symposium on Dermatology and Psychiatry*. Vienna: ESDaP, 1987.
3 Condé-Salazar L, Gomez J, Meza B. Artefactual irritant dermatitis. *Contact Dermatitis* 1993; **28**: 246.
4 Stoberi C, Musalek M, Partsch H. Artificial oedema of the extremity. *Hautartz* 1994; **45**: 149–53.

Dermatitis simulata

Apparent skin disease can be represented by patients who are ingenious enough to use external disguise to simulate disease. Make up has been used to paint on a rash [1], sugar to simulate chronic cheilitis, drugs to induce skin discoloration [2] and topical printing dyes to produce discoloured sweat [3]. These deceptions were clever enough to confuse their doctors for months. Most of these patients were young and immature, but a somatizing illness was recorded in one older patient and previous treated depression in another.

REFERENCES

1 King MC, Chalmers RJG. Another aspect of contrived disease: 'dermatitis simulata'. *Cutis* 1984; **34**: 463–4.
2 Sneddon IB. Simulated disease: problems in diagnosis and management. *J R Coll Physicians Lond* 1983; **17**: 199–205.
3 McSween R, Perkins W, Millard L. A green man: a case of sweat artefact. *Arch Dermatol* (in press).

Dermatitis passivata

The cessation of normal skin cleansing will produce an accumulation of keratinous crusts. This is commonly seen in geriatric or demented patients who suffer from self-neglect and has been called the Diogenes syndrome [1]. Lesions are usually found on the chest, back or groin; however, a group of patients were described [2] who showed lesions on the face or arms. Notably, they were young adults who were invariably accompanied by parents or family. Significant psychopathology such as schizoid thought disorder or hysterical limb palsy was present. Specialist psychological therapy was usually necessary.

REFERENCES

1 Clark ANG, Mankikar GD, Gray I. Diogenes syndrome: a study of neglect in old age. *Lancet* 1975; **i**: 366–8.
2 Millard LG. Dermatitis passivata: the young Diogenes syndrome. *Cutis* (in press).

Munchausen's syndrome [1]

Asher used this term to describe the notorious hospital hopper who presents with a dramatic and untruthful story of illness. The patients are usually male, and travel widely from hospital to hospital complaining of abdominal pain, haemorrhage or some neurological incapacity. Skin lesions such as non-healing wounds, widespread blistering and multiple excoriations may be part of the syndrome of simulated disease [2]. The secondary gain is prolonged medical attention, although serious consequences such as septicaemia and paraplegia have occurred [3] from induced cutaneous ulceration.

Meadow [4] has described the syndrome of Munchausen by proxy where the illness is fabricated by the parent, usually mother, or someone *in loco parentis*. Rarely, the parent exhibits the syndrome herself and produces proxy lesions on the child (polle syndrome) [5]. Skin lesions are one of the less common presentations and are usually crude forms of dermatitis artefacta [4,6]. Munchausen by proxy may also be seen in the elderly, mentally handicapped or other dependent persons.

REFERENCES

1 Asher R. Munchausen's syndrome. *Lancet* 1951; **1**: 339–41.
2 Gorman WF, Winograd M. Crossing the border from Munchausen to malingering. *J Fla Med Assoc* 1988; **75**: 147–50.
3 Burket JM, Burket BA. Factitial dermatitis resulting in paraplegia. *J Am Acad Dermatol* 1987; **17**; 306–7.
4 Meadow SR. Munchausen syndrome by proxy. *Arch Dis Child* 1982; **57**: 92–8.
5 Verity CM, Winkworth C, Bruman D. Polle syndrome: children of Munchausen. *Br Med J* 1979; **2**: 422–3.
6 Meadow SR. Who's to blame—mothers, Munchausen or medicine? *J R Coll Physicians Lond* 1994; **28**: 332–7.

Malingering [1]

Asher [1] defined malingering as the imitation, production or encouragement of illness for a deliberate end. Fear, desire and escape are the three main motives to produce false or grossly exaggerated physical or psychological symptoms. Soldiers feigning disease and disability hope to avoid duty, suspend transfer or be discharged from the service. Workers can prolong sick leave, delay corporate change of job or seek to obtain early retirement with an apparently extended illness. Some patients may seek compensation for some contrived illness, for example alleged burns or aggravate and continue an existing disease, for example industrial dermatitis, out of a sense of grievance or retribution. Prolonged cases of supposed medical negligence, for example non-healing wounds, are common in those with imagined dissatisfaction with their doctors or the care they have been given.

Cutaneous lesions are usually crude forms of artefact dermatitis [2]. Chronic non-healing postoperative scars are manipulated with instruments, or even faecal injection to maintain sepsis [3]. Hand dermatitis, both irritant and allergic contact dermatitis may be perpetuated to seek higher compensation awards [4].

Most patients are male with borderline or paranoid personality. A past history of conflict with the law is common. Treatment is difficult and compliance erratic [5].

REFERENCES

1 Asher R. Malingering. In: *Talking Sense*. Bath: Pitman Press, 1973: 145–7.
2 Lyell A. Cutaneous artefactual disease. *J Am Acad Dermatol* 1979; **1**: 391–407.
3 Reich P, Gottfreid LA. Factitious disorders in a teaching hospital. *Ann Intern Med* 1983; **99**: 240–7.
4 Condé-Salazar L, Gomez J, Meza B. Artefactual irritant dermatitis. *Contact Dermatitis* 1993; **28**: 246–7.
5 Szaz T. Malingering. Diagnosis or social condemnation. *Arch Neurol Psychiatry* 1967; **195**: 432–43.

Self-mutilation

Dermatologists are seldom asked to manage patients who admit to self-mutilation. Most common among these are young women with borderline personality [1] without intellectual deficiency who are wrist slashers [2]. They are described further as usually attractive, unmarried, easily addicted and unable to relate to others. The patient slashes her wrist at the slightest provocation but does not commit suicide. The performance of the act brings some relief. Another group of female non-psychotic patients perform delicate self-cutting, which leaves fine, linear, non-sutured scars on the wrist and forearm [3]. It has been suggested that this reflects a more obsessional personality with a compulsive ritualized act to relieve tension. Other studies have also shown that a substantial number of patients who cut themselves were depressed. Child abuse and family psychiatric history were frequent [4]. Anorexia nervosa was also present. The more severe forms of self-mutilation leading to autocastration or enucleation of an eye are usually reported in association with schizophrenia [5].

REFERENCES

1 Schaffer CB, Carroll J, Abramovitz SI. Self mutilation and the borderline personality. *J Nerv Ment Dis* 1982; **170**: 468–70.
2 Graff H, Mallin R. The syndrome of the wrist-cutter. *Am J Psychiatry* 1967; **124**: 36–4.
3 Gardner AR, Gardner AJ. Self mutilation, obsessionality and narcissism. *Br J Psychiatry* 1975; **127**: 127–32.
4 Ghaziuddin M, Tsai L, Naylor M, Ghaziuddin N. Mood disorder in a group of self cutting adolescents. *Acta Paedopsychiatr* 1992; **55**: 103–5.
5 Simpson MA. Self-Mutilation. *Br J Hosp Med* 1976; **16**: 430–8.

Miscellaneous conditions

Psychic possession

Another example of dermatological deception was described by McGuire [1], who in 1978 saw two separate outbreaks of skin disorders among factory workers in a small northern English town. In each outbreak a central female figure with non-industrial dermatological problems fuelled an epidemic of what was thought to be dermatitis among several employees in a ceramics factory and a second epidemic in a textile factory. In the first outbreak, 10 employees were affected and in the second, 17. No significant dermatological pathology of industrial origin was found. More recently, a similar outbreak occurred in a warehouse, triggered by two severe cases of non-occupational eczema, combined with the idea that incoming aircraft parts to the warehouse from foreign countries might be 'dirty' in some way. This caused a heightened perception of the risk of skin disease with increased frequency of hand washing. Overfrequent hand washing in a few employees resulted in precisely what the warehouse staff had been trying to avoid [2]. A similar outbreak in the pottery industry was described as 'epidemic hysteria dermatologica' [3].

In the UK, where the word 'compensation' and the word 'dermatitis' are closely linked, this type of reaction is common, and it is clearly important, if possible, to visit a factory very early and examine all the complainants in an outbreak of alleged 'epidemic' industrial dermatitis.

REFERENCES

1 McGuire A. Psychic possession among industrial workers. *Lancet* 1978; **i**: 376–8.
2 Ashworth J, Rycroft RJ, Waddy RS, Irvine D. Irritant contact dermatitis in warehouse employees. *Occup Med* 1993; **43**: 32–4.
3 Ilchyshyn A, Smith AG. Gum arabic sensitivity and epidemic hysteria dermatologica. *Contact Dermatitis* 1985; **13**: 282–3.

Sick building syndrome

Various skin complaints ('dryness', itching, etc.), which may reach epidemic proportions, have been attributed by workers to a so-called 'sick' building, in which ventilation and humidity are found to be suboptimal. Optimizing both humidity and ventilation may be helpful in managing these symptoms in an office environment. There was a high level of facial skin complaints in Swedish women working at visual display units [1]. However, half the patients referred for dermatological examination because of facial skin complaints had rosacea and their skin lesions were found to be mild, despite pronounced symptoms. Many with symptoms had no visible skin pathology. Symptoms were more common in those lower down the office hierarchy than in managers, but women had more symptoms than men, irrespective of their status [2].

REFERENCES

1 Berg M. Facial skin complaints and work at visual display units. Epidemiological clinical and histopathological studies. *Acta Derm Venereol (Stock)* 1989; **69** (Suppl. 150): 6–9.
2 Editorial. Sick building syndrome. *Lancet* 1991; **338**: 1493–4.

Habituation to dressings

Liddell and Cotterill [1] described a group of patients who became habituated to occlusive bandages, which had been initially applied many years before as treatment for either gravitational ulcers or eczema of the legs. Although the skin in all patients had returned to complete normality, it was impossible to persuade the patients to abandon their occlusive therapy. The patients tended to be elderly, single, lonely and inadequate, and most were male.

It was thought that the behaviour in this group may be regarded as 'attention seeking' in that they derive some sympathy from others because of their problem. Avoidance of work may have been successfully accomplished by four of the male patients.

Some patients seem to enjoy the social contact that regular attendance at the clinic brings and are reluctant to be discharged. Thus, it appears that occlusive dressings may support not only the legs, but in a minority of patients, the psyche too.

REFERENCE

1 Liddell K, Cotterill JA. Habituation to occlusive dressings. *Lancet* 1973; **i**: 1485–6.

Psychogenic pruritus

Musaph [1] pointed out that one mechanism for relieving everyday irritations is to scratch a little. The motorist stopped at a red traffic light almost invariably scratches some accessible site such as the neck and most of us develop a small itch from time to time during the day that is relieved by slight scratching. Musaph calls this the 'traffic-light phenomenon' and sees it as a common way of relieving minor frustrations. Individuals who develop localized or generalized neurodermatitis may begin in this way, but their itch–scratch cycle gets out of hand. In some individuals, intense scratching can induce an ultimate feeling of pleasure and this may be related to the release of opioids centrally. The calcitonin gene-related peptide may be important in the pathogenesis of nodular prurigo, but not in localized neurodermatitis [2]. Some regard pruritus vulvae and pruritus ani, for which no organic cause such as *Candida* infection can be found, as a form of localized neurodermatitis.

There are data to suggest that enkephalins and endorphins are important as neurotransmitters in the CNS in mediating the sensation of itch because it has been recognized for many years that, although morphine may alleviate pain, it may aggravate itch. As itch and pain are thought to share common neurological pathways, the central elicitation of itch by morphine may result from binding to opioid receptors and this binding may mimic normal physiological binding of endorphins and enkephalins at these receptor sites [3]. Moreover, naloxone, an opioid antagonist, has been found to reduce or abolish histamine-provoked itch [3]. It has been shown that naloxone can relieve itching experienced by patients with intrahepatic cholestasis and may also be effective in patients with generalized pruritus due to chronic liver disease. This drug, however, did not produce a uniform reduction in itching in all patients. Patients with generalized pruritus who had responded well to placebo reported greater itching after naloxone, probably due to the abolition of the placebo response. Conversely, the placebo non-responders reported less itch after naloxone than the placebo responders, suggesting that naloxone may be competing with an endorphin system, thus modulating the individual perception of itch [3,4].

From the more practical point of view, it has been demonstrated that the degree of pruritus in psoriasis correlates well with the degree of depressive psychopathology present [5]. In this study, the severity of pruritus correlated with neither stress nor alcohol intake.

A psychiatric and psychodynamic investigation of patients with prurigo nodularis demonstrated an extraordinary propensity for these patients to suffer from psychological trauma, and a distinct correlation was claimed between the outbreak of the disease and the preceding loss of a human relationship detrimental to self-esteem [6]. A significant proportion of patients with generalized pruritus may be suffering from depression. Using the Beck depression inventory, significantly more patients with generalized pruritus (32.4%) had depressive symptomatology than controls [7].

An episode of explosive spread of pruritus and rash was described as a manifestation of epidemic hysteria in 57 out of 159 rural elementary school students. The symptoms occurred only at sites readily accessible to the hands and disappeared promptly when the children left school in the evening but recurred each morning on return. It was thought that the onset on the outbreak was related to academic stresses [8].

Telepathic pruritus was described in a paranoid schizophrenic man who suffered from a delusion that others used mental telepathy to make him itch [9].

REFERENCES

1 Musaph H. Psychogenic pruritus. *Semin Dermatol* 1983; **2**: 217–22.
2 Valaasti A, Suomalainen H, Rechardt L. Calcitonin gene-related peptide immunoactivity in prurigo nodularis: a comparative study with neurodermatitis circumscripta. *Br J Dermatol* 1989; **120**: 619–23.
3 Bernstein JE, Swift R. Relief of intractable pruritus with naloxone. *Arch Dermatol* 1979; **115**: 1366–7.
4 Summerfield JA. Naloxone modulates the perception of itching. *Br J Clin Pharmacol* 1980; **10**: 180–3.
5 Gupta MA, Gupta K, Kirkby S *et al*. Pruritus in psoriasis: a prospective study of some psychiatric and dermatologic correlates. *Arch Dermatol* 1988; **124**: 1052–7.
6 Valtola J. A psychiatric and psychodynamic investigation of LCO (prurigo nodularis Hyde) patients. *Acta Derm Venereol Suppl (Stockh)* 1991; **156**: 49–52.
7 Sheehan-Dare RA, Henderson MJ, Cotterill JA. Anxiety and depression in patients with chronic urticaria and generalized pruritus. *Br J Dermatol* 1990; **123**: 769–74.
8 Robinson P, Swewczyk M, Haddy L *et al*. Outbreak of itching and rash. Epidemic hysteria in an elementary school. *Arch Intern Med* 1984; **144**: 1959–62.
9 Bernhard JD, Gardner MR. Telepathic pruritus. *Cutis* 1990; **55**: 59–60.

Cutaneous disease and alcohol misuse [1]

The psychosocial effects of chronic and disfiguring skin disease commonly produce feelings of stigma and rejection. Tension-lessening and oblivion-producing substances such as alcohol are commonly used by affected patients [1]. A study of a large urban population suggested that male as well as female psoriatics showed an excess rate of alcoholism [2]. However, further studies suggested that, whilst alcohol abuse was not a factor in the onset of psoriasis, it became significant in women after the disease was present and was significantly associated with the area of skin surface involvement [3]. Other work confirmed the relationship between the severity of psoriasis and alcohol excess in men but not in women [4]. Furthermore, in a prospective study Gupta *et al*. [5] showed that a daily intake of alcohol of more than 80 g was more frequently associated with less treatment-induced inpatient improvement in the percentage of the total body surface area affected by psoriasis in men but not in women. In a wide review, Higgins and du Vivier [6] suggest that the changed character and distribution of psoriasis make it more difficult to treat. Discoid eczema appears to be related to alcohol excess, as are exacerbations in rosacea, postadolescent acne and superficial skin infections. They postulate that these changes may be the result of the profound effects of alcohol on immune function and skin vasculature.

REFERENCES

1 Ginsburg IH, Link BG. Feelings of stigmatization in patients with psoriasis. *J Am Acad Dermatol* 1989; **20**: 53–60.
2 Lidegaard B. Disease associated with psoriasis in a population of middle aged urban native Swedes. *Dermatologica* 1986; **172**: 298–304.
3 Poikolinen K, Reunala T, Karvonen J. Smoking, alcohol and life events related to psoriasis among women. *Br J Dermatol* 1994; **130**: 473–7.
4 Monk BE, Neill SM. Alcohol consumption and psoriasis. *Dermatologica* 1986; **173**: 57–60.
5 Gupta MA, Schnork NJ, Gupta AK, Ellis CN. Alcohol intake and treatment responsiveness in psoriasis. *J Am Acad Dermatol* 1993; **28**: 730–5.
6 Higgins EM, du Vivier AW. Cutaneous disease and alcohol misuse. *Br Med Bull* 1994; **50**: 85–98.

AIDS, HIV infection and psychological illness (see Chapter 26)

Most CNS involvement complicating HIV infection occurs in the late phase of the disease. Such patients have been usefully classified firstly into those with headache or meningitic symptoms, secondly those with focal CNS symptoms or signs and lastly those with non-focal cerebral and/or motor dysfunction [1]. This latter group present with mental illness where alertness is characteristically impaired because of metabolic or toxic encephalopathy, or as a disorder in which alertness is preserved despite cognitive decline, and this distinct entity is defined as the AIDS dementia complex (ADC) [2]. This syndrome is also known as HIV-1-associated cognitive/motor complex (HACC) and both terms refer to a distinct subcortical dementia characterized by retarded and imprecise cognition and motor control. It develops in patients with late HIV infection and immunosuppression, and has been shown to have a higher incidence in those with CD4 counts less than 100 than in those with counts over 500 [3]. In a controlled study Grant and Atkinson [3] showed that the neuropsychological deficit as measured by a broad range of cognitive functions was 44% in seropositive patients and up to 87% in those with AIDS. The presence of the ADC usually indicates a poor prognosis with a 6-month cumulative mortality in those with most psychological deficit of 67%. A prospective controlled study of high-dose zidovudine improved performance on neuropsychological testing [4], but similar information is not available on newer drugs such as protease inhibitors.

REFERENCES

1 Price RW. Neurological complications of HIV infection. *Lancet* 1996; **348**: 445–52.
2 Price R. Management of AIDS dementia complex and HIV-1 infection of the nervous system. *AIDS* 1995; **9** (Suppl. A): S221–36.
3 Grant I, Atkinson JH. The evolution of neurobehavioural complications of HIV infection. *Psychol Med* 1990; **20**: 747–54.
4 Sidtis JJ, Gatsonis C, Price RW et al. Zidovudine treatment of the AIDS dementia complex. *Ann Neurol* 1993; **33**: 343–9.

Suicide in dermatological patients

Some dermatological patients become so disturbed that they do commit suicide successfully [1–5].

In a recent study of 217 patients with psoriasis, 10% of patients reported a death wish and 6% reported active suicidal ideation at the time of the study [6]. Moreover, suicide ideation was found in seven of 11 patients with Darier's disease [7]. A group of 16 patients—seven males and nine females—who committed suicide successfully after presenting with dermatological problems to two dermatologists working in the same skin department, have recently been described [1]. The majority of these patients had either body-image disorders (dysmorphophobia; body dysmorphic disorder) or acne. In addition, patients with long-standing and debilitating skin disease, such as psoriasis or systemic sclerosis, may become depressed enough to commit suicide, and there is always an attendant risk of suicide in patients with established, severe psychiatric problems who are referred to dermatologists. This becomes more common with the increasing number of drugs now available to treat psychiatric disorders, whilst established drugs, such as lithium, which can induce a wide variety of skin problems, but most commonly acne, psoriasis and hair disorders, continue to be used relatively commonly [8].

It is important to recognize that patients with dermatological non-disease, and particularly females with facial complaints, may be extremely depressed and at risk of suicide [9]. Acne scarring can have just as profound an effect, or even a more profound effect, on body image, self-esteem and confidence as inflammatory acne. The positive therapeutic role of isotretinoin was emphasized in this study [1], and funding problems in the UK in regard to the provision of isotretinoin could have potential fatal consequences.

There is a definite risk of suicide in patients with active HIV disease [3], and rates of suicide for people with AIDS were 66 times higher than in the general population in New York City. Men with AIDS aged 20–59 years were 36 times more likely to commit suicide than their counterparts without such a diagnosis. Half of the people in this particular sample had expressed suicidal intents and one-quarter killed themselves by jumping from the windows of medical units in general hospitals [4]. Assisted suicide has occurred in up to 23% of patients with AIDS [10].

REFERENCES

1 Cotterill JA, Cunliffe WJ. Suicide in dermatological patients. *Br J Dermatol* 1997; **137**: 246–50.

2 Ive FA, Magnus A, Warin RP, Wilson Jones E. 'Actinic reticuloid': a chronic dermatosis associated with severe photosensitivity and the histological resemblance to lymphoma. *Br J Dermatol* 1969; **81**: 469–85.

3 King MB. *AIDS, HIV and Mental Health.* Cambridge: Cambridge University Press, 1993: 32–6.

4 Marzuk PM, Tieney H, Tardiff K *et al.* Increased risk of suicide in persons with AIDS. *JAMA* 1988; **259**: 1333–7.

5 Monk BE, Rao YJ. Delusions of parasitosis with fatal outcome. *Clin Exp Dermatol* 1994; **19**: 341–2.

6 Gupta MA, Schork NJ, Gupta AK *et al.* Suicidal ideation in psoriasis. *Int J Dermatol* 1993; **33**: 188–90.

7 Denicoff KD, Lehman ZA, Rubinow DR *et al.* Suicidal ideation in Darier's disease. *J Am Acad Dermatol* 1990; **22**: 196–8.

8 Heng MCY. Lithium carbonate toxicity. Acneform eruption and other manifestations. *Arch Dermatol* 1982; **118**: 246–8.

9 Cotterill JA. Skin and the psyche. *Proc R Coll Physicians Edin* 1995; **25**: 29–33.

10 Van den Boom FMLG, Mead C, Gremmen T, Roozenburg H. AIDS, euthanasia and grief. 1991. Paper presented at the VIIth International Conference on AIDS, Florence, Book of Abstracts, v.i, MD 55.

Treatment of psychocutaneous disorders [1]

General management

'Disease' is a perception of ill health rather than a physical entity. The same degree of physical damage will be translated into different 'diseases' by different patients. In many patients, psoriasis does not itch; in a few it is very itchy. The condition is the same; the perception and interpretation differ so that it is necessary first to understand the language in which the disease is expressed. Once translated, the key is provided for an understanding of a patient's particular concern, and for a valid channel of therapeutic communication.

When a rapid cure is possible, there is no great problem in management. However, where a disease is of unknown origin and unpredictable duration, it is likely to assume undue proportions in the patient's thoughts. In diseases of the skin, as in other spheres of life, the unknown is feared. The spots of acne are magnified in any mirror. The patient and the dermatologist see two different images. It is the patients rather than the spots that must be treated.

Psychiatry is not an exact science. Some anxiety or depression will be felt by many of the patients seen by a dermatologist. This may be unrelated to their skin disease but more often plays some part in it or occasionally is the reason for its presentation. When the anxiety is reasonable and openly expressed—fear of cancer, ignorance of prognosis, anxiety about scarring and so on—it is sufficient to reassure the patient with a clear explanation, in easily understood terms. When anxiety is obviously present but at first denied, its nature must be elicited by careful questioning. Those whose conflicts are fully repressed, but whose skin lesions, often factitious in type, leave no doubt about the cause, present the most difficult problems.

All patients with skin disease respond to a receptive and sympathetic approach. Visible illness has a particularly disturbing emotional effect. Itching intensifies this. The physician must have patience, sympathy and insight into human behaviour, and must inspire the patient to talk freely. Advice should be given sparingly and without expecting it always to be taken. The dermatologist must know when a psychological situation is out of control and must recognize organic mental disease and endogenous depression as such, and seek psychiatric help.

The therapeutic effect of the physician's personality is often underrated. The stronger this is, the less necessary are drugs. Even the act of touching a patient with skin disease relieves the anxiety of those who have marked feelings of guilt and ostracism. When it is necessary to draw out the patient's emotional difficulties, the 'listening ear' is as important as the 'seeing eye'. Tones of voice, hesitancy, a temporary stammer or an unguarded or ambiguous remark may provide the key to an important emotional difficulty. Initial explanations given by a patient are often 'cover stories' and are not intended to be believed.

The first aim in management must be to determine whether any significant emotional situation is present, then whether the reaction is one of anxiety, depression or hysteria, and then how the environmental stresses can be reduced or the patient's frustration, guilt or aggression be eased or rechannelled. Hidden fears can often be remedied once they are expressed; anxiety about a child, spouse or parent may lie behind apparent rudeness. Fatigue alone may provide a 'stressful situation' and the adjustment of household burdens, insistence on holidays or proper periods of rest, and the provision of 'emotional bunkers' when the situation cannot be avoided, are matters of common sense and experience of what is feasible. Feelings of guilt, 'dirtiness' and inadequacy, frequently components of a depressive state, are more difficult to dispel and may require expert help. Obsessional behaviour and phobias are also usually beyond the reach of superficial psychotherapy.

The English language is weak in words that are not themselves emotive but can be used to describe emotional disturbances. To ask if a patient has 'any worries' is to invite a denial, which is often misleading. It may be more fruitful to ask about tiredness or depression. The manner of the reply matters more than the phrasing.

When a fuller assessment of the social and domestic situation is required, the services of a trained medical social worker are called for to extract information about family relationships and stresses and to indicate where these can be helped or eased.

The help of relatives must also often be enlisted, although their concern is not always disinterested if they are themselves part of the emotional situation. The parents of children with hair pulling or adolescents with artefacts must be approached tactfully. It is not they who have raised the cry for help, but they are often the cause of it. They may feel their honour impugned and their pride at stake.

Employers, schoolteachers and rehabilitation officers can give further information or material help in particular situations. To some patients, a priest's aid is invaluable.

Three further general points have to be made. The patient may present with a dermatosis that represents only one facet of a complex psychocutaneous situation. It serves its function in expressing an emotional disturbance. If 'cured' too quickly, without attention being paid to the underlying emotional problem, the patient may develop other less accessible ills. Secondly, psychiatrists themselves are of different persuasions. Their views on aetiology and their approach to treatment differ considerably. It is well for the dermatologist to be aware of this lest the patient loses confidence by being given different explanations and advice. Finally, there is a small but important group of patients who do not want to get better [2]. They are skilled at deceiving their doctors, their spouses and their friends. They suffer from 'too-good' husbands and 'too-kind' doctors. Many have an histrionic personality. Once recognized, certain principles of management should be followed; even then the prognosis is not good. The patient has too much to lose by recovering.

Drugs [3,4]

There has been a healthy reaction in recent years against the overuse of drugs in the management of patients with psychoneurotic disorders, and some patients may refuse to take them. However, short-term therapy with anxiolytics or sedatives may be as helpful to anxious itching patients as analgesics are to those in pain. Sleep deprivation is common, and the restoration of a normal pattern is an adequate reason for giving hypnotics. Those anxious to avoid giving or receiving such therapy will have to resort, with an easy conscience, to antihistamines with sedative side-effects.

Some patients will respond well to placebos, but others will develop adverse reactions even to these.

The primary indications for antipsychotic drugs are schizophrenia, acute mania and other psychotic states including paranoid disorders. In dermatology, these drugs, particularly pimozide, may help with other monosymptomatic hypochondriacal syndromes such as delusions of parasitosis or onychotillomania [5].

The antidepressants most often used by dermatologists are the tricyclics [6], either for a frank depressive illness, perhaps in association with a chronic skin disorder, or for patients with symptoms such as burning or itching that seem to have no physical basis. Some of these drugs have other useful actions [7]: some affect serotonin metabolism, others, such as doxepin, have antihistamine activity which may be helpful in pruritus. Doxepin therapy has also been found helpful in neurotic excoriations [8].

REFERENCES

1 Sarti MG, Cossidente A. Therapy in psychosomatic dermatology. *Clin Dermatol* 1984; **2**: 255–73.
2 Sneddon J. Patients who do not want to get better. *Semin Dermatol* 1983; **2**: 183–7.
3 Gupta MA, Gupta AK, Haberman HF. Psychotrophic drugs in dermatology. *J Am Acad Dermatol* 1986; **14**: 633–45.
4 Koo J, Gamba C. Psychopharmacology for dermatologic patients. *Dermatol Clin* 1996; **14**: 509–25.
5 Haman K. Onychotillomania treated with pimozide. *Acta Derm Venereol (Stockh)* 1982; **62**: 364–6.
6 Gupta MA, Gupta AK, Ellis CN. Anti-depressant drugs in dermatology. *Arch Dermatol* 1987; **123**: 647–52.
7 Newbold PCH. Antidepressants and the skin. *Br Med J* 1988; **296**: 379.
8 Harris BA, Sherertz EF, Flowers FP. Improvement of chronic neurotic excoriations with doxepin therapy. *Int J Dermatol* 1987; **26**: 541–3.

Hypnosis [1]

Hypnosis has always had its adherents and detractors but until recently there has been little attempt at scientific evaluation. Thus, there have been claims that hypnosis could induce inflammatory change and blisters in skin [2], and more than 30 years ago it was shown that immediate type 1 reactions, and even a Mantoux reaction, could be modified by hypnotic suggestion. The diminution in the Mantoux response was shown to be due to a reduction in oedema rather than in the cellular response [3]. Hypnotic suggestion has been used to treat various types of ichthyosis 7 [4–7]. It was claimed that the depth of the trance-like state could be important in determining the response to therapy, at least as far as patients with ichthyosis are concerned and that best results were obtained in deep-trance rather than light-trance subjects [5].

There are also many case reports detailing the response of warts to hypnosis, the most striking case being that where only a half of each subject's body was treated. Disappearance of the warts on the treated side was observed whilst other warts on the control side remained unchanged [8].

Recently, 18 adults with extensive atopic dermatitis, resistant to conventional treatment, were treated with hypnotherapy with statistically significant benefit, measured both subjectively and objectively [13]. More encouragingly, the benefit was maintained at follow-up for up to 2 years. Moreover, 20 children with severe resistant atopic dermatitis were also treated by hypnosis and all but one showed immediate improvement, which was maintained subsequently. In 12 of the 20 children whose families replied to a questionnaire up to 18 months after treatment, 10 of them maintained improvement in mood. It may be that improvement was achieved more by anxiety reduction and stress management than direct suggestion, but whatever the mechanism of action, hypnotherapy is both effective, economical and free from any harmful side-effects. The age range in this study of the children was 2–15 years, so the technique can be employed successfully in quite young children.

Relaxation techniques, which approximate to light hypnotic states, led to some improvement in patients with chronic urticaria, although the number of their weals did not lessen [14].

REFERENCES

1 Cotterill JA. Hypnosis in dermatology. In: Champion RH, ed. *Recent Advances in Dermatology*, Vol 7. Edinburgh: Churchill Livingstone, 1986; 256–7.
2 Wittkower E, Russell B. *Emotional Factors in Skin Disease*. London: Cassell, 1953: 13.
3 Black S. Inhibition of the immediate type hypersensitivity by direct suggestion under hypnosis. *Br Med J* 1963; **1**: 925–8.
4 Bethune HD, Kidd CD. Psychophysiological mechanisms in skin disease. *Lancet* 1961; **2**: 1419–22.
5 Kidd CD. Congenital ichthyosiform erythroderma treated by hypnosis. *Br J Dermatol* 1996; **78**: 101–5.
6 Mason AA. Ichthyosis and hypnosis. *Br Med J* 1955; **2**: 57–8.
7 Winck CAS. Congenital ichthyosiform erythroderma treated by hypnosis: a report of two cases. *Br Med J* 1961; **2**: 741–3.
8 French AP. Treatment of warts by hypnosis. *Am J Obstet Gynecol* 1973; **116**: 887–8.
9 Sinclair-Gieben AHC, Chalmers D. The treatment of warts by hypnosis. *Lancet* 1959; **2**: 480–2.
10 Surman OS, Gottlieb SK, Hackett TP, Silverberg BL. Hypnosis in the treatment of warts. *Arch Gen Psychiatry* 1973; **28**: 439–41.
11 Tasini MF, Hackett TP. Hypnosis and the treatment of warts in immunodeficient children. *Am J Clin Hypnosis* 1977; **17**: 152–4.
12 Ullman M, Budek S. On the psyche of warts. Hypnotic suggestion and warts. *Psychosom Med* 1960; **22**: 68–76.
13 Stewart AC, Thomas SE. Hypnotherapy as a treatment for atopic dermatitis in adults and children. *Br J Dermatol* 1995; **113**: 778–83.
14 Hertzer CL, Lookingbill DP. Effects of relaxation therapy and hypnotisability in chronic urticaria. *Arch Dermatol* 1987; **123**: 913–16.

Miscellaneous therapies

Biofeedback techniques

In recent years interest has grown in biofeedback techniques, during which patients are given visual or auditory information about the level of a particular autonomic function and then learn, through mechanisms that are not yet clear, to exercise some voluntary control over it. Biofeedback has been used for dyshidrotic eczema [1] and for hyperhidrosis [2].

Behaviour therapy

Behaviour therapy has sometimes been useful for patients who scratch repeatedly. In one study [3], parents were trained to withdraw their attentions when their child scratched; in another [4], a patient was required to monitor his own scratching, and, to gain his therapist's attention, intervals without scratching were required. Habit-reversal therapy helped a group of patients with atopic eczema [5–7].

Group therapy

Group therapy has been tried in psoriasis [8]. Small groups of psoriatics met to discuss their problems with a trained fellow sufferer and a physician; illness behaviour, anxiety and feelings of depression all decreased. Help along similar lines can come from self-help groups [9].

REFERENCES

1 Miller RM, Coger RW. Skin conductance conditioning with dyshidrotic eczema patients. *Br J Dermatol* 1979; **101**: 435–40.
2 Duller P, Gentry WD. Use of biofeedback in treating chronic hyperhidrosis—a preliminary report. *Br J Dermatol* 1980; **103**: 143–6.
3 Allen K, Harris FR. Elimination of a child's excessive scratching by training the mother in reinforcement procedures. *Behav Res Ther* 1966; **4**: 79–84.
4 Cataldo MF, Varni JW, Russo DC *et al.* Behaviour therapy techniques in treatment of exfoliative dermatitis. *Arch Dermatol* 1980; **116**: 919–22.
5 Bridgett C, Noren P, Staughton R. *Atopic Skin Disease: A Manual for Practitioners.* Petersfield: Wrightson Biomedical, 1996.
6 Melin L, Frederiksen T, Noren P *et al.* Behavioural treatment of scratching in patients with atopic dermatitis. *Br J Dermatol* 1986; **115**: 467–74.
7 Noren P, Melin L. The effect of combined topical steroids and habit-reversal treatment in patients with atopic dermatitis. *Br J Dermatol* 1989; **121**: 359–66.
8 Schulte MB, Cormane RH, van Dijk E *et al.* Group therapy of psoriasis. *J Am Acad Dermatol* 1985; **12**: 61–6.
9 Logan RA. Self-help groups for patients with chronic skin diseases. *Br J Dermatol* 1988; **118**: 505–8.

Psychiatric problems caused by dermatological treatment

It is well-known that systemic glucocorticoid therapy can induce either depression or hypomania. Indeed, particular care must be taken with corticosteroids in patients with a past history of manic–depressive illness. It is less well known that antimalarials and dapsone can induce psychosis [1,2]. Aciclovir-induced psychosis has also been described in patients with impaired renal function [3]. There is also a report of a man who applied 70% diethyltoluamide, the commonest insect repellant, immediately before a sauna, and developed an acute manic psychosis after 2 weeks [4].

REFERENCES

1 Daneshmend TK. The neurotoxicity of dapsone; adverse drug reactions. *Acute Poisoning Rev* 1984; **3**: 53–8.
2 Evans RL, Khalid S, Kinney JL. Antimalarial psychosis revisited. *Arch Dermatol* 1984; **120**: 765–7.
3 Thomson CR, Goodship THJ, Rodger RSC. Psychiatric side-effects of acyclovir in patients with chronic renal failure. *Lancet* 1985; **ii**: 385–6.
4 Snyder JW, Poe RO, Stubbins JF *et al.* Acute manic psychosis following the dermal application of N,N-diethyl-m-toluamide (DEET) in an adult. *Clin Toxicol* 1986; **24**: 429–39.

Skin disease in patients with learning disability

Mental deficiency is not a disease in its own right but a condition resulting from a variety of causes, some inborn and others acquired. As a rough guide, some 3% of the population are mentally defective, with an IQ of below 70, but the terms idiot, imbecile and moron are now obsolete in the professional sense. The class of higher-grade learning disabled subjects shades into that of the duller members of the ordinary population [1].

The number of syndromes in which cutaneous lesions and mental deficiency may be associated is large, and many of them have been delineated only during the last few years. Although many of these genetic or developmental conditions are rare, when put together they constitute a formidable part of present-day paediatrics [2]. In addition, there are a number of other skin abnormalities that seem to affect those with learning disabilities in particular.

However, the available statistics must be interpreted with caution as they relate to patients in special institutions to which admission is largely determined by social factors. The proportion of disabled patients of the lowest grade, and of those of any grade with associated severe physical difficulties, is likely to be higher in such institutions than in the learning disabled population as a whole. In addition, institutional life itself may influence the prevalence of skin disease by allowing the rapid spread of infections, and other conditions may be favoured by unsuspected nutritional deficiencies.

The skin abnormalities of learning disabled people fall into three broad groups as outlined below.

Cutaneous lesions specifically associated with syndromes of genetic or developmental origin

Many of the numerous associations of this type are dealt with in detail elsewhere. Sometimes, the nature of the defect is understood at biochemical level (Table 64.1) and sometimes chromosomal abnormalities have been demonstrated (Table 64.2), but in most cases the mechanism of both the cutaneous changes and mental impairment remains obscure (Table 64.3). The severity of the mental defect and of the cutaneous involvement may run more or less in parallel as in epiloia, but in most of these conditions there is no such relationship and the prevalence and severity of the mental impairment are highly variable.

Table 64.1 Some metabolic disorders that may be associated with mental defect and skin changes.

Anginosuccinic amino aciduria	Trichorrhexis nodosa
Cretinism	Coarse, dry skin and hair
Gangliosidosis (type 1) [5]	Extensive Mongolian spots
Hartnup disease	Photosensitivity
Homocystinuria	Fine hair, livedo reticularis
Hunter's syndrome [6]	Ivory white papules
Lesch–Nyhan syndrome	Self-mutilation
Lipoid proteinosis	Skin nodules and plaques
Phenylketonuria	Eczema, long eyelashes
Menke's syndrome	Hair defects

Table 64.2 Some conditions in which chromosomal abnormalities may be associated with mental defect and skin changes.

Down's syndrome	Ichthyosis
Familial X/Y translocation [7]	Facial hypertrichosis
Partial trisomy 2P	Scalp defect, haemangiomas
Patau syndrome (trisomy 13)	Depigmented spots, café-au-lait
Ring chromosome 14 [8]	patches
	Nail hypoplasia, lymphoedema
Trisomy 18	Preauricular skin tags, scalp
Wolf–Hirschorn syndrome	defects, flame naevi
(4P deletion)	Acne
XYY syndrome (see Chapter 12)	

Table 64.3 Some other conditions in which mental defect may be associated with skin abnormalities.

Albinism	Monilethrix
Alopecia/retardation	Moynahan's syndrome
syndromes [9]	Naevus sebaceous syndrome
Anhidrotic ectodermal dysplasia	Netherton's disease
Apert's syndrome	Neurofibromatosis
Ataxia–telangiectasia	Onchotrichodysplasia with
Basal cell naevus syndrome	neutropenia [10]
Cockayne's syndrome	Papillon–Leage syndrome
Coffin–Siris syndrome [3]	Poikiloderma congenitale
Dystrophia myotonica	Richner–Hanhart's syndrome [11]
De Sanctis–Cacchione syndrome	Rubinstein–Taybi syndrome [12]
Fanconi's anaemia	Russell–Silver dwarfism
Focal dermal hypoplasia	Sjögren–Larsson syndrome [13]
Hallerman–Streiff syndrome	Spina bifida
IBIDS syndrome [1]	Sturge–Weber syndrome
Incontinentia pigmenti	Treacher–Collins syndrome
Leprechaunism	Werner's syndrome
Marfan's syndrome	Wyburn–Mason syndrome

IBIDS, ichthyosis, brittle hair, impaired intelligence, decreased fertility and short stature.

Non-specific cutaneous lesions showing an increased prevalence in patients with learning disability

Moniliform hamartoma (Chapter 15). Beaded strands of papules, mainly on the forehead and temples, develop at puberty in some patients, more often in black people than in white people.

Atypical keratosis pilaris. A symmetrical eruption of erythematous follicular papules extending from the base of the neck to the lumbar region is seen in young adults in institutions for the learning disabled [14]. This might represent pityrosporum folliculitis.

Abnormal hair patterns [4]. The frequency of abnormal patterns of hair growth has been emphasized and is confirmed by our experience. Fusion of the eyebrows and a low frontal hairline are often seen; the latter is characteristic of true microcephalics but occurs in other defectives.

Hypertrichosis of the trunk or limbs is not unusual. The significance of the abnormal patterns is unknown and further surveys are required.

Atopic dermatitis. Only one patient with atopic dermatitis was found among over 200 defective children examined (A.J. Rook, unpublished, 1953). Others have noticed a low prevalence of eczema [4], but atopic dermatitis is frequent in patients with Down's syndrome and phenylketonuria.

Traumatic keratoses and hypertrichosis [15]. The severely disabled develop the habit of biting or chewing the forearm, hand, fingers or lips when excited or angry. Repeated biting at the same site induces thickening, hyperpigmentation and hypertrichosis. More rarely, there may be atrophic scarring, particularly on the hands. Keratoses in unusual sites may result from the repeated adoption of the same posture.

Traumatic alopecia. This is the result of a hair-pulling tic, and is also not uncommon. The patch selected for plucking is usually in the frontoparietal region, but may be anywhere on the scalp and even in the pubic region (A.J. Rook, unpublished, 1953). Multiple self-mutilations including traumatic alopecia are seen in children with familial sensory neuropathy (Chapter 63).

Crusted scabies. The crusted form of scabies [16] (Chapter 33) is particularly frequent in those with severe learning disability.

Bacterial infections. Pyogenic infections accounted for 34% of patients referred from an institution for a dermatologist's opinion. The high incidence suggests a low resistance to pyogenic organisms but the part played by the unhygienic habits of the patients is difficult to evaluate. Folliculitis of the thighs occurred in children and adolescents of both sexes, predominantly in the males. Chronic suppurative hidradenitis was seen exclusively in adolescent boys. Erythrasma has a high prevalence [17].

Mycoses. Trichophyton infections are often common and refractory in colonies of mental defectives. It is possible that enzyme induction by other drugs administered reduces the efficacy of griseofulvin.

Intertrigo and perleche. Genitocrural intertrigo is common in incontinent patients, especially those who are bed-ridden. Perleche, frequently complicated by fissuring and secondary infection, is seen in a large proportion of patients who dribble constantly.

Primary irritant dermatitis. The failure to take reasonable care in the use of disinfectants and cleansing agents is responsible for a relatively high incidence of primary irritant dermatitis in those patients who are encouraged to carry out simple domestic duties. Allergic contact dermatitis is said to be uncommon [4], perhaps because exposure to potential sensitizing agents is limited.

Drug reactions. The higher incidence of epilepsy in mental defectives accounts for the relative frequency of reactions to drugs.

Non-specific cutaneous lesions, the prevalence and cause of which are not proved to differ significantly from those of the general population

There is no reliable evidence that the other common dermatoses are either more or less frequent in the learning disabled than in normal individuals [16]. Doubt has been cast upon the widely accepted association between epilepsy and acne [18].

REFERENCES

1 Jorizzo JL, Atherton DJ, Crounse RG *et al.* Ichthyosis, brittle hair, impaired intelligence, decreased fertility and short stature (IBIDS syndrome). *Br J Dermatol* 1982; **106**: 705–10.
2 Ousted C. In: Salmon MA, ed. *Developmental Defects and Syndromes.* Aylesbury: HM & M, 1978.
3 Carey JC. Hall BD. The Coffin–Siris syndrome. *Am J Dis Child* 1978; **132**: 667–71.
4 Butterworth T, Wilson M, Jr. Incidence of disease of the skin in feebleminded persons. *Arch Dermatol Syphilol* 1938; **38**: 203–9.
5 Weissbluth M, Esterly NB, Caro WA. Report of an infant with GMI gangliosidosis type 1 and extensive and unusual mongolian spots. *Br J Dermatol* 1981; **104**: 195–200.
6 Prystowsky SD, Maumenee IH, Freeman RG *et al.* A cutaneous marker in the Hunter syndrome: a report of four cases. *Arch Dermatol* 1977; **113**: 602–5.
7 Metaxotou C, Ikkos D, Panagiotopoulou P *et al.* A familial X/Y translocation in a boy with ichthyosis, hypogonadism and mental retardation. *Clin Genet* 1983; **24**: 380–3.
8 Schmidt R, Eviator L, Nitowsky HM *et al.* Ring chromosome 14: a distinct clinical entity. *J Med Genet* 1981; **18**: 304–20.
9 Baraitser M, Carter CO, Brett EM. Case reports of a new alopecia/mental retardation syndrome. *J Med Genet* 1983; **20**: 64–75.
10 Hernandez A, Olivares F, Cantu JM. Autosomal recessive onychotrichodysplasia, chronic neutropenia and mild mental retardation: delineation of the syndrome. *Clin Genet* 1979; **15**: 147–52.
11 Bohnert A, Anton-Lamprecht I. Richner–Hanhart's syndrome: ultrastructural abnormalities of epidermal keratinization indicating a causal relationship to high intracellular tyrosine levels. *J Invest Dermatol* 1982; **79**: 68–74.
12 Selmanowitz VJ, Stiller MJ. Rubinstein–Taybi syndrome: cutaneous manifestations and colossal keloids. *Arch Dermatol* 1981; **117**: 504–6.
13 Jagell S, Linden S. Ichthyosis in the Sjögren–Larsson syndrome. *Clin Genet* 1982; **21**: 243–52.
14 Coombs FP, Butterworth T. Atypical keratosis pilaris. *Arch Dermatol* 1950; **62**: 305–13.
15 Ressmann A, Butterworth T. Localized acquired hypertrichosis. *Arch Dermatol Syphilol* 1952; **65**: 458–63.
16 Kidd CB, Meenan JC. The neurodermatoses and intelligence. *Br J Dermatol* 1961; **73**: 134–6.
17 Savin JA, Somerville DA, Noble WC. The bacterial flora of trichomycosis axillaris. *J Med Microbiol* 1970; **3**: 352–6.
18 Greenwood R, Fenwick PBC, Cunliffe WJ. Acne and anti-convulsants. *Br Med J* 1983; **287**: 1669–70.

Chapter 65
Disorders of Nails

R.P.R.DAWBER, R.BARAN & D.de BERKER

Introduction

The epithelial part of the nail apparatus develops *in utero* from the primitive epidermis. In generalized integumentary diseases, such as psoriasis, the nail apparatus, hair follicle and epidermis may all be structurally and functionally affected, presumably because of their common tissue of origin.

The main function of the nail apparatus is to produce a strong, relatively inflexible, keratinous nail plate over the dorsal surface of the end of each digit. The nail plate acts as a protective covering for the fingertip. By exerting counter-pressure over the volar skin and pulp, the flat nail plate adds to the precision and delicacy of both the ability to pick up small objects and many other subtle finger functions [1,2]. Fingernails typically cover approximately one-fifth of the dorsal surface, whereas on the great toe the nail may cover up to 50% of the dorsum of the digit.

REFERENCES

1 Baran R, Dawber RPR, eds. *Diseases of the Nail and their Management*, 3rd edn. Oxford: Blackwell Scientific Publications, 1994.
2 Scher RK, Daniel CR, eds. *Nails: Therapy, Diagnosis, Surgery*. Philadelphia: WB Saunders, 1990.

Anatomy and biology of the nail unit

Structure

Gross anatomy [1–5]

The component parts of the nail apparatus are shown diagrammatically in Fig. 65.1. The rectangular nail plate is the largest structure, resting on and firmly attached to the nail bed; it is less adherent proximally, apart from the posterolateral corners. Approximately one-quarter of the nail is covered by the proximal nail fold, and a narrow margin of the sides of the nail plate is often occluded by the lateral nail folds. Underlying the proximal part of the nail is the white lunula (half-moon lunule); this area represents the most distal region of the matrix [6]. It is most prominent on the thumb and great toe and may be partly or completely concealed by the proximal nail fold in other digits. The reason for the white colour is not known [7–9]. The natural shape of the free margin of the nail is the same as the contour of the distal border of the lunula. The nail plate distal to the lunula usually appears pink, due to its translucency, which allows the redness of the vascular nail bed to be seen through it. The proximal nail fold has two epithelial surfaces, dorsal and ventral; at the junction of the two, the cuticle projects distally onto the nail surface. The lateral nail folds are in continuity with the skin on the

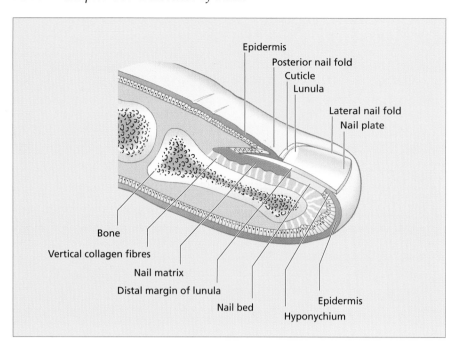

Fig. 65.1 Longitudinal section of a digit showing the dorsal nail apparatus.

sides of the digit laterally, and medially they are joined by the nail bed. Some authorities term the lateral nail fold and adjacent tissue lateral to the nail fold the nail wall.

The definition of nail matrix is controversial [10]. There is common acceptance that there is a localized region beneath proximal nail which produces the major part of the normal nail plate. For those who consider this the sole source of nail it is termed simply the matrix, or germinal matrix. However, there is some evidence that other epithelial parts of the nail unit also contribute to the nail plate, and these are then also attributed matrix status. According to the histological criteria of Lewis [4] (Fig. 65.2), matrix can be subdivided into dorsal (ventral aspect of the proximal nail fold), intermediate (germinal matrix or simply matrix) and ventral (nail bed) sections. The nail bed is also termed the sterile matrix and its role in the production of nail is unclear. Although it appears that the nail plate may thicken by up to 30% as it passes from the distal margin of the lunula to the end of the nail bed [2],

this is not associated with an increase in cell numbers and may represent compaction of the nail from distal tip trauma rather than nail-bed or nail-plate production [11]. The situation may change in disease, where the nail-bed changes its histological appearance to gain a granular layer and may contribute a false nail of cornified epithelium to the undersurface of the nail [5].

At the point of separation of the nail plate from the nail bed, the proximal part of the hyponychium may be modified as the *solehorn* [12]. This is a central thickened structure with a dermal core. It is usually found on the toes of elderly people, where there are often associated vascular abnormalities. Beyond the solehorn region, the hyponychium terminates at the distal nail groove; the tip of the digit beyond this ridge assumes the structure of the epidermis elsewhere.

When the attached nail plate is viewed from above, two distinct areas may be visible: the proximal lunula and the larger pink zone. On close examination, two further

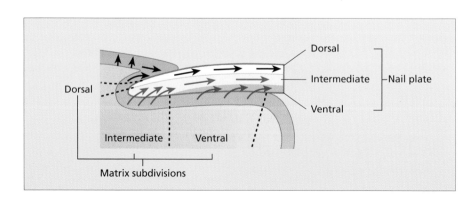

Fig. 65.2 Diagram to show the direction of differentiation and cell movement within the nail apparatus.

distal zones can often be identified: the distal yellowish-white margin and immediately proximal to this the onychodermal band [13]. Terry describes this as a barely perceptible, narrow, transverse band 0.5–1.5 mm wide and more prominent in acrocyanosis. The exact anatomical basis for the onychodermal band is not known, but it appears to have a different blood supply to the main body of the nail bed; if the tip of the finger is pressed firmly, the band and an area just proximal to it blanch, and if the pressure is repeated several times the band reddens. Many changes in colour have been described in the onychocorneal band in health and disease [13]. Histologically, it is defined as the most distal attachment of cornified epithelium to the undersurface of the nail. As such, it is structurally significant for the adherence of nail plate to the nail bed. Once breached, as in conditions such as psoriasis, separation of the nail bed from the nail plate can be progressive.

Microscopic anatomy [14]

Nail folds

The proximal nail folds are similar in structure to the adjacent skin but are normally devoid of dermatoglyphic markings and pilosebaceous glands. There is a normal granular layer. From the distal area of the proximal nail folds the cuticle adheres to the upper surface of the nail plate; it is composed of modified stratum corneum and serves to protect the structures at the base of the nail, particularly the germinal matrix, from environmental insults such as irritants, allergens and bacterial and fungal pathogens.

Nail matrix (intermediate matrix)

Nail matrix produces the major part of the nail plate (Fig. 65.2). The basal compartment of the matrix is broader than the same region in normal epithelium or in other parts of the nail unit, such as the nail bed [10]. There is no granular layer, and cells differentiate with the expression of trichocyte 'hard' keratin as they become incorporated into the nail plate. During this process, they may retain their nuclei until more distal in the nail plate. These retained nuclei are called *pertinax bodies*. Apart from this, the detailed cytological changes seen in the matrix epithelium under the electron microscope are essentially the same as in the epidermis [15,16].

The nail matrix contains melanocytes in the lowest three cell layers and these donate pigment to the keratinocytes. A count of 6.5 melanocytes per millimetre of matrix basement membrane can be used as a guide to a normal matrix melanocyte population [17]. The appearance of melanocytes separate from the basement membrane distinguishes them from those found in the nail folds, which are primarily basal [18]. Matrix melanocytes are further distinguished from those elsewhere by their failure to produce melanin in normal circumstances in white people. This can change with melanotic streaks presenting in local inflammatory, naevoid or neoplastic disease. In non-white people, brown streaks are common, and they are almost universal in Afro-Caribbeans by the age of 60 years.

Langerhans' cells are detectable in the matrix by CD1a staining, and the matrix appears to contain basement membrane components indistinguishable from normal skin [19].

Nail bed

Nail bed consists of an epidermal part (ventral matrix) with underlying connective tissue closely apposed to the periosteum of the distal phalanx. There is no subcutaneous fat in the nail bed, although scattered dermal fat cells may be visible microscopically.

The nail bed epidermal layer (ventral matrix) is usually no more than two or three cells thick, and the transitional zone from living keratinocyte to dead ventral nail-plate cell is abrupt, occurring in the space of one horizontal cell layer; in this regard it closely resembles the Henle layer of the internal root sheath of the epidermis [20]. Nail bed cells do not have any independent movement, and it is yet to be clearly demonstrated whether they are incorporated into an overlying nail plate as it grows distally [21]. The process of nail-bed keratinization has been likened to that seen in rat-tail epidermis, possibly being affected by pressure changes. The loss of the overlying nail results in the development of a granular layer, which is otherwise present only in disease states [22,23].

The nail bed dermal collagen is mainly orientated vertically, being directly attached to the phalangeal periosteum and the epidermal basal lamina. Within the connective tissue network lie blood vessels, lymphatics, a fine network of elastic fibres and scattered fat cells; at the distal margin, eccrine sweat glands have been seen [1].

Nail plate

The nail plate comprises three horizontal layers: a thin dorsal lamina, the thicker intermediate lamina and a ventral layer from the nail bed [4]. This is not always apparent with normal light microscopy using routine stains, where the nail demonstrates a transition between flattened cells dorsally and thicker cells on the ventral aspect. Electron microscopy shows squamous cells with tortuous, interlocking plasma membranes [15,16]. At high magnification, the contents of each cell show a uniform fine granularity similar to the hair cuticle [20].

In older age groups, acidophilic masses representing nuclear fragments are occasionally seen—the so-called pertinax bodies [4].

The nail plate contains significant amounts of phospholipid, mainly in the dorsal and intermediate layers, which contribute to its flexibility. The detectable free fats and long-chain fatty acids may be of extrinsic origin. For further details of these and other histochemical changes in the component parts of the nail apparatus, the reader is referred to more detailed texts [8,24].

The nail plate is rich in calcium, found as the phosphate in hydroxyapatite crystals; it is bound to phospholipids intracellularly [25]. The relevance of other metals, which are present in smaller amounts, including copper, manganese, zinc, iron and others, is not known [22]. Calcium exists in a concentration of 0.1% by weight, 10 times greater than in hair. It is possible that calcium is not an intrinsic part of the nail but is incorporated from extrinsic sources. Calcium does not significantly contribute to the hardness of the nail [6].

Nail keratin

Nail keratin analysis shows essentially the same fractions as in hair:
1 fibrillar, low-sulphur protein;
2 globular, high-sulphur matrix protein;
3 high glycine–tyrosine-rich matrix protein.
Amino-acid analysis shows higher cysteine, glutamic acid and serine and less tyrosine in nail compared with hair and wool [26,27].

An alternative classification of keratins defines them as 'soft' epithelial keratins or 'hard' trichocyte keratins. The latter are characteristic of hair and nail differentiation, where their high sulphur content is probably responsible for their rugged physical qualities. This is matched by the resistance of trichocyte keratins to dissolution in strong solvent.

Trichocyte and epithelial keratins are intermediate filaments representing the major cytoskeletal protein of epithelial cells. They share the normal classification into type I or type II based on gene hybridization, which reflects segregation on two-dimensional electrophoresis into acidic and basic proteins. Each acidic keratin is expressed in a tissue with a corresponding basic keratin to form specific heterodimers, which are assembled into higher-order protofibrils and protofilaments.

Keratin distribution in the nail and associated epithelium has been studied in adult [28,29], infant [28] and embryonic digits [30,31]. Immunohistochemistry of the epithelial structures of normal nail demonstrates that the suprabasal keratin pair K1/K10 is found on both aspects of the proximal nail fold and to a lesser degree in the matrix. However, it is absent from the nail bed. This is reversed when there is nail bed disease, such as onychomycosis or psoriasis, where a granular layer develops and K1/K10 becomes expressed at corresponding sites [23]. The nail bed contains keratin synthesized in normal basal layer epithelium, K5/K14, which is also found in nail

matrix. An antibody marking the epitope characteristically associated with keratin expressed in the basal layer is found throughout the thickness of the nail bed, but only basally in the matrix [23].

Recent examination of the nail bed using monospecific monoclonal antibodies to the keratin pair K6/K16 demonstrates this in the nail bed, but not in the germinal matrix [28]. This is paradoxical given our understanding of this keratin pair as being characteristic of psoriasis and wound healing, where proliferation is a prominent feature. It has been shown that the nail bed has very low rates of proliferation [10,32], and it may be that K6/K16 are more precisely illustrating a loss of differentiation, often associated with proliferation in skin, but representing the resting state of nailbed epithelium.

The location of K6/K16 is reflected in the localization of the features of pachyonychia congenita. In this group of autosomal dominant disorders, there is thickening of the nail plate attributed to disease of the nail plate. In some forms of pachyonychia congenita, there is a missense mutation of the initiation peptide of K16 [33].

Trichocyte keratins can also be detected immunohistochemically within the epithelial structures of the nail unit. A monospecific antibody to Ha-1 has been created and characterized on nail, hair and skin. In the nail, it demonstrates a well-demarcated suprabasal region corresponding to the matrix [28]. Proximally, it does not extend onto the ventral aspect of the proximal nail fold, sometimes described as the dorsal matrix. Distally, the keratin expression is limited to a margin taken as corresponding to the lunula. Ha-1 is only one of at least 10 trichocyte keratins, but quantitatively it probably represents a large fraction of nail keratin. According to its distribution it appears to define a matrix consistent with the classic description of the germinal matrix.

REFERENCES

1 Gonzalez-Serva A. The normal nail: structure and function. In: Scher RK, Daniel CR, eds. *Nails: Therapy, Diagnosis and Surgery*. Philadelphia: WB Saunders, 1990: 11–30.
2 Johnson M, Comaish JS, Shuster S. Nail is produced by the normal nail bed: a controversy resolved. *Br J Dermatol* 1991; **125**: 27–9.
3 Lewin K. The normal fingernail. *Br J Dermatol* 1965; **77**: 421–4.
4 Lewis BL, Montgomery H. The senile nail. *J Invest Dermatol* 1955; **24**: 11–18.
5 Samman PD. Anatomy and physiology. In: Samman PD, Fenton D, eds. *The Nails in Disease*. London: Heinemann, 1986: 1–20.
6 Cohen PR. The lunula. *J Am Acad Dermatol* 1996; **34**: 943–53.
7 Achten G. L'ongle normal et pathologique. *Dermatologica* 1963; **126**: 229–34.
8 Baran R, Dawber RPR, eds. *Diseases of the Nails and their Management*, 2nd edn. Oxford: Blackwell Scientific Publications, 1994: 4–5.
9 Burrows MT. The significance of the lunula of the nail. *Johns Hopkins Hosp Rep* 1919; **18**: 357–61.
10 de Berker D, Angus B. Markers of epidermal proliferation are limited to nail matrix in normal nail. *Br J Dermatol* 1996; **135**: 555–9.
11 de Berker DAR, MaWhinney B, Sviland L. Quantification of regional matrix nail production. *Br J Dermatol* 1996; **134**: 1083–6.
12 Pinkus F. In: Jadassohn J, ed. *Handbuch der Haut und Geschlechtskrankheiten*. Berlin: Springer-Verlag, 1927: 267–89.

13 Terry RB. The onychodermal band in health and disease. *Lancet* 1955; **i**: 179–81.

14 Lewis BL. Microscopic studies of foetal and mature nail and surrounding soft tissue. *Arch Dermatol* 1954; **70**: 732–6.

15 Hashimoto K. Ultrastructure of the human toenail. 1. Proximal nail matrix. *J Invest Dermatol* 1971; **56**: 235–46.

16 Hashimoto K. Ultrastructure of the human toenail. *Ultrastruct Res* 1971; **36**: 391–410.

17 Tosti A, Cameli N, Piraccini BM *et al*. Characterisation of nail matrix melanocytes with anti-PEP1, anti-PEP8, TMH-1 and HMB-45 antibodies. *J Am Acad Dermatol* 1994; **31**: 193–6.

18 de Berker D, Graham A, Dawber RPR, Thody A. Melanocytes are absent from the normal nail bed: the basis of a clinical dictum. *Br J Dermatol* 1996; **134**: 564.

19 Sinclair RD, Wojnarowska F, Leigh IM, Dawber RPR. The basement membrane zone of the nail. *Br J Dermatol* 1994; **131**: 499–505.

20 Achten G. L'ongle normal. *J Med Esth Chir Dermatol* 1988; **XV**: 193–200.

21 Zaias N. The movement of the nail bed. *J Invest Dermatol* 1967; **48**: 402–3.

22 Zaias N. *The Nail in Health and Disease*. New York: Spectrum Press, 1990: 6–7.

23 de Berker D, Sviland L, Angus BA. Suprabasal keratin expression in the nail bed: a marker of dystrophic nail bed differentiation. *Br J Dermatol* 1995; **133** (Suppl. 45): 16.

24 Sayag J, Jancovici E. Physiologie de l'ongle. In: Meynadier J, ed. *Précis de Physiologie Cutané*. Paris: Editions de le Porte Verte, 1980: 121–3.

25 Cane AK, Spearman RIC. A histochemical study of keratinisation in the domestic fowl. *J Zool* 1967; **153**: 337–44.

26 Baden HP, Goldsmith LA, Flemming BC. A comparative study of the physicochemical properties of human keratinised tissue. *Biochem Biophys Acta* 1973; **322**: 269–78.

27 de Berker D, Westgate G, Leigh IM. Pattern of hard keratin (Ha-1) expression in nail matrix corresponds to nail plate morphology. *Br J Dermatol* 1996; **134**: 584.

28 de Berker D, Leigh I, Wojnarowska F. Patterns of keratin expression in the nail unit—an indicator of regional matrix differentiation. *Br J Dermatol* 1992; **127**: 423.

29 Haneke E. The human nail matrix—flow cytometric and immuno-histochemical studies. *Clinical Dermatology in the Year 2000*. London: Book of Abstracts, 1990.

30 Heid WH, Moll I, Franke WW. Patterns of expression of trichocytic and epithelial cytokeratins in mammalian tissues. II Concomitant and mutually exclusive synthesis of trichocytic and epithelial cytokeratins in diverse human and bovine tissues. *Differentiation* 1988; **37**: 215–30.

31 Moll I, Heid HW, Franke WW, Moll R. Patterns of expression of trichocytic and epithelial cytokeratins in mammalian tissues. *Differentiation* 1988; **39**: 167–84.

32 Zaias N, Alvarez J. The formation of the primate nail plate. An autoradiographic study in the squirrel monkey. *J Invest Dermatol* 1968; **51**: 120–36.

33 McLean WHI, Rugg EL, Lunny DP *et al*. Keratin 16 and keratin 17 mutations cause pachyonychia congenita. *Nature Genet* 1995; **9**: 273–8.

Development and comparative anatomy [1–3]

The nail apparatus develops and matures from the primitive epidermis between the ninth and 20th weeks of intrauterine growth. At 20 weeks, the matrix cells show postnatal-type cell division, differentiation and keratinization, and the nail plate begins to form and move distally [4,5]; the nail bed loses its granular layer at this stage [6]. By 36 weeks, the complete nail plate reaches the tip of the digit and is surrounded by prominent lateral nail folds and a well-formed cuticle.

The structure of claws and hooves and their evolutionary relationship to humans has been well reviewed [2,3,7]. In higher primates, nails have evolved with the acquisition of manual dexterity; other mammals do not possess such flattened claws from which nails have evolved. Claws and talons are harder than human nails, probably because of their high content of calcium phosphate as crystalline hydroxyapatite within keratinized cells compared with human nails [8]. The hard 'soft plate' under hooves is produced from an area equivalent to the subungual part of the claw. In some animals, cloven hooves have only developed on the 'digits' that touch the floor; in horses, the single large hoof is produced from the third digit. The keratin biochemistry of the human nail has many similarities to that of the anteater or pangolin [6,9].

REFERENCES

1 Breathnach AS. *An Atlas of the Ultrastructure of Human Skin*. London: Churchill Livingstone, 1971.

2 Moore K. *The Developing Human*, 4th edn. Philadelphia: WB Saunders, 1988.

3 Spearman RIC. The physiology of the nail. In: Jarrett A, ed. *The Physiology and Pathophysiology of the Skin*, Vol. 5. New York: Academic Press, 1978: 1827–41.

4 Zaias N. Embryology of the human nail. *Arch Dermatol* 1963; **87**: 37–42.

5 Zaias N. *The Nail in Health and Disease*. New York: Spectrum Press, 1990.

6 Baden HP, Kubilus J. A comparative study of the immunologic properties of hoof and nail fibrous proteins. *J Invest Dermatol* 1984; **83**: 327–31.

7 Chapman RE. Hair, wool, quill, nail, claw, hoof, horn. In: Bereiter Hahn J, Matoltsy AG, Richards KS, eds. *Biology of the Integument*, Vol. 2. Berlin: Springer-Verlag, 1986.

8 Pautard FGE. Calcification of keratins. In: Rook AJ, Champion RH, eds. *Progress in the Biological Sciences in Relation to Dermatology*. Cambridge: Cambridge University Press, 1964: 227–9.

9 Spearman RIC. On the nature of the horny scales of the pangolin. *J Linn Soc Zool* 1967; **46**: 267–9.

Blood supply [1]

There is a rich arterial blood supply to the nail bed and matrix derived from paired digital arteries, a large palmar and small dorsal digital artery on either side. The palmar arteries are supplied from the large superficial and deep palmar arcades [2]. The main supply passes into the pulp space of the distal phalanx before reaching the dorsum of the digit (Fig. 65.3). Distally, the arteries are extremely tortuous and coiled, which allows them to be distorted without kinking to occlude supply. An accessory supply arises further back on the digit and does not enter the pulp space [3]. There are two main arterial arches (proximal and distal) supplying the nail bed and matrix, formed from anastomoses of the branches of the digital arteries. In the event of damage to the main supply in the pulp space, such as may occur with infection or scleroderma, there may be sufficient blood from the accessory vessels to permit normal growth of the nail.

There is a capillary loop system to the whole of the nail fold but the loops to the roof and matrix are flatter than those below the exposed nail [4] (see Chapter 49 for observations on capillaries of the posterior nail fold). There are many arteriovenous anastomoses beneath the nail—glomus bodies—which are concerned with heat regulation. Glomus bodies are important in maintaining

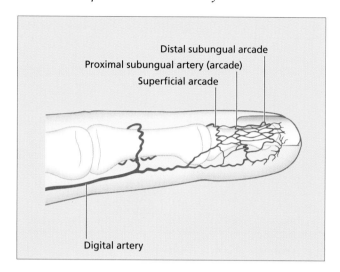

Fig. 65.3 Arterial supply of the distal finger.

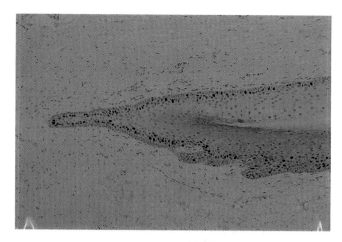

Fig. 65.4 Proliferating epithelial cells of the matrix and ventral aspect of the proximal nail fold, staining with the antibody MIB-1.

acral circulation under cold conditions—arterioles constrict with cold but glomus bodies dilate [5]. These occupy the subdermal tissues and increase in number in a gradient towards the distal nail bed [6].

REFERENCES

1 Baran R, Dawber RPR. Structure, embryology, comparative anatomy and physiology. In: Baran R, Dawber RPR, eds. *Diseases of the Nail and their Management,* 2nd. Oxford: Blackwell Scientific Publications, 1994.
2 Smith DO, Oura C, Kimura C, Toshimuri K. Arterial anatomy and tortuosity in the distal finger. *J Hand Surg* 1991; **16A**: 297–302.
3 Flint MH. Some observations on the vascular supply of the nail bed and terminal segments of the finger. *Br J Plast Surg* 1955; **8**: 186–94.
4 Samman PD. The human toenail. Its genesis and blood supply. *Br J Dermatol* 1959; **71**: 296–301.
5 Ryan TJ. The arteriovenous anastomoses. In: Jarrett A, ed. *The Physiology and Pathophysiology of the Skin,* Vol. 2. London: Academic Press, 1973: 612–14.
6 Wolfram-Gabel R, Sick H. Vascular networks of the periphery of the fingernail. *J Hand Surg* 1995; **20B**: 488–92.

Nail growth and morphology

Clinicians used to observing the slow rate of growth of diseased or damaged nails are apt to view the nail apparatus as inert, although it is biochemically and kinetically active throughout life. In this respect, it differs from the hair follicle, which undergoes periods of quiescence as part of the follicular cycle.

Cell kinetics

The kinetic activity of the matrix has been examined using many techniques. These include immunohistochemistry, autoradiography and direct measurement of matrix product (i.e. nail plate) by ultrasound [1], micrometer or histology.

There is a broad basal compartment of proliferating cells in the matrix, which can be detected immuno-

histochemically with antibodies to proliferating cell nuclear antigen and Ki-67 (Fig. 65.4); both antigens are associated with proliferating cells [2]. The matrix is also the site of maximal inclusion of tritiated thymidine if injected into the peritoneum of squirrel monkeys and followed subsequently by autoradiography [3]. Although there was some inclusion of thymidine into the nail bed, Zaias and Alvarez interpreted the findings as indicating that the nail bed had no role in creation of the nail plate. Norton [4] drew a similar conclusion from work with live human subjects where both labelled thymidine and glycine were injected locally to act as markers of proliferating and metabolically active keratinocytes, and primarily labelled the matrix.

However, the earlier work of Lewis [5] suggested on histological grounds that the nail plate is a trilaminar structure originating from three separate matrix zones: the dorsal matrix (ventral aspect of proximal nail fold), intermediate matrix (germinal matrix) and ventral matrix (nail bed). In support of this, Johnson and coworkers [6,7] demonstrated that 21% of the nail thickness is gained as it passes over the nail bed, implying that the nail bed is generating this fraction of the nail plate. De Berker *et al.* noted that the increase in nail thickness did not coincide with corresponding increases of nail-plate cells [2]. This challenges the interpretation that nail thickens over the nail bed through the contribution from underlying structures. An alternative explanation may be appropriate, such as compaction arising through repetitive distal trauma. Others have also argued this debate [8], and, although the nail bed may have a significant contribution to make in disease [9], the evidence for its contribution at other times is conflicting.

Nail morphology

Why the nail grows flat, rather than as a heaped-up

keratinous mass, has generated much thought and discussion [10–14]. Several factors probably combine to produce a relatively flat nail plate: the orientation of the matrix rete pegs and papillae; the direction of cell differentiation [15]; and moulding of the direction of nail growth between the proximal nail fold and distal phalanx [16]. Containment laterally within the lateral nail folds assists this orientation, and the adherent nature of the nail bed is likely to be important. In diseases such as psoriasis, the nail bed can lose its adherent properties, exhibiting onycholysis. In addition, there may be subungual hyperkeratosis. These combined factors make psoriasis the most common pathology in which up-growing nails are seen. Onychogryphosis is characterized by upward growth of thickened nail. In this condition, the nail matrix may become bucket shaped and the effect of the overlying proximal nailfold is lost.

Linear nail growth [17–19]

Over the last century, many studies have been carried out on the linear growth of the nail plate in health and disease; these have been reviewed [20,21] and are listed in Tables 65.1 and 65.2 [22]. Most of these studies have been performed by observing the distal movement of a reference mark etched on the nail plate over a fixed period of time; this may well correlate with matrix germinative cell kinetics but there is no direct proof that it does. However, studies on nail growth in psoriasis, and its inhibition by cytostatic drugs [23,24], suggest that cell kinetics and linear growth rate do have a direct correlation.

Fingernails grow at approximately 1 cm per 3 months and toenails at one-third of this rate.

Table 65.1 Physiological and environmental factors affecting the rate of nail growth.

Faster	Slower
Daytime	Night
Pregnancy [25]	First day of life [14]
Minor trauma/nail biting [26,27]	
Right hand nails	Left hand nails [28,29]
Youth, increasing age	Old age [18,23,30]
Fingers	Toes [31]
Summer [18]	Winter or cold environment [32,33]
Middle, ring and index	Thumb and little [28,31,34,35]
Male gender	Female gender [27,35]

Table 65.2 Pathological factors affecting the rate of nail growth.

Faster	Slower

Psoriasis [36]
   Normal nails [23]
   Pitting
   Onycholysis [37]
	Finger immobilization [41]

Pityriasis rubra pilaris [21,38]	Fever [42]
	Beau's lines [43]
Etretinate, rarely [39]	Methotrexate [24] Azathioprine [24] Etretinate [39]
Idiopathic onycholysis of women [37]	Denervation [44]
Bullous ichthyosiform erythroderma [13]	Poor nutrition Kwashiorkor [45]
Hyperthyroidism [28]	Hypothyroidism [28]
Levodopa [40]	Yellow nail syndrome [13]
Arteriovenous shunts [28]	Relapsing polychondritis [46]

REFERENCES

1 Finlay AY, Moseley H, Duggan TC. Ultrasound transmission time: an *in vivo* guide to nail thickness. *Br J Dermatol* 1987; **117**: 765–70.
2 de Berker D, MaWhinney B, Sviland L. Quantification of regional matrix nail production. *Br J Dermatol* 1996; **134**: 1083–6.
3 Zaias N, Alvarez J. The formation of the primate nail plate. An autoradiographic study in squirrel monkeys. *J Invest Dermatol* 1968; **51**: 120–36.
4 Norton LA. Incorporation of thymidine 3H and glycine-2 H³ in the nail bed matrix and bed of humans. *J Invest Dermatol* 1971; **56**: 61–8.
5 Lewis BL. Microscopic studies of foetal and mature nail and surrounding soft tissue. *Arch Dermatol* 1954; **70**: 732–7.
6 Johnson M, Comaish JS, Shuster S. Nail is produced by the normal nail bed: a controversy resolved. *Br J Dermatol* 1991; **125**: 27–9.
7 Johnson M, Shuster S. Continuous formation of nail along the nail bed. *Br J Dermatol* 1993; **128**: 277–80.
8 Pinkus F. In: Jasassohn J, ed. *Handbuch der Haut und Geschlechtskrankheiten.* Berlin: Springer-Verlag, 1927: 267–89.
9 Samman PD. The ventral nail. *Arch Dermatol* 1961; **84**: 192–5.
10 Baran R. Nail growth direction revisited. *J Am Acad Dermatol* 1981; **4**: 78–83.
11 Kligman AM. Nail growth direction revisited. *J Am Acad Dermatol* 1981; **4**: 82.
12 Kligman AM. Why do nails grow out instead of up? *Arch Dermatol* 1961; **84**: 181–3.
13 Samman PD. *The Nails in Disease,* 3rd edn. London: Heinemann, 1978: 14.
14 Schmiegelow P, Lindner J, Puschmann M. Autoradiographische Quantifizierung dosisabhängiger 35S CystinbZW. *Aktuelle Dermatol* 1983; **2**: 62.
15 Hashimoto K. Ultrastructure of the human toenail. *Arch Dermatol Forsch* 1971; **240**: 1–22.
16 Kelikian H. *Congenital Deformities of the Hand and the Forearm.* Philadelphia: WB Saunders, 1974: 210–12.
17 Baran R, Dawber RPR, eds. *Guide Médico-Chirurgical des Onychopathies.* Paris: Arnette, 1990: 12.
18 Bean WB. Nail growth: 30 years of observations. *Arch Intern Med* 1974; **134**: 497–502.
19 Dawber R, Baran R. Nail growth. *Cutis* 1987; **39**: 99–102.
20 Baran R, Dawber RPR, eds. *Diseases of the Nail and their Management,* 2nd edn. Oxford: Blackwell Scientific Publications, 1994: 1–34.

21 Runne U, Orfanos CE. The human nail. *Curr Probl Dermatol* 1981; **9**: 102–49.

22 de Doncker P, Pierard GE. Acquired nail beading in patients receiving itraconazole—an indicator of faster nail growth? A study using optical profilometry. *Clin Exp Dermatol* 1994; **19**: 404–6.

23 Dawber RPR. Fingernail growth in normal and psoriatic subjects. *Br J Dermatol* 1970; **82**: 454–7.

24 Dawber RPR. The effect of methotrexate, corticosteroids and azathioprine on fingernail growth in psoriasis. *Br J Dermatol* 1970; **83**: 680–8.

25 Hewitt D, Hillman RW. Relation between rate of nail growth in pregnant women and estimated previous general growth rate. *Am J Clin Nutr* 1966; **19**: 436–9.

26 Gilchrist ML, Buxton LHD. The relation of fingernail growth to nutritional status. *J Anat* 1939; **73**: 575–81.

27 Hamilton JB, Tereda H, Mestler GE. Studies of growth throughout the lifespan in Japanese. *Gerontology* 1955; **10**: 401–10.

28 Orentreich N, Markofsky J, Vogelman JH. The effect of ageing on the rate of linear nail growth. *J Invest Dermatol* 1979; **73**: 126–30.

29 Pfister R. Das normale Onychodiagramm. *Z Haut Geschlechtskr* 1955; **18**: 132–7.

30 Lavelle CE. Nail growth. *Curr Probl Dermatol* 1981; **9**: 102–4.

31 Pfister R, Henera J. Wachstum und Gestaltung der Zehennagel bei Gesunden. *Arch Klin Exp Dermatol* 1965; **223**: 263-74.

32 Donovan KM. Antarctic environment and nail growth. *Br J Dermatol* 1977; **96**: 507–10.

33 Roberts DF, Sandford MR. A possible climatic effect on nail growth. *Appl Physiol* 1958; **13**: 135–7.

34 Knobloch VH. Das normale Wachstum der Fingernagel. *Deutsch Med Wochenschr* 1953; **78**: 743–5.

35 Le Gros-Clark WE, Buxton LHD. Studies in nail growth. *Br J Dermatol* 1938; **50**: 221–9.

36 Landherr G, Braun-Falco O, Hofmann C *et al*. Fingernagel Wachstum bei Psoriatitern unter PUVA-Therapie. *Hautarzt* 1982; **33**: 210–13.

37 Dawber RPR, Samman PD, Bottoms E. Fingernail growth in idiopathic and psoriatic onycholysis. *Br J Dermatol* 1971; **85**: 558–67.

38 Dawber RPR. The ultrastructure and growth of human nails. *Arch Dermatol Res* 1980; **269**: 197–204.

39 Baran R. Action thérapeutique et complications du rétinoid aromatique sur l'appareil unguéal. *Ann Dermatol Vénéréol* 1982; **109**: 367–70.

40 Miller E. Levodopa and nail growth. *N Engl J Med* 1973; **288**: 916–19.

41 Dawber RPR. Effects of immobilisation on fingernail growth. *Clin Exp Dermatol* 1981; **6**: 1–4.

42 Sibinger MS. Observations on growth of fingernails in health and disease. *Pediatrics* 1959; **24**: 225–33.

43 Weismann K. Beau and his description of transverse depressions on nails. *Br J Dermatol* 1977; **97**: 571–2.

44 Head H, Sherrin J. The consequence of injury to peripheral nerves in man. *Brain* 1905; **28**: 116–18.

45 Babcock MJ. Methods of measuring fingernail growth in nutritional studies. *J Nutr* 1955; **55**: 323–38.

46 Estes SA. Relapsing polychondritis. *Cutis* 1983; **32**: 471–6.

Nails in childhood and old age

Childhood [1,2]

In early childhood, the nail plate is relatively thin and may show temporary koilonychia. This is particularly prominent on the great toes. Under the age of 5 years, nails are also prone to terminal onychoschizia (lamellar splitting). This can be most prominent on the sucked thumb, but is also seen on the toes. Sucking may also lead to paronychia, which can be a troublesome condition in childhood, with pain and nail dystrophy. Ingrowing can also cause pain and may present in different forms. At birth, there is often a degree of distal ingrowing, particularly in the great toe, as the nail has not surmounted the tip of

the digit in its development [3]. In a more gross form, this may present as congenital hypertrophic lip of the hallux, where soft-tissue overgrowth may resemble fibrous tumours of the digit before spontaneously disappearing [4]. Painful distal embedding can lead to infection, but as long as the toenail is properly orientated with respect to the underlying phalanx, the condition subsides. The changes associated with congenital malalignment of the great toe may also subside within 5–10 years in about 50% of children. In this condition, there is deviation of the tip of the great toe nail laterally, rotating on the distal phalanx. The nail is yellow, triangular, thickened and has transverse ridges [5].

In one study [6], 92% of normal infants between 8 and 9 weeks of age showed a single transverse line (Beau's line) on the fingernails. One child demonstrated a transverse depression through the whole nail thickness on all 20 digits [7]. Normal surface markings of the nail can differ in children from those seen in adults. A herring-bone pattern is common and gradually diminishes with time [8], which may reflect a gradual change in the pattern of matrix maturation.

Old age

Many of the changes seen in old age may occur in younger age groups in association with impaired arterial blood supply. Elastic tissue changes diffusely affecting the nail bed epidermis are often seen histologically [9]; these changes may be due to the effects of UV radiation, although it has been stated that the nail plate is an efficient filter of UVB radiation [10]. The whole subungual area in old age may show thickening of blood-vessel walls with vascular elastic tissue fragmentation. Pertinax bodies are often seen in the nail plate. Nail growth is inversely proportional to age [11]; related to this slower growth, corneocytes are larger in old age [12].

The nail plate becomes paler, dull and opaque with advancing years, and white nails similar to those seen in cirrhosis, uraemia and hypoalbuminaemia may be seen in normal subjects. Longitudinal ridging is present to some degree in most people after 50 years of age and this may give a 'sausage links' or beaded appearance.

For details of the common traumatic abnormalities and changes due to inadequate pedicure or neglect, detailed texts should be consulted [1,11].

REFERENCES

1 Baran R, Barth J, Dawber RPR, eds. *Nail Disorders*. London: Dunitz, 1991: 78–101.

2 Barth JH, Dawber RPR. Diseases of the nails in children. *Paediatr Dermatol* 1987; **12**: 275–90.

3 Silverman RA. Pediatric disease. In: Scher RK, Daniel CR, eds. *Nails: Therapy, Diagnosis and Surgery*. Philadelphia: WB Saunders, 1990.

4 Hammerton MD, Shrank AB. Congenital hypertrophy of the lateral nail folds of the hallux. *Pediatr Dermatol* 1988; **5**: 243–5.

5 Baran R. Congenital malalignment of the toe nail *Arch Dermatol* 1980; **116**: 1346.
6 Turano AF. Beau's lines in infancy. *Pediatrics* 1968; **41**: 996–4.
7 Wolf D. Beau's lines in childhood. *Cutis* 1982; **29**: 191–4.
8 Parry EJ, Morley WN, Dawber RPR. Herringbone nails: an uncommon variant of nail growth in childhood. *Br J Dermatol* 1995; **132**: 1021–2.
9 Baran R. Nail care in the 'golden years' of life. *Curr Med Res Opin* 1982; **7**: 96–101.
10 Parker SG, Diffey BL. The transmission of optical radiation through human nails. *Br J Dermatol* 1983; **108**: 11–14.
11 Baran R, Dawber RPR, eds. *Diseases of the Nail and their Management*, 2nd edn. Oxford: Blackwell Scientific Publications, 1994: 105–20.
12 Germann H, Barran W, Plewig G. Morphology of corneocytes from human nail plates. *J Invest Dermatol* 1980; **74**: 115–18.

Nail signs and systemic disease

It is important for clinicians to understand and accurately describe nail findings if they are to communicate accurately with their colleagues and avoid the vagueness that often surrounds nail pathology. Signs fall into categories of shape, surface and colour.

Abnormalities of shape

Clubbing

In clubbing there is increased transverse and longitudinal nail curvature with hypertrophy of the soft-tissue components of the digit pulp.

Hyperplasia of the fibrovascular tissue at the base of the nail allows the nail to be 'rocked' and in causes associated with cardiopulmonary disease there may be local cyanosis.

There are three forms of geometric assessment that can be performed. *Lovibond's angle* is found at the junction between the nail plate and the proximal nail fold, and is normally less than 160°. This is altered to over 180° in clubbing (Fig. 65.5). *Curth's angle* at the distal interphalangeal joint is normally approximately 180°. This is diminished to less than 160° in clubbing (Fig. 65.6).

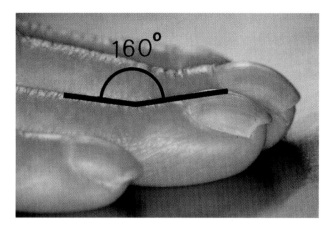

Fig. 65.6 Clubbing: Curth's modified profile sign.

Schamroth's window is seen when the dorsal aspects of two fingers from opposite hands are apposed, revealing a window of light, bordered laterally by the Lovibond angles. As this angle is obliterated in clubbing, the window closes [1].

Clubbing appears to be related to increased blood flow through the vasodilated plexus of nail unit vasculature, more than to vessel hyperplasia. Altered vagal tone and microvascular infarcts have been implicated [2,3].

Pathological associations of clubbing include inflammatory bowel disease, carcinoma of the bronchus and cirrhosis. In forms associated with bronchiectasis or neoplasm, prominent inflammatory joint signs may also be seen, resulting in hypertrophic pulmonary osteoarthropathy. In some cases of bronchiectasis, a variant of clubbing, *shell-nail syndrome*, can be seen. This is distinguished from clubbing by the presence of atrophy of underlying bone and nail bed [4] and may have more in common with yellow-nail syndrome than with clubbing.

REFERENCES

1 Lampe RM, Kagan A. Detection of clubbing—Schamroth's sign. *Clin Pediatr* 1983; **22**: 125.
2 Currie AE, Gallagher PJ. The pathology of clubbing: vascular changes in the nail bed. *Br J Dis Chest* 1988; **82**: 382–5.
3 Silveri F, Carlino G, Cervini C. The endothelium/platelet unit in hypertrophic osteoarthropathy. *Clin Exp Rheum* 1992; **10** (Suppl. 7): 61–6.
4 Cornelius CE, Shelley WB. Shell nail syndrome associated with bronchiectasis. *Arch Dermatol* 1967; **96**: 694–5.

Koilonychia

In koilonychia (Greek: *Koilos* hollow, *onyx* nail), there is reverse curvature in the transverse and longitudinal axis giving a concave dorsal aspect to the nail [1]. Fingers and toes may be affected with signs most prominent in the thumb or great toe. The nail may be thickened, thinned,

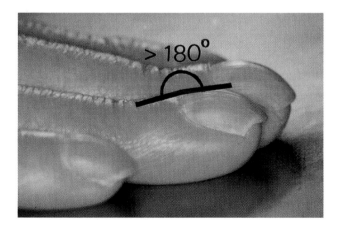

Fig. 65.5 Clubbing: Lovibond's profile sign. The angle is normally less than 160°, but exceeds 180° in clubbing.

softened or unchanged in quality. Koilonychia is common in infancy as a benign feature of the great toenail, although in some infants its persistence may be associated with a deficiency of cysteine-rich keratin [2] in trichothiodystrophy. The most common systemic association is with iron deficiency [3] and haemochromatosis, although the majority of adults with koilonychia demonstrate a familial pattern which may be autosomal dominant [4]. In dermatoses such as psoriasis and dermatophyte infection, nailbed hyperkeratosis may push the nail up distally to produce a spoon-shaped nail, and in mechanics softening of the nail with oil may be a factor [5].

REFERENCES

1 Stone OJ. Spoon nails and clubbing: significance and mechanisms. *Cutis* 1975; **16**: 235–41.
2 Jalili MA, Al-Kassab S. Koilonychia and cystine content of nails. *Lancet* 1959; **ii**: 108–10.
3 Hogan GR, Jones B. The relationship of koilonychia and iron deficiency in infants. *J Pediatr* 1970; **77**: 1054.
4 Bergeron JR, Stone OJ. Koilonychia. A report of familial spoon nails. *Arch Dermatol* 1967; **95**: 351.
5 Dawber RPR. Occupational koilonychia. *Br J Dermatol* 1974; **91** (Suppl.10): 11.

Macronychia and micronychia

Macronychia and micronychia nails are considered too large or small in comparison with other nails on nearby digits. The nail disorder is usually associated with an abnormal digit, arising from underlying bony abnormalities such as local gigantism causing macronychia or megadactyly [1]. This is also the basis of racket thumb (Fig. 65.7), the most common form of benign, dominantly inherited macronychia. Plexiform neurofibromas may cause nail changes and duplication of the terminal phalanges may cause bifid or small nails [2].

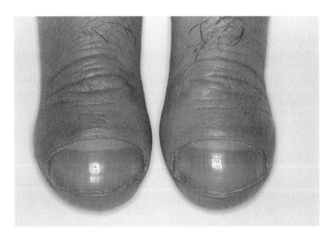

Fig. 65.7 Racket nail associated with clubbing.

REFERENCES

1 Barsky AJ. Macrodactyly. *J Bone Joint Surg* 1967; **49**: 1255–6.
2 Millman AJ, Strier RP. Congenital onychodysplasia of the index fingers. *J Am Acad Dermatol* 1982; **7**: 57–65.

Anonychia

Anonychia is absence of all or part of one or several nails [1]. The term implies a permanent state which can be congenital and associated with underlying bony changes [2]. If there is residual nail matrix, there may be some vestigial nail or hyperkeratosis. Temporary anonychia may arise from onychomadesis (nail loss) associated with transient local or systemic upset. If local, the appearance of the nail unit may reflect the precipitating cause.

REFERENCES

1 Solammedivi SV. Simple anonychia. *South Med J* 1981; **74**: 1555.
2 Baran R, Juhlin L. Bone dependent nail formation. *Br J Dermatol* 1986; **114**: 371–5.

Abnormalities of nail attachment

Nail shedding

Nails can be lost through different mechanisms, as follows.
1 Complete loss of the nail plate due to proximal nail separation extending distally [1] is called onychomadesis and is a progression of profound Beau's lines. This may reflect local or systemic disease and in the latter may result in temporary loss of all nails.
2 Local dermatoses such as the bullous disorders and paronychia may cause nail loss. Generalized dermatoses may be manifest, for example toxic epidermal necrolysis (TEN) and severe/rapid onset of pustular psoriasis. Scarring of the nail unit is seen in lichen planus and following TEN, which may both provoke nail loss.
3 Trauma is a common cause of recurrent loss and may reflect the nature of the activity, such as football, some underlying abnormality of footwear [2] or pedal mechanics. It is often associated with subungual haemorrhage [3].
4 Temporary loss has also been described due to retinoids [4], and large doses of cloxacillin and cephaloridine during the treatment of two anephric patients [5].
5 Onychoptosis defluvium or alopecia unguium describes atraumatic, familial, non-inflammatory nail loss [6]. It may be periodic and associated with dental amelogenesis imperfecta.

Trauma in athletes may cause nail loss mainly affecting the great toe.

REFERENCES

1 Runne U, Orfanos CE. The human nail. *Curr Probl Dermatol* 1981; **9**: 102.

2 Almeyda J. Platform nails (Letter). *Br Med J* 1973; i: 176.
3 Baran R, Barth J, Dawber RPR, eds. Splinter haemorrhage and subungual haematoma. In: *Nail Disorders*. London: Dunitz, 1991: 84–8.
4 Baran R. Retinoids and the nails. *J Dermatol Treat* 1990; **1**: 151–4.
5 Eastwood JB, Curtin JR, Smith EKM *et al.* Shedding of the nails apparently induced by large amounts of cephaloridine and cloxacillin in 2 anephric patients. *Br J Dermatol* 1969; **81**: 750–2.
6 Oliver WJ. Recurrent onychoptosis occurring as a family disorder. *Br J Dermatol* 1927; **26**: 59–68.

Onycholysis

Onycholysis is the distal and/or lateral separation of the nail from the nail bed [1,2]. Psoriatic onycholysis can be considered the reference point for other forms of onycholysis where it is typically distal, with variable lateral involvement. Areas of separation appear white or yellow due to air beneath the nail and sequestered debris, shed squames and glycoprotein exudate. Isolated islands of onycholysis present as 'oily spots' or 'salmon patches' in the nail bed. At the border of onycholysis, the nail bed is usually reddish-brown, reflecting the underlying psoriatic inflammatory changes. All the common causes are associated with diminished adherence of nail to nailbed as a primary (idiopathic) or secondary event and include trauma, fungal infection, eczema and photo-onycholysis [3].

Idiopathic onycholysis

This is a painless separation of the nail from its bed, which occurs without apparent cause. Overzealous manicure, frequent wetting and cosmetic 'solvents' may be the cause and they may not be admitted by the patient. There may, however, be a minor traumatic element, as the condition occurs rather more often in persons who keep their nails abnormally long. Maceration with water may also be a factor [3]. It must be distinguished from other causes of onycholysis (see below). The affected nails grow very quickly [4].

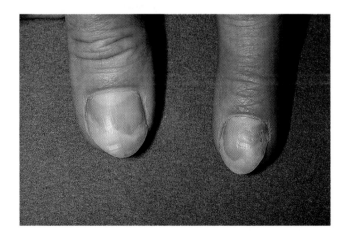

Fig. 65.8 Onycholysis: idiopathic type.

The condition usually starts at the tip of one or more nails and extends to involve the distal third of the nail bed (Fig. 65.8). Persistent manicure is attempted to remove the debris which accumulates within the onycholytic space, and this can result in a crescentic margin of onycholysis matching the onychocorneal band and appearing similar in all involved digits. Pain occurs only if there is further extension as a result of trauma or if active infection supervenes. More often there is microbial colonization of a mixed nature, including *Candida albicans* and several bacteria, of which *Pseudomonas pyocyanea* is the most common. If the condition persists for several months, the nail bed becomes dark and irregularly thickened.

The condition is mostly seen in women and many cases return to normal after a few months. The longer it lasts the less likely is the nail to become reattached, due to keratinization of the exposed nailbed.

Treatment [5]. The patient should be advised to cut away as much as possible of the loosened nail and to apply a topical steroid preparation containing antibiotics and nystatin, for example Triadcortyl cream, to the nail bed two or three times a day, or to use miconazole hydrocortisone cream twice a day [1]. Reattachment is slow, and the loosened nail should be recut several times if necessary. The object of treatment is to prevent infection becoming established below the loosened nail, because this leads to thickening of the nail bed and prevents reattachment. Four per cent thymol in chloroform (not available in the USA) is still recommended by some authorities as a means of preventing infection and further maceration of the nail bed [6]; 2% thymol is often as strong as the patient can tolerate, however, and is usually effective.

Secondary onycholysis

There are many other causes of onycholysis, which is one of the commonest nail signs [5,7–9]. They may be grouped as follows.

1 Dermatological disorders: psoriasis, fungal infections and dermatitis are common causes; congenital ectodermal defect is a rare one.
2 General medical conditions: impaired peripheral circulation, hypothyroidism [10], hyperthyroidism [11], hyperhidrosis, yellow-nail syndrome and shell-nail syndrome.
3 Trauma: minor trauma is a common cause and many occupational cases are due to trauma [6,12]. Immersion of the hands in soap and water may be considered traumatic, as also may the use of certain nail cosmetics. It has also been described after the application of 5% 5-fluorouracil to the fingertips [13].
4 Hereditary partial onycholysis associated with hard nails [14].
5 Photo-onycholysis (Fig. 65.9) may occur during

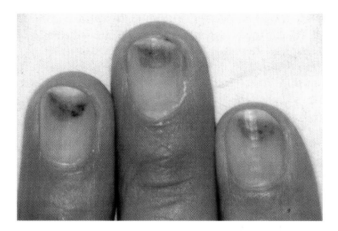

Fig. 65.9 Photo-onycholysis with a uniform pattern of discoloured onycholysis in the midline.

treatment with psoralens, demethylchlortetracycline and doxycycline [15,16], and rarely other antibiotics. This is sometimes associated with cutaneous photosensitivity (Chapter 25).

REFERENCES

1 Ray L. Onycholysis: a classification and study. *Arch Dermatol* 1963; **88**: 181–5.
2 Taft EH. Onycholysis; a clinical review. *Aust J Dermatol* 1968; **2**: 345–51.
3 Baran R. Juhlin L. Drug-induced photo-onycholysis. Three subtypes identified in a study of 15 cases. *J Am Acad Dermatol* 1987; **17**: 1012–16.
4 Dawber RPR, Samman PD, Bottoms E. Fingernail growth in idiopathic and psoriatic onycholysis. *Br J Dermatol* 1971; **85**: 558–60.
5 Wilson JW. Paronychia and onycholysis: aetiology and therapy. *Arch Dermatol* 1965; **92**: 726–30.
6 Forck G, Kastner N. Onycholysis. *Hautarzt* 1967; **18**: 85–8.
7 Baran R, Barth J, Dawber RPR, eds. Onycholysis. In: *Nail Disorders*. London: Dunitz 1991: 69–73.
8 Baran R, Dawber RPR, eds. *Diseases of the Nails and their Management*. Oxford: Blackwell Scientific Publications, 1994: 58.
9 Kechijian P. Onycholysis of the fingernails: evaluation and management. *J Am Acad Dermatol* 1985; **12**: 552–60.
10 Fox EC. Diseases of the nails: report of cases of onycholysis. *Arch Dermatol Syphilol* 1940; **44**: 426–8.
11 Luria MN, Asper SP. Onycholysis in hyperthyroidism. *Ann Intern Med* 1958; **42**: 102–8.
12 Heinmann H, Silverberg MG. Onycholysis in fur workers. *Arch Dermatol Syphilol* 1941; **44**: 426–8.
13 Shelley WB. Onycholysis due to 5-fluorouracil. *Acta Derm Venereol (Stockh)* 1972; **52**: 320–2.
14 Schultz HD. Hereditary partial onycholysis and hard nails. *Dermatol Wochenschr* 1966; **152**: 766–8.
15 Franks SB, Coton HJ, Mirkin W. Photo-onycholysis due to tetracycline. *Arch Dermatol* 1971; **103**: 520.
16 Orentreich N, Harber LC, Tromovitch TH. Photosensitivity and photo-onycholysis due to demethylchlortetracycline. *Arch Dermatol* 1961; **83**: 730–7.

Pterygium

The term pterygium describes the winged appearance achieved when a central fibrotic band divides a nail proximally into two. However, the fibrotic tissue may not always grossly alter the nail and can extend from the lateral nail fold as well as the more typical proximal nail fold. A large pterygium may destroy the whole nail.

An inflammatory destructive process precedes pterygium formation. There is fusion between the nail fold and underlying nail bed. The fibrotic band then obstructs normal nail growth. Superficial abnormal vessels may be seen and there are no skin markings. The feature most typically develops in trauma or lichen planus or its variants, such as idiopathic atrophy of the nail [1] and graft-versus-host disease [2]. It can also occur in leprosy, where it may represent scarring secondary to neuropathic damage and secondary purulent infection [3].

REFERENCES

1 Samman PD. Idiopathic atrophy of the nails. *Br J Dermatol* 1969; **81**: 746–9.
2 Little BJ, Cowan MA. Lichen planus-like eruption and nail changes in a patient with graft-versus-host disease. *Br J Dermatol* 1990; **122**: 841–3.
3 Patki AH, Mehta JM. Pterygium unguis in a patient with recurrent type 2 lepra reaction. *Cutis* 1989; **44**: 311–12.

Ventral pterygium [1]

Ventral pterygium or pterygium inversum unguis [2] occurs on the distal undersurface of the nail with forward extension of the nail-bed epithelium dislocating the hyponychium and obscuring the distal groove. Causes include trauma, systemic sclerosis [2,3], Raynaud's phenomenon, lupus erythematosus, familial [4] and infective [5]. The overlying nail may be normal, but adjacent soft tissues can be painful.

REFERENCES

1 Drake L. Pterygium inversum unguis. *Arch Dermatol* 1976; **112**: 255–6.
2 Caputo R, Cappio F, Rigoni C *et al.* Pterygium inversum unguis. Report of 19 cases and review of the literature. *Arch Dermatol* 1993; **129**: 1307–9.
3 Patterson JW. Pterygium inversum unguis-like changes in scleroderma. *Arch Dermatol* 1977; **113**: 1429–30.
4 Amblard P, Reymond JL. Familial subungual pterygium. *Ann Dermatol Vénéréol* 1980; **107**: 949–50.
5 Patki AH. Pterygium inversum unguis in a patient with leprosy. *Arch Dermatol* 1990; **126**: 1110.

Subungual hyperkeratosis

Subungual hyperkeratosis entails hyperkeratosis of the nail bed and hyponychium and may occur in a range of conditions, including those where the primary diagnosis is not clear. Nail-plate changes are variable, but thickening is common. Dry, white or yellow hyperkeratosis may crumble away from the overhanging nail. Hyperkeratosis may extend on to the digit pulp. Features of onychomycosis and wart virus infection (mainly toes) or psoriasis, pityriasis rubra pilaris and eczema (mainly fingers) may be found elsewhere to determine the aetiology.

The nail bed is an epithelium of low proliferative turnover. Any disease process which affects it is likely to result in an excess of squamous debris. The overlying nail prevents simple loss. The initial outcome is compaction of debris into layers of subungual hyperkeratosis. The only route of loss is by emerging distally with the growing nail.

Focal subungual keratoses are seen with Darier's disease, and keratotic debris beneath the nail in Norwegian (crusted) scabies may contain mites and eggs.

Nail thickening

Isolated thickening of the nail is associated with yellow discoloration as the nail bed vasculature is obscured. Common causes include psoriasis, eczema, trauma and onychomycosis, some of which may be associated with subungual hyperkeratosis. The shape of the nail may alter depending upon the underlying cause, such as in yellow-nail syndrome, where there is increased curvature in the longitudinal and transverse axes.

In toenails in the elderly and yellow-nail syndrome, retarded longitudinal growth of the nail is compensated for by increased thickness [1]. Yellow nail may also develop where the nail bed produces abnormal nail [2]. Onychogryphosis describes thickened nails, usually the great toenail, which commonly grow upwards in a spiral. It is attributed to chronic distorting trauma and can be treated surgically or by conservative methods. These include trimming with an electric drill, chemical destruction with 40% urea paste, phenolization of the matrix to achieve total ablation (reduced phenol time to 2 min) or carbon dioxide laser.

REFERENCES

1 Higashi N, Matsumura T. The aetiology of onychogryphosis of the great toe nail and of ingrowing nail. *Hifu* 1988; **30**: 620–3.
2 Schönfeld PHIR. The pachyonychia congenita syndrome. *Acta Derm Venereol (Stockh)* 1980; **60**: 45–9.

Changes in nail surface

Longitudinal grooves

Longitudinal grooves may run all or part of the length of the nail in the longitudinal axis and need to be distinguished from ridges which are proud of the nail surface [1]. Grooves may be full or partial thickness.

The median canaliform dystrophy of Heller [2] is the most distinctive form [3], split usually in the midline, with fir-tree-like appearance of ridges angled backwards. The thumbs are most commonly affected and the involvement may be symmetrical. The cuticle may be normal, as distinct from the cuticle in habit tic deformity (washboard nails). After a period of months or years the nails often return to normal, but relapse may occur [4] and a ridge may replace the original defect. Some patients give a definite history of

trauma [1], or the disorder can be attributed to oral retinoids [5]. Familial cases have been recorded. Sutton [6] described involvement of a toenail in which a flabby filament of fleshy tissue was present in the canal. Treatment is unnecessary, but the patient should be advised to apply an emollient cream to the nail fold.

Physiological furrows and ridges are accentuated in lichen planus, rheumatoid arthritis, peripheral vascular disease, old age and Darier's disease. *Onychorrhexis* may occur where there are superficial grooves in the nail which lead to a distal split.

Tumours (warts, myxoid cysts) pressing on the matrix, or a proximal nail-fold pterygium, may produce a longitudinal groove.

REFERENCES

1 Ronchese F. Peculiar nail anomalies. *Arch Dermatol* 1951; **63**: 565–9.
2 Heller J. Dystrophia unguium mediana canaliformis. *Dermatol Z* 1928; **51**: 416–17.
3 Zelger J, Wohlfarth P, Putz R. Dystrophia unguium mediana canaliformis Heller. *Hautarzt* 1974; **25**: 629.
4 Sweet RD. Dystrophia unguium mediana canaliformis. *Arch Dermatol Syphilol* 1951; **64**: 61–2.
5 Bottomley W, Cunliffe W. Median canaliform dystrophy associated with isotretinoin therapy. *Br J Dermatol* 1992; **127**: 447.
6 Sutton RJ, Jr. Solenonychia: canaliform dystrophy of the nails. *South Med J* 1965; **58**: 1143–6.

Transverse grooves and Beau's lines [1]

Transverse grooves may be full or partial thickness through the nail. When they are endogenous they have an arcuate margin matching the lunula. If exogenous, such as those

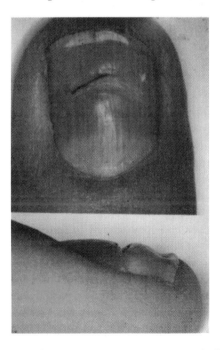

Fig. 65.10 Beau's lines present as transverse grooves in the nail matching the proximal margin of the nail matrix and lunula.

due to manicure, the margin may match the proximal nail fold and the grooves may be multiple as in washboard nails associated with a habit tic [2,3]. When multiple, it may be difficult to distinguish a habit tic from psoriasis. Transverse grooves may be on isolated diseased digits (trauma, inflammation or neurological events), or generalized, reflecting a systemic event such as coronary thrombosis, measles, mumps or pneumonia. If endogenous, they are usually referred to as *Beau's lines* [4,5]. They arise through temporary interference with nail formation and become visible on the nail surface (Fig. 65.10) some weeks after the precipitant. The distance of the groove from the nail fold is related to the time since the onset of growth disturbance. The depth and width of the groove may be related to the severity and duration of disturbance, respectively. In many cases, grooves are seen on all 20 nails but are most prominent on the thumb and great toenail, and are deeper in the midline of the nail. Full-thickness grooves can be associated with distal extension of the plane of separation of the nail plate. This can lead to nail loss, termed *onychomadesis*.

REFERENCES

1 Runne V, Orfanos CE. The human nail. *Curr Probl Dermatol* 1981; **9**: 102–49.
2 de Berker DAR. What is a Beau's line? *Int J Dermatol* 1994; **33**: 545–6.
3 Macaulay WL. Transverse ridging of the thumbnails. *Arch Dermatol* 1966; **93**: 421–3.
4 Beau JHS. Note sur certain caractères de séméiologie rétrospective présentés par les ongles. *Arch Gén Méd* 1846; **11**: 447–9.
5 Weismann K. Lines of Beau: possible markers of zinc deficiency. *Acta Derm Venereol (Stockh)* 1977; **57**: 88–90.

Pitting

Pitting presents as punctate erosions in the nail surface. Individual pits may be shallow or deep, with a regular or irregular outline. The individual pits of psoriasis are said to be less regular in form and in overall pattern than those of alopecia areata, but this is not always the case. When numerous, they appear randomly distributed upon the nail surface, or have a geometric pattern. The latter may cause rippling or create a grid of pits. Extensive pitting combined with other surface irregularities results in the appearance of *trachyonychia*. An isolated large pit may produce a localized full-thickness defect in the nail plate termed *elkonyxis*, which is found in Reiter's disease, psoriasis and following trauma.

Histologically, pits represent foci of parakeratosis, reflecting isolated nail malformation [1].

REFERENCE

1 Zaias N. Psoriasis of the nail. A clinicopathologic study. *Arch Dermatol* 1969; **99**: 567–79.

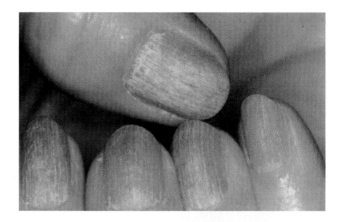

Fig. 65.11 Trachyonychia: roughened surface of up to 20 nails.

Trachyonychia

Trachyonychia presents as a rough surface affecting all of the nail plate and up to 20 nails [1] (20-nail dystrophy). The original French term was sand-blasted nails, which evokes the main clinical feature of a grey, roughened surface (Fig. 65.11). It is mainly associated with alopecia areata [2], psoriasis and lichen planus, although the most common presentation is as an isolated nail abnormality. In the isolated form, histology shows spongiosis and a lymphocytic infiltrate [3] of the nail matrix. It may present as a self-limiting condition in childhood or as a more chronic problem in adulthood. There is some response to potent topical, locally injected and systemic steroids, but this may be temporary. Childhood forms normally resolve spontaneously.

REFERENCES

1 Samman PD. Trachyonychia (rough nails). *Br J Dermatol* 1979; **101**: 701.
2 Baran R. Twenty nail dystrophy of alopecia areata. *Arch Dermatol* 1981; **117**: 1.
3 Tosti A, Fanti PA, Morelli R *et al.* Spongiotic trachyonychia. *Arch Dermatol* 1991; **127**: 584–5.

Onychoschizia

Onychoschizia is also known as lamellar dystrophy and is characterized by transverse splitting into layers at or near the free edge (Fig. 65.12) in fingers and toes, especially in infants [1]. This can result in discoloration because of sequestration of debris between the layers. Variants include splitting at the lateral margins alone and multiple crenellated splits at the free edge. It is seldom associated with any systemic disorder, although it has been reported with polycythaemia [2].

Scanning electron microscopy illustrates the tendency of the lamellar structure of nail to separate after repeated immersion in water [3], but case–control studies show that

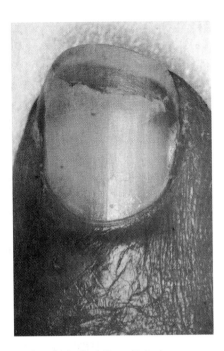

Fig. 65.12 Onychoschizia (lamellar splitting).

occupation is not a major determinant of the condition [4]. However, efforts at retaining hydration (gloves, emollient and base coat with nail varnish) may help reverse clinical changes. Biotin has been used as systemic therapy, but the evidence for its efficacy is weak [5].

REFERENCES

1 Scher RK. Brittle nails. *Int J Dermatol* 1989; **28**: 515–16.
2 Graham-Brown RAC, Holmes R. Lamellar nail dystrophy with poly-cythaemia. *Clin Exp Dermatol* 1980; **5**: 209–12.
3 Wallis MS, Bowen WR, Guin JR. Pathogenesis of onychoschizia (lamellar dystrophy). *J Am Acad Dermatol* 1991; **24**: 44–8.
4 Lubach D, Beckers P. Wet working conditions increase brittleness of nails but do not cause it. *Dermatology* 1992; **185**: 120–2.
5 Colombo VE, Gerber F, Bronhofer M *et al.* Treatment of brittle fingernails and onychoschizia with biotin: scanning electron microscopy. *J Am Acad Dermatol* 1990; **23**: 1127–32.

Brittle nails

Brittle nails [1–3] are often associated with onychoschizia and frequent immersion of the hands in water, especially if alkaline. Treatment is the same as for onychoschizia. Other common causes are iron deficiency anaemia and impaired peripheral circulation. A rare cause is disturbance of arginine metabolism, when it is also associated with diffuse alopecia [4].

REFERENCES

1 Baran R, Barth J, Dawber RPR, eds. Fragile, brittle and soft nails. In: *Nail Disorders*. London: Dunitz, 1991: 137–44.
2 Kechijian P. Brittle fingernails. *Dermatol Clin* 1985; **3**: 421–9.
3 Scher RK. Brittle nails. *Int J Dermatol* 1989; **28**: 515–16.
4 Shelley WB, Rawnsley HM. Aminogenic alopecia: loss of hair associated with arginosuccinic aciduria. *Lancet* 1965; **ii**: 1327–8.

Beading and ridging

Beading and ridging have been described as occurring more often than normal in patients with rheumatoid arthritis [1]. More recently, increased beading has been examined using optical profilometry in patients taking itraconazole for onychomycosis [2]. Itraconazole is known to increase the rate of nail growth, and it was proposed that beading may be a feature of this increase. As beading is more commonly a feature of old age, when nail growth rate slows down, one would not expect beading to correspond directly to faster linear nail growth. Both beading and ridging are common signs in normal ageing patients and at present their significance remains unclear.

REFERENCES

1 Hamilton EDB. Nail studies in rheumatoid arthritis. *Ann Rheum Dis* 1960; **19**: 167–73.
2 de Doncker P, Pierard GE. Acquired nail beading in patients receiving itraconazole—an indicator of faster nail growth? A study using optical profilometry. *Clin Exp Dermatol* 1994; **19**: 404–6.

Changes in colour [1–7]

Alteration in nail colour may arise through changes affecting the dorsal nail surface, the substance of the nail plate, the undersurface of the nail or the nail bed.

Exogenous pigment

Exogenous pigment on the upper surface is easy to demonstrate by scraping the nail. If the proximal margin of the pigment is an arc matching the proximal nail fold, that is a further clue confirming an exogenous source. Often, the cuticle is less absorbent than nail and there will be a narrow proximal margin of unstained nail. This margin will broaden as the period since exposure lengthens. Hence the 'quitters' nail, demonstrating the cessation of smoking and nicotine-free fingers for 2 months.

Exogenous pigment on the undersurface of the nail is less easy to demonstrate and may mean that part or all of the nail needs to be avulsed in order to scrape the undersurface and examine it separate from the nail bed. The green pigment of *Pseudomonas* infection [6] in association with onycholysis is a typical situation where partial avulsion is the best way to demonstrate the site of pigmentation, although it may not always be the best treatment.

Nail-plate changes

The substance of the nail plate can be changed by the

addition of pigment or the alteration of the normal cellular and intercellular organization such that there is loss of normal lucency. Pigment is typically added in the form of melanin produced by matrix melanocytes during nail formation. This produces a brown longitudinal streak the entire length of the nail. In white people this is abnormal and requires thorough assessment and, in some instances, biopsy. In darker-skinned races it is a common variant. The inclusion of heavy metals and some drugs into the nail via the matrix can also produce altered nail-plate colour, such as a grey colour associated with silver. The disruption of normal nail-plate formation by disease, chemotherapy, poisons or trauma can result in waves of parakeratotic nail cells or small splits between cells within the nail. Both make the nail less lucent and produce the white marks of true *leukonychia*. Transmission electron microscopy suggests that there is a change in collagen fibre organization, which might provide an intracellular basis for altered diffractive properties. This disruption can be achieved at nail formation or subsequently in the case of fungal nail infection, where discoloration may start distolaterally, rather than via the matrix.

Nail-bed changes

In addition to generalized vascular changes in the nail bed, there can be localized changes, as seen with nail bed tumours. In the instance of a glomus tumour, this may be the sole method of localization and arises because of the differential blood supply in the tumour and surrounding nail bed. Subungual hyperkeratosis, or the inclusion of drugs (antimalarials, phenothiazines) may also change the apparent colour of the nail. Splinter haemorrhages, representing ruptured nail-bed vessels, deposit haemoglobin on the undersurface of the nail, which grows out.

REFERENCES

1 Baran R. Longitudinal melanotic streaks as a clue to Laugier–Hunziker syndrome. *Arch Dermatol* 1979; **115**: 1448–9.
2 Daniel CR. Nail pigmentation abnormalities. *Dermatol Clin* 1985; **3**: 431–43.
3 Daniel CR, Zaias N. Pigmentary abnormalities of the nails with emphasis on systemic diseases. *Dermatol Clin* 1988; **6**: 305–13.
4 Higashi N. Melanonychia due to tinea unguium. *Hifu* 1990; **32**: 379–80.
5 Lovemann AB, Fliegelman MT. Discoloration of the nails. *Arch Dermatol* 1955; **72**: 153.
6 Shellow WVR, Koplon BS. Green striped nails: chromonychia due to *Pseudomonas aeruginosa*. *Arch Dermatol* 1963; **97**: 149.
7 Zaias N. Onychomycosis. *Arch Dermatol* 1972; **105**: 263–74.

True leukonychia

White discoloration of the nail attributable to matrix dysfunction occurs in a variety of patterns [1,2]. There is the rare, inherited form called total leukonychia, in which all nails are milky porcelain white [3]. In subtotal

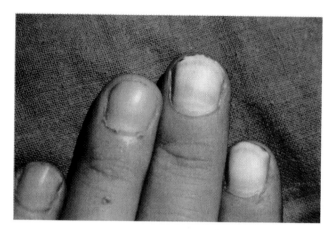

Fig. 65.13 True leukonychia with white nail in the distal free edge.

leukonychia, the proximal two-thirds are white, becoming pink distally. This is attributed to a delay in keratin maturation, and the nail may still appear white at the distal overhang (Fig. 65.13).

Transverse leukonychia (Mees' line) reflects a systemic disorder, such as chemotherapy or poisoning [4], affecting matrix function. The 1–2-mm-wide transverse band is in the arcuate form of the lunula and is analogous to a Beau's line, with which it is occasionally found. Punctate leukonychia is comprised of 1–3-mm-diameter white spots attributed to minor matrix trauma (e.g. manicure) and is also seen in alopecia areata. The pattern and number of spots may change as the nail grows. With longitudinal leukonychia, there is a parakeratotic focus in the matrix, sometimes attributable to Darier's disease or a small tumour.

REFERENCES

1 Albright SD, Wheeler CE. Leukonychia: total and partial leukonychia in a single family with review of the literature. *Arch Dermatol* 1964; **90**: 392–9.
2 Grossman M, Scher RK. Leukonychia: review and classification. *Int J Dermatol* 1990; **29**: 535–41.
3 Baran R, Dawber RPR, eds. *Diseases of the Nails and their Management*. Oxford: Blackwell Scientific Publications, 1994: 72.
4 Marino MT. Mees' lines. *Arch Dermatol* 1990; **126**: 827–8.

Apparent leukonychia

In apparent leukonychia, changes in the nail bed are responsible for the white appearance [1,2]. Nail-bed pallor may be a non-specific sign of anaemia, oedema or vascular impairment. It may occur in particular patterns which have become associated with certain conditions.

Terry's nail

This is white proximally and normal distally and is attributed to cirrhosis, congestive cardiac failure and adult-onset diabetes mellitus [3]. Nail-bed biopsy reveals only mild changes of increased vascularity. This is similar to *half-and-half nails*, where there is a proximal white zone and distal (20–60%) brownish sharp demarcation, the histology of which suggests an increase of vessel wall thickness and melanin deposition. It is seen in 9–50% of chronic renal failure patients and after chemotherapy. It is unclear whether the variant *Neapolitan nails*, where there are bands of white, brown and red, is a version of half-and-half or Terry's nails, or a feature of old age.

Muehrcke's paired white bands

These bands are parallel to the lunula in the nail bed, with pink between two white lines. They are commonly associated with hypoalbuminaemia, the correction of which by albumin infusion can reverse the sign.

REFERENCES

1 Albright SD, Wheeler CE. Leukonychia: total and partial leukonychia in a single family with review of the literature. *Arch Dermatol* 1964; **90**: 392–9.
2 Grossman M, Scher RK. Leukonychia: review and classification. *Int J Dermatol* 1990; **29**: 535–41.
3 Holzberg M, Walker HK. Terry's nails: revised definition and new correlations. *Lancet* 1984; **i**: 896–9.

Colour changes due to drugs [1]

There are a number of colour changes which are due to drugs. Yellowing of the nail is a rare occurrence in prolonged tetracycline therapy, which can also produce a pattern of dark distal photo-onycholysis associated with photo-sensitivity [2]. The whole nail is affected and returns to normal when the drug is discontinued. A similar effect, but of a bluish colour, is seen with mepacrine [3], the nails fluorescing yellow–green or white when viewed under Wood's light. Normal nails show slight fluorescence of violet–blue colour.

Chloroquine may produce blue–black pigmentation of the nail bed [4]. Other antimalarials may produce longitudinal or vertical bands of pigmentation on the nail bed or in the nail [5,6]. A fixed drug eruption of the nail bed can be dark blue [7]. Argyria may discolour the nails slate blue [8], and inorganic arsenic may produce longitudinal bands of pigment or transverse white stripes (*Mees' stripes*) across the nail.

Hyperpigmentation due to increase in melanin in the nail and nail bed has been noted in children after 6 weeks of treatment with doxorubicin (adriamycin) [9,10]. Other similar cytotoxic drugs may cause a variety of patterns of increased pigmentation [1]. However, in acquired immunodeficiency syndrome (AIDS), longitudinal melanonychia may be seen in untreated cases [11,12] as well as those receiving zidovudine [9,13].

REFERENCES

1 Baran R, Dawber RPR, eds. *Diseases of the Nails and their Management*. Oxford: Blackwell Scientific Publications, 1994: 63.
2 Orentreich N, Harber LC, Tromovitch TH. Photosensitivity and photo-onycholysis due to demethylchlortetracycline. *Arch Dermatol* 1961; **83**: 730–7.
3 Mallon E, Dawber RPR. Longitudinal melanonychia induced by minocycline. *Br J Dermatol* 1994; **130**: 794–5.
4 Tuffanelli D, Abraham RK, Dubois E. Pigmentation from antimalarial drugs. *Arch Dermatol* 1963; **88**: 419–26.
5 Colomb D. Antimalarial nail pigmentation. *Bull Soc Fr Dermatol Syphiligr* 1975; **82**: 319–22.
6 Maguire A. Antimalarial nail pigmentation. *Lancet* 1963; **i**: 667–71.
7 Wise F, Sulzberger MB. Drug eruptions. *Arch Dermatol Syphilol* 1933; **27**: 549–67.
8 Ramelli G. Argyria. *Cutis* 1972; **10**: 155–9.
9 Goark SP, Hood AF, Nelson K. Nail pigmentation associated with zidovudine. *J Am Acad Dermatol* 1984; **5**: 1032–3.
10 Pratt CB, Shanks EC. Hyperpigmentation of the nails due to doxorubicin. *JAMA* 1974; **228**: 460.
11 Fisher BK, Warner LC. Cutaneous manifestations of AIDS. *Int J Dermatol* 1987; **16**: 615–30.
12 Panwalker A. Nail pigmentation in AIDS. *Ann Intern Med* 1987; **107**: 943–4.
13 Gallais V, Lacour JPh, Perrin C *et al*. Acral hyperpigmented macules and longitudinal melanonychia in AIDS patients. *Br J Dermatol* 1992; **126**: 387–91.

Yellow-nail syndrome

The nails in yellow-nail syndrome are yellow due to thickening, sometimes with a tinge of green possibly due to secondary infection. The lunula is obscured and there is increased transverse and longitudinal curvature and loss of cuticle (Fig. 65.14). Occasionally, there is chronic paronychia with onycholysis and transverse ridging [1]. The condition usually presents in adults, but may occur as early as the age of 8 years [2]. The features are usually accompanied by lymphoedema [3] at one or more sites and respiratory or nasal sinus disease. The nails grow at a greatly reduced rate: 0.1–0.25 mm/week for fingernails compared with the lowest normal 0.5 mm/week. All 20 nails may be involved, although often a few are spared.

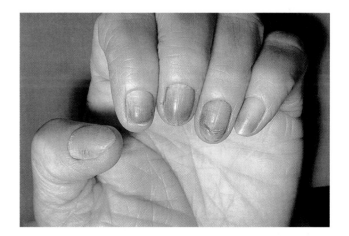

Fig. 65.14 Yellow-nail syndrome.

Histologically, in the nail bed and matrix, dense fibrous tissue is found replacing subungual stroma, with numerous ectatic, endothelium-lined vessels [4]. A foreign-body reaction has been noted [5]. It has been suggested that obstruction of lymphatics by this dense stroma leads to the abnormal lymphatic function found in the affected digits in some instances [6], but not all [7].

The oedema most frequently affects the legs, and may not be seen for some months after the nail change has been noted. Less often it affects the face or hands and occasionally it is universal. Recurrent pleural effusions have been noted in a few cases [8,9]. Chronic bronchitis and bronchiectasis may also occur [10]. The oedema has been shown to be due to abnormalities of the lymphatics, either atresia, or varicosity in some cases [9]. As some cases seem to have normal lymphatics, it is possible that a functional rather than an anatomical defect may be present [11], or perhaps only the smallest lymph vessels are defective. Although the nail changes may draw attention to the underlying lymphatic abnormality, they are found only in a minority of patients with congenital abnormality of the lymphatics. The condition may be associated with an increased incidence of malignant neoplasms [9,12,13]. Other associations include D-penicillamine therapy [3] and nephrotic syndrome [14]. In hypothyroidism and AIDS [15] there may be yellow nails, but it is debatable whether these represent yellow-nail syndrome, or simply the discoloration of nail associated with retarded growth [16].

Although the nail changes, once established, are usually permanent, complete reversion to normal may occur at times. Attempted treatments include oral [17] and topical vitamin E [18], oral zinc [19] and treatment of chronic infection at other sites [20].

REFERENCES

1 Samman PD, White WF. The 'yellow nail' syndrome. *Br J Dermatol* 1964; **76**: 153–7.
2 Magid M, Esterly NB, Prendiville J, Fujisaki C. The yellow nail syndrome in an 8 year old girl. *Pediatr Dermatol* 1987; **4**: 90–3.
3 Ilchyshin A, Vickers CFH. Yellow nail syndrome associated with penicillamine therapy. *Acta Derm Venereol (Stockh)* 1983; **63**: 554–5.
4 De Coste SD, Imber MJ, Baden HP. Yellow nail syndrome. *J Am Acad Dermatol* 1990; **22**: 608–11.
5 Mallon E, Dawber RPR. Nail unit histopathology in the yellow nail syndrome. *Br J Dermatol* 1995; **133** (Suppl. 45): 55.
6 Fenton DA, Bull R, Gane J et al. Abnormal lymphatic function assessed by quantitative lymphoscintigraphy in the yellow nail syndrome. *Br J Dermatol* 1990; **123** (Suppl. 37): 32.
7 Ellis JP, Marks R, Pery BJ. Lymphatic function: the disappearance rate of ^{131}albumin from the dermis. *Br J Dermatol* 1970; **82**: 593–9.
8 Emerson PA. Yellow nails, lymphoedema and pleural effusions. *Thorax* 1966; **21**: 247–53.
9 Miller E, Rosenow EC, Olsen AM. Pulmonary manifestations of the yellow nail syndrome. *Chest* 1972; **61**: 452–8.
10 Dilley JJ, Kierland RR, Randall RV et al. Primary lymphoedema associated with yellow nails and pleural effusions. *Br J Med* 1968; **204**: 670–3.
11 Bull RH, Fenton DA, Mortimer PS. Lymphatic function in the yellow nail syndrome. *Br J Dermatol* 1996; **134**: 307–12.
12 Burrows NP, Russell Jones R. Yellow nail syndrome in association with carcinoma of the gall bladder. *Clin Exp Dermatol* 1991; **16**: 471–3.
13 Stosiek N, Peters KP, Hiller D et al. OP. Yellow nail syndrome in a patient with mycosis fungoides. *J Am Acad Dermatol* 1993; **28**: 792–4.
14 Cockram CS, Richards P. Yellow nails and nephrotic syndrome. *Br J Dermatol* 1979; **101**: 707–9.
15 Chernosky ME, Finley VK. Yellow nail syndrome in patients with AIDS. *J Am Acad Dermatol* 1985; **13**: 731–6.
16 Scher RK. Acquired immunodeficiency syndrome and yellow nails. *J Am Acad Dermatol* 1988; **18**: 758–9.
17 Ayres S, Mihan R. Yellow nail syndrome. Response to vitamin E. *Arch Dermatol* 1973; **108**: 267–8.
18 Williams HC, Buffham R, du Vivier A. Successful use of topical vitamin E solution in the treatment of nail changes in yellow nail syndrome. *Arch Dermatol* 1991; **127**: 1023–8.
19 Arroyo JF, Cohen ML. Yellow nail syndrome cured by zinc supplementation. *Clin Exp Dermatol* 1993; **18**: 62–4.
20 Pang SM. Yellow nail syndrome resolution following treatment of pulmonary tuberculosis. *Int J Dermatol* 1993; **32**: 605–6.

Red lunulae

Erythema of all or part of the lunula may affect all digits, but most prominently the thumb. Erythema is less intense in the distal lunula, where it can merge with the nail bed or be demarcated by a pale line, and can be obliterated by pressure on the nail plate. The appearance can fade over a few days. A single report of histological features failed to reveal vascular or epidermal changes [1]. Dotted red lunulae have been reported in psoriasis and alopecia areata, but otherwise changes the list of associations is so broad as to be unconvincing [2].

REFERENCES

1 Cohen PR. Red lunulae: case report and review of the literature. *J Am Acad Dermatol* 1992; **26**: 292–4.
2 Wilkerson MG. Wilkin JK. Red lunulae revisited: a clinical and histopathologic examination. *J Am Acad Dermatol* 1989; **20**: 453–7.

Splinter haemorrhages

Splinter haemorrhages represent longitudinal haemorrhages in the nail bed conforming to the pattern of subungual vessels [1–4]. They are most frequently seen in the distal nail bed and on the fingers of the dominant hand reflecting trauma as the cause. In dermatological practice, they are often found in association with psoriasis, dermatitis and fungal infection of the nails. As they occur under so many conditions, their importance as a sign of disease is often exaggerated.

Large numbers of proximal haemorrhages with no obvious traumatic origin may indicate a systemic cause [5], such as bacterial endocarditis or antiphospholipid syndrome [6]. Unilateral splinters may arise after arterial catheterization on the involved side. Examination under oil with an ophthalmoscope may reveal greater detail.

REFERENCES

1 Heath D, Williams DR. Nail haemorrhages. *Br Heart J* 1978; **40**: 1300–5.
2 Kilpatrick ZM, Greenberg PA, Sanford JP. Splinter haemorrhages, their clinical significance. *Arch Intern Med* 1965; **115**: 730–5.
3 Monk BE. The prevalence of splinter haemorrhages. *Br J Dermatol* 1980; **103**: 183–5.
4 Young JB, Will EJ, Mulley GP. Splinter haemorrhages: facts and fiction. *J R Coll Phys Lond* 1988; **22**: 240–3.
5 Gross NJ, Tall R. Clinical significance of splinter haemorrhages. *Br Med J* 1963; **ii**: 1496–8.
6 Ames DE, Asherson RA, Aynes B *et al*. Bilateral adrenal infarction, hypoadrenalism and splinter haemorrhages in the primary antiphospholipid syndrome. *Br J Rheumatol* 1994; **31**: 117–20.

Developmental abnormalities of the nails [1,2]

Anonychia

Absence of the nails from birth is a rare congenital anomaly. It may occur as an isolated sign or be accompanied by other defects of the digits and other structures. Littman and Levin [3] described a girl with seven nails missing, and reported that her brother was similarly affected; it was suggested that this was a recessive trait. The mode of inheritance of most of these disorders has not yet been established with certainty. The condition described as anonychia with ectrodactylia [4] has been investigated more fully, however, and has been shown to be inherited as a dominant trait without sex linkage. In this condition, there is usually complete absence of the nails on the index and middle fingers, and when there is any nail on the thumb it is often present on the proximal lateral corners of the nail fold. On the ring fingers, the radial half of the nail is often absent, and the nail bed is also missing. In a minority of affected individuals there are striking and bizarre defects of the digits, sometimes restricted to one hand or foot. The defects usually take the form of absence of one or more digits. Two sisters in a sibship of five, whose parents were first cousins, are recorded as having rudimentary nails associated with congenital deafness. The parents showed neither abnormality [5]. Bart *et al*. [6] described a family with congenital absence of areas of skin, blistering of skin and mucous membranes, and absence or deformity of the nails inherited as an autosomal dominant trait. It is now classified as a subtype of dominantly inherited dystrophic epidermolysis bullosa, with the responsible gene mapped to chromosome 3p [7]. Verbov [8] described a case with bizarre flexural pigmentation and anonychia, thought to be an autosomal dominant condition.

REFERENCES

1 Juhlin L, Baran R. In: Baran R, Dawber RPR, eds. *Diseases of the Nails and their Management*, 2nd edn. Oxford: Blackwell Scientific Publications, 1994: 297–9.
2 Telfer NR, Barth JH, Dawber RPR. Congenital and hereditary nail dystrophies—an embryological approach to classification. *Clin Exp Dermatol* 1988; **13**: 160–3.
3 Littman A, Levin S. Autosomal recessive anonychia. *J Invest Dermatol* 1964; **42**: 177–80.
4 Lees DH. Anonychia and ectrodactylia. *Ann Hum Genet* 1957; **22**: 69–71.
5 Feinmesser M, Zelig S. Anonychia and congenital deafness. *Arch Otolaryngol* 1962; **74**: 507–10.
6 Bart BJ, Gorlin RJ, Anderson E *et al*. Congenital localised absence of skin; associated abnormalities resembling epidermolysis bullosa. *Arch Dermatol* 1966; **93**: 296–304.
7 Zelickson B, Matsumara K, Kist D *et al*. Bart's syndrome. *Arch Dermatol* 1995; **131**: 663–8.
8 Verbov J. Anonychia with bizarre flexural pigmentation—an autosomal dominant dermatosis. *Br J Dermatol* 1975; **92**: 469–74.

Nail–patella syndrome

This uncommon condition is of special interest because it involves abnormalities of ectodermal and mesodermal structure. It is inherited as an autosomal dominant trait with linkage between the locus controlling the syndrome and that of the ABO blood groups [1]. In a typical case, the nails are grossly defective, being only one-third or half the normal size and never reaching the free edge of the finger [2]. In other cases, the thumbnails alone may be defective or only the ulnar half of each may be missing [3]. In every case, the thumbnails are most affected [4] and the remaining nails, if involved, are progressively less damaged from index to little finger. The half moons may be triangular, with a distal peak (Fig. 65.15) in the midline [5]. Even when the nail is completely missing, the nail bed is present. In addition to the nail changes, the patellae are smaller than normal and may be rudimentary, so that the knees are unstable. There are also bony spines arising

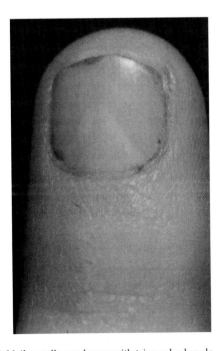

Fig. 65.15 Nail–patella syndrome with triangular lunula.

from the posterior aspect of the iliac bones, visible on X-ray examination.

Other recorded features include hyperextension of the joints, skin laxity, hyperhidrosis [6] and renal abnormalities [7,8].

In 1965 there were 255 patients with this syndrome known to be living in the UK, and the prevalence is estimated at one per 22 million. The mutation rate is estimated at one per 1.9 million alleles per generation [9].

The condition must be distinguished from congenital ectodermal defects and pachyonychia congenita.

REFERENCES

1 Renwick JH. *The genetics of the nail–patella syndrome.* MD thesis, London University, 1956.
2 Renwick JH, Izatt MM. Some genetic parameters of the nail–patella locus. *Ann Hum Genet* 1965; **28**: 369–78.
3 Levan NE. Congenital defect of thumbnails. *Arch Dermatol Syphilol* 1961; **83**: 938–40.
4 Guidera KJ, Satterwhite Y, Ogden JA *et al*. Nail patella syndrome: a review of 44 orthopaedic patients. *J Paediatr Orthop* 1991; **11**: 737–42.
5 Daniel CR, Osment LS, Noojin RO. Triangular lunulae; a clue to nail patella syndrome. *Arch Dermatol* 1980; **116**: 448–9.
6 Pechman KJ, Bergfield WF. Hyperhidrosis in nail–patella syndrome. *J Am Acad Dermatol* 1980; **3**: 627–30.
7 Ben Bassat M. The glomerulo-basement membrane in nail–patella syndrome. *Arch Pathol* 1971; **92**: 350–5.
8 Goodman RM. Hereditary congenital deafness with onychodystrophy. *Arch Otolaryngol* 1959; **90**: 474–7.
9 Renwick JH, Lawler SD. Genetic linkage between the ABO and nail–patella loci. *Ann Hum Genet* 1955; **19**: 312–31.

Congenital onychodysplasia of the index fingers

SYN. ISO KIKUCHI SYNDROME [1,2]

In this condition, the nail of the index finger is absent, small or represented by two nails of unequal size. There may be a family history suggestive of autosomal dominant inheritance, but there is frequently no clear genetic pattern, and involvement of other digits has been reported [1,3,4]. Underlying changes in the distal phalanx can usually be demonstrated by lateral X-ray, where bifurcation of the distal phalanx is the norm [4]. Syndactyly is an associated hand anomaly in some cases [2].

REFERENCES

1 Baran R. Syndrome d'Iso Kikuchi (COIF syndrome); 2 cas avec revue de la littérature. *Acta Derm Venereol (Stockh)* 1980; **107**: 431–5.
2 Miura T, Nakamura R. Congenital onychodysplasia of the index fingers. *J Hand Surg* 1990; **15A**: 793–7.
3 Kikuchi I, Horikawa S, Amano F. Congenital onychodysplasia of the index fingers. *Arch Dermatol* 1974; **110**: 743–6.
4 Kikuchi I. Congenital onychodysplasia of the index fingers: a case involving the thumb nails. *Semin Dermatol* 1991; **10**: 7–11.

Pachyonychia congenita (Fig. 65.16)

This is a rare genodermatosis in which hypertrophy of the nails occurs, in some cases associated with nail bed

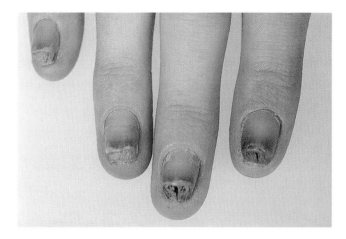

Fig. 65.16 Pachyonychia congenita.

and hyponychial hyperkeratosis [1,2]. It is important to establish the site of abnormal nail plate production if therapy is to be directed at surgical removal or ablation of the responsible tissue. Autosomal dominant inheritance is the rule, although Haber and Rose [3] described cases transmitted in an autosomal recessive form. A heterozygous missense mutation in the helix initiation motif for keratin 17 is found in Jackson–Lawler pachyonychia congenita (MIM #167210, PC-2) and there is a similar fault in the keratin 16 gene in the Jadassohn–Lewandosky (MIM #167200, PC-1) form of the disease [4]. This form is also reported as suffering a heterozygous deletion in a keratin 6 isoform (K6a) in the affected members of a Slovenian family [5].

The thickened nails can be treated surgically in some instances [6,7].

Type 1. Jadassohn–Lewandosky type. The nails are normal at birth but within months they become discoloured and progressively thicken, more so on the hands than feet. Typical associated findings include palmar and plantar hyperkeratosis and warty skin lesions at various sites: knees, elbows, buttocks, legs, ankles and popliteal region. Acral bullae may be crippling and hyperhidrosis may be severe. Mouth and corneal dyskeratosis are less common findings.

Type 2. Uniform nail thickening occurs; *Candida* colonization may be found in some of the nails associated with chronic mucosal candidiasis, suggesting an immune defect.

Type 3. Jackson–Lawler type. In this type, with less severe nail thickening and keratoses than type 1, many associations have been described: erupted teeth at birth; multiple epidermal cysts; sebocystomatosis; dry, lustreless and kinky scalp hair; eyebrows that stand straight out; hamartomas.

Type 4. Nail thickening and keratoses are associated with widespread macular pigmentation, mainly flexural. Cutaneous amyloidosis was noted in one pedigree [8].

The single case described by Sharma *et al.* [9], in which convulsions and fundal phakomas occurred, also had tuberous sclerosis.

REFERENCES

1 Feinstein A, Friedman J, Schwach-Millet M. Pachyonychia congenita. *J Am Acad Dermatol* 1988; **19**: 705–11.
2 Samman PD. Developmental abnormalities. In: Samman PD, Fenton DA, eds. *The Nails in Disease*. London: Heinemann, 1986: 168–93.
3 Haber RM, Rose TH. Autosomal recessive pachyonychia congenita. *J Am Acad Dermatol* 1986; **122**: 919–23.
4 McLean WHI, Rugg EL, Lunny DP *et al.* Keratin 16 and keratin 17 mutations cause pachyonychia congenita. *Nature Genet* 1995; **9**: 273–8.
5 Bowden PE, Haley JL, Kansky A *et al.* Mutation of a type II keratin gene (K6a) in pachyonychia congenita. *Nature Genet* 1995; **10**: 363–78.
6 Cosman B, Symonds FC, Crikelair GF. Plastic surgery in pachyonychia congenita and other dyskeratoses. *Plast Reconstr Surg* 1964; **33**: 226–41.
7 Thomsen RJ, Zuehlke RL, Beckman BL. Pachyonychia congenita. Surgical management of the nail changes. *J Dermatol Surg Oncol* 1982; **8**: 24.
8 Tidman MJ, Wells RS, MacDonald DM. Pachyonychia congenita with cutaneous amyloidosis and hyperpigmentation: a distinct variant. *J Am Acad Dermatol* 1987; **16**: 935–40.
9 Sharma VK, Sharma R, Kaus S. Pachyonychia congenita with tuberous sclerosis. *Int J Dermatol* 1989; **28**: 332–3.

Infections of the nail and nail folds

Fungal nail infections

See Chapter 31.

Paronychia

Bacterial paronychia

Acute paronychia is a common complaint and is usually due to staphylococcal infection. It may result from local injuries, splits, splinters or nail biting, or there may be no preceding injury. It also occurs frequently as a complication of chronic paronychia, when other organisms may be involved, including streptococci, *Pseudomonas pyocyanea*, coliform organisms and *Proteus vulgaris*.

The condition presents as a painful swelling of the nail fold. If superficial it may point close to the nail and can easily be drained by incision with a size 11 scalpel, without anaesthesia [1]. Deeper lesions are best treated by antibiotics in the first place, but if they do not improve within 2 days, incision under local anaesthesia is required, particularly in childhood. A broad-spectrum antibiotic is preferred because it is unlikely that the organisms can be identified in advance. Some authorities recommend removing the proximal one-third of the nailplate without initial incisional drainage. This gives more rapid relief and more sustained drainage.

REFERENCE

1 Keyser JJ, Littler JW, Eaton RG. Surgical treatment of infections and lesions of the perionychium. *Hand Clin* 1990; **6**: 137–53.

Chronic paronychia

This is one of the commonest specific nail complaints met within dermatological practice. It ranks in importance with fungal infections and psoriasis as a cause of nail disease, but presents more commonly and is often misdiagnosed and mistreated. It occurs in those who have chronically wet hands, especially if the hands are also cold [1,2]. Wet foods are a combined source of factors, where the food may be an irritant [3]. It is predominantly a disease of domestic workers, bar staff, canteen workers and fishmongers [4]. The majority of cases are in patients between 30 and 60 years of age [1], although chronic paronychia is also seen in children, especially as a result of finger- or thumbsucking [5].

A background of endogenous eczema is common such that irritant reactions are easily initiated and made chronic. It is also common in diabetes [2]. Any finger may be involved, most often the index and middle fingers of the right hand and the middle finger of the left [4]. These fingers may be more subject to minor trauma than the remainder. The condition begins as a slight swelling at the base of one or more nails (Fig. 65.17), which is tender, but much less so than in acute paronychia. The cuticle is soon lost and pus may form below the nail fold. Inflammation adjacent to the matrix disturbs nail growth, resulting in irregular transverse ridges and other surface irregularities, which may be combined with discoloration (Fig. 65.17). There is some evidence that the darkening is due to the pigment from *Pseudomonas* infection of the nail [6]. In long-standing cases, the size of the nail may be reduced, and this reduction is exaggerated by bolstering of the fold all around the nail. Most of the nail deformity is due to the inflammation interfering with the formation of the nail, but a true *Candida* infection of the nail plate is occasionally seen.

There is a complex relationship with *Candida*, usually *Candida albicans* [7], which may be identified by swabs or scraping. Stone and Mullins [8] showed that chronic paronychia can be produced by non-viable *C. albicans* introduced into a relatively sterile nail fold. Much of the chronic inflammation seen in this disorder probably arises from an irritant reaction to material sequestered beneath the proximal nail fold. The loss of the cuticle means that detergent and other solvents may gain access to this tight space and act like a prolonged irritant patch test. This chronic non-infective inflammatory component is why topical steroids are useful in addition to antimicrobials as part of the treatment. Acute exacerbations occur from time to time and are due to secondary bacterial infection. Various

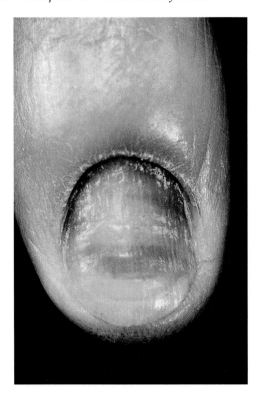

Fig. 65.17 Chronic paronychia with nail-plate discoloration due to *Pseudomonas pyocyanea*.

organisms may be found, including *Staphylococcus aureus* or *albus*, *Proteus vulgaris*, *Escherichia coli* and *Pseudomonas pyocyanea*. Barlow *et al.* [9] consider *Staphylococcus aureus* plays a more active part in initiating the process by penetrating the keratin at the base of the nail and opening up the nail fold. The role of *S. aureus* as a superantigen may also be relevant. Ingested allergens may also play a part [10].

Treatment. Treatment is a combination of avoidance of precipitants, hand care and medication. Perhaps the most important part of the treatment, but the one most difficult to achieve, is to keep the hands dry. For all wet work the patients should be advised to wear cotton gloves under rubber gloves and avoid manicure of the proximal nail folds. Covering the affected fingers with a porous surgical tape may afford some protection, but normal occlusion aggravates the problem. General hand care with emollient and protection during rough work is useful. If this stage of the therapy is not adequately pursued, the condition is likely to fail to settle whatever medical treatment is provided.

Topical therapy requires a combination of steroid and antimicrobial. The former may be very potent for short periods when there is adequate antimicrobial cover. Injected triamcinolone (2.5 mg/ml) is useful in some instances. Topical imidazoles are usually sufficient to treat *Candida*

and may provide a modest therapy against some bacteria. More potent topical antibacterials may be needed. Barlow *et al.* [9] suggest using gentamicin ointment during the day and nystatin ointment at night. When features are marked, oral antibiotics appropriate for *Staphyloccocus aureus* should be used. Because of the 'mixed' aetiology of the inflammation, many clinicians use antiseptic or antibiotic–anticandida–steroid creams in the chronic phase. However, Wilson [11] recommends 4% thymol in chloroform (not available in the USA) inserted into the groove with a dropper and advocates avoidance of creams.

Incision is not indicated unless the condition enters an acute tender purulent phase, where removal of the proximal third of the nail may help. Attempting to clean out the nail fold with a sharpened orange stick is not recommended. If there is obvious candidal infection elsewhere, or *Candida* onychomycosis, this must also be treated. Cryosurgery, using liquid nitrogen spray to the nail folds, or surgical removal of the proximal nail fold and adjacent part of the lateral nail folds, may cure recalcitrant cases [12–14].

REFERENCES

1 Esteves J. Chronic paronychia. *Dermatologica* 1959; **119**: 229–31.
2 Hellier FF. Chronic paronychia: aetiology and treatment. *Br Med J* 1955; **ii**: 1358–60.
3 Tosti A, Buerra L, Mozelli R *et al.* Role of food in the pathogenesis of chronic paronychia. *J Am Acad Dermatol* 1992; **27**: 706–10.
4 Frain-Bell W. Chronic paronychia. Short review of 590 cases. *Trans St John's Hosp Dermatol Soc* 1957; **38**: 29–35.
5 Stone OJ, Mullins JF. Chronic paronychia in childhood. *Clin Pediatr* 1968; **7**: 104–7.
6 Samman PD. Management of disorders of the nails. *Clin Exp Dermatol* 1982; **7**: 189–94.
7 Marten RH. Chronic paronychia: a mycological and bacteriological study. *Br J Dermatol* 1959; **71**: 422–6.
8 Stone OJ, Mullins JF. Role of *Candida albicans* in chronic disease. *Arch Dermatol* 1965; **91**: 70–2.
9 Barlow AJE, Chattaway FW, Holgate ML *et al.* Chronic paronychia. *Br J Dermatol* 1970; **82**: 448–53.
10 Zaias N. *The Nail in Health and Disease.* Stanford NJ, USA: Appleton & Lange, 1990.
11 Wilson JW. Paronychia and onycholysis; aetiology and therapy. *Arch Dermatol* 1965; **92**: 726–30.
12 Baran R, Bureau H. Surgical treatment of recalcitrant chronic paronychias of the fingers. *J Dermatol Surg Oncol* 1981; **7**: 106–9.
13 Daniel CR. Paronychia. *Dermatol Clin* 1988; **3**: 461–4.
14 Baran R, Barth J, Dawber RPR, eds. Paronychia. In: *Nail Disorders.* London: Dunitz, 1991: 93–101.

Pseudomonas infection

This is almost always a complication of onycholysis or chronic paronychia and is usually restricted to one or two nails (Fig. 65.17). The nail plate has a characteristic bluish-black or green colour [1–3] and smells infected. This colour is due to accumulation of debris below the nail and the pigment pyocyanin adhering to the undersurface of the nail plate. Pigment may remain after the organism has been removed. In some cases, the nail plate appears to be invaded by the bacillus [2]. Treatment [4] is as described for onycholysis or paronychia, whichever appears to be the prominent predisposing state. In addition, it is possible to treat with gentamicin or sulphacetamide eye drops to eradicate the colonization where onycholysis is resistant to therapy.

REFERENCES

1 Bauer MF, Cohen BA. The role of *Pseudomonas aeruginosa* infections about the nails. *Arch Dermatol* 1957; **75**: 394–6.
2 Chernosky ME, Dukes CD. Green nails: importance of *Pseudomonas aeruginosa* in onychia. *Arch Dermatol* 1963; **88**: 548–53.
3 Goldman L, Fox H. Greenish pigmentation of nail plates from *Bacillus pyocyaneus*. *Arch Dermatol* 1944; **49**: 136–7.
4 Samman PD. Topical sulphacetamide for onycholysis. *Clin Exp Dermatol* 1982; **7**: 189–90.

Herpetic paronychia [1,2]
SYN. HERPETIC WHITLOW

This uncommon condition is due to primary inoculation of the herpes simplex virus and presents as single or grouped blisters close to the nail; it may give a honeycomb appearance. Clear at first, the blisters soon become purulent and may break and be replaced by crusts. It is usually very painful and takes about 3 weeks to resolve, with pain settling in half that time. Lymphangitis sometimes occurs and may precede vesiculation. Diagnosis may be established by recovering the virus from a recent blister and by cytological examination of the blister floor. Contact cases may occur.

Treatment probably does little to shorten the course of the disorder, but cleaning with 1/6000 potassium permanganate followed by the application of a bland cream is recommended. Relapse may occur as with other primary herpetic infections. The value of thymidine analogues, such as 5% topical idoxuridine and oral or topical aciclovir, remains unproven at this site; if the lesion is seen within 2 days of onset, topical aciclovir may inhibit progression.

Numbness of the finger has been reported following infection [1] and persistent lymphoedema may occur.

REFERENCES

1 Chang T, Gorbach SL. Primary and recurrent herpetic whitlow. *Int J Dermatol* 1977; **16**: 752–4.
2 Stern H, Elek SD, Millar DM *et al*. Herpetic whitlow; cross-infection in hospitals. *Lancet* 1958; **ii**: 871–4.

Human immunodeficiency virus infection

The nail appears more prone to infection from dermatophytes, yeasts and herpesvirus in those with human immunodeficiency virus (HIV) infection [1]. The patterns of infection may alter, such that proximal subungual white fungal infection is said to be a pointer to immunodeficiency and particularly HIV [2]. The nail folds may be red in the absence of infection [3] and the nail can manifest various patterns of melanonychia, which is usually attributed to zidovudine therapy [4].

REFERENCES

1 Daniel R, Norton LA, Scher RK. The spectrum of nail disease in patients with human immunodeficiency virus infection. *J Am Acad Dermatol* 1992; **27**: 93–7.
2 Dompmartin D, Dompmartin A, Deluol AM *et al*. Onychomycosis and AIDS: clinical and laboratory findings in 62 patients. *Int J Dermatol* 1990; **29**: 337–9.
3 Itin PH, Gilli L, Nüesch R *et al*. Erythema of the proximal nail fold in HIV-infected patients. *J Am Acad Dermatol* 1996; **35**: 631–3.
4 Bendick C, Heinrich R, Steigleder GK. Azidothymidine induced pigmentation of skin and nails. *Arch Dermatol* 1989; **125**: 1285–6.

Dermatoses affecting the nails

Psoriasis

Psoriasis is probably the most common disorder affecting fingernails with consequent dystrophy. Between 1.5 and 3% of the population have psoriasis, and up to 50% of psoriatics have nail involvement [1]. Over a lifetime, this may cumulatively increase to 80–90% [2]. In children, nail involvement ranges from 7% [3] to 39% [4], and pitting has been observed in the first week of life in the offspring of a mother severely affected with psoriasis [5].

Clinical features. When the diagnosis of psoriatic nail dystrophy is in doubt, the main differential diagnoses are onychomycosis and lichen planus. In onychomycosis, the features usually present in the toes, whereas the fingernails are more commonly affected in psoriasis. Equally, there are often changes on the nail surface alone in psoriasis, whereas in onychomycosis, features are usually within or beneath the nail plate. If there is fingernail involvement in onychomycosis, it is usually of only one or a minority of digits, in contrast with psoriasis where there are usually several digits affected.

Some forms of fingernail lichen planus and psoriasis are very difficult to distinguish. Both may result in roughened nails (trachyonychia) with subungual hyperkeratosis. If pits are prominent the diagnosis of psoriasis can be made, but if they are subtle and difficult to distinguish from other surface changes, they may be part of lichen planus. The nails in Reiter's disease and pityriasis rubra pilaris can also be difficult to distinguish from psoriasis [6,7], where distal subungual hyperkeratosis and splinter haemorrhages are common [8]. Aggressive forms of atypical nail psoriasis presenting in later life may represent acrokeratosis paraneoplastica. The patient is usually male, with subungual hyperkeratosis and scaling of the periunguium, ears and nose associated with malignancies of the upper gastrointestinal or respiratory tract [9–11].

Arthritis of the distal interphalangeal joint suggests a psoriatic cause of any associated dystrophy [12], with the exception of changes due to a myxoid pseudocyst associated with adjacent osteoarthritis. Baker *et al.* [13] found that there was no strict relationship between which joints are arthritic and which nails are dystrophic, although Jones *et al.* [14] noted that in a group of 100 psoriatics with arthritis, where there was nail involvement there was a significantly greater chance of there being joint disease in the adjacent distal interphalangeal joint. There was also a

significant correlation between PASI (Psoriasis Area and Severity Index) score and scoring of nail disease, and nail disease increased with the duration of psoriasis. A variant of nail psoriasis presents with pain and soft-tissue swelling of the distal digit associated with psoriatic nail changes and underlying bone erosion and periosteal reaction. This can be in the absence of joint involvement and has been termed psoriatic onychopachydermoperiostitis [15].

In order of reducing frequency, nail signs include pits, onycholysis, subungual hyperkeratosis, nail-plate discoloration, uneven nail surface, splinter haemorrhages, acute and chronic paronychia and transverse midline depressions in the thumb nails.

Pits. Pits more commonly affect fingers than toes (Fig. 65.18). They represent punctate surface depressions arising from proximal matrix disease (Table 65.3). Zaias [1,15] has demonstrated small columns of pathological parakeratotic nail falling off the upper surface of the nail plate to produce a pit. The origin of pits means that they can be influenced by disease in the proximal nail fold and it is thought that injection of triamcinolone into the nail fold alone can suppress this clinical feature. The pattern of pitting may be disorganized, or in transverse/longitudinal rows as seen in alopecia areata [2]. Pits may be shallow or large [16], to the point of leaving a punched-out hole in the nail plate (elkonyxis).

Onycholysis. Focal nail-bed parakeratosis produces an 'oily spot' or 'salmon patch'. Extension of this area to the free

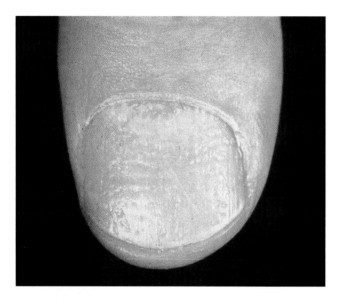

Fig. 65.18 Psoriasis: diffuse pitting.

Clinical feature	Area of disease	Duration of disease
Changes in nail plate	*Matrix*	
Pits	Proximal matrix	Episodic: short
Transverse furrows	Proximal matrix; distal extension depends upon depth of furrow	1–2 weeks
Crumbling nail plate	Entire matrix	Prolonged
Leukonychia with rough surface	Proximal matrix; leukonychia may involve distal matrix	Variable
Changes in nail bed and hyponychium	*Nail bed*	
Splinter haemorrhages	Nail bed dermal ridge haemorrhage	Short duration
Oily spot/onycholysis	Nail bed psoriasis	Prolonged
False nail following onychomadesis	Nail bed psoriasis	Prolonged
Subungual hyperkeratosis	Nail bed psoriasis	Prolonged
Yellow/green discoloration of nail bed	Secondary infection by yeasts or *Pseudomonas*	Prolonged

Table 65.3 Relationship between clinical features and site of disease activity in psoriasis of the nail. (From Zaias [1].)

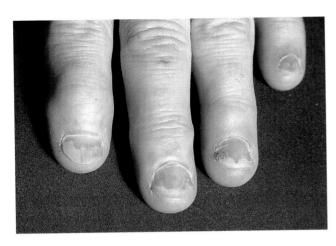

Fig. 65.19 Psoriasis: onycholysis.

edge gives onycholysis, which typically has a reddish brown margin. Alternatively, onycholysis may commence at the distal edge (Fig. 65.19), representing disruption of the onychocorneal band [17]. Once this band of firm attachment has been breached, the condition is often progressive. Minor manicure, wet work and leverage from long nails exacerbates the condition.

Discoloration. Discoloration in psoriasis is multifactorial. The major factors are nail thickening and subungual hyperkeratosis. Both of these contribute to a yellow appearance particularly common in the toes. It is possible that at this site repeated trauma elicits the isomorphic reaction with local exacerbation of psoriasis. The coincidence of onychomycosis and psoriasis is also seen in the toenails [18] and can add to the pathological appearance. *Candida* species and *Pseudomonas* infection can result in green discoloration. While non-dermatophytes and bacteria are common, dermatophytes are rare [1].

Subungual hyperkeratosis. Subungual hyperkeratosis represents nail-bed disease (Fig. 65.20). Substantial nail-plate thickening may result from subungual hyperkeratosis, which is most marked distally and extends proximally. The fingertip may become very tender where there is gross subungual hyperkeratosis, as the nail-plate attachment is greatly reduced and the nail can easily be caught and tug on the matrix attachment. Subungual hyperkeratosis is a prominent feature when pityriasis rubra pilaris affects the nail and is often seen with splinter haemorrhages [6,19].

Nail-plate abnormalities. Splits, atrophy and fragility may be seen. The nail may also thicken, independent of subungual hyperkeratosis. Transverse midline depressions resembling the nail changes seen in 'washboard nails' [20] are also seen. Normally, they are attributed to the habit tic of disrupting the cuticle (Fig. 65.21) and, although this may play a part in psoriasis, it appears that there is a lower

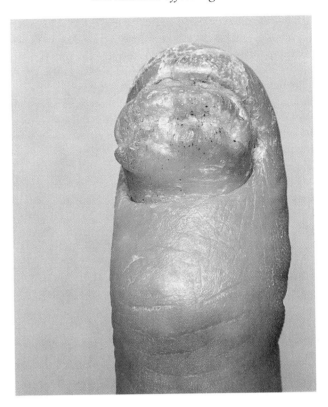

Fig. 65.20 Psoriasis: subungual hyperkeratosis.

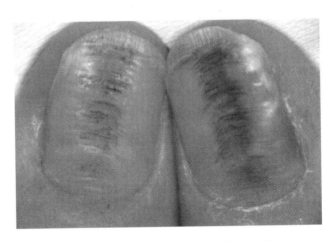

Fig. 65.21 Multiple transverse grooves of the thumb nails.

threshold for the development of this midline feature in the presence of psoriasis.

Splinter haemorrhages. Splinter haemorrhages are seen in the nailbed of 42% of fingernails and 6% of toenails [21]. This may be due to the increased capillary prominence and fragility in nail-bed dermis in psoriasis and the presence of dystrophy. Where transverse overcurvature occurs for reasons other than psoriasis, splinter haemorrhages are also common, suggesting that mechanical factors may contribute to splinter haemorrhage formation.

Subacute and chronic paronychia. Periungual involvement may be dramatic and inflammatory, giving rise to gross disruption of nail matrix. Loss of the nail may follow with scaling of the nail bed, or a deep transverse furrow.

Chronic psoriatic paronychia causes loss of the cuticle. The nail plate can become thin [22], although this may be offset by matrix disease, which can result in thickened nail. The nail fold may be scaly, in the form of psoriasis seen elsewhere.

Acropustulosis. This form of psoriasis involves destructive pustulation of the nail unit. It may present as part of pustular psoriasis, acrodermatitis continua of Hallopeau [23] or parakeratosis pustulosa (typically in young girls) on isolated digits. The nail plate may be lifted off by sterile pustules in the nail bed and matrix. There is associated erythema and discomfort of the end of the digit. There may be long-term nail loss, except in parakeratosis pustulosa, which usually resolves spontaneously. Parakeratosis pustulosa may affect only part of one digit. There is pitting and ridging combined with fine scaling erythema of the periunguium and only very rarely pustules. It is usually interpreted as a form of psoriasis, although it shares histological features with eczema [24], and some consider it a variant of eczema [25].

Acrodermatitis continua of Hallopeau can be very aggressive and result in resorptive osteolysis [26] or loss of toes and distal parts of fingers [27]. In a study of 20 patients with the condition, seven were male, 13 female, with a mean age of 46 years, and all had involvement of only one digit, with no features of psoriasis elsewhere [28].

Histopathology. Histopathology varies according to the clinical focus of the disease [1,29]. The matrix and nail bed develop a granular layer. Conversely, the hyponychium, where a granular layer is normally present, no longer has one [1]. Where there is subungual hyperkeratosis, there are mounds of parakeratotic keratinocytes beneath the nail plate. Neutrophils may be found throughout these mounds and Munro microabscesses may form. Similar features are seen in acrodermatitis continua of Hallopeau [28]. Amorphous material interpreted as glycoprotein may accumulate within the keratotic mass [1]. Acanthosis and elongation of the rete ridges is present, with increased dilatation and tortuosity of the capillaries of the dermal papillae. Where the nail is lost, the nail bed may form a false nail of compacted hyperkeratosis [30]. The matrix can become quiescent, which can be demonstrated immunohistochemically by the absence of synthesis of the hard keratin Ha-1, which is normally a major constituent of nail [31].

The nail plate may show faults, clinically manifest as transverse splits and pits, which are lined with para-keratotic cells. These probably originate from the most proximal part of the matrix, or the ventral aspect of the proximal nail fold [1].

Treatment. General hand care is important to avoid evocation of the isomorphic (Köbner) response, whereby minor trauma may elicit psoriasis. These measures include: avoid manicure, keep the nails short, wear gloves for wet work and heavy or greasy manual work, avoid direct exposure to solvents and encourage emollient usage. Concealment with nail lacquer is a reasonable approach to milder forms of psoriasis, and surface irregularities can be smoothed by the use of nail gel. This is a polymer, applied by a beautician and hardened by exposure to a table-top UVA source. The gel can then be shaped and buffed. Gel or other forms of sculptured or adherent artificial nails have the potential for aggravating onycholysis and are not usually recommended if this is a prominent feature.

Active treatments are mainly directed at the more dystrophic forms of nail involvement and may sometimes help with onycholysis. Often the focus of therapy is the proximal nail fold, where active psoriasis is disturbing the underlying matrix and lack of cuticle is promoting chronic paronychia. Medical treatments include the following.

Local steroids. Clobetasol propionate ointment may be used without occlusion, rubbed into the nail fold. Duration of treatment is limited by local atrophy. It is useful for psoriatic paronychia where there are secondary nail-plate changes. Onycholysis may benefit if the nail is clipped back to the point of nail-plate attachment and the nail bed treated topically. *Candida* is a frequent colonizer of this space and warrants treatment at the same time. Triamcinolone acetonide may be used by injection into the nail fold or nail bed with regional or digital ring block. Using 0.1 ml injections of 10 mg/ml triamcinolone acetonide at matrix and nail bed sites, on no more than two or three occasions, de Berker and Lawrence report a good response in subungual hyperkeratosis, nail-plate thickening and ridging. However, onycholysis and pitting improved in only 50% of nails [32]. Alternative regimens employ more dilute triamcinolone (2.5–5 mg/ml) and are routinely used more than two or three times per digit, infiltrating the proximal nail fold alone and making a ring block optional. Triamcinolone has also been used with the Port-O-Jet or Dermojet, with improvement of pitting as well as other features [33]. There is a single anecdotal report that use of these devices has been associated with implantation epidermoid cysts, and many reports that local infection is more likely with this form of steroid delivery than with injection [34].

Photochemotherapy. Subjects may improve as part of their general psoralen and UVA (PUVA) therapy [35] or may have psoralen and UVA combined solely in the nail unit [36]. This can be done with topical or systemic psoralen. Specific high-dose handsets of UVA lamps have been advocated. As part of whole-body PUVA, 18 of 26 patients showed a greater than 50% improvement in nail changes, although pitting was unresponsive. With local therapy, four of five patients showed improvement, with pitting also responding.

Retinoids. The nail plate is made thin by acetretin and etretinate. This reduces subungual hyperkeratosis. Pitting or onycholysis may be exacerbated [37,38]. Pustulation may be improved.

Others. Systemic methotrexate and cyclosporin may both help the nail unit but would not usually be advocated as therapy for this area of disease alone. Acrodermatitis continua of Hallopeau is the exception and may respond to methotrexate.

Topical cyclosporin has been reported as useful in a single case report [39].

5-Fluorouracil 1% has been used topically in 20% urea [40] and also in propylene glycol [41]. Pitting and subungual hyperkeratosis were thought to respond well to the former. Both are contraindicated in onycholysis.

Calcipotriol under occlusion has been used, with moderate benefit.

Superficial radiotherapy [42] and electron-beam therapy [43] have been shown to be only of temporary benefit and are not usually recommended.

Treatment of coincident fungal infection may provide clinical benefit, although it is seldom a dermatophyte and positive cultures may only represent colonization.

REFERENCES

1 Zaias N. Psoriasis of the nail. A clinical pathological study. *Arch Dermatol* 1969; **99**: 567–79.
2 Samman PD. *The Nails in Disease*, 3rd edn. London: Heinemann, 1978.
3 Puissant A. Psoriasis in children under the age of 10: a study of 100 observations. *Gaz Sanita* 1970; **19**: 191.
4 Nanda A, Kaur S, Kaur I et al. Childhood psoriasis: an epidemiologic survey of 112 patients. *Pediatr Dermatol* 1990; **7**: 19–21.
5 Stankler L. Foetal psoriasis. *Br J Dermatol* 1988; **119**: 684.
6 Griffiths WAD. Pityriasis rubra pilaris: an historical approach. 2—Clinical features. *Clin Exp Dermatol* 1976; **1**: 37.
7 Lovy M, Bluhm G, Morales A. Occurrence of pitting in Reiter's syndrome. *J Am Acad Dermatol* 1980; **2**: 66.
8 Sonnex TS, Dawber RPR, Zachary CB et al. The nails in adult type I pityriasis rubra pilaris. A comparison with Sezary syndrome and psoriasis. *J Am Acad Dermatol* 1986; **15**: 956–60.
9 Bazex A, Griffiths A. Acrokeratosis paraneoplastica. A new cutaneous marker of malignancy. *Br J Dermatol* 1980; **102**: 304.
10 Richard M, Giroux JM. Acrokeratosis paraneoplastica (Bazex syndrome). *J Am Acad Dermatol* 1987; **16**: 178–83.
11 Handfield-Jones S, Matthews CNA, Ellis JP et al. Acrokeratosis paraneoplastica of Bazex. *J R Soc Med* 1992; **85**: 548–50.
12 Wright V, Roberts MC, Hill AGS. Dermatological manifestations in psoriatic arthritis. A follow up study. *Acta Derm Venereol (Stockh)* 1979; **59**: 235.
13 Baker H, Golding DN, Thompson M. The nails in psoriatic arthritis. *Br J Dermatol* 1964; **76**: 549–54.
14 Jones SM, Armas JB, Cohen MG et al. Psoriatic arthritis: outcome of disease subsets and relationship of joint disease to nail and skin disease. *Br J Rheumatol* 1994; **33**: 834–9.
15 Boisseau-Garsaud AM, Beylot-Barry M, Doutre MS et al. Psoriatic onycho-pachydermo-periostitis. *Arch Dermatol* 1996; **132**: 176–80.
16 Zaias N. Psoriasis of the nail unit. *Dermatol Clin* 1984; **2**: 493–505.
17 Sonnex TS, Griffiths WAD, Nicol WJ. The nature and significance of the transverse white band of human nails. *Semin Dermatol* 1991; **10**: 12–16.
18 Szepes E. Mycotic nail fold infection of psoriatic nails. *Mykosen* 1986; **29**: 82–4.
19 Cohen PR, Prystowsky JH. PRP: a view of diagnosis and treatment. *J Am Acad Dermatol* 1989; **20**: 801–7.
20 Macaulay WL. Transverse ridging of the thumbnails. *Arch Dermatol* 1966; **93**: 421–3.
21 Calvert HT, Smith MA, Wells RS. Psoriasis and the nails. *Br J Dermatol* 1963; **75**: 415–18.
22 Ganor S. Chronic paronychia and psoriasis. *Br J Dermatol* 1975; **92**: 685–8.
23 Baran R. Hallopeau's acrodermatitis. *Arch Dermatol* 1979; **115**: 815–18.
24 Dulanto P, Armijo-Morens M, Camacho-Martinez F. Histological finding in parakeratosis pustulosa. *Acta Derm Venereol (Stockh)* 1974; **54**: 365–7.
25 Hjorth N, Thomsen K. Parakeratosis pustulosa. *Br J Dermatol* 1967; **79**: 527–32.
26 Miller JL, Soltani K, Toutellotte CD. Psoriatic acrosteolysis without arthritis. *J Bone Joint Surg Am* 1971; **53**: 371–4.
27 Mahowald ML, Parrish RM. Severe osteolytic arthritis mutilans pustular psoriasis. *Arch Dermatol* 1982; **118**: 434.
28 Pirracini BM, Fanti PA, Morelli R, Tosti A. Hallopeau's acrodermatitis continua of the nail apparatus: a clinical and pathological study of 20 patients. *Acta Derm Venereol (Stockh)* 1994; **74**: 65–7.
29 Lewin K, Dewit S, Ferrington RA. Pathology of the fingernail in psoriasis. *Br J Dermatol* 1972; **86**: 555–63.
30 Samman PD. The ventral nail. *Arch Dermatol* 1961; **84**: 192–5.
31 de Berker D, Westgate G, Leigh I. Patterns of hard keratin (Ha-1) expression in nail matrix correspond to nail plate morphology. *Br J Dermatol* 1996; **134**: 584.
32 de Berker D. Lawrence CM. A simplified protocol of nail steroid injection for psoriatic nail dystrophy. *Br J Dermatol* 1995; **133** (Suppl. 45): 15.
33 Gottlieb NL, Riskin WG. Complications of local corticosteroid injections. *JAMA* 1980; **243**: 1547–8.
34 Peachey RDG, Pye RJ, Harman RR. The treatment of psoriatic nail dystrophy with intradermal steroid injections. *Br J Dermatol* 1976; **95**: 75–8.
35 Marx JL, Scher RK. The response of psoriatic nails to photochemotherapy. *Arch Dermatol* 1980; **110**: 1023–4.
36 Handfield-Jones SE, Boyle J, Harman RRM. Local PUVA treatment for nail psoriasis. *Br J Dermatol* 1987; **116**: 280–1.
37 Baran R. Retinoids and the nails. *J Dermatol Treat* 1990; **1**: 151–4.
38 Ellis IN, Voohees JJ. Etretinate therapy. *J Am Acad Dermatol* 1987; **16**: 291–9.
39 Tosti A, Guerra L, Bardazzi F, Lanzarini M. Topical cyclosporin in nail psoriasis. *Dermatologica* 1990; **180**: 110.
40 Fritz K. Psoriasis of the nail. Successful topical treatment with 5-fluorouracil. *Z Hautkr* 1988; **64**: 1083–8.
41 Friedriekson T. Topically applied fluorouracil in the treatment of psoriatic nails. *Arch Dermatol* 1974; **110**: 735–6.
42 Yu RCH, King CM. A double blind study of superficial radiotherapy in psoriatic nail dystrophy. *Acta Derm Venereol (Stockh)* 1992; **72**: 134–6.
43 Kwang TY, Nee TS, Seng KTH. A therapeutic study of nail psoriasis using electron beams. *Acta Derm Venereol (Stockh)* 1995; **75**: 90.

Darier's disease [1–5]

Nail involvement is common in Darier's disease. Ninety-six per cent are reported to have acral changes, of which nail changes are the most common [2]. These include red and/or white longitudinal streaks in the nail, often terminating in a V-shaped nick (Fig. 65.22). The streak may represent a zone of fragile or thinned nail, which makes it prone to fragmentation at the tip with the consequent nick. In severe cases, the nails are almost lost by extension of the fragmentation process to involve the entire matrix. Subungual hyperkeratotic papules can be found in the hyponychium. Histologically, matrix and nail-bed changes resemble the acantholysis seen in involved skin with

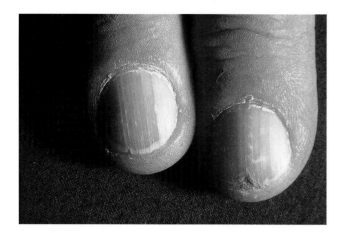

Fig. 65.22 Darier's disease: white and red longitudinal lines and distal notching.

the addition of multinucleate giant cells and epithelial hyperplasia in the nail bed [5]. These histological features make it possible to diagnose Darier's disease when it is confined to the nail [1]. Excess ridging and a rough nail surface may also be found, as may total leukonychia. Occasionally, marked thickening of the nail plate occurs. It is probable that the nail is sometimes affected in the absence of disease elsewhere [1].

Hailey–Hailey disease has some histological similarities and may also present with longitudinal white streaks [2]. However, the disease does not have the same destructive effect and is not associated with hyperkeratoses or symptoms of the nail apparatus.

REFERENCES

1 Bingham EA, Burrows D. Darier's disease. *Br J Dermatol* 1984; **111** (Suppl. 26): 88–9.
2 Burge SM, Wilkinson JD. Darier–White disease: a review of the clinical features in 163 patients. *J Am Acad Dermatol* 1992; **27**: 40–50.
3 Ronchese F. The nail in Darier's disease. *Arch Dermatol* 1965; **91**: 617–18.
4 Schubert H. Darier's disease. *Z Haut Geschlechskr* 1966; **41**: 239–44.
5 Zaias N, Ackerman AB. The nail in Darier–White disease. *Arch Dermatol* 1973; **107**: 193–9.

Eczema

Nail changes in eczema may be seen in the context of eczema elsewhere or as an isolated finding. Endogenous and exogenous factors may contribute. The nail changes may reflect this division, in that they may be in response to a systemic atopic disposition, with pitting in the absence of inflammation, or may demonstrate the effects of local eczema in the nail unit influencing nail formation.

The common allergens such as nickel, fragrance and medicaments rarely have particular bearing on nail abnormalities. However, rubber, chrome and irritant dermatitis are significant factors in hand dermatitis. These materials, and hand dermatitis in general, are associated with particular occupations. Selective exposure to such allergens or strong irritants is as important as chronic low-grade irritation from milder agents, such as water, seen in catering workers.

Cyanoacrylates used in prosthetic nails can provoke local and distant allergic reactions. Formaldehyde, occasionally used as a nail hardener, can provoke painful onycholysis if the patient becomes sensitized, or sometimes when acting solely as an irritant. Some allergens may cause nail dystrophy without associated inflammation.

A combination of atopy and an exogenous irritant or allergic contact reaction is common.

Clinical features. Nail matrix disturbance is reflected in thickening, pits, nail loss, transverse ridges and furrows in a pattern similar to psoriatic nail disease (Table 65.4).

Nail-bed disease can produce subungual hyperkeratosis, splinter haemorrhages, onycholysis and pain. Allergens and irritants can be sequestered beneath the free edge of the nail to achieve high concentrations and prolonged exposure.

Nail changes may betray eczema elsewhere and the nails may be buffed smooth and shiny, indicating their use as a tool for rubbing.

Associated hand dermatitis may show vesicles, scaling, erythema, cracks and swollen fingers, although the presence of vesicles will not always distinguish the condition from psoriasis, which should be sought at other sites. The distribution on the hand or foot may give some clues as to possible local causes, such as gloves, shoes, prosthetic nails or nail varnish. Hands and feet should always be examined together, as the presence of disease in both diminishes the likelihood of a contact dermatitis.

Defining the presence of atopy may be useful, with prick tests or a total IgE. Patch testing can be useful even in the absence of active eczema as subungual hyperkeratosis and discomfort may be disproportionate to the cutaneous features [1].

Treatment. General hand care is important, with the avoidance of soap, irritants, wet work and any identified cause. Protective gloves should be used, with copious emollient application. Barrier creams are not usually adequate protection once features have developed. Potent topical steroids may be needed, sometimes with additional topical or systemic antimicrobial therapy. These should be rubbed in around the nail folds. In the young, steroids may precipitate premature closure of the phalangeal epiphyses if too potent or used for too long [2]. Osteomyelitis has also been reported in children using potent topical steroids in this area.

Hand or foot PUVA can help.

REFERENCES

1 Marren P, de Berker DAR, Powell S. Occupational contact dermatitis due to Quaternium 15 presenting as nail dystrophy. *Contact Dermatitis* 1991; **25**: 253–5.

Table 65.4 Differential diagnosis between four common nail disorders: fungal infections, psoriasis, chronic paronychia and dermatitis.

	Colour	Onycholysis	Pitting	Filaments or spores in potash preparations	Cross-ridging	Other
Fungal infections	Often yellow or brown: part or whole of nail	Frequent	Infrequent	Filaments, usually abundant	Absent	Associated fungal infections elsewhere
Psoriasis	May be normal or yellow or brown	Frequent	Often present and fine	Absent	Uncommon	Associated psoriasis elsewhere or family history of psoriasis
Chronic paronychia	Edge of nail often discoloured brown or black	Usually absent	Uncommon	May be spores in edge of nail: filaments and spores in scrapings from nail fold	Frequent	Predominantly women; wet work and cold hands cause predisposition
Dermatitis	May be normal	Confined to tip or absent	Coarse pits frequent	Absent	Frequent	Recent history of dermatitis on hands

2 Boiko S, Kaufman RA, Lucky AW. Osteomyelitis of the distal phalanges in three children with severe atopic dermatitis. *Arch Dermatol* 1988; **124**: 418–23.

Lichen planus

Nails are involved in about 10% of cases of disseminated lichen planus [1]. In a study of 24 adults with nail lichen planus, nail changes were the sole manifestation of the disease in 75% [2,3] and the figure may be higher in children [4,5], in whom lichen planus of all types is rare. This suggests only a modest degree of overlap between the disease process in the nail unit and at other sites. Although the skin lesions may itch intensely, nail disease may be relatively asymptomatic except when nails are shed.

Clinical features. The disease can involve the proximal nail-folds with bluish-red discoloration. Nail-plate changes include thinning, onychorrhexis, brittleness, crumbling or fragmentation, and accentuation of surface longitudinal ridging. All these features are secondary to disease affecting the matrix, which can also produce transient or permanent longitudinal melanonychia [6] or leukonychia as a postinflammatory phenomenon (Fig. 65.23). When inflammation is intense and widespread within the nail apparatus, nails may be shed. Single longitudinal depressions in the nail, with a distal notch or entire split may arise from a pterygium. This is a fibrotic band of tissue fusing the proximal nail fold with the nail bed and matrix following destructive local inflammation. Surviving proximal matrix is unable to push growing nail through the scar tissue, with a consequent split.

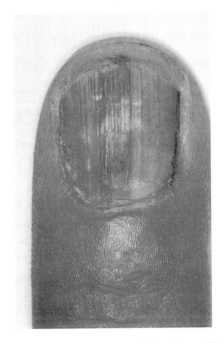

Fig. 65.23 Lichen planus with longitudinal melanonychia.

Nail-bed disease can produce subungual hyperkeratosis and onycholysis. Bullous lichen planus may affect the soles of the feet and in particular the toenails. Permanent anonychia may follow [7] (Fig. 65.24).

Twenty-nail dystrophy, with stippling of the nail plate (see Fig. 65.11) in up to 20 nails, is seen in a range of autoimmune diseases [8], alopecia areata [3], primary

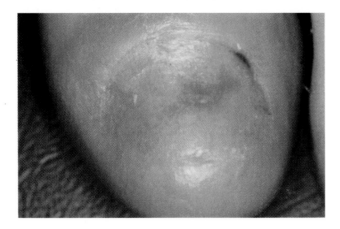

Fig. 65.24 Anonychia following lichen planus.

biliary cirrhosis and possibly in pemphigus [9]. In itself, it does not indicate the diagnosis of lichen planus, but is one of the recognized forms of the disease. It is one of the more common childhood patterns of presentation in which the nails feel rough, and lose their lustre. It has a reasonably good prognosis, in contrast with idiopathic atrophy of the nails, which may also occur in children. In this form, the surface change is less marked and the change in overall nail morphology greater, with thinning and shrivelling of the nail plate.

In the related disorder, lichen nitidus, numerous pits giving a fine rippling effect have been reported [11]. Longitudinal ridging, beads and thickening may occur and nails become brittle.

In keratosis lichenoides chronica, although the skin condition may resemble hyperkeratotic lichen planus, the nail changes may mimic psoriasis. Thirty per cent have nail involvement, with hyperkeratotic hypertrophy of periungual tissues.

Lichen planus nail changes are seen in graft-versus-host disease [12] and in the disseminated lichenoid papular dermatosis of AIDS. There can be an overlap between lichen planus and discoid lupus erythematosus, both in the skin and nails.

The differential diagnosis for the range of appearances of lichen planus in the nail unit includes Stevens–Johnson syndrome, infection, peripheral vascular disease, trauma and radiodermatitis.

Histology. In 20-nail dystrophy, there is a granular layer in the nail bed and matrix, with marked spongiosis [3]. The hypergranulosis is believed to reflect the disordered keratinization that causes both subungual hyperkeratosis and the poor nail-plate formation. In other forms of nail lichen planus, in addition to hypergranulosis, there is occasionally saw-toothing of the rete pattern, and colloid bodies are rarely seen [2,13,14].

In 20-nail dystrophy it may be useful to perform a screen for organ-specific antibodies because of the association with alopecia areata and the related autoimmune diathesis [3].

Treatment. Potent topical steroids may help when rubbed into the nail folds in the active stage. Triamcinolone acetonide may be instilled into the proximal nail fold under local anaesthetic. In children, potent steroid therapy puts them at risk of premature closure of the phalangeal epiphyses. Oral steroids at up to 60 mg/day have been used to arrest severe scarring nail lichen planus [2]. Failure to do this will result in nail loss or permanent dystrophy. Ulcerative lichen planus of the nail unit may benefit from grafting the nail bed.

REFERENCES

1 Samman PD. The nails in lichen planus. *Br J Dermatol* 1961; **73**: 288–92.
2 Tosti A, Peluso AM, Fanti PA *et al*. Nail lichen planus. Clinical and pathological study of 24 patients. *J Am Acad Dermatol* 1993; **28**: 724–30.
3 Tosti A, Fanti PA, Morelli R *et al*. Trachyonychia associated with alopecia areata. A clinical and pathological study. *J Am Acad Dermatol* 1991; **25**: 266–70.
4 de Berker D, Dawber RPR. Childhood lichen planus. *Clin Exp Dermatol* 1991; **16**: 233.
5 Milligan A, Graham-Brown RAC. Lichen planus in childhood: a review of six cases. *Clin Exp Dermatol* 1990; **15**: 340–2.
6 Baran R, Jancovici E, Sayag J, Dawber RPR. Longitudinal melanonychia in lichen planus. *Br J Dermatol* 1985; **113**: 369–74.
7 Cornelius CE, Shelley WB. Permanent anonychia due to lichen planus. *Arch Dermatol* 1967; **96**: 434–5.
8 Wilkinson JD, Dawber RPR, Bowers RP, Flemming K. Twenty nail dystrophy of childhood. *Br J Dermatol* 1979; **100**: 217–21.
9 de Berker D, Dalziel K, Dawber RPR, Wojnarowska F. Pemphigus associated with nail dystrophy. *Br J Dermatol* 1993; **129**: 461–4.
10 Samman PD. Idiopathic atrophy of the nails. *Br J Dermatol* 1985; **81**: 746–9.
11 Munro CS, Cox NH, Marks JM *et al*. Lichen nitidus presenting as palmoplantar hyperkeratosis and nail dystrophy. *Clin Exp Dermatol* 1993; **18**: 381–3.
12 Saurat JH. Gluckman E. Lichen planus-like eruption following bone marow transplantation: a manifestation of the graft-versus-host disease. *Clin Exp Dermatol* 1977; **2**: 335–44.
13 Barth JH, Millard PR, Dawber RPR. Idiopathic atrophy of the nails. A clinicopathological study. *Am J Dermatopathol* 1988; **10**: 514–17.
14 Zaias N. The nail in lichen planus. *Arch Dermatol* 1970; **101**: 264–71.

Tumours under or adjacent to the nail

Tumours of the nail apparatus and adjacent structures are relatively common. Neoplasms of the nail area can be divided into benign, benign but aggressive lesions (e.g. keratoacanthoma, recurring digital fibrous tumours of childhood and some warts) and malignant tumours.

Clinical diagnosis is often difficult because of traumatic factors, infection, pigmentation, and because the translucent nail-plate masks physical signs in the nail bed. Also, common tumours, easily recognized at other sites, may behave differently in the nail apparatus. An X-ray investigation should be carried out on all swellings in or around the nail apparatus, particularly those affecting a single digit, to exclude osteoma. Where changes are primarily in soft tissues, magnetic resonance imaging (MRI) may be preferable [1].

Benign tumours

Viral warts

This is the most common tumour involving the nail, usually found in one of the nail folds, but also seen in the digit pulp and less commonly on the nail bed. In the lateral nail folds, there may be no nail-plate changes, but proximal nail fold warts can result in longitudinal ridging and nail-plate distortion (Fig. 65.25) and nail bed warts may cause onycholysis (Fig. 65.26). Erosion of underlying bone has also been reported.

The causal human papillomavirus is usually type 1, 2 or 4. Nail biting and certain occupations, such as butcher, may predispose to warts and complicate therapy. Warts are more common and difficult to eradicate in the immunosuppressed, particularly in organ-transplant recipients.

The most significant lesion from which warts need to be distinguished is squamous cell (epidermoid) carcinoma. However, this malignancy often destroys part of the matrix and nail bed and is usually painful; both features are

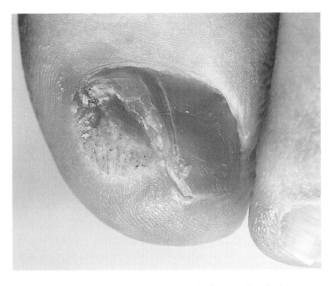

Fig. 65.26 Nail-bed warts can cause onycholysis and nail-plate disruption.

uncommon in benign viral warts, unless aggressive cryosurgery has been used or there has been bacterial infection. Other diagnoses, such as syringometa-plasia, amyloid, subungual corn and verrucous epidermal naevus [2], may mimic viral warts.

Most warts remit spontaneously, but a wide range of therapies are available and include topical salicylic acid (paste, on plaster or in collodion), combined with abrasion [3], cryosurgery [3–6], bleomycin [7,8], cantharidin [9], curettage and carbon dioxide laser therapy [10,11], and interferon [12].

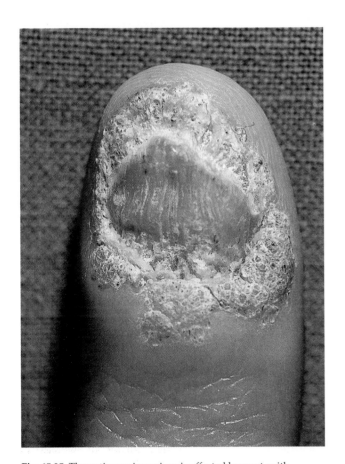

Fig. 65.25 The entire periunguium is affected by wart, with secondary nail changes.

REFERENCES

1 Drapé JL, Idy-Peretti I, Goettmann S *et al.* Standard and high resolution MRI in glomus tumours of toes and fingertips. *J Am Acad Dermatol* 1996; **35**: 550–5.
2 Solomon LM, Fretzin DF, Dewald RL. The epidermal naevus syndrome. *Arch Dermatol* 1968; **97**: 273–85.
3 Bunney MH, Nolan MW, Williams DA. An assessment of methods of treating viral warts by comparative trials based on a standard design. *Br J Dermatol* 1976; **94**: 667–79.
4 Colver GB, Dawber RPR. Cryosurgery—the principles and simple practice. *Clin Exp Dermatol* 1989; **14**: 1–6.
5 Dawber RPR, Colver GB, Jackson A. *Cutaneous Cryosurgery*, 2nd edn. London: Dunitz, 1997: 38–48.
6 Kuflik E. Cryosurgical treatment of periungual warts. *J Dermatol Surg Oncol* 1984; **10**: 673–6.
7 Munn SE, Higgins E, Marshall M, Clement M. A new method of intralesional bleomycin therapy in the treatment of recalcitrant warts. *Br J Dermatol* 1996; **135**: 969–72.
8 Shelley WB, Shelley ED. Intralesional bleomycin sulphate therapy for warts: a novel bifurcated needle puncture technique. *Arch Dermatol* 1991; **127**: 234–6.
9 Tkach JR. Finding and inventing alternative therapies. How I do it. *Dermatol Clin* 1989; **7**: 1–18.
10 Logan RO, Zachary CB. Outcome of carbon dioxide laser therapy for persistent cutaneous warts. *Br J Dermatol* 1989; **121**: 99–105.
11 Street ML, Roenigk RK. Recalcitrant periungual verrucae: the role of carbon dioxide laser vaporisation. *J Am Acad Dermatol* 1990; **23**: 115–20.
12 Stadler R, Mayer-da-Silva A, Bratzke B *et al.* Interferons in dermatology. *J Am Acad Dermatol* 1989; **20**: 650–6.

Fibrous tumours

There are several types of fibrous tumours of the nail apparatus, which can be differentiated on clinical and histological grounds [1,2]. Koenen tumours are associated with tuberous sclerosis and present at puberty as periungual fibromas. They are often multiple, large or small, elongated or nodular, and may produce a longitudinal groove in the nail plate due to matrix compression. Histologically, they show loose collagen with numerous small vessels distally, but with dense collagen and few vessels proximally.

Acquired periungual fibrokeratoma [3] is probably the same as acquired digital fibrokeratoma and garlic clove fibroma (Fig. 65.27). They are all benign, asymptomatic fibromas with a hyperkeratotic tip and narrow base arising in the periunguium, especially at the proximal aspect of the matrix. They grow out along the nail resulting in a longitudinal groove. There are three histological variants:
1 thick, dense, closely packed collagen bundles;
2 similar to 1, but with increased fibroblasts in the cutis;
3 oedematous and loose dermis.

Fibrous dermatofibroma is a true fibroma presenting as a smooth-edged tumour, commonly in the periungual tissues rather than within the nail unit. There is no collar of elevated skin as is often seen in acquired fibrokeratomas and it lacks the hyperkeratotic tip. It is hypocellular, but with prominent collagen bundles and rarely has a histiocytic dermal component. Occasionally, fibromas can be confused with other lesions, such as Bowen's disease, exostosis, keloid, dermatofibrosarcoma, eccrine poroma, neurofibroma and verruca. Multiple soft fibromas presenting on the dorsal aspect of digits in childhood may be infantile digital fibromatosis. These are benign and resolve with age [4,5].

Treatment is by excision. In acquired periungual fibrokeratoma arising in the proximal matrix, great care is needed to remove the origin of the tumour without damaging the matrix: there is a fine balance between allowing recurrence and producing long-term nail dystrophy. Koenen tumours are particularly prone to relapse, probably because of their dermal origin.

REFERENCES

1 Baran R, Perrin C, Baudet J, Requena L. Clinical and histological patterns of dermatofibromas (true fibromas) of the nail apparatus. *Clin Exp Dermatol* 1994; **19**: 31–5.
2 Kint A. Baran R. Histopathologic study of Koenen tumours. *J Am Acad Dermatol* 1988; **18**: 369–72.
3 Bart RS, Andrade R, Kopf AW, Leider M. Acquired digital fibrokeratomas. *Arch Dermatol* 1968; **97**: 120–9.
4 Cohen MM, Hayden PW. A newly recognised hamartomatous syndrome. *Birth Defects* 1979; **5B**: 291–6.
5 Reye RDK. Recurring fibrous digital tumours of childhood. *Arch Pathol* 1965; **80**: 228–31.

Subungual exostosis

A subungual exostosis is a benign bony outgrowth of the distal part of the terminal phalanx. It is usually found on the great toe [1] or rarely a finger [2] in subjects between the age of 10 and 35 years (Fig. 65.28). It is not clear whether trauma is causal. Pain, arising from trauma, is common, because the tumour protrudes and is easily knocked. The nail plate is elevated laterally but rarely damaged by the tumour. X-ray reveals an outgrowth of trabeculated bone

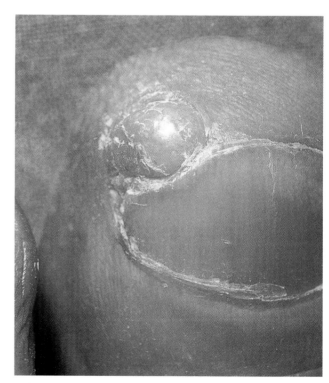

Fig. 65.28 Subungual exostosis.

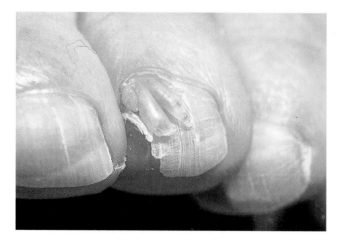

Fig. 65.27 Garlic clove fibroma.

[3], which may seem modest in comparison with the clinical complaint because of the large radiolucent cartilaginous cap.

Distinction from a subungual osteochondroma may be possible histologically because fibrous cartilage caps the bony outgrowth in exostosis and hyaline cartilage in osteochondroma [4,5]. Whereas this rule is often stated, it is not clear whether an absolute distinction can be made between the two lesions.

Where multiple exostoses exist, autosomal dominant multiple exostosis syndrome must be considered. The tumours in this condition are 'near the knee and far from the elbow' and can be destructive to nail [6]. The importance of making the diagnosis lies in the remote possibility of transformation of individual tumours to chondrosarcoma [7]. Older patients may have a different variety of exostosis, which represents hyperostosis of the distal tuft. This can cause elevation of the nail and pincer deformity, whereby the distal and lateral borders of the nail curve downward and inward to act as a pincer upon the nail bed.

Treatment. Treatment of subungual exostosis is by partial nail avulsion and removal of the tumour using bone nibblers or a chisel. A margin of normal bone needs to be removed at the base to prevent recurrence. There is a 10% relapse rate following surgery and children are more prone to relapse than adults [5,8]. Permanent matrix damage may follow surgery if tumours undermine the matrix.

REFERENCES

1 Landon GC, Johnson KA, Dahlin DC. Subungual exostoses. *J Bone Joint Surg Am* 1979; **61**: 256–9.
2 Carroll RE, Chance JT, Inan Y. Subungual exostoses of the hand. *J Hand Surg* 1992; **17B**: 569–74.
3 Evison G, Price CHG. Subungual exostoses. *Br J Radiol* 1966; **39**: 451–5.
4 Apfelberg D, Druker D, Maser MR, Lash H. Subungual osteochondroma: differential diagnosis and treatment. *Arch Dermatol* 1979; **115**: 472–3.
5 Eliezri YD, Taylor SC. Subungual osteochondroma: diagnosis and management. *J Dermatol Surg Oncol* 1992; **18**: 753–8.
6 Baran R, Bureau H. Multiple exostoses syndrome presenting with anonychia on a single finger. *J Am Acad Dermatol* 1991; **25**: 333–5.
7 Solomon L. Chondrosarcoma in hereditary multiple exostoses. *S Afr Med J* 1974; **48**: 671–6.
8 de Berker D, Lawrence CM, Dahl MGC. Outpatient surgery for subungual exostoses. *Br J Dermatol* 1994; **131** (Suppl. 44): 44.

Other bone tumours

Enchondromas

An enchondroma is a cartilage tumour, which may present as a painful solitary tumour of the distal phalanx with clubbing, paronychia, nail thickening, discoloration, ridging and elevation of the nail, and pathological fractures [1]. In Ollier's disease, multiple digits are usually affected. In Maffuci's syndrome there are multiple subcutaneous angiomas and hard cartilaginous nodules of the epiphyseal line, which may distort the entire hand or foot [2].

X-ray shows lucent expansion of distal phalanges alone, with spotty calcification in simple enchondromas. In Maffuci's syndrome there is widespread lucency in many phalanges of all the digits. Treatment is by enucleation of the tumour and autologous cancellous bone grafting. All these tumours can be associated with chondrosarcoma, angiosarcoma being an additional risk in Maffuci's syndrome [3].

Osteoid osteoma [4–6]

Osteoid osteomas of the distal phalanx present with enlargement of the entire digit tip in a young adult, with thickening of nail, clubbing, and increased local sweating. Violaceous skin changes, and a tender tumour may be palpated within the diffuse swelling and the tumour may cause a nagging pain, characteristically relieved by non-steroidal anti-inflammatory drugs.

X-ray reveals a small area of rarefaction surrounded by sclerosis, but symptoms may precede this appearance and an isotope bone scan or MRI may show the focus earlier. Arteriography and thermography demonstrate the hypervascularity. Surgical treatment of this benign condition is by *en bloc* resection through a fishmouth incision.

Implantation epidermoid cyst

Implantation epidermoid cyst may produce gradual enlargement of the tip of the digit, with the appearance of clubbing, or pincer nail. Pain may arise due to disturbance of the underlying bone where there is erosion, with distortion of cortical bone seen on X-ray, or a cyst may be demarcated on MRI. There is sometimes a history of previous trauma or surgery. Surgery is generally curative [7,8].

Metastases

Metastatic tumours present as inflamed swellings at the tip of a digit, with relatively few symptoms. X-ray reveals an osteolytic lesion, and systemic examination and investigation may reveal the primary focus; 50% will be from carcinoma of the lung [9].

REFERENCES

1 Yaffee HW. Peculiar nail dystrophy caused by an enchondroma. *Arch Dermatol* 1965; **91**: 361.
2 Monses B, Murphy WA. Distal phalangeal erosive lesions. *Arthritis Rheum* 1984; **27**: 449–55.
3 Lewis RJ, Ketcham AS. Maffuci's syndrome; functional and neoplastic significance. *J Bone Joint Surg Am* 1973; **55**: 1465–79.
4 Bowen CVA, Dzus AK, Hardy DA. Osteoid osteomata of the distal phalanx. *J Hand Surg* 1987; **12B**: 387–90.
5 Brown RE, Russel JB, Zook EG. Osteoid osteoma of the distal phalanx of

the finger: a diagnostic challenge. *Plast Reconstr Surg* 1991; **90**: 1016–21.
6 Jaffé HL. Osteoid osteoma. A benign osteoblastic tumour composed of osteoid and atypical bone. *Arch Surg* 1935; **31**: 709–28.
7 Baran R, Broutard JC. Epidermoid cyst of the thumb presenting as a pincer nail. *J Am Acad Dermatol* 1989; **19**: 143–4.
8 Schajowicz F, Alello CA, Slullitel I. Cystic and pseudo-cystic lesions of the terminal phalanx with special reference to epidermoid cyst. *Clin Orthop Rel Res* 1970; **68**: 84–92.
9 Baran R, Tosti A. Metastatic carcinoma to the terminal phalanx of the big toe: report of two cases and review of the literature. *J Am Acad Dermatol* 1994; **31**: 259–63.

Vascular tumours

Glomus tumour

Glomus tumours are the most characteristic of vascular nail bed tumours. There is pain, which may be spontaneous or evoked by mild trauma or temperature change. Nail-plate changes depend on the location of the tumour. Matrix tumours cause splitting and distortion of the nail plate. Nail bed lesions are most likely to appear as bluish or red foci of 1–5mm diameter beneath the nail. On X-ray, 50% show a depression in the underlying phalanx; MRI can reveal the exact site of the tumour [1–3]. High-resolution ultrasound has also been used with some success [4].

Histology is the definitive investigation and reveals vascular channels lined with endothelium and cuboidal glomus cells. These have dark nuclei and pale cytoplasm. Myelinated and non-myelinated nerves are found, which may account for the associated symptoms; neuromas must be considered in the differential diagnosis [5].

Treatment. Excision is the treatment of choice. It is usually possible to remove the lesion completely without risk of relapse [6]. Residual scarring of the nail may remain, depending on the nature of the surgery and the extent of preoperative damage.

REFERENCES

1 Drapé JL, Idy-Peretti I, Goettmann S *et al.* Standard and high resolution MRI in glomus tumours of toes and fingertips. *J Am Acad Dermatol* 1996; **35**: 550–5.
2 Goettmann S, Drape JL, Idy-Peretti I *et al.* Magnetic resonance imaging: a new tool in the diagnosis of tumours of the nail apparatus. *Br J Dermatol* 1994; **130**: 701–10.
3 Jablon M, Horowith A, Bernstein DA. Magnetic resonance imaging of a glomus tumour of the fingertip. *J Hand Surg* 1990; **15A**: 507–9.
4 Fornage BD, Schernberg FL, Rifkin MD, Touche DH. Sonographic diagnosis of glomus tumour of the finger. *J Ultrasound Med* 1984; **3**: 523–4.
5 Shelley ED, Shelley WB. Exploratory nail plate removal as a diagnostic aid in painful subungual tumours: glomus tumour, neurofibroma and squamous cell carcinomas. *Cutis* 1986; **38**: 310–12.
6 Carroll RE, Berman AT. Subungual glomus tumours of the hand. *J Bone Joint Surg Am* 1972; **54**: 691–703.

Pyogenic granuloma

Pyogenic granulomas are benign eruptive haemangiomas.

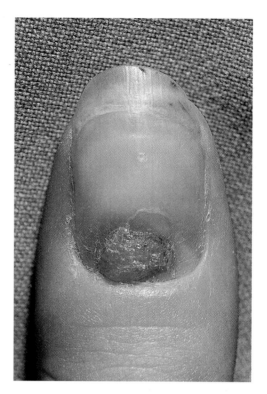

Fig. 65.29 Pyogenic granuloma penetrating the nail plate.

They may involve the nail fold, with a prominent collar of epithelium, or be subungual and penetrate the nail plate (Fig. 65.29). In this location, they almost invariably arise from the matrix and produce a localized deformity of the nail plate, visible as the nail grows distally. Mild penetrating injury, retinoids [1] and cyclosporin [2] may be initiating factors, but most commonly there is no obvious cause. Pyogenic granulomas bleed easily and must be distinguished from an amelanotic malignant melanoma, histiocytoid haemangioma [3], granulation tissue reaction to ingrowing nail and cavernous angioma. The possibility of melanoma makes histological examination mandatory. Bacteriology is also required and may help with the diagnosis of coccal nail fold angiomatosis, which may resemble a pyogenic granuloma arising from the matrix. This can relapse locally and on other digits [4].

Treatment. Once histology is available, if the lesion persists, destructive therapy such as carbon dioxide laser or suppressive therapy such as a potent topical steroid can be used. The latter is preferable and adequate for matrix lesions where infection has been adequately treated.

REFERENCES

1 Baran R. Retinoids and the nails. *J Dermatol Treat* 1990; **1**: 151–4.
2 Higgins EM, Hughes JR, Snowden S, Pembroke AC. Cyclosporin-induced periungual granulation tissue. *Br J Dermatol* 1995; **132**: 829–30.
3 Tosti A, Peluso AM, Fanti PA *et al.* Histiocytoid haemangioma with prominent fingernail involvement. *Dermatology* 1994; **189**: 87–9.
4 Davies MG. Coccal nail fold angiomatosis. *Br J Dermatol* 1995; **132**: 162–3.

Arteriovenous abnormalities

Periungual and subungual arteriovenous tumours (cirsoid aneurysms) are firm, bluish, non-pulsatile nodules in a nail fold or penetrating the nail [1]. Treatment by excision reveals histology of thick-walled vascular channels with fibrous tissue boundaries and no internal elastic lamina. In the presence of a digital arteriovenous malformation, the digit and nail bed are purple, with gradual shrinkage and overcurvature of the nail plate [2]. Growth may be rapid in young people in whom the digit may become bulbous and painful. X-ray may reveal aneurysmal destruction of the terminal phalanx, and more precise detail may be gained by MRI.

REFERENCES

1 Burge SM, Baran R, Dawber RPR, Verret JL. Periungual and subungual arteriovenous tumours. *Br J Dermatol* 1986; **115**: 361–6.
2 Enjolras O, Riché MC. *Hémangiomes et malformations vasculaires superficielles.* New York: Medsi/McGraw Hill, 1990.

Myxoid cyst

SYN. MYXOID OR MUCOID PSEUDOCYST

This benign cystic swelling has many names and is often termed a pseudocyst because a cellular cyst wall can seldom be demonstrated. It is usually located between the crease of the distal interphalangeal joint on the dorsal surface and the proximal nail fold. Less commonly it is found between the proximal nail fold and the nail plate, beneath the nail matrix or in the digit pulp. Pressure on the matrix results in a longitudinal groove or gutter in the nail plate (Fig. 65.30), which may have transverse ridges within it reflecting episodes of decreased matrix pressure when the cyst is decompressed through discharge of its contents. When the tumour occupies the space between the nail and proximal nail fold, it may protrude from beneath the nail fold with what appears to be a keratotic tip, mimicking a fibrokeratoma. When located beneath the matrix, the nail becomes misshapen, with increased transverse curvature, and the lunula appears red.

Myxoid cysts are more common in the fingers than the toes. They contain a clear gelatinous fluid that may discharge spontaneously or on minor trauma. This fluid may be the product of mucoid degeneration of connective tissue or be derived directly from the adjacent distal interphalangeal joint with which a communication is usually demonstrable by injection of methylene blue into the joint [1,2]. The condition of the joint is a major factor in the origin of the tumour, with osteoarthritic osteophytes damaging the joint capsule and provoking the flaw through which synovial fluid escapes. Infection of the ruptured pseudocyst may cause septic arthritis or local paronychia, although this is uncommon.

High-resolution ultrasound or MRI provides non-

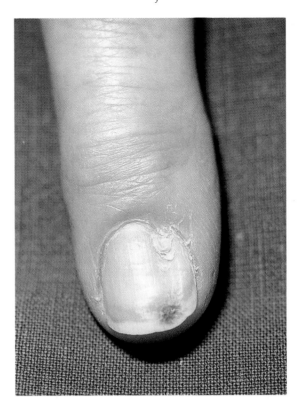

Fig. 65.30 Nail-plate groove due to proximal myxoid cyst.

invasive visualization to confirm the diagnosis or to localize the pedicle in recurrent cases. However, it may be more practical to attempt transillumination with a pen torch. This will distinguish it from a giant-cell tendon sheath tumour, which is usually found overlying the dorsal distal interphalangeal crease in women with osteoarthritis [3,4]. Giant-cell tendon sheath tumours are often rubbery and fail to transilluminate. Alternatively, a myxoid cyst will easily puncture using a size 11 scalpel, with sterile technique, revealing the diagnostic gelatinous contents.

Histology usually reveals a pseudocyst cavity within a fibrous capsule containing a myxomatous stroma with scattered fibroblasts. Areas of myxomatous change may merge to form a multilobular pseudocyst. Some workers report a mesothelial lining to the pseudocyst, consistent with continuity with the synovial joint space. This is not always confirmed and may mean that there are different histological forms of myxoid pseudocysts.

Treatment. There are many conservative approaches to cure [5,6], none of which is definitive. These include incision and drainage (pricking with a sterile blade or needle), which may be repeated by the patient [7], injected sclerosant [8] or steroid [9,10], cryosurgery [11,12], laser [13] and infrared photocoagulation [14].

Surgical therapy may entail removal of osteophytes involving the distal interphalangeal joint [15–17], excising the distal margin of the proximal nail fold if the tumour is located there [18] or tracing the communication between the joint and cyst with methylene blue and tying it off [2].

There is a high relapse rate after single treatments with less invasive therapies. More detailed surgical therapies are more effective [17,18].

REFERENCES

1 Kleinert HE, Kutz JE, Fishman JH *et al.* Etiology and treatment of the so-called mucous cyst of the finger. *J Bone Joint Surg* 1972; **54A**: 1455–8.
2 Newmeyer WL, Kilgore ES, Graham WP. Mucous cyst: the dorsal distal interphalangeal joint ganglion. *Plast Reconstr Surg* 1974; **53**: 313–15.
3 Averill RM, Smith RJ, Campbell CJ. Giant cell tumours of the bones of the hand. *J Hand Surg* 1980; **5**: 39–50.
4 Wright CJE. Benign giant-cell synovioma. An investigation of 85 cases. *Br J Surg* 1951; **38**: 257–71.
5 Baran R, Haneke E. Tumours of the nail apparatus and adjacent tissues. In: Baran R, Dawber RPR, eds. *Diseases of the Nails and their Management*, 2nd edn. Oxford: Blackwell Scientific Publications, 1994: 474–6.
6 de Berker DAR. Treatment of myxoid cysts. *J Dermatol Treat* 1995; **6**: 55–7.
7 Epstein E. A simple technique for managing digital mucous cysts. *Arch Dermatol* 1979; **115**: 1315–16.
8 Audebert C. Treatment of mucoid cysts of fingers and toes by injection of sclerosant. *Dermatol Clin* 1989; **7**: 179–81.
9 Epstein E. Steroid injection of myxoid finger cysts. *JAMA* 1965; **194**: 98–9.
10 Johnson WC, Graham JH, Helwig EB. Cutaneous myxoid cyst. A clinicopathological and histochemical study. *JAMA* 1965; **191**: 15–20.
11 Dawber RPR, Colver G, Jackson A. In: *Cutaneous Cryosurgery. Principles and Clinical Practice.* London: Dunitz, 1992: 71–2.
12 Dawber RPR. Myxoid cysts of the finger: treatment by liquid nitrogen spray cryosurgery. *Clin Exp Dermatol* 1983; **8**: 153–7.
13 Huerter CJ, Wheeland RG, Bailin PL, Ratz JL. Treatment of digital myxoid cysts with carbon dioxide laser vaporization. *J Dermatol Surg Oncol* 1987; **13**: 723–7.
14 Kemmett D, Colver GB. Myxoid cysts treated by infra-red photocoagulation. *Clin Exp Dermatol* 1994; **19**: 118–20.
15 Brown RE, Zook EG, Russell RC *et al.* Fingernail deformities secondary to ganglions of the distal interphalangeal joint (mucous cysts). *Plast Recontr Surg* 1991; **87**: 718–25.
16 Gingrass MK, Brown RE, Zook EG. Treatment of fingernail deformities secondary to ganglions of the distal interphalangeal joint. *J Hand Surg* 1995; **20A**: 502–5.
17 Kasdan ML, Stallings SP, Leis V, Wolens D. Outcome of surgically treated mucous cysts of the hand. *J Hand Surg* 1994; **19A**: 504–7.
18 Salasche SJ. Myxoid cysts of the proximal nail fold, a surgical approach. *J Dermatol Surg Oncol* 1984; **10**: 35–9.

Squamous cell carcinoma

SYN. EPIDERMOID CARCINOMA

Squamous cell carcinoma of the nail unit includes *in situ* (Bowen's disease) and invasive forms (Fig. 65.31). A single biopsy may fail to make a distinction between them. A tumour that appears *in situ* at one site may be invasive elsewhere [1]. Periungual features include hyperkeratotic, warty changes, erosions and fissuring, macerated cuticle, periungual swelling, erythema and occasional secondary infection. Subungual changes include onycholysis with a friable or warty nail bed, longitudinal melanonychia, nail dystrophy, ingrowing or loss. Nodular change with ulceration and bleeding is a late development. The condition may affect many digits [2]. Common misdiagnoses include onycho-mycosis, periungual warts, recurrent paronychia, pyogenic granuloma and subungual

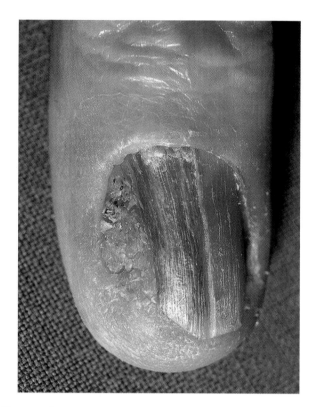

Fig. 65.31 Bowen's disease with melanonychia.

exostosis. As some of these conditions do not warrant biopsy and clinicians seldom think of squamous cell carcinoma at this site, the diagnosis is frequently delayed. Mean periods of 52 months [3], 9 years [4] and 5 years [5] have been reported.

Predisposing factors include radiation exposure [2,6], human papillomaviruses 16, 18 and 34 [3,4,6,7] and possibly ectodermal dysplasias and chronic trauma. Features of chronic radiation damage to the periunguium may precede the onset of malignancy [8]. Examination and history should include a note of genital wart infection or cervical dysplasia in the patient or partner [6]. Appropriate investigation includes X-ray and biopsy of a large and representative area. Failed diagnosis can also be attributed to poor diagnostic biopsy technique. Prognosis is good and there are only five cases of metastatic disease in the literature [9], one of which was in a patient with ectodermal dysplasia [10]. Another case was reported by Mauro *et al.* [11].

Treatment. Mohs micrographic surgery is the treatment of choice as long as there is no evidence of bone involvement [1,5,12], allowing the digit to be preserved in most instances. Alternatives include digit amputation, local excision and radiotherapy [13].

REFERENCES

1 Mikhail G. Subungual epidermoid carcinoma. *J Am Acad Dermatol* 1984; **11**: 291–8.
2 Baran RL, Gormley DE. Polydactylous Bowen's disease of the nail. *J Am Acad Dermatol* 1987; **17**: 201–4.
3 Sau P, McMarlin S, Sperling LC, Katz R. Bowen's disease of the nail bed and periungual area. *Arch Dermatol* 1994; **130**: 204–9.
4 Moy RL, Eliezri YD, Nuovo GJ *et al.* Human papillomavirus type 16 DNA in periungual squamous cell carcinomas. *JAMA* 1989; **261**: 2669–73.
5 Godlminz D, Bennett RG. Mohs micrographic surgery of the nail unit. *J Dermatol Surg Oncol* 1992; **18**: 721–6.
6 Guitart J, Bergfeld WF, Tuthull RJ *et al.* Squamous cell carcinoma of the nail bed: a clinicopathological study of twelve cases. *Br J Dermatol* 1990; **123**: 215–22.
7 Ashinoff R, Jumli J, Jacobson M *et al.* Detection of HPV DNA in squamous cell carcinoma of the nail bed and finger determined by polymerase chain reaction. *Arch Dermatol* 1991; **127**: 1813–18.
8 Richert B, de la Brassine M. Subungual chronic radiodermatitis. *Dermatology* 1993; **186**: 290–3.
9 McHugh RW, Hazen P, Eliezri YD, Nuovo GJ. Metastatic periungual squamous cell carcinoma: detection of human papillomavirus type 35 RNA in the digital tumour and axillary lymph node metastases. *J Am Acad Dermatol* 1996; **34**: 1080–2.
10 Campbell J, Keokarn T. Squamous cell carcinoma of the nail bed in epidermal dysplasia. *J Bone Joint Dis* 1966; **48**: 92–9.
11 Mauro JA, Maslyn R, Stein AA. Sqramous cell carcinoma of the nail bed in hereditary ectodermal dysplasia. *NY State J Med* 1972; **72**: 1065–6.
12 de Berker DAR, Dahl MGC, Malcolm AJ, Lawrence CM. Micrographic surgery for subungual squamous cell carcinoma. *Br J Plast Surg* 1996; **49**: 414–19.
13 Attiyeh FF, Shah J, Booker RJ *et al.* Subungual squamous cell carcinoma. *JAMA* 1979; **241**: 262–3.

Epithelioma cuniculatum [1,2]

Epithelioma cuniculatum is a slow-growing, locally destructive, low-grade tumour, histologically related to squamous cell carcinoma. It is typically found on the sole of the foot, but may involve the periunguium. It is warty, with discharge of foul-smelling yellow material from nail bed sinuses. The overlying nail is disrupted by onycholysis or destruction at the matrix, and there may be paronychia. The underlying bone is usually affected. X-ray reveals destruction of the terminal phalanx in most cases and biopsy confirms the diagnosis. A system of epithelium-lined channels within the tumour form fistulae extruding keratinous debris. Mitoses and dyskeratotic cells are rare and the benign appearance may lead to the misdiagnosis of pseudoepitheliomatous hyper-plasia. Mohs micrographic surgery is a useful treatment.

REFERENCES

1 McKee P, Wilkinson JD, Black MM *et al.* Carcinoma (epithelioma) cuniculatum: a clinicopathological study of nineteen cases and review of the literature. *Histopathology* 1986; **5**: 425–36.
2 Tosti A, Morelli R, Fanti PA *et al.* Carcinoma cuniculatum of the nail apparatus; report of 3 cases. *Dermatology* 1993; **186**: 217–21.

Keratoacanthoma

Subungual or periungual keratoacanthomas are typically painful, rapidly enlarging lesions, which are usually solitary. The name is misleading as there is no indication that the tumour follows the same pattern of involution seen in keratoacanthomas elsewhere; also, there is no apparent relationship with sun exposure. Although trauma and wire wool have been implicated [1], in most cases there is no obvious precipitating factor. Erosion of bone is seen on X-ray, which is an essential preliminary investigation [2–5]. This feature is likely to represent a pressure effect of rapid subungual expansion, rather than bone invasion. The diagnosis is made partly on the history but largely from the histology, which closely resembles that of a keratoacanthoma seen elsewhere, but showing little or no squamous dysplasia [4]. Subungual wart, squamous cell carcinoma and subungual exostosis are among the differential diagnoses. Clinically, subungual keratotic incontinentia pigmenti tumours fall between the appearance of fibroma and keratoacanthoma [6,7]. They resemble the latter in often being painful and causing underlying bone changes. They are commonly multiple and seen with the other features of incontinentia pigmenti, which is lethal in males.

Treatment. Treatment of subungual keratoacanthoma can be by Mohs micrographic surgery or curettage. More aggressive treatments, including amputation of the digit, have been employed in the past, but are not warranted. Given the concern that the tumour may represent a form of squamous cell carcinoma, micrographic surgery may be the treatment of choice.

REFERENCES

1 Fisher AA. Subungual keratoacanthoma: possible relationship of exposure to steel wool. *Cutis* 1990; **46**: 26–8.
2 Cramer SF. Subungual keratoacanthoma. A benign bone eroding neoplasm of the distal phalanx. *Am J Clin Pathol* 1981; **75**: 425–9.
3 Keeney GL, Banks PM, Linscheid RL. Subungual keratoacanthoma. Report of a case and review of the literature. *Arch Dermatol* 1990; **124**: 1074–6.
4 Oliwiecki S, Peachey RDG, Bradfield JWB *et al.* Subungual keratoacanthoma— a report of four cases and review of the literature. *Clin Exp Dermatol* 1994; **19**: 230–5.
5 Patel MR, Desai SS. Subungual keratoacanthoma in the hand. *J Hand Surg* 1989; **14A**: 139–42.
6 Adeniran A, Townsend PLG, Peachey RDG. Incontinentia pigmenti (Bloch–Sulzberger syndrome) manifesting as painful periungual and subungual tumours. *J Hand Surg* 1993; **18B**: 667–9.
7 Bessems PJM, Jagtman BA, Van de Staak W. Progressive, persistent, hyperkeratotic lesions in incontinentia pigmenti. *Arch Dermatol* 1988; **124**: 29–30.

Melanocytic lesions

Benign melanocytic lesions usually present as longitudinal melanonychia (LM). This is also a common appearance of early malignant melanoma of the nail matrix [1]. An understanding of the causes of benign nail pigmentation is important in order to judge when biopsy is indicated to exclude melanoma.

Benign causes of LM

Laugier–Hunziker syndrome

Laugier–Hunziker syndrome gradually evolves with pale-brown LM on one or more digits [2,3]. There may be periungual involvement resembling Hutchinson's sign and the oral and genital mucosae may be affected with pigmented macules.

Subungual naevi

Subungual naevi may present in adulthood or early in life with LM, or naevoid melanosis of the nail plate [4] (Fig. 65.32). This has been described in Mediterranean [5] and Japanese [6] populations and it is not clear how often it occurs in northern white populations.

Drug therapy

Drug therapy with minocycline, zidovudine [7] and antimalarials may produce brown streaks in the nail (see p. 2831), as may dermatoses such as lichen planus [8] and onychomycosis [9], trauma [10] and non-melanocytic tumours such as squamous cell carcinoma *in situ* [11] (Fig. 65.31). Subungual blood pigment may resemble melanin, but associated features in the history and appearance usually make it possible to distinguish the two.

Benign racial pigmentation

The most common cause of LM is racial variation. Seventy-seven per cent of Afro-Caribbeans over 20 years of age have LM and this prevalence rises to almost 100% by the age of 50 years [12]. It is present in 10–20% of Japanese [13] and is more common in Mediterranean races than in northern Europeans. However, in this context, the percentage of malignant melanomas presenting in the nail unit is higher in Afro-Caribbeans (15–20%) [14] than in any other group (3% in white populations [15]). This contrasts with the low incidence of malignant melanoma at other skin sites in Afro-Caribbeans.

Malignant melanoma [16–18]

There are many features of LM that should suggest the possibility of malignant melanoma. These include the presence of brown–black periungual pigmentation (Hutchinson's sign) [19], especially when the pigmentation develops in a single digit in adult life and is evolving to become darker and broader and has blurred edges. Hutchinson's sign needs careful assessment and does not necessarily carry a bad prognosis [2,20]. The suspicion of melanoma is raised further if the individual has any other risk factors for melanoma, if the involved digit is a thumb, great toe or index finger, and if the nail has become dystrophic.

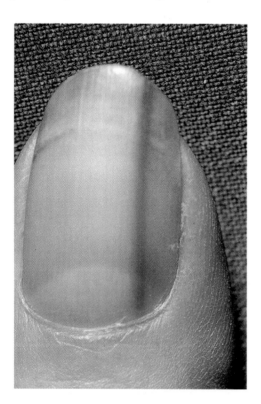

Fig. 65.32 Benign longitudinal melanonychia due to a subungual naevus.

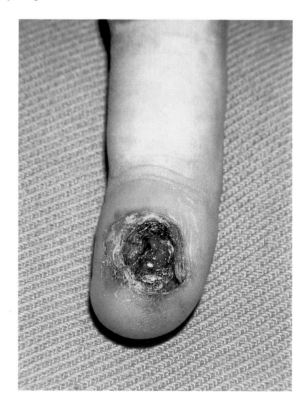

Fig. 65.33 Malignant melanoma arising in the nail matrix and invading the nail bed.

In spite of the importance of LM as a warning sign, 25% of subungual melanomas present as amelanotic tumours. This exceeds the percentage of melanomas presenting as an amelanotic tumour elsewhere. It is difficult to determine whether these tumours were always amelanotic [21] or whether loss of pigment is due to development of the disease process (Fig. 65.33). This form of melanoma usually has associated nail-plate damage and easily bleeds. With this appearance, the differential diagnosis includes pyogenic granuloma, chronic paronychia and vascular tumour.

The significance of preceding trauma is unclear [21]. Such a history is present in a large number of cases. It is thought that primary nail-unit malignant melanoma arises only from within the matrix and not from the nail bed. This is consistent with the absence of antigenically identifiable melanocytes in the nail bed [22] and can provide some reassurance when assessing pigmented lesions which are not arising from the matrix. However, such lesions may be arising from the nail folds, or be secondary malignant melanomas.

Biopsy of LM

Given the gravity of the potential cause of melanonychia, there should be a low threshold for biopsy. The type of biopsy can be determined by a range of factors [10], as follows.

1 Periungual pigmentation present. This indicates high risk of malignancy. If there are no other factors to account for this pigmentation, the whole area of affected nail unit should be removed *en bloc* down to bone with a 1-mm margin of normal tissue. Cosmetic considerations are secondary.

2 Lateral third of nail plate involved. This indicates lateral longitudinal biopsy. The cosmetic outcome is reasonable and the assurance provided by complete removal of the affected area is usually worthwhile.

3 Mid portion of the nail plate involved. The cosmetic outcome of complete excision at this site is potentially bad. This is particularly so if the origin of melanocytes is proximal in the matrix. This may be determined by sampling the free edge of the nail plate and performing a Masson–Fontana stain. Pigment in the lower part of the nail reflects a distal matrix origin, compared with ventral nail pigment reflecting an origin in the proximal matrix. The latter carries a high risk of scarring following excision.

For lesions less than 3 mm wide. The potential for postoperative dystrophy in midline lesions warrants preliminary investigation of thin (less than 3mm) pigmented streaks with a matrix punch biopsy unless the clinical evidence of malignancy is overwhelming. This technique involves:

1 reflection of proximal nail fold to visualize the origin of the pigment;
2 a 3-mm punch biopsy through the nail down to bone at the pigment origin, but leaving the biopsy *in situ*;
3 proximal hemiavulsion, which will leave the 3-mm biopsy of nail remaining;
4 examination of fully exposed matrix;
5 careful removal of 3-mm biopsy of matrix and nail with iris scissors;
6 after gentle undermining, partial approximation and suture of the wound with 7/0 monofilament may be attempted for proximal matrix wounds.

Removal of the nail plate before biopsy can mean one loses the site of pigment origin once the clue of melanonychia has gone. Removal of the 3-mm biopsy without hemiavulsion of the surrounding nail is difficult and may result in damage to the specimen, which compromises histological interpretation. For these reasons, the method outlined above is preferred.

For lesions 3–6 mm wide. If the pigment arises from distal matrix, a transverse matrix biopsy can be performed. Proximal matrix pigment requires an *en bloc* removal and repair using a Schernberg and Amiel flap.

For lesions greater than 6 mm wide. Matrix punch or transverse biopsy is usually adequate as the preliminary investigation.

The most common pattern is of acral lentiginous melanoma [15], although one series reported the superficial spreading type as being marginally more common [23]. In the acral lentiginous form, there is lentiginous spread of pleomorphic, often dendritic, atypical melanocytes in the basal and suprabasal layers of the epidermis. Epidermal melanoma cells may be incorporated into the nail plate and seen on stained clippings of nail taken from the free edge. Dermal melanoma cells are pleomorphic, with spindle, epithelioid, polygonal, dendritic and bizarre shapes.

Hutchinson's sign is represented histologically by atypical melanocytes mainly in the basal layer, with a few higher in the epidermis.

In situ subungual melanoma has junctional nests of melanoma cells.

Nodular patterns of melanoma are rare.

Amputation of the digit is the routine treatment, although local excision is occasionally practised for small, shallow lesions. Adjuvant isolated limb perfusion has failed to show benefit in stage 1 subungual melanoma [24], but use of a more aggressive regimen has possibly been associated with improved survival [25].

Recent British surveys suggest that the poor prognosis of subungual melanoma is related to the depth of invasion at diagnosis (4.7 mm). This reflects late diagnosis (3 months to 12 years) [23]. The mean 5-year survival was 41% compared with 61% for a control group of primary cutaneous malignant melanomas in the same study [26]. Other series have produced similar results, although recent Japanese evidence supports the idea that diagnosing subungual melanoma early, with a lower Breslow thickness, improves prognosis, with an 87% 5-year survival rate [25].

REFERENCES

1 Saida T, Oshima Y. Clinical and histopathologic characteristics of early lesions of subungual malignant melanoma. *Cancer* 1989; **63**: 556–60.
2 Baran R, Bariere H. Longitudinal melanonychia with spreading pigmentation in Laugier–Hunziker syndrome: a report of 2 cases. *Br J Dermatol* 1986; **115**: 707–10.
3 Veraldi S, Cavicchini S, Benelli C, Gasparini G. Laugier–Hunziker syndrome: a clinical, histopathologic and ultrastructural study of four cases and review of the literature. *J Am Acad Dermatol* 1991; **25**: 632–6.
4 Tosti A, Baran R, Piraccini BM *et al.* Nail matrix naevi: a clinical and histopathologic study of twenty-two patients. *J Am Acad Dermatol* 1996; **34**: 765–71.
5 Léauté-Labrèze C, Bioulac-Sage P, Taïeb A. Longitudinal melanonychia in children. *Arch Dermatol* 1996; **132**: 167–9.
6 Kikuchi I, Inoue S, Sakaguchi E *et al.* Nevoid nail area melanosis in childhood (cases which showed spontaneous regression). *Dermatology* 1993; **186**: 88–93.
7 Gallais V, Lacour JPH, Perrin C *et al.* Acral hyperpigmented macules and longitudinal melanonychia in AIDS patients. *Br J Dermatol* 1992; **126**: 387–91.
8 Juhlin L, Baran R. Longitudinal melanonychia after healing of lichen planus. *Acta Derm Venereol (Stockh)* 1989; **69**: 338–9.
9 Matsumoto T, Matsuda T, Padhye AA *et al.* Fungal melanonychia: ungual phaeohyphomycosis caused by *Wangiella dermatitidis. Clin Exp Dermatol* 1992; **17**: 83–6.
10 Baran R, Kechijian P. Longitudinal melanonychia (melanonychia striata). Diagnosis and management. *J Am Acad Dermatol* 1989; **21**: 1165–75.
11 Baran R, Simon C. Longitudinal melanonychia: a symptom of Bowen's disease. *J Am Acad Dermatol* 1988; **6**: 1359–6.
12 Monash S. Normal pigmentation in the nails of the negro. *Arch Dermatol* 1932; **25**: 876–81.
13 Kopf AW, Waldo E. Melanonychia striata. *Australas J Dermatol* 1980; **21**: 59–70.
14 Collins RJ. Melanomas in the Chinese among south western Indians. *Cancer* 1984; **55**: 2899–902.
15 Blessing K, Kernohan NM, Park KGM. Subungual malignant melanoma—clinicopathological features of 100 cases. *Histopathology* 1991; **19**: 425–9.
16 Baran R, Haneke E. Tumours of the nail apparatus and adjacent tissues. In: Baran R, Dawber RPR, eds. *Diseases of the Nails and their Management*, 3rd edn. Oxford: Blackwell Scientific Publications, 1994: 483–97.
17 Daly JM, Berlin R, Urmacher C. Subungual melanoma. *Ann Surg* 1987; **161**: 545–52.
18 Feibleman CE, Stoll H, Maize JC. Melanomas of the palm, sole and nailbed: a clinicopathologic study. *Cancer* 1980; **46**: 2492–504.
19 Kopf AW. Hutchinson's sign of subungual malignant melanoma. *Am J Dermatopathol* 1981; **3**: 201–2.
20 Baran R, Kechijian P. Hutchinson's sign: a reappraisal. *J Am Acad Dermatol* 1996; **34**: 87–90.
21 Miura S, Jimbow K. Clinical characteristics of subungual melanomas in Japan. *J Dermatol* 1985; **12**: 393–402.
22 de Berker D, Dawber RPR, Thody A, Graham A. Melanocytes are absent from normal nail bed; the basis of a clinical dictum. *Br J Dermatol* 1996; **134**: 564.
23 Rigby HS, Briggs JC. Subungual melanoma: a clinicopathological study of 24 cases. *Br J Plast Surg* 1992; **45**: 275–8.
24 Vrouenraets BC, Kroon BBR, Klaase JM *et al.* Regional isolated perfusion with melphalan for patients with subungual melanoma. *Eur J Surg Oncol* 1993; **19**: 37–42.
25 Kato T, Suetake T, Sugiyama Y *et al.* Epidemiology and prognosis of subungual melanoma in 34 Japanese patients. *Br J Dermatol* 1996; **134**: 383–7.
26 McLaren KM, Hunter JAA, Smyth JF *et al.* The Scottish Melanoma Group: a progress report. *J Pathol* 1989; **158**: 335A.

Nail surgery [1,2]

Nail surgery is delicate and requires attention to detail. It is important that anyone performing a nail biopsy appreciates the principles outlined in the preliminary section of this chapter on anatomy and physiology and that they obtain tuition in detailed technique. Once in this position, the outcome of nail-unit surgery is usually excellent and provides useful and definitive diagnostic material [3].

For many procedures, the routine skin surgery pack needs to be supplemented by specialized instruments. These include a Freer septum elevator for finger work and a larger elevator for the great toenail. English nail splitters are essential for performing partial avulsion. They have a flat undersurface, which can be introduced beneath the nail to act as an anvil and a sharp upper part which cuts down upon the nail to meet the other half of the instrument. For bone surgery, such as removal of exostoses, bone rongeurs and McKindoes are needed.

Indications

A nail biopsy may perform several functions. It may provide useful positive diagnostic information, or help exclude a malignant condition, such as squamous cell carcinoma of the nail bed. Painful conditions may be relieved by the drainage of pus with proximal hemiavulsion, or ablation of an ingrowing toenail. Focal pathology, such as a glomus tumour or the origin of melanonychia can be completely excised and provide the diagnosis. If a positive diagnostic and therapeutic attitude is taken to the nail disorder, a good outcome can be expected.

Diagnostic nail biopsy may be undertaken as part of the investigation of nail dystrophy of unknown cause in the presence of more than one negative mycology sample.

Biopsy of the nail plate alone, or with associated nail bed and occasionally matrix, may be needed to confirm fungal infection in atypical cases, but biopsies are more commonly directed at distinguishing between dermatoses affecting the nail, such as lichen planus, psoriasis or infiltrative disease. In instances of nail dystrophy of a single digit, it is appropriate to biopsy to exclude a neoplasm once necessary imaging has been performed.

Caution is needed in patients with relevant medical and circulatory problems. The latter are subject to poor reperfusion following the tourniquet and it may be necessary to abbreviate the procedure to ensure no inadvertent damage is done. The wound must be seen to bleed and the digit colour return before the dressing is applied in these cases, and this can take several minutes.

This contrasts with the usual pace at which dressings are applied to prevent bleeding in a healthy digit. Diabetics may have ischaemia combined with immune impairment and frequently need attention to toenail problems. Paradoxically, they are cited as a group in whom cold steel surgery for nail problems is preferable to other techniques such as phenolic ablation or cryosurgery. This is because the course of healing in these wounds is predictable and often shorter than wounds produced by other therapies.

Preoperatively

It is essential to prepare the patient for the procedure by a discussion on a day separate from surgery. In this discussion, the patient must appreciate the potential benefits and problems of the biopsy. It is useful to make it clear that it will be painful and that they will have a degree of disability postoperatively for which they must make provision at home and at work. The best surgical technique can be utterly confounded by a patient who goes back to work in a dirty place the next day. Much of the information concerning scarring, the need for elevation, dressings and analgesia needs to be repeated on the day of the procedure. The patient should have a means of transport home which does not involve them driving or standing for prolonged periods.

The affected digit should be soaked in warm antiseptic and scrubbed in a manner similar to that used by the surgeon prior ro gloving. This will diminish the bacterial load beneath the free edge of the nail, which is a source of potential pathogens. Soaking for 10 min softens the nail and facilitates removal of parts of the nail plate, so avoiding

complete avulsion. During this period, the local anaesthetic can take effect.

Anaesthetic (Fig. 65.34) [4–6]

Lignocaine 1–2% or equivalent can be used. Bupivacaine can be used to provide prolonged analgesia. There should be no adrenaline in the anaesthetic because of the risk of provoking prolonged peripheral ischaemia. A 30-gauge needle causes less discomfort during injection than larger needles, and minimizes the risk of damage to digital nerves when inserting a ring block. Risk of nerve trauma may be reduced further by the use of nerve-block needles, which have less traumatic tips.

The most common form of anaesthetic is delivered as a ring block (digital nerve block) by injection into the dorsolateral aspect of the digit at the base, with about 1–2 ml on each side of the phalanx. Greater than 5 ml may impair circulation, but this can be assessed visually during the procedure and is very variable according to the bulk of individual digits. Anaesthesia may take 10–20 min to become total. In the great toe, additional anaesthetic should be placed ventrally. After 10 min, efficacy of the block can be assessed at the digit tip with the same needle; if the anaesthesia is incomplete, it can be supplemented by a small local injection at the site of surgery. However, this can increase tissue turgor and render fine manipulation difficult.

An alternative is the distal 'wing' block given 2–3 mm proximal to the junction of the proximal and lateral nail folds. The injection is first directed distally into the lateral nail fold. After partial withdrawal, it is redirected over the proximal nail fold. Sufficient is used to produce blanching in both nail folds. The procedure is repeated on the other side to achieve complete block. The digit is more sensitive distally than proximally and it is often more comfortable to provide the traditional proximal digital nerve block.

Fig. 65.34 Diagram to show digital sites of injection for a ring block.

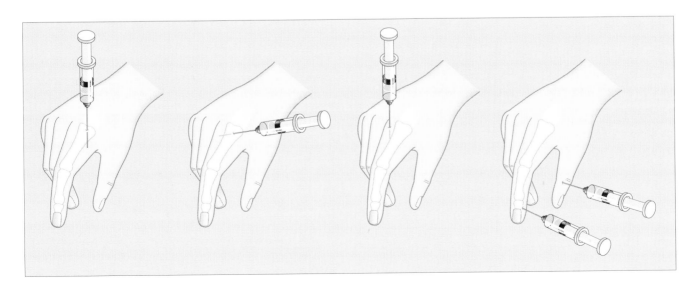

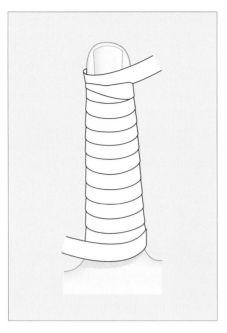

(a)

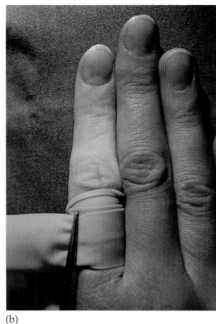

(b)

Fig. 65.35 (a) A Penrose drain is applied from the tip and wound down the digit achieving exsanguination. (b) The drain is then unwound from the top, with the base maintained secure with artery forceps.

For invasive procedures on many digits concurrently, more proximal or regional blocks can be employed.

Tourniquet

It is important that the area of applied pressure beneath the tourniquet is as broad as possible to avoid pressure damage to underlying structures. In particular, neuritis may be a long-term complication of a narrow, tight, prolonged tourniquet. This effect can be exacerbated by topping up anaesthetic near the tourniquet after it is in place. Ischaemia can be tolerated in a normal digit for 20 min and possibly longer, with no complications as long as there is no local trauma from the tourniquet.

The standard tourniquet for local anaesthetic is the Penrose drain (Fig. 65.35), which may be wound around the digit from the tip proximally. This exsanguinates the digit and provides a tourniquet effect which can be maintained with a pair of artery forceps. A sterile glove is an alternative. It is worn by the patient and the tip of the glove digit at the site of surgery is snipped off. It is then rolled back to the base of the digit, exsanguinating it, providing a tourniquet and avoiding contamination from adjacent digits peroperatively. With general anaesthetic, an exsanguinating cuff can be used on the forearm or calf.

Specimen

The specimen must be delivered to the pathologist undistorted and with the maximum of clinical and operative information. It is useful to allow the specimen to adhere lightly to a piece of paper before immersion in fixative, or to enclose it in a small plastic mesh cassette. This should be matched with a detailed drawing on the histopathology request form. It is helpful to work regularly with the same pathologist for nail specimens as processing requires specialized understanding of specimen preparation and histological interpretation.

Postoperatively

Dressings should be ready before removal of the tourniquet. They must be firm and moderately bulky. An acceptable dressing includes an antimicrobial ointment under a greasy tulle, padding and a small bandage. This should be held in place with oblique or longitudinal sticky tape to avoid a tourniquet effect if the digit swells. A sling or plastic overshoe should be provided.

The frequency of dressings is determined by the nature of the procedure and the patient. An antiseptic soak is normally needed to remove the dressing and clean the wound. Infection should be treated vigorously with systemic antibiotics combined with daily antiseptic soaks.

It is good practice to provide a moderately strong analgesic and to recommend taking it regularly in the first 48 h. It may prove unnecessary, but the distress of unrelieved pain in the few who suffer warrants caution. Some patients need night-time sedation.

In most cases, it is wise to see the patient within 2 days of surgery to personally supervise a change of dressing, review the wound and answer any questions which have arisen.

REFERENCES

1 Haneke E, Baran R. Nail Surgery and traumatic abnormalities. In: Baran R, Dawber RPR, eds. *Diseases of the Nail and their Management*, 2nd edn. Oxford: Blackwell Scientific Publications, 1994: 345–410.
2 Salasche SJ, Peters VJ. Tips on nail surgery. *Cutis* 1985; **35**: 428–38.
3 de Berker D, Dahl MGC, Comaish JS, Lawrence CM. The value of nail unit surgery in dermatology. *Acta Derm Venereol (Stockh)* 1996; **76**: 484–7.
4 Abadir A. Use of local anaesthetics in dermatology. *J Dermatol Surg* 1975; **1**: 68–72.
5 Chiu DTW. Transthecal digital block: flexor tendon sheath used for anaesthetic infusion. *J Hand Surg* 1990; **15A**: 471–3.
6 Cohen SJ, Roegnik RK. Nerve blocks for cutaneous surgery on the foot. *J Dermatol Surg Oncol* 1991; **17**: 527–34.

Patterns of nail biopsy

Nail avulsion [1,2]

Nail avulsion can be performed in order to examine underlying tissues or to provide temporary relief in cases of soft-tissue trauma. In isolation, it is not a treatment for ingrowing toenails. The procedure requires a distal or ring block and an elevator in addition to the routine instrument pack. For a partial avulsion, nail splitters are also needed.

To minimize the trauma of the procedure, soft-tissue nail attachments need to be loosened at all sites prior to removal. This minimizes tearing damage to the nail folds. The cuticle may need disrupting with fine scissors or a blade, but all other detachments can be performed with a septum elevator. Once this is done, the nail is gripped with a pair of rugged artery forceps and removed by a mixed twisting and lifting action (Fig. 65.36).

With a lateral partial avulsion, the nail splitter is used to define the medial margin and only the attachments of the piece of nail to be removed need to be interrupted.

Proximal hemiavulsion of the nail plate entails the following technique.
1 The origin of the nail and its proximal lateral aspects are undermined with a septum elevator.

Fig. 65.36 The three stages of standard nail avulsion.

2 In nails with a shallow lateral nail fold, a nail splitter may be inserted and the nail transversely bisected.
3 In nails with a deep lateral nail fold, a deep transverse score is placed with a scalpel across the nail halfway down.
4 The septum elevator is then fully inserted through the transverse score to loosen and elevate the proximal nail.

REFERENCES

1 Albom MJ. Avulsion of a nail plate. *J Dermatol Surg Oncol* 1977; **3**: 34–5.
2 Baran R. More on avulsion of nail plate. *J Dermatol Surg Oncol* 1981; **7**: 854.

Nail-bed biopsy [1–4]

Biopsy of the nail bed is usually performed to investigate a focal abnormality of nail bed or changes in the nail plate arising distally. Occasionally, it may be appropriate to biopsy

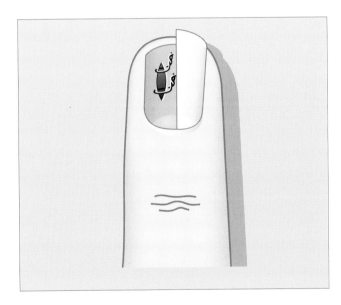

Fig. 65.37 After partial nail avulsion, the nail bed can be seen and biopsied along the longitudinal access.

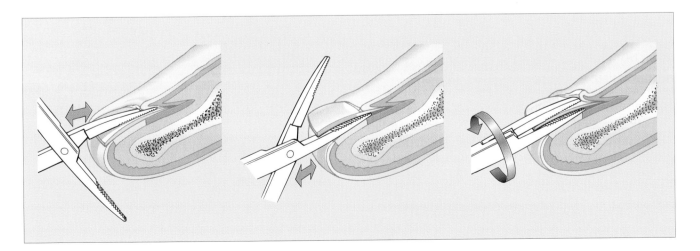

through the nail plate where the histological relationship between nail bed and plate is under investigation. More commonly, the nail bed is visualized first, following complete or partial avulsion. A thin ellipse is taken down to bone in the long axis of the digit (Fig. 65.37). An alternative is to employ a double punch technique, where a 6-mm hole can be made in the nail plate with a biopsy punch over the area of nail bed to be examined. The nail bed may then be sampled using a smaller punch.

If there has been nail avulsion, it is possible to close the wound, which may require gentle undermining. In small biopsies, this may be unnecessary, and the wound will heal well by secondary intention. When the nail is left *in situ* or if the double punch technique is used, closure is not possible. After a double punch, as long as there is complete haemostasis, the original disc of nail plate can be returned after soaking in antiseptic; it may reattach or at least provide a natural dressing during the early healing phase.

No scarring is anticipated from this biopsy if it is small and does not extend into the nail matrix.

REFERENCES

1 Baran R, Sayag J. Nail biopsy. Why, when, where, how? *J Dermatol Surg Oncol* 1976; **2**: 322–4.
2 Haneke E, Baran R. Nail surgery and traumatic abnormalities. In: Baran R, Dawber RPR, eds. *Diseases of the Nail and their Management*, 2nd edn. Oxford: Blackwell Scientific Publications, 1994: 345–416.
3 Hanno R, Mathes BM, Krull EA. Longitudinal nail biopsy in evaluation of acquired nail dystrophies. *J Am Acad Dermatol* 1986; **14**: 803–9.
4 Rich P. Nail biopsy: indications and methods. *J Dermatol Surg Oncol* 1992; **18**: 673–82.

Matrix biopsy

Lateral longitudinal nail biopsy [1,2]

Lateral longitudinal nail biopsy is the definitive method for sampling all the tissues of the nail unit. It is most commonly required when there is dystrophy affecting the whole nail or for the excision of a melanonychia. If focal matrix pathology occurs laterally, longitudinal biopsy may be warranted to preserve the shape of the nail, which can otherwise be altered by local matrix surgery. Early literature suggested that longitudinal biopsies of less than 3 mm in width could be taken from the midline of the nail without scarring [3] but it is now accepted that this may produce long-term nail dystrophy.

The first incision starts in the lateral nail sulcus, between the nail and nail fold. The distal limit is just beneath the distal groove, in the tip of the digit. Proximally, the incision extends almost to the first of the transverse skin markings of the distal interphalangeal joint. The medial margin of the ellipse is formed by an incision through the nail plate, which has been softened by an antiseptic soak. Both incisions are down to bone and separated by 3 mm at the widest point. The specimen is released from its deep

attachment from the distal point proximally. The nail can be lifted at the free edge with forceps, allowing the bottom of the specimen to be released with curved iris scissors. Particular care is needed at the proximal end to ensure that the matrix is fully sampled without damage.

A 3/0 or 4/0 monofilament suture is used for closure. One suture closes the wound through the proximal nail fold. One or two further sutures are needed through the nail plate and lateral nail fold. The suture is designed to

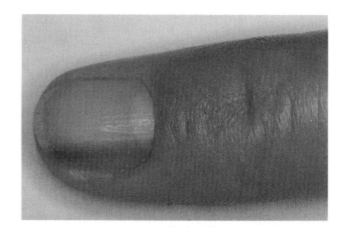

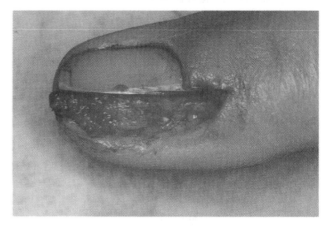

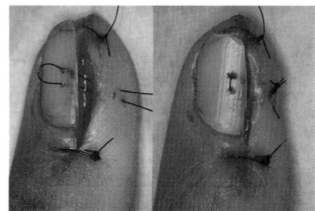

Fig. 65.38 A large, lateral, longitudinal nail biopsy is closed with sutures designed to reconstruct the lateral nail fold.

elevate the lateral nail fold and enhance the embedding of the new nail edge in the nail fold (Fig. 65.38).

The nail will be permanently narrowed following this procedure and the contour of the lateral and proximal nail fold intersection is altered to provide a more acute angle. In spite of the specialized suture to elevate the lateral nail fold, the nail is seldom fully embedded in a new lateral sulcus. Where biopsies of greater than 3 mm width are taken, the nail may develop malalignment, with distal deviation towards the side of the biopsy [4].

REFERENCES

1 Rich P. Nail biopsy: indications and methods. *J Dermatol Surg Oncol* 1992; **18**: 673–82.
2 Salasche SJ, Peters VJ. Tips on nail surgery. *Cutis* 1985; **35**: 428–38.
3 Zaias N. The longitudinal nail biopsy. *J Invest Dermatol* 1967; **49**: 406–8.
4 de Berker D, Baran R. Acquired malalignment of the nail following broad lateral longitudinal nail biopsy. *Acta Derm Venereol (Stockh)* 1997 (in press).

Transverse matrix biopsy (Fig. 65.39)

A transverse matrix biopsy may be performed to investigate focal matrix abnormality of a nail dystrophy arising from the matrix.

The proximal nail fold is reflected following an oblique incision at the junction with the lateral nail folds and gentle separation of the proximal nail fold from the dorsal aspect of the nail plate. The matrix is then visualized by performing a proximal hemiavulsion. A thin ellipse is taken from the distal matrix with the distal margin of the excision matching the shape of the lunula.

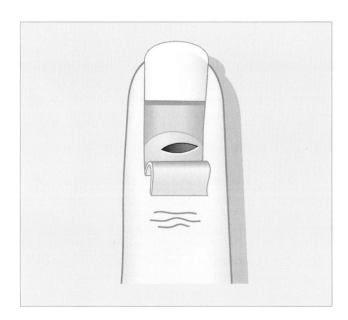

Fig. 65.39 Crescentic or narrow elliptical transverse matrix biopsy, which can be performed after removal of the proximal half of the nail plate alone.

The wound may be gently undermined, taking care with the extremely fragile matrix epithelium and undermining most on the distal nail bed margin. Loose sutures with resorbable 6/0 monofilament can be used.

Once healed, a blemish may remain in the margin of the lunula. The nail plate will show changes in thickness proportional to the extent of the biopsy.

Nail-fold biopsy [1–4]

Proximal nail-fold biopsy

It may be necessary to biopsy the proximal nail fold to investigate a local dermatosis, connective tissue disease or focal tumour. The biopsy can be taken in different axes, but preservation of the symmetry and curvature of the proximal nail fold is a priority. If sutures are to be used, a distal wing block should be avoided, as the tissues will become turgid and difficult to manipulate.

Transverse nail-fold biopsy

A transverse ellipse (for connective tissue disease), a 2-mm punch (far from the free edge) or a shave biopsy are simple nail fold procedures. The transverse ellipse and punch biopsies are down to the dorsal aspect of the nail plate. The matrix may require protection from cutting trauma and this can be achieved by inserting a septum elevator between the nail fold and the nail.

The transverse biopsy requires 4/0 monofilament suture. Wounds from other biopsy methods can be left to heal by secondary intention. Postoperatively, a thin line may remain in the nail fold after the transverse biopsy; otherwise, these techniques leave little or no scarring. There is no nail-plate change.

Crescentic nail-fold biopsy

A larger nail-fold biopsy can be taken as a distal crescentic wedge. A crescentic incision is performed just proximal to the cuticle with the blade bevelled to direct trauma away from the proximal matrix if the nail is penetrated. Additional matrix protection may be provided by inserting a septum elevator beneath the proximal nail fold. The distal fraction of the proximal nail fold (including the cuticle) can be removed, although the width of the specimen should not exceed 4–5 mm in the midline. The contour is aimed at recreating a new edge to the entire nail fold. The wound heals by secondary intention and a new cuticle usually reforms, depending upon the original problem. The amount of exposed nail is permanently enlarged, but the nail surface is unchanged unless ridging or grooves produced by the original pathology are reversed.

This technique can be used for the excision of chronic paronychia resistant to routine therapy. It has also been

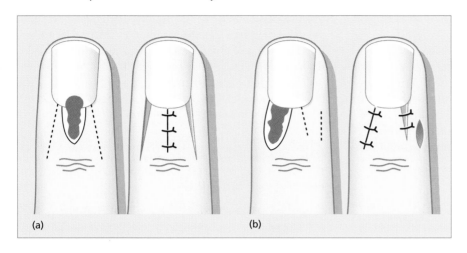

Fig. 65.40 Method for removing a small lesion from the proximal nail fold.

recommended for the excision of digital mucous cysts occupying the most distal margin of the nail fold. At this site, it is argued that the lesions are solely degenerative and do not communicate with the joint space [3,4].

Focal nail-fold biopsy

Focal pathology in the nail fold can be excised by a V-shaped incision into the nail fold. The excision is through the entire thickness of the nail fold, but should not penetrate underlying nail. Relaxing incisions are made at one or both of the lateral margins of the proximal nail fold (Fig. 65.40). The primary defect is closed with 4/0 monofilament and the relaxing incisions heal by secondary intention. Wounds in the midline of the nail fold can leave some scarring, but the nail plate is usually unaffected.

REFERENCES

1 Baran R. Removal of the proximal nail fold. Why, when, how? *J Dermatol Surg Oncol* 1986; **12**: 234–6.
2 Haneke E, Baran R. Nail surgery and traumatic abnormalities. In: Baran R, Dawber RPR, eds. *Diseases of the Nail and their Management*, 2nd edn. Oxford: Blackwell Scientific Publications, 1994: 345–416.
3 Salasche SJ. Myxoid cysts of the proximal nail fold: a surgical approach. *J Dermatol Surg Oncol* 1984; **10**: 35–9.
4 Schnitzler L, Baran R, Civatte J et al. Biopsy of the proximal nail fold in collagen diseases. *J Dermatol Surg Oncol* 1976; **2**: 313–15.

Nail-plate biopsy [1]

It is sometimes useful to biopsy the nail plate, with or without a small piece of the hyponychium. This may help differentiate between onychomycosis and psoriasis. If hyponychium is included, a small bleb of anaesthetic will be needed or a distal wing block can be performed. A chunk of distal nail plate of at least 3 mm width is then removed with large nail clippers. Subungual debris should also be obtained and a scalpel may be needed if hyponychium is attached. Hyponychial wounds heal by secondary intention after cautery haemostasis and leave no scarring.

REFERENCE

1 Suarez SM, Silvers DN, Scher RK. Histologic evaluation of nail clippings for diagnosing onychomycosis. *Arch Dermatol* 1991; **127**: 1517–19.

Lateral matrix phenolization [1,2]

Ingrowing nails, and particularly toenails, are treated in many different ways [1–5]. However, phenolization is quick, relatively painless and has a high success rate. Any area of matrix may be phenolized, including total ablation. The procedure yields no specimen other than the nail plate.

After anaesthetic, antiseptic soak and tourniquet, the margin of lateral ingrowing nail is avulsed using nail splitters to separate it from the rest of the nail plate. The nail folds are then protected with a layer of yellow soft paraffin and 85% aqueous phenol is applied on the end of an orange stick to the exposed matrix. This is done for 3 min (one stick per minute), before douching with 70% alcohol to neutralize the chemical cautery. Although 3 min is common practice [1], in a recent series of phenolization of 537 ingrowing nails phenol was applied for 5–6 min and a 99% 1-year cure rate was achieved, with a mean healing period of 20 days [2].

As a result of this chemical burn, there is some ooze from the wound, which can occasionally last several weeks, but it is seldom infected and often pain free. If the ooze is prominent, the toe should receive daily potassium permanganate or povidone–iodine soaks, after culture for specific microbes. The nail is permanently narrowed.

There is occasionally a small element of lateral nail regrowth, but further surgery is only indicated if there is repeated symptomatic ingrowing. Complete nail ablation can be achieved using the same technique applied to the entire matrix.

REFERENCES

1 Dagnall JC. The history, development and current status of nail matrix phenolisation. *Chiropodist* 1981; **36**: 315–24.
2 Kimata Y, Uetake M, Tsukada S, Harii K. Follow up study of patients treated for ingrown nails with the nail matrix phenol method. *Plast Reconstr Surg* 1995; **95**: 719–24.
3 Bose B. A technique for excision of nail fold for ingrowing toenail. *Surg Gynecol Obstet* 1971; **132**: 511.
4 Haneke E. Surgical treatment of ingrown toenails. *Cutis* 1986; **37**: 251–6.
5 Johnson DB, Ceilley RI. A revised technique for the ablation of the matrix of a nail. *J Dermatol Surg Oncol* 1979; **5**: 642.

Other surgical modalities

Mohs micrographic surgery

This technique applied to the nail unit exploits the principle of maximum conservation of healthy tissue while ensuring tissue clearance of tumour. It is particularly useful in squamous cell carcinoma of the nail unit (see p. 2850), where it should be offered as an alternative to digit amputation when there is no evidence of invasion of bone by tumour [1,2]. At this site, the conservation of normal tissue is of considerable functional significance.

Cryosurgery

Cryosurgery is widely used for the treatment of periungual warts. There is a small risk of damage to the tendons in the finger with aggressive freezing techniques. It is also used for myxoid cysts [3,4]. The cysts should be evacuated of their mucoid contents before a double 20-s freeze–thaw cycle. EMLA (eutectic mixture of local anaesthetics) or injected local anaesthetic may sometimes be needed. This regimen produces cure in approximately 30% of cases [4], although more aggressive freezing can produce better results [3].

Infrared photocoagulation

This has been used as a treatment for myxoid cysts of the proximal nail fold [5]. The contents are evacuated through a puncture wound before treatment.

Carbon dioxide laser

There is a range of indications for carbon dioxide laser [6-8], and its virtue may be in provision of a bloodless wound which allows a good view of the surgical procedure. This can only normally be provided in cold-steel surgery by an effective tourniquet.

The bulk of laser work on the nail unit is for subungual and periungual warts. This uses the defocused mode with a 1–2-mm spot at 5–10 W output. This can be intermittent, in 0.05-sec bursts, or continuous. Haemostasis may not be complete, and both anaesthetic and tourniquet are usually used with the laser.

It is also useful as a focused destructive instrument in the treatment of myxoid cysts and ablation of abnormal nail in irreversible nail disorders. This includes partial destruction of the matrix of nails in pachyonychia congenita to reduce nail thickness.

REFERENCES

1 de Berker DAR, Dahl MGC, Malcolm AJ, Lawrence CM. Micrographic surgery for subungual squamous cell carcinoma. *Br J Plast Surg* 1996; **49**: 414–19.
2 Goldminz D, Bennett RG. Mohs micrographic surgery of the nail unit. *J Dermatol Surg Oncol* 1992; **18**: 721–6.
3 Dawber RPR, Sonnex T, Leonard J, Ralfs I. Myxoid cysts of the finger: treatment by liquid nitrogen spray cryosurgery. *Clin Exp Dermatol* 1983; **8**: 153.
4 de Berker DAR, Lawrence CM. Cryosurgery for myxoid cysts. *Br J Dermatol* 1997 (Suppl. 50): 27.
5 Kemmett D, Colver GB. Myxoid cysts treated by infra-red coagulation. *Clin Exp Dermatol* 1994; **19**: 118–20.
6 Apfelberg D, Maser M, Lash H, White D. Efficacy of the carbon dioxide laser in hand surgery. *Ann Plast Surg* 1984; **13**: 320–6.
7 Street M, Roegnik R. Recalcitrant periungual verrucae: the role of carbon dioxide laser vaporization. *J Am Acad Dermatol* 1990; **12**: 115–20.
8 Bennett G. Laser use in foot surgery. *Foot Ankle* 1989; **10**: 110–14.

Traumatic nail disorders

Nails may show signs of acute trauma, scars following acute trauma or chronic repetitive trauma.

Acute trauma

Acute trauma is classified with respect to severity, ranging from a small haematoma to digit amputation (Table 65.5).

Table 65.5 Classification of acute trauma. (From [1].)

Type	Effect	Therapy
I	Small haematoma associated with a small break in the nail bed	Fenestration of nail over the haematoma
II	Large haematoma (25%) of nail) with significant nail-bed injury	Remove nail in order to identify site and nature of subungual damage
III	Large haematoma, nail plate displaced	X-ray may reveal fracture of terminal phalanx, usually in association with nail-bed laceration which requires resorbable 6/0 suture
IV	Severe crush injury	Avulsion needed to reveal matrix, with multiple lacerations requiring careful reconstruction
V	Amputation of tip of digit, may include parts of matrix	If tip can be retrieved it should be used as a graft. Otherwise nail bed from other sites may provide autologous grafts

Nail-bed laceration

The nail bed may be lacerated by different forms of trauma, including incisions, crush and avulsion injuries. In simple injuries there is displacement of the nail plate, which may be found proximally avulsed, but retaining distal attachment to the nail bed. In this form of trauma, and in many others, the nail plate can be used as a useful splint [1]. Initially, the nail bed damage needs to be assessed by avulsion, and then the nail can be replaced after any necessary nail bed repair has been performed; a small window for drainage of blood and exudate is made in the nail [2]. More complicated injuries may require flap or graft reconstructions and, in some instances, vascularized composite nail grafts are used with microvascular anastomoses. When the wounds arise from crush injury, fracture is relatively common. If the distal tuft has been fractured to leave fragments of bone dispersed in the soft tissues, it may prevent long-term morbidity if these are removed [3].

REFERENCES

1 Van Beek AL, Kassan MA, Adson MH *et al*. Management of acute fingernail injuries. *Hand Clin* 1990; **6**: 23–38.
2 Zook EG. Discussion of 'Management of acute nail bed avulsions.' *Hand Clin* 1990; **6**: 57–8.
3 Zook EG. The perionychium. In: Green DP, ed. *Operative Hand Surgery*. New York: Churchill Livingstone, 1982: 1331–75.

Delayed trauma

The most common kind of chronic deformity following an acute injury is a split nail or reduction in the length of the nail bed with consequent overcurvature of the tip of the nail.

Cure of a split-nail deformity is difficult, with only a modest chance of success [1]. Sometimes, there is an associated pterygium. Treatment entails excision of the nail bed and matrix scar, and in the case of a pterygium, a split-skin graft may be placed on the ventral aspect of the proximal nail fold to help prevent recurrence of the pterygium. It is important to keep the wounded aspects of nail bed or matrix separate from the overlying nail fold after surgery, and this is often best done by returning the nail plate after soaking it in antiseptic during the procedure.

If treatment is required for a shortened distal phalanx with nail bed changes, there are two choices [2]: the entire nail can be phenolized, or a V–Y advancement flap can be performed based on two neurovascular pedicles.

REFERENCES

1 Hoffman S. Correction of a split nail deformity. *Arch Dermatol* 1973; **108**: 568–9.
2 Baran R, Dawber RPR, eds. *Diseases of the Nail and their Management*, 2nd edn. Oxford: Blackwell Scientific Publications, 1994: 378–9.

Haematoma [1,2]

Subungual bleeding is a common sign. It may present as a feature of acute trauma, with pain due to the recent event in combination with pain arising from the pressure exerted by the subungual accumulation of blood. Haematoma arising within the matrix will be incorporated into the nail plate [3]. The only treatment which can be offered is to relieve the pressure, and if seen soon after the injury this can be done by puncturing the nail, for instance with a hot, pointed implement, cautery or a small drill. This procedure will relieve pain and may save the nail. The possibility of an underlying fracture must be considered for larger haematomas [1]. As a general rule, if more than 25% of the visible nail is affected, the nail plate should be removed. With less extreme trauma, haematoma may not develop immediatlely and may be painless. This is most common in the toes and may give rise to clinical uncertainty as to whether it represents early subungual melanoma. A history of traumatic hobbies is useful, and signs of symmetrical nail trauma and inappropriate footwear all point towards trauma as the cause of the appearance. In this situation, making a small punch in the surface of the nail may reveal old blood as the source of pigment. Malignancies can bleed and so confirmation of blood does not refute the possibility of a tumour; but as an isolated finding in the absence of other clues, this test should be sufficient to obviate the need for surgical exploration. An alternative is to score a transverse groove in the nail at the proximal margin of the pigment and observe over a few weeks as the discoloration grows out. If pigment continues to spread proximal to the groove, surgical exploration is needed.

REFERENCES

1 Farrington H. Subungual haematoma—an evaluation of treatment. *Br Med J* 1964; **i**: 742–4.
2 Mortimer PS, Dawber RPR. Trauma of the nail unit including sports injuries. *Dermatol Clin* 1985; **3**: 415–20.
3 Stone OJ, Mullins JF. The distal course of nail haemorrhage. *Arch Dermatol* 1963; **88**: 186–7.

Chronic repetitive trauma

Chronic repetitive trauma may take several forms. Some have been considered in other sections detailing transverse ridges produced by a habit tic (Fig. 65.21; p. 2839), the canaliform dystrophy of Heller (Fig. 65.41; p. 2863) and chronic paronychia (Fig. 65.17; p. 2836).

Nail biting

The nail plate, periunguium and nail bed are all subject to nail biting and picking. Although fingers are most commonly involved, rarely toenails are also bitten [1].

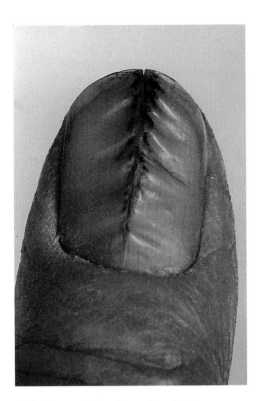

Fig. 65.41 Median canaliform dystrophy of Heller.

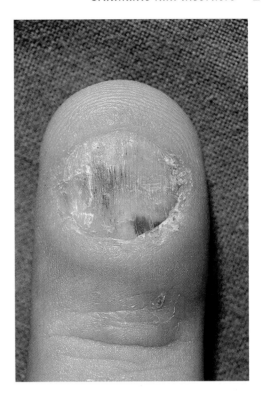

Fig. 65.42 Nail biting can be extensive, with damage to the nail folds and nail plate causing subungual haemorrhage.

This produces distinctive features, which are found in 60% of children, 45% of adolescents and 10% of adults [2]. The majority of moderate nail biters have no associated psychiatric disorder [3,4]. Focal abnormalities, such as viral warts, are often a complication, whether as a cause or as a result of the Köbner effect after biting. Aggressive forms may be associated with self-mutilating disorders such as Lesch–Nyhan syndrome.

The nails are typically short, with up to 50% of the nail bed exposed. The free edge may be even or ragged. Surface change may include splitting of the nail into layers or a sand-papered effect, and the nail may acquire a brown longitudinal streak [5]. The most aggressive nail biting (onychotillomania/onychophagia) can produce subungual haemorrhage, strips of nail loss, with residual spurs or loss of the entire nail (Fig. 65.42). Onychotillomania may be allied to parasitophobia when the patient picks off pieces claiming that they contain parasites [6]. A rough and irregular nail and nail fold may result. Many fingernails are involved. Oral pimozide may be beneficial [7].

Direct damage and secondary infection may make nail loss permanent or result in pterygium formation. The nail folds are sometimes bitten, in addition to, or as a substitute for, the nail. This can lead to bleeding and chronic paronychia with acute infective exacerbations. This in turn may lead to nail-plate damage or ridging and nail-fold scarring. In cases associated with infection, osteomyelitis of the terminal phalanx can develop [8,9]. Subjects will sometimes deny nail biting and attribute the appearance

to a disease which stops nail growth. Transverse grooves scored proximally in the nail plate will confirm that the nail is growing by moving distally with time. In aggressive nail biting, the groove may be eroded from the surface.

Trauma is sometimes inflicted by other nails, with pushing back of the proximal nail fold as part of a habit tic (see p. 2839). This results in serial transverse ridges and depressions running up the midline of the nail, associated with loss of the cuticle. In more conscious forms of self-damage, sharp instruments are used to produce dermatitis artefacta of the nail unit, and the nail fold is commonly preserved [10].

Treatment. Treatment is often unsuccessful and cure relies largely on the motivation of the patient. Local antiseptics and antimicrobial ointments may help settle the infection secondary to nail-unit damage. Those with the most bitter taste are often prescribed in the belief that this will discourage biting. This is seldom the case. Antidepressants [11] and behavioural therapy [12] have been used with some success in limited studies.

REFERENCES

1 Hurley PT, Balu V. Self-inflicted anonychia. *Arch Dermatol* 1982; **118**: 956–7.
2 Malone AJ, Massler M. Index of nail biting in children. *J Abnorm Social Psychol* 1952; **47**: 193–202.

3 Ballinger BR. The presence of nail-biting in normal and abnormal populations. *Br J Psychol* 1970; **117**: 445–6.

4 Colver GB. Onychotillomania. *Br J Dermatol* 1987; **117**: 397–9.

5 Baran R. Nail biting and picking as a possible cause of longitudinal melanonychia. *Dermatologica* 1990; **181**: 126–8.

6 Combes FC, Scott MJ. Onychotillomania. *Arch Dermatol Syphilol* 1951; **63**: 778–80.

7 Hamann K. Onychotillomania treated with pimozide (Orap). *Acta Derm Venereol (Stockh)* 1982; **62**: 364–7.

8 Tosti A, Peluso AM, Bardazzi F *et al*. Phalangeal osteomyelitis due to nail biting. *Acta Derm Venereol (Stockh)* 1994; **74**: 206–7.

9 Waldmann BA. Osteomyelitis caused by nail biting. *Pediatr Dermatol* 1991; **7**: 189–90.

10 Norton L. Self-induced trauma to the nails. *Cutis* 1987; **40**: 223–7.

11 Leonard HL, Lenane MC, Swedo SC *et al*. A double blind comparison of clomipramine and desipramine treatment of severe onychophagia (nail biting). *Arch Gen Psychiatry* 1991; **48**: 821–7.

12 Silber KP, Haynes CE. Treating nailbiting: a comparative analysis of mild aversion and competing response therapies. *Behav Res Ther* 1992; **30**: 15–22.

Hang nails

These are due to hard pieces of epidermis breaking away from the lateral nail folds. Although often due to nail biting, they may result from many other minor injuries. The splits may be painful when they penetrate to the underlying dermis. They should be removed with sharp, pointed scissors.

Nutcracker nails

Under this heading, Cohen [1] described splitting and onycholysis caused by the habit of separating the two halves of cracked walnuts over a period of 10 years.

REFERENCE

1 Cohen BH. Nutcracker nails. *Cutis* 1975; **16**: 141.

Damage from nail manicure instruments

Metal instruments, such as a nail file or scissors, wooden or plastic orange sticks, or nail whitener pencils may create acute or chronic injuries in the nail area. Onycholysis may result from using the sharp point for cleaning under the nail plate. Nails, however, are best cleaned with a nail brush and soap, because overzealous manicure, pushing back the cuticles, may result in white streaks across several nails. Cleaning around the nail with contaminated instruments may lead to acute or chronic paronychia. According to Brauer and Baran [1], it is not advisable to cut or clip the nail plate, as this produces a shearing action that weakens the natural layered structure and promotes fracturing and splitting. An emery board is preferred for shaping the fingernail by filing from the sides of the nail towards the centre.

REFERENCE

1 Brauer E, Baran R. Cosmetics: the care and adornment of the nail. In: Baran R, Dawber RPR, eds. *Diseases of the Nails and their Management*, 3rd edn. Oxford: Blackwell Scientific Publications, 1994: 285–95.

Trauma from footwear

Onychogryphosis and nail hypertrophy [1–5]

Onychogryphosis is an acquired dystrophy usually affecting the great toenail, which is thickened, yellow and twisted. It is most commonly seen in the elderly [1,2,4], although trauma and biomechanical foot problems may precipitate similar changes in middle age or before.

At one time, onychogryphosis was known as ostlers' nail, owing to the fact that some cases could be traced to injury caused by a horse trampling on the foot of the ostler. Competitive sport is a more contemporary cause. The injury once sustained is aggravated by footwear and, as the nail becomes longer and thicker, the damage from the footwear becomes progressively more important. Nail hypertrophy implies thickening and increase in length, whereas onychogryphosis implies curvature also.

Some cases of nail hypertrophy are intrinsic, and this applies especially to toenails other than the nail of the great toe. The nail becomes thick and circular in cross-section instead of flat, and thus comes to resemble a claw. There are two possible explanations for this formation.

1 There is insufficient matrix under cover of the posterior fold to exert a flattening effect.

2 The nail bed is contributing a greater quantity of keratin to the nail than usual.

Hypertrophy of fingernails is usually traumatic in origin and is often the result of a single injury.

In onychogryphosis, one or more nails become greatly thickened (Fig. 65.43), and with neglect, increase in length, becoming curved like a ram's horn. The nails of the great

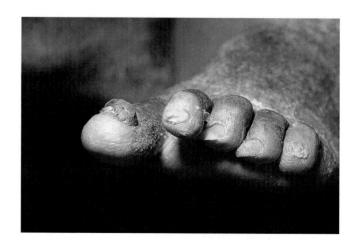

Fig. 65.43 Early onychogryphosis of the left great toenail.

toes are most often involved, but no toenail is exempt. It is possible that the nail-plate distortion produced by chronic untreated onychomycosis may be partly responsible for onychogryphosis at a later stage. In extreme cases, the free edge may press on or even re-enter the soft tissues of the foot.

Treatment of onychogryphosis and nail hypertrophy is either radical or palliative. Radical treatment consists of surgical removal of the nail and matrix and is recommended in young persons with good circulation. Palliative treatment requires regular paring and trimming of the affected nails, usually by a chiropodist using nail clippers and a file or mechanical burr. The thickened nails are extremely hard and trimming is difficult. Not infrequently, the nail is invaded by granulation tissue from the nail bed, and incision of this during trimming will result in pain and haemorrhage.

Other causes of thickened nails are psoriasis, pityriasis rubra pilaris, Darier's disease, fungal infections, pachyonychia congenita, congenital ectodermal defects and congenital malalignment of the great toenails [6].

REFERENCES

1 Cohen PR, Scher RK. Geriatric nail disorders: diagnosis and management. *J Am Acad Dermatol* 1992; **26**: 521–31.
2 Dawber RPR, Bristow I, Mooney J. *The Foot: Problems in Podiatry and Dermatology*. London: Dunitz, 1996.
3 Douglas MA, Krull EA. Diseases of the nails. In: Conn WB, ed. *Current Therapy*. Philadelphia: WB Saunders, 1981: 712.
4 Gilchrist AK. Common foot problems in the elderly. *Geriatrics* 1979; **34**: 67–70.
5 Lubach D. Erbliche onychogryphosis. *Hautarzt* 1982; **33**: 331–3.
6 Baran R, Bureau H. Congenital malignment of the great toenail as a cause of ingrowing toenail in infancy. *Clin Exp Dermatol* 1983; **6**: 619–23.

Ingrowing toenail [1–3]

The soft tissue at the side of the nail (lateral nail fold) is penetrated by the edge of the nail plate, resulting in pain, sepsis and, later, the formation of granulation tissue [4]. Penetration is often caused by spicules of nail at the edge of the nail plate, which have been separated from the main portion of the nail. The great toes are those most often affected. The main cause for the deformity is compression of the toe from the side due to ill-fitting footwear, and the main contributory cause is cutting the toenails in a half-circle instead of straight across. Anatomical features, such as an abnormally long great toe and prominent lateral nail folds, are important in some cases. In recent years, the condition may have been caused in a minority of cases by the successful therapy of fungal infections of the nails with griseofulvin: a nail which has been infected for a long time is reduced in size, and the nail bed shrinks around it; when the infection is even partly overcome the nail plate is increased in size, the nail bed is no longer large enough to accommodate the whole of the new nail, and the lateral nail fold may be penetrated on each side.

In infancy, ingrowing toenail most commonly occurs before shoes are worn, associated with crawling, 'pedalling' or wearing undersized 'jumpsuits' [5]; acute paronychia may be associated [6]. Rarely, it is congenital [7] and even familial [2].

The first symptoms are pain and redness, shortly followed by swelling and pus formation. Granulation tissue then forms and adds to the swelling and discharge. More severe infection may follow. There is seldom any difficulty with diagnosis.

Treatment. Treatment may be difficult and prolonged [4,8]. The first essential is to insist on the patient wearing shoes sufficiently wide and pliable to remove lateral pressure [9]. Any abnormality of the foot/toe function should be corrected. The patient must also be instructed to cut the nail straight across instead of in a semicircle. The nail must be allowed to grow until its edges are clear of the end of the toe before it is cut; this prevents the further formation of marginal spicules. In the early stages, the infection may be overcome by the application of antiseptics and by inserting a pledget of cotton-wool under the edge of the nail. Twice-daily warm-water baths followed by careful drying and powdering are helpful. If the infection is more severe and there is local cellulitis, an appropriate systemic antibiotic should be administered. When granulation tissue forms this should be destroyed by cauterization with a silver nitrate stick. If these conservative measures fail, operative intervention will be necessary. The granulation tissue should be excised and the nail fold may require removal at the same time. In some cases, avulsion of the nail will be required, and indications for this are continuing cellulitis, severe pain and failure to improve with less radical treatment. The time-honoured removal of part of the nail is not now considered satisfactory treatment. It is important, however, to remove the spicule, which may be quite large, from its embedded site.

If recurrence occurs after conservative therapy, then removal of the nail and matrix is required. A variety of operations have proponents but lateral matricectomy is usually adequate (see p. 2860) [4,8]. This operation is suitable for young persons, but in the elderly and especially in association with diabetes or impaired peripheral circulation, conservative treatment employing a skilled podiatrist is recommended.

REFERENCES

1 Baran R, Bureau H. Congenital malalignment of the great toenail as a cause of ingrowing toenail in infancy. *Clin Exp Dermatol* 1983; **6**: 619–23.
2 Cambiaghi S, Pistritto G, Gelmeti C. Congenital hypertrophy of the lateral nail folds of the hallux in twins. *Br J Dermatol* 1997; **136**: 635–6.
3 Samman PD. Nail deformities due to trauma. In: Samman PD, Fenton DA, eds. *The Nails in Disease*. London: Heinemann, 1986: 148–9.
4 Baran R. L'ongle incarné. *Ann Dermatol Vénéréol* 1987; **114**: 1597–604.
5 Verbov J. Ingrowing toenails in infancy. *Br Med J* 1978; **ii**: 1087.
6 Walker S. Paronychia of the great toe of infants. *Clin Pediatr* 1979; **18**: 247–8.

7 Katz A. Congenital ingrown toenails. *J Am Acad Dermatol* 1996; **34**: 519–20.
8 Salasche S. Nail surgery. In: Scher RK, Daniel CR, eds. *Nails: Therapy, Diagnosis, Surgery*. Philadelphia: WB Saunders, 1990: 258–80.
9 Wernick J, Gibbs RC. Pedal biomechanics and toenail disease. In: Scher RK, Daniel CR, eds. *Nails: Therapy, Diagnosis, Surgery*. Philadelphia: WB Saunders, 1990: 244–9.

The nail and cosmetics [1–3]

Dermatologists need to know the therapeutic options open to a patient when drugs may not provide the ideal aesthetic or functional solution to a medical problem. Professional cosmetic advice may be the most appropriate step in some cases. However, the dermatologist may gain most experience of nail cosmetic products through their adverse effects, as they occasionally cause injury to the nail and surrounding tissues and may cause reactions at distant sites. In this section, the basic ingredients of nail preparations are considered together with the pathological changes sometimes induced by them [1,2,4]. In assessing eczematous and other periungual reactions, it is important also to realize that nail tissues, particularly the subungual and paronychial areas, may be 'reservoirs' for small amounts of cosmetic preparations applied by hand to other parts of the skin; these may cause nail-apparatus abnormalities.

Nail polish

The term nail lacquer is sometimes used to include enamels, top coats and base coats, either as separate entities or combined in one product. Chemically, they are similar, although they contain different ratios of the same constituents to lend different characteristics. The base coat is a material used to improve the adhesion or bonding of enamel to the nail. A top coat improves the depth and lustre of the enamel and increases its resistance to chipping and abrasion. Nail polishes consist of solids and solvent ingredients, the former representing about 30%, the latter 70% of the product. Essentially, the ingredients can be divided into six principal groups.
1 Cellulose film formers, such as nitrocellulose. These give gloss, body and gel structure.
2 Resins, such as toluene sulphonamide formaldehyde resin, to improve the gloss and adhesion of the film.
3 Plasticizers, such as dibutylphthalate, added to give the film pliability, to minimize shrinkage, and soften and plasticize the cellulose.
4 Thixotropic suspending agents, such as bentonite, for non-settling and flow. They keep pigments in suspension on shaking.
5 Solvents (such as butyl) and diluents (such as toluene), which keep nitrocellulose, resin and plasticizer in a liquid state and control the application and drying time.
6 Colour substances. These are either inorganic (iron oxides) or a variety of certified organic colours (D and C yellow, A1 lakes). In principle, they require to be insoluble in a nail lacquer system.

'Pearls' or 'frosts' are produced by bismuth oxychloride and titanium dioxide coated with mica and guanine (obtained from fish scales). 'Clears' contain a small tint.

The base coat is formulated in a manner similar to standard lacquer, but it has a lower non-volatile content (less nitrocellulose) and a lower viscosity, because a thinner film is desirable; it may also contain hydrolysed gelatin. In the top coat the nitrocellulose content is increased, and the resin is reduced. A slight increase in plasticizer content improves elasticity of the film. There is no pigment. The top coat often has an added sunscreen.

Reactions such as nail polish dermatitis of allergic origin frequently appear on any part of the body accessible to the nails, with no signs in or around the nail apparatus [3]. The commonest areas involved are the eyelids [5], the lower half of the face, the sides of the neck and the upper chest. Generalized dermatitis may rarely occur. Sometimes the use of nail polish on stockings to stop 'runs' or on nickel-plated costume jewellery to prevent nickel dermatitis may induce nail-polish dermatitis respectively on the legs or at the site of the metal contact. Nail-polish dermatitis may occur in the user's partner or other close contacts. Although any ingredient may account for distant allergic contact dermatitis, toluene sulphonamide formaldehyde resin is the most common culprit [6]. After the nail polish is removed, the dermatitis usually clears rapidly unless secondary infection or lichenification has occurred. Metal pellets put in some bottles to maintain a liquid state may cause nickel reactions and onycholysis.

Nail-plate staining from the use of polish is most commonly yellow–orange in colour. It typically starts near the cuticle, extends to the nail tip and becomes progressively darker from base to tip. With the leaking out of the varnish, the dyes penetrate the nail too deeply to be removed. Injury to the nail plate from nail lacquers is rare. However, 'granulation' of nail keratin, a superficial friability, can be observed in some instances where individuals leave nail lacquer on for many weeks, or due to poor formulation of the product. For patch testing, several nail lacquers should be used and tested 'as is'; they should be allowed to dry for 15 min because the solvents and diluents may cause false-positive reactions. The following substances should be included in the test battery.

Toluene sulphonamide formaldehyde resin (10% petrolatum)
Nickel (0.5% petrolatum) DMG spot test for nickel
Glyceryl phthalate resin (polymer resin) (10% petrolatum)
Pearly material—guanine powder (pure)
Formaldehyde (1–2% in aqua)
Colophony (resin) 10% petrolatum (Fisher) 20% (Cronin), drometrizole (Tunuvin P) 1% petrolatum to 5%

The resin contains no free formaldehyde. Formaldehyde is merely the chemical moiety on which the resin is formed. Usually, formaldehyde-sensitive individuals do not cross-react with this resin. However, it has been suggested that there is always a small amount of free formaldehyde present in many preparations [7]. Various cosmetic companies make varnishes which are formulated without the sensitizing resin, using alkyl resin as a substitute; unfortunately this tends to peel and chip.

Nail polish removers

These are composed of various solvents such as acetone. Occasionally, nail polish removers cause trouble by excessive drying of the nail plate and may be responsible for some inflammation of nail folds.

Acrylic nails

SYN. SCULPTURED NAILS; GEL NAILS

There are three forms of sculptured acrylic nails, with a range of possible adverse reactions [8]. The basic kit is sold as a set containing a template, a liquid monomer and a powdered polymer. Self-curing acrylic resins are created by polymerization of methyl methacrylate monomer and polymethyl methacrylate powder with an organic peroxide and an accelerator. They harden at room temperature. The compound has to be moulded on the natural nail. The acrylic compound is applied to a nail which has been roughened on the surface. When hardened, the compound produces a prosthetic nail which is enlarged and elongated by repeated applications. The prosthesis can be filed and manicured to shape, and as the nail plate grows out, further applications of acrylic can be made to maintain a regular contour.

Gel nails are the second form of acrylic nail. The acrylate monomer is painted onto the nail before exposure to a UV source, which induces polymerization and photo-bonding of the gel to the nail plate. The hardened surface can then be filed, polished and coated.

The final form is cyanoacrylate 'Krazy glue' or 'Super glue' preparations, which are painted onto the nail and polymerize directly in air.

Allergic contact dermatitis may occur, typically 2–4 months after the first application [9]. The reaction may involve the face, eyelids and dorsal aspect of some of the involved fingers as well as paronychial tissues. All affected individuals complain of severe onychial and paronychial pain, sometimes associated with persistent paraesthesia, and uncommonly nail discoloration is seen. The nail bed can be dry and thickened. The nail dystrophy usually consists of onycholysis with thinning and splitting of the true nail. It may be several months before the nails return to normal. Positive sculptured artificial nail patch tests most commonly show reactions to the acrylic liquid

monomer and not to the polymer—this is similar to denture allergy. Suggested allergens for testing should include: methyl methacrylate monomer (10% in olive oil) and methacrylate acid esters (1 and 5% in olive oil and petrolatum). As acrylic monomers may cross-react, the newer products seem just as likely to cause allergic dermatitis.

Preformed plastic nails

Preformed plastic nails are packaged in several shapes and sizes to conform to the normal nail-plate configuration. Such nails are trimmed to fit the fingertip and are fixed with specific adhesive supplied with the kit. The usefulness of these prosthetic nails is limited by the need for some normal nail to be present for attachment. Normal physical and chemical insults to the nails cause the preformed plastic nails to loosen unless the ethyl 2-cyanoacrylate adhesive is used. If the preformed nails remain in place for 3 or 4 days they may cause onycholysis and nail-surface damage; less commonly, complete disruption of the nail may occur if the plastic nail is left *in situ* for 3 or more days. The changes may be indistinguishable from those caused by formaldehyde nail hardeners. In some cases, distant allergic eczematous contact dermatitis of the face and eyelids has occurred. On patch testing, the patients react far more often to the adhesive than to the prosthetic nails. Suggested test substances are paratertiary butyl phenol resin (1% petrolatum); tricresyl ethyl phthalate (5% petrolatum); cyanoacrylates; other glues (5% methyl ethyl ketone).

Nail hardeners

Nail keratin can be hardened by tissue fixatives such as formaldehyde preparations. These are not commercially available in the USA because of their toxic effects. Nail changes caused by such nail hardeners may include subungual haemorrhage and bluish discoloration of the nail. The nail returns to normal when the offending agent is discontinued. Formaldehyde nail hardeners have been reported as causing onycholysis and allergic contact dermatitis; they may also act as irritants. Patch testing should be with formaldehyde (1–2% in aqua). Because of its irritant qualities, reactions should be interpreted with caution.

Stick-on nail dressing, 'press-on' nail polish, synthetic nail covers

Stick-on nail dressings consist of a thin, coloured synthetic film with an adhesive which fixes them firmly to the nail. The pathological changes produced in nails vary considerably in intensity from patient to patient, and may include flaking, roughness, ridging, onycholysis, disappearance of the lunula, disorganization of the nail plate, delaminated and broken nails, mild paronychial inflammation, and often disappearance of the cuticle. In some instances the nail only returns to normal after a year. The effects on the nail are traumatic, possibly irritant, but rarely allergic.

Nail-mending kits

These include paper strips of a basic film-forming product to create a 'splint' for the partially fractured nail plate.

Nail wrapping

In nail wrapping, the free edge of each nail is splinted with layers of a fibrous substance, such as cotton-wool, paper or plastic film; it is fixed with a variety of nitrocellulose glues. After drying, the edge is shaped, and the nail is coated with enamel. The entire procedure needs to be repeated approximately every 2 weeks.

Cuticle removers or softeners

These contain sodium or potassium hydroxide. If they are left in place for more than approximately 20 min, minor degrees of irritation may result. Triethanolamine can be a sensitizing agent (5% in petrolatum for patch testing). Cuticle removers contain substances such as quaternary ammonium or urea.

Nail cream

This is an ordinary water-in-oil moisturizing cream, with low water (30%) and high lipid content. It is applied, after cleaning the hands, to prevent or diminish brittleness.

Nail buffing

Weekly buffing may be indicated for removing small particles of nail debris, thus enhancing the lustre and smoothness of the nail plate. Buffing creams, which contain waxes and finely ground pumice, and buffing powders, are abrasive and should not be overused on thin nails.

REFERENCES

1 Baran R, Barth J, Dawber RPR, eds. Cosmetic treatment of nail dystrophies. In: *Nail Disorders*. London: Dunitz, 1991: 181–2.
2 Brauer E, Baran R. Cosmetics: the care and adornment of the nail. In: Baran R, Dawber RPR, eds. *Diseases of the Nails and their Management*. Oxford: Blackwell Scientific Publications, 1994: 285–95.
3 Dobes WL, Nippert PH. Contact eczema due to nail polish. *Arch Dermatol* 1944; **49**: 183–7.
4 Cronin E. *Contact Dermatitis*. Edinburgh: Churchill Livingstone, 1980: 792.
5 Shah M, Lewis F, Gawkrodger DJ. Facial dermatitis and eyelid dermatitis: a comparison of patch test results and final diagnoses. *Contact Dermatitis* 1996; **34**: 140–1.
6 Liden C, Berg M, Färv G, Wrangsjö K. Nail varnish allergy with far-reaching consequences. *Br J Dermatol* 1993; **68**: 57–62.
7 Nater JP, de Groot AC, Liem DH. Nail cosmetics. In: Nater JP, de Groot AC, eds. *Unwanted Effects of Cosmetics and Drugs Used in Dermatology*. Amsterdam: Excerpta Medica, 1983: 277.
8 Rosenzweig R, Sher RK. Nail cosmetics: adverse reactions. *Am J Contact Dermatitis* 1993; **4**: 71–7.
9 Fisher AA, Franks A, Glick H. Allergic sensitization of the skin and nails; acrylic plastic nails. *J Allergy* 1957; **28**: 84–8.

Chapter 66
Disorders of Hair

R. P. R. DAWBER, D. de BERKER &
FENELLA WOJNAROWSKA

Anatomy and physiology

Introduction [1–12]

Hair has no vital function in humans, yet its psychological functions are extremely important, as any clinical dermatologist or cosmetician can readily attest from routine daily practice. If the inevitability of scalp baldness makes it reluctantly tolerable to genetically disposed men, in women, loss of hair from the scalp is even more distressing than the growth of body or facial hair in excess of the culturally acceptable norm.

The evolutionary history of hair is no less enigmatic. Whatever its origin, it is clear that the warm-blooded mammals owe much of their evolutionary success to the properties of the hairy pelage as a heat insulator. Paradoxically, Man's movement from the ancestral forest home to populate the globe is linked with a reversion to relative nudity and an ability to keep cool (Chapter 2). Moreover, hair serves other purposes: in particular, it is concerned with sexual and social communication by constructing adornments such as the mane of the lion or the beard of the human male, or assisting in the dispersal of scents secreted by complexes of sebaceous or apocrine glands.

For these evolutionary reasons, hair follicles are not all under identical control mechanisms. To match the animal 'coat' to seasonal changes in ambient temperature or environmental background requires moulting and replacement of the hairs. The process appears to involve an inherent follicular rhythm, modified by circulating hormones such as androgens or thyroxine, whose secretion is, in turn, geared to environmental cues through the hypothalamus and hypophysis.

The control of sexual hair growth must be clearly differentiated from that of the moult cycle. The development of pubic, axillary and other body hair is delayed until puberty because it is dependent upon androgens in both sexes: that 'male' hormones are, in contrast, also a prerequisite for the manifestation of androgenetic alopecia still defies adequate explanation.

Hair grows from follicles, which are stocking-like infoldings of the superficial epithelium, each of which encloses at its base a small stud of dermis known as the dermal papilla. The cylinder of hair may be regarded as a holocrine secretion arising by division of cells surrounding the papilla, in the region known as the bulb. The follicles are sloped in the dermis, and the longer ones extend into the subcutaneous layer. An oblique muscle, the arrector pilorum, runs from a point in the mid-region of the follicle wall to the dermo-epidermal junction. Above the muscle, one or more sebaceous glands, and in some regions of the body an apocrine gland also, open into the follicle.

In all mammals, including humans, but with the possible exception of the merino sheep, and the poodle dog, hair follicles show intermittent activity. Thus, each hair grows to a maximum length, is retained for a time without further growth, and is eventually shed and replaced.

REFERENCES

1 Ebling FJG. Hair. *J Invest Dermatol* 1976; **67**: 98–105.
2 Hamilton JB. The growth, replacement and types of hair. *Ann NY Acad Sci* 1950; **53**: 461–752.
3 Lubowe II. Hair growth and hair regeneration. *Ann NY Acad Sci* 1959; **83**: 359–511.
4 Lyne AG, Short BF, eds. *Biology of the Skin and Hair Growth*. Sydney: Angus & Robertson, 1965.
5 Montagna W, Ellis RA, eds. *The Biology of Hair Growth*. New York: Academic Press, 1958.
6 Montagna W, Dobson RL, eds. *Advances in Biology of Skin*, Vol. IX. *Hair Growth*. Oxford: Pergamon, 1969.
7 Orfanos CE, ed. *Haar und Haarkrankheiten*. Stuttgart: Gustav Fischer-Verlag, 1979.
8 Orfanos CE, Happle R, eds. *Hair and Hair Diseases*. Berlin: Springer-Verlag, 1990.
9 Orfanos CE, Montagna W, Stüttgen G, eds. *Hair Research: Status and Future Aspects*. Berlin: Springer-Verlag, 1981.
10 Dawber R, ed. *Diseases of the Hair and Scalp*, 3rd edn. Oxford: Blackwell Science, 1997.
11 Hardy MH. The secret life of the hair follicle. *Trends Genet* 1992; **8**: 55–9.
12 Dawber RPR, Van Neste D. *Hair and Scalp Disorders*. London: Dunitz, 1995.

Development and distribution of hair follicles

Hair follicles appear first in the regions of the eyebrows, upper lip and chin at about 9 weeks of embryonic development, and in other regions in the fourth month [1]; by 22 weeks, the full complement of follicles is established. A fuller account of embryonic development is given in Chapter 3. As the body surface increases, there is a decrease in the actual density of follicles [2,3]. It has been generally accepted that under normal circumstances new follicles do not develop in adult skin; the evidence for and against neogenesis of follicles has been reviewed [4]. Recent work on transplanting dermal papillae below hairless epithelium has cast doubt on this concept. The total number of follicles in an adult man has been estimated at about 5 million, of which about 1 million are on the head and perhaps 100 000 in the scalp. There appear to be no significant sexual or racial differences in follicle number [2,3].

On the cheek and forehead, the average density of follicles of all types has been recorded as around 800/cm^2, whereas on the thigh and leg, it was only 50/cm^2 [2].

The greatest density of vellus hairs occurs on the forehead where there are on average 400–450/cm^2 in young adults of both sexes. Females have a similar density on the cheek. Lower densities of 50–100/cm^2 are found on the chest and back in both sexes [5,6].

In the scalp, a significant loss of hair follicles occurs with advancing age [7]; in adults aged 20–30 years an average of 615/cm^2 has been noted, but between 30 and 50 years the mean density falls to 485/cm^2, and by 80–90 years it is only 435/cm^2 [8]. There is undoubtedly a long-term decrease in follicles in baldness: a comparison of bald with hairy scalps for the whole range of 30–90 years gave means of 306/cm^2 and 459/cm^2 respectively [8].

REFERENCES

1 Pinkus H. Embryology of hair. In: Montagna W, Ellis RA, eds. *The Biology of Hair Growth*. New York: Academic Press, 1958: 1–32.
2 Szabo G. The regional frequency and distribution of hair follicles in human skin. In: Montagna W, Ellis RA, eds. *The Biology of Hair Growth*. New York: Academic Press, 1958: 33–8.
3 Szabo G. The regional anatomy of the human integument with special reference to the distribution of hair follicles, sweat glands and melanocytes. *Philos Trans R Soc Lond Biol* 1967; **252**: 447–85.
4 Muller SA. Hair neogenesis. *J Invest Dermatol* 1971; **56**: 1–9.
5 Blume U, Ferracin J, Verschoore M *et al*. Physiology of the vellus follicle: hair growth and sebum excretion. *Br J Dermatol* 1991; **124**: 21–8.
6 Blume U, Verschoore M, Poncet M. The vellus hair follicle in acne: hair growth and sebum excretion. *Br J Dermatol* 1993; **129**: 23–6.
7 Barman JM, Astore I, Pecoraro V. The normal trichogram of people over 50 years but apparently not bald. In: Montagna W, Dobson RL, eds. *Advances in Biology of Skin*, Vol. IX. *Hair Growth*. Oxford: Pergamon Press, 1969: 211–20.
8 Giacometti L. The anatomy of the human scalp. In: Montagna W, ed. *Advances in the Biology of Skin*, Vol. VI. *Ageing*. Oxford: Pergamon, 1965: 97–120.

The active follicle

Dynamics [1–3]

The bulk of any hair fibre is composed of a thick cortex made up of elongated keratinized cells cemented together, which in pigmented hairs contain granules of melanin. The cortex is surrounded by a cuticle and may also have a continuous or discontinuous core or medulla (Figs 66.1 & 66.2). Although the cuticle is formed as a single cell layer, the cells become progressively imbricated (tile-like) as they move peripherally. The outer cells overlap, their free edges directed towards the tip; these cells interlock with the cuticle of the surrounding inner root sheath. The latter consists of three layers, its outer cuticle and the Henle and Huxley layers; it is formed in pace with the hair and its keratinized cells are ultimately desquamated (Figs 66.1 & 66.3). Investing it is the outer root sheath, which is continuous with the superficial epithelium, and this is itself enclosed in a non-cellular partition known as the vitreous or 'glassy' layer of fibrous connective tissue, formed of collagenous fibres, a few elastic fibres and fibroblasts.

Cell formation in hair follicles has been studied by intracutaneous injection of 10µCi of tritiated thymidine into sites on the human scalp [4]. In biopsy samples taken 40 min later, labelling of cells was observed in the lower half of the hair bulb but not elsewhere. However, labelled cells were distributed diffusely within the area and not in a well-defined basal layer along the papilla, and no labelled

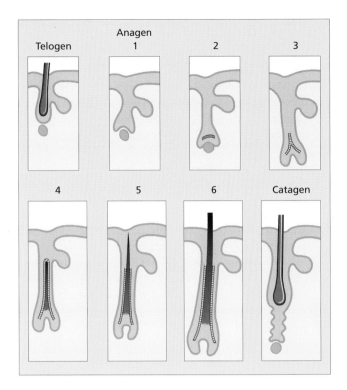

Fig. 66.1 The hair cycle. In stage 1 of anagen, cells at the base of the epithelial sac—the secondary germ—begin to show mitotic activity. In stage 2, the lower part of the follicle grows down, partly enclosing the dermal papilla. The inner root sheath appears as a keratinized plate-like structure overlying the matrix. At the same time, cells in the dermal papilla enlarge and begin to become separated by an extracellular matrix. As the follicle enters anagen 3 the keratinizing inner root sheath assumes a conical shape and the cortex starts to differentiate beneath it. Tyrosinase activity and melanogenesis becomes apparent in melanocytes in the matrix. In anagen 4, the cortex is keratinizing but has not yet penetrated the inner root sheath. Pigment donation to cortical cells is evident at this stage. In anagen 5, the developing hair shaft finally penetrates the inner root sheath at the level of the sebaceous duct, and anagen 6 represents the fully developed follicle. Stages 1–5 of anagen are sometimes known collectively as proanagen and stage 6 as metanagen. (Courtesy of Dr A. Messenger, Sheffield.)

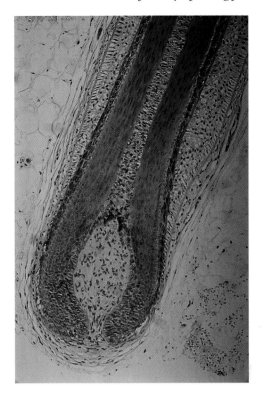

Fig. 66.2 Anagen (stage VI) scalp hair follicle. H & E stain. (Courtesy of Dr A. McDonagh, Royal Hallamshire Hospital, Sheffield, UK.)

mitotic figures were observed. Six hours after injection, the number of labelled cells had increased, labelled mitotic figures were seen and some movement was detected in cells of the outer bulb destined to become inner root sheath. Subsequently, a stream of cells moving into the cortex could also be perceived, but it moved much more slowly. In general, these results confirm earlier suggestions that new cells are formed by division in the region of the bulb surrounding the lower two-thirds of the dermal papilla; this does not answer the question of whether only cells adjacent to the dermal papilla are capable of division [5]. The fact that the number of grains per cell is reduced as labelled cells move peripherally suggests that further divisions take place, and the assumption that at each division one daughter cell remains capable of further

division and attached to the dermal papilla is also questionable in the light of studies of the behaviour of cells in the basal layer of the superficial epidermis [6].

REFERENCES

1 Forslind B. The growing anagen hair. In: Orfanos CE, Happle R, eds. *Hair and Hair Diseases*. Berlin: Springer-Verlag, 1990: 73–97.
2 Montagna W, van Scott EJ. The anatomy of the hair follicle. In: Montagna W, Ellis RA, eds. *The Biology of Hair Growth*. New York: Academic Press, 1958: 39–64.
3 Odland GF. Structure of the skin. In: Goldsmith LA, ed. *Biochemistry and Physiology of the Skin*. Oxford: Oxford University Press, 1983: 3–63.
4 Epstein WL, Maibach HT. Cell proliferation and movement in human hair bulbs. In: Montagna W, Dobson RL, eds. *Advances in Biology of Skin*, Vol. IX. *Hair Growth*. Oxford: Pergamon, 1969: 83–7.
5 Bullough WS, Laurence EB. The mitotic activity of the follicle. In: Montagna W, Ellis RA, eds. *The Biology of Hair Grwoth*. New York: Academic Press, 1958: 171–87.
6 Greulich RC. Aspects of cell individuality in the renewal of stratified squamous epithelium. In: Montagna W, Lobitz WC, Jr, eds. *The Epidermis*. New York: Academic Press, 1964: 117–33.

Composition of hair keratin [1–6]

Keratins are a group of insoluble cysteine-containing proteins produced in the epidermal tissues of vertebrates. Hair contains hard keratin, which differs from the soft keratin of desquamating tissues by its higher sulphur content.

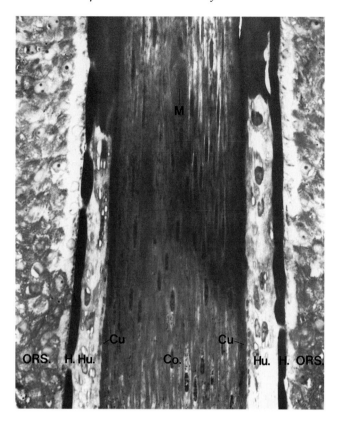

Fig. 66.3 Concentric layers of the hair follicle (resin embedded section). Within the cortex (Co) only occasional medullary cells are present (M). Within the outer root sheath (ORS), all layers show keratinization, which in the Huxley layer (Hu) is only evident in the upper area.

X-ray crystallography of hair gives a so-called α-diffraction pattern indicating an axial repeat of 0.51 nm units. If the hair is stretched or heated in water it gives the β-pattern with an axial repeat of 0.33 nm. This bears some similarity to the 'feather pattern' characteristic of keratin in avian and reptilian tissues, which has a repeat of 0.31 nm. A fourth pattern, described as amorphous because it lacks discrete reflections, occurs in the keratin of the hair cuticle. It is of interest that this is the site of the most dense concentration of high sulphur protein.

It was concluded from the X-ray diffraction pattern that the polypeptide chains of α-keratin had a geometrically regular secondary structure. The hypothesis was proposed that they were arranged in an α-helix with 3.6 amino-acid residues in each turn of 0.54 nm. The 0.51-nm repeat could be explained if the helices were tilted, which led to the suggestion that they were intertwined to form a rope of two or three strands [2], and possibly even seven [7]. The change to the β-pattern when hair is stretched can be explained by assuming that the helix is pulled into a straight-chain configuration.

Filaments known as microfibrils have long been recognized in keratinizing cells and are believed to bind up to form macrofibrils. It is now realized that all cells contain filaments of several size ranges, including six major types of intermediate filaments, 7–10 nm in diameter. Keratins fall within this category. The current view is that there are several stages of organization as keratin filaments are progressively assembled from polypeptides, namely a protofilament 2 nm in diameter consisting of 2 strands, a 3-nm protofilament of 2 × 2 strands, a 4–5-nm protofibril of 2 × 4 strands, and a 10-nm filament of 4 × 8 strands (Chapter 1).

Chemical analysis of keratin is complicated because the earlier procedures to render it soluble by breaking the disulphide links of an interchain, intramolecular or intermolecular nature can also cleave the peptides. Three soluble fractions are obtained from wool, a low sulphur of molecular weight 45 000–50 000, a high sulphur of molecular weight 10 000–28 000, and a high glycine-tyrosine. The complete amino-acid sequences have been determined for at least 21 wool proteins [3]. Low sulphur fractions contain the α-helices and account for the keratin filaments. The high sulphur proteins are not keratins but are associated with the filaments to create a fibre–matrix complex.

Within the last 15 years considerable advances have been made in understanding the biochemistry of keratins and the mechanisms of their alignment into macrofibrils, especially in relation to the epidermis. The keratins of the hair and hair follicle are discussed in Chapter 1, and by Lane *et al.* [8].

REFERENCES

1 Baden HP. Hair keratin. In: Orfanos CE, Happle R, eds. *Hair and Hair Diseases*. Berlin: Springer-Verlag, 1990: 45–71.
2 Fraser RDB, McRae TP, Rogers GE, eds. *Keratins: Their Composition, Structure and Biosynthesis*. Springfield: Thomas, 1972.
3 Gillespie JM. The structural proteins of hair: isolation, characterization and regulation of biosynthesis. In: Goldsmith LA, ed. *Biochemistry and Physiology of the Skin*. Oxford: Clarendon Press, 1983: 475–510.
4 Mercer EH. Electron microscopy and the biosynthesis of fibers. In: Montagna W, Ellis RA, eds. *The Biology of Hair Growth*. New York: Academic Press, 1958: 113–33.
5 Mercer EH, ed. *Keratin and Keratinization*. Oxford: Pergamon, 1961.
6 Rudall KM. The biomolecular structure of hair keratin. In: Rook A, Champion RH, eds. *Progress in the Biological Sciences in Relation to Dermatology*, Vol. 2. Cambridge: Cambridge University Press, 1964: 355–68.
7 Swanbeck G. A theory for the structure of α-keratin. In: Montagna W, Lobitz WC, Jr, eds. *The Epidermis*. New York: Academic Press, 1964: 339–50.
8 Lane EB, Wilson CA, Hughes BR, Leigh IM. Stem cells in hair follicles. *Ann NY Acad Sci* 1991; **642**: 197–213.

Ultrastructure [1–25]

The medulla

The cells of the medulla begin to show vesicles within their cytoplasm in the suprabulbar region. Such cells contain high concentrations of glycogen and may rarely include melanosomes (Fig. 66.4). Ultimately, above the level of the

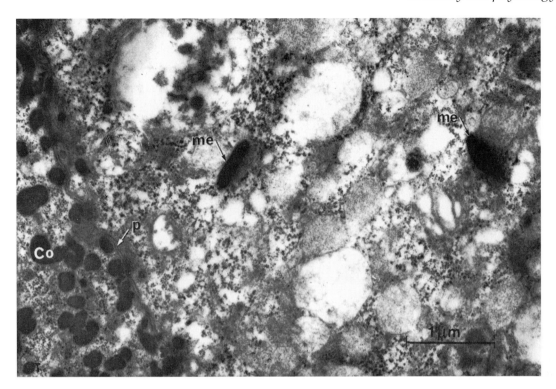

Fig. 66.4 Transverse section of adult hair, just above the bulb. Part of a cortical cell (Co) is separated by a plasma membrane (p) from a cell of the medulla containing vesicles and melanosomes (me).

epidermis, the cells appear to dehydrate and the large vacuoles become air-filled.

The cortex [1]

In the zone just below the tip of the dermal papilla, the microfibrils can already be seen in the cells which give rise to the cortex. They rapidly aggregate to form clusters; in the upper bulb region, aggregates a few tenths of a micron wide can be seen as fibrils with the light microscope. At this level the fibrils are birefringent and give the oriented α-type X-ray diffusion pattern; thus, the synthesis of the basic structure is virtually complete. Subsequently, the denser sulphur-rich matrix develops, coincident with the intense sulphydryl reaction, which indicates the presence of cysteine links. In contrast with the superficial epidermis (Chapter 3) and the inner root sheath, keratohyalin granules do not appear at any stage. On transmission electron microscopy the fully mature cortex is seen to consist of closely packed spindle-shaped cells with their boundaries separated by a narrow gap (20–25 nm) containing a dense, central plasma membrane or intercellular lamella (10–15 nm), generally believed to be proteinaceous and to cement the cells together. Within the cells, most of the microfibrils are closely packed and orientated longitudinally in lamellae, although some remain in loose bundles. In transverse section these concentric lamellae have a characteristic 'fingerprint' appearance (Fig. 66.5).

The cortex is the largest component of the mature hair fibre [26].

The cuticle of the hair [2,17]

The cuticle consists of five to 10 overlapping cell layers, each 350–450 nm thick. The mature cells are thin scales consisting of compact cuticular keratin which shows outer and inner zones of different densities (Fig. 66.6). Between the cell boundaries is a narrow gap (30 nm) containing a dense central intercellular lamella. From the outside, the scales can be seen to be imbricated like the tiles on a roof. Over the newly formed part of the hair the cell margins are intact, but as the hair emerges from the skin they become ragged (Fig. 66.7) and progressively break off ('weathering').

The 'environmental' outer surface of each cuticular cell has a very clear A-layer, which is rich in high sulphur protein; this protects the cuticular cells from premature breakdown due to chemical and physical 'insults'.

The inner, less dense part of the exocuticle also has a high concentration of sulphur-rich protein.

Inner root sheath [3]

Each of the three layers of the inner root sheath keratinizes, and although the rates of maturation are different, the patterns of change are identical. Filaments are about 7 nm thick and, in contrast with the hair cortex, amorphous

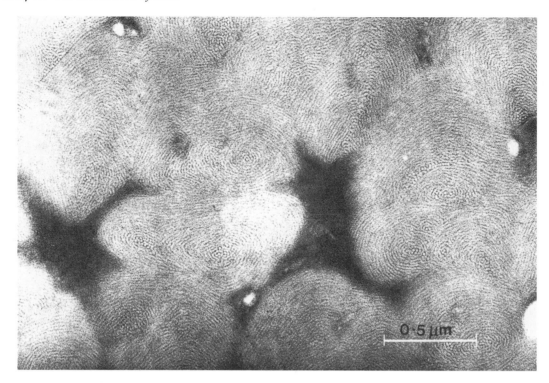

Fig. 66.5 Transverse section of transformed cortical cells of human hair. The relatively translucent filaments, set in a more dense, sulphur-rich matrix, appear as concentric lamellae (macrofibrils) giving a characteristic 'fingerprint' pattern.

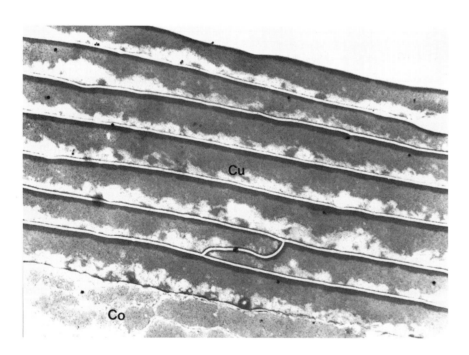

Fig. 66.6 Hair cuticle layers (Cu) surrounding the central cortex (Co) (electron micrograph). Silver methenamine stain.

trichohyalin granules appear in the cytoplasm. As the cells move up the follicle towards the surface, the filaments become more abundant and the number and size of the granules increase. In the hardened cytoplasm, however, only filaments can be seen. The changes occur first in the outermost Henle layer, then in the innermost cuticle and lastly in Huxley's layer, which is situated between them (Fig. 66.8).

The inner root sheath hardens before the presumptive hair within it, and it is consequently thought to control the

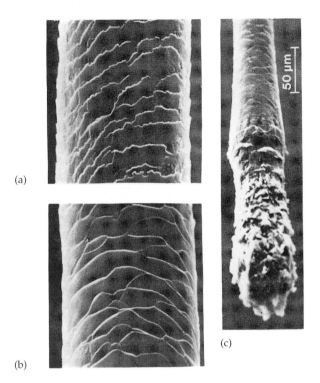

(a)

(b)

(c)

Fig. 66.7 (a) Surface view of jagged cuticular scales in the distal portion of the hair. (b) Surface view of cuticular scales in the region adjacent to the club. (c) Surface view of the proximal part of a club hair from the human scalp. (Courtesy of Dr D. Jackson, University of Sheffield, Sheffield, UK.)

Fig. 66.8 Transverse section of adult human terminal hair to show transformed Henle layer (He) with nuclear remnant (n), and Huxley layer (Hu) with trichohyalin (t) and filaments (f) in cytoplasm.

definitive shape of the hair shaft in health and in many genetic diseases with abnormal hair morphology.

Outer root sheath

As shown in both mice [9] and humans [8,10,11], the outer root sheath is composed of two layers. In the outer, the cells gradually increase in number, produce membrane-limited granules, or cementosomes, and keratinize in the region of the hair canal. The inner layer consists of single cells in which tonofilaments and keratohyalin, but not cementosomes, accumulate. Staining by antihair keratin monoclonal antibodies [10] has suggested that the differentiating cells of the medulla, cortex, cuticle and inner root sheath display similar keratin expression, but the innermost cell layer of the outer root sheath displays a unique expression.

REFERENCES

1 Birbeck MSC, Mercer EH. The electron microscopy of the human hair follicle. Part I. Introduction and the hair cortex. *J Biophys Biochem Cytol* 1957; **3**: 203–14.

2 Birbeck MCS, Mercer EH. The electron microscopy of the human hair follicle. Part II. The hair cuticle. *J Biophys Biochem Cytol* 1957; **3**: 215–22.

3 Birbeck MCS, Mercer EH. The electron microscopy of the human hair follicle. Part III. The inner root sheath and trichohyaline. *J Biophys Biochem Cytol* 1957; **3**: 223–30.

4 Breathnach AS. *An Atlas of the Ultrastructure of Human Skin.* London: Churchill, 1971.

5 Forslind B. The growing anagen hair. In: Orfanos CE, Happle R, eds. *Hair and Hair Diseases.* Berlin: Springer-Verlag, 1990: 73–97.

6 Forslind B, Swanbeck G. Keratin formation in the hair follicle. I. An ultrastructural investigation. *Exp Cell Res* 1966; **43**: 191–209.

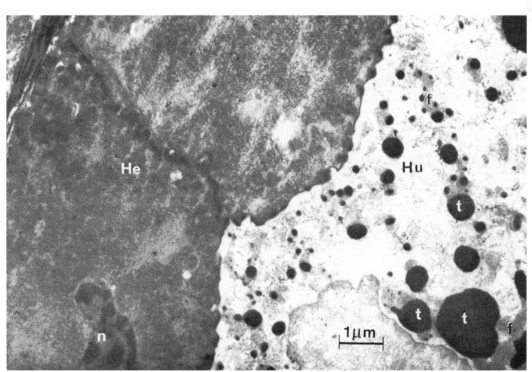

7 Fraser RDB, McRae TP, Rogers GE. *Keratins. Their Composition, Structure and Biosynthesis.* Springfield: Thomas, 1972.

8 Ito M. The innermost layer of the outer root sheath in human anagen hair follicle. Light and electron microscopic study. *Arch Dermatol Res* 1986; **279**: 112–19.

9 Ito M. Electron microscopic study on cell differentiation in anagen follicles in mice. *J Invest Dermatol* 1988; **90**: 65–72.

10 Ito M, Tazawa T, Ito K *et al.* Immunological characteristics and histological distribution of human hair fibrous proteins: studied with anti-hair monoclonal antibodies, HKN-2, HKN-4 and HKN-6. *J Histochem Cytochem* 1986; **34**: 269–75.

11 Ito M, Tazawa T, Shimaza N *et al.* Cell differentiation in human anagen hair follicles studied with anti-hair keratin monoclonal antibodies. *J Invest Dermatol* 1986; **86**: 563–9.

12 Mahrle G, Christenhusz R, Orfanos C. (Haar und Haarcuticula im Raster-Electronenmikroskop). Observations on hair and hair cuticle employing a stereoscan electron microscope. *Arch Klin Exp Dermatol* 1969; **235**: 295–300.

13 Mercer EH. Electron microscopy of keratinized tissues. In: Montagna W, Ellis RA, eds. *The Biology of Hair Growth.* New York: Academic Press, 1958: 91–111.

14 Mercer EH. *Keratin and Keratinization.* Oxford: Pergamon, 1961.

15 Odland GF. Structure of the skin. In: Goldsmith LA, ed. *Biochemistry and Physiology of the Skin.* Oxford: Oxford University Press, 1983: 3–63.

16 Orfanos C, Ruska H. Die Feinstruktur des menschlichen Haares. I. Die Haar-Cuticula. *Arch Klin Exp Dermatol* 1968; **231**: 97–110.

17 Orfanos C, Ruska H. Die Feinstruktur des menschlichen Haares. II. Der Haar-Cortex. *Arch Klin Exp Dermatol* 1968; **231**: 264–78.

18 Orfanos C, Ruska H. Die Feinstruktur des menschlichen Haares. III. Das Haarpigment. *Arch Klin Exp Dermatol* 1968; **231**: 279–92.

19 Parakkal PF, Matoltsy AG. A study of the differentiation products of the hair follicle cells with the electron microscope. *J Invest Dermatol* 1964; **43**: 23–4.

20 Puccinelli VA, Caputo R, Ceccarelli B. The structure of the human hair follicle and hair shaft: an electron microscope study. *G Ital Dermatol Sifilol* 1967; **108**: 453–98.

21 Rogers GE. Structural and biochemical features of the hair follicle. In: Montagna W, Lobitz WC, Jr, eds. *The Epidermis.* New York: Academic Press, 1964: 179–236.

22 Roth SI, Clark WH, Jr. Ultrastructural evidence related to the mechanism of keratin synthesis. In: Montagna W, Lobitz WC, Jr, eds. *The Epidermis.* New York: Academic Press, 1964: 303–37.

23 Swift JA. The electron histochemistry of cystine-containing proteins in thin transverse sections of human hair. *J R Microscop Soc* 1967; **88**: 449–60.

24 Van Scott EJ. Keratinization and hair growth. *Annu Rev Med* 1968; **19**: 337–50.

25 Zelickson AS. *Ultrastructure of Normal and Abnormal skin.* Philadelphia: Lea & Febiger, 1967.

26 Hashimoto K. Structure of human hair. *Clin Dermatol* 1988; **6**: 7–15.

Cyclic activity of the follicle [1]

The duration of activity of follicles, or anagen, varies greatly between species, in any species from region to region, and with age [1–5]. For example, in the rat the dorsal hair is fully formed in 3 weeks and the shorter ventral hair in only 12 days [6], whereas in the guinea-pig, anagen lasts for 20–40 days [7].

In human vellus follicles [8] of both sexes, the periods of activity ranged from about 40 to 80 days (Table 66.1). For terminal hairs in young Japanese males, the length of anagen has been estimated at 19–26 weeks on the leg, 6–12 weeks on the arm, 4–13 weeks on the finger, 4–14 weeks in the moustache and 8–24 weeks in the region under the temple [5]. Seago and Ebling [9] estimated averages of 54 and 28 days, respectively, for the thighs and arms of white males, and 22 days for each of these sites in females (Fig. 66.9). On the vertex of a 60-year-old Japanese man, the growing period for coarse hairs ranged between 19 and 94 weeks, and that of finer hairs between 7 and 22 weeks [5]. However, it is clear that in the human scalp, anagen may last as long as 3 years and sometimes much longer [10,11].

Activity is followed by a relatively short transitional phase, catagen (see Figs 66.1 & 66.10), occupying about 2 weeks in the human scalp, and a resting phase or telogen (see Fig. 66.1). Towards the end of anagen, scalp follicles show a gradual thinning and lightening of pigment at the base of the hair shaft [10,12]. The melanocytes in the region of the tip of the dermal papilla cease to produce melanin, resorb their dendrites and become indistinguishable from the matrix cells. The middle region of the bulb now starts to become constricted; distal to the constriction the

Table 66.1 Parameters of vellus hair growth.

Area	Sex	Follicles in anagen (%)	Rate of growth (mm/day)	Duration of anagen (days)	Definitive length (mm), age 15–20 years	Definitive length (mm), age 25–30 years
Forehead	F	49	0.04	58	2.2	1.6
	M	50	0.03	63	1.7	1.5
Cheek	F	46	0.06	79	4.1	3.4
	M	—	—	—	—	—
Shoulder	F	—	—	—	—	—
	M	33	0.12	51	6.0	4.3
Chest	F	42	0.11	41	4.1	3.4
	M	35	0.11	51	5.1	4.4
Back	F	31	0.15	42	5.9	4.9
	M	32	0.12	49	6.4	5.0

Data from Blume U *et al.* [8]. It may be observed that the difference in definitive length of the vellus between the back and the forehead is accounted for entirely by the rates of growth; that between male and female chests is entirely explained by the periods of anagen.

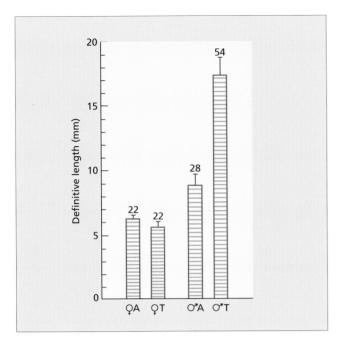

Fig. 66.9 Definitive length (mean ± SE) of hairs on the upper arm (A) and thigh (T) of 11 females and nine males aged 20–30 years. The average duration of anagen is also shown, and each segment represents the average growth per day.

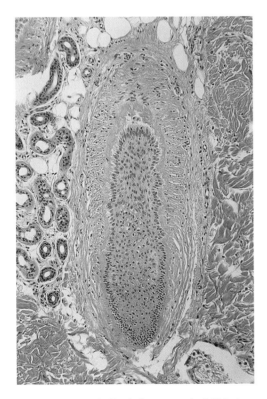

Fig. 66.10 The regressing bulb of a human scalp follicle in catagen. The thickened and corrugated vitreous membrane lies immediately peripheral to the central epithelial column. Outside it is a wide connective tissue sheath with an inner layer of radial and an outer layer of longitudinal fibres. (Courtesy of Dr A. McDonagh, Royal Hallamshire Hospital, Sheffield, UK.)

expanded base of the hair becomes keratinized as a 'club' (Figs 66.1, 66.11 & 66.12) and below the epithelial column can be seen the dermal papilla, which becomes released from its surrounding epidermis. From the onset of catagen [13], the connective tissue sheath of the follicle, in particular the 'vitreous' membrane, thickens enormously and causes characteristic corrugation of the epithelial strand (see Fig. 66.10). Subsequently, the club hair moves towards the skin surface so that the epithelial column lengthens. After the ascent of the presumptive club, the epithelial strand shortens progressively from below and finally is reduced to a small, nipple-like structure, the secondary germ. This resting stage, or telogen, lasts only a few weeks in the human scalp. When the next hair cycle starts, the secondary germ elongates by cell division, grows downwards, becomes invaginated by the papilla and gives rise to a new bulb, from which arises the keratinized dome of a new hair (Fig. 66.12). The old club is ultimately shed but, in the rat at least, it may be retained after emergence of the new hair.

Changes in the extracellular matrix of the dermal papilla may offer a clue as to what dermal–epidermal interactions are involved in the cyclic activity of the hair follicle [14,15].

In the adult human scalp, the activity of each follicle is independent of its neighbours [10,16,17]; such a pattern is known as a mosaic. At any one time, on average up to 13% of the follicles are in telogen, although the range is large; it has been recorded as 4–24% [10,16,18,19]. Only 1% or fewer are in catagen. If there are about 100000 follicles in the scalp and their period is about 1000 days, about 100 hairs ought to be lost each day; in practice, the average recovery of shed hairs is usually rather less, and over 100 can be regarded as high [10,11]. Follicles throughout the body, as well as those on the scalp, are out of synchrony and, indeed, have different periodicities. It is of particular interest, however, that the cycles of the hair comprising each 'Meijéres trio group' are in phase [5] (Figs 66.13 & 66.14).

The guinea-pig has been said to resemble the human in that moulting of the adult appears to take place in a mosaic pattern. However, in the newborn animal all follicles are simultaneously active [7], and it seems that for at least 50 days after birth, and probably for much longer, follicles producing a single fibre type show a measure of synchrony with each other but are out of phase with those producing different fibre types. The finding is of interest, because in humans there is frequently a more or less synchronous moult of scalp hairs during the early months of life as well as the shed of lanugo in development [11], and there is evidence of the passage of a growth wave from front to back in the scalp of newborn infants [11,18,20]. Thus, it may be that in both the guinea-pig and human, asynchrony gradually develops from synchrony.

Many animals moult in a characteristic wave pattern; in the rat, for example, replacement of hairs starts in the venter and bands of activity and shedding move over the flanks to the dorsum, subsequently spreading to the head and

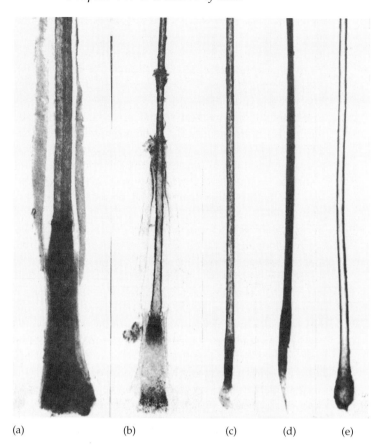

(a)   (b)   (c)   (d)   (e)

Fig. 66.11 Appearance of the hair root in plucked hairs. (a) Normal anagen hair; (b) dysplastic anagen hair with the root sheath still attached to it, from a female scalp showing chronic diffuse alopecia; (c) dysplastic anagen hair without root sheath; (d) dystrophic hair without root sheath and lacking matrix, but with pointed proximal end; (e) club hair. (Courtesy of O. Braun-Falco and H. Zaun.)

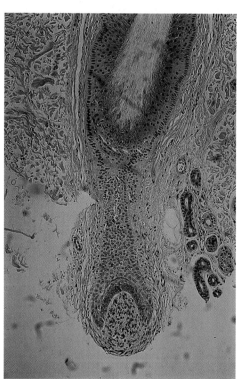

Fig. 66.12 Scalp hair follicle. Early anagen (stage II) showing dermal papilla partly engulfed by the epidermal matrix, but no sign of a keratinizing hair. (Courtesy of Dr A. McDonagh, Royal Hallamshire Hospital, Sheffield, UK.)

tail regions. Initially, while the animal is growing, the moults are correlated with age, and such spontaneous cycles continue throughout life in laboratory rodents [3,21–23]. However, in wild mammals, at least in temperate zones, the adult moult becomes seasonal, so that by altering the nature and colour of the pelage, the animal becomes adapted to ambient temperature, background or other environmental changes [23]. The skin cycle seems to resemble the sexual cycle in that it is influenced by the environment through the hypothalamus, the anterior hypophysis and the endocrine system [3,22]. An important environmental cue is the changing photoperiod as monitored by the pineal, which secretes melatonin during the hours of darkness. Ambient temperature appears to exert a modifying effect [3,22]. Hair growth in humans shows seasonal fluctuations [24]; this is discussed below.

Undoubtedly, changes in the hair cycle may be involved in transient hair loss in humans. Some of the conditions formerly grouped under the description 'alopecia symptomatica', which can result from a variety of mental and physical stresses, involve the simultaneous precipitation of many follicles into catagen. Kligman [11] described several cases of postfebrile alopecia in which shedding of club hairs began about 3–4 months after the fever and continued for several weeks. At the height of shedding, the telogen counts made from scalp biopsies ranged from

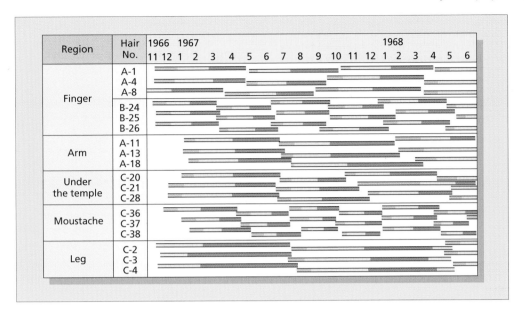

Region	Hair No.	1966 11	12	1967 1	2	3	4	5	6	7	8	9	10	11	12	1968 1	2	3	4	5	6
Finger	A-1 A-4 A-8 B-24 B-25 B-26																					
Arm	A-11 A-13 A-18																					
Under the temple	C-20 C-21 C-28																					
Moustache	C-36 C-37 C-38																					
Leg	C-2 C-3 C-4																					

Fig. 66.13 Cycles of three hairs in a Meijéres trio group. The pink bar indicates the time for the emergence of a new hair from the shedding of the club. The yellow bar indicates the period of activity of the follicle subsequent to emergence and the green bar indicates the resting period. (From Saitoh M *et al.* [5].)

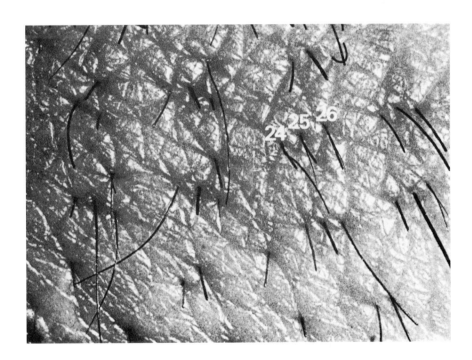

Fig. 66.14 Meijéres trio group from the finger of a man aged 30 years. (From Saitoh M *et al.* [5].)

34 to 53%; regeneration was well under way 6 weeks later. Similarly, a prisoner who underwent a series of trials for murder began to lose hairs at the rate of over 1000 per day about 10 weeks after conviction; there were no histological abnormalities except for an increased proportion of follicles in telogen. The phenomenon has been given the name 'telogen effluvium' (syn. telogen defluvium). The nature of the neuroendocrine or other mechanisms by which it is brought about remains to be elucidated. The condition bears some similarity to postpartum alopecia, which is presumed to follow hormonal changes and is considered further below (p. 2881).

REFERENCES

1 Ebling FJ, Johnson E. The control of hair growth. *Symp Zool Soc Lond* 1964; **12**: 97–130.
2 Ebling FJ. The hair follicle. In: Rook AJ, Champion RH, eds. *Progress in the*

Biological Sciences in Relation to Dermatology. Cambridge: Cambridge University Press, 1964: 303–23.

3 Ebling FJ. Comparative and evolutionary aspects of hair replacement. In: Rook AJ, Walton GS, eds. *Comparative Physiology and Pathology of the Skin.* Oxford: Blackwell Scientific Publications, 1965: 87–102.

4 Johnson E. Environmental influences on the hair follicle. In: Orfanos CE, Montagna W, Stüttgen G, eds. *Hair Research; Status and Future Aspects.* Berlin: Springer-Verlag, 1981: 183–94.

5 Saitoh M, Uzuka M, Sakamoto M. Human hair cycle. *J Invest Dermatol* 1970; **54**: 65–81.

6 Johnson E. Quantitative studies of hair growth in the albino rat. I Normal males and females. *J Endocrinol* 1958; **16**: 337–50.

7 Jackson D, Ebling FJ. The guinea-pig hair follicle as an object for experimental observation. *J Soc Cosmet Chem* 1971; **22**: 701–9.

8 Blume U, Ferracin J, Verschoore M *et al.* Physiology of the vellus follicle; hair growth and sebum excretion. *Br J Dermatol* 1991; **124**: 21–8.

9 Seago SV, Ebling FJG. The hair cycle on the human thigh and upper arm. *Br J Dermatol* 1985; **113**: 9–16.

10 Kligman AM. The human hair cycle. *J Invest Dermatol* 1959; **33**: 307–16.

11 Kligman AM. Pathologic dynamics of human hair loss. I Telogen effluvium. *Arch Dermatol* 1961; **83**: 175–98.

12 Parakkal PF. Morphogenesis of the hair follicle during catagen. *Z Zellforsch Mikros Anat* 1970; **107**: 174–86.

13 Sugiyama S, Takahashi M, Kamimura M. The ultrastructure of the hair follicle in early and late catagen, with special reference to the alteration of the junction structure between the dermal papilla and epithelial component. *J Ultrastruct Res* 1976; **54**: 359–73.

14 Couchman JR. Rat hair follicle dermal papillae have an extracellular matrix containing basement membrane components. *J Invest Dermatol* 1986; **87**: 762–7.

15 Couchman JR, King JL, McCarthy KJ. Distribution of two basement membrane proteoglycans through hair follicle development and the hair growth cycle in the rat. *J Invest Dermatol* 1990; **94**: 65–70.

16 Barman JM, Astore I, Pecoraro V. The normal trichogram of the adult. *J Invest Dermatol* 1965; **44**: 233–6.

17 Pecoraro V, Astore I, Barman JM *et al.* The normal trichogram in the child before the age of puberty. *J Invest Dermatol* 1964; **42**: 427–30.

18 Pecoraro V, Astore I, Barman JM. Cycle of the scalp hair of the new-born child. *J Invest Dermatol* 1964; **43**: 145–7.

19 Pecoraro V, Barman JM, Astore I. The normal trichogram of pregnant women. In: Montagna W, Dobson RL, eds. *Advances in Biology of Skin,* Vol IX. *Hair Growth.* Oxford: Pergamon, 1969: 203–10.

20 Barman JM, Pecoraro V, Astore I *et al.* The first stage of the natural history of the human scalp-hair cycle. *J Invest Dermatol* 1967; **48**: 138–41.

21 Chase HB, Rauch H, Smith VW. Critical stages of hair development and pigmentation in the mouse. *Physiol Zool* 1951; **24**: 1–8.

22 Ebling FJ, Hale PA. The control of the mammalian moult. *Mem Soc Endocrinol* 1970; **18**: 215–37.

23 Ling JK. Pelage and moulting in wild mammals with special reference to aquatic forms. *Q Rev Biol* 1970; **45**: 16–54.

24 Randall VA, Ebling FJ. Seasonal changes in human hair growth. *Br J Dermatol* 1991; **124**: 146–50.

Hormonal influences [1]

It is important to make a clear distinction between the effects of a range of hormones on the follicular cycle, in evolutionary terms related to the adaptive function of moulting, and the particular role of androgens in the induction of sexual and other adult hair which is an adaptation for delaying until puberty the associated sociosexual signals [2]. Most dermatological problems centre around androgen-dependent hair, which will be considered separately below. Knowledge of other hormonal mechanisms is, however, relevant not only to understanding the control of the moult cycle but also to the problems of human hair loss in thyroid dysfunction and following pregnancy.

Each hair follicle appears to have an intrinsic rhythm. In rats, this has been shown to continue when the site is changed [3] or even, under some circumstances, when the follicle is transplanted to another animal in a different phase of the moult [4]. Plucking of hairs from resting follicles brings forward the next period of activity, and such follicles continue out of phase with their neighbours, at least for a time [5]. The nature of this intrinsic control and the mechanism by which epilation or wounding affect it are unknown. One hypothesis is that a mitotic inhibitor accumulates during anagen and is gradually used up or dispersed during telogen [6,7]; another is that growth-promoting wound hormones are released by epilation [8]. The finding that removal of residual club hairs after follicular activity has commenced does not affect the anagen in progress but does advance the next eruption of hairs [9,10] appears to be out of keeping with the inhibitor hypothesis.

Plucking rat hairs during telogen has been shown to induce high levels of ornithine decarboxylase within 4 h [11], although during the first 60 min the enzyme actually decreases in activity [12]. This decrease is at first very rapid, and about 30% of the activity is lost within 5 min. There is no great change in other enzymes or in the protein synthetic capacity of the skin. It appears that an inhibitor of ornithine decarboxylase is produced, and the extraction of such an enzyme from epilated skin [13] raises the possibility that it is involved in the intrinsic mechanism.

Irrespective of intrinsic control, the overall timing of the cyclic events also appears to be influenced by systemic factors, for follicles on homografts gradually come into phase with their hosts [4], and parabiotic rats gradually come to moult in phase with each other [14]. This systemic control mechanism may embody components as yet unknown, but it could be accounted for by facts that can be demonstrated. In rats, oestradiol, testosterone and adrenal steroids delay the initiation of follicular activity [15,16] and oestradiol also delays the shedding of club hairs [15], so that the moult is accelerated by gonadectomy or adrenalectomy; conversely, thyroid hormone advances onset of follicular activity and thyroidectomy or inhibition of the thyroid delays passage of the moult [17,18]. Oestradiol has similarly been shown to delay the onset of follicular activity in the guinea-pig [19]. In the rat, hypophysectomy advances it, so the influence of the gonadal system appears to override that of the thyroid [18]. The hypothalamus and the hypophysis may thus exert their influence by way of the thyroid, with the adrenal cortex and the gonads forging a link between environmental, reproductive and moulting cycles [17,20].

Hormones also influence follicles in anagen. Studies in which rat hairs were pulse labelled with ^{35}S-cysteine [9] showed that oestradiol or thyroxine each similarly reduced the duration of the active phase, their effects being additive when they were administered simultaneously. In contrast, whereas oestradiol decreased the rate of hair growth, thyroxine had the opposite effect. These findings suggest that the two hormones do not have the same site of action.

Human hair is profoundly affected by thyroid hormones. In studies carried out in Sheffield [21], 16 out of 150 women who complained of hair loss were diagnosed as hypothyroid on the basis of serum protein-bound iodine levels confirmed by radioiodine tracer studies. Mean hair diameter was reduced [22]; whereas diameters in normal subjects had a symmetrical distribution with a marked peak at 0.08 mm, in all subjects with hair loss, and especially in those with hypothyroidism, the spread was much wider, with separate peaks at 0.04 mm and 0.06 mm. The proportion of roots in telogen has been shown to be abnormally high in hairs plucked from the occipital and parietal areas of hypothyroid subjects; treatment with thyroid hormone restored it to normal after 8 weeks [23].

The phenomenon of postpartum hair loss also appears to result from a hormonally mediated change in the cycles of scalp follicles. A loss of hairs at about two to three times the normal rate gives rise to a transient alopecia about 4–6 months after parturition. At this time, the proportion of hairs in telogen can be as much as 15% [24], whereas in late pregnancy it may be less than 5%, which is only about one-third of normal (Fig. 66.15). This suggests that the passage of follicles into catagen, followed by shedding of club hairs, is slowed down by pregnancy, but occurs precipitously after parturition when hormonal conditions are altered, particularly by a rapid fall in oestrogen levels. The pattern of fluctuation in the anagen/telogen ratio has been observed over three consecutive pregnancies in one subject over a period of 9 years; the change became less marked in each successive pregnancy [25].

REFERENCES

1 Messenger AG, Dawber RPR. The physiology and embryology of hair growth. In: Dawber RPR, ed. *Diseases of the Hair and Scalp*, 3rd edn. Oxford: Blackwell Science, 1997: 25–7.
2 Ebling FJG, Hale PA, Randall VA. Hormones and hair growth. In: Goldsmith LA, ed. *Biochemistry and Physiology of the Skin*, 2nd edn. Oxford: Oxford University Press, 1991.
3 Ebling FJ, Johnson W. Hair growth and its relation to vascular supply in rotated skin grafts and transposed flaps in the albino rat. *J Embryol Exp Morphol* 1959; **7**: 417–30.
4 Ebling FJ, Johnson E. Systemic influence on activity of hair follicles in skin homografts. *J Embryol Exp Morphol* 1961; **9**: 285–93.
5 Johnson E, Ebling FJ. The effect of plucking hairs during different phases of the follicular cycle. *J Embryol Exp Morphol* 1964; **12**: 465–74.
6 Chase HB. Growth of the hair. *Physiol Rev* 1954; **34**: 113–26.
7 Chase HB, Eaton GT. The growth of hair follicles in waves. *Ann NY Acad Sci* 1959; **85**: 365–8.
8 Argyris TS. Hair growth induced by damage. In: Montagna W, Dobson RL, eds. *Advances in Biology of Skin*, Vol. IX. *Hair Growth*. Oxford: Pergamon, 1969: 339–56.
9 Hale PA, Ebling FJ. The effects of epilation and hormones on the activity of rat hair follicles. *J Exp Zool* 1975; **191**: 49–62.
10 Hale PA, Ebling FJ. The effect of a single epilation of successive hair eruptions in normal and hormone-treated rats. *J Exp Zool* 1979; **207**: 49–72.
11 Morrison DM, Goldsmith LA. Ornithine decarboxylase in rat skin. *J Invest Dermatol* 1978; **70**: 309–13.
12 Lesiewicz J, Morrison DM, Goldsmith LA. Ornithine decarboxylase in rat skin: 2. Differential response to hair plucking and a tumor promoter. *J Invest Dermatol* 1980; **75**: 411–16.
13 Lesiewicz J, Goldsmith LA. Antizyme release is an early event in ornithine decarboxylase induction by hair plucking. *J Invest Dermatol* 1983; **80**: 97–100.
14 Ebling FJ, Hervey GR. The activity of hair follicles in parabiotic rats. *J Embryol Exp Morphol* 1964; **12**: 425–38.
15 Johnson E. Quantitative studies of hair growth in the albino rat. II. The effect of sex hormones. *J Endocrinol* 1958; **16**: 351–9.
16 Johnson E. Quantitative studies of hair growth in the albino rat. III. The role of the adrenal glands. *J Endocrinol* 1958; **16**: 360–8.
17 Ebling FJ, Johnson E. The control of hair growth. *Symp Zool Soc Lond* 1964; **12**: 97–130.
18 Ebling FJ, Johnson E. The action of hormones on spontaneous hair growth cycles in the rat. *J Endocrinol* 1964; **29**: 193–201.
19 Jackson D, Ebling FJ. The activity of the hair follicles and their response to oestradiol in the guinea-pig *Cavia porcellus* L. *J Anat* 1972; **111**: 303–16.
20 Ebling FJ, Hale PA. The control of the mammalian moult. *Mem Soc Endocrinol* 1970; **18**: 215–37.
21 Eckert J, Church RE, Ebling FJ *et al.* Hair loss in women. *Br J Dermatol* 1967; **79**: 543–8.
22 Jackson D, Church RE, Ebling FJ. Hair diameter in female baldness. *Br J Dermatol* 1972; **87**: 361–7.
23 Freinkel RK, Freinkel N. Hair growth and alopecia in hypothyroidism. *Arch Dermatol Syphilol* 1972; **106**: 349–52.
24 Lynfield YL. Effect of pregnancy on the human hair cycle. *J Invest Dermatol* 1960; **35**: 323–7.
25 Pecoraro V, Barman JM, Astore I. The normal trichogram of pregnant women. In: Montagna W, Dobson RL, eds. *Advances in Biology of Skin*, Vol. IX. *Hair Growth*. Oxford: Pergamon, 1969: 203–20.

Androgen-dependent hair [1]

The growth of obvious facial, trunk and extremity hair in the male, and of pubic and axillary hair in both sexes, is clearly dependent on androgens. The development of such

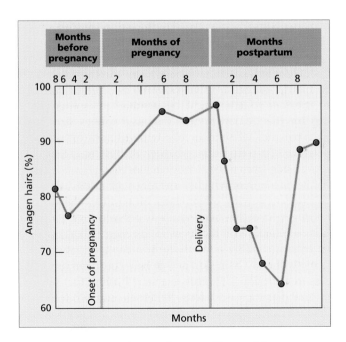

Fig. 66.15 Percentage of anagen hairs in a 25-year-old woman before, during and after pregnancy. (From Lynfield [24].)

hair at puberty is, in broad terms and at least initially, in parallel with the rise in levels of androgen from testicular, adrenocortical and ovarian sources, which occurs in both sexes and is somewhat steeper in males [2].

That testosterone from the interstitial cells of the testis is responsible for growth of beard and body hair in male adolescence and that testicular activity is itself initiated by gonadotrophic hormones of the pituitary is unquestioned. However, the findings that growth-hormone deficient boys and girls are less than normally responsive to androgens, and that growth hormone is necessary as a synergistic factor to allow testosterone to be fully effective with respect to protein anabolism, growth promotion and androgenicity [3], suggest that hypophysial hormones might also play a more direct role. In support of such a view is the evidence that the pubertal spurt in human body growth requires both growth hormone and androgen [4], and that the change from infantile to adult pelage can be prevented by hypophysectomy in both the dog [5] and the rat, in which it can be restored by prolactin [6]. Moreover, the response of the rat sebaceous glands to testosterone is also reduced by hypophysectomy and can be restored by hypophysial hormones (Chapter 42).

Direct evidence of the role of testicular androgen is that castration reduces growth of the human beard [7], whereas testosterone stimulates it in eunuchs and elderly men [8]. As facial and body hair is normally absent from women, it appears to require high levels of the hormone and, because it is usually deficient in cases of 5α-reductase deficiency [9], it seems that metabolism of the testosterone to 5α-dihydrotestosterone is mandatory (Chapter 4). This view is further supported by the finding that in patients with coeliac disease, the rate of beard growth was correlated with the level of 5α-dihydrotestosterone in the plasma but not with that of testosterone [10]. The role of androgen is further demonstrated in the treatment of hirsute women with the antiandrogen cyproterone acetate [11,12], which reduces the definitive length, rate of growth, diameter and extent of medullation of the thigh hairs [13,14]. Although the plasma androgen levels are lowered, the major part of the action appears to be by competition for the androgen receptors in the hair follicle [15–17].

Growth of pubic and axillary hair is also undoubtedly androgen dependent. This hair is deficient in testicular feminization, a condition in which genetic males develop as females because of a lack of intracellular androgen receptor, and in women suffering from adrenal insufficiency [18]. However, it appears to be present in the condition type II incomplete hermaphroditism, in which genetic males lack 5α-reductase even though their plasma testosterone is normal [9]. Therefore, it seems probable that growth of the pubic hair requires only low levels of androgen and is not dependent on 5α-reductase.

Scalp hair differs in that its growth does not require any androgenic stimulus. However, in genetically ordained subjects, androgen is paradoxically responsible for post-pubertal hair deficiency on the vertex of the scalp [19–21]. The existence of testosterone receptors in scalp hair follicles is implied by the fact that female diffuse alopecia can be alleviated by oral antiandrogens [22,23], and has been directly demonstrated in cultured dermal papilla cells [24]. The additional necessity for 5α-reductase is suggested by the evidence that male bald scalp has a greater capacity than non-bald scalp to convert testosterone to 5α-dihydrotestosterone [25], that isolated hair roots have a similar capacity [26] and that recession of the frontal hairline does not occur in cases of familial male pseudo-hermaphroditism involving 5α-reductase deficiency [18]. However, the oxidative pathway may also be important, as the major metabolite produced by isolated hair roots *in vitro* is androstenedione [27,28].

If growth of hair on the face and body and deficiency of hair on the scalp are both androgen dependent, the question arises whether hirsutism and baldness are provoked by excess androgen or by an enhanced peripheral response. When hirsutism is associated with other gross signs of virility or with menstrual disorder, it clearly has an endocrine pathology. Much more frequently, the hirsutism is described as idiopathic because there is no obvious 'central' hormonal disturbance. In idiopathic hirsutism the concentration of plasma testosterone is usually within or only slightly above the normal range; androstenedione is more often found to be elevated [29–31]. The possibility that free androgen may be higher is suggested by the finding that sex hormone binding globulin (SHBG) is, on average, lower [17]. However, although such minor abnormalities are frequently associated with hirsutism, they cannot account for every case, because about 40% of all patients appear to show all hormonal parameters within the normal range [32]. The finding that hirsute women with no evidence of ovarian or adrenal dysfunction excreted about four times as much 5α-androstenediol as non-hirsute women [33] suggested that increased 5α-reductase activity in the hair follicle might be involved; this was borne out by the demonstration that suprapubic skin from such patients, when incubated with tritiated testosterone, produced 5α-reduced metabolites at about four times the rate of skin from normal women [34–36].

The question of whether androgenetic alopecia in men is associated with other signs of virility or abnormal androgen levels has been similarly debated. Evidence that it is correlated with hairiness of the chest [37] appears to be contradicted by a failure to find any association with density of body hair, skin and muscle thickness or rate of sebum excretion [38]. However, the finding that despite normal plasma testosterone, bald men tend to have lower SHBG and higher salivary testosterone does suggest that they might enjoy more available androgen [39].

Most female diffuse alopecia is androgenetic. Although it may be associated with virilism and high androgen levels resulting from disorders of the adrenal cortex, pituitary or ovaries, plasma androgens are more usually within normal limits. However, as in males, there is a tendency for SHBG to be lower, but with a considerable overlap of the normal range [40].

As human hair so clearly differs between regions in its response to androgens, it is obvious that any possible animal models must be viewed with caution. Growth of the vibrissae of rats [41], the hairs of the gerbil ventral gland [42] and, presumably, the mane of the lion, are all androgen dependent. Even if male baldness is truly mimicked by the stump-tailed macaque, the model is not particularly accessible [43,44], and the wattled starling, which loses feathers from its head, can hardly be considered as a greatly superior alternative [45].

REFERENCES

1 Messenger AG, Dawber RPR. The physiology and embryology of hair growth. In: Dawber RPR, ed. *Diseases of the Hair and Scalp*, 3rd edn. Oxford: Blackwell Science, 1997: 23–5.
2 Winter JSD, Faiman C. Pituitary–gonadal relations in female children and adolescents. *Pediatr Res* 1973; **7**: 948–53.
3 Zachmann M, Aynsley-Green A, Prader A. Interrelations of the effect of growth hormone and testosterone in hypopituitarism. In: Pecile A, Muller EE, eds. *Growth Hormone and Related Peptides*. Amsterdam: Excerpta Medica, 1976: 286–96.
4 Tanner JM, Whitehouse RH. The pattern of growth in children with growth hormone deficiency before, during and after treatment. In: Pecile A, Muller EE, eds. *Growth and Growth Hormone*. Amsterdam: Excerpta Medica, 1972: 429–51.
5 Houssay BA. Extirpación de la hipófisis en el perro. *Endocrinology* 1918; **2**: 497–8.
6 Rennels EG, Callahan WP. The hormonal basis for pubertal maturation of hair in the albino rat. *Anat Rec* 1959; **135**: 21–32.
7 Hamilton JB. Age, sex and genetic factors in the regulation of hair growth in man: a comparison of Caucasian and Japanese populations. In: Montagna W, Ellis RA, eds. *The Biology of Hair Growth*. New York: Academic Press, 1958: 399–433.
8 Chieffi M. Effect of testosterone administration on the beard growth of elderly males. *J Gerontol* 1949; **4**: 200–4.
9 Griffin JE, Wilson JD. Studies on the pathogenesis of the incomplete forms of androgen resistance in man. *J Clin Endocrinol Metab* 1977; **45**: 1137–43.
10 Farthing MJG, Mattei AM, Edwards CRW *et al*. Relationship between plasma testosterone and dihydrotestosterone concentrations and male facial hair growth. *Br J Dermatol* 1982; **107**: 559–64.
11 Hammerstein J, Cupceancu B. Behandlung des Hirsutismus mit Cyproteronacetat. *Dtsch Med Wochenschr* 1969; **94**: 829–34.
12 Hammerstein J, Meckies J, Leo-Rossberg I *et al*. Use of cyproterone acetate (CPA) in the treatment of acne, hirsutism and virilism. *J Steroid Biochem* 1975; **6**: 827–36.
13 Ebling FJ, Thomas AK, Cooke ID *et al*. Effect of cyproterone acetate on hair growth, sebaceous secretion and endocrine parameters in a hirsute subject. *Br J Dermatol* 1977; **97**: 371–81.
14 Ebling FJ, Cooke ID, Randall VA *et al*. The influence of cyproterone acetate on the activity of hair follicles and sebaceous glands in man. In: Hammerstein J, Lachnit-Fixson U, Neumann F *et al*., eds. *Androgenization in Women*. Amsterdam: Excerpta Medica, 1979: 239–45.
15 Barnes EW, Irvine WJ, Hunter WM *et al*. Cyproterone acetate: a study involving two volunteers with idiopathic hirsutism. *Clin Endocrinol* 1975; **4**: 65–73.
16 Cittadini E, Barreca P. Uses of antiandrogens in gynecology. In: Martini L, Motta M, eds. *Androgens and Antiandrogens*. New York: Raven Press, 1977: 309–19.
17 Sawers RS, Randall VA, Iqbal MJ. Studies on the clinical and endocrine effects of anti-androgens. In: Jeffcoate SL, ed. *Androgens and Anti-androgen Therapy*. New York: Wiley, 1982: 145–68.
18 Leshin M, Wilson JD. Mechanisms of androgen-mediated hair growth. In: Orfanos CE, Montagna W, Stüttgen G, eds. *Hair Research*. Berlin: Springer-Verlag, 1981: 205–9.
19 Hamilton JB. Male hormone stimulation is a prerequisite and an incitant in common baldness. *Am J Anat* 1942; **71**: 451–80.
20 Hamilton JB. Patterned loss of hair in man: types and incidence. *Ann NY Acad Sci* 1951; **53**: 708–28.
21 Hamilton JB. Effect of castration in adolescent and young adult males upon further changes in the proportions of bare and hairy scalp. *J Clin Endocrinol Metab* 1960; **20**: 1309–18.
22 Dawber RPR, Sonnex T, Ralfs I. Oral anti-androgen treatment of common baldness in women. *Br J Dermatol* 1982; **106** (Suppl. 22): 20.
23 Zaun H. In: Kukita A, Seiji M, eds. *Proceedings of the 16th International Congress on Dermatology*. Tokyo: University of Tokyo Press, 1983: 113–16.
24 Randall VA, Thornton MJ, Elliott K *et al*. A comparison of androgen receptor levels in cultured dermal papilla cells from human hair follicles with varying sensitivities to androgens. *J Endocrinol* 1989; **121** (Suppl.) Abstract 67.
25 Bingham KD, Shaw DA. The metabolism of testosterone by human male scalp skin. *J Endocrinol* 1973; **57**: 111–21.
26 Schweikert HV, Wilson JD. Androgen metabolism in isolated hair roots. In: Orfanos CE, Montagna W, Stüttgen G, eds. *Hair Research*. Berlin: Springer-Verlag, 1981: 210–14.
27 Sansone-Bazzano G, Reisner RM, Bazzano G. Conversion of testosterone-1,2-^{3}H to androstenedione-^{3}H in the isolated hair follicle of man. *J Clin Endocrinol* 1972; **34**: 512–15.
28 Schweikert HV, Wilson JD. Regulation of human hair growth by steroid hormones. I Testosterone metabolism in isolated hair. *J Clin Endocrinol Metab* 1974; **38**: 811–19.
29 Bardin CW, Lipsett MB. Testosterone and androstenedione blood production rates in normal women and women with idiopathic hirsutism or polycystic ovaries. *J Clin Invest* 1967; **46**: 891–902.
30 James VHT, Andre CM. In: Curry AS, Hewlett JV, eds. *Biochemistry in Women; Clinical Concepts*. Boca Raton: CRC Press, 1974: 23.
31 Rosenfield RL. Plasma testosterone binding globulin and indexes of the concentration of unbound plasma androgens in normal and hirsute subjects. *J Clin Endocrinol Metab* 1971; **32**: 717–28.
32 Lucky AW, McGuire J, Rosenfield RL *et al*. Plasma androgens in women with acne vulgaris. *J Invest Dermatol* 1983; **81**: 70–4.
33 Mauvais-Jarvis P, Charransol G, Bobas-Masson F. Simultaneous determination of urinary androstanediol and testosterone in an evaluation of human androgenicity. *J Clin Endocrinol Metab* 1973; **36**: 452–9.
34 Kuttenn F, Mowszowicz I, Schaison G *et al*. Androgen production and skin metabolism in hirsutism. *J Endocrinol* 1977; **75**: 83–91.
35 Kuttenn F, Mowszowicz I, Mauvais-Jarvis P. Androgen metabolism in human skin. In: Mauvais-Jarvis P, Vickers CFH, Wepierre J, eds. *Percutaneous Absorption of Steroids*. London: Academic Press, 1980: 99–121.
36 Mauvais-Jarvis P. Androgen metabolism in human skin: mechanisms of control. In: Martini L, Motta M, eds. *Androgens and Antiandrogens*. New York: Raven Press, 1977: 229–45.
37 Šalamon T. Genetic factors in male pattern alopecia. In: Baccaredda-Boy A, Moretti G, Frey JR, eds. *Biopathology of Pattern Alopecia*. Basel: Karger, 1968: 39–49.
38 Burton JL, Ben Halim MM, Meyrick G *et al*. Male-pattern alopecia and masculinity. *Br J Dermatol* 1979; **100**: 567–71.
39 Cipriani R, Ruzza G, Foresta C *et al*. Sex-hormone-binding globulin and saliva testosterone levels in men with androgenetic alopecia. *Br J Dermatol* 1983; **109**: 249–52.
40 Miller JA, Darley CR, Karkavitas K *et al*. Low sex-hormone binding globulin levels in young women with diffuse hair loss. *Br J Dermatol* 1982; **106**: 331–6.
41 Ibrahim L, Wright EA. Effect of castration and testosterone propionate on mouse vibrissae. *Br J Dermatol* 1983; **108**: 321–6.
42 Mitchell OG, Butcher EO. Growth of hair in the ventral glands of castrate gerbils following testosterone administration. *Anat Rec* 1966; **156**: 11–17.
43 Montagna W, Machida H, Perkins E. The skin of primates: XXVIII. The stump tail macaque (*Macaca speciosa*). *Am J Phys Anthropol* 1966; **24**: 71–86.
44 Uno H, Adachi K, Montagna W. Morphological and biochemical studies of hair follicle in common baldness of stump-tailed macaque (*Macaca speciosa*). In: Montagna W, Dobson RL, eds. *Advances in Biology of Skin*, Vol. IX. *Hair Growth*. Oxford: Pergamon, 1969: 221–45.
45 Hamilton JB. A male pattern baldness in wattled starlings resembling the condition in man. *Ann NY Acad Sci* 1959; **83**: 429–47.

Energy metabolism in hair follicles [1–3]

Studies in which freshly plucked hair follicles from the human scalp were incubated with ^{14}C-labelled glucose or other substrates indicate that, in common with many other tissues and organs, hair follicles utilize glucose via the Emden–Meyerhoff pathway, the pentose cycle and the tricarboxylic acid cycle. However, hair follicles differ from muscle in several respects. They have a faster glycolytic rate, a slower respiration rate and considerable pentose cycle activity, although this is insignificant in muscle.

Active and resting follicles differ remarkably. In active follicles, compared with resting follicles, glucose utilization is increased by 200%, glycolysis by 200%, activity of the pentose cycle by 800%, metabolism by other pathways by 150% and adenosine triphosphate (ATP) production via the respiratory chains by 270% [1].

REFERENCES

1 Adachi K, Uno H. Some metabolic profiles of human hair follicles. In: Montagna W, Dobson RL, eds. *Advances in Biology of Skin*, Vol. IX. *Hair Growth*. Oxford: Pergamon, 1969: 511–34.
2 Adachi K, Takayasu S, Takashima I *et al.* Human hair follicles: metabolism and control mechanisms. *J Soc Cosmet Chem* 1970; **21**: 901–24.
3 Uno H, Adachi K, Montagna W. Morphological and biochemical studies of hair follicle in common baldness of stump-tailed macaque (*Macaca speciosa*). In: Montagna W, Dobson RL, eds. *Advances in Biology of Skin*, Vol. IX. *Hair Growth*. Oxford: Pergamon, 1969: 221–45.

Types of hair [1]

Different types of hair may be produced by different kinds of follicle, and the type of hair produced in any particular follicle can change with age or under the influence of hormones. Animals characteristically have both an overcoat of stiff guard hairs and an undercoat of fine hairs [2], but many kinds of follicle and fibre have been described. Many species also have large vibrissae or sinus hairs, which are sensory and are produced from special follicles containing erectile tissue. There are no strictly comparable follicles in humans, but there are occasional large so-called tylotrich follicles [3] with a structure suggesting a sensory function; they are most numerous in abdominal skin [4].

The infantile pelage of animals is usually fine, and such 'puppy' fur is retained in the adult if the young animal is hypophysectomized [5]. In the absence of precise knowledge about species differences in pituitary hormones, the question of whether growth hormone or prolactin induces the change to adult pelage may be unrealistic [6]; moreover, steroid hormones also influence the type of hair produced [7].

In humans, a prenatal coat of fine, soft, unmedullated and usually unpigmented hair, known as *lanugo*, is normally shed *in utero* in the eighth to ninth month of gestation; however, lanugo may be retained throughout life in the rare hereditary syndrome hypertrichosis lanuginosa

(p. 2890). Postnatal hair may be divided at the extreme into two kinds: vellus, which is soft, unmedullated, occasionally pigmented and seldom more than 2 cm long; and terminal hair, which is longer, coarser, and often medullated and pigmented. However, there is a range of intermediate kinds [8]. Before puberty, terminal hair is normally limited to the scalp, eyebrows and eyelashes. After puberty, secondary sexual 'terminal' hair is developed from vellus hair in response to androgens.

REFERENCES

1 Dawber RPR, Van Neste D. Hair science. In: Dawber RPR, Van Neste D, eds. *Hair and Scalp Disorders*. London: Dunitz, 1995: 19–20.
2 Dry FW. The coat of the mouse. *J Genet* 1926; **16**: 287–340.
3 Straile WE. Sensory hair follicles in the mammalian skin: the tylotrich follicle. *Am J Anat* 1960; **106**: 133–47.
4 Winkelmann RK. The innervation of a hair follicle. *Ann NY Acad Sci* 1959; **83**: 400–7.
5 Houssay BA. Extirpación de la hipófisis en el perro. *Endocrinology* 1918; **2**: 497–8.
6 Rennels EG, Callahan WP. The hormonal basis for pubertal maturation of hair in the albino rat. *Anat Rec* 1959; **135**: 21–32.
7 Mohn MP. The effect of different hormonal states on the growth of hair in rats. In: Montagna W, Ellis RA, eds. *The Biology of Hair Growth*. New York: Academic Press, 1958: 335–98.
8 Rook A. Endocrine influences on hair growth. *Br Med J* 1965; **i**: 609–14.

Racial and individual variation

Wide genetically determined variations in the patterns and amount of hair growth can be observed both between races and between individuals [1]. The most striking differences are seen in scalp hair. It is a common observation that Mongoloids tend to have coarse straight hair, Negroids curly hair (at the extreme, the intertwined shafts give rise to the 'peppercorn' pattern) and Caucasoids a range of textures and curl. According to several authors, the macroscopic appearance of hair is related to its cross-section. Thus, Mongoloid hair is the most massive and is circular; Negroid hair is oval, and Caucasoid hair is moderately elliptical and finer than Mongoloid [2–4]. Other evidence suggests that the shape of the follicle determines hair form: the Negroid follicle is helical, the Mongoloid follicle completely straight, and the Caucasoid follicle varies between these extremes. However, even a straight Caucasoid follicle may produce a hair with an oval cross-section [5]. Significant variations between populations can be shown for a number of other measurements such as medullation, cuticular scale count, kinking and average curvature [6].

A hypothesis [7] that hair form is controlled by only three or four genes (straight, wavy, spiral and peppercorn) is not currently accepted. Dyer [8], while accepting that the genes have major as opposed to biometric or polygenic effects, concludes that a number of genes are involved. In contrast, Hrdy [6] states that hair form is undoubtedly polygenic, but suggests that relatively few genes are involved.

Mongoloids, both male and female, have less pubic, axillary, beard and body hair than Caucasoids. The surface area covered by coarse beard hairs and the weight of hairs grown per day are less in Japanese than Caucasians, as are the mean number of axillary hairs and their daily growth [9]. Not only amounts of hair but also the patterns of distribution may vary between populations. Thus, Setty [10,11] has shown that absence of hair on the foot combined with presence of hair on the thighs and lower leg is three times more frequent in Negroids than in Caucasoids.

The growth of coarse hairs on the rim of the helix (*hypertrichosis of the pinna*) occurs between the ages of 17 and 45 in many males among the Bengali and Sinhalese [12–15]. The character is well known to geneticists as a possible example of Y-linked inheritance. In other races, few or many coarse hairs may grow on the helix or on the other regions of the pinna, usually after the third decade. The patterns have been classified [16] but their modes of inheritance are unknown.

A syndrome of 'hairy elbows' (*hypertrichosis cubiti*) [17] has been described in two of five siblings [18]. The mode of inheritance is uncertain. Hypertrichosis of the elbow region was noticed soon after birth. It reached its greatest extent and severity at the age of 5 years and then slowly regressed.

Such individual variations in the patterns of hair growth can now be accurately recorded and correlated with other hereditary traits. They will be of undoubted genetic interest and may, like certain variations in the pattern of the eyebrows, prove to have clinical implications.

REFERENCES

1 Dawber RPR, Van Neste D. Hair science. In: Dawber RPR, Van Neste D, eds. *Hair and Scalp Disorders*. London: Dunitz, 1995: 19–20.
2 Steggerda M. Cross sections of human hair from four racial groups. *J Hered* 1940; **31**: 475–6.
3 Steggerda M, Seibert HC. Size and shape of head hair from six racial groups. *J Hered* 1941; **32**: 315–18.
4 Vernall DG. A study of the size and shape of cross sections of hair from four races of men. *Am J Phys Anthropol* 1961; **19**: 345–50.
5 Lindelof B, Forslind B, Hedblad MA *et al*. Human hair form. *Arch Dermatol* 1988; **124**: 1359–63.
6 Hardy D. Quantitative hair form variation in seven populations. *Am J Phys Anthropol* 1973; **39**: 7–18.
7 Fischer E. Versucheiner Phänogenetik der normalen korperlichen Eigenschaften des Menschen. *Z Induct Abstamm Vererb* 1939; **76**: 47.
8 Dyer KF, ed. *The Biology of Racial Integration*. Bristol: Scientechnica, 1974.
9 Hamilton JB. Age, sex and genetic factors in the regulation of hair growth in man: a comparison of Caucasian and Japanese populations. In: Montagna W, Ellis RA, eds. *The Biology of Hair Growth*. New York: Academic Press, 1958: 399–433.
10 Setty LR. A comparative study of the distribution of hair of the hand and foot of white and negro males. *Am J Phys Anthropol* 1966; **25**: 131–8.
11 Setty LR. The distribution of hair of the lower limb in white and negro males. *Am J Phys Anthropol* 1968; **29**: 51–5.
12 Dronamraju KR. A note on the age of onset of hypertrichosis pinnae auris in Orissa, West Bengal and Ceylon. *J Genet* 1963; **53**: 324–7.
13 Dronamraju KR, Haldane JBS. Inheritance of hairy pinnae. *Am J Hum Genet* 1962; **14**: 102–3.
14 Sarkar SS, Banerjee AR, Bhattacharjee P *et al*. A contribution to the genetics of hypertrichosis of the ear rims. *Am J Hum Genet* 1961; **13**: 214–23.
15 Stern C, Centerwall WR, Sarkar SS. New data on the problem of Y-linkage of hairy pinnae. *Am J Hum Genet* 1964; **16**: 455–71.
16 Setty LR. Hair patterns of the pinna of white and negro males. *Am J Phys Anthropol* 1969; **31**: 153–62.
17 Barth JH, Dawber RPR. Hypertrichosis. In: Dawber RPR, ed. *Diseases of the Hair and Scalp*, 3rd edn. Oxford: Blackwell Science, 1997: 490–3.
18 Beighton P. Familial hypertrichosis cubiti: hairy elbows syndrome. *J Med Genet* 1970; **7**: 158–60.

Changes with age [1]

At puberty, terminal hair gradually replaces vellus, starting in the pubic regions. In both sexes [2] the first pubic hair is sparse, long, downy, slightly pigmented and almost straight. It later becomes darker, coarser, more curled and extends in area to form an inverse triangle. A British study [3,4] showed that boys had the first recognizable pubic hair at an average age of 13.4 years, and the full adult 'female' pattern at 15.2 years, about $3\frac{1}{2}$ years after the start of development of the genitalia. The corresponding mean ages for girls were considerably earlier, namely 11.7 years and 13.5 years. In about 80% of men and 10% of women the pubic hair continues spreading until the mid-twenties or later; there is no absolute distinction between male and female patterns, only one of degree [5]. Of 3858 normal young men, 4.7% were found to have a horizontal upper border to the pubic hair, and a further 10.3% had a convex border [6]. In another study, 3% of women aged 25–34 were found to have an acuminate upper border [7].

Axillary hair first appears about 2 years after the start of pubic hair growth. The amount, as measured by the weight of the fully grown mass, continues to increase until the late twenties in males as well as in females, in whom, however, it is less at any age [8]. The mean amounts grown per day increase from late puberty until the mid-twenties and thereafter decrease steadily.

Facial hair in boys first appears at about the same time as the axillary hair, starting at the corners of the upper lip, and spreading medially to complete the moustache and then the cheeks and beard.

Terminal hair development is continued in regular sequence on the legs, thighs, forearms, abdomen, buttocks, back, arms and shoulder [9]. The patterns of distribution of terminal hair on the neck, chest, back and limbs have been effectively differentiated and classified by Setty [10–14]. The extent of terminal hair tends to increase throughout the years of sexual maturity, but most patterns occur over a wide age range. The adult pattern is not achieved until the fourth decade, when the androgen levels are already somewhat lower than in early adult life. Moreover, aural hairs do not appear until late middle-age, and a detailed study [15] of coarse sternal hair in men showed that the hairs continue to increase in length and number from puberty to the fifth or sixth decade.

Certain follicles of the scalp may regress (miniaturize) with age to produce only fine, short vellus hair [16]. This condition of patterned baldness, androgenetic alopecia, is inherited and requires male hormone [17]; it is prevented by castration before puberty [17], although not substantially reversed by castration in maturity [18]. Some 35% of men of caucasoid stock [19] develop, during the third and fourth decades, sharply defined patches of alopecia in the peroneal area of the lower leg and, often, smaller patches on the calves; this may be a 'weathering' effect from friction and pressure.

REFERENCES

1 Dawber RPR, Van Neste D. *Hair and Scalp Disorders*. London: Dunitz, 1995: 19–20.
2 Tanner JM, ed. *Growth at Adolescence*, 2nd edn. Oxford: Blackwell Scientific Publications, 1962.
3 Marshall WA, Tanner JM. Variations in pattern of pubertal changes in girls. *Arch Dis Child* 1969; **44**: 291–303.
4 Marshall WA, Tanner JM. Variations in pattern of pubertal changes in boys. *Arch Dis Child* 1970; **45**: 13–23.
5 Thomas PK, Ferriman DG. Variation in facial and pubic hair growth in white women. *Am J Phys Anthropol* 1957; **15**: 171–80.
6 McGregor D. Distribution of pubic hair in a sample of fit men. *Br J Dermatol* 1961; **73**: 61–4.
7 Beek CH. A study of extension and distribution of human body hair. *Dermatologica* 1950; **101**: 317–31.
8 Hamilton JB. Age, sex and genetic factors in the regulation of hair growth in man: a comparison of Caucasian and Japanese populations. In: Montagna W, Ellis RA, eds. *The Biology of Hair Growth*. New York: Academic Press, 1958: 399–433.
9 Reynolds EL. The appearance of adult patterns of body hair in man. *Ann NY Acad Sci* 1951; **53**: 576–84.
10 Setty LR. The distribution of chest hair in caucasoid males. *Am J Phys Anthropol* 1961; **19**: 285–7.
11 Setty LR. Hair patterns on the back of white males. *Am J Phys Anthropol* 1962; **20**: 365–73.
12 Setty LR. The distribution of hair of the upper limb in caucasoid males. *Am J Phys Anthropol* 1964; **22**: 143–8.
13 Setty LR. The distribution of anterior cervical hair in white and negro males. *Am J Phys Anthropol* 1966; **24**: 321–4.
14 Setty LR. The distribution of hair of the lower limb in white and negro males. *Am J Phys Anthropol* 1968; **29**: 51–5.
15 Hamilton JB, Terada H, Mestler GE *et al.* I Coarse sternal hairs, a male secondary sex character that can be measured quantitatively; the influence of sex, age and genetic factors. II Other sex-differing characters: relationship to age, to one another, and to values for coarse sternal hairs. In: Montagna W, Dobson RL, eds. *Advances in Biology of Skin*, Vol. IX. *Hair Growth*. Oxford: Pergamon, 1969: 129–51.
16 Hamilton JB. Patterned loss of hair in man: types and incidence. *Ann NY Acad Sci* 1951; **53**: 708–28.
17 Hamilton JB. Male hormone stimulation is a prerequisite and an incitant in common baldness. *Am J Anat* 1942; **71**: 451–80.
18 Hamilton JB. Effect of castration in adolescent and young adult males upon further changes in the proportions of bare and hairy scalp. *J Clin Endocrinol Metab* 1960; **20**: 1309–18.
19 Ronchese F, Chace RR. Patterned alopecia about the calves and its apparent lack of significance. *Arch Dermatol Syphilol* 1937; **40**: 416–22.

The trichogram

The proportion of active to resting follicles in the scalp can be determined from plucked hairs and is a useful clinical parameter [1]. Barman *et al.* [2] first described such an analysis as a 'trichogram' but included within the term data on the density of hair follicles, thickness of hair and rate of growth. In fact, the systematized use of epilation to study

hair roots originated with Van Scott [3,4] and has been exploited by several other workers [1,5–15], each of whom has developed individual techniques.

For the prospective investigator, the literature is confusing, because in addition to the normal phases of the hair-follicle cycle, dysplastic and dystrophic hair roots have been described not only in pathological conditions but also in some healthy persons. If the hair is pulled out slowly, more such roots will be seen, so it seems that some, at least, must be artefactual. This is of considerable relevance in some conditions of the scalp and in systemic diseases of which hair changes are a manifestation, in which anagen/telogen studies are used to assess progress of the disease or its treatment. However, for monitoring the status and progress of androgenetic alopecia, whether the hair thinning is patterned or diffuse, only the simple determination of anagen-to-telogen ratios in the vertex and occipital regions is necessary, i.e. the proportion of telogen hairs in the sample (the telogen count), which is easy to use in clinical practice [12].

Examination should be carried out at a standard time (at least 4 days) after the last washing of the hair [5,14]. The areas should be carefully selected and specified. The hair should be cut to about 0.5 cm above the scalp surface and about four to seven hairs extracted with a rapid tug by tightly closing spade-ended epilating forceps placed as close to the skin as possible. The procedure must be repeated in contiguous areas to obtain a sample of not less than 50 hairs [16,17]. The hairs can be immediately examined in water, but are better mounted on glass slides under a cover slip using a medium such as Depex; for telogen count analysis alone, the hairs can be mounted dry.

For diagnosis of the hair root status, the overall shape is of primary importance, but the presence or absence of root sheaths and the external contours are also useful evidence [10,14]. The principal features are as follows.
1 *Anagen* (see Fig. 66.11a). The root is usually largest at its base, although it may have an equal diameter throughout. The inner root sheath is usually present and firm. The plucked roots may show an angle of 20° or more with the shaft, which is presumably artefactual [14].
2 *Telogen* (Fig. 66.11e). The root is clearly characterized by its club shape with smooth contours, lack of angulation and loose sheath.
3 *Dysplastic* (Figs 66.11b,c). The matrix is diminished in diameter and often deformed; the root sheath is loose or absent.
4 *Dystrophic* (Fig. 66.11d). The changes are so severe that the root has broken off at the narrowest level and tapers to a point; root sheaths are never present.

The highest ratio of anagen to telogen hairs, over 90%, occurs in children. In adult men, even those not clinically bald, the ratio is lowest in the frontovertical region, but non-bald women—as distinct from those with alopecia androgenetica—show no regional differences [5]. A study of scalp hairs from 146 clinically normal subjects [18] revealed that the overall proportion of hairs in anagen was 83% in men and 86% in women; the corresponding figures for telogen were 15% and 11%. Catagen hairs accounted for only 2.9% of the total in men and 2.1% in women, and were only demonstrable in 31% of men and 19% of women. Dystrophic anagen hairs were found in 46% of men, where they accounted for 3.2% of the total, and in 48% of women, where they accounted for 2.5%.

For assessment of the degree of androgenetic alopecia, Rushton *et al.* [19] have proposed the 'unit area trichogram', in which the root status and shaft diameter are determined for all of the hairs plucked from a small, defined area. In their view, only hairs over 40 μm in diameter are likely to grow longer than 80 mm and thus provide meaningful hair in the cosmetic sense.

In all the hair treatment trials of the last decade, phototrichograms have mainly been used [20].

REFERENCES

1 Braun-Falco O, Heilgemeir GP. Hair root microscopy. In: Dawber R, Rook A, eds. *Seminars in Dermatology*, Vol. 4. New York: Thieme–Stratten, 1985: 19.
2 Barman JM, Pecoraro V, Astore I. Method, technic and computations in the study of the trophic state of the human scalp hair. *J Invest Dermatol* 1964; **42**: 421–5.
3 Van Scott EJ. Response of hair roots to chemical and physical influence. In: Montagna W, Ellis RA, eds. *The Biology of Hair Growth*. New York: Academic Press, 1958: 441–9.
4 Van Scott EJ, Reinertson RP, Steinmuller R. The growing hair roots of the human scalp and morphological changes therein following amethopterin therapy. *J Invest Dermatol* 1957; **29**: 197–204.
5 Braun-Falco O. Dynamik des normalen und pathologischen Haarwachstums. *Arch Klin Exp Dermatol* 1966; **227**: 419–52.
6 Braun-Falco O, Fischer C. Über den Einfluss des Haarwaschens auf des Haarwurzelmuster. *Arch Klin Exp Dermatol* 1966; **226**: 136–43.
7 Braun-Falco O, Rassner B. Über den Einfluss der Epilations-technik auf normale und pathologische Haarwurzelmuster. *Arch Klin Exp Dermatol* 1965; **223**: 501–8.
8 Braun-Falco O, Zaun H. Über die Beteiligung des gesamten Capilitiums bei Alopecia areata. (Involvement of the entire scalp hair in alopecia areata). *Hautarzt* 1962; **13**: 342–8.
9 Braun-Falco O, Zaun H. Zum Wesen der Chronischen diffusen Alopecie bei Frauen. *Arch Klin Exp Dermatol* 1962; **215**: 165–80.
10 Ebling FJG, Randall VA. Hormonal actions on hair follicles and associated glands. In: Skerrow D, Skerrow CJ, eds. *Methods in Skin Research*. New York: John Wiley and Sons, 1984: 297–327.
11 Meiers HG. Die Methode des Trichogrammes. *Artz Kosmetol* 1967; **6**: 22.
12 Mortimer CH, Rushton H, James KC. Effective medical treatment for common baldness in women. *Clin Exp Dermatol* 1984; **9**: 342–50.
13 Orfanos CE. Alopecia androgenetica. In: Orfanos CE, ed. *Haar und Haarkrankheiten*. Stuttgart: Gustav-Fischer, 1979: 573–604.
14 Peereboom-Wynia JDR. Hair root characteristics of the human scalp hair in health and disease. University of Rotterdam, 1982 (thesis).
15 Rook A, Dawber R, eds. *Diseases of the Hair and Scalp*, 2nd edn. Oxford: Blackwell Scientific Publications, 1991.
16 Bosse K. Vergleichende Untersuchungen zur Physiologie und Pathologie des Haarwechsels unter besonderer Berücksicktigung seiner Synchronisation II. *Hautarzt* 1967; **18**: 35–41.
17 Bosse K. Der Einfluss der Entzundigung auf das Haarwachstum. *Hautarzt* 1967; **18**: 218–24.
18 Witzel M, Braun-Falco O. Uber den Haarwurzelstatus am Menschlichen Capillitium unter physiologischen Bedingungen. *Arch Klin Exp Dermatol* 1963; **216**: 221–30.
19 Rushton H, James KC, Mortimer CH. The unit area trichogram in the assessment of androgen-dependent alopecia. *Br J Dermatol* 1983; **109**: 429–37.
20 Jacobs JP, Szpunar CA, Warner ML. Use of topical minoxidil therapy for androgenetic alopecia in women. *Int J Dermatol* 1993; **32**: 758–61.

Seasonal changes

Evidence that human hair growth varies with season [1] has been advanced by several authors and was reviewed by Saitoh *et al.* [2] who add some observations on Japanese subjects. Orentreich [3] reported that three women in New York experienced maximal hair fall in November. Clear and statistically significant data on seasonal variation was provided by a study of 14 young white men in Sheffield, UK, at a latitude of 53.4°N [4].

Scalp

The proportion of scalp follicles in anagen, as determined by plucking hairs, reached a single peak of over 90% around March and fell steadily to a trough in September (Fig. 66.16a). This pattern appeared to be shared by all areas of the scalp.

The numbers of shed hairs collected by the subjects (Fig. 66.16b) closely followed the pattern of activity of the follicles. Hair loss reached a peak around August/September, when the fewest follicles were in anagen. At this time, the average loss of hairs was about 60/day, more than double that during the previous March and compatible with the observed increase from 10 to 20% in the proportion of follicles in telogen.

The diameter of growing scalp hairs exhibited no significant seasonal fluctuations, although the variations showed a similar pattern to that of thigh hair diameter (see below).

Beard

The rate of beard growth (Fig. 66.17a) showed very significant seasonal variation. It was lowest in January and February and from March it increased steadily to reach a peak about 60% higher in July.

Thigh

The rate of growth of thigh hair (Fig. 66.17b) showed a similar seasonal pattern to that of the beard. The mean rate from February to March was 0.27 mm/day. It then rose to reach a plateau of about 0.3 mm/day from June to September and then declined steadily for 6 months.

The percentage of follicles in anagen (Fig. 66.18a) showed a remarkable and quite different pattern. It appeared to be lowest in March and August, and highest in May/June and November/December. The pattern is exactly what would

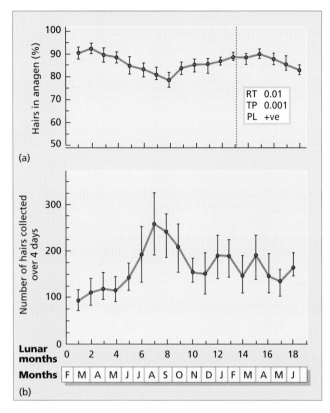

(a)

(b)

Fig. 66.16 (a) Monthly measurements of the percentage of plucked scalp hairs in anagen in 14 white men in Sheffield, UK (mean ± SEM). The probabilities of significant seasonal variation, assessed by the non-parametric runs test (RT), turning point (TP) and phase length (PL). Chi-squared tests are also shown. (b) The number of scalp hairs shed over a 4-day period each lunar month by 14 white men from Sheffield, England (mean ± SEM). (Courtesy of V.A. Randall and J. Ebling, Bradford, UK.)

be expected if the follicles were undergoing a spring moult and an autumn moult, in common with many other mammals of the temperate zone. The diameter of thigh hair (Fig. 66.18b) showed a pattern similar to that of the follicular changes, although the differences were less pronounced.

The seasonal variation in the rate of growth of beard and thigh hair probably reflects circannual changes in circulating androgens. It is possible that the peak in hair fall associated with the increase in the percentage of follicles in telogen in the scalp is similarly related to testosterone levels, but such an explanation is insufficient to account for the apparent changes in the hair follicles in the thigh [4].

REFERENCES

1 Dawber RPR, Van Neste D. Hair science. In: Dawber RPR, Van Neste D, eds. *Hair and Scalp Disorders*. London: Dunitz, 1995: 20–21.
2 Saitoh M, Uzuka M, Sakamoto M. Human hair cycle. *J Invest Dermatol* 1970; **54**: 65–81.
3 Orentreich N. Scalp hair replacement in man. In: Montagna W, Dobson RL, eds. *Advances in Biology of Skin*, Vol. IX. *Hair Growth*. Oxford: Pergamon, 1969: 99–108.

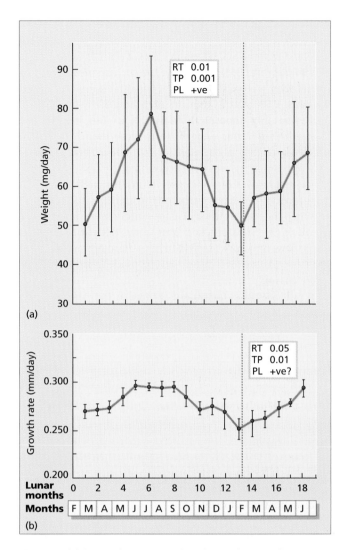

(a)

(b)

Fig. 66.17 (a) Seasonal variation in beard growth in 14 white men (mean ± SEM). (b) Thigh hair growth rate calculated from samples removed every 28 days from a specific area of the left thighs of 14 white men (mean ± SEM). (Courtesy of V.A. Randall and J. Ebling, Bradford, UK.)

4 Randall VA, Ebling FJG. Seasonal changes in human hair growth. *Br J Dermatol* 1991; **124**: 146–51.

Rate of hair growth

The rate of hair growth varies from species to species, and within one species from region to region, as well as with sex and age. For example, in the rat it can be more than 1 mm in 24 h [1–3] and in the guinea-pig up to 0.6 mm in 24 h [4], whereas in humans it is much less. The rate has been determined by direct measurement of marked hairs *in situ* [5,6], by shaving and clipping at selected intervals [2,7–10] or by pulse labelling with ^{35}S-cysteine [1,3,4,11–13]. In experimental mammals, parenteral doses of 0.1 μCi of ^{35}S-DL-cysteine per kilogram body weight at daily

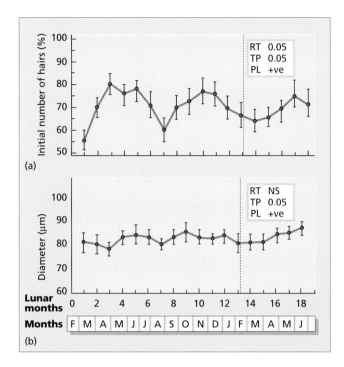

(a)

(b)

Fig. 66.18 (a) Percentage of hairs in anagen on the thigh in 14 white men (mean ± SEM). (b) Diameter of thigh hair in 14 white men (mean ± SEM). (Courtesy of V.A. Randall and J. Ebling, Bradford, UK.)

intervals have given satisfactory autoradiographs of hairs exposed for 3 or 4 weeks, but up to 20 times this amount with exposures of only 3 days has been used [1,3,12]. In the human scalp, results have been obtained by giving eight intradermal injections, each containing $0.05\,\mu$Ci ^{35}S-L-cysteine in $0.05\,$ml isotonic saline, over an area of about $2\,$cm^2, and repeating the process after 3 or 4 weeks [13].

Computer image analysis of photographs has also been proposed for quantification of hair. The technique appears feasible for assessment of hair density [14] or hair diameters [15], and it has been applied to measurement of the lengths and growth rates of vellus hairs [16].

Comparable measurements are obtained by all methods. The average rate of growth of human hair has been stated to be about $0.03\,$mm/24 h for the vellus [16] on the male forehead (see Table 66.1), $0.21\,$mm/24 h on the female thigh [7] and $0.38\,$mm/24 h on the chin of a young male [7]. On the crown of the scalp it averaged about $0.5\,$mm per 24 h, being slightly less on the margins [7]. In another study [5] in which graduated capillary tubes were fitted around the growing hairs, the average growth per 24 h in males was as follows: vertex $0.44\,$mm; temple $0.39\,$mm; chest $0.44\,$mm; beard $0.27\,$mm. The average rate on the vertex of women was $0.45\,$mm/24 h and there were no variations diurnally or during the menstrual cycle [5]. Although scalp hair grows faster in women than in men [5,17], the rate before puberty is greater in boys than in girls [18]. The average

rate over the whole body is greater in men than in women [10]. Irrespective of sex, growth appears to be highest in the two decades between 50 and 69 years of age [10]. Some workers believe that the growth rate remains constant in any individual follicle [5], whereas others have found that most hairs either increase or decrease their growth rates [11]. From studies on the guinea-pig [4], it seems clear that the growth rate depends upon the time for which the activity of the follicle has been in progress.

There is agreement that shaving has no effect on the rate of growth [5,19]. Various endocrine factors have been shown to influence the rate of hair growth in animals; for example, oestrogens reduce it [1,20,21] and thyroxine increases it [8].

Hair diameter, as well as the rate of growth, has proved a useful measure of follicular output [22,23].

REFERENCES

1 Hale PA, Ebling FJ. The effect of epilation and hormones on the activity of rat hair follicles. *J Exp Zool* 1975; **191**: 49–62.
2 Johnson E. Quantitative studies of hair growth in the albino rat. I. Normal males and females. *J Endocrinol* 1958; **16**: 337–50.
3 Priestley GC. Rates and duration of hair growth in the albino rat. *J Anat* 1966; **100**: 147–57.
4 Jackson D, Ebling FJ. The guinea-pig hair follicle as an object for experimental observation. *J Soc Cosmet Chem* 1971; **22**: 701–9.
5 Saitoh M, Uzuka M, Sakamoto M *et al*. Rate of hair growth. In: Montagna W, Dobson RL, eds. *Advances in Biology of Skin*, Vol. IX. *Hair Growth*. Oxford: Pergamon, 1969: 183–201.
6 Trotter M. Life cycles of hair in selected regions of the body. *Am J Phys Anthropol* 1924; **7**: 427–37.
7 Barman JM, Pecoraro V, Astore I. Method, technic and computations in the study of the trophic state of the human scalp hair. *J Invest Dermatol* 1964; **42**: 421–5.
8 Ebling FJ, Johnson E. The action of hormones on spontaneous hair growth cycles in the rat. *J Endocrinol* 1964; **29**: 193–201.
9 Ebling FJ, Thomas AK, Cooke ID *et al*. Effect of cyproterone acetate on hair growth, sebaceous secretion and endocrine parameters in a hirsute subject. *Br J Dermatol* 1977; **97**: 371–81.
10 Pelfini C, Cerimele D, Pisanu G. Aging of the skin and hair growth in man. In: Montagna W, Dobson RL, eds. *Advances in Biology of Skin*, Vol. IX. *Hair Growth*. Oxford: Pergamon, 1969: 153–60.
11 Comaish S. Autoradiograph studies of hair growth in various dermatoses; investigation of a possible circadian rhythm in human hair growth. *Br J Dermatol* 1969; **81**: 283–7.
12 Johnson E. Inherent rhythms of activity in the hair follicle and their control. In: Lyne AG, Short BF, eds. *Biology of the Skin and Hair Growth*. Sydney: Angus & Robertson, 1965: 491–505.
13 Munro D. Hair growth measurement using intradermal sulfur^{35} cystine. *Arch Dermatol* 1966; **93**: 119–22.
14 Gibbons RD, Fiedler-Weiss VC, West DP *et al*. Quantification of scalp hair–a computer-aided methodology. *J Invest Dermatol* 1986; **86**: 78–82.
15 Van Neste D, Dumortier M, De Coster W. Phototrichogram analysis: technical aspects and problems in relation to automated quantitative evaluation of hair growth by computer-assisted image analysis. In: Van Neste D, Lachapelle JM, Antoine JL, eds. *Hair Growth and Alopecia Research*. Dordrecht: Kluwer Academic Publishers, 1989: 155–65.
16 Blume U, Ferracin J, Verschoore M *et al*. Physiology of the vellus follicle: hair growth and sebum excretion. *Br J Dermatol* 1991; **124**: 21–8.
17 Myers RJ, Hamilton JB. Regeneration and rate of growth of hairs in men. *Ann NY Acad Sci* 1951; **53**: 562–8.
18 Pecoraro V, Astore I, Barman J *et al*. The normal trichogram in the child before the age of puberty. *J Invest Dermatol* 1964; **42**: 427–30.
19 Lynfield YL, MacWilliams P. Shaving and hair growth. *J Invest Dermatol* 1970; **55**: 170–2.

20 Jackson D, Ebling FJ. The effect of oestradiol on moulting in the guinea-pig (*Cavia porcellus* L.). *J Endocrinol* 1970; **48**: lv–lvi.
21 Johnson E. Quantitative studies of hair growth in the albino rat. II. The effect of sex hormones. *J Endocrinol* 1958; **16**: 351–9.
22 Ebling FJG, Randall VA. Hormonal actions on hair follicles and associated glands. In: Skerrow D, Skerrow CJ, eds. *Methods in Skin Research*. New York: John Wiley and Sons, 1984: 297–327.
23 Sims RT. The measurement of hair growth as an index of protein synthesis in malnutrition. *Br J Nutr* 1968; **22**: 229–36.

Cultivation *in vitro*

Whole follicles or cells derived from them can be maintained *in vitro* for the study of hair growth, the behaviour of dermal and epidermal constituents or the binding of hormones [1,2].

Hair follicles have been isolated from rat skin by repeated shearing with fine scissors [3] and from human scalp by microdissection [4]. Human scalp follicles in culture for a period grew hair at 0.3 mm/24 h, about the same rate as *in vivo*, and they became transformed into catagen by addition of epidermal growth factor (EGF).

Dermal papilla cells have been cultured from a range of mammals [5] following the initial work in rats [6] and humans [7]. Such cells are distinguishable from other fibroblasts by their capacity for aggregation, a property which is particularly marked when they are grown on collagen gels [8]. Their biosynthetic capabilities show some similarities to those of dermal fibroblasts, but there are also some differences [9].

Both dermal papilla cells and fibroblasts have been shown to possess specific androgen receptors. Papilla cells have higher levels in the beard and moustache but not in areas of scalp insensitive to androgens [10].

Cells of epithelial as well as dermal origin have been cultured from plucked human scalp hairs [11]. Differentiation has been followed in hair keratinocytes grown on collagen plated glass slips [12] and keratinocytes from the outer root sheath have been serially cultivated [13].

REFERENCES

1 Philpott MP, Sanders DA, Kealey T. Effects of insulin and insulin-like growth factors on cultured human hair follicles. *J Invest Dermatol* 1994; **102**: 857–61.
2 Philpott MP, Sanders DA, Kealey T. Whole hair follicle culture. *Dermatol Clin* 1996; **14**: 595–607.
3 Green MR, Clay CS, Gibson WT *et al.* Rapid isolation in large numbers of intact, viable, individual hair follicles from skin: biochemical and ultrastructural characterization. *J Invest Dermatol* 1986; **87**: 768–70.
4 Philpott MP, Green MR, Kealey T. An *in vitro* model for the study of human hair growth. *J Invest Dermatol* 1990; **95**: 483.
5 Randall VA. The use of dermal papilla cells in studies of normal and abnormal hair follicle biology. *Dermatol Clin* 1996; **14**: 585–94.
6 Jahoda CAB, Oliver RF. Vibrissa dermal papilla cell aggregative behaviour *in vivo* and *in vitro*. *J Embryol Exp Morphol* 1984; **79**: 211–24.
7 Messenger AG, Senior HJ, Temple A *et al.* *In vitro* properties of dermal papilla cells cultured from human hair follicles. *Br J Dermatol* 1985; **113**: 768–9.
8 Messenger AG, Senior HJ, Bleehen SS. The *in vitro* properties of dermal papilla cell lines established from human hair follicles. *Br J Dermatol* 1986; **114**: 425–30.

9 Katsuoka K, Mauch C, Schell H *et al.* Collagen type synthesis in human hair papilla cells in culture. *Arch Dermatol Res* 1988; **280**: 140–4.
10 Randall VA, Thornton MJ, Elliott K *et al.* Androgen receptors in cultured dermal papilla cells and dermal fibroblasts from scalp, beard and sexual skin. *J Invest Dermatol* 1989; **92**: 503.
11 Wells J, Seiber VK. Morphological characteristics of cells derived from plucked human hair *in vitro*. *Br J Dermatol* 1985; **113**: 669–75.
12 Imcke E. Mayer-da-Silva A, Detmar M *et al.* Growth of human hair follicle keratinocytes *in vitro*. *J Am Acad Dermatol* 1987; **17**: 779–84.
13 Limat A, Noser FK. Serial cultivation of single keratinocytes from the outer root sheath of human scalp hair follicles. *J Invest Dermatol* 1986; **87**: 485–8.

Excessive growth of hair [1–4]

Growth of hair which in any given site is coarser, longer or more profuse than is normal for the age, sex and race of the individual is regarded as excessive. The terms hirsutism and hypertrichosis are often applied interchangeably and indiscriminately to excessive hair growth of any type in any distribution. On phylogenetic grounds, and on the basis of its specific androgenic induction, the growth in the female of coarse terminal hair in the male adult sexual pattern should be differentiated clearly from the numerous other forms of excessive hair growth of widely varying aetiology. The term hirsutism will be restricted to androgen-dependent hair patterns and the term hypertrichosis will be applied to other patterns of excessive hair growth.

There is much confusion in the literature concerning generalized congenital hypertrichosis because of a plethora of names such as apeman, bearman, dogman, manlion, wildman, etc. [5].

REFERENCES

1 Breckwoldt M. Hirsutism. In: Orfanos C, Happle R, eds. *Hair Diseases*. Berlin: Springer-Verlag, 1989: 777–91.
2 Brooksbank BWL. Endocrine aspects of hirsutism. *Physiol Rev* 1961; **41**: 623–76.
3 Fenton DA. In: Dawber R, Rook A, eds. *Seminars in Dermatology*, Vol. 4. New York: Thieme–Stratton, 1985: 43–52.
4 Simpson NB, Barth JH. Hirsutism: In: Rook AJ, Dawber RPR, eds. *Diseases of the Hair and Scalp*, 2nd edn. Oxford: Blackwell Scientific Publications, 1991: 71–135.
5 Bondeson J, Miles AEW. The hairy family of Burma. *J R Soc Med* 1996; **89**: 403–5.

Hypertrichosis

Hypertrichosis lanuginosa

In congenital hypertrichosis, the fetal pelage is not replaced by vellus and terminal hair but persists, grows excessively and is constantly renewed throughout life. In the acquired form, the previously normal follicles of all types revert at any age to the production of hair with lanugo characteristics [1].

Congenital hypertrichosis lanuginosa
SYN. HYPERTRICHOSIS UNIVERSALIS CONGENITA

Aetiology. Only about 60 cases of this rare syndrome have

been reported. Traditionally, they have been classified into two groups—'dog faced' and 'simian'—but a survey [2] suggests that there may be only a single genotype, with considerable interfamily variation in the phenotype. With one exception [3], all published pedigrees suggest autosomal dominant inheritance.

Clinical features [2,4–7]. The child is usually noticed to be excessively hairy at birth (Fig. 66.19). The hair gradually lengthens until by early childhood the entire skin, apart from the palms and soles, is covered by silky hair, which may be 10 cm or more long. Long eyelashes and thick eyebrows are conspicuous features. Some affected individuals are normal at birth and sometimes for the first few years of life, before the universal replacement of other hair types by lanugo. Once established, the hypertrichosis is permanent, but some diminution of hairiness of trunk and limbs may be noted in later childhood. At puberty, axillary, pubic and beard hairs retain their downy character. Hypodontia or anodontia and deformities of the external ear are apparently associated in some families, but the physical and mental development of most patients has been normal. In a Mexican family, hypertrichosis was associated with an osteochondral dysplasia [8].

The status of the apparently recessive form is still more uncertain. Three children of a normal mother were densely hairy at birth and died within a week. Neonatal shaving was of cosmetic benefit in one rare case [6].

Gingival hyperplasia may be associated [9].

REFERENCES

1 Barth JH, Dawber RPR. Hypertrichosis. In: Dawber RPR, ed. *Diseases of the Hair and Scalp*, 3rd edn. Oxford: Blackwell Science, 1997: 490–3.
2 Felgenhauer WR. Hypertrichosis lanuginosa universalis. *J Génet Humaine* 1969; **17**: 10–13.
3 Jansen TAE, De Lange C. Familial hypertrichosis totalis. *Acta Paediatr Scand* 1945; **33**: 69–85.

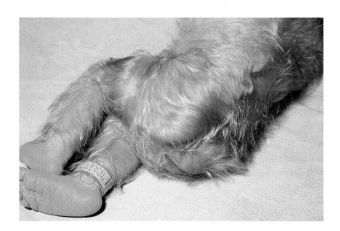

Fig. 66.19 Congenital hypertrichosis lanuginosa. (Courtesy of Dr Partridge, Leamington, UK.)

4 Barth JH, Wilkinson JD, Dawber RPR. Prepubertal hypertrichosis. *Arch Dis Child* 1987; **63**: 666–70.
5 Beighton P. Congenital hypertrichosis lanuginosa. *Arch Dermatol* 1970; **101**: 669–72.
6 Partridge JW. Congenital hypertrichosis lanuginosa: neonatal shaving. *Arch Dis Child* 1987; **62**: 623–6.
7 Tourain A, ed. *L'Hérédité en Médecine*. Paris: Masson, 1995: 525–34.
8 Cantu JM, Sanchez-Corona J, Hernandez A. A distinct osteochondrodysplasia with hypertrichosis. *Hum Genet* 1982; **60**: 36–40.
9 Lee IJ, Im SB, Kim D-K. Hypertrichosis universalis congenita: a separate entity or the same disease as gingival fibromatosis. *Paediatr Dermatol* 1993; **10**: 263–5.

Acquired hypertrichosis lanuginosa

Aetiology. In the dramatic severe forms this syndrome is rare. It usually accompanies a serious and often fatal illness. Fine, downy hair grows over a large area of the body, replacing normal hair and primary and secondary vellus. About 60 cases have been reported and all except two (of which there has been no follow-up) were suffering from malignant disease of the gastrointestinal tract, bronchus, breast, gall bladder, uterus, bladder or other organs [1–5]. One patient with lymphatic leukaemia had acquired ichthyosis as well as hypertrichosis, and one had a lymphoma. The hypertrichosis may precede the diagnosis of a neoplasm by several years.

Pathology. In one case [6] the lanugo follicles lay almost parallel to the surface, and were apparently derived from mantle follicles.

Clinical features [7–9]. In the milder forms ('malignant down' [6]) hair is confined to the face, where it attracts attention by its appearance on the nose and eyelids and other sites that normally are clinically hairless. As the growth of hair continues, it may ultimately involve the entire body, apart from the palms and soles. Existing terminal hair of scalp, beard and pubes may not be replaced, and may contrast in colour and texture with the very fine white or blonde lanugo. Such hair may grow abundantly even on the previously bald scalp. The hair may grow exceedingly rapidly, up to 2.5 cm/week, and may be more than 10 cm long.

REFERENCES

1 Hegedus SI, Schorr WF. Acquired hypertrichosis lanuginosa and malignancy. *Arch Dermatol* 1970; **106**: 84–8.
2 Hensley GT, Glynn KP. Hypertrichosis lanuginosa as a sign of internal malignancy. *Cancer* 1969; **24**: 1051–3.
3 Jemec GBE. Hypertrichosis lanuginosa acquisita: report of a case and review of the literature. *Arch Dermatol* 1986; **122**: 805–8.
4 Knowling MA, Meakin JW, Hradsky NS. Hypertrichosis associated with carcinoma of the lung. *Can Med Assoc J* 1982; **126**: 1308–10.
5 Ricken KH. Hypertrichosis lanuginosa bei chronische lymphatische Leukämie. *Z Hautkr* 1979; **54**: 819–24.
6 Davis RA, Newman DM, Phillips MJ. Acquired hypertrichosis lanuginosa. *Can Med Assoc J* 1978; **118**: 1090–6.
7 Gonzales JJ, Ungaro PC, Hooper JW. Acquired hypertrichosis lanuginosa. *Arch Intern Med* 1980; **140**: 969–70.

8 Goodfellow A, Calvert H, Bohn G. Hypertrichosis lanuginosa acquisita. *Br J Dermatol* 1980; **103**: 431–3.
9 Sindhupak W, Vibhagool A. Acquired hypertrichosis lanuginosa. *Int J Dermatol* 1983; **21**: 599–603.

Universal hypertrichosis

This term describes a condition in which the hair pattern is normal but in any site the hairs are larger and coarser than usual. The eyebrows may be double. Inheritance is determined by an autosomal dominant gene. The condition is not very rare, and modern fashions exposing more of the traditionally covered areas are bringing to hospital patients who would previously have been content to keep their bodies covered.

The condition is most often seen in dark-skinned Mediterranean and Middle Eastern subjects.

Naevoid hypertrichosis

The growth of hair abnormal for the site and the age of the patient in its length, shaft diameter and colour may occur as a circumscribed developmental defect, either isolated or associated with other naevoid abnormalities [1].

Melanocytic naevi (Chapter 38) may be accompanied by a vigorous growth of coarse hair. The hair may be present from infancy or may develop at puberty. Less often, circumscribed hypertrichosis may occur as the only clinical abnormality. Histologically, the epidermis is acanthotic and the follicles are large, but there is no excess of melanocytes.

Hypertrichosis is a characteristic feature of Becker's naevus (Chapter 15). The coarse hairs develop in the same body regions as the pigmentation, usually the thoracic or pelvic girdle, but pigmentation and hypertrichosis are not coextensive. It has been suggested that this naevus is a functional one, being androgen dependent; acne may also occur in the same site.

A tuft of hair in the lumbosacral region, the so-called faun-tail naevus, is often associated with diastematomyelia (Fig. 66.20).

Symptomatic hypertrichosis

Hypertrichosis, symmetrical and usually widespread, occurs as a sequel to, or manifestation of, a wide variety of pathological states. In none is the mechanism by which the growth of hair is induced fully understood. In some, an endocrine mechanism can be assumed. In others, an abnormality of dermal connective tissue, including the hair papilla, provoked by some biochemical agency can be postulated with some degree of probability; in the remaining conditions, the pathogenesis of the hypertrichosis is even more obscure.

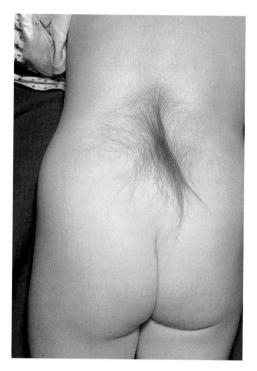

Fig. 66.20 Lumbosacral hypertrichosis ('faun tail'), here associated with diastematomyelia.

Hereditary disorders [2]

Porphyria (Chapter 59). Hypertrichosis of exposed skin is a common feature of the very rare erythropoietic porphyria; appearing first on the forehead, it later extends to the cheeks and chin, and, to a lesser degree, to other exposed areas. It is also present in many cases of the much more common erythropoietic protoporphyria [3].

In porphyria cutanea tarda, hypertrichosis is an inconstant finding, but may accompany the pigmentation, blistering and scleroderma-like changes on exposed skin, and is well marked in some children with the disease [4]. In black people, hypertrichosis and pigmentation may be present without blistering [5]. The most extreme degree of hypertrichosis is seen in children with hepatic porphyria induced by haxachlorobenzene or other chemicals. Hypertrichosis is frequent in porphyria variegata. The temples, forehead and cheeks are covered with downy hair. There is also increased pigmentation.

Epidermolysis bullosa. Gross hypertrichosis of the face and limbs has occurred in association with epidermolysis bullosa of the dystrophic type, although this is rare (Chapter 40).

Hurler's syndrome and other mucopolysaccharidoses (Chapter 12). Hypertrichosis is usually present from early infancy or early childhood on the face, trunk and limbs and may be a conspicuous feature. The eyebrows are often bushy and confluent. In abortive forms, the hair growth may first appear after puberty and be more limited in extent.

Congenital macrogingivae [6] (Chapter 69). Exuberant overgrowth of the gingivae as an isolated congenital defect is not uncommon. The association with profuse hypertrichosis of trunk, limbs and lower face has been reported on several occasions. Some patients have markedly acromegaloid features [7].

Cornelia de Lange syndrome (Chapter 12). These mildly microcephalic mentally defective children have a low hairline and profuse overgrowth of the eyebrows. The forehead is covered with long, fine hair. Hypertrichosis is usually also conspicuous on the lower back and may be generalized.

Winchester syndrome. This rare hereditary disorder is characterized by dwarfism, joint destruction and corneal opacities. The skin in many parts of the body becomes thickened, hyperpigmented and hypertrichotic [8,9].

Trisomy 18 (Chapter 12). Generalized hypertrichosis of variable degree is present in these patients.

Endocrine disturbances

Hypothyroidism [10]. A profuse growth of hair on the back and the extensor aspects of the limbs develops in some children with hypothyroidism.

Hyperthyroidism. Coarse hair often grows over the plaques of pretibial myxoedema.

Berardinelli's syndrome [11]. From early life, growth and maturation are accelerated and there is lipodystrophy with muscular hypertrophy. Enlargement of the liver and hyperlipidaemia are other constant features. The skin is coarse and often hypertrichotic.

Possible diencephalic or pituitary mechanisms. Severe generalized hypertrichosis has been reported in young children after encephalitis [12] and after mumps followed by the sudden onset of obesity [13]. A diencephalic disturbance is postulated. Generalized hypertrichosis occurred in a girl after traumatic shock [14] and remitted in 6 months. There are many reports of hypertrichosis after head injuries, especially in children [2]. The hair growth is first noticed 4–12 weeks after the injury (which seems to be of no consistent type) and appears as fine silky hair on the forehead, cheeks, back, arms and legs and may be asymmetrical. It is sometimes shed after a few months, but may persist.

Hypertrichosis has been reported in the rare hereditary globoid leukodystrophy, Krabbe's disease. Most patients die in infancy [8].

Teratogenic syndromes

Fetal alcohol syndrome [15]. Mental and physical retardation affects the infants of many mothers with chronic alcoholism. The cutaneous changes include hypertrichosis and capillary haemangiomatosis.

Other conditions

Malnutrition [16]. Gross malnutrition, which may be primary or occur in coeliac disease or other malabsorption states or in severe infections, may cause profuse generalized hypertrichosis in children.

Anorexia nervosa [17]. An increased growth of fine, downy hair on face, trunk and arms, sometimes of severe degree, has been reported in about 20% of cases, but is now rarely seen.

Acrodynia [16]. Some increased growth of hair on the limbs is common. In severe cases, the hypertrichosis is very conspicuous on the face, trunk and limbs. One child was described as monkey-like.

Dermatomyositis [18]. Excessive hair growth has been noted mainly in children and principally on the forearms, legs and temples, but it may be more extensive.

REFERENCES

1 Rupert LS, Bechtel M, Pellegrini A. Naevoid hypertrichosis. *Paediatr Dermatol* 1994; **11**: 49–50.
2 Barth JH. Hypertrichosis. In: Rook RJ, Dawber RPR, eds. *Diseases of the Hair and Scalp,* 2nd edn. Oxford: Blackwell Scientific Publications, 1991: 256–82.
3 Dean G, ed. *The Porphyrias.* London: Pitman, 1963.
4 Pinol Aguade J, Lecha M, Almeida J *et al*. Porfiria cutanea tarda en miños. *Med Cutanea* 1973; **7**: 37–42.
5 Zeligman J. Patterns of porphyria in the American Negro. *Arch Dermatol* 1963; **88**: 616–26.
6 Byars LT, Jurkiewicz M. Congenital macrogingivae and hypertrichosis. *Plast Reconstr Surg* 1962; **27**: 608–12.
7 Vontobel F. Idiopathic gingival hyperplasia and hypertrichosis associated with acromegaloid features. *Helv Paediatr Acta* 1973; **28**: 401–11.
8 Cohen AH, Hollister DW, Reed WB. The skin and the Winchester syndrome. *Arch Dermatol* 1975; **111**: 230–6.
9 Winchester P, Grossman H, Lim WN *et al.* A new acid mucopolysaccharidosis with skeletal deformities. *Am J Roentgenol* 1969; **106**: 121–8.
10 Perloff WH. Hirsutism—a manifestation of juvenile hypothyroidism. *JAMA* 1955; **157**: 651–2.
11 Berardinelli W. An undiagnosed endocrinopathy syndrome. *J Clin Endocrinol Metab* 1954; **14**: 193–204.
12 Stegano G, Vignetti P. Considerazione su di ipertricosi con cerebropatia. *Arch Ital Pediatr Puericolt* 1955; **17**: 421–4.
13 Lesne E. Mumps hypertrichosis. *Bull Soc Pediatr* 1930; **28**: 94–6.
14 Robinson RCV. Temporary acquired hypertrichosis following traumatic shock. *Arch Dermatol* 1955; **71**: 401–2.
15 Hanson JW, Jones KL, Smith DW. Fetal alcohol syndrome. *JAMA* 1976; **235**: 1458–60.
16 Holzel A. Hypertrichosis in childhood. *Acta Paediatr Scand* 1951; **40**: 59–69.
17 Ryle JA. Anorexia nervosa. *Lancet* 1936; **ii**: 140–4.
18 Reich MG, Reinhart JB. Dermatomyositis associated with hypertrichosis. *Arch Dermatol Syphilol* 1948; **57**: 725–32.

Iatrogenic hypertrichosis

In iatrogenic hypertrichosis, there is a uniform growth of fine hair increased over extensive areas of the trunk, hands and face, i.e. unrelated to androgen-dependent hair growth.

The mode of action of the offending drugs on hair follicles is not known; the same mechanism is not involved in all cases. Cortisone, diphenylhydantoin and penicillamine are all known to affect connective tissue, but in different ways. Psoralens presumably induce hypertrichosis in predisposed subjects by accentuating the tendency of sunlight to induce this temporary change. The stimulation of hair growth on sun-exposed sites by benoxaprofen may have a similar mechanism. Existing vellus hairs increase in length and less so in diameter. The hairs are seldom more than 3 cm in length and are considerably finer than terminal hair.

Diphenylhydantoin induces hypertrichosis after 2–3 months. It affects the extensor aspects of the limbs, then the face and trunk and clears within a year of cessation of therapy [1].

Diazoxide produces hypertrichosis in all of those treated but it seems to be a cosmetic problem in only one-half [2,3]; in adults, the anagen phase may last longer [4]. There are no associated changes in the sebaceous glands [2].

Minoxidil commonly induces hypertrichosis [5]. It is apparent after a few weeks' therapy [6].

Hypertrichosis of some degree develops in 60% of patients treated with cyclosporin [7–9]. Keratosis pilaris may precede the appearance of thick, pigmented hair on the face, trunk and limbs. Changes in other parts of the pilosebaceous unit occur; keratosis pilaris (21%), sebaceous hyperplasia (10%) and acne (15%) [8].

Benoxaprofen induces a fine, downy growth of hair on the face and exposed extremities after only a few weeks [10].

Streptomycin caused hypertrichosis in 22 of 27 children who had received 1 g daily for miliary tuberculous meningitis [11]. Buffoni [12] observed hypertrichosis in about 66% of cases of meningitis so treated, and postulated that the streptomycin did not act directly on the follicles.

Prolonged administration of cortisone may induce hypertrichosis, most marked on the forehead, the temples and the sides of the cheeks, but also on the back and the extensor aspects of the limbs.

Penicillamine appears to cause lengthening and coarsening of hair on the trunk and limbs.

Psoralens, used in the treatment of vitiligo and psoriasis, may induce temporary hypertrichosis of light-exposed skin [13].

REFERENCES

1 Livingstone S, Peterson D, Bohs LL. Hypertrichosis occurring in association with dilantin therapy. *J Pediatr* 1955; **47**: 351–2.
2 Koblenzer PJ, Baker L. Hypertrichosis lanuginosa associated with diazoxide therapy in prepubertal children; a clinicopathological study. *Ann NY Acad Sci* 1968; **150**: 373–9.
3 Prigent F, Gantzer A, Romain O *et al*. Hypertrichose diffuse acquisé au cours d'un traitment par diazoxide chez un nouveau-né. *Ann Dermatol Vénéréol* 1988; **115**: 191–2.
4 Burton JL, Schutt WH, Caldwell IW. Hypertrichosis due to diazoxide. *Br J Dermatol* 1975; **93**: 707–9.
5 Burton JL, Marshall A. Hypertrichosis due to minoxidil. *Br J Dermatol* 1979; **101**: 593–5.
6 Lorette G, Nivet H. Hypertrichose diffuse au minoxidil chez un enfant de deux ans et demi. *Ann Dermatol Vénéréol* 1985; **112**: 527–8.
7 Bencini PL, Montagnino G, Sala F *et al*. Cutaneous lesions in 67 cyclosporin-treated renal transplant recipients. *Dermatologica* 1986; **172**: 24–31.
8 Bencini PL, Montagnino G, Crosti C *et al*. Acne in a kidney transplant patient treated with cyclosporin A. *Br J Dermatol* 1986; **114**: 396.
9 Griffiths CEM, Powles AV, Leonard JN *et al*. Clearance of psoriasis with low dose cyclosporin. *Br Med J* 1986; **293**: 731–3.
10 Fenton DA, English JS, Wilkinson JD. Reversal of male pattern baldness, hypertrichosis, and accelerated hair and nail growth in patients receiving benoxaprofen. *Br Med J* 1982; **248**: 1228–9.
11 Fono R. Appearance of hypertrichosis during streptomycin treatment. *Ann Paediatr* 1950: **174**: 389–92.
12 Buffoni L. Streptomicini e ipertricosi. *Minerva Pediatr* 1951; **3**: 710–12.
13 Singh G, Lal S. Hypertrichosis and hyperpigmentation with systemic psoralen treatment. *Br J Dermatol* 1967; **79**: 501–2.

Acquired circumscribed hypertrichosis

Cutting or shaving the hair influences neither its rate of growth nor the calibre of the hair shaft. However, repeated or long-continued inflammatory changes involving the dermis, whether or not clinically evident scarring is produced, may result in the growth of long and coarse hair at the site. The cause of the hair growth is usually obvious but may be overlooked when the trauma is occupational; for example, circumscribed patches of hypertrichosis on the left shoulder in people frequently carrying heavy sacks [1]. A patch of hypertrichosis on one forearm is sometimes seen in mental defectives who have acquired the habit of chewing this site [2]. Sometimes the hypertrichosis, which may involve too few follicles to have attracted the patient's attention, develops at the site of an accidental wound or a vaccination scar [3]. It has developed on the back of the hand and fingers 3 months after the excision of warts [4]. It has been reported also in an irregular pattern on the legs in chronic venous insufficiency [5], around the edges of a burn [6] and at the site of multiple clusters of excoriated insect bites [7]. Hypertrichosis of this type may occur near inflamed joints and has been reported particularly in association with gonococcal arthritis [8] and in the skin overlying chronic osteomyelitis of the tibia [9]. Very exceptionally, inflammatory dermatoses, especially in children, may induce a temporary overgrowth of hair, for example after eczema [10] (Fig. 66.21) and varicella [11]. A linear pattern of hypertrichosis on the leg has been described after recurrent thrombophlebitis which persisted for a year [12]. Hypertrichosis may occur in the indurated skin in melorheostotic scleroderma [13]; the diagnosis is established by radiological examination when the skin has completely healed. The damaged skin in epidermolysis bullosa may also become hypertrichotic [14]. Children have

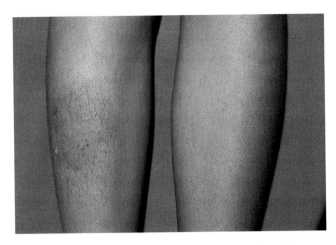

Fig. 66.21 Circumscribed hypertrichosis in an area of steroid-treated lichen simplex.

developed itching eczema and local hypertrichosis at the site of injection of diphtheria/tetanus vaccine adsorbed on aluminium chloride [15].

Hypertrichosis of one leg after a prolonged period of occlusion by plaster of Paris is a phenomenon well known to orthopaedic surgeons. It occurs mainly in children. The hypertrichosis may be attributed either to protection of the skin by the plaster from normal weathering or to increased skin temperature. The hair returns to normal within a few weeks of removal of the plaster.

A similar phenomenon is seen with localized hypertrichosis affecting the dorsum of the hand and wrist after local fractures. This is usually associated with reflex sympathetic dystrophy where there is pain, change in skin temperature and altered sweating.

REFERENCES

1 Csillag J. Über Beruishypertricose. *Arch Dermatol Syphilol* 1921; **134**: 147–8.
2 Ressmann AC, Butterworth T. Localized acquired hypertrichosis (as a result of biting in mentally deficient). *Arch Dermatol Syphilol* 1952; **65**: 458–60.
3 Linser A. Demonstrationen: Patient mit einer Hypertrichosis irritative. *Klin Wochenschr* 1926; **115**: 149–50.
4 Friederich HC, Gloor M. Postoperativ 'irritative' Hypertrichose. *Zeitschr Haut Geschlechts* 1970; **45**: 10–11.
5 Schraibman IG. Localized hirsutism. *Postgrad Med J* 1967; **43**: 545–6.
6 Shafir R, Tsur H. Local hirsutism at the periphery of burned skin. *Br J Plast Surg* 1979; **32**: 93–5.
7 Tisocco LA, Del Campo DV, Bennin B et al. Acquired localised hypertrichosis. *Arch Dermatol* 1981; **117**: 129–31.
8 Heidemann H. Et tifaelde af hypertrichose opstaalt i tilknytning til en gonorrhoisk ledaffektasion. *Ugeskrift Laeger* 1934; **96**: 553–5.
9 Schuller PA, Frost JA. Osteomilitis cronica de perone e hipertrichosis localizada. *Medicina* 1956; **24**: 360–1.
10 Edel K. Hypertrichosis als verwikkeling bij eczeem. *Neaerland Tijdschr Geneesk* 1938; **82**: 2466–7.
11 Naveh Y, Friedman A. Transient circumscribed hypertrichosis following chicken pox. *Paediatrics* 1972; **50**: 487–8.
12 Soyuer U, Aktas E, Ozesmi M. Post phlebitic localized hypertrichosis. *Arch Dermatol* 1988; **124**: 30–1.
13 Miyachi Y, Hori T, Yamada A et al. Linear melorheostotic scleroderma and hypertrichosis. *Arch Dermatol* 1979; **115**: 1233–4.
14 Cofano AR. Su un caso di epidermolisi bollosa distrofica con accentuada ipertricosi. *Ann Ital Dermatol* 1995; **10**: 195–6.
15 Pembroke HC, Marten RH. Unusual reactions following diphtheria and tetanus immunization. *Clin Exp Dermatol* 1979; **4**: 345–7.

Hirsutism

Perception of hirsuties is by definition subjective, and women present with a wide variation in severity [1]. Both the severity of the hirsuties and the degree of acceptance are dependent on racial, cultural and social factors. Even the criteria for the definition of hirsuties used by physicians vary widely [2–6]. In order to solve this issue, different groups have evolved different grading schemes for hair growth. The study by Ferriman and Gallwey [3], which has become the standard grading system, has defined hirsuties purely on quantitative grounds. Other physicians have examined women complaining of hirsuties and compared them with controls; they have demonstrated that there is a considerable overlap in the grades of hirsuties between those women who consider themselves to be hirsute and control women [4,6]. Hair on the face, chest or upper back is a good discriminating factor between hirsute women and controls with similar hair growth scores. In clinical practice, it has often been suggested that 'real' hirsutism is simply that which the woman thinks is excessive in herself.

Hair is second only to the skin colour as a feature of racial difference. Facial and body hair is less commonly seen on oriental people [7], black people and native Americans than on white people [8]. Even among white people there are differences; hair growth is heavier on those of Mediterranean than those of Nordic ancestry [9]. The pattern of hair growth in hirsuties within different racial groups is identical [3–6]; however, different criteria have made the determination of the comparative incidence and severity within these groups difficult to assess. Only one study of a random population stated how many women considered themselves to be hirsute. McKnight [5] examined 400 unselected students, 60% of whom were Welsh: 9% were considered by both the women and investigator to be hirsute and 4% were considered to be disfigured by their facial hair growth. This investigation also included studies of hair growth in women who were not complaining of hirsuties. These studies have been rigorously performed and confirm ethnic variations in density of hair growth. It is important to the definition of hirsuties that a sizeable proportion of normal women have some terminal hairs on their face, breasts or lower abdomen.

Lorenzo [10] studied 90 hirsute women and found an increased incidence of hirsutism in their female relatives compared with control populations. McKnight [5] reported that 14% of hirsute Welsh women gave a positive family history. This tendency to familial clustering in hirsutism might have been anticipated, as some of the underlying disorders which result in hyperandrogenism may have a familial basis; for example, congenital adrenal hyperplasia is linked to the major histocompatibility complex [11] and a very strong family relationship has been reported in the polycystic ovary syndrome (PCOS) [12].

In hirsuties, one role of society is to determine the threshold level for normality and this is now determined by the media. Women receive a barrage of advertisements for cosmetics that are based on the premise that only a woman with a hairless body can be both normal and healthy.

There have been few studies on the psychological status of hirsute women. Meyer and Zerssen [13] concluded on the basis of a small sample of patients studied within a psychoanalytic framework that many suffered reactive psychic disturbances. A small controlled study [14] revealed increased levels of anxiety. In contrast, Callan *et al.* [15] were unable to detect significant differences in comparison with normative data.

Another approach to the psychological aspect of hirsuties has been to implicate 'stress' as an aetiological factor for hirsuties. Segre [16] states, in his monograph on the hirsute female, that: 'Lack of peace of mind appears at the core of the problem. We believe it to be both a cause and result of hirsutism'. This view has been endorsed [17]. The onset of hirsutism in four of 10 hirsute women was noted to coincide with a period of emotional stress [18]. Bush and Mahesh [19] reported stress-induced hirsutism in a young woman whose unstressed twin was not hirsute.

REFERENCES

1 Hughes CL. Hirsutism. In: Olsen EA, ed. *Disorders of Hair Growth*. New York: McGraw-Hill, 1994: 337–52.
2 Editorial. Endocrine treatment in hirsutism. *Br Med J* 1975; ii: 461–2.
3 Ferriman D, Gallwey JD. Clinical assessment of body hair growth in women. *J Clin Endocrinol* 1961; **21**: 1440–9.
4 Lunde O, Grottum P. Body hair growth in women; normal or hirsute. *Am J Phys Anthropol* 1984; **64**: 307–12.
5 McKnight E. The prevalence of 'hirsutism' in young women. *Lancet* 1964; i: 410–12.
6 Shah PN. Human body hair—a quantitative study. *Am J Obstet Gynecol* 1957; **73**: 1255–61.
7 Hamilton JE. Age, sex and genetic factors in the regulation of hair growth in men: a comparison of Caucasian and Japanese populations. In: Montagna W, Ellis RA, eds. *The Biology of Hair Growth*. New York: Academic Press, 1958: 399–417.
8 Danforth CH, Trotter M. The distribution of body hair in white subjects. *Am J Phys Anthropol* 1922; **5**: 259–65.
9 Greenblatt RB. Hirsutism—ancestral curse or endocrinopathy. In: Mahesh VB, Greenblatt RB, eds. *Hirsutism and Virilism*. Boston: John Wright, 1983: 1–9.
10 Lorenzo EM. Familial study of hirsutism. *J Clin Endocrinol Metab* 1970; **31**: 556–60.
11 Gordon MT, Conway DI, Anderson DC *et al.* Genetics and biochemical variability of variants of 21 hydroxylase deficiency. *J Med Genet* 1985; **22**: 354–7.
12 Hague WM, Adams J, Reeders ST *et al.* Familial polycystic ovaries: a genetic disease? *Clin Endocrinol* 1988; **29**: 593–6.
13 Meyer AE, Zerssen DV. Frauen mit sogenanntem idiopathischem Hirsutismus. *J Psychosom Res* 1960; **4**: 206–10.
14 Rabinowitz S, Cohen R, Le Roith D. Anxiety and hirsutism. *Psychol Rep* 1983; **53**: 827–33.
15 Callan A, Dennerstein L, Burrows GD *et al.* The psychoendocrinology of hirsutism. In: Dennerstein L, Burrows GD, eds. *Obstetrics, Gynaecology and Psychiatry*. Melbourne: University of Melbourne, 1980: 43–51.
16 Segre EJ, ed. *Androgens, Virilization and the Hirsute Female*. Springfield: Thomas, 1967: 92–4.
17 Rook AJ. Aspects of cutaneous androgen-dependent syndromes. *Int J Dermatol* 1980; **19**: 357–60.
18 Merivale WH. The excretion of pregnanediol and 17-ketosteroids during the menstrual cycle in benign hirsutism. *J Clin Pathol* 1951; **4**: 78–83.
19 Bush IE, Mahesh VB. Adrenocortical hyperfunction with sudden onset of hirsutism. *J Endocrinol* 1959; **18**: 1–7.

Androgens and hirsutism

There have been several attempts to correlate hair growth in women with plasma androgen levels but these reports have yielded conflicting results. Reingold and Rosenfield [1] noted a considerable variability between hair growth scores and free testosterone, but no significant relationship. Ruutiainen *et al.* [2] have calculated a complex formula for multiple plasma androgen levels:

Testosterone/SHBG + androstenedione/100 + dehydroepiandrosterone sulphate/100

This correlates with hair growth only in women with idiopathic hirsuties. In a further study, the same group [3] found a relationship between hair growth and salivary testosterone levels, but in this study no selection of patients was required. A different ratio has been determined for female baldness [4]:

3α-androstanediol glucuronide/SHBG

These relationships are clearly unsatisfactory because they cannot explain the differential response to androgens by hair follicles at different sites on the body. The development of hair follicle and dermal papilla models *in vitro* should help answer these questions [5].

The physiological mechanisms for androgenic activity may be considered in three stages:
1 production of androgens by the adrenals and ovaries;
2 their transport in the blood on carrier proteins—principally SHBG;
3 their intracellular modification and binding to the androgen receptor.

The first sign of androgen production in women occurs 2–3 years before the menarche and is due to adrenal secretion [6]. The signal for this development is unknown; there may be increased activity of C_{17-20} lyase, which redirects glucocorticoid precursors towards the androgen pathway, or there may be a reduced forward metabolism of dehydroisoandrosterone (DHA) as a result of reduced activity of Δ^5-3β-hydroxysteroid dehydrogenase; this process represents a maturation of the adrenal zona reticularis. The major androgens secreted by the adrenal are androstenedione, DHA and DHA sulphate (DHAS). Their control during postpubertal life is unknown but it is thought that androstenedione and DHA may be controlled by adrenocorticotrophic hormone (ACTH), as their serum levels mirror those of cortisol [7,8].

Ovarian androgen production begins under the influence of the pubertal secretion of luteinizing hormone (LH) and takes place in the theca cells. The predominant androgen secreted by the ovaries is androstenedione during the reproductive years, and testosterone after the menopause. Androgen secretion continues throughout the menstrual cycle but peaks at the middle of an ovulatory cycle [9]. Androstenedione secretion is greater from the ovary containing the dominant follicle [10].

In normal women, the majority of testosterone production (50–70%) is derived from peripheral conversion of androstenedione in skin and other extrasplanchnic sites [11–13]. The remaining proportion is secreted directly by the adrenals and ovaries. The relative proportion estimated from each gland varies between reported studies, from 5 to 20% from the ovary and 0–30% from the adrenal [13,14]. DHA is the source of less than 10% of circulating androstenedione and 1% of circulating testosterone [15,16].

Androgen transport proteins

In non-pregnant women, the majority of circulating androgens are bound to a high-affinity β-globulin, SHBG. A further 20–25% is transported loosely bound to albumin, and about 1% circulates freely. The free steroid is believed to be active, and the binding protein is therefore of paramount importance. The affinity of the androgens for SHBG is proportional to their biological activity.

The function of SHBG is unknown. It is probable that its main role is to buffer acute changes in unbound androgen levels and to protect androgens from degradation. Burke and Anderson [17] suggested that it also acts as a biological amplifier. High oestrogen levels increase SHBG and therefore reduce available androgen; high androgen levels reduce SHBG and increase available free androgen.

REFERENCES

1 Reingold SB, Rosenfield RL. The relationship of mild hirsutism or acne in women to androgens. *Arch Dermatol* 1987; **123**: 209–14.
2 Ruutiainen K, Erkola R, Kaihola HL *et al*. The grade of hirsutism correlated to serum androgen levels and hormonal indices. *Acta Obstet Gynecol Scand* 1985; **64**: 629–34.
3 Ruutiainen K, Sannika E, Santii R *et al*. Salivary testosterone in hirsutism: correlations with serum testosterone and the degree of hair growth. *J Clin Endocrinol Metab* 1987; **64**: 1015–20.
4 De Villez RL, Dunn J. Female androgenic alopecia; the 3 alpha, 17-beta-androstanediol glucuronide/sex hormone binding globulin ratio as a possible marker for female pattern baldness. *Arch Dermatol* 1986; **122**: 1011–17.
5 Randall VA. The use of dermal papilla cells in studies of normal and abnormal hair follicle biology. *Dermatol Clin* 1996; **14**: 585–94.
6 Reiter EO, Fuldauer VG, Root AW. Secretion of the adrenal androgen dehydroepiandrosterone sulphate, during normal infancy, childhood, and adolescence, in sick infants and children with endocrinological abnormalities. *J Pediatr* 1977; **90**: 766–70.
7 James VHT, Tunbridge D, Wilson GA *et al*. Central control of steroid hormone secretion. *J Steroid Biochem* 1978; **9**: 429–34.
8 Rosenfeld RS, Rosenburg BJ, Fukushima DK *et al*. 24-Hour secretory pattern of dehydroisoandrosterone and dehydroisoandrosterone sulphate. *J Clin Endocrinol Metab* 1975; **40**: 850–8.
9 Vermeuler A, Verdonck L. Plasma androgen levels during the menstrual cycle. *Am J Obstet Gynecol* 1976; **125**: 491–8.
10 Baird DT, Burger PE, Heaven-Jones GD *et al*. The site of secretion of androstenedione in non-pregnant women. *J Endocrinol* 1974; **63**: 201.
11 Horton R. Markers of peripheral androgen production. In: Serio M, Motta M, Martini L, eds. *Sexual Differentiation; Basic and Clinical Aspects*. New York: Raven Press, 1984: 261–85.
12 Horton R, Tait JF. Androstenedione production and interconversion rates measured in peripheral blood and studies on the possible site of its conversion to testosterone. *J Clin Invest* 1966; **45**; 301–6.
13 Kirschner MA, Bardin CW. Androgen production and metabolism in normal and virilised women. *Metabolism* 1972; **21**: 667–73.
14 Moltz L, Sorensen R, Schwartz U *et al*. Ovarian and adrenal vein steroids in healthy women with ovulatory cycles—selective catheterization findings. *J Steroid Biochem* 1984; **20**: 901–8.
15 Horton R, Tait JF. *In vivo* conversion of dehydroisoandrosterone to plasma androstenedione and testosterone in man. *J Clin Endocrinol Metab* 1967; **27**: 79–85.
16 Kirschner MA, Sinhamahapatra S, Zucker IR *et al*. The production, origin and role of dehydro-epiandrosterone and 5-androstenediol as androgen prehormones in hirsute women. *J Clin Endocrinol Metab* 1973; **37**: 183–8.
17 Burke CW, Anderson DC. Sex-hormone binding globulin is an oestrogen amplifier. *Nature* 1972; **240**; 38.

Androgen pathophysiology in hirsuties [1,2]

Hirsuties is a response of the hair follicles to androgenic stimulation, and increased hair growth is therefore often seen in endocrine disorders characterized by hyperandrogenism. These disorders may be due to abnormalities of either the ovaries or adrenal glands. It is likely that many hirsute women have underlying PCOS (Table 66.2). A small proportion of hirsute women have no detectable hormonal abnormality and are usually classified as 'idiopathic' hirsuties. This subgroup is gradually becoming smaller as diagnostic techniques become more refined, and is probably due to more subtle forms of ovarian or adrenal hypersecretion, or alterations in serum androgen binding proteins or in the cutaneous metabolism of androgens.

Although many hirsute women are obese, the role of adipose tissue is undefined but it is clinically recognized,

Table 66.2 Causes of hirsuties.

Ovarian causes
Polycystic ovary syndrome
Ovarian tumours
Adrenal causes
Congenital adrenal hyperplasia
Cushing's disease
Prolactinoma
Gonadal dysgenesis
Androgen therapy
Idiopathic hirsuties
?? Stress

although undocumented, that weight loss by obese hirsute women with menstrual irregularities may result in regulation of menses and a reduction in body hair growth.

Polycystic ovary syndrome [3,4]. The perception of PCOS has changed dramatically since it was first described by Stein and Leventhal in 1935 [5]. They defined a syndrome consisting of obesity, amenorrhoea, hirsutism and infertility associated with enlarged polycystic ovaries. This disorder has been a controversial diagnosis, as it is defined by the appearance of organs that are difficult to visualize. This has led to the use of multiple diagnostic formulations based on clinical and biochemical abnormalities. A more fundamental issue has been raised by modern imaging techniques, which have revealed the presence of polycystic ovaries in apparently normal women [6]. Ideas concerning the pathogenesis of PCOS have been as controversial as the diagnosis, and different authorities embrace the belief that it is primarily due to an ovarian abnormality, inappropriate gonodotrophin secretion, a disorder of the adrenal glands or increased peripheral aromatase activity resulting in hyperoestrogenaemia [7]. Whether the increased androgen is of adrenal or ovarian origin remains controversial [8].

The pattern of clinical features of patients with PCOS will depend to an extent on the diagnostic definition of the disorder and upon the presenting symptom, be it dermatological, endocrine or gynaecological. Using ultrasound visualization of polycystic ovaries as the diagnostic criterion, Conway *et al.* [9] found the following clinical features in a series of 556 patients: hirsuties (61%), acne (24%), alopecia (8%), acanthosis nigricans (2%), obesity (35%), menorrhagia (1%), oligomenorrhoea (45%), amenorrhoea (26%) and infertility (over 29%). However, those patients who present to a dermatologist will almost invariably have acne and/or hirsuties.

Laboratory investigations in PCOS usually reveal an elevated level of LH, often with an increased LH/FSH (follicle-stimulating hormone) ratio, and testosterone, androstenedione and oestradiol levels are often raised [10]. The demonstration by ultrasound examination of multiple peripheral ovarian cysts around a dense central core will depend on the expertise of the operator [11].

Ovarian tumours. Hirsuties is a nearly universal feature in virilizing ovarian tumours; however, functioning tumours that cause virilization represent approximately 1% of ovarian tumours [12]. Amenorrhoea or oligomenorrhoea develop in all premenopausal patients, and alopecia, cliteromegaly, deepening of the voice and a male habitus develop in about half of the patients [13,14]. The majority of patients with virilizing ovarian tumours have raised plasma testosterone levels [12,14].

Hirsuties in pregnancy. Hirsuties has only rarely been reported to develop during pregnancy; it may be due to the development of PCOS or a virilizing tumour. PCOS has been reported to present with virilization during the first or third trimester and may regress postpartum [15]. Androgens freely cross the placenta and virilization of a female fetus may occur [16]. The range of tumours occurring during pregnancy has been reviewed by Novak *et al.* [17].

Congenital adrenal hyperplasia. Cholesterol is metabolized in the adrenal cortex, via a complex pathway, into aldosterone, cortisol, androgens and oestrogens. A defect in a pathway results in a reduction of the product of the pathway involved, with a redistribution of the precursors to other pathways, which results in overproduction of the other hormones. Complete absence of a particular enzyme may be incompatible with life, and severe reduction in enzyme activity is usually apparent at birth or in early childhood due to dehydration with a salt-losing state and/or virilization.

Partial reduction in enzyme activity may present after childhood and, during the past decade, a small proportion of women presenting with postpubertal hirsuties have been demonstrated to have subtle forms of 'late-onset' congenital adrenal hyperplasia (CAH). The diagnosis cannot be made clinically, and dynamic endocrine investigations are required to differentiate between PCOS and idiopathic hirsuties. Women with late-onset CAH may have normal menstrual cycles; however, approximately 80% will have polycystic ovaries [18].

21-hydroxylase deficiency [19] is the commonest defect associated with late-onset CAH. As many as 3–6% of women presenting with hirsuties may be affected with this form. This form is an allelic variant of the classic childhood salt-wasting type; the classic form is associated with HLA-Bw47 and the late onset form with HLA-B14. Of women with this abnormality, 75% will present with hirsutism, with or without menstrual irregularities.

3β- and 11β-hydroxylase deficiencies are less common forms of CAH and are consequently less frequently found in hirsute women [20].

Acquired adrenocortical disease. Adrenal carcinomas usually present with abdominal swelling or pain; however, 10% of both adenomas and carcinomas may present with isolated virilization [21]. The combination of virilization and Cushing's syndrome strongly suggests the presence of a carcinoma. The testosterone level is usually markedly raised in the latter.

Patients with Cushing's syndrome are said to have both hypertrichosis, a generalized diffuse growth of fine hair due to hypercortisolaemia, and androgen-induced coarse hair in the usual male pattern [22].

Gonadal dysgenesis. Moltz *et al.* [23] described six patients with 46XY gonadal dysgenesis. All had unambiguously female genitalia but male skeletal characteristics: wide span, broad shoulders and chest; two were hirsute, two had temporal recession and three had deep voices. Rosen *et al.* [24] reported a further 30 patients with gonadal dysgenesis, of whom three (with Y chromosome material) presented with slowly progressive hirsuties and secondary amenorrhoea.

Hyperprolactinaemia. The exact relationship between prolactin and hirsuties is not clear. The incidence of hirsuties in the amenorrhea–galactorrhoea syndrome has been reported as 22–60% [25]. This may be due to a direct effect of prolactin on adrenal androgen production or to PCOS, with which it is frequently associated; prolactin has also been reported to attenuate cutaneous 5α-reductase activity both *in vivo* and *in vitro* [26].

Idiopathic hirsuties (Fig. 66.22). Idiopathic hirsuties is the diagnostic category given to those hirsute women in whom no overt underlying endocrine disorder can be detected. There are a number of subtle dynamic alterations in the androgen metabolism of hirsute women compared with non-hirsute women: daily testosterone production is increased by 3.5–5-fold; the majority of androgen is secreted as testosterone (hirsute 75% versus normal, less than 40%) rather than as androstenedione [27]; increased androgens in hirsute women are associated with lower levels of SHBG, which binds less testosterone and increases its free level [28]. More free testosterone is, therefore, available for peripheral metabolism and clearance; these two factors disguise the increased rates of testosterone production. Free testosterone is a more sensitive measure of testosterone status and is approximately threefold greater in hirsute than non-hirsute women [29].

Normal values for total testosterone are found in 25–60% of hirsute women and in 80% of those with regular menstrual cycles [30]. This may be due to the effect of SHBG or to the wide fluctuations in plasma testosterone seen in hirsute women. Consequently, multiple measurements are often required to detect the increased levels. However, some women will not demonstrate elevations of testosterone despite exhaustive investigation. Paradoxically, in these women, the growth of hair by their skin is the only, and most sensitive, androgen bioassay.

REFERENCES

1 Oake RJ, Davies SJ, McLachlan MSF *et al.* Plasma testosterone in adrenal and ovarian vein blood of hirsute women. *Q J Med* 1974; **43**: 603–14.
2 Simpson NB, Barth JH. Hair patterns: hirsuties and androgenetic alopecia. In: Dawber RPR, ed. *Diseases of the Hair and Scalp*, 3rd edn. Oxford: Blackwell Science, 1997: 140–55.
3 Stahl NL, Teeslink CR, Greenblatt RB. Ovarian, adrenal, and peripheral testosterone levels in the polycystic ovary syndrome. *Am J Obstet Gynecol* 1973; **117**: 194–9.
4 Balen AH, Conway GS, Kaltsas G *et al.* Polycystic ovary syndrome: the spectrum of the disorder in 1741 patients. *Hum Reprod* 1995; **10**: 2107–11.
5 Stein IF, Leventhal MC. Amenorrhoea associated with bilateral polycystic ovaries. *Am J Obstet Gynecol* 1935; **29**: 181–4.
6 Polson DW, Adams J, Wadsworth J *et al.* Polycystic ovaries—a common finding in normal women. *Lancet* 1988; **i**: 870–2.
7 McKenna TJ. Current concepts: pathogenesis and treatment of polycystic ovary syndrome. *N Engl J Med* 1988; **318**: 558–69.
8 Polson DW, Reed MJ, Franks S *et al.* Serum 11-beta-hydroxyandros-tenedione as an indicator of the source of excess androgen production in women with polycystic ovaries. *J Clin Endocrinol Metab* 1988; **66**: 946–50.
9 Conway GS, Honour JW, Jacobs HS. Heterogeneity of the polycystic ovary syndrome: clinical, endocrine and ultrasound features in 556 patients. *Clin Endocrinol* 1989; **30**: 459–64.
10 Coney P. Polycystic ovarian disease: current concepts of patho-physiology and therapy. *Fertil Steril* 1984; **42**: 667–72.
11 Adams J, Polson DW, Franks S. Prevalence of polycystic ovaries in women with anovulation and idiopathic hirsutism. *Br Med J* 1986; **293**: 355–7.
12 Woodruff JD, Parmley TH. Virilizing ovarian tumors. In: Mahesh VB, Greenblatt RB, eds. *Hirsutism and Virilism: Pathogenesis and Management.* Boston: John Wright, 1983: 129–45.
13 Sandberg EC, Jackson JR. A clinical analysis of ovarian virilising tumors. *Am J Surg* 1963; **105**: 784–95.
14 Moltz L, Pickartz H, Sorensen R *et al.* Ovarian and adrenal vein steroids in seven patients with androgen-secreting ovarian neoplasm: selective catheterization findings. *Fertil Steril* 1984; **42**: 585–96.
15 Shortle BE, Warren MP, Tsin D. Recurrent androgenicity in pregnancy; a case report and literature review. *Obstet Gynecol* 1987; **70**: 462–8.
16 Fayez JA, Bunch TR, Miller GL. Virilization in pregnancy associated with polycystic ovary disease. *Obstet Gynecol* 1974; **44**: 511–15.
17 Novak DJ, Lauchlan SC, McCawley JC *et al.* Virilization during pregnancy: case report and review of literature. *Am J Med* 1970; **49**: 281–90.
18 Hague WM, Adams J, Rodda C *et al.* Prevalence of ultrasonically detected polycystic ovaries in females with congenital adrenal hyperplasia. *J Endocrinol* 1986; **111** (Suppl.): 46–7.
19 Dewailly D, Vantyghem-Haudiquet MC, Saintard C *et al.* Clinical and biological phenotypes in late-onset 21-hydroxylase deficiency. *J Clin Endocrinol Metab* 1986; **63**: 418–23.
20 Pang S, Lerner AJ, Stoner E *et al.* Late onset adrenal steroid 3 beta hydroxysteroid dehydrogenase deficiency. I. A cause of hirsutism in pubertal and postpubertal women. *J Clin Endocrinol Metab* 1985; **60**: 428–33.
21 King DR, Lack EE. Adrenal cortical carcinoma: a clinical and pathologic study of 49 cases. *Cancer* 1979; **44**: 239–49.
22 Griffing GT, Melby JC. Cushing's syndrome. In: Mahesh VB, Greenblatt RB, eds. *Hirsutism and Virilism*. Boston: John Wright 1983: 63–78.

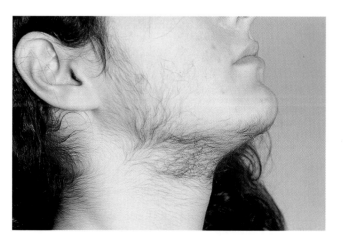

Fig. 66.22 Facial hirsutism: in this case not associated with any systemic disease or detectable biochemical endocrine abnormality.

23 Moltz L, Schwartz U, Pickartz H *et al.* XY gonadal dysgenesis: aberrant testicular differentiation in the presence of H-Y antigen. *Obstet Gynecol* 1981; **58**: 17–23.

24 Rosen GF, Kaplan B, Lobo RA. Menstrual function and hirsutism in patients with gonadal dysgenesis. *Obstet Gynecol* 1988; **71**: 677–83.

25 Robyn C, Tukumbane M. Hyperprolactinemia and hirsuties. In: Mahesh VB, Greenblatt RB, eds. *Hirsutism and Virilism*. Boston: John Wright, 1983: 189–211.

26 Serafini P, Lobo RA. Prolactin modulates peripheral androgen metabolism. *Fertil Steril* 1986; **45**: 41–50.

27 Kirschner MA, Bardin CW. Androgen production and metabolism in normal and virilised women. *Metabolism* 1972; **21**: 667–77.

28 Hauner H, Ditschuneit SB, Pal SB *et al.* Fat distribution, endocrine and metabolic profile of obese women with and without hirsutism. *Metabolism* 1988; **37**: 281–6.

29 Cummings DC, Wall SR. Non sex-hormone binding globulin-bound testosterone as a marker for hyperandrogenism. *J Clin Endocrinol Metab* 1985; **61**: 873–80.

30 Wils RA, Umstsot EA, Andersen RN *et al.* Androgen parameters and their correlation with body weight in 138 women thought to have hyperandrogenism. *Am J Obstet Gynecol* 1983; **146**: 602–10.

Cutaneous virilism

Alterations in the cutaneous sensitivity to androgens is the reason cited for the existence of hirsuties in the presence of normal serum androgens and the lack of hirsuties in women with raised androgens. However, there has been no systematic study of hyperandrogenized non-hirsute women to determine whether or not they have other cutaneous features of androgen excess. The skin is a complex structure containing many different tissues and it is now recognized that most of the structures within the skin are modified by androgens. The eccrine and sebaceous glands are more active and the skin is thicker and contains more collagen in men than in women [1]. Inflammation of the apocrine glands in hidradenitis suppurativa is associated with hyperandrogenism [2], as is occlusion of the follicular duct both in vellus and terminal hairs [3]. It is possible, therefore, that the skin of non-hirsute hyperandrogenized women does respond to androgens, but not by the development of terminal hairs.

Shuster [1] has proposed a primary role for the skin. He suggested that in some individuals, the genetically determined level of cutaneous enzymes is sufficient to produce a negative feedback on the ovaries and adrenals and so enhance androgen production; he offered no evidence to support this hypothesis. However, studies by Toscano *et al.* [4] have provided data for a primary increase in cutaneous androgen metabolism. They noted that the only androgen abnormality in women who have a very short history of hirsuties (less than 1 year) is an increase in the cutaneous androgen products (dihydrotestosterone (DHT) and 3α-androstanediol). The metabolic activity of skin in hirsuties is increased both in direct incubation assays of skin and by measurements *in vivo* of, for example, 3α-androstanediol glucuronide. Whole skin homogenates from genital [5] and pubic skin of hirsute women have been demonstrated to express increased conversion of testosterone to DHT. However, isolated hair follicles from hirsute women do not appear to have different enzyme activities from controls [6]. As the pilosebaceous units contain considerable androgen metabolizing ability, the increased conversion of testosterone by whole skin homogenates may merely reflect the increased mass of pilosebaceous tissue in hirsute women.

3α-Androstanediol glucuronide has been proposed to be a specific marker of cutaneous androgen metabolism; early studies suggested that it was raised only in hirsute women with polycystic ovaries but not in controls or non-hirsute women with polycystic ovaries; there has been little confirmatory work and a recent study has cast doubt on its infallibility [7].

Hirsute women have a number of metabolic and systemic abnormalities, which suggest that hirsuties is not only a cosmetic disability but may have a more serious prognosis. Hirsute women have body shapes that tend towards the male form [8] and with this, they have altered lipid profiles that would suggest an increased risk of cardiovascular disease [9]. A relationship between diabetes and hyperandrogenism in women or 'diabetes of bearded women' has been recognized for many years [10]. However, it has now been established that the disordered carbohydrate metabolism is due to insulin resistance (IR). Furthermore, acanthosis nigricans (AN) acts as a cutaneous marker for the IR. The combination of AN and IR occurs in 5% of women with hyperandrogenism (HA) [11] and in 7% of women presenting with hirsuties [12]. Women with HAIR-AN have marked features of virilism, namely muscular physique, acne, alopecia and hidradenitis suppurativa [12].

Insulin may have an important role in the pathogenesis of hyperandrogenism. Studies *in vitro* have demonstrated that insulin exerts a stimulatory effect on ovarian androgen production and that it inhibits the synthesis of SHBG by the liver [13]. Its mode of action may be through the receptors for insulin-like growth factors, which are present both in the ovaries and in the skin. Stimulation of the latter may result in AN. It is, however, unknown whether the hyperinsulinaemia and insulin resistance are primary or secondary.

REFERENCES

1 Shuster S. The sebaceous glands and primary cutaneous virilism. In: Jeffcoate SL, ed. *Androgens and Anti-androgen Therapy*. Chichester: John Wiley and Sons, 1982: 1.

2 Mortimer PS, Dawber RPR, Gales MA *et al.* Mediation of hidradenitis suppurativa by androgens. *Br Med J* 1986; **292**: 245–9.

3 Barth JH, Wojnarowska F, Dawber RPR. Is keratosis pilaris another androgen-dependent dermatosis? *Clin Exp Dermatol* 1988; **13**: 240–4.

4 Toscano V, Adamo MV, Caiola S *et al.* Is hirsutism an evolving syndrome? *J Endocrinol* 1983; **97**: 379–87.

5 Serafini P, Lobo RA. Increased 5-alpha-reductase activity in idiopathic hirsutism. *Fertil Steril* 1985; **43**: 74–8.

6 Glickman SP, Rosenfield RL. Androgen metabolism by isolated hairs from women with idiopathic hirsutism is usually normal. *J Invest Dermatol* 1984; **82**: 62–9.

7 Scanlon MJ, Whorwood CB, Franks S *et al*. Serum androstanediol glucuronide in normal hirsute women and patients with thyroid dysfunction. *Clin Endocrinol* 1988; **29**: 529–34.
8 Evans DJ, Barth JH, Burke CW. Body fat topography in women with androgen excess. *Int J Obesity* 1988; **12**: 157–62.
9 Hauner H, Ditschuneit SB, Pal SB *et al*. Fat distribution, endocrine and metabolic profile in obese women with and without hirsuties. *Metabolism* 1988; **37**: 281–6.
10 Achard C, Thiers S. Insuffisance glycolytique associée au virilisme pilaire (diabète des femmes à barbe). *Bull Acad Nat Méd* 1921; **cxxxvi**: 58–63.
11 Flier JS, Eastman RC, Minaker KL *et al*. Acanthosis nigricans in obese women with hyperandrogenism: characterization of an insulin-resistant state distinct from the type A and B syndromes. *Diabetes* 1985; **34**: 101–5.
12 Barth JH, Wojnarowska F, Dawber RPR. Acanthosis nigricans, insulin resistance and cutaneous virilism. *Br J Dermatol* 1988; **118**: 613–20.
13 Plymate SR, Matej LA, Jones RE *et al*. Inhibition of sex hormone-binding globulin production in the human hepatoma (Hep G2) cell line by insulin and prolactin. *J Clin Endocrinol Metab* 1988; **67**: 460–7.

Diagnostic approach to the hirsute woman

Most hirsute women have probably been aware of excess hair since puberty; some will give a shorter history but it will be in the order of years. Some women are so good at cosmetic procedures that they do not appear hirsute at all. It is important to obtain facts from the history regarding patterns of hirsuties and alopecia or other features of cutaneous virilism and evidence for PCOS, for example, irregular menses or infertility. A family history of childhood dehydration or precocious puberty in a brother might be a feature of CAH. A drug history may point to an ingested source of androgens, for example glucocorticoid or anabolic steroids, and those used to enhance athletic performance. The progestogenic components of many contraceptive preparations are relatively androgenic and this is often cited as a cause of hirsuties, but this has not been a relevant factor in our experience.

The cutaneous examination will include the pattern and severity of hair growth and the associated presence of acne, androgenetic alopecia and acanthosis nigricans. Features suggestive of systemic virilization will include a deepening of the voice, increased muscle bulk and loss of the smooth skin contours, hypertension, striae distensae and cliteromegaly. Cliteromegaly is probably the most important physical sign pointing towards systemic virilization. The implication of systemic virilization, especially where there is a short history (for example, less than 1 year) is that there is a tumour causing it, which is quite different from 'cutaneous virilism'.

The extent to which it is necessary for hirsute women to be investigated is debatable. The main reason for the depth of investigation of hirsute women is the inability to differentiate between idiopathic hirsuties, PCOS and CAH on clinical grounds, and it is out of this quagmire that the standard of overinvestigation has arisen. The therapeutic tools available at present are too clumsy to warrant such diagnostic definition [1,2].

REFERENCES

1 Crosignani PG, Rubin B. Strategies for the treatment of hirsutism. *Hormone Res* 1989; **4**: 651–9.
2 Marshburn PB, Carr BR. Hirsutism and virilization: a systematic approach to benign and potentially serious causes. *Postgrad Med* 1995; **97**: 99–106.

Therapy

Most women will be satisfied with the assurance that they are not 'turning into men' and may not require any medical help or may only need advice about local destructive measures; however, many women will already have tried these methods.

Cosmetic measures

The easiest measure is to bleach the hair with hydrogen peroxide. This produces a yellow hue due to the native colour of keratin and may be as unacceptable as the original colour. Hair plucking is widely performed, but the act of plucking not only removes the hair shaft but also stimulates the root into the anagen phase and there is only a brief delay while the shaft grows through the epidermis. Shaving avoids this problem by removing all the hairs but is followed by growth only of the hairs that were previously in anagen.

Waxing is performed by the application of a sheet of soft wax onto the skin and, as soon as it has hardened with the hair shafts embedded, it is abruptly peeled off the skin, removing all the shafts. This is a painful method and is often complicated by folliculitis. Certain natural sugars, long used in parts of the Middle East, are becoming popular in place of waxes as they appear to depilate as effectively, but with less trauma.

Electrolysis is the only permanent method for removal of hair [1]. A fine electrical wire is introduced down the hair shaft to the papilla which is destroyed by an electrical current. Laser thermolytic hair removal is now widely used, but its long-term efficacy is not yet known [2].

Systemic antiandrogen therapy

Because hirsuties is a condition mediated by androgens, attempts have been made to ameliorate the growth of hair with drugs with antiandrogenic properties. The complete spectrum of therapeutic agents evaluated in the treatment of hirsuties is described in the following text. It is, however, our practice to use cyproterone acetate as first-line therapy for those women whose hirsuties is so severe as to warrant systemic therapy.

It is important that hirsute women are carefully selected prior to initiating therapy for the following reasons. First, the effect on hair growth takes several months to become apparent and only partial improvement may be expected.

Second, antiandrogens feminize male fetuses and it is essential that the women do not become pregnant. Third, these drugs only have a suppressive, and not curative, effect that wears off a few months after cessation of therapy, and therapy may need to be taken indefinitely if a favourable improvement occurs. Finally, the long-term safety of these drugs is unknown and tumours in laboratory animals have been reported with several of the following agents.

Cyproterone acetate [3,4]. Cyproterone acetate (CPA) is both an antiandrogen and an inhibitor of gonadotrophin secretion. It reduces androgen production, increases the metabolic clearance of testosterone and binds to the androgen receptor; in addition, long-term therapy is associated with a reduction in the activity of cutaneous 5α-reductase. Cyproterone acetate is a potent progestogen but does not reliably inhibit ovulation. It is usually administered with cyclical oestrogens in order to maintain regular menstruation and to prevent conception in view of the risk of feminizing a male fetus.

Several dose regimens have been advocated. Low-dose therapy (Dianette; Schering AG) is an oral contraceptive containing 35 μg ethinyl oestradiol and 2 mg CPA, taken daily for 21 days in every 28. However, many of the dose-ranging and efficacy studies have been performed using the preparation which contained 50 μg ethinyl oestradiol; this may be relevant, as only the higher dose of oestrogen increases SHBG. Current dosage recommendations for CPA usually advise that 50 mg or 100 mg CPA should be administered for 10 days/cycle. However, there have now been many dose-ranging studies which suggest that there is no dose effect. Objective studies comparing Dianette with and without extra CPA found no difference, either in the reduction of the overall hirsuties grades or in the reduction in hair-shaft diameters [5].

Side-effects of CPA include weight gain, fatigue, loss of libido, mastodynia, nausea, headaches and depression. All these side-effects are more frequent with a higher dose. Contraindications to its use are the same as for the contraceptive pill and include cigarette smoking, age, obesity and hypertension.

Spironolactone [6,7]. Spironolactone has several anti-androgenic pharmacological properties. It reduces the bioavailability of testosterone by interfering with its production and increases its metabolic clearance. It binds to the androgen receptor and, like cyproterone acetate, long-term therapy is associated with a reduction in cutaneous 5α-reductase activity [8]. It was an act of serendipity that demonstrated its therapeutic advantage in hirsuties. A 19-year-old hirsute woman with PCOS was treated with spironolactone (200 mg/day) for concurrent hypertension and she noted after 3 months that she needed to shave less frequently. This report was soon followed by studies demonstrating that spironolactone reduced testosterone production and subjectively reduced hair growth in hirsute women. Different dose schedules of spironolactone have been studied, varying between 50 and 200 mg taken either daily or cyclically (daily for 3 weeks in every 4). Within this dose range, the one chosen will depend on the severity of the hirsuties.

There have been no formal clinical trials between the two treatments, but comparative reports claim that both agents are equally effective; Rubens and Vermeulen [9] reported that 50 mg cyproterone acetate given in the reverse sequential regimen is similar to spironolactone (100 mg/day). It is not known whether the two agents have an additive effect.

Spironolactone may feminize a male fetus. Long-term, high-dose spironolactone has been shown to produce tumours in rodents. Some clinicians feel that this finding makes long-term use inappropriate in healthy young patients with hirsutism.

5α-reductase inhibitors. 5α-reductase inhibitors are a potential systemic therapy for hirsutism. Finasteride inhibits the type 2 isoenzyme and has been assessed in small placebo-controlled trials with promising results after 6 months therapy [10]. Other similar drugs are likely to be available in the near future. This group of drugs feminizes a male fetus, which is a drawback in the therapy of women of child-bearing potential.

Corticosteroids. These are first-line therapy for congenital adrenal hyperplasia and were the first endocrine therapy to be employed in the treatment of hirsuties with the rationale of suppressing the production of adrenal androgens. Corticosteroids are effective in reducing plasma androgen levels but there are contradictory reports regarding their therapeutic effect on hair growth [11].

Medroxyprogesterone acetate. Medroxyprogesterone acetate (MPA) is a synthetic progestogen, which was introduced as an anovulatory agent due to its ability to block gonadotrophin secretion. It reduces androgen levels by reducing the production of testosterone and increasing its metabolic clearance.

A comparison of a topical (0.2% ointment) with systemic therapy either by intramuscular injection of MPA (150 mg every 6 weeks) or subcutaneous injection (100 mg every 6 weeks) was said to give a beneficial response in most patients [12]. MPA given alone may result in menorrhagia.

Desogestrel. This is the progestogen used in the Marvelon contraceptive pill (Organon Ltd), which contains 30 μg ethinyl oestradiol and 150 mg desogestrel. All the studies undertaken have reported subjective and/or objective reductions in hair growth of 20–25% after 6–9 months' therapy, with a high degree of patient satisfaction [13].

Ketoconazole. This is a potent inhibitor of adrenal and ovarian steroid synthesis. There have been only isolated reports of its use in hirsuties but these have demonstrated a marked reduction in hair growth after 6 months [14]. This treatment cannot be recommended in view of the risks of hepatic toxicity during long-term therapy.

Flutamide [15]. This acts as a pure antiandrogen and works by binding to androgen receptors. However, it has no antigonadotrophic effect, and the result of binding to central androgen receptors is that it prevents the negative feedback effect of testosterone and consequently androgen levels rise. There has been a single study in hirsuties in which flutamide (250 mg twice a day) was administered with an oral contraceptive for 7 months; 12 out of 13 patients demonstrated a subjective improvement in hair growth and acne [16].

Gonadotrophin-releasing hormone agonists. Gonadotrophin-releasing hormone (GnRH) agonists inhibit LH production and this results in profound suppression of androgen production. These agents are presently under investigation, but preliminary studies suggest that they effectively reduce hair growth and acne in women with PCOS [17].

Cimetidine. This is a weak antiandrogen as indicated by androgen receptor-binding studies. A study of patients with idiopathic hirsuties demonstrated a marked reduction in hair growth using hair weight, whereas no such effect was seen in controls given only a placebo [18].

Bromocriptine. This is a dopamine agonist, and long-term therapy with bromocriptine regulates menstrual cycle length, but 12 months' therapy produced no measurable effect on linear hair growth in women with polycystic ovaries [19].

REFERENCES

1 Richards R, McKenzie MA, Meharg GE. Electroepilation in hirsutism. *J Am Acad Dermatol* 1986; **15**; 693–8.
2 Grossman MC, Dierickx C, Farinelli W *et al.* Damage to hair follicles by normal mode ruby laser pulses. *J Am Acad Dermatol* 1996; **35**: 889–94.
3 Jones DB, Ibraham I, Edwards CRW. Hair growth and androgen responses in hirsute women treated with continuous cyproterone acetate and cyclical ethinyl oestradiol. *Acta Endocrinol* 1987; **116**: 497–503.
4 Jones KR, Katz M, Keyzer C *et al.* Effect of cyproterone acetate on rate of hair growth in hirsute females. *Br J Dermatol* 1981; **105**: 685–91.
5 Barth JH, Cherry CA, Wojnarowska F *et al.* Cyproterone acetate for severe hirsutism; results of a double-blind dose-ranging study. *J Clin Endocrinol Metab* 1991; **35**: 5–10.
6 Barth JH, Cherry CA, Wojnarowska F *et al.* Spironolactone is an effective and well tolerated systemic anti-androgen therapy for hirsute women. *J Clin Endocrinol Metab* 1989; **68**: 96–102.
7 Ober KP, Hennessy JF. Spironolactone therapy for hirsutism in a hyperandrogenic woman. *Ann Intern Med* 1987; **98**: 643–51.
8 Serafini P, Catalino J, Lobo RA. The effect of spironolactone on genital skin 5α-reductase. *J Steroid Biochem* 1985; **23**: 191.
9 Rubens R, Vermeulen A. Clinical assessment of two antiandrogen treatments, cyproterone acetate combined with ethinyl estradiol and spironolactone in hirsutism. In: Schindler AE, ed. *New Developments in Biosciences 3*. Berlin: de Gruyter, 1987: 133–40.
10 Tolino A, Petrone A, Sarnacchiaro F *et al.* Finasteride in the treatment of hirsutism: new therapeutic perspectives. *Fertil Steril* 1996; **66**: 61–5.
11 Rittmaster RS, Givner ML. Effect of daily and alternate day low dose prednisolone on serum cortisol and adrenal androgens in hirsute women. *J Clin Endocrinol Metab* 1988; **67**: 400–6.
12 Schmidt JB, Huber J, Spona J. Medroxyprogesterone acetate therapy in hirsutism. *Br J Dermatol* 1985; **113**: 161–6.
13 Ruutianen K. The effect of an oral contraceptive containing ethinyl-estradiol and desogestrel on hair growth and hormonal parameters of hirsute women. *Int J Gynaecol Obstet* 1986; **24**: 361–70.
14 Martikainen H, Heikkinen J, Ruokonen A *et al.* Hormonal and clinical effects of ketoconazole in hirsute women. *J Clin Endocrinol Metab* 1988; **66**: 987–94.
15 Erenus M, Gurbuz O, Durmusoglu E. Comparison of the efficacy of spironolactone versus flutamide in the treatment of hirsutism. *Fertil Steril* 1994; **61**: 613–16.
16 Cusan L, Dupont A, Tremblay R *et al.* Treatment of hirsutism with the pure antiandrogen flutamide. *Proc Int Soc Gynaecol Endocrinol* 1988: 74–95.
17 Rittmaster RS. Differential suppression of testosterone and estradiol in hirsute women with the superactive gonadotrophin-releasing hormone agonist leuprolide. *J Clin Endocrinol Metab* 1988; **67**: 651–6.
18 Grandesso R, Spandri P, Gangemi M *et al.* Hormonal changes and hair growth during treatment of hirsutism with cimetidine. *Clin Exp Obstet Gynaecol* 1984; **11**: 105–10.
19 Murdoch AP, McClean KG, Watson MJ *et al.* Treatment of hirsutism in polycystic ovary syndrome with bromocriptine. *Br J Obstet Gynaecol* 1987; **94**: 358–67.

Alopecia

Androgenetic alopecia

SYN. COMMON BALDNESS; MALE-PATTERN ALOPECIA

Nomenclature. Androgenetic alopecia is widely referred to as male-pattern alopecia, but this term is too restrictive and leads to missed diagnoses, especially in females [1].

Aetiology. The human is not the only primate species in which baldness is a natural phenomenon associated with sexual maturity. The orangutan and the chimpanzee both show some degree of baldness when they reach maturity. Other species showing this phenomenon include the uakari and the stump-tailed macaque. Studies in these animals have demonstrated clearly that androgenetic alopecia is a physiological process in genetically predisposed individuals whether simian or human. Terminal follicles are progressively transformed into 'vellus' follicles, i.e. a 'miniaturization' process.

The prevalence of androgenetic alopecia in any population has not been accurately recorded, but it probably approaches 100% in the Caucasoid races. In other words, the replacement of some terminal follicles by vellus-type follicles from puberty onwards is a universal phenomenon.

Hair patterns [2]. Hamilton [3] produced the first useful grading scale after examining 312 white males and 214 white females aged 20–89 years (Fig. 66.23). This classification was modified by Norwood [4] who added grades IIIa, III vertex, IVa and Va to the Hamilton scale. The Norwood

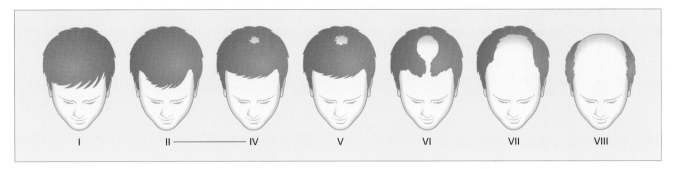

Fig. 66.23 Hamilton classification of androgenetic alopecia (types II–IV overlap).

scoring system has been used extensively in clinical trials of regrowth, particularly with regard to topical minoxidil.

Hamilton described the natural progression of the normal prepubertal scalp pattern (type I) in both sexes to type II in 96% of men and 79% of women after puberty. He also observed patterns type V and VIII (Fig. 66.24) in 58% of men aged over 50 years, with the extent of baldness tending to increase to the age of 70 years. About 25% of women developed type IV scalps by the age of 50 years, after which there was no further increase in balding. Indeed, after 50, some women who had developed type II

at puberty, revert to type I. Types V to VIII were not found in any women.

Although, as these figures show, androgenetic alopecia occurs in women with some frequency, it more often assumes a diffuse form [5] (Figs 66.25 & 66.26).

Venning and Dawber [6] have shown a change of patterning in 100% of 564 women over 20 years old. In this study, these workers carefully wetted the vaultal hair and observed from above. They analysed their patients by decade and found that 87% of premenopausal women showed vaultal thinning of the Ludwig pattern I–III and 13% had Hamilton type II–IV. Postmenopausal women showed an increased tendency to the male patterning, with 63% of Ludwig I–III and 37% of Hamilton II–V, including some women with deep M-shaped bitemporal frontoparietal recession.

Other observations, much less accurately recorded, tended to group together Hamilton's types II, III and IV, and are therefore of interest only in confirming the great frequency of androgenetic alopecia in other populations of Caucasoids.

It has been suggested that separating hair patterns into the eight Hamilton and three Ludwig types is only of use in defining a population for the purpose of clinical trial evaluation. The grades are imprecise measures of a continuum of hair patterns that are seen in adults of both sexes. The single consistent finding is a change from the prepubertal pattern in all adults. The magnitude and rate of that change are influenced by genetic predisposition and by sex hormone levels in both sexes [6].

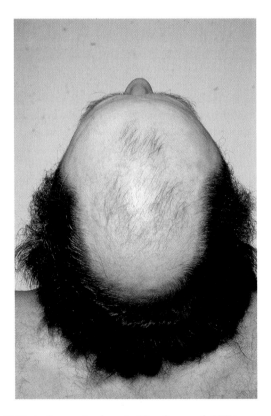

Fig. 66.24 Androgenetic alopecia. Hamilton grade VIII in a normal man.

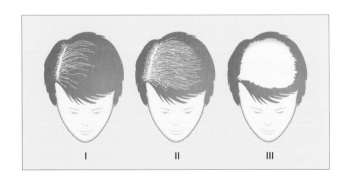

Fig. 66.25 Androgenetic alopecia. Ludwig grades, most typically seen in women.

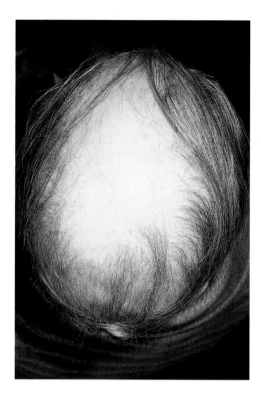

Fig. 66.26 Androgenetic alopecia. Ludwig grade III in a normal postmenopausal woman.

Inheritance. The very high frequency of androgenetic alopecia has complicated the many attempts to establish its mode of inheritance. Moreover, it is by no means clear that androgenetic alopecia is genetically homogeneous, and some authorities differentiate between early onset (before the age of 30 years in men) and the same pattern 20 years later. Some think that it is determined by a single pair of sex-influenced factors. Both gene frequency studies and family histories support this hypothesis.

In a small study of first-degree relatives of 56 women with androgenetic alopecia, Smith and Wells [7] showed that 54% of males and 25% of females over the age of 30 years were similarly affected. These authors considered that baldness could apparently develop in the heterozygous female, and they postulated that this resulted from dominant inheritance with increased penetrance in the male, or by multifactorial inheritance. The concept of multifactorial inheritance was supported by Šalamon [8], although the question remains unanswered. It is still unclear whether early and late-onset androgenetic alopecia are inherited separately. It is nevertheless certain that both are inherited and that both depend upon androgenic stimulation of susceptible follicles. In a search for a biochemical marker of baldness, Hodgins *et al.* [9] plucked scalp hair follicles from young adults not yet expressing baldness but with a strong family history of androgenetic alopecia and found two populations, one with high 17β-

hydroxysteroid activity and one with low enzyme activity. Low enzyme activity seemed to be related to retention of hair and a family history of hair retention. Extension of this type of work is essential to arrive at a precise definition of the mode of inheritance.

There is no association between androgenetic alopecia and dense hair patterns on the trunk and limbs [10]; nor is there an association between hair loss and increased fertility [11].

REFERENCES

1 Simpson NB, Barth J. Hair patterns: hirsuties and androgenetic alopecia. In: Dawber RPR, ed. *Diseases of the Hair and Scalp*, 3rd edn. Oxford: Blackwell Science, 1997: 177–88.
2 Olsen E. Androgenetic alopecia. In: Olsen E, ed. *Disorders of Hair Growth*. New York: McGraw-Hill, 1994: 257–84.
3 Hamilton JB. Patterned long hair in man; types and incidence. *Ann NY Acad Sci* 1951; **53**: 708–14.
4 Norwood O'TT. Male pattern baldness. Classification and incidence. *South Med J* 1975; **68**: 1359–70.
5 Ludwig E. Classification of the types of androgenic alopecia (common baldness) arising in the female sex. *Br J Dermatol* 1977; **97**: 249–56.
6 Venning VA, Dawber R. Patterned androgenic alopecia. *J Am Acad Dermatol* 1988; **18**: 1073–8.
7 Smith MA, Wells RS. Male type alopecia, alopecia areata and normal hair in women. *Arch Dermatol* 1964; **89**: 95–101.
8 Šalamon T. Genetic factors in male pattern alopecia. In: Baccaredda-Boy A, Moretti G, Frey JR, eds. *Biopathology of Pattern Alopecia*. Basle: Karger, 1968: 39–56.
9 Hodgins MB, Murad S, Simpson NB. A search for variation in hair follicle androgen metabolism which might be linked to male pattern baldness. *Br J Dermatol* 1985; **113**: 794–5.
10 Burton JL, Ben Halim MM, Meyrick G. Male pattern alopecia and masculinity. *Br J Dermatol* 1979; **100**: 507–12.
11 Damon A, Burr WA, Gerson DE. Baldness, fertility and number and sex ratio of children. *Hum Biol* 1965; **37**: 366–74.

Pathology [1]. The earliest histological change is focal perivascular basophilic degeneration in the lower third of the connective tissue sheath of otherwise normal anagen follicles. This is followed by a perifollicular lympho-histiocytic infiltrate at the level of the sebaceous duct. The basophilic sclerotic remains of the connective tissue sheath can be seen in the process as 'streamers' [1]. The destruction of the connective tissue sheath may account for the irreversibility of hair loss. In about a third of biopsies, multinucleate giant cells are seen surrounding fragments of hair [2]. The erector pili muscle decreases in size more slowly than the follicle [3]. In the scalp that appears totally bald, most of the follicles are short and small, with some quiescent terminal follicles.

As the balding scalp loses its protective covering of hair, so solar degenerative changes may be seen. The reduction of blood supply has been confirmed by modern methods [4], but whether it follows or precedes the hair loss is unknown.

The development of baldness is associated with shortening of the anagen phase of the hair cycle and consequently with an increase in the proportion of telogen hairs, which may be detected in trichograms of the frontovertical region before baldness is evident [5].

The reduction in the size of the affected follicles, which is the essential histological feature of androgenetic alopecia, necessarily results in a reduction in the diameter of the hairs they produce. This reduction is said to be greater in women than in men [6]. Balding patients showed a wide spread of hair-shaft diameters, with peaks at 0.04 mm and 0.06 mm, whereas non-bald subjects showed a symmetrical distribution with a single peak at 0.08 mm.

REFERENCES

1 Kligman AM. The comparative histopathology of male-pattern baldness and senescent baldness. In: De Villez RL, ed. *Clinics in Dermatology*, Vol. 6, No. 4. Philadelphia: Lippincott, 1988: 108–13.
2 Domnitz JM, Silvers DN. Giant cells in male pattern alopecia—a histological marker and pathogenic clue. *J Cutan Pathol* 1979; **6**: 108–13.
3 Maguire HC, Kligman AM. The histopathology of common male baldness. *Proc XII Int Congr Dermatol*, Washington, 1962: 1438–41.
4 Klemp P, Peters K, Hansted B. Subcutaneous blood flow in early male pattern baldness. *J Invest Dermatol* 1989; **92**: 725–30.
5 Vogelsberg H, Klarner W, Rupec M. Einige Beobachtungen zur Frage der androgenetischen Alopezie der Frau. *Zeitschr Hautkrank* 1980; **55**: 125–30.
6 Jackson D, Church RE, Ebling FJ. Hair diameter in female baldness. *Br J Dermatol* 1972; **87**: 361–7.

Pathogenesis. Any unifying hypothesis for androgenetic alopecia has to explain all of the following: the occurrence in humans and simian species; strong autosomal inheritance; the involvement of both sexes; geographical patterning of hair loss on the scalp, and the coexistence of greasy skin, acne and hirsutism in some women.

Hamilton [1] showed that baldness did not develop in 10 eunuchoids, 10 men castrated at puberty and 34 men castrated during adolescence. Following administration of testosterone, baldness developed in those who were genetically predisposed; when testosterone was discontinued the baldness did not progress, although it did not reverse. In further studies, Hamilton [2] showed that the time interval between puberty and castration was crucial to the development of the beard in males. Castration before puberty prevented the development of a beard, between 16 and 20 years of age it partially prevented the full development of a beard, and after the age of 20 years it had no effect on beard development. Testosterone administration at any stage following castration allowed full growth of beard. Very high doses of testosterone caused some virilization, with beard growth [3], but there is no record of change in scalp hair pattern. It appears that the magnitude of the response of hair to androgens may be set permanently by modification of gene expression following puberty.

The discovery of the importance of exposure to androgen in the pathogenesis of baldness led to claims for increased sexuality and androgens in balding males. Scientific support for this fanciful hypothesis is lacking. Pitts [4] found elevated serum dehydroepiandrosterone sulphate but normal testosterone levels in 18 balding males

compared with non-balding controls. The improvement in technology and the ability to measure free and bound androgens has shown that normal male levels of androgen are sufficient to make manifest the degree of baldness determined genetically for the individual. The situation in women is different, and it has become apparent that the degree of baldness may, in part, be related to circulating androgen levels [5–7]. In addition, up to 48% of women presenting to an endocrine clinic with diffuse vaultal alopecia had evidence of polycystic ovarian disease [8].

All adult women show a change from the prepubertal hair pattern [9]. The maximum change in hair pattern occurs after the menopause, when oestrogen levels decline and a more 'androgenic' environment exists. Androgens, in the normal female range, induce baldness only in premenopausal women with a strong genetic predisposition. In women with a less strong genetic predisposition, baldness develops only when androgen production is increased or drugs with androgen-like activity are taken, such as some progestogens in the oral contraceptive. In some women, even grossly abnormal levels of androgen cause no clinically significant baldness, although all such patients are necessarily hirsute.

The association of seborrhoea and androgenetic alopecia led to some erroneous theories in the 19th century. The 'seborrhoea' probably has more to do with the refatting kinetics of fine hair than with any change in sebaceous gland activity except in a few women. During the course of androgenetic alopecia, the total number of sebaceous glands decreases significantly.

Sebaceous glands are under androgenic control and in men seem to be under maximal stimulation from normal circulating androgen levels. In women, however, increased sebum production occurs following a small increase in circulating androgens. It is not surprising, therefore, that many young women with higher grades of baldness, who have demonstrable abnormalities in circulating androgens, also have greasier skin. Maibach *et al.* [10] found no differences in the casual level or hourly production of sebum on the bald or hairy scalp of balding men and the scalp of fully haired subjects.

The weight of evidence strongly supports the opinion that the essential inherited factor responsible for androgenetic alopecia concerns the manner in which certain follicles in the frontovertical region of the scalp react to androgens. The ability of the pilosebaceous unit to metabolize a wide range of androgens has been established beyond doubt [11,12]. The enzyme 5α-reductase plays an important part in this process, converting testosterone to dihydrotestosterone (DHT). Adult males with a genetically determined deficiency of 5α-reductase demonstrate normal circulating levels of testosterone but reduced DHT. Phenotypically, they lack any tendency to androgenetic alopecia and have sparse facial and body hair [13].

There are two isoenzymes of 5α-reductase, and type 2 is lacking in congenital 5α-reductase deficiency. Paradoxically, type 1 appears more widely distributed in the skin and hair follicles. Immunohistochemistry reveals type 1 5α-reductase in the dermal papilla, outer root sheath and sebaceous glands of the hair follicle, and basal layer of the epidermis. Type 2 5α-reductase is found predominantly in the prostate, but antibodies to the type 2 enzyme stain the inner root sheath of the hair follicle and sweat glands [14].

The type 2 isoenzyme is more widespread in the skin in infancy, at which stage it could play a conditioning role, programming follicles to respond to postpubertal androgens in a genetically determined manner [15].

These aspects of androgen metabolism are important in the light of new drugs capable of inhibiting both forms of 5α-reductase, thereby offering a new therapeutic avenue in androgenetic alopecia and hirsutism.

The interconversion of androgens within the pilo-sebaceous unit has also been discussed in Chapter 42. The same androgens are responsible for the seborrhoea of acne, the conversion of vellus to terminal hair in the beard, pubic area and axillae, and, paradoxically, the opposite effect on hair in the balding process in both sexes. Sebaceous gland androgen metabolism has been studied extensively, but even with the pilosebaceous unit we cannot with certainty extrapolate results from the sebaceous gland to the hair follicle or vice versa. The presence of androgen receptors has been established in sebocytes of the hamster flank organ but it has been much more difficult to localize androgen receptors or androgen metabolizing enzyme systems in the hair follicle. The presence of androgen receptors on dermal papillary cells in culture [16] and the ability of dermal papilla cells to metabolize a range of androgens [17] suggest that this area holds much promise for further investigation.

Differences in sebaceous gland 3β-hydroxysteroid dehydrogenase Δ^{4-5} isomerase activity between bald and non-bald scalps may be due to geographical influences in the balding areas or related to slight elevations of plasma dehydroepiandrosterone and dehydroepiandrosterone sulphate in some balding males [4].

If individual variation in androgen metabolism is linked causally to hair loss or retention it should be apparent in women and in young men before the onset of baldness. Hodgins *et al.* [18] have reported two populations of high- and low-activity variants of the enzyme 17β-hydroxysteroid dehydrogenase in plucked hair roots. Enzyme activity appeared to be linked to the presence or absence of a strong family history of baldness.

In androgenetic alopecia, therefore, a change occurs in genetically prone follicles following exposure to androgens at puberty. From this time, a 'genetic clock' is set running, which eventually leads the follicle to undergo cycles of decreasing length, producing finer and finer hair, until full

vellus change occurs (miniaturization). The genetic 'switch' would appear to be an irreversible process; however, the tendency for some follicles to appear to regrow during treatment with minoxidil and antiandrogens has cast some doubt on the irreversibility of androgenetic alopecia.

REFERENCES

1 Hamilton JB. Male hormone stimulation is a prerequisite and an incitement in common baldness. *Am J Anat* 1942; **71**: 451–60.
2 Hamilton JB. Age, sex and genetic factors in the regulation of hair growth in man; a comparison of Caucasian and Japanese populations. In: Montagna W, Ellis, RA, eds. *The Biology of Hair Growth.* New York: Academic Press, 1958: 399–413.
3 Price P, Wass JAH, Griffin JE *et al.* High dose androgen therapy in male pseudohermaphroditism due to 5α-reductase deficiency and disorders of the androgen receptor. *J Clin Invest* 1984; **74**: 1496–501.
4 Pitts RL. Serum elevation of dehydroepiandrosterone sulfate associated with male pattern baldness in young men. *J Am Acad Dermatol* 1987; **16**: 571–9.
5 De Villez RL, Dunn J. Female androgenic alopecia. The 3α,17β-androstanediol glucuronide/sex hormone binding globulin ratio as a possible marker for female pattern baldness. *Arch Dermatol* 1986; **122**: 1011–14.
6 Miller JA, Darley CR, Karkavitas K *et al.* Low sex-hormone binding globulin levels in young women with diffuse hair loss. *Br J Dermatol* 1982; **106**: 331–5.
7 Moltz L. Hormonale Diagnostik der sogenannten androgenetischen Alopezie der Frau. *Geburts Frauenheil* 1988; **48**: 203–6.
8 Futteweit W, Dunif A, Yeh HC *et al.* The prevalence of hyperandrogenism in 109 consecutive female patients with diffuse alopecia. *J Am Acad Dermatol* 1988; **19**: 831–7.
9 Venning VA, Dawber R. Patterned androgenic alopecia. *J Am Acad Dermatol* 1988; **18**: 1073–8.
10 Maibach HI, Feldman R, Payne B *et al.* Scalp and forehead sebum production in male pattern alopecia. In: Baccaredda-Boy A, Moretti G, Frey JR, eds. *Biopathology of Pattern Alopecia.* Basle: Karger, 1968: 171–90.
11 Fazekas AG, Sandor T. The metabolism of dehydroepiandrosterone by human scalp hair follicles. *J Clin Endocrinol* 1973; **36**: 582–7.
12 Hay JB, Hodgins MB. Distribution of androgen metabolism enzymes in isolated tissues of human forehead and axillary skin. *J Endocrinol* 1978; **79**: 29–35.
13 Imperato-McGinley J, Guerrero L, Gautier T *et al.* Steroid 5α-reductase deficiency in man: an inherited form of male pseudohermaphroditism. *Science* 1974; **186**: 1213–15.
14 Eicheler W, Dreher M, Hoffman R *et al.* Immunohistochemical evidence for differential distribution of 5 alpha-reductase isoenzyme in human skin. *Br J Dermatol* 1995; **113**: 371–6.
15 Kaufman KD. Androgen metabolism as it affects hair growth in androgenetic alopecia. *Dermatol Clin* 1996; **14**: 697–711.
16 Messenger AG, Thornton MJ, Elliott K *et al.* Androgen responses in cultured human hair papilla cells. *J Invest Dermatol* 1988; **91**: 382–3.
17 Murad S, Hodgins MB, Simpson NB *et al.* Androgen receptors and metabolism in cultured dermal papilla cells from human hair follicles. *Br J Dermatol* 1986; **113**: 768–9.
18 Hodgins MB, Murad S, Simpson NB. A search for variation in hair follicle androgen metabolism which might be linked to male pattern baldness. *Br J Dermatol* 1985; **113**: 794.

Clinical features. The essential clinical feature of androgenetic alopecia in both sexes is the replacement of terminal hairs by progressively finer hairs, which are eventually short and virtually unpigmented. This process may begin at any age after puberty and may become clinically apparent by the age of 17 years in the normal male and by 25–30 years in the endocrinologically normal female. The reduction in the size of the follicles is accompanied by shortening of anagen and by increased shedding of telogen hairs. Miniaturized hairs become increasingly evident, replacing coarser intermediate or terminal hairs.

Males. The replacement of terminal by smaller hairs occurs characteristically in a distinctive pattern, which spares the posterior and lateral scalp margins, even in the most advanced cases, and even in old age. The sequence of patterns in the male has been described by Hamilton (see Figs 66.23 & 66.24). Bitemporal recession is followed by balding of the vertex. Variations in the pattern are governed at least in part by genetic factors. The rate of progression is probably determined by heredity.

Females. The use of the term male-pattern alopecia must be held partly responsible for the frequent failure to appreciate that in its earlier stages androgenetic alopecia in women need not conform to the 'male pattern' (Figs 66.25 & 66.26). As in the male, increased shedding of telogen hairs accompanies the reduction of shaft diameter, but the follicles first affected are more widely distributed over the frontovertical region. As a result, many secondary vellus hairs are interspersed with hairs which are still normal and others only slightly reduced in diameter. Partial baldness is sometimes first apparent on the vertex, but the most frequent presentation of androgenetic alopecia in women is as a diffuse alopecia [1]. Ludwig [2] has classified the succession of patterns which occur in women to produce the distinctive clinical features of 'female pattern alopecia'. However, Venning and Dawber [3] have shown that all women display a change of scalp hair pattern after puberty. The rate of change of patterning is very slow but accelerates during and after the menopause. These workers also showed that hair patterns of the classical 'male type' shown by Hamilton (see Figs 66.23 & 66.24) occur with increasing frequency after the menopause. The occurrence of Ludwig pattern III or Hamilton pattern V or greater in a premenopausal woman is unlikely [4]. Androgens also stimulate sebaceous gland activity. A full medical history and examination are essential, and in many cases endocrinological investigation is desirable in all women with androgenetic alopecia of rapid onset, even if it be an isolated abnormality, and in women with baldness of gradual onset but accompanied by menstrual disturbance, hirsutism or recrudescence of acne. Hair loss of Hamilton type IV may occur in women without hirsutism but more extensive baldness (types VI–VII) is always accompanied by hirsutism.

Whiting [5] has described a pattern of diffuse hair loss in women often interpreted as androgenetic alopecia, but which may technically be a form of chronic telogen effluvium. Features include a history of sudden onset in a woman in her fourth to sixth decade. The amount of hair shed is often more impressive than the resultant alopecia, which is diffuse with mild thinning at the temples.

Histologically, although there may be a slight increase in telogen hairs, the major feature distinguishing the condition from androgenetic alopecia is the relative absence of vellus hairs in chronic telogen effluvium and their abundance in androgenetic alopecia. This is best demonstrated by performing horizontal sections of a 4-mm punch biopsy.

The condition may continue and fluctuate for years without progressive alopecia. In the absence of a precise cause, no specific treatment is advocated.

REFERENCES

1 Maguire HC, Kligman AM. Common baldness in women. *Geriatrics* 1963; **18**: 329–34.
2 Ludwig E. Classification of the types of androgenic alopecia (common baldness) occurring in the female sex. *Br J Dermatol* 1977; **97**: 247–54.
3 Venning VA, Dawber R. Patterned androgenic alopecia. *J Am Acad Dermatol* 1988; **18**: 1073–8.
4 Futterweit W, Dunif A, Yeh HC *et al*. The prevalence of hyperandrogenism in 109 consecutive female patients with diffuse alopecia. *J Am Acad Dermatol* 1988; **19**: 831–9.
5 Whiting DA. Chronic telogen effluvium. *Dermatol Clin* 1996; **14**: 723–32.

Therapy. There is now partially effective treatment that prevents further transformation of terminal into vellus hair for many women in whom the severity of baldness is the result of abnormal androgen metabolism. For those in whom the thinning or shedding is a major concern [1], inhibition of the process is possible with modern treatments.

Surgery. All surgical procedures are attempts to spread parietal and occipital hairs thinly over the rest of the scalp. Hair can be redistributed using autografts or flaps. Either can be performed in combination with reduction of the bald area by excision and closure. Grafts may be as large as a 4-mm punch biopsy, but better results are achieved with much smaller 'micrografts', which can be manipulated to produce a natural-looking frontal hair line. Rotation flaps from the parietal to the frontal area may give a better appearance [2]. Reduction of the bald area by removal of an ellipse from the vault or repeated such operations may cover the top of the head by stretching the remaining parietal scalp. Expansion techniques have been used successfully to restore post-traumatic alopecia and more recently for common baldness in men [3]. In theory, surgery is definitive, but it is often performed long before the ultimate pattern of hair loss is clear. This can produce a peculiar appearance after a few years, and further surgery may be required.

Wigs. In women, hair loss is usually too diffuse for transplantation surgery to be possible. If it is extensive, only a wig will conceal it. In addition, there are various procedures by which small wigs are interwoven with the pre-existing terminal hair, and the cosmetic result is sometimes satisfactory. The patient who seeks advice from a doctor before embarking on some such procedure should be assessed in the same way as a patient considering surgery, and the issue must be addressed as to whether baldness is really the problem.

Antiandrogens. The side-effects of antiandrogens in general preclude their use in men. In women, there is some scientific evidence for regrowth of hair with cyproterone acetate, but in general this drug, in doses of 50–100 mg/ day with ethinyl oestradiol, may be said to prevent further progression [4]. Burke and Cunliffe [5] reported subjective improvement with oral spironolactone, and Aram [6] claimed success with high-dose cimetidine, which also has antiandrogenic activity.

Oral type 2 5α-reductase inhibitors, which have specificity of action on the prostate and the vertex of the scalp, have given optimistic results in androgenetic alopecia in men. Longer-term studies are necessary before their use can be fully justified.

Non-hormonal therapy. Many therapies given systemically for other reasons may produce general hypertrichosis and concurrent improvement in androgenetic alopecia, i.e. benoxaprofen, cyclosporin A and PUVA, but these cannot be used as treatment. Only minoxidil has been shown to enhance regrowth significantly when used topically. Minoxidil is a piperidinopyrimidine derivative and a potent vasodilator which is effective orally for severe hypertension. When applied topically as a 2% solution in an alcohol and water base containing 10% propylene glycol, minoxidil has shown conversion of vellus to terminal hair in up to 30% of individuals [7,8]. Terminal hair appeared to regrow at the margins, but complete covering of the bald areas was seen in less than 10% of responders. De Villez [9] suggested that bald men who responded best to minoxidil were those in whom the balding process was at an early stage, with a maximum diameter of the bald area less than 10 cm and in whom the pretreatment hair density was in excess of 20 hairs/cm^2. There was an increasing dose response up to 2% minoxidil using the recommended 1 ml twice-daily regimen [10]. There is a slight increase in benefit if the concentration is increased to 5%. Minoxidil sulphate may be the active metabolite; following oral administration the skin demonstrates sulphates and sulphotransferase activity, but this aspect has yet to be fully explored scientifically.

Topical minoxidil appears to be a safe therapy with side-effects only of local irritation and a low incidence of contact dermatitis [11]. Clinical regression occurs, after 3 months, to the state of baldness that would have existed if treatment had not been applied [10]. Patients should be warned that in order to maintain any beneficial effect, applications must continue twice a day for the rest of their lives [8]. The effectiveness of topical minoxidil in women with androgenetic alopecia is equivalent to that in men.

The availability of a topical treatment that appears to some extent to reverse the problem of androgenetic alopecia in males has encouraged many young men to seek medical help. These men should be counselled carefully and made aware of the need for continuous use to maintain any effect. It is preferable that advice be given by qualified medical practitioners who are fully aware of the pitfalls of treatment so that these often vulnerable individuals may be kept away from commercial centres where profit is the only motivation. Each patient needs careful medical assessment to ensure that the diagnosis is beyond doubt. He or she should then be given a detailed explanation of the nature and significance of the alopecia. However, when baldness first becomes manifest at a stressful stage of their career, many may attempt to lay the blame for any lack of success, socially or at work, on their baldness, even when this is of minimal extent. Such patients should be encouraged to discuss their problem in full. In the course of doing so, they often become aware that they have not seen their baldness in its proper perspective, but may be enabled to do so. However, in some patients this lack of insight is only one of the many manifestations of a depressive illness, which may require treatment.

REFERENCES

1 Cash TF, Price VH, Savin RC. Psychological effects of androgenetic alopecia in women. *J Am Acad Dermatol* 1993; **29**: 568–70.
2 Dardour JC. Treatment of male pattern baldness with a one stage flap. *Aesthet Plast Surg* 1985; **9**: 109–16.
3 Masser MR. A twin tissue expander used in the elimination of alopecia. *Plast Reconstr Surg* 1988; **81**: 444–50.
4 Mortimer CH, Rushton H, James KC. Effective medical treatment for common baldness in women. *Clin Exp Dermatol* 1984; **9**: 342–8.
5 Burke B, Cunliffe WJ. Oral spironolactone therapy for female patients with acne, hirsutism or androgenic alopecia (Correspondence). *Br J Dermatol* 1985; **112**: 124–8.
6 Aram H. Treatment of female androgenetic alopecia with cimetidine. *Int J Dermatol* 1987; **26**: 128–33.
7 Reitschel RL, Duncan SH. Safety and efficacy of topical minoxidil in the management of androgenetic alopecia. *J Am Acad Dermatol* 1987; **16**: 677–85.
8 Olsen EA, Weiner MS, Amara LA *et al*. Five year follow-up of men with androgenetic alopecia treated with topical minoxidil. *J Am Acad Dermatol* 1990; **22**: 643–9.
9 De Villez RL. Topical minoxidil therapy in hereditary androgenetic alopecia. *Arch Dermatol* 1985; **121**: 197–202.
10 Olsen EA, Delong ER, Weiner MS. Long-term follow-up of men with male pattern baldness treated with topical minoxidil. *J Am Acad Dermatol* 1987; **16**: 688–95.
11 Tosti A, Bardazzi F, De Padova MP *et al*. Contact dermatitis to minoxidil. *Contact Dermatitis* 1985; **13**: 275–7.

Congenital alopecia and hypotrichosis

Total or partial absence of hair of developmental origin

occurs in a bewildering variety of clinical forms, either as an apparently isolated defect or in association with a wide range of other anomalies. A logical classification must be based on detailed histological and genetic investigations and these, unfortunately, are seldom carried out. Provisionally, a purely clinical classification is useful to enable the clinician at least to understand the clearly defined types [1].

REFERENCE

1 Sinclair R, de Berker D. Hereditary and congenital alopecia and hypotrichosis. In: Dawber RPR, ed. *Diseases of the Hair and Scalp*, 3rd edn. Oxford: Blackwell Science, 1997: 252–397.

Total alopecia
SYN. ATRICHIA CONGENITA

As an isolated abnormality [1,2]

Aetiology. Total alopecia as an apparently isolated defect is usually determined by an autosomal recessive gene. Some pedigrees have been traced back to the early 19th century [1]. Dominant or irregular dominant inheritance has occurred in some families [3,4]. The two genotypes seem to be phenotypically indistinguishable, but detailed investigation would probably reveal differences. The term 'total' is relative, but if any hairs are present they are extremely few. Many isolated cases and families reported under the diagnosis of congenital alopecia are found on review of the original reports to be unquestionably examples of other syndromes; many were hidrotic ectodermal dysplasia.

Pathology. The hair follicles are absent in adult life, even when the fetal hair coat has been normal. Sebaceous glands are smaller than normal. When a few stray hairs have survived, the structure of the shaft appears to be normal.

Clinical features [4,5]. The scalp hair is often normal at birth but is shed between the first and sixth months, after which no further growth occurs. In some cases the scalp has been totally hairless at birth and has remained so [5]. Eyebrows, eyelashes and body hair may also be absent [6], but more often there are a few straggling pubic and axillary hairs and scanty eyebrows and eyelashes. Teeth and nails are normal, and general health, intelligence and life expectancy are unimpaired.

With associated defects

Total or almost total alopecia is unusual in hereditary syndromes.

Progeria. Scalp and body hair is totally deficient.

Hydrotic ectodermal dysplasia. Total or almost total alopecia is associated with palmoplantar keratoderma and thickened discoloured nails. Any hairs which are present are structurally normal but are often finer than the average.

Moynahan's syndrome [7]. This autosomal recessive syndrome, reported in male siblings, is associated with mental retardation, epilepsy and total baldness of the scalp; the hair may regrow in childhood between 2 and 4 years of age.

Atrichia with keratin cysts [6]. This rare syndrome, comparable with the condition found in certain hairless mice, has been reported only in girls, but the mode of inheritance is unknown. Total and permanent alopecia develops after the first hair coat is shed. At any age between 5 and 18 years, numerous small, horny papules appear, first on the face, neck and scalp, and then gradually over the greater part of the limbs and trunk. Histologically, the papules are thick-walled keratin cysts [8].

Baraitser's syndrome [9]. This autosomal recessive syndrome presents as almost total alopecia following the loss of some downy scalp hair present at birth.

Three cases are reported in an inbred family [9]: all had almost total alopecia of all sites, including eyebrows and lashes. There were occasional isolated hairs. Mental and physical retardation were associated.

REFERENCES

1 Calvo Melendro J. Atriquia Congenita total y permanente. *Med Clin* 1955; **24**: 253–7.
2 Dawber RPR, ed. *Diseases of the Hair and Scalp*, 3rd edn. Oxford: Blackwell Science, 1997: 260–2.
3 Birke G. Über Atrichia congenita und Erbgang. *Arch Dermatol Syphilol* 1954; **197**: 322–5.
4 Tillman WG. Alopecia congenita. *Br Med J* 1952; **ii**: 428–9.
5 Linn HW. Congenital atrichia. *Australas J Dermatol* 1964; **7**: 223–5.
6 Friederich HC. Zur Kenntnis der Kongenitale Hypertrichosis. *Dermatol Wochenschr* 1950; **121**: 408–10.
7 Moynahan EJ. Familial congenital alopecia. *Proc R Soc Med* 1962; **55**: 411–12.
8 Delprat A, Bonafé JL, Lugardon Y. Atrichie congenitale avec kystes. *Ann Dermatol Vénéréol* 1994; **121**: 802–4.
9 Baraitser M, Carter C, Brett EM. A new alopecia/mental retardation syndrome. *J Med Genet* 1983; **20**: 64–75.

Hypotrichosis [1,2]

Aetiology and pathology. Congenital hypotrichosis of sufficient degree to cause social embarrassment is not uncommon, and is probably determined by an autosomal dominant gene. Severe degrees of congenital hypotrichosis without associated defects are rare. Dominant inheritance has been recorded [3,4] but many cases have occurred sporadically. There are a number of distinct syndromes.

Hypotrichosis is a relatively common feature of many hereditary syndromes, usually in association with other ectodermal defects. In the majority, the hair is not only sparse but is structurally abnormal. Where hypotrichosis is the most prominent manifestation and the structural defect is distinctive and well characterized, it has given its name to the syndrome, as in monilethrix and pili torti. In other syndromes, the scanty scalp hair is a minor and sometimes inconstant manifestation, and the shaft defect is usually less specific, although often gross. The follicles are sparse and are reduced in size, and the hair shafts are brittle and deficient in pigment. The nature of the disturbance in keratinization is not known.

Clinical features [5]. When hypotrichosis occurs as an isolated abnormality the scalp hair at birth is normal in quantity and quality, but is shed during the first 6 months and never adequately replaced. It is sparse, fine, dry and brittle and seldom exceeds 10 cm in length. The eyebrows, eyelashes and vellus may be absent, sparse or normal. In exceptional cases, improvement or recovery has taken place at puberty, but the condition is usually permanent.

In some families, the hair is normal until the age of 5 years or later, when growth becomes retarded and the scalp is progressively denuded so that baldness is almost total by the age of 25 years [4].

Many of the hereditary syndromes of which hypotrichosis is a constant or frequent feature are listed in Table 66.3. In the majority, the hair is not only sparse but fine and brittle, and is often hypopigmented. The hair shafts are often

Table 66.3 Alopecia or hypotrichosis in hereditary syndromes. (Data from Happle [1] and Sinclair & de Berker [2].)

	Main features of syndrome	Characteristics of hair
Hidrotic ectodermal dysplasia	Nails thickened, striated, discoloured. Palmoplantar keratoderma	Scalp hair sparse and fine; may be completely absent
Progeria	Normal first year, then gross retardation of physical growth. Senile appearance; thin, dry, wrinkled skin, bird-like features	Total alopecia
Monilethrix	Keratosis pilaris, especially on occiput and nape	Normal at birth; later brittle, beaded hair 1–2 cm in length. Microscopy diagnostic
Pili torti	Hair defect main manifestation	Onset usually in second or third year. Hair sparse and brittle; spangled in reflected light. Microscopy diagnostic
Anhidrotic ectodermal dysplasia	Usually male. Reduced sweating. Sunken nose, conical teeth. Smooth, finely wrinkled skin	Sparse, dry, fine, short, scalp hair and eyelashes; hair may sometimes be normal
Rothmund–Thomson syndrome	Erythema cheeks, hands, feet from 3 to 6 months, followed by poikiloderma. Light sensitivity	Scalp hair sparse; eyebrows, eyelashes and body hair very sparse
Werner's syndrome	Sclerodermiform changes face and extremities. Cataracts	Premature greying at 14–18 years. Progressive alopecia from adolescence
Hallermann–Streiff syndrome	Dyscephaly. Aplasia of mandible. Proportionate dwarfism	Normal at birth; later sparse with patchy alopecia, often sutural
Marinesco–Sjögren syndrome	Cerebellar ataxia. Mental retardation. Cataract. Small stature	Scalp hair fine, sparse, short; deficient in pigment
Netherton's syndrome	Females, males. Eczema	Sparse, brittle; often bamboo-hairs; trichorrhexis invaginata or nodosa
Cartilage–hair hypoplasia	Dwarfism, skeletal abnormalities	Sparse, brittle, fine and light in colour, but hair may be normal
Trichorhinophalangeal syndrome	Pear-shaped nose	Hair sparse, fine, brittle (may be normal)
AEC syndrome*	Ankyloblepharon, ectodermal dysplasia, cleft lip and palate	Hair sparse, coarse, wiry
EEC syndrome*	Ectrodactyly, ectodermal dysplasia, cleft lip and/or palate	Hair sparse
Follicular atrophoderma	Depressions at follicular orifices. Basal cell naevi	Sparse and fine
Menkes' syndrome	Retarded growth. Symptoms of cerebral and cerebellar degeneration	Sparse, brittle, poorly pigmented

*AEC and EEC syndromes are described in Chapter 12.

defective but may show no consistent well-characterized structural abnormality. As the hypotrichosis is not the most prominent feature of these syndromes, they are described more fully in other chapters.

There are also other syndromes, as yet incompletely investigated, in which hypotrichosis is associated with other defects.

Hypotrichosis with keratosis pilaris [6]. The hair is apparently normal at birth but after the birth coat has been shed, between the second and sixth months, it fails to grow satisfactorily and remains sparse, short, brittle and poorly pigmented. Eyebrows and eyelashes may be normal or sparse. Keratosis pilaris is present in the occipital region and neck, and sometimes on the trunk and limbs. Nails, teeth and general physical development are normal. The hairs show no beading or other distinctive abnormality.

Hypotrichosis with keratosis pilaris and lentiginosis [6]. Seven females in three generations in a family of three males and 13 females developed hypotrichosis at or just after puberty, which progressed until the menopause. Axillary and pubic hair was completely lost. There was keratosis pilaris of the scalp and axillae, brittleness and longitudinal striation of the nails and centrofacial lentiginosis.

Eyelid cysts, hypodontia and hypotrichosis. See [7].

Hypomelia, hypotrichosis, facial haemangioma syndrome [8]. This 'pseudothalidomide' syndrome, which is probably determined by an autosomal recessive gene, associates gross reduction defects of the limbs, a mid-facial capillary naevus and sparse, silver–blonde hair.

Hypotrichosis, Marie–Unna type [9–11]. This rare but very distinctive syndrome is determined by an autosomal dominant gene. Affected individuals may be normal at birth or be completely or almost completely hairless. Hair becomes or remains sparse or absent until about the third year when coarse, flattened, irregularly twisted hair appears on the scalp. This coarse hair is gradually lost with the approach of puberty as follicles are progressively destroyed by a scarring process. The hair loss is greatest around the scalp margins and on the vertex, but may be patchy. Lashes, eyebrows and body hair are sparse, and often virtually absent from birth. General physical and mental development are normal. Scanning electron microscopy shows that the hair shafts are coarse, irregularly twisted and fluted [9].

Hypotrichosis in disorders of amino-acid metabolism. In many disorders with amino aciduria, the hair is hypopigmented and is often also fine, friable and sometimes sparse. Fine, sparse hair has been reported in phenylketonuria, arginosuccinic aciduria and hyperlysinaemia.

A number of case reports associate hypotrichosis with a variety of ectodermal defects. Some such cases may represent partial forms of recognized syndromes but it is probable that many additional distinct syndromes remain to be identified and characterized.

Differential diagnosis. Microscopy of plucked hairs will exclude the more distinctive structural defects (pili torti, monilethrix and pili annulati). Other ectodermal defects should be carefully sought and relatives should be examined.

REFERENCES

1 Happle R. Genetic defects involving the hair. In: Orfanos CE, Happle R, eds. *Hair and Hair Diseases*. Berlin: Springer-Verlag, 1989: 325–62.
2 Sinclair R, de Berker D. Hereditary and congenital alopecia and hypotrichosis. In: Dawber RPR, ed. *Diseases of the Hair and Scalp*, 3rd edn. Oxford: Blackwell Science, 1997: 252–394.
3 Brain RT. Hereditary hypotrichosis. *Proc R Soc Med* 1938; **32**: 87.
4 Toribo J, Quinones PA. Hereditary hypertrichosis simplex of the scalp. *Br J Dermatol* 1974; **91**: 687–96.
5 Dawber RPR, Van Neste D. Congenital alopecia. In: Dawber RPR, Van Neste D. *Hair and Scalp Disorders*. London: Dunitz, 1995: 41–51.
6 Greither A. Hypotrichosis with keratosis pilaris and lentiginosis. *Arch Klin Exp Dermatol* 1960; **210**: 123–7.
7 Burkett JM. Eyelid cysts, hypodontia and hypotrichosis. *J Am Acad Dermatol* 1984; **10**: 922–5.
8 Hall BD, Greenberg MH. Hypomelia, hypotrichosis, facial haemangioma syndrome. *Am J Dis Child* 1972; **123**: 602–6.
9 Peachey RDG, Wells RS. Hereditary hypotrichosis (Marie–Unna type) *Trans St John's Hosp Dermatol Soc* 1971; **57**: 157–66.
10 Solomon LM, Esterly M, Medenica M. Hereditary trichodysplasia: Marie–Unna syndrome. *J Invest Dermatol* 1971; **57**: 389–400.
11 Stevanovic DV. Hereditary hypertrichosis congenita: Marie–Unna syndrome. *Br J Dermatol* 1970; **83**: 331–3.

Circumscribed alopecia of congenital origin [1,2]

The differential diagnosis of circumscribed alopecia of developmental origin presents little difficulty if a reliable history is available. Without it, alopecia areata and the acquired cicatricial alopecias must be considered.

The commonest forms are naevoid. Epidermal naevi are usually devoid of hair and present as warty or smooth but slightly indurated plaques. A zone of non-cicatricial alopecia sometimes develops around melanocytic naevi.

Aplasia of all layers of the skin gives rise to a congenital defect, usually a circular or rectilinear area of scarring somewhat depressed below the scalp surface and commonly on the vertex.

Irregular areas of cicatricial alopecia not preceded by clinically apparent inflammatory changes produce the syndrome known as pseudopelade. Pseudopelade may develop during early infancy in association with certain hereditary syndromes, for example incontinentia pigmenti and Conradi's syndrome.

Circumscribed non-cicatricial alopecia is uncommon. It is the result of hypoplasia or aplasia of a group of follicles. The scalp is clinically normal and histologically shows no change other than a reduced number of follicles. Any follicles present are usually small and of vellus rather than terminal type. The first hair coat is normal and the patches develop between the third and sixth months, although if they are small and not completely bald, they may not be noticed by the parents until considerably later.

Several clinical forms occur [1,2]. In *vertical alopecia*, a small and often irregular patch of alopecia is present on the vertex at birth. It has been confused with aplasia cutis, but the skin is normal apart from the absence of appendages. In *sutural alopecia*, which is one component of the Hallermann–Streiff syndrome, multiple patches overlie the cranial sutures. *Triangular alopecia* [3–6] was first recognized by Sabouraud. In the usual form, a triangular area overlying the frontotemporal suture just inside the anterior hairline, and with its base directed forwards, is completely bald or covered by sparse vellus hairs. Rarely, similar triangular patches have occurred on the nape of the neck.

Single or multiple small patches of total alopecia or hypotrichosis may occasionally occur in other sites but are often inconspicuous.

REFERENCES

1 Barth JH. Circumscribed alopecia of infancy. In: Dawber RPR, ed. *Diseases of the Hair and Scalp*, 3rd edn. Oxford: Blackwell Science, 1997.
2 Frieden IJ. Aplasia cutis congenita. *J Am Acad Dermatol* 1986; **14**: 646–60.
3 Canizares O. Alopecia triangularis congenita. *Arch Dermatol Syphilol* 1941; **44**: 1106–9.
4 Fuerman EJ. Congenital triangular alopecia. *Cutis* 1981; **28**: 196–7.
5 Kubba R, Rook A. Congenital triangular alopecia. *Br J Dermatol* 1976; **95**: 657–9.
6 Tosti A. Congenital triangular alopecia. *J Am Acad Dermatol* 1987; **16**: 991–3.

Disturbances of hair cycle: telogen effluvium

SYN. TELOGEN DEFLUVIUM

Aetiology [1]. In the normal young adult scalp, 80–90% of follicles are in the anagen phase of the hair cycle, although there is some variation with site and age. Kligman [2] introduced the term telogen effluvium to describe the shedding of normal club hairs, which follows the premature precipitation of anagen follicles into telogen, a process which may be regarded as the common response of the follicles to many different types of 'stress'. Fever, prolonged and difficult childbirth [3], surgical operations [4], haemorrhage (including blood donation), sudden severe reduction of food intake ('crash' dieting) and emotional stress, including perhaps that of prolonged jet flights, may all induce this response; the proportion of follicles affected, and hence the severity of the subsequent alopecia, depends partly on the duration and severity of the precipitating cause and partly on unexplained individual variation in susceptibility. The club hairs may be retained for about 3 months until the affected follicles are well advanced in a new anagen, or may be shed

prematurely. The most frequent form of postpartum effluvium is probably due to the withdrawal of factors that have inhibited normal entry to catagen during later pregnancy. It is universal to some degree, but is often subclinical. A similar state of affairs prevails when the contraceptive pill is discontinued after it has been taken continuously for some time [5,6].

Pathology. Histological examination shows no abnormality other than an increase in the proportion of follicles in telogen. The shed hairs are normal 'clubs'.

Clinical features [7,8]. Diffuse shedding of hairs is the only symptom. The patient may be aware of increased loss on the brush or comb or during shampooing. The daily loss ranges from under 100 to over 1000. If the lower rates of shedding are continued for only a short period there may be no obvious baldness in the previously normal scalp, because loss of over 25% of the total complement of hairs is never attained. In the patient of either sex with androgenetic alopecia, previously inapparent, the added diffuse loss may deceptively unveil it, or a previously recognized slight baldness may become more conspicuous. If shedding occurs at higher rates, or is long continued, obvious diffuse baldness is produced (Fig. 66.27). It

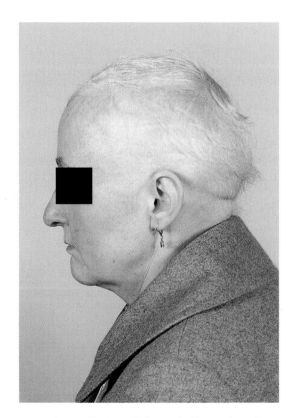

Fig. 66.27 Telogen effluvium (defluvium). Chronic form due to iron deficiency anaemia (analgesic 'abuse' with gastro-intestinal blood loss).

may be severe but is seldom, if ever, total. Unless the 'stress' is repeated, spontaneous complete regrowth takes place almost invariably in about 6 months. Exceptionally, prolonged or high fevers, such as typhoid, may destroy some follicles completely so that only partial recovery is possible. If postpartum effluvium is severe and recurs after successive pregnancies, regrowth may ultimately be incomplete [5].

Diagnosis. The diagnosis is usually simple. Increased shedding of hair is clearly related to the stressful episode that preceded it by 6–16 weeks. Plucked hairs show a large proportion of normal club hairs until the shedding is complete. The alopecia induced by heparin is very similar but the time interval is often shorter. Other chemical alopecias are discussed on page 2915. They can sometimes be excluded by the examination of plucked hairs. Alopecia areata of very rapid onset is usually patchy at first but may become total within a week. Telogen effluvium is always diffuse and never total [7]. Acute syphilitic alopecia is patchy. Increased shedding of club hairs is, of course a variable but often very obvious symptom of early androgenetic alopecia. Loose anagen hair syndrome can be differentiated by root microscopy.

Whiting [9] proposes a form of chronic telogen effluvium to explain the non-progressive hair loss in middle-aged women who present with shedding as the main complaint.

REFERENCES

1 Headington JT. Telogen effluvium: new concepts and review. *Arch Dermatol* 1993; **129**: 556–8.
2 Kligman AM. Pathologic dynamics of human hair loss. I. Telogen effluvium. *Arch Dermatol* 1961; **83**: 175–98.
3 Schiff BL, Kern AB. Study of postpartum alopecia. *Arch Dermatol* 1963; **87**: 609–11.
4 Desai SP, Peat ER. Telogen effluvium after anaesthesia and surgery. *Anesth Analg* 1984; **63**: 83–5.
5 Dawber RPR, Connor BL. Pregnancy, hair loss and the pill. *Br Med J* 1971; **iv**: 234–5.
6 Griffiths WAD. Diffuse hair loss and oral contraceptives. *Br J Dermatol* 1973; **88**: 31–6.
7 Steigleder GK, Mahrle G. Haarausfall als polyätiologisches Symptom. *Fortschr Praktisch Dermatol Venereol* 1973; **7**: 237–81.
8 Steck WD. Telogen effluvium. *Cutis* 1978; **21**: 543–4.
9 Whiting DA. Chronic telogen effluvium. *Dermatol Clin* 1996; **14**: 723–31.

Diffuse alopecia of endocrine origin

Diffuse alopecia occurs in many endocrine syndromes, but the mechanisms have not been fully investigated in humans [1]. In many case reports, the criteria for the diagnosis of the endocrine disorder have been inadequate.

Hypopituitary states

The hypopituitary dwarf is usually hairless. In pitu-

itary deficiency beginning after puberty, as in Sheehan's syndrome, the scalp hair becomes very thin, and pubic and axillary hair is totally lost. The skin is yellowish, dry and lacks turgidity.

Hypothyroidism [2–5]

Diffuse loss of scalp hair and later of body hair is frequent in hypothyroidism. Sparsity of the eyebrows may be conspicuous and a decrease in axillary hair is evident in about 50% of cases [5]. The trichogram shows the proportion of roots in telogen to be abnormally high, suggesting either prolonged telogen or premature catagen, or both [6]. Regrowth is usual when the hypothyroidism is controlled, but may be incomplete. Reports to the contrary probably apply to the association of androgenetic alopecia, possibly owing to more 'free' androgen due to decreased SHBG. Diffuse alopecia may be the only clinical manifestation of hypothyroidism. The diagnosis of hypothyroidism must be based on critical clinical assessment, together with estimation of the thyroxine level and thyroid-stimulating hormone (TSH). Alopecia has occurred in iodine-induced hypothyroidism [7] in which the serum protein-bound iodine level was high.

Hyperthyroidism [2]

In hyperthyroidism, diffuse alopecia develops in 40–50% of cases, but is rarely severe. It is reversible if 'miniaturization' is not extreme. Alopecia areata (p. 2919) and vitiligo occur with increased frequency.

Hypoparathyroidism

The scalp hair is coarse, sparse and dry. It is easily shed with slight trauma and the alopecia may appear irregularly patchy. Similar changes have been reported in pseudo-hypoparathyroidism [8].

Diabetes mellitus

In poorly controlled diabetes, diffuse alopecia may occur, probably of telogen effluvium type.

Pregnancy

The hair changes in pregnancy are described on page 2881.

Oral contraceptives

Diffuse alopecia has been attributed to oral contraceptives [9] but the evidence is conflicting. Studies of anagen–telogen counts [10,11] showed a variable response: some women showed a temporary and some a more prolonged increase in telogen ratio, and in others no change was observed. In general, no clinically significant changes are induced, but in some women diffuse hair shedding follows 3–4 weeks after the contraceptive is discontinued, as after pregnancy [12]; recovery occurs spontaneously, usually within a few months of onset.

REFERENCES

1 Rook A. Endocrine influences on hair growth. *Br Med J* 1965; **i**: 609–14.
2 Comaish JS. Hair loss in thyroid disease. In: Dawber R, ed. *Seminars in Dermatology*, Vol. 4. New York: Thieme–Stratton, 1985: 32–40.
3 Holt PJA, Marks R. The epidermal response to change in thyroid status. *J Invest Dermatol* 1977; **68**: 299–301.
4 Saito R, Hori Y, Kuribayashi T. Alopecia in hypothyroidism. In: Kobori T, Montagna W, eds. *Biology and Diseases of Hair*. Baltimore: University Park Press, 1976: 279–85.
5 Williams RH. Thyroid and adrenal interrelations with special reference to hypotrichosis axillaris. *Clin Endocrinol Metab* 1947; **7**: 52–6.
6 Freinkel RK, Freinkel N. Hair growth and alopecia in hypothyroidism. *Arch Dermatol* 1972; **106**: 349–52.
7 Chapman RS, Main RA. Diffuse thinning of hair in iodine-induced hypothyroidism. *Br J Dermatol* 1967; **79**: 103–5.
8 Corea L, Lupattelli L. Hair loss in pseudohypoparathyroidism. *Folio Endocrinol* 1972; **25**: 347–50.
9 Cormia FA. Alopecia from oral contraceptives. *JAMA* 1967; **201**: 635–7.
10 Zaun H, Ruffing H. Untersuchungen über den Einfluss anti-konzeptiver zweiphasen-Hormonpräparate auf das Wachstum der Kopfhaare. *Arch Klin Exp Dermatol* 1970; **238**: 197–206.
11 Zaun H, Gerber T. Die Wirkung Monophasischer Ovulations-hemmer auf das Wachstum der Kopfhaare. *Arch Klin Exp Dermatol* 1969; **234**: 355–61.
12 Griffiths WAD. Diffuse hair loss and oral contraceptives. *Br J Dermatol* 1973; **88**: 31–6.

Alopecia of chemical origin [1]

Many chemicals which are capable of inducing alopecia are in frequent use in therapeutics [2]. Humans are only rarely and accidentally exposed to others. Together, they account for a small but increasing proportion of cases of diffuse alopecia [3,4]. In many instances, their mode of action is uncertain and a logical classification is therefore impracticable.

Thallium

Thallium salts are no longer prescribed in the UK for the depilation of the scalp infected with ringworm, and are not contained in any preparation on sale to the public. In many other countries, they are still used as pesticides, and serious outbreaks of poisoning have followed the contamination of grain stores and other food [5,6]. Thallium salts are tasteless and have been used in homicide and suicide [7]. Thallium is rapidly taken up by anagen follicles and disturbs keratinization [8,9]. Many hairs break within the follicle; irregularity of the dark keratogenous zone and air bubbles within the shaft near the tapered tip give a distinctive appearance. Many other follicles enter catagen prematurely. Surface keratinization is also disturbed [10]. Alopecia is the most constant symptom. The loss of hair begins after 10 days as diffuse shedding of abnormal anagen hairs. It may rapidly become complete or, with lower doses, may be followed by the gradual shedding of club hairs over a period of 3 or 4 months. In severe poisoning, death may result from acute cerebral and renal damage before hair loss can occur. In less severe cases, the associated symptoms are very variable [5,8]; ataxia, weakness, somnolence, tremor, headache, nausea and vomiting are among the most constant. In mild poisoning, alopecia may be the only feature [11]. In all cases, the hair regrows completely within 6 months, but there may be persistent signs of residual cerebral damage. The diagnosis may be suspected on clinical grounds but can be confirmed only by the detection of thallium in the urine and faeces in which it may continue to be excreted for 4 or 5 months [12]. There is no specific treatment.

Thyroid antagonists [13]

Some patients with thyrotoxicosis treated with thiouracil or carbimazole develop a diffuse alopecia. Long continued administration of iodides has induced hypothyroid alopecia [14].

Anticoagulants

All the anticoagulant drugs (heparin, heparinoids and coumarins) will induce alopecia [3,15,16]. Coumarins such as warfarin are widely used as rodent poisons and are sometimes accidentally ingested by children [4]. The highest dose, and not the duration of the exposure, determines the degree of hair loss. Apparently normal club hairs are shed some 2–3 months after the effective blood level is achieved. There is often moderately increased shedding without obvious alopecia, but with high dosage moderate or severe alopecia may occur. Full recovery follows cessation of the drug.

Cytostatic agents [17]

Many cytostatic agents employed therapeutically [18] or given with criminal intent can cause hair loss. Diffuse, often total, alopecia of anagen effluvium type is the rule in most tumour chemotherapy. Experimental and clinical studies with cyclophosphamide [19] show that some anagen follicles enter catagen prematurely; in others the inhibition of mitosis in the matrix results in a constriction in the shaft or a complete break. A similar constriction is produced by aminopterin [20]. Clinically, alopecia is frequently observed after cyclophosphamide therapy. It has also been reported after therapeutic doses of colchicine [21,22], after an abortifacient dose of aminopterin [23] and after cantharidin. Hairs with broken constricted shafts may be shed diffusely as early as 4–6 days after the first effective dose, and shedding of apparently normal telogen hairs may continue for some months.

When cytostatic drugs are indicated, the expected loss of hair will be minimized to some degree by scalp hypothermia, for example applying ice packs to the scalp for 30 min before the drug is injected [18].

Triparanol

Triparanol [24], and the chemically unrelated antipsychotic drug fluorobutyrophenone [25], disturb keratinization by inhibiting cholesterol synthesis. Scalp and body hair becomes dry and sparse, and light in colour. The skin is generally dry and ichthyotic. Cataracts develop later in some cases.

Hypervitaminosis A

Excessive consumption of vitamin A gives rise to a variable syndrome [26] in which the principal features are dryness, irritability and sometimes pigmentation of the skin, and slowly progressive thinning of scalp and body hair, eyebrows and eyelashes. Loss of weight, fatigue, anaemia and bone pain are frequent, and the liver and spleen are sometimes enlarged. The symptoms develop insidiously after doses in excess of 50 000 units daily have been ingested for many months. The mode of action of vitamin A on hair growth is unknown [3]. Diagnosis is established by estimation of the fasting blood level of the vitamin. Slow recovery takes place when the vitamin A is discontinued.

Dry skin, xerostomia, hair kinking [27] and diffuse hair loss [28] are seen with systemic retinoids, which share the metabolic pathways involved in vitamin A poisoning.

Boric acid

Occupational exposure to sodium borate has caused diffuse alopecia [29]. Boric acid mouthwashes have caused a similar pattern of hair loss. Serum boric acid levels were elevated. Boric acid taken with suicidal intent caused total alopecia after 10 days [30].

Other chemicals

Reversible alopecia is occasionally induced by other chemicals [2]; potassium thiocyanate formerly prescribed for hypertension [31]; trimethadione employed in the control of epilepsy [20]; bismuth after prolonged overdosage; industrial exposure to the cyclic condensation products of monomeric chloroprene in the manufacture of rubber [32]. The possible effects of oral contraceptives are discussed on page 2914. Other drugs described as inducing hair loss include lithium carbonate, pyridostigmine [33], dixarazine [34] and etretinate [28].

Propranolol [35], metoprolol, levodopa [36] and cimetidine [37] have all been suspected of causing diffuse alopecia after several months of administration, as has ibuprofen [1].

The amino acid mimosine in *Leucaena glauca* and some other leguminous plants and the toxic substance in the nut *Lecythus* [38], which appears to be selenocystathionine [31], have also caused alopecia. Seleniferous plants are a well-known cause of hair loss in cattle, and there are occasional reports of a similar effect in humans.

There are many anecdotal and unsubstantiated cases of alopecia thought to be related to specific drugs—amiodarone, cimetidine, danazol, gentamicin, itraconazole, metyrapone, pyridostigmine, sulphasalazine and terfenadine [1,39].

REFERENCES

1 Simpson N. Diffuse alopecia. In: Dawber RPR, ed. *Diseases of the Hair and Scalp*, 3rd edn. Oxford: Blackwell Science 1997: 164–9.
2 Stroud JD. Drug-induced alopecia. In: Maibach H, Rook AJ, eds. *Seminars in Dermatology*, Vol. 4. New York: Thieme–Stratton, 1985: 37.
3 Flesch P. Inhibition of keratinizing structure by systemic drugs. *Pharmacol Rev* 1963: 653–77.
4 Rook A. Some chemical influences on hair growth and pigmentation. *Br J Dermatol* 1965; **77**: 115–29.
5 Chamberlain PH, Stavincha WB, Davis H. Thallium poisoning. *Pediatrics* 1958; **22**: 1170–82.
6 Hollander L. Multiple cutaneous effects of potassium sulfocyanate. *Arch Dermatol Syphilol* 1949; **59**: 112–17.
7 Heyroth EF. Thallium. *Rep US Publ Health Serv* (Suppl.) 197–206.
8 Reed D, Crawley J, Faros N. Thallotoxicosis. *JAMA* 1963; **183**: 516–22.
9 Thyresson N. Effect of thallium on hair growth in the white rat. *Acta Derm Venereol Suppl. (Stockh)* 1952; **29**: 370–6.
10 Schwartzman RM, Kirschbaum JO. Cutaneous histopathology of thallium poisoning. *J Invest Dermatol* 1962; **39**: 169–75.
11 Hubler WR. Hair loss as a symptom of chronic thallotoxicosis. *South Med J* 1966; **59**: 436.
12 Arnold W. Die Dynamik des Haarausfalls bei Thallium-Vergiflung. *Arch Klin Exp Dermatol* 1964; **218**: 396–9.
13 Lundbaek K. Toxic, allergic and 'myxedematoid' symptoms in the treatment of thyrotoxicosis. *Acta Med Scand* 1946; **124**: 266–81.
14 Chapman RS, Main RA. Diffuse thinning of hair in iodine-induced hypothyroidism. *Br J Dermatol* 1967; **79**: 103–5.
15 Fischer R, Burcher R, Reith T. Der Haarausfall nach antikoaguliender Therapie. *Schweiz Med Wochenschr* 1983; **83**: 509–13.
16 Tudhope GR, Cohen H, Meikle RW. Alopecia following treatment with dextran sulphate and anticoagulant drugs. *Br Med J* 1958; **i**: 1034.
17 Crounse RG, van Scott EJ. Changes in scalp hair roots as a measure of toxicity from cancer chemotherapeutic drugs. *J Invest Dermatol* 1960; **35**: 83–90.
18 Dean JC, Salmon SE, Griffith KS. Prevention of doxorubicine-induced hair loss with scalp hypothermia. *N Engl J Med* 1974; **301**: 1427–9.
19 Braun-Falco O. Klinik und Pathomechanismus der EndoxanAlopecie als Beitrag zur Wesen cytostatischer Alopecie. *Arch Klin Exp Dermatol* 1961; **212**: 194–9.
20 Holowach J, Sanden HV. Alopecia as a side effect of treatment of epilepsy with trimethadione. *N Engl J Med* 1960; **263**: 1187–8.
21 Malkinson ED, Lynfield YL. Colchicine alopecia. *J Invest Dermatol* 1959; **33**: 371–8.
22 Mikkleson WM. Alopecia totalis after colchicine treatment of acute gout. *N Engl J Med* 1956; **255**: 766–70.
23 Maibach HI, Maguire HC. Acute hair loss from drug-induced abortion. *N Engl J Med* 1959; **220**: 1112–13.
24 Winkelmann RK, Perry HO, Archer RWP. Cutaneous syndromes produced as side effects of triparanol. *Arch Dermatol* 1963; **87**: 372–7.
25 Simpson GM, Blair JH, Cranswick CH. Cutaneous effects of a new butyrophenone drug. *Clin Pharmacol Ther* 1964; **5**: 310–13.
26 Soler-Bechara J, Soscia JL. Chronic hypervitaminosis A. *Arch Intern Med* 1963; **112**: 462–6.

27 Bunker CB, Maurice PDL, Dowd PM. Isotretinoin and curly hair. *Clin Exp Dermatol* 1990; **15**: 143–5.
28 Berth-Jones J, Shuttleworth D, Hutchinson PE. A study of etretinate alopecia. *Br J Dermatol* 1990; **122**: 751–6.
29 Tan TG. Occupational toxic alopecia due to borax. *Acta Derm Venereol (Stockh)* 1970; **50**: 55–8.
30 Schillinger BM. Boric acid induced total alopecia. *J Am Acad Dermatol* 1982; **7**: 667–8.
31 Aronow L, Kerdel-Vegas F. Seleno cystathione, a pharmacologically active factor in the seeds of *Lecythus allaria. Nature* 1965; **205**: 1185–6.
32 Lijhancova G. Berufsbedingte Haarausfall durch Chloroprene. *Berufs-dermatosen* 1967; **15**: 280–2.
33 Falkson G, Schulz EJ. Skin changes caused by cancer chemotherapy. *Br J Dermatol* 1964; **76**: 309–24.
34 Poulsen J. Hair loss, depigmentation of hair, ichthyosis produced by dixarazine. *Acta Derm Venereol (Stockh)* 1981; **61**: 85–8.
35 Hilder MJ. Propranolol hair loss. *Cutis* 1979; **24**: 63–5.
36 Marshall A, Williams MJ. Alopecia and levodopa (Letter). *Br Med J* 1971; **ii**: 47.
37 Khalse JH. Cimetidine associated alopecia. *Int J Dermatol* 1983; **22**: 202–3.
38 Kerdel-Vegas F. Generalised hair loss due to ingestion of 'Coco de Mono'. *J Invest Dermatol* 1964; **42**: 91–4.
39 Field LM. Toxic alopecia caused by pyridostigmine bromide (Letter). *Arch Dermatol* 1980; **116**: 1103.

Alopecia of nutritional and metabolic origin [1]

Hair is affected early in protein deficiency, as protein is conserved for more essential purposes. Malnutrition influences the structure of the hair shaft and, sometimes, the colour of the hair. Short-term experimental protein deprivation causes atrophy of the bulb and loss of internal and external root sheaths but no changes in the anagen/telogen ratio, although these would probably develop if the protein deprivation was continued [2].

Marasmus is the result of protein–calorie deficiency, usually in the first year of life. The hair is fine and dry; the diameter of the hair bulbs is reduced to one-third of normal and almost all follicles are in telogen [3]. Kwashiorkor occurs during the second year of life in children suddenly weaned to a diet very low in protein and high in carbohydrate. The hair changes are grossly similar to those in marasmus, but there are more anagen follicles although most are atrophic [2]. The differences between the findings in these two states of malnutrition may be related to the degree and rapidity of protein deprivation. In both states, the hair is brittle and easily shed, and partial or complete alopecia may occur; the hair is lustreless and if normally black, may assume a reddish tinge [4,5]. Many hair shafts may show constrictions, which increase their vulnerability to trauma. Hair cuticle changes which are observed in the electron microscope appear not to contribute usefully to nutritional assessment [6].

Hair changes have been reported in anorexia nervosa, where low calorie intake is usually associated with a diet high in vegetables containing vitamin A. Lurie [7] described acquired pili torti and hair loss in a group of 17 anorexic teenagers.

Surveys of hair-root morphology may provide a simple and inexpensive way of assessing the nutritional status of a community [8,9], but root changes reflect only relatively gross differences [10].

Iron deficiency is occasionally associated with diffuse alopecia, even in the absence of anaemia. The association is often difficult to prove because it is not always easy to evaluate other possible factors, but in some cases the apparent response to the administration of iron is convincing [11].

Zinc deficiency resulting from a failure in absorption gives rise to alopecia and cutaneous changes in acrodermatitis enteropathica. Zinc deficiency may result from prolonged parenteral alimentation, giving rise to erythema, scaling, bullae and hair loss [12]. Parenteral alimentation may also cause deficiency of essential fatty acids. This results in erythema, scaling of the scalp and eyebrows, and diffuse alopecia. The remaining hair is dry and unruly, but this may be reversed by the topical application of safflower oil.

Defects of hair growth occur in certain metabolic disorders but the alleged finding of arginosuccinic acid in the urine of patients with monilethrix has been proved to be due to technical error [13,14], and a similar finding claimed in other defects of the hair shaft requires confirmation. Changes resembling trichorrhexis nodosa have been more reliably related to arginosuccinic aciduria.

In homocystinuria [15], which is an inborn error in the metabolic pathways of methionine, the hair is sparse, fine and fair. It appears normal on microscopy but shows an orange–red fluorescence when stained with acridine orange and examined under UV light. Affected children are mentally retarded, have a shuffling, duck-like gait, a malar flush and a wide variety of skeletal defects.

In hereditary orotic aciduria [16], which is a rare inborn error of pyrimidine metabolism characterized by retarded physical and mental development and macrocytic anaemia, the hair is fine, short and sparse.

A genetically determined defect in the incorporation of histidine, tyrosine and arginine into hair keratin has been found in a syndrome in which dry, lustreless, tightly curled hair is associated with flat, fragile, dystrophic nails and enamel hypoplasia of the teeth [17].

REFERENCES

1 Gummer CL. Diet and hair loss. In: Maibach H, Rook AJ, eds. *Seminars in Dermatology*, Vol. 4. New York: Thieme–Stratton, 1985: 53–64.
2 Bradfield RB, Bailey MA. Hair root response to under-nutrition. In: Montagna W, Dobson RL, eds. *Hair Growth*. Oxford: Pergamon, 1968: 109–19.
3 Bradfield RB, Cordario A, Graham GG. Hair root adaptation to marasmus. *Lancet* 1969; **ii**: 1395–6.
4 El-Hefnawi H, Shukri AS, Rashed A. Kwashiorkor in the United Arab Republic. *Br J Dermatol* 1965; **77**: 137–50.
5 Sims RT. Hair growth in kwashiorkor. *Arch Dis Child* 1967; **42**: 397–400.
6 Bradfield RB, Montagna W. Scanning electron microscopy in assessment of protein-calorie malnutrition (Letter). *Lancet* 1974; **ii**: 1026.
7 Lurie R, Danziger Y, Kaplan Y *et al.* Acquired pili torti—a structural hair shaft defect in anorexia nervosa. *Cutis* 1996; **57**: 151–6.

8 Bradfield RB. Hair tissue as a medium for the differential diagnosis of protein-calorie malnutrition. *J Pediatr* 1974; **89**: 294.

9 Bradfield RB, Gray SO. Simplified procedure for field preparation of hair DNA specimens (Letter). *Lancet* 1975; **i**: 406.

10 Johnson AA, Lotham MC, Rue DA. Hair root morphology in the assessment of protein-calorie malnutrition. *J Invest Dermatol* 1975; **65**: 311–14.

11 Comaish JS. Metabolic disorders and hair growth. *Br J Dermatol* 1971; **84**: 83–5.

12 Weismann K. Zinc metabolism and skin. In: Rook A, Savin J, eds. *Recent Advances in Dermatology.* Edinburgh: Churchill Livingstone, 1980: 109–14.

13 Comaish JS. Aminogenic alopecia (Letter). *Lancet* 1966; **i**: 97.

14 Efron ML, Hoefnagel D. Arginosuccinic acid in monilethrix. *Lancet* 1966; **i**: 321–2.

15 Carson NAJ, Dent CE, Field CMB. Homocystinuria. *J Pediatr* 1965; **66**: 565–83.

16 Becroft DNO, Phillips LI. Hereditary orotic aciduria and megaloblastic anaemia. *Br Med J* 1965; **i**: 546–52.

17 Robinson GC, Miller JR, Worth JR. Hereditary enamel hypoplasia with characteristic hair structure. *Pediatrics* 1966; **37**: 498–502.

Chronic diffuse alopecia [1,2]

More or less evenly distributed loss of hair occurring continuously, but sometimes fluctuating in severity, is common in both sexes. It is seen more frequently in women over the age of 25 years, either because certain forms occur more often in women or because women are more eager to seek advice.

'Chronic diffuse alopecia' is not an acceptable diagnosis. This clinical state may be brought about by a number of different factors, singly or in combination; in many cases no fully convincing cause can be established, but the majority are probably variants of androgenetic alopecia.

A factor that is usually ignored, but which probably makes a significant if small contribution in many cases, is the diffuse reduction in follicle density which occurs from the third decade onwards.

Other factors that must be carefully assessed in each case are as follows:

1 *Androgenetic alopecia.* Endocrine investigations, notably the estimation of plasma testosterone levels (free and total) have shown that androgenetic alopecia is common in women. The diagnosis has tended to be overlooked when, as is usually the case, the pattern of loss is a diffuse frontovertical thinning differing from the typical, more sharply bitemporal and vertical alopecia seen in men. The latter occurs in women only when androgen output approaches the male levels. In the authors' experience, the great majority of women presenting with chronic diffuse alopecia have androgenetic alopecia as the principal or only defect.

2 *Other endocrine factors.* Hypothyroidism is a relatively frequent factor in some series of cases but there are regional variations in its prevalence and it is often diagnosed on inadequate evidence. Hyperthyroidism, hypopituitarism and perhaps diabetes mellitus are occasionally incriminated. Diffuse hair loss has appeared to be related to oophorectomy, but there is no evidence that it follows a normal menopause.

3 *Telogen effluvium.* Acute telogen effluvium following 3 or 4 months after a clearly defined episode such as childbirth or severe stress is not a diagnostic problem, but it is uncertain whether prolonged emotional stress can maintain an increased rate of hair loss by the regular precipitation of small numbers of follicles prematurely into telogen. A high telogen count alone does not establish this diagnosis, for high counts may be found in hypothyroidism, protein deficiency and in other conditions, including androgenetic alopecia.

4 *Chemical agents.* The chemicals known to produce hair loss are mentioned on page 2915. It is probable that others may have a similar effect; amphetamines have been suspected.

5 *Nutritional deficiency.*

6 *Impaired liver function.* In many patients with impaired liver function from hepatitis or cirrhosis, the telogen ratio is increased and in some there is clinically evident alopecia. Disturbed amino-acid metabolism has been postulated as its cause.

7 *Severe chronic illness* may be associated with alopecia. Neoplastic disease may result in mild or moderate alopecia, the severity of which cannot as yet be related to such factors as the degree of anaemia or of cachexia, and which may prove to be determined by secondary endocrine effects. Occasionally, alopecia may be a presenting symptom of neoplasia, for example Hodgkin's disease, either owing to increased telogen shedding or from specific tumour infiltration, i.e. alopecia neoplastica.

8 *Chronic diffuse alopecia of unknown origin.* When all these factors have been excluded, many cases remain unexplained, the majority of them in women aged 30–50 years. The age group concerned, the occasional association with seborrhoea and the reduction in hair-shaft diameter, of which the patient herself is sometimes aware, suggest that further studies of androgen metabolism may be informative, but in some cases testosterone excretion has already been shown to be within normal limits. However, the intermediary metabolism of androgen may prove to be abnormal.

This group of unexplained cases certainly does not represent a single uniform entity. In some, the alopecia fluctuates in severity over months or years but eventually recovers more or less completely. In others, notably those in whom the hair is becoming finer, the alopecia tends to be progressive, although often occurring extremely slowly.

This group of cases includes what may be a distinct clinical entity and which has been so regarded in some countries for many years under the name of 'widow's cap alopecia'. The patients are postmenopausal women, and the alopecia, which has been shown not to be androgen dependent, is markedly accentuated on the vertex rather than in the whole frontovertical region as in androgenetic alopecia.

Some women who are deeply distressed about 'loss of hair' show no evidence of alopecia or at least no greater sparsity than their uncomplaining contemporaries; this is known as the dysmorphophobic state. Some such women are often depressed and others are in need of help with other psychological or psychiatric problems; the psychiatric diagnosis, dysmorphophobia, must always be considered—this is important because suicide may be a sequel.

REFERENCES

1 Simpson NR. Diffuse alopecia. In: Dawber RPR, ed. *Diseases of the Hair and Scalp*, 3rd edn. Oxford: Blackwell Science, 1997.
2 Fiedler V, Hafeez A. Diffuse alopecia. In: Olsen E, ed. *Disorders of Hair Growth*. New York: McGraw-Hill, 1994: 241–56.

Alopecia in central nervous system disorders

Alopecia has been described in association with a number of diseases of the central nervous system but in many instances the association was probably fortuitous. There are four forms of hair loss in which the association appears to be valid, although the mechanism is unknown.
1 Total and permanent alopecia has accompanied lesions of the mid-brain and brainstem [1]—a glioma in the region of the hypothalamus or post-encephalitic damage to the mid-brain.
2 Temporary diffuse alopecia may follow head injuries, particularly in children [2] and may be associated with reversible hirsutism.
3 Total loss of hair occurred at about annual intervals for 20 years in a patient with syringomyelia and syringobulbia [3].
4 Androgenetic baldness occurs early in myotonic dystrophy [4]. A genetic linkage rather than a direct effect of the neurological changes is probably concerned.

Piloerection [5]

Episodes of piloerection may occur in patients with lesions close to the hypothalamus or involving some portion of the limbic system, but the symptom has no precise localizing value.

REFERENCES

1 Hoff H, Riehl G. Alopecia in lesions of the midbrain and brain stem. *Arch Dermatol Syphilol* 1937; **176**: 196–9.
2 Tarnow G. Diffuse alopecia following a head injury. *Neurovis Relat* 1971; **X** (Suppl.): 549–51.
3 Mikula F, Stiedl L. Total alopecia in syringomyelia and syringobulbia. *Dermatol Wochenschr* 1961; **143**: 543–5.
4 Waring JJ, Walker CE. Studies in dystrophia myotonica. *Ann Intern Med* 1940; **65**: 763–99.
5 Brody LA. Piloerection associated with hypothalamic lesions. *Neurology* 1960; **10**: 993–4.

Alopecia areata

Aetiology [1]. Alopecia areata (AA) accounts for about 2% of new dermatological outpatient attendances in the UK and the USA. It is not at present possible to attribute all or indeed any case of AA to a single cause. Among the many factors that appear to be implicated in at least a proportion of cases are the patient's genetic constitution, the atopic state, non-specific immune and organ-specific autoimmune reactions, and possibly emotional stress. The process can be inhibited to a variable extent by several very different therapeutic measures: corticosteroids; local irritants; photochemotherapy; induction of contact dermatitis, or by cyclosporin [2]. The different chemistries and modes of action of these therapies have opened new channels of research. However, the subsequent studies have done little more than reinforce the generally held belief that both genetic predisposition and the atopic state influence prognosis, but the triggering mechanisms remain obscure.

Genetic factors. The incidences of a family history of AA have been reported as 4–27% [3,4]. The mode of inheritance is thought to be autosomal dominant with variable penetrance. Racial factors may also be important, as Arnold [5] found AA disproportionately common among Japanese in Hawaii.

There have been several studies of AA in twins, with some pairs showing concurrence of onset [6]. HLA studies have shown conflicting results. Orecchia *et al.* [7] showed increased prevalence of HLA-DR5, which was linked to disease severity in 127 patients, but these workers failed to demonstrate any difference in class I HLA markers when compared with a control population [8]. Association with DR5, and more frequently DR4, has been noted in subsequent studies [9]. Colombe *et al.* [10] have recently demonstrated that the HLA associations are most pronounced with chronic forms of AA. Long-standing patchy AA is associated with DQ3, and long-standing alopecia totalis or universalis have additional associations with DR4, DR5, DR11 and DQ7.

The association between AA and the atopic state was noted by Robinson and Tasker [11]. Many other studies have since confirmed this link [12,13].

Du Vivier and Munro [14] found 60 cases of AA among 1000 patients with Down's syndrome but only one in 1000 of mentally retarded controls; in 25 of the 60 cases, the alopecia was total or universal. Down's syndrome patients are known to be susceptible to autoimmunity in general.

Autoimmunity [15]. There is widespread agreement with the hypothesis that AA is an autoimmune disease despite the fact that the evidence is at best circumstantial. Support has come from three main areas of research: association with autoimmune diseases, humoral immunity and cell-mediated immunity.

Thyroid disease is the most frequently described disease in association with AA, but the published figures are contradictory. Muller and Winkelmann [12], in the largest study reported to date, found evidence of thyroid disease in 8% of 736 cases compared with less than 2% in the control population in North America. Milgraum *et al.* [16] found 24% of 45 children under 16 years with AA to have abnormal thyroid function tests and/or elevation of thyroid microsomal antibody levels. Reliable statistics based on the prospective study of large numbers of patients are lacking. Kern [17] has found a statistically significant association between AA and Hashimoto's disease, pernicious anaemia and Addison's disease. Brown *et al.* [18] have suggested an increased incidence of autoimmune and gonadal disease in male AA patients, but these findings remain unconfirmed. The association of vitiligo with AA is accepted by most authors. Muller and Winkelmann [12] reported an incidence of 4%.

The following disorders, all of a possible immunological nature, have also been reported in association with AA: pernicious anaemia, systemic lupus erythematosus and rheumatoid arthritis, polymyalgia rheumatica, myasthenia gravis, ulcerative colitis, lichen planus and the *Candida* endocrinopathy syndrome [3,19].

1 *Humoral immunity.* Studies of organ-specific antibodies in AA have given conflicting results, perhaps due to small groups of patients and controls and differing methodology [20]. Galbraith *et al.* [21] also found an increase in thyroid autoantibodies. Friedmann [3,20], in a controlled study of 229 cases, reported increased frequencies of thyroid antibodies in 30% of females and 10% of males, and an increased frequency of gastric parietal cell antibodies, which tended to be more common in males. In 45 children under 16 years of age with AA, Milgraum *et al.* [16] found detectable antibody levels to thyroid microsomal elements (11%), smooth muscle (16%) and parietal cells (4%). Using the DEBR rat model of AA, McElwee *et al.* [22] demonstrated follicular autoantibodies evolving in parallel with clinical disease.

2 *Cell-mediated immunity.* Studies of cell-mediated immunity in AA also yield an inconsistent picture; again, small studies have led to conflicting results. Circulating total T-cell numbers have been reported as reduced [23] or normal [24]. Suppressor T-cell numbers have been variously reported as reduced, normal, or increased [24]. Gu *et al.* [25] also reported an increase in non-antigen-specific spontaneous and antibody-dependent cell-mediated cytotoxic responses of peripheral blood lymphocytes. Friedmann [20] attempted to resolve this conflict by suggesting that while there is general agreement that a reduction in numbers of circulating T cells occurs in AA, the level of reduction is related to disease severity. Similarly, the impairment of helper T-cell function and the change in suppressor T-cell numbers may also reflect changes in disease activity.

The strongest direct evidence for autoimmunity comes from the consistent findings of a lymphocytic infiltrate in and around hair follicles, and Langerhans' cells have also

been seen in the peribulbar region [26]. Biopsies from scalps of patients treated with the contact allergen diphencyprone, or oral and topical minoxidil [27] have shown a reduction in the peribulbar T-cell population in regrowing AA, but no change in the absence of regrowth. Direct immunofluorescent examination has failed to demonstrate antifollicle antibodies in affected scalps. Friedmann [23] was unable to demonstrate a response of lymphocytes from patients with AA to crude scalp extract *in vitro*. Messenger and Bleehen [28] reported ectopic expression of MHC type II antigen HLA-DR by epithelial cells in the presumptive cortex and root sheaths of hair follicles in active lesions of AA. This is thought to represent a mechanism through which cells may present their own specific surface antigens to sensitized MHC-restricted T-inducer cells.

Therefore, AA appears to belong to the group of organ-specific autoimmune diseases [29]. There is a shared hereditary susceptibility, organ-specific antibodies occur with increased frequency in patients with AA, and there is altered T-cell regulation of the immune response. However, unlike most organ-specific autoimmune diseases, direct activity against hair follicle components has yet to be demonstrated. Further research in this area is obviously required. Prospective long-term studies and the relationship between lymphocyte and disease activity [20] are worthy of further attention.

Infection. Recent work examining the possibility of cytomegalovirus infection in AA has been inconclusive, with both positive [30] and negative findings [31].

Emotional stress. A wealth of case-lore suggests that stress may be an important precipitating factor in some cases of AA. Attempts at objective evaluation using standard psychiatric procedures such as the Rorschach test showed over 90% of patients with AA to be psychologically abnormal and up to 29% to have psychological factors and family situations that may have affected the onset or course of the disease [4]. Alleged cures by suggestion or sleep therapy [32] have been claimed to support the stress hypothesis. The findings of Ferraro [33] using the Bernereuter personality index in AA showed 'feelings of inferiority, introspection and a need for encouragement'.

REFERENCES

1 Messenger A, Simpson NB. Alopecia areata. In: Dawber RPR, ed. *Diseases of the Hair and Scalp*, 3rd edn. Oxford: Blackwell Science, 1997: 545–85.
2 Gupta AK, Ellis CN, Cooper KD *et al.* Oral cyclosporine for the treatment of alopecia areata. A clinical and immuno-histochemical analysis. *J Am Acad Dermatol* 1990; **22**: 242–8.
3 Friedmann PS. Alopecia areata and autoimmunity. *Br J Dermatol* 1981; **105**: 153–7.
4 De-Waard-Van der Spek FB, Oranje AP, De Raeymaecker DM *et al.* Juvenile versus maturity-onset alopecia areata—a comparative retrospective clinical study. *Clin Exp Dermatol* 1989; **14**: 429–36.

5 Arnold HL. Alopecia areata; prevalence in Japanese and prognosis after reassurance. *Arch Dermatol Syphilol* 1952; **66**: 191–7.

6 Weidmann AI, Zion LS, Mamelok AE. Alopecia areata occurring simultaneously in identical twins. *Arch Dermatol* 1956; **74**: 424–32.

7 Orecchia G, Belvedere MC, Martinetti M *et al.* Human leukocyte antigen region involvement in the genetic predisposition to alopecia areata. *Dermatologica* 1987; **175**: 10–15.

8 Kuntz BM, Selzle D, Braun-Falco O *et al.* HLA antigens in alopecia areata. *Arch Dermatol* 1977; **113**: 1716.

9 Devic 1991.

10 Colombe BW, Price VH, Khoury EL *et al.* HLA Class II antigen associations help to define two types of alopecia areata. *J Am Acad Dermatol* 1995; **33**: 757–61.

11 Robinson SS, Tasker S. Alopecia areata associated with neuro-dermatitis. *Urol Cutan Rev* 1948; **52**: 468–73.

12 Muller SA, Winkelmann RK. Alopecia areata. *Arch Dermatol* 1963; **88**: 290.

13 Young E, Bruns HM, Berrens L. Alopecia areata and atopy (Proceedings). *Dermatologica* 1978; **156**: 308–16.

14 Du Vivier A, Munro DD. Alopecia areata, autoimmunity and Down's syndrome. *Br Med J* 1975; **1**: 191–4.

15 Muller HK, Rook AJ, Kubba R. Immunohistology and autoantibody studies in alopecia areata. *Br J Dermatol* 1980; **102**: 609–15.

16 Milgraum SS, Mitchell AJ, Bacon GE *et al.* Alopecia areata, endocrine function and autoantibodies in patients 16 years of age or younger. *J Am Acad Dermatol* 1987; **17**: 57–61.

17 Kern F. Laboratory evaluation of patients with alopecia areata. In: Brown AC, ed. *First Human Hair Symposium*. New York: Medcom, 1974: 222–40.

18 Brown AC, Follard ZF, Jarrett WH. Ocular and testicular abnormalities in alopecia areata. *Arch Dermatol* 1982; **118**: 546–9.

19 Brenner W, Diem E, Gschnait F. Coincidence of vitiligo, alopecia, onychodystrophy, localised scleroderma and lichen planus. *Dermatologica* 1979; **159**: 356–60.

20 Friedmann PS. Clinical and immunologic associations of alopecia areata. *Semin Dermatol* 1985; **4**: 9–24.

21 Galbraith GMP, Thiers BH, Vasaly DV *et al.* Immunological profiles in alopecia areata. *Br J Dermatol* 1984; **110**: 163–70.

22 McElwee KJ, Pickett P, Oliver RF. The DEBR rat, alopecia areata and autoantibodies to the hair follicle. *Br J Dermatol* 1996; **134**: 55–63.

23 Friedmann PS. Decreased lymphocyte reactivity and autoimmunity in alopecia areata. *Br J Dermatol* 1981; **105**: 145–52.

24 Hordinsky MK, Hollgren H, Nelson D *et al.* Suppressor cell number and function in alopecia areata. *Arch Dermatol* 1984; **120**: 188–95.

25 Gu SQ, Ros AM, Thyresson N *et al.* Spontaneous cell-mediated cytotoxicity (SCMC) in patients with alopecia universalis. *Acta Derm Venereol (Stockh)* 1981; **61**: 434–9.

26 Wiesner-Menzel L, Happle R. Intrabulbar and peribulbar accumulation of dendritic OKT 6-positive cells in alopecia areata. *Arch Dermatol Res* 1984; **276**: 333.

27 Fiedler-Weiss VC, Buys CM. Response to minoxidil in severe alopecia areata correlates with T lymphocyte stimulation. *Br J Dermatol* 1987; **117**: 759–65.

28 Messenger AG, Bleehen SS. Expression of HLA-DR by anagen hair follicles in alopecia areata. *J Invest Dermatol* 1985; **85**: 569–76.

29 Hordinsky MK. Alopecia areata. In: Olsen EA, ed. *Disorders of Hair Growth*. New York: McGraw-Hill, 1994: 195–222.

30 Skinner RB, Jr, Light WH, Bale GF *et al.* Alopecia areata and the presence of cytomegalovirus DNA. *JAMA* 1995; **273**: 1419–20.

31 Tosti A, Gentilomi G, Venturoli S *et al.* No correlation between cyto-megalovirus and alopecia areata. *J Invest Dermatol* 1996; **107**: 443.

32 Martin P, Levy A, Minvielle H *et al.* Application de la médecine psychosomatique à la dermatologie. *Presse Méd* 1959; **67**: 461–5.

33 Ferraro S. Il Bernereuter Personality Inventory in ammelati di area Celsi. *Clinical Dermatol* 1979; **10**: 51–5.

Experimental AA. There have been many unsuccessful attempts to induce patches of alopecia areata experimentally [1]. Friedmann [2] proposed that the athymic nude mouse might be a useful model in which to study alopecia areata. Sawada *et al.* [3] showed that cyclosporin, a potent modulator of T-cell activity, stimulated hair growth of nude mice. Gilhar [4] reported that hair grafts from patients with alopecia areata and alopecia universalis were transplanted successfully onto athymic nude mice and that hair growth within the grafts could be stimulated by cyclosporin. Interesting work in progress includes the alopecia (DEBR) rat [5], which loses hair in association with a marked perifollicular and intrafollicular infiltrate.

REFERENCES

1 Thiers W, Klaschka F. Tierexperimentelle Sensibilisingsstudien als Beitrag zur Pathogenese der Alopecia areata. *Arch Klin Exp Dermatol* 1970; **237**: 51–8.

2 Freidmann PS. Clinical and immunologic associations of alopecia areata. *Semin Dermatol* 1985; **4**: 9–24.

3 Sawada M, Terada N, Taniguchi R *et al.* Cyclosporin A stimulates hair growth in nude mice. *Lab Invest* 1987; **56**: 684–91.

4 Gilhar A, Pillar T, Etzioni A. The effect of topical cyclosporin on the immediate shedding of human scalp hair grafted onto nude mice. *Br J Dermatol* 1988; **119**: 767–74.

5 Michie HJ, Jahoda CAB, Oliver RF, Johnson BE. The DEBR rat: an animal model of human alopecia areata. *Br J Dermatol* 1991; **125**: 94–100.

Pathology and pathodynamics. Eckert *et al.* [1] proposed that AA progresses as a wave of follicles which enter telogen prematurely, and this has become the generally accepted view. Anagen/telogen ratios vary considerably with the stage and duration of the disease process. Biopsy specimens taken early in the course of the disease show the majority of follicles in telogen or late catagen. Some anagen hair bulbs are situated at a higher level in the dermis than normal [2]; a peribulbar lymphocytic infiltrate is seen around follicles, this being more dense in early lesions; the infiltrate consists predominantly of T cells, with increased numbers of Langerhans' cells. The infiltrate disappears during regrowth but the sequence of events is unknown. Established lesions show no decrease in follicle numbers. Anagen development is halted when the inner root sheath

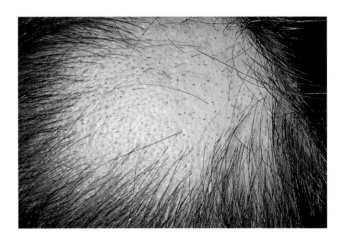

Fig. 66.28 Alopecia areata. A single scalp patch with many marginal short, broken 'exclamation-mark' hairs (see also Fig. 66.29)

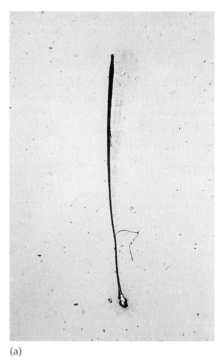

(a)

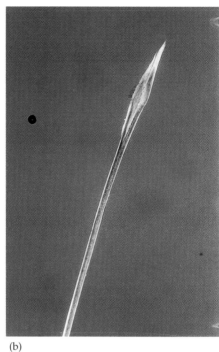

(b)

Fig. 66.29 Alopecia areata. (a) A plucked 'exclamation-mark' hair (see Fig. 66.28) from an active progressing area. (b) The distal end of an exclamation-mark hair has a greater calibre than proximally.

has assumed a conical shape, with evidence of early cortical differentiation but no cortical keratinization. This stage is equivalent to anagen III. Characteristic abnormalities of the hair shaft in AA have been recognized for over a century. Exclamation-mark hairs (Figs 66.28 & 66.29) are the main feature, although they are not invariably present. They are thought to be club hairs of normal calibre and pigmentation, but the distal ends are ragged and frayed [3,4]. Below their broken tips they taper towards a small but otherwise normal club. Similar hairs can be found in trichotillomania, although the imprecise diagnostic criteria of trichotillomania can make it difficult to distinguish from alopecia areata in some instances. In areas showing early regrowth, some follicles contain multiple fine hair shafts. The single consistent histological feature is the presence of a dense, peribulbar and intrafollicular lymphocytic infiltrate. The upper, permanent portion of the hair follicle may also be involved in the infiltrate either in anagen or telogen. Messenger and Bleehen [5] found that lesional anagen follicles demonstrated injury, which was confined to keratinocytes in the presumptive cortex. In an extension of this work, Messenger *et al.* [6] proposed a hypothetical model that satisfied the histological evidence to explain the formation of exclamation-mark hairs and the non-destructive nature of the disease.

In an electron-microscopic study of AA, Messenger and Bleehen [5] showed the lesional anagen follicles had evidence of non-specific injury to matrix cells around the upper pole of the dermal papilla and to cells of the presumptive cortex. These workers also confirmed the presence of degenerative changes in the suprapapillary

matrix. Messenger and Bleehen [7] demonstrated aberrant expression of HLA-DR in cells of the precortical matrix and presumptive cortex. Messenger *et al.* [6] suggested that the presence of HLA-DR antigen in cells of the precortical matrix provided evidence that this site could be of fundamental importance in the pathogenesis of AA and may be the primary target for the disease process.

The concept of fundamental damage occurring in the cells of the precortical matrix and the presumptive cortex does permit explanation of the alterations in the hair cycle. AA affects the follicle in anagen but does not cause an abrupt cessation of mitotic activity in the matrix. Once in telogen the follicle is thought to be 'safe' but when re-entry into anagen takes place the attack is resumed, anagen development can go no further, and the follicle returns prematurely to telogen. There is therefore a cyclical process, which may explain why follicles are not destroyed permanently. The variations observed in the number of normal telogen hairs, dystrophic hairs and exclamation-mark hairs were interpreted by Messenger *et al.* [6], who postulated that the follicle can respond in three different ways to pathological trauma depending on the severity of the insult. At its most severe, the process damages and weakens the hair in the keratogenous zone and at the same time precipitates the follicle into catagen and then telogen. Such hairs break when the keratogenous zone reaches the surface of the scalp; these are later extruded as exclamation-mark hairs. Alternatively, a follicle may simply be precipitated into normal catagen and subsequently be shed as a club hair. Such follicles may then produce dystrophic anagen hairs. Finally, it is possible that some follicles are injured just sufficiently to induce dystrophic changes, while they continue to grow in the anagen phase.

REFERENCES

1 Eckert J, Church RE, Ebling FJ. The pathogenesis of alopecia areata. *Br J Dermatol* 1968; **80**: 203–11.
2 Van Scott EJ, Ekel TM. Geometric relationships between the matrix of the hair bulb and its dermal papilla in normal and alopecia scalp. *J Invest Dermatol* 1958; **31**: 281–90.
3 Jackson D, Church RE, Ebling FJ. Alopecia areata hairs. A scanning electron microscopic study. *Br J Dermatol* 1971; **85**: 242–6.
4 Peereboom-Wynia JDR, Koerten HK, van Joost TH *et al*. Scanning electron microscopy comparing exclamation mark hairs in alopecia areata with normal hair fibres mechanically broken by traction. *Clin Exp Dermatol* 1989; **14**: 47–56.
5 Messenger AG, Bleehen SS. Alopecia areata: light and electron microscopic pathology of the regrowing white hair. *Br J Dermatol* 1984; **110**: 155–64.
6 Messenger AG, Slater DN, Bleehen SS. Alopecia areata: alterations in the hair growth cycle and correlation with the follicular pathology. *Br J Dermatol* 1986; **114**: 337–46.
7 Messenger AG, Bleehen SS. Expression of HLA-DR by anagen hair follicles in alopecia areata. *J Invest Dermatol* 1985; **85**: 569–80.

Heterogeneity. Most authorities have regarded AA as a clinicopathological entity, but the bewildering variety of its associated diseases and unpredictability of its course would be more readily explained if AA was a heterogeneous clinical syndrome. This view was shared by Mitchell and Krull [1]. Ikeda [2] proposed a classification that takes into account other clinical features in addition to the alopecia itself. Studies in the Netherlands [3] and in the UK [4] have in general supported Ikeda's hypothesis and suggested that there may be considerable geographical variation in the relative incidence of the various types of AA.

Ikeda's four types may be categorized as follows (as recorded in Japan).

Type I. The common type accounted for 83% of patients. It occurred mainly between the ages of 20 and 40 years, and usually ran a total course of less than 3 years. Individual patches tended to regrow in less than 6 months, and alopecia totalis developed in only 6%.

Type II. The atopic type accounted for 10% of patients. The onset was usually in childhood and the disease ran a lengthy course in excess of 10 years. Individual patches tended to persist for a year and alopecia totalis developed in 75%.

Type III. The prehypertensive type (4%) occurred mainly in young adults and ran a rapid course with an incidence of alopecia totalis in 39% of patients.

Type IV. The 'combined' type (5%) occurred mainly in patients over 40 years and ran a prolonged course, but resulted in alopecia totalis in only 10% of patients.

There has been little support for Ikeda's prehypertensive type, but most authors agree that the presence of atopy confers a poor prognosis and slow rate of remission. Almost all the published work on AA considers it to be a single entity. The clinical description below follows this convention, as Ikeda's approach to the disease has not

yet been applied sufficiently widely for its validity to be established.

REFERENCES

1 Mitchell AJ, Krull EA. Alopecia areata: pathogenesis and treatment. *J Am Acad Dermatol* 1984; **11**: 763–74.
2 Ikeda T. A new classification of alopecia areata. *Dermatologica* 1965; **113**: 421–45.
3 De-Waard Van der Spek FB, Oranje AP, De Raeymaecker DM *et al*. Juvenile versus maturity-onset alopecia areata—a comparative retrospective clinical study. *Clin Exp Dermatol* 1989; **14**: 429–36.
4 Rook AJ. Common baldness and alopecia areata. In: Rook AJ, ed. *Recent Advances in Dermatology*, Vol. 4. Edinburgh: Churchill Livingstone, 1977: 223–44.

Age and sex incidence [1–3]. The available statistics are all based on hospital attendance figures and therefore do not reflect the true incidence of AA. The reported sex incidence has varied widely, from males outnumbering females by 3 to 1 [4], through equality [5], to twice as common in females [6]. In an investigation in Italy confined to children with AA [7], less than 1% of 213 cases began in the first year, and the peak incidence was in the fourth and fifth years. Onset before the age of 2 years was recorded in under 2% of 736 cases in North America [5].

In summary, if all clinical variants of AA are grouped together, the hospital statistics of most countries show that the sexes are approximately equally affected, and that the onset occurs at any age, with a peak decade lying at some point between the ages of 20 and 50 years.

REFERENCES

1 Anderson I. Alopecia areata: a clinical study. *Br Med J* 1950; **ii**: 250–4.
2 Gip L, Lodin A, Molin L. Alopecia areata. *Acta Derm Venereol (Stockh)* 1969; **49**: 180–4.
3 Lopez B. Contribucíon al conocimiento de la etiopatogenia y tratamiento de la pelada. *Actas Derm Siffilogr* 1951; **42**: 589–94.
4 Bastos Araujo A, Poiares Baptista A. Algunas consideracions sobre 300 casos de pelada. *Trab Soc Portuges Dermatol Venereol* 1967; **15**; 135–9.
5 Muller SA, Winkelmann RK. Alopecia areata. *Arch Dermatol* 1963; **88**: 290–7.
6 Friedmann PS. Clinical and immunologic associations of alopecia areata. *Semin Dermatol* 1985; **4**: 9–14.
7 Bessone L. Rilievi statistici sull'alopecia nell'infanzia. *Aggiornament Pediatr* 1965; **16**: 1.

Clinical features. The characteristic initial lesion of AA is commonly a circumscribed, totally bald, smooth patch (Fig. 66.28); it is often noticed by chance by a parent, hairdresser or friend. Exclamation-mark hairs (Fig. 66.29) may be present at its margin, where hairs that appear normal may also be very readily extracted [1]. Subsequent progress is very varied; the initial patch may regrow within a few months, or further patches may appear after an interval of 3–6 weeks and then in a cyclical fashion. These intervals are of varying duration. A succession of discrete patches may rapidly become confluent by the diffuse loss of remaining hair. In some cases, the initial hair loss is diffuse and total denudation of the scalp has been reported

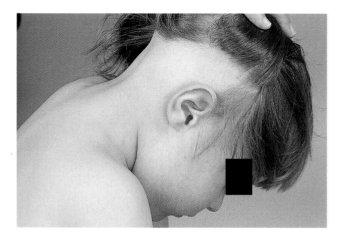

Fig. 66.30 Marginal alopecia areata. Poor prognostic ophiasis ('serpentine') pattern.

within 48 h. However, diffuse hair loss may occur over part or the whole of the scalp without the development of bald areas. Regrowth is often at first fine and unpigmented, but usually the hairs gradually resume their normal calibre and colour. Regrowth in one region of the scalp may occur while the alopecia is extending in others.

The scalp is the first affected site in over 60% of cases. In dark-haired men, patches in the beard are conspicuous and in such individuals are often the first to be noticed. The eyebrows and eyelashes are lost in many cases of AA and may be the only sites affected. The term alopecia totalis is applied to total or almost total loss of scalp hair and alopecia universalis is the loss of all body hair. The extension of alopecia along the scalp margin is known as ophiasis (Fig. 66.30). AA strictly confined to one-half of the body has been reported after a head injury [2].

Progress. Rook [3] highlighted the gloomy outlook for the sufferer of AA. Further evidence of heterogeneity in AA is provided by the difference in prognosis reported from various countries. In Chicago [4], the duration of the initial attack was less than 6 months in 33% of patients and less than 1 year in 50%, but 33% never recovered from the initial attack. The incidence of relapse in the whole of this series of 230 patients was 86%, but in those followed up for 20 years it was 100%. Of those patients developing AA before puberty, 50% became totally bald and none recovered. In contrast, only 25% of those developing AA after puberty became totally bald and 5.3% recovered. Muller and Winkelmann [5] from the Mayo Clinic reported that only 1% of the children and 10% of adults with alopecia totalis showed complete regrowth. Schmitt [6] reported complete recovery of alopecia universalis in only 10 of 50 patients, the poorer prognosis being in cases of prepubertal onset. In no case of AA is a completely confident prognosis justifiable; one woman, who lost all her hair at 16 years of age, failed to regrow it despite eight pregnancies, but recovered it almost completely at the age of 50 [7].

Undoubtedly, AA in the atopic state has a poor prognosis, and if hair loss is total before puberty it is unlikely to regrow permanently. AA at any age in a non-atopic subject may be given a reasonably good prognosis providing it has remained circumscribed for over 6 months. The ophiasic pattern of AA deserves its bad reputation, associated with atopy [8].

White hair in alopecia areata. Klingmüller [2] showed that white hairs were spared initially by the disease process. Patients with sudden diffuse onset of AA would appear to 'go white' over the course of a few days [9] (see below); this has been reported in several famous historical personalities [9]. Regrowing hair is often temporarily unpigmented (Fig. 66.31).

Associated clinical changes. Nail involvement in AA has been reviewed by Baran and Dawber [10]. The reported incidence of nail dystrophy (Chapter 65) in AA ranges from 7 to 66%. The nail involvement varies from marked alteration of the nails to diffuse, fine pitting (Fig. 66.32). It may involve the majority of nails, but solitary nail involvement may also occur. Gross nail dystrophy is said to be proportional to the degree of hair loss [8]. Onychodystrophy may precede or follow resolution of the AA. Surface modifications include ridging with frequent onychorrhexis, cross fissures, Beau's lines or transverse lines of uniform pits which are similar to those seen in psoriasis.

There are many reports of cataracts in association with alopecia totalis. However, Summerly *et al.* [11] found symptomless punctate lens opacities with equal frequency in 58 patients with AA and normal controls. Horner's syndrome, ectopia of the pupil, iris atrophy or tortuosity of the fundal vessels, were reported by Langhof and Lenke [12].

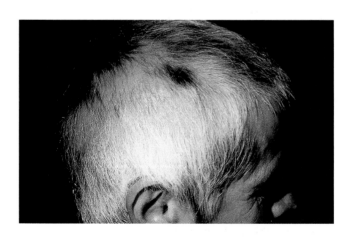

Fig. 66.31 Alopecia areata. Patchy, regrowing, unpigmented hair.

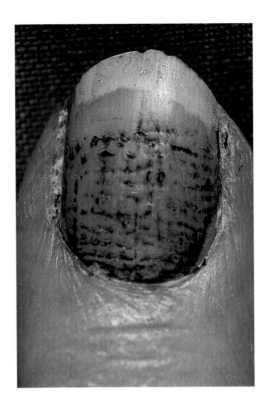

Fig. 66.32 An organized pattern of pitting present on all fingernails 8 months prior to onset of alopecia areata. The pits are highlighted with mascara.

REFERENCES

1 Peereboom-Wynia JDR, Koerten HK, van Joost T *et al*. Scanning E.M. comparing exclamation mark hairs in alopecia areata with normal hair fibres mechanically broken by traction. *Clin Exp Dermatol* 1989; **14**: 47–52.
2 Klingmüller G. Über 'plötzliches Weissworden' und psychische Traumen bei der Alopecia areata. *Dermatologica* 1958; **117**: 84–8.
3 Rook AJ, ed. Common baldness and alopecia areata. In: *Recent Advances in Dermatology*, Vol. 4. Edinburgh: Churchill Livingstone, 1977: 223–44.
4 Walker SA, Rothman S. Alopecia areata. A statistical study and consideration of endocrine influences. *J Invest Dermatol* 1950; **14**: 403–12.
5 Muller SA, Winkelmann RK. Alopecia areata. *Arch Dermatol* 1963; **88**: 290–7.
6 Schmitt CL. Trauma as a factor in the production of alopecia universalis (preliminary report). *Pennsyl Med J* 1953; **56**: 975–7.
7 Freeman KL. Alopecia areata. *Can Med Assoc J* 1952; **67**: 6–10.
8 De-Waard-Van der Spek FB, Oranje AP, De Raeymaecker DM *et al*. Juvenile versus maturity-onset alopecia areata—a comparative retrospective clinical study. *Clin Exp Dermatol* 1989; **14**: 429–35.
9 Helm F, Milgrom H. Can scalp hair suddenly turn white? *Arch Dermatol* 1970; **102**: 162–7.
10 Baran R, Dawber RPR, eds. *Diseases of the Nails and their Management*. Oxford: Blackwell Scientific Publications, 1984: 192–5.
11 Summerly R, Watson DM, Copeman PWM. Alopecia areata and cataracts. *Arch Dermatol* 1966; **93**: 411–14.
12 Langhof H, Lenke L. Ophthalmologische Befunde bei Alopecia areata. *Dermatol Wochenschr* 1962; **146**: 585–8.

Treatment [1–3]. The variable and uncertain natural history of AA accounts for the multiplicity of uncritical claims for a large variety of therapeutic procedures. In order to overcome this problem, workers have tended to choose patients with alopecia totalis or alopecia universalis because these conditions tend to run a more stable course and are traditionally more difficult to treat. Although there is an undoubted relationship between AA and alopecia totalis or alopecia universalis, the latter conditions are not necessarily good models in which to test for therapeutic efficacy in AA. This approach treats AA as a homogeneous entity, which may not be justified [4]. Ikeda's type I might be expected to run a relatively benign course with a high natural remission rate and only 6% developing alopecia totalis, whereas Ikeda's original type II (atopic) group were much less fortunate, with 75% developing alopecia totalis. It seems reasonable, therefore, that future clinical trial designs should, at least, separate the atopic subjects before randomization rather than during analysis.

The sad fact that there is no universally proven treatment for AA is evident from the multiplicity of claims for therapeutic success. The analysable evidence can be divided into four main areas:
1 non-specific irritants, for example dithranol and phenol;
2 'immune inhibitor', for example systemic steroids, PUVA, cyclosporin;
3 'immune enhancers', for example contact dermatitis induction, inosiplex;
4 of unknown action, for example minoxidil.

Counter-irritants. Many have been employed in AA but most studies predate the modern era of clinical trials; therefore, claims of effectiveness for phenol, benzyl benzoate and UVB in erythema doses cannot be substantiated. However, claims for dithranol have some scientific support. Fiedler-Weiss and Buys [5] reported a good cosmetic response in 25% of their patients with severe AA, but all experienced pruritus, local erythema and scaling.

Systemic corticosteroids [6]. Systemic corticosteroids will restore normal hair growth in many cases of AA. The hairs show abrupt repigmentation and thickening without discontinuity of the shaft [7]. Controversy remains, however, as to the justification for prescribing these potentially hazardous drugs, because most cases relapse at some stage during or after withdrawal of treatment. Very high doses up to 100 mg prednisolone daily [8] have been recommended, but universal side-effects due to the steroids were noted, and in this clinical trial more than two-thirds of the patients experienced hair loss after stopping treatment. These problems have prompted other dermatologists to try mixed regimens of systemic, topical and intralesional steroids [9].

Topical and intralesional steroids. Attempts to reduce the hazard of systemic steroids have included both topical and intralesional administration. There have been a number of claims for the effectiveness of topical application using fluocinolone and halcinonide [10]. At best, persistent regrowth occurs in those cases in which it might have been expected to occur spontaneously. In some cases, a troublesome folliculitis may result.

Intralesional steroids have proved more helpful but the positive indications for their use remain limited. Intralesional triamcinolone suspension is preferred either by needle injection or by jet injection [11]. Intralesional corticosteroids have a small but useful role in the management of AA. They can be used to accelerate regrowth in a circumscribed patch of AA that is cosmetically disfiguring or difficult to conceal, and can be useful for maintaining regrowth of the eyebrows in alopecia totalis; but great care must be exercised to avoid steroid side-effects in the eye. Atrophy may be an unsightly complication of intralesional corticosteroids and is usually confined to the injection site [12].

Topical immunotherapy. The use of potent sensitizing chemicals to induce and maintain contact dermatitis of the scalp has produced regrowth of hair in some sufferers of AA with both localized and severe forms. Variable success has been attributed to dinitrochlorobenzene (DNCB), squaric acid dibutyl ester (SADBE) and diphencyprone (DCP), with sporadic reports of success with the plant *Primula obconica* [13–15]. The first report of regrowth after DNCB is attributed to Rosenberg and Drake [16]. Sensitization was induced by painting the skin with a 2% solution of DNCB. The application 10 days later of a 0.1% solution provoked a dermatitis reaction in those patients (the majority) who became sensitized. Weekly applications were then made to the bald areas using the minimum concentration to induce mild inflammatory changes (often as low as 0.0001%). Many clinical trials followed and reported variable success with this drug from 10% up to 78%, the effect being greatest in localized AA and least in alopecia totalis and alopecia universalis. Patients with a family history of AA [17], a personal or family history of atopy, and those who failed to produce a dermatitis reaction, all failed to produce good regrowth. SADBE and DCP are potent sensitizers and free from mutagenic activity (unlike DNCB [18]), and are not likely to be encountered in everyday life or in the workplace. Most authors have used a 2% solution of SADBE in acetone as the sensitizing dose followed by application of the minimum dose to achieve contact dermatitis. Happle *et al.* [3,15] have been the leading advocates for SADBE, with good results in up to 70% of patients. Tosti *et al.* [19] found SADBE no better than placebo in patchy AA. Happle *et al.* [13] have also reported encouraging results with DCP. However, Ashworth *et al.* [20] were less successful.

In recent years, topical DCP has been used as a sensitizer, with much promise in the short term; its limitations are similar to those of other sensitizers [14,21].

The mechanism of action of contact sensitization in AA remains speculative. Two concepts of local immune modulation have been advanced. First, it is proposed that effector T cells are attracted into the area; Happle [17] suggested the occurrence of localized antigen competition and Bröker *et al.* [22] extended this theory to claim that repeated application activates non-specific suppressor mechanisms to suppress the effector cells responsible for AA.

The role for topical contact sensitization in the treatment of AA is limited. Side-effects include pruritus, blistering, secondary infection and urticaria. The rate of response of alopecia totalis seems to be so disappointing long-term that the risks of uncomfortable side-effects probably outweigh any benefits. These methods may be worth trying in patients with tufted, almost total, alopecia and long-standing patchy alopecia.

Photochemotherapy. Rollier and Warcewski [23] reported induction of hair regrowth in AA with 8-methoxypsoralen (8-MOP) and sunlight. Further reports using 8-MOP plus UVA (PUVA) have claimed success for up to 60% of patients [24]. Claudy and Gagnaire [25] reported good responses only when total body irradiation was employed. Lassus *et al.* [24] reported good results in 30% of patients, but 20–40 treatment exposures were necessary to achieve benefit, and all series showed a high relapse rate of 50–90% on stopping therapy. There is a poor response in alopecia totalis. PUVA has many effects on the local immune response within skin, and these may be important in the action of PUVA in AA. One report of successful treatment with topical haematoporphyrin plus UVA [26] has yet to be confirmed. Total body PUVA is probably more effective than local irradiation, but the dose needs to exceed several hundred joules, therefore the treatment is rarely justified [27].

Minoxidil. Minoxidil (2,4-diamino-6-piperidinopyrimidine-3-oxide) is a potent vasodilator widely used in the past for the treatment of severe hypertension. Its oral use is limited because of a reversible but cosmetically unacceptable hypertrichosis of the face, arms and legs [28]. Preliminary reports of a high success rate with topical minoxidil in AA [29] have been followed by double-blind and dose–response studies, which were less encouraging [30]. Tosti *et al.* [19], however, found no difference between a 3% solution of minoxidil and placebo in moderate patchy AA. In a continuation study, a better response was seen after 64 weeks, and Price [31] commented that the outcome was dependent on initial severity. The highest rate has been obtained by 5% topical minoxidil solution [32].

The mechanism of action of minoxidil in AA is also unknown. Evidence points towards an effect on circulating and tissue lymphocytes and hair follicle keratinocytes [32,33]. Topical minoxidil is yet another therapy whose initial promise has not been substantiated.

Immune modulation. Drugs which alter the immune state might be expected to shed some light on the pathogenesis of AA and may also be of therapeutic benefit. Oral cyclosporin, a powerful modulator of T-cell function, produced regrowth in alopecia totalis [34]. However, oral cyclosporin is potentially both nephrotoxic and hepatotoxic. Topical cyclosporin has been tried in concentrations from 5 to 10% (w/v) in various oily excipients and produced sporadic patchy regrowth which was little better than placebo [35]. Lowy and coworkers [36] reported success with oral inosiplex but the effect was lost within 2–3 weeks of cessation. A further double-blind placebo-controlled study showed a better response than placebo; however, only partial regrowth was seen, but growth was maintained in the majority after crossover to placebo [37].

Summary. The decision whether or not to treat AA should be made at an early age. Nothing can justify the prolonged use of expensive placebos. If the prognosis is poor, for example, in a prepubertal atopic with total alopecia, a full explanation and help in adjusting to the problems of wearing a wig will be of far greater value to the child than the false raising of unwarranted hopes. However, in the majority of cases in which the prognosis is good, reassurance, aided if necessary by topical or intralesional corticosteroids, can be advised. Systemic corticosteroids are justifiable only in exceptional circumstances. Of the newer therapies, topical diphencyprone currently seems to show the most promise. It is most logical to treat those patients with an apparently good prognosis (!), to lessen the chances of any relapse after response.

REFERENCES

1 Messenger A, Simpson NR. Alopecia areata. In: Dawber RPR, ed. *Diseases of the Hair and Scalp*, 3rd edn. Oxford: Blackwell Science, 1997.
2 Fiedler VC, Alaiti S. Treatment of alopecia areata. *Dermatol Clin* 1996; **14**; 733–8.
3 Hoffmann R, Happle R. Topical immunotherapy in alopecia areata. *Dermatol Clin* 1996; **14**: 739–44.
4 Ikeda T. A new classification of alopecia areata. *Dermatologica* 1965; **131**: 421–45.
5 Fiedler-Weiss VC, Buys CM. Evaluation of anthralin in the treatment of alopecia areata. *Arch Dermatol* 1987; **123**: 1491–7.
6 Sharma VK. Pulsed administration of corticosteroids in the treatment of alopecia areata. *Int J Dermatol* 1996; **35**: 133–5.
7 Berger RA, Orentreich N. Abrupt changes in hair morphology following corticosteroid therapy in alopecia areata. *Arch Dermatol* 1960; **82**: 408–12.
8 Winter RJ, Kern F, Blizzard EM. Prednisolone therapy for alopecia areata. *Arch Dermatol* 1976; **122**: 1549–83.
9 Unger WP, Schemmer RJ. Corticosteroids in the treatment of alopecia totalis. *Arch Dermatol* 1978; **114**: 1486–92.
10 Montes LF. Topical halcinonide in alopecia areata and in alopecia totalis. *J Cutan Pathol* 1977; **4**: 47–53.
11 Abell E, Munro DD. Intralesional treatment of alopecia areata with triamcinolone acetonide by jet injection. *Br J Dermatol* 1973; **88**: 55–81.
12 Gupta AK, Rasmussen JE. Perilesional linear atrophic streaks associated with intralesional corticosteroid injections in a psoriatic plaque. *Pediatr Dermatol* 1987; **4**: 259–60.
13 Happle R, Hausen BM, Wiesner-Menzel L. Diphencyprone in the treatment of alopecia areata. *Acta Derm Venereol (Stockh)* 1983; **63**: 49–57.
14 Naldi L, Parazzini F, Cainelli T. Role of topical immunotherapy in the treatment of alopecia areata. *J Am Acad Dermatol* 1990; **22**: 654–61.
15 Happle R, Kalvaran KJ, Büchner U *et al*. Contact allergy as a therapeutic tool for alopecia areata; application of squaric acid dibutyl ester. *Dermatologica* 1980; **161**: 289–94.
16 Rosenberg E, Drake L. Discussion of Dunaway DA. Alopecia areata. *Arch Dermatol* 1976; **112**: 256.
17 Happle R. Antigenic competition as a therapeutic concept for alopecia areata. *Arch Dermatol Res* 1980; **267**: 109–14.
18 Krakta J, Gorez G, Vizethum W *et al*. Dinitrochlorobenzene influence on the cytochrome P-450 system and mutagenic effects. *Arch Dermatol Res* 1979; **266**: 315–26.
19 Tosti A, De Padova MP, Minghetti G *et al*. Therapies versus placebo in the treatment of patchy alopecia areata. *J Am Acad Dermatol* 1986; **15**: 209–16.
20 Ashworth J, Tuyp E, MacKie R. Allergic and irritant contact dermatitis compared in the treatment of alopecia totalis and universalis. A comparison of the value of topical diphencyprone and tretinoin gel. *Br J Dermatol* 1989; **120**: 397–403.
21 Gordon PM, Aldridge RD, McVittee E, Hunter JAA. Topical diphencyprone for alopecia areata: evaluation of 48 cases after 30 months' follow-up. *Br J Dermatol* 1996; **134**: 869–72.
22 Bröker EB, Echernacht-Happle K, Hamm H *et al*. Abnormal expression of class I and class II major histocompatibility antigens in alopecia areata: modulation by topical immunotherapy. *J Invest Dermatol* 1987; **88**: 564–9.
23 Rollier R, Warcewski Z. Le traitement de la pelade par la méladinine. *Bull Soc Fr Dermatol Syphiligr* 1974; **81**: 97–101.
24 Lassus A, Eskwlinen A, Johansson E. Treatment of alopecia areata with three different PUVA modalities. *Photodermatology* 1984; **1**: 141–50.
25 Claudy AL, Gagnaire D. PUVA treatment of alopecia areata. *Arch Dermatol* 1983; **119**: 975–82.
26 Monfrecola G, D'Anna F, Delfino M. Topical hematoporphyrin plus UVA for treatment of alopecia areata. *Photodermatology* 1987; **4**: 305–10.
27 Taylor CR, Hawk JLM. PUVA treatment of AA partialis, totalis and universalis: audit of 10 years' experience at St. John's Institute of Dermatology. *Br J Dermatol* 1995; **133**: 914–18.
28 Linas SL, Nies AS. Minoxidil. *Ann Intern Med* 1981; **94**: 61–74.
29 Fenton DA, Wilkinson JD. Alopecia areata treated with topical minoxidil. *J R Soc Med* 1982; **75**: 963–5.
30 Weiss VC, West DO, Fu TS *et al*. Alopecia areata treated with topical minoxidil. *Arch Dermatol* 1984; **120**: 457–66.
31 Price VH. Topical minoxidil (3%) in extensive alopecia areata, including long-term efficacy. *J Am Acad Dermatol* 1987; **16**: 737–47.
32 Fiedler-Weiss VC. Potential mechanisms of minoxidil-induced hair growth in alopecia areata. *J Am Acad Dermatol* 1987; **16**: 653–8.
33 Fiedler-Weiss VC, Buys CM. Response to minoxidil in severe alopecia areata correlates with T lymphocyte stimulation. *Arch Dermatol* 1987; **123**: 1491–7.
34 Gupta AK, Ellis CN, Cooper KD *et al*. Oral cyclosporin for the treatment of alopecia areata. *J Am Acad Dermatol* 1990; **22**: 242–8.
35 De Prost Y, Teillac D, Plaquez F *et al*. Placebo controlled trial of topical cyclosporin in severe alopecia areata. *Lancet* 1986; **ii**: 803–4.
36 Lowy M, Ledoux-Corbusier M, Achten G *et al*. Clinical and immunologic response to Isoprinosine in alopecia areata and alopecia universalis: association with auto-antibodies. *J Am Acad Dermatol* 1985; **12**: 78–84.
37 Galbraith GMP, Thiers BH, Jensen J *et al*. A randomised double-blind study of inosiplex (Isoprinosine) therapy in patients with alopecia. *J Am Acad Dermatol* 1987; **16**: 977–81.

Traumatic alopecia

The term traumatic alopecia is applied to alopecia induced by physical trauma. These cases fall into three main categories.

1 Alopecia resulting from the deliberate, although at times unconscious, efforts of the patient, who is under tension or is psychologically disturbed—trichotillomania.

2 Alopecia resulting from cosmetic procedures applied incorrectly or with misguided and excessive vigour or frequency—cosmetic alopecia.

3 Alopecia resulting from accidental trauma—accidental alopecia.

Trichotillomania [1–4]

Introduction. The term trichotillomania was suggested by Hallopeau in 1889 [5] for the compulsive habit that induces an individual to pluck hair repeatedly. There are obvious objections to this overdramatic term for what is often a trivial problem, particularly in childhood. The term mania was a more general term in the 19th century, in contrast to the very specific modern psychiatric term which is not relevant in this context.

Pathology [6]. The histological changes vary according to the severity and duration of the hair plucking. Numerous empty canals are the most consistent feature. Some follicles are severely damaged; there are clefts in the hair matrix, the follicular epithelium is separated from the connective tissue sheath, and there are intraepithelial and perifollicular haemorrhages and intrafollicular pigment casts [7]. Injured follicles may form only soft, twisted hairs—a process which has been described as a separate entity under the name of trichomalacia [8]. Many follicles are in catagen, with very few or no follicles in telogen. Some dilated follicular infundibula contain horny plugs [2].

Aetiology and psychopathology. Trichotillomania occurs more than twice as frequently in females as in males, but below the age of 6 years boys outnumber girls by 3:2 and the peak incidence in boys is in the 2–6 age group [2]. It is seven times more frequent in children than adults. The child develops the habit of twisting hair round its fingers and pulling it. The act is only partially conscious and may replace the habit of thumb-sucking. Various psychiatric studies are not in complete agreement, but emotional deprivation in the maternal relationship is considered by some authorities to be important in initiating the habit.

The rarer and more severe form occurs predominantly in females of any age from early adolescence onwards, and most are aged 11–40 years; the peak incidence in females is between 11 and 17 years [2]. The hair-pulling begins in a provocative social situation in a subject who is often greatly disturbed psychologically [8]. Exceptionally severe forms may be seen in young patients and the minor forms in older patients [9].

Clinical features. In the younger patients, the hair pulling tic develops gradually and unconsciously but is not usually denied by the patient. Hair is plucked most frequently from one frontoparietal region. There results an ill-defined patch on which the hairs are twisted and broken at various distances from the clinically normal scalp. The texture and colour of the broken hairs are of course unaffected. One young child plucked the hair of her contemporaries as well as her own [10].

In the more severe form, the patient usually consistently denies touching his or her hair. The patient presents with

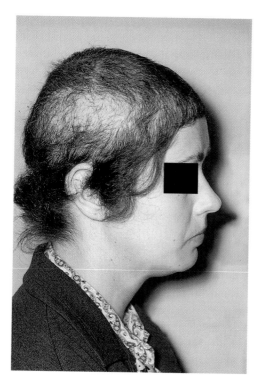

Fig. 66.33 Trichotillomania. Characteristic 'tonsure' pattern with scalp margin hair spared (Orentreich sign).

an extensive area of scalp on which the hair has been reduced to a coarse stubble uniformly 2.5–3 mm long. Most characteristically, the plucked area covers the entire scalp apart from the margin (Fig. 66.33), hence the validity of the term 'tonsure alopecia' [8]. The hair plucking may be continued for years and the disfiguring baldness is held by the patient to be responsible for the psychological problems. A mother and daughter have been affected at the same time [11].

Much more unusual is the habit of plucking the eyelashes, eyebrows and beard [7,12]. Very exceptionally the patient may pluck hair also, or only, from other regions of the body, such as the mons pubis and perianal region.

The child may also suck and even eat the hair (trichophagy) [9]. In such cases, examination of the mouth may reveal hairs [13] and enquiry should be made for systemic symptoms related to the presence of a hairball, for example dysphagia, vomiting, anaemia, abdominal pain or constipation. This symptom was present in 10% of children with trichotillomania [13].

Differential diagnosis. The minor form in young children is often confused with ringworm or with AA. In ringworm, the texture of the infected hairs is abnormal and the scalp surface may be scaly. It is wise to examine all cases under Wood's light and also to examine broken hairs under the microscope. AA may be difficult to exclude with certainty at the first examination, but the course of the condition soon establishes the correct diagnosis; histology may be very useful in early lesions [2]. We have known the hair-pulling tic to develop in a child recovering from typical AA.

Treatment and prognosis. The habit tic in young children is usually eradicated, except in the mentally retarded. The child's problem should be discussed with them and their parents. The diagnosis is often rejected by the parents who have not observed the child pulling the hair and find it unacceptable to believe that the problem is self-inflicted. In a recent series, over 50% required psychiatric referral [13]. Usually, support from the dermatologist is sufficient; behaviour therapy is also said to be helpful.

Tonsure trichotillomania is a very different proposition. Some patients recover, but many fail to do so, despite skilled psychiatric care, which may involve the use of major or minor tranquillizers and psychotherapy.

REFERENCES

1 Greenberg H, Sarner CA. Trichotillomania. *Arch Gen Psychiatr* 1965; **12**: 482–7.
2 Muller SA. Trichotillomania; a study of 66 patients. *J Am Acad Dermatol* 1990; **23**: 56–62.
3 Muller SA, Winkelmann RK. Trichotillomania. *Arch Dermatol* 1972; **105**: 535–43.
4 Schneides D, Janniger CK. Trichotillomania. *Cutis* 1994; **53**: 293–5.
5 Hallopeau H. Alopécie par grattage (trichomanie ou trichotillomanie). *Ann Dermatol Syphiligr* 1889; **10**: 440–6.
6 Lachapelle JM, Pierard GE. Traumatic alopecia in trichotillomania; a pathologic interpretation of histologic lesions in the pilosebaceous unit. *J Cutan Pathol* 1977; **4**: 57–63.
7 Mehregan AH. Trichotillomania; a clinicopathological study. *Arch Dermatol* 1970; **102**: 129–35.
8 Sanderson KV, Hall-Smith P. Tonsure trichotillomania. *Br J Dermatol* 1970; **82**: 342–9.
9 Monroe JT, Jr, Abse DW. The psychopathology of trichotillomania and trichophagy. *Psychiatry* 1963; **26**: 95–100.
10 Reuter K. Ein besonderer Fall von Trichotillomanie. *Zeitschr Haut Geschlechts* 1951; **10**: 287.
11 Hall-Smith SP. Familial trichotillomania. *Trans St John's Hosp Dermatol Soc* 1966; **52**: 135–41.
12 Jillson OF. Alopecia. II Trichotillomania (trichotillohabitus). *Cutis* 1983; **31**: 383–6.
13 Oranje AP, Peereboom-Wynia JDR, De Raeymaecker DMJ. Trichotillomania in childhood. *J Am Acad Dermatol* 1986; **15**: 614–21.

Cosmetic alopecia

The dictates of religion, custom and fashion have imposed an immense variety of physical stresses on human hair. The nomenclature of the resulting patterns of baldness inevitably lacks any consistency. It is possible only to list the clinical syndromes most widely reported; any new hairdressing technique may give rise to new patterns [1].

Pathology. Two processes are responsible for most of the pathological changes observed. Hair, sometimes already weakened by chemical applications, may be broken by friction or tension. Prolonged tension may induce follicular inflammatory changes which may eventually lead to scarring. Traction alopecia is induced particularly readily in subjects with incipient common baldness, for the telogen hairs, which make up a higher proportion of the total, are more readily extracted than anagen hairs.

Traumatic and marginal alopecia. The essential changes in the many variants of this syndrome are the presence of short, broken hairs, folliculitis and some scarring in circumscribed patches at the scalp margins.

In one form, which is caused by the tension imposed by procedures intended to straighten kinky hair [2], alopecia commonly begins in triangular areas in front of and above the ears, but may involve other parts of the scalp margin, or even linear areas in other parts of the scalp. Itching and crusting may be pronounced. The so-called 'pony-tail' hair style may cause similar changes in the frontal hair margin [3]. Keratin cylinders—'hair casts'—may surround many hairs just above the scalp surface [4].

Frontal and parietal traction alopecia may occur in young Sikh boys as a result of twisting their uncut hair tightly on top of the head [5], and tight braiding and wooden combs produce traction alopecia in the Sudan; frontal loss is reported in Libyan women as a result of traction from a tight scarf [6].

Afro-Caribbean hair styles with tight braiding of the hair into rows known variously as corn, cain or cane rows or braids may cause marginal alopecia and central alopecia with widening of the partings.

Brush roller alopecia. Brush rollers, if applied frequently and with too much vigour, may cause irregular patches of more or less complete alopecia, surrounded by a zone of erythema with broken hairs [7].

Hot-comb alopecia [8]. Black women who use hot combs to straighten the hair may develop a progressive cicatricial alopecia, slowly extending centrifugally from the vertex. This procedure is now rarely carried out.

Massage alopecia. The overenthusiastic application of medication to the scalp, with firm massage, may cause baldness and excessive 'weathering' (trichorrhexis nodosa).

Brush alopecia. Vigorous brushing may cause significant damage to hair that is already fragile as the result of a developmental defect. The bristles with square or otherwise angular tips, present in some brushes made of synthetic fibres, may prove particularly traumatic.

Alopecia secondary to hair weaving. Patchy traction alopecia has been reported to result from the cosmetic procedure of weaving additional hair into persistent terminal hair in order to camouflage common baldness.

Deliberate alopecia. The authors have seen a family from Pakistan in which three sisters during childhood were subjected to tight plaiting and traction of the central V of the frontal hair [9]. The resulting V alopecia was considered desirable.

Diagnosis. The traumatic cosmetic alopecias do not present any diagnostic difficulties, provided the possibility is considered. Their cause is rarely recognized by the patient and is often accepted with suspicion.

REFERENCES

1 Wilborn WS. Disorders of hair growth in African Americans. In: Olsen E, ed. *Disorder of Hair Growth.* New York: McGraw-Hill, 1994: 389–407.
2 Costa OC. Traumatic negroid alopecia. *Br J Dermatol* 1946; **58**: 280–2.
3 Slepyan AH. Traction alopecia. *Arch Dermatol* 1958; **78**: 395–9.
4 Rollins TG. Traction folliculitis with hair casts and alopecia. *Am J Dis Child* 1961; **101**: 609–13.
5 Singh G. Traction alopecia in Sikh boys. *Br J Dermatol* 1975; **92**: 232–8.
6 Malhotra YK, Kanwar AJ. Traumatic alopecia among Libyan women. *Arch Dermatol* 1980; **116**: 987–90.
7 Lipnik MJ. Traction alopecia from brush rollers. *Arch Dermatol* 1961; **84**: 493–6.
8 Lo Presti P, Papa CM, Kligman AM. Hot comb alopecia. *Arch Dermatol* 1968; **98**: 234–6.
9 Anstey AV, Wojnarowska FT. Traumatic alopecia with discoid lupus erythematosus (Letter). *Clin Exp Dermatol* 1991; **16**: 231–2.

Accidental traumatic alopecia

Alopecia secondary to accidental mechanical trauma to the scalp is usually not a diagnostic problem, but in some circumstances the trauma may be unperceived and the cause of the hair loss undetected.

Women who had undergone prolonged pelvic operations in the Trendelenburg position developed, 12–26 days later, a vertical patch of alopecia, which was preceded by oedema, exudation and crusting. Pressure ischaemia during the operation was considered to be the cause of the alopecia [1]. In one large clinic, over a period of 3 years, 60 cases of occipital pressure alopecia were observed after open-heart surgery [2]. In 29 of these cases, the hair loss was permanent. Temporary alopecia followed prolonged pressure on the scalp by a foam rubber ring used to prevent such an occurrence [3].

REFERENCES

1 Abel RR. Postoperative (pressure) alopecia. *Anesthesiology* 1964; **25**: 869–71.
2 Lawson NW, Mills NL, Ochsner NL. Occipital alopecia following cardiopulmonary bypass. *J Thorac Cardiovasc Surg* 1976; **71**: 342–5.
3 Patel KD, Henschel EO. Postoperative alopecia. *Anaesth Analg* 1980; **59**: 311–14.

Cicatricial alopecia

Cicatricial alopecia is the generic term applied to alopecia which accompanies or follows the destruction of hair follicles, whether by a disease affecting the follicles themselves or by some process external to them. The follicles may be absent as the result of a developmental defect or may be irretrievably injured by trauma, as in burns or radiodermatitis. They may be destroyed by a specific and identifiable infection—favus, tuberculosis or syphilis, for example—or by the encroachment of a benign or malignant tumour. In other cases, their destruction can be reliably attributed to a named, although still mysterious, disease process such as lichen planus, lupus erythematosus or sarcoidosis. When all the clinically and histologically acceptable causes have been eliminated, two named syndromes of cutaneous origin remain, *pseudopelade* and the less well defined *folliculitis decalvans*. Once these too have been excluded, there still remain cases in which any greater precision of diagnosis than 'cicatricial alopecia' may be unwarranted. Once the preliminary diagnosis of cicatricial alopecia has been made, the scalp should be searched for other changes—folliculitis, follicular plugging or broken hairs—and hairs, even if grossly normal in appearance, should be extracted from the edge of the bald area for microscopy and culture. If no firm diagnosis is achieved, general skin examination and systemic studies should be carried out where appropriate.

If the decision is made to take a biopsy, its site must be carefully selected and an early lesion should be preferred. Several punch biopsies are preferable to a single elliptical biopsy; in this way, the biopsies can be orientated along follicles, and different stages of the disease process can be investigated.

Classification [1,2]. The causes of cicatricial alopecia are classified here into broad groups, and the individual causes then considered in greater detail. Many of the causes are discussed in other chapters where appropriate.

1 Developmental defects and hereditary disorders
 Aplasia cutis
 Facial hemiatrophy (Romberg's syndrome)
 Epidermal naevi
 Hair follicle hamartomas
 Incontinentia pigmenti
 Focal dermal hypoplasia of Goltz
 Porokeratosis of Mibelli
 Scarring follicular keratosis
 Ichthyosis
 Darier's disease
 Epidermolysis bullosa
 Polyostotic fibrous dysplasia
 Conradi's syndrome (chondrodystrophia calcificans)
2 Physical injuries
 Mechanical trauma
 Scalp necrosis after embolization surgery
 AIDS—secondary infections (various)
 Burns
 Radiodermatitis

3 Medicaments
4 Fungal infections
Kerion
Trichophyton violaceum
T. sulphureum
Favus
5 Bacterial infections
Tuberculosis
Syphilis
6 Pyogenic infections
Carbuncle
Furuncle
Folliculitis
Acne necrotica
7 Protozoal infections
Leishmaniasis
8 Virus infections
Herpes zoster.
9 Tumours
Basal cell epithelioma
Squamous cell epithelioma
Syringoma
Metastatic tumours
Lymphomas
Adnexal tumours
10 Dermatoses of uncertain aetiology
Lichen planus
Graham–Little syndrome
Tufted folliculitis
Dermatomyositis
Lupus erythematosus
Scleroderma; morphoea
Necrobiosis lipoidica
Pyoderma gangrenosum
Lichen sclerosus
Mastocytosis
Sarcoidosis
Cicatricial pemphigoid
Follicular mucinosis
Temporal arteritis
Erosive pustular dermatosis
Eosinophilic cellulitis
11 Clinical syndromes
Dissecting cellulitis of the scalp (Chapter 27)
Pseudopelade
Folliculitis decalvans and tufted folliculitis
Alopecia parvimacularis

Clinical syndromes [1]. In the 19th century and earlier there were descriptions of cases of cicatricial alopecia probably conforming to these clinical syndromes. In 1885, Brocq [3] described what later became known as pseudopelade [4], but as he subsequently admitted [5], it continues to confuse the nomenclature. Pseudopelade is now regarded as a syndrome in which destruction of follicles leading to permanent patchy baldness is not accompanied by any clinically evident inflammatory pathology—probably a specific entity, which may be an autoimmune atrophy.

Quainquad [6] described a form of scarring alopecia in which pustular folliculitis of the advancing margin was a conspicuous feature. To this condition the term folliculitis decalvans is now commonly applied.

Alopecia parvimacularis as described by Dreuw [7] is a questionable entity. It has been regarded as pseudopelade occurring in childhood, but it differs from that syndrome in several respects; it may represent scarring lichen planus.

Histology. Pinkus [8], using acid alcoholic orcein stain, studied the elastic fibres around the hair follicles in many sections from cicatricial alopecia of a variety of types. He found that the fibrous strands which replaced destroyed follicles in lichen planus and lupus erythematosus consist of collagen without elastic-like bodies or elastic fibres. In lupus erythematosus there is, in addition, widespread destruction of elastic fibres in the interfollicular dermis. The cases included 180 which satisfied the diagnostic criteria of pseudopelade: absence of sebaceous glands, more or less normal epidermis, no significant follicular plugging, small areas of subepidermal loss of elastic fibres, collagenous and elastic fibrosis at sites of destroyed follicles. Of these 180 cases, 106 showed additional features which led Pinkus to differentiate them provisionally as 'fibrosing alopecia'. The most striking of these features is the development of elastic fibres around the lower part of the follicle, even at an early stage in the process. The features of fibrosing alopecia were a general hyperplasia of elastic fibres in the interfollicular dermis and the presence of less perifollicular cellular infiltrate than in pseudopelade.

Treatment. Whatever the type of scarring alopecia, once the process has been shown to have become arrested, or is in a static phase, surgical removal of the affected area should be considered. This has become more relevant in recent times because of the ability to remove even large areas with good cosmetic results [9].

REFERENCES

1 Dawber RPR, ed. Cicatricial alopecia. In: *Diseases of the Hair and Scalp*, 3rd edn. Oxford: Blackwell Science, 1997: 588–90.
2 Elston DM, Bergfeld WF. Cicatricial alopecia. In: Olsen E, ed. *Disorders of Hair Growth*. New York: McGraw-Hill, 1994: 285–314.
3 Brocq L. Alopecia. *J Cutan Vener Dis* 1885; **3**: 49–56.
4 Brocq L, Lenglet E, Ayrignac J. Recherches sur l'alopecie atrophiante, varieté pseudopelade. *Ann Dermatol Syphiligr* 1905; **6**: 1, 97, 209–15.
5 Brocq L, ed. Pseudopelade. In: *Traité Elementaire de Dermatologie Pratique*, Vol. 2. Paris: Doin, 1907: 648–58.
6 Quainquad E. Folliculite epilante decalvante. *Ann Dermatol Syphiligr* 1889; **10**: 99–105.
7 Dreuw H. Über epidemische Alopecie. *Monatsch Prak Dermatol* 1910; **51**: 18–24.
8 Pinkus H. Differential patterns of elastic fibres in scarring and non-scarring alopecia. *J Cutan Pathol* 1978; **5**: 93–101.

9 Roenigk RK, Wheeland RG. Tissue expansion in cicatricial alopecia. *Arch Dermatol* 1987; **123**: 641–52.

Pseudopelade [1]

The term pseudopelade is used here to designate a slowly progressive cicatricial alopecia, without clinically evident folliculitis and no marked inflammation. There is no doubt that lichen planus can produce a very similar clinical picture and there are some authorities who maintain on the basis of associated skin lesions and histopathological findings that 90% of cases of 'pseudopelade' are caused by lichen planus [2]. At a later stage, lupus erythematosus also can cause similar changes. However, some patients with pseudopelade never show any clinical or histological evidence of lichen planus [1]. Pseudopelade is therefore generally regarded as a clinical syndrome which may be the end result of any one of a number of different pathological processes (known and unknown) [3], although a specific clinically uninflamed type has always been recognized.

Pathology [3]. If clinically normal scalp at the edge of a plaque of pseudopelade is examined, numerous lymphocytes are seen around the upper two-thirds of the follicles [4]. Later, the follicles are destroyed and the epidermis becomes thin and atrophic, and the dermis densely sclerotic. Follicular 'ghosts' without inflammatory changes are seen.

Clinical features [1]. Although both sexes may be affected, and the condition has occurred in childhood [5], the patient is usually a woman and over 40 years of age. She may complain of slight irritation at first, but more often a small bald patch or patches (Fig. 66.34) discovered by chance by the patient or by her hairdresser, is the first evidence of the disease. The initial patch is most often on the vertex, but may occur anywhere on the scalp. The course thereafter is extremely variable. In a majority of cases, extension of the process takes place only very slowly; indeed, after 15 or 20 years the patient may still be able to arrange her hair to conceal the patches effectively. In some cases, extension occurs more rapidly, and exceptionally there may be almost total baldness after 2 or 3 years.

On examination, the affected patches are smooth, soft and slightly depressed. At an early stage in the development of any individual patch there may be some erythema. The patches tend to be small and round or oval, but irregular bald patches may be formed by confluence of many lesions (Fig. 66.35). The hair in uninvolved scalp is normal, but if the process is active the hairs at the edges of each patch are very easily extracted. Detailed studies by Braun-Falco *et al.* [1] strongly support the idea that pseudopelade is a distinct entity with the diagnostic criteria as follows:

1 Clinical criteria:
  (a) irregularly defined and confluent patches of alopecia;
  (b) moderate atrophy (late stage);
  (c) mild perifollicular erythema (early stage);
  (d) female/male = 3:1;
  (e) long course (more than 2 years);
  (f) slow progression with spontaneous termination possible

2 Direct immunofluorescence negative or at least only IgM [4].

3 Histological criteria [6]:
  (a) absence of marked inflammation;
  (b) absence of widespread scarring;
  (c) absence of significant follicular plugging;
  (d) absence, or at least decrease, of sebaceous glands;
  (e) presence of normal epidermis (only occasionally atrophy);
  (f) fibrotic streams into subcutis.

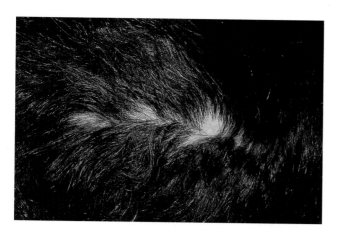

Fig. 66.34 Pseudopelade. Early, small patches.

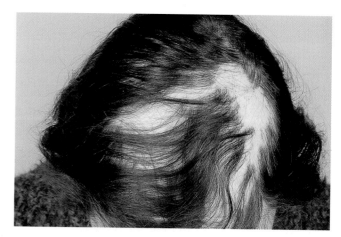

Fig. 66.35 Pseudopelade. Late stage in which many small patches have coalesced into larger lesions.

Treatment. If the scarring alopecia can be shown to be secondary to lichen planus or lupus erythematosus, the treatment appropriate for these conditions may be prescribed. However, whether the baldness is of known or unknown origin, it is irreversible. If the disfigurement is considerable and no active inflammatory changes are present, autografting from unaffected to scarred scalp may be considered [7], or surgical 'expansion' techniques in severe cases.

The intradermal injection of corticosteroids does not seem to influence the extension of the disease process in cases of unknown origin.

REFERENCES

1 Braun-Falco, Imei S, Schmoeckel C *et al.* Pseudopelade of Brocq. *Dermatologica* 1986; **172**: 18–26.
2 Gay Prieto J. Pseudopelade of Brocq; its relationship to some forms of cicatricial alopecia and to lichen planus. *J Invest Dermatol* 1955; **24**: 323–34.
3 Degos R, Rabut R, Duperrat B *et al.* L'etat pseudopeladique. *Ann Dermatol Syphiligr* 1954; **81**: 5–12.
4 Pincelli C, Girolomoni G, Benassi L. Pseudopelade of Brocq: an immunologically mediated disease? *Dermatologica* 1987; **176**: 49–57.
5 Reinertson RP. Pseudopelade with nail dystrophy. *Arch Dermatol* 1958; **78**: 282–7.
6 Headington JT. Cicatricial alopecia. *Dermatol Clin* 1996; **14**: 773–82.
7 Stough DB, Berger RA, Orentreich N. Surgical improvement of cicatricial alopecia of diverse etiology. *Arch Dermatol* 1968; **97**: 331–5.

Folliculitis decalvans and tufted folliculitis

Under the general term folliculitis decalvans we group together the various syndromes in which clinically evident chronic folliculitis leads to progressive scarring. This is probably a heterogeneous group.

Aetiology. The cause of folliculitis decalvans is still uncertain. *Staphylococcus aureus* may be grown from the pustules. Some abnormality of the host must be postulated. Some authors have emphasized the possible role of the seborrhoeic state and some use the term 'cicatrizing seborrhoeic eczema'; but folliculitis decalvans is rare and the seborrhoeic state is common, therefore the association probably has no special significance.

Shitara *et al.* [1] reported severe folliculitis decalvans in two siblings who also had chronic candidiasis; defective cell-mediated immunity was demonstrated. It seems probable that a local failure in the immune response or in leukocyte function may be the essential abnormality in most cases. Folliculitis decalvans of the scalp occurs in both sexes. It typically affects women aged 30–60 years and men from adolescence onwards.

Pathology. Follicular abscesses with a polymorphonuclear infiltrate are directly succeeded by scarring, or there may be a prolonged intermediate stage of granulomatous

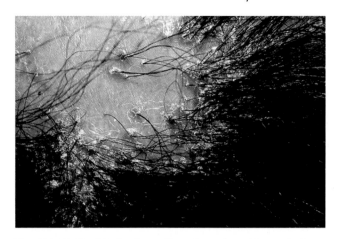

Fig. 66.36 Folliculitis decalvans. Central scarring with marginal pustules on the scalp.

folliculitis with numerous lymphocytes, and some plasma cells and giant cells [2].

Clinical features. Any or all hair regions may be involved, and in the syndrome sometimes referred to as 'atrophic folliculitis in seborrhoeic dermatitis', the beard, pubes, axillae and inner thighs may be involved, and less often the scalp as well. The severity of the inflammatory changes fluctuates, but the course is prolonged.

The scalp alone may be involved or the scalp together with pubes and axillae. There are multiple rounded or oval patches, each surrounded by crops of follicular pustules (Fig. 66.36). There may be no other changes, but successive crops of pustules, each followed by destruction of the affected follicles, produce slow extension of the alopecia.

Tufted folliculitis [3–5] may be a variant of this entity—an upper follicular acute inflammatory polymorphonuclear infiltrate is associated clinically with close grouping or 'tufting' of hairs.

Treatment. All patients should be investigated for underlying defects of immune response and of leukocyte function, as a possible guide to effective treatment.

Systemic antibiotics will often prevent further extension of the disease, but only for as long as they are administered. Brozena *et al.* [6] reported a single patient who improved after 10 weeks of rifampicin therapy and had no new lesions up to 1 year later.

REFERENCES

1 Shitara A, Igareshi R, Morohashi M. Folliculitis decalvans and cellular immunity—two brothers with oral candidiasis (in Japanese). *Jpn J Dermatol* 1974; **28**: 133.
2 Headington JT. Cicatricial alopecia. *Dermatol Clin* 1996; **14**: 773–82.
3 Dalziel K, Telfer N, Dawber RPR. Tufted folliculitis. *Am J Dermatopathol* 1990; **12**: 37–41.
4 Tong AKF, Baden H. Tufted folliculitis. *J Am Acad Dermatol* 1989; **21**: 1096–9.

5 Khalifen L, Todd DJ. Tufted folliculitis in Jordanian patients. *Int J Dermatol* 1996; **35**: 280–2.
6 Brozena SJ, Cohen LE, Fenske NA. Folliculitis decalvans—response to rifampicin. *Cutis* 1988; **42**: 512.

Alopecia parvimacularis

Dreuw [1] reported an outbreak of alopecia affecting 60 of the 85 boys in two schools. The patches of alopecia were small, irregularly round or angular, and appeared atrophic, but in 90% of cases the hair regrew satisfactorily. Permanent scarring alopecia developed in the remaining 10% of cases. There were no inflammatory changes and no fungus or other organisms could be discovered. Many similar outbreaks have been described [2].

Pathology. Non-specific inflammatory changes are seen involving some follicles, but sparing others. The degree of scarring depends on the number of contiguous follicles destroyed. In some cases, the pathological changes eventually resemble those of pseudopelade [3].

Clinical features [4]. All reported cases have been children. The patches of alopecia are of rapid onset, quickly reaching their greatest extent, and are usually numerous. They seldom exceed 1–2 cm in diameter, and are characteristically irregularly angular in shape. Over the course of a few weeks, the hair regrows in most cases to leave no clinically evident alopecia, but in some patients cicatricial alopecia results.

Diagnosis. Mycotic infection must be excluded by microscopy and by culture. The multiple bites of insects, scratched and secondarily infected, can give rise to small patches of alopecia, but the history should exclude this diagnosis, as well as secondary syphilis.

REFERENCES

1 Dreuw H. Klinische Beobachtungen bei 101 haarkrankten Schulknaber. *Monats Prakt Dermatol* 1910; **51**: 103–7.
2 Davis H. Epidemic alopecia areata. *Br J Dermatol* 1914; **26**: 207–10.
3 Loewenthal LJA, Lurie HI. An outbreak of linear scarring alopecia. *Br J Dermatol* 1956; **68**: 88–94.
4 Hofer W. Sporadisches Auftreten von Alopecia parvimacularis. *Dermatol Wochenschr* 1964; **149**: 381–8.

Dermatoses of uncertain aetiology

Lichen planus (Chapter 41)

Aetiology. Lichen planus is a disease or, more probably, a 'reaction pattern', of unknown origin but belonging to the autoimmune group of conditions. It occurs throughout the world, but there are marked regional variations in its incidence and in its clinical manifestations. These variations probably result from relative differences in the importance of various aetiological agents.

Pathology [1]. The initial abnormality is in the epidermis: fibrillar changes in the basal cells lead to the formation of colloid bodies and at an early stage these, and macrophages containing pigment, may be seen in the dermis. By immunofluorescence, fibrin and IgM may be detected in the upper dermis, and various components of complement in the basement-membrane zone. The wounded basal cells are continually replaced by the migration of cells from neighbouring normal epidermis. In the established lesion, the horny layer and granular layer are thickened and there is irregular acanthosis. Flattening of the rete pegs gives rise to a saw-tooth configuration. There is liquefaction degeneration of the basal cells. Close up against the epidermis is a dense infiltrate of lymphocytes and some histiocytes. In many sections, some colloid bodies can be seen. If the process involves hair follicles, the infiltrate extends around them and the hairs are replaced by keratin plugs. The follicles may ultimately be totally destroyed.

Clinical features [2]. Lichen planus occurs at any age, but in over 80% of cases the onset is between 30 and 70 years [3]. Significant involvement of the scalp is relatively infrequent—only 10 of 807 patients in one series [3]—but the incidence is probably rather higher than such figures suggest, because they tend to exclude those patients in whom alopecia, classified as pseudopelade, was the only manifestation of the disease. Scalp involvement occurs in over 40% of patients with either of two unusual variants of lichen planus: the bullous or erosive form and lichen planopilaris. Most patients seen with scalp lesions are middle-aged women, but a girl aged 13 years with scarring has been reported [4]. In the experience of the authors, scarring lichen planus of the scalp is disproportionately common in individuals of Indian extraction in comparison with other racial groups.

Recent scalp lesions may show violaceous papules, erythema and scaling [5], but before long, follicular plugs become conspicuous and scarring replaces all other changes. Eventually, the plugs are shed from the scarred area which remains white and smooth. If the patch is extending, horny plugs may still be present in follicles around its margins.

More often, the scalp lesions are well established by the time the patient attends hospital, and the irregular white patches are not clinically diagnostic and indeed may not show any distinctive histological features. This is the clinical picture known as pseudopelade. The diagnosis of lichen planus can be made only in the presence of unquestionable lesions elsewhere and lichen planus histology. These may take the form of bullous lichen planus with shedding of nails [6], of bullous lesions associated with typical lichen planus of the skin and mucous membranes [7], or of lichen planus of very limited extent involving, for example, the nails only [8].

In a clinical syndrome that has caused much controversy (see Graham-Little syndrome), groups of horny follicular papules on the trunk and limbs either precede or follow the development of scarring alopecia. The evidence that this syndrome is at least in many cases a manifestation of lichen planus is based on its occasional association with typical lichen planus and the presence in early lesions of histological changes acceptable as lichen planus [9].

Prognosis. In some patients, the course of lichen planus of the scalp is slow and only a few inconspicuous patches are present after many years. However, particularly if the skin lesions are of bullous or planopilaris type, they may rapidly result in extensive and permanent baldness. The rare childhood cicatricial lichen planus has a very poor prognosis.

Treatment. In some cases, a short course of systemic treatment with a corticosteroid may be desirable. In other cases, intralesional corticosteroids are helpful but only at a stage when active inflammatory changes are still present. Potent topical steroids such as clobetasol propionate ointment twice a day may slightly inhibit the process.

REFERENCES

1 Headington JT. Cicatricial alopecia. *Dermatol Clin* 1996; **14**: 773–82.
2 Mehregan DA, Van Hale HM, Muller SA. Lichen planopilaris. *J Am Acad Dermatol* 1992; **27**: 935–7.
3 Altman J, Perry HO. The variations and course of lichen planus. *Arch Dermatol* 1961; **84**: 179–88.
4 Borda JM, Mazzini RHE, Ruiz DA. Liquen del cuero cabelludo. *Arch Argentin Dermatol* 1961; **11**: 257–61.
5 Sannicandro G. Etudes sur le lichen ruber planus typique et atypique ulcero-erosif, ulcerohemorragique, sclero-cicatriciel, alopecique et sur ses rapports avec les modifications de la protidopoiese. *Ann Dermatol Syphiligr* 1954; **81**: 380–6.
6 Cram DL, Kierland RR, Winkelmann RK. Ulcerative lichen planus of the feet. *Arch Dermatol* 1966; **93**: 692–5.
7 Ebner H. Lichen ruber planus mit Onychatrophie und narbiger Alopezie. *Dermatologica* 1973; **147**: 219–24.
8 Corsi H. Atrophy of hair follicle and nail matrix in lichen planus. *Br J Dermatol* 1937; **49**: 376–88.
9 Waldorf DS. Lichen planopilaris. *Arch Dermatol* 1966; **93**: 684–9.

Graham-Little syndrome [1,2]

In 1915, Graham-Little reported the case of a woman aged 55 years, who had suffered for 10 years from slowly progressive cicatricial alopecia and for 5 months from groups of horny papules [3]. Since then, many further cases have been reported. Whether this syndrome is or is not a form of lichen planus is still unresolved, although the immunofluorescent findings in typical cases strongly suggest lichen planus [4]. However, whatever its cause or causes, the syndrome is distinctive. It is known eponymously and variously as the Graham-Little, Lassueur–Graham-Little, or Piccardi–Lassueur–Little syndrome.

Pathology. In the scalp, the mouths of affected follicles are filled by horny plugs. The underlying follicle is progressively destroyed and eventually an atrophic epidermis covers sclerotic dermis. In the axillae and pubic region, the follicles are likewise destroyed, although the skin does not appear clinically to be atrophic.

Clinical features. Most patients are women between the ages of 30 and 70 years. The essential features of the syndrome are progressive cicatricial alopecia of the scalp, loss of pubic and axillary hair without clinically evident scarring, and the rapid development of keratosis pilaris [5].

In most patients the earliest change has been patchy cicatricial alopecia of the scalp. In general [6] the scalp alopecia precedes the widespread keratosis pilaris by months or years. In some patients [7], the alopecia and the keratosis pilaris appear to have developed more or less simultaneously, or the keratosis pilaris has preceded the discovery of the alopecia.

The scalp changes are commonly described simply as patches of cicatricial alopecia. Some authors specifically mention associated follicular plugging of the scalp [7], and others refer to 'scaly red patches'.

The keratosis pilaris is referred to in early case reports as lichen spinulosus, which emphasizes that the horny papules are prolonged into conspicuous spines. In most cases they have developed aggressively over a period of weeks or months and have been grouped into plaques, often on the trunk, or the trunk and limbs, but occasionally involving the eyebrows and the sides of the face. Pruritus is an inconstant symptom; it was noted in several reported cases [8]. Thinning and ultimately total loss of pubic and axillary hair has been noted in many cases.

Treatment. None is known. Surgical treatment may be considered as in other cicatricial alopecias.

REFERENCES

1 Arnozan X. Folliculite depilantes des partier glabres. *Bull Soc Fr Dermatol Syphiligr* 1982; **3**: 187–94.
2 Brocq L, Langlet E, Agrinac J. Recherches sur alopecie atrophisante, varieté pseudopelade. *Ann Dermatol Syphiligr* 1905; **6**: 1, 97, 209–13.
3 Graham-Little. Folliculitis decalvans et atrophicans. *Br J Dermatol* 1915; **27**: 183–90.
4 Horn RT, Goette DK, Odom RB *et al*. Immunofluorescent findings and clinical changes in two cases of follicular lichen planus. *J Am Acad Dermatol* 1982; **7**: 203–6.
5 Rongioletti F, Ghigliotti G, Gambina C *et al*. Agminate lichen follicularis with cysts and comedones. *Br J Dermatol* 1990; **122**: 844–9.
6 Pages F, Lapyre J, Misson R. Syndrome de Lassueur–Graham-Little. *Ann Dermatol* 1961; **88**: 272–80.
7 Reiss F, Reisch M, Buncke CM. Keratodermatitis folliculitis decalvans. *Arch Dermatol* 1958; **78**: 616–22.
8 Kubba R, Rook A. The Graham-Little syndrome. *Br J Dermatol* 1975; **93** (Suppl. 11): 53.

Circumscribed scleroderma

Circumscribed scleroderma is rare in the scalp, but may

occur there as single or multiple lesions. The early stages of morphoea are rarely seen in the scalp unless a bald area is affected. Morphoea tends to regress spontaneously after 3–5 years, but the plaque may continue to enlarge for much longer periods. The hair is shed at an early stage to leave a cicatricial alopecia. The diagnosis must be confirmed histologically. Linear circumscribed morphoea in the frontal region—'en coup de sabre' morphoea—has been associated with hereditary deficiency of complement C2 [1].

REFERENCE

1 Hulsmans RFHJ, Asghar SS, Siddiqui AH, Cormane RH. Hereditary deficiency of C2 in association with linear slceroderma, 'en coup de sabre'. *Arch Dermatol* 1986; **122**: 76–80.

Developmental defects and hereditary disorders

Scarring follicular keratosis

Numerous syndromes have been described and elaborately named, all of them characterized by keratosis pilaris associated with some degree of inflammatory change leading to destruction of the affected follicles [1].

Only detailed clinical and genetic studies can provide the essential facts to allow reliable differentiation of syndromes which some authorities regard as forms or degrees of a single state and others accept as distinct entities. Temporarily, the reported cases can be conveniently classified in three groups; in addition, certain apparently well-defined entities can be recognized.
1 Atrophoderma vermiculata (acne vermiculata, folliculitis ulerythematosa reticulata). There is honeycomb atrophy of the cheeks. Scarring alopecia may occur, but rarely.
2 Keratosis pilaris atrophicans faciei (ulerythema oophryogenes). The process is more or less confined to the eyebrow region.
3 Keratosis pilaris decalvans (keratosis follicularis spinulosa decalvans, follicular ichthyosis). Keratosis pilaris of variable extent is associated with cicatricial alopecia [2].

All these conditions are assumed to be genetically determined, although many cases occur sporadically. Such genetic data as are available are considered under the individual forms.

The follicles are initially distended by horny plugs, the dermis is oedematous and there is some lymphocytic infiltration around follicles and vessels. Later, the follicles are destroyed. Small epithelial cysts may be numerous, particularly in keratosis pilaris atrophicans faciei.

Clinical features. Atrophoderma vermiculata usually begins in childhood. Follicular plugs, often in the pre-auricular regions, are gradually shed to leave reticulate atrophy. On the face, the extent of the process is variable. Exceptionally, cicatricial alopecia of the scalp may be associated [3].

Keratosis pilaris atrophicans faciei (ulerythema oophryogenes) is present from early infancy. Erythema and horny plugs begin in the outer halves of the eyebrows, which they eventually destroy, and then advance medially and to a variable extent on the cheeks. Involvement of the scalp has apparently not been reported in cases in which the eyebrows are predominantly involved. However, there are case histories to which this diagnosis has been applied, but which appear to be more rationally classified in one of the other categories in which alopecia has occurred. Such cases emphasize the need for improved diagnostic criteria.

Keratosis pilaris decalvans is also such a variable syndrome that several genotypes must be considered. Keratosis pilaris begins in infancy or childhood, often on the face. Its ultimate extent may be confined to the face or to face and limbs, or may be more or less universal. It is often succeeded by atrophy on the face, but rarely on the limbs or trunk. Cicatricial alopecia is noted from early childhood or later, and may be localized or extensive [4].

Three members of one family developed keratosis pilaris of the face in early childhood [5] and then extensively on the back and limbs, and on the scalp, where horny papules replaced hairs. A similar syndrome was reported [6] in a young man who had keratosis pilaris and severe cicatricial alopecia. The occurrence of cases similar to those reported by MacLeod [5] in other siblings, born of normal parents, suggested recessive inheritance but the evidence was incomplete. The pattern of hair loss in the family reported by Ullmo [7] was in the distribution of the Marie–Unna type of congenital alopecia, apart from the presence of keratosis pilaris on the face.

What may be another distinct syndrome associates extremely severe keratosis pilaris—'closely woven bristles'—with almost complete alopecia, reduced sweating and deafness [8].

Treatment. Only symptomatic measures are available. Retinoic acid deserves a trial. The status of oral retinoids remains controversial, although anecdotal response has been noted.

REFERENCES

1 Rand RE, Arndt KA. Follicular syndromes with inflammation and atrophy. In: Fitzpatrick TB, Eisen AZ, Wolff K *et al.*, eds. *Dermatology in General Medicine*, 3rd edn. New York: McGraw-Hill, 1987: 717–32.
2 Rand RE, Baden H. Keratosis follicularis spinulosa decalvans: report of two cases and review of the literature. *Arch Dermatol* 1983; **119**: 22–9.
3 Fisher AA. Keratosis pilaris rubra atrophicans faciei with diffuse alopecia of the scalp. *Arch Dermatol* 1957; **75**: 283–9.
4 Dawber RPR, Van Neste D. *Hair and Scalp Disorders*. London: Dunitz, 1995: 118–39.
5 MacLeod JMH. Three cases of 'ichthyosis follicularis' associated with baldness. *Br J Dermatol* 1909; **21**: 165–71.
6 Kubba R, Mitchell JNS, Rook A. Keratosis pilaris with recurrent folliculitis decalvans. *Br J Dermatol* 1975; **93** (Suppl. 11): 55.

7 Ullmo A. Un nouveau type d'agenesie et de dystrophie pilaire familiale et hereditaire. *Dermatologica* 1944; **90**: 74–8.
8 Morris J, Ackerman AB, Koblenzer PJ. Generalized spiny hyperkeratosis, universal alopecia and deafness. *Arch Dermatol* 1969; **100**: 692–7.

Porokeratosis of Mibelli

This is a rare disorder of keratinization characterized by extending plaques of hyperkeratosis succeeded by atrophy. The rapid extension of a previously minimal lesion in a patient receiving immunosuppressive agents suggested that in porokeratosis there is a mutant clone of cells in the epidermis, the proliferation of which is normally controlled by immune processes [1].

Porokeratosis of Mibelli commonly begins in childhood but may first appear at any age. It is most frequent on limbs, particularly the hands and feet, the neck, the shoulders and the face but may occur anywhere including the scalp [2]. The initial lesion is a crateriform horny papule which gradually extends to form a circinate or irregular atrophic plaque with a raised horny margin, which may be surmounted by a furrow from which the lamina of horn projects. In the scalp there is loss of hair in the atrophic phase.

REFERENCES

1 Macmillan AL, Roberts SOB. Porokeratosis of Mibelli. *Br J Dermatol* 1974; **90**: 45–8.
2 Sehgal VM, Dube B. Porokeratosis (Mibelli) in a family. *Dermatologica* 1967; **134**: 269–72.

Incontinentia pigmenti

This rare syndrome occurs almost exclusively in females; its inheritance is probably determined by an X-linked gene usually lethal in the male [1].

Cicatricial alopecia has been present in at least 25% of reported cases; it appears in early infancy and ceases to extend after a variable period of up to 2 years, but the loss of hair is of course permanent. Other hair defects present in some cases have been hypoplasia of the eyebrows and eyelashes, and woolly hair naevus of the scalp [2].

REFERENCES

1 Carney RG, Carney RG, Jr. Incontinentia pigmenti. *Arch Dermatol* 1970; **102**: 157–62.
2 Wiklund DA, Weston WL. Incontinentia pigmenti. *Arch Dermatol* 1960; **115**: 701–5.

Generalized follicular hamartoma

Cicatricial alopecia beginning in childhood was a feature of a syndrome described by Mehregan and Hardin [1]. Their patient was a woman aged 23 years. From infancy, she had widespread horny plugs over the trunk and limbs and small pits on the palms and soles. She later developed cicatricial alopecia, in which, from the age of 8 years, appeared follicular tumours. The tumours of the scalp were proliferating tricholemmal cysts. The lesions of palms and soles showed funnel-shaped dilatation of sweat ducts, which were plugged with parakeratotic material containing acid mucopolysaccharide. Ridley and Smith [2] described this entity with alopecia and myasthenia gravis.

REFERENCES

1 Mehregan AH, Hardin I. Generalized follicular hamartoma. *Arch Dermatol* 1973; **107**: 435–40.
2 Ridley CM, Smith NP. Generalized hair follicle hamartoma associated with alopecia and myasthenia gravis. *Clin Exp Dermatol* 1981; **6**: 283–6.

Epidermolysis bullosa

The term epidermolysis bullosa is applied to a group of distinct genetically determined disorders characterized by the formation of bullae of skin, and often also of mucous membranes, in response to trauma, or spontaneously (Chapter 40). Only one of these diseases is accompanied by abnormalities of scalp or hair—recessive dystrophic epidermolysis bullosa; however, Gamborg Nielsen and Sjolund [1] described a new syndrome of localized epidermolysis bullosa simplex associated with hair, nail and teeth abnormalities. Alopecia may also occur in junctional epidermolysis bullosa.

Bullae form at the dermo-epidermal junction and fragments of dermis may adhere to the roof.

The inexorable blistering of skin and mucous membranes dominates the picture. The blisters are followed by atrophic scarring. This may give rise to more or less extensive cicatricial alopecia of the scalp [2,3]. Of 30 cases studied by Videl [4], three had cicatricial alopecia.

REFERENCES

1 Gamborg Nielsen P, Sjolund E. Epidermolysis bullosa simplex: localisation associated with anodontia, hair and nail abnormalities. *Acta Derm Venereol (Stockh)* 1985; **65**: 526–31.
2 Wagner W. Alopezia und Nagelveranderungen bei Epidermolysis bullosa hereditaria. *Zeitschr Haut Geschlechtskr* 1956; **20**: 270–4.
3 Vuorinen E. Uber ein Zwillingspaar mit Epidermolysis bullosa dystrophica polydysplastica. *Dermatologica* 1970; **140** (Suppl.): 3–5.
4 Videl J. Epidermolysis ampollares. *Acta Derm Sifiliogr* 1974; **65**: 3–7.

Cleft lip-palate, ectodermal dysplasia and syndactyly

This rare or rarely recognized syndrome is probably hereditary, and determined by an autosomal recessive gene.

The constant features of the syndrome are mental retardation, cleft palate, genital hypoplasia, cicatricial alopecia, defective teeth and syndactyly [1].

REFERENCE

1 Brown P, Armstrong HB. Ectodermal dysplasia, mental retardation, cleft lip/palate and other anomalies in three sibs. *Clin Genet* 1976; **9**: 35–40.

Polyostotic fibrous dysplasia

The progressive enlargement over a eriod of 10 years of a bald patch present since childhood was shown histologically to be due to the replacement of the follicles by coils of fibrous tissue. The patient had polyostotic fibrous dysplasia [1].

REFERENCE

1 Shelley WB, Wood MG. Alopecia with fibrous dysplasia and osteomas of the skin. *Arch Dermatol* 1976; **112**: 715–19.

Cicatricial pemphigoid
SYN. BENIGN MUCOSAL PEMPHIGOID

Cicatricial pemphigoid affects predominantly the elderly, and women more than men [1,2], and is associated with autoantibodies to the basement membrane zone adhesion complex (see Chapter 40).

Bullae are formed at the dermo-epidermal junction. Direct immunocytochemical studies show that linear deposits of IgG, IgA, C3 and C4 may be found in the basement-membrane zone, but circulating basement-membrane zone antibodies (IgG or IgA) are not always demonstrable [3].

The skin is involved in 40–50% of cases, and the disease affects predominantly the ocular and/or genital mucous membrane. However, the skin lesions may precede the mucosal lesions by months or years [4]. The skin lesions repeatedly recur and leave scars. The favoured sites are the face, and upper trunk, the scalp being involved in approximately 10% of cases [5]. Skin lesions, predominantly on the head and neck, are the major feature of the Brunsting–Perry variant.

Management will often be dictated by the need to control mucosal lesions. If recurrent bullae in a localized area of skin are troublesome, excision and grafting may be successful [5]. Whether to prescribe oral corticosteroids or immunosuppressive drugs for skin lesions alone is controversial, but topical clobetasol propionate cream may inhibit the process to some degree.

REFERENCES

1 Pearson RW. Advances in the diagnosis and treatment of blistering diseases: a selective review. In: Malkinson F, Pearson RW, eds. *Year Book of Dermatology*. Chicago: Year Book Publications, 1977: 7.
2 Kurzhals G, Stolz W, Maciejewski W, Kurpati S. Localized cicatricial pemphigoid. *Arch Dermatol* 1995; **131**: 580–1.
3 Holubar K, Honigsmann H, Wolff K. Cicatricial pemphigoid. *Arch Dermatol* 1973; **108**: 50–6.
4 Leenutaphong V, von Kries R, Plewig G. Localised cicatricial pemphigoid (Brunsting–Perry) electron microscopic study. *J Am Acad Dermatol* 1989; **21**: 1089–93.
5 Slepyan AH, Burks JW, Fox J. Persistent denudation of the scalp in cicatricial pemphigoid. Treatment by skin grafting. *Arch Dermatol* 1961; **84**: 444–51.

Erosive pustular dermatosis of the scalp

This clinical entity [1,2] particularly affects women over 70 years of age. Its cause is unknown but Grattan *et al.* [3] suggested that local trauma and sun damage are important in their study of 12 cases.

Pathology. Histological examination shows areas of epidermal erosion, a chronic inflammatory cell infiltration in the dermis consisting predominantly of lymphocytes and plasma cells and, sometimes, small foci of foreign-body giant cells where hair follicles have been destroyed.

Clinical features. Initially, a small area of scalp becomes red, crusted and irritable; crusting and superficial pustulation overlie a moist eroded surface. As the condition extends, areas of activity coexist with areas of cicatricial alopecia. Squamous carcinoma has developed in the scars [4].

Differential diagnosis. Pyogenic and yeast infection is excluded by bacteriological examination and the lack of response to antibacterial or antifungal agents. Biopsy may be necessary to exclude pustular psoriasis, cicatricial pemphigoid, 'irritated' solar keratosis or squamous cell carcinoma.

Treatment. The stronger topical corticosteroids such as 0.05% clobetasol propionate will suppress the inflammatory changes. Gradual reduction in the potency of topical steroid over a 6-month period may result in cure. Maintenance therapy with sun protection and intermittent moderate potency steroid can provide long-term relief. Ikeda *et al.* [5] suggested oral zinc sulphate can be curative in some cases.

REFERENCES

1 Caputo R, Veraldi S. Erosive pustular dermatosis of the scalp. *J Am Acad Dermatol* 1993; **28**: 96–7.
2 Pye RJ, Peachey RDG, Burton JL. Erosive pustular dermatosis of the scalp. *Br J Dermatol* 1979; **100**: 559–63.
3 Grattan CEH, Peachey RD, Boon A. Evidence for a role of local trauma in the pathogenesis of erosive pustular dermatosis of the scalp. *Clin Exp Dermatol* 1988; **13**: 7–12.
4 Lovell CR, Harman RRM, Bradfield JWB. Cutaneous carcinoma arising in erosive pustular dermatosis of the scalp. *Br J Dermatol* 1980; **102**: 325–30.
5 Ikeda M, Arata J, Isaka H. Erosive dermatosis of the scalp successfully treated with oral zinc sulphate. *Br J Dermatol* 1983; **105**: 742–7.

Necrobiosis lipoidica

Necrobiosis occurs in 0.2–0.3% of cases of diabetes mellitus, and approximately 70% of patients with necrobiosis have diabetes. The diabetic cases begin in childhood or early adult life and the non-diabetic cases rather later and usually in women.

The oval atrophic plaques classically occur on the shins

but may be seen in other parts of the body including the scalp. The patches are glazed and yellowish, often with conspicuous telangiectases. Scarring may be dense. The clinical features in the scalp have varied from large plaques of cicatricial alopecia to multiple small areas of scarring resembling alopecia parvimacularis [1].

An atrophic form affecting predominantly the forehead and the scalp has been described [2,3]. In general, the differential diagnosis is from sarcoidosis [4].

REFERENCES

1 Gertmann H, Dickmans-Burmeister D. Ungewohnliche Hautveran-derungen bei einem 4 jahrigen Kinde mit Diabetes mellitus. 'Nekrobiosis diabetica acute parvimaculata'. *Hautarzt* 1969; **20**: 265–72.
2 Navaratnam A, Hodgson CA. Necrobiosis lipoidica presenting on the face and scalp. *Br J Dermatol* 1973; **89** (Suppl. 9): 100–1.
3 Wilson Jones E. Necrobiosis lipoidica presenting on the face and scalp. *Trans St John's Hosp Dermatol Soc* 1971; **57**: 202–9.
4 Maurice DDL, Goolamali SK. Sarcoidosis of the scalp presenting as scarring alopecia. *Br J Dermatol* 1988; **119**: 116–18.

Lichen sclerosus et atrophicus

This disease affects females ten times more often than males [1]. Lichen sclerosus of the scalp appears to be rare. In one case [2], an elderly woman, it caused extensive cicatricial alopecia; there were also lesions of the trunk and vulva.

REFERENCES

1 Wallace HI. Lichen sclerosis et atrophicus. *Trans St John's Hosp Dermatol Soc* 1972; **57**: 148–60.
2 Foulds IS. Lichen sclerosus et atrophicus of the scalp. *Br J Dermatol* 1980; **103**: 197–9.

Lumpy scalp syndrome [1]

The inheritance of this syndrome is determined by an autosomal dominant gene of variable expressivity. Raw areas are present in the scalp at birth. They heal to leave irregular nodules of connective tissue which, on histological examination, are not keloidal in structure. The pinnae are deformed: the tragus, antitragus and lobule are small or rudimentary. The nipples are rudimentary or absent, and only areolae are present.

REFERENCE

1 Finlay AY, Marks R. An hereditary syndrome of lumpy scalp, odd ears and rudimentary nipples. *Clin Exp Dermatol* 1989; **15**: 240.

Lipo-oedematous alopecia [1,2]

This syndrome has been recognized only in black women, in whom an increase in thickness of the subcutis of the scalp, affecting particularly the subcutaneous fat, is associated with atrophy and fibrous replacement of many hair follicles. Clinically, there is slowly progressive diffuse alopecia and obvious thickening of the scalp.

REFERENCES

1 Coskey RJ, Fosnaugh R, Fire G. Lipoedematous alopecia. *Arch Dermatol* 1961; **84**: 619–22.
2 Curtis JW, Heising RA. Lipoedematous alopecia associated with skin hyperelasticity. *Arch Dermatol* 1964; **89**: 819–20.

Physical trauma

The diagnosis and treatment of the consequences of physical injuries of the scalp will seldom confront the dermatologist, but he may be consulted as to the cause of an apparent physical injury, for example aplasia cutis may be falsely attributed to forceps injury at childbirth.

The attachment of an electrode to the scalp for monitoring the fetal heartbeat during labour may occasionally cause some superficial damage to the scalp and this may be followed by a small scar. Aplasia cutis has sometimes been mistaken for such a lesion [1].

An unusual case of cicatricial alopecia in a boy aged 13 years was due to injury to the scalp by an intravenous infusion given in infancy for gastroenteritis [2].

Exceptionally, self-inflicted injuries may involve the scalp and leave scars.

Halo scalp ring [3]

A type of alopecia, which may be temporary or permanent, is an area of scalp hair loss due to prolonged pressure on the vertex by the uterine cervix during or prior to delivery, resulting in a haemorrhagic form of caput succedaneum.

Scalp necrosis after surgical embolization

Adler *et al.* [4] described a case in which ischaemic necrosis of the occipital scalp occurred following embolization and surgery for a large convexity meningioma.

REFERENCES

1 Brown ZA, Jung AL, Stenehuver MA. Aplasia cutis congenita and the fetal scalp electrode. *Am J Obstet Gynecol* 1977; **129**: 351–60.
2 Strong AMM. Extensive cicatricial alopecia following a scalp vein infusion. *Clin Exp Dermatol* 1979; **4**: 197–9.
3 Prendiville JS, Esterly NB. Halo scalp ring: a cause of scarring alopecia. *Arch Dermatol* 1987; **123**: 992–4.
4 Adler JR, Upton J, Wallman J *et al.* Management and prevention of necrosis of the scalp after embolization and surgery for meningioma. *Surg Neurol* 1988; **25**: 357–66.

Chronic radiodermatitis [1,2]

Roentgen discovered X-rays in 1895. X-ray epilation of the face for hirsutism was frequently employed during the first two decades of the 20th century, and although Schultz [3] condemned this treatment, it continued to be so widely used that Cipollaro and Einhorn [4] entitled their paper: 'The use of X-rays for the treatment of hypertrichosis is dangerous'.

X-ray epilation for the treatment of scalp ringworm was introduced in Paris in 1904. The discovery of griseofulvin in 1958 gradually made X-ray epilation unnecessary, but it has been estimated that between 1904 and 1959 some 300 000 children throughout the world were treated with X-rays for ringworm of the scalp. Correct dosage did not cause toxicity; however, technical errors were frequent, from inadequate and poorly calibrated apparatus. The treatment produced complete epilation in about 3 weeks and regrowth after 2 months. The follow-up of 2043 patients treated in childhood showed a higher incidence of cancer in the patients than in a control group [1]. Radiodermatitis of the scalp may occur also as an unavoidable consequence of skin damage during the treatment of both internal malignant disease and malignant disease of the skin.

The use of X-rays for epilation depends on the high susceptibility of anagen hairs to radiation. Epilating and subepilating doses produced dystrophic changes in human hairs as early as the 4th day after exposure [5]. Chronic radiodermatitis may follow acute radiodermatitis, but may develop only slowly as degenerative changes induced by sun exposure and ageing become superimposed. In chronic radiodermatitis, the epidermis is generally atrophic with loss of hair follicles and sebaceous glands, but there are also irregular areas of acanthosis. Degenerative changes and nuclear abnormalities are frequent in the epidermis. Dermal collagen stains irregularly. Superficial small vessels are telangiectatic, but deeper vessels are partially or completely occluded by fibrosis.

Clinical features. The development of a basal cell carcinoma in middle age or later in an area of the scalp should lead the dermatologist to enquire about X-ray epilation for ringworm in childhood [6]. In other cases, the patient complains of hair loss, which is apparently accentuated in certain areas and these areas are found to show both androgenetic alopecia and reduction of follicle population as a result of the earlier radiation.

Chronic radiodermatitis produced by radiation therapy of a malignant tumour of the scalp presents a circumscribed area of cicatricial alopecia. Radiation necrosis may simulate a recurrence of carcinoma, but the edges of the necrotic ulcer are not raised. The diagnosis should be confirmed by a biopsy. Superficial X-ray of Grenz ray type does not penetrate deeply enough to damage scalp follicles. Malignant tumours arising in radiodermatitis should be excised [7].

REFERENCES

1 Albert RE, Omran AR. Follow-up study of patients treated with X-ray epilation for tinea capitis. I. Population characteristics, post-treatment illness and mortality experience. *Arch Environ Health* 1968; **17**: 899–905.
2 Getzrow PL. Chronic radiodermatitis and skin cancer. In: Andrade R, Gumport SL, Popkin GL *et al.*, eds. *Cancer of the Skin*. Philadelphia: WB Saunders, 1976: 458–67.
3 Schultz F, ed. *The X-ray Treatment of Skin Diseases*. London: Rebman, 1912: 135–51.
4 Cipollaro AC, Einhorn MB. The use of X-rays for the treatment of hypertrichosis is dangerous. *JAMA* 1947; **135**: 349–54.
5 Van Scott EJ, Reinertson RP. Detection of radiation effects on hair roots of the human scalp. *J Invest Dermatol* 1957; **29**: 205–16.
6 Ridley CM. Basal cell carcinoma following X-ray epilation of the scalp. *Br J Dermatol* 1962; **74**: 222–7.
7 Conway H, Hugo NE. Radiation dermatitis and malignancy. *Plast Reconstruct Surg* 1966; **38**: 255–9.

Non-cicatricial scalp disorders

Pruritic syndromes

Pruritus of the scalp may occur as an isolated symptom in the absence of any objective changes. The patient is often middle-aged, the pruritus is spasmodic and may be intense, and exacerbations are frequently related to periods of stress or fatigue.

Pruritus is also the predominant manifestation of acne necrotica, in which scattered vesicles followed by small crusts are a source of severe discomfort. Dermatitis herpetiformis may involve the scalp. Grouped papules and vesicles in recurrent crops may be associated with similar lesions of the trunk and limbs.

Lichen simplex is a frequent cause of pruritus of the nape and occipital region in women, and may also be localized above one or both ears. In the affected region, the scalp is thickened and scaly.

The protection provided by the hair accounts for the rarity of contact dermatitis, and even reactions to hair dyes and other hair cosmetics more commonly involve the ears, neck, forehead or face than the scalp itself. However, intense irritation of the scalp is sometimes the initial symptom of a sensitization reaction and, rarely, eczematous changes may affect the whole or part of the scalp. Apart from hair cosmetics and medicaments, hats should be suspected.

Seborrhoeic and atopic dermatitis and other inflammatory disorders may be pruritic, but pruritus is seldom a presenting symptom. Psoriasis is not usually pruritic but may occasionally be so.

In children and in women of any age, pediculosis should be excluded no matter what the social status of the patient. Multiple insect bites are sometimes a puzzling source of irritation in children, and are usually rapidly complicated by infection as a result of excoriation. In infants, in old age and in the immunosuppressed, scabies may cause scalp irritation.

Pityriasis capitis

It now seems reasonable to accept pityriasis as near-physiological scaling of the scalp or other hairy regions, which may or may not be fortuitously associated with 'seborrhoea' or with baldness. Pityriasis simplex or furfuracea is popularly known as dandruff.

Aetiology. Pityriasis is a cosmetic affliction of adolescence and adult life and is relatively rare and mild in children. Its peak incidence and severity are reached at the age of about 20 years and it becomes less frequent after 50 years. At age 20 years, some 50% of white people are affected in some degree.

The age incidence suggests that an androgenic influence is important, and the level of sebaceous activity may be a factor. However, gross seborrhoea may occur without pityriasis and commonly severe pityriasis may be present without clinically apparent excessive sebaceous activity.

The microbial origin of pityriasis was accepted by Sabouraud in the 19th century, but a number of later authors could establish no correlation between the degree of pityriasis and the population of *Pityrosporum ovale*. However, the role of *P. ovale* is still disputed. This yeast increases in number at puberty and it elaborates substances that inhibit the growth of dermatophytes. The large numbers of *P. ovale* in scalps with pityriasis have been regarded as secondary to the increased scaling [1]. In another investigation of yeasts in subjects with and without pityriasis [2], it was concluded that although no specific organism was significantly related to pityriasis, an increase in the total microbial flora was a factor in the increase of pityriasis. It had previously been demonstrated that the application of yeast inhibitors to one half of the scalp produced a greater reduction in pityriasis than did the application of a bacterial inhibitor to the other half of the same scalp [3]. When the scalp flora of 11 subjects was almost completely eliminated by the application of nystatin and neomycin, the production of pityriasis was reduced by over 50%; and when a nystatin-resistant strain of *P. ovale* was then introduced, the severity of the pityriasis increased by over 80% [4]. However, some antimicrobial agents will decrease the flora without affecting the severity of pityriasis [1]. Further quantitative studies of the microflora have not finally resolved the problem of their precise role in the production of pityriasis; *P. ovale* is more abundant in pityriasis than in the normal scalp, and still more so in seborrhoeic dermatitis, whereas *Corynebacterium acnes* is less abundant in pityriasis than in normal scalps, and almost disappears in seborrhoeic dermatitis [5]; these changes could be influenced by increased blood flow as *C. acnes* is strictly anaerobic.

Some of the investigations mentioned above, tending to attribute a pathogenic role to microorganisms, were not well controlled. The balance of evidence [6] suggests that scalp organisms do not play any role in causing pityriasis capitis but are present in abundance because of the increased availability of scalp nutrients. Shuster [7], on historical and scientific grounds, presented the contrary view, particularly stressing the importance of the beneficial effects of antipityrosporum agents as supporting the infection aetiology.

Pathology. In the normal scalp the horny layer consists of 25–35 fully keratinized and closely coherent cells; in pityriasis there are usually fewer than 10 layers of cells, and these are often parakeratotic and irregularly arranged, with deep crevices resulting in the formation of the flakes visible clinically [1]. Autoradiographic studies [8,9] showed a high labelling index and stratum corneum transit time of 3–4 days. Application of selenium sulphide reduced the labelling index and slowed down the transit time.

Clinical features. Small, white or grey scales accumulate on the surface of the scalp in localized, more or less segmental patches or more diffusely. After removal with an effective shampoo, the scales form again within 4–7 days. The condition first becomes a cosmetic problem during the second and third decades, but there are long-term and short-term variations in its severity, without obvious cause. There are also variations in the ease with which the scales become detached and drift unaesthetically among the hair shafts or fall on the collar and shoulders. Although pityriasis usually clears spontaneously during the fifth or sixth decade, it may persist in old age.

In those subjects whose scalps become greasy at or after puberty, the seborrhoea binds the scale in a greasy 'paste' and it is no longer shed, but accumulates in small adherent mounds—as so-called pityriasis steatoides. The development of clinically evident inflammatory changes in such individuals leads to seborrhoeic dermatitis. Pruritus is not a feature of simple pityriasis. It is very much more common when inflammatory changes develop in the seborrhoeic scalp, and such recurrent episodes may be clearly related to periods of stress. Acne necrotica, which may be intensely irritable, also can complicate pityriasis.

Diagnosis. The presence of more than very mild pityriasis in a young child throws doubt on the diagnosis. Extreme and persistent scaling, even though it lacks the characteristic features of psoriasis, is always suspect, particularly if there is a family history of this disease. Widespread scaling, sometimes with scarring, may occur in some forms of ichthyosis. At any age, if pruritus is troublesome, pediculosis must be carefully excluded.

Small areas of scaling with dull broken hair shafts are typical of *Microsporum* ringworm. Localized scaling in children is therefore an indication for examination of the scalp under Wood's light, and of the broken hairs under the microscope. A nervous hair-pulling tic may result in twisted and broken hairs of normal texture in a patch of postinflammatory scaling.

Profuse, adherent silvery scale should suggest pityriasis amiantacea.

Treatment. Pityriasis in its milder forms is a physiological process. The object of treatment is to control it at the lowest possible cost and inconvenience to the patient, appreciating that any procedure found to be effective will need to be repeated at regular intervals.

In the average case, one of the many proprietary shampoos may be found effective. Selenium sulphide, which has been shown to reduce epidermal turnover [8,9], is very useful for many patients but fails inexplicably in others. The same may be said of preparations containing zinc pyrithione or zinc omadine, which are said to reduce the yeast population [10].

The evidence presented by Shuster [7] and Shuster and Blachford [11] has converted many clinicians away from the above to specific antipityrosporum therapy with imidazole compounds, for example ketoconazole shampoo [12].

REFERENCES

1 Ackerman AB, Kligman AM. Some observations on dandruff. *J Soc Cosmet Chem* 1969; **20**: 81–6.
2 Roia FC, Vanderwyk RW. Residual microbial flora of the human scalp and its relationship to dandruff. *J Soc Cosmet Chem* 1969; **20**: 113–19.
3 Vanderwyk RW, Hechemey KE. A comparison of the bacterial and yeast flora of the human scalp and their effect upon dandruff production. *J Soc Cosmet Chem* 1967; **18**: 629–36.
4 Gosse RM, Vanderwyk RW. The relationship of a nystatin-resistant strain of *Pityrosporum ovale* to dandruff. *J Soc Cosmet Chem* 1969; **20**: 603–9.
5 McGinley KJ, Leyden JJ, Marples RR *et al*. Quantitative microbiology of the scalp in non-dandruff, dandruff and seborrhoeic dermatitis. *J Invest Dermatol* 1975; **64**: 401–13.
6 Leyden JJ, McGinley KJ, Kligman AM. Role of microorganisms in dandruff. *Arch Dermatol* 1976; **112**: 333–40.
7 Shuster S. The aetiology of dandruff and the mode of action of therapeutic agents. *Br J Dermatol* 1984; **111**: 235–42.
8 Plewig G, Kligman AM. The effect of selenium sulphide on epidermal turnover of normal and dandruff scalps. *J Soc Cosmet Chem* 1969; **20**: 767–71.
9 Plewig G, Kligman AM. Zellkinetische Untersuchungen bei Kopfschuppenerkrankung. *Arch Klin Exp Dermatol* 1970; **236**: 406–10.
10 Brauer EW, Opdyke DL, Burnett CM. The anti-seborrhoeic qualities of zinc pyrithione in a cream vehicle. *J Invest Dermatol* 1966; **47**: 174–82.
11 Shuster S, Blachford N. Seborrhoeic dermatitis and dandruff—a fungal disease. *R Soc Med Publ Lond* 1988: 1–30.
12 Cutsen JV, Gerven FV, Cauwenbergh G. The inflammatory effects of ketoconazole. *J Am Acad Dermatol* 1991; **25**: 257–9.

Pityriasis amiantacea

Pityriasis amiantacea is a reaction of the scalp often without evident cause. It may complicate seborrhoeic dermatitis, psoriasis or lichen simplex. Its association with these and other conditions is difficult to evaluate. It depends on the initial clinical diagnosis. Cases which some dermatologists would accept as early psoriasis are labelled pityriasis amiantacea by others. If such cases are excluded then there is no definite association between pityriasis amiantacea and psoriasis [1]. In Knight's study of 71 patients [2], two had associated psoriasis and nine had eczema; he pointed out that pityriasis amiantacea may occur at any age but the average age was 25 years (range 5–40 years).

Pathology. Biopsies from 18 patients were examined by Knight [2]. The most consistent findings were spongiosis, parakeratosis, migration of lymphocytes into the epidermis, and a variable degree of acanthosis. The essential features responsible for the asbestos-like scaling are diffuse hyperkeratosis and parakeratosis together with follicular keratosis, which surrounds each hair with a sheath of horn.

Clinical features [2]. Masses of adherent, silvery scales, overlapping like the tiles on a roof, adhere to the scalp and are attached in layers to the shafts of the hairs which they surround (Fig. 66.37). The underlying scalp may be red and moist or may show simple erythema and scaling, or the features of psoriasis, seborrhoeic dermatitis or of lichen simplex.

A relatively common form seen mainly in young girls complicates recurrent or chronic fissuring behind one or both ears. The scales extend some distance into the neighbouring scalp. Another form extends upwards from patches of lichen simplex and is seen mainly in middle-aged women. The disease is usually confined to small areas of the scalp, but may be very extensive, either involving a large area diffusely, or affecting a number of small patches. The latter form in children often proves to be psoriasis by its subsequent course. The majority of patients notice some hair loss in areas of severe scaling. The hair regrows when the scaling is effectively treated. If scarring alopecia occurs, it may well be related to secondary infection, i.e. mixed bacterial and pityrosporum.

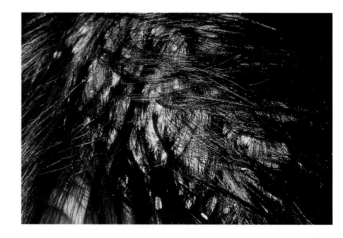

Fig. 66.37 Pityriasis amiantacea.

Diagnosis. Usually, the distinctive clinical appearance makes the diagnosis easy, but the identification of the underlying disease may not be straightforward; indeed, none may be established.

Treatment. Where pityriasis complicates lichen simplex or psoriasis, the underlying condition must be treated, but it may be useful initially to eliminate the abundant scale by the use of oil of Cade ointment or a topical tar/salicylic acid ointment, which is also effective in many cases where no preceding disease of the scalp is discovered. Either preparation should be washed out of the scalp after 4–5 h with a suitable shampoo, for example tar or imidazole shampoo. Even then, the condition tends to recur sometimes.

If psoriasis is associated, then the same local or systemic treatment principles used in general may be effective in treating the scalp [3]. Potent topical corticosteroid scalp liquids, or short courses of systemic corticosteroid, may be beneficial in some cases.

REFERENCES

1 Hersle K, Lindholm A, Mobaeken H *et al*. Relationship of pityriasis amiantacea to psoriasis. *Dermatologica* 1979; **159**: 245–50.
2 Knight AG. Pityriasis amiantacea; a clinical and histopathologic investigation. *Clin Exp Dermatol* 1977; **2**: 137–44.
3 Dawber RPR. Aspects of treatment of scalp psoriasis. *J Dermatol Treat* 1989; **1**: 103–8.

Folliculitis

See Chapter 27.

Keloidalis nuchae

See Chapter 27.

Dissecting cellulitis

See Chapter 27.

Pseudofolliculitis

See Chapter 27.

Cutis verticis gyrata [1,2]

The term cutis verticis gyrata (CVG) describes the hypertrophy and folding of the skin of the scalp, to present a gyrate or cerebriform appearance. Dermatologists use the term to describe a morphological syndrome with many causes.

Pathology. The essential abnormality appears to be overgrowth of the scalp in relation to the underlying skull.

Some predisposing factor must be postulated, as it occurs in only a small proportion of cases of each of the conditions with which it is associated. The naevoid forms usually prove to be melanocytic. Biopsies in the primary form [3] showed possible sebaceous hyperplasia, but no obvious excess of collagen.

Aetiology and clinical features. Primary CVG, which occurs almost exclusively in males, is probably genetically determined, but its mode of inheritance is uncertain [4]; most cases appear to be sporadic. It has been reported in association with Darier's disease and with tuberous sclerosis. It accounts for 0.5% of the retarded population in Sweden [4], Scotland [5] and the USA [6]. The prevalence of the condition may be still higher, as there is evidence that at least some patients with the Lennox–Gastart syndrome (retardation with an electroencephalograph showing slow and irregular space and wave complexes) later develop CVG [6].

The longitudinal and irregularly parallel folds of the scalp may appear in late childhood or at puberty and slowly become more accentuated. The IQ is rarely over 35 and cerebral palsy (spastic diplegia) and epilepsy are present [4,7].

Pachydermoperiostosis. This genetically determined syndrome also occurs mainly in men and has often been confused with CVG. It differs from it in several particulars. The scalp is folded but the skin of the face is affected, as is that of the hands and feet. The cutaneous changes, which are accompanied by thickening of the phalanges and of the long bones of the limbs, progress for 10–15 years, then become static.

Acromegaly. Mild degrees of CVG are not uncommon in acromegaly, but more severe forms have been reported [8,9].

Other endocrine disorders. Rarely, CVG has been associated with cretinism or myxoedema, but the significance of these case reports is uncertain.

Naevi. Naevi may assume a folded or cerebriform structure and thus simulate CVG. The naevus is present at birth and usually covers only a relatively small area [10] but may slowly increase in size to cover most of the scalp. Most of the reported cases have been naevi of melanocytic type, but neurofibromas and fibromas can assume this form [11].

Treatment. In the majority of cases only symptomatic measures are practicable. Plastic surgery was helpful in CVG in acromegaly [1] and may of course be indicated in cerebriform naevi.

REFERENCES

1 Abu-Jamra F, Dinsich DF. Cutis verticis gyrata. *Am J Surg* 1966; **111**: 274–9.
2 Diven DG, Tanus T, Raimer S. Cutis verticis gyrata. *Int J Dermatol* 1991; **30**: 710–11.
3 Paulson G, Dudley AW. Cutis verticis gyrata. *Confinia Neurolog* 1966; **28**: 432.
4 Akesson HO. Cutis verticis gyrata and mental deficiency in Sweden. II Genetic aspects. *Acta Med Scand* 1964; **177**: 459–63.
5 MacGillvray RC. Cutis verticis gyrata and mental retardation. *Scott Med J* 1967; **12**: 450–6.
6 Paulson GW. Cutis verticis gyrata and the Lennox syndrome. *Dev Med Child Neurol* 1974; **16**: 196–200.
7 Kratten FI. The incidence of cutis verticis gyrata in three low-grade mental defectives. *J Med Sci* 1958; **104**: 850–6.
8 Zeisler EP, Wieder LJ. Cutis verticis gyrata and acromegaly. *Arch Dermatol Syphilol* 1940; **42**: 1092–9.
9 Serfling HJ, Foelsche W. Extensive Form einer Cutis verticis gyrata bei Hypophysenadenome. *Zentralblatt Chirurg* 1959; **84**: 473–9.
10 Hammond G, Ransome HK. Cerebriform nevus resembling cutis verticis gyrata. *Arch Surg* 1937; **35**: 309–16.
11 McConnell LH, Davies AJM. Massive fibroma of the scalp. *Ann Surg* 1943; **118**: 154–8.

Abnormalities of hair shaft

Structural defects of the hair shaft may be sufficient in degree to cause significant cosmetic disability, or they may render the hair abnormally susceptible to injury by minor degrees of trauma (excessive weathering). They may also be the result of hereditary or acquired metabolic disorders, affording valuable clues to the diagnosis of these disorders [1].

Price [2] classified anomalies of the shaft into those which are associated with increased fragility, and those which are not. This distinction is useful because only the former present clinically as patchy or diffuse alopecia. Price's classification will be followed throughout the present chapter. Whiting [3] has published a detailed and authoritative outline of all the major structural defects. Birnhaum and Baden [4] have also carefully reviewed the rarer structural abnormalities.

REFERENCES

1 de Berker D, Sinclair R. Defects of the hair shaft. In: Dawber RPR, ed. *Diseases of the Hair and Scalp*, 3rd edn. Oxford: Blackwell Science Limited, 1997: 396–489.
2 Price VH. Strukturanomalien des Haarschaftes. In: Orfanos CE, ed. *Haar und Haarkrankheiten*. Stuttgart: Fischer, 1979: 387–446.
3 Whiting DA. Structural abnormalities of the hair shaft. *J Am Acad Dermatol* 1987; **16**: 1–34.
4 Birnhaum PS, Baden HP. Heritable disorders of hair. *Dermatol Clin* 1987; **5**: 137–53.

Structural defects with increased fragility

Monilethrix (beading of hair) (Fig. 66.38)

Smith [1] initially called this condition 'a rare nodose condition of the hair'. Radcliffe Crocker subsequently suggested the term monilethrix. Nevertheless, some early reports, and even some more recent ones, confuse moni-

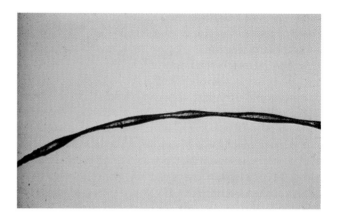

Fig. 66.38 Monilethrix, showing characteristic 'beading', node formation.

lethrix with other shaft defects, for example trichorrhexis nodosa, when 'weathering' is severe.

Aetiology. The hereditary nature of monilethrix was recognized soon after the condition was first identified. Autosomal dominant transmission has been demonstrated in numerous large pedigrees [2–4]. The alleged occurrence of normal carriers of the dominant gene has not been proven, for a parent with only 5% of abnormal follicles is easily passed as normal [5]. The gene appears to have high penetrance but variable expressivity. Several pedigrees have suggested an autosomal recessive trait [6]. Monilethrix may be a heterogeneous condition [7], but in some families studies have linked it to the gene cluster at 12q13 [8].

Pathology. The hair shaft is beaded and breaks easily. Elliptical nodes 0.7–1 mm apart, are separated by narrower internodes. The widths of the nodes and the distances between them show some variation within a single family. By scanning electron microscopy, the nodes and some of the internodes show a normal imbricated scale pattern, but most internodes show longitudinal ridging [9,10].

Histologically, the follicle shows wide and narrow zones corresponding to the nodes and internodes [11], but the general structure of the follicle is otherwise normal. Salamon and Schneyder [3] and Gummer and Dawber [12] noted that changes were visible in the zone of keratinization; the cell membranes of the deeper hair shaft cuticular cells are thrown into folds, particularly at the narrower internodes where breakage occurs.

Attempts have been made to investigate the mechanism of node formation and to relate it to the diurnal rate of hair growth. Klingmuller [13] claimed to have found a 48-h cycle in two patients. Baker [14] studied four cases in which he found that a complete nodal complex was formed in 24 h. Comaish [9] found no daily rhythm and no simple time cycle. Lubach and Traintos [15] showed no regular rhythm of node formation.

Intermittent administration of an antimitotic agent can give rise to zones of constriction alternating with zones of normal diameter [16].

Studies with the electron microscope [17] have shown that increased susceptibility of the hair shaft to the effects of the trauma—premature weathering—is an important factor in the failure of the hair to attain a normal length.

Clinical features. Monilethrix shows considerable variation in age of onset, severity and course [18]. There is not yet sufficient information to establish whether these variations are in part consistently correlated with different genotypes. There is, however, much variation even within the more commonly reported autosomal dominant form, but some of it is merely apparent.

The hair may be obviously abnormal at birth but is most commonly normal, and is progressively replaced by abnormal hair during the first months of life; in other cases, the normal hair is succeeded by horny follicular papules from the summit of which emerge fragile beaded hairs. The follicular keratoses and the abnormal hairs are most frequent on the nape and occiput but may involve the entire scalp. In a typical case, the short stubble of brittle hairs and rough horny plugs give a distinctive appearance (Fig. 66.39). In some cases, the eyebrows and eyelashes, pubic and axillary hair and general body hair may be affected.

In many patients, the condition persists with little change throughout life [4]. Spontaneous improvement or complete recovery has occurred [1] and has been reported during pregnancy [19]. Griseofulvin also has temporarily restored normal hair growth [20].

Associated defects. Some investigators [3] thought the association with oligophrenia and with nail and tooth defects was significant. It is possible that such associations may be a feature of the recessive phenotype, as oligophrenia and poor physical development were noted also in two siblings with monilethrix [21]. Association with juvenile cataract has been reported [22].

Reports of abnormalities of amino-acid metabolism are conflicting. Argininosuccinic aciduria has been reported [23], but a technical error was subsequently detected [24]. No abnormality in the urinary amino-acid pattern was found in the autosomal dominant type [19] or in an isolated case [25]. An apparent excess of aspartic acid and arginine in the urine of an affected mother and daughter was described by Marques Llagaria *et al.* [26].

Treatment. None is available but Tamayo [27] has suggested that oral retinoids can induce some hair regrowth. This may be due to a therapeutic effect on the keratosis pilaris, which lessens in combination with a reduction of shaft beading and modest increase in overall hair length [28]. Reduction of hairdressing trauma may be followed by some improvement, thus lessening the 'weathering' from chemical and physical insults.

REFERENCES

1 Smith WG. A rare nodose condition of the hair. *Br Med J* 1879; **11**: 291–6.
2 Rodemund OE. Zur Monilethrix. *Zeitschr Haut Geschlectskrank* 1969; **44**: 291–9.
3 Salamon T, Schneyder UW. Über die Monilethrix. *Arch Klin Exp Dermatol* 1962; **215**: 105–10.
4 Solomon IL, Green OC. Monilethrix. *N Engl J Med* 1963; **269**: 1279–85.
5 Deraemaeker R. Monilethrix: report of a family with special reference to some problems concerning inheritance. *Am J Hum Genet* 1957; **9**: 195–201.
6 Hanhert E. Erstmaliger Hinweis auf das Vorkommen einer Monohybrid-rezessivere Erbgangs bei Monilethrix (Moniletrichosis). *Arch Julius-Klaus Stift Verebungsforsch* 1955; **30**: 1.
7 Richard G, Itin P, Lin JP *et al.* Evidence for genetic heterogeneity in monilethrix. *J Invest Dermatol* 1996; **107**: 812–14.
8 Stevens HP, Kelsall DP, Dawber RPR *et al.* Linkage of monilethrix to the trichocyte and keratin gene cluster on 12q11–q13. *J Invest Dermatol* 1996; **106**: 795–9.
9 Comaish S. Autoradiographic studies of hair growth and rhythm in monilethrix. *Br J Dermatol* 1969; **81**: 443–9.
10 Dawber RPR. Weathering of hair in some genetic hair shaft abnormalities. In: Brown A, Crosin RG, eds. *Hair: Trace Elements and Human Illness.* New York: Praeger, 1980: 95–102.
11 de Berker D, Ferguson DJP, Dawber RPR. Monilethrix: a clinicopathological demonstration of the defect. *Br J Dermatol* 1993; **128**: 327–9.
12 Gummer CL, Dawber RPR, Swift JA. Monilethrix: an electron microscopic and electron histochemical study. *Br J Dermatol* 1981; **105**: 529–36.
13 Klingmuller G. Monilethrix mit 48 Studen-Rhythmus. *Hautarzt* 1954; **5**: 23–7.
14 Baker H. An investigation of monilethrix. *Br J Dermatol* 1962; **74**: 24–30.
15 Lubach D, Triantos N. Untersuchungen uber die Monilethrix. *Hautarzt* 1979; **30**: 253–9.
16 Van Scott EJ, Reinhertson RP, Steinmuller R. The growing hair roots of the human scalp and morphologic changes therein following aminopterin therapy. *J Invest Dermatol* 1957; **29**: 197–209.
17 Dawber RPR. Weathering of hair in monilethrix and pili torti. *Clin Exp Dermatol* 1977; **2**: 271–80.
18 Amichai B, Grunwald MH, Halevy S. Hair loss in a 6-month-old child. *Arch Dermatol* 1996; **132**: 577–8.
19 Summerly R, Donaldson EM. Monilethrix. *Br J Dermatol* 1962; **74**: 387–94.
20 Keipert JA. The effect of griseofulvin on hair growth in monilethrix. *Med J Aust* 1973; **ii**: 1236–8.

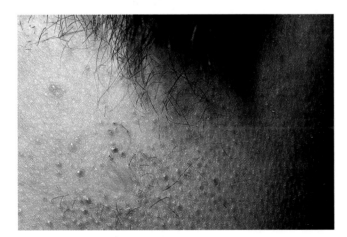

Fig. 66.39 Monilethrix. Nape of the neck showing follicular keratoses and short broken hairs; beading was only clearly visible in this case with a × 8 magnifying lens and by light microscopy (see Fig. 66.38).

21 Sfaello H, Hariga J. Monilothrix associé à la debilité mental; étude d'une famille. *Arch Belges Derm Syph* 1967; **23**: 363.
22 Thiel E. Monilethrix und Fruhstar. *Hautarzt* 1959; **10**: 271–9.
23 Grosfeld JCM, Mighorst JA, Moolhuysen TMGF. Argininosuccinic aciduria in monilethrix. *Lancet* 1964; **ii**: 789–91.
24 Efron ML, Hoefnagel D. Argininosuccinic acid in monilethrix. *Lancet* 1966; **i**: 321.
25 Mader AK, Rose JH. Monilethrix und Argininbersteinsaure-Ausscheidung. *Dermatol Monatschr* 1969; **155**: 409–16.
26 Marques Llagaria E, Calap Calatynd J, Torres Peris V. Monilethrix: Estudio apropositio de dos casos familares. *Acta Derm Sifiligr* 1973; **64**: 203–12.
27 Tamayo L. Monilethrix—treated with the oral retinoid Ro-10-9359 (Tigason). *Clin Exp Dermatol* 1983; **8**: 393–6.
28 de Berker DAR, Dawber RPR. Monilethrix treated with oral retinoids. *Clin Exp Dermatol* 1990; **16**: 226–8.

Pseudomonilethrix

It is not uncommon to see patients who complain that their hair is of poor quality or brittle, and if the patient in question is a young child, microscopy of the hair to exclude the classical shaft defects is a routine procedure. It should be a routine procedure also in the older child or adult. Bentley-Phillips and Bayles [1] described a syndrome which they termed 'pseudomonilethrix' in South Africans of European or Indian descent. The status of the syndrome is uncertain; some of the shaft deformities may be artefactual.

The patients present with alopecia from the age of 8 years onwards and their lack of hair can be shown to be the result of a defect whose inheritance is determined by an autosomal dominant gene. The defect renders the hair so fragile that it readily breaks with the trauma of brushing, combing or other hairdressing procedures.

On microscopy, one, or occasionally two, of three abnormalities can be seen. These are:

1 pseudomonilethrix—irregular nodes, which on electron microscopy prove to be the protruding edges of depressions in the shaft;
2 irregular twists of 25–200° without flattening of the shaft;

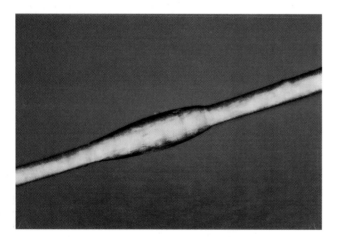

Fig. 66.40 Hair lacquer can cause fusiform bulges along the hair shaft.

3 breaks with brush-like ends in an apparently normal shaft.

There is no keratosis pilaris. Most authorities now believe that pseudomonilethrix microscopic changes are artefactual. They can be produced in normal hairs by trauma from tweezers or forceps, or compressing overlapping hairs between two glass slides: the indentation in one shaft caused by another overlying hair exactly mimics the appearance of pseudomonilethrix [2]. Hair lacquer and gel can also cause beading visible under the light microscope [3] (Fig. 66.40).

REFERENCES

1 Bentley-Phillips B, Bayles MAH. Pseudomonilethrix. *Br J Dermatol* 1975; **92**: 113–20.
2 Zitelli JA. Pseudomonilethrix: an artefact. *Arch Dermatol* 1986; **122**: 688–92.
3 Itin PH, Schiller P, Mathys D, Guggenheim R. Cosmetically induced hair beads. *J Am Acad Dermatol* 1997; **36**: 260–1.

Pili torti (twisting of hair)

The first definite description of pili torti was given by Schutz [1], although earlier authors had referred to the condition. Ormsby and Mitchell [2] twice presented the same patient to the Chicago Dermatological Society; on the first occasion the diagnosis was 'atrophia pilorum'; monilethrix. In discussion, attention was drawn to the fact that the hairs were twisted and not beaded! Galewsky [3] suggested the term 'pili torti', which was also adopted by Ronchese [4] in America.

In pili torti, the hairs are flattened and at irregular intervals completely rotated through 180° around their long axis (Fig. 66.41). The increasing use of the scanning electron microscope has made it clear that twisted hairs occur in many distinct forms, and that the twisting may be associated with a number of other shaft defects. Occasional twists of varying angle should not be taken to be this distinctive genetically 'fixed' abnormality of pili torti—many dystrophies and distortions of the follicular zone of keratinization will vary the hair shaft 'bore', sometimes showing < 180° irregular twists.

Syndromes of which twisted hair is a feature

Menkes' syndrome. Light-coloured, twisted hair is a manifestation of a hereditary defect of intestinal copper transport; the inheritance is of sex-linked recessive type. The twisting of the hair microscopically is generally exactly the same as in pili torti [5,6].

Bjornstad's syndrome. Twisted hair with sensorineural deafness: probable autosomal dominant inheritance.

Bazex syndrome. Twisted hair, with basal carcinomas of the face and follicular atrophoderma.

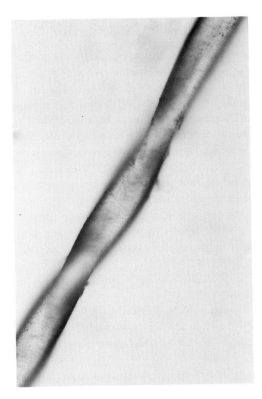

Fig. 66.41 Pili torti. Light micrograph showing 180° twists.

Crandall's syndrome. Twisted hair and deafness are associated with hypogonadism; probable sex-linked recessive inheritance.

Hypohidrotic ectodermal dysplasia. Twisted hairs associated with characteristic facies and dental defects.

Pseudomonilethrix. Twisted hair is associated, in the individual or the family, with apparently beaded hairs of autosomal dominant inheritance.

When patients with these syndromes are excluded, only pili torti remains, but there is evidence that they do not constitute a homogeneous entity: the hairs show considerable variation from patient to patient in their ability to withstand breaking and pulling, i.e. the hairs in some patients weather badly, but in others they do not [7].

Pollitt *et al.* [8] reported siblings with mental retardation, pili torti and trichorrhexis nodosa; their hair keratin was deficient in cysteine. However, dystrophic pili torti may occur with a normal cysteine content [9]; this case developed less weathered hair after puberty but the twists remained—possibly due to hair sebum 'protecting' the hair shafts from weathering [10].

Aetiology. In those cases in which classical pili torti of early onset appears to have occurred as an isolated defect, inheritance has usually been determined by an autosomal dominant gene [11,12]. There are many reports of apparently sporadic cases [13]. However, there are also cases in which the siblings of consanguineous parents have been affected and in which recessive inheritance must be suspected [14].

Local inflammatory processes which distort the follicles can result in distorted and twisted hairs, such as may be found around the edges of patches of cicatricial alopecia [15]. Acquired pili torti-type changes were produced by retinoids [16]; this is more 'kinked' rather than twisted. Non-scarring acquired pili torti has also been recorded in anorexia nervosa [17].

Pathology. The earlier reports emphasized that the affected hairs were flattened and twisted through 180° around their long axis at irregular intervals along the shaft. The load-extension curve (breaking stress analysis) resembles that of the wool of merino sheep; the hairs breaking more easily than normal. Histologically, the only abnormality is some curvature of the hair follicles. With the scanning electron microscope, the cuticle of the hair shaft appears normal [18], although severe weathering changes are not uncommon.

Clinical features. The hair is usually normal at birth, but is gradually replaced by abnormal hair, which becomes clinically evident as early as the third month, or not until the second or third year. There is a wide variation from case to case in the fragility of the hair, and hence in the clinical picture. Affected hairs are brittle and may break off at a length of 5 cm or less, or grow longer in areas of the scalp less subject to trauma. There may therefore be only a short, coarse stubble over the whole scalp or there may be circumscribed baldness, irregularly patchy or occipital. Affected hairs have a spangled appearance in reflected light.

Other ectodermal defects may be associated with pili torti. Keratosis pilaris is the most recently reported, but nail dystrophies, dental abnormalities, corneal opacities and mental retardation have all been described [19]. The syndrome described as corkscrew hair [20] is microscopically separate.

The diagnosis should be suspected if the hair is brittle and dry. The typical spangled appearance in reflected light is present only if the hair is at least moderately severely affected, yet is not so brittle that it breaks to leave only a sparse stubble. Microscopic examination of several hairs must be made to confirm the diagnosis.

REFERENCES

1 Schutz J. Pili moniliformis. *Arch Dermatol Syphilol* 1946; **53**: 69–73.
2 Ormsby OS, Mitchell JH. Atrophia pilorum. *Arch Dermatol Syphilol* 1925; **12**: 146–52.
3 Galewsky E. Pili torti. *Arch Dermatol Syphilol* 1932; **26**: 659–66.
4 Ronchese F. Twisted hairs (pili torti). *Arch Dermatol Syphilol* 1932; **26**: 98–104.

5 Dupre A, Enjolras O. Syndrome de Menkes avec pilotortoge alternante. *Ann Dermatol Vénéréol* 1980; **102**: 269–71.

6 Menkes JH, Alter M, Steigleder GK *et al.* A sex-linked recessive disorder with retardation of growth, peculiar hair and focal cerebral and cerebellar degeneration. *Paediatrics* 1962; **29**: 764–79.

7 Dawber RPR. Weathering of hair in monilethrix and pili torti. *Clin Exp Dermatol* 1977; **2**: 271–9.

8 Pollitt RJ, Jenner FA, Davis M. Sibs with mental and physical retardation, with abnormal amino-acid composition of the hair. *Arch Dis Child* 1968; **43**: 211–20.

9 Lyon JB, Dawber RPR. A sporadic case of dystrophic pili torti. *Br J Dermatol* 1977; **96**: 197–8.

10 Telfer N, Cutler TP, Dawber RPR. The natural history of pili torti. *Br J Dermatol* 1989; **120**: 323–5.

11 Gedda L, Cavalieri R. Relievi genetici delle Distrofie congenita dei capelli. *Cronache Inst Dermopat Immacol* 1962; **17**: 3–8.

12 Rief PH, Patrizi A, Piraccini BM. Autosomal dominant pili torti. *Eur J Dermatol* 1996; **6**: 385–7.

13 Laub D, Horan RF, Yaffe H *et al.* A child with hair loss: pili torti, apparently unassociated with other abnormalities. *Arch Dermatol* 1987; **123**: 1071–7.

14 Pierini LE, Borda JMC. Pili torti. *Rev Argentina Dermatosifilog* 1947; **31**: 75–9.

15 Kurwa AR, Abdel-Aziz AHM. Pili torti—congenital and acquired. *Acta Derm Venereol (Stockh)* 1973; **10**: 34–8.

16 Hays SC, Camisa C. Acquired pili torti in 2 patients treated with synthetic retinoids. *Cutis* 1985; **35**: 466–70.

17 Lurie R, Danziger Y, Kaplan Y. Acquired pili torti in anorexia nervosa. *Cutis* 1996; **57**: 151–2.

18 Dawber RPR, Comaish S. Scanning electron microscopy of normal and abnormal hair shafts. *Arch Dermatol* 1970; **101**: 316–23.

19 Friederich HC, Seitz R. Uber eine forme der ektodermalen Dysplasie unter dem Bilde der Pili torti mit Augenbeteiligung und Storung der Schweissekretion. *Dermatol Wochenschr* 1955; **131**: 277–81.

20 Whiting DA. Structural abnormalities of the hair shaft. *J Am Acad Dermatol* 1987; **16**: 1–24.

Bjornstad's syndrome [1,2]

SYN. CRANDALL'S SYNDROME

In this syndrome, pili torti is associated with sensorineural hearing loss. The loss of hair usually begins in infancy but in one case it was not noticed until the age of 8 years. There is a correlation between the severity of the hair defect and the degree of hearing loss. On microscopy, the hair shafts show longitudinal ridging and irregular twisting. A further affected brother and sister suggests that the mode of inheritance is probably autosomal recessive [3].

Two brothers were investigated after they had reached puberty and were found to have secondary hypogonadism [4] with deficiency of luteinizing and of growth hormones.

REFERENCES

1 Bjornstad RT. Pili torti and sensory neural loss of hearing. *Proc Fennoscand Assoc Dermatol.* Copenhagen, 1965: 3–6.

2 Petit A, Dontenwille MM, Blanchet-Bardon C, Civatte J. Pili torti with congenital deafness (Bjornstad's syndrome)—report of three cases in one family suggesting autosomal dominant transmission. *Clin Exp Dermatol* 1993; **18**: 94–6.

3 Voigtlander V. Pili torti with deafness (Bjornstad syndrome). *Dermatologica* 1979; **159**: 50–7.

4 Crandall BF, Samec L, Sparkes RS *et al.* A familial syndrome of deafness, alopecia and hypogonadism. *J Pediatr* 1973; **82**: 461–5.

Netherton's syndrome (bamboo hair) [1–4]

Netherton [5] observed bamboo-like nodes in the fragile hairs of a girl with 'erythematous scaly dermatitis'. It has gradually become apparent that ichthyosis linearis circumflexa and 'bamboo hairs' (trichorrhexis invaginata) (Fig. 66.42) are two features of a single syndrome [6]. Most cases of Netherton's syndrome have had ichthyosis linearis circumflexa (ILC) but some have ichthyosis vulgaris [7] or both conditions, or ichthyosiform erythroderma. All cases of ILC in which hair changes have been carefully sought have been found to show them.

ILC is thus an almost constant feature of the syndrome, with hair shaft defects of various types and degrees of severity. Until the nature of the underlying abnormality is fully understood, the eponym Netherton's syndrome is acceptable. Some authorities [8] question the variability of the syndrome.

The inheritance of Netherton's syndrome appears to be determined by an autosomal recessive gene of variable expressivity. Girls are affected more than boys.

Pathology. The histological changes have, until recently, not been considered diagnostic, but it has now been shown that in the figurate lesions there is eosinophilic degeneration of cells in the upper malpighian layers. The eosinophilic material, probably a glycoprotein, is seen also in the overlying parakeratotic horny layer. Using the electron microscope, the severity of the localized disturbance of keratinization is confirmed; the desmosome–tonofilament complex is reduced, membrane coating granules and keratolysation are lacking, and dense round bodies are present. The horny layer has lost its lamellar structure.

Scanning electron microscopy of the hair shafts shows focal defects which produce the development of torsion nodules, invaginated nodules (trichorrhexis invaginata) and trichorrhexis nodosa [9,10].

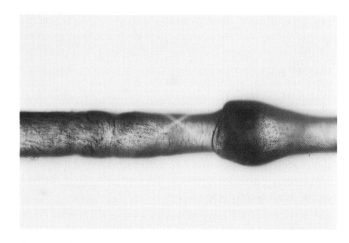

Fig. 66.42 Light microscopy revealing a trichorrhexis invaginata node likened to bamboo.

Clinical features [11]. The patient may present primarily either with cutaneous changes or complaining of sparse and fragile hairs. Generalized scaling and erythema are present from birth or early infancy, but the degree, extent and persistence of the erythema are very variable. In some cases the erythema may be slight and transient. On the trunk and limbs, the fine, dry scales are associated with a polycyclic and serpiginous eruption whose horny margin slowly changes its pattern.

Atopic manifestations are superimposed in some patients [12].

The hair defects may be detected only if deliberately sought, but in most cases are readily apparent clinically [10]. The hair is short, dry, lustreless and brittle, and the eyebrows and lashes are sparse or absent. Jones *et al.* [13] described two cases in which neonatal hypernatraemia occurred.

There is no specific treatment. Nagata [14] described some response to photochemotherapy.

REFERENCES

1 Altman J, Stroud J. Netherton's syndrome and ichthyosis linearis circumflexa. *Arch Dermatol* 1969; **100**: 550–5.
2 Ito M, Ito K, Hashimoto K. Pathogenesis of trichorrhexis invaginata (bamboo hair). *J Invest Dermatol* 1984; **83**: 1–7.
3 Šalamon T, Lazovic O, Stenek S. Über das Netherton-Syndrome. *Hautarzt* 1972; **23**: 66–72.
4 de Berker D, Paige DG, Ferguson DJP, Dawber RPR. Golf-tee hairs in Netherton disease. *Pediatr Dermatol* 1995; **12**: 7–8.
5 Netherton GW. A unique case of trichorrhexis nodosa—'bamboo hairs'. *Arch Dermatol* 1958; **78**: 482–90.
6 Mevorah B, Frenk E, Brooke EM. Ichthyosis linearis circumflexa Comel. *Dermatologica* 1974; **149**: 201–6.
7 Brodin MMB, Porter PS. Netherton's syndrome. *Cutis* 1980; **26**: 185–92.
8 Hurwitz S, Kirsch N, McGuire J. Reevaluation of ichthyosis and hair shaft anomalies. *Arch Dermatol* 1971; **103**: 266–73.
9 Murphy GM, Griffiths WAD, Grice K. Netherton's syndrome. *J R Soc Med* 1989; **82**: 683–5.
10 Orfanos CE, Mahrle G, Šalamon T. Netherton-Syndrome. *Hautarzt* 1971; **22**: 397–404.
11 Judge MR, Morgan G, Harper JL. A clinical and immunological study of Netherton's syndrome. *Br J Dermatol* 1994; **131**: 615–19.
12 Porter PS, Starke JC. Netherton's syndrome. *Arch Dis Child* 1968; **43**: 319–26.
13 Jones SK, Thomason LM, Surbrugg SK et al. Neonatal hypernatraemia in 2 siblings with Netherton's syndrome. *Br J Dermatol* 1986; **114**: 741–4.
14 Nagata T. Netherton's syndrome which responded to photochemotherapy. *Dermatologica* 1980; **161**: 51–60.

Trichorrhexis nodosa

Trichorrhexis is best regarded as a distinctive response of the hair shaft to injury [1]. If the degree or frequency of the injury is sufficient, it can be induced in normal hair [2]. The cuticular cells become disrupted, allowing the cortical cells to splay out to form nodes [3]. If, however, the hair is abnormally fragile, trichorrhexis may follow relatively trivial injury. The trauma of hairdressing procedures has often been incriminated [4]. Scratching may produce identical changes in the hairs in the genitocrural region [4]; and the severity of experimentally induced trichorrhexis nodosa is related to the degree of trauma, in patients with or without pre-existing trichorrhexis. The cumulative effect of shampooing, brushing, sea bathing and sunlight led to seasonal recurrences each summer [5].

That congenital and hereditary defects of the hair shaft can predispose to trichorrhexis nodosa is well established. Trichorrhexis nodosa may occur in pseudomonilethrix, in Netherton's syndrome or with pili annulati. Trichorrhexis nodosa is a feature of the rare metabolic defect argininosuccinic aciduria, in which it is associated with mental retardation [6]; there is a deficiency of the enzyme argininosuccinase. Some 20 patients have been reported [7,8]. The hair tends to be dry, brittle and lustreless and may show trichorrhexis nodosa, but not all patients with this metabolic disorder develop it.

Trichorrhexis nodosa may occur in certain families as an apparently isolated defect of the hair; node formation and fracture are induced by minimal trauma and develop during the early months of life. Wolff *et al.* [9] described as trichorrhexis congenita the presence from birth of trichorrhexis nodosa confined to the scalp, with normal teeth and nails.

In a case of generalized trichorrhexis nodosa in a male adult [10], electron histochemical study showed evidence of a disorder in the formation of α-keratin chains within the globular matrix of the hair cortex with respect to cystine.

Pathology. In simple trichorrhexis nodosa, the shaft may appear normal with the light or electron microscope except at the nodes; or the shaft, apart from the proximal 1 cm, may show signs of abnormal wear and tear [3]. At the nodes, the cuticle bulges and is split by longitudinal fissures (Fig. 66.43). If fracture occurs transversely through a node, i.e. trichoclasis, the end of the hair resembles a small paintbrush.

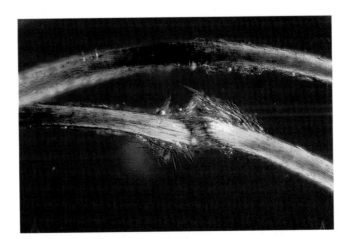

Fig. 66.43 Trichorrhexis node. Polarized light examination demonstrates the splayed cortical fibres radiating from the transverse fracture in a trichorrhexis node.

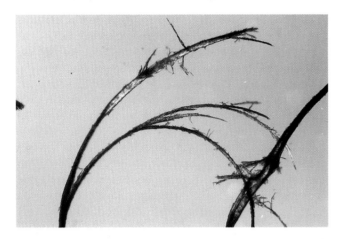

Fig. 66.44 Proximal trichorrhexis nodes and dramatic split ends (trichoptilosis) are visible in hair from an Afro-Caribbean woman.

Clinical features. In trichorrhexis nodosa complicating a congenital defect of the hair shafts, the hair breaks so easily that large or small portions of the scalp show only broken stumps and alopecia may be quite gross. In the much commoner conditions in which trauma plays a proportionately larger role and the predisposing inadequacy of the shaft a proportionately smaller one, there are three principal clinical presentations [11].

1 Distal trichorrhexis nodosa occurs in all races. Often it is discovered incidentally and only a few whitish nodules are seen near the ends of scattered hairs. If many hairs are affected the patient may complain that the hair is dry, dull or brittle.

2 There is a generalized variant seen in Afro-Caribbean women called proximal trichorrhexis nodosa. The scalp hair is universally short and brittle and demonstrates severe weathering on light microscopic examination (Fig. 66.44).

3 The third clinical form was well described by Sabouraud [12] but it appears now to be rare. In a localized area of scalp, moustache or beard, some hairs are broken, and others show from one to five or six nodules [13].

Diagnosis. The congenital forms must be differentiated from other shaft defects. The distal acquired form may simulate dandruff or even pediculosis. In all cases, diagnosis depends on careful microscopy. Excessive physical and chemical (cosmetic) trauma must be avoided, apart from shampooing.

REFERENCES

1 Whiting DA. Structural abnormalities of the hair shaft. *J Am Acad Dermatol* 1987; **16**: 1–24.
2 Dawber RPR, ed. *Diseases of the Hair and Scalp*, 3rd edn. Oxford: Blackwell Science, 1997: 401–13.
3 Dawber RPR, Comaish JS. Scanning electron microscopy of normal and abnormal hair shafts. *Arch Dermatol* 1970; **101**: 316–22.
4 Chernosky ME, Owens DW. Trichorrhexis nodosa. *Arch Dermatol* 1966; **94**: 577–81.
5 Papa CM, Mills OH, Hanshaw W. Seasonal trichorrhexis nodosa. *Arch Dermatol* 1972; **106**: 888–92.
6 Allan JD, Cusworth DC, Dent CE *et al.* A disease, probably hereditary, characterized by severe mental deficiency and a constant gross abnormality of amino acid metabolism. *Lancet* 1958; **i**: 182–7.
7 Brenton DP, Cusworth DC, Harley S *et al.* Argininosuccinic aciduria: clinical, metabolic and dietary study. *J Mental Defic Res* 1974; **18**: 1–13.
8 Shih VE. Early dietary management in an infant with arginino-succinase deficiency: preliminary report. *J Pediatr* 1972; **80**: 645–51.
9 Wolff HH, Vigl E, Braun-Falco O. Trichorrhexis congenita. *Hautarzt* 1975; **26**: 576–81.
10 Leonard JN, Gummer CL, Dawber RPR. Generalised trichorrhexis nodosa. *Br J Dermatol* 1980; **103**: 85–8.
11 Price V. Office diagnosis of structural hair anomalies. *Cutis* 1975; **15**: 213–39.
12 Sabouraud R. Trichoclasie, trichorrhexie et trichopilose. *Ann Dermatol Syphiligr* 1921; **2**: 445–50.
13 Camacho-Martinez FF. Localised trichorrhexis nodosa. *J Am Acad Dermatol* 1989; **20**: 696–8.

Trichothiodystrophy

The term trichothiodystrophy (TTD) was coined [1,2] to describe brittle hair with an abnormally low sulphur content [3]. It is not yet certain whether the different syndromes of which it is a feature represent a single rather variable entity, or distinct entities sharing this feature [4–7].

Various syndrome complexes accompanied by brittle hair have been associated with trichothiodystrophy [8].

1 Brittle hair, intellectual impairment, decreased fertility, short stature (BIDS).

2 Ichthyosis and BIDS (IBIDS).

3 Photosensitivity and IBIDS (PIBIDS) [9]. Van Neste *et al.* [5] described the association of TTD with xeroderma pigmentosum (Table 66.4).

Where it has been possible to establish the mode of inheritance, this has been of autosomal recessive type.

Pathology. The hair is brittle and weathers badly [11]. With

Table 66.4 Guidelines for classification of trichothiodystrophy. (From Dawber [10]. Courtesy of *Dermatologic Clinics*.)

A	Isolated congenital hair defect
B As type A +	Nail dystrophy (unreported by 1995)
C As type B +	Mental retardation
D As type C +	Growth retardation
D¹ As type D +	Decreased fertility in family studies
E As type D +	Ichthyosis
E1	Lamellar ichthyosis (congenital type)
E2	Ichthyosis vulgaris (acquired type, as usual in F)
F As type E2 +	Light sensitivity
	Evaluation of DNA repair
	Complementation studies with xeroderma pigmentosum cells
	Defect similar to that in xeroderma pigmentosum complementation group D

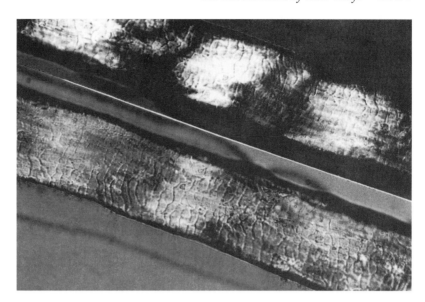

Fig. 66.45 Trichothiodystrophy. Alternating bright and dark zones in the polarizing microscope. (Courtesy of D. Van Neste, Brussels.)

trauma it may break cleanly (trichoschisis) or may form nodes somewhat resembling trichorrhexis nodosa but without conspicuous release of individual spindle cells [1,2]. The hairs are flattened and can be twisted into various appearances—rather like a ribbon or shoe lace.

With the scanning electron microscope the hairs are seen to be flattened, and sometimes folded over themselves (ribbon-like). The shaft is irregular with ridging and fluting and the cuticular scales are patchily absent. With the polarizing microscope the hairs show alternating bright and dark zones (Fig. 66.45).

Gummer and Dawber [12], using transmission electron microscopic methods, showed a quantitative decrease in high-sulphur protein in the hair shaft and a failure of this protein to migrate to the exocuticular part of the cuticle cells. Gillespie and Marshall [13] showed that the low sulphur and cysteine were related to a decrease in high-sulphur protein.

Clinical features. The hair is sparse, short and brittle, but the degree of alopecia varies considerably. There may be lamellar ichthyosis. The nails may be dystrophic. Mental and physical development may be normal but one or both may be slightly, moderately or severely retarded. Until further cases have been studied, the relationship between the syndromes showing trichothiodystrophy is a matter for speculation.

Photosensitivity is a variable factor and provides overlap with xeroderma pigmentosum group D. The overlap extends to some common faults in repair of photodamaged DNA. Analogous disorders in mutant rodents suggest an abnormality in the ERCC2 DNA-repair gene. The product of this gene has a dual function in nucleotide excision repair as a helicase and as a transcription factor. The latter could entail influence over many diverse proteins, accounting

for the varied nature of trichothiodystrophy syndromes [14].

REFERENCES

1 Price VH, Odom RB, Jones FT *et al.* Trichothiodystrophy: sulfur-deficient brittle hair. In: Brown AC, Crounse RG, eds. *Hair, Trace Elements and Human Illness.* New York: Praeger, 1980: 22–7.
2 Price VH, Odom RB, Ward WH *et al.* Trichothiodystrophy; sulfur deficient brittle hair as a marker for a neuroectodermal symptom complex. *Arch Dermatol* 1980; **166**: 1375–86.
3 Van Neste D, Degreef H, van Haute N *et al.* High sulfur protein deficient hair. *J Am Acad Dermatol* 1989; **20**: 195–202.
4 Itin PH, Pittelkow MR. Trichothiodystrophy: review of sulfur-deficient brittle hair syndromes and association with ectodermal dysplasias. *J Am Acad Dermatol* 1990; **22**: 705–19.
5 Van Neste D, Miller X, Bohner E. Clinical symptoms associated with trichothiodystrophy. In: *Trends in Human Hair Growth and Alopecia Research*, No. 19. Dortrecht: Kluwer Academic Publishing, 1989: 183–99.
6 Tolmie JL, de Berker DAR, Dawber RPR *et al.* Syndromes associated with trichothiodystrophy. *Clin Dysmorph* 1994; **3**: 1–14.
7 Van Neste D, Gillespie JM, Marshall RC *et al.* Morphological and biochemical characteristics of trichothiodystrophy-variant hair. *Br J Dermatol* 1993; **128**: 384–8.
8 Crovato F, Borrore C, Rebora A. Trichothiodystrophy: BIDS, IBIDS & PIBIDS? *Br J Dermatol* 1983; **108**: 247–53.
9 Rebora A, Guarrera M, Crovato F. Amino-acid analysis in hair from PIBI (D) S syndrome. *J Am Acad Dermatol* 1986; **15**: 109–15.
10 Dawber RP. *Dermatol Clin* 1996; **14**: 765.
11 Venning VA, Dawber RPR, Ferguson JDP *et al.* Weathering of hair in trichothiodystrophy. *Br J Dermatol* 1986; **114**: 591–9.
12 Gummer CL, Dawber RPR. Trichothiodystrophy; an ultrastructural study of the hair follicle. *Br J Dermatol* 1985; **113**: 273–80.
13 Gillespie JM, Marshall RC. Comparison of the proteins of normal and trichothiodystrophic human hair. *J Invest Dermatol* 1983; **80**: 195–205.
14 de Berker D, Sinclair R. Defects of the hair shaft. In: Dawber RPR, ed. *Diseases of the Hair and Scalp*, 3rd edn. Oxford: Blackwell Science, 1997: 396–489.

Marinesco–Sjögren syndrome

This rare syndrome, of autosomal recessive inheritance, has as its principal features [1] cerebellar ataxia, dysarthria, retarded physical and mental development and congenital cataracts. The teeth are abnormally formed and the lateral incisors may be absent. The nails are flat, thin and fragile.

The hair is sparse, fine, light in colour, short and brittle. On microscopy, transverse fractures—trichoschisis—can be seen at the sites of impending fractures. In polarized light the hair is irregularly birefringent. Scalp biopsy shows normal anagen follicles, but with incomplete keratinization of the internal root sheath [2].

REFERENCES

1 Norwood WF. The Marinesco–Sjögren syndrome. *J Pediatr* 1964; **65**: 431–7.
2 Porter PS. The genetics of human hair growth. *Birth Defects* (Original Article Series) 1971; **7**: 69–81.

Structural defects without increased fragility

Pili annulati (ringed hair) [1,2]

Aetiology. This abnormality is characterized by hair showing alternate light and dark bands along its length, but which is otherwise normal. The inheritance of ringed hair has been shown in many extensive pedigrees to be determined by an autosomal dominant gene [3,4]. One pedigree [5] was compatible with autosomal recessive inheritance; sporadic cases have been described [6]. Blue naevus and ringed hair were associated in some members of a family, but the two conditions segregated [3].

Pathology and pathogenesis [7]. With the light microscope the abnormal dark bands alternating with normal light bands are reversed. The bright appearance of the abnormal bands in reflected light is due to air spaces in the cortex [8] (Fig. 66.46). The rate of growth has been measured in one case [3] and found to be 0.16 mm/day, which is less than half the average normal rate. Breaking stress analysis showed no significant abnormality in ringed hair, but fractures were always in the normal bands.

Electron-microscopic studies [9] showed that the clusters of air-filled cavities, randomly distributed throughout the cortex in the abnormal bands, lie partly within cortical cells and between macrofibrils, or in the case of larger cavities appear to replace cortical cells. Hairs from the family described by Dawber [3] showed an abnormal surface cuticle which appeared 'cobble-stoned' on scanning electron microscopy. Electron histochemical methods confirmed this finding: cuticle cells are thrown into folds [10]. The pathogenesis of ringed hair remains uncertain. The abnormal alternating bands appear to be produced at random and not cyclically in relation to specific periods of growth [3].

Clinical features. Ringed hair may be associated with a very variable degree of fragility. When the fragility is slight

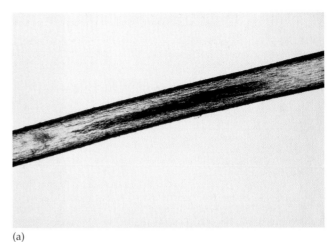

(a)

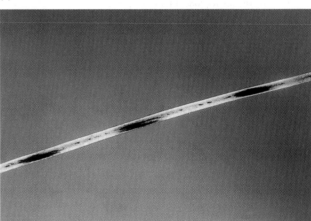

(b)

Fig. 66.46 (a) Pili annulati. Hair shaft by transmitted light showing an abnormal dark band (central part) due to multiple cortical air spaces. This corresponds to a bright region as seen by reflected light. (b) The abnormality is intermittent, causing the beaded or ringed appearance.

and relatively few hairs are affected, the condition may be discovered only when deliberately sought. If many hairs are affected and fragility is great, then short hair may attract attention in early life and the 'banded' and sandy appearance of the shafts in reflected light can be readily detected. The axillary hair is occasionally affected [11].

The diagnosis is readily established on microscopy of affected hair. A defect in which partially twisted shafts have an elliptical cross section has been named pseudo pili annulati because such hair may give an impression of alternating light and dark bands [12].

Prognosis and treatment. The prognosis is good in the sense that severity of the defect does not increase with age.

REFERENCES

1 Karsch A. De Capillitiri humani coloiebus quardan. Cited by Landois, 1866.

2 Landois L. Das plötzliche Ergrauen der Haupthaare. *Arch Pathol Anat Physiol* 1866; **35**: 575–99.
3 Dawber R. Investigation of a family with pili annulati associated with blue naevus. *Trans St John's Hosp Dermatol Soc* 1972; **58**: 51–62.
4 Tomedei M, Ghetti P, Puiatti P *et al*. Pili annulati: family study. *G Ital Dermatol Venereol* 1987; **122**: 427–36.
5 Ebbing HC. Gibt es auch bei Ringelhaaren (pili annulati) einen einfach-rezessiven Erbgang? *Homo* 1957; **8**: 35–43.
6 Dini G, Casigliani R, Rindi L *et al*. Pili annulati. *Int J Dermatol* 1988; **27**: 256–61.
7 Amichai B, Grunwald MH, Halevy S. Hair abnormality present since birth. *Arch Dermatol* 1996; **132**: 577–8.
8 Cady LOP, Trotter M. Study of ringed hair. *Arch Dermatol Syphilol* 1922; **6**: 301–11.
9 Price VH, Thomas RS, Jones FT. Pili annulati. *Arch Dermatol* 1968; **98**: 640–8.
10 Gummer CL, Dawber RPR. Pili annulati: electron histochemical studies on affected hairs. *Br J Dermatol* 1981; **105**: 303–10.
11 Montgomery RM, Binder AI. Ringed hair. *Arch Dermatol Syphilol* 1948; **58**: 177–91.
12 Price VH, Thomas RS, Jones FT. Pseudo pili annulati. *Arch Dermatol* 1970; **102**: 54–8.

Woolly hair

History and nomenclature. Woolly hair is more or less tightly coiled hair occurring over the entire scalp or part of it, in an individual not of negroid origin [1]. It is a feature that has been much confused by many authors. The investigation by Hutchinson *et al*. [2] has done much to clarify the clinical types; the classification proposed by these authors is as follows.
1 Hereditary woolly hair. The inheritance of this disorder is determined by an autosomal dominant gene.
2 Familial woolly hair. The genetic evidence is inconclusive but the condition has occurred in siblings whose parents were normal. Autosomal recessive inheritance is probable [3].
3 Symmetrical circumscribed allotrichia appears to be a distinct syndrome.
4 Woolly hair naevus. This is a circumscribed developmental defect, present at birth, and apparently not genetically determined.

Hereditary woolly hair

In some pedigrees the shaft diameter in affected individuals is reduced [2]; the hair is fragile and may show trichorrhexis nodosa. Excessively curly hair is evident at birth or in early infancy; it has sometimes been described as negroid in appearance. Anderson [4] considered that the hair, although tightly coiled, was not negroid. The degree of variation in severity within a family is inconstant [2]. The hair shaft may be twisted [5]. In some cases the hair is brittle and breaks readily.

Familial woolly hair

There is a marked reduction in the diameter of hair shafts, which may be poorly pigmented. The hair is brittle and on scanning electron microscopy shows signs of cuticular wear and tear [2]. So few cases have been reported that generalizations are unwarranted. In three cases [2], fine, tightly curled, poorly pigmented hair was present from birth; in two of them the hair never achieved a length of more than 2 or 3 cm. Eyebrows and body hair were sparse.

Symmetrical circumscribed allotrichia

Among cases reported as woolly hair naevus are some for which Norwood [6] has proposed the term 'whisker hair' but which are identical to the cases previously reported as symmetrical circumscribed allotrichia. From adolescence onwards, the hair, in an irregular band extending around the edge of the scalp from above the ears towards the occipital region, becomes coarse and whisker-like. A similar case was recorded by Bovenmyer [7]. Many people believe that whisker hair is synonymous with acquired progressive kinking (p. 2954).

Woolly hair naevus [8,9]

The hair in the affected region of the scalp is finer than elsewhere. Electron microscopy of the abnormal hair showed the absence of cuticle; trichorrhexis nodosa was present [10]. The hair in a circumscribed area of the scalp is tightly curled from birth to infancy. The size of the affected areas usually increases only proportionately with general growth. The abnormal hair may be slightly paler in colour than that of the rest of the scalp. In over half of the reported cases, a pigmented or epidermal naevus has been present, but not always at the same site. A woolly hair naevus has been associated also with ocular defects [11]. Other cases have been reported [12,13].

REFERENCES

1 Neild VS, Pegum JS, Wells RS. The association of keratosis pilaris atrophicans and woolly hair, with and without Noonan's syndrome. *Br J Dermatol* 1984; **110**: 357–61.
2 Hutchinson PE, Cairns RJ, Wells RS. Woolly hair. *Trans St John's Hosp Dermatol Soc* 1974; **60**: 160–76.
3 Furando J, Gertalos MR, Fontarnau R. Woolly hair. Estudo histologica y ultrastructurale en quatro casos. *Acta Dermosiphiligr* 1979; **70**: 203–10.
4 Anderson E. An American pedigree for woolly hair. *J Hered* 1936; **27**: 444–9.
5 Verbov J. Woolly hair: study of a family. *Dermatologica* 1978; **157**: 42–8.
6 Norwood CT. Whisker-hair—an update. *Cutis* 1981; **27**: 651–5.
7 Bovenmyer DA. Woolly hair naevus. *Cutis* 1979; **24**: 322–4.
8 Reda AM, Rogers RS, Peters MS. Woolly hair naevus. *J Am Acad Dermatol* 1990; **22**: 377–81.
9 Amichai B, Grunwald MH, Halevy S. A child with a localized hair abnormality. *Arch Dermatol* 1996; **132**: 577–8.
10 Crosti C, Menni S. Woolly hair naevus. Osservazioni su tre casi clinici. *G Ital Dermatol/Minerva Dermatol* 1979; **114**: 45–8.
11 Jacobson KV, Lewis M. Woolly hair naevus with ocular involvement. *Dermatologica* 1975; **151**: 249–56.
12 Anderson NP. Woolly haired naevus of the scalp. *Arch Dermatol Syphilol* 1943; **47**: 286–90.
13 Domonkos AN. Woolly hair naevus. *Arch Dermatol* 1962; **85**: 568–71.

Acquired progressive kinking of the hair

Acquired progressive kinking (APK) of the scalp hair appears to be extremely rare, but in many cases may not be recorded. It is probably synonymous with whisker hair [1]. Some cases have been confused with the woolly hair naevus, but APK is differentiated clinically by its onset in adolescence or adult life and its progressive extension over a period of years [2,3].

Aetiology and pathology. The aetiology of APK is unknown; there is as yet no evidence that it is genetically determined. The hairs in the affected region of the scalp may be finer or coarser than in the normal scalp; they show irregularly distributed kinks and half twists. The duration of anagen is reduced.

Clinical features. The patient gradually becomes aware that the hair in one region of the scalp is becoming kinky and that a progressive change in texture is occurring. On examination the hair on one or more regions of the scalp is wiry, kinky and unruly, dry and lustreless. There are no sharply defined boundaries between normal and abnormal hair. In some of the cases described, the acquired kinking preceded the development of androgenetic alopecia [2].

REFERENCES

1 Norwood OT. Whisker hair. *Arch Dermatol* 1979; **115**: 930–5.
2 Mortimer PS, Gummer CL, English J *et al*. Acquired progressive kinking of hair. Report of 6 cases and review of the literature. *Arch Dermatol* 1985; **121**: 1031–7.
3 Cullen SI, Fulghum DD. Acquired progressive kinking of hair. *Arch Dermatol* 1989; **125**: 252–7.

Uncombable hair syndrome

SYN. SPUN-GLASS HAIR; CHEVEUX INCOIFFABLES; PILI TRIANGULI ET CANALICULI

Aetiology [1]. This very distinctive hair-shaft defect appears to have been first described by Dupre *et al.* [2]. Since then, many more cases have been reported, some of them under the name of 'spun-glass hair'. The mode of inheritance is probably autosomal dominant [3].

Pathology. Microscopically, the hairs may appear more or less normal. On histological (horizontal sections) examination of the scalp hair in the scanning electron microscope (Fig. 66.47), the triangular configuration of the shaft is clearly seen, and also a well-defined longitudinal depression [4,5]. The term 'pili trianguli et canaliculi' has been proposed for these defects. The pili canaliculi are present in all cases, pili trianguli in the majority and pili torti in a few [6]. Van Neste *et al.* [7] have suggested that the misshapen dermal papilla alters the shape of the internal root sheath, which hardens (before the hair within)

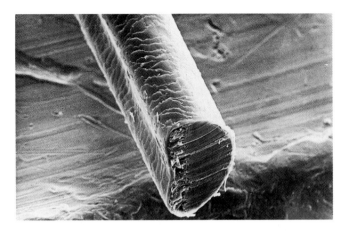

Fig. 66.47 Uncombable hair syndrome. Scanning electron micrograph showing essentially triangular cross-section and canalicular depression or gutter along one side.

in a triangular cross-sectional shape; the hair then hardens into a shape complementing the root sheath. The defect resembles the 'straight hair naevus' of which it may be a diffuse form.

Clinical features [4,5]. The abnormality may first become obvious from 3 months to 12 years of age. The hair is normal in quantity and sometimes also in length, but its wild, disorderly appearance totally resists all efforts to control it with brush or comb. In some cases, these efforts lead to the hair breaking, but increased fragility is not a constant feature [8]. The hair is often a rather distinctive silvery blonde colour. The eyebrows and eyelashes are normal.

The clinical appearance is usually distinctive. With light microscopy the diagnosis cannot be reliably established unless triangular hairs are seen. The appearances in the electron microscope are distinctive. No treatment is known, although oral biotin therapy has been suggested [9].

REFERENCES

1 Mallon E, Dawber RPR, de Berker DAR, Ferguson DJP. Cheveux incoiffables—diagnostic, clinical and hair microscopic findings, and pathogenetic studies. *Br J Dermatol* 1994; **131**: 608–14.
2 Dupre A, Rochiccidi P, Bonafe J-L. 'Cheveux incoiffables': anomalie congenitale des cheveux. *Bull Soc Fr Dermatol Syphiligr* 1973; **80**: 111–17.
3 Herbert AA, Charrow J, Esterly NB *et al*. Uncombable hair (pili trianguli et canaliculi); evidence for dominant inheritance with complete penetrance. *Am J Med Genet* 1987; **28**: 185–91.
4 Dupre A, Bonafe J-L. Le syndrome des cheveux incoiffables. Pili trianguli et canaliculi. *Ann Dermatol Vénéréol* 1978; **105**: 627–32.
5 Dupre A, Bonafe J-L. A new type of pilar dysplasia. The uncombable hair syndrome with pili trianguli et canaliculi. *Arch Dermatol Res* 1978; **261**: 217–23.
6 Ferrando J, Fontarnau R, Gratacos MR *et al*. Pili canaliculi ('cheveux incoiffables' ou 'cheveux en fibre de verre') Dix nouveaux cas avec etude au microscope electronique a balayage. *Ann Dermatol Vénéréol* 1989; **107**: 243–7.
7 Van Neste D, Armijo-Subieta F, Tennstedt D *et al*. The uncombable hair syndrome; four non-familial cases. *Arch Dermatol Res* 1981; **217**: 223–4.

8 Baden HP, Schoenfeld RJ, Stroud JD *et al.* Physicochemical properties of spunglass hair. *Acta Derm Venereol (Stockh)* 1981; **61**: 441–6.
9 Shelley WB, Shelley ED. Uncombable hair syndrome; observations on response to biotin. *J Am Acad Dermatol* 1985; **13**: 97–100.

Straight-hair naevus

In the straight-hair naevus, the hairs in a circumscribed area of a negroid scalp are straight, and are round in cross section. The abnormal hair may be associated with an epidermal naevus [1,2]. With the scanning electron microscope, the cuticular scales may appear small and their pattern disorganized.

This has been suggested as a localized form of cheveux incoiffables.

REFERENCES

1 Downham TF, Chapel TA, Lupulescu AP. Straight hair naevus syndrome: a case report with scanning electron microscope findings of hair morphology. *Int J Dermatol* 1976; **15**: 498–501.
2 Gibbs RL, Berger RA. The straight hair naevus. *Int J Dermatol* 1970; **9**: 47–9.

Loose anagen hair syndrome [1]

This distinctive condition [2–4] features anagen hairs that are loosely anchored and easily pulled from the scalp. The majority of cases are fair-haired children, aged 2–9 years, mostly girls. They typically have slightly unruly hair, which is of uneven length. There may be areas of alopecia, leading to a misdiagnosis of alopecia areata, but which, in fact, represent modest hair pulling. The child is well, and there are no other ectodermal abnormalities. There may be a positive family history, suggestive of autosomal dominant inheritance.

Hair is easily and painlessly plucked with the hair-pull test. Microscopy of plucked hair may show ruffling of the cuticle adjacent to the anagen bulb, giving the appearance of a 'floppy sock'. The hair shaft may have twists and grooves, and be angular in cross-section. There is neither an inner nor outer root sheath.

The hair becomes more normal with age, although the pull test may still yield abnormally large numbers of hairs into adulthood [5].

There have been isolated reports of loose anagen syndrome associated with hypohidrotic ectodermal dysplasia [6] and ocular coloboma [7].

Histology shows premature keratinization of the inner root sheath layers of Huxley and Henle. Trichograms show 98–100% anagen hairs with no telogen hairs.

REFERENCES

1 Li VW, Baden HP, Kvedar JC. Loose anagen syndrome and loose anagen hair. *Dermatol Clin* 1996; **14**: 745–51.
2 Price VH, Gummer CL. Loose anagen syndrome. *J Am Acad Dermatol* 1989; **20**: 249–58.
3 Hamm H, Traupe H. Loose anagen hair of children. *J Am Acad Dermatol* 1989; **20**: 242–8.
4 Baden HP, Kvedar C, Magro CM. Loose anagen hair syndrome as a cause of hereditary hair loss in children. *Arch Dermatol* 1992; **128**: 1349–50.
5 Chapman DM, Miller RA. An objective measurement of the anchoring strength of anagen hair in an adult with loose anagen hair syndrome. *J Cutan Pathol* 1996; **23**: 288–92.
6 Azon-Masoliver A, Ferrando J. Loose anagen hair in hypohidrotic ectodermal dysplasia. *Pediatr Dermatol* 1996; **13**: 29–32.
7 Murphy MF, McGinnity FG, Allen GE. New familial association between ocular coloboma and loose anagen syndrome. *Clin Genet* 1995; **47**: 214–16.

Other abnormalities of the shaft

Trichoclasis

Trichoclasis is the common 'greenstick' fracture of the hair shaft. Transverse fractures of the shaft occur, partly splinted by intact cuticle; cuticle, cortex and sulphur content are normal. This sign may be seen in a variety of congenital and acquired 'fragile' hair states.

The condition termed trichorrhexis blastysis [1]—unusual facies, failure to thrive, unexplained diarrhoea and abnormal hairs—showed scanning electron micrographs resembling trichoclasis.

REFERENCE

1 Stankler L, Lloyd D, Pollitt RJ *et al.* Unexplained diarrhoea and failure to thrive in 2 siblings with unusual hair. *Arch Dis Child* 1982; **57**: 212–14.

Trichoptilosis

History and nomenclature

The term trichoptilosis describes longitudinal splitting of the hair shaft. The patient will often refer to the condition as 'split ends'.

Aetiology. Trichoptilosis is the commonest macroscopic response of the hair shaft to the cumulative effects of chemical and physical trauma. It can readily be produced experimentally by vigorous brushing of normal hair, and it occurs in the nodes of pili torti. It is one component of the 'weathering' process particularly seen in long hair in normal individuals and in any congenital 'brittle hair' syndrome.

Pathology. The distal end of the hair shaft is split longitudinally into two or several divisions. Other microscopic evidence of hair damage may be present.

Clinical features. Trichoptilosis is often an incidental finding in a person who complains that his or her hair is dry and brittle. Trichorrhexis nodosa and trichoclasis are often present in the same patient. Central trichoptilosis, a longitudinal split in the hair shaft without involvement of the tip, sometimes occurs [1].

Treatment. Careful explanation is necessary to encourage the patient to avoid further chemical trauma, because otherwise the condition will inevitably recur.

REFERENCE

1 Burkhart CG, Huttner JJ, Bruner J. Central trichoptilosis. *J Am Acad Dermatol* 1981; **5**: 703–8.

Circle hairs [1]

Circle and spiral hairs occur in middle-aged men on the back, abdomen and thighs as small dark circles next to hair follicles. They are an unusual form of ingrown hair lying in a coiled track just below the stratum corneum and can be easily extracted. Keratin follicular plugging is not associated (cf. scurvy, which may demonstrate keratosis pilaris with rolled and 'corkscrew' hairs).

REFERENCE

1 Levit F, Scott MJJR. Circle hairs. *J Am Acad Dermatol* 1983; **8**: 423–7.

Trichomalacia

Miescher [1] described as trichomalacia a patchy alopecia in which some follicles are plugged and contain soft, deformed, swollen hairs. The changes have been attributed to the repeated trauma resulting from a hair-pulling tic [2,3], and subsequent histological studies in trichotillomania confirm this opinion.

Pathology. Above the bulb, the cells of the hair shaft appear to be disconnected and the hair is shapeless or partially disintegrated. High in the follicle, the shaft is thin and may be coiled. Whiting [4] described biopsy specimens as showing partially avulsed hair roots which are deformed and twisted; clefting occurs between matrix cells and between hair bulb and outer connective tissue sheath. There is no inflammatory reaction; these changes are said to be pathognomonic of trichotillomania. The clinical features are also those of trichotillomania.

REFERENCES

1 Miescher G. Trichomalacie. *Arch Dermatol Syphilol* 1942; **183**: 117–29.
2 Haensch R, Blaich W. Trichomalacia und Trichotillomania. *Arch Klin Exp Dermatol* 1960; **210**: 447–52.
3 Miescher G, Schmuziger P. Trichomalacie und Trichotillomanie. *Dermatologica* 1957; **114**: 199–206.
4 Whiting DA. Structural abnormalities of the hair shaft. *J Am Acad Dermatol* 1987; **16**: 1–24.

Trichoschisis [1]

Trichoschisis is a clean, transverse fracture across the hair shaft through cuticle and cortex; the fracture is associated with localized absence (loss) of cuticular cells. It is said to be a characteristic microscopic finding of the many syndromes associated with trichothiodystrophy. It probably represents a clean fracture through hair with decreased high-sulphur matrix protein content and, particularly, a similar decrease in the exocuticle and A layer of cuticular cells. It may be prominent in the sulphur-deficiency syndromes but it should not be considered as specific or pathognomonic.

REFERENCES

1 Brown AC, Belsher RB, Crounse RG *et al*. A congenital hair defect; trichoschisis and alternating birefringence and low-sulfur content. *J Invest Dermatol* 1970; **54**: 496–504.

Pohl-Pinkus constriction [1]

In some individuals, a zone of decreased shaft diameter coincides in time with a surgical operation, an illness, or the administration of folic acid antagonists or other drugs that inhibit mitosis; it was first described by Pohl in 1894—he later changed his name to Pinkus. The proportion of hairs so affected is variable and it seems probable that hairs in early anagen are most susceptible to a period of hypoproteinaemia or disturbed protein synthesis. This phenomenon was present in 21 of 100 hospitalized patients [2]; whether the illness or operation had been associated with pyrexia was not a relevant factor.

These constrictions in the hair shaft have been considered to be analogous to the transverse furrows in the nails (Beau's lines) which also coincide with episodes of ill health. Longer narrowings, resembling monilethrix, may occur with 'bolus' doses of cytotoxic drugs that do not lead to anagen effluvium.

REFERENCES

1 Pinkus H, ed. *Die Einwirkung von Krankheiten auf das Kopfhaar des Menschen*. Berlin: Karger, 1971.
2 Sims RT. Reduction of hair shaft diameter associated with illness. *Br J Dermatol* 1967; **79**: 43–50.

Tapered hairs

Tapered hairs may occur in association with many other structural abnormalities of the hair shaft. They may arise in association with any process inhibiting cell division in the hair matrix; severe inhibition may lead to fracture if the narrowing of the fibre is marked. If the matrix inhibitory influence is temporary, the shaft may widen again, giving a local 'dumbbell-like' appearance in the emerging shaft, for example due to cytotoxic drugs not leading to complete anagen effluvium. An alternative type of tapered hair is the so-called 'embryonic' anagen hair—short hairs with tapered pointed tips seen in trichotillomania but also in acquired progressive kinking [1] and regrowing hair in AA.

REFERENCE

1 Coupe RL, Johnston MM. Acquired progressive kinking of hair: structural changes and growth dynamics. *Arch Dermatol* 1969; **100**: 191–9.

Bayonet hairs

Bayonet hairs are characterized by a 2–3 mm spindle-shaped, hyperpigmented expansion of the hair cortex just proximal to a tapered tip and may be associated with hyperkeratinization of the upper third of the follicle. They are probably related to the first type of tapered hair described above.

Trichonodosis

Michelson [1] first proposed the term *noduli laqueati*, and noted that naturally curly hair was most frequently affected. The term trichonodosis was popularized later by Kren [2], who found the condition in 35 out of 64 consecutively examined patients with skin disease.

Aetiology. The knotting of the hair shafts is induced by trauma. Short, curly hair of relatively flat diameter is most readily affected [3]. Knots were found most frequently in negroid hair and in short, curly caucasoid hair; none was seen in long, straight hair.

Pathology. The only abnormalities are secondary to the knotting and are localized to that part of the shaft which forms the knot [3]. With the scanning electron microscope, the cuticle shows longitudinal fissuring and fractures, and cuticle scales are lost.

Clinical features [3]. Trichonodosis is usually an incidental finding, for it is inconspicuous and must be deliberately sought. One or few hairs are affected. The trauma of brushing or combing may cause the shaft to break at the site of the knot.

REFERENCES

1 Michelson P. Anomalien des Haarwachstums und der Haarfarbung. In: *Handbuch der speziellen Pathologie und Therapie* 1884; **14**: 89–93.
2 Kren O. Trichonodosis. *Wien Klin Wochenschr* 1907; **20**: 916–23.
3 Dawber RPR. Knotting of scalp hair. *Br J Dermatol* 1974; **91**: 169–74.

Trichostasis spinulosa

This is probably a normal, age-related phenomenon— easily overlooked—in which successive telogen hairs are retained in predominantly sebaceous follicles [1]. When it was specifically sought, 51 cases were seen in 1 month in Madras [2].

Aetiology. Ladany [3] thought trichostasis was no more than a variant of the comedo, and pointed out that 85% of comedones contain from one to 10 or more vellus hairs. Trichostasis is found most commonly in the middle-aged or elderly and is said by most authors to occur particularly on the nose and face [3]. Other sites were perhaps not always examined, for others have found it to be not uncommon on the trunk and limbs [4].

Pathology. The affected follicles contain up to 50 vellus hairs embedded in a keratinous plug. A mild perifolliculitis is often present. The condition must be differentiated from the 'multiple hairs' of Flemming—Giovannini in which up to seven hairs grow from a composite papilla with a common outer root sheath [5].

Clinical features [6]. Those reported to be affected have ranged in age from 17 to over 60 years. The lesions, which closely resemble comedones, may occur predominantly on the nose, forehead and cheeks, or the face may be spared and the nape, back, shoulders, upper arms and chest may be affected. The lesions vary greatly in number. On inspection with a hand lens the 'comedones' seem to be unusually prominent and in some cases a tuft of hairs may be seen projecting through the horny plug.

Treatment. Keratolytic preparations have often been recommended but we have found them of little value. The most effective treatment is topical retinoic acid [7] which should be used as in the treatment of acne. Depilatory wax has also been successfully employed [6].

REFERENCES

1 Goldschmidt H, Hajyo-Tomoka MJ, Kligman AM. Trichostasis spinulosa: a common inapparent follicular disorder of the aged. In: Brown AC, ed. *First Human Hair Symposium*. New York: Medcom Press, 1974: 50–6.
2 Kailasam V, Kailasam A, Thambiah AS. Trichostasis spinulosa. *Int J Dermatol* 1979; **18**: 297–300.
3 Ladany E. Trichostasis spinulosa. *J Invest Dermatol* 1954; **23**: 33–4.
4 Young MC, Jorizzo JL, Sanchez RL *et al*. Trichostasis spinulosa. *Int J Dermatol* 1985; **24**: 575–80.
5 Pinkus H. Multiple hairs (Flemming–Giovannini). *J Invest Dermatol* 1951; **17**: 291–7.
6 Sarkany I, Gaylarde PM. Trichostasis spinulosa and its management *Br J Dermatol* 1971; **84**: 311–16.
7 Mills OH, Kligman AM. Topically applied tretinoin in the treatment of trichostasis spinulosa. *Arch Dermatol* 1973; **108**: 378–81.

Pili multigemini
SYN. PILI BIFURCATI

The term pili multigemini [1] describes an uncommon

developmental defect of hair follicles as a result of which multiple matrices and papillae form hairs which emerge through a single pilosebaceous canal. The incidence of multigeminate hairs in the general population is unknown. Numerous follicles showing this defect have been seen in a patient with cleidocranial dysostosis [2].

Pathology. From 2–8 matrices and papillae, each with its internal root sheath, form hairs which are often flattened, ovoid or triangular in configuration and may be grooved. In the follicular canal, contiguous hairs may adhere, bifurcate and then re-adhere.

Clinical features. Multigeminate follicles occur mainly on the face, especially along the lines of the jaw. Tufts of hair may be seen emerging from a few or many follicles. Their discovery is often a matter of chance but the patient may complain of recurrent inflammatory nodules, leaving scars.

Treatment. This is unsatisfactory. If the hairs are plucked, they regrow [2].

REFERENCES

1 Pinkus H. Multiple hairs (Flemming–Giovannini). *J Invest Dermatol* 1951; **17**: 291–7.
2 Mehregan AH, Thompson WS. Pili multigemini. Report of a case in association with cleidocranial dysotosis. *Br J Dermatol* 1979; **100**: 315–20.

Hair casts

Hair casts (peripilar keratin casts) are firm, yellowish white accretions ensheathing, but not attached to, scalp hairs and freely movable up and down the affected shafts [1]. Such lesions are often found in scaly and seborrhoeic disorders of the scalp, and in children with hairstyles requiring traction [2].

Pathology. In cross-section, casts are composed of a central layer of retained internal root sheath and an outer, thick keratinous layer. Scalp histology shows the follicular openings packed with parakeratotic squames, which break off at intervals to form hair casts.

Casts are found quite commonly in scaly, mainly parakeratotic conditions of the scalp such as psoriasis and pityriasis amiantacea [3]. Cases have been described in association with traction hairstyles [2,4,5] and hair sprays [6].

Clinical findings. Hair casts (Fig. 66.48) may occur as an isolated abnormality unrelated to any overt scalp disease; such cases may mimic pediculosis capitis [7] and have been termed pseudonits [8,9]. Girls and young women are most commonly affected; hundreds of casts may develop within a few days. No cause is known, but sex-linked inheritance has been suggested [1]. It is possible

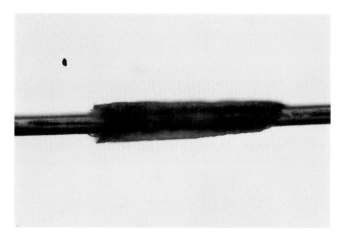

Fig. 66.48 Circumferential keratin cast resembling a cuff around the hair shaft.

that this type may represent an unusual manifestation of psoriasis.

If patients with scaly parakeratotic diseases of the scalp complain of persistent dandruff, which resists apparently adequate treatment, this is likely to be due to multiple hair casts.

Diagnosis. In the absence of associated scalp disease, casts may be mistaken for pediculosis capitis, trichorrhexis nodosa or hair knots [10]. Of these nodal shaft abnormalities, only hair casts are freely movable along the hair.

Treatment. Any causative scalp disease must be treated. Keratolytic preparations and shampoos that readily improve scalp scaling frequently fail to remove casts; prolonged brushing and combing is necessary to slide casts off the affected hairs [3,11].

REFERENCES

1 Kligman AM. Hair casts. *Arch Dermatol* 1957; **75**: 509–13.
2 Zhang W. Epidemiological and aetiological studies on hair casts. *Clin Exp Dermatol* 1995; **20**: 202–7.
3 Dawber RPR. The scalp and hair care in psoriasis. *J Psorias Assoc* 1979; **16**: 5–13.
4 Crovato F, Rebora A, Crosti C. Hair casts. *Dermatologica* 1980; **160**: 281–6.
5 Rollins TG. Traction folliculitis with hair casts and alopecia. *Am J Dis Child* 1961; **101**: 131–6.
6 Scott MJ. Peripilar keratin casts. *Arch Dermatol* 1959; **79**: 654–8.
7 Brunner MJ, Facq JM. A pseudoparasite of scalp hair. *Arch Dermatol* 1957; **75**: 583–7.
8 Kohn SR. Hair casts or pseudonits. *JAMA* 1977; **238**: 2058–9.
9 Keipert JA. Peripilar keratin casts (pseudonits) and psoriasis. *Med J Aust* 1974; **1**: 218–22.
10 Dawber RPR. Knotting of scalp hair. *Br J Dermatol* 1974; **91**: 169–74.
11 Bowyer A. Peripilar keratin casts. *Br J Dermatol* 1974; **90**: 231–6.

Weathering of the hair shaft [1,2]

All hair fibres undergo some degree of cuticular and

secondary cortical breakdown from root to tip before being shed during the telogen or early anagen phase of the hair cycle. The term weathering of hair has been limited by some authorities to structural changes in the hair shaft due to cosmetic procedures; indeed, both *in vivo* and *in vitro* studies carried out by cosmetic scientists have shown the type of damage that factors such as combing, brushing, bleaching and permanent waving can cause [3,4]. However, in considering the degeneration of hair fibres, cosmetic and other influences such as natural friction, wetting and UV radiation are so interwoven that it is more useful in practice to define weathering as the degeneration of hair from root to tip due to a variety of environmental and cosmetic factors. Scalp hair, having a long anagen phase and being subject to more frictional damage and cosmetic treatment, shows more deep cuticular and cortical degeneration than fibres from other sites.

Weathering of scalp hair has been studied in greater detail than hair from other sites. At the root end, surface cuticle cells are closely apposed to deeper layers. Within a few centimetres of the scalp, the free margin of these cells lifts up and breaks irregularly [5]. Increasing scale loss leads to surface areas denuded of cuticle. Many fibres show complete loss of overlapping scales well proximal to the tip. This is particularly common on long hair shafts, which frequently have a frayed tip. Proximal to terminal fraying, longitudinal fissures may be present between exposed cortical cells. Hairs subjected to considerable friction damage may show transverse fissures and some nodes of the type seen in trichorrhexis nodosa [6,7]. Hair that has been bleached or permanently waved may show shaft distortion. The severest changes are mostly seen near the distal part of the hair shaft in normal scalp hair.

Trichorrhexis nodosa is the severest form of weathering. Many of the changes seen in normal hair towards the tip are visible more proximally in congenitally weakened hair [8,9] and in trichorrhexis nodosa caused by overuse of cosmetic treatments [10].

In some hair structural abnormalities such as monilethrix and pili torti, specific weathering patterns may be seen.

REFERENCES

1 de Berker D, Sinclair R. Defects of the hair shaft. In: Dawber RPR, ed. *Diseases of the Hair and Scalp*, 3rd edn. Oxford: Blackwell Science, 1997: 427–9.
2 Dawber RPR. Weathering of hair in some genetic hair dystrophies. In: Brown AC, Crounse RG, eds. *Hair, Trace Elements and Human Illness*. New York: Praeger, 1980.
3 Brown AG, Swift JA. Hair breakage; the scanning electron microscope as a diagnostic tool. *J Soc Cosmet Chem* 1985; **26**: 289–98.
4 Robinson VNE. A study of damaged hair. *J Soc Cosmet Chem* 1976; **27**: 155–62.
5 Garcia ML, Epps JH, Yare RS. Normal cuticle wear patterns in human hair. *J Soc Cosmet Chem* 1978; **29**: 155–64.
6 Chernosky ME. Acquired trichorrhexis nodosa. In: Brown AC, ed. *The First Human Hair Symposium*. New York: Medcom Press, 1974.
7 Dawber RPR, Comaish S. Scanning electron microscopy of normal and abnormal hair shafts. *Arch Dermatol* 1970; **101**: 316–23.
8 Politt RJ, Jenner FA, Davies M. Sibs with mental and physical retardation and trichorrhexis nodosa with abnormal amino-acid composition of the hair. *Arch Dis Child* 1968; **42**: 211–20.
9 Lyon JB, Dawber RPR. A sporadic case of dystrophic pili torti. *Br J Dermatol* 1977; **96**: 197–9.
10 Camacho-Martinez F. Localised trichorrhexis nodosa. *J Am Acad Dermatol* 1989; **20**: 696–700.

Longitudinal ridging and grooving

One or several longitudinal grooves and ridges can occur along the hair shaft; the overlying cuticle is usually intact in the absence of severe weathering influences. It is a microscopic sign that may occur in many different forms in Marie–Unna syndrome, uncombable hair syndrome, the narrow internodes of monilethrix and many other hereditary and congenital abnormalities, and may represent altered moulding of hair by misshapen internal root sheath.

Bubble hair

Brown [1] reported an unusual case of an acquired localized reversible hair shaft defect with intrinsic 'bubbles' within hairs, thought to be due to repeated cosmetic trauma. Subsequent reports [2,3] have demonstrated that the bubbles are a sign of thermal injury, particularly of damp hair [3]. This may be due to poor thermostat control of a hair dryer, but most of us suffer bubble hairs by singeing over the cooker (Fig. 66.49).

REFERENCES

1 Brown VM, Crounse RG, Abele DC. An unusual new hair shaft abnormality, 'bubble hair'. *J Am Acad Dermatol* 1986; **15**: 1113–16.
2 Detwiles SP, Carson JL, Woosley JT *et al*. Bubble hair. *J Am Acad Dermatol* 1994; **30**: 54–60.
3 Gummer CL. Bubble hair: a cosmetic abnormality caused by brief, focal heating of damp hair fibres. *Br J Dermatol* 1994; **131**: 901–3.

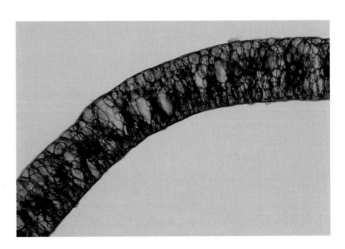

Fig. 66.49 Appearance of normal scalp hair after exposure to naked flame. Bubbles form within the cortex.

Hair pigmentation [1–4]

Melanin literally means black but scientists have long used the term to describe a range of pigments from yellow to black [5]. Animal biologists usually define melanin as pigment derived from the melanophore—the melanocyte. The superficial structures of most vertebrates contain such melanin pigments—skin, hair, scales and feathers.

If one is to understand and study the nature of the basic mechanisms that regulate pigmentation in humans, one should consider the process in sequence [3].

Four major classes of factors regulate mammalian melanin pigmentation:
1 those regulating the number and position of melanocytes in the hair and skin;
2 those regulating tyrosinase and melanin synthesis;
3 those governing the morphology and distribution of melanosomes in melanocytes; and
4 factors modulating the transfer of melanosomes from melanocytes to keratinocytes and the distribution of melanosomes in the latter cells.

Many of the disease states described later in this chapter illustrate specific defects within this overall scheme of events.

In humans, hair pigmentation depends entirely on the presence of melanin from melanocytes, but the actual colour perceived may sometimes depend also on physical phenomena. The range of colours produced by melanins is limited to shades of grey, yellow, brown, red and black. In contrast, many other animals display colours due to such pigments as porphyrins and carotenoids in addition to melanins.

It is important to remember that much of the research done on melanogenesis and its cellular control is in relation to cells in other epithelial surfaces, mainly the epidermis. There is no reason to believe that the biochemical events in hair-bulb melanocytes are different, and the work that has been carried out suggests they are similar.

Melanin chemistry [6]

Many problems remain to be resolved regarding the structure of natural melanins. The whole range of human hair colour is due to two types of melanin: eumelanins, which are mainly in black and brown hair, and phaeomelanins, which are yellow or red and give auburn and blonde hair [7]. Whatever the hair colour seen by the eye, isolated melanin is brown in colour and gives a dark brown solution in aqueous alkaline hydrogen peroxide [8].

Lloyd *et al.* [9] have shown that, in general, hair bulb tyrosinase activity does not decline linearly with age but tends to be maximal in middle age. A probable relationship of specific tyrosinases to human hair colours is still controversial [10]. There seems little doubt that the hair bulb produces eumelanin similar to that found in other sites [11].

It has been traditional to believe that each individual produces only eumelanin or phaeomelanin throughout life. This is probably untrue. Juhlin and Ortonne [12], for example, described a 57-year-old man whose red scalp hair began to turn dark brown at 50 years of age, and suggested a change from phaeomelanogenesis to eumelanogenesis as the basis for this. Many other natural hair-colour changes may reflect similar biochemical changes.

Melanocytes and melanogenesis

The melanocyte is the site of pigment production in the hair bulb. Functional melanocytes are situated in the bulb at the apex of the dermal papilla among the cells of the hair matrix, the main body of the cell being in contact with the basement membrane. Melanocytes are also present in the external root sheath and other parts of the follicle.

In black hair follicles, deposition of melanin within melanosomes continues until the whole unit is uniformly dense. Lighter-coloured hair shows less melanin deposition, and blonde hair follicles show melanosomes with a moth-eaten appearance. Red and blonde hair follicles have spherical melanosomes; those in brown and black hair are ellipsoidal [13].

Melanocytes in the hair bulb (and epidermis) differ from those found in internal structures in donating pigment to receptor cells, i.e. the hair matrix cells (keratinocytes) that ultimately differentiate to produce the hair cortex. No pigment is donated to presumptive cuticular and internal root sheath cells [14], although pigment granules have been detected in the cuticle of human nostril hair and in the coats of many animals [15]. In the epidermis, each melanocyte has a relationship to a determined pool of adjacent keratinocytes to which, under certain circumstances, melanocytes without dendrites may transfer pigment [16]. At present, there is no evidence to show whether a similar defined pool of receptor cells exists for each melanocyte in the hair follicle, but it remains a probability.

Melanocytes are functionally active only during the anagen phase of the hair cycle. They were formerly thought to disappear during telogen but it is now known that they remain at the surface of the papilla in a shrunken adendritic form. Jimbow *et al.* [17] found melanocytes with mature melanosomes in resting (telogen) feather follicles [18]. It is possible that the full complement of melanocytes present during successive anagen phases is the result not only of reactivation of 'dormant' cells, but also of new cells due to melanocyte replication [19].

Melanin granules are distributed throughout the hair cortex but in greater concentration toward the periphery. The pigment granules of black and brunette hair have oval pigment grains with a more or less homogeneous inner structure, and sharp boundaries; the surface is finely grained, with a thin surrounding membrane-like layer of osmophilic material [14]. Black hair granules are also relatively hard as judged from ultramicrotome sectioning, and have a high refractive index [15]. A greater absolute number of such granules are present in dark hair compared with lighter shades. Blonde hair granules are smaller, partly ellipsoid and partly rod-shaped in longitudinal section, and frequently have a rough, irregular and pitted surface.

Hair colour due to physical phenomena

The white colour of hair seen when melanin is absent is an optical effect due to reflection and refraction of incident light from various interfaces at which zones of different refractive index are in contact. Thus, in general, non-pigmented hair with a broad medulla appears paler than nonmedullated hair. Normal 'weathering' of hair along its length may lead to the terminal part appearing lighter than the rest due to a similar mechanism—the cortex and cuticle become disrupted and form numerous interfaces from internal reflection and refraction of light. This also applies in trichorrhexis nodosa (excessive 'weathering'), in which patients often note a lightening in colour of the brittle hair, and in the white bands of pili annulati. Because these optical lightening effects are due to reflection and refraction of incident light, when such hairs are viewed by transmitted light microscopy they appear dark. Newly formed unpigmented hair with no medulla appears yellowish rather than white. This is probably the intrinsic colour of dense keratin as orientated in hair fibres. Findlay [20] showed that the perceived colour is affected by the physical characteristics of the hair shaft and may bear little relationship to the true chromaticity of the shaft.

Hair colour in humans appears to be purely decorative and has no essential biological function. The racial and genetic colour differences that have evolved are probably related to the UV radiation protective colours seen in the skin, i.e. dark-skinned races have dark hair. Hair pigment, however, is not important in protection against the effects of sunlight, and hair with less natural amounts of melanin 'weathers' less well, i.e. the structure of hair colour appears to be a matter of serendipity.

Lanugo hair present *in utero* is unpigmented. Vellus hair is also typically unpigmented but, in men in particular, some vellus fibres may pigment slightly after puberty. Hair colour varies according to body site in most people [21]. Eyelashes are usually the darkest. Scalp hair is generally lighter than genital hair, which often has a reddish tint even in subjects having essentially brown hair. Grobbelaar [22] showed that hair on the lower and lateral scrotal surfaces is lighter than on the pubes. Apart from individuals with red scalp hair, a red tint to axillary hair is commonest in brown-haired individuals.

Hairs on exposed parts may be bleached by sunlight. Very dark hair first lightens to a brownish red colour but rarely becomes blonde even after strong sunlight exposure; brown hair, however, may be bleached white.

Control of hair colour

Hair colour is primarily under close genetic supervision; however, the exact hormonal and cellular mechanisms that control melanocyte function are not clearly worked out. An intimate relationship must exist between the factors controlling melanocyte and matrix cell activity, as melanocyte mitosis and melanosome production and transfer occur only during the anagen phase of the hair cycle. A negative feedback system has been postulated. Enzyme degradation products of melanosomes within matrix cells may cross cell membranes to melanocytes and control further melanin production or transfer [19]. A melanocyte-specific 'chalone' acting within a negative-feedback system may well exist for follicular melanocytes.

Follicular melanocytes are known to respond like epidermal melanocytes to melanocyte-stimulating hormone (MSH), which can darken light-coloured hair. A summary of current knowledge of the structure and function of MSH is provided in [2]. Three forms of MSH have been described: α, β and γ. These are small peptide hormones consisting of 12–18 amino acids. In vertebrates they are produced from the intermediate lobe of the pituitary gland. All three melanotrophins are cleavage products of a common precursor peptide, pro-opiomelanocortin. ACTH and α-MSH contain homologous internal sequences. Thus, the hyperpigmentation that occurs in Addison's disease, Nelson's syndrome and ectopic ACTH syndrome may be the result of ACTH, α-MSH and even other peptides with common sequences. The effects of hormones other than MSH on hair pigmentation have yet to be clearly elucidated. Oestrogens and progestogens may increase hair colour in view of their effect on the epidermis during pregnancy.

REFERENCES

1 Messenger AG. Control of hair growth and pigmentation. In: Olsen E, ed. *Disorders of Hair Growth*. New York: McGraw-Hill, 1994: 39–58.
2 Bolognia JL, Pawelek JM. Biology of hypopigmentation. *J Am Acad Dermatol* 1988; **19**: 217–25.
3 Prunieras M. Melanocytes, melanogenesis and inflammation. *Int J Dermatol* 1986; **25**: 624–9.
4 Zviak C, Dawber RPR. Hair colour. In: Zviak C, ed. *The Science of Hair Care*. New York: Marcel Dekker, 1986: 23–45.
5 Robin CP, ed. *Anatomic et Physiologie Cellulaire*. Paris: Baillière et Fils, 1873.
6 Prota G, Crescenzi S, Miscuraca G *et al.* New intermediates in phaeomelanogenesis *in vitro*. *Experimentia* 1970; **26**: 1058–70.
7 Prota G. Structure and biogenesis of phaeomelanins. In: Riley V, ed. *Pigmentation, its Genesis and Biological Control*. New York: Appleton–Century–Crofts, 1972.
8 Arnaud JC, Bore P. Isolation of melanin pigments from human hair. *J Soc Cosmet Chem* 1981; **32**: 137–45.
9 Lloyd T, Garry FL, Manders EK *et al.* The effect of age and hair colour on human hair bulb tyrosinase activity. *Br J Dermatol* 1987; **116**: 485–95.
10 King RA, Olds DP. Electrophoretic patterns of human hair bulb tyrosinase. *J Invest Dermatol* 1981; **77**: 201–17.
11 Nicholaus RA, Piattelli M, Fattorusso E. The structure of melanins

and melanogenesis. IV. On some natural melanins. *Tetrahedron* 1964; **20**: 1163–7.

12 Juhlin L, Ortonne JP. Red scalp hair turning dark-brown at 50 years of age. *Acta Derm Venereol (Stockh)* 1986; **66**: 71–7.

13 Montagna W, Parakkal PK. *The Structure and Function of Skin*. New York: Academic Press, 1974: 232–9.

14 Orfanos C, Ruska H. Die Feinstruktur des menschlichen Haares. III Das Haarpigment. *Arch Klin Exp Dermatol* 1968; **231**: 279–80.

15 Swift JA. The histology of keratin fibres. In: Asquith RS, ed. *The Chemistry of Natural Protein Fibres*. London: John Wiley and Sons, 1977.

16 Hadley ME, Quevado WC. Vertebrate epidermal melanin unit. *Nature* 1966; **209**: 1334–7.

17 Jimbow K, Roth S, Fitzpatrick TB. Ultrastructural investigation of autophagocytosis of melanosomes and programmed death of melanocytes in white Leghorn feathers. *Dev Biol* 1974; **36**: 8–14.

18 Silver AF, Chase HB, Potten CF. Melanocyte precursor cells in the hair follicle germ during the dormant stage (telogen). *Experimentia* 1969; **25**: 209–16.

19 Jimbow K, Roth S, Fitzpatrick TB *et al.* Mitotic activity in non-neoplastic melanocytes *in vivo* as determined by histochemical, autoradiographic and electron microscopic studies. *J Cell Biol* 1975; **66**: 663–77.

20 Findlay G. An optical study of human hair colour in normal and abnormal conditions. *Br J Dermatol* 1982; **107**: 517–23.

21 Wasserman HP. *Ethnic Pigmentation: Historical, Physiological and Clinical Aspects*. Excerpta Medica: Amsterdam.

22 Grobbelaar CS. The distribution of, and correlation between eye, hair and skin colour in male students at the University of Stellenbosch. *Ann Univ Stellenbosch* 1952; **28**: Sect a/1; 12.

Variation in hair colour

Genetic and racial aspects [1,2]

Mammalian hair colour has long been a subject of considerable interest to geneticists and, in a variety of species including humans, a number of genetic variants have been described. Genetic studies of hair colour not only provide us with knowledge of gene function, they also give insight into the mechanisms of hair pigmentation [3]. From laboratory and animal studies, a general conformity has been shown in the complement of genes affecting hair colour [4] and it is reasonable to assume that an essentially similar complex of genes may be involved in humans. Human hair (and skin) colour is influenced by at least four gene loci, which are probably allelic [5]. The chief obstacle to more detailed studies of hair colour inheritance in humans is the absence of clear data on crosses between individuals with 'pure' Caucasoid, Negroid and Mongoloid skin. Ethnic differences in hair colour are very conspicuous, as are the differences in hair morphology, although colour and hair form are inherited separately [6]. Dark hair predominates in the world. Among Caucasoids there is wide variation in colour within geographical regions. Blonde hair is most frequent in northern Europe and black hair in Southern and Eastern Europe; foci of blondeness are to be found even in North Africa, the Middle East and in some Australoids. Congoid, Capoid, Mongoloid and Australoid hair is mainly black.

Red hair (rutilism)

This has attracted more attention than other colours because it is less common and because it is so distinctive. The melanin pigment is phaeomelanin, not eumelanin. In Italy, and in the UK excluding East Anglia, the distribution of red hair is similar to that of blood group O [7]. The incidence of red hair varies from 0.3% in northern Germany to as high as 11% in parts of Scotland. Like hair of many other colours, red hair often darkens with age from red through brown to sandy or auburn in the adult. The skin of redheads is generally pale, burns easily in sunlight and pigments very little even after prolonged and frequent sun exposure.

Heterochromia

This implies the growth of hair of two distinct colours in the same individual. A colour difference between scalp and moustache is not uncommon. In fair-haired individuals, pubic and axillary hair, eyebrows and eyelashes are much darker than scalp hair. In humans, eyelashes are generally the most darkly pigmented hairs. Black- and brown-haired subjects often have red or auburn sideburns. In those other than the fair-haired, genital hair is usually lighter than scalp hair and it may have a reddish tint even in those with brown pubic hair; 33% of a series of South African white people had red axillary hair whereas this was only occasionally seen in black people; also, hair on the lower and lateral aspect of the scrotum was lighter than on the pubes [8]. In brown-haired individuals, a reddish tint is more common in axillary hair than on the scalp.

In general, scalp hair darkens with age. Rarely, a circumscribed patch of hair occurs of different colour. This generally has a genetic basis, although the type of inheritance is not known in humans. Patchy differences of hair colour are of five types.

1 Tufts of very dark hair growing from a melanocytic naevus.
2 Hereditary, usually autosomal dominant heterochromia, for example tufts of red hair at the temples in a black-haired subject or a single black patch in a blonde.
3 Perhaps as a result of somatic mosaicism; partial asymmetry of hair and eye colour may occur sporadically.
4 The white forelock of piebaldism.
5 The 'flag' sign in kwashiorkor.

Greying of hair (canities)

Greying of hair is usually a manifestation of the ageing process and is due to a progressive reduction in melanocyte function [9]. The larger medullary spaces of older people may contribute to the process.

There is a gradual dilution of pigment in greying hairs, i.e. the full range of colour from normal to white can be seen both along individual hairs and from hair to hair. Loss of hair-shaft colour is associated with decrease and eventual cessation of tyrosinase activity in the lower bulb [10]. In white hairs, melanocytes are infrequent or absent [11] or possibly dormant. It has been suggested that autoimmunity plays a part in the pathogenesis of greying; grey hair certainly has an association with the autoimmune disease pernicious anaemia [12,13].

The age of onset of canities is primarily dependent on the genotype of the individual although acquired factors may play a part. The visual impression of greyness is more obvious (seen earlier) in the fair-haired. In Caucasoid races, white hair first appears at the age of 34.2 ± 9.6 years, and by the age of 50 years 50% of the population have at least 50% grey hairs [14]. The onset in black people is 43.9 ± 10.3 years, and in Japanese between 30 and 34 years in men and between 35 and 39 years in women. The beard and moustache areas commonly become grey before scalp or body hair. On the scalp the temples usually show greying first, followed by a wave of greyness spreading to the crown and later to the occipital area.

Rapid onset allegedly 'overnight' greying of the hair has excited the literary, medical and anthropological worlds for centuries [15]. Many reports have been overdramatized but it certainly occurs. Historical examples often quoted include Sir Thomas More and Marie Antoinette whose hair became grey over the night preceding their execution. The probable mechanism for rapid greying is the selective shedding of pigmented hairs in diffuse AA, the non-pigmented hairs being retained (Figs 66.50 & 66.51).

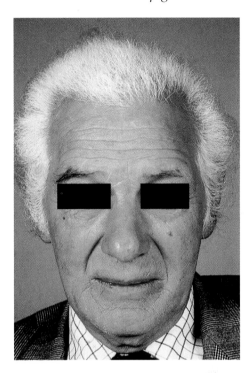

Fig. 66.51 Rapid greying of hair. Same patient as Fig. 66.50 taken 1 week later. Due to alopecia areata. (Courtesy of Dr D. Fenton, St Thomas' Hospital, London,UK.)

Despite occasional reports to the contrary, in general, greying of hair is progressive and permanent, although melanogenesis during anagen may be intermittent for a time before finally stopping. Most of the reports of the return of normal hair colour from grey are examples of a pigmented regrowth following AA, which eventually repigments in many cases. The reported repigmentation of grey hair in association with Addisonian hypoadrenalism may result from a mechanism similar to that in AA or vitiligo, in view of the known association between these diseases [16–18]. Darkening of grey hair may occur following large doses of *p*-aminobenzoic acid [19].

Premature greying (Fig. 66.52)

Premature greying of hair has been defined as onset of greying before 20 years of age in white people and 30 years of age in black people. It probably has a genetic basis and occasionally occurs as an isolated autosomal dominant condition. The association between premature greying and certain organ-specific autoimmune diseases is well documented. The relationship is probably not one of common pathogenesis, but on the basis of genetic linkage. It is often stated that premature greying may be an early sign of pernicious anaemia, hyperthyroidism and, less commonly, hypothyroidism, and all autoimmune diseases that have a genetic predisposition. In a controlled study of the integumentary associations of pernicious anaemia, 11%

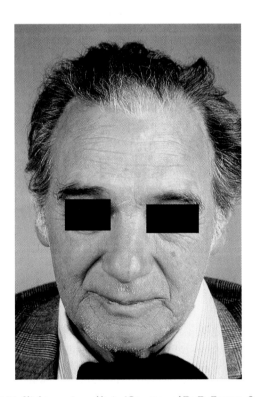

Fig. 66.50 Slight greying of hair. (Courtesy of Dr D. Fenton, St Thomas' Hospital, London, UK.)

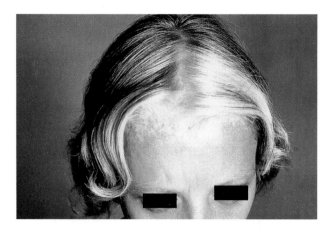

Fig. 66.52 Premature greying of hair, which commenced at 19 years of age in this individual.

had premature greying [12]. In Book's syndrome, an autosomal dominant trait, premature greying is associated with premolar hypodontia and palmoplantar hyperhidrosis [20]. In the early stages, it may be partially reversible [21].

The premature ageing syndromes, progeria and Werner's syndrome (pangeria), may have very early greying as a prominent feature. It does not occur in metageria, or total lipodystrophy [22]. In progeria it is associated with marked loss of scalp hair as early as 2 years of age.

In dystrophia myotonica the onset of grey hair may precede the myotonia and muscle wasting.

Premature canities is an inconstant feature of the Rothmund–Thomson syndrome; when present, it typically commences in adolescence.

One-third of patients with chromosome 5p syndrome (cri du chat syndrome) have prematurely grey hair [23].

Poliosis

Poliosis is defined as the presence of a localized patch of white hair due to the absence or deficiency of melanin in a group of neighbouring follicles. Essentially, the changes in melanogenesis are the same in the hair follicle as in the affected epidermis.

Hereditary defects [24]

Piebaldism (white spotting or partial albinism) is an autosomal dominant abnormality with patches of skin totally devoid of pigment, which remain unchanged throughout life. Most commonly, a frontal white patch occurs—the white forelock—which may be the only sign. Melanocytes are decreased in number, but are morphologically abnormal and contain normal non-melanized premelanosomes, and also premelanosomes and melanosomes of abnormal appearance [25]. Similar pathological changes are seen in Tiez's syndrome of generalized 'white

spot' loss of skin and hair pigment, complete deaf mutism and eyebrow hypoplasia [26]. Whether or not melanocytes are present in the affected areas remains controversial.

Waardenburg's syndrome [27,28] shows skin changes so similar to piebaldism that they are presumed to have a similar pathogenesis. Symptoms and signs are present from birth and include dystopia canthorum with lateral displacement of the medial canthi, hypertrophy of the nasal root and hyperplasia of the inner third of the eyebrows with confluent brows. Total or partial iridial heterochromia may occur, as may perceptive deafness. The white forelock is present in 20% of cases. Premature greying may develop with or without the white forelock [29]; a minority have piebaldism and congenital nerve deafness but no other overt signs of Waardenburg's syndrome, suggesting that this association may be genetically distinct.

In vitiligo, the white patches of skin frequently have white hairs within them. The histological changes are consistent with an 'autoimmune injury' to the melanocytes.

The Vogt–Koyanagi–Harada syndrome [30] consists of a postfebrile condition comprising bilateral uveitis, labrynthine deafness, tinnitus and vitiligo, poliosis and AA [31].

Alezzandrini's syndrome combines unilateral facial vitiligo, retinitis and poliosis of eyebrows and eyelashes [32]; perceptive deafness is rarely associated.

In AA, regrowing hair is frequently white. It may remain so, particularly in cases of late onset. Although absent hair pigment is only evident at the stage of resolution, melanocytes are lost from the hair bulb quite early and migrate to the dermal papilla.

Poliosis occurs in 60% of cases of tuberous sclerosis. Depigmented hair may be the earliest sign [33].

The pathognomonic signs of Von Recklinghausen's multiple neurofibromatosis relate to hyperpigmented areas—café au lait macules and axillary and perineal freckling. Scalp hypopigmented patches must not be mistaken for vitiliginous changes.

Acquired defects [34]. Permanent pigmentary loss may be induced by inflammatory processes which damage melanocytes, for example herpes zoster. X-irradiation often causes permanent hair loss but less intense treatment leads to hypopigmented and, rarely, hyperpigmented hair. Patchy white hair may develop on the beard area after dental treatment.

Albinism [26]

In autosomal recessive oculocutaneous albinism (complete, perfect, or generalized albinism) similar changes are found in the hair bulb melanocytes as in the epidermis [26]. This applies to tyrosine positive and negative types. Melanocytes are structurally normal and active in producing melanosomes of grades I and II. They are, however, enzymically inactive. The melanocyte system is never completely devoid of melanin. In Caucasoids, the hair is typically yellowish-white though it might be cream, yellow, yellowish-red or vibrant red. This range of colour parallels that seen in normal blonde Caucasoids. In Negroid albinos the hair colour is white or yellowish-brown.

Chediak–Higashi syndrome

This syndrome is basically an autosomal recessive defect of the membrane-bound organelles of several cell types [35]. It combines oculocutaneous hypopigmentation with a lethal defect of leukocytes. The hair is silvery grey or light blonde and may be sparse.

Colour changes induced by drugs and other chemicals

Some topical agents temporarily change hair colour. Dithranol and chrysarobin stain light coloured or grey hair mahogany brown. Resorcin, formerly used a great deal in a variety of skin diseases, colours black or white hair yellow or yellowish-brown.

Some systemic drugs alter hair colour by interfering with the eumelanin or phaeomelanin pathway; in others, the mechanism is not known. Chloroquine interferes with phaeomelanin synthesis [36], i.e. it affects only blonde and red-haired individuals; the changes are completely reversible. Mephenesin, a glycerol ether used for diseases with muscle spasms, causes pigmentary loss in dark-haired people [3]. Triparanol, an anticholesterolaemic drug, and fluorobutyrophenone, an antipsychotic drug, both interfere with keratinization and cause hypopigmentation and sparse hair. Minoxidil and diazoxide [27,38], two potent antihypertensive agents, both cause hypertrichosis and darkening of hair. The colour produced by diazoxide is reddish, whereas minoxidil darkens hair mainly by converting vellus hair to terminal hair. Hydroquinone and phenylthiourea interfere with tyrosine activity, causing hypopigmentation of skin and hair [39].

Darkening of white hair occurred in a patient with Parkinson's disease following the addition of carbidopa and bromocriptine therapy [40].

Colour changes due to nutritional deficiencies

Because specific dietary deficiencies are rare in humans, most clinical knowledge of their effects is derived from laboratory and animal studies. Copper deficiency in cattle causes achromotrichia because it is the prosthetic group of tyrosinase; loss of hair colour from this mechanism occurs in humans as Menkes' kinky hair syndrome. In protein malnutrition, exemplified by kwashiorkor, hair colour changes are a prominent feature; normal black hair becomes brown or reddish, and brown hair becomes blonde [41,42]. Intermittent protein malnutrition leads to the 'flag' sign of kwashiorkor (signe de la bandera). Alternating white (abnormal) and dark bands occur along individual hairs. Similar changes to kwashiorkor have been described in severe ulcerative colitis and after extensive bowel resection.

The lightening of hair colour from black to brown described in severe iron-deficiency anaemia may be an effect on keratinization rather than on melanocytic function [43].

Noppakun and Swasdikul [44] described a case of reversible white hair in vitamin B_{12} deficiency and commented on a variety of reversible and other hair colour changes in adult coeliac disease.

Hair colour in metabolic disorders

Phenylketonuria is an autosomal recessive disorder in which the tissues are unable to metabolize phenylalanine to tyrosine because of phenylalanine hydroxylase deficiency. Mental retardation, fits and decreased pigmentation of the skin, eyes and hair occur with eczema and dermographism. Black hair may become brown, and older institutionalized patients with phenylketonuria may have pale blonde or grey hair. Tyrosine treatment causes darkening towards normal colour within 1–2 months.

The paling of hair seen in homocystinuria is probably due to keratinization changes resulting from the error in methionine metabolism.

Light, almost white hair and recurrent oedema are the surface manifestations of the hair condition, 'oast house' disease. Methionine concentration in the blood is raised.

Accidental hair discoloration

Hair avidly binds many inorganic elements and thus hair colour changes are occasionally seen after exposure to certain substances.

Exposure to high concentrates of copper in industry or from inadvertently high concentrations in tap water [45] or in swimming pools may cause green hair, particularly visible in blonde-haired subjects [46,47]. Cobalt workers get bright blue hair and a deep blue tint may be seen in indigo handlers [48]. A yellowish hair colour is not uncommon in white- or grey-haired heavy smokers due to tar in cigarette smoke; yellow staining may also occur from picric acid and dithranol. Trinitrotoluene (TNT) workers sometimes develop yellow skin and reddish-brown hair.

REFERENCES

1 Dawber R, ed. *Diseases of the Hair and Scalp*, 3rd edn. Oxford: Blackwell Science, 1997.
2 Baker JR. *Race*. London: Oxford University Press, 1974.
3 Takeuchi T. Genetic control of mammalian hair colour. In: Kobori T, Montagna W, eds. *Biology and Diseases of the Hair*. Baltimore: University Park Press, 1975: 110–33.

4 Fitzpatrick TB, Brunet P, Kukita A. The nature of hair pigmentation. In: Montagna W, Ellis RA, eds. *Biology of Hair Growth*. New York: Academic Press, 1958: 144–54.

5 Harrison GA. Differences in human pigmentation; measurement, geographical variation and causes. *J Invest Dermatol* 1973; **60**: 418–30.

6 Trotter M, Duggins OH. Age changes in head hair from birth to maturity. *Am J Phys Anthropol* 1950; **8**: 467–77.

7 Harrison GA, Weiner JS, Tanner JM *et al. Human Biology, An Introduction to Human Evolution, Variation and Growth*. London: Oxford University Press, 1964.

8 Grobbelaar CS. The distribution of and correlation between eye, hair and skin colour in male students at the University of Stellenbosch. *Ann Univ Stellenbosch* 1952; **28** sect, A1; 12.

9 Kligman AM. Pathologic dynamics of human hair loss. *Arch Dermatol* 1961; **83**: 175–82.

10 Kukita A, Fitzpatrick TB. The demonstration of tyrosinase in melanocytes of the human hair matrix by autoradiography. *Science* 1955; **121**: 893–904.

11 Hertzberg J, Gusck W. Das Ergrauen des Kapfhaares. Eine histo-und fermentschemische sowie elektronen-mikroskopische Studie. *Arch Klin Exp Dermatol* 1970; **236**: 368–75.

12 Dawber RPR. Integumentary associations of pernicious anaemia. *Br J Dermatol* 1970; **82**: 221–6.

13 Klaus SN. Acquired pigment dilution of the skin and hair; a sign of pancreatic disease in the tropics. *Int J Dermatol* 1980; **19**: 508–11.

14 Keough EV, Walsh RJ. Rate of greying human hair. *Nature* 1965; **207**: 877–80.

15 Jelinek JE. Sudden whitening of hair. *Bull NY Acad Med* 1972; **48**: 1003–6.

16 Cunliffe WJ, Hall R, Newell DJ *et al.* Vitiligo, thyroid disease and autoimmunity. *Br J Dermatol* 1968; **80**: 135–42.

17 Dunlop D. Eighty-six cases of Addisons's disease. *Br Med J* 1963; **ii**: 887–99.

18 Main RA, Robbie RB, Gray ES *et al.* Smooth muscle antibodies and alopecia areata. *Br J Dermatol* 1975; **92**: 289–95.

19 Sieve BF. Darkening of grey hair following para-aminobenzoic acid. *Science* 1941; **94**: 257–60.

20 Book JA. Clinical and genetic studies of hypodontia. I Premolar aplasia, hyperhidrosis and canities prematura: a new hereditary syndrome in man. *Am J Hum Genet* 1950; **2**: 240–5.

21 Tobin DJ, Cargnello JA. Partial reversal of canities in a 22-year-old normal Chinese male. *Arch Dermatol* 1993; **129**: 789–90.

22 Gilkes JJH, Sharvill DE, Wells RS. The premature ageing syndromes. Report of eight cases and descriptions of a new entity named metageria. *Br J Dermatol* 1974; **91**: 243–52.

23 Breg WR. Abnormalities of chromosomes 4 and 5. In: Gardner LI, ed. *Endocrine and Genetic Diseases of Childhood and Adolescence*. Philadelphia: WB Saunders, 1975.

24 Mosher DB, Fitzpatrick TB. Piebaldism. *Arch Dermatol* 1988; **124**: 245–350.

25 Grupper C, Prunieras M, Hincky M *et al.* Albinisme partiel familial (piebaldisme): étude ultrastructurale. *Ann Dermatol Syphilol* 1970; **97**: 267–86.

26 Witkop CJ, Jr. Albinism. In: Harris H, Hirschom K, eds. *Advances in Human Genetics*. New York: Plenum Press, 1971.

27 Burton JL, Marshall A. Hypertrichosis due to minoxidil. *Br J Dermatol* 1979; **101**: 593–6.

28 Waardenburg PJ. New syndrome combining developmental abnormalities of the eyelid, eyebrows, nose root, with pigmentary defects of the iris and head hair and with congenital deafness. *Am J Hum Genet* 1951; **3**: 195–202.

29 Rugel SJ, Keats EU. Waardenburg's syndrome in six generations of one family. *Am J Dis Child* 1965; **109**: 579–89.

30 Koyanagi Y. Dysacusis, alopecia, und poliosis bei schwerer Uveitis nicht traumatischen Ursprungen. *Klin Monats Augenheik* 1929; **82**: 194–8.

31 Howsden HM. Vogt–Koyanagi–Harada syndrome and psoriasis. *Arch Dermatol* 1973; **108**: 395–9.

32 Alezzandrini AA. Manifestations unilaterales de degenerescence tapetoretinienne de vitiligo, de poliose, de cheveux blancs et hypoacousie. *Ophthalmologica* 1964; **147**: 409–15.

33 McWilliam TS, Stephenson JBP. Depigmented hair; the earliest sign of tuberose sclerosis. *Arch Dis Child* 1978; **53**: 961–9.

34 Prunieras M. Melanocytes, melanogenesis and inflammation. *Int J Dermatol* 1986; **25**: 624–8.

35 White JG, Clawson CC. The Chediak–Higashi syndrome: the nature of the giant neutrophil granules and their interaction with cytoplasm and foreign particles. *Am J Pathol* 1980; **48**: 151–9.

36 Saunders TS, Fitzpatrick LE, Seji M *et al.* Decrease in human hair colour,

and feather pigment of fowl following chloroquine diphosphate. *J Invest Dermatol* 1959; **33**: 87–98.

37 Spillane JD. Brunette to Blond. Depigmentation of hair during treatment with oral mephenesin. *Br Med J* 1963; **i**: 997–8.

38 Ridgley GV, Kassassieh SD. Minoxidil. *Lahey Clin Foundation Bull* 1979; **28**: 80–6.

39 Dieke SH. Pigmentation and hair growth in black rats as modified by the chronic administration of thiourea, phenylthiourea and alpha-naphthylthiourea. *Endocrinology* 1947; **40**: 123–30.

40 Reynolds NJ, Crossley J, Ferguson I *et al.* Darkening of white hair in Parkinson's disease. *Clin Exp Dermatol* 1989; **14**: 317–20.

41 Bradfield RB. Hair tissue as a medium for the differential diagnosis of protein-calorie malnutrition: a commentary. *J Pediatr* 1974; **84**: 294–9.

42 Bradfield RB, Jellife DB. Hair colour changes in kwashiorkor. *Lancet* 1974; **i**: 461–3.

43 Sato S, Jitsukawa K, Sato H *et al.* Segmental heterochromia in black scalp hair associated with Fe-deficiency anaemia. *Arch Dermatol* 1989; **125**: 531–8.

44 Noppakun N, Swasdikul D. Hyperpigmentation of skin and nails with white hair due to vitamin B_{12} deficiency. *Arch Dermatol* 1986; **122**: 896–904.

45 Goldschmidt H. Green hair. *Arch Dermatol* 1979; **115**: 1288–90.

46 Blanc D, Zultak M, Rochefort A. Les cheveux vert; étude clinique, chimique et epidemiologique. *Ann Dermatol Vénéréol* 1988; **115**: 807–12.

47 Melnik BC, Plewig G, Daldrup T. Green hair; guidelines for diagnosis and therapy. *J Am Acad Dermatol* 1986; **15**: 1065–9.

48 Beigel H. Blue hair in indigo handlers. *Arch Pathol Anat Physiol* 1965; **83**: 324–8.

Hair cosmetics

Women and men have always been concerned about their hair, and have sought to modify it by grooming, colouring, cutting and wigs. There are references in Egyptian papyruses to the importance of arranging the hair prior to seduction [1,2].

Twentieth-century woman has continued this concern at modifying her appearance by cosmetic preparations and nowhere is this concern more strongly manifest than in connection with the hair; no doubt a measure of its psychological and sexual importance. The production of shampoos, dyes, waving and other hair applications has become big business in every Western country. Science has benefited enormously from this industry as many of the advances have come from cosmetic science laboratories [3,4].

REFERENCES

1 Pomey-Rey D. Hair and psychology. In: Zviak C, ed. *The Science of Hair Care*. New York: Marcel Dekker Inc, 1986.

2 Gummer C, Dawber RPR. Hair cosmetics. In: Dawber RPR, ed. *Diseases of the Hair and Scalp*, 3rd edn. Oxford: Blackwell Science, 1997: 732–59.

3 Zviak C, Dawber RPR. Hair structure, function and physicochemical properties. In: Zviak C, ed. *The Science of Hair Care*. New York: Marcel Dekker Inc, 1986: 1–34.

4 Schoen LA, ed. *Skin and Hair Care*, 1st English edn. Harmondsworth: Penguin Books, 1978.

Shampoos [1–4]

In modern terms, a shampoo may be defined as a suitable detergent for washing hair, which leaves the hair in good condition. Originally, shampoos were used solely for cleansing hair, but their range of function has extended in recent years to include conditioning, and the treatment of some hair and scalp diseases.

In principle, to wash hair a shampoo must remove grease, as it is the latter which attracts dirt and other particulate matter. The polar group of a detergent achieves this by displacing oil from the hair surface. The evaluation of shampoo detergency is difficult and complicated. The consumer tends to equate detergency with foaming; in Western society, few shampoos sell unless they possess good foaming power. In the evaluation of detergents as shampoos no single criterion can be used, although instrumental methods have been devised. Efficacy can be based only on the subjective impression of the consumer. The factors taken into consideration include:

1 ease of distribution of shampoo over the hair;
2 lathering power;
3 ease of rinsing and combing of wet hair;
4 lustre of hair;
5 speed of drying;
6 ease of combing and setting.
Safety is of paramount importance.

Shampoo formulations

These vary enormously but the basic ingredients can be resolved into a few groups—water, detergent and some fatty material. Soap shampoos are made from vegetable or animal fats and remove dirt and grease as efficiently as detergents; however, a scum forms with hard water and the trend has therefore been increasingly towards detergents as the principal washing ingredient. Detergents are synthetic petroleum products and form no hard-water scum.

Shampoos contain:

1 principal surfactants for detergency and foaming power;
2 secondary surfactants to improve and 'condition' hair;
3 additives which both complete the formulation and add 'special' effects.
Whatever the claims of some manufacturers, most special additives end up down the sink [5]!

In general, cosmetic shampoos can be dry (powder types), liquid, solid cream, aerosol or oily. Antidandruff, 'medicated' and scalp treatment shampoos contain antiseptics and active agents such as coal- and wood-tar fractions. Clear liquid shampoos are the most popular, including 'cleansing' types, sold for treating greasy hair, and 'cosmetic' types having good conditioning action and popular among women with dry or 'normal' hair. For details of other specific formulas, the reader is recommended to read more specialized texts [3,4,6]

Shampoo safety

Shampoos obviously must be non-toxic, and at concentrations used by the consumer not irritate either skin or eyes. New shampoo formulations are tested exhaustively prior to marketing, particularly to assess their propensity to cause eye irritation, scarring and corneal opacities. Skin irritation is not usually encountered from shampoos that have low eye irritancy potential. Eye safety is assessed by the technique known as the Draize test; standard solutions of shampoo are instilled into the conjunctival sac of an albino rabbit. In general, the eye irritancy of detergents is greatest with cationics, followed by anionics, and least with non-anionics. There are exceptions to this, suggesting that shampoo irritancy may be due to properties other than detergency including surface activity, pH, wetting power, foaming power (Ross–Miles test), and wetting and foaming power together. Most shampoos are, in fact, irritant but not dangerously so. Allergic contact dermatitis due to biocides does occur (Chapters 20 and 21).

Conditioners

Dry hair lacks gloss and lustre and is difficult to style. This results from natural weathering and is worsened by chemical and physical processes applied to the hair. Conditioners comprise fatty acids and alcohols: natural triglycerides, for example almond, avocado, corn and olive oil; waxes, for example beeswax, jojoba oil, mink oil, lanolin; phospholipids, for example egg yolk and soya bean; vitamins A, B and E, protein hydrolysates of silk, collagen, keratin (horn and hoof), gelatin and other proteins; and cationic polymers. Conditioners are available in a variety of forms and are widely used. They provide lubrication and gloss and render the hair easier to comb and style. The most commonly used are creams and emulsions applied for a few minutes after washing and then rinsed off. Deep conditioners are left on for up to 30 min, often with damp heat. Fluids, gels and aerosol foams have become popular recently and aid styling. Hair oils are traditional conditioners. Men may use brilliantines, greases or oils to leave the hair glossy and sleek [3].

REFERENCES

1 Corbett JP. The chemistry of hair-care products. *J Soc Dyers Colourists* 1976; **92**: 285–93.
2 Robbins CR, ed. *Chemical and Physical Behaviour of Human Hair*, 1st edn. New York: Van Nostrand Reinhold, 1979.
3 Zviak C, Bouillon C. Hair treatment and hair care products. In: Zviak C, ed. *The Science of Hair Care*. New York: Marcel Dekker, 1986: 210–24.
4 Zviak C, Vanderberghe G. Scalp and hair hygiene: shampoos. In: Zviak C, ed. *The Science of Hair Care*. New York: Marcel Dekker, 1986: 224–41.
5 Spoor HJ. Shampoos. *Cutis* 1973; **12**: 671–6.
6 Gummer C, Dawber RPR. Hair cosmetics. In: Dawber RPR, ed. *Diseases of the Hair and Scalp*, 3rd edn. Oxford: Blackwell Science, 1997: 732–59.

Cosmetic hair colouring [1–4]

Since the days of the pharaohs, women in particular have used hair dyes both to hide grey hair and for reasons of fashion. The latter use has increased enormously during the past 50 years and now men are using hair dyes.

The penetration of dyes into hair depends on molecular size and the aqueous swelling of the hair at the time of application of the dye; basicity of the dye is also important. The most successful dyes are relatively small molecules.

Excluding bleaches, hair-colouring materials can be divided into three groups: vegetable, metallic and synthetic organic dyes. In advanced countries, vegetable and metallic hair colourants are almost obsolete because of the more 'natural' colours obtained with synthetic organic materials.

Vegetable dyes

Henna may be used to give reddish auburn shades. It is obtained from shrubs found in North Africa and the Middle East—*Lawsonia alba*, *L. spinosa* and *L. inermis*. The dye is produced from dried leaves, which are removed before the plant flowers. The active principle is an acidic naphthoquinone (lawsone); it is still to be found in some hair rinses. Traditionally, it is applied as a thick paste 'pack', which is left *in situ* for 5–60 min. The effects last for up to 10 weeks. This process is non-toxic but messy, and fingernails may become stained. Henna rinses are mixtures of henna and powdered indigo leaves that produce blue–black shades. A wide range of products containing compound henna exist [5]. Ground flower heads of a Roman or German chamomile yield a yellow dye: 1,3,4,-trihydroxyflavone (apigenin). It stains only the cuticle and can be used to lighten or brighten hair. Other vegetable dyes include extracts from logwood and walnut shell and these can be used by patients who are paraphenylenediamine sensitive. These products are obtainable at herbalists and beauty shops.

Metallic dyes

Traditionally, hair dyes for men have been of this type, as the colour changes occur less rapidly and are not as immediately obvious as with the oxidative dyes. Inorganic salts are used, which are altered by the hair and coat the surface as either oxides from reduction of the metal salts by keratin, or sulphides from the action of the sulphur in keratin on the metal. They all give a rather dull (metallic) appearance and may cause brittle or damaged hair if used too often.

Lead acetate, with precipitated sulphur or sodium thiosulphate, gives brown to black shades; grey hair may be changed through yellow to brown or black. Silver nitrate used alone produces a greenish-black colour; pyrogallol is used as developer. Colours from ash blonde to black are possible by mixing silver nitrate variously with copper, cobalt or nickel; brownish-black skin staining is the great disadvantage. Bismuth salts give shades of brown. Newer metallic dyes, containing a metal plus an organic ligand,

are used on textile fibres and in some hair-dye patents. Metallic dyes cannot be removed without hair damage and should be left to grow out.

Synthetic organic dyes

This group has now been in use for more than 40 years. They are the most important type because of the comprehensive range of 'natural' colours which can be obtained. Most penetrate the hair cuticle, i.e. they are potentially permanent, but in recent years less permanent types have been introduced.

Synthetic organic colourants are of three types:
1 *Temporary*. These wash out with one shampoo and last no longer than 1 week. Many temporary rinses belong to this group, including fashionable unnatural colours used by avant-garde sects and groups! They are available in aerosol sprays by incorporation into transparent polymeric plastics such as PVP; the disadvantage of such vehicles is their tendency to flake off onto clothing.
2 *Semipermanent*. In the UK, these have the widest appeal. They are used frequently at home and also in salons to brighten or subdue a natural colour, modify a permanent or bleached colour, or modify white or grey. They are of sufficiently small molecular size to penetrate the cortex. They are intrinsically coloured, i.e. no developing is required, cf. the oxidative permanent group. They are relatively easy to wash out with shampoos containing ammonia; other shampoos must be used six to 10 times to remove them. Some semipermanent dyes have an affinity for thioglycollate-waved hair. Many are now used in colour shampoos.
3 *Permanent* (developed or oxidation dyes). These do not rely on the natural colour of a single chemical dye stuff, cf. semipermanents, but require an oxidative developer—hydrogen peroxide—to produce the final colour:

Paraphenylenediamine (PPD) and/or
paratoluenediamine (PTD)

+

Hydrogen peroxide
↓
Applied to hair
↓
Quinone diamine (small molecule)
↓
Penetrate hair—to cortex
↓
Large molecules produced
(by diamine 'self' condensation and modifiers, e.g. pyrogallol)

Other substances may be included in specific formulations to give greater intensity to the dye, for example resorcinol and polyhidric phenols.

Oxidative dyes are potentially hazardous. The need for hydrogen peroxide enables lighter shades to be obtained and is chiefly responsible for the structural damage to hair which may occur if care is not exercised. Additives such as pyrogallol and resorcinol are potential irritants. The greatest problem is the potential of PPD (less so with PTD) to cause allergic dermatitis. Up to 10% of users may develop type IV allergy [6,7]. All dyes in this group are therefore sold with instructions to carry out preliminary patch testing 24–48 h before the proposed dye is used. Thus, the dye system is applied to skin either behind one ear or on the forearm—any redness, swelling or blistering implies allergy and the dyeing should not therefore proceed. A negative patch test does not mean that subsequent allergy cannot develop; it simply shows the subject is not allergic at the time the test is carried out. If allergy is shown, it is not sufficient merely to stop all future use of oxidative dyes; unfortunately, cross-sensitization also occurs with other aromatic benzenes, for example, sulphonamides and some local anaesthetics, which must also be avoided for life. Modern formulations seem to cause less problems with allergy [8]. Hair dyes of this group have been incriminated as possible carcinogens [9]. Chromosome breaks have occurred under experimental conditions [10] and an increased incidence of tumours has been found in regular users [11]. It has also been intimated that aplastic anaemia could be produced by hair dyes [12]. None of these reports is sufficiently conclusive to warrant the withdrawal of such dyes.

Permanent dyes last for several months; they must not be applied more frequently than every 2–3 weeks because hair damage will occur. Permanently dyed hair must therefore be allowed to grow out. However, if a light shade has been produced and the subject wishes a darker shade, then temporary rinses may safely be used as these only coat the hair surface and have no propensity to cause structural damage.

For less commonly used permanent dye formulations, such as 'highlights', the reader is referred to specialized texts [4].

Bleaches [13–15]

Women have bleached their hair since Roman times. Bleaching is used both to lighten hair and to prepare it to take up hair dyes. Bleaching is an oxidative alkaline treatment which oxidizes and bleaches melanin. The hair lightens to reddish or yellow tones depending on the underlying hair colour, and ultimately to platinum. Bleaching is very damaging to the hair, rendering it dry, porous and more prone to tangle. Overuse may cause disruption and fracture of the hair. Thus, it is advisable to perform permanent waving before bleaching. Home bleaching is usually performed with 6% hydrogen peroxide (20 volumes) with ammonia to speed the reaction, which

otherwise takes 12 h. Salons use more powerful bleaching creams, powders and pastes, which are much faster. They are often applied to individual strands of hair, others being left untreated to give highlights, which lessens the problem of the darkened roots. Bleaching is terminated by shampooing or an acid rinse. The human eye perceives a more aesthetically acceptable blonde ('platinum' blonde) when the bleached hair is treated with a blue or lilac colourant.

REFERENCES

1 Corbett JF, Menkart T. Hair colouring. *Cutis* 1973; **12**: 190–5.
2 Kalopesis G. Toxicology and hair dyes. In: Zviak C, ed. *The Science of Hair Care*. New York: Marcel Dekker, 1986.
3 Zviak C. Hair coloring: non-oxidation coloring. In: Zviak C, ed. *The Science of Hair Care*. New York: Marcel Dekker, 1986.
4 Zviak C. Oxidation coloring. In: Zviak C, ed. *The Science of Hair Care*. New York: Marcel Dekker, 1986.
5 Natow AJ. Henna. *Cutis* 1986; **38**: 21–5.
6 Blohm SG, Rajka G. The allergenicity of paraphenylene diamine. *Acta Derm Venereol (Stockh)* 1970; **50**: 49–55.
7 Lubowe I. Allergic dermatitis and cosmetics. *Cutis* 1973; **11**: 431–5.
8 Calnan C. Adverse reactions to hair products. In: Zviak C, ed. *The Science of Hair Care*. New York: Marcel Dekker, 1986.
9 Burnett CM. Evaluation of toxicity and carcinogenicity of hair dyes. *J Toxicol Environ Health* 1980; **6**: 247–51.
10 Kirkland DJ, Lawler SD, Venitt S. Chromosome damage and hair dyes. *Lancet* 1978; **ii**: 124–6.
11 Burnett CM, Menkart T. Hair dyes and breast cancer. *N Engl J Med* 1978; **299**: 1253–60.
12 Burnett CM, Corbett JF, Lanman BM. Hair dyes and aplastic anaemia. *Drug Chem Toxicol* 1978; **1**: 45–7.
13 Natow AJ. Hair bleach. *Cutis* 1986; **37**: 28–31.
14 Wolfram LJ, Hall K, Hui I. The mechanism of hair bleaching. *J Soc Cosmet Chem* 1970; **21**: 875–85.
15 Zviak C. Hair bleaching. In: Zviak C, ed. *The Science of Hair Care*. New York: Marcel Dekker, 1986.

Permanent waving [1,2]

Permanent waving has been defined as the process of changing the shape of the hair so that the new shape persists through several shampoos. During the last 70 years, increasing knowledge of keratin chemistry has enabled semipermanent chemical methods to be developed. Whatever the process used, three stages are involved in hair waving: (1) physical or chemical softening of the hair; (2) reshaping; and (3) hardening of fibres to retain the reshaped position.

Softening

Water can extend the hydrogen bonds between adjacent polypeptides in the keratin molecule, allowing temporary reshaping to be carried out—exposure to high humidity or rewetting immediately reverses the process. To obtain a more durable effect from water, steam may be used which, in a limited way, disrupts disulphide bonds. Heat and steam alone are rarely acceptable to modern women because their effects are temporary and the treatment is uncomfortable. Heat can be more effectively employed in conjunction with ammonium hydroxide and potassium bisulphite or triethanolamine as agents to reduce disulphide bonds; great skill is involved in this process as failure to judge the time of application of chemicals and heat may cause severe damage. Chemical heat pads are still rarely used, for example, employing heat produced from an exothermic reaction, such as quicklime.

Since 1945, cold wave processes using substituted thiosulphates, i.e. thioglycolates, have largely superseded hot waving. Thioglycolates are potent reducers of disulphide bonds in the keratin molecule:

$$-S = S- \rightarrow 2-SH$$

A typical cold waving lotion contains thioglycolic acid plus ammonia or monoethanolamine.

Acid permanent waves have recently become popular for salon use. They contain glyceryl monothioglycolate and produce a softer curl, and can be used on damaged and bleached hair. Their disadvantage is the high frequency of sensitization in the hairdressers using the product and, occasionally, sensitization of the client [3].

Reshaping

The type of rollers or curlers used to reshape the softened hair depends on the training of the hairdresser and the fashion desired. The degree of curl or tightness of the permanent wave depends both on the diameter of the roller and the size of the strand wound round the roller. Increasing the time of the exposure to the perming solution up to 20 min increases the curl, but longer times do not give a further increase. The strength of the solution used depends on the hair type, texture and previous bleaching. Home permanent waves are weaker and cannot achieve the same degree of curl. 'Tepid' waving involves using a weaker thioglycolate solution plus warm air. Neutralization is carried out initially with the curlers in place and again after they have been carefully removed. The reshaping stage is thus a great test of hairdressing skill and experience.

Hardening (neutralizing or setting)

In general, this process involves a reversal of the softening (reduction) stages:

$$2-SH \xrightarrow{\text{oxidation}} -S = S-$$

It is important to note that complete reversal to presoftened 'strength' cannot occur because many free SH groups may not be in a position for oxidation to be effective, for example:

$$2-SH \rightarrow -S-C-S- \qquad (C = carbon)$$
$$2-SH \rightarrow -S-Ba-S- \qquad (Ba = barium)$$

Atmospheric oxidation may efficiently neutralize the waving process. This method is slow and rollers must be left in position for several hours overnight. Chemical oxidation is now the rule. Hairdressers generally use hydrogen peroxide whereas most solutions for home use contain sodium perborate or percarbonate (UK) or sodium or potassium bromate (USA). This is why hair is lighter after permanent waving. Some neutralizers contain shellac, which may react with alcohol groups to cause hair discoloration.

Practical procedures

Hot waving

This is almost never used. The procedure is:
1 shampooing;
2 hair divided and rollers or curlers applied under slight tension;
3 waving solution applied;
4 heating.

Heating varies according to the solution used or the type of wave required. Electric rollers or exothermic reactive chemicals may be used. The latter allow free head movement during the waving. The skill of this procedure lies in good hair sectioning, judging the right amount of solution, correct winding tension and appropriate steaming time.

Cold waving

This also involves initial shampooing, hair division into locks, moistening with waving lotion and application of croquignole curlers. Further solution may then be applied. The softening time is 10–20 min. Occasionally, mild heat is included, using exothermic chemicals or the natural heat from the head by enclosing the scalp in a plastic bag. These may add to the comfort of the process. Rinsing then takes place, followed by neutralization with the oxidizing solution for up to 10 min. After removing the curlers, further 'hardening' solution is usually applied. 'Loose' curl waves last for no more than a few weeks but 'tight' curl styles may persist for 4–12 months.

REFERENCES

1 Zviak C. Permanent waving and hair straightening. In: Zviak C, ed. *The Science of Hair Care.* New York: Marcel Dekker, 1986.
2 Wickett RR. Permanent waving and straightening of hair. *Cutis* 1987; **39**: 496–500.
3 Morrison LH, Storrs FJ. Persistence of an allergen in hair after glyceryl monothioglycolate-containing permanent wave solutions. *J Am Acad Dermatol* 1988; **19**: 52–9.

Hair straightening [1,2]

In principle, the methods used to straighten hair are similar to those used in permanent waving. The practice is almost exclusively used to straighten negroid hair.

Pomades

These are mostly used by men with relatively short hair. They are greasy and act by 'plastering' hair into position.

Hot-comb methods

Shampooing is carried out and the hair is towelled dry; oil is then applied, for example petroleum jelly or liquid paraffin, which act as heat-transferring agents. Heat pressing with hot combing is then used (148–260°F), causing breakage and reforming of disulphide bonds, allowing the hair to be moulded straight. Structural damage (and breakage) of hair is common with this process and scarring alopecia may occur as a result of hot waxes entering the follicles. Sweating and rain reverse this procedure.

Cold methods

The chemical methods employed use alkaline reducing agents (caustics), thioglycolates, ammonium carbonate or sodium bisulphite. Caustic soda preparations are usually creams and require the application of protective scalp oil or wax. They are combed through the hair and left for 15–20 min; the hair is combed and straightened again, then rinsed and neutralized. These preparations are limited to salon use because of their potential to cause irritant dermatitis and damage the hair. Thioglycolate creams are the commonest agents used; the cream is applied liberally to the hair, which is then combed until it is straight. The cream is then washed off and a neutralizer (oxidizing agent) applied. Other straighteners ('relaxers') do not contain thioglycolates, for example sodium bisulphite and ammonium carbonate, acidic ethylene glycol or 1,3-propylene glycol. Bisulphite straighteners are suitable for home use in combination with alkaline stabilizers.

REFERENCES

1 Wickett RR. Permanent waving and straightening of hair. *Cutis* 1987; **39**: 496–500.
2 Zviak C. Permanent waving and hair straightening. In: Zviak C, ed. *The Science of Hair Care*. New York: Marcel Dekker, 1986.

Hair setting [1]

Setting lotions have changed considerably in recent years. The traditional semiliquid gels based on watersoluble gums, for example, tragacanth, karaya and acasia, have been replaced by various synthetic polymers in a bewildering array of forms—aerosol foams and sprays, liquids and gels.

Most are based on PVP in a gelled aqueous solution and give an attractive glossy, non-greasy appearance [2]. Some preparations incorporate other ingredients to condition or to add antistatic action, lustre or sheen.

Setting lotion and spray formulations are considered safe, after early reports of foreign-body granulomatous inflammation [3,4] had been questioned and not supported by further cases. Hair sprays were incriminated as a possible cause of peripilar casts [5] but this was not confirmed by later work [6].

REFERENCES

1 Zviak C. Hair setting. In: Zviak C, ed. *The Science of Hair Care*. New York: Marcel Dekker, 1986.
2 Friefeld M, Lyons J, Martinelli AT. Polyvinylpyrrolidone in cosmetics. *Am Perfumery* 1962; **77**: 25.
3 Edelson BG. Thesaurosis following inhalation of hair spray (Letter). *Lancet* 1959; **ii**: 465–6.
4 Bergmann M, Flance IJ, Blumenthal AT. Thesaurosis following inhalation of hair spray; a clinical and experimental study. *N Engl J Med* 1958; **258**: 471–6.
5 Scott MJ. Peripilar keratin casts. *Arch Dermatol* 1959; **79**: 654–9.
6 Dawber RPR. Hair cast. *Br J Dermatol* 1979; **100**: 417–20.

Methylolated compounds

Many cosmetic preparations, by their action on the keratin molecule, irreversibly weaken the hair. The cosmetic scientist has produced chemicals that attempt to combat this problem. The formulations contain methylolated compounds of varying strength depending on the type of hair under treatment and the solubility of the compound. Most preparations containing alkylated methylol compounds have greater stability and release very little formaldehyde [1].

REFERENCE

1 Zviak C, Bouillon C. Hair treatment and hair care products. In: Zviak C, ed. *The Science of Hair Care*. New York: Marcel Dekker, 1986.

Hair removers

The terms 'epilation' and 'depilation' have varied in their exact definition over the years. It is more convenient to define the exact process used, or the principle behind it, under the general term 'hair removers'. Superfluous hair may be masked by bleaching or removed by a variety of methods such as plucking, waxing, shaving, chemical processes and electrolysis—only the latter is permanent. No method is entirely satisfactory and the one adopted will depend on personal preference and the character, area and amount of hair growth.

Recent work on laser thermolysis suggests that, with refinement, this technique may provide rapid and permanent hair follicle destruction.

Bleaching is widely used for hair, particularly on the upper lip and the arms. It is painless, and when repeated often inflicts sufficient damage to cause hair breakage. However, bleached hair can look very obvious against dark skin. Some individuals develop an irritant reaction to bleach; it is therefore advisable to carry out a preliminary test—if irritation occurs within 30–60 min, the peroxide strength and duration of application should be reduced.

Shaving is unacceptable to some women as being too 'masculine'; however, the majority are happy to shave axillary and leg hair. Modern bathing costumes are very brief and require the wearer to shave the inner thighs and even part of the pubic region. In these sites it is common to experience folliculitis during regrowth, sometimes also due to infection with *Staphylococcus aureus*.

Waxing is one of the oldest methods known. Typically, the wax is preheated, applied to the area to be treated, allowed to cool, then stripped off taking the embedded hair with it. Some 'cold' waxes are available which act in the same way. Glucose and zinc oxide waxing has the advantage of lasting up to several weeks before a repeat is required. Only relatively long hair can be treated in this way. Some women find it painful and irritating. It is more often used by beauticians than in the home [1].

Plucking is really satisfactory only for individual or small groups of scattered coarse hairs. It is useful for sparse nipple or abdominal hairs. It is usually done with tweezers. As with waxing, it requires to be repeated only every few weeks.

Chemical hair removers are now widely used for superfluous hair removal from most sites, including the face. Their use on the face is limited by their irritancy potential. Sulphides and stannites, widely used in the past, have now been largely superseded by substituted mercaptans. Sulphides were unsatisfactory both because of skin irritancy and because of their odour—hydrogen sulphide—generated particularly when the preparation was washed off; strontium sulphide preparations are still available. Substituted mercaptans form the basis of virtually all modern chemical depilatory preparations. They are slower in action than the sulphides but are safe enough for facial use if necessary. Thioglycolates are used in a concentration of 2–4% and typically act within 5–15 min. Of the thioglycolates, the calcium salt is most favoured as it is the least irritant—the pH is maintained by an excess of calcium hydroxide which also acts to prevent the excess alkalinity known to irritate skin. Attempts to formulate products which accelerate the rather slow thioglycolate action have not been particularly successful. Modern preparations are available in foam, cream, liquid and aerosol forms, the one chosen depending on personal preference. Because thioglycolates attack keratin, not specifically hair, they may have adverse effects on the epidermis if manufacturers' recommendations are not adhered to; it is generally suggested that a small test site should first be treated in order to prevent more extensive irritant reactions in susceptible individuals.

Electrolysis [2,3]

All the above methods are temporary, the only practical permanent procedure being electrolysis. This involves passing a fine wire needle into the hair follicle and destroying the bulb with an electric current passed along it—the hair is loosened and plucked from each treated follicle. Disposable needles should be used to prevent transmission of infection. Either a galvanic or modified high-frequency electric current is used. Galvanic electrolysis is slower but destroys more follicles in one treatment. High-frequency current (electrocoagulation) is quicker but more regrowth is seen with this method. Relatively cheap, battery-operated machines have been developed for home use. These have all the disadvantages and potential hazards of those used by electrolysists with the added problem of an amateur operator.

The limitations of electrolysis in skilled hands are those of cost and time; even the best operators can only deal with 25–100 hairs per sitting, and hair regrows in up to 40% of the follicles treated. Shaving, a few days prior to electrolysis, increases the number of hairs in anagen and these are more easily destroyed [3]. In general, electrolysis is mostly used for localized, coarse facial hair and alternative methods employed for excess hair on other body sites. Apart from regrowth of hair, the problems which can occur with this mode of hair removal include discomfort during treatment, perifollicular inflammation and scarring, punctate hyperpigmentation and, rarely, bacterial infection.

A controlled investigation was carried out comparing the results of electrolysis with those of diathermy. Permanent destruction of the hairs could be achieved by either method and the time required for the total destruction of all hair roots in a given area was the same, but the diameter of hairs regrowing after diathermy was greater than that of hairs regrowing after electrolysis [4]. The results of depilation depend on the skill and dexterity of the operator. In countries such as the UK, in which a Diploma in Medical Electrolysis exists, patients should wherever possible be referred to technicians who have obtained this certification of their proficiency. In the USA, the American Electrolysis Association regulates professional standards. Similar regulations will be required for laser thermolysis.

REFERENCES

1 Rentoul JR, Aitken AA. The cosmetic treatment of hirsutism. *Practitioner* 1980; **24**: 1171–84.
2 Blackwell G. Permanence in electrolysis epilation. *Cutis* 1973; **11**: 753–8.
3 Richards RN, McKenzie MA. Electroepilation (electrolysis) in hirsutism. *J Am Acad Dermatol* 1986; **15**: 693–9.

4 Peereboom-Wynia JDR. The effect of electrical epilation on the beard hair of women with idiopathic hirsutism. *Arch Dermatol* 1975; **254**: 15–20.

Complications

Matting of scalp hair is most commonly a sudden, usually irreversible, tangling of scalp hair due to shampooing [1]. Excessive bleaching, permanent waving and straightening procedures may induce excessive weathering and fragility of hair.

REFERENCE

1 Wilson CL, Ferguson DJ, Dawber RPR. Matting of scalp hair during shampooing—a new look. *Clin Exp Dermatol* 1990; **15**: 139–41.

Chapter 67
The Skin and the Eyes

J.L.BURTON & R.A.HARRAD

Introduction

A knowledge of ophthalmology as it relates to the skin is important to the dermatologist for several reasons.
1 It is essential to recognize and treat immediately any dermatosis, such as herpes simplex or malignancy of the eyelid, which might threaten visual acuity.
2 The eyes and the periorbital tissues are of great cosmetic importance, and patients are often extremely concerned about cosmetic blemishes in this region. Even minor problems such as milia or wrinkles will often provoke great anxiety.
3 The skin around the eyes is modified in several ways to protect the eyeball, for example by the presence of mobile eyelids, eyelashes, Meibomian glands, etc., and these modifications predispose the skin in these areas to certain dermatoses.
4 Like the skin, the conjunctiva and cornea are exposed to potentially damaging environmental factors such as irritants, allergens and infective agents, and in some cases the dermatologist must collaborate with the ophthalmologist in the investigation and management of these conditions.
5 The eye is derived in part from the embryonic ectoderm, and as a result there are many congenital syndromes which affect both the skin and the eyes.
6 Many acquired systemic diseases also affect the skin, and in some of these a full examination of the eyes, including the retina, will provide important diagnostic information.
7 The dermatologist must be aware of any ocular complications which therapy might produce.

The 'overlap' between dermatology and ophthalmology is so large that only a superficial account of the subject can be given in this chapter. For further ophthalmological details, the references listed below should be consulted.

BIBLIOGRAPHY

Duane TD, Jaeger EA. External diseases and diseases of the uvea. In: Wilson FM, ed. *Clinical Ophthalmology*, Vol. 4. Philadelphia: Harper and Row, 1986.
Griffiths DG, Salasche SJ, Clemons DE, eds. *Cutaneous Abnormalities of the Eyelid and Face; an Atlas with Histopathology.* New York: McGraw-Hill, 1987.

Kanski JJ. *Clinical Ophthalmology*. Oxford: Butterworth, 1989.
Mannis MJ, MacSai MS, Huntley AC. *Eye and Skin Disease*. Philadelphia: Lippincott–Raven, 1996.
Thiers BH, Grant-Kels JM, Rothe MJ *et al. Dermatologic Clinics: Oculocutaneous Diseases, I and II*, Vol. 10, Nos. 3, 4, 1992.

The appendages of the eye

These include the eyebrows, the eyelids, the lacrimal apparatus and the conjunctiva.

The eyebrows

These consist of thickened arches of skin, which bear numerous short, thick hairs directed obliquely to the surface. The eyebrows are connected with the facial muscles of expression, and in humans they serve as an organ of communication by emphasizing facial expressions of surprise, anger, etc. They also help to prevent sweat from the forehead running into the eyes.

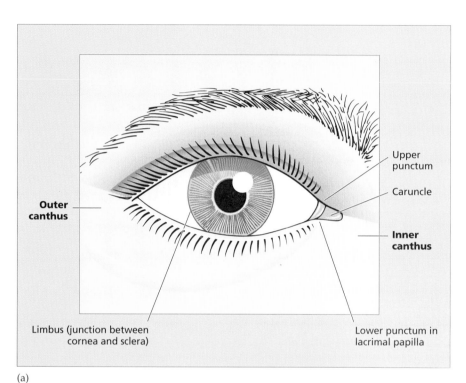

(a)

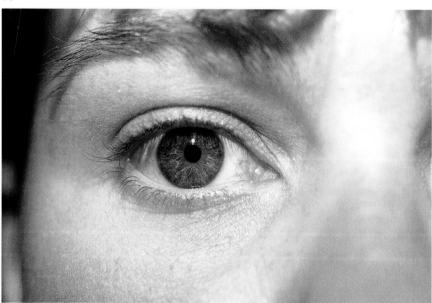

(b)

Fig. 67.1 The external appearance of the right eye. The lacrimal punctum lies in close apposition to the eyeball and cannot be seen unless the eyelid is everted.

The eyelids [1,2]

The skin of the eyelids is extremely thin, and is continuous with the conjunctiva at the margin of the lids. The subcutaneous tissue, which contains little or no fat, is lax and delicate, and is very susceptible to oedema formation. The *tarsal plates* are elongated areas of dense connective tissue, one in each lid, which contribute to the support of the eyelids. The upper eyelid has its own elevator muscle, the *levator palpebrae superioris*, the aponeurosis of which is attached to the anterior surface of the upper tarsal plate.

The *palpebral fissure* is the almond-shaped space between the lids formed when the eyes are open. The angles at the junction of the upper and the lower lids are called the *canthi*. At the inner canthus, nearest the nose, each eyelid bears a small conical elevation at its margin, the *lacrimal papilla*, the summit of which is pierced by a small orifice, the *lacrimal punctum*, which is the beginning of the lacrimal canaliculus (Fig. 67.1).

The eyelashes (*cilia*) are thick, curved hairs arranged in a double or a triple row at the margin of the lids. The upper lashes curve upwards, and the lower lashes curve downwards, so that they do not interlace when the eyelids are closed.

The *glands of Moll* are large, modified sweat glands, which are arranged in several rows close to the free margin of the lids. The *glands of Zeis* are sebaceous glands which open into the follicles of the lashes.

The *Meibomian glands* are modified sebaceous glands which open on the eyelid margin between the eyelashes and the conjunctiva. Each gland consists of a single straight tube with numerous secondary follicles opening into it. The deeper parts of the tube, and the secondary follicles, are lined by lipid-filled polyhedral cells, and the mouth of the tube is lined by stratified epithelium. There are about 30 glands in each eyelid. They can be seen through the mucous membrane by everting the eyelids. Their oily secretion helps to produce an airtight closure of the eyelids, prevents the overflow of tears and reduces their evaporation. Its composition resembles that of sebum [3]. The mucocutaneous junction of the lid is sometimes known as the grey line.

The lacrimal apparatus

The lacrimal apparatus both produces the tears and conducts them away via the nasolacrimal ducts (Fig. 67.2).

The lacrimal gland, a modified sweat gland, is lodged in a depression at the outer angle of the orbit. Its anterior margin is closely adherent to the posterior part of the upper eyelid. The gland has six to 12 ducts, which open by a series of minute orifices on the upper and outer half of the palpebral conjunctiva. The orifices are arranged in a row so that the tear fluid is dispersed over the surface of the globe. In addition, there are a variable number (four to 35) of much smaller accessory lacrimal glands in the upper conjunctiva.

It is thought that these accessory glands provide the basic continual tear production of the eye, and the function of the main lacrimal gland is to provide a gush of tears when the eye is injured in any way [4].

The tear film consists of three layers: a superficial lipid layer (from the Meibomian glands), which retards evaporation and prevents spillage from the lid margins; a middle, watery layer (from the lacrimal glands); and a deep layer, which is mucoid, produced by the goblet cells of the conjunctiva [5].

The tears drain via the puncta and the lacrimal canals into the common canalicula and lacrimal sac and thence via the nasolacrimal duct, into the nose.

The conjunctiva

The conjunctiva lines the inner surface of the eyelids, and it is then reflected over the anterior portion of the eyeball, up to the edge of the cornea. The folds formed by the reflection of the conjunctiva from the lids onto the globe of the eye are called the *superior* and *inferior palpebral fornix*, respectively.

The tarsal portion, lining the eyelids, is thick, opaque and highly vascular. The bulbar portion, overlying the sclera, is much thinner and less vascular.

The conjunctiva in the palpebral folds also contains numerous mucous glands, in addition to a rich nerve plexus. There are also accumulations of lymphoid tissue, which are probably analogous to lymphoid follicles, like the Peyer's patches in the intestine.

The *lacrimal caruncle* is a small, red, conical body, which fills up the triangular space at the inner canthus. It is a small island of skin which contains sweat and sebaceous glands. At the outer side of this lacrimal caruncle is a small fold of mucous membrane, the *plica semilunaris*, which is the rudiment of the third eyelid seen in birds (the nictitating membrane).

Protective mechanisms

A number of specific mechanisms help to prevent the eye from being damaged by trauma or infection.
1 The eyelids protect the eye from mechanical damage during the blink reflex, which is one of the quickest reflexes in the body. In addition, the regular closure of the lids over the eye every few seconds helps to detach any foreign particles from the surface of the globe.
2 The presence of any foreign body on the cornea or conjunctiva induces a copious flow of tears, which washes the foreign matter away.
3 The epithelial cells on the surface of the eye have a rapid turnover rate, so that any damage quickly heals.
4 The epithelial cells possess tight junctions between them, so that bacterial invasion is hindered.
5 Immunological protective mechanisms are most important.

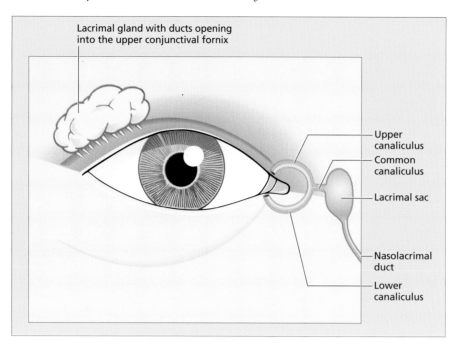

Lacrimal gland with ducts opening
into the upper conjunctival fornix

Upper
canaliculus

Common
canaliculus

Lacrimal sac

Nasolacrimal
duct

Lower
canaliculus

Fig. 67.2 The lacrimal apparatus of the right eye.

Specific and non-specific mechanisms, involving both cell-mediated and humoral immunity, confer protection both at a local level and via systemic responses. Tears contain lysozyme, an enzyme which attacks mucopeptides in bacterial cell walls, and another bacteriostatic protein called lactoferrin [6]. Immunoglobulins, including IgG and secretory IgA, are present in the tears and in the corneal stroma [7–11]. Complement components (from both the classical and the alternative pathways) are also found in human tears, and Langerhans' cells are present in the corneal and conjunctival epithelium [12]. Large numbers of mast cells are found in the conjunctiva and eyelids.

It is a tribute to the protective mechanisms described above that severe infection of the cornea is relatively uncommon, although obviously any conjunctival infection poses a threat to the cornea, and must be regarded by the clinician as potentially serious.

Factors which predispose to conjunctival or corneal infection are listed in Table 67.1.

Table 67.1 Factors which predispose to external ocular infections.

Chronic infection of the lids (blepharitis)
Poor eyelid closure, e.g. due to ectropion or facial palsy
Corneal anaesthesia
Contact lens wear
Other ocular disease including tear-film anomalies, sicca
 syndrome, corneal melting syndrome, mucous membrane
 pemphigoid
Immunosuppression (congenital or acquired)
Topical therapy, e.g. glucocorticoid or prolonged antibiotic
Corneal or subtarsal foreign body
Entropion

REFERENCES

1 Burns RP. Eyelids, lacrimal apparatus and conjunctiva. *Arch Ophthalmol* 1968; **79**: 211–25.
2 Montagna W, Ford DM. Histology and cytochemistry of human skin. XXXIII. The eyelid. *Arch Dermatol* 1980; **100**: 328–35.
3 Cory CC, Hinks W, Burton JL *et al.* Meibomian gland secretion in the red eyes of rosacea. *Br J Dermatol* 1973; **89**: 25–7.
4 Allansmith MR, Kajiyama G, Abelson MB *et al.* Plasma cell content of main and accessory lacrimal glands and conjunctiva. *Am J Ophthamol* 1976; **82**: 819–26.
5 Bron A. Prospects for the dry eye. *Trans Ophthalmol Soc UK* 1986; **104**: 801–10.
6 Broekhuyse RM. Tear lactoferrin, a bacteriostatic and complexing protein. *Invest Ophthalmol* 1974; **13**: 550–5.
7 Allansmith MR, Whitney CR, McLellan *et al.* Immunoglobulins in the human eye. Location, type and amount. *Arch Ophthalmol* 1973; **89**: 36–45.
8 Allansmith MR, de Ramus A, Maurice D. The dynamics of IgG in the cornea. *Invest Ophthalmol Vis Sci* 1979; **18**: 947–55.
9 Allansmith MR. Defense of the ocular surface. *Int Ophthalmol Clin* 1979; **19**: 93–109.
10 Allansmith MR, Gillette TE. Secretory component in the human ocular tissues. *Am J Ophthalmol* 1980; **89**: 353–61.
11 Bluestone J, Easty DL, Golberg LS. Lacrimal immunoglobulins and complement quantified by counter-immuno-electrophoresis. *Br J Ophthalmol* 1975; **59**: 279–82.
12 Rodrigues MM, Rowden G, Hackett J *et al.* Langerhans cells in the normal conjunctiva and peripheral area of selected species. *Invest Ophthalmol Vis Sci* 1981; **21**: 759–65.

BIBLIOGRAPHY

Allansmith MR, ed. *The Eye and Immunology*. St Louis: CV Mosby, 1982.
Easty DL. Manifestations of immunodeficiency diseases in ophthalmology. *Trans Ophthalmol Soc UK* 1977; **97**: 8–17.
Easty DL. Infection of the eye. *Practitioner* 1980; **226**: 593.
Grant-Kels JM, Kels BD. Human ocular anatomy. *Dermatol Clin* 1992; **10**: 473–82.
Sevel D. A reappraisal of the development of the eyelids. *Eye* 1988; **2**: 123–9.

Table 67.2 Hereditary causes of synophrys (hypertrophy and fusion of the eyebrows).

Familial, as an isolated characteristic
Hypertrichosis lanuginosa
Cornelia de Lange syndrome [3]
Mucopolysaccharidosis
Waardenburg's syndrome
Broad-thumb hallux syndrome
Del(3p) syndrome [4]
Frydman syndrome
Pachyonychia congenita

The eyebrows

There is a wide variation in the colour, distribution and density of the eyebrow hairs. The inheritance of the form of the eyebrows is polygenic. Some hereditary variations are of no known significance, but others are associated with other developmental defects, or are part of a recognized syndrome [1].

Synophrys

This term is applied when the eyebrows are profuse, with a tendency to meet in the centre of the face. Table 67.2 lists some hereditary causes of synophrys.

In Cornelia de Lange syndrome (also known as the Brachmann de Lange syndrome) the eyebrows meet in the centre, but they are neat, arched and well-defined, as though they have been pencilled in. The lips are thin, with a long philtrum and a crescent-shaped mouth [2].

The eyebrows also tend to become more bushy in the ageing male, often in association with increased hairiness of the ears. The cause of this increased hair growth at a time when androgen levels are decreasing is unknown. Bushy eyebrows may also occur in other acquired forms of hypertrichosis, for example due to drugs, such as diazoxide, and fusion of the eyebrows has been reported in kwashiorkor.

Congenital erythropoietic porphyria and porphyria cutanea tarda also cause hypertrichosis of the eyebrows. Congenital erythropoietic porphyria can also cause other ocular changes including scleromalacia, keratomalacia and pigmentary chorioretinopathy [5].

REFERENCES

1 Waardenburg PJ. *Genetics and Ophthalmology*. Oxford: Blackwell Scientific Publications, 1961.
2 Ireland M, Donnai B, Burn J. Brachmann de Lange syndrome. *Am J Med Genet* 1993; **47**: 959–61.
3 Levin AV, Seidman DJ, Nelson LB, Jackson LG. Ophthalmologic findings in the Cornelia de Lange syndrome. *J Pediatr Ophthalmol Strabismus* 1990; **27**: 94–102.
4 Narahara K, Kikkewa K. Loss of the 3p-25.3 band is critical in the manifestations of the del(3p) syndrome. *Am J Med Genet* 1990; **32**: 269–73.
5 Sevel D, Burger D. Ocular involvement in cutaneous porphyria. *Arch Ophthalmol* 1971; **85**: 280.

Hypoplasia

Table 67.3 lists some inherited diseases in which there is hypoplasia of the eyebrows.

Many acquired conditions also cause sparsity of the eyebrows. In alopecia areata, the eyebrows may be the only site affected. Thinning of the eyebrows also occurs in hypothyroidism, erythroderma, follicular mucinosis, secondary syphilis and leprosy.

Lepromatous leprosy causes thinning of the outer third of the eyebrows in the early stages, often with depigmentation, and this progresses to total loss of the brows and lashes. Eventually, there is likely to be more serious involvement of the eye, including corneal changes or granulomatous iritis [2]. Tuberculoid leprosy, by contrast, produces loss of corneal sensation and neuroparalytic keratitis, but does not cause loss of the eyebrows.

Table 67.3 Hereditary causes of hypoplasia of the eyebrows.

Familial, as an isolated characteristic
Ectodermal dysplasia (e.g. the anhidrotic type; Fig. 67.3)
Polydysplastic epidermolysis bullosa
Keratosis pilaris atrophicans
Ulerythema ophryogenes
Oculomandibular dysostosis
Oculovertebral dysplasia
Monilethrix
Pili torti (Fig. 67.4)
Popliteal web syndrome
Progeria
Atrichia congenita
Ablepharon–macrostomia syndrome [1]

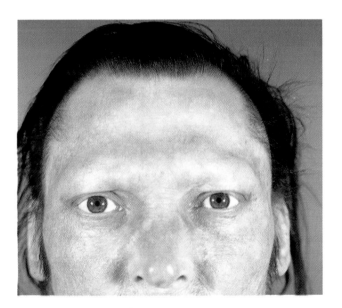

Fig. 67.3 Characteristic supraorbital bossing and absence of eyebrows and lashes in congenital anhidrotic ectodermal dysplasia.

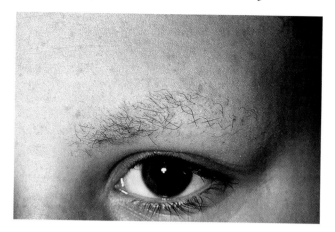

Fig. 67.4 Sparse eyebrows in pili torti. (Courtesy of Dr C.Y. Tan, Dudley Road Hospital, Birmingham, UK.)

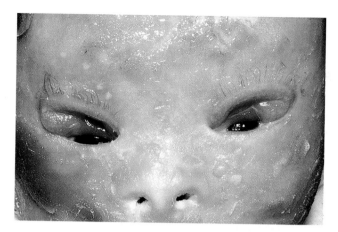

Fig. 67.5 A harlequin fetus, showing pronounced eclabion (eversion of the eyelids). (Courtesy of Dr F. Lawlor, St Thomas' Hospital, London, UK.)

Plucking of the eyebrows for cosmetic reasons is common, but true trichotillomania of the eyebrows is unusual.

The eyebrows are often involved in seborrhoeic dermatitis, and sometimes in psoriasis, and these and similar inflammatory dermatoses can produce temporary thinning.

Postinflammatory cicatricial alopecia may involve the eyebrows. It may follow discoid lupus erythematosus, or specific infections such as lupus vulgaris or tertiary syphilis, and is occasionally seen in folliculitis decalvans. Scarring, with loss of eyebrows or eyelashes, may also follow chemical or thermal burns or radiation.

Loss of eyebrows can be camouflaged by the use of eyebrow pencils, permanent tattooing or a hair prosthesis glued in place daily [3].

Depigmentation

The eyebrows share in the hypopigmentation of albinism and phenylketonuria, and they may be affected in vitiligo, leprosy, piebaldism, Waardenburg's syndrome, Vogt–Koyanagi syndrome and Allezandrini's syndrome.

REFERENCES

1 Price NJ, Pugh RE, Farndon PA, Willshaw ME. Ablepharon–macrostomia syndrome. *Br J Ophthalmol* 1991; **25**: 317–19.
2 Shields J, Waring GO, Monte LG. Ocular findings in leprosy. *Am J Ophthalmol* 1974; **77**: 880–90.
3 Draelos ZK, Yeatts RP. Eyebrow loss, eyelash loss and dermatochalasis. *Dermatol Clin* 1992; **10**: 793–8.

The eyelids

Numerous developmental defects such as mandibulo-facial dysostosis or the Goldenhar syndrome can affect the palpebral fissure, or the size and shape of the eyelids, but these are mainly of interest to the paediatrician and ophthalmologist.

Several hereditary dermatoses also affect the eyelids. In ichthyosiform erythroderma, the early development of ectropion is a characteristic feature, and scarring and tumour formation of the eyelids is an important and distressing complication of xeroderma pigmentosum. The eyelids are severely affected in the harlequin fetus (Fig. 67.5), often with severe ectropion.

Hereditary dermatoses associated with absent or hypoplastic eyelids (ablepharon) include the following.

Ablepharon macrostomia. This rare disorder is characterized by absent eyelids, ectropion, abnormal ears, rudimentary nipples, dry, redundant skin, macrostomia and ambiguous genitalia [1]. Patients with the *Barber–Say syndrome* also have severe hypertrichosis and atrophic skin [2].

Ablepharon with follicular ichthyosis and hairy pinnae has been recorded [3].

Neu–Laxova syndrome. This rare, lethal condition is inherited as an autosomal recessive. The features include polyhydramnios, growth retardation, microcephaly and ichthyosis with thick, hyperkeratotic skin. The eyes protrude and the eyelids are rudimentary [4,5].

REFERENCES

1 Pellegrino JE, Schnur RE, Boghosian-Sell LE *et al*. Ablepharon macrostomia syndrome with associated cutis laxa: possible localization to 18q. *Hum Genet* 1996; **97**: 532–6.
2 Martinez Santana S, Perez Alvarez FP, Frias JL, Martinez M-L. Hypertrichosis, atrophic skin, ectropion and macrostomia (Barber–Say syndrome): report of a new case. *Am J Med Genet* 1993; **47**: 20–3.
3 Chausaria BD, Goswami HK. Congenitally malformed female infant with hairy pinnae. *Clin Genet* 1971; **2**: 111–14.
4 Schapiro I, Borochowitz Z, Degani S *et al*. Neu–Laxova syndrome: prenatal ultrasonographic diagnosis, clinical and pathological studies and new manifestations. *Am J Med Genet* 1992; **43**: 602–5.

5 Kuseyri F, Bilgic L, Apak MY. Neu–Laxova syndrome: report of a case from Turkey. *Clin Genet* 1993; **43**: 267–9.

Ptosis

Drooping of the eyelid on one or both sides is a common congenital defect. Mild ptosis commonly develops in the elderly due to laxity of the connective tissue and dehiscence of the levator aponeurosis, but in these cases the eye movements and pupils are normal. There are many important acquired causes, such as third-nerve palsy, Horner's syndrome and myasthenia gravis, which require neurological referral. Dystrophia myotonica may be recognized by the characteristic facies, the recession of the frontal hair line and the delayed relaxation phase of the handshake.

Ptosis may be associated with other ocular abnormalities. Ptosis, ectopia lentis and high myopia may be dominantly inherited and have been described in association with Ehlers–Danlos syndrome and also in families without the Ehlers–Danlos syndrome [1]. Ptosis may also be associated as a syndrome with blepharophimosis, epicanthus inversus and telecanthus, and is a feature of Frydman syndrome (see below).

Pseudoptosis occurs when the upper eyelid skin is so lax that it sags and droops down over the eyelid margin. This defect is readily corrected by plastic surgery. Laxity of the eyelid skin is common in the elderly, and many ophthalmologists call this *dermatochalasia* to distinguish it from *blepharochalasia*, which occurs at a younger age due to cutis laxa or Ascher's syndrome.

Dermatochalasia and blepharochalasia must be distinguished from laxity of the eyelid, which is the ability to pull the eyelid further than 8 mm from the globe. Lid laxity predisposes to entropion, ectropion, epiphora and ocular irritation [2].

Blepharophimosis syndrome

This distinctive autosomal dominant syndrome is characterized by blepharophimosis, ptosis, epicanthus inversus and telecanthus [3]. The first three features of the syndrome tend to accentuate each other, so that the palpebral fissure is markedly reduced in both height and width, and the patient has to compensate for the ptosis by tilting the head backwards. The fourth feature of the syndrome, telecanthus, is an increased distance between the inner canthi (hypertelorism is similar, but refers to radiological evidence of an increased distance between the orbits).

Surgery, usually a brow-suspension procedure, should be undertaken to prevent disuse amblyopia due to stimulus deprivation.

Frydman syndrome

Frydman described six patients with an autosomal recessive condition in which prognathism, syndactyly and short stature were associated with blepharophimosis, weakness of the extraocular and frontal muscles and synophrys [4].

Telecanthus

This term refers to an increased distance between the medial canthi of the eyelids, i.e. the eyes appear widely spaced. Telecanthus is almost always present in Waardenburg's syndrome [5].

Blepharospasm

This is a form of focal dystonia (sustained muscle contraction), which causes disabling closure of the eyelids due to spasm of the periorbital muscles. Long-standing blepharospasm may lead to functional blindness, and it can also cause overhanging eyebrows or excess eyelid tissue, which may require plastic surgery [6]. Disabling blepharospasm can now be treated successfully by injection of botulinum toxin into the periorbital muscles. This causes weakness to develop over the next week or so, reducing the dystonic spasm, and the effect lasts for 2–4 months. The injections can be repeated, and the treatment appears to be safe and effective [7]. However, ptosis is a common complication of this treatment [7].

Botulinum toxin has also been used to treat vertical frown lines by injecting it into the corrugator muscle, which runs from the medial eyebrow to the nasal root. The injections have to be repeated every 4–6 months, but the results appear to be superior to those obtained with collagen injection [8].

Epicanthus

This term is used to describe a vertical skin fold at the inner canthus [9]. Such folds are normal in the fetus, but in white individuals they usually disappear before birth. In Mongolian races, the condition persists into adult life. White children with a mild persistent epicanthic fold will often improve at puberty, when the nose enlarges, but in severe cases plastic surgery may be needed. Some cases will appear to have a convergent squint, but this is usually an optical illusion. A cover test is the simplest way to exclude the presence of convergent squint. The light reflexes of a torch in the corneae will be symmetrical and the apparent squint will disappear if the skin over the bridge of the nose is picked up to eliminate the epicanthic fold.

Epiblepharon is an exaggeration of epicanthus tarsalis in which the horizontal skin fold is associated with inversion of the lashes. It occurs in over 40% of Japanese babies, but decreases with age. Most cases are asymptomatic, but it can produce discomfort, epiphora or photophobia [10], and in these cases excision of an ellipse of the skin is curative.

Dennie–Morgan infraorbital fold

Morgan [11] described two patients with atopic eczema with an accentuated linear fold in the lower eyelids, and he quoted Dennie, who had previously observed the same sign. There is no doubt that this fold is commonly seen in atopic patients, but opinions are divided as to its significance. Some authors believe that it is a marker of atopy, even in the absence of eczema [12,13]; others believe that it is merely a non-specific effect of eczema affecting the eyelid [14], and there are those that believe that, although a single fold is non-specific, a double fold is a more reliable sign of atopy. Uehara [15] found the fold in 83% of atopic patients with lower eyelid dermatitis, and in only 7% of atopics with no dermatitis of the eyelids. The fold was also present in eight of 11 patients with contact dermatitis of the eyelids.

REFERENCES

1 Gillum WN, Anderson RL. Predominantly inherited blepharoptosis, high myopia and ectopia lentis. *Arch Ophthalmol* 1982; **100**: 282–4.
2 Draelos ZK, Yeatts RP. Eyebrow loss, eyelash loss, and dermatochalasis. *Dermatol Clin* 1992; **10**: 793–8.
3 Kohn R, Romano PE. Blepharoptosis, blepharophimosis, epicanthus inversus and telecanthus—a syndrome with no name. *Am J Ophthalmol* 1971; **72**: 625–31.
4 Frydman M, Curran HA, Carmon G, Savir H. Autosomal recessive blepharophimosis, ptosis, V-esotropia, syndactyly and short stature. *Clin Genet* 1992; **41**: 57–61.
5 da Silva EO. Waardenburg's syndrome: a clinical and genetic study of two large kindreds and literature review. *Am J Med Genet* 1991; **40**: 65–74.
6 Grandas F, Elston J, Quinn N. Blepharospasm: a review of 264 patients. *J Neurol Neurosurg Psychiatry* 1988; **51**: 767–72.
7 Denistic M, Pirtosek Z, Vodusek DB *et al*. Botulinum toxin in the treatment of neurological disorders. *Ann NY Acad Sci* 1994; **710**: 76–87.
8 Elston JS. The clinical use of botulinum toxin. *Semin Ophthalmol* 1988; **3**: 249–60.
9 Johnson CC. Epicanthus and epiblepharon. *Arch Ophthalmol* 1978; **96**: 1030–3.
10 Noda S, Hayasaka S, Setogawa T. Epiblepharon with inverted eyelashes in Japanese children. 1: Incidence and symptoms. *Br J Ophthalmol* 1989; **73**: 126–7.
11 Morgan DB. A suggestive sign of allergy. *Arch Dermatol & Syph* 1948; **57**: 1050.
12 Holzegel K. Unterlidfalte beim endogenen Ekzem. *Hautarzt* 1977; **28**: 45.
13 Meenan FOC. The significance of Morgan's fold in children with atopic dermatitis. *Acta Derm Venereol Suppl (Stockh)* 1980; **12**: 42–3.
14 Mevorah B. Minor clinical features of atopic dermatitis. Evaluation of their clinical significance. *Dermatologica* 1988; **177**: 360–4.
15 Uehara M. Infra-orbital fold in atopic dermatitis. *Arch Dermatol* 1981; **117**: 627–9.

The floppy eyelid syndrome

This syndrome develops in patients who sleep face down [1,2], and, contrary to previous reports, it is not confined to obese or male patients [3].

The upper eyelids become rubbery and floppy so that they evert spontaneously during sleep. As a result of this nocturnal conjuctival exposure, the patients develop chronic papillary conjunctivitis of the upper tarsus. Histological examination shows a marked decrease in tarsal elastin, although collagen is normal [4].

The condition has been described in association with a variety of other ocular defects, including blepharochalasis, tapetoretinal degeneration, keratoconus, and also with pachydermoperiostosis [5–7].

Surgical eyelid shortening may be required, and horizontal eyelid shortening and levator aponeurosis repair is usually effective.

REFERENCES

1 Culbertson WW, Ostler HB. The floppy eyelid syndrome. *Am J Ophthalmol* 1981; **92**: 5666–75.
2 Dannenfeld ED, Parry HD, Gibraltar RP *et al*. Keratoconus associated with the floppy eyelid syndrome. *Ophthalmology* 1991; **98**: 1674–8.
3 Culbertson WW, Tseng SC. Corneal disorders in the floppy eyelid syndrome. *Cornea* 1994; **13**; 330–42.
4 Netland PA, Sugrue SP, Albert DM *et al*. Histopathologic features of the floppy eyelid syndrome. *Ophthalmology* 1994; **101**: 174–81.
5 Parunovic A. Floppy eyelid syndrome. *Br J Ophthalmol* 1983; **67**: 264–6.
6 Parunovic A. Floppy eyelid syndrome, associated with keratoconus. *Br J Ophthalmol* 1988; **72**: 634–5.
7 Downes RN, Minini F, Collins JRO *et al*. Floppy eyelid syndrome in pachydermoperiostosis. *Orbit* 1989; **8**: 93–9.

Ectropion

In this condition, the lower eyelid falls away from the eyeball and tends to become everted. The lacrimal punctum loses its close apposition to the globe, and so the tear fluid is unable to drain through the usual channels, resulting in epiphora. The exposed conjunctiva becomes chronically inflamed and unsightly, and the constant flow of tears over the cheeks may irritate the skin.

Ectropion is common in elderly people, probably due to a lessening of tone in the periorbital muscles, a decrease in the orbital fat [1] and loss of elasticity of connective tissue (Fig. 67.6). It also occurs in inflammatory conditions of the periorbital skin, especially in chronic erythroderma, ichthyosis and sun-damaged skin. Cicatricial ectropion may complicate scarring of the cheeks, for example as scar tissue contracts

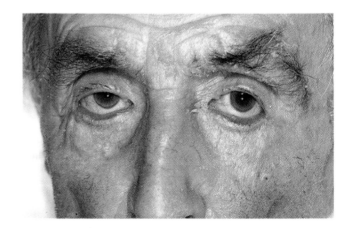

Fig. 67.6 Senile ectropion.

after treatment of a basal cell carcinoma. Mild ectropion is also common in facial paralysis. It may also occur in some rare syndromes, such as the *Kabuki makeup syndrome*, with cleft lip and palate [2].

Senile ectropion and paralytic ectropion respond well to surgery to produce horizontal eyelid shortening, sometimes with the addition of inverting sutures.

Cicatricial ectropion usually requires excision of the scar tissue and a skin graft [3].

Eyelid imbrication

This term refers to overriding of a lax upper eyelid, allowing the lower eyelid lashes to rub the upper tarsal conjunctiva to produce chronic inflammation (see also trichiasis, p. 2994).

The condition may be treated by ocular lubricants and night-time shielding of the eye, particularly in patients with floppy eyelids. In severe cases, surgical eyelid shortening may be considered.

Entropion

In this condition, the upper or lower eyelid turns inward, and the lashes cause irritation by rubbing on the cornea or conjunctiva. Corneal abrasions or ulceration may result. In entropion, there is anterior displacement of the mucocutaneous junction (recognized by conversion of the squamous epithelium into conjunctival epithelium with microvilli). It is thought that the tear film is the stimulus for this histological change [4]. In ectropion the situation is reversed, with keratinization of the epithelium taking place posterior to the Meibomian gland openings [1].

Entropion, like ectropion, is common in the elderly, probably due to a combination of horizontal laxity of the lower eyelid and spasm of the marginal fibres of the orbicularis muscle. It may be present only intermittently, but can be elicited by asking the patient to squeeze the eye tightly shut, and on subsequent opening of the eye, the eyelid will remain folded inward. Scarring of the tarsal plate can also cause entropion. This may follow trauma, or it may be secondary to a disease such as trachoma.

The defect may be corrected by plastic surgery, usually a transverse eyelid split and everting sutures (Wies operation) sometimes combined with horizontal eyelid shortening. Temporary improvement may be achieved by taping down the lower eyelid and applying chloramphenicol ointment, or by subcutaneous injection of botulinum toxin [5].

REFERENCES

1 Stefanszyn MA, Hiyadat AA, Flanagan JC. The histopathology of involutional ectropion. *Ophthalmology* 1985; **92**: 120–7.
2 Hauda Y, Maeda K, Toida M *et al*. Kabuki make-up syndrome (Niikawa–Kuroki syndrome) with cleft lip and palate. *J Craniomaxillofac Surg* 1991; **19**: 99–101.
3 Collin JRO. *A Manual of Systematic Eyelid Surgery*, 2nd edn. Edinburgh: Churchill Livingstone, 1989.
4 Barber K, Dabbs T. Morphological observations on patients with presumed trichiasis. *Br J Ophthalmol* 1988; **72**: 17–22.
5 Hoh HB, Steel D, Potts MJ, Harrad RA. The use of botulinum toxin for lower lid entropion. *Orbit* 1995; **14**: 131–6.

Periorbital oedema

There are many systemic causes of oedema of the eyelids and periorbital tissues (Table 67.4), and dermatologists occasionally have the satisfaction of diagnosing hypothyroidism or thyrotoxicosis in a patient referred from a general physician (Fig. 67.7).

Many dermatological diseases also cause eyelid oedema (Table 67.5), but the commonest are angio-oedema, lymphoedema and contact dermatitis (usually contact allergy).

Table 67.4 Systemic causes of periorbital oedema.

Angio-oedema
Glomerulonephritis (especially nephrotic syndrome)
Other causes of hypoalbuminaemia
Cardiac failure
Hypo- or hyperthyroidism
Dermatomyositis
Lupus erythematosus
Leukaemia
Superior vena caval syndrome
Fixed drug eruption
Bacterial or viral infections (especially in early stages)
    Scarlatina
    Infectious mononucleosis
Parasites or protozoal infections
    Trichiniasis
    Filariasis
    Onchocerciasis
    Trypanosomiasis
    Malaria

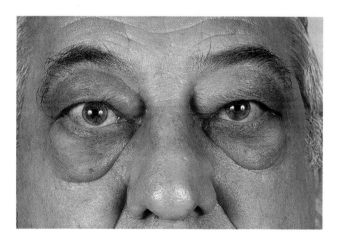

Fig. 67.7 Periorbital oedema due to thyrotoxicosis. The swelling cleared completely following treatment with antithyroid medication.

Table 67.5 Local causes of periorbital oedema.

Trauma (including dermatitis artefacta)
Infection
   Stye
   Chancre
   Dacryocystitis
   Erysipelas
   Herpes simplex
   Herpes zoster
   Anthrax
   Cat-scratch disease
   Deep mycoses
   Orbital cellulitis
   Intraocular infections (TB, etc.)
   Sinusitis
Contact dermatitis and other eczemas
Lymphoedema (including rosacea and acne vulgaris)
Insect bites
Oleogranuloma
Chalazion
Orbital tumour
Cavernous sinus thrombosis
Blepharochalasis syndrome

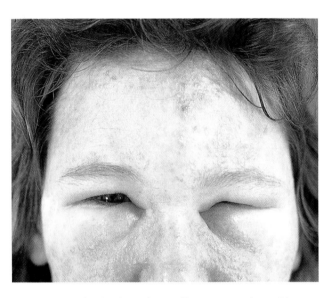

Fig. 67.8 Periorbital oedema due to allergic contact dermatitis.

These three are usually readily differentiated, even from the history alone, as angio-oedema is transient, lymphoedema is permanent and contact dermatitis is accompanied by redness and itching, followed by scaling in the recovery phase (Fig. 67.8). However, angio-oedema can be complicated by epidermal changes induced by rubbing, or by topical medicaments.

Dermatomyositis classically causes eyelid swelling with a violaceous hue. Rarely, there may also be weakness of the extrinsic ocular muscles or a retinopathy. A few cases of unilateral periorbital oedema due to lupus erythematosus have occurred (p. 3008)

In trichinosis, the eyelids are red and swollen, and the associated fever, malaise and myalgia may suggest a diagnosis of dermatomyositis. Marked eosinophilia is almost invariable in trichinosis.

In some patients with recurrent 'puffiness' of the eyes, mainly middle-aged females, no cause can be identified, but it is probable that some of these patients have intermittent lymphoedema, possibly secondary to occult rosacea. Acne vulgaris has also been described as a cause of periorbital lymphoedema, which was responsive to isotretinoin [2].

Loss of fenestration of the orbital septum with age gives the appearance of eyelid oedema, but is in fact prolapsed fat.

In one young man, swelling of the lower eyelids was due to oleogranuloma caused by the injection of petroleum jelly to counteract what he perceived as distressing wrinkles [3].

In South and Central America, Chagas' disease due to *Trypanosoma cruzi* is an important cause of eyelid swelling. Severe urticated eyelid oedema associated with preauricular lymphadenopathy (*Romano's sign*) is almost pathognomonic in endemic areas.

In loa-loa, conjunctivitis due to the worm crossing the eye may be associated with eyelid oedema.

Dermatitis

The eyelid is a frequent site of contact dermatitis, possibly because the skin is so thin and it is touched many times a day by the fingers. The condition is much commoner in women, and in one large series of patients with eyelid dermatitis, 46% had contact allergy, 15% had exposure to an irritant and 23% had atopic dermatitis [4].

The allergens most often incriminated in contact dermatitis of the eyelids are cosmetics (especially nail varnish), aerosol sprays, red-headed matches, plants (especially *Primula obconica*), occupational hazards and topical ophthalmic medicaments. The eczema is often of the acute type, and the cause, often unsuspected by the patient, must be confirmed by patch testing. Nickel dermatitis may be associated with secondary dermatitis of the eyelids.

Maibach *et al.* [5] have emphasized that discomfort of the eyelids, with or without dermatitis, may have many causes, and not all cases are due to intolerance to eye cosmetics.

Chronic eczema of the eyelids with thickening due to repeated rubbing occasionally occurs without discernible cause. This is sometimes labelled as neurodermatitis of the eyelids, but it is probable that some cases are due to unrecognized contact dermatitis.

Pigmentation

There is considerable racial and familial variation in the degree of pigmentation of the eyelids [6–8]. Many people with coffee-coloured skin appear to have marked periorbital melanosis as a genetic trait (Fig. 67.9). The skin below the

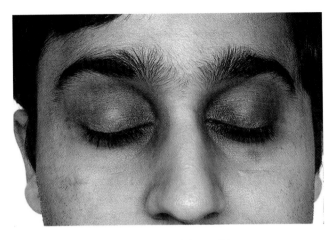

Fig. 67.9 Familial hypermelanosis of the eyelids.

eyes also becomes darker during periods of exhaustion, dehydration or illness (especially sinusitis), but this is presumably a vascular change, as it can quickly disappear.

Pigmentation of the periorbital skin can also be post-traumatic, for example after a haematoma ('black eye'), or postinflammatory, or it can accompany melanocyte-stimulating hormone (MSH)-induced melanosis of any cause.

Severe periorbital haematoma can be treated by the application of leeches, but there is a risk of infection with the gut commensal of the leech, *Aeromonas hydrophila* [9].

Chemical pigmentation. The prolonged use of mercurial or silver preparations can produce a permanent slate-blue or grey–brown discoloration. Local hypermelanosis may also be due to cosmetics containing phototoxic agents, usually psoralens.

Lichen planus may present as violaceous papules on the eyelids, or as reticulate brown pigmentation.

Ochronosis (Chapter 59). In this metabolic condition, the sclera as well as the eyelids may show a brownish discoloration.

Depigmentation

The eyelids may be involved in a general depigmenting disorder (Chapter 39), but the Vogt–Koyanagi syndrome (Chapter 39) classically involves the eyelids [10,11]. The condition occasionally develops in sympathetic ophthalmia, secondary to a penetrating injury of the contralateral eye.

Thiotepa eyedrops instilled into the eyes after ocular surgery have also caused periocular depigmentation, as have mercurial ointments [12].

Dilated veins

If these cause a cosmetic problem, they can be treated by laser therapy or by fine skin incisions and interruption of the vessels by bipolar cautery [13].

Naevi

Pigmented naevi of the eyelids are fairly common. Early surgical treatment is advised for large congenital naevi of the eyelids because of the risk of malignancy. Surgery in the first few months of life can give a good cosmetic result [14].

The rare *divided naevus* (kissing naevus) is a melanocytic naevus in adjacent areas of the upper and lower eyelids, which appears to be a single lesion when the eyelids are closed. The precursor cells must have been present at the time when the fused eyelids separated at around the 24th week of gestation [14].

The *naevus of Ota*, which affects the eyelids, conjunctiva and sclera, may be thought of as an aberrant Mongolian spot. Occasionally, the pigmentation is confined to the eye, with no cutaneous involvement (melanosis oculi). Naevus of Ota carries an increased risk of ocular melanoma and glaucoma [15,16].

Strawberry naevi are relatively common on the eyelids and no treatment is usually required, although intradermal triamcinolone may be used if the naevus is so large that the child is in danger of amblyopia [17]. Surgical debulking is done if necessary at a later stage. Occasionally, a deep component in the orbit produces proptosis, and this may require treatment with high-dose prednisolone.

Port-wine stains also commonly affect the eyelids. Some cases are associated with structural anomalies in the anterior segment of the eye, which may lead to congenital or infantile glaucoma. About 8% of patients with port-wine stains in the trigeminal dermatome have glaucoma and/or central nervous system involvement [18]. The onset of the glaucoma may be delayed until adult life.

REFERENCES

1 Harrison SM. Retinopathy in childhood dermatomyositis. *Am J Ophthalmol* 1973; **76**: 786–90.
2 Connelly MG, Winkelmann RK. Solid facial edema as a complication of acne vulgaris. *Arch Dermatol* 1985; **121**: 87–90.
3 Boynton JR. Eyelid oleogranulomas caused by petroleum jelly injection. *Arch Ophthalmol* 1988; **106**: 550–1.
4 Nethercott JR, Nield G, Holness DL. A review of 79 cases of eyelid dermatitis. *J Am Acad Dermatol* 1989; **21**: 223–30.
5 Maibach HI, Engasser P, Ostler B. Upper eyelid dermatosis syndrome. *Dermatol Clin* 1992; **10**: 549–54.
6 Aguilera Diaz L. Hyperpigmentation of the eyelids. *Ann Dermatol Syphilol* 1972; **99**: 43–6.
7 Goodman RM. Periorbital hyperpigmentation: an overlooked genetic disorder of pigmentation. *Arch Dermatol* 1969; **100**: 169.
8 Hunziker N. Apropos of familial hyperpigmentation of the eyelid. *J Genet Hum* 1962; **11**: 16–21.
9 Ménage MJ, Wright G. Use of leeches in a case of periorbital haematoma. *Br J Ophthalmol* 1991; **75**: 755–6.
10 Cowan CL, Halder RM, Grimes PE. Ocular disturbances in vitiligo. *J Am Acad Dermatol* 1986; **15**: 17–24.
11 Wagoner MD, Albert DM, Lerner AB. New observations on vitiligo and ocular disease. *Am J Ophthalmol* 1983; **96**: 16–26.

12 Harben DJ, Cooper PH, Rodman OG. Thiotepa-induced leukoderma. *Arch Dermatol* 1979; **115**: 973–4.
13 Kersten RC, Kulwin R. Management of cosmetically objectionable veins in the lower eyelids. *Arch Ophthalmol* 1989; **107**: 278–80.
14 McDonnell PJ, Mayou B. Congenital divided naevus of the eyelids. *Br J Ophthalmol* 1988; **72**: 198–201.
15 Dutton JJ, Anderson RL, Schelper RL *et al.* Orbital malignant melanoma and oculodermal melanocytosis: report of 2 cases and review of the literature. *Ophthalmology* 1984; **91**: 497–507.
16 Gonder JR, Shields JA, Albert DM. Uveal malignant melanoma associated with ocular and oculodermal melanocytosis. *Ophthalmology* 1982; **89**: 953–60.
17 Boyd MJ, Collin JRO. Capillary haemangiomas: an approach to their management. *Br J Ophthalmol* 1991; **75**: 298–300.
18 Tallman B, Tan OT, Morelli JG *et al.* Location of port-wine stain and the likelihood of ophthalmic and/or CNS complications. *Pediatrics* 1991; **87**: 323–7.

Benign tumours, papules and cysts

Almost any neoplastic or infiltrative lesion of the skin can occasionally occur on the eyelids, but the following are worthy of special mention, either because of their predilection for this region, or because they may involve the eye.

Xanthelasma (Fig. 67.10)

The yellow plaques on the eyelids may be an isolated finding or associated with xanthomas elsewhere (Chapter 59). Xanthelasma palpebrarum is often a sign of familial hypercholesterolaemia, but in 40–70% of cases the lipid levels are normal [1,2]. Even in normolipidaemic patients, however, there may be a decrease in the high-density lipoprotein levels [1]. A large study in Iceland of more than 8000 subjects showed no association with heart disease [3]. The prevalence of xanthelasma rises with age, being about 1.5% in octagenarians [4].

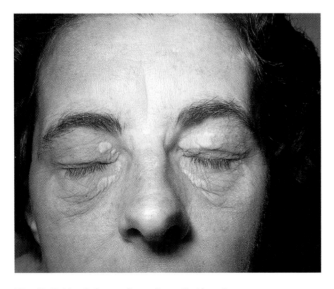

Fig. 67.10 Xanthelasma due to hyperlipidaemia.

Xanthelasma may be treated for cosmetic reasons by the careful application of 90% trichloracetic acid, using a cotton-wool applicator. The treatment causes stinging and an immediate white discoloration of the treated area, but the subsequent inflammatory reaction eventually causes a marked decrease in the xanthelasma, presumably because the lipid is removed by macrophages. Care is needed to prevent the trichloracetic acid trickling down the face or into the eyes. The treatment can be repeated after a few weeks if necessary.

REFERENCES

1 Tosti A, Varotti C, Tosti G *et al.* Bilateral extensive xanthelasma palpebrarum. *Cutis* 1988; **41**: 113–14.
2 Watanabe A. Serum lipids, lipoprotein lipids and coronary heart disease in patients with xanthelasma palpebrarum. *Atherosclerosis* 1981; **38**: 283–90.
3 Jonsson A, Sigfusson N. Significance of xanthelasma palpebrarum in the normal population. *Lancet* 1976; **i**: 372.
4 Roederer GO. Xanthelasma palpebrarum and corneal arcus in octagenarians. *N Engl J Med* 1987; **317**: 1740.

Necrobiotic xanthogranuloma

When it occurs on the eyelids, this condition (Chapter 52) resembles xanthelasma, although it is usually thicker, with a nodular surface. The lesions may become inflamed or necrotic and may ulcerate. There may be yellow plaques on the conjunctiva or sclera, and orbital infiltration may lead to exophthalmos [1–3].

Juvenile xanthogranuloma

These lesions (Chapter 53) occasionally involve the eyelids, conjunctiva, iris or ciliary body, either alone or in combination with skin tumours elsewhere [4–6]. Other ocular findings may include glaucoma, hyphaema, heterochromia iridis and iritis. Although uveal lesions are rare, the complications are serious, and review by an ophthalmologist is recommended [5].

Amyloidosis

Amber-coloured papules of the eyelids, with intralesional haemorrhage, have been reported as an early sign of systemic amyloidosis [7].

Lipoid proteinosis

Pearly nodules of the eyelid margins (Fig. 67.11) are a distinc-tive feature of lipoid proteinosis [8].

Syringomas, milia, trichoepitheliomas and tricholemmomas

These also tend to produce pearly papules on the eyelids,

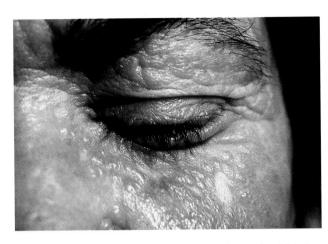

Fig. 67.11 Yellowish papules of the eyelids and periorbital skin in lipoid proteinosis. (Courtesy of Dr C. Tapadhinas, Hospital Curry Cabral, Lisbon, Portugal.)

and can be difficult to distinguish from each other without histology [9]. Syringomas, the commonest adnexal tumours of the lids, are usually multiple. Multiple tricholemmomas can occur on the eyelids in Cowden's syndrome. Retinal glioma and *Drusen* of the optic disc have also been reported in this syndrome.

Mucosal neuroma syndrome

This syndrome also produces lumpy papules along the ciliary margin, but the condition can be recognized clinically by the other features of the syndrome (Chapter 70).

Melanoacanthoma

Minute, shining, black papules may develop in the eyelid margin along the line of the lashes. Histologically, these are similar to dermatosis papulosa nigra [10].

Pilomatrixoma

This is often located on the eyelid or eyebrow, but is rarely diagnosed clinically [11].

Neurofibromatosis

This condition may affect the eyelids. In some cases, plexiform neuromas may produce gross enlargement of the eyelid, and there may be penetration of the mass into the orbit.

Oncocytoma

This is a benign tumour of the oxyphil epithelial cells, which can arise in the eyelid, caruncle or conjunctiva. It presents as a bright-red or yellowish tumour with a smooth or lobulated surface [12,13].

Marginal cysts

The glands of Moll (apocrine sweat glands in the eyelid margin) may become blocked to form a translucent cystic swelling. The lesion usually presents as a painless white or yellowish cyst on the lower eyelid close to the lacrimal punctum. Similar retention cysts may arise from the glands of Zeis (sebaceous glands associated with the lashes). Marginal cysts are best treated by excision.

Chalazion

SYN. MEIBOMIAN CYST

This painless, red swelling on the conjunctival surface of the eyelid is caused by a granulomatous reaction in a Meibomian gland, and may follow an infection of the gland (Fig. 67.12). There is a firm lump in the eyelid, which is clearly visible when the eyelid is everted. Some cases settle with conservative treatment, but if large or persistent the lesion can be treated surgically by incision and curettage through the conjunctival surface of the eyelid [14].

Dermoid cysts

These occur in the upper outer or upper inner angle of the orbit and they often have a deep extension into the orbit, so the surgeon must be prepared for this. A preoperative computed tomography (CT) scan of the orbit is advisable. Dermoid cysts can be up to 5 cm in diameter and may close the eyelid, or press on the globe [15]. They may become infected or inflamed.

Mucocoele

When this lesion arises from the frontal or ethmoidal sinus, it erodes the bone and extends into the orbit or the subcutaneous tissues of the eyelid. It presents as a smooth

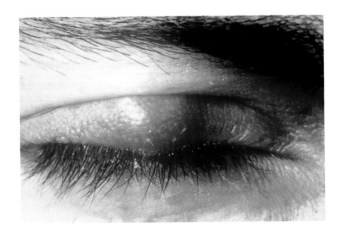

Fig. 67.12 Chalazion of the upper eyelid.

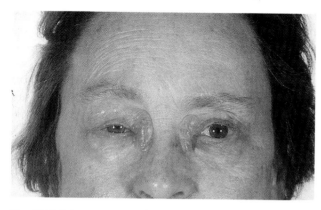

Fig. 67.13 Subcutaneous emphysema presenting as blistering around the eyes. In this case, the subcutaneous emphysema was a complication of endotracheal intubation. (Courtesy of Dr C. Hinds, Royal Liverpool Hospital, Liverpool, UK.)

fluctuant immobile mass, which may become inflamed [16]. Mucocoele of the lacrimal sac is associated with epiphora and commonly becomes infected. Lacrimal drainage surgery, comprising a dacryocystorhinostomy, is usually required.

Eyelid emphysema

If there is a communication between the paranasal spaces and the eyelid, blowing the nose can produce a sudden swelling of the eyelid due to subcutaneous emphysema (Fig. 67.13). The eyelid becomes puffy, with crepitus on palpation due to air in the tissues.

There is usually a history of blunt trauma to the face, causing a defect in the bony orbit. Patients with a fractured orbit should be warned against noseblowing, and treated with systemic antibiotics.

REFERENCES

1 Codere F, Lee RD, Anderson RL. Necrobiotic xanthogranuloma of the eyelid. *Arch Ophthalmol* 1983; **101**: 60–3.
2 Robertson DM, Winkelmann RK. Ophthalmic features of necrobiotic xantho-granuloma with paraproteinaemia. *Am J Ophthalmol* 1984; **97**: 173–5.
3 Kossard S, Winkelmann RK. Necrobiotic xanthogranuloma with paraprotein-aemia. *J Am Acad Dermatol* 1980; **3**: 257–70.
4 Hadden OB. Bilateral juvenile xanthogranuloma of the iris. *Br J Ophthalmol* 1975; **59**: 669–702.
5 Dapling RB, Nelson ME. Ocular lesions in patients with cutaneous juvenile xanthogranuloma. *Br J Dermatol* 1994; **130**: 260–1.
6 Wertz FD, Zimmerman LE, McKeown CA *et al.* Juvenile xanthogranuloma of the iris, optic nerve, disc, retina and choroid. *Ophthalmology* 1982; **89**: 1331–5.
7 Natelson EA, Duncan WC, Macossay CR *et al.* Amyloidosis palpebrarum. *Arch Intern Med* 1970; **125**: 304–7.
8 Jensen AD, Khodadoust AA, Emery JM. Lipoid proteinosis. *Arch Ophthalmol* 1972; **88**: 273–7.
9 Hidayat AA, Font RC. Trichilemmoma of eyelid and eyebrow. A clinico-pathologic study of 31 cases. *Arch Ophthalmol* 1980; **98**: 844–6.
10 Spott D, Heaton CL, Wood MG. Melanoacanthoma of the eyelid. *Arch Dermatol* 1972; **105**: 898–9.
11 Seitz B, Holbach LM, Naumann GF. Pilomatrixoma of the eyelids—clinical differential diagnosis and follow-up of 17 patients. *Ophthalmologica* 1993; **90**: 766–9.
12 Biggs SL, Font RL. Oncocytic lesions of the caruncle and other ocular adnexa. *Arch Ophthalmol* 1977; **95**: 474–8.
13 Lamping KA, Albert DM, Ni C. Oxyphil cell adenomas: 3 case-reports. *Arch Ophthalmol* 1984; **102**: 263–5.
14 Smythe D, Hurwitz J, Tayfour F. The management of chalazion. *Can J Ophthalmol* 1990; **2**: 252–9.
15 Jakobiec FA, Bonanno PA, Siegelmann J. Conjunctival adnexal cysts and dermoids. *Arch Ophthalmol* 1978; **96**: 1404–9.
16 Jarrett WH, Gutman FA. Ocular complications of infection of the paranasal sinuses. *Arch Ophthalmol* 1969; **81**: 683–8.

Malignancy

Precancerous lesions

Actinic keratosis and Bowen's disease occurring on the eyelids should be treated vigorously because of the risk of later malignancy. The intraepidermal carcinoma of the eyelid margin may be warty and misleadingly innocent in appearance (Fig. 67.14). It is easily mistaken for a viral or seborrhoeic wart. An adequate biopsy must include at least one entire eyelash follicle [1].

Cryotherapy is probably the treatment of choice, although careful use of the hyfrecator can also give good results. In severe cases, plastic surgery may be indicated.

Malignant tumours

Malignant tumours of the eyelids obviously pose a difficult problem, both because of their close proximity to the eyeball, and the difficulty of ensuring adequate tissue excision without losing the function of the eyelids. It is essential to remove the whole of the malignant tissue, even if a large tissue defect is left. If necessary, plastic surgery can be undertaken as a secondary procedure to repair the defect, once histological clearance is confirmed.

The vast majority of malignant tumours of the eyelids are *basal cell carcinomas*, and 70% of them occur on the lower eyelid. Basal cell carcinoma at this site can easily be mis-

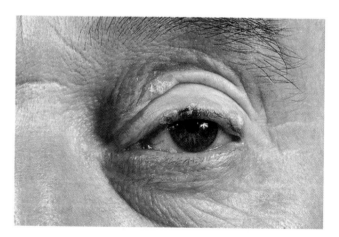

Fig. 67.14 Intraepidermal squamous carcinoma of the upper eyelid margin and an actinic keratosis just above the eyelid.

taken for a benign condition, such as a skin-coloured 'mole', or a marginal cyst [2]. Lesions near the medial canthus can spread deeply into the orbit and sinuses and can be devastating. Inadequate treatment can lead to the later necessity for heroic surgery, such as orbitectomy and transcranial ethmoidectomy [3]. Early referral to an oculoplastic surgeon is advisable. Prior biopsy is not recommended, as this may distort tumour margins.

Mohs' chemosurgery gives the best outcome for basal cell cancer in this area (Chapter 81). If this is not available, excision biopsy followed by plastic surgical repair after confirmation of histological clearance is recommended. Curettage is not advisable, as the tumour margins are deceptive, the thin eyelid skin tears easily and there is no firm base on which to scrape. Radiotherapy and cryotherapy have been used successfully, but the recurrence rate is likely to be higher than with excision (as high as 30%), and there is some evidence that tumours which recur after radiotherapy are more aggressive subsequently than those which recur after surgery [4,5]. Careful follow-up for many years is necessary.

For *squamous cell cancer, keratoacanthoma* or *malignant melanoma* of the eyelids, excision biopsy and plastic surgical repair is the treatment of choice.

Gorlin's syndrome (Chapter 36)

The eyelid is a site of predilection for the naevoid basal cell tumours (Fig. 67.15) and in adult life these may become aggressive [6]. Associated ocular findings in this syndrome include hypertelorism, strabismus, epicanthus, coloboma of the choroid and congenital cataract.

Xeroderma pigmentosum

The eyelids share in the skin damage of xeroderma pigmentosum, and this may result in blepharospasm, epiphora, entropion, ectropion or symblepharon [7]. Photophobia is almost universal [8]. Conjunctival tumours may occur, and keratitis with vascularization and scarring may lead to blindness. In order to conserve eyelid tissue, cryotherapy is the preferred mode of treatment for basal cell cancers in these patients.

Sebaceous cell carcinoma

Sebaceous cancer is rare in other sites, but is more common on the eyelids. It originates from the Meibomian glands or the glands of Zeis, and 70% of cases affect the upper eyelid [9]. It can mimic a chalazion and ulcerates only at a late stage. It can also present as blepharoconjunctivitis due to intraepithelial spread. Metastasis is common, so that the mortality rate is around 15% [10,11]. Any 'chalazion' persisting for more than a few months should be biopsied. Histological misdiagnosis is frequent unless a sample of adequate size is taken [2,12]. Radiotherapy is not advised. Wide local excision with frozen section control and immediate reconstruction is the treatment of choice [9]. Where conventional histology is used, fresh tissue must be stained specifically for fat before alcohol processing. Orbital exenteration may be required to prevent metastasis [13].

Eccrine sweat-gland carcinoma

Two sweat-gland carcinomas have a predilection for the eyelids, namely the mucous adenocarcinoma and the primary 'signet-ring' carcinoma, which causes an indurated thickening of the eyelid. Both are commoner in middle-aged or elderly men, and tend to recur following excision [14–16].

Merkel cell carcinoma

This can occur on the upper eyelid, presenting as a hard, painless, rapidly growing mass. It is an aggressive lesion, which requires wide excision, as recurrence can be fatal [17]. It can mimic chalazion [18].

Metastatic cancer

This is fairly rare, accounting for less than 1% of all eyelid malignancy. It presents in several ways: as a diffuse leathery induration of the eyelid, which may cause ptosis or lid lag, or as an ulcer, or a painless nodule [19,20].

Malakoplakia (Chapter 53)

This is a rare histiocytic skin tumour which appears to have a predilection for the eyelids [21].

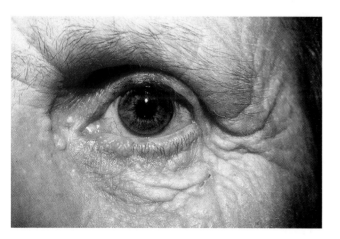

Fig. 67.15 Small naevoid basal cell cancers around the eyelids in Gorlin's syndrome.

REFERENCES

1 MacCallum DI, Kinmont PD, Williams DW *et al*. Intraepidermal carcinoma of the eyelid margin. *Br J Dermatol* 1975; **93**: 239–52.

2 Lober CW, Fenske NA. Basal cell, squamous cell and sebaceous gland carcinomas of the periorbital region. *J Am Acad Dermatol* 1991; **25**: 685–90.

3 Rosen HM. Periorbital basal cell cancer requiring ablative craniofacial surgery. *Arch Dermatol* 1987; **123**: 376–8.

4 Matthaus W. Fifteen years experience with cryotherapy of eyelid, facial and conjunctivial tumours in 2745 cases. *Fortschr Ophthalmol* 1987; **84**: 568–76.

5 Rodriguez-Sains RS, Robins P, Smith B *et al.* Radiotherapy of periocular basal cell carcinomas: recurrence rates and treatment, with special reference to the medial canthus. *Br J Ophthalmol* 1988; **72**: 134–8.

6 Southwick J, Schwartz RA. The basal cell naevus syndrome. Disasters seen among a series of 36 patients. *Cancer* 1979; **44**: 2296–9.

7 Ginsberg J. Present status of Meibomian gland carcinoma. *Arch Ophthalmol NY* 1965; **73**: 271–7.

8 Kraemer KH. Xeroderma pigmentosum: cutaneous ocular and neurologic abnormalities in 830 published cases. *Arch Dermatol* 1987; **123**: 241–50.

9 Tan KC, Lee ST, Cheah ST. Surgical treatment of sebaceous carcinoma of the eyelids with clinico-pathological correlation. *Br J Plast Surg* 1991; **44**: 117–21.

10 Doxanas MT, Green WR. Sebaceous gland carcinoma. *Arch Ophthalmol* 1984; **102**: 245–8.

11 Rao NA, Hidayat AA, McLean IW *et al.* Sebaceous gland carcinoma of the ocular adnexa: a clinico-pathologic study of 104 cases. *Hum Pathol* 1982; **13**: 113–22.

12 Kahn JA, Doane JF, Grove AS. Sebaceous and meibomian carcinomas of the eyelid. Recognition, diagnosis and management. *Ophthalmic Plast Reconstr Surg* 1991; **7**: 61–6.

13 Gurin DM, Rapini R. Aggressive sebaceous carcinoma of the eyelid: an elusive diagnosis. *Cutis* 1993; **52**: 40–2.

14 Boi S, de Concini M, Detassis C. Mucinous sweat gland adenocarcinoma of the inner canthus. *Ann Ophthalmol* 1988; **20**: 189–90.

15 Glatt HJ, Proia AD, Tsoy EA *et al.* Malignant syringoma of the eyelid. *Ophthalmology* 1984; **91**: 987–90.

16 Ni C, Dryja TP, Albert DM. Sweat gland tumours of the eyelids. A clinico-pathologic analysis of 55 cases. *Int Ophthalmol Clin* 1982; **22**: 1–22.

17 Searl SS, Boynton JR, Markowitch W *et al.* Malignant Merkel cell neoplasm of the eyelid. *Arch Ophthalmol* 1984; **102**: 907–11.

18 White IF, Orrell JM, Roxborough ST. Merkel cell tumour of the eyelids, masquerading as chalazion. *J R Coll Surg Edin* 1991; **36**: 129–30.

19 Ferry AP, Font RL. Carcinoma metastatic to the eye and orbit. I. A clinico-pathologic study of 227 cases. *Arch Ophthalmol* 1974; **92**: 276–86.

20 Rosenblum GA. Metastatic breast cancer in the eyelid. *Cutis* 1983; **31**: 411–15.

21 Font RL. Malakoplakia of the eyelid. Clinical, histopathologic and ultrasound characteristics. *Ophthalmology* 1988; **95**: 61–8.

Eyelid surgery

Small tumours of the eyelid are excised as a full-thickness wedge with a small margin of healthy tissue. The wound can often be closed directly. Where there is substantial tissue loss, it is usually necessary to rebuild the eyelid, reconstituting the tarsal plate and the skin separately. A defect in the lower eyelid may be repaired using a tarsoconjunctival flap [1] to reconstitute the tarsus of the lower eyelid. A flap of tarsus and conjunctiva is fashioned from the upper lid and sutured into the defect; the blood supply from the conjunctiva and Muller's muscle is left intact. A free skin graft is taken from the contralateral upper eyelid and sutured onto the anterior surface of the graft. The eyelid remains sutured in the closed position until the flap is divided after about 6 weeks. An alternative approach is the Mustardé cheek rotation flap [2]. Defects of the lateral half of the lower eyelid may be left to granulate with excellent results. Upper eyelid defects may be repaired using a lower bridge flap. When grafting skin on to the eyelids, it is best to use skin from the contralateral upper

eyelid, as this is a good match for colour and texture. Postauricular or supraclavicular skin are the next best sources. An approachable account of eyelid surgery may be found in Collin's *Manual of Systematic Eyelid Surgery* [3].

REFERENCES

1 Hughes WL. *Reconstructive Surgery of the Eyelids.* St Louis: CV Mosby, 1954.

2 Mustardé JC. *Repair and Reconstruction of the Orbital Region*, 2nd edn. Edinburgh: Churchill Livingstone, 1980.

3 Collin JRO. *A Manual of Systematic Eyelid Surgery*, 2nd edn. Edinburgh: Churchill Livingstone, 1989.

Blepharitis

Definition. Chronic inflammation of the eyelid margins.

Aetiology. The condition is associated with seborrhoeic dermatitis in about one-third of cases, although some cases begin in early childhood, before there is any evidence of sebaceous activity. In the UK, staphylococcal infection is thought to play a part in about one-third of cases, although in warmer countries staphylococcal infection is more prevalent [1]. It was shown many years ago that the topical application of a filtrate from a culture of *Staphylococcus aureus* can produce toxic conjunctivitis [2]. Meibomian gland dysfunction may also be important [3,4].

Clinical features. This is a common, chronic and troublesome condition. The severity varies from mild hyperaemia and scaling (Fig. 67.16) to destructive inflammatory changes, with swollen eyelids, distorted lashes, and deformity or ulceration of the eyelid margins (ulcerative blepharitis). Hard, brittle crusts or scales are said to be characteristic of staphylococcal infection. The eyes often appear red-rimmed,

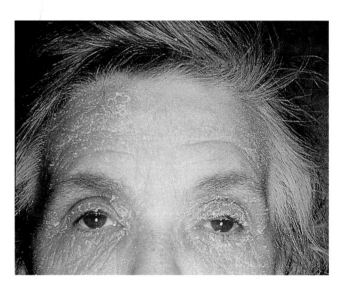

Fig. 67.16 Seborrhoeic dermatitis with blepharitis.

and the conjunctiva appears 'bleary', with a diffuse reddish tinge. Complications of staphylococcal blepharitis include chronic conjunctivitis, internal or external hordeola, chronic Meibomian adenitis, trichiasis, ulceration of the corneal margin, epithelial keratitis and phlyctenular conjunctivitis [5].

Treatment. This is often unsatisfactory, and relapse is common. It is important to treat the condition early, because successful treatment is difficult in old, well-established cases. The eyelid margins should be rubbed gently with a moist cotton-tipped applicator soaked in diluted baby shampoo or a new proprietary product (I-Scrub, a mixture of ionic and non-ionic surfactants), which is claimed to be less irritant [6]. Scrapings of crust should be examined for staphylococci and, if present, tested for antibiotic sensitivity. Antibiotic ointments such as chloramphenicol, sulphacetamide, bacitracin or mupirocin are useful, but 2% ketoconazole cream appears to be little better than a placebo [7].

For acute exacerbations not due to staphylococci, chloramphenicol eye ointment with added hydrocortisone should be applied to the eyelid margins at frequent intervals for a week or so, with vigorous removal of the accumulated scales. Any coexisting dandruff and seborrhoeic dermatitis must be treated simultaneously. Some patients benefit from tetracycline.

Differential diagnosis. The condition should be distinguished from the sicca syndrome, the 'red eye' of rosacea and from phthiriasis of the lashes (p. 2993). Infection with *Moraxella* can cause angular blepharitis, but the lesions are usually moister.

Psoriasis of the eyelid margin, which is uncommon, can cause confusion, and lupus erythematosus, dermatomyositis and contact dermatitis can also cause scaling of the eyelid margins.

If there is ulceration, herpetic infection must be considered.

REFERENCES

1 Smolin G, Okumoto M. Staphylococcal blepharitis. *Arch Ophthalmol* 1977; **95**: 812–16.
2 Allen JH. Staphylococcic conjunctivitis. *Am J Ophthalmol* 1937; **20**: 1025–7.
3 Mathers WD, Shields WJ, Sachdev MS *et al.* Meibomian gland dysfunction in chronic blepharitis. *Cornea* 1991; **10**: 277–85.
4 McCulley JP, Dougherty BS, Deneau EG. Classification of chronic blepharitis. *Ophthalmology* 1982; **89**: 1173–80.
5 Thygeson P. Complications of *Staphylococcus* blepharitis. *Am J Ophthalmol* 1969; **68**: 446–9.
6 Leibowitz HM, Capino D. Treatment of chronic blepharitis. *Arch Ophthalmol* 1988; **106**: 720.
7 Nelson ME, Midgley G, Blatchford NR. Ketoconazole in the treatment of blepharitis. *Eye* 1990; **4**: 151–9.

Ocular rosacea

The typical cutaneous lesions of rosacea (Chapter 46) may extend onto the eyelids, causing desquamation and erythema, but the eye itself may also be involved. The ocular involvement may precede the skin lesions by many years, and in some cases the lesions may be confined to the eye [1].

Rarely, local steroids applied to the eyelids for some other cause can produce lesions resembling rosacea, akin to perioral dermatitis [2].

Clinical features [1,3–5]. Chronic conjunctival hyperaemia and blepharitis are common, but many other ocular problems have been described, including iritis, iridocyclitis, chalazion, Meibomian adenitis, scleritis, episcleritis, corneal thinning, neovascularization and corneal scarring. Rosacea keratitis, which produces a triangular peripheral vascularization of the cornea, has a poor prognosis and may lead to blindness.

At least one-third of rosacea patients have some degree of blepharitis or conjunctivitis [5]. Many patients have keratoconjunctivitis sicca and some 40% of patients have decreased tear production [6]. Meibomian gland inflammation occurs much more commonly than it does in other types of blepharitis [7–9].

The aetiology of ocular rosacea is unknown, but instability of the tear film and changes in lipid composition of the Meibomian gland secretion have been suggested as possible causes [10].

Treatment. Tetracycline is the drug of choice, and has been shown to be effective against blepharitis, Meibomian keratoconjunctivitis and even progressive rosacea keratitis [11]. Warm compresses and artificial tears are helpful. Weak topical steroid preparations have also been used, although they can cause side-effects (p. 3010). Retinoids do not seem to help ocular rosacea and may even aggravate the situation [12].

REFERENCES

1 Borrie P. Rosacea with special reference to its ocular manifestations. *Br J Dermatol* 1953; **65**: 458–63.
2 Fisher AA. Periocular dermatitis akin to the perioral variety. *J Am Acad Dermatol* 1986; **15**: 642–4.
3 Jenkins MS, Brown SI, Lempert SL *et al.* Ocular rosacea. *Am J Ophthalmol* 1979; **88**: 618–22.
4 Donshik PC, Hoss DM, Ehlers WH. Inflammatory and papulosquamous disorders of the skin and eye. *Dermatol Clin* 1992; **10**: 533–47.
5 Browning DJ, Proia AD. Ocular rosacea. *Surv Ophthalmol* 1986; **31**: 145–58.
6 Lemp MA, Mahmood MA, Weiler HH. Association of rosacea and keratoconjunctivitis sicca. *Arch Ophthalmol* 1984; **102**: 556–7.
7 McCulley JP, Dougherty JM. Blepharitis associated with acne rosacea and seborrhoeic dermatitis. *Int Ophthalmol Clin* 1985; **21**: 159–72.
8 McCulley JP, Dougherty M. Bacterial aspects of chronic blepharitis. *Arch Ophthalmol* 1986; **105**: 314–17.
9 McCulley JP, Dougherty JM. Classification of chronic blepharitis. *Ophthalmology* 1982; **89**: 1173–80.
10 Cory CC, Hinks W, Burton JL *et al.* Meibomian gland secretion in the red eyes of rosacea. *Br J Dermatol* 1973; **89**: 25–7.
11 Knight A, Vickers CFH. A follow-up of tetracycline treated rosacea with special reference to rosacea keratitis. *Br J Dermatol* 1975; **93**: 577–80.
12 Hoting E, Paul E, Plewig G. Treatment of rosacea with isotretinoin. *Int J Dermatol* 1986; **25**: 660–3.

Demodectic blepharitis

This condition [1–3] is not universally accepted as a distinct entity, as *Demodex* can be found in normal eyelash follicles, but some authors maintain that the organism can cause inflammation of the eyelash follicles. Objective changes are slight: there may be some redness, and some eyelashes may be shed, but there is no scaling. Clifford and Fulk [4] found that 16% of 256 subjects had infestation of the eyelids with *Demodex*, and increased numbers of *Demodex* were associated with a loss of eyelashes and also with diabetes mellitus. Frequent bathing with boric acid, or benzalkonium 1/7000 is helpful, as is topical sulphur [3].

REFERENCES

1 Morgan RJ, Coston TO. Demodectic blepharitis. *South Med J* 1964; **57**: 694 –7.
2 Post CF, Juhlin E. *Demodex folliculorum* and blepharitis. *Arch Dermatol* 1963; **88**: 298–302.
3 Ayres S, Jr, Ayres S III. Demodectic eruptions. *Arch Dermatol* 1961; **83**: 154–65.
4 Clifford CW, Fulk GW. Association of diabetes, lid loss and *Staphylococcus aureus* with infestation of the eyelids by *Demodex folliculorum* (Acari, Demodicidae). *J Med Entomol* 1990; **27**: 467–70.

Infection

Most infections of the skin may occasionally involve the eyelids, but the following are of particular importance.

Viral infections

Molluscum contagiosum [1]

This viral disease commonly affects the eyelids, and, although many cases resolve spontaneously, there may be follicular conjunctivitis, which is believed to be caused by a reaction to the toxic products of the virus. A superficial punctate keratitis may develop, and if allowed to persist this can lead to a vascular pannus overgrowing the cornea. Although typical molluscum lesions are easy to recognize, those on the eyelid margins may be hidden by the base of the lashes, and they may have an atypical appearance, perhaps because of frequent bathing by the tear fluid.

If the patient is cooperative, molluscum lesions on the eyelid may be incised and the contents curetted out, or the eyelid may be everted and the lesions treated by a careful, light application of liquid nitrogen. In less cooperative patients, such as young children, it may be necessary to use a general anaesthetic.

The infection is much more aggressive in acquired immune deficiency syndrome (AIDS) patients [2].

Warts

These commonly occur on the eyelid margins as a filiform projection. They can usually be successfully treated by careful cryotherapy, using liquid nitrogen on a cotton-wool swab applied to the end of the warty lesion.

Herpes simplex

See ocular herpes, page 3003.

Herpes zoster ophthalmicus [3–6]

Ocular complications are likely when herpes zoster involves the ophthalmic division of the trigeminal nerve, particularly if the nasociliary branch is affected.

Often, the periorbital tissue is so swollen that the eyelids are closed, but in some cases mild cutaneous disease may be accompanied by severe ocular disease. The effects of herpes zoster ophthalmicus range from the trivial to the devastating, and almost any tissue of the orbital contents may be affected. The corneal disease takes many forms and can pose considerable management problems. The microdendritic type of keratitis is transitory and self-limiting and needs no treatment. The mucous plaque keratitis shows only a poor response to aciclovir and steroids are often required. In neuroparalytic keratitis, steroids must be avoided. Steroids should only be used sparingly in exposure keratitis [4,5]. Urgent ophthalmological consultation is required for all patients with herpes zoster ophthalmicus. Any patient under the age of 50 years who presents with herpes zoster ophthalmicus should be suspected of having human immunodeficiency virus (HIV) infection [2].

REFERENCES

1 Vannas S, Lapinleimu K. Molluscum contagiosum in the skin, caruncle and conjunctiva. *Acta Ophthalmol* 1967; **45**: 314–16.
2 Sarraf D, Ernest JT. AIDS and the eyes. *Lancet* 1996; **348**: 525.
3 Easty D. Ocular disease in varicella-zoster infections. In: *Virus Diseases of the Eye*. London: Lloyd-Luke, 1985: 228–56.
4 Liesegang TJ. Corneal complications from herpes zoster ophthalmicus. *Ophthalmology* 1985; **92**: 316–24.
5 Marsh RJ. Ophthalmic zoster. *Lancet* 1991; **338**: 1527.
6 Marsh RJ, Cooper M. Double-masked trial of topical acyclovir and steroids in the treatment of herpes zoster ocular inflammation. *Br J Ophthalmol* 1991; **75**: 542–6.

Bacterial infections

Bacterial infection of the eyelids generally produces marked swelling because the skin is lax, and the lesions are usually painful because of the abundant nerve supply of the region. Such infection must be treated urgently because of the risk of intracranial spread via the cavernous sinus.

Hordeolum (stye)

Hordeolum externum is a common condition due to a staphylococcal infection of the eyelash follicle, and corresponding to a furuncle elsewhere in the skin. The whole eyelid may become red, swollen and painful, but eventually the lesion points and discharges pus. The application of local heat will speed resolution and antibiotic eye ointment should be applied to prevent recurrence.

Hordeolum internum affects Meibomian glands rather than eyelashes. As the Meibomian gland is embedded in the tough, fibrous tarsal plate, with no room for expansion, this condition is more painful than the ordinary stye, and the pus eventually discharges through the conjunctival surface of the eyelid rather than on the eyelid margin. This condition may be followed by chalazion, and some ophthalmologists consider hordeolum internum may be regarded as an infected chalazion.

Meibomian adenitis
SYN. MEIBOMITIS

Infection of the Meibomian glands causes a burning sensation, and the patient may notice an intermittent film over the eye. On inspection, the gland orifices appear dilated and inflamed. Slit-lamp examination shows a foamy tear film with suspended particles. The condition is treated by daily expression of the Meibomian glands, followed by application of an appropriate antibiotic ointment.

Periorbital cellulitis

It is vitally important that this condition should be recognized and treated as soon as possible with an appropriate systemic antibiotic because of the risk of spread of infection into the orbit, with consequent severe or even fatal complications [1].

Necrotizing fasciitis (Chapter 27)

This is a particularly dangerous condition when it involves the skin around the eyes, for it must be treated by wide surgical excision of the infected tissues, and there is a natural reluctance for surgeons to remove the eyelids for a non-neoplastic disease [2–5]. The diagnosis is based on the clinical features, with a spreading purple discoloration of the eyelid, and progression to blistering and ulceration (Fig. 67.17). The patient is pyrexial, with a tachycardia, and the white-cell count shows a neutrophilia. The anti-deoxyribonuclease (DNase) titre is usually very high, but the anti-streptolysin-O (ASO) titre is not helpful [6]. Intravenous antibiotics such as cephalosporins in high dosage should be given. Early surgery is mandatory, as the mortality in some series is as high as 50%. In some cases, the eye may have to be sacrificed. This potentially fatal infection is often wrongly diagnosed [5,6].

Chancriform pyoderma

See Chapter 27.

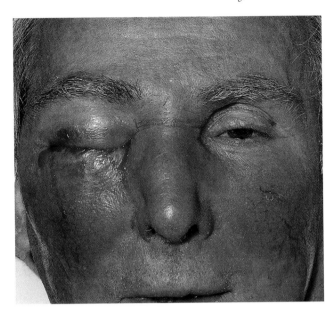

Fig. 67.17 Necrotizing fasciitis of the periorbital tissue. (Courtesy of Dr B. Leppard, Southampton General Hospital, Southampton, UK.)

REFERENCES

1 Jackson K, Baker SR. Periorbital cellulitis. *Head Neck Surg* 1987; **9**: 227–34.
2 Galosi AF, Hermann WP. Fasciitis necroticans. *Deutsch Med Wochenschrift* 1979; **104**: 1095–9.
3 Rosenthal WN, Insler MS. Periorbital necrotizing fasciitis. *Ann Ophthalmol* 1987; **19**: 426–7.
4 Seal DV, Leppard BJ, Widdowson J *et al*. Necrotizing fasciitis due to *Streptococcus pyogenes*. *Br Med J* 1980; **280**: 1419–20.
5 Walters R. A fatal case of necrotizing fasciitis of the eyelid. *Br J Ophthalmol* 1988; **72**: 428–31.
6 Leppard BJ, Seal DV. The value of bacteriology and serology in the diagnosis of necrotizing fasciitis. *Br J Dermatol* 1983; **109**: 37–44.

Parasitic infection

Myiasis (Chapter 33)

Flies of the order Diptera may deposit their eggs or larvae in the eyelid skin or conjunctiva, where they may resemble a furuncle or hordeolum. Some types such as *Hypoderma bovis*, prevalent near herds of cattle, can bore through the sclera to produce severe ocular damage ('fly-blown eye').

Phthiriasis (lice) of the eyelashes [1–5]

The crab louse (*Pthirus pubis*) can infest the eyelashes because the distance between the contiguous lashes, like the distance between the pubic hairs, is just right to allow the louse to grasp adjacent hair shafts. The adult lice are difficult to see without a slit-lamp, as they lurk at the base of the lashes, but their egg cases are easily seen as tiny 'pearls' adhering to the eyelashes. Sometimes the skin near the base of the lashes may show small bluish spots (*maculae caeruleae*) due to the lice bites.

The condition may be treated by the application of 20% fluorescein, which is non-irritant [6]. Malathion is also effective, but to avoid irritation the aqueous rather than the alcoholic solution should be used [3]. One application is usually sufficient.

REFERENCES

1 Alexander JO'D. *Phthirus pubis* infestation of the eyelashes. *JAMA* 1983; **250**: 32.
2 Baker RS. *Phthirus pubis* (pubic louse) blepharitis. *Am J Dis Child* 1984; **138**: 1079–80.
3 Burns DA. The treatment of *Pthirus pubis* infestation of the eyelids. *Br J Dermatol* 1987; **117**: 741–3.
4 Kirschner MH. *Phthirus pubis* infestation of the eyelashes. *JAMA* 1982; **248**: 428–9.
5 Perlman HH, Fraga S, Medina M. Phthiriasis palpebrarum. *J Pediatr* 1956; **49**: 88–90.
6 Mathew M, D'Souza P, Mehta DK. A new treatment of pthiriasis palpebrarum. *Ann Ophthalmol* 1982; **14**: 439–41.

The eyelashes

Trichomegaly
SYN. LONG LASHES

This may be due to a genetic trait. Increased growth of the eyelashes has also been described in HIV infection [1,2] (Fig. 67.18), following treatment with leukocyte A interferon for non-Hodgkin's lymphoma [3], and also after cyclosporin to prevent graft rejection [4]. Long lashes also occur in some patients with phenylketonuria or kala-azar [5].

Distichiasis
SYN. DOUBLE LASHES

This term applies when there is a second row of lashes on the posterior border of the eyelid margins, arising from

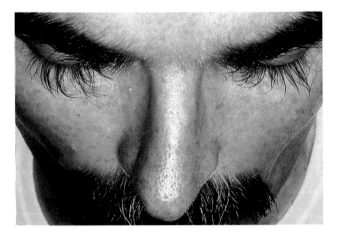

Fig. 67.18 Long eyelashes in a patient with acquired immunodeficiency syndrome. (Courtesy of Professor C. Farthing, New York, USA.)

the orifices of the Meibomian glands. It is an uncommon condition, inherited as a dominant trait [6–8], but it can occasionally be acquired, for example in the Stevens–Johnson syndrome. It has also been linked with familial lymphoedema [9] and with congenital heart defects [10].

Trichiasis (aberrant lashes, ingrowing lashes, pseudocilia)

Trichiasis is used as an 'umbrella term' for conditions which cause the lashes to come into contact with the eyeball. The growth of the lashes is often misdirected. There may be other abnormalities of the eyelids, such as blepharitis (or trachoma in endemic areas). Around 70% of patients with trichiasis have some degree of entropion [11].

The troublesome lashes can be pulled out, but they tend to regrow, and electrolysis of the hair roots may be necessary to prevent regrowth.

REFERENCES

1 Casanova JM, Puig T, Rubio M. Hypertrichosis of the eyelashes in acquired immuno-deficiency syndrome. *Arch Dermatol* 1987; **123**: 1599–601.
2 Jasnier M. Hypertrichosis des cils au cours de SIDA. *Ann Dermatol Vénéréol* 1987; **114**: 490–1.
3 Foon KA, Dougher G. Increased growth of the lashes in a patient given leukocyte A interferon. *N Engl J Med* 1984; **311**: 1259.
4 Weaver DT, Bartley GB. Cyclosporine-induced trichomegaly. *Am J Ophthalmol* 1990; **109**: 293–4.
5 Velez A, Kindelan JM, Garcia-Herola A *et al.* Acquired trichomegaly and hypertrichosis in metastatic adenocarcinoma. *Clin Exp Dermatol* 1995; **20**: 237–9.
6 Fox SA. Distichiasis. *Am J Ophthalmol* 1962; **53**: 14–18.
7 Scheie HG, Albert DM. Distichiasis and trichiasis: origin and management. *Am J Ophthalmol* 1966; **61**: 718–19.
8 Shammas HF. A family with congenital distichiasis. *J Med Genet* 1976; **13**: 514–15.
9 Pap Z. Syndrome of lymphoedema and distichiasis. *Hum Genet* 1980; **53**: 309–10.
10 Goldstein S. Distichiasis, congenital heart defects and mixed peripheral vascular anomalies. *Am J Med Genet* 1985; **20**: 283–94.
11 Barber K, Dabbs T. Morphological observations on patients with presumed trichiasis. *Br J Ophthalmol* 1988; **72**: 17–22.

Madarosis
SYN. LOSS OF LASHES

Alopecia areata, trichotillomania and blepharitis, both idiopathic and infective, are common causes of madarosis, but many other causes of hair loss can occasionally affect the lashes.

Madarosis occurs in 46% of leprosy patients in the USA [1]. Leprosy patients also develop subconjunctival fibrosis, punctate keratopathy, cataract and corneal hypoaesthesia. Madarosis has been reported in familial acanthosis [2].

Madarosis can be camouflaged by eyeliner, artificial lashes affixed by methacrylate-based adhesive or permanent pigment tattooing [3].

REFERENCES

1 Dana MR, Hochman MA, Viana MA *et al*. Ocular manifestations of leprosy in the USA. *Arch Ophthalmol* 1994; **112**: 626–9.
2 Chuang S-D, Jee S-H, Chiu H-C *et al*. Familial acanthosis nigricans with madarosis. *Br J Dermatol* 1995; **133**: 104–8.
3 Draelos ZK, Yeatts RP. Eyebrow loss, eyelash loss and dermatochalasis. *Dermatol Clin* 1992; **10**: 793–8.

Depigmentation

Like the eyebrows, the lashes may be depigmented as part of more widespread depigmenting diseases, such as albinism, vitiligo or phenylketonuria. Depigmentation may also occur during regrowth following loss of lashes in alopecia areata. Inflammatory diseases, such as blepharitis, can also cause loss of pigmentation.

Vogt–Koyanagi–Harada disease (Chapter 39)

This mysterious condition causes severe loss of central vision, and may be accompanied by iritis and meningism. There is usually a large exudative retinal detachment. As the acute phase settles, atrophy of the pigment epithelium develops, and in the later stages there is depigmentation of the eyelids and lashes, often with symmetrical vitiligo on other parts of the body.

Antibodies to uveal pigment have been demonstrated in this disease, but the correlation with disease activity is not good.

Sympathetic ophthalmia

Vitiligo and poliosis of the eyebrows and lashes also develop in *sympathetic ophthalmia*, a granulomatous uveitis which very rarely occurs in both eyes about 10 days to 8 weeks after a unilateral perforating injury of the eye, although it can sometimes occur several years later.

The lacrimal apparatus

Keratoconjunctivitis sicca

Deficiency of tear secretion is common in the elderly. It also occurs in a more severe form as a manifestation of Sjögren's syndrome (Chapter 58), although there may be a paradoxical increase in tear secretion in the early stages. The patient complains that the eyes feel dry and gritty. The corneal mucous secretions become tenacious, and this tends to pull strips of epithelium from the cornea when the patient blinks. This is called filamentous keratitis. Other complications may include bacterial infection due to lack of lysozyme in the tears, ulceration and scarring.

About 10% of AIDS patients experience a dry-eye syndrome [1], but the aetiology is unclear [2].

Staining with 1% Rose Bengal allows the dry areas on the cornea and conjunctiva to be seen as pink patches of keratitis. The Rose Bengal eyedrops must be washed out thoroughly as they are irritant. Local anaesthetic may be helpful. *Schirmer's test* provides a crude screening test for keratoconjunctivitis sicca. A 30-mm strip of filter paper is placed in the lower conjunctival sac, and the tear secretion runs along the length of the paper. Less than 10 mm after 5 min is suggestive of keratoconjunctivitis sicca.

Treatment includes the use of methylcellulose or hypromellose artificial tears, applied as necessary. Simple ointments provide lubrication at night. Severely affected patients may need to have their tear ducts artificially blocked to retain their tears. Acetyl cysteine eyedrops are useful for clumping of corneal mucus, but many patients complain that these drops make their eyes sting.

REFERENCES

1 Khadem M, Kalish SB, Goldsmith J *et al*. Ophthalmologic findings in AIDS. *Arch Ophthalmol* 1984; **102**: 201–6.
2 Sarraf D, Ernest JT. AIDS and the eyes. *Lancet* 1996; **348**: 525–8.

Acute dacryo-adenitis
SYN. LACRIMAL GLAND INFLAMMATION

This condition is rare, but can complicate mumps or herpes simplex infections. It presents as a painful swelling in the outer half of the upper eyelid, and on raising the eyelid the swollen gland can be seen bulging under the conjunctiva.

Chronic enlargement of the lacrimal gland

This condition may be due to chronic inflammation (50%) or to benign or malignant tumour (50%). In sarcoidosis, there may be associated uveitis and parotid enlargement.

Gustatory lacrimation
SYN. CROCODILE TEARS SYNDROME

Paroxysmal lacrimation during mastication, especially with salty foods, occasionally occurs during the recovery phase of facial palsy, probably due to misdirection of the salivary nerve fibres to the lacrimal gland. Ectropion may be present, and the annoying epiphora produces sore, red skin on the cheeks.

The lacrimal drainage apparatus

Dacryocystitis
SYN. INFLAMMATION OF THE LACRIMAL SAC

This condition is generally due to obstruction of the nasolacrimal duct. It presents with epiphora, swelling and redness at the inner canthus of the eye. Treatment consists of antibiotic drops and systemic antibiotics. For recurrent attacks, a drainage operation (dacryocystorhinotomy) may be required.

Congenital mucocele

Some authors apply the term congenital mucocele to a distension of the lacrimal sac due to obstruction, which presents at birth as a smooth, blue–grey swelling inferior to the inner canthus. This is best treated with massage and topical antibiotics.

The conjunctiva

Conjunctivitis

The 'red eye' is a common and important problem. The first step in diagnosis is to decide whether the dilated vessels are conjunctival or ciliary. If the vessels supplying the conjunctiva only are dilated, the redness will be superficial and more obvious towards the fornices (palpebral folds). If the deeper vessels supplying the cornea and ciliary body are dilated, the redness will be less bright, and will be worse in the limbal area surrounding the cornea. Most cases of simple conjunctivitis show the typical 'conjunctival' injection, but if there is associated keratitis the injection will extend to the limbal vessels.

Foreign-body conjunctivitis

Small particles of grit or other foreign material commonly irritate the conjunctival surface. They can usually be seen, surrounded by injected vessels, and they can be removed by irrigating the eye with normal saline, or by using fine forceps. Examination should include eversion of the upper eyelid. If the conjunctiva or cornea has been scratched, it is wise to apply an antibiotic eye ointment for a day or two.

A type of foreign-body conjunctivitis of particular interest to dermatologists is that due to the irritant hairs of the gypsy moth caterpillar, which can cause eyelid dermatitis [1]. The hairs can get into the conjunctival sac and cause severe painful inflammation, with late ocular sequelae.

Hayfever conjunctivitis

This is a type 1 hypersensitivity reaction which produces transient conjunctival itching, redness and lacrimation within minutes of exposure to an air-borne allergen such as grass pollen. It is accompanied by nasal mucosal itching and paroxysmal sneezing and there may be mild photophobia. The lids may become slightly swollen and in a few cases there may be true urticaria or angio-oedema. The cornea is not affected, and the eyes appear normal between attacks.

There is a marked seasonal distribution when the disease is caused by pollen, but *perennial allergic conjunctivitis* is a variant caused by allergens such as animal dander or industrial chemicals, which are present throughout the year.

The allergen reaches the conjunctiva via the tear film and then makes contact with the IgE antibody affixed to mast cells, which then discharge their granules, as they do in urticaria. Strangely enough, however, the level of histamine in the tears is not increased in hayfever conjunctivitis [2], although when histamine is dropped into the normal eye, it produces symptoms indistinguishable from those of hayfever.

In some cases, prick tests may be used to identify the allergen, and a variety of desensitizing injections are commercially available, but these are less effective for the ocular than the nasal symptoms. The hayfever should be treated in the usual way with antihistamines or cromoglycate. The beneficial effect of treatment with cromoglycate or lodoxamide drops may be delayed by several days. Levocabastine is a new topical antihistamine with a more rapid onset of action. The application of ice-cold compresses to the eyes may give some symptomatic relief, and in severe cases topical steroid eyedrops may be used for a limited period, provided there is no risk of herpes simplex infection and no history of glaucoma in close relatives.

REFERENCES

1 Beaucher WN, Farnham JE. Gypsy-moth caterpillar dermatitis. *N Engl J Med* 1982; **306**: 1301–2.
2 Allansmith MR, Baird RS, Higgenbotham EJ. Technical aspects of histamine determination in human tears. *Am J Ophthalmol* 1980; **90**: 719–24.

Contact lens intolerance

Intolerance of contact lenses manifests itself as stinging (either on insertion or after several hours of wearing the lens), itching, blurred vision or photophobia. The affected eyes are often red, with conjunctival oedema, and fluorescein staining may show superficial punctate keratitis. There may or may not be evidence of dermatitis of the eyelids.

Contact lens wearers who develop conjunctivitis should seek the advice of an ophthalmologist, but dermatologists are occasionally called upon to advise on possible allergic causes of contact lens intolerance.

The chemicals found in contact lenses and contact lens solutions are listed elsewhere [1]. Lens care products generally consist mainly of water with various added preservatives, surface-active wetting agents, lubricating agents, proteolytic cleansers and buffers.

Thiomersal, widely used as a disinfectant, has in the past been a common cause of allergic intolerance [2], but its use has now declined. Sorbic acid and papain are still common causes of stinging, and affected patients may show contact urticaria to these compounds on patch testing [3].

Podmore and Storrs [1] studied 20 patients with contact lens intolerance and found that eight gave positive delayed patch tests, six had immediate hypersensitivity (contact urticaria) and nine showed no reaction to the test battery.

Some of the latter group may have suffered from other eye conditions such as giant papillary conjunctivitis, or there may have been allergens which were not tested.

REFERENCES

1 Podmore P, Storrs FJ. Contact lens intolerance: allergic conjunctivitis? *Contact Dermatitis* 1989; **20**: 98–103.
2 Reitschel RL, Wilson LA. Ocular inflammation in patients using soft contact lenses. *Arch Dermatol* 1982; **118**: 147–50.
3 Santucci B, Cristardo A, Picardo M. Contact urticaria from papain in a soft lens solution. *Contact Dermatitis* 1985; **12**: 233.

Atopy

Diseases of the eye which are more common in atopic subjects include eyelid eczema, severe blepharitis, allergic conjunctivitis, allergic keratitis, keratoconus, corneal infections (especially herpes simplex), cataract and retinal detachment [1–5]. Some atopic patients can be recognized by their facial appearance, and this is partially due to the Dennie–Morgan infraorbital fold (p. 2982).

The management of allergic eye disease in patients with atopy is complicated by their predisposition to herpes simplex infections. Vernal catarrh normally requires topical steroid therapy, which is contraindicated in patients with ocular herpes simplex, and in some cases it seems that vernal conjunctivitis can trigger off a recrudescence of a herpetic infection.

Atopic keratoconjunctivitis

In atopic eczema, the eyelids are scaly, lichenified, crusted and inflamed, and there is often increased wrinkling of the periorbital skin. In severe cases, there may be some degree of ectropion, with maceration of the inner and outer canthi due to overflow of tears.

The conjunctiva is sometimes hyperaemic, and the appearances can be difficult to distinguish from marginal blepharitis. There may also be keratitis, and repeated attacks can produce scarring and vascularization of the cornea, leading to visual loss. The immunopathology of this reaction is not known, but it is presumably not due simply to IgE-mediated histamine, as these complications do not occur in hayfever conjunctivitis. Atopic keratoconjunctivitis must also be distinguished from contact blepharokeratoconjunctivitis, and early vernal conjunctivitis.

Atopic eczema with eye involvement also predisposes to keratoconus (p. 3004). This is hard to treat, because keratoconjunctivitis is not conducive to wearing contact lenses, and it also makes corneal grafting a riskier procedure.

Cataract occurs in about 10% of atopic subjects who have had keratoconjunctivitis for 10 years or more, although many of these cataracts are of little clinical significance [6]. Steroid therapy may cause progression of the cataract in such cases, however, and some authors recommend examination by slit-lamp before starting therapy with systemic steroids or psoralen and UVA (PUVA) in atopic eczema patients. The opacities are usually bilateral and symmetrical. They form in the anterior cortex of the lens, and are characteristically shaped like a bearskin rug. The mechanism which provokes them is puzzling, because the avascular lens is remote from immunological influences.

Atopic eczema patients also have an increased risk of retinal detachment.

Treatment. Atopic keratoconjunctivitis is a serious disease because of its potential for causing vision loss. For acute punctate keratitis without vascularization, a mild steroid should be applied topically every few hours for several days. Patients must be encouraged not to scratch their eyes, and cotton gloves should be worn at night. Once the condition has been controlled by a topical steroid, maintenance therapy is with cromoglycate or lodoxamide drops.

Atopic retinal detachment

There have been over 130 reported cases of retinal detachment in patients with atopic dermatitis, mainly from Japan [4]. The pathogenesis is unknown, but it occurs at a young age and both eyes may be affected.

REFERENCES

1 Bloch-Michel *et al.* Atopy and herpetic keratitis. In: Sundmacher R, ed. *Herpetic Eye Diseases*. Munich: Bergmann Verlag, 1981.
2 Easty DL, Entwistle C, Funk A *et al.* Herpes simplex keratitis and keratoconus in the atopic patient. *Trans Ophthalmol Soc UK* 1975; **95**: 267–76.
3 Roussus J, Denis J. Interference between ocular herpes and allergic diseases. An epidemiological approach. In: Sundmacher R, ed. *Herpetic Eye Diseases*. Munich: Bergmann Verlag, 1981.
4 Yoneda K, Okamoto H, Wada Y *et al.* Atopic retinal detachment. Report of 4 cases and a review of the literature. *Br J Dermatol* 1995; **133**: 586–91.
5 Donshik PC, Hoss DM, Ehlers WH. Inflammatory and papulosquamous disorders of the skin and eye. *Dermatol Clin* 1992; **10**: 33–47.
6 Norris PG, Rivers JK. Screening for cataracts in patients with severe atopic eczema. *Clin Exp Dermatol* 1987; **12**: 21–2.

Vernal catarrh (conjunctivitis)

This is a chronic disease of unknown origin which produces intense irritation, lacrimation, photophobia and ropy mucus. It is characterized by bilateral conjunctivitis, with giant papillae in the upper tarsal conjunctiva, and in the limbal form of the disease by papillary hypertrophy of the limbic conjunctiva. White, chalky concretions may occur in the region of the limbus. There may be a punctate keratitis, and a persistent epithelial defect in the anterior layers of the cornea. This may be followed by the development of a fixed corneal plaque, which requires surgical removal.

The condition is worse in the spring, but may persist in a milder form throughout the year. It rarely appears before the age of 3 years or after 25 years, and it is commoner in males than in females. About 75% of cases occur in association with some other manifestation of atopy such as atopic eczema, asthma, or allergic rhinitis.

The differential diagnosis includes giant papillary (foreign-body) conjunctivitis [1], hayfever conjunctivitis, atopic conjunctivitis and trachoma.

Treatment is similar to that of atopic keratoconjunctivitis, with topical steroids and sodium cromoglycate. Nearly all patients eventually make a full recovery.

REFERENCE

1 Richmond PP, Allansmith MR. Giant papillary conjunctivitis. *Int Ophthalmol Clin* 1981; **21**: 65–82.

Phlyctenular conjunctivitis

This condition occurs in children who live in crowded poverty. In some cases, it is thought to be due to a reaction to a staphylococcal antigen or to an endogenous tuberculoprotein.

Phlyctens are raised, white nodules, usually seen near the limbus, accompanied by a leash of dilated conjunctival vessels. The nodules eventually ulcerate and disappear, but new phlyctens may appear at a different site. The condition is often fairly asymptomatic, but if the cornea is involved there may be marked lacrimation and photophobia.

Treatment is with local steroid eyedrops, and improved diet and hygiene.

Chronic conjunctivitis

Low-grade chronic inflammation of the conjunctiva is common, but the cause is often difficult to establish.

Possible causes include chronic blepharitis, allergy to cosmetics or topical medication, overtreatment with antibiotics, unsuspected foreign-body or intermittent entropion, exogenous irritants, such as chemical fumes or insecticide powders, and deficiency of tear production.

As many as 10% of AIDS patients develop non-specific conjunctivitis [1].

Infections

Bacterial infections

Acute purulent conjunctivitis

This is characterized by conjunctival injection and a mucopurulent discharge from the eyes. It may be caused by a variety of microorganisms. The most common causative organisms are *Staphylococcus*, *Haemophilus* and *Streptococcus*. Treatment is by irrigation and the application of antibiotic eyedrops. The newer fluoroquinolones such as ciprofloxacin offer no advantage over the cheaper chloramphenicol [2].

Gonorrhoeal conjunctivitis

Gonorrhoea can cause conjunctivitis with a very profuse, purulent discharge. The eyelids are swollen and red, and the conjunctivae are swollen and haemorrhagic. This condition should be treated as an emergency, as it can cause ulceration and severe eye damage within 24h, especially in the newborn, in whom it can occur after passage through an infected birth canal.

REFERENCES

1 Sarraf D, Ernest JT. AIDS and the eyes. *Lancet* 1996; **348**: 525–8.
2 Editorial. Fluoroquinolones for the eye. *Drug Therap Bull* 1994; **32**: 78–9.

Chlamydial infections

Psittacosis, lymphogranuloma venereum, trachoma and inclusion conjunctivitis are caused by organisms of the genus *Chlamydia*, known collectively as trachoma inclusion conjunctivitis (TRIC) agents. *Chlamydia* are not true viruses. Unlike viruses they multiply by binary fission, they possess ribosomes, and their growth is inhibited by several antimicrobial drugs.

Trachoma

This condition is serious because it produces scarring of the conjunctiva and the cornea. It causes more cases of preventable blindness throughout the world than any other disease. The patient complains of pain, lacrimation and photophobia, with a sticky mucoid discharge. In the early stages, the upper tarsal conjunctiva shows follicles, with marked injection, and the cornea shows punctate keratitis with pannus formation, especially in the upper half. There is progressive scarring, entropion and trichiasis.

The disease occurs in overcrowded unhygienic conditions in hot, dry countries where flies buzz around the eyes to obtain moisture. Secondary bacterial infection is common, and this contributes to the corneal scarring. In many cases blindness results.

Treatment is with systemic tetracycline, local antibiotics to prevent secondary infection, and improvement in hygiene. Surgical procedures may be required to correct the damage to the cornea and the lids.

Paratrachoma

This term is applied to several diseases, including *TRIC inclusion conjunctivitis of the newborn*, which originates from the maternal genital mucosa, and *TRIC punctate keratoconjunctivitis* in the adult, which is a sexually transmitted disease.

Paratrachoma responds well to topical tetracycline therapy. If there is a genital reservoir causing repeated infection, it may be necessary to give a systemic antibiotic for up to 6 weeks.

Viral infections

Viral attack tends to produce a follicular conjunctivitis with a superficial punctate keratitis, usually with enlargement of the pre-auricular lymph nodes.

Adenovirus

This is the most common form of infectious conjunctivitis. There are several subtypes, which can cause different clinical pictures.

Epidemic keratoconjunctivitis is highly contagious, and is common in institutions such as schools and hospitals. The onset is sudden, with acute conjunctivitis and painless preauricular lymphadenopathy. Both eyes are affected. There is no effective therapy other than antibiotic drops to prevent secondary infection.

Herpes simplex

This can produce acute follicular conjunctivitis with painful swelling of the pre-auricular nodes. It is usually unilateral. There may be small herpetic vesicles on the adjoining eyelids, and a superficial punctate keratitis.

The treatment is as for dendritic ulcers (p. 3003).

Miscellaneous diseases

Conjunctivitis is a common feature of the Stevens–Johnson syndrome (Fig. 67.19), Reiter's disease and some types of vasculitis, particularly the allergic granulomatous vasculitis of Churg and Strauss. It is also a prominent feature of some systemic infections, particularly measles.

Loiasis can cause conjunctival pain and lacrimation associated with painful facial swellings (calabar swellings). Conjunctival lesions occur occasionally in several other systemic diseases, such as sarcoidosis and lupus erythematosus, but these are usually an incidental finding rather than a dominant or presenting symptom.

Parinaud's oculoglandular syndrome

This term refers to the association of granulomatous conjunctivitis with enlarged pre-auricular lymph nodes. Many infections will produce this combination, for example leptothrix, cat-scratch disease and tuberculosis, but sarcoidosis is another important cause. The presence of an enlarged pre-auricular node is helpful in distinguishing infective conjunctivitis from that due to toxins or allergy.

Ligneous conjunctivitis [1–4]

This is a rare type of membranous conjunctivitis of unknown cause, which is sometimes familial. It is most common in young children, especially girls, but it can occur at any age. The eyelids feel woody to palpation, and there is an irregular mass of hyalinized connective tissue arising from the tarsal conjunctiva. It can affect other mucous membranes to produce oral plaques, or vaginal crusting with intermenstrual bleeding and discharge. Involvement of the larynx, vocal cords, trachea and nasopharynx has also been recorded, as has hydrocephalus [1]. Histology shows extensive deposits of amorphous eosinophilic material in the upper dermis interspersed with inflammatory cells. The immune responses are exaggerated, with an increase in activated T cells and plasma cells in the lesions [2].

Treatment is unsatisfactory, as regrowth of the membrane follows fairly rapidly after surgical removal, although cyclosporin or azathioprine may help [1,2].

REFERENCES

1 Editorial. Ligneous conjunctivitis. *Lancet* 1990; **i**: 84.
2 Holland EJ, Chan C. Immunohistologic findings and results of treatment with cyclosporin in ligneous conjunctivitis. *Am J Ophthalmol* 1989; **107**: 160–6.
3 Hidayat ASA, Riddle PJ. Ligneous conjunctivitis—a clinicopathologic study of 17 cases. *Ophthalmology* 1987; **94**: 949–59.
4 Marcus DM, Walton D, Donshik P *et al*. Ligneous conjunctivitis with ear involvement. *Arch Ophthalmol* 1990; **108**: 514–19.

Ataxia–telangiectasia

In this rare condition (Chapter 45), conjunctival telangiectasia occurs in virtually all cases, and may also be present on the eyelids. Involvement of the central nervous system produces a variety of abnormal eye movements, for example nystagmus, convergence weakness and strabismus.

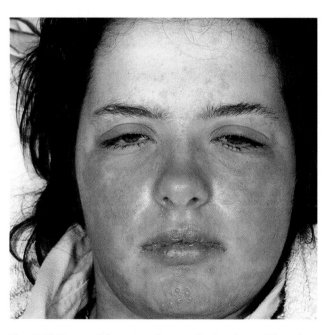

Fig. 67.19 Stevens–Johnson syndrome, affecting the eyelids and conjunctiva. Note the involvement of the oral mucosa and the blisters on the chin.

Conjunctival Kaposi's sarcoma

This presents as a reddish plaque which can mimic subconjunctival haemorrhage or chalazion.

Subconjunctival haemorrhage

A sudden appearance of blood under the conjunctiva commonly follows slight trauma or a cough or sneeze, and is usually of little significance. It may occasionally be a manifestation of hypertension or a bleeding diathesis, and these conditions must be excluded. The blood is gradually absorbed and no treatment is required unless some underlying cause is discovered.

Pingueculae

Degenerative changes sometimes occur in the interpalpebral conjunctiva of the elderly, probably as a result of environmental trauma such as UV radiation and dust. The elastic tissues proliferate to form a yellowish nodule, usually on the nasal side of the cornea. This pinguecula is often scarcely visible unless the patient develops a coincidental conjunctivitis, when it may stand out as a pale avascular area against a red background. A pinguecula is harmless and no treatment is required. It must be distinguished from a pterygium (p. 3005).

Immunobullous diseases

Cicatricial pemphigoid
SYN. BENIGN MUCOUS MEMBRANE PEMPHIGOID

This condition (Chapter 40), which is indistinguishable from bullous pemphigoid on laboratory tests [1–3], can lead to serious ocular complications, including blindness. Rupture of the conjunctival bullae leads to symblepharon (fusion of the bulbar and palpebral conjunctiva). Other important complications include dry eye due to blocked teargland openings, conjunctival scarring and inverted lashes. These complications tend to lead to corneal opacification, which is eventually bilateral. There is a predisposition to conjunctival infection [4]. In a review of 457 cases of cicatricial pemphigoid, ocular lesions were found in 64% [5].

A snip biopsy of the conjunctiva can be used to establish the diagnosis, but caution is required, as any form of ophthalmic surgery can precipitate an acute inflammatory reaction in untreated patients with cicatricial pemphigoid. The biopsy should be taken from a site distant from the 'active' disease. Topical antibiotics must be applied following the biopsy. Although IgG is the dominant immunoglobulin class in direct immunofluorescence of the skin, linear IgA deposition occurs in 47% of conjunctival biopsies in patients with ocular cicatricial pemphigoid [6]. Indirect immunofluorescence is less reliable, but the positive yield can be increased substantially by using undiluted serum and salt-split human skin as the substrate [7].

Treatment. Expert ophthalmological advice is always required. Artificial tears are used to treat dry eyes, if necessary with surgical occlusion of the puncta. Blepharitis is treated with regular eyelid hygiene, including compresses, scrubs and topical antibiotics. Contact lenses may be used in suitable cases to protect the cornea. Topical corticosteroids are relatively ineffective in cicatricial pemphigoid. Systemic therapy is with prednisolone and a concomitant agent, for example dapsone, azathioprine or cyclophosphamide. Dapsone is probably the first-line therapy for mild or moderate cases, with cyclophosphamide being reserved for the more severe cases [8]. Topical tretinoin ointment (0.01%) may also reverse the squamous metaplasia of the ocular epithelium [9]. Mast-cell stabilizers, such as ketotifen, have also been tried. Trichiasis may be treated by electrodesiccation.

Drug-induced ocular pemphigoid

Various topical antiglaucoma medications (pilocarpine, timolol, etc.) and topical idoxuridine have been reported to cause conjunctival scarring. The clinical features closely resemble cicatricial pemphigoid [10,11].

Histopathology is also virtually identical in the two conditions, but immunofluorescence is negative or nonspecific in drug-induced cases. It can be difficult to distinguish the two conditions, however, especially if the drug has been used in both eyes, as immunofluorescence is not reliably positive or negative in either condition and, because patients with cicatricial pemphigoid have an increased incidence of glaucoma even before diagnosis, they may have used an antiglaucoma drug coincidentally [3]. Some authors believe that antiglaucoma drugs can provoke true cicatricial pemphigoid [12]. A similar condition has been described in association with practolol therapy [13].

Pemphigus vulgaris (Chapter 40)

Conjunctivitis with associated mucoid discharge is common [12], but bullae and erosions are rare, and cicatrization and keratopathy do not generally occur [14]. Erosions of the medial end of the eyelid have been reported [15].

Paraneoplastic pemphigus vulgaris (Chapter 40)

Severe ocular involvement with cicatrizing conjunctivitis is common in this condition. Conjunctival biopsies generally show the classic changes of pemphigus vulgaris [12].

Linear IgA disease (Chapter 40)

Around 50% of patients show cicatrizing conjunctivitis on careful examination, which is clinically identical to cicatricial

Table 67.6 Bullous eruptions involving the conjunctiva.

	Age	Clinical features	Associated lesions
Bullous erythema multiforme (syn. Stevens–Johnson syndrome)	Children; young adults	Acute onset; intense oedema; large bullae	Bullae of mouth, genital skin
Benign mucous membrane pemphigoid	Usually over 60, F>M	Insidious onset; soreness; scarring	Erosions and scarring in mouth; skin bullae few, inconstant
Linear IgA disease	Children or adults	Cicatrizing conjunctivitis	Tense blisters, often in annular distribution in genital area
Pemphigus vulgaris	40–60, often Jewish	Eyes involved infrequently	Erosions of oral mucous membrane; skin bullae
Recessive dystrophic epidermolysis bullosa	Children	Onset from birth; eyes involved infrequently; bullae and scarring	Extensive bullae of skin and mucous membranes
Acquired epidermolysis bullosa	Adults	Eyes rarely involved	Trauma-induced blisters, which heal with milia
Dermatitis herpetiformis	Adults	Ocular involvement rare; vesicles and erosions of conjunctiva have been reported	Irritable papules and vesicles of limbs and trunk
Hydroa vacciniforme	Children	Vesiculo-ulcerative or hypertrophic conjunctivitis in 20%	Vesicles on light-exposed skin

pemphigoid [2,16]. In seven patients who had conjunctival biopsy performed, four had linear IgG deposits, but none showed positive immunofluorescence with IgA [2].

Lichen planus (Chapter 41)

Involvement of the conjunctiva has rarely been reported in this condition [17].

Epidermolysis bullosa acquisita (Chapter 40)

Mucosal involvement occurs in most patients with epidermolysis bullosa acquisita, and the ocular lesions resemble those in cicatricial pemphigoid. Conjunctival scarring may lead to blindness. Milia of the eyelids can also occur [18–21]. Table 67.6 lists some bullous diseases which occasionally affect the conjunctiva.

REFERENCES

1 Venning VA, Allen J, Millard PR *et al.* The localization of the bullous pemphigoid and cicatricial pemphigoid antigens. *Br J Dermatol* 1989; **120**: 305–15.
2 Kelly SE, Frith PA, Millard PR *et al.* A clinicopathological study of mucosal involvement in linear IgA disease. *Br J Dermatol* 1988; **119**: 161–70.
3 Venning VA, Frith PA, Bron AJ *et al.* Mucosal involvement in bullous and cicatricial pemphigoid: clinical and immunopathological study. *Br J Dermatol* 1988; **118**: 7–10.
4 Mondino BJ, Brown SI. Ocular cicatricial pemphigoid. *Ophthalmology* 1981; **88**: 95–100.
5 Ahmed AR, Hombal SM. Cicatricial pemphigoid. *Int J Dermatol* 1986; **25**: 90–6.
6 Leonard JN, Hobday CM, Haffenden GP *et al.* Immunofluorescence studies in ocular cicatricial pemphigoid. *Br J Dermatol* 1988; **118**: 209–17.
7 Sarret Y, Hall R, Cobo LM *et al.* Salt-split human skin substrate for the immunofluorescent screening of sera of patients with cicatricial pemphigoid, and a new method of immunoprecipitation of IgA antibodies. *J Am Acad Dermatol* 1991; **24**: 952–8.
8 Tauber J, Sainz de la Maza C, Foster CS. Systemic chemotherapy for ocular pemphigoid. *Ophthalmology* 1991; **10**: 185–95.
9 Tseng SCG. Topical tretinoin treatment for severe dry eye disorders. *J Am Acad Dermatol* 1986; **15**: 860–6.
10 Lass JH, Thoft RA, Dohlman CH. Idoxuridine-induced conjunctival cicatrization. *Arch Ophthalmol* 1983; **101**: 747–50.
11 Fiore PM, Jacobs IH, Goldberg DB. Drug-induced pemphigoid: a spectrum of diseases. *Arch Ophthalmol* 1987; **105**: 1660–3.
12 Camisa C, Meisler DM. Immunobullous disease with ocular involvement. *Dermatol Clin* 1992; **10**: 557–71.
13 Van Joost T, Crone RA, Overdijk AD. Ocular cicatricial pemphigoid associated with practolol therapy. *Br J Dermatol* 1976; **74**: 447–50.
14 Hodak E, Kremer I, David M *et al.* Conjunctival involvement in pemphigus vulgaris. A clinical, histopathological and immunofluorescent study. *Br J Dermatol* 1990; **123**: 615–20.
15 Nelson ME, Rennie IG. Symmetrical lid margin erosions: a condition specific to pemphigus vulgaris? *Arch Ophthalmol* 1988; **106**: 1651–2.
16 Leonard JN, Wright P, Williams DM *et al.* The relationship between linear IgA disease and benign mucous membrane pemphigoid. *Br J Dermatol* 1984; **110**: 307–14.
17 Dhermy P, Hie C, Pouliquen Y *et al.* Lichen planus of the conjunctiva. *J Fr Ophtalmol* 1983; **6**: 51–7.
18 Aurora AL. Ocular changes in epidermolysis bullosa lethalis. *Am J Ophthalmol* 1975; **79**: 464–70.
19 Lang PG, Jr, Taput MJ. Severe ocular involvement in a patient with epidermolysis bullosa acquisita. *J Am Acad Dermatol* 1987; **16**: 439–43.
20 Kurzhals G, Stolz W, Meurer M *et al.* Epidermolysis bullosa acquisita. *Arch Dermatol* 1991; **127**: 391–5.
21 Zierhut M, Thiel HJ, Weidle EJ *et al.* Ocular involvement in epidermolysis bullosa acquisita. *Arch Ophthalmol* 1989; **107**: 398–401.

Stevens–Johnson syndrome and toxic epidermal necrolysis

There may be severe sequelae for the eye in erythema multiforme, Stevens–Johnson syndrome and toxic epidermal necrolysis, and the ocular changes may be indistinguishable in these conditions [1–3]. In the acute stages, the conjunctivae may be inflamed and the eyelids are red, swollen and crusted. Distinct vesicles may develop, and the eyelashes may be lost. Secondary bacterial infection is common. More severe involvement may progress to membranous conjunctivitis, due to coalescence of fibrin and cellular debris. If this is pulled off, there may be bleeding of the underlying tissue, with resulting cicatrization.

Visual acuity may also be diminished by corneal vesiculation, or acute anterior iritis. In the later stages, there may be scarring, symblepharon, ectropion or entropion and trichiasis.

Scarring of the upper lid can also cause poor eyelid closure (lagophthalmos), which leads to corneal damage, keratitis and accumulation of debris.

Destruction of the conjunctival goblet cells causes a relative mucin deficiency in the tears. Mucin is required for tear film stability, and this deficiency therefore produces dry spots in the cornea, due to the tear film breaking up in less than 10 sec. The resulting corneal exposure produces punctate epithelial keratitis, epithelial defects, corneal infection, ingrowth of new blood vessels, scarring, corneal opacity, and even perforation with panophthalmitis.

Details of treatment are beyond the scope of this text, but expert ophthalmological advice is urgently required for any patient with erythema multiforme, Stevens–Johnson syndrome or toxic epidermal necrolysis who develops ocular involvement. Corticosteroids and the 'blind' use of antibiotics are best avoided [1]. Botulinum toxin has been used to rest the eye and to diminish corneal scarring.

REFERENCES

1 Roujeau JC, Revuz J. Intensive care in dermatology. In: Champion RH, Pye RJ, eds. *Recent Advances in Dermatology* Vol. 8. Edinburgh: Churchill Livingstone, 1990; 85–99.
2 Avakian R, Flowers FP, Araujo OE, Ramos-Caro FA. Toxic epidermal necrolysis: a review. *J Am Acad Dermatol* 1991; **25**: 69–79.
3 Wilkins J, Morrison L, White CR. Oculocutaneous manifestations of the erythema multiforme/Stevens–Johnson syndrome/toxic epidermal necrolysis spectrum. *Dermatol Clin* 1992; **10**: 571–82.

Epidermolysis bullosa

The conjunctiva and cornea may be affected in both the congenital [1–4] and the acquired [5,6] forms of epidermolysis bullosa (EB).

More than two-thirds of patients with recessive dystrophic EB have potentially serious ocular involvement. The conjunctiva lacks anchoring fibrils and is therefore, like the skin, liable to suffer bullous and cicatricial changes following minor trauma [7].

Ophthalmological advice is needed to prevent deformity of the eyelids and ectropion. Exposure of the cornea when the eye is shut (lagophthalmos) is a major threat, as it leads to drying and infection of the cornea. Scarring around the tear ducts can further reduce lubrication of the cornea, and

artificial tears may be required. Oculoplastic surgery may be needed in some cases.

Corneal abrasion and scarring is also common, with the risk of loss of visual acuity.

REFERENCES

1 McDonnell PJ, Spalton DJ. The ocular signs and complications of epidermolysis bullosa. *J R Soc Med* 1988; **81**: 576–8.
2 McDonnell PJ. The eye in dystrophic epidermolysis bullosa. *Eye* 1989; **3**: 79–83.
3 Gans LA. Eye lesions of epidermolysis bullosa. *Arch Dermatol* 1988; **124**: 762–4.
4 Granek H, Baden HP. Corneal involvement in epidermolysis bullosa simplex. *Arch Ophthalmol* 1980; **79**: 464–70.
5 Zierhut M, Thiel H-J, Weidle EG *et al*. Ocular involvement in epidermolysis bullosa acquisita. *Arch Ophthalmol* 1989; **107**: 398–401.
6 Richter BJ, McNutt S. The spectrum of epidermolysis bullosa acquisita. *Arch Dermatol* 1979; **115**: 1325–8.
7 Iwamoto M, Haik BG, Iwamoto T. The ultrastructural defect in conjunctiva from a case of recessive dystrophic epidermolysis bullosa. *Arch Ophthalmol* 1991; **109**: 1382–6.

Incontinentia pigmenti

Ocular changes are quite common in this rare genodermatosis [1]. As they are generally not severe and over 90% of patients appear to have normal vision, they may not be recognized by dermatologists. Squints with refractive errors occur in over one-third of patients, and they can result in mild unilateral visual impairment. Abnormalities of the developing retinal vessels and underlying pigment cells occur in 40% of cases. New vessel formation, bleeding and fibrosis can occur, as in the retinopathy of prematurity. In some patients, there may be intraocular scarring and even blindness. Other recorded associations include microphthalmos, cataracts and optic atrophy.

Regular screening by an ophthalmologist is recommended, as photocoagulation and cryotherapy have been shown to cause regression of new vessel formation [2,3]. Squint and amblyopia may also develop as the child grows older.

REFERENCES

1 Landy SJ, Donnai D. Incontinentia pigmenti (Bloch–Sulzberger syndrome). *J Med Genet* 1993; **30**: 53–9.
2 Nishimura M, Oka Y, Tagaki I *et al*. The clinical features and treatment of the retinopathy of Bloch–Sulzberger disease (incontinentia pigmenti). *Jpn J Ophthalmol* 1980; **24**: 310–19.
3 Rahi J, Hungerford J. Early diagnosis of the retinopathy of incontinentia pigmenti: successful treatment by cryotherapy. *Br J Ophthalmol* 1990; **74**: 377–9.

The cornea

Slit-lamp microscopy is a most useful technique for examining the transparent media of the eye, i.e. the cornea, aqueous humour, lens and vitreous.

The instrument consists of a horizontally mounted microscope, and a lamp that produces a variable slit of light, which illuminates the point of focus of the microscope. The narrow slit beam gives the effect of an optical section, and allows differences in optical density to be visualized. In the normal eye, the anterior and posterior surfaces of the cornea show clearly and the corneal stroma reflects some light, but the aqueous humour is optically empty.

Corneal inflammation (keratitis) produces a white rather than a red opacity, because of the cornea's avascularity.

Ocular herpes simplex infection

This important viral infection is the commonest cause of corneal opacities in developed countries [1]. As in the case of the skin, the infection may be primary or secondary. The majority of isolates from adults with ocular herpes simplex are herpes simplex virus type 1 (HSV-1) but HSV-2 infection can occur in infants who acquire the primary infection from the maternal genital tract.

Primary herpes simplex infection. Primary ocular infection can occur in infancy with minimal involvement of the eyelids. It generally causes a follicular conjunctivitis, which persists for 2–3 weeks, and involvement of the cornea occurs in about 30% of cases. The prognosis is very good unless topical steroids are used [2,3].

Recurrent herpetic conjunctivitis. This condition can occur in the absence of cutaneous or corneal lesions, when it is difficult to diagnose, and is readily mistaken for an adenoviral infection [4]. It causes acute follicular conjunctivitis with painful swelling of the pre-auricular lymph nodes. There may be small herpetic vesicles on the adjoining lids, or a superficial punctate keratitis. It is important to avoid topical steroid therapy for this condition because of the risk of provoking a dendritic ulcer.

Dendritic ulcer (recurrent herpetic keratitis). Herpes simplex infection of the cornea starts with an acutely painful eye, lacrimation and photophobia. The earliest visible changes consist of fine, linear, epithelial opacities. These later form small vesicles, which break down to leave raw areas that stain with fluorescein or Rose Bengal. The latter is preferable as it does not diffuse so readily into the corneal stroma and mask any underlying oedema or cellular infiltrate. It also outlines the whole of the infected area, rather than just the ulcer. Dendritic ulcers have a characteristic pattern of irregular, zig-zag-shaped, branched lines with rounded tips. The corneal sensation is diminished, and the lesions are often slow to heal.

If left untreated, the dendritic ulcer may heal in 5–10 days, but the epithelial defect may remain for a longer period. Persistent lesions may be due to continuing viral activity, but they may also result from the effect of topical antiviral agents, which can slow the rate of epithelial regeneration.

Dendritic ulcers are usually unilateral and there is not usually any associated conjunctivitis. Bilateral ulcers can, however, occur in immunodeficient or atopic subjects [5].

A patient who has had an attack of herpetic keratitis has almost a 50% chance of recurrence in the next 2 years.

Corneal trophic (metaherpetic ulcers). After a dendritic ulcer has healed, the epithelium sometimes breaks down again to form a chronic ulcer with a heaped-up edge. This raised margin is composed of cells that are apparently unable to migrate across the damaged epithelium. The condition is not due to continuing viral activity, and antiviral therapy can damage the epithelium and make matters worse. This type of ulcer can persist for several weeks and there may be secondary bacterial invasion of the ulcerated surface.

Stromal herpes simplex keratitis. In about 30% of patients with dendritic ulcers, the infection spreads into the corneal stroma. Deep invasion of this type is a serious complication and there are several patterns of clinical activity, for details of which specialist texts must be consulted [6].

Herpes keratitis tends to be more severe in atopic patients, and stromal keratitis can cause severe ulceration or perforation of the cornea [5].

Herpes simplex uveitis. This condition may complicate herpetic stromal keratitis, but it occasionally presents without any evidence of corneal involvement [7]. In many cases of uveitis that follow herpes simplex infection of the eye, the virus cannot be isolated, and immunological factors are thought to play an important part in causing the damage [8,9].

Treatment. Many problems may arise in the management of ocular herpes, and an ophthalmologist should be consulted in all cases. It is vital to prevent the virus entering the corneal stroma, from whence it may be impossible to eradicate. Antiviral therapy should be given early in the course of the disease, and in cases with recurrent keratitis where 'trigger' factors such as fever or menstruation are recognized, it is wise to give prophylactic antiviral therapy after exposure to the 'trigger', even before symptoms have developed.

Current therapy is with antiviral drugs such as 3% topical aciclovir, idoxuridine, adenine arabinoside, or trifluorothymidine [6,10]. Where medical treatment has failed, surgical treatment such as keratoplasty should be considered, although the results are sometimes poor, especially in atopic subjects [5,11].

Topical steroid therapy can have a disastrous effect in herpes simplex infections of the eye. Dendritic ulcers treated with steroid eye drops rapidly lose their characteristic outline and become much more extensive and map-like in appearance [12]. As a result of better medical education, however, the severe management problems which were encountered in the 1960s are becoming less common [6].

REFERENCES

1 Liesegang TJ, Melton J III, Daly PJ. Epidemiology of ocular herpes simplex: incidence in Rochester, Minnesota, 1950 through 1982. *Arch Ophthalmol* 1989; **107**: 1155–9.
2 Nahmias AJ, Visintine AM, Caldwell DR *et al.* Eye infections with herpes simplex in neonates. *Surv Ophthalmol* 1976; **21**: 100–5.
3 Poirer RH. Herpetic ocular lesions in childhood. *Arch Ophthalmol* 1980; **98**: 704–6.
4 Darouger S, Woodland RM. Acute follicular conjunctivitis and kerato-conjunctivitis due to herpes simplex infection in London. *Br J Ophthalmol* 1978; **62**: 834–9.
5 Easty DL, Entwistle C, Funk A *et al.* Herpes simplex keratitis and keratoconus in the atopic patient. *Trans Ophthalmol Soc UK* 1975; **95**: 267–76.
6 Easty DL, ed. *Virus Disease of the Eye*. London: Lloyd Luke, 1985.
7 Sundmacher R, Neumann-Haefelin D. Herpes simplex infection. In: Silverstein AM, O'Connor R, eds. *International Symposium on Immunology and Immunopathology of the Eye*. New York: Masson; 1979: 255.
8 Oh JO. Primary and secondary herpes simplex uveitis in rabbits. *Surv Ophthalmol* 1976; **21**: 178–84.
9 Oh JO. Role of immunity in the pathogenesis of herpes simplex uveitis. In: Silverstein AM, O'Connor R, eds. *International Symposium on Immunology and Immunopathology of the Eye*. New York: Masson, 1979.
10 Collum LMT, O'Connor M, Logan P. Oral acyclovir in herpetic keratitis. *Trans Ophthalmol Soc UK* 1985; **104**: 629–34.
11 Witmer R. Results of keratoplasty in metaherpetic keratitis. In: Sundmacher R, ed. *Herpetic Eye Diseases*. Munich: Bergmann Verlag, 1981: 419–21.
12 Thygeson P. Historical observations on herpetic keratitis. *Surv Ophthalmol* 1976; **21**: 82–90.

Miscellaneous diseases

Punctate epithelial keratitis

This condition is a common complication of several viral infections including adenovirus, TRIC, varicella–zoster and primary herpes simplex. The condition presents with painful eyes and epiphora. Examination by the slit-lamp microscope after staining with fluorescein will reveal the characteristic small opacities on the surface of the cornea.

Superficial stromal keratitis

SYN. NUMMULAR KERATITIS

This condition may be caused by herpes zoster or by recurrent herpes simplex infections. It presents with blurring of vision and photophobia, and is characterized by areas of cellular infiltrate surrounded by haloes of stromal haze just below Bowman's membrane.

It responds to topical steroid therapy, but antiviral cover is also recommended.

Suppurative keratitis

Most patients with this serious condition have had some previous abnormality of the eye. It is due to secondary bacterial infection of the cornea, usually following some other cause of ulceration such as a herpetic infection or incorrect use of contact lenses. The eye is very painful, and on examination there is an abscess in the corneal stroma, which may extend into a hypopyon ulcer, with pus and fibrin in the anterior chamber. Common bacterial causes include staphylococci, streptococci, pneumococci and pseudomonas. Urgent treatment with the appropriate systemic antibiotic in high dosage is required. Infection with *Acanthamoeba* may be encountered in contact lens wearers.

Keratoconus

This is a condition of uncertain aetiology in which the apex of the cornea bulges progressively to produce visual deterioration (myopic astigmatism). It is more common in atopic subjects. Contact lenses can produce a dramatic improvement in the vision, but in severe cases corneal grafting may be necessary.

Band keratopathy

A band-like opacity in the cornea may be produced by an area of subepithelial calcium deposition. It is most commonly seen in the presence of chronic inflammation such as Still's disease.

Corneal changes in other dermatoses

The ichthyoses

Numerous ocular changes have been reported in various ichthyotic disorders [1–3].

In ichthyosis vulgaris, there may be corneal changes, including stromal opacities, punctate erosions, and band keratopathy. X-linked ichthyosis is associated with the same changes, but in addition there may be corneal opacities in the region of Desçemet's membrane. In lamellar ichthyosis, the conjunctiva may be keratinized, and in more than 50% of cases there is some degree of ectropion, which may cause exposure keratitis. Keratitis also occurs in the keratitis, ichthyosis, deafness syndrome (KIDS), and there are pigmentary retinal changes in Refsum's disease and in the Sjögren–Larrson syndrome.

Darier's disease

In this condition, the cornea may show irregular deposits peripherally, with linear whorls in the centre, but these are asymptomatic [4].

REFERENCES

1 Jay B, Blach RK, Wells RS. Ocular manifestations of ichthyosis. *Br J Ophthalmol* 1968; **52**: 217–26.
2 Rand RE, Baden HP. The ichthyoses—a review. *J Am Acad Dermatol* 1983; **8**: 285–305.
3 Sever R, Frost P, Weinstein G. Eye changes in ichthyoses. *JAMA* 1968; **206**: 2283–6.
4 Blackman HJ, Rodrigues R, Peck GL. Corneal lesions in keratosis follicularis. *Ophthalmology* 1980; **87**: 931–43.

UV radiation

UV irradiation of all wavelengths can damage the eye [1–5], and the damage depends on the wavelength of the irradiation. The conjunctiva and cornea absorb UV rays of less than 300 nm, and the lens absorbs rays of 300–400 nm. Some forms of cataract and senile macular degeneration may be related to UV exposure [6–9].

Pterygium

This is a degenerative condition of the anterior lamina of the cornea (*Bowman's membrane*) and the superficial corneal lamellae, which results in vascular tissue extending over the epithelium. The condition is probably due to excessive exposure to UV radiation [10], and in northern Australia pterygium affects 15% of men over 60 years of age [11].

The process begins at the lateral edges of the cornea and extends towards the centre, taking a continuation of the conjunctival epithelium with it. The pterygium commonly stops growing before it causes significant visual impairment. Vision is impaired if the pterygium encroaches on the pupil. Such cases require surgical treatment.

Photokeratitis

UVB irradiation causes conjunctivitis and photokeratitis, and it may be involved in other corneal and conjunctival diseases [1,6]. Epidemiological evidence suggests it is an important cause of carcinoma of the conjunctiva [12].

PUVA therapy has been shown to cause cataracts in both animals and humans [13,14]. It is important that suitable sunglasses should be worn on the day of PUVA therapy until the psoralen has been eliminated. Moseley *et al.* [15] found that of 58 types of glasses tested only 66% gave adequate protection, and 19% of the sunglasses allowed dangerous levels of UV transmission. McKinlay [5] has reviewed the safety limits for various types of irradiation of the eye. Ophthalmologists in Wisconsin treated more than 150 patients in a 12-month period for ocular damage, mainly photokeratitis, due to tanning devices [16].

REFERENCES

1 Lerman S, van Voorhees A. Cutaneous and ocular ramifications of ultraviolet radiation. *Dermatol Clin* 1992; **10**: 483–504.
2 Absolon MJ. Effect of ultra-violet light on the eye. *Trans Ophthalmol Soc UK* 1985; **104**: 522–3.
3 Collier R *et al.* Effects of ambient near-UV exposure. *ARVO Abstracts* 1984; 18.
4 Jackson EM. *Photobiology of the Skin and the Eye*. New York: Marcel Dekker, 1986.
5 McKinlay AF, ed. *Hazards of Optical Radiation*. Bristol: Hilger, 1988.
6 Bochow TW. UV exposure and risk of posterior subcapsular cataracts. *Arch Ophthalmol* 1989; **107**: 369–72.
7 Cheng H. Causes of cataract. *Br Med J* 1989; **298**: 1470–1.
8 Taylor HR, West SK, Rosenthal FS. Effect of ultraviolet radiation on cataract formation. *N Engl J Med* 1988; **319**: 1429–33.
9 Cruickshank CJ, Klein R, Klein B. Sunlight and age-related macular degeneration: the Beaver Dam study. *Arch Ophthalmol* 1993; **111**: 514–18.
10 Karai I, Horiguchi S. Pterygium in welders. *Br J Ophthalmol* 1984; **68**: 347–9.
11 Moran DJ, Hollows FC. Pterygium and UV radiation. A positive correlation. *Br J Ophthalmol* 1984; **68**: 343–6.
12 Newton R, Ferlay J, Reeves G *et al.* Effect of ambient solar ultra-violet radiation on incidence of squamous-cell carcinoma of the eye. *Lancet* 1996; **347**: 1450–1.
13 Hammersley O, Jessen F. A retrospective study of cataract formation in 96 patients treated with PUVA. *Acta Derm Venereol (Stockh)* 1982; **62**: 444–6.
14 Lafond G, Roy PE, Grenier R. Lens opacities appearing during therapy with methoxsalen and long-wave UV radiation. *Can J Ophthalmol* 1984; **19**: 173–5.
15 Moseley H, Lever R, Jones SK. The suitability of sunglasses used by patients following ingestion of psoralens. *Br J Dermatol* 1988; **118**: 247–53.
16 Morbidity and Mortality Report Centers for Disease Control. Injuries associated with ultraviolet tanning devices—Wisconsin. *Arch Dermatol* 1989; **125**: 887–8.

The sclera

The sclera is composed of collagen and elastic tissue, and therefore it can be involved in many diseases of connective tissue.

Blue sclerae

If the sclera becomes thin, the underlying melanin lining the retina shows on the surface as a blue colour, just as melanin in the skin can shine through the connective tissue in a blue naevus. Osteogenesis imperfecta is a classical cause of blue sclerae[1]. Blue–black discoloration of the sclerae can also follow minocycline therapy [2] (Fig. 67.20).

If the sclera is weakened or thinned sufficiently it may form a localized bulge called a *staphyloma*.

Ochronosis

A black pigment derived from homogentisic acid is deposited in the connective tissue, and this is sometimes visible as blue–black patches in the sclera (Chapter 59). This pigmentation does not usually appear before middle age (Fig. 67.21).

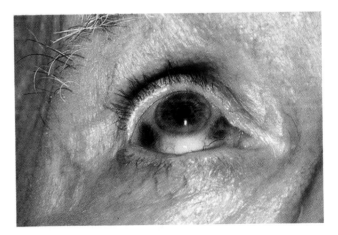

Fig. 67.20 Blue–black discoloration of the sclera due to minocycline therapy. (Courtesy of Dr C. Archer, Bristol Royal Infirmary, Bristol, UK.)

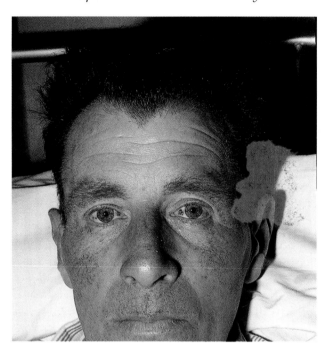

Fig. 67.21 Pigmented sclerae and nose due to ochronosis in a patient with alkaptonuria.

Episcleritis

Inflammation of the superficial layer of the sclera is called episcleritis. The eye is red and uncomfortable, but in contrast to scleritis the dilated vessels can be moved over the eyeball. The cause is unknown, but it is presumed to be an immunological disease. Approximately 30% of cases have an associated medical condition such as herpes zoster, rheumatoid arthritis, tuberculosis or a hypersensitivity disorder (e.g. the 'desert bumps' reaction of coccidiodomycosis, San Joaquim Valley Fever). Episcleritis is a benign, recurring condition and it does not progress to scleritis except when it is due to herpes zoster [3].

In nodular episcleritis, the affected area is raised and localized, and is usually situated near the limbus.

Most cases resolve within 3 weeks and so treatment is usually unnecessary, but for persistent or uncomfortable cases sodium chloride eye drops are helpful.

Scleritis

Inflammation of the deeper layers of the collagen is called scleritis. It is commonly due to an underlying medical or dermatological condition (Table 67.7) [4,5].

Scleritis is a serious condition, which is often bilateral and recurrent and may lead to blindness. It causes severe pain with swelling of the eyelids, tenderness of the globe, and marked dilatation of the deep and superficial episcleral vessels. Scleritis is always accompanied by episcleritis, but if there is any doubt about whether scleritis is present,

Table 67.7 Diseases associated with scleritis.

Rheumatoid disease
Polyarteritis nodosa
Wegener's disease
Relapsing polychondritis [6,7]
Herpes zoster
Gout
Erythema nodosum

adrenaline eyedrops can be instilled, which will constrict the episcleral vessels only. The dilated scleral vessels are then visible as a purple discoloration.

In nodular scleritis, there is a localized painful lesion with scleral oedema. When the attack settles, the sclera becomes transparent, leaving a slate-grey area where the choroid shines through.

In diffuse scleritis, the pain is less severe, but the cornea may be involved causing keratitis and keratolysis ('corneal melt').

Scleromalacia perforans

This condition is a form of nodular scleritis, which is often free from pain and inflammation. The nodule slowly breaks down to leave a hole in the sclera, with the choroid visible beneath.

All types of scleritis may lead to further ocular complications including keratitis, uveitis, glaucoma, cataract and retinal detachment. Treatment is with topical steroids, in combination with systemic glucocorticoids or non-steroidal anti-inflammatory agents.

The sclera is formed of collagen, and in some ways the eye resembles a ball-and-socket joint. It will be seen from Table 67.7 that many of the diseases which cause scleritis are also associated with arthritis. About 50% of cases of scleritis have rheumatoid disease, and scleritis predicts a poor prognosis for the arthritis. Treatment is with high-dose systemic steroids in conjunction with immunosuppressive therapy.

REFERENCES

1 Kaiser-Kupffer MI, Podgor MJM, McClain L *et al.* Correlation of ocular rigidity and blue sclerae in osteogenesis imperfecta. *Trans Ophthalmol Soc UK* 1985; **104**: 191–5.
2 Sabroe RA, Archer CB, Harlow D *et al.* Minocycline-induced discolouration of the sclerae. *Br J Dermatol* 1996; **135**: 314–16.
3 Watson PG, Hayreh SS. Scleritis and episcleritis. *Br J Ophthalmol* 1976; **60**: 163–91.
4 McGavin DD, Williamson J, Forrester JV *et al.* Episcleritis and scleritis. A study of their clinical manifestations and association with rheumatoid disease. *Br J Ophthalmol* 1976; **60**: 192–226.
5 Watson PG. Diseases of the sclera and episclera. In: Duane TD, ed. *Clinical Ophthalmology* Vol. 4. *External Diseases: the Uvea.* Hagerstown, MD: Harper and Row, 1986.
6 Stiles MC. Relapsing polychondritis. *Arch Ophthalmol* 1989; **107**: 277–9.
7 Isaak BL, Liesegang TJ, Michet CJ, Jr. Ocular and systemic findings in relapsing polychondritis. *Ophthalmology* 1986; **93**: 681–9.

The uveal tract

This tract is formed from the iris, the ciliary body and the choroid.

The iris

Flecks of pigment or freckles on the iris are common and are of no importance. Melanocytic naevi occasionally occur in otherwise normal people and, as in the skin, they may rarely undergo malignant transformation.

Lisch nodules

These are small melanocytic naevi of the iris, which occur in 95% of cases of generalized neurofibromatosis [1,2]. They are best detected by slit-lamp examination. In segmental neurofibromatosis Lisch nodules may be confined to the affected side. Other ocular manifestations of neurofibromatosis include plexiform neuroma of the lids (often with associated glaucoma), thickening of the corneal nerves, and retinal astrocytic hamartomas. The latter are flat, pale lesions, which may gradually expand into a 'mulberry' form.

Leiomyoma of the iris

Leiomyoma of the iris, which arises from the muscle cells, resembles a malignant melanoma clinically, but it does not metastasize.

Waardenburg's syndrome

This syndrome (Chapter 39) can be associated with heterochromasia or hypopigmentation of the iris.

REFERENCES

1 Jakobiec FA. Neurofibromatosis. In: Duane TD *et al.* ed *Clinical Ophthalmology*, Vol. 2. Hagerstown, MD: Harper and Row, 1984.
2 Weleber RG, Zonana J. Iris hamartoma in segmental neurofibromatosis. *Am J Ophthalmol* 1983; **96**: 740–2.

Acute uveitis
SYN. INFLAMMATION OF THE UVEAL TRACT

The classical symptoms are pain, photophobia, lacrimation and blurred vision. There is conjunctival injection of the ciliary type, with injected vessels around the limbus. The iris pattern is blurred, due to exudation of protein and cells into the anterior chamber. Clumps of exudate and cells may settle on the posterior surface of the cornea to form precipitates. The pupil constricts and may become adherent to the anterior surface of the lens (posterior synechiae). These adhesions may cause the pupil to become irregular, and this is particularly noticeable after the application of mydriatics.

In many cases of uveitis, no underlying disease is found, but possible associations include ankylosing spondylitis, inflammatory bowel disease, sarcoidosis, Reiter's disease, Behçet's disease, viral illnesses and syphilis.

Ocular Behçet's disease

Behçet's disease affects the eye, the mouth and the skin (Chapter 69). In the eye, it classically produces a relapsing iritis with hypopyon, but conjunctivitis, episcleritis, keratitis, cellular infiltrates of the vitreous body, retinitis, retinal thrombosis, optic atrophy and papilloedema have also been reported [1–3]. Ocular involvement occurs in about 50% of patients with Behçet's disease, and if the retina is involved the long-term prognosis for vision is poor, with complete blindness ensuing in many cases [4].

In the past, the disease was suppressed with prednisolone, although chlorambucil and colchicine have also been used successfully [4,5]. Cyclosporin with low-dose prednisolone is now used for severe cases. It can produce a rapid improvement in visual acuity, although its use is limited by its side-effects, and some cases have a severe relapse when the cyclosporin is withdrawn [6–8].

REFERENCES

1 Bietti GB, Bruna F. An ophthalmic report on Behçet's disease. In: Monacelli M, ed. *International Symposium on Behçet's Disease*. Basel: Karger, 1966: 79–92.
2 Kalbian VV, Challis MT. Behçet's disease: report of 12 cases with 3 manifesting as papilloedema. *Am J Med* 1970; **49**: 823–9.
3 Pazarh H. Ocular involvement in Behçet's disease. In: Lehner T, Barnes CG, eds. *Recent Advances in Behçet's Disease*. London: RSM International Congress Symposium Series 103, 1986.
4 Benezra D, Cohen E. Treatment and prognosis in ocular Behçet's disease. *Br J Ophthalmol* 1986; **70**: 589–95.
5 Lightman S. Uveitis management. *Lancet* 1991; **338**: 1501–4.
6 Masuda K, Nakajima A, Urayama A *et al.* Double masked study of cyclosporin versus colchicine, and long-term open study of cyclosporin in Behçet's disease. *Lancet* 1989; **i**: 1094–6.
7 Muftuoglu A, Pazarli H, Yurdakul S *et al.* Short-term cyclosporin treatment of Behçet's disease. *Br J Ophthalmol* 1987; **71**: 387–90.
8 Nussenblatt RB, Palestine AG. Cyclosporin: immunology, pharmacology and therapeutic uses. *Surv Ophthalmol* 1986; **31**: 159–69.

Sarcoidosis

Ocular lesions occur in about 40% of black patients and in about 20% of white patients. Uveitis and small granulomatous lesions of the conjunctiva are common, but choroiditis and dry eye also occur [1–3]. Conjunctival lesions offer a useful site for biopsy.

REFERENCES

1 Karcioglu ZA, Brear R. Conjunctival biopsy in sarcoidosis. *Am J Ophthalmol* 1985; **99**: 68–70.
2 Obendorf CD. Sarcoidosis and its ophthalmologic manifestations. *Am J Ophthalmol* 1978; **86**: 648–52.
3 Weinreb RN, Kimura SJ. Uveitis associated with sarcoidosis or angiotension converting enzyme. *Am J Ophthalmol* 1980; **89**: 180–2.

The lens

Cataract

A small opacity in the lens may be asymptomatic in the early stages. Cataracts may be detected by looking at the pupil through the ophthalmoscope held about 20 cm from the eye. The cataract will be seen silhouetted against the 'red reflex'. Dermatologists need to be aware that systemic steroid therapy can cause cataracts in the back of the lens, and if they occur the drug should, if possible, be withdrawn. Other causes of cataract of relevance to dermatologists include UV or X-irradiation, atopic eczema and Refsum's disease. Congenital varicella can cause microphthalmia with cataracts.

Ectopia lentis

If the suspensory ligament of the lens is absent, the lens may become displaced and its edge may be seen through the ophthalmoscope. In Marfan's syndrome, ectopia lentis is often associated with myopia and astigmatism, and the weakened zonule predisposes to traumatic dislocation of the lens.

The choroid and retina

Many general medical conditions produce characteristic changes, which can be seen on fundoscopy. Some conditions not mentioned above which are of particular interest to the dermatologist are as follows.

Tuberous sclerosis (Chapter 12)

Astrocytic hamartoma is a common complication, and vision is affected if it involves the optic disc. It starts as a grey patch with poorly defined edges, and progresses to a lobulated, yellowish 'mulberry' tumour. Other ocular complications include ocular nerve palsy, conjunctivitis, keratoconus and glaucoma [1,2].

Sturge–Weber syndrome (Chapter 15)

Cavernous angioma of the choroid is common in this syndrome, either as a small, flat lesion in the posterior fundus, or as a more diffuse red area, looking like velvet. Conjunctival and episcleral angiomas also occur. Glaucoma is a complication in about 30% of cases.

In the past, the term *phakomatosis* has been used to describe various conditions characterized by hamartomas of the skin and the eyes, for example neurofibromatosis, tuberous sclerosis and Sturge–Weber syndrome. The term is unsatisfactory for several reasons, however, and its use is now discouraged.

Epidermal naevus syndrome (Chapter 15)

This affects the eye in one-third of cases. The most common lesion is involvement of the eyelid or conjunctiva, but many internal problems have been reported.

Pseudoxanthoma elasticum (Chapter 44)

Angioid streaks in the retina are an important diagnostic feature of this condition.

Focal dermal hypoplasia of Goltz (Chapter 12)

Numerous ocular abnormalities have been reported in this condition, including corneal opacities, opaque vitreous humour, lens subluxation, coloboma, blue sclera, strabismus, microphthalmos and anophthalmos [3]. The eyes are affected in about 20% of cases.

Oculocerebrocutaneous syndrome (Chapter 15)
SYN. DELLEMAN–ORTHRYS SYNDROME

This rare condition is the differential diagnosis of Goltz disease (above). The syndrome includes various malformations, including focal dermal hypoplasia, preorbital or postauricular skin tags, orbital cysts, microphthalmia, eyelid coloboma, cerebral defects, epilepsy and developmental delay [4].

Systemic lupus erythematosus

Retinal changes are not uncommon, including flame-shaped haemorrhages, and 'cotton-wool' spots (cytoid bodies) due to small retinal infarcts. Other ocular complications include keratoconjunctivitis sicca and band keratopathy [5,6].

Episcleritis occurs in about 10% of patients with systemic lupus erythematosus, although it is often asymptomatic [7]. Episcleritis does not seem to occur in chronic cutaneous lupus erythematosus, although erythematous plaques on the eyelids and conjunctival involvement are relatively common in this condition [7]. Discoid lupus erythematosus affects the eyelids, and is occasionally confined to that region [8].

The bulbar conjunctival mucosa is a suitable tissue for the lupus band test, using a 3 mm punch biopsy [9]. In systemic lupus erythematosus, the conjunctival test was positive in five of 12 cases, and in chronic cutaneous lupus erythematosus the test was positive in 10 of 20 cases. These positive results were higher than those obtained using forearm skin and lip, and the conjunctival test sometimes gave a positive result when both the skin and lip were negative.

Periorbital oedema with bruising occurs rarely, especially with lupus erythematosus profundus [10].

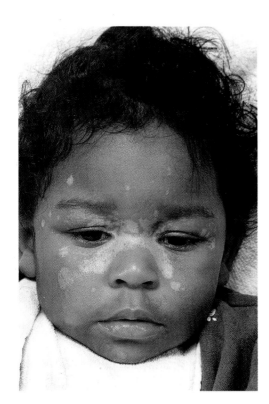

Fig. 67.22 Depigmented patches around the eyes in a child who had neonatal lupus erythematosus. (Courtesy of Dr D. Atherton, Great Ormond Street Hospital for Sick Children, London, UK.)

Neonatal lupus (Chapter 14). Periorbital pigmentation in this condition classically gives a raccoon-like appearance. At a later stage, the skin may be depigmented (Fig. 67.22).

Acute leukaemia

Most patients with acute leukaemia will develop eye lesions at some stage. Haemorrhagic retinopathy or infiltrate are common, and there may be asymptomatic deposits in the choroid. Proptosis also occurs due to dense infiltrates in the orbit [11].

Mycosis fungoides

There may be a wide range of eye problems, ectropion secondary to erythroderma being the commonest. Other problems may include conjunctival or lacrimal gland tumours, keratitis, uveitis, optic atrophy, retinopathy and proptosis [12].

Wegener's granulomatosis

Ocular involvement is common, including keratoconjunctivitis, granulomatous scleritis or uveitis, orbital granuloma and retinal detachment [13,14].

Candida of the eye

Cutaneous *Candida* infection rarely affects the eye, but in chronic mucocutaneous candidosis associated with immunodeficiency there may be blepharitis, keratoconjunctivitis and corneal ulceration. In *Candida* septicaemia complicating debilitation, drug abuse or prolonged use of indwelling catheters, etc., there may be *Candida* endophthalmitis affecting almost any of the ocular tissues. There may be white lesions of the choroid or retina, with filamentous extensions into the vitreous [15,16].

Noonan's syndrome (Chapter 12)

Ocular features of this condition include hypertelorism, slanting palpebral fissures and epicanthic folds. Bilateral orbital oedema can also occur, possibly due to lymphatic hypoplasia [17].

A detailed account of the retinal changes in these and other diseases is given in the reference text by Gass [18].

REFERENCES

1 Grover WD. Early recognition of tuberous sclerosis by fundoscopic examination. *J Pediatr* 1969; **75**: 991–2.
2 Schwartz PL, Beards JA, Maris PJ *et al.* Tuberous sclerosis associated with retinal angioma. *Am J Ophthalmol* 1980; **90**: 485–8.
3 Thomas JV, Yoshizemi MO, Beyer CK *et al.* Ocular manifestations of focal dermal hypoplasia syndrome. *Arch Ophthalmol* 1977; **95**: 1977–2001.
4 Wilson RD, Traverse L, Hall JG *et al.* Oculo-cerebro-cutaneous syndrome. *Am J Ophthalmol* 1985; **99**: 142–8.
5 Huey C, Jakobiec FA, Iwamoto PR *et al.* Discoid lupus erythematosus of the eyelids. *Ophthalmology* 1983; **90**: 1389–98.
6 Kearns W, Wood W, Marchese A. Chronic cutaneous lupus including the eyelid. *Ann Ophthalmol* 1982; **14**: 1009–10.
7 Burge SM, Frith PA, Frith RP, Juniper RP *et al.* Mucosal involvement in systemic and chronic cutaneous lupus erythematosus. *Br J Dermatol* 1989; **121**: 727–41.
8 Tosti A, Tosti G. Discoid lupus erythematosus solely involving the eyelids: report of 3 cases. *J Am Acad Dermatol* 1987; **16**: 1259–60.
9 Burge SM, Frith PA, Millard PR *et al.* The lupus band test in oral mucosa, conjunctiva and skin. *Br J Dermatol* 1989; **121**: 743–52.
10 Lodi A, Pozzi M, Agostoni A *et al.* Unusual onset of lupus erythematosus profundus. *Br J Dermatol* 1993; **129**: 96–7.
11 Allen R, Straatsma B. Ocular involvement in leukaemia and allied disorders. *Arch Ophthalmol* 1961; **66**: 490–4.
12 Stenson S, Ramsay DL. Ocular findings in mycosis fungoides. *Arch Ophthalmol* 1981; **99**: 272–4.
13 Fauci AS, Haynes BF, Katz P *et al.* Wegener's granulomatosis. Prospective clinical and therapeutic experience in 85 patients for 21 years. *Ann Intern Med* 1983; **98**: 76–85.
14 Koyama T, Matsuo N, Watanake Y *et al.* Wegener's granulomatosis with destructive ocular manifestations. *Am J Ophthalmol* 1984; **98**: 736–40.
15 Aguilar GL, Blumenkrantz MS, Egbert PR *et al.* Candida endophthalmitis after intravenous drug abuse. *Arch Ophthalmol* 1979; **97**: 96–100.
16 Edwards JE, Jr, Foos RY, Montgomerie JZ. Ocular manifestations of *Candida* septicaemia. Review of 76 cases of haematogenous spread of *Candida* endophthalmitis. *Medicine* 1974; **53**: 47–55.
17 Phillips WG, Dunnill MGS, Kurwa AR, Black MM. Orbital oedema: an unusual presentation of Noonan's syndrome. *Br J Dermatol* 1993; **129**: 190–2.
18 Gass JDM. *The Stereoscopic Atlas of Macular Disease.* St Louis: Mosby, 1987.

The orbit

Proptosis

Thyrotoxic exophthalmos

The staring appearance of patients with exophthalmos is usually due to eyelid retraction, with only a relatively mild degree of protrusion of the globe (Fig. 67.23). These cases generally improve when the hyperthyroidism (if present) is corrected, but many cases of 'dysthyroid' eye disease have normal thyroid function tests.

A much more serious form of proptosis associated with ophthalmoplegia occurs in some cases. This may follow thyroidectomy, but it also occurs in euthyroid patients. This is due to involvement of the extraocular muscles, which become thickened and swollen by a lymphocytic infiltrate and deposition of mucopolysaccharides. Cases occasionally present to the dermatologist with marked puffiness of the periorbital tissues or with associated pretibial myxoedema.

The management of exophthalmos associated with ophthalmoplegia is best carried out by an ophthalmologist working closely with an endocrinologist.

Orbital cellulitis

Infection of the facial skin or nasal sinuses may spread to the orbit, producing acute swelling with proptosis and marked oedema of the conjunctiva and lids. The patient is unwell, and eye movements are restricted. If untreated, this condition may progress to cavernous sinus thrombosis, with visual loss and papilloedema. Urgent treatment with high-dose antibiotics is required, and attempts should be made to culture the organism from the nose, conjunctiva, throat and any septic lesions on the skin. CT scan should be performed to detect sinus disease, which may require urgent referral to an ear, nose, and throat specialist.

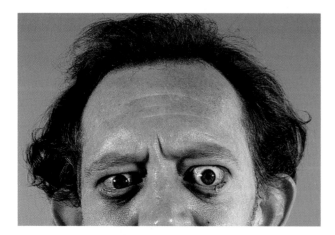

Fig. 67.23 Exophthalmos due to thyrotoxicosis.

Orbital cellulitis is particularly important in children, in whom blindness may ensue in hours. The differential diagnosis in a child includes acute leukaemic infiltrate and neuroblastoma.

Subacute or chronic orbital inflammation

This may occur with sarcoid, syphilis or 'orbital pseudo-tumour' (a non-neoplastic infiltration of the orbit by lymphocytes and plasma cells).

Other causes

Other orbital causes of proptosis include benign or malignant tumours of the orbit, malignant infiltrates (e.g. from leukaemia or lymphoma) and mucocele.

Microphthalmos

Several congenital syndromes cause a small eyeball associated with a cutaneous defect.

In the Hallerman–Streiff syndrome (Chapter 15), bilateral microphthalmos is associated with cataracts, sparse eyebrows and eyelashes, and various cutaneous, skeletal and dental defects.

In the Cross syndrome, there is hypopigmentation, microphthalamos, an opaque cornea, nystagmus, mental deficiency and spasticity (Chapter 39).

Microphthalmos also occurs in the congenital rubella syndrome.

Complications of dermatological therapy

Glucocorticoids

Both topical and systemic glucocorticosteroids can have adverse effects on the eye [1].

Systemic steroids predispose to glaucoma, posterior subcapsular cataract and ocular infection, especially a flare-up of herpetic keratitis.

Topical steroid eyedrops are often used to suppress inflammatory disease of the eye that is not infective in origin. They can cause numerous problems, as can potent steroid preparations applied to the eyelids.

Superinfection

Ocular infection is more likely to develop because of the suppression of the inflammatory response, and if it does occur the characteristic signs will be masked. Bacterial infections may progress, or may be complicated by fungal or viral infection, especially herpes simplex. Perforation of dendritic ulcers was a rare occurrence before the advent of local steroid preparations.

Topical steroids may predispose to *Pseudomonas* corneal ulcers, *Chlamydia trachomatis* activation, and fungal keratitis. Systemic steroids predispose to *Candida* endophthalmitis [1].

Glaucoma

Open-angle glaucoma is usually a genetic disorder with recessive inheritance. About one-third of the USA population is heterozygous for this gene and possession of only one of the glaucoma genes makes the subject more liable to develop steroid-induced glaucoma [2].

Patients requiring long-term steroid eye drops should have their ocular pressures measured at regular intervals, particularly if they have a first-degree relative who has suffered from glaucoma [3].

Unsupervised self-medication with steroid eye drops (e.g. for hayfever) is dangerous and has caused blindness [4].

Some of the newer steroid preparations such as fluorometholone appear less likely to increase intraocular pressure [3,5].

Cataract

Posterior subcapsular cataract occasionally follows the use of steroid eye drops, although it is much more likely after the use of systemic steroid therapy [6,7].

Rebound inflammation

Rapid tapering of topical steroid therapy for ocular inflammation in erythema multiforme, Reiter's syndrome, etc. may lead to rebound inflammation, which may cause corneal ulceration or even perforation. Most cases of rebound uveitis will respond to treatment with a cycloplegic and topical steroids within 3–10 days [1].

Retarded healing

Both topical and systemic steroids will retard corneal epithelial healing.

Other ocular complications of steroids

These include ptosis, mydriasis, exophthalmos (in euthyroid patients), blue sclerae in children, refractive changes and pseudotumour cerebri [1].

Retinoids

Isotretinoin frequently causes ocular side-effects [8–11] and in one series of 237 patients, 261 adverse ocular effects were recorded [12]. Blepharoconjunctivitis and subjective complaints of blurred vision or dry eyes are common, and many patients cannot tolerate contact lenses while receiving isotretinoin. More serious reactions include papilloedema, pseudotumour cerebri (raised intracranial pressure), and white or grey corneal opacities, although all these are reversible when the drug is stopped. Mild disturbances of retinal function (poor night vision and excessive glare sensitivity) have also been reported [13].

Etretinate causes the same ocular side-effects as isotretinoin, but in addition it can cause impaired colour vision [14].

Antimalarials

Chloroquine selectively accumulates in the eye due to binding to melanin, and it can cause retinal damage [15]. The classical 'bull's eye' maculopathy is associated with severe and irreversible loss of vision, but this is now rarely seen. There is no certain way to detect early retinal damage, despite the use of various screening tests such as the electro-oculogram and colour-vision testing [16]. Most cases of retinopathy have been reported in patients receiving long-term high doses of chloroquine.

Other eye changes reported with chloroquine therapy have included decreased colour vision, scotomas, retinal oedema, macular pigmentation, loss of the corneal reflex and corneal deposits.

Ocular toxicity is rare with daily doses less than 4 mg/kg (lean body weight) of chloroquine or 6.5 mg/kg of hydroxychloroquine sulphate, provided renal function is normal. Patients should have an initial baseline examination by an ophthalmologist before starting treatment with antimalarials, but most experts now feel that regular monitoring is not necessary, although treatment should be stopped and an ophthalmological opinion obtained if any visual abnormality develops.

The Amsler grid, a white grid superimposed on a black background, can be used by the patient for regular testing at home. The development of wavy, grey or indistinct lines during monocular fixation on the central white spot may indicate incipient visual field defects.

Retinal crystals due to carotenoids

Beta-carotene and canthaxanthine are plant pigments which tend to deposit in the stratum corneum to produce an orange or bronze discoloration [17,18]. They have a potential photo-protective effect and have been used in some countries to produce an artificial 'tan'. About 10–40% of people who take canthaxanthine for tanning develop small, bright-yellow crystals in the retinae, easily visible on fundoscopy [19]. The crystals have little or no effect on retinal function, although a few patients have asymptomatic field defects. The crystalline retinopathy tends to persist for at least a year after the canthaxanthine is stopped.

REFERENCES

1 Renfro L, Snow JS. Ocular effects of systemic steroids. *Dermatol Clin* 1992; **10**: 505–12.
2 Becker B, Hahn KA. Topical steroids and heredity in primary open angle glaucoma. *Am J Ophthalmol* 1964; **57**: 543–51.
3 Morrison E, Archer DB. Effect of fluorometholone on the intraocular pressure of corticosteroid responders. *Br J Ophthalmol* 1984; **68**: 581–4.
4 Roberts W. Rapid progression of cupping in glaucoma precipitated by topical corticosteroids. *Am J Ophthalmol* 1968; **66**: 520–2.
5 Mindel JS, Goldberg J, Travitian HO. Comparative ocular pressure elevation by medrysone, fluorometholone and dexamethasone phosphate. *Arch Ophthalmol* 1980; **98**: 1577–8.
6 Spaeth GL, von Smallman L. Corticosteroids and cataracts. *Int Ophthalmol Clin* 1966; **6**: 915–29.
7 Urban RC, Cotlier E. Corticosteroid-induced cataracts. *Surv Ophthalmol* 1986; **31**: 102–10.
8 Caffery BE, Josephson J. Ocular side-effects of isotretinoin therapy. *J Am Optometric Assoc* 1988; **59**: 221–4.
9 Lebowitz MA, Berson DS. Ocular effects of oral retinoids. *J Am Acad Dermatol* 1988; **19**: 209–11.
10 Gross EG, Helfgott MA. Retinoids and the eye. *Dermatol Clin* 1992; **10**: 521–32.
11 Gold JA, Shupack JL, Nemec MA. Ocular side effects of the retinoids. *Int J Dermatol* 1989; **28**: 218–25.
12 Fraunfelder FT, Meyer SM. Adverse ocular reactions possibly associated with isotretinoin. *Am J Ophthalmol* 1985; **100**: 534–7.
13 Weleber RG, Denman ST, Hanifin J *et al.* Abnormal retinal function associated with isotretinoin therapy for acne. *Arch Ophthalmol* 1986; **104**: 831–7.
14 Brown RD, Grattan C. Etretinate and vision. *Lancet* 1988; **i**: 585–6.
15 Kerdel F, Grant-Kels JM, Rothe MJ *et al.* Antimalarial agents and the eye. *Dermatol Clin* 1992; **10**: 513–20.
16 Easterbrook M. The sensitivity of Amsler grid testing in early chloroquine retinopathy. *Trans Ophthalmol Soc UK* 1985; **104**: 204–6.
17 Ros AM, Leyon H, Wennersten G. Retinal crystals due to canthaxanthine. *Photodermatol* 1985; **2**: 183–5.
18 Rousseau A. Canthaxanthine deposits in the eye. *J Am Acad Dermatol* 1983; **8**: 123–4.
19 Harnois C. Canthaxanthine retinopathy. Anatomic and functional reversibility. *Arch Ophthalmol* 1989; **107**: 539–40.

Allergy to topical eye preparations [1]

Almost all drugs used topically in the eye may occasionally cause a local contact reaction. In most, but not all, cases this will be of the delayed hypersensitivity type. Neomycin and idoxuridine are common culprits. The affected eyes have a 'bleary' look and the eyelids usually become red and puffy, wrinkled or scaly. In some cases, the swelling may be so marked that the eyelids are completely closed, and the oedema spreads to the neighbouring cheeks (see also 'Eyelid dermatitis', p. 2984).

REFERENCE

1 Wilson FM. Adverse external ocular effects of topical ophthalmic medications. *Surv Ophthalmol* 1989; **24**: 57–88.

Chapter 68
The External Ear

C.T.C.KENNEDY

Anatomy and physiology [1,2]

The external ear consists of the auricle, the external auditory canal and the outer layer of the tympanic membrane.

The auricle, or pinna (Fig. 68.1), is a convoluted, elastic and cartilaginous plate covered by skin which is continuous medially with the lining of the external auditory canal. Except on the lobe and at the back of the ear, the skin is bound firmly to the cartilage. The auricle is attached to the head by fibrous ligaments and three vestigial auricularis muscles. The size and general detail of the auricle can vary greatly between individuals, and may be characteristically affected in a number of congenital syndromes. In humans, the auricle is largely functionless and motionless.

The epidermis of the ear has a complex dermo-epidermal junction, a conspicuous stratum granulosum and a thick, compact stratum corneum [3]. The dermis contains abundant elastic tissue. Sebaceous glands are numerous, particularly on the tragus and lobe, and fine vellus or terminal hairs occur over the entire surface, but are especially prominent on the helix and tragus. Coarser terminal hair is seen in some men as a Y-linked and androgen-dependent inherited trait (Fig. 68.2). Eccrine sweat glands are sparsely and irregularly distributed except in the external auditory canal, which has, instead, a large number of modified apocrine or ceruminous glands. The pinna has a variably thick fatty layer that extends between perichondrium and reticular dermis and that also forms the main fibrofatty core of the lobe of the ear.

The blood supply to the auricle is provided by anastomosing branches of the superficial temporal and posterior auricular arteries, which drain via posterior auricular and superficial temporal veins into the external jugular vein and via the superficial temporal, maxillary and facial veins into the internal jugular vein. Lymphatic drainage is to the superficial parotid, retro-auricular and superficial cervical lymph nodes. Embryonic fusion planes and minute deficiencies in the cartilaginous portion of the external auditory canal provide potential pathways for the spread of infection and tumours.

There is a complex nerve supply to the ear involving elements of the Vth, VIIth, IXth and Xth cranial nerves as well as cervical branches of the greater and lesser auricular nerves. The back of the ear is supplied by the greater auricular nerve (C2,3), the concha by the auricular branch of the vagus (X) and the anterior part of the ear by the auriculotemporal branch of the Vth cranial nerve. Intercommunicating branches of the VIIth, IXth and Xth supply the deeper parts of the ear. With this complicated nerve supply, otalgia is more commonly due to referred pain than to disease in the ear itself [4]. Within the dermis, the nerve supply is abundant, especially around hair follicles where there are complicated basket-like networks of acetyl- and butylcholinesterase nerve fibres [3]. Free nerve endings are also present but there are no organized nerve endings, as occur on glabrous skin elsewhere [5].

The external auditory canal extends upwards and backwards in an S-shaped curve from the concha to the tympanic membrane. The angle of curvature varies between races and individuals, being more marked in white people than in black people or Polynesians. This has a bearing on trauma, infection and the retention of moisture. The length of the canal is 2.5 cm as measured from the concha to drum. The outer third of the canal is cartilaginous and is lined by a thicker layer of skin than the inner portion within the temporal bone. Subcutaneous tissue is scanty, and the epithelium is firmly bound to the perichondrium. Sebaceous glands are plentiful, and open into the follicles of extremely fine vellus hairs. Occasionally, larger terminal hairs (tragi) arise in the canal or around the meatus and these, if they become matted with wax or debris, may interfere with normal epidermal 'migration' and ventilation of the ear and hence may play a part in the development of 'hot-weather ear'.

Eccrine sweat glands are not present in the auditory canal but modified apocrine (ceruminous) glands are numerous.

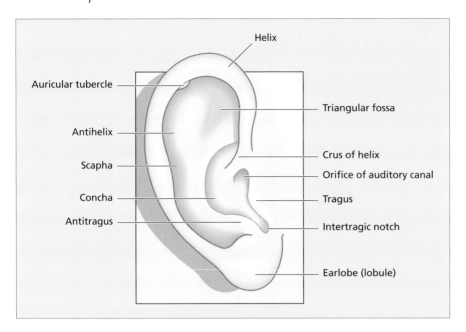

Fig. 68.1 Anatomical landmarks of the auricle.

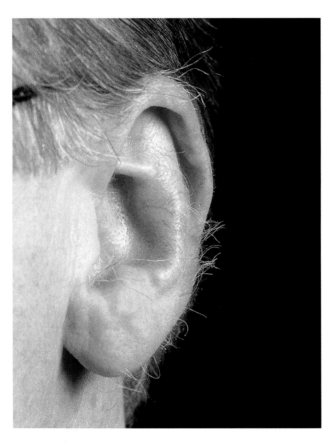

Fig. 68.2 Coarse terminal hair on the auricle: a trait associated with the Y-chromosome.

They increase in size and activity at puberty. There is great individual and racial variability, and, although concentrated in the cartilaginous part of the canal, they may also occur, albeit sparsely, in the osseous portion.

The inner osseous part of the acoustic canal constitutes two-thirds of its total length. The skin is firmly bound to the periosteum, subcutaneous tissue being nearly absent and is only 0.2 mm thick. The epidermis in this situation is thin and easily traumatized, and rete ridges are absent [1]. The skin of the external auditory canal and tympanic membrane is unique in that there is no frictional squame loss; cerumen (wax) and epithelial debris have therefore to be removed by a special 'migratory' property of the external ear canal epithelium [6]. A slight narrowing of the canal, the isthmus, occurs at or just medial to, the junction of the two parts. When marked, it may impede the flow of cerumen to the exterior. Just medial to the isthmus, inferiorly and anteriorly, is the tympanic sulcus. Debris often collects here, especially in patients with chronic external otitis.

The surface pH of the auditory canal varies [7] from 5.6–5.8 at the concha to 7.3–7.5 at 5–10 mm within the canal. With inflammation, the pH becomes slightly more acid.

Cerumen

Cerumen is the combined product of sebaceous and apocrine glands. It contains both squalene and insoluble fatty acids. Its extrusion is aided by mastication and by the peripheral movement and desquamation of the epithelial cells of the canal. It is impeded if the ear canal is too narrow or tortuous, or when inflammation interferes with the normal process of 'migration'.

There are two varieties of cerumen: a dark, hard variety more common in males, and a soft, lighter variety normally found in females. Although not bactericidal, cerumen does not encourage bacterial or fungal growth. An increased secretion of cerumen occurs with excessive sweating, stress or inflammation and has also been reported in patients treated with aromatic retinoids [8,9]. If wax becomes impacted or adherent, it may be removed either manually or by syringing. Both its presence and its removal may cause inflammation due to trauma, infection or contact dermatitis from medicaments or irritant cerumenolytics [10]. Inflammation interferes with normal epidermal migration and tends therefore both to induce and to encourage the retention of scale. The pruritus associated with excess cerumen, and the low-grade inflammation that often accompanies this, frequently leads to a persistent form of low-grade neurodermatitis.

REFERENCES

1 Perry ET. *The Human Ear Canal.* Springfield: Thomas, 1957.
2 Lucente FE. Anatomy, histology and physiology. In: Lucente FE, Lawson W, Novick NL, eds. *The External Ear.* Philadelphia: WB Saunders, 1995: 1–17.
3 Montagna W, Giacometti L. Histology and cytochemistry of human skin: XXXII. The external ear. *Arch Dermatol* 1969; **99**: 757–67.
4 Al-Sheikhli ARJ. Pain in the ear—with special reference to referred pain. *J Laryngol Otol* 1980; **94**: 1433–40.
5 Sinclair DC, Weddell G, Zander E. The relationship of cutaneous sensibility to neurohistology in the human pinna. *J Anat* 1952; **86**: 402–11.
6 Alberti PWRM. Epithelial migration on the tympanic membrane *J Laryngol Otol* 1964; **78**: 808–30
7 Fabricant ND. The pH factor in the treatment of otitis externa. *Arch Otolaryngol* 1957; **65**: 11–12.
8 Burge SM, Wilkinson JD, Miller AJ *et al.* The efficacy of an aromatic retinoid, Tigason, in the treatment of Darier's disease. *Br J Dermatol* 1981; **104**: 675–9.
9 Kramer M. Excessive cerumen production due to the aromatic retinoid Tigason in a patient with Darier's disease. *Acta Derm Venereol (Stockh)* 1981; **62**: 267–8.
10 Holmes RC, Johns AN, Wilkinson JD *et al.* Medicament contact dermatitis in patients with chronic inflammatory ear disease. *J R Soc Med* 1982; **75**: 27–30.

Examination [1]

As well as examining the pinna, the dermatologist may need to examine the ear canal. Equipment available should include a headlight or equivalent, otoscope, several sizes of ear specula, ear curettes, metal applicators, bayonet forceps, ear irrigation apparatus and cotton.

General inspection of the auricles should take account of their symmetry, size, shape and position, and completeness of development.

The ear canal is best inspected when the auricle is pulled gently upwards, outwards and backwards, and the largest possible speculum is used. It is essential to avoid traumatizing the thin skin of the canal, particularly beyond the isthmus. If inspection reveals accumulation of cerumenous debris, this can sometimes be removed carefully using a curette or wire loop along the posterior wall. If the material is against the drum, gentle suction may be feasible. Irrigation should only be used if the drum is known to be intact.

Samples may need to be taken for bacteriology, mycology and histology. If a biopsy is required from the canal, this should be devolved to a surgeon with the necessary expertise.

REFERENCE

1 Lucente FE. Techniques of examination. In: Lucente FE, Lawson W, Novick NL, eds. *The External Ear.* Philadelphia: WB Saunders, 1995: 18–24.

Developmental defects

The auricle begins to develop at the end of the fifth week of embryonic life in the first branchial groove, contributed to by the first (mandibular) and second (hyoid) arches [1]. Six hillocks appear on these arches and later fuse to form the complex shape of the fully developed auricle.

Developmental defects are considered in detail in Chapter 15. Only those defects of the ear that are sufficiently common to constitute a part of general dermatological practice are therefore considered here, together with some general principles relating to congenital ear abnormalities and their more important medical and otological associations [2–6]. Pinna abnormalities are sufficiently often associated with conductive hearing loss that screening tests should be carried out [7].

Many developmental defects are of unknown aetiology. Some, however, are associated with chromosomal abnormalities, for example those occurring in Down's syndrome or associated with syndromes that have well-recognized Mendelian inheritance patterns, for example the *ecto*dactyly, *ectodermal dysplasia* and *cleft lip–palate (EEC)* syndrome. Environmental factors may be implicated as in the fetal alcohol syndrome and the fetal hydantoin syndrome, and maternal exposure to isotretinoin and thalidomide.

Congenital ear abnormalities exhibit great variability, even within syndromes or families, and any one aetiological factor may be associated with a variety of ear malformations. External ear malformations as part of a genetic syndrome account for less than 10% of all external ear abnormalities; isolated cases of ear malformation may be either non-genetic in origin or associated with poor gene penetrance [8].

Microtia (small ears)

Small ears are often associated with hearing deficit and may be a feature of many syndromes. In addition to being small, the pinna may be rudimentary, resembling the hillocks from which it is embryologically derived. The more primitive the appearance, the greater the likelihood of hearing abnormalities, usually due to defects or atresia of the ossicles. There may also be a narrowing or atresia of the auditory canal [9] and various abnormalities of the inner ear [5]. A wide variety of non-aural abnormalities are associated with small ears, multiple malformations occurring in 56% in one large series [10]. Small ears are a feature of many syndromes including Down's syndrome, the Treacher–Collins syndrome, Goldenhar syndrome,

Apert's syndrome, various first and second branchial arch and first branchial cleft syndromes, Mohr's orofaciodigital syndrome, the Duane retraction syndrome and thalidomide embryopathy [5,6,11].

Macrotia (large ears)

Macrotia is a developmental variation in which the amount of tissue between the helix and antihelix is increased, causing the ears to wing out. The ear may also be diffusely enlarged, or elongated. Such changes are common in Turner's syndrome, and there may be associated sensorineural deafness. Generally enlarged ears are sometimes seen in patients with the XXXXY chromosome defect. The cartilaginous parts of the ears are enlarged and soft in the Laband syndrome [12,13]. In this rare disorder the ears are large and floppy, in association with a bulbous soft nose, gingival fibromatosis and a variety of other findings including absence or dysplasia of nails and/or terminal phalanges, hyperextensibility of joints, hepatosplenomegaly, and rarely hypertrichosis and mental retardation.

Low-set ears

Normally, the top of the helix is at the same level as the eyebrow, the earlobe is above the angle of the mandible and the external auditory meatus is at the level of the ala nasi. Low-set ears may in addition be posteriorly rotated, and are often small. The condition is usually bilateral. Although it may be isolated, it is often associated with major middle-ear or systemic malformations, appearing, for example, in Turner's, Noonan's, Patau's and Crouzon's syndromes.

Variations in the shape of the pinna

Minor variations in size and shape are common and not usually associated with any other abnormality. These include the '*bat ear*' or protruding ear, in which the antihelix lacks the usual bulge; the '*lop ear*', in which there is an unrolled helix, a poorly developed antihelix and scapha, and a large concha resulting in a somewhat floppy ear; and the *prominent auricular (Darwin's) tubercle*. Variations in the contour of the helix and antihelix to produce a bulge of the antero-superior part of the pinna account for so-called *Mozart's* ear, and in '*Wildemuth's ear*' the antihelix is prominent and the formation of the helix is poor. These minor ear anomalies can be a syndromic feature or can be associated with conductive and occasionally sensorineural hearing loss, but in most instances they are isolated. They may, however, be inherited, as in the Mozart family. A distinctive '*railroad track*' *abnormality* with marked prominence of the crus of the helix is said to occur in up to 30% of children with fetal alcohol syndrome [11] and a protruding auricle may, rarely, be a sign of neuromuscular

disease [14]. Various abnormalities of the configuration of the pinna have been described in the distinctive '*lumpy scalp syndrome*', in which other features include absent or rudimentary nipples and dermal nodules on the scalp [15,16]. The lobule can show isolated abnormalities, for example pits and clefts. Absence of the lobule is, however, usually associated with a syndrome of a more serious nature [6]. Diagonal linear creases in the lobule are seen in the Beckwith–Wiedemann syndrome, and in adult life in association with some degenerative diseases (see p. 3017), although they are a common finding in normal individuals.

Peri-auricular anomalies

Pre-auricular pits, sinuses (Fig. 68.3) and tags are relatively common, with an incidence of approximately 1% [4,8]. Accessory auricles occur as small, firm elevations of skin and cartilage just anterior to the tragus or ascending crus of the helix. They may be single or multiple and may occur anywhere in a line from the tragus to the angle of the mouth. Accessory auricles, congenital fistulae and other external ear manifestations may occur alone or may be associated with more widespread first and second branchial arch abnormalities [3,4,8] or with developmental abnormalities of the genito-urinary tract [17].

Dermatological associations

Sebaceous cysts, often multiple, occur on the lobe and on

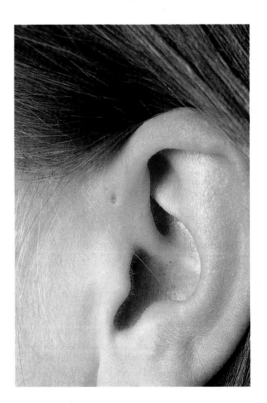

Fig. 68.3 Pre-auricular sinus.

the posterior auricular skin, and epidermoid cysts are also fairly common. Retro-auricular, follicular and keratotic plaques containing multiple follicular cysts have been reported [18]. Haemangiomas are fairly common.

Congenital arteriovenous fistula of the pinna has been described. There is gradual enlargement of the ear, which becomes pulsatile and warmer than the opposite ear. Ulceration and necrosis can occur.

Developmental anomalies of ear hair

Hypertrichosis of the ears has been described in infants born of diabetic mothers [19,20].

REFERENCES

1 Bowden REM. Development of the middle and external ear in man. *Proc R Soc Med* 1977; **70**: 807–15.
2 Anson BJ, Donaldson JA. In: *Surgical Anatomy of the Temporal Bone and Ear, Part II. The Ear: Developmental Anatomy,* 2nd edn. Philadelphia: WB Saunders, 1973: 17–150.
3 Bellucci RJ. Congenital aural malformations: diagnosis and treatment: Symposium on Congenital Disorders in Otolaryngology. *Otolaryngol Clin N Am* 1981; **14**: 95–124.
4 Melnick M. The etiology of external ear malformations and its relation to abnormalities of the middle ear, inner ear, and other organ systems. In: *Birth Defects: Original Article Series, March of Dimes Birth Defects Foundation,* Vol. XVI New York: Alan R. Liss, 1980: 303–31.
5 Bergstrom LB. Anomalies of the ear. In: English GM, ed. *Otolaryngology,* Vol. 1. Philadelphia: Lippincott, 1990.
6 Sakashita T, Sando I, Kamerer DB. Congenital anomalies of the external and middle ears. In: Bluestone CD, Stool SE, Kenna MA, eds. *Pediatric Otolaryngology,* 3rd edn. Philadelphia: WB Saunders, 1996: 333–70.
7 Jaffe BF. Pinna anomalies associated with congenital conductive hearing loss. *Pediatrics* 1976; **57**: 332–41.
8 Melnick M, Myrianthopoulos NC. External ear malformations: epidemiology, genetics and natural history. In: *Birth Defects: Original Article Series, March of Dimes Birth Defects Foundation,* Vol. XV. New York: Alan R. Liss, 1979: 1–139.
9 Jahrsdoerfer RA. Congenital atresia of the ear. *Laryngoscope* 1978; **88** (Suppl. 13): 1–48.
10 Jafek BW, Nager GT, Stife J *et al.* Congenital aural atresia: an analysis of 311 cases. *Trans Am Acad Ophthalmol Otolaryngol* 1975; **80**: 588–95.
11 Aase JM. Microtia—clinical observations. In: Gorlin RJ, ed. *Birth Defects: Original Article Series, March of Dimes Birth Defects Foundation,* Vol. XVI. New York: Alan R. Liss, 1980: 289–97.
12 Laband PF, Habib G, Humphreys GC. Hereditary gingival fibromatosis. Report of an affected family with associated splenomegaly and soft tissue abnormalities. *Oral Surg Oral Med Oral Pathol* 1964; **17**: 339–51.
13 Bazopoulou-Kyrkanidou E, Papagianoulis L, Papanicolaou S, Mavrou A. Laband syndrome: a case report. *J Otol Pathol Med* 1990; **19**: 385–7.
14 Smith DW, Takashima H. Protruding auricle: a neuromuscular sign. *Lancet* 1978; **i**: 747–9.
15 Finlay AY, Marks R. An hereditary syndrome of lumpy scalp, odd ears and rudimentary nipples. *Br J Dermatol* 1978; **99**: 423–30.
16 Steinberg RD, Ethington J, Esterly NB. Lumpy scalp syndrome. *Int J Dermatol* 1990; **29**: 657–8.
17 Melnick M. Hereditary hearing loss and ear dysplasia—renal adysplasia syndromes: syndrome delineation and possible pathogenesis. In: Levin LS, ed. *Birth Defects: Original Article Series, March of Dimes Birth Defects Foundation,* Vol. XVI. New York: Alan R. Liss 1980: 59–72.
18 de Auda G, Viguale R, Carlevaro A *et al.* Cysts in retroauricular infundibulopapillary plaques. *Med Cutan Ibero Lat Am* 1985; **13**: 331–4.
19 Woods DL. Malan AF, Coetzee EJ. Intra-uterine growth in infants of diabetic mothers. *S Afr Med J* 1980; **58**: 441–3.
20 Rafaat M. Hypertrichosis pinnae in babies of diabetic mothers. *Pediatrics* 1981; **68**: 745–6.

Ageing changes

Many changes seen on the skin of the pinna attributed to ageing are a result of its exposure to environmental factors, especially UV radiation, cold (perniosis) and infrared radiation. The elderly exposed pinna often shows varying degrees of dermal and epidermal atrophy, solar keratoses and lentigines, solar elastosis, telangiectasia and venous lakes. If the pinna is at least partially light protected, as in many women, the skin may still appear somewhat thinned due to intrinsic ageing changes.

Ear length

It is recognized in Chinese culture that length of the ear in men is a predictor for longevity [1]. Two studies would appear to confirm this: one from Kent, UK [2] and one from Japan [3]. The increase in length of the male ear from the age of 30 years onwards may have a 7-year periodicity [4].

Earlobe creases

First described in 1973 [5], and now known as Frank's sign, a diagonal crease in the earlobes of adults has been associated in many studies with an increased risk for atherosclerotic coronary artery disease. A meta-analysis in 1983 gave a relative risk of 2.06 for heart disease if there are bilateral creases [6] and there is approximately double the risk for death from heart disease [7,8]. The crease can be graded in terms of length and depth, and deeper, longer creases have the strongest association. The ear crease

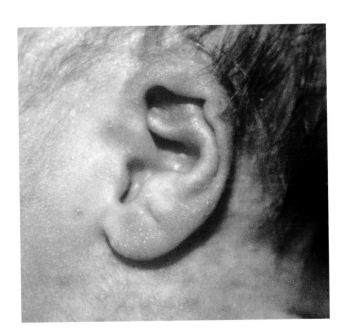

Fig. 68.4 Diagonal earlobe crease in an infant with Beckwith–Wiedemann syndrome.

appears to be separate from other risk factors for coronary artery disease, and is not simply a function of age [9]. Earlobe creases and atheroma have been speculatively linked with alterations in macrophage function [10].

Ear-canal hair has also been associated with coronary artery disease in Indians [11].

Diagonal earlobe creases are seen in other contexts, for example the Beckwith–Wiedemann syndrome [12] (Fig. 68.4), and do not seem to be associated with coronary artery disease in Hawaians [13], native Americans [14] or Chinese [15].

Earlobe creases have also been associated with primary open-angle glaucoma [16].

REFERENCES

1 Woo Pick-Ngor, Lip Peck-Lin. Why do old men have big ears? (Letter.) *Br Med J* 1996; **312**: 586.
2 Heathcote JA. Why do old men have big ears? (Letter.) *Br Med J* 1996; **311**: 1668.
3 Asai Y, Yoshimura M, Nago N, Yamada T. Correlation of ear length with age in Japan (Letter.) *Br Med J* 1996; **312**: 582.
4 Verhulst J, Onghena P. Circaseptennial rhythm in ear growth. *Br Med J* 1996; **313**: 1597–8.
5 Frank ST. Aural sign of coronary artery disease. *N Engl J Med* 1973; **289**: 327–8.
6 Elliott WJ. Earlobe crease and coronary artery disease: 1000 patients and review of the literature. *Am J Med* 1983; **75**: 1024–32.
7 Kirkham N, Murrells T, Melcher DH, Morrison EA. Diagonal earlobe creases and fatal cardiovascular disease: a necropsy study. *Br Heart J* 1989; **61**: 361–4.
8 Patel V, Champ C, Andrews PS *et al*. Diagonal earlobe creases and atheromatous disease: a post mortem study. *J R Coll Physicians Lond* 1992; **26**: 274–7.
9 Tranchesi B, Barbosa V, de Albuquerque CP *et al*. Diagonal earlobe creases as a marker of the presence and extent of coronary atherosclerosis. *Am J Cardiol* 1992; **70**: 1417–20.
10 Sapira JD. Earlobe creases and macrophage receptors. *South Med J* 1991; **84**: 537–8.
11 Verma SK, Khamesra R, Bordia A. Earlobe crease and ear-canal hair as predictors of coronary artery disease in Indian populations. *Indian J Chest Dis Allied Sci* 1988; **30**: 189–96.
12 Weidemann HR. Earlobe creases, congenital and acquired. (Letter.) *N Eng J Med* 1979; **301**: 111.
13 Rhoads GG, Klein K, Yano K, Preston H. The earlobe crease sign of obesity in middle-aged Japanese men. *Hawaii Med J* 1977; **36**: 74–7.
14 Fisher JR, Sievers ML. Earlobe crease in American Indians (Letter.) *Ann Intern Med* 1980; **93**: 512.
15 Cheng TO. Diagonal earlobe creases. (Letter.) *J R Coll Physicians Lond* 1992; **26**: 460.
16 Hawksworth NR. Diagonal earlobe creases; an association with primary open angle glaucoma (Letter.) *J R Coll Physicians Lond* 1992; **26**: 459–60.

Traumatic conditions

Contusion and haematoma

Bruises of the ear are usually due to blunt trauma and are common in contact sports, such as boxing, wrestling and rugby. In children, physical abuse may need to be excluded [1,2]. A distinctive condition known as the 'tin ear' syndrome has been considered pathognomonic of child abuse: a triad of isolated ear bruising, haemorrhagic retinopathy and a small ipsilateral subdural haematoma [3].

Following trauma, blood and serum collects in the plane between perichondrium and cartilage, and will undergo fibrosis if not removed early. The patient should be carefully examined for concurrent auditory canal, middle ear, parotid and central nervous system trauma.

Repeated trauma may result in the distorted nodular deformity known as *cauliflower ear,* due to varying degrees of cartilage necrosis, fibrosis and dystrophic calcification.

Treatment. Subperichondrial haematomas must be treated promptly, with full aseptic technique to avoid secondary perichondritis. Small collections of fluid can be aspirated by syringe, or drained through a small incision and a laterally placed pressure dressing applied to prevent reaccumulation [4]. Another useful technique is to use a through-and-through suture technique to maintain bolsters over the area where the haematoma has been evacuated [5]. Other approaches include a posterior incision and suction drainage [6] and fenestrations in the cartilage to promote adhesion of the opposing perichondral layers [7]. Prophylactic antibiotics are sometimes given. Improvement of the cauliflower ear usually requires multiple corrective procedures.

REFERENCES

1 Manning SC, Casselbrant M, Lammers D. Otolaryngologic manifestations of child abuse. *Int J Pediatr Otorhinolaryngol* 1990; **20**: 7–16.
2 Willner A, Ledereich PS, de Vries EJ. Auricular injury as a presentation of child abuse. *Arch Otolaryngol Head Neck Surg* 1992; **118**: 634–7.
3 Hanigan WC, Peterson RA, Njus G. Tin ear syndrome: rotational acceleration in pediatric head injuries. *Pediatrics* 1987; **80**: 618–22.
4 Germon WH. The care and management of acute haematoma of the external ear. *Laryngoscope* 1980; **90**: 881–5.
5 Schuller DE, Dankle SD, Strauss RH. A technique to treat wrestler's auricular hematoma without interrupting training or competition. *Arch Otolaryngol Head Neck Surg* 1989; **115**: 202–6.
6 Bull PD, Lancer JM. Treatment of auricular haematoma by suction drainage. *Clin Otolaryngol* 1984; **9**: 355–60.
7 Tenta LT, Keyes GR. Reconstructive surgery of the external ear. *Otolaryngol Clin N Am* 1981; **14**: 917–38.

Laceration and avulsion

Lacerations of the pinna vary from the trivial to amputation [1]. Because of the risk of cartilage infection, potentially dirty wounds should always be carefully cleaned and a course of prophylactic antibiotic given. It is probably best to avoid suturing the cartilage itself unless pieces overlap or are severely displaced [2]. Injuries that expose cartilage will need to be covered with a skin graft, for example taken from behind the ear or the upper eyelid. If the perichondrium is destroyed, cartilage may need to be excised so that the graft can be placed on the posterior perichondrium. If the postauricular area is not injured, a pedicled island flap of postauricular skin may be pulled through the area of excised cartilage and sutured into place. If the helix or antihelix is exposed, it may be possible to cover it with an advancement or rotation flap from the posterior surface of the auricle. Large areas may need to be covered with a pedicled flap of temporoparietal fascia, which in turn is covered with a split skin graft. The lobule of the ear can be repaired by direct closure, but a cosmetically superior result may be obtained by a broken line repair or Z-plasty [3]. Many techniques have been described for repair of major trauma, including even complete avulsion of the pinna [1,4] but these are likely to be beyond the scope of the dermatologist.

REFERENCES

1 Templer J, Renner GJ. Injuries of the external ear. *Otolaryngol Clin N Am* 1990; **23**: 1003–18.
2 Mladick RA. Salvage of the ear in acute trauma. *Clin Plast Surg* 1978; **5**: 427–35.
3 Walike J, Larrabee WF. Repair of the cleft earlobe. *Laryngoscope* **95**: 876–7.
4 Lawson W. Management of acute trauma. In: Lucente FE, Lawson W, Norvick NL, eds. *The External Ear*. Philadelphia: WB Saunders, 1996: 177–82.

Ear piercing

Earrings have been worn by men and women since antiquity, and tend to follow the dictates of fashion. Current trends include using earrings in almost all parts of the body, the use of up to 10 or more in a single ear, and the piercing of cartilage. So-called 'high' ear piercing has a significant risk for perichondritis [1] and chondritis [2].

Complications are very common, with rates of about 30% whether the procedure is carried out by medical personnel, friend or relative, or in a store, and is independent of technique, there being little difference whether needle, staple gun or sharpened stud is used [3]. Contact dermatitis, inflammation, bleeding, non-purulent draining and infection are the commonest adverse effects [4].

The ear is also pierced in acupuncture as used in traditional medicine, and complications have been reported [5,6].

Complications. Various infections and reactions may occur after ear piercing as follows.

Localized bacterial infection, usually with Gram-positive cocci, is common; predisposing factors include skin disease, such as atopic or contact dermatitis. Life-threatening septicaemia has been described [7]. Infants with unsuspected immunodeficiency and individuals with valvular heart disease may be at particular risk. Other bacterial infections described include *Pseudomonas aeruginosa* perichondritis and chondritis due to high ear piercing [1,2], and primary tuberculosis [8].

Viral hepatitis may also be a hazard [9,10].

Oedema and haematoma [3,4,11] usually respond to cold compresses, pressure and removal of the earring. Haematoma may require incision and drainage [12].

Trauma can occur from pressure on the lobe and postauricular skin, and inaccurate insertion of the post of the earring. Heavy earrings can tear the earlobe, sometimes making it bifid. Repair of the latter is probably best by excision of the cleft and simple closure with eversion of the edges [13], although a staggered repair such as a Z-plasty may be appropriate in some cases.

Sensitization to nickel from earrings remains a major cause of this common problem, and is one explanation for the higher incidence in females [14]. Even stainless steel studs and clasps, which can produce irritant as well as allergic effects, may release sufficient nickel to elicit contact dermatitis [15]. Gold sensitization, although less common, can be a protracted cause of dermatitis even after the earrings are removed [16]. Contact dermatitis from other materials used in earrings such as olive wood [17], copper [18], cobalt [19,20] and chromium [21] have been described, and may also occur from the use of topical antiseptics, antibiotics and dressings used to treat infection.

Granulomatous and lymphoid reactions. Reddish brown and purple papules and nodules at sites of ear piercing may denote a granulomatous response to gold [22,23] and a lymphocytoma cutis-like reaction has been described [24–26]. Sarcoidosis has presented after ear piercing [27].

Embedded earrings. The spring-loaded gun method of ear piercing can result in the earring backing becoming embedded in the back of the ear [28]. The 'vanishing earring' [29] can resemble a keloid [30]. The embedded metal can usually be pulled out, or if necessary an incision made to locate it.

Epidermal cyst formation. Implantation epidermal cysts due to ear piercing often present as tender, chronic, inflammatory swellings, sometimes with drainage. There is usually an epithelial lined track as well as cysts, and all epithelial tissue must be removed, for example with a skin punch [31].

Keloids quite commonly follow ear piercing, especially in those ethnic groups with a predisposition (Fig. 68.5). The keloids seem to occur more on the back surface than the front of the earlobe [32]. As well as being unsightly, they can itch and be painful.

Treatment options include intralesional steroid, pressure, and excision with or without concurrent use of intralesional steroid or radiotherapy [33,38]. Prospective controlled trials are needed to assess these approaches.

Localized argyria. Bluish macules have been described on the posterior surface of the earlobe [39,40].

Frostbite has followed the use of ethyl chloride topical anaesthesia [41].

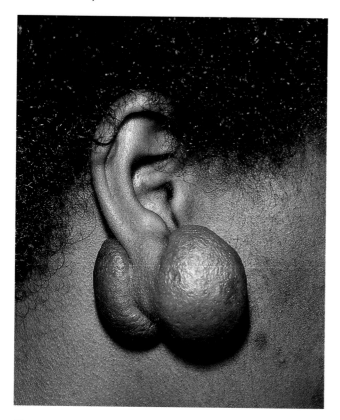

Fig. 68.5 Keloids following ear piercing.

Measures to prevent complications [42]. Many of the complications of ear piercing are avoidable. The procedure is best not carried out on children under the age of 5 years, those with immunodeficiency, valvular heart disease or sarcoidosis, and there is clearly a risk if the individual has a tendency to keloid formation. It has been recommended that a surgical grade, stainless steel, one-piece earring with an interlocking groove is preferable. Gold-plated or gold-alloy earrings should be avoided for at least 6 weeks after the ear has been pierced. Sterile technique is important. Piercing of cartilage should be avoided. Only nickel-free earrings should be used. Large or heavy earrings should be removed prior to activities that may result in tearing the earlobes.

REFERENCES

1 Cumberworth VL, Hogarth TB. Hazards of ear-piercing procedures which traverse cartilage: a report of pseudomonas perichondritis and review of other complications. *Br J Clin Pract* 1990; **44**: 512–13.
2 Turkeltaub SH, Habal MB. Acute pseudomonas chondritis as a sequel to ear piercing. *Am Plast Surg* 1990; **24**: 279–82.
3 Biggar RJ, Haughie GE. Medical problems of ear piercing. *NY State J Med* 1975; **75**: 1460–2.
4 Cortese TA, Dickey RA. Complications of ear piercing. *Am Fam Physician* 1971; **4**: 66–72.
5 Allison G, Kravitz E. Auricular chondritis secondary to acupuncture. *N Engl J Med* 1975; **293**: 780.
6 Davis O, Powell M. Auricular perichondritis secondary to acupuncture. *Arch Otolaryngol* 1985; **111**: 770–1.
7 Lovejoy FH, Jr, Smith DH. Life-threatening staphylococcal disease following ear piercing. *Pediatrics* 1970; **46**: 301–3.
8 Morgan LG. Primary tuberculosis inoculation of an earlobe: report of an unusual case and review of the literature. *J Pediatr* 1952; **40**: 482–5.
9 Van Sciver AE. Hepatitis from ear piercing. *JAMA* 1969; **207**: 2285.
10 Johnson CJ, Anderson H, Spearman J. Viral hepatitis in young women after ear piercing. *MMWR* 1973; **22**: 390–5.
11 Jay AL. Ear piercing problems. *Br Med J* 1977; **2**: 574–5.
12 Ellis DAF. Complication and correction of the pierced ear. *J Otolaryngol* 1976; **5**: 247–50.
13 Apesos J, Kane M. Treatment of traumatic earlobe clefts. *Aesth Plast Surg* 1993; **17**: 253–5.
14 Larsson-Stymne B, Widstrom L. Ear piercing—a cause of nickel allergy in school girls? *Contact Dermatitis* 1985; **13**: 289–93.
15 Fischer T, Fregert S, Gruvberger B. Nickel release from ear-piercing kits and earrings. *Contact Dermatitis* 1984; **10**: 39–41.
16 Fisher AA. Allergic contact dermatitis due to gold earrings. *Cutis* 1990; **39**: 473–5.
17 Hausen BM, Rothenborg HW. Allergic contact dermatitis caused by olive wood jewelry. *Arch Dermatol* 1981; **17**: 732–4.
18 Karlberg AT, Boman A, Wahlberg JE. Copper—a rare sensitizer. *Contact Dermatitis* 1983; **9**: 134–9.
19 Menné T. Relationship between cobalt and nickel sensitization in females. *Contact Dermatitis* 1980; **3**: 337–40.
20 Lammintausta K, Pitkanen OP, Kalino K *et al.* Interrelationship of nickel and cobalt contact sensitization. *Contact Dermatitis* 1985; **13**: 148–52.
21 Burrows D. The dichromate problem. *Int J Dermatol* 1984; **23**: 215–20.
22 Fisher AA. Metallic gold; the cause of a persistent allergic 'dermal' contact dermatitis. *Cutis* 1974; **14**:177–80.
23 Aoshima T, Oguchi M. Intracytoplasmic crystalline inclusions in dermal infiltrating cells of granulomatous contact dermatitis due to gold earrings. *Acta Derm Venereol (Stockh)* 1988; **68**: 261–4.
24 Iwatsuki K, Tagami H, Moriguichi T *et al.* Lymphadenoid structure induced by gold hypersensitivity. *Arch Dermatol* 1982; **118**: 608–11.
25 Iwatsuki K, Yamada M, Tagigawa M *et al.* Benign lymphoplasia of the earlobes induced by gold earrings: immunohistologic study on the cellular infiltrates. *J Am Acad Dermatol* 1987; **16**: 83–8.
26 Zilinsky I, Tsur H, Trau H, Orenstein A. Pseudolymphoma of the earlobes dueto ear piercing. *J Dermatol Surg Oncol* 1989; **15**: 666–8.
27 Mann RJ, Peachey RDG. Sarcoidal tissue reaction—another complication of ear piercing. *Clin Exp Dermatol* 1983; **8**: 199–200.
28 Muntz HR, Cui DJ, Asher BA. Embedded earrings: a complication of the ear-piercing gun. *Int J Ped Otorhinolaryngol* 1990; **19**: 73–6.
29 de San Lazaro C, Jackson RH. Vanishing earrings. *Arch Dis Child* 1986; **61**: 606–7.
30 Saleeby ER, Rubin MG, Youshock E *et al.* Embedded foreign bodies presenting as earlobe keloids. *J Dermatol Surg Oncol* 1984; **10**: 902–4.
31 Ellis DAF. Complications and corrections of the pierced ear. *J Otolaryngol* 1976; **5**: 247–50.
32 Slobodkin D. Why more keloids on back than front of earlobe? *Lancet* 1990; **335**: 335–6.
33 Brent B. The role of pressure therapy in the management of earlobe keloids: a preliminary report of a controlled study. *Ann Plast Surg* 1978; **1**: 579–81.
34 Weimar VM, Ceilley RI. Treatment of keloids on earlobes. *J Dermatol Surg Oncol* 1979; **5**: 522–3.
35 Pollack SV, Goslen JB. The surgical treatment of keloids. *J Dermatol Surg Oncol* 1982; **8**: 1045–9.
36 Salasche SJ, Grabski WJ. Keloids of the earlobes: a surgical technique. *J Dermatol Surg Oncol* 1983; **9**: 552–6.
37 Rauscher GE, Kolmer WL. Treatment of recurrent earlobe keloids. *Cutis* 1986; **37**: 67–8.
38 Chaudry MR, Akhtar S, Duvalsaint F *et al.* Ear lobe keloids, surgical excision followed by radiation therapy: a 10-year experience. *Ear Nose Throat J* 1994; **73**: 779–81.
39 van den Nieuwenhuijsen IJ, Calame JJ, Brynzeel DP. Localised argyria caused by silver earrings. *Dermatologica* 1988; **177**: 189–91.
40 Shall L, Stevens A, Millard LG. An unusual case of acquired localised argyria. *Br J Dermatol* 1990; **123**: 403–7.
41 Noble DA. Another hazard of pierced ears. *Br Med J* 1979; **1**: 125.
42 Hendricks WM. Complications of ear piercing: treatment and prevention. *Cutis* 1991; **48**: 386–94.

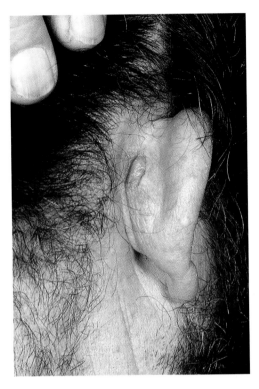

Fig. 68.6 Acanthoma fissuratum. Nodular thickening behind the pinna superficially resembling basal cell carcinoma.

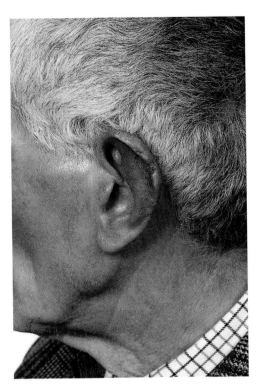

Fig. 68.7 Perniosis. Purple discoloration, soft-tissue loss and crusting due to acute-on-chronic cold injury.

Acanthoma fissuratum

This chronic response to friction and pressure from the spectacle frame can present with papules or nodules, sometimes with ulceration, in the supra- or retro-auricular folds (Fig 68.6). Even when bilateral, basal cell carcinoma is a differential diagnosis. Acanthoma fissuratum is discussed in Chapter 23.

Cold injury

The ears are extremely susceptible to cold, and the pinna may be affected by chilblains in winter (Fig. 68.7). Extreme cold will cause frostbite (Chapter 24). Similar changes have also been reported as a consequence of using excessive amounts of ethylchloride spray for ear piercing [1]. Frost-bite may result in vesiculation, blisters and ischaemic necrosis of both skin and cartilage. Ears that have previously been damaged by cold may subsequently become calcified.

Cold is also a provoking factor in patients with 'juvenile spring eruption' [2], chondrodermatitis nodularis helicis, chillblain lupus erythematosus and cryoglobulinaemia.

The ear subjected to frostbite should be thawed rapidly by the application of wet, sterile cotton pledgets warmed to 38–42°C for about 20 min [3] with adequate analgesic cover.

REFERENCES

1 Noble DA. Another hazard of pierced ears (use of ethylchloride spray anaesthetic with children). (Letter.) *Br Med J* 1979; **1**: 125.
2 Berth-Jones J, Norris PG, Graham-Brown RA *et al.* Juvenile spring eruption of the ears. *Clin Exp Dermatol* 1989; **14**: 462–3.
3 Sessions DG, Stallings JO, Mills WJ, Beal DD. Frostbite of the ear. *Laryngoscope* 1971; **81**: 1223–32.

Solar damage

The external ear is often exposed to solar radiation, and therefore liable to acute and chronic sequelae. A significant hazard from severe sunburn is the development of perichondritis (see below). Many photosensitivity disorders will present on the ear, for example polymorphic light eruption, lupus erythematosus and porphyria (see Chapter 25).

The full gamut of chronic solar damage is frequently seen on the ears, including erythema, telangiectasia, atrophy, blotchy pigmentation, solar keratoses and cutaneous malignancies. As on the lower lip, venous lakes may be seen (Fig. 68.8). Solar elastosis is often evident, and distinctive elastotic nodules may be seen particularly on the anterior crus of the antihelix [1–3]. These lesions are usually bilateral, asymptomatic, and present as pale papules or nodules. Occasionally, they can occur on the helix and be painful, simulating chondrodermatitis nodularis. They differ from 'weathering' nodules (Fig. 68.9), which, like chondrodermatitis nodularis, occur on the helix of the ear [4].

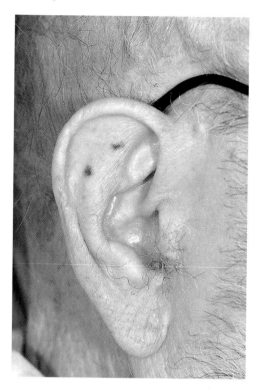

Fig. 68.8 Venous lakes on a sun-damaged pinna.

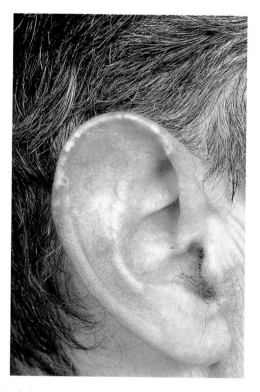

Fig. 68.9 Several firm, white 'weathering' nodules on the helical rim.

For treatment of mild, acute sunburn, cold compresses may be sufficient. More severe cases may benefit from a course of systemic corticosteroid, given for 5 days and then tapered. Preventive measures are discussed in Chapter 25.

REFERENCES

1 Carter VH, Constantine VS, Poole WL. Elastotic nodules of the antihelix. *Arch Dermatol* 1969; **100**: 282–5.
2 Kocsard E, Ofner F, Turner B. Elastotic nodules of the antihelix. *Arch Dermatol* 1970; **101**: 370.
3 Weedon D. Elastotic nodules of the ear. *J Cutan Pathol* 1980; **8**: 429–33.
4 Kavanagh GM, Bradfield JWB, Collins CMP, Kennedy CTC. Weathering nodules of the ear: a clinicopathological study. *Br J Dermatol* 1996; **135**: 550–4.

Altitude injury

A distinctive presentation of petechiae and haemorrhagic bullae in the skin of the external auditory canal and tympanic membrane has been described in air pilots descending from high altitudes or in pressure chambers while wearing well-sealed earplugs as noise protectors [1].

For treatment, a steroid–antibiotic eardrop has been advised, and if sizeable clots are present they can be gently dislodged by suction after the application of hydrogen peroxide. Preventive methods include the use of perforated earplugs on high-altitude descent.

REFERENCE

1 Senturia BH, Peugnet HB. Aero-otitis externa. *Laryngoscope* 1946; **56**: 225–36.

Radiation injury

Therapeutic use of radiation may result in characteristic acute and chronic changes (see Chapter 79). The cartilage can be susceptible to destruction if inappropriate techniques are used. Postradiation changes on the external auditory canal include thickening of the canal epithelium, subepithelial fibrosis and resorption of underlying bone, as well as ulceration of the epithelium and the development of cholesteatoma [1].

REFERENCE

1 Adler M, Hawke M, Berger G *et al.* Radiation effects on the external auditory canal. *J Otolaryngol* 1985; **14**: 226–32.

Foreign bodies

A variety of vegetable, animal and mineral substances may be encountered lodged in the external ear and external auditory canal, and are frequently unsuspected. Presenting symptoms include pain, hearing loss, inflammation and discharge.

Vegetable matter, such as beans, peas and cotton, tends to absorb water and swell, impacting in the ear canal. Arthropods are the commonest animal material. While alive, their motion within the ear can produce distinctive symptoms, even vertigo. Flies can deposit eggs in the external auditory canal and the resulting myiasis has produced severe complications [1]; larvae in the triangular fossa of the pinna can also cause marked inflammation [2]. Mineral materials include beads, sand and pebbles, fragments of plaster and metallic substances. Even batteries have been found lodged in the ear and can produce serious consequences [3–5]. Impacted cerumen can behave like a foreign body in the ear canal. Loose hairs in the ear canal have been reported as a cause of noise [6].

Retrieval of foreign bodies should only be undertaken if appropriate instrumentation and expertise is available. For children, with whom the problem is more common, general anaesthesia is required. Small foreign bodies can usually be extracted with a curette or alligator forceps. Live insects should first be killed by drowning or by the installation of ether, chloroform or spirit. If some vegetable materials have absorbed water and become impacted, it may be necessary to divide the foreign body 'in situ' and remove the fragments. It may be necessary to control bleeding from the skin of the canal, for example with adrenalin-soaked gauze, and the canal should then be packed with an antibiotic-impregnated dressing. In cases of a battery lodged in the ear canal, it is essential that an ENT surgeon is involved in the management, because of the likelihood of serious destructive change to the middle ear and beyond.

REFERENCES

1 Mendivil JA, El Shammaa NA. Aural myiasis caused by *Cochliomyia hominivorax*: case report. *Milit Med* 1979; **144**: 261–2.
2 Kron MA. Human infestation with *Cochliomyia hominivorax*, the New World screwworm. *J Am Acad Dermatol* 1992; **27**: 264–5.
3 Rachlin LS. Assault with battery. *N Engl J Med* 1984; **311**: 921–2.
4 Kavanagh KT, Litovitz T. Miniature battery foreign bodies in auditory and nasal cavities. *JAMA* 1986; **255**: 1470–2.
5 Capo JM, Lucente FE. Alkaline battery foreign bodies of the ear and nose. *Arch Otolaryngol Head Neck Surg* 1986; **112**: 562–3.
6 Goldman G, Toher L. A hair in the ear as a cause of noise. (Letter.) *N Engl J Med* 1982; **306**: 1553.

Chondrodermatitis nodularis

This painful condition usually involves the superior portion of the helix, but may appear on the antihelix, concha, tragus and antitragus. It has formerly been known as painful nodule of the ear [1].

Aetiology. The principal factors in its pathogenesis are pressure and a compromised local blood supply. It is more common in patients who habitually sleep on one side at night but can be triggered off by other factors including cold and pressure from headgear, earphones, etc. The age of onset is over 40 years in most cases and the condition is commoner in males than females. We have encountered chondrodermatitis nodularis in juveniles, but only when

there is an abnormality such as marked prominence of the antihelix. Alteration of connective tissue by chronic sun exposure is also thought to be a factor [2]. Chondrodermatitis nodularis has been reported in a series of cases of systemic sclerosis [3].

Pathology [4,5]. A typical lesion of chondrodermatitis nodularis consists of a nodule of degenerate, homogeneous collagen surrounded by vascular granulation tissue with an overlying acanthotic epidermis, and there may be a central ulcer through which the damaged collagen is extruded. In nearly all cases there is inflammation and fibrosis of the underlying perichondrium, and degenerative changes may be seen in the cartilage. Although many authors view the condition as an example of transepidermal elimination of altered connective tissue, it has been suggested that the infundibular portion of the hair follicle is primarily involved, with perforation of the follicular contents into the dermis [6,7].

Clinical features. The patient, usually a middle-aged to elderly man, seeks advice on account of pain. The more stoical may postpone consultation until the lesion interferes with sleep. The pain, which is sometimes severe, is initiated by pressure and occasionally by cold. It may be brief but

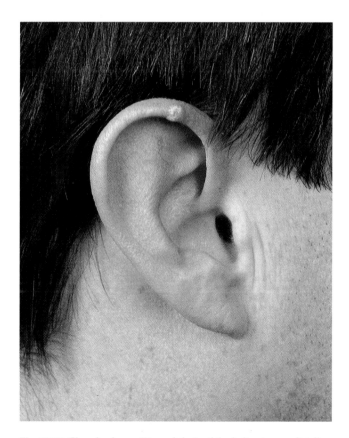

Fig. 68.10 Chondrodermatitis nodularis of the helix. A superficially ulcerated exquisitely tender nodule.

can persist and throb for an hour or more. Occasionally, and particularly in women, there is little discomfort. The lesion is a globular or oval nodule, about 0.5–2cm in diameter, raised above the often hyperaemic surrounding skin (Fig. 68.10). The surface is frequently scaly or crusted, concealing a small ulcer.

In men, nearly 90% of nodules are situated on the helix, usually at the upper pole and more frequently on the right, but may occur on the antihelix [8], tragus, concha and antitragus, in order of decreasing frequency [9]. Occasionally, there are multiple nodules or lesions, and they may occur bilaterally [10]. In women, the left and right ears are affected equally and the proportion of lesions on the antihelix and tragus is greater [11]. The nodules attain a maximum size in a few months and then remain unchanged indefinitely.

Diagnosis. Although the associated pain and tenderness are characteristic, the lesion is often misdiagnosed. Differential diagnosis includes basal and squamous cell carcinomas, solar keratosis, calcification of the pinna, elastotic nodules and 'weathering nodules' [12].

Treatment. Excision, with a narrow margin of normal skin, is the treatment of choice [13,14]. This approach can usefully be modified by the additional use of a curette, to define the extent of necrotic cartilage [15]. Removal of cartilage only can provide excellent results and be cosmetically superior [16]. On the antihelix it is usually necessary to raise a small flap of skin in order to shave-excise or curette the underlying cartilage. Other treatments used include intralesional steroid therapy [17], liquid nitrogen cryotherapy, and carbon dioxide laser [18,19]. In more severe or recurrent cases, a larger, wedge resection of the helix may be needed. In all patients, efforts must be made to reduce pressure or trauma to the helix.

REFERENCES

1 Forster OH. Painful nodular growth of the ear. *Arch Dermatol* 1925; **11**: 149–65.
2 Goette DK. Chondrodermatitis nodularis chronica helicis: a perforating necrobiotic granuloma. *J Am Acad Dermatol* 1980; **2**: 148–54.
3 Bottomley WW, Goodfield MDJ. Chondrodermatitis nodularis helicis occurring with systemic sclerosis—an under-reported association? *Clin Exp Dermatol* 1994; **19**: 219–20.
4 Shuman R, Helwig EB. Chondrodermatitis nodularis helicis chronica. *Am J Clin Pathol* 1954; **24**: 126–44.
5 Santa Cruz DJ. Chondrodermatitis nodularis helicis: a transepidermal perforating disorder. *J Cutan Pathol* 1980; **7**: 70–6.
6 Hurwitz RM. Painful papule of the ear: a follicular disorder. *J Dermatol Surg Oncol* 1987; **13**: 270–4.
7 Hurwitz RM. Pseudocarcinomatous or infundibular hyperplasia. *Am J Dermatopathol* 1989; **11**: 189–91.
8 Burns DA, Calnan CD. Chondrodermatitis nodularis antihelicis. *Clin Exp Dermatol* 1978; **3**: 207–8.
9 Barker LP, Young AW, Sachs W. Chrondrodermatitis of the ears: a differential study of nodules of the helix and antihelix. *Arch Dermatol* 1960; **81**: 53–63.
10 Cannon CR. Bilateral chondrodermatitis helicis: case presentation and review of the literature. *Am J Otol* 1985; **6**: 164–6.
11 Yaffee HS. Perichondritis in nuns caused by a change of head-dress. *Arch Dermatol* 1963; **87**: 735.
12 Kavanagh GM, Bradfield JWB, Collins CMP, Kennedy CTC. Weathering nodules of the ear; a clinicopathological study. *Br J Dermatol* 1996; **135**: 550–4.
13 Zimmerman MC. Removal of chondrodermatitis nodularis helicis. In: Epstein E, Epstein E, Jr, eds. *Skin Surgery*, 5th edn. Springfield: Thomas, 1982: 1137–9.
14 Ceilly RI. Surgical treatment of chondrodermatitis nodularis chronica helicis. In: Roenigk RK, Roenigk HH, Jr, eds. *Dermatologic Surgery: Principles and Practice*. New York: Marcel Dekker, 1988: 373–5.
15 Coldiron BM. The surgical management of chondrodermatitis nodularis helicis chronica. *J Dermatol Surg Oncol* 1991; **17**: 902–4.
16 Lawrence CM. The treatment of chondrodermatitis nodularis with cartilage removal alone. *Arch Dermatol* 1991; **127**: 530–5.
17 Wade TR. Chondrodermatitis nodularis helicis: a review with emphasis on steroid therapy. *Cutis* 1979; **24**: 406–9.
18 Karam F, Bauman T. Carbon dioxide laser treatment for chondrodermatitis nodularis chronica helicis. *Ear Nose Throat J* 1988; **67**: 757–63
19 Taylor MB. Chondrodermatitis nodularis chronica helicis: successful treatment with the carbon dioxide laser. *J Dermatol Surg Oncol* 1991; **17**: 862–4.

Pseudocyst of the ear

SYN. ENDOCHONDRIAL PSEUDOCYST;
IDIOPATHIC CYSTIC CHONDROMALACIA

A non-inflammatory, fluid-filled cavity within the cartilage of the ear.

Aetiology. Although the cause is unknown in most cases, trauma is likely to be important at least in some, as in fracture in the ear cartilage [1], habit-twisting of the ears [2], and rubbing due to atopic eczema [3]. Most speculations about the pathogenesis include an underlying malformation of the cartilage and degeneration due to release of lysosomal enzymes from chondrocytes. A role for cytokines has also been suggested [4].

Pathology. There is a cavity within the cartilage, the walls of which show the presence of eosinophilic amorphous material [5,6]. There may be focal fibrosis, especially in older lesions.

Clinical features. Most cases are young men, although the condition is seen over a wide age range [7] including infants [8]. Occasional cases have been recorded in females [9]. All races are affected [10]. There may be a predilection for Chinese, although this could be reporting bias [11,12]. The condition is usually unilateral and presents as an asymptomatic swelling, which is non-tender and fluctuant. Occasionally, there are signs of inflammation and some tenderness. The commonest location is on the upper half of the ear (Fig. 68.11), on the scapha, less commonly over the helix and antihelix. Sometimes, coalescent swellings are seen. Aspiration usually yields serous fluid, which soon reaccumulates.

Diagnosis. The differential diagnosis includes traumatic perichondritis, relapsing polychondritis (Chapter 44), haematoma, dermoid cyst and epidermoid cyst, benign and malignant tumours, but these can if necessary be excluded by a histological examination.

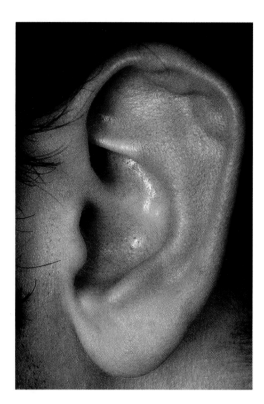

Fig. 68.11 Pseudocyst. Asymptomatic fluctuant swellings on the upper pinna.

Treatment. Needle aspiration followed by the introduction of a few drops of 1% tincture of iodine then application of a contour pressure bandage is often successful [10]. For recurrences, excision of the anterior wall of the cyst, suturing the skin flap back and use of a pressure dressing can produce a cosmetically satisfactory result in most cases [12]. Intralesional corticosteroid is sometimes helpful [13].

REFERENCES

1 Grabski WJ, Salasche SJ, McCollough ML, Angeloni VL. Pseudocyst of the auricle associated with trauma. *Arch Dermatol* 1989; **125**: 528–30.
2 Gonzales M, Raton JA, Manzano D *et al.* Pseudocyst of the ear. *Acta Derm Venereol (Stockh)* 1993; **73**: 212–13.
3 Devlin J, Harrison CJ, Whitby DJ, David TJ. Cartilaginous pseudocyst of the external auricle in children with atopic eczema. *Br J Dermatol* 1990; **122**: 699–704.
4 Yamamoto T, Yokoyama A, Umeda T. Cytokine profile of bilateral pseudocyst of the auricle (Letter). *Acta Derm Venereol (Stockh)* 1995; **76**: 92–3.
5 Glamb R, Kim R. Pseudocyst of the auricle. *J Am Acad Dermatol* 1984; **11**: 58–63.
6 Heffner DK, Hyams VJ. Cystic chondromalacia (endochondral pseudocyst) of the auricle. *Arch Pathol Lab Med* 1986; **110**: 740–3.
7 Lazar RH, Heffner DK, Hughes GB, Hyams VK. Pseudocyst of the auricle: a review of 21 cases. *Otolaryngol Head Neck Surg* 1986; **94**: 360–1.
8 Santos AD, Kelley PE. Bilateral pseudocyst of the auricle in an infant girl. *Pediatr Dermatol* 1995; **12**: 152–5.
9 Santos VD, Polisar IA, Ruffy ML. Bilateral pseudocysts of the auricle in a female. *Ann Otol* 1976; **83**: 9–11.
10 Cohen PR, Grossman ME. Pseudocyst of the auricle: case report and world literature review. *Arch Otolaryngol Head Neck Surg* 1990; **116**: 1202–4.
11 Engel D. Pseudocyst of the auricle in Chinese. *Arch Otolaryngol* 1996; **83**: 29–34.
12 Choi S, Lam K, Chan K, Ghadially F. Enchondral pseudocyst of the auricle in Chinese. *Arch Otolaryngol Head Neck Surg* 1984; **110**: 792–6.
13 Myamoto H, Dida M, Onuma S, Uchiyama M. Steroid injection therapy for pseudocyst of the auricle. *Acta Derm Venereol (Stockh)* 1994; **74**: 140–2.

Dermatoses and the external ear

Atopic dermatitis

A crusted eczematous fissure at the junction of the earlobe and the face is a common finding in atopics, and can be regarded as a reliable feature of atopy [1–3]. In the series of Tada *et al.* [3], 45 of their 46 patients with severe atopic dermatitis had infra-auricular fissures. In addition to involvement of the infra-auricular crease, the tragal notch and sometimes the whole of the pinna may be commonly involved. Treatment of eczema and the secondary infection that often accompanies it is discussed in Chapter 17.

REFERENCES

1 Voss M, Voss E, Schubert H. Schuppung der Ohren—ein Leitsymtom der Ichthyosis gruppe? *Dermatol Monatsschr* 1982; **168**: 394–7.
2 Sampson HA. Atopic dermatitis. *Ann Allergy* 1992; **69**: 469–81.
3 Tada J, Toi Y, Akiyama H, Arata J. Infra-auricular fissures in atopic dermatitis. *Acta Derm Venereol (Stockh)* 1994; **74**: 129–31.

Seborrhoeic dermatitis

In its mildest form, seborrhoeic dermatitis simply causes a little scaling and inflammation at the entrance to the external auditory meatus, in the concha or in the auricular folds. When severe, the whole pinna may be affected and there may be infective eczematoid dermatitis both in and around the ear or postauricularly. The relationship between seborrhoeic dermatitis and otitis externa is discussed in Chapter 17.

Asteatotic eczema

The exposed position of the ear renders it vunerable to the climatic changes that can induce asteatotic eczema (see Chapter 17). This common cause of a dry, itchy ear is mainly seen in the elderly. Aggravating factors include overzealous cleansing, cold, windy weather, low humidity indoors and air-conditioned air during the summer. There may be little to see other than slight scaling. Similar changes can occur in the ear canal, where additional factors include drying vehicles used in eardrops, for example alcohol and acetone. Management will include avoidance of provocative factors, and use of emollients.

Contact dermatitis

The external ear is commonly affected by both irritant and allergic contact dermatitis [1]. Causes of contact allergy may be grouped as follows.

1 Products used for the hair and scalp: hairspray, shampoos, hair dyes, hair nets, bathing caps.
2 Items worn or placed in or on the ear: jewellery, especially nickel alloys (see ear piercing p. 3019).
3 Plastic, rubber or metal ear appliances, for example hearing aids, spectacles, headphones, telephone receivers, earplugs, hair nets.
4 Objects used to clean or scratch the ear, for example hairpins, matches.
5 Cosmetics and toiletries: make-up, perfumes, soaps and creams.
6 Topical medicaments.
7 Others (transferred to the ear by fingers): nail varnish, plant resins (e.g. poison ivy, oak or sumac).

The role of occult allergic contact dermatitis in patients with otitis externa is discussed on page 3034.

REFERENCE

1 Jones EH. Allergy of the external ear and canal. *Otolaryngol Clin N Am* 1974; **7**: 735–48.

Psoriasis

Both guttate and plaque psoriasis involve the external ear. Sometimes this is by extension from the scalp, face or neck. Like seborrhoeic dermatitis, it often involves the concha and distal part of the external auditory canal, but usually its colour, the nature of the scaling and the presence of psoriasis elsewhere allow it to be differentiated. Sometimes both conditions appear to coexist.

Acne

Comedones frequently involve the concha, and they are occasionally found on the helix, tragus or earlobe. Inflammatory cysts may be found on the lobe, at the entrance to the external auditory canal, in both the pre- and post-auricular areas. Pressure from spectacle frames, telephone receivers or headsets can aggravate acne lesions.

Darier's disease

Occasionally, Darier's disease can present with involvement of the external ear as the principal affected site, with erythema, oedema and crusting mimicking an eczematous reaction [1].

REFERENCE

1 Thompson AC, Shall L, Moralee SJ. Darier's disease of the external ear. *J Laryng Otol* 1992; **106**: 725–6.

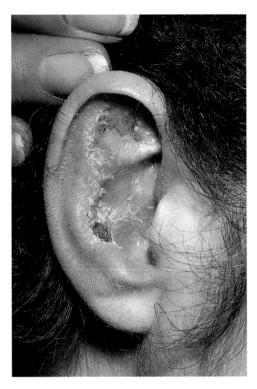

Fig. 68.12 Cutaneous lupus erythematosus. Acute erythema and erosions following sun exposure.

Transepithelial elimination disorders

The ear may occasionally be the site for lesions of Kyrle's disease, elastosis perforans serpiginosa, perforating folliculitis and perforating papules of diabetic dialysis patients. These conditions are discussed in Chapter 44.

Lupus erythematosus (Fig. 68.12)

Although most parts of the pinna may be involved in lupus erythematosus, pits and scarring in the concha are distinctive features [1,2]. Atrophy often occurs, and even perforation of the pinna [3].

REFERENCES

1 Shuster S. A simple sign of discoid lupus erythematosus. (Letter.) *Br J Dermatol* 1981; **104**: 350–1.
2 Rebora A. Scarring of the concha as a sign of lupus erythematosus. (Letter.) *Br J Dermatol* 1982; **106**: 122.
3 Lucky PA. Lupus erythematosus with perforation of the pinna. *Cutis* 1983; **32**: 554–7.

Mudi-chood

This distinctive dermatosis, which typically affects the nape of the neck and upper shoulders of girls and young women in the Kerala state of South India, can occur on the ears. It is thought to be the result of the frictional and occlusive effects of moist, oily hair in a hot and humid environment. Individual lesions are hyperpigmented papules with a thin surrounding rim of scale, occurring on the posterolateral aspects of the pinnae [1].

REFERENCE

1 Sugathan P. Mudi-chood on the pinnae. *Br J Dermatol* 1976; **95**; 197–8.

Lymphocytoma cutis

When the ear is involved, the lobe is characteristically affected, often with a large single nodule. Possible causative factors include *Borrelia burgdorferi* infection [1] and gold earrings [2,3].

REFERENCES

1 Albrecht A, Hofstadter S, Artsob H *et al.* Lymphadenosis benigna cutis resulting from *Borrelia* infection (*Borrelia* lymphocytoma). *J Am Acad Dermatol* 1991; **24**: 621–5.
2 Murata J, Toyoda H, Nogita T *et al.* A case of lymphadenosis benigna cutis of the earlobe: an immunohistochemical study. *J Dermatol* 1992; **19**: 186–9.
3 Kobayashi J, Nanko H, Nakamura J, Mizoguchi M. Lymphocytoma cutis induced by gold earrings. *J Am Acad Dermatol* 1992; **27**: 457–8.

Jessner's benign lymphocytic infiltration

This condition occasionally involves the ear and post-auricular region, and sunlight may precipitate or worsen the eruption.

Granuloma annulare

Typical papular and annular dermal lesions of granular annulare may involve the pinna, sometimes in the absence of lesions elsewhere [1].

REFERENCE

1 Muhlbauer JE. Granuloma annulare. *J Am Acad Dermatol* 1980; **3**: 217–30.

Primary cutaneous amyloidosis

Asymptomatic papules on the helix and concha of the ear have been described as the sole manifestation of cutaneous amyloidosis [1]; such lesions can also occur with more generalized papular amyloid [2] and with macular amyloid of the back [3].

REFERENCES

1 Hicks BC, Weber PJ, Hashimoto K *et al.* Primary cutaneous amyloidosis of the auricular concha. *J Am Acad Dermatol* 1988; **18**: 19–25.
2 Bakos L, Weissbluth ML, Pires AKS, Muller LFB. Primary amyloidosis of the concha (Letter.) *J Am Acad Dermatol* 1989; **3**: 524–5.
3 Barnadas M, Perez M, Esquius J *et al.* Papules in the auricular concha: lichen amyloidosus in a case of biphasic amyloidosis. *Dermatologica* 1990; **181**: 149–51.

Angiolymphoid hyperplasia with eosinophilia

SYN. PSEUDOPYOGENIC GRANULOMA; ATYPICAL PYOGENIC GRANULOMA; EPITHELIOID HAEMANGIOMA; HISTIOCYTOID HAEMANGIOMA INTRAVENOUS ATYPICAL VASCULAR PROLIFERATION; NODULAR ANGIOBLASTIC HYPERPLASIA WITH EOSINOPHILIA; LYMPHOFOLLICULOSIS [1–4]

This is a reactive proliferative disorder of blood vessels with a variable component of inflammatory cells. It occurs in both a dermal [5] and a subcutaneous form [6], and is most commonly found on the head and neck. The two forms are regarded as variants of the same condition [7–9].

Aetiological factors include trauma, pregnancy and immunization procedures [10].

Histology. There are circumscribed collections of vessels whose endothelial cells are epithelioid, i.e. have abundant eosinophilic cytoplasm and large nuclei. These cells sometimes proliferate into the lumen, and may occur in solid clumps. The associated inflammatory infiltrate consists of lymphocytes, sometimes lymphoid follicles, and there are varying numbers of eosinophils.

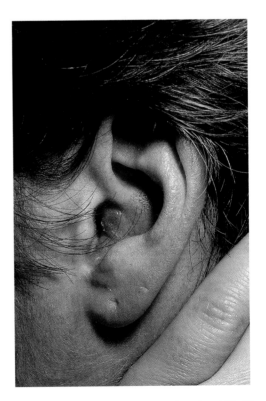

Fig. 68.13 Angiolymphoid hyperplasia with eosinophilia. Firm, red–brown nodules at the entrance to the external auditory canal.

Clinical features. The dermal form commonly affects the pinna, external auditory meatus (Fig. 68.13) and postauricular area. The lesions are red–brown papules or nodules. Occasionally, they itch and can be painful or pulsatile [10,11]. The condition mainly affects young to middle-aged adults, and in some series there is a female preponderance [12].

Differential diagnosis includes pyogenic granuloma (rare at this site), bacillary angiomatosis and angiosarcoma.

Treatment. The treatment of choice is surgical excision, although recurrence often occurs. Intralesional corticosteroids, laser, for example of the argon type [13], and radiotherapy have been used in some cases with benefit.

REFERENCES

1 Enzinger FM, Weiss SW. *Soft Tissue Tumors*. St Louis: CV Mosby, 1983; 391–7.
2 Rosai J. Angiolymphoid hyperplasia with eosinophilia of the skin. *Am J Dermatopathol* 1982; **4**: 175–84.
3 Rosai J, Akerman LR. Intravenous atypical vascular proliferation. A cutaneous lesion simulating a malignant blood vessel tumour. *Arch Dermatol* 1974; **109**: 714–17.
4 Bendl BJ, Asano K, Lewis RJ. Nodular angioblastic hyperplasia with eosinophilia and lymphofolliculosis. *Cutis* 1977; **19**: 327–9.
5 Wilson Jones E, Bleehen SS. Inflammatory angiomatous nodules with abnormal blood vessels occurring about the ears and scalp (pseudo and atypical pyogenic granuloma). *Br J Dermatol* 1969; **81**: 804–16.
6 Wells GC, Whimster IW. Subcutaneous lymphoid hyperplasia with eosinophilia. *Br J Dermatol* 1969; **81**: 1–15.
7 Kandil E. Dermal angiolymphoid hyperplasia with eosinophilia versus pseudopyogenic granuloma. *Br J Dermatol* 1970; **83**: 405–8.
8 Mehregan AH, Shapiro L. Angiolymphoid hyperplasia with eosinophilia. *Arch Dermatol* 1971; **103**: 50–7.
9 Reed RJ, Terezakis N. Subcutaneous angioblastic lymphoid hyperplasia with eosinophilia (Kimura's disease). *Cancer* 1972; **29**: 489–97.
10 Olsen TG, Helwig EB. Angiolymphoid hyperplasia with eosinophilia. A clinicopathologic study of 116 patients. *J Am Acad Dermatol* 1985; **12**: 781–96.
11 Leonard JN, Ryan TJ, Dawber RP. Pseudopyogenic granuloma. *Clin Exp Dermatol* 1981; **6**: 215–18.
12 Henry PG, Burnett JW. Angiolymphoid hyperplasia with eosinophilia. *Arch Dermatol* 1978; **114**: 1168–72.
13 Vallis RC, Garfield Davies D. Angiolymphoid hyperplasia of the head and neck. *J Laryngol Otol* 1988; **102**: 100–1.

Skin reactions to osseo-integrated implants

Restoration of the pinna, following traumatic loss or congenital absence may be achieved using an osseo-integrated skin-penetrating titanium fixture. About 10% of such patients have skin reactions [1,2]. The reaction consists of erythema and crusting, sometimes with significant infection, which should be adequately treated.

REFERENCES

1 Jacobsson M, Tjellstrom A, Fine L, Andersson H. A retrospective study of osseointegrated skin-penetrating titanium fixtures used for retaining facial prostheses. *Int J Oral Maxillofac Implants* 1992; **7**: 523–8.
2 Gitto CA, Plata WG, Schaaf NG. Evaluation of the peri-implant epithelial tissue of percutaneous implant abutments supporting maxillofacial prostheses. *Int J Oral Maxillofac Implants* 1994; **9**: 197–206.

Elephantiasis of the external ears

Chronically red swollen ears may occur for a number of reasons including long-standing eczema, psoriasis [1] and chronic streptococcal infection. Long-standing head louse infection has also been reported as a cause [2].

REFERENCES

1 Grant JM. Elephantiasis nostras verrucosa of the ears. *Cutis* 1982; **29**: 441–4.
2 Mahzoon S, Azadeh B. Elephantiasis of external ears: a rare manifestation of pediculosis capitis. *Acta Derm Venereol (Stockh)* 1983; **63**: 363–5.

Psychocutaneous disorders

Dermatitis artefacta and delusions of parasitosis (see Chapter 64) may occasionally result in self-induced lesions on the ears and even in the ear canals.

Granuloma faciale

The ear is an occasional site for this distinctive disorder [1].

REFERENCE

1 Foss MH. Granuloma faciale: report on a case. *Acta Derm Venereol (Stockh)* 1957; **37**: 473–82.

Immunobullous diseases

Pemphigus, pemphigoid, dermatitis herpetisformis and epidermolysis bullosa aquisita may all involve the ear, and occasionally the auditory canal.

Systemic disease and the external ear

Many conditions described more fully elsewhere will occasionally present on the external ear with lesions of diagnostic value.

Granulomatous disorders

These include sarcoidosis [1,2] especially the lupus pernio variety. Metastatic Crohn's disease may rarely involve the ear [3]. Atypical facial necrobiosis may involve the ear, as well as the more typical location on the face and scalp. Wegener's granulomatosis can present with serous or suppurative otitis and conductive or sensory neural deafness [4,5]. A similar allergic granulomatosis affected both ears in a young black South African who died from glomerulonephritis [6]. Infective granulomatous diseases involve the ear, notably leprosy, in which the earlobe is a valuable site for taking smears [7]. Lupus vulgaris, other manifestations of tuberculosis, atypical mycobacterial infection (e.g. *Mycobacterium marinum* from swimming-pool injuries), deep fungal infections and even syphilis [8] can involve the ear.

Collagen vascular diseases

As well as discoid lupus, subacute cutaneous lupus erythematosus and systemic lupus erythematosus may also involve the ears. Scleroderma can produce pallor and telangiectasia of the auditory canal. Rheumatoid disease is characterized by nodules, which can occur on the ear, where they may ulcerate due to pressure from the pillow or spectacles.

Pyoderma gangrenosum [9]

The ear is an occasional presenting site for this primary ulcerative disorder, discussed in Chapter 49. Vasculitis and factitial disease may be mimicked.

Metabolic disorders

Xanthomas occasionally occur on the ears, presenting as yellow nodules. Gouty tophi frequently involve the pinna (Fig. 68.14), and may antedate the onset of joint disease or appear decades after the initial attack. The helix and the antihelix are typical sites. Histology is distinctive. Porphyria cutanea tarda (Fig. 68.15) may present with vesicles and

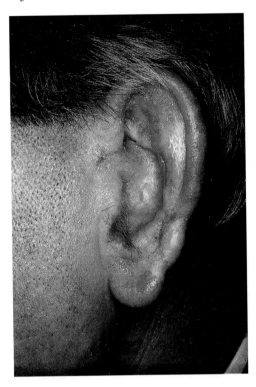

Fig. 68.15 Porphyria cutanea tarda. Firm, whitish sclerodermoid changes, at the site of repeated blistering.

bullae, often on a background of scarring, hyperpigmentation, milia, sclerodermoid plaques and hypertrichosis. Pseudocysts of the auricle and perichondritis may be simulated [10].

Diseases of connective tissue

Cutis laxa may result in distinctive pendulous earlobes [11].

Alkaptonuria

SYN. OCHRONOSIS

This is typically associated with a bluish discoloration of the auricular cartilage due to oxidization of bound homogentisic acid (Fig. 68.16). The cerumen in such patients may be very dark, a finding that can precede other clinical manifestations.

Calcium deposition

Calcium deposition may occur in many circumstances (see Chapter 59) and occasionally the ear is involved. Usually, calcium deposits in the ear occur for local reasons, for example degenerative changes in the cartilage. In infants, congenital nodular calcification of Winer should be considered [12].

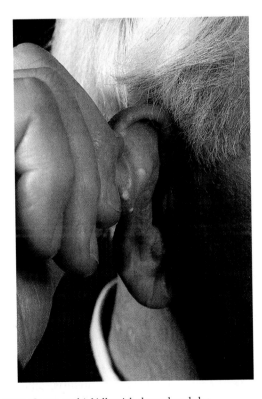

Fig. 68.14 Gouty tophi. Yellowish dermal nodules.

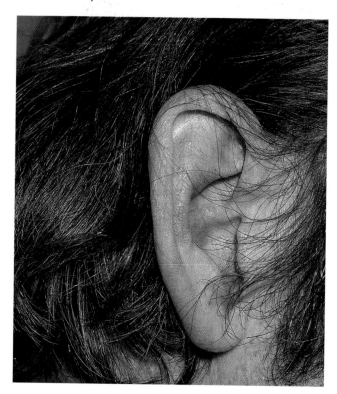

Fig. 68.16 Alkaptonuria. The auricular cartilage has a distinctive blue colour. (Courtesy of Dr P. Hollingworth, Southmead Hospital, Bristol, UK.)

Endocrine disorders

In Addison's disease, the pigmentary changes may involve the ear, and ossification of the auricular cartilage may occur [13]. In acromegaly, there is usually enlargement of the auricular cartilage and coarsening of the overlying skin.

Paraneoplastic syndromes

Bazex' syndrome (acrokeratosis paraneoplastica) (Chapter 61) commonly affects the ears and is an important marker for internal malignancy [14].

Drug-related effects

Hypertrophy of the retro-auricular folds may be seen as a consequence of phenytoin therapy [15]. Hypertrichosis of the ear canal due to minoxidil therapy can be a predisposing factor for external otitis [16].

REFERENCES

1 Nova A. Sarcoidosis of the ear. *Ear Nose Throat J* 1981; **60**: 307–8.
2 Swansson-Beck H, Goos M, Christophers E. Ohrlappchengranulom. *Hautarzt* 1982; **33**: 115–16.
3 McCallum DI, Gray WM. Metastatic Crohn's disease. *Br J Dermatol* 1976; **95**: 551–4.
4 McCaffrey TU, McDonald TJ, Facer GW *et al*. Otologic manifestation of Wegener's granulomatosis. *Otolaryngol Head Neck Surg* 1980; **88**: 586–93.
5 Kornblut AD, Wolffs M, Fauci AS. Ear disease in patients with Wegener's granulomatosis. *Laryngoscope* 1982; **92**: 713–17.
6 Bentley-Phillips B, Bayler MA. Destructive granuloma of the ear. *Int J Dermatol* 1980; **19**: 336–9.
7 Mansfield RE, Storkan MA, Cliff IS. Evaluation of the earlobe in leprosy. A clinical and histopathological study. *Arch Dermatol* 1969; **100**: 407–12.
8 Wilcox JR. An atypical case of secondary syphilis. *Br J Venereol Dis* 1981; **57**: 30–2.
9 Lysy J, Zimmerman J, Ackerman Z, Reifen E. Atypical auricular pyoderma gangrenosum simulating fungal infection. *J Clin Gastroenterol* 1989; **11**: 561–4.
10 Bukachevsky R, Kimmelman CP. Otolaryngologic manifestations of porphyria cutanea tarda *Otolaryngol Head Neck Surg* 1989; **101**: 402–3.
11 Ghigliotti G, Parodi A, Borgiani L *et al*. Acquired cutis laxa confined to the face. *J Am Acad Dermatol* 1991; **24**: 504–5.
12 Azon-Masoliver A, Ferrando J, Navarra E, Mascaro JE. Solitary congenital nodular calcification of Winer located on the ear: report of two cases. *Pediatr Dermatol* 1989; **6**: 191–3.
13 Chadwick JM, Downham TF. Auricular calcification. *Int J Dermatol* 1978; **17**: 799–801.
14 Bazex A, Griffiths A. Acrokeratosis paraneoplastica—a new cutaneous marker of malignancy. *Br J Dermatol* 1980; **102**: 301–6.
15 Trunnell TN, Waisman M. Hypertrophied retroauricular folds attributable to diphenylhydantoin therapy. *Cutis* 1982; **30**: 207–9.
16 Toriumi DM, Konior RJ, Berktold RE. Severe hypertrichosis of the external ear canal during minoxidil therapy. *Arch Otolaryngol Head Neck Surg* 1988; **114**: 918–19.

Infection

The anatomy of the ear with its many folds and the semi-occluded nature of the external auditory canal make it particularly susceptible to intertriginous infection, especially with Gram-negative organisms. A close anatomical relationship between the middle and external ear means that infections can pass relatively easily from one to the other, and the eardrum should always be examined. The cartilaginous and bony structures close to the skin are particularly vulnerable to infection. Although chondritis and perichondritis may have other causes, they are included in this section.

Infections of the pinna

Staphylococcus aureus, alone or in association with group A β-haemolytic *Streptococcus*, may cause impetigo contagiosum of the ear. This is a relatively common site for infection in infants and young children. *S. aureus* is also the most common causative organism of furuncles (boils) and carbuncles, which are more common in the external auditory canal than on the pinna. Cracks and fissures around the auricle are often the portal of entry for β-haemolytic streptococcal infection manifesting as erysipelas. This is more common in the elderly, the newborn and those suffering from malnutrition, disability, alcoholism, diabetes or immune deficiency states.

Erysipelas typically begins with high fever, constitutional upset including malaise, vomiting and headache, and there is rapidly spreading erythema and oedema from the pinna on to the face. There is often lymphadenopathy. Recurrent attacks of cellulitis of the face may have the same predisposing factors as at other body sites (Chapter 27). Recurrent attacks of cellulitis lead to fibrosis and lymphoedema. Treatment of erysipelas and cellulitis is discussed in Chapter 27. The term *infective eczematoid dermatitis* is still used for an oozing, crusted, eczematous condition occurring on and often below the pinna in association with chronic discharge from the ear. Coagulase-positive staphylococci are the most frequently isolated bacteria. The ear canal is oedematous and erythematous, and purulent discharge may be seen coming from a perforated tympanic membrane.

The condition should be differentiated from impetigo, secondarily infected contact dermatitis, seborrhoeic dermatitis and atopic dermatitis.

Treatment. Primary infection of the ear must be treated appropriately, usually with a systemic antibiotic; any associated chronic otitis media or mastoiditis is likely to be managed by an otologist. Involved skin can be cleansed with saline, 1:10000 potassium permanganate or dilute aluminium acetate soaks and then treated with a topical steroid.

Perichondritis and chondritis

Inflammation of the cartilage itself (chondritis), or more commonly the vascularized lining (perichondritis), can be indistinguishable from infection of these structures, and infection is a common complication whatever the cause [1,2].

Aetiology. There are many causes, including physical trauma (Fig. 68.17), thermal and chemical burns, frostbite, acupuncture, pressure (e.g. from tight headphones and head-dresses [3] and ear piercing, including acupuncture [4,5]. Perichondritis may occasionally follow superficial infections of the ear such as furunculosis or otitis externa. The most common infecting organism is *Pseudomonas aeruginosa*, although other Gram-negative organisms and *Staphylococcus* may at times be responsible.

Clinical features. Chondritis and perichondritis are typically painful. The pinna becomes hot, painful and swollen, with loss of normal contour due to oedema, and there may be accumulation of pus in the subperichondrial layer. Constitutional symptoms are common. The inflammation can spread back to the adjoining face. The destruction of cartilage results in deformity of the ear, which may be severe. Necrotizing fasciitis can follow perichondritis of the pinna [6], and if suspected must be treated by urgent debridement.

Diagnosis. Perichondritis may be difficult to distinguish from cellulitis, although perichondritis is usually more painful and does not involve the lobule of the ear, which lacks cartilage. Relapsing polychondritis (Chapter 44) usually involves cartilage elsewhere and is often recurrent.

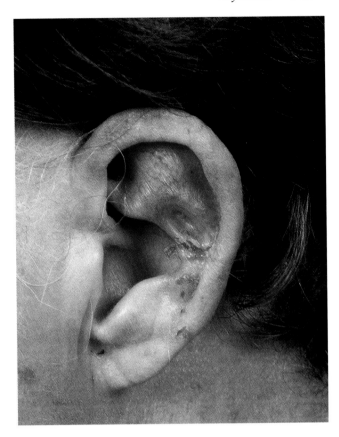

Fig. 68.17 Pressure ulcer exposing cartilage, a potential cause of chondritis.

Treatment. Treatment should be instituted promptly. If an abscess has developed, early drainage is necessary. Ciprofloxacin or other quinolones are probably the treatment of choice [7,8]. Necrotic cartilage may subsequently need to be excised, and fluid collections aspirated.

REFERENCES

1 Martin R, Yonkers AJ, Yarington CT, Jr. Perichondritis of the ear. *Laryngoscope* 1976; **86**: 664–73.
2 Bassiouny A. Perichondritis of the auricle. *Laryngoscope* 1981; **91**: 422–31.
3 Williams HC. Turban ear. *Arch Dermatol* 1994; **130**: 117–19.
4 Allison G, Kravitz E. Auricular chondritis secondary to acupuncture. *N Engl J Med* 1975; **293**: 780.
5 Davis O, Powell M. Auricular perichondritis secondary to acupuncture. *Arch Otolaryngol* 1985; **111**: 770–1.
6 Skorina J, Kaufman D. Necrotizing fasciitis originating from pinna perichondritis. *Otolaryngol Head Neck Surg* 1995; **113**: 467–73.
7 Noel SB, Scattan P, Meadors MC *et al.* Treatment of *Pseudomonas aeruginosa* auricular perichondritis is with oral ciprofloxacin. *J Dermatol Surg Oncol* 1989; **15**: 633–7.
8 Thomas JN, Swanson N. Treatment of perichondritis with a quinolone derivative—norfloxacin. *J Dermatol Surg Oncol* 1988; **14**: 447–9.

Other bacterial infections of the pinna

Mycobacterial infection can rarely involve the external ear. Lupus vulgaris can produce extensive destruction [1].

Secondary involvement from underlying lymph-node disease (scrofuloderma) can present with hearing loss, tinnitus and periauricular lymphadenopathy, with only minimal secretion in the ear canal [2].

Atypical mycobacteria that may involve the ear include *Mycobacterium marinum* acquired from swimming-pool injuries.

In *leprosy*, the ear is almost always involved in the lepromatous type, and there may be evident infiltration of the skin. The earlobe is often used before taking smears [3].

Syphilis may occasionally involve the ear, usually in the secondary stage [4].

REFERENCES

1 Fasal P. But it was not leprosy. *Cutis* 1975; **15**: 499–509.
2 Hunsaker DH. Conchomeatoplasty for chronic otitis externa. *Arch Otolaryngol Head Neck Surg* 1988; **114**: 395–8.
3 Mansfield RE, Storkan MA, Cliff IS. Evaluation of the earlobe in leprosy. A clinical and histopathological study. *Arch Dermatol* 1969; **100**: 407–12.
4 Wilcox JR. An atypical case of secondary syphilis. *Br J Venereol Dis* 1981; **57**: 30–2.

Viral infections

Herpes simplex occasionally involves the ear. It is often transmitted during contact sports such as rugby and wrestling. Herpes zoster may present as an isolated herpetiform eruption of the external ear or may be associated with ipsilateral facial palsy and auditory symptoms (Ramsay–Hunt syndrome; geniculate herpes). The condition usually begins with pain and may initially be mistaken for erysipelas. Vesicles usually appear on about the fifth day and involve the pinna, the external auditory meatus and, rarely, the tympanic membrane. There is usually malaise, pyrexia and lymphadenopathy. Facial palsy, when it occurs, is usually transient, but more severe and persistent cases do occur. Taste and lacrimation may also be affected. Compression damage to the VIIIth cranial nerve may lead to tinnitus, vertigo, nystagmus, nausea and deafness. Management of herpes zoster is discussed in Chapter 26.

Superficial and deep mycoses

Dermatophyte fungi may rarely involve the ear, but when present can simulate granulomatous disease [1] and chondritis [2].

Pityriasis versicolor may involve the ears, but is usually easy to diagnose.

In cases of ulcerative granulomatous disease of the ear, deep fungal infections, for example sporotrichosis [3] should be considered. Biopsy, examination of smears, cultures and serological studies should enable accurate diagnosis. Deep fungal infection may prompt an enquiry for underlying immune deficiency.

Otomycosis is discussed under otitis externa.

REFERENCES

1 Verbov J. Granulomatous *Trichophyton rubrum* infection of the pinnae. *Br J Dermatol* 1973; **89**: 212–13.
2 Bishop M, Rist TE. Tinea of the ear mimicking chondritis. *Cutis* 1979; **23**: 638–9.
3 Cox RL, Reller LB. Auricular sporotrichosis in a brick mason. *Arch Dermatol* 1979; **115**: 1229–30.

Infections of the external auditory canal and meatus

External otitis
SYN. OTITIS EXTERNA [1]

Otitis externa is a loose term that embraces more than one disease process. Aetiologically, it is rarely unifactorial [2] and constitutional, traumatic, environmental and microbial factors usually coexist. The condition is characterized by inflammation of the canal epithelium and by varying degrees of pain, itch, deafness and discharge.

Pathogenesis. Otitis externa can be divided, for convenience, into two main groups [3]: (i) a *'reactive' group* consisting of patients suffering from eczema, psoriasis or seborrhoeic dermatitis; and (ii) a *predominantly 'infective' group* in which either bacteria or fungi are involved. The two components often, however, coexist. The cause in many cases is not apparent [4] but the following predisposing factors appear to be important.

Genetic and constitutional. There are significant racial and individual differences in susceptibility to otitis externa. This may be due to anatomical differences in the curvature of the external auditory canal or narrowing of the isthmus—natives of New Guinea with wide, straight canals only rarely suffer from external otitis [5]—or, possibly, to differences in the type, amount or composition of cerumen, whose waxy constituency and low pH are protective against bacteria. *Pseudomonas aeruginosa*, the commonest bacterial pathogen in external otitis, binds to cells by a lectin-mediated process, and binding occurs more in individuals expressing blood group A on their epithelial cells [6].

Abundant tragal hair or plugs of wax and debris increase the relative humidity and reduce ventilation of the external auditory canal so that the canal epithelium becomes macerated and more susceptible to infection. Hypertrichosis of the canal due to minoxidil has been associated with external otitis [7]. Dental abnormalities and poor mastication [8] may also retard expulsion of wax and epithelial squames.

The atopic and seborrhoeic states predispose to external otitis not only by interfering with the integrity of the auricular epithelium but also by encouraging scratching and secondary infection [9]. Both too much and too little cerumen and alterations in skin pH have at times been held responsible [10].

Environmental. Heat, humidity and moisture are undoubtedly important in 'hot-weather ear' or 'swimmers' ear' [11,12]. This condition is common, especially among white people in tropical and subtropical regions. High temperature, high relative humidity and swimming [13] all encourage maceration and secondary bacterial or fungal infections of the canal epithelium. Fresh-water swimming appears to be a particular risk factor [14]. Failure to dry the ears completely after swimming, shampooing or showering may also be a factor in some cases [15].

Traumatic. Trauma, in the opinion of many investigators [2,9,13,16,17], is one of the prime factors in both the initiation and the persistence of many cases. In one series of 113 patients, 58 admitted using wool-tippped matches, two admitted using bare matches and seven used hairgrips to relieve itching [2]. Patients suffering from eczema or those with neurodermatitis tend to scratch, rub or 'fiddle' with their ears; other patients appear obsessed about cleaning their ears and by doing so excessively they interfere with the normal homeostatic and self-cleaning properties [18]. Impacted cerumen may cause irritation, which is often increased by inexpert attempts to remove it; so may pressure from hearing aids and transistor ear pieces and, especially with the 'internal' hearing aid, a combination of pressure and occlusion often leads to the development of external otitis.

Pyococcal and mycotic infection. The epidermis of the external auditory canal is normally fairly resistant to infection. The bacterial flora, although varying with race, geography and season, tends to resemble that of the skin but with a higher likelihood of finding *Pseudomonas aeruginosa* [19]. In hot, humid environments, however, and particularly among swimmers, whose ears are habitually wet, the incidence of *Pseudomonas aeruginosa* and other Gram-negative infections rises substantially [20,21] as does the frequency with which *Aspergillus* or *Candida* species are isolated [16]. An outbreak of *Pseudomonas* otitis has been reported in association with contaminated pool water [22] but a source has rarely been found in other series, and it is assumed that *Pseudomonas* infections are of endogenous origin.

In more temperate climates, *Staphylococcus aureus* is often isolated [2, 9]. This may be associated with evidence of skin disease elsewhere or with staphylococcal carriage. Certainly, recurrent cases of staphylococcal otitis externa should have nasal and perianal swabs; occasionally it may be necessary to swab and 'destaph' the whole family. Staphylococcal carriage has also been observed following the use of airline headsets [23]. In other cases, there may be an underlying tympanic perforation or coexistent otitis media. The ear drums should therefore always be examined, especially in patients with unilateral or recurrent disease. Occasionally, infection spreads out from the ear canal and causes impetigo or infective eczema of the auricle and surrounding skin.

In the tropics, mycotic infections of the external ear canal are relatively common [24,25]. Aspergillus [11,26–28], *Candida* [27], *Penicillium* [26] and *Mucor* are the species most often incriminated, most cases being due to either *Aspergillus niger* or *Candida albicans*. There is some debate, however, as to whether these fungi are pathogenic, opportunistic, saprophytic or simply commensal [25–27,29].

REFERENCES

1 Lucente FE. Diseases due to infection. In: Lucente FE, Lawson W, Novick NL, eds. *The External Ear.* Philadelphia: WB Saunders, 1996: 48–97.
2 McKelvie M, McKelvie P. Some aetiological factors in otitis externa. *Br J Dermatol* 1966; **78**: 227–31.
3 Mawson SR, Ludman H, eds. *Diseases of the Ear,* 4th edn. London: Edward Arnold, 1979.
4 Russell JD, Donnelly M, McShane DP *et al*. What causes acute otitis externa? *J Laryngol Otol* 1993; **107**: 898–901.
5 Quayle AF. Otitis externa in New Guinea. *Med J Aust* 1944; **2**: 228–31.
6 Steuer MK, Hofstadter F, Probster L *et al*. Are ABH antigenic determinants on human outer ear canal epithelium responsible for *Pseudomonas aeruginosa* infections? *Otorhinolaryngol* 1995; **57**: 148–52.
7 Toriumi DM, Konior RJ, Berktold RE. Severe hypertrichosis of the external ear canal during minoxidil therapy. *Arch Otolaryngol Head Neck Surg* 1988; **114**: 918–19.
8 Dunn B. Otitis externa and malposed third molars. *J Laryngol Otol* 1962; **76**: 981–4.
9 Keogh C, Russell B. The problem of otitis externa. *Br Med J* 1956; **i**: 1068–72.
10 McLaurin JW, Raggio TP, Simmons M. Persistent external otitis. *Laryngoscope* 1965; **75**: 1699–707.
11 Yassin A, Mostafa MA, Moawad MK. Fungus infection of the ear (clinical and cultural studies). *J Laryngol Otol* 1964; **78**: 591–602.
12 Calderon R, Mood EW. An epidemiological assessment of water quality and 'swimmers' ear'. *Arch Environ Health* 1982; **37**: 300–5.
13 Strauss NB, Dierker RL. Otitis externa associated with aquatic activities (swimmer's ear). *Clin Dermatol* 1987; **5**: 103–11.
14 Springer GL, Shapiro EA. Fresh water swimming as a risk factor for otitis externa: a case-control study. *Arch Environ Health* 1985; **40**: 202–6.
15 Russell JD, Donnelly M, McShane DP *et al*. What causes acute otitis externa? *J Laryngol Otol* 1993; **107**: 898–901.
16 Wright DN, Alexander JM. Effect of water on the bacterial flora of swimmers' ears. *Arch Otolaryngol* 1974; **99**: 15–18.
17 Hirsch BE. Infections of the external ear. *Am J Otolaryngol* 1992; **13**: 145–55.
18 Alberti PWRM. Epithelial migration on the tympanic membrane. *J Laryngol* 1964; **78**: 808–30.
19 Brook I. Microbiological studies of bacterial flora of the external auditory canal in children. *Acta Otolaryngol* 1981; **91**: 285–7.
20 Hoadley AW, Knight DE. External otitis among swimmers and nonswimmers. *Arch Environ Health* 1975; **30**: 445–8.
21 Lambert IJ. A comparison of the treatment of otitis externa with 'Otosporin' and aluminium acetate: a report from a services practice in Cyprus. *J R Coll Gen Pract* 1981; **31**: 291–4.
22 Weingarten MA. Otitis externa due to *Pseudomonas* in swimming pool bathers. *J R Coll Gen Pract* 1977; **27**: 359–60.
23 Brook I. Bacterial flora of airline headset devices. *Am J Otolaryngol* 1985; **6**: 111–14.
24 Beaney GRE, Broughton A. Tropical otomycosis. *Laryngol Otol* 1967; **81**: 987–97.
25 Youssef YA, Abdou MH. Studies on fungus infection of the external ear: I. Mycological and clinical observations. *J Laryngol Otol* 1967; **81**: 401–12.
26 Haley LD. Etiology of otomycosis II. Bacterial flora of the ear. *Arch Otolaryngol* 1950; **52**: 208–13.
27 Gregson AEW, La Touche CJ. Otomycosis: a neglected disease. *J Laryngol Otol* 1961; **75**: 45–69.
28 Ismail HK. Otomycosis. *J Laryngol Otol* 1962; **76**: 713–19.
29 Smyth GDL. Fungal infection in otology. *Br J Dermatol* 1964; **76**: 425–8.

Histopathology [1–4]. In most cases of external otitis, there is acanthosis, elongation of the rete ridges and an increase in orthokeratosis and parakeratosis. Spongiosis occurs in eczematous and seborrhoeic forms. The nature of the dermal infiltrate varies with both cause and chronicity. The histopathology is seldom diagnostic except when fungal mycelia are seen.

Clinical features. The condition can be acute, subacute or chronic. In patients seen at hospital, it tends to be severe, chronic or chronic relapsing, but in the community it is less severe and recalcitrant [5,6].

Mild attacks may present with pain or itching without discharge and with a minimally congested or swollen meatus. The degree of irritation or discomfort is often out of all proportion to the appearance. This stage probably represents early damage to the meatal skin [7]. Most cases of this type will resolve with simple therapeutic measures, but a minority, perhaps due to trauma, secondary infection or failure to keep the ear dry and clean, progress to more severe disease.

Fully developed acute external otitis (diffuse otitis externa) is characterized by a sudden onset of ear pain, itching, a sense of fullness or stuffiness if there is significant oedema, and a variable degree of hearing loss. The otalgia is often exacerbated by jaw movements. With progression, there is usually drainage of pus, which tends to be bluish green in colour if *Pseudemonas* is the dominant infecting organism. Examination shows erythema and swelling, which may spread from the external auditory meatus to involve the concha or beyond. The external auditory canal shows erythema and oedema, and there is macerated debris and perhaps greenish pus present. In severe cases, inflammation can extend to involving the tympanic membrane. Hearing loss is due to oedema of the canal, and this may be sufficient to obscure vision of its full length. Traction on the pinna to examine the canal and pressure over the tragus characteristically elicit pain. The discharge from the ear is often malodorous, and if *Pseudomonas* is present will be musty bluish green. There may be associated fever, malaise and regional lymphadenopathy.

It is important to gently remove debris in the process of a full examination, and to try to determine whether the disease is secondary to otitis media, and whether or not the tympanic membrane is intact.

Bullous external otitis [8] is an uncommon variant in which there is a sudden onset of severe pain followed by discharge of blood from the ear canal. Bluish-red haemorrhagic bullae are visible on the osseous canal walls.

In granular external otitis the lining of the meatus and canal is replaced in part or whole by granulation tissue, which can project inwards as pedunculated masses. These are usually found near the tympanic membrane, arising from the osseous end of the canal. Granular external otitis is associated with a severe or neglected course [9,10].

The term chronic external otitis is sometimes used for cases that have had persistent symptoms for more than 2 months [11]. Microbiological assessment has shown a significant organism in 82% in one series: *Staphylococcus aureus* in one-third; *Pseudomonas* in one-third and various other Gram-negative and Gram-positive organisms in the remainder. In addition, 17 of the 99 patients had fungal disease alone [12]. It is likely that in most cases of chronic otitis externa, particularly when treatment has been used for the acute attack and symptoms have continued, concurrent dermatological disorders are present. Cases that behave in a recalcitrant manner may have an underlying systemic disease such as acquired immune deficiency syndrome (AIDS), malnutrition, uncontrolled diabetes mellitus, or be on high-dose steroids or chemotherapeutic agents [13].

Seborrhoeic dermatitis, atopic dermatitis and psoriasis usually occur only at the meatus but may sometimes extend further into the canal. Seborrhoeic otitis externa is extremely common and has been regarded by some dermatologists as the basis for most cases of otitis externa. The symptoms and signs, however, are normally mild unless complicated by secondary factors and usually consist of no more than superficial scaling and a little discomfort or itching. Signs of pityriasis capitis or of seborrhoeic dermatitis elsewhere are usually present. The condition may deteriorate at times of stress or fatigue. Secondary bacterial infection is common. In this 'reactive' group the appearance is often that of a dermatitis spreading into the ear in contrast with those cases with a primarily 'infective' aetiology where infection and/or inflammation often appears to be spreading out from the ear and where the entire length of the canal is often affected. The clinical appearance, however, is often non-diagnostic.

In infective eczema there is usually intense pruritus associated with exudate. The condition may complicate both otitis media and otitis externa and is usually associated with some degree of otorrhoea. In others it appears to develop from seborrhoeic dermatitis that has become secondarily infected. The condition may affect the meatus, concha, lobe and peri-auricular skin and often spreads widely. The postauricular fold is commonly affected. The symptoms and signs are those of eczema with an accompanying or preceding aural discharge. In seborrhoeic individuals, other areas may be involved at the same time. Fissures and cellulitis are common complications.

Contact dermatitis is often occult [14] and easily overlooked. Sensitivity to topically applied medicaments is common in chronic otitis externa. Occlusion, the recurrent nature of the disease and frequent usage of antibiotics on an already damaged skin probably account for the high incidence of contact dermatitis at this site. Other sensitivities include nickel from hair pins, metal implements, etc., chromate and phosphorus sesquisulphide in matches, and nail varnish. It is characteristic that the degree of itching and burning is often markedly out of proportion to the amount of erythema and oedema present. Contact dermatitis may also rarely occur with ear moulds [15]. Clinically, it is often difficult to differentiate neurodermatitis from contact dermatitis.

Lichen simplex (neurodermatitis) may be localized to one area of the meatus or may occur more diffusely over the tragus, triangular fossa and adjoining skin. The condition is usually diagnosed by the history rather than the signs. Itching is intense, but often intermittent. The need to scratch or rub is compulsive, although often denied. Signs of inflammation are often minimal, but some degree of oedema and scaling is common. Complications from trauma, infection and sensitization are frequent. Intermittent itching of the external auditory canal—non-specific external otitis [2]—can also occur, irregularly and over a long period, without any obvious cause and with minimal signs of disease.

Whatever the primary aetiology, with the passage of time chronic external otitis becomes an increasingly complex diagnostic and therapeutic problem.

REFERENCES

1 Senturia BH. *Disease of the External Ear*. Springfield: Charles C. Thomas, 1957.
2 Jones EH. *External Otitis*. Springfield: Charles C. Thomas, 1965.
3 Perry ET. *The Human Ear Canal*. Springfield: Charles C. Thomas, 1957.
4 Peterkin GAG. Otitis externa. *J Laryngol Otol* 1974; **88**: 15–21.
5 Price J. Otitis externa in children. *J Roy Coll Gen Prac* 1976; **26**: 610–15.
6 Lambert IJ. A comparison of the treatment of otitis externa with 'Otosporin' and aluminium acetate: a report from a services practice in Cyprus. *J Roy Coll Gen Prac* 1981; **31**: 291–4.
7 Wright DN, Alexander JM. Effect of water on the bacterial flora of swimmers' ears. *Arch Otolaryngol* 1974; **99**: 15–18.
8 Senturia BH. External otitis, acute diffuse. *Ann Otol Rhinol Laryngol* 1973; **82** (Suppl 8): 1–23.
9 Moffett AJ. Granulating myringitis: unusual affection of the eardrum. *J Laryngol Otol* 1943; **58**: 453–6.
10 Lucente FE. Diseases due to infection. In: Lucente FE, Lawson W, Novick NL, eds. *The External Ear*. Philadelphia: WB Saunders, 1996: 48–97.
11 Hirsch BE. Infections of the external ear. *Am J Otolaryngol* 1992; **13**: 145–55.
12 Hawke M, Wong J, Krajden S. Clinical and microbiological features of otitis externa. *J Otolaryngol* 1984; **13**: 289–95.
13 Selesnick SH. Otitis externa: management of the recalcitrant case. *Am J Otol* 1994; **15**: 408–12.
14 Holmes RC, Wilkinson JD, Johns AN *et al.* Medicament contact dermatitis in patients with chronic inflammatory ear disease. *J Roy Soc Med* 1982; **75**: 27–30.
15 Cockerill D. Allergies to ear moulds. A study of reactions encountered by hearing aid users to some ear mould materials. *Br J Audiol* 1987; **21**: 145.

Differential diagnosis. The part played by trauma, environment, infection, sensitization and altered physiology and anatomy must be assessed and evaluated as accurately as possible. Difficulties often arise in the interpretation of bacteriological and mycological findings. 'Hearing-aid dermatitis' is more often due to traumatic and physical factors than to allergic sensitivity. Antibiotics, especially when prescribed in combination with corticosteroids, may cause occult sensitivity and are one cause of chronicity. The importance of perineal and nasal transfer of infection should not be underestimated and mechanical interference with the external auditory canal in patients with otitis externa tends to be the rule rather than the exception.

External otitis is unlikely to be confused with any other condition except perhaps psoriasis and eczema, and these, of course, may coexist. Middle-ear disease, past and present, should always be excluded.

Swabs should be taken for bacteriological culture and epithelial debris examined and sent for mycological culture. Potassium hydroxide preparations showing evidence of epithelial invasion with hyphae are probably more important in this respect than a positive culture, which may simply indicate commensal or saprophytic infection.

In any long-standing or resistant case, patch testing with a special 'ear battery' [1] should be undertaken to rule out unsuspected contact dermatitis. If there is excess granulation, middle-ear disease should be ruled out, and if the patient is diabetic, debilitated, very young, elderly or immunosuppressed, malignant otitis externa must also be excluded.

Another condition that may need to be considered is *bullous myringitis*, an uncommon condition probably due to upper respiratory tract viral infection, such as influenza virus, which presents with single or multiple bullae on the tympanic membrane and adjacent canal wall. It can resemble bullous external otitis, which is usually due to *Pseudomonas*. Sudden severe pain is a feature, but resolves rapidly after rupture of the bullae. Furuncles of the external auditory canal are described below. Other bacteria may be a rare cause, for example gonococcal otitis externa [2].

Complications. Recurrent otitis externa may also develop into hypertrophic otitis externa or localized elephantiasis nostra [3] of the ears as a result of the effects of chronic lymphatic obstruction. The resultant narrowing of the external acoustic canal coupled with the underlying lymphoedema makes recurrent and repeated infections even more likely.

Secondary trauma. Once an irritable focus occurs in the canal, energetic attempts to remove wax or debris or to satisfy the urge to rub or scratch the infected area often intensify the inflammation. Cotton buds, although frequently regarded as safe, are a common cause of tympanic perforation [4].

Secondary sensitization. This is usually a consequence of treatment or a reaction to objects placed in the ear to alleviate itching. Therapeutic agents may therefore enhance and perpetuate the condition for which they were prescribed. Penicillin, neomycin, framycetin (Soframycin) and chloramphenicol are all well-known topical sensitizers, but even gentamicin, Vioform (chinoform), polymyxin and bacitracin may sensitize at times [1]. Allergy to topical medicaments is found in as many as 40% of patients with chronic or treatment-resistant otitis externa [1,5]. Sensitivity to nail varnish may be misconstrued as lichen simplex and, in women who are nickel sensitive, otitis externa may be aggravated by using metal objects to alleviate itching or to clear the ear. Otoscopes themselves may release nickel.

Another source of contact dermatitis is chromate [6] or phosphorus sesquisulphide in match heads, which some people use to scratch their ears.

Benign non-necrotizing otitis externa. This usually presents as chronic, non-painful otorrhoea with an ulcer present in the floor of the external canal. Surgery may be a better alternative to long-term medical management [7].

Allergic and 'ide' reactions [8,9]. A few well-documented cases have been reported in which recurrent pruritus, oedema and scaling of the ear canal have occurred with or without involvement of the hands or other areas in response to fungal infections elsewhere or with food or drug allergies.

Treatment. The general principles of treatment of otitis externa are to relieve pain, reduce itching, prevent trauma and avoid known or potential sensitizers. Significant infective organisms should be identified and treated appropriately.

Many mild cases of otitis externa will respond to simple aural toilet, antiseptic wicks and the use of appropriate antiseptic or antibiotic drops.

When there is coexistent eczema, combined steroid–antiseptic or steroid–antibiotic drops or wicks can be used. It should be noted, however, that many of the common infecting organisms are frequently antibiotic resistant, and swabs for culture and sensitivity should therefore be taken before prescribing topical or systemic antibiotics. In chronic cases, a great variety of treatments will already have been given and medicament contact dermatitis will therefore be more likely. Because this is often occult, patch testing should be done in all patients with chronic disease.

Pain is often severe, especially with acute staphylococcal infections, and strong analgesics may be required. Local heat also often helps. Bed rest and daily wicks or dressing may be needed in the more severe case. Oral antibiotics may be given if necessary once sensitivities are known.

Topical treatment. This is the essential part of therapy and the most difficult to carry out satisfactorily. Eardrops are of less value than regular cleaning of the ear, and this initially needs to be done daily by a doctor or an experienced nurse. Less severe cases may be treated once a week. Having cleaned the ear of debris and wax, a wick may be inserted or the patient instructed to apply eardrops regularly. When the cartilaginous portion of the canal alone is involved, the patient can be shown how to apply the prescribed medicament by holding a loose wool-tipped orange stick 2.5 cm from its end and inserting this until the fingers touch the tragus.

If wax is impacted, this can be softened with oil, glycerine or sodium bicarbonate eardrops and then removed either manually or by syringing, as long as the drum can be visualized and there is no perforation. Obstinate cases should be referred to an otologist. Some proprietary cerumenolytics

are irritant and should be left in the ear for only 15–30 min before syringing.

In most chronic or complicated cases, treatment must be continued regularly for some weeks after apparent cure. Care must be taken to prevent cross-infection from other body sites, especially the anterior vestibule of the nose and the perineum, and the ear should be kept as dry and as clean as possible. A very large number of medicaments have been used in the treatment of otitis externa. Alcohol 70–85% (isopropyl alcohol), 1–2% acetic acid, aluminium subacetate solution and 2% salicylic acid in 60% spirit are all safe and useful. Wicks with 8–13% aluminium acetate, 0.25–0.50% silver nitrate or glycerine and ichthyol are used to treat hypertrophic otitis externa. Wicks may also be impregnated with corticosteroids. Although the use of corticosteroids in the form of lotions, paints, creams and ointments is a common practice, the choice of an associated bacterial agent is more difficult. Neomycin, framycetin (Soframycin), gentamicin and polymyxin are probably acceptable as short-term treatments for acute otitis externa but the risk of sensitization and cross-sensitization increases with more protracted usage. The combination of neomycin with polymyxin will cover both *Staphylococcus aureus* and *Pseudomonas aeruginosa* [10]. For patients with chronic or chronic relapsing otitis externa, iodochlorhydroxyquinoline (Vioform, chinoform) can be used alone or in combination with corticosteroids. This has a broad range of action but sensitivity can still occur. Old remedies, such as the aniline dyes, 0.5–1% in 70% spirit (e.g. gentian violet), may be useful.

The imidazoles have largely replaced nystatin and amphotericin as antifungal agents, as they are active against *Aspergillus* as well as *Candida,* but acetic acid, boric acid and 25% m-cresyl acetate may still at times be useful: 2% salicylic acid in spirit is useful for prophylaxis. Several eardrops, for example the aminoglycosides, chlorhexidine, polymyxin and chloramphenicol, are potentially ototoxic [11,12] and should be avoided in the presence of tympanic perforation.

In all cases of external otitis, treatment should be prolonged beyond the time of apparent recovery and patients should be advised how best to avoid recurrence and about the dangers of indiscriminate or prolonged self-medication.

Surgical treatments. Occasionally, chronic otitis externa is due to narrowing of the external auditory meatus. Surgical enlargement of the meatus can then bring about resolution [13].

REFERENCES

1 Holmes RC, Wilkinson JD, Johns AN *et al.* Medicament contact dermatitis in patients with chronic inflammatory ear disease. *J R Soc Med* 1982; **75**: 27–30.
2 Pareek SS. Gonococcal otitis externa. (Letter.) *N Engl J Med* 1979; **300**: 1490.
3 Grant JM. Elephantiasis nostra verrucosa of the ears. *Cutis* 1982; **29**: 441–4.
4 Robertson MS. A critical comment on the use of cotton buds. *N Z Med J* 1971; **86**: 102–3.

5 Fraki JE, Kalimo K, Tuohimaa P *et al.* Contact allergy to various components of topical preparations for treatment of external otitis. *Acta Otolaryngol* 1985; **100**: 414–18.

6 McKelvie M, McKelvie P. Some aetiological factors in otitis externa. *Br J Dermatol* 1966; **78**: 227–31.

7 Wormald PJ. Surgical management of benign necrotizing otitis externa. *J Laryngol Otol* 1994; **108**: 101–5.

8 Brown WH. Some observations on neurodermatitis of the scalp, with particular reference to tinea amiantacea. *Br J Dermatol Syphil* 1948; **60**: 81–90.

9 Jones EH. *External Otitis*. Springfield: Thomas, 1965.

10 Fairbanks DNF. Otic topical agents. *Ear Nose Throat J* 1981; **60**: 239–42.

11 Brummett RE, Harris RF, Lindgren JA. Detection of ototoxicity from drugs applied topically to the middle ear space. *Laryngoscope* 1976; **86**: 1177–87.

12 Mittelman H. Ototoxicity of 'ototopical' antibiotics: past, present, and future. *Trans Am Acad Ophthalmol Otolaryngol* 1977; **76**: 1432–43.

13 Hunsaker DH. Conchomeatoplasty for chronic otitis externa. *Arch Otolaryngol Head Neck Surg* 1988; **114**: 395–8.

Invasive external otitis [1]

SYN. MALIGNANT EXTERNAL OTITIS [2]; NECROTIZING EXTERNAL OTITIS

This is an infection of the skin of the external ear canal which spreads to deeper structures and causes necrosis.

Aetiology. In most cases, the infecting organism is *Pseudomonas aeruginosa*, although occasionally other organisms have been involved: *Staphylococcus aureus* [3], *Staphylococcus epidermidis* [4], *Klebsiella oxytoca* [5], *Aspergillus* [6–10] and *Actinomycetes*. The condition characteristically occurs in elderly diabetics [1,11–13] but is also seen with some frequency in the immunocompromised [1,14,15] and has been reported in association with diabetes insipidus [16]. Cases have been reported in children [17,18]. In diabetics, microangiopathy may be important in the pathogenesis [1]. It is possible that abnormalities of cellular immunity and polymorphonuclear function are important in some cases [19,20], but in many instances the pathogenesis is poorly understood.

Pathology. In most cases, there is evidence of osteomyelitis [5]. An early event is acellular necrosis of cartilage [21].

Clinical features. Quite often there is a preceding history of irrigation of the ear. The commonest presenting symptom is pain, which is usually very severe and persistent. It may spread from the region of the ear to the vertex, temporal or occipital areas, and there may be temporomandibular joint pain. The second most common symptom is discharge from the ear. In up to 50% there is some degree of hearing loss. Systemic symptoms, including fever, are uncommon [1]. There may be symptoms due to involvement of cranial nerves, particularly dysphagia.

On examination the external auditory canal is always abnormal, with varying degrees of oedema and erythema, and extensive granulation tissue formation is evident. This is particularly seen on the posterior and inferior aspect of the wall and at the junction between the bony and cartilaginous segments of the canal. There may be swelling of the soft tissues around the ear. Cranial neuropathies may be found in up to 40% of patients [1,15]. Facial palsy is the most common finding but involvement of cranial nerves IV, VI, VIII, IX, X and XII may be variably present. When such nerve involvement is found, the disease is more extensive.

Investigations usually show elevation of the erythrocyte sedimentation rate, but the white-cell count is often normal.

Diagnosis. Invasive external otitis is usually diagnosed on clinical suspicion. It is essential to obtain material for culture to determine the infective cause, and samples should be taken from the ear canal, the granulations, soft tissue and bone, depending on the case. Blood cultures may also be valuable.

Imaging techniques can be helpful, particularly in diagnosing bony involvement and following progress of the disease, and should enable granular external otitis to be distinguished from the much more serious invasive external otitis. Plain films, computed tomography (CT) scans, bone scans and magnetic resonance imaging (MRI) have all been used. MRI with or without gadolinium enhancement is probably the best technique for soft-tissue involvement, evaluation of the meninges and changes within the osseous medullary cavity, although CT is preferred for the initial diagnosis and recognition of cortical bone erosion [22,23].

Complications. Spread of the disease can produce parotitis, mastoiditis or osteomyelitis of the base of the skull and thence spread to the contralateral side. Meningitis can occur, and is an important cause of death. Cranial nerve paralysis may result in aspiration pneumonia. Overall, there is a mortality of 10–20%, and in the presence of cranial neuropathies the mortality is 70% [1,15].

Treatment. Because of the range of possible infections, it is essential to base treatment on the result of culture. For *Pseudomonas*, the traditional approach has been to use an extended spectrum antipseudomonal penicillin for 4–8 weeks and an aminoglycoside for 4–6 weeks [1]. Ciprofloxacin [24,25] can be successful if used early in the course of disease. When there is evidence of extensive bone destruction, removal of necrotic material is necessary. Some cases fail to respond to antibiotic therapy, and if the facility is available, hyperbaric oxygen can improve the outlook [26]. Ascorbic acid has also been recorded as an adjuvant therapy [19].

When the infective cause is bacteria other than *Pseudomonas* or a fungus, advice on the choice of antimicrobial agent should be taken from a microbiologist.

REFERENCES

1 Doroghazi RM, Nadol JB, Jr, Hyslop NE, Jr *et al.* Invasive external otitis. Report of 21 cases and review of the literature. *Am J Med* 1981; **71**: 603–14.

2 Chandler JR. Malignant external otitis. *Laryngoscope* 1967; **78**: 1257–94.

3 Keay DG, Murray AM. Clinical records: malignant external otitis due to *Staphylococcus* infection. *J Laryngol Otol* 1988; **102**: 926–7.

4 Barrow HN, Levenson MJ. Necrotizing 'malignant' external otitis caused by *Staphylococcus* epidermidis. *Arch Otolaryngol Head Neck Surg* 1992; **118**: 94–6.

5 Bernheim J, Sade J. Histopathology of the soft parts in 50 patients with malignant external otitis. *J Laryngol Otol* 1989; **103**: 366–8.

6 Cunningham M, Yu VL, Turner J *et al.* Necrotizing otitis externa due to *Aspergillus* in an immunocompetent patient. *Arch Otolaryngol Head Neck Surg* 1988; **114**: 554–6.

7 Bickley LS, Betts RF, Parkins CW. Atypical invasive external otitis. *Arch Otolaryngol Head Neck Surg* 1988; **114**: 1024–8.

8 Phillips P, Bryce G, Sheperd J *et al.* Invasive external otitis caused by *Aspergillus. Rev Infect Dis* 1990; **12**: 277–81.

9 Gordon G, Giddings NA. Invasive otitis externa due to *Aspergillus* species: case report and review. *Clin Infect Dis* 1994; **19**: 866–70.

10 Anderson LL, Giandoni MB, Keller RA, Grabski WJ. Surgical wound healing complicated by *Aspergillus* infection in a non-immunocompromised host. *Dermatol Surg* 1995; **21**: 799–801.

11 Meyerhoff WL, Gates GA, Montalbo PJ. *Pseudomonas* mastoiditis. *Laryngoscope* 1977; **87**: 483–92.

12 Johnson MP, Ramphal R. Malignant external otitis. Report on therapy with ceftazidime and review of therapy and prognosis. *Rev Infect Dis* 1990; **12**: 173–80.

13 Lang R, Goshen S, Kitzes-Cohen R *et al.* Successful treatment of malignant external otitis with oral ciprofloxacin: report of experience with 23 patients. *J Infect Dis* 1990; **161**: 537–40.

14 Kielhofner M, Atmar RL, Hamill RJ. Life-threatening *Pseudomonas aeruginosa* infections in patients with human immunodeficiency virus infection. *Clin Infect Dis* 1992; **14**: 403–11.

15 Rubin J, Yu VL. Malignant external otitis: insights into pathogenesis, clinical manifestations, diagnosis and therapy. *Am J Med* 1988; **85**: 391–8.

16 Giguere P, Rouillard G. Otite externe maligne bilatérale chez une fillete de 10 ans. *J Otolaryngol* 1976; **5**: 159–66.

17 Coser PL, Stamm AEC, Lobo RC *et al.* Malignant external otitis in infants. *Laryngoscope* 1980; **90**: 312–16.

18 Joachims HZ. Malignant external otitis in children. *Arch Otolaryngol* 1976; **102**: 236–7.

19 Corberand J, Nguyen F, Fraysse B *et al.* Malignant external otitis and polymorphonuclear leukocyte migration impairment: improvement with ascorbic acid. *Arch Otolaryngol* 1982; **108**: 122–4.

20 Yust I, Radiano C, Tartakovsky B *et al.* Impairment of cellular immunity in patients with malignant external otitis. *Acta Otolaryngol* 1980; **90**: 398–403.

21 Ostfeld E, Segal M, Czernobilsky B. Malignant external otitis: early histopathologic changes and pathogenic mechanism. *Laryngoscope* 1981; **91**: 965–70.

22 Gherini SG, Brackmann DE, Bradley WG. Magnetic resonance imaging and computerized tomography in malignant otitis externa. *Laryngoscope* 1986; **96**: 542–8.

23 Grandis JR, Curtin HD, Yu VL. Necrotizing (malignant) external otitis: prospective comparison of CT and MR imaging in diagnosis and follow-up. *Radiology* 1995; **196**: 499–504.

24 Brody T, Pensak ML. The fluoroquinolones. *Am J Otol* 1991; **12**: 477–9.

25 Morrison GAJ, Bailey CM. Relapsing malignant otitis externa successfully treated with ciprofloxacin. *J Laryngol Otol* 1988; **102**: 872–6.

26 Davis JC, Gates GA, Lerner C *et al.* Adjuvant hyperbaric oxygen in malignant external otitis. *Arch Otolaryngol Head Neck Surg* 1992; **118**: 89–93.

27 Rubin J, Stoehr G, Yu VL *et al.* Efficacy of oral ciprofloxacin plus rifampicin for treatment of malignant external otitis. *Arch Otolaryngol Head Neck Surg* 1989; **115**: 1063–9.

Furunculosis

A furuncle is a staphylococcal infection of a hair follicle [1]. It may occur in the canal at the junction of the conchal and canal skin.

The patient presents with pain, which can be aggravated by chewing if there is involvement of the anterior canal wall. There may be sufficient swelling to obstruct the entrance to the canal. There is often regional lymphadenopathy.

Furunculosis can usually be distinguished from external otitis by the normal appearance of the canal epithelium and an absence of discharge; the two conditions can, however, coexist. If possible the tympanic membrane should be examined, in order to exclude otitis media and mastoiditis.

Localized lesions associated with mild swelling usually respond to an oral antistaphylococcal antibiotic [1]. If an abscess or carbuncle is present, incision and drainage may be necessary. The latter can be achieved with a wick.

REFERENCE

1 Hirsch BE. Infection of the external ear. *Am J Otolaryngol* 1992; **13**: 145–55.

Otomycosis

Otomycosis is an inflammatory process due to a variety of yeast and fungal organisms as the primary aetiological agent. The same range of fungi may be found in patients with multifactorial or bacterial external otitis (see above).

Aetiology. The species of fungus and yeast involved vary somewhat depending on ambient climate, but in most parts of the world *Aspergillus species* account for the majority of isolates, and *Candida albicans* is the next most frequent. Others include phycomycetes, *Rhizopus*, *Actinomyces* and *Penicillium*. The fact that these organisms can be pathogenic as well as saprophytic has been confirmed in a number of studies [1–4].

The factors that convert organisms that are normally saprophytic into pathogens are similar to those that apply to bacterial external otitis. Heat and humidity are foremost, and account for the frequency of otomycosis in the tropics, in those using hearing aids and occlusive ear moulds. Diabetes mellitus, immunosuppression, both systemic and topical antibiotics and steroids are also important.

Clinical features. The principal symptom is itching, which can have a quality of being deep inside the ear. This is usually accompanied by a sensation of fullness. Pain is uncommon, in contrast to bacterial external otitis. Discharge, if any, is usually slight. There may be hearing loss of a conductive type. Because of the irritation, patients are liable to traumatize the canal and may then initiate the symptoms and signs of bacterial external otitis.

On examination the dominant feature is the presence of wispy, filamentous masses, which may be isolated or diffusely present in the canal. These masses are white, grey or stippled black if *Aspergillus* is present. Inflammation of the canal epithelium is usually mild. There may be some epithelial debris, which may be either moist or dry.

Diagnosis. The clinical appearance is usually distinctive. As always with external canal disorders it is important to check for other pathology. Material can be taken for mycological examination and culture.

Treatment [5]. Careful cleaning followed by drying is a prerequisite to successful management. The canal can then be wiped out, for example with m-cresyl acetate or 1% thymol in 70% alcohol, and the specific treatment applied on a wick. Treatment should be changed daily until a satisfactory result has been achieved. Many agents have been advocated for otomycosis, but there is little evidence to promote one above the others. They include aluminium acetate, acetic acid, m-cresyl acetate, thiomersal, gentian violet, clioquinol, nystatin, amphotericin B and the imadazoles.

In rare situations, usually in the immunosuppressed, there may be cellulitis of the surrounding soft tissues directly due to fungal infection. In such cases, itraconazole is likely to be the treatment of choice.

REFERENCES

1 Nielsen PG, Fungi isolated from chronic external ear disorders. *Mykosen* 1985; **28**: 234–7.
2 Sood VB, Sinha A, Mohaoatra LN. Otomycosis: a clinical entity—clinical and experimental study. *J Laryngol Otol* 1988; **81**: 999–1173.
3 Stern JC, Lucente FE. Otomycosis. *Ear Nose Throat J* 1988; **67**: 804–10.
4 Talwar P, Chakrabarti A, Kaur P *et al.* Fungal infection of ear with special reference to chronic suppurative otitis media. *Mycopathologia* 1988; **104**: 47–50.
5 Lucente FE. Diseases due to infection. In: Lucente FE, Lawson W, Novick NL, eds. *The External Ear.* Philadelphia: WB Saunders, 1995; 81–6.

AIDS and the external ear [1]

The consequences of human immunodeficiency virus (HIV) infection will at times be seen on the pinna and in the external auditory canal. The ear is a relatively common site for manifestation of Kaposi's sarcoma. Florid seborrhoeic dermatitis is often a presenting feature of AIDS. The occurrence of molluscum contagiosum lesions in an adult should prompt a suspicion of immunodeficiency, and on the ear the lesions can resemble basal cell carcinoma. Bacillary angiomatosis may produce vascular papules and nodules on the ear. Herpes simplex and zoster can be more florid in patients with AIDS. Polyps in the external auditory canal due to *Pneumocystis carinii* have been described [2].

REFERENCES

1 Lucente FE. Diseases due to infection. In: Lucente FE, Lawson W, Novick NL, eds. *The External Ear.* Philadelphia: WB Saunders, 1995; 95–6.
2 Gherman CR, Ward RR, Bassis ML. *Pneumocystis carinii* otitis media and mastoiditis as the initial manifestation of the acquired immunodeficiency syndrome. *Am J Med* 1988; **85**: 250–2.

Tumours of the pinna and external auditory canal [1]

Benign tumours

On the pinna, these will present as papules or nodules, sometimes with distinctive morphology. In the external auditory canal, benign tumours tend to present with hearing loss, and may predispose to infection.

Benign tumours found on the pinna include melanocytic naevus, seborrhoeic keratosis (Fig. 68.18), squamous cell

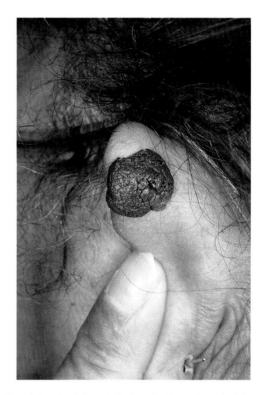

Fig. 68.18 Seborrhoeic keratosis (basal cell papilloma) of the pinna.

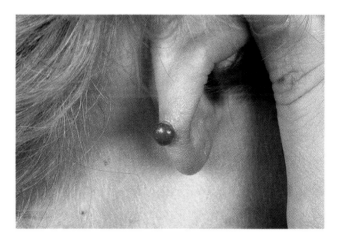

Fig. 68.19 Lobulated capillary haemangioma (pyogenic granuloma). A bright-red nodule with a surrounding collarette of keratin.

papilloma, pilomatrixoma [2,3], trichoepithelioma [4] and trichofolliculoma [5,6], myoma, chondroma, osteoma, fibroma [7], neurofibroma [8], neurilemmoma [9], granular cell tumour, haemangioma (Fig. 68.19) and lymphangioma [10]. Benign glandular tumours may occur on the pinna, but are more common in the canal, especially sebaceous adenoma. Occasional unique lesions have been described [11].

Extra-adrenal paraganglioma (glomus jugulare tumour) of the temporal bone can manifest in the external ear canal as a friable, haemorrhagic neoplasm and can cause conductive hearing loss [1]. This tumour can be locally aggressive, and there are rare instances of metastasis.

Osteoma and exostosis

Exostoses of the external auditory canal are usually bilateral, symmetrical, multiple, diffuse, broadly based growths of bone arising from the tympanic bone in the external auditory canal [12,13]. Frequent exposure to cold water is an aetiological factor in nearly all cases [14].

Osteomas can usually be differentiated by their solitary and unilateral distribution. They are often attached by a narrow pedicle to the tympanosquamous or tympanomastoid suture line [12]. Osteomas and exostoses are normally asymptomatic unless they enlarge sufficiently to block the external auditory canal [15].

Various conditions can mimic benign tumours. On the pinna, these include cysts of various types, viral warts and molluscum contagiosum, chondrodermatitis, elastotic and weathering nodules, keloids, congenital malformations such as accessory tragi, nodular calcinosis [17], gouty tophi, deposits of amyloid, angiolymphoid hyperplasia with eosinophilia and 'pseudolymphoma', inflammatory polyps, hamartomas [16], choristomas [18] and congenital cysts of branchial arch origin in the external auditory canal. Cholesteatoma may also occur in the external canal.

REFERENCES

1 Hyams VJ. Pathology of tumours of the external ear. In: Lucente FE, Lawson W, Novick NL, eds. *The External Ear.* Philadelphia: WB Saunders, 1995: 108–48.
2 Vinayak BC, Cox GJ, Ashton-Key M. Pilomatrixoma of the external auditory meatus. *J Laryngol Otol* 1993; **107**: 333–4.
3 Sevin K, Can Z, Yilmaz S, Saray A, Yormuk E. Pilomatrixoma of the earlobe. *Dermatol Surg* 1995; **21**: 245–6.
4 Ferlito A, Recher G, Polidero F *et al.* Solitary trichoepithelioma and epithelioma adenoides cysticum of Brooke involving the external auditory meatus. *J Laryngol Otol* 1981; **95**: 835–41.
5 O'Mahony JJ. Trichofolliculoma of the external auditory meatus. Report of a case and review of the literature. *J Laryngol Otol* 1981; **95**: 623–5.
6 Srivastava RN, Ajwani KD. Trichofolliculoma. *Ear Nose Throat J* 1979; **58**: 159–60.
7 Varletzides E, Grigoriades S, Tsiliguri E. An unusual localization of fibroma on the lobe of the ear. *Pamminerva Med* 1980; **22**: 37–9.
8 Trevisani TP, Pohl AL, Matloub HS. Neurofibroma of the ear: function and aesthetics. *Plast Reconstr Surg* 1982; **70**: 217–19.
9 Fodor RI, Pastore PN, Frable MA. Neurilemmoma of the auricle: a case report. *Laryngoscope* 1977; **87**: 1760–4.
10 Grabb WC, Dingman RO, Oneal RM *et al.* Facial hamartomas in children:

neurofibroma, lymphangioma and hemangioma. *Plast Reconstr Surg* 1980; **66**: 509–27.
11 Donati P, Balus L. Folliculosebaceous cystic hamartoma: reported case with a neural component. *Am J Dermatopathol* 1993; **15**: 277–9.
12 Graham MD. Osteomas and exostoses of the external auditory canal. A clinical, histopathologic and scanning electron microscopic study. *Ann Otol Rhinol Laryngol* 1979; **88**: 566–72.
13 Sheehy JL. Diffuse exostoses and osteomata of the external auditory canal: a report of 100 operations. *Otolaryngol Head Neck Surg* 1982; **90**: 337–42.
14 di Bartolomeo JR. Exostoses of the external auditory canal. *Ann Otol Rhinol Laryngol* 1979; **88** (Suppl. 61): 2–20.
15 Kemink JL, Graham MD. Osteomas and exostoses of the external auditory canal—medical and surgical management. *J Otolaryngol* 1982; **11**: 101–6.
16 Kacker SK, Dasgupta G. Hamartomas of the ear and nose. *J Laryngol Otol* 1973; **87**: 801–5.
17 Hansen KK, Segura AD, Esterly NB. Solitary congenital nodule on the ear of an infant. *Pediatr Dermatol* 1993; **10**: 88–90.
18 Braun GA, Lowry D, Meyers A. Bilateral choristomas of the external auditory canals. *Arch Otolaryngol* 1978; **104**: 467–8.

Glandular tumours

Tumours of the ceruminous glands are rare. It is often difficult to distinguish between adenoma and carcinoma on histological grounds [1–3] and the term ceruminoma [4] is probably best avoided. The tumours comprise benign and pleomorphic adenomas, locally malignant mucoepidermoid carcinomas, malignant adenocarcinomas and adenoid cystic carcinomas (cylindromas) [2]. Tumours of the cerumen glands have been reported in association with other sweat-gland tumours elsewhere [5].

Isolated cases of syringocystadenoma papilliferum, apocrine cystadenoma, benign eccrine cylindroma, hidradenoma papilliferum and carcinomas of eccrine and sebaceous origin have also been reported [6,7].

Benign tumours produce symptoms of obstruction and hearing loss. Pain is the usual presenting feature of the more malignant tumours. Other symptoms include bleeding, otorrhea and with spread of the neoplasm, nerve palsies occur. Treatment is in the province of the otorhinolaryngologist.

REFERENCES

1 Wetli CV, Pardo V, Millard M, Gerston K. Tumors of ceruminous glands. *Cancer* 1972; **29**: 1169–78.
2 Pulec JL. Glandular tumours of the external auditory canal. *Laryngoscope* 1977; **87**: 1601–12.
3 Lynde CW, McLean DI, Wood WS. Tumors of the ceruminous glands. *J Am Acad Dermatol* 1984; **11**: 841–7.
4 Neldner KH. Ceruminoma. *Arch Dermatol* 1968; **98**: 344–8.
5 Habib MA. Ceruminoma in association with other sweat gland tumours. *J Laryngol Otol* 1981; **95**: 415–20.
6 Dehner LP, Chen KTK. Primary tumours of the external and middle ear: benign and malignant glandular neoplasms. *Arch Otolaryngol* 1980; **106**: 13–19.
7 Nissim F, Czernobilsky B, Ostfeld E. Hidradenoma papilliferum of the external auditory canal. *J Laryngol Otol* 1981; **95**: 843–8.

Premalignant epithelial neoplasms of the auricle

Because of its high level of exposure to UV radiation [1],

especially in men, the auricle is a common site for premalignant and malignant lesions of epidermal origin. Other predisposing factors include prior ionizing radiation, a chronic dermatosis such as lupus vulgaris and genetic factors such as xeroderma pigmentosum and Gorlin's syndrome.

The commonest premalignant lesion is the solar keratosis, which can occur on all sun-exposed aspects of the auricle, but is especially common on the upper surface of the helix [2,3]. The clinical presentations include an erythematous telangiectatic patch, a focal area of scaling or hyperkeratosis, and cutaneous horn. Solar keratoses on the auricle are often multiple. Solar elastosis may be evident in the surrounding skin. On the auricle, progression to squamous carcinoma from solar keratosis may occur more readily than at other sites [4].

Other premalignant lesions include Bowen's disease, radiation and tar keratoses, and, rarely, keratoacanthoma [5].

Treatment. Several forms of treatment can eradicate premalignant lesions from the auricle, but there are no adequate data to compare them. They include excision, curettage, electrosurgery, cryotherapy, 5-fluorouracil and photodynamic therapy. The choice will depend on a number of factors including the need for a tissue diagnosis, size and location of the lesion, likely cosmetic outcome and the available facilities. Follow-up is important for detection of recurrences and the appearance of new lesions.

Squamous carcinoma of the auricle

In most instances, squamous cell carcinoma evolves from a premalignant lesion, usually a solar keratosis, and occurs predominantly in elderly white men, although at a younger age in the immunosuppressed. Early on, squamous cell carcinoma may be suspected when there is induration of the base of a scaly papule, nodule or cutaneous horn. With progression, squamous cell carcinoma usually ulcerates and with invasion of cartilage can become grossly destructive (Fig. 68.20). Local spread along perichondrial, periosteal and neurovascular planes can make squamous cell carcinoma of the auricle very difficult to control. With the exception of the lip, auricular squamous cell cancer is more likely to metastasize than is squamous cell cancer at any other sun-exposed site (11% compared with 2%) [6]. There is a small but significant mortality [2,3]. Adverse prognostic factors for both local recurrence and metastasis of squamous cell carcinoma include size (more than 2 cm), depth of invasion (more than 4 mm, Clark levels 4 and 5), perineural involvement, and poor differentiation of the tumour [7]. It is not clear, however, to what extent these are independent variables; shallow lesions with large surface area, i.e. more than 2 cm diameter, do not seem to have a poor prognosis. If squamous cell carcinoma recurs after primary treatment, there is a much greater risk for further recurrence and metastasis [7].

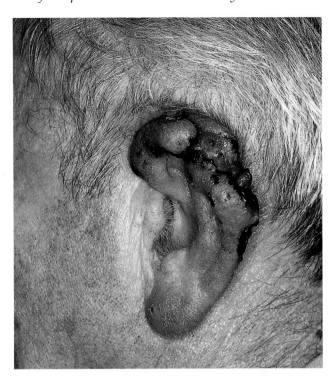

Fig. 68.20 Squamous carcinoma of the auricle. An advanced tumour with extensive destruction of the ear cartilage. (Courtesy of Mr D. Baldwin, Southmead Hospital, Bristol, UK.)

Treatment. It is important to achieve control of the disease with the initial treatment for squamous cell carcinoma. For small, minimally invasive lesions, simple excision, cryotherapy or curettage with cautery/electrodesiccation may be adequate. For larger lesions, and especially those with adverse prognostic factors, the choice is likely to be between surgery, Mohs' micrographic surgery and radiation therapy.

The surgical procedure used will depend on the location and extent of the tumour. Smaller lesions can often be removed by wedge excision with primary repair by advancement flaps. Larger and ill-defined lesions are best closed by temporary grafts pending a histopathological assessment of the margins before definitive repair is carried out. Partial or total amputation may be needed for large tumours. If there is spread beyond the pinna, resection of the parotid, temporal bone, temporomandibular joint or mandibular ramus may be be required, with appropriate repair.

Several authors have recommended minimal resection margins, for example 1 cm [8], 6 mm with frozen section control [9], 8 mm for 1-cm-diameter tumours and 1.5 cm for 3-cm-diameter tumours [10], all with removal of the underlying cartilage. Overall, there is an incidence of 18.7% recurrence during follow-up for 5 years or more with non-Mohs' modalities compared with 5.3% for Mohs' micrographic surgery, suggesting that the latter is the treatment of choice [7].

Squamous cell carcinomas in the tragal and pretragal location appear to have a greater tendency to spread along embryonic fusion planes and may only be curable by radical surgery, for example parotidectomy in association with removal of the tumour [11].

Radiotherapy can be successful as a primary treatment for squamous cell carcinoma of the auricle [12], with megavoltage electron-beam therapy having therapeutic and cosmetic advantages over conventional orthovoltage X-ray treatment [13]. There may, however, be a higher recurrence rate [4,14] compared with surgery, particularly for large tumours [13,15]. Radiation therapy can be complicated by damage to the cartilage and associated chronic infection; deformity of the pinna is another long-term consequence. Radiotherapy may improve the outlook for cases with extensive local spread requiring radical surgery.

The management of squamous cell carcinoma with metastasis to regional lymph nodes and beyond is outside the scope of the dermatologist.

Basal cell carcinoma of the auricle

Basal cell carcinoma of the auricle is somewhat less common than squamous cell carcinoma (Fig. 68.21). It is also mainly due to the effects of solar radiation, but is much less liable to metastasize [4,16].

The approach to treatment is essentially similar to that

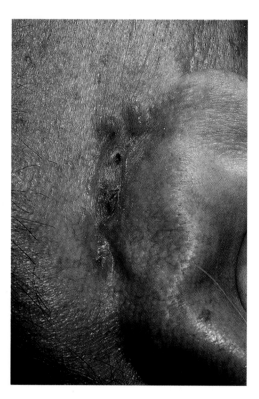

Fig. 68.21 Basal cell carcinoma. Translucent ulcerated nodules in the retro-auricular fold.

outlined for squamous cell carcinoma. Mohs' micrographic surgery is the most likely modality to achieve cure with lesions which are extensive, deeply invasive or recurrent, and those with a morphoeic growth pattern.

REFERENCES

1 Green A, Williams G. Ultraviolet radiation and skin cancer: epidemiological data from Australia. In: Young AR, Moan J, Bjorn LO, Nultsch W, eds. *Environmental UV Photobiology.* New York: Plenum Press, 1993; 233–54.
2 Byers R, Kesler K, Redman B, *et al.* Squamous carcinoma of the external ear. *Am J Surg* 1983; **146**: 447–50.
3 Freedlander E, Chung FF. Squamous cell carcinoma of the pinna. *Br J Plast Surg* 1983; **36**: 171–5.
4 Blake GB, Wilson SP. Malignant tumours of the ear and their treatment: 1. Tumours of the auricle. *Br J Plast Surg* 1974; **27**: 67–76.
5 Patterson HC. Facial keratoacanthoma. *Otolaryngol Head Neck Surg* 1983; **91**: 263–70.
6 Johnson TM, Rowe DE, Nelson BR, Swanson NA. Squamous carcinoma of the skin (excluding lip and oral mucosa). *J Am Acad Dermatol* 1992; **26**: 467–84.
7 Rowe DE, Carroll RJ, Day CL. Prognostic factors for local recurrence, metastasis and survival rates in squamous carcinoma of the skin, ear and lip. *J Am Acad Dermatol* 1992; **26**: 976–90.
8 Pless J. Carcinoma of the external ear. *Scand J Plast Reconstr Surg* 1976; **10**: 147–51.
9 Kitchens GD. Auricular wedge resection and reconstruction. *Ear Nose Throat J* 1989; **21**: 552–4.
10 Levine HL, Kinney SE, Bailin PL, Roberts JK. Cancer of the periauricular region. *Dermatol Clin* 1989; **7**: 781–95.
11 Niparko JK, Swanson NA, Baker SR *et al.* Local control of auricular, periauricular, and external canal malignancies with Mohs' surgery. *Laryngoscope* 1990; **100**: 1047–51.
12 Avila J, Bosch A, Aristizabal S *et al.* Carcinoma of the pinna. *Cancer* 1977; **40**: 2891–5.
13 Hunter RD, Pereira DTM, Pointon RCS. Megavoltage electron beam therapy in the treatment of basal and squamous cell carcinomata of the pinna. *Clin Radiol* 1982; **33**: 341–5.
14 Schewe EJ, Pappalardo C. Cancer of the external ear. *Am J Surg* 1962; **104**: 753–5.
15 Mazeron JJ, Ghalie R, Zeller J *et al.* Radiation therapy for carcinoma of the pinna using iridium 192 wires; a series of 70 patients. *In J Radiat Oncol Biol Phys* 1986; **12**: 1757–63.
16 Small CS, Hawkins FD. Basal cell carcinoma with metastases. *Arch Pathol* 1949; **47**: 196–204.

Squamous and basal cell carcinoma of the external auditory canal

Non-glandular carcinomas of the external auditory canal are uncommon. Most are squamous in type (Fig. 68.22). They affect a younger age group (50–65 years) and, in contrast to squamous cell carcinoma of the auricle, there is much less of a male preponderance. A preceding history of chronic otitis is common [1,2].

Most squamous carcinoma of the canal has an infiltrative growth pattern. It tends to grow along the canal, escaping anteriorly through Santorini's fissures in the cartilaginous segment and Huschke's foramen in the bony portion, into the temporomandibular joint and parotid. Spread also occurs posteriorly into the mastoid, and through the tympanic membrane into the middle ear and thence to the carotid canal, apex of the petrous temple bone, the internal auditory canal, base of the skull and the dura. Metastasis to lymph nodes and distantly is common.

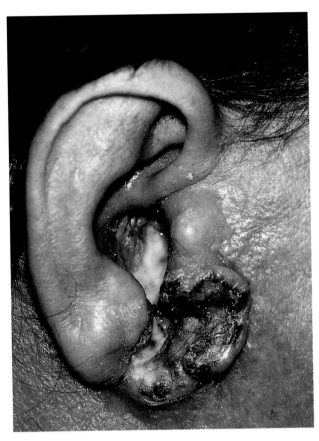

Fig. 68.22 Squamous carcinoma of the external auditory canal. Purulent discharge, inflammation and destruction of the meatus. (Courtesy of Mr D. Baldwin, Southmead Hospital, Bristol, UK.)

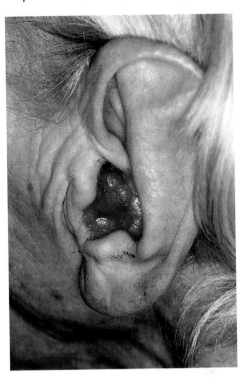

Fig. 68.23 Basal cell carcinoma of the external auditory canal. An erythematous tumour presenting as obstruction at the entrance of the canal. (Courtesy of Mr M. Birchill, Southmead Hospital, Bristol, UK.)

Overall, there is a much poorer prognosis than for squamous cell carcinoma of the pinna, with 5-year survival rates of about 40% [3]. Adverse factors are a large lesion, invasion of cartilage or bone, facial nerve palsy, spread to the middle ear and beyond, and lymph-node metastasis. The extent of the disease can be determined accurately by CT scanning [4].

Verrucous carcinoma of the external auditory canal is an uncommon variant that can appear cytologically banal but nevertheless invade bone, by a pushing rather than infiltrative growth pattern [5,6].

Basal cell carcinoma of the external auditory canal can be locally destructive (Fig. 68.23), but does not metastasize and has a much better prognosis than squamous cell carcinoma [7].

The most common symptoms of invasive squamous carcinoma of the canal are purulent and bloody discharge from the ear, followed by pain, hearing loss and facial paralysis. Examination reveals a friable tumour, partially or completely obstructing the external auditory canal.

Treatment. Surgery is the treatment of choice, the extent determined by an assessment of the limits of tumour growth.

Postoperative radiotherapy improves the outlook [8–11], but for lesions that have spread deeply or metastasized cure is most unlikely.

REFERENCES

1 Lederman M. Malignant tumours of the ear. *J Laryngol Otolaryngol* 1965; **79**: 85–119.
2 Paaske PB, Witten J, Schwer S, Hansen HS. Results in treatment of carcinoma of the external auditory canal and middle ear. *Cancer* 1987; **59**: 156–60.
3 Chen KTK, Dehner LP. Primary tumors of the external and middle ear. I. Introduction and clinicopathologic study of squamous cell carcinoma. *Arch Otolaryngol* 1978; **104**: 244–52.
4 Arriaga M, Curtin H, Takashi H, *et al.* Staging proposal for external auditory meatus carcinoma based on pre-operative clinical examination and computed tomography findings. *Ann Otol Rhinol Laryngol* 1990; **99**: 714–21.
5 Stafford DN, Frootko NJ. Verrucous carcinoma in the external auditory canal. *Am J Otol* 1986; **7**: 443–5.
6 Proops DW, Hawke WM, Van Nostrand AW *et al.* Verrucous carcinoma of the ear. Case report. *Ann Otol Rhinol Laryngol* 1984; **93**: 385–8.
7 Stell PM. Basal cell carcinoma of the external auditory meatus. *Clin Otolaryngol* 1984; **9**: 187–90.
8 Hahn SS, Kim JA, Goodchild N, Constable WD. Carcinoma of the middle ear and external auditory canal. *Radiat Oncol Biol Phys* 1983; **9**: 1103–7.
9 Lewis JS. Cancer of the ear. *Cancer* 1987; **37**: 78–87.
10 Kinney SE. Squamous cell carcinoma of the external auditory canal. *Am J Otol* 1989; **10**: 111–16.
11 Shih L, Crabtree JA. Carcinoma of the external auditory canal; an update. *Laryngoscope* 1990; **100**: 1215–18.

Malignant melanoma

Malignant melanoma of the external ear is relatively uncommon. It accounted for 4.8% of all auricular malignancies in one series [1] and represented 7% of all melanomas in another series [2]. Melanomas are about three times more common in males than females [2,3], and are found in a similar frequency distribution on the ear as squamous carcinoma and its precursors, i.e. about half occur on the helix and a quarter on the antihelix [2] but they are rarely found in the external auditory canal. Most melanomas are of superficial spreading or nodular type. The major determinant for prognosis is Breslow thickness [3]. Treatment is no different from malignant melanoma elsewhere (see Chapter 38).

REFERENCES

1 Blake GB, Wilson SP. Malignant tumours of the ear and their treatment: 1. Tumours of the auricle. *Br J Plast Surg* 1974; **27**: 67–76.
2 Pack GT, Conley J, Oropeza R. Melanoma of the external ear. *Arch Otolaryngol* 1970; **92**: 106–13.
3 Cox NH, Aitchison TC, Sirel JM, MacKie RM. Comparison between lentigo maligna melanoma and other histogenetic types of malignant melanoma of the head and neck. *Br J Cancer* 1996; **73**: 940–4.

Other malignant tumours

Other malignant tumours involving the external ear or the external auditory canal are all rare. The pathology is reviewed in Friedman and Arnold's monograph [1]. The dermatologist may encounter Merkel-cell tumour [2], Kaposi's sarcoma [3] or rhabdomyosarcoma (mainly in children) [4–6]. Angiosarcoma of the pinna has the same gloomy outlook as it does on the scalp [7]. Other sarcomas have been recorded but are exceptionally rare. Lymphomas may occur on the external ear, particularly mycosis fungoides. The ear may be involved by direct extension from tumours nearby, for example the parotid and also by metastases from distant sites [8].

REFERENCES

1 Friedman I, Arnold W. *Pathology of the Ear.* Edinburgh: Churchill Livingstone, 1993.
2 Hanna GS, Ali MH, Akosa AB, Maher EJ. Merkel-cell carcinoma of the pinna. *J Laryngol Otol* 1988; **102**: 607–11.
3 Gnepp DR, Chandler W, Hyams VJ. Primary Kaposi's sarcoma of the head and neck. *Ann Med* 1984; **100**: 107–14.
4 Jaffe N, Fuller RM, Farber S. Rhabdomyosarcoma in children: improved outlook with a multidisciplinary approach. *Am J Surg* 1973; **125**: 482–7.
5 Maurer HM. Rhabdomyosarcoma in childhood and adolescence. *Current Probl Cancer* 1978; **2**: 3–36.
6 Feldman BA. Rhabdomyosarcoma of the head and neck. *Laryngoscope* 1982; **92**: 424–40.
7 Leighton SE, Levine TP. Angiosarcoma of the external ear: a case report. *Am J Otol* 1991; **12**: 54–6.
8 Golding-Wood DG, Quiney RE, Cheesman AD. Carcinoma of the ear: retrospective analysis of 61 patients. *J Laryngol Otol* 1989; **103**: 653–6.

Miscellaneous conditions

Cholesteatoma of the external auditory canal

Cholesteatoma of the middle ear space is accumulation of keratinous debris within a sac-like squamous epithelial lining. It can grow at the expense of normal structures and if it ruptures, the associated foreign body-type inflammatory reaction can produce serious damage.

A similar condition occurs rarely in the external auditory canal, although its status as a true cholesteatoma is disputed [1,2]. The accumulation of stratum corneum occurs within a cyst-like penetration of the bony portion of the canal wall by the epithelial lining. There is localized ulceration of the skin of the floor of the canal, with underlying osteitis and sometimes necrosis of bone. A necrotic sequestrum may become incorporated into the cholesteatoma. The cause is unknown, but trauma, for example from hard wax and manipulation of the canal seems important in some cases [3].

Cholesteatoma usually occurs in patients over the age of 40 years. Symptoms are a dull pain in one ear, and otorrhea. Examination shows a white cystic mass protruding into the canal. The main differential diagnosis is from neoplasms and keratosis obturans [4,5]. External auditory canal cholesteatoma can occasionally behave aggressively, and erode into the mastoid cavity, middle ear, temporomandibular joint and adjacent soft tissue. CT scans can be useful to assess the extent of the disease. Treatment is within the province of the otorhinolaryngologist.

Keratosis obturans

This uncommon condition of unknown cause consists of a localized accumulation of desquamated keratin in the ear canal. It is usually bilateral, and typically occurs in younger patients than external auditory canal cholesteatoma. There is conductive hearing loss, sometimes with otalgia. Keratosis obturans can be associated with paranasal sinus disease and bronchitis. Treatment consists of careful removal of the accumulated keratin. Irrigation with water should be avoided [4,5].

REFERENCES

1 Friedman I, Arnold W. *Pathology of the Ear.* Edinburgh, Churchill Livingstone 1993: 30–1.
2 Sismanis A, Williams GH, Abedi E. External auditory meatus cholesteatoma. In: Tos M, Thomas J, Peitersen E, eds. *Cholesteatoma and Mastoid Surgery* Amsterdam: Kugler and Ghedini, 1984: 577–82.
3 Holt JJ. Ear canal cholesteatoma. *Laryngoscope* 1992; **102**: 608–13.
4 Piepergerdes JC, Kramer BM, Behnke EE. Keratosis obturans and external auditory canal cholesteatoma. *Laryngoscope* 1980; **90**: 383–90.
5 Shire JR, Donegan JO. Cholesteatoma of the external auditory canal and keratosis obturans. *Am J Otol* 1986; **7**: 361–4.

Referred pain

Due to the complicated nerve supply to the ear, referred

pain is commoner than pain due to lesions in the ear itself [1]. Non-otological causes of such pain include the otomandibular syndrome [2] due to dysfunction of the temporomandibular joint, cervical arthritis with involvement of the cervical nerves, tonsillitis and carcinoma of the pharynx. Hair in the ear canal is an occasional cause [3]. Psychogenic otalgia has also been reported [4].

REFERENCES

1 Sheikhi AARJ. Pain in the ear—with special reference to referred pain. *J Laryngol Otol* 1980; **94**: 1433–40.
2 Arlen H. The otomandibular syndrome: diagnosis. *Ear Nose Throat J* 1978; **57**: 553–6.
3 Papay FA, Levine HL, Schiavone WA. Facial fuzz and funny feelings. *Cleveland Clin J Med* 1989; **56**: 273–6.
4 Dight R. Psychogenic earache. An unusual cause of otalgia. *Med J Aust* 1980; **i**: 76–7.

Chapter 69
The Oral Cavity

CRISPIAN SCULLY

Introduction

Oral lesions are usually the result of local disease but may be the early signs of systemic disease, including dermatological disorders, and in some instances may cause the main symptoms. This chapter mainly discusses disorders of the oral mucosa that may present at a dermatology clinic and dental and periodontal defects that may be related to skin disease.

The chapter is divided into a brief discussion of the biology of the mouth, an overview of the more common signs and symptoms affecting specific oral tissues, discussion of the disorders of the oral mucosa of most relevance to dermatology and a tabulated review of oral manifestations of systemic diseases. Only the more classic lesions are illustrated. About 20 of the colour illustrations are from the *Colour Atlas of Oral Disease*, 1996 (reproduced by kind permission of C. Scully, S. Flint and S.R. Porter, and publishers Martin Dunitz, London). More detail of histology is available elsewhere [1].

Biology of the mouth

The oral epithelium

The oral epithelium consists of a *functional compartment*— the progenitor cells (basal and parabasal cells)—which is the site of cell division; a *maturation compartment* (spinous and granular cells) where the cells become more terminally differentiated; and a superficial *cornified compartment* of squames and areas of keratinization, either orthokeratotic or parakeratotic. In the non-keratinized regions such as the buccal (cheek) and floor-of-mouth mucosae, overt keratinization and granular cells are absent and the surface cells are flattened, with elongated nuclei [2].

Regional differences in the mucosa

The mucosa is divided into masticatory, lining and specialized types: *masticatory mucosa* (hard palate, gingiva) is adapted to the forces of pressure and friction and keratinized with numerous tall rete ridges and connective tissue papillae and little submucosa. *Lining mucosa* (buccal, labial and alveolar mucosa, floor of mouth, ventral surface of tongue, soft palate, lips) is non-keratinized with broad rete ridges and connective tissue papillae and abundant elastic fibres in the lamina propria [3,4].

Specialized mucosa on the dorsum of the tongue, adapted for taste and mastication, is keratinized, with numerous rete ridges and connective tissue papillae, abundant elastic and collagen fibres in the lamina propria and no submucosa. The tongue is divided by a V-shaped groove, the *sulcus terminalis*, into an anterior two-thirds and a posterior third. Various papillae on the dorsum include the *filiform papillae*, which cover the entire anterior surface and form an abrasive surface to control the food bolus as it is pressed against the palate, and the *fungiform papillae*. The latter are mushroom-shaped, red structures covered by non-keratinized epithelium. They are scattered between the filiform papillae and have taste buds on their surface. Adjacent and anterior to the sulcus terminalis are eight to 12 large *circumvallate papillae*, each surrounded by a deep groove into which open the ducts of serous minor salivary glands. The lateral walls of these papillae contain taste buds.

The *foliate papillae* consist of four to 11 parallel ridges, alternating with deep grooves in the mucosa, on the lateral margins on the posterior part of the tongue. There are taste buds on their lateral walls.

The lingual tonsils are round or oval prominences with intervening lingual crypts lined by non-keratinized epithelium. They are part of *Waldeyer's oropharyngeal ring* of lymphoid tissue.

The teeth

The teeth develop from ectoderm [5]. At around the sixth week of intrauterine life the oral epithelium proliferates over the maxillary and mandibular ridge areas to form primary epithelial bands which project into the mesoderm, and produce a dental lamina in which discrete swellings appear—the enamel organs of developing teeth. Each enamel organ eventually produces tooth enamel, and the mesenchyme, which condenses beneath the enamel organ (actually neuroectoderm), forms a dental papilla which produces the dentine and pulp of the tooth. The enamel organ together with the dental papilla constitute the tooth germ, and this becomes surrounded by a mesenchymal dental follicle, from which the periodontium forms, ultimately to anchor the tooth in its bony socket.

There are 10 deciduous (primary or milk) teeth in each jaw: all are fully erupted by the age of about 3 years (Fig. 69.1). The secondary or permanent teeth begin to erupt at about the age of 6–7 years and the deciduous teeth begin to be slowly lost by normal root resorption. However, some milk teeth may still present at the age of 12–13 years. The full permanent dentition consists of 16 teeth in each jaw: normally most have erupted by about 12–14 years of age but the last molars (third molars or wisdom teeth), if present, often erupt later or may impact and never appear in the mouth.

Teething

'Teething' in infancy is a poorly understood condition and the soreness and fever is often due to infection such as herpes simplex stomatitis. Nevertheless, there may be a

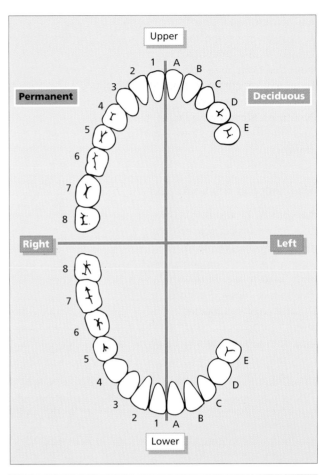

DENTITION	TOOTH	DESIGNATION	ERUPTION TIMES
Deciduous	Central incisors	A	6 to 9 months
	Lateral incisors	B	7 to 10 months
	Canines	C	16 to 20 months
	1st molars	D	12 to 16 months
	2nd molars	E	20 to 30 months
Permanent	Central incisors	1	6 to 8 years
	Lateral incisors	2	7 to 9 years
	Canines	3	9 to 12 years
	1st premolar	4	10 to 12 years
	2nd premolar	5	10 to 12 years
	1st molars	6	6 to 7 years
	2nd molars	7	11 to 13 years
	3rd molars	8	17 to 25 years

Fig. 69.1 Tooth eruption times.

very minor degree of pyrexia around the time of tooth eruption [6].

The junction of the mucosa with the teeth

The dentogingival junction represents a unique anatomical feature concerned with the attachment of the gingival (gum) mucosa to the tooth. Non-keratinized gingival epithelium forms a cuff surrounding the tooth, and at its lowest point on the tooth is adherent to the enamel or cement. This 'junctional' epithelium is unique in being bounded both on its tooth and lamina propria aspects by basement membranes. Above this is a shallow sulcus or crevice (up to 2 mm deep), the gingival sulcus or crevice. Neutrophils continually migrate into the gingival crevice, and there is also a slow exudate of plasma (crevicular fluid).

Immunity in the oral cavity

Movement of the soft tissues during speech and swallowing, and salivation, ensures that much foreign material is swallowed. The need for this cleaning mechanism is clearly apparent in patients with facial paralysis, or those with xerostomia, in whom there is accumulation of oral debris and subsequent infection.

Saliva also aggregates bacteria and deters their attachment to surfaces. Salivary lysozyme, thiocyanate, peroxides and various mucins and other components may be antimicrobial and saliva is inhibitory to various microbial agents including, for example, human immunodeficiency virus (HIV).

Salivary tissue derives its B cells from the gastrointestine-associated lymphoid tissue (GALT) system [7]. Salivary acinar cells produce secretory component (transport piece) needed for transport of IgA into the saliva and its stability in the presence of salivary or gastric proteolytic enzymes. Although the exact contribution to oral defence made by salivary IgA antibodies is difficult to assess, some patients who have IgA deficiency suffer from oral infections, and in animals it is possible to induce protective salivary IgA antibodies to caries-producing organisms such as *Streptococcus mutans*.

Neutrophils and other leukocytes are particularly essential for oral health as shown by the fact that patients with HIV infection, neutropenia, agranulocytopenia, leukaemia or chronic granulomatous disease are predisposed to severe gingivitis and rapid periodontal breakdown, as well as mouth ulceration and infections.

REFERENCES

1 Eveson JW, Scully C. *Colour Atlas of Oral Pathology*. London: Mosby, 1995.
2 Hume WJ, Potten CS. Advances in epithelial kinetics—an oral view. *J Oral Pathol* 1979; **8**: 3–22.
3 Meyer J, Squier CA, Gerson SJ. *The Structure and Function of Oral Mucosa*. Oxford: Pergamon Press, 1984.
4 Prime SS. Development, structure and function of oral mucosa. In: Scully C, ed. *The Mouth in Health and Disease*. Oxford: Heinemann Medical, 1989: 124–44.
5 Ten Cate AR. *Oral Histology*, 2nd edn. St Louis, Missouri: CV Mosby, 1985.
6 Jaber L, Cohen IJ, Mor A. Fever associated with teething. *Arch Dis Child* 1992; **67**: 233–4.
7 Lamey PJ, Scully C. Salivary gland development, anatomy and physiology. In: Scully C, ed. *The Mouth in Health and Disease*. Oxford: Heinemann Medical, 1989: 283–8.

Signs and symptoms affecting specific oral tissues

Oral pain

Most oral pain is local in origin, usually a consequence of dental caries or sometimes trauma. Neurological, vascular, psychogenic and referred pains are less common.

Premature eruption of teeth

Erupted teeth, particularly in the mandibular central incisor region, rarely may be present at birth (natal teeth), or appear within the first few days or weeks of life (neonatal teeth). This rare event (about 0.1% of live births) occasionally has a familial basis or is associated with some other developmental anomaly. Such teeth occasionally cause ulceration of the infant's tongue or mother's nipple but usually they can be safely left *in situ*.

Retarded eruption of teeth

Congenital hypopituitarism, congenital hypothyroidism (cretinism), Down's syndrome, cleidocranial dysplasia, cytotoxic drugs and radiotherapy may cause retarded eruption of teeth, but most cases are of local aetiology (e.g. impactions).

Dental aplasia
SYN. HYPODONTIA; ANODONTIA

Wisdom teeth (third molars), second premolars and upper lateral incisors are sometimes absent in otherwise normal individuals, probably because of some unidentified genetic trait. Up to 25% of white people lack a third molar. Absence of several teeth may indicate systemic disease such as cleidocranial dysplasia, incontinentia pigmenti or ectodermal dysplasia.

Hypodontia is often associated with microdontia and is often bilaterally symmetrical. It is important to remember that teeth may be apparently missing simply because they are unerupted.

Loosening and early loss of teeth (Table 69.1)

Early loss of teeth is usually caused by trauma, dental caries or destructive periodontal disease [1]. Congenital disorders such as Down's syndrome, Papillon–Lefèvre syndrome, neutropenia, other immune defects, or acquired disorders such as diabetes mellitus or immune defects may predispose to periodontal disease. Teeth are also lost early in other rare systemic disorders, for example eosinophilic granuloma or hypophosphatasia.

Table 69.1 Pathological causes of loosening and early loss of the teeth.

Local causes
Trauma
Periodontitis
Neoplasms

Systemic causes
Disorders with some immune deficit
  Down's syndrome
  Diabetes mellitus
  Leukopenia or leukocyte defects
  HIV disease
  Juvenile periodontitis
  Rapidly progressive periodontitis
  Papillon–Lefèvre syndrome
Hypophosphatasia
Ehlers–Danlos syndrome (type VIII)

Others
Acrodynia
Neoplasms
Eosinophilic granuloma

Table 69.2 Causes of discoloration of teeth.

Extrinsic
Poor oral hygiene
Smoking
Beverages/food
Drugs, e.g. iron, chlorhexidine, sweetened medication
Stains, e.g. from betel chewing

Intrinsic
Trauma
Caries
Restorative materials, e.g. amalgam
Pink spot (internal resorption)
Drugs—mainly tetracyclines
Fluorosis
Dentinogenesis imperfecta
Amelogenesis imperfecta
Porphyria
Kernicterus (severe neonatal jaundice)

REFERENCE

1 Watanable K. Prepubertal periodontitis: a review of diagnostic criteria, pathogenesis and differential diagnosis. *J Periodont Res* 1990; **25**: 31–48.

Extra teeth

Extra (supernumerary) teeth are uncommon and usually of an unknown cause. They are generally found in the premaxilla. Supernumerary teeth are common in cleidocranial dysplasia.

Malformed and discoloured teeth (Table 69.2)

There is a wide range of normal variation in tooth morphology and colour, especially between races.

Local infection or trauma, or unknown factors, may cause malformation of a single tooth (or a few). The lower premolars are usually affected because there is caries and periapical infection related to their deciduous predecessors; such hypoplastic teeth are termed *Turner's teeth*. The upper permanent incisors may be malformed if there is trauma to the deciduous incisors. Radiotherapy or cytotoxic therapy may cause hypoplasia, as may congenital rubella or cytomegalovirus infection. However, classical *Hutchinsonian* (screwdriver-shaped) *incisors* and *Moon's* (or mulberry) *molars* of congenital syphilis are extremely rare. Hypoplasia is also seen in early onset malabsorption syndromes, many severe childhood illnesses (Fig. 69.2) and organ transplantation [1,2] and in some forms of epidermolysis bullosa [3–5]. Peg-shaped teeth may be normal variants (Fig. 69.3) or may be found in some ectodermal

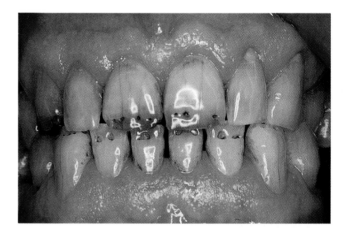

Fig. 69.2 Hypoplasia of teeth related to severe childhood respiratory infection.

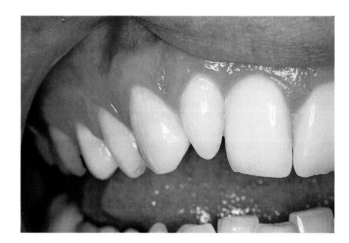

Fig. 69.3 A peg-shaped maxillary lateral incisor—a fairly common variant.

dysplasias (p. 3052). Taurodontism (see below) can be found in a range of dermatological disorders [3].

Erosion of teeth may occur because of the repeated use of acidic drinks or sucking citrus fruits, or as a feature of gastric regurgitation in bulimia, anorexia nervosa or alcoholism.

Most dental discoloration is caused by smoking, foods and beverages (such as tea), medicines such as iron or chlorhexidine or poor oral hygiene. Tetracyclines given to a pregnant or lactating mother may discolour the child's teeth and, if given to a child, particularly one under the age of 8 years, may cause significant brown intrinsic tooth staining (Fig. 69.4). The regular use of sweetened medication at night (e.g. trimeprazine syrup in a child with eczema) can cause discoloration due to dental caries.

Fluoride, at the concentrations present in water supplies in Western countries, or given prophylactically, may occasionally produce inconsequential minute white flecks but concentrations over 2p.p.m. may produce significant fluorosis.

Genetic defects that may cause tooth discoloration include dentinogenesis imperfecta (Fig. 69.5) which may

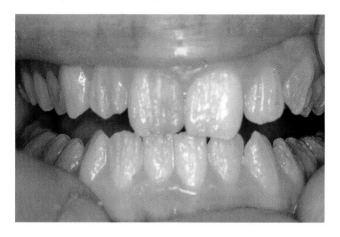

Fig. 69.6 Amelogenesis imperfecta: one variant showing longitudinal ridging of teeth.

be seen in some patients with osteogenesis imperfecta, and amelogenesis imperfecta (Fig. 69.6) [3,4].

REFERENCES

1 Hosey MT, Gordon G, Kelly DA, Shaw L. Oral findings in children with liver transplants. *Int J Paediatr Dent* 1995; **5**: 29–34.
2 Morisaki I, Abe K, Tong LS, *et al.* Dental findings of children with biliary atresia. *J Dent Child* 1990; **57**: 220–3.
3 Hill FJ, Winter GB. The teeth in dermatological diseases. In: Champion RH, ed. *Recent Advances in Dermatology*. London: Livingstone, 1986: 103–26.
4 Scully C, Welbury R. *Colour Atlas of Oral Disease in Children and Adolescents*. London: Mosby–Wolfe, 1994
5 Seow WK. Enamel hypoplasia in the primary dentition: a review. *J Dent Child* 1991; **58**: 441–52.

Taurodontism

Taurodont teeth are most readily diagnosed on radiographs

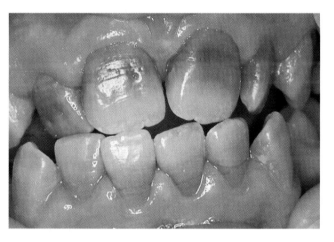

Fig. 69.4 Pronounced intrinsic tooth discoloration from use of tetracyclines in childhood.

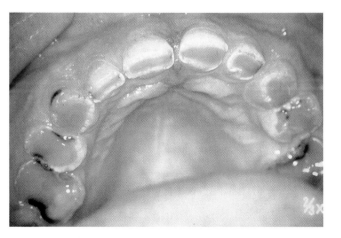

Fig. 69.5 Dentinogenesis imperfecta: staining and severe attrition.

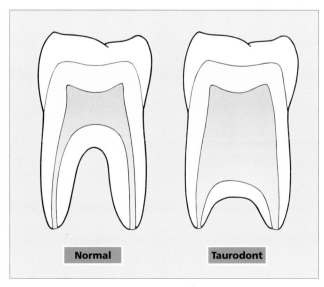

Normal   Taurodont

Fig. 69.7 Taurodontism.

Table 69.3 Dermatological disorders in which taurodontism may occasionally be found.

Some ectodermal dysplasias
Trichodento-osseous syndrome
Tricho-onychodental syndrome
Epidermolysis bullosa
Dental oculocutaneous syndrome
Otodental dysplasia
Orofacial digital syndrome type II
Dyskeratosis congenita

---

since their most obvious features, the increased pulp chamber and a more inferiorly placed root bifurcation in premolars and molars, are not detectable on clinical examination (Fig. 69.7). However, on clinical examination, lack of constriction of the tooth at the neck may be suggestive of taurodontism.

Taurodontism is generally most obvious in molars of both deciduous and permanent dentitions, and may be found in single or several teeth, with or without evidence of other disorders. Most studies have shown an overall prevalence of the order of 2% with no sex predilection, but oriental people are especially affected.

Dermatological conditions with which taurodontism may be associated are shown in Table 69.3 [1].

REFERENCE

1 Ogden GR. Taurodontism in dermatologic disease. *Int J Dermatol* 1988; **27**: 360–4.

Ectodermal dysplasia

Ectodermal dysplasia is typically characterized by development abnormalities in at least two different ectodermally derived systems. Oral abnormalities are common, especially missing teeth and abnormally shaped teeth

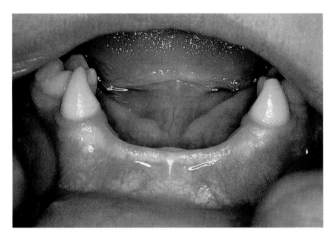

Fig. 69.8 Hypodontia and malformed teeth are common in ectodermal dysplasia.

(Fig. 69.8). There are many variations, as discussed in the following sections, and in Chapter 12.

X-linked hypohidrotic ectodermal dysplasia [1,2]

Hypodontia is common in X-linked hypohidrotic ectodermal dysplasia. Some anterior teeth are usually present but their crowns are typically conical or peg shaped. The posterior teeth, when present, are smaller but otherwise normal. Overclosure of the jaws, together with maxillary hypoplasia and frontal bossing give a characteristic facial appearance. There may be a degree of impaired salivary gland function.

Female carriers of this syndrome may have hypodontia and/or microdontia.

Autosomal recessive ectodermal dysplasia [1,3]

Dental and oral anomalies in this condition are identical to those in the X-linked form of ectodermal dysplasia, although relatives may have a normal dentition.

Hypodontia, taurodontism and sparse hair [4]

There are a few reports of a variant of ectodermal dysplasia where there is taurodontism, and somewhat lesser hypodontia than in the more classic forms of ectodermal dysplasia.

Autosomal dominant hypodontia with nail dysgenesis [5]

Hypodontia, conical deciduous and permanent teeth, and dysplastic nails characterize this variant of ectodermal dysplasia.

Incontinentia pigmenti [6]

SYN. BLOCH–SULZBERGER SYNDROME [6]

Hypodontia and retarded eruption affect both dentitions and the anterior teeth are small. The teeth tend also to be conical, often with accessory cusps.

Chondroectodermal dysplasia [7]

SYN. ELLIS–VAN-CREVELD SYNDROME

Natal teeth, mild hypodontia or hyperdontia, malformed or small teeth are seen in chondroectodermal dysplasia. Accessory cusps are common. However, the most obvious oral anomalies are the multiple fraeni extending from the lips and buccal mucosae to the alveolar ridges of both jaws.

Cranioectodermal dysplasia [8]

Deciduous teeth are small and may have dysplastic enamel, although the condition is so rare that the permanent teeth have not been clearly described. There may be hypodontia or taurodontism. Dolicocephaly, hair anomalies and shortened arms, fingers and toes are associated.

Nance–Horan syndrome [9]

X-linked congenital cataracts with supernumerary teeth constitute the Nance–Horan syndrome. The incisor teeth may also be morphologically abnormal and can resemble Hutchinson's incisors of congenital syphilis.

Trichodental syndrome [10,11]

The trichodental syndrome is a rare dominantly inherited condition in which there is fine, short hair, thinning of the lateral ends of the eyebrows, hypodontia and/or conical teeth.

Trichodento-osseous syndrome [12,13]

Tight, curly hair, sclerotic cortical bone and oral anomalies (especially thin enamel) are found in this autosomal dominant condition. The hypoplasia–hypomaturation type of amelogenesis imperfecta, enamel hypoplasia, unerupted teeth and taurodontism may be associated.

Trichonychodental syndrome [14]

This autosomal dominant trait of fine, curly hair and thin, dysplastic nails may be associated with taurodontism and enamel or dentinal developmental defects.

Curry–Hall syndrome [15]

Deciduous teeth are small and conical, and the incisors are often retained since their permanent successors may be congenitally absent. The remaining permanent teeth do erupt but are small. Other features include short limbs, polydactyly and nail dysplasia.

Otodental dysplasia [16,17]

Globe-shaped posterior teeth (globodontia) in both dentitions are the most common oral feature of this autosomal dominant condition which is associated with sensorineural hearing loss. Other oral anomalies include taurodontism, microdontia and hypodontia. The incisors are not affected and the patients are otherwise well.

REFERENCES

1 Levin LS. Dental and oral abnormalities in selected ectodermal dysplasia syndromes. *Birth Defects* 1988; **24**: 205–27.
2 Sofaer JA. Hypodontia and sweat pore counts in detecting carriers of X-linked hypohidrotic ectodermal dysplasia. *Br Dent J* 1981; **151**: 327–30.
3 Bartlett RC, Eversole LR, Adkins RS. Autosomal recessive hypohidrotic ectodermal dysplasia: dental manifestations. *Oral Surg* 1972; **33**: 736–42.
4 Stenvik A, Zachrisson BU, Svatum B. Taurodontism and concomitant hypodontia in siblings. *Oral Surg* 1972; **33**: 841–5.
5 Hudson CD, Witkop CJ. Autosomal dominant hypodontia with nail dysgenesis. Report of twenty-nine cases in six families. *Oral Surg* 1975; **39**: 409–23.
6 Gorlin RJ, Anderson JA. The characteristic dentition of incontinentia pigmenti: a diagnostic aid. *J Pediatr* 1960; **57**: 78–85.
7 Sarnant H, Amir E, Legum CP. Development dental anomalies in chondro-ectodermal dysplasia (Ellis–Van-Creveld syndrome). *J Dent Child* 1980; **47**: 28–31.
8 Levin LS, Perrin JCS, Ose L *et al.* A heritable syndrome of craniosynostosis, short thin hair, dental abnormalities, and short limbs: cranioectodermal dysplasia. *J Pediatr* 1977; **90**: 55–61.
9 Bixler D, Higgins M, Hartsfield J. The Nance–Horan syndrome: a rare X-linked ocular–dental trait with expression in heterozygous females. *Clin Genet* 1984; **26**: 303–35.
10 Kersey PJW. Tricho-dental syndrome: a disorder with a short hair cycle. *Br J Dermatol* 1987; **116**: 259–63.

Table 69.4 Oral features in rare ectodermal dysplasia variants [1–3].

Syndrome	Oral manifestations	Facial manifestations	Other features
GAPO (*growth retardation, alopecia, pseudoanodontia, and optic atrophy*)	Failure of both dentitions to erupt	Frontal bossing Midface hypoplasia	*See left-hand column*
Johanson-Blizzard	Hypodontia in both dentitions. Roots of deciduous teeth are short and deformed, crowns are conical	Microcephaly Hypoplastic alae nasi	Hearing loss, pancreatic dysfunction, mental retardation
Waardenburg	–	Cleft lip/palate	Deafness Hair depigmentation
LEOPARD (*lentigines, electrocardiographic anomalies, ocular hypertelorism, pulmonary stenosis, abnormal genitalia, retarded growth, deafness*)	No mucosal lentigines but there may be granular cell myoblastomas	Triangular face with hypertelorism and ptosis	*See left-hand column*
Congenital erythrokeratoderma with sensorineural hearing loss	Hyperkeratosis Occasional carcinoma	–	*See left-hand column*

3054 *Chapter 69: The Oral Cavity*

11 Salinas CF, Spector M. Tricho-dental syndrome. In: Brown AC, Crounse RG, eds. *Hair, Trace Elements and Human Illness*. Praeger: New York, 1980: 240–56.
12 Jorgenson RJ, Warson RW. Dental abnormalities in the trichodento-osseous (TDO) syndrome. *Oral Surg* 1973; **36**: 696–700.
13 Wright JT, Roberts MW, Wilson AR, Kudhail R. Tricho-dento-osseous syndrome. *Oral Surg* 1994; **77**: 487–493.
14 Koshiba H, Kimura O, Nakata M. Clinical, genetic and histologic features of the trichonychodental (TOD) syndrome. *Oral Surg* 1978; **46**: 376–85.
15 Shapiro SD, Jorgenson RJ, Salinas CF. Brief clinical report: Curry–Hall syndrome. *Am J Med Genet* 1984; **17**: 579–83.
16 Levin LS, Jorgenson RJ, Cook RA. Otodental dysplasia: a 'new' ectodermal dysplasia. *Clin Genet* 1975; **8**: 136–44.
17 Witkop CJ, Gudlach KH, Street WJ *et al*. Globodontia in the otodental syndrome. *Oral Surg* 1976; **41**: 472–83.

Other rare ectodermal dysplasias, pachonychia congenita and Clouston syndrome are discussed in Chapter 12. Others are summarized in Table 69.4.

REFERENCES

1 Gorlin RJ. Selected ectodermal dysplasias. *Birth Defects* 1988; **24**: 123–48.
2 Gorlin RJ, Anderson RC, Moller JH. The leopard (multiple lentigines) syndrome revisited. In: Bergsman D, McKusick V, Konigsmark B, eds. *The Clinical Delineation of Birth Defects*, Part IX. *Ear*. New York: Alan R. Liss, 1971: 110–15.
3 Johanson A, Blizzard R. A syndrome of congenital aplasia of the alae nasi, deafness, hypothyroidism, dwarfism, absent permanent teeth and malabsorption. *J Pediatr* 1971; **79**: 982–7.

Periodontal disease

Periodontal breakdown is usually a consequence of inflammatory destruction (periodontitis) as a result of poor oral hygiene and the subsequent accumulation of dental bacterial plaque. It is seen mainly in adults. The host defences are extremely important in maintaining periodontal health, as is demonstrated well in the periodontal breakdown that may accompany leukaemias, leukocyte defects, diabetes and HIV infection. Periodontal breakdown is also a feature of Down's syndrome, Ehlers–Danlos syndrome type VIII, and the Papillon–Lefèvre syndrome. Periodontal breakdown in a child who is capable of maintaining good oral hygiene almost invariably suggests an immune or other systemic defect.

Papillon–Lefèvre syndrome (Chapter 34)

This is a rare, autosomal recessive condition of palmoplantar hyperkeratosis with periodontoclasia (periodontosis or periodontal breakdown) which appears in childhood [1–3].

There is chronic inflammation and degeneration of the periodontium affecting both dentitions. There are no obvious abnormalities in either the tooth cementum or dentine. The affected skin shows diffuse hyperkeratosis, hypergranulosis and acanthosis. There is defective polymorphonuclear leukocyte function and abnormal fibroblast production of collagen in some cases [4,5].

The major oral feature of Papillon–Lefèvre syndrome is premature periodontal breakdown in both the deciduous and permanent dentitions. The teeth develop and erupt normally but the gingiva become red, swollen and bleed easily with the formation of periodontal pockets, loss of alveolar bone, loosening and shedding of the teeth. The deciduous teeth are often lost by the age of 5 years and the permanent teeth are almost invariably lost by the age of 16 years. The teeth are involved roughly in the order they erupt.

Hyperkeratosis of the palms and particularly the soles appears at about the age of 3–5 years, concurrent with the periodontal breakdown in the deciduous dentition. Similar plaques may also be seen on the lips, cheeks and eyelids. There may also be calcification of the dura and some patients have recurrent pyogenic infections [6].

Similar syndromes with late-onset Papillon–Lefèvre syndrome [7] or including arachnodactyly and acro-osteolysis have also been described [8].

Diagnosis is on clinical and radiographic grounds. Prognosis is poor. Intensive dental care is needed. Retinoids may be useful in suppressing peridontal and skin lesions and minimizing the pyogenic infections [6,9,10].

REFERENCES

1 Efeoglu J, Porter SR, Mutlu S *et al*. Papillon–Lefèvre syndrome affecting two siblings. *Br J Pediatr Dent* 1990; **6**: 115–20.
2 Haneke E. The Papillon–Lefèvre syndrome: keratosis palmoplantaris with periodontopathy: report of a case and review of cases in the literature. *Hum Genet* 1979; **51**: 1–35.
3 Smith P, Rosenzweig KA. Seven cases of Papillon–Lefèvre syndrome. *Periodontics* 1967; **5**: 42–6.
4 Cheung HS, Landow RK, Bauer M. Increased collagen synthesis by gingival fibroblasts derived from a Papillon–Lefèvre patient. *J Dent Res* 1982; **61**: 378–81.
5 Van Dyke TE, Taubman MA, Ebersole JL *et al*. The Papillon–Lefèvre syndrome: neutrophil dysfunction with severe periodontal disease. *Clin Immunol Immunopathol* 1984; **31**: 419–29.
6 Bergman R, Friedman-Birnbaum R. Papillon–Lefèvre syndrome: a study of the long term clinical course of recurrent pyogenic infections and the effects of etretinate treatment. *Br J Dermatol* 1988; **119**: 731–6.
7 Brown RS, Hays GL, Flaitz CM *et al*. A possible late-onset variation of Papillon–Lefèvre syndrome. *J Periodontol* 1993; **64**: 379–86.
8 Puliyel JM, Sridharanlyer KS. A syndrome of keratosis palmoplantaris congenita, pes planus, onychogryphosis, periodontosis, arachnodactyly and a peculiar acrosteolysis. *Br J Dermatol* 1986; **115**: 243–8.
9 El Darouti MA, Al Raubaie SM, Eiada MA. Papillon–Lefèvre syndrome: successful treatment with oral retinoids in three patients. *Int J Dermatol* 1988; **27**: 63–6.
10 Gelmetti C, Nazzaro V, Cerri D, Fracasso L. Long-term preservation of permanent teeth in a patient with Papillon–Lefèvre syndrome treated with etretinate. *Pediatr Dermatol* 1989; **6**: 222–5.

Leukocyte adhesion deficiency

Defects in cell-surface receptors on neutrophils and other leukocytes result in a range of disorders, especially recurrent cutaneous, respiratory and middle-ear infection, as well as periodontal destruction in both dentitions.

Local efforts to preserve the dentition, using debridement together with antimicrobials have been of little value [1,2].

REFERENCES

1 Meyle J. Leukocyte adhesion deficiency and prepubertal periodontitis. *Periodontol 2000*; 1994; **6**: 26–36.
2 Waldrop TC, Anderson DC, Hallmon WW *et al*. Periodontal manifestations of the heritable Mac-1, LFA-1 deficiency syndrome. *J Periodontol* 1987; **58**: 400–16.

Hereditary palmoplantar keratoderma

The Unna–Thost variety of hereditary palmoplantar kerato-derma may be associated with oral keratosis or periodontosis. [1,2].

Ehlers–Danlos syndrome [3]

Early-onset periodontitis is seen in type VIII Ehlers–Danlos syndrome (Chapter 44).

Down's syndrome [4]

Periodontitis is common in Down's syndrome.

Prader–Willi syndrome [5]

Periodontitis has been recorded in Prader–Willi syndrome, presumably as a consequence of the diabetes.

REFERENCES

1 Ergorov HA. Unna–Thost syndrome in four generations. *Vestn Dermatol Venerol* 1978; **7**: 68–71.
2 Nikolov D, Lazarevska B, Arsovski T. Hereditary palmo-plantar kera-toderma Unna–Thost with periodontitis. *God Med Fak Skopje* 1976; **22**: 415–24.
3 Stewart RE, Hollister DW, Rimoin DL *et al*. A new variant of Ehlers–Danlos syndrome: an autosomal dominant disorder of fragile skin, abnormal scarring and generalized periodontitis. *Birth Defects* 1977; **13**: 85–93.
4 Saxen L, Aula S. Periodontal bone loss in patients with Down's syndrome. *J Periodontol* 1982; **53**: 158–62.
5 Greenwood RE, Small ICB. Case report of the Prader–Willi syndrome. *J Clin Periodontol* 1990; **17**: 61–3.

Gingival disorders

Bleeding

Bleeding from the gingival margins is common, usually a consequence of gingivitis because of inadequate oral hygiene leading to the accumulation of dental bacterial plaque (Table 69.5). The tendency to gingivitis is slightly increased in patients taking oral contraceptives and in some pregnant women (especially during the second trimester).

Gingival haemorrhage, however, may be an early feature in some vascular or platelet disorders and is commonly a problem in leukaemic patients.

Table 69.5 Causes of gingival bleeding.

Local
Chronic gingivitis
Chronic periodontitis
Acute necrotizing gingivitis

Systemic
Any condition causing exacerbation of gingivitis (e.g. pregnancy)
Leukaemia
Human immunodeficiency virus infection
Other causes of purpura
Clotting defects
Drugs, e.g. anticoagulants
Scurvy

Swelling

Gingival swelling is seen in chronic gingivitis and may be produced by drugs such as phenytoin, cyclosporin, nife-dipine and diltiazem (Fig. 69.9). Gingival swelling is seen with hypertrichosis both in drug-induced hyperplasias and in hereditary gingival fibromatosis.

A degree of gingival swelling may be seen in herpetic stomatitis, pregnancy, leukaemia, Crohn's disease, scurvy, Wegener's granulomatosis, sarcoidosis, amyloidosis, lipoid proteinosis, mucopolysaccharidoses and other disorders. Localized swellings (epulides) may be of local aetiology or can be manifestations of pregnancy or systemic disease (Table 69.6).

Pigmentation

Gingival pigmentation is usually seen in dark-skinned races (but may be seen even in white people) (Fig. 69.10).

Addison's disease, Kaposi's sarcoma, and melanoma are the most important acquired causes of pigmented lesions

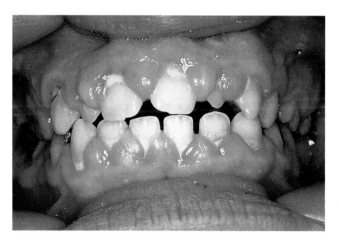

Fig. 69.9 Gingival hyperplasia in phenytoin therapy. Concomitant folate deficiency in this patient also caused mouth ulcers, seen in the maxillary buccal vestibule.

Table 69.6 Causes of gingival swelling.

	Generalized	Localized

Local	Chronic gingivitis
	Hyperplastic gingivitis
	  due to mouth breathing
		Abscesses
		Cysts
		Pyogenic granuloma
		Neoplasms and warts
		  (various)

Systemic	Hereditary gingival
	  fibromatosis
	  and associated syndromes
	Drugs
	  Phenytoin
	  Cyclosporin
	  Nifedipine, diltiazem
	Pregnancy
	Sarcoidosis
	Crohn's disease
	Leukaemia
	Wegener's granulomatosis
	Scurvy
	Amyloidosis
	Mucopolysaccharidoses
	Mucolipidosis
	Juvenile hyaline fibromatosis
	Lipoid proteinosis
		Pregnancy
		Sarcoidosis
		Orofacial granulomatosis
		Crohn's disease
		Wegener's granulomatosis
		Amyloidosis
		Neoplasms (various)

but drugs such as hydroxychloroquinine and minocycline may also cause hyperpigmentation.

Redness

Chronic marginal gingivitis is the usual cause of gingival redness, and then is usually restricted to the gingival margins and interdental papillae.

More widespread erythema, particularly if associated with soreness, is usually caused by primary herpes simplex stomatitis, or desquamative gingivitis, usually due to lichen planus or mucous membrane pemphigoid, rarely by

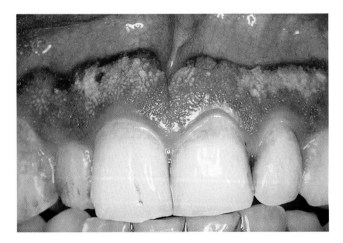

Fig. 69.10 Gingival hyperpigmentation of racial origin. The white lesion is due to accumulated oral debris—oral hygiene is very poor.

pemphigus or other dermatoses, or occasionally by allergic responses. Red lesions may also represent erythroplasia, haemangiomas or neoplasms such as carcinoma, Wegener's granulomatosis or Kaposi's sarcoma [1,2].

Ulcers

Acute ulcerative (necrotizing) gingivitis or a similar disorder is a rare complication of HIV infection, neutropenia or leukaemia and, in the malnourished or some immunosuppressed patients, may spread to the cheek (*noma* (cancrum oris)). Aphthae (sometimes) and other causes of mouth ulcers (rarely) involve the gingiva. Gingival ulcers are sometimes self-induced (artefactual) in psychologically disturbed or mentally handicapped patients [1,2].

REFERENCES

1 Scully C, Porter SR. Disorders of the gums and periodontium. *Med Int* 1990; **76**: 3150–3153.
2 Scully C, Porter SR. Oral Medicine 1: Teeth and the periodontium. *Postgrad Dent* 1992; **2**: 93–100.

Oral mucosa

Blisters

Blisters may be seen as a result of burns but the most important vesiculobullous disorders affecting the oral mucosa are pemphigoid (including cicatricial pemphigoid) and pemphigus (Table 69.7). The bullae of mucous membrane pemphigoid may or may not be bloodfilled and, in

Table 69.7 Main causes of mouth ulcers associated with systemic disease.

Microbial disease
  Herpetic stomatitis
  Chickenpox
  Herpes zoster
  Hand, foot and mouth disease
  Herpangina
  Infectious mononucleosis
  HIV disease
  Tuberculosis
  Syphilis
  Rarely fungal infections
Malignant neoplasms
Cutaneous disease
  Erosive lichen planus and chronic ulcerative stomatitis
  Pemphigus
  Pemphigoid
  Erythema multiforme
  Dermatitis herpetiformis and linear IgA disease
  Epidermolysis bullosa
  Other dermatoses

Continued.

Table 69.7 *(continued)*

Blood disorders
  Anaemia
  Leukaemia
  Neutropenia
  Other white cell dyscrasias
Gastrointestinal disease
  Coeliac disease
  Crohn's disease
  Ulcerative colitis
Rheumatic diseases
  Lupus erythematosus
  Behçet's syndrome
  Sweet's syndrome
  Reiter's disease
Drugs
  Cytotoxic and other agents
  Acrodynia
Radiotherapy
Disorders of uncertain pathogenesis
  Angina bullosa haemorrhagica
  Hypereosinophilic syndrome
  Eosinophilic ulcer
  Necrotizing sialometaplasia

the former case, a bleeding tendency must be excluded. Blood-filled blisters may also be caused by localized oral purpura (angina bullosa haemorrhagica) or amyloidosis. The bullae of pemphigus are rarely seen as they break down rapidly to produce ulcers. Epidermolysis bullosa and erythema multiforme may present with oral bullae or vesicles, but ulcers are more common. Vesicles may be seen in viral infections, especially in herpes simplex stomatitis, chickenpox, herpangina and hand, foot and mouth disease.

Mucoceles, caused by extravasation of mucus from minor salivary glands, produce isolated blisters, typically in the lower labial mucosa.

Oral purpura

Oral petechiae are usually caused by trauma or suction. More widespread purpura is most frequently a manifestation of a bleeding tendency caused by thrombocytopenia and may also be seen in infectious mononucleosis, rubella, HIV infection, leukaemia or scurvy. Petechiae may also occur in amyloidosis.

Oral pigmentation

Race is the most important cause of oral pigmentation. Addison's disease, melanoma, Laugier–Hunziker syndrome, pigmentary incontinence and other causes must be excluded. Peutz–Jegher's disease is the association of circumoral and sometimes intraoral melanosis with small-intestinal polyposis (Chapter 39).

Red areas

Telangiectasia may be a manifestation of hereditary haemorrhagic telangiectasia, primary biliary cirrhosis or systemic sclerosis, or may follow radiotherapy. Haemangiomas are usually isolated but may occasionally extend deeply and rarely involve the ipsilateral meninges, producing a facial angioma and epilepsy, sometimes with mental handicap (Sturge–Weber syndrome). Intraoral haemangiomas may be seen in Maffucci's syndrome.

Localized red areas may represent erythroplasia, carcinoma, candidiasis, lichen planus or lupus erythematosus. Kaposi's sarcoma may present as a red, purple, brown or bluish macule or nodule as may epithelioid angiomatosis. Hereditary mucoepithelial dysplasia is a rare cause of oral erythema.

Lingual depapillation in deficiencies of iron, folate or vitamin B_{12} may produce the red tongue termed glossitis. Geographical tongue may also produce red patches.

Irradiation-induced mucositis is a further cause of a red, sore mouth.

Ulcers

Oral ulcers are often caused by trauma or recurrent aphthae (p. 3069). Malignant neoplasms may present as ulcers. Various infections or systemic disorders, particularly those of blood, gastrointestinal tract or skin, also produce mouth ulcers, as may drugs and irradiation (Table 69.7).

White patches (Table 69.8)

Thrush (acute candidiasis) is a 'disease of the diseased' and produces oral white patches.

HIV infection causes hairy leukoplakia, a white lesion on the tongue (p. 3099).

Table 69.8 Main causes of oral white lesions.

Local
Frictional keratosis
Smoker's keratosis
Idiopathic keratosis
Carcinoma
Burns
Skin grafts

Systemic
Candidiasis
Lichen planus
Lupus erythematosus
Papillomas (some)
Hairy leukoplakia (mainly HIV disease)
Syphilitic keratosis
Chronic renal failure
Inherited lesions (e.g. white-sponge naevus)

Leukoplakia is often associated with friction or smoking, occasionally with syphilis, candidiasis or chronic renal failure but most cases are idiopathic. Lichen planus and lupus erythematosus may present as white lesions. Rarely, lichenoid lesions are associated with various drugs, liver disease or graft-versus-host disease (GVHD). Carcinoma may present as a white lesion.

Inherited causes of white patches, such as white sponge naevus and dyskeratosis congenita, are rare [1,2].

REFERENCES

1 Scully C, Porter SR. Diseases of the oral mucosa. *Med Int* 1990; **76**: 3154–62.
2 Scully C, Porter SR. Oral Medicine 2. Disorders affecting the oral mucosa. *Postgrad Dent* 1992; **2**: 109–13.

Salivary glands

Dry mouth
SYN. XEROSTOMIA

The complaint of a dry mouth is by no means always supported by objective evidence, and not infrequently has a psychogenic basis. Drugs with anticholinergic or sympathomimetic activity are the most common cause of xerostomia

Table 69.9 Causes of dry mouth.

Drugs with anticholinergic effects
Atropine and analogues
Tricyclic antidepressants
Antihistamines
Antiemetics
Phenothiazines
Antihypertensives
Lithium

Drugs with sympathomimetic effects
Ephedrine and other decongestants
Bronchodilators
Amphetamines and appetite suppressants

Dehydration
Diabetes mellitus
Diarrhoea and vomiting

Organic disease of glands
Sjögren's syndrome
Sarcoidosis
Human immunodeficiency virus infection

Psychogenic
Anxiety states
Depression
Hypochondriasis

Iatrogenic
Radiotherapy
Graft-versus-host disease

Table 69.10 Causes of salivary gland swelling.

Local	
Inflammatory	Ascending bacterial sialadenitis
Neoplasms	Various
Duct obstruction	Usually by a calculus
Systemic	
Inflammatory	Mumps
	Sjögren's and sicca syndrome
	Sarcoidosis
	Actinomycosis
	Human immunodeficiency virus infection
Others	Sialosis
	Mikulicz's disease (lymphoepithelial lesion and syndrome)
Drugs	Chlorhexidine
	Phenylbutazone
	Iodine compounds
	Thiouracil
	Catecholamines
	Sulphonamides
	Phenothiazines
	Methyldopa

(Table 69.9). Tricyclic antidepressants, phenothiazines and lithium are most commonly implicated.

Sjögren's syndrome and sarcoidosis are the systemic disorders most commonly associated with this complaint. Severe dehydration from any cause, irradiation of the major salivary glands and, rarely, HIV infection, ectodermal dysplasia, cystic fibrosis and GVHD may produce xerostomia.

Swelling

Mumps is the most common cause of salivary gland swelling, particularly in children. Duct obstruction, bacterial sialadenitis, Sjögren's syndrome, sarcoidosis, sialoadenosis (sialosis), neoplasms and HIV infection usually affect adults (Table 69.10). Sialosis may be a feature of diabetes or alcoholic cirrhosis.

Sialorrhoea
SYN. PTYALISM

Sialorrhoea (excessive salivation) is a very uncommon complaint and is rarely confirmed objectively. Psychogenic 'causes' are more common than organic disease.

Painful oral lesions or foreign bodies (e.g. new dentures) may cause sialorrhoea, as may cholinergic drugs such as anticholinesterases and the analgesics buprenorphine and meptazinol.

Drooling of saliva may occur in normal infants, in 'teething', and in persons with pharyngeal obstruction or in various disorders in which there is poor neuromuscular coordination (mentally handicapped, Parkinsonism, facial palsy) and, very rarely, rabies [1,2].

REFERENCES

1 Lamey PJ, Scully C. Diseases of the salivary glands. *Medicine Int* 1990; **76**: 54–62.
2 Scully C, Porter SR. Oral Medicine 3. Salivary disorders. *Postgrad Dent* 1993; **3**: 150–3.

Cacogeusia and halitosis [1,2]

Cacogeusia (an unpleasant taste in the mouth) and halitosis are usually a consequence of poor oral hygiene, oral or nasal infections, starvation, smoking, some foods, xerostomia, drugs or psychogenic disorders, but may appear in various

Table 69.11 Causes of unpleasant taste and halitosis.

Local
Oral infections
    Chronic periodontitis
    Acute necrotizing gingivitis
    Pericoronitis
    Dental abscess
    Dry socket
Nasal disease
    Sinusitis
    Oroantral fistula
    Foreign body in nose
    Neoplasms

Systemic
Salivary gland disorders causing xerostomia
    Sjögren's syndrome
    Irradiation damage
Psychogenic causes
    Depression
    Anxiety states
    Psychoses
    Hypochondriasis
Foods
    Garlic
    Curries
    Onions
Drugs
    Smoking
    Drugs causing dry mouth
    Metronidazole
    Solvent abuse
    Alcohol
    Chloral hydrate
    Nitrites and nitrates
    Dimethyl sulphoxide
    Cytotoxic drugs
    Phenothiazines
    Amphetamines
Respiratory tract infections or neoplasms
Liver failure and cirrhosis
Renal failure
Diabetic ketosis
Gastrointestinal disease

systemic disorders such as suppurative respiratory infections, hepatic or renal failure, diabetic ketosis or gastrointestinal disease (Table 69.11).

REFERENCE

1 Scully C, Porter SR, Greenman J. What to do about halitosis. *Br Med J* 1994; **308**: 217–18.
2 Van Steenberghe D, Rostenberg M. *Bad Breath*. Leuven: Leuven University Press, 1996.

Neurological disorders

Loss of sense of taste
SYN. AGEUSIA

Lingual nerve trauma (usually from wisdom-tooth surgery), xerostomia, some drugs such as penicillamine, psychotic disorders and neurological disease such as cerebral metastases, and lesions affecting the chorda tympani or central connections may be responsible for loss of the sense of taste. Anosmia commonly produces an apparent loss of sense of taste.

Sensory disturbances

Sensory disturbances about the mouth usually result from damage to the lingual or inferior alveolar nerves during removal of wisdom or other teeth, jaw fractures or orthognathic surgery. However, peripheral or central neuropathies may be responsible.

Genetic disorders affecting the oral mucosa

White or whitish lesions

Sebaceous glands

Fordyce spots
SYN. FORDYCE'S GRANULES

Fordyce spots are sebaceous glands beneath the oral mucosa containing neutral lipids similar to those found in skin sebaceous glands [1]. They are not associated with hair follicles.

Fordyce spots are extremely common: probably 80% of the population have them. They are usually seen in the buccal mucosa, particularly inside the commissures (Fig. 69.11), and sometimes in the retromolar regions and upper lip as soft, yellowish granules [1–4]. Fordyce spots are often not noticeable in children until after puberty (although they are present histologically), and they seem to be more obvious in males, in patients with greasy skin and in the elderly. They may be increased in some rheumatic disorders [5].

The spots are totally benign, although the occasional patient or physician becomes concerned about them or

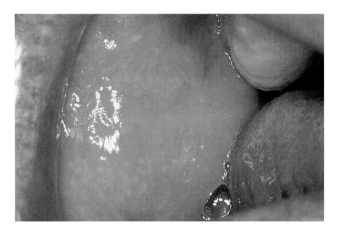

Fig. 69.11 Fordyce spots: sebaceous glands in the buccal mucosa.

misdiagnoses them as thrush or lichen planus. No treatment is indicated, other than reassurance. The spots may become less prominent if isotretinoin is given [6].

REFERENCES

1 Nordstrom KM, McGinley KJ, Lessin SR *et al*. Neutral lipid composition of Fordyce's granules. *Br J Dermatol* 1989; **121**: 669–70.
2 Batsakis JG, Littler ER, Leahy MS. Sebaceous cell lesions of the head and neck. *Arch Otolaryngol* 1972; **95**: 151–7.
3 Daley TD. Pathology of intraoral sebaceous glands. *J Oral Pathol Med* 1993; **22**: 241.
4 Sewerein I. The sebaceous glands in the vermilion border of the lips and the oral mucosa of man. *Acta Odontol Scand* 1975; **33** (Supp. 68): 13–226.
5 Vilpoula AH, Vli-kerttula UI, Terho PE *et al*. Sebaceous glands in the buccal mucosa in patients with rheumatic disorders. *Scand J Rheumatol* 1983; **12**: 337–42.
6 Monk BE. Fordyce spots responding to isotretinoin therapy. *Br J Dermatol* 1994; **131**: 335.

Sebaceous adenoma

Sebaceous adenomas are exceedingly rare in the mouth, except in association with salivary glands but have been described in the buccal mucosa [1,2].

Nevus sebaceus of Jadassohn

Oral manifestations may rarely occur as fibroepitheliomatous nodules in patients with a sebaceous naevus of the skin but are extremely rarely seen in isolation [3–5].

REFERENCES

1 Daley TD. Pathology of intraoral sebaceous glands. *J Oral Pathol Med* 1993; **22**: 241.
2 Miller AS, McCrea MW. Sebaceous gland adenoma of the buccal mucosa. *J Oral Surg* 1968; **26**: 593–5.
3 Kelley JE, Hibbard E, Giansanti J. Epidermal nevus syndrome: report of a case with unusual oral manifestations. *Oral Surg* 1972; **34**: 774–80.
4 Morency R, Labelle H. Nevus sebaceus of Jadassohn: a rare oral presentation. *Oral Surg* 1987; **64**: 460–2.
5 Reichart PA, Lubach D, Becker J. Gingival manifestation in linear nevus sebaceus syndrome. *Int J Oral Surg* 1983; **12**: 437–43.

Epithelium

Leukoedema

This is not a mucosal disease but simply the name given to the faint whitish lines seen in some normal buccal mucosae, often prominent in black people. The whitish lines disappear if the mucosa is stretched—a diagnostic test [1–3].

REFERENCES

1 Axell T, Henricsson V. Leukoedema—an epidemiologic study with special reference to the influence of tobacco habits. *Community Dent Oral Epidemiol* 1981; **9**: 142–6.
2 Duncan SC, Su WPD. Leukoedema of the oral mucosa (possibly an acquired white sponge naevus). *Arch Dermatol* 1980; **116**: 906–8.
3 Van Wyk CW, Ambrosio SC. Leukoedema: ultrastructural and histochemical observations. *J Oral Pathol* 1983; **12**: 29–35.

White-sponge naevus

SYN. CANNON'S DISEASE; PACHYDERMIA ORALIS; WHITE FOLDED GINGIVOSTOMATOSIS

Aetiology. A rare familial disorder usually inherited as an autosomal dominant trait [1]; there appears to be abnormal tonofilament aggregation [2].

Pathology. There is hyperplastic acanthotic epithelium in which gross oedema causes a basket-weave appearance. The superficial epithelium has a 'washed-out' appearance as it stains only very lightly.

Clinical features. The oral mucosa is almost invariably involved in white-sponge naevus. Painless shaggy or folded white lesions typically affect the buccal mucosa bilaterally but may also involve other areas, although rarely the gingival margins.

Similar lesions may also affect the upper respiratory tract, genitalia and anus [3].

This is a benign condition with an excellent prognosis.

Diagnosis. The family history and clinical examination are usually adequate to differentiate this from other white lesions such as cheek biting, lichen planus and candidiasis.

Treatment. Reassurance is all that is required, although some have suggested that antimicrobial therapy clears the lesions [4,5].

REFERENCES

1 Ciola B. White sponge naevus of the oral mucosa. *J Conn State Dent Assoc* 1976; **51**: 122–6.
2 Frithiof L, Banoczy J. White sponge naevus (leukoedema exfoliativum mucosae oris): ultrastructural observations. *Oral Surg* 1976; **41**: 607–22.
3 Jorgenson RJ, Levin LS. White sponge naevus. *Arch Dermatol* 1981; **117**: 73–6.

4 Lim J, Keting S. Oral tetracycline rinse improves symptoms of white sponge naevus. *J Am Acad Dermatol* 1992; **26**: 1003–5.
5 McDonagh AJG, Gawkrodger DJ, Walker AE. White sponge naevus successfully treated with tetracycline. *Clin Exp Dermatol* 1990; **15**: 152–3.

Chronic mucocutaneous candidiasis (Chapter 31)

Chronic mucocutaneous candidiasis (CMC) includes a range of congenital disorders characterized by chronic candidiasis involving mouth, nails, and other sites. Persistent, adherent, white lesions are seen in the mouth often with angular stomatitis [1–3] and, in candidiasis–endocrinopathy syndrome, there may also be enamel hypoplasia [3].

REFERENCES

1 Cleary TG. Chronic mucocutaneous candidiasis. In: Bodey GP, ed. *Candidiasis: Pathogenesis, Diagnosis and Treatment*. New York: Raven Press, 1993: 241–52.
2 Porter SR, Scully C. Candidiasis endocrinopathy syndrome. *Oral Surg* 1986; **61**: 573–8.
3 Porter SR, Eveson JW, Scully C. Enamel hypoplasia secondary to candidiasis endocrinopathy syndrome. *Pediatr Dent* 1995; **17**: 216–19.

Dyskeratosis congenita (Chapter 12)

SYN. ZINSSER–ENGMAN–COLE SYNDROME

Oral lesions appear between the ages of 5 and 10 years, when the tongue and possibly the buccal mucosa and palate develop diffuse white lesions with a premalignant potential. These lesions resemble leukoplakia or lichen planus. The oral epithelium shows non-specific hyperkeratosis, a prominent granular cell layer and mild acanthosis [1–4].

Other rare oral features include taurodont or hypocalcified teeth and mucosal hyperpigmentation. Other manifestations include lesions of other mucosae, skin and appendages and bone-marrow dysfunction.

REFERENCES

1 Cannell H. Dyskeratosis congenita. *Br J Oral Surg* 1971; **9**: 8–10.
2 Koch HF. Effect of retinoids on precancerous lesions of the oral mucosa. In: Orfanos CE, Braun-Falco O, Farber EM *et al.*, eds. *Retinoids: Advances in Basic Research and Therapy*. Berlin: Springer-Verlag, 1981: 307–12.
3 Loh HS, Koh ML, Giam YC. Dyskeratosis congenita in two male cousins. *Br J Oral Surg* 1987; **25**: 492–9.
4 Ogden GR, Connor E, Chisholm D. Dyskeratosis congenita: report of a case and review of the literature. *Oral Surg* 1988; **65**: 586–91.

Pachyonychia congenita [1] (Chapter 65)

About 60% of patients with this syndrome have oral keratosis, 10% have angular stomatitis, and 16% have natal or neonatal teeth. Some patients also develop chronic oral candidiasis.

The keratosis is usually benign and requires no treatment. Dental advice should be sought regarding natal or neonatal teeth.

Clouston syndrome [2] (Chapter 12)

Palmoplantar hyperkeratosis, hair defects, nail dysplasia and oral white lesions have been described in this autosomal dominant form of ectodermal dysplasia. There may be diffuse white lesions in the buccal mucosa, palate, tongue and elsewhere but reports of malignancy are rare.

Tylosis [3–6] (Chapter 34)

This autosomal dominant syndrome of palmoplantar hyperkeratosis may predispose to oesophageal carcinoma. Oral white lesions have also been described, but there is little evidence that these are premalignant.

Focal palmoplantar and oral hyperkeratosis syndrome

Focal hyperkeratosis at weight-bearing areas of the palms and soles with hyperkeratosis of the attached gingiva and occasionally other sites is an autosomal dominant trait. [7,8].

Olmsted syndrome [9] (Chapter 34)

Perioral keratoderma may be seen in this syndrome.

REFERENCES

1 Feinstein A, Friedman J, Schewach-Millet M. Pachyonychia congenita. *J Am Acad Dermatol* 1988; **19**: 705–11.
2 George DI, Escobar VH. Oral findings of Clouston's syndrome (hidrotic ectodermal dysplasia). *Oral Surg* 1984; **57**: 258–62.
3 O'Mahoney MY, Ellis JP, Hellier M. Familial tylosis and carcinoma of the oesophagus. *J R Soc Med* 1984; **77**: 514–17.
4 Tyldesley WR. Oral leukoplakia associated with tylosis and esophageal carcinoma. *J Oral Pathol* 1974; **3**: 62–70.
5 Tyldesley WR, Osborne-Hughes R. Tylosis, leukoplakia and oesophageal carcinoma. *Br Med J* 1973; **4**: 427.
6 Ellis A, Field JK, Field EA *et al.* Tylosis associated with carcinoma of the oesophagus and oral leukoplakia in a large Liverpool family: a review of six generations. *Oral Oncol* 1994; **30B**: 102–12.
7 Fred HL, Gieser RG, Berry WR, Eiband JM. Keratosis palmaris et plantaris. *Arch Intern Med* 1964; **113**: 866–87.
8 Laskaris G, Vareltzidis H, Augernou G. Focal palmoplantar and oral mucosa hyperkeratosis syndrome. *Oral Surg* 1980; **50**: 250.
9 Judge MR, Misch K, Wright P, Harper JI. Palmoplantar and periorificial keratoderma with corneal epithelial dysplasia: a new syndrome. *Br J Dermatol* 1991; **125**: 186–8.

Hereditary benign intraepithelial dyskeratosis [1]

SYN. WITKOP–VON SALLMANN SYNDROME

Aetiology. This is a very rare autosomal dominant condition found mainly in some groups of mixed ethnic origin, predominantly in North Carolina.

Pathology. There is pronounced epithelial acanthosis, vacuolization in the stratum spinosum and eosinophilic cells apparently engulfed by normal squamous cells ('tobacco cells').

Clinical features. Oral lesions appear in childhood and become more obvious by adolescence. Milky white, smooth, somewhat translucent plaques affect predominantly the buccal mucosae, the lips and ventrum of the tongue.

Ocular lesions include conjunctivitis with gelatinous conjunctival plaques which become evident in infancy. There may be photophobia and eventual corneal involvement.

Oral biopsy is usually indicated in order to differentiate this disease from white-sponge naevus and other white lesions.

Treatment. No treatment is required.

REFERENCE

1 Witkop CJ, Shankle CM, Graham JB. Hereditary benign intraepithelial dyskeratosis. II. Oral manifestations and hereditary transmission. *Arch Pathol* 1960; **70**: 696–711.

Epstein's pearls
SYN. GINGIVAL CYSTS OF THE NEWBORN

Epstein's pearls are superficial, white, keratin-containing cysts seen on the palatal or alveolar mucosa of about 80% of neonates. They are symptomless and inconsequential, usually being shed within a few weeks [1].

REFERENCE

1 Gilhar A, Winsterstein G, Godfried E. Gingival cysts of the newborn. *Int Dent J* 1988; **27**: 261–2.

Darier's disease [1–4] (Chapter 34)

Oral lesions, typically flattish, coalescing, red plaques that eventually turn white and affect the keratinized mucosa of the dorsum of the tongue, palate and gingiva, are seen in up to 50% of patients with skin lesions of Darier's disease

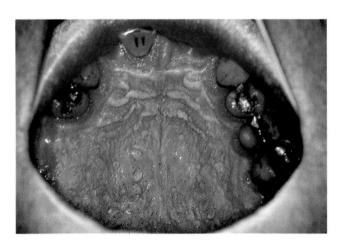

Fig. 69.12 Darier's disease: oral white lesions resemble those of nicotinic stomatitis (see Fig. 69.43).

(Fig. 69.12). They resemble nicotinic stomatitis clinically. The oral changes are most marked in patients with the most severe skin changes.

Warty dyskeratoma [5,6] (Chapter 34)

Warty dyskeratoma or focal acantholytic dyskeratosis is rare in the oral cavity but typically presents as a nodule or papule on the gingiva, palate or alveolar ridge. The histology is similar to that of Darier's disease and transient acantholytic dermatosis, with suprabasal epithelial splits and 'corps ronds'.

REFERENCES

1 Ferris T, Lamey PJ, Rennie JS. Darier's disease: oral features and genetic aspects. *Br Dent J* 1990; **168**: 71–3.
2 Macleod RI, Munro CS. The incidence and distribution of the oral lesions in patients with Darier's disease. *Br Dent J* 1991; **171**: 133–6.
3 Spouge JD, Trott JR, Chesko G. Darier–White's disease: a cause of white lesions of the oral mucosa. Report of four cases. *Oral Surg* 1966; **21**: 441–57.
4 Tegner E, Jonsson N. Darier's disease with involvement of both submandibular glands. *Acta Derm Venereol (Stockh)* 1990; **70**: 451–2.
5 Laskaris G, Sklavounou A. Warty dyskeratoma of the oral mucosa. *Br J Oral Surg* 1985; **23**: 371–5.
6 Leider AS, Eversole LR. Focal acantholytic dyskeratosis of the oral mucosa. *Oral Surg* 1984; **58**: 64–70.

Keratitis, ichthyosis and deafness syndrome (Chapter 34)
SYN. KID SYNDROME

Dental dysplasia, persistent oral ulceration, chronic mucocutaneous candidiasis and occasional carcinoma may be seen in the KID syndrome [1,2].

REFERENCES

1 Baden HP, Alper JC. Ichthyosiform dermatosis, keratitis and deafness. *Arch Dermatol* 1977; **113**: 1701–4.
2 Cremers CWRJ, Philipsen VMJG, Mali JWH. Deafness, ichthyosiform erythroderma, cornea involvement, photophobia and dental dysplasia. *J Laryngol Otol* 1977; **91**: 585–7.

Pigmented lesions

Most oral hyperpigmentation is racial in origin and is particularly noticeable on the labial anterior gingivae (see Fig. 69.10).

Naevi

Pigmented naevi are much less common in the oral mucosa than in skin. The intramucosal type of naevus is most common (about 60%) and another 25% are blue naevi. Compound and junctional naevi and combined naevi are rare in the mouth.

Pathology. The intramucosal naevus consists of a collection of melanocytic cells in the lamina propria without involvement of the epithelium. The blue naevus consists of spindle cells at any level in the lamina propria. The junctional naevus consists of clusters of benign naevus cells at the epithelio-mesenchymal junction and the lamina propria is otherwise not involved.

Clinical features. Pigmented naevi are seen particularly on the vermilion border of the lip and on the palate or buccal mucosa [1]. These lesions are usually brown, macular, do not change rapidly in size or colour and are painless. The prognosis is good.

Excision biopsy is recommended both for cosmetic reasons and to exclude malignancy, especially melanoma [2].

REFERENCES

1 Buchner A, Hansen LS. Pigmented nevi of the oral mucosa. *Oral Surg Oral Med Oral Pathol* 1980; **49**: 55–62.
2 Hansen LS, Buchner A. Changing concepts of the junctional naevus and melanoma. Review of the literature and report of a case. *J Oral Surg* 1981; **39**: 961–5.

Peutz–Jegher syndrome (Chapter 39)

Oral brown or black macules may appear in infancy, but unlike the circumoral lesions, these do not fade after puberty.

Laugier–Hunziker syndrome
See Chapter 39.

Complex myxomas, spotty pigmentation and endocrine overactivity

SYN. CARNEY SYNDROME

Carney syndrome differs clinically from Peutz–Jegher syndrome in that hyperpigmentation is less common intraorally but more common on the conjunctiva than in Peutz–Jegher syndrome, and other manifestations are also present. This autosomal dominant trait causes cardiac and cutaneous myxomas, with mammary myxoid fibro-adenomas, spotty cutaneous hyperpigmentation, primary pigmented nodular adrenocortical disease, testicular Sertoli-cell tumours and growth-hormone-secreting pituitary adenoma. It may present with oral hyperpigmentation and myxomas [1–3].

Cases previously described as the NAME syndrome (*n*aevi, *a*trial myxoma, *m*yxoid neurofibromas, and *e*phelides), and the LAMB syndrome (*l*entigines, *a*trial myxoma, *m*uco-cutaneous myxoma, *b*lue naevi) may represent this complex, which also has close similarities to the LEOPARD syndrome and the syndrome of arterial dissections with lentiginosis (Chapter 39).

The hyperpigmentation in the Carney syndrome is facial and occurs on the vermilion of the lips in about 35%, but about 8% have pigmented lesions on the oral mucosa, and about 2% have oral myxomas, usually on the palate or tongue [2].

REFERENCES

1 Carney JA, Gordon H, Carpenter PC *et al.* The complex of myxomas, spotty pigmentation and endocrine overactivity. *Medicine* 1985; **64**: 270–83.
2 Cook CA, Lund BA, Carney JA. Mucocutaneous pigmented spots and oral myxomas: the oral manifestations of the complex of myxomas, spotty pigmentation and endocrine overactivity. *Oral Surg* 1987; **63**: 175–83.
3 Stratakis CA, Carney JA, Lin J-P *et al.* Carney complex, a familial multiple neoplasia and lentiginosis syndrome. *J Clin Invest* 1996; **97**: 699–705.

Red lesions

Hereditary haemorrhagic telangiectasia (Chapter 45)
SYN. OSLER–RENDU–WEBER SYNDROME

This syndrome is characterized by multiple telangiectasia on the lips, perioral skin, and in the mouth [1].

Haemangioma

An oral haemangioma is usually deep red or blue–purple. It blanches on pressure, and is fluctuant to palpation. It may be level with the mucosa or have a lobulated or raised surface [2]. Most haemangiomas are seen in isolation but a few may be multiple and/or part of a wider syndrome such as Maffucci syndrome [3]. Haemangiomas are at risk from trauma and prone to excessive bleeding if damaged (e.g. during tooth extraction). Oral lesions suspected of being haemangiomatous should not be routinely biopsied; aspiration is far safer. Kaposi's sarcoma and epithelioid angiomatosis should be excluded. Occasionally, oral haemangiomas develop phlebolithiasis.

Oral haemangiomas are left alone unless causing symptoms, when they are best treated with cryosurgery, if small, or by litigation or embolization of feeding vessels if large.

Sturge–Weber syndrome (Chapter 15) [2,4]

The haemangioma in the trigeminal area in this syndrome is usually unilateral and may involve the mouth. The oral haemangioma fortunately rarely involves bone but may be associated with hypertrophy of affected tissues. If the patient is treated with phenytoin, gingival hyperplasia may follow [4,5].

Klippel–Trenaunay–Weber syndrome (Chapter 15)

Haemangiomas of the buccal mucosa and tongue, macro-glossia, maxillary hyperplasia and an anterior open bite have been recorded in this syndrome [6,7].

Blue rubber–bleb naevus syndrome [8]

See Chapter 15.

Maffucci syndrome [3]

See Chapter 15.

REFERENCES

1 Flint SR, Keith O, Scully C. Hereditary haemorrhagic telangiectasia: family study and review. *Oral Surg* 1988; **66**: 440–4.
2 Stal S, Hamilton S, Spira M. Haemangioma, lymphangioma and vascular malformations of the head and neck. *Otolaryngol Clin North Am* 1986; **19**: 769–96
3 Laskaris G, Skouteris C. Maffucci syndrome: report of a case with oral haemangiomas. *Oral Surg* 1984; **57**: 263–6.
4 Uram M, Zubillaga C. The cutaneous manifestations of Sturge–Weber syndrome. *J Clin Neuroophthalmol* 1982; **2**: 245–8.
5 Scully C. Orofacial manifestations of the neurodermatoses. *J Dent Child* 1980; **47**: 255–60.
6 Sciubba JJ, Brown AM. Oral–facial manifestations of Klippel–Trenaunay–Weber syndrome. *Oral Surg* 1977; **43**: 227–32.
7 Steiner M, Gould AR, Graves SM *et al.* Klippel–Trenaunay–Weber syndrome. *Oral Surg* 1987; **63**: 208–15.
8 Crosher RF, Blackburn CW, Dinsdale RCW. Blue rubber–bleb naevus syndrome. *Br J Oral Surg* 1988; **26**: 160–4.

Hereditary mucoepithelial dysplasia

Hereditary mucoepithelial dysplasia is a dyskeratotic epithelial syndrome involving mucosa, skin, hair, eyes and lungs [1,2].

Aetiology. Autosomal dominant inheritance.

Pathology. There is some acantholysis as well as benign dyskeratosis of individual cells [2]. Electron microscopy shows an abnormality in desmosomes and gap junctions.

Clinical features. The oral lesions are painless, red macules or maculopapules and are seen predominantly on the palate and gingiva. They appear in infancy and may persist throughout life.

In addition there may be follicular keratosis, alopecia, photophobia, cataracts, corneal vascularization and various cardiorespiratory complications, especially potentially lethal bullous lung disease, spontaneous pneumothorax and bullous emphysema.

REFERENCES

1 Scheman AJ, Ray DJ, Witkop CJ *et al.* Hereditary mucoepithelial dysplasia. *J Am Acad Dermatol* 1989; **21**: 351–7.
2 Witkop CJ, White JG, Sank JJ *et al.* Clinical, histologic, cytologic and ultrastructural characteristics of the oral lesions from hereditary mucoepithelial dysplasia. *Oral Surg* 1978; **46**: 645–57.

Wiskott–Aldrich syndrome (Chapter 14)

Oral petechiae may occur [1].

REFERENCE

1 Porter SR, Sugermann PB, Scully C *et al.* Orofacial manifestations in the Wiskott–Aldrich syndrome. *J Dent Child* 1994; **61**: 404–7.

Vesiculoerosive disorders

Epidermolysis bullosa (Chapter 40)

Oral mucosal lesions are found in about 30% of patients with epidermolysis bullosa [1–5]. They are fairly common in dystrophic and lethal forms of epidermolysis bullosa but are rare in most simplex types except the superficial type, where they are found in 70% [2,6–8].

Blisters, sometimes preceded by white patches, develop rapidly, particularly where there is trauma. They rupture to produce ulcers, often with eventual scarring, particularly in the recessive dystrophic types. There is a predisposition to oral squamous cell carcinoma, mainly in the Hallopeau–Siemens type.

Dental hypoplasia and other defects may also be a feature especially of junctional epidermolysis bullosa (Table 69.12) and, with the difficulty in maintaining adequate oral hygiene, there is a predisposition to caries [4].

The oral manifestations in the various inherited forms of this condition are summarized in Table 69.13 and epidermolysis bullosa acquisita is discussed in Chapter 40.

Table 69.12 Possible dental findings in epidermolysis bullosa. (From Nowak [8].)

Enamel	Dentine	Cementum
Pitting hypoplasia Hypomineralization Abnormal prism structure Abnormally thin	Normal thickness and structure	Normal thickness Mainly acellular

REFERENCES

1 Album MM, Gaisin A, Leek WT *et al.* Epidermolysis bullosa dystrophica polydysplastica. *Oral Surg* 1977; **43**: 859–72.
2 Fine JD, Johnson L, Wright T. Epidermolysis bullosa simplex superficialis. *Arch Dermatol* 1989; **125**: 633–8.
3 Sedano HO, Gorlin RJ. Epidermolysis bullosa. *Oral Surg* 1989; **67**: 555–63.
4 Wright JT, Capps J, Johnson LB *et al.* Oral and ultrastructural dental manifestations of epidermolysis bullosa. *J Dent Res* 1988; **67**: 249.
5 Wright JT, Fine JD, Johnson L. Hereditary epidermolysis bullosa: oral manifestations and dental management. *Pediatr Dent* 1993; **15**: 242–7.
6 Pearson RW. Clinicopathologic types of epidermolysis bullosa and their non-dermatological complications. *Arch Dermatol* 1988; **124**: 718–25.
7 Rubenstein R, Esterly NB, Fine JD. Childhood epidermolysis bullosa acquisita. *Arch Dermatol* 1987; **123**: 772–6.
8 Nowak AJ. Oropharyngeal lesions and their management in epidermolysis bullosa. *Arch Dermatol* 1988; **124**: 742–5.

Immune defects

Mouth ulcers can feature in congenital immune defects [1–7] including Chediak–Higashi syndrome, Papillon–Lefèvre syndrome, familial neutropenia, cyclic neutropenia, Job's syndrome, chronic granulomatous disease, and glycogen-storage disease type 1b.

Table 69.13 Oral manifestations in epidermolysis bullosa. (EB) (From Sedano and Gorlin [3] and Pearson [6].)

Type	EB subtype	Mucosal lesions	Dental hypoplasia
I Epidermolytic (simplex); autosomal dominant	Generalized (Köbner)	±	–
	Localized (Weber–Cockayne)	–	–
	Localized (Kallin)	–	Anodontia
	With mottled pigmentation and punctate keratoderma	+	–
	With bruising (Ogna)	–	±
	Herpetiform (Dowling–Meara)	+	–
	Superficial	+	–
II Junctional; autosomal recessive	Generalized, severe (Herlitz)	+	++
	Generalized, mild	+	+
	Localized	±	+
	Inverse	±	+
	Progressive	+	–
III Dermolytic (dystrophic) Autosomal dominant	Hyperplastic (Cockayne–Touraine)	±	–
	Albopapuloid (Pasini)	+	–
	Pretibial (Kuske–Portugal)	–	–
Autosomal recessive (Hallopeau-Siemens)	Localized	+	±
	Generalized	++	++
	Mutilating	+++	+++
	Inverse	+	–
VI Acquired type	Adult form	±	–
	Child form	+	–

–, Absent; +, mild; ++, moderate; +++, severe.

REFERENCES

1 Dougherty N, Galaletto MA. Oral sequelae of chronic neutrophil defects; case report of a child with glycogen storage disease type 1b. *Pediatr Dent* 1995; **17**: 224–9.
2 Porter SR, Scully C. Orofacial manifestations in primary immunodeficiencies: polymorphonuclear leukocyte defects. *J Oral Pathol Med* 1993; **22**: 310–11.
3 Porter SR, Scully C. Orofacial manifestations in primary immunodeficiencies: T lymphocyte defects. *J Oral Pathol Med* 1993; **22**: 308–9.
4 Porter SR, Scully C. Orofacial manifestations in primary immunodeficiencies involving IgA deficiency. *J Oral Pathol Med* 1993; **22**: 117–19.
5 Scully C. Orofacial manifestations in chronic granulomatous disease of childhood. *Oral Surg* 1981; **51**: 148–51.
6 Scully C, Macfadyen E, Campbell A. Oral manifestations in cyclic neutropenia. *Br J Oral Surg* 1982; **20**: 96–101.
7 Scully C, Porter SR. Orofacial manifestations in primary immunodeficiencies: common variable immunodeficiencies. *J Oral Pathol Med* 1993; **22**: 157–8.

Lumps and swellings

Hereditary gingival fibromatosis

Aetiology. An autosomal dominant condition [1–3].

Pathology. The gingival connective tissue is mainly composed of thick, interlacing collagen fibres forming a dense, almost avascular, mass in which many fibrocytes have dark, shrunken nuclei. Mucoid material and some giant cells may be found.

Clinical features. There is generalized gingival enlargement, especially obvious over the anterior maxilla and during the transition from deciduous to permanent dentitions [1,4–6]. If the enlargement is gross, it may move or cover the teeth and even protrude from the mouth. The changes initially involve the gingival papillae and later the attached gingiva. The affected gingiva is usually of normal colour but firm in consistency, and the surface becomes coarsely stippled. Patients may also be hirsute, as may patients with drug-induced gingival hyperplasia. The prognosis is good, but gingival surgery is often indicated [2].

Although most patients have only gingival fibromatosis, there are occasional associations with supernumerary teeth [7] or with the Zimmermann–Laband, Murray–Puretic–Drescher, Rutherford, Cowden and Cross syndromes [2,6].

REFERENCES

1 Bozzo L, Almeida O, Scully C, Aldred M. Familial gingival fibromatosis; report of an extensive four generation pedigree. *Oral Surg* 1994; **78**: 452–4.
2 Clark D. Gingival fibromatosis and related syndromes. *J Can Dent Assoc* 1987; **53**: 137–40.
3 Gould AR, Escobar VH. Symmetrical gingival fibromatosis. *Oral Surg* 1981; **51**: 62–7.
4 Bazoupoulou-Kyrkanidou E, Papagianoulis L, Papanicoliou S, Mavrou A. Laband syndrome: a case report. *J Oral Pathol Med* 1990; **19**: 385–7.
5 Bakaeen G, Scully C. Hereditary gingival fibromatosis and the Zimmermann–Laband syndrome. *J Oral Pathol Med* 1991; **20**: 456–9.
6 Chadwick B, Hunter B, Hunter L *et al*. Laband syndrome: report of two cases, review of the literature and identification of additional manifestations. *Oral Surg* 1994; **78**: 57–63.
7 Wynne SE, Aldred ME, Bartold M. Hereditary gingival fibromatosis associated with hearing loss and supernumerary teeth—a new syndrome. *J Periodontol* 1995; **66**: 75–9.

Juvenile hyaline fibromatosis (Chapter 44)

SYN. MURRAY–PURETIC–DRESCHER SYNDROME

Gingival enlargement may be seen in juvenile hyaline fibromatosis [1,2]. It may precede tooth eruption or may present only in the first decade. It increases with age. Histology shows dilated capillaries in a hyaline periodic acid Schiff–positive matrix with pseudocartilaginous cells.

REFERENCES

1 Aldred MJ, Crawford PJM. Juvenile hyaline fibromatosis. *Oral Surg* 1987; **63**: 71–7.
2 Sciubba JJ, Nieblom T. Juvenile hyaline fibromatosis (Murray–Puretic–Drescher syndrome): oral and systemic findings in siblings. *Oral Surg* 1986; **62**: 397.

Congenital epulis

SYN. GRANULAR CELL MYOBLASTOMA

Congenital epulis is a rare benign swelling on the maxillary alveolus in an infant [1,2]. It is probably a reactive mesenchymal lesion. There is an 8 : 1 female predominance.

This is usually a pedunculated firm pink swelling, which is treated by excision. Histology shows large polygonal cells with a fine granular eosinophilic cytoplasm.

REFERENCES

1 Fuhr AH, Krogh PHJ. Congenital epulis of the newborn: centennial review of the literature and case report. *J Oral Surg* 1972; **30**: 30–5.
2 Webb JD, Wescott WB, Corell RW. Firm swelling on the anterior maxillary gingiva in an infant. *J Am Dent Assoc* 1984; **109**: 307–8.

Focal dermal hypoplasia (Chapter 12)

SYN. GOLTZ'S SYNDROME

Focal dermal hypoplasia is a rare, presumably X-linked, genodermatosis [1]. Papillomas, usually of the oral mucosa and lips, dental anomalies and occasional cleft lip and palate are the main oral features [2,3]. The dental anomalies, seen in about one-half of affected individuals, include hypodontia and enamel defects.

REFERENCES

1 Greer RO, Reissner MW. Focal dermal hypoplasia: current concepts and differential diagnosis. *J Periodontol* 1989; **60**: 330–5.
2 Ishibashi A, Kurihara Y. Goltz's syndrome: focal dermal dysplasia syndrome (focal dermal hypoplasia). Report of a case and its etiology and pathogenesis. *Dermatologia* 1972; **144**: 156–60.
3 Valerius NH. A case of focal dermal hypoplasia syndrome (Goltz) with bilateral cheilo-gnatho-palatoschisis. *Acta Paediatr Scand* 1984; **63**: 287–90.

Acanthosis nigricans (Chapter 34)

Oral papilliferous lesions may be a feature of both familial and malignant acanthosis nigricans [1].

REFERENCE

1 Bazopoulou E, Laskaris G, Katsabas A *et al*. Familial benign acanthosis nigricans with predominant early oral manifestations. *Clin Genet* 1991; **50**: 160.

Lymphangioma (Chapter 51)

At least some lymphangiomas are hamartomas.

Lymphangioma is uncommon in the mouth. It is of similar structure to a haemangioma, but contains lymph rather than blood. It often has a 'frogspawn' appearance (Fig. 69.13).

Lymphangiomas are usually solitary and affect the tongue predominantly. They are occasionally associated with cystic hygroma [1]. One study has found blue, domed lymphangiomas on the alveolar ridges of about 4% of newborn black children [2]. These lesions, which were usually bilateral, often regressed spontaneously.

Small lymphangiomas need no treatment. Larger lesions may require excision although cryotherapy can be useful.

REFERENCES

1 Karmody CS, Fortson JK, Calcaterra VE. Lymphangiomas of the head and neck in adults. *Otolaryngol Head Neck Surg* 1982; **90**: 283.
2 Levin LS, Jorgenson RJ, Jarvey BA. Lymphangiomas of the alveolar ridge in neonates. *Pediatrics* 1976; **56**: 881.

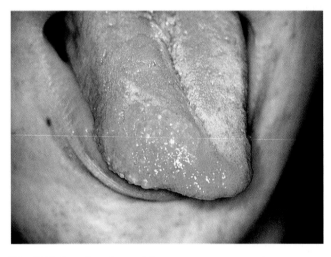

Fig. 69.13 Lymphangioma of the tongue—a common site.

Dermoid cyst (Chapter 15)

This developmental cyst commonly arises above the mylohyoid muscle in the midline of the neck. It usually becomes clinically obvious in the second decade of life and causes elevation of the tongue.

Occasionally dermoid cysts become infected and then painful. Treatment is by surgical excision.

Lingual thyroid

Ectopic thyroid tissue may rarely present in the mouth. Typically, there is an asymptomatic smooth-surfaced lump in the midline of the base of the tongue, between the sulcus terminalis and epiglottis at the site of the foramen caecum [1]. Occasionally, a lingual thyroid may produce dysphagia, cough or pain [1,2]. Some 10% of cadaver tongues contain thyroid tissue but clinical presentation is much less common.

Not all lingual thyroid tissue is functional and function tends to decline with age. Where thyroid-stimulating hormone levels are high, thyroid hormone supplements are indicated [2]. Scintiscanning is important to ensure the presence of normal thyroid tissue in the neck before considering any removal of a lingual thyroid.

Malignant change is rare in lingual thyroids though follicular carcinomas have been recorded.

REFERENCES

1 Jones JAH. Lingual thyroid. *Br J Oral Surg* 1986; **24**: 58–62.
2 Weider DJ, Parker W. Lingual thyroid. Review, case reports and therapeutic guidelines. *Ann Otol Rhinolaryngol* 1977; **86**: 841–5.

Lingual tonsil

The lingual tonsil is a mass of lymphoid tissue in the posterior third of the tongue, between the epiglottis posteriorly and the circumvallate papillae anteriorly. It is usually divided in the midline by a ligament (Fig. 69.14). Although usually small and asymptomatic, it may become enlarged, especially in atopic patients. It may be so prominent that it fills the vallecula and impinges against the epiglottis. It tends to involute with increasing age.

If the lingual tonsil is large it may cause a globus sensation, alteration of the voice, dyspnoea or obstructive sleep apnoea. Occasionally there may be lingual tonsillitis

with a red, swollen, painful tongue, fever and neutrophilia [2].

The condition must be distinguished from benign and malignant tumours of the tongue, including lingual thyroid, but the symmetry of the lingual tonsil and its midline division are helpful diagnostic pointers.

Treatment may be required if the enlarged tonsil causes symptoms. Surgery may be hazardous because of the copious blood supply to the tongue base. Electrocautery and cryotherapy are generally regarded as safer procedures [1].

REFERENCES

1 Golding-Wood DG, Whittet HB. The lingual tonsil. A neglected symptomatic structure? *J Laryngol Otol* 1989; **103**: 922–5.
2 Joseph M, Reardon E, Goodman M. Lingual tonsillectomy: a treatment for inflammatory lesions of the lingual tonsil. *Laryngoscope* 1984; **94**: 179–84.

Other anomalies

Oral hair

Oral hair is a rare, innocuous anomaly [1], which is not to be confused with hairy tongue (p. 3104).

Scrotal (fissured) tongue

The cause of a fissured tongue (plicated or scrotal tongue) is unclear, but it is a common condition affecting more than 5% of the population [2]. It is occasionally associated with geographical tongue (Fig. 69.15). Patients with Down's syndrome often have a fissured tongue and it is a feature of the rare Melkersson–Rosenthal syndrome.

Ankyloglossia

Ankyloglossia or tongue-tie, is an uncommon isolated anomaly in which the lingual fraenum is tight and the

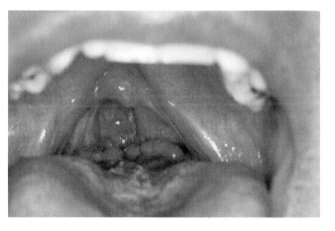

Fig. 69.14 Lingual tonsil showing a well-demarcated midline groove. (Courtesy of Dr C.T.C. Kennedy, Bristol Royal Infirmary, Bristol, UK.)

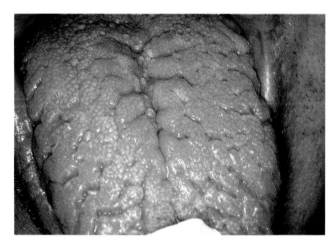

Fig. 69.15 Fissured or scrotal tongue.

tongue cannot be fully protruded. There may be a family history and sometimes deviation of the epiglottis or larynx [3,4]. Speech is not usually affected but the ability to suckle [5], and to cleanse the buccal sulcus with the tongue may be. If necessary, surgery to the fraenum will relieve ankyloglossia.

REFERENCES

1 Baughman RA, Heidrich PD. The oral hair: an extremely rare phenomenon. *Oral Surg* 1980; **49**: 530–1.
2 Kullaa-Mikkonen A, Sorvari T, Kotilainen R *et al.* Morphological variations on the dorsal surface of the human tongue. *Proc Finn Dent Soc* 1985; **81**: 104–10.
3 Kern I. Tongue-tie. *Med J Aust* 1991; **155**: 3–34.
4 Mukai S, Mukai C, Asaoka K. Ankyloglossia with deviation of the epiglottis and larynx. *Ann Otol Rhinol Laryngol* 1991; **100**: 3–19.
5 Notestine GE. The importance of the identification of ankyloglossia (short lingual frenulum) as a cause of breast feeding problems. *J Hum Lact* 1990; **6**: 113–15.

Various orocutaneous syndromes

Neurofibromatosis (Chapter 12)

SYN. VON-RECKLINGHAUSEN'S SYNDROME

Oral lesions are not uncommon in generalized neurofibromatosis [1]. About two-thirds of patients have intraoral neurofibromas affecting predominantly the tongue, lips, buccal mucosa, or palate. Enlarged fungiform papillae are found in about 50% of patients. About 60% have radiographic evidence of disease, especially enlargement of the mandibular canal or foramen, or branching of the canal [2,3].

Malignant transformation is rare in intraoral neurofibromas [4].

REFERENCES

1 Scully C. Orofacial manifestations of the neurodermatoses. *J Dent Child* 1980; **47**: 255–60.
2 D'Ambroso JA, Langlais RP, Young RS. Jaw and skull changes in neurofibromatosis. *Oral Surg* 1988: **66**: 391–6.
3 Shapiro S, Abramovitch K, van Dis ML. Neurofibromatosis: oral and radiographic manifestations. *Oral Surg* 1984; **58**: 493–8.
4 Shotton JC, Stafford ND, Breach NJ. Malignant triton tumour of the palate—a case report. *Br J Oral Surg* 1988; **26**: 120–3.

Gorlin's syndrome (naevoid basal-cell carcinoma syndrome) (Chapter 36)

Odontogenic keratocysts (primordial cysts) of the jaws are a common feature of this syndrome [1–3]. These cysts should be surgically removed but have a tendency to recur. There are also occasional reports of oral neoplasms, notably fibrosarcoma, ameloblastoma and squamous carcinoma [4].

REFERENCES

1 Gorlin RJ. Nevoid basal-cell carcinoma syndrome. *Medicine* 1987; **66**: 98–113.

2 Howell JB. Nevoid basal cell carcinoma syndrome: profile of genetic and environmental factors in oncogenesis. *J Am Acad Dermatol* 1984; **11**: 98–104.
3 MacIntyre DR, Hislop SWG, Ross JW *et al.* The basal cell naevus syndrome. *Dental Update* 1985; **12**: 630–5.
4 Moos KF, Rennie JS. Squamous cell carcinoma arising in a mandibular keratocyst in a patient with Gorlin's syndrome. *Br J Oral Surg* 1987; **25**: 280–4.

Gardner's syndrome (Chapter 12)

Multiple jaw osteomas are a feature of Gardner's syndrome. Some 80% of patients with familial adenomatosis coli have osteomas and 30% have dental anomalies such as supernumerary or impacted teeth, or odontomes [1–3].

REFERENCES

1 Gardner EJ. Familial polyposis coli and Gardner's syndrome—is there a difference? *Prog Clin Biol Res* 1983; **115**: 39–43.
2 Sondergaard JO, Bulow S, Jarvinen H *et al.* Dental anomalies in familial adenomatous polyposis coli. *Acta Odontol Scand* 1987; **45**: 61–3.
3 Wolfe J, Jarvinen HJ, Hietanen J. Gardner's dento-maxillary stigmas in patients with familial adenomatosis coli. *Br J Oral Maxillofac Surg* 1986; **24**: 410–16.

Cowden's syndrome (Chapter 12)

Oral mucosal lesions in Cowden's disease may be found in the absence of cutaneous stigma. They are typically smooth pink or whitish papules found especially on the palatal, gingival and labial mucosae. These are benign fibromas. Oral squamous carcinoma is a rare complication [1–5].

REFERENCES

1 Rosenberg-Gertzman CB, Clark M, Gaston B. Multiple hamartoma and neoplasia syndrome (Cowden's syndrome). *Oral Surg* 1980; **49**: 314–16.
2 Shapiro SD, Lambert WC, Schwartz RA. Cowden's disease: a marker for malignancy. *Int J Dermatol* 1988; **27**: 232–7.
3 Starink TM, van Der Veen JP, Arwert F. The Cowden syndrome: a clinical and genetic study in 21 patients. *Clin Genet* 1986; **29**: 222–33.
4 Swart JGN, Lekkas C, Allard RHB. Oral manifestations in Cowden's syndrome. *Oral Surg* 1985; **59**: 264–8.
5 Porter SR, Cawson RA, Scully C, Eveson JW. Multiple hamartoma syndromes presenting with oral lesions. *Oral Surg* 1996; **82**: 295–301.

Tuberous sclerosis (Chapter 12)

SYN. EPILOIA

Oral manifestations in tuberous sclerosis include pit-shaped enamel defects in both dentitions, and gingival fibromatosis [1–4].

REFERENCES

1 Lygidakis NA, Lindenbaum RH. Oral fibromatosis in tuberous sclerosis. *Oral Surg* 1989; **68**: 725–8.
2 Scully C. The orofacial manifestations of tuberous sclerosis. *Oral Surg* 1977; **44**: 706–16.
3 Smith D, Porter SR, Scully C. Gingival and other oral manifestations in tuberous sclerosis. *Periodont Clin Invest* 1993; **15**: 13–18.
4 Weits-Binnerts JJ, Hoff M, van Grunsven MF. Dental pits in deciduous teeth: an early sign in tuberous sclerosis. *Lancet* 1982; **ii**: 1344–5.

Acquired disorders of the oral mucosa

This section discusses the main causes of mouth ulcers, other causes of oral soreness, white lesions and pigmented or red lesions, and lumps and swellings.

Mouth ulcers

The causes of mouth ulcers are diverse (Tables 69.7, 69.14), partly because lesions such as vesicles rapidly break down in the mouth as a result of trauma, moisture and infection.

Mouth ulcers of local aetiology

It is surprising that oral ulceration due to local factors is not more frequent. Accidental cheek biting or facial trauma may cause ulceration in any individual; the history is usually quite clear and a single ulcer of short duration (5–10 days) is present. Ulceration due to biting an anaesthetized lower lip or tongue following a dental local analgesic injection is a fairly common problem in young children.

Orthodontic appliances or, more commonly, dentures (especially if new) are responsible for many traumatic oral ulcers. These ulcers are usually clearly related to the appliance and have been a problem in the care of cleft-palate patients [1]. Chronic trauma may cause a well-defined ulcer with a whitish keratotic halo [2].

Other local causes of ulceration include thermal burns, especially of the tongue and palate (e.g. 'pizza burn') and chemical burns from the holding of medicaments or drugs (e.g. aspirin) against the mucosa.

The possibility of some other aetiology of ulcers of apparently local cause, should always be borne in mind. Child abuse may cause ulcers, especially over the upper labial fraenae. Self-mutilation may be seen in some psychologically disturbed patients [3,4], in mentally handicapped patients, individuals with sensory impairment and in the Lesch–Nyhan syndrome [5–8]. Oral purpura or ulceration may be seen on the lingual fraenum or palate from cunnilingus or fellatio, respectively [9].

Prognosis. Most ulcers of local cause heal spontaneously within 7–10 days if the cause is removed.

Table 69.14 Causes of mouth ulcers (see also Table 69.7).

Local causes (e.g. trauma)
Recurrent aphthae (and Behçet's syndrome)
Malignant neoplasms
Ulcers associated with systemic disease
Drugs
Irradiation of the oral mucosa
Disorders of uncertain pathogenesis

Treatment. Maintenance of good oral hygiene and the use of hot saline mouthbaths and 0.2% aqueous chlorhexidine gluconate mouthwash aid healing. A 0.1% benzydamine mouthwash may help give relief. Occasionally mechanical protection with an acrylic guard may help [7].

Patients should be reviewed within 3 weeks to ensure healing has occurred. Any ulcer lasting more than 2–3 weeks should be regarded with suspicion and biopsied—it may be a neoplasm or other serious disorder.

REFERENCES

1 Bacher M, Goz G, Pham T *et al*. Congenital palatal ulcers in newborn infants with cleft lip and palate; diagnosis, frequency and significance. *Cleft Palate J* 1996; **33**: 37–42.
2 Reade PC, Rich AM, Steidler NE. Peripheral keratosis on oral mucosal ulcers: a clinical sign of non-neoplastic disease. *Br J Oral Surg* 1984; **22**: 372–7.
3 Kotansky K, Goldberg M, Tenenbaum HC, Mock D. Factitious injury of the oral mucosa; a case series. *J Periodontol* 1995; **66**: 241–5.
4 Lamey PJ, McNab L, Lewis MAO, Gibb R. Oral artefactual disease. *Oral Surg* 1994; **77**: 131–4.
5 Scully C. The orofacial manifestations of the Lesch–Nyhan syndrome. *Int J Oral Surg* 1981; **10**: 380–3.
6 Stewart DJ, Kernohan DC. Self-inflicted gingival injuries: gingivitis artefacta, factitial gingivitis. *Dent Pract Dent Rec* 1972; **22**: 418–26.
7 Sugahara T, Mishima K, Mori Y. Lesch–Nyhan syndrome: successful prevention of lower lip ulceration caused by self-mutilation by use of mouth guard. *Int J Oral Maxillofac Surg* 1994; **23**: 37–8.
8 Symons AL, Rowe PV, Romanink K. Dental aspects of child abuse. *Aust Dent J* 1987; **32**: 42–7.
9 Van Wyk CW. An oral lesion caused by fellatio. *Am J Forensic Med Pathol* 1981; **2**: 217–19.

Recurrent aphthous stomatitis

Recurrent aphthous stomatitis (RAS) is characterized by recurring episodes of ulcers, typically from childhood or adolescence, each lasting from 1 to about 4 weeks before healing. Aphthae typically are small, round or ovoid ulcers with a circumscribed margin, erythematous halo and a yellow or grey floor (Fig. 69.16). The term recurrent oral ulcer is rather imprecise and should be avoided [1–8].

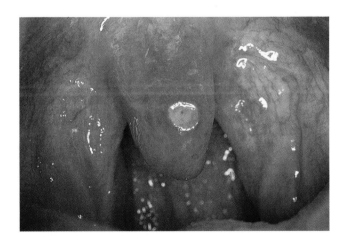

Fig. 69.16 Recurrent aphthae on the uvula.

Aetiology. The aetiology of RAS is not clear. A positive family history is found with about one-third of patients and there is an increased frequency of human leukocyte antigen (HLA)-A2, -A11, -B12 and -DR2 supporting a genetic basis for susceptibility in some patients.

There are identifiable predisposing factors in some patients (Table 69.15). A minority (about 10–20%) of patients attending outpatient clinics with RAS have an underlying haematological abnormality, usually a low serum iron or ferritin, or deficiency of folate or vitamin B_{12}. A few have multiple deficiencies [2]. Up to 3% of RAS patients have coeliac disease but in others a gluten-free diet is of no value [9]. Patients with deficiency states often, but not always, have gastrointestinal symptoms, and their RAS are often of recent onset. Other aetiological factors in RAS include stress and trauma. Aphthae are also seen in Behçet's syndrome, Sweet's syndrome, HIV infection and, rarely, in children in association with fever and pharyngitis [10]. Orogenital ulceration with aphthae is probably a forme fruste of Behçet's syndrome,

There is no evidence that RAS is an autoimmune disease [1,3,8]. There is no known association with systemic autoimmune disorders, none of the common autoantibodies is found, and RAS tend to resolve or decrease spontaneously with increasing age. The serum immunoglobulin levels are usually normal, although IgA and IgG may be increased, and immune complexes may be found.

It now seems likely that there is a minor degree of immunological dysregulation underlying aphthae. Attempts to implicate a variety of viruses or bacteria in the aetiology of RAS have largely been unsuccessful, but there may be cross-reacting antigens between the oral mucosa and microorganisms such as *Streptococcus sanguis* or its L form, such as heat-shock protein [4,8,11].

Cell-mediated immune mechanisms appear to be involved in the pathogenesis of RAS. In the lesions, helper T-cells predominate early on, with some natural killer (NK) cells. Cytotoxic cells then appear and there is evidence for an antibody-dependent cellular cytotoxicity reaction.

Clinical features. RAS is a common disease which probably afflicts at least 20% of the population. There is a high prevalence in higher socio-economic classes.

There are three main clinical types of RAS. Most common are minor aphthous ulcers which account for 80% of all RAS. Some 10% of patients with RAS have major aphthous ulcers, and a further 10% suffer from a herpetiform type of ulceration (Table 69.16).

Minor aphthous ulcers (syn. Mikulicz ulcers). Minor RAS (MiRAS) occur mainly in the 10–40-year age group, and often cause minimal symptoms. MiRAS are usually 2–4 mm in diameter, found mainly on the non-keratinized mobile mucosa of the lips, cheeks and floor of the mouth, sulci or ventrum of the tongue. They are uncommon on the gingiva, palate or dorsum of the tongue. Only a few ulcers (one to six) appear at a time; they heal in 7–10 days and recur at variable intervals. MiRAS are usually round or ovoid, but are often more linear when in the buccal sulcus, a common site. The ulcer floor is initially yellowish but becomes greyish as epithelialization proceeds. There is an erythematous halo and some oedema but MiRAS heal with little or no evidence of scarring.

Major aphthous ulcers (syn. Sutton's ulcers). Previously known as a periadenitis mucosa necrotica recurrens (PMNR), major RAS (MaRAS), are larger, recur more frequently, last longer and are more painful than MiRAS. They reach a large size, even more than 1 cm in diameter. MaRAS are found on any area of the oral mucosa, including the dorsum of the tongue or palate. Usually only a few ulcers (one to six) occur at one time; they heal slowly over 10–40 days, and recur frequently. The MaRAS are round or ovoid with an inflammatory halo, and may heal with scarring. Occasionally a raised erythrocyte sedimentation rate or plasma viscosity is found.

Herpetiform ulceration. Herpetiform ulceration (HU) is found in a slightly older age group and there is a female predominance. HU are often extremely painful and recur so frequently that ulceration may be virtually continuous. HU begins with vesiculation which passes rapidly into multiple, minute (2-mm), discrete ulcers at any oral site. The ulcers increase in size and coalesce to leave large,

Table 69.15 Systemic and other factors that may occasionally underlie or be associated with recurrent aphthous stomatitis (RAS).

Factor	Comments
Behçet's syndrome	Association of RAS with ocular lesions; genital ulcers and multisystem disease
Sweet's syndrome	See p. 2192
Haematinic deficiency	In some studies, 10–20% of patients with RAS have deficiencies of iron, folic acid or vitamin B_{12}
Gastrointestinal disease	Malabsorption states (pernicious anaemia, coeliac disease and Crohn's disease) may precipitate RAS in a small minority
Endocrine factors	In some women, RAS are clearly related to a fall in progestogens in the luteal phase of the menstrual cycle; hormone therapy may be beneficial
Immunodeficiency	A few patients with RAS have an immune defect such as HIV disease
Other factors	Trauma, certain foods, stress and cessation of smoking may play a part

Table 69.16 Main features of recurrent aphthous stomatitis.

	Minor aphthae	Major aphthae	Herpetiform ulcers
Age of onset	Childhood or adolescence	Childhood or adolescence	Young adult
Ulcer size	2–4 mm	May be 10 mm or larger	Initially tiny but ulcers coalesce
Number of ulcers	Up to about six	Up to about six	10–100
Sites affected	Mainly vestibule, labial, buccal mucosa and floor of mouth; rarely dorsum of tongue, gingiva or palate	Any site	Any site but often on ventrum of tongue
Duration of each ulcer	Up to 10 days	Up to 1 month	Up to 1 month
Other comments	The most common type of aphthae	May heal with scarring	Affect females predominantly

ragged ulcers which heal in 10 days or longer. Their similarity to herpetic stomatitis gives HU their name, but there is no evidence that herpes simplex virus is involved.

Prognosis. RAS in most patients resolve or abate spontaneously with age. An underlying identifiable predisposing cause is particularly likely where RAS commence or worsen in adult life.

Diagnosis. This is a clinical diagnosis. Biopsy is indicated only where some other cause of ulceration is suspected. Episodic mouth ulcers are also seen in cyclical neutropenia.

Treatment. It is important to exclude systemic lesions of Behçet's or other syndromes (p. 3072), and systemic predisposing factors. Investigation should include full blood count, iron studies and, possibly, red-cell folate, serum vitamin B$_{12}$ and calcium, since RAS may be the only clinical manifestation of coeliac or other gastrointestinal disease.

Predisposing factors should be corrected where possible [2]. Therapy is not always satisfactory. Good oral hygiene should be maintained by the use of 0.2% aqueous chlorhexidine gluconate mouthwash. A topical tetracycline mouthwash such as a Mysteclin capsule emptied into 5 ml of water (tetracycline 250 mg plus nystatin 250 000 units) or Mysteclin elixir may be especially useful in those with HU but, in most cases of RAS, topical corticosteroids are more useful. Hydrocortisone hemisuccinate (Corlan) pellets 2.5 mg four times daily, and triamcinolone acetonide in carboxymethyl cellulose (Adcortyl in Orabase) four times daily are useful and do not cause adrenocortical suppression. Occasionally, stronger topical corticosteroids (beclomethasone, fluocinonide) are required. Rarely are systemic corticosteroids or other immunosuppressants required.

The occasional patient who relates ulcers to the menstrual cycle or to an oral contraceptive may benefit from suppression of ovulation with a progestogen, or a change of oral contraceptive. If there is an obvious relationship to certain foods, these should be excluded from the diet [12].

Thalidomide, in doses of up to 300 mg daily can often induce remission, especially in major aphthae, but its important teratogenic effects and the risk of neuropathy must be considered [13,14]. Other therapies for RAS such as benzydamine, carbenoxolone, dapsone, dicromoglycate, levamisole, colchicine, pentoxifylline or sucralfate may have a role in individual cases, but are not generally very effective, or have adverse effects [5,8,15,16,17].

REFERENCES

1 Eversole LR. Immunopathology of oral mucosal ulcerative, desquamative and bullous diseases. *Oral Surg* 1994; **77**: 555–71.

2 Porter SR, Flint S, Scully C, Keith O. Recurrent aphthous stomatitis: the efficacy of replacement therapy in patients with underlying haematinic deficiencies. *Ann Dent* 1992; **L1**: 14–16.

3 Porter SR, Petersen A. Recurrent aphthous stomatitis. *Crit Rev Oral Biol Med* (in press).

4 Porter SR, Scully C, Flint SR. Haematological status in recurrent aphthous stomatitis compared with other oral disease. *Oral Surg* 1988; **66**: 41–4.

5 Rattan J, Schneider M, Arber N *et al*. Sucralfate suspension as a treatment of recurrent aphthous stomatitis. *J Intern Med* 1994; **236**: 341–3.

6 Rennie JS, Reade PC, Hay KD *et al*. Recurrent aphthous stomatitis. *Br Dent J* 1985; **159**: 361–7.

7 Rogers RS. Recurrent aphthous stomatitis and Behçet's syndrome. In: Safai R, Good RA, eds. Immunodermatology. New York: Plenum Press, 1981: 345.

8 Scully C, Porter S. Recurrent aphthous stomatitis: current concepts of aetiology, pathogenesis and management. *J Oral Pathol Med* 1989; **18**: 21–7.

9 Hunter IP, Ferguson MM, Scully C *et al*. Effects of dietary gluten elimination in patients with recurrent minor aphthous stomatitis and no detectable gluten enteropathy. *Oral Surg* 1993; **75**: 595–8.

10 Marshall GS, Edwards KM, Butler J *et al*. Syndrome of periodic fever, pharyngitis and aphthous stomatitis. *J Pediatr* 1987; **110**: 43–6.

11 Hasan A, Childerstone A, Pervink T *et al*. Recognition of a unique peptide epitope of the mycobacterial and human heat shock protein 65–60 antigen by T cells of patients with recurrent oral ulcers. *Clin Exp Immunol* 1995; **99**: 392–97.

12 Hay KD, Reade PC. The use of an elimination diet in the treatment of recurrent aphthous ulceration of the oral cavity. *Oral Surg* 1984; **57**: 504–7.

13 Grattan CEH, Scully C. Oral ulceration: a diagnostic problem. *Br Med J* 1986; **292**: 1093–4.

14 Grinspan D, Blanco GF, Aguero S. Treatment of aphthae with thalidomide. *J Am Acad Dermatol* 1989; **20**: 1060–3.

15 Katz J, Langevitz P, Shemer J *et al*. Prevention of recurrent aphthous stomatitis with colchicine: an open trial. *J Am Acad Dermatol* 1994; **31**: 459–61.

16 Scully C, Flint S, Porter SR. *A Colour Atlas of Oral Disease*. London: Martin Dunitz, 1996.

17 Wahba-Yahav AV. Severe idiopathic recurrent aphthous stomatitis: treatment with pentoxifylline. *Acta Derm Venereol (Stockh)* 1995; **75**: 157.

Behçet's syndrome

Definition. Behçet's syndrome is the association of RAS with genital ulceration and eye disease (especially iridocyclitis and retinal vasculitis) [1–3]. There may be a number of other systemic or cutaneous manifestations (Table 69.17).

Aetiology. The aetiology of Behçet's syndrome is uncertain but it appears to be becoming more common. There is a genetic background with a high prevalence of Behçet's syndrome in people from around the Mediterranean, the Middle East, China and Japan and, as in RAS, there are occasional familial cases and associations with HLA types, in this case particularly with HLA-B5 (Bw51 split) [3,4].

There are immunological changes similar to those seen in patients with RAS, with various T-lymphocyte abnormalities (especially suppressor T-cell dysfunction), changes in serum complement and increased polymorphonuclear leukocyte motility. There is also evidence that mononuclear cells may initiate antibody-dependent cellular cytotoxicity to oral epithelial cells, and evidence of disturbed NK-cell activity [5].

Many of the features of Behçet's syndrome (erythema nodosum, arthralgia, uveitis) are common to established immune-complex disease and indeed, circulating immune complexes (usually antigen–antibody complexes) and vasculitis are found. The antigen responsible has not been reliably identified but may include herpes simplex virus or streptococcal antigens [3,6].

Clinical features. Most patients are males, usually in their third or fourth decade. RAS is found in up to 98% of patients with Behçet's syndrome and is the initial manifestation in 30–75% (Fig. 69.17), but only a very small percentage of all patients with RAS progress to Behçet's syndrome. Recent HLA findings, such as the association of Behçet's syndrome with HLA-B5, -Bw51 and -DR7 and immunological findings may eventually help determine which patients are at risk and

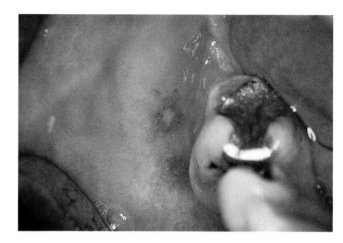

Fig. 69.17 Minor aphthae in Behçet's syndrome.

Table 69.17 Behçet's syndrome.

	Features	Incidence (%)
Major criteria		
Oral	Aphthae	90–100
Genital	Ulcers	64–88
Neuro-ocular	Iridocyclitis Retinal vasculitis Optic atrophy Syndromes resembling disseminated sclerosis, pseudobulbar palsy or neurosyphilis Meningoencephalitis Others	10–90
Dermatological	Pustules Erythema nodosum Pathergy	48–88
Minor criteria	Proteinuria and haematuria Thrombophlebitis Aneurysms Arthralgias	

when the transition to Behçet's syndrome may occur [3,4].

Genital ulcers are especially painful in females with Behçet's syndrome, and resemble RAS but may recur less frequently, although they may scar on healing. Recurrent orogenital ulceration (Neumann's bipolar aphthosis) may also be seen as an isolated entity, although it is unclear whether these patients suffer a forme fruste of Behçet's syndrome, or will, with time, develop systemic disease.

Up to 90% of patients with Behçet's syndrome have eye involvement, most commonly relapsing iridocyclitis, but anterior and posterior uveitis, retinal vascular changes, optic atrophy and other lesions may occur. Both eyes are eventually involved and blindness may result.

Skin lesions may also occur. Venepuncture is, in some patients, followed by pustulation, but this phenomenon (*pathergy*), said to be characteristic of Behçet's syndrome, is rarely seen in patients from the UK. A range of skin lesions can be seen, including papules, vesicles, pustules, folliculitis, pyoderma, acneiform eruptions, necrotizing vasculitis and erythema nodosum-like lesions.

Neurological involvement is uncommon but carries a poor prognosis: patterns include meningomyelitis, a brainstem syndrome, a syndrome typified by pyramidal and extrapyramidal signs and a confusional state culminating in dementia.

Large-joint arthropathies are common, usually subacute, self-limiting and non-deforming. One variant (MAGIC syndrome) is associated with *m*outh *a*nd *g*enital ulcers and *i*nflamed *c*artilage [7].

Prognosis. Unlike RAS, Behçet's syndrome is not self-limiting. It causes morbidity (especially in terms of ocular and neurological disease) and mortality. Most patients present with oral and ocular disease but there follows a relapsing and remitting but variable course. Central nervous system involvement, thromboses of major vessels and gastrointestinal perforation result in a poor prognosis.

Diagnosis. Behçet's syndrome is diagnosed on clinical grounds alone. Although there are no universally accepted diagnostic criteria, the concurrence of three major or two major and one minor criteria (see Table 69.17) are generally accepted as diagnostic. Activity of Behçet's disease may be assessed by serum levels of acute-phase proteins or antibodies to intermediate filaments. Both are raised in active disease, as is the erythrocyte sedimentation rate. Peripheral blood T4/T8 cell ratios are decreased. There may also be cryoglobulinaemia, leukocytosis and eosinophilia.

Management. Other causes of oculomucocutaneous syndromes (Table 69.18) should be excluded [8,9]. Systemic therapy includes colchicine, cyclophosphamide, chlorambucil, corticosteroids, azathioprine, levamisole, dapsone, aciclovir and cyclosporin. This multiplicity confirms their overall low level of reliability. Thalidomide at a dose of up to 400 mg daily may be of value in recalcitrant orogenital ulceration, although it can be difficult to obtain. It is teratogenic and must be used with extreme caution [10,11]. Oral ulcers may respond to topical corticosteroids, tetracycline or 5-amino-salicylic acid [12]. Ocular lesions usually respond to cyclosporin, but tend to relapse when treatment is stopped.

REFERENCES

1 Arbesfeld SJ, Kurban AK. Behçet's disease: new perspectives on an enigmatic syndrome. *J Am Acad Dermatol* 1988; **19**: 767–79.
2 Jorizzo JL. Behçet's syndrome. *Arch Dermatol* 1986; **122**: 556–8.
3 Lehner T, Barnes CG, eds. *Recent Advances in Behçet's Disease.* London: Royal Society of Medicine, 1989.
4 Okuyama T, Kunikane H, Kasahara M *et al.* Behçet's disease. In: Albert ED, Baur MP, Mayer WR, eds. *Histocompatibility Testing.* Berlin: Springer Verlag, 1984: 397.
5 Bang DS, Lee S, Kim DH *et al.* Investigation of cell-mediated immunity in patients with Behçet's syndrome, using the DNCB sensitization. *Korean J Dermatol* 1985; **23**: 769–73.

Table 69.18 Oculomucocutaneous syndromes.*

| Disease | Main lesions | | |
	Oral and genital	Ocular	Skin
Behçet's syndrome	Aphthae	Uveitis	Erythema nodosum
Sweet's syndrome	Aphthae	Conjunctivitis episcleritis	Inflamed papule or nodule
Erythema multiforme	Erosions	Erosions	Target lesions
Cicatricial pemphigoid	Bullae Erosions	Erosions Scarring	Occasional dome-shaped bullae
Pemphigus	Erosions	Erosions	Multiple, flaccid bullae
Reiter's syndrome	Ulcers	Conjunctivitis	Keratoderma blenorrhagica

* Ulcerative colitis, herpes simplex, syphilis, lupus erythematosus, mixed connective tissue disease and other disorders may also cause oral, cutaneous and ocular lesions.

6 Behçet's disease research committee of Japan. Skin hypersensitivity to streptococcal antigens and the induction of systemic symptoms by the antigens in Behçet's disease—a multicenter study. *J Rheumatol* 1989; **16**: 506–11.

7 Firestein GS, Gruber HC, Weisman MH *et al.* Mouth and genital ulcers with inflamed cartilage: MAGIC syndrome. *Am J Med* 1985; **79**: 65–72.

8 Grattan CEH, Scully C. Oral ulceration: a diagnostic problem. *Br Med J* 1986; **292**: 1093–4.

9 Hamza M. Orogenital ulcerations in mixed connective tissue disease. *J Rheumatol* 1985; **12**: 643–4.

10 Bowers PW, Powell RJ. Effect of thalidomide on oral ulceration. *Br Med J* 1983; **287**: 799–800.

11 Jenkins JS, Powell RJ, Allen BR *et al.* Thalidomide in severe orogenital ulceration. *Lancet* 1984; **ii**: 1424–6.

12 Ranzi T, Campanini M, Bianchi RA. Successful treatment of genital and oral ulceration in Behçet's disease with topical 5-aminosalicylic acid. *Br J Dermatol* 1989; **120**: 471–2.

Sweet's syndrome (Chapter 49)

Pustular lesions leading to aphthous-like ulcers may be found in Sweet's syndrome and there are occasional associations with Behçet's syndrome and with Sjögren's syndrome, each of which has oral manifestations. About 5% of patients in the UK with Sweet's syndrome have oral aphthae, although up to 30% of Japanese patients suffer aphthae [1,2].

REFERENCES

1 Driban NE, Alvarez MA. Oral manifestations of Sweet's syndrome. *Dermatologica* 1984; **169**: 102–3.

2 Mizoguchi M, Chikakane K, Goh K *et al.* Acute febrile neutrophilic dermatosis (Sweet's syndrome) in Behçet's disease. *Br J Dermatol* 1987; **116**: 727–34.

Malignant neoplasms

More than 90% of malignant neoplasms in the mouth are squamous cell carcinomas. Nearly 30% of all oral cancers affect the lip: some 25% affect the tongue—the common intraoral site [1–5]. Most intraoral cancers involve the lateral border of the tongue and/or the floor of the mouth (the graveyard area), although why this site appears predisposed to tumour development is unclear.

Although in Western countries oral cancer accounts for less than 3% of all malignant tumours, it is a significant world health problem and overall is the sixth most common malignant neoplasm. In parts of South-East Asia, for example, particularly India, some 40% of malignancy is oral cancer. High levels are also seen in other parts of the developing world such as Brazil, but also in parts of Europe such as areas of northern France and eastern Europe.

Oral carcinoma

Aetiology. The incidence of oral cancer varies widely in different areas and in different races within one geographical area [6]. Newfoundland, for example, has the highest incidence of oral carcinoma in the West, with about 10 times the UK incidence. In the UK, oral cancer is most prevalent among Celts. Oral cancer is twice as common in Scotland as it is in England and Wales and the incidence appears to be increasing [7–10].

Oral cancer in the West predominantly affects males between the ages of 55 and 75 years, although it is occasionally seen in younger persons. Smoking, tobacco and alcohol appear to have a synergistic effect in the aetiology of oral cancer [6,7,9,10]. Smokers of more than 40 cigarettes per day appear to be about five times more likely than non-smokers to develop oral cancer, but many heavy smokers also drink alcohol. Studies of those who abstain from such habits (e.g. Mormons, Seventh Day Adventists) reveal a lower incidence of oral cancer in those groups. The increasing incidence of smoking since World War II may be responsible for the rising prevalence of oral cancer [4,7,8,11].

Reverse smoking—where the lighted end is held in the mouth, as in parts of India—is linked with a high incidence of oral cancer, particularly of the hard palate, an otherwise unusual site. Cigar smoking has shown an association with floor-of-mouth leukoplakia in women. Bidi (a type of cigarette made of tobacco rolled in a dried temburni leaf) which is smoked in India, is associated with a high incidence of leukoplakia, particularly at the commissures, and oral cancer.

Tobacco chewing also predisposes to oral cancer especially in parts of Asia where tobacco is chewed or held in the mouth for long periods, in a betel quid which often also contains betel vine leaf, areca nut, catechu and slaked lime. Betel chewing, together with smoking, increases the risk of oral cancer by about 25 times.

Women in the southeast USA who place snuff in the buccal sulcus are predisposed to gingival and alveolar carcinoma. Currently there is concern that the use of smokeless tobacco may predispose to oral cancer.

Several studies have shown an association between high alcoholic beverage consumption and oral cancer. For example, Brittany has the highest incidence of oral cancer in western Europe and there is a close relationship between the consumption of Calvados (a pot-stilled spirit) and cancer of the mouth (and oesophagus).

Although there is evidence that chronic mucosal irritation enhances chemically induced oral carcinoma in animals, there is no unequivocal evidence that this is aetiological in human oral cancer. Patients who drink and smoke heavily may have poor oral hygiene.

Some workers in the UK textile industry are at risk from oral cancer, apparently related to exposure to dust from carding raw cotton and wool.

Tertiary syphilis may cause a diffuse glossitis or keratosis which may be premalignant but, although some early studies showed positive syphilis serology in a few patients with oral carcinoma, this rate was not higher than in controls. Many patients with tertiary syphilis were also heavy smokers and drinkers, factors equally likely to be incriminated in the aetiology of oral cancer.

Some other leukoplakias, especially commissural and speckled leukoplakias (the more highly premalignant forms), may be infected with *Candida albicans* which appears not to be simply a secondary invader of a damaged, already dysplastic, epithelium, but may, by the production of carcinogens, induce dysplasia [11].

There are associations between liver dysfunction and oral cancer. Animal studies have shown that liver damage (by various factors, including alcohol) can enhance chemically induced oral cancer.

Iron deficiency in humans, as in the Patterson–Kelly (Plummer–Vinson) syndrome of sideropenia, achlorhydria and glossitis, appears to predispose to oral, pharyngeal and oesophageal carcinoma. In animals, iron deficiency appears to accelerate chemically induced oral carcinogenesis. Other dietary factors, such as vitamin A, may be protective [12].

The evidence at present does not necessarily implicate or exonerate herpes simplex virus in the aetiology of oral carcinoma, although the virus can induce malignant transformation *in vitro*. Papillomaviruses have been detected in some leukoplakias and some oral cancers but are also found in non-malignant lesions, and their role, if any, in oncogenesis of oral cancer is also unclear [13].

Premalignant oral lesions. In some patients who develop oral cancer, the tumour arises from clinically definable premalignant lesions such as erythroplasia, some types of leukoplakia, oral submucous fibrosis or erosive lichen planus [13]. In India, most oral cancers are preceded by premalignant lesions but in Western societies many arise from clinically normal mucosa.

Pathology. The essential features distinguishing oral carcinoma are invasion through the basement membrane and epithelial dysplasia. In more highly differentiated tumours, premature keratinization results in concentric rings of keratin (cell nests). The tumour infiltrates locally and metastasizes primarily via the lymphatics, and usually locally to cervical lymph nodes [14]. Significant systemic metastases are seen only late in the disease.

Pseudoepitheliomatous hyperplasia may be seen in benign conditions, particularly in median rhomboid glossitis, granular cell tumour and necrotizing sialometaplasia, all of which must be differentiated from carcinoma.

Clinical features. Carcinoma often presents as a mouth ulcer, although even then it is not always painful [5,15]. The appearance of carcinomas, however, is highly variable and they may also be in the form of a red or white area, a lump or fissuring (Figs 69.18–69.20). Lymph-node examination is of paramount importance to detect metastases, although most oral cancer presents at a stage

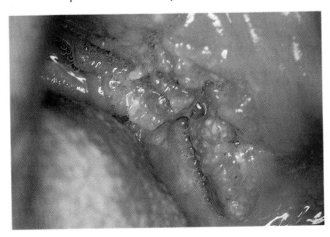

Fig. 69.18 Squamous cell carcinoma: pebbly surface.

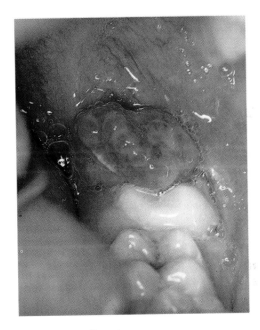

Fig. 69.19 Squamous cell carcinoma.

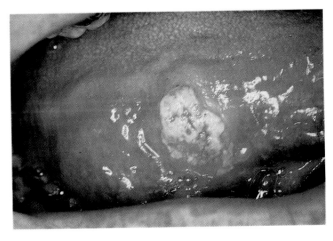

Fig. 69.20 Squamous cell carcinoma presenting as a mainly white lesion.

when there is little clinical evidence of local metastases to lymph nodes.

Any chronic oral lesion should be regarded with suspicion, especially if there is induration, fixation to underlying tissues, any recent change in appearance, associated lymphadenopathy or no obvious explanation for the lesion.

Prognosis. Despite the fact that oral cancer should be one of the most readily detected neoplasms because of the easy access for clinical and biopsy examination, the 5-year survival for intraoral tumours is only about 30%. The prognosis is worst where the floor-of-mouth, alveolus, posterior tongue or maxilla is involved. Most tumours are relatively advanced (T2 or more) and this and the presence of metastases also adversely affect prognosis.

The prognosis is also usually worse for male and elderly patients—possibly because of the somewhat later presentation for treatment, or because of associated medical problems. Many patients with oral cancer are heavy smokers and drinkers, and some have cirrhosis and nutritional defects.

Diagnosis [12]. Clinical features which suggest malignancy include:
1 the presence of erythroplasia;
2 a granular appearance of an ulcer with fissuring or raised exophytic margins;
3 the presence of abnormal blood vessels supplying a lump;
4 induration;
5 fixation of the lesion to deeper tissues or to overlying skin or mucosa;
6 enlarged regional cervical lymph nodes.

The whole mucosa should be examined as there may be widespread dysplastic mucosa ('field change') or even a second neoplasm.

Incisional biopsy, which is invariably required, should be sufficiently large to include enough suspect and apparently normal tissue. Red, rather than white, areas are most likely to show dysplasia, and hence should be biopsied.

Attempts to highlight probable dysplastic areas before biopsy, for example by the use of toluidine blue dye, are unfortunately not reliable, but may be of some help in deciding which area is best to biopsy where there is widespread 'field change' [1].

An excisional biopsy should be avoided unless the lesion is extremely small since this is unlikely to have excised an adequately wide margin of tissue if the lesion is malignant, but will have destroyed for the surgeon or radiotherapist clinical evidence of the site and character of the lesion.

Exfoliative cytology of oral mucosal lesions is, by and large, valueless and time consuming as a diagnostic procedure and cannot be depended upon to give a reliable diagnosis in this or any of the serious oral mucosal disorders.

Treatment. The major impact that treatment has had on the prognosis of oral cancer to date has been in relation to improved anaesthetic and medical care. Surgical reconstruction has also been markedly improved and there are fewer side-effects from modern radiotherapy. There is now evidence that vitamin A derivatives may be of benefit in patients with premalignant lesions, and in preventing second primary neoplasms.

The treatment of oral cancer involves one or a combination of [5,16,17]:
1 radiotherapy;
2 surgery; and very occasionally
3 chemotherapy.

The many variables, such as local resources, expertise and referral patterns, as well as the variable nature of oral cancer patients in terms of site, stage of disease and medical problems, mean that there have been few large unequivocal controlled trials of treatment.

Patients who die of their disease almost always do so either because of failure to control the primary tumour or because of metastatic spread to cervical lymph nodes which enlarge and invade adjacent tissues.

REFERENCES

1 Epstein JB, Scully C, Spinelli JJ. Toluidine blue and Lugol's iodine application in the assessment of oral malignant disease and lesions at risk of malignancy. *J Oral Pathol Med* 1992; **21**: 160–3.
2 Langdon J, Henk J. Malignant tumours of the mouth, jaws and salivary glands. London: Edward Arnold, 1995.
3 Scully C, Malamos D, Levers BGH *et al*. Sources and patterns of referrals of oral cancer: the role of general practitioners. *Br Med J* 1986; **293**: 599–601.
4 Scully C, Prime SS, Boyle P. Oral cancer (leading article). *Lancet* 1989; **ii**: 311–12.
5 Scully C, Ward-Booth P. Detection and treatment of early cancers of the oral cavity. *Crit Rev Oncol Hematol* 1995; **21**: 63–75.
6 Scully C, Flint S, Porter SR. *A Colour Atlas of Oral Disease*. London: Martin Dunitz, 1996.
7 MacFarlane GJ, Boyle P, Scully C. Rising mortality from cancer of the tongue in young Scottish males. *Lancet* 1987; **ii**: 912.
8 MacFarlane GJ, Boyle P, Scully C. Oral cancer in Scotland: changing incidence and mortality. *Br Med J* 1992; **305**: 1121–3.
9 Baden E. Prevention of cancer of the oral cavity and pharynx. *Cancer* 1987; **37**: 49–62.
10 Davis S, Severson RK. Increasing incidence of cancer of the tongue in the United States among young adults. *Lancet* 1987; **ii**: 910–11.
11 Cawson RA, Binnie WH. Candida leukoplakia and carcinoma: a possible relationship. In: Mackenzie IE, Dabelsteen E, Squier CA, eds. *Oral Premalignancy*. Iowa: University of Iowa Press, 1982.
12 Scully C. Oral precancer: preventive and medical approaches to management. *Oral Oncol* 1995; **31B**: 16–26.
13 Scully C, Cawson RA. Oral potentially malignant lesions. *J Epidemiol Biostat* 1996; **1**: 3–12.
14 Carter RL, Pittman MR. Squamous carcinomas of the head and neck: some patterns of spread. *J R Soc Med* 1980; **73**: 420–7.
15 Scully C. Clinical diagnostic methods for the detection of premalignant and early malignant oral lesions. *Community Dent Health* 1993; **1**(Suppl.1): 43–52.
16 Beetham KW, Williams RG. The curative potential of surgery in the management of advanced mouth cancer. *Clin Oncol* 1980; **6**: 337–41.
17 Peterson DE, Elias EG, Sonis ST *et al*. *Head and Neck Management of the Cancer Patient*. Nijhoff: The Hague, 1986.

Verrucous carcinoma [1]

Verrucous carcinoma is an uncommon, warty, white neoplasm which is rarely ulcerated [2]. Some verrucous carcinoma develops as a result of the local use of snuff or tobacco. Confirmation of diagnosis by biopsy is particularly important as verrucous carcinoma responds well to excision but, if irradiated, may undergo anaplastic change, with subsequent acceleration of growth and invasiveness.

Keratoacanthoma [3]

Intraoral keratoacanthomas are very rare. They usually appear as an ulcer with a rolled margin, clinically indistinguishable from squamous carcinoma usually on the anterior or maxillary gingiva [1,3,4]. It is unclear as to whether intraoral keratoacanthomas regress spontaneously, as all have been excised for diagnosis.

REFERENCES

1 Hume WJ, Quayle AA. An unusual epithelial neoplasm of gingiva resembling the keratoacanthoma. *Br J Oral Surg* 1985; **23**: 366–70.
2 McDonald JS, Crissman JD, Gluckman JL. Verrucous carcinoma of the oral cavity. *Head Neck Surg* 1982; **5**: 22–8.
3 Eversole LR, Leider AS, Alexander G. Intraoral and labial keratoacanthomas. *Oral Surg* 1982; **54**: 663–7.
4 Whyte AM, Hansen LS, Lee C. The intraoral keratoacanthoma: a diagnostic problem. *Br J Oral Surg* 1986; **24**: 438–41.

Oral malignant primary neoplasms other than oral squamous cell carcinoma

The following comprise up to 10% of all oral malignant tumours:

1 salivary gland tumours;
2 malignant melanoma;
3 lymphomas—non-Hodgkin's lymphomas are increasingly seen in the fauces in HIV disease and immunocompromised persons;
4 sarcomas;
5 neoplasms of bone and connective tissue;
6 some odontogenic tumours;
7 maxillary antral carcinoma (or other neoplasms);
8 Langerhans' cell histiocytosis;
9 Kaposi's sarcoma—oral Kaposi's sarcoma is typically now seen in HIV disease or other immunocompromised persons and especially in the posterior palate as a brown or purple macule that becomes nodular and ulcerates;
10 other neoplasms.

Metastatic oral neoplasms

Metastases to the oral tissues are rare, accounting for only 1% of all oral tumours and most appear in bone, especially the mandibular premolar or molar area or condyle. Most oral metastases originate from carcinomas of breast, lung, kidney, stomach or liver [1,2].

Metastases may present with pain, paraesthesia, sensory loss, loosening of teeth, delayed healing of an extraction wound or pathological fracture. Metastases may occasionally appear as an alveolar or gingival swelling or ulcer.

REFERENCES

1 Keller EE, Gunderson LL. Bone disease metastatic to the jaw. *J Am Dent Assoc* 1987; **115**: 697–701.
2 Nishimura Y, Yakata H, Kawasaki T *et al.* Metastatic tumours of the mouth and jaws: a review of the Japanese literature. *J Maxillofac Surg* 1982; **10**: 253–8.

Ulcers in association with systemic disease

Aphthae (p. 3069) are occasionally associated with systemic disease. However, a wide range of systemic diseases, especially haematological, gastrointestinal and dermatological disorders, may cause other oral lesions which, because of the moisture, trauma and infection in the mouth, tend to break down to leave ulcers or erosions. Oral ulceration is also frequently caused by infections and can be caused by drugs or irradiation (see Table 69.7).

Haematological diseases

Deficiency states

Low iron, folate or vitamin B_{12} levels may predispose to aphthae (Fig. 69.21). A few of these patients also have anaemia, sometimes with other oral features such as glossitis or angular stomatitis, but many have a deficiency state with no established anaemia [1,2]. Occasionally, patients with deficiency of B vitamins may develop other types of oral ulcer, and sometimes epithelial dysplasia [3].

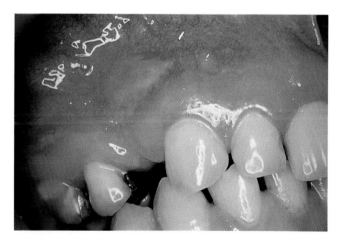

Fig. 69.21 Aphthous-like ulceration in the maxillary buccal sulcus in folate deficiency.

REFERENCES

1 Field EA, Speechley JA, Rugman FR *et al.* Oral signs and symptoms in patients with undiagnosed vitamin B12 deficiency. *J Oral Pathol Med* 1995; **24**: 468–70.
2 Tyldesley WR. Oral signs and symptoms in anaemias. *Br Dent J* 1985; **139**: 232–6.
3 Theaker JM, Porter SR, Fleming KA. Oral epithelial dysplasia in vitamin B12 deficiency. *Oral Surg* 1989; **67**: 81–3.

Leukopenias and agranulocytosis

White-cell dyscrasias and HIV infection are also often complicated by oral ulceration (Fig. 69.22). Oral ulceration may be a major symptom in patients with leukopenias, and may be the first manifestation of drug-induced agranulocytosis. Painful, deep, irregular ulcers, often with only a minimal inflammatory halo, involve the mouth and/or pharynx and tend to extend and penetrate slowly. In cyclical neutropenia, ulcers appear episodically at 21-day intervals in association with the neutropenic episodes. Severe periodontitis is often also a feature of leukocyte and other immune defects and the patients may suffer from recurrent infections elsewhere [1–3]. Methotrexate can cause oral ulceration in the absence of leukopenia.

REFERENCES

1 Baehni PC, Payot P, Tsai CC *et al.* Periodontal status associated with chronic neutropenia. *J Clin Periodontol* 1983; **10**: 222–30.
2 Porter SR, Scully C, Standen G. Autoimmune neutropenia manifesting as recurrent oral ulceration. *Oral Surg* 1994; **78**: 178–80.
3 Scully C, Gilmour G. Neutropenia and dental patients. *Br Dent J* 1986; **160**: 43–6.

Leukaemias

Oral ulceration may be a prominent feature, especially in the acute leukaemias and myelodysplasia [1]. Other oral manifestations of leukaemia include mucosal pallor, gingival haemorrhage, gingival swelling, petechiae and ecchymoses [2–5]. Oral infections with *Candida albicans* and Gram-negative bacteria including *Pseudomonas* species,

Escherichia coli, *Proteus*, *Klebsiella* and *Serratia* species are common, especially in acute leukaemias, and may act as a portal for septicaemia [6]. Herpes simplex or zoster–varicella virus ulcers are also common (Fig. 69.23). Chemotherapy complicates the situation because it, too, can produce oral ulceration [2,7].

Other findings include paraesthesia (particularly of the lower lip), extrusion of teeth, painful swellings over the mandible and parotid swelling (Mikulicz's syndrome).

REFERENCES

1 Porter SR, Scully C. Gingival and oral mucosal ulceration associated with the myelodysplastic syndrome. *Oral Oncol* 1994; **30B**: 346–50.
2 Barrett AP. A long term prospective clinical study of oral complications during conventional chemotherapy for acute leukemia. *Oral Surg* 1987; **63**: 313–16.
3 Dreizen S, McCredie KB, Body GP *et al.* Quantitative analysis of the oral complications of anti-leukemia chemotherapy. *Oral Surg* 1986; **62**: 650–3.
4 Dreizen S, McCredie KB, Keating MJ *et al.* Malignant gingival and skin infiltrates in adult leukemia. *Oral Surg* 1983; **55**: 572–8.
5 Scully C, MacFarlane TW. Orofacial manifestations in childhood malignancy: clinical and microbiological findings during remission. *ASDC J Dent Child* 1983; **50**: 121–5.
6 Dreizen S, McCredie KB, Bodey GP *et al.* Microbial mucocutaneous infections in acute adult leukaemia. *Postgrad Med* 1986; **79**: 107–18.
7 Dreizen S, McCredie KB, Keating MJ. Chemotherapy-associated oral haemorrhages in adults with acute leukaemia. *Oral Surg* 1983; **55**: 572–8.

Management of oral lesions in white-cell dyscrasias

Microbiological investigations, with specimens for anaerobic culture, are essential. Oral hygiene should be carefully maintained with 0.2% aqueous chlorhexidine mouthwashes and the use of a soft toothbrush. Prophylactic antifungal therapy such as nystatin mouthwashes (10 ml of nystatin, 100 000 units/ml) used four times daily, nystatin pastilles (same dose), or amphotericin lozenges (10 mg four times daily) is also indicated. Viral infections should be treated with topical or systemic aciclovir; some haematologists use aciclovir prophylactically.

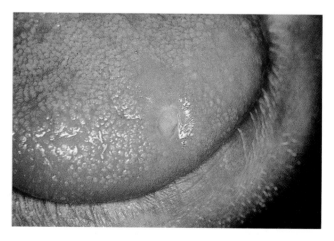

Fig. 69.22 Aphthous-like ulceration in human immunodeficiency virus disease.

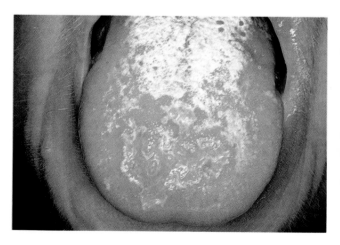

Fig. 69.23 Herpes simplex lingual recurrence, and candidiasis in leukaemia: similar lesions may be seen in human immunodeficiency virus infection.

Granulocytic sarcoma

SYN. CHLOROMA

Granulocytic sarcomas are rare in the oral cavity. Most present with swelling or symptoms related to skeletal involvement [1,2]. The maxilla is particularly involved [1].

REFERENCES

1 Barker GR, Sloan P. Maxillary chloroma: a myeloid leukaemic deposit. *Br J Oral Surg* 1988; **26**: 124–8.
2 Ficarra G, Silverman S, Quivey JM *et al*. Granulocytic sarcoma (chloroma) of the oral cavity: a case with aleukaemic presentation. *Oral Surg* 1987; **63**: 709–14.

Myelodysplastic syndrome

Oral manifestations in myelodysplastic syndrome include particularly ulceration but also paraesthesiae, petechiae, burning mouth, gingival hyperplasia, xerostomia and herpes labialis [1–4].

REFERENCES

1 Epstein JB, Priddy RW, Sparling T *et al*. Oral manifestations in myelodysplastic syndrome. *Oral Surg* 1986; **61**: 466–70.
2 Flint SR, Sugerman P, Scully C *et al*. The myelodysplastic syndromes: case report and review. *Oral Surg* 1990; **70**: 579–83.
3 Gibson J, Lamey P-J, Watson WH *et al*. The myelodysplastic syndrome presenting with oral symptoms. *Br Dent J* 1987; **163**: 234–5.
4 Porter SR, Scully C. Gingival and oral mucosal ulceration associated with the myelodysplastic syndrome. *Oral Oncol* 1994; **30B**: 346–50.

Lymphomas

Lymphomas may appear as oral swellings which sometimes ulcerate. They occur on the pharynx or palate, or occasionally tongue, gingivae or lips and may cause pain, or sensory disturbance. Herpes zoster and simplex infections are common.

Some 2–10% of lymphomas present first in the oral cavity and, in one series lymphomas were the third most common oral malignancy seen. Eighty per cent of oral lymphomas are composed of follicular centre cells or postfollicular cells [1–5.] There is an increased incidence of oral lymphomas in HIV disease [6].

Cutaneous T-cell lymphoma. Oral lesions are late in cutaneous T-cell lymphoma and may be plaques, lumps or ulcers [7].

Lethal midline granuloma. Lethal midline granuloma is the term sometimes used to include a spectrum of conditions including Wegener's granulomatosis, polymorphic reticulosis (PMR or lymphomatoid granulomatosis), and idiopathic midline destructive disease (IMDD) [1,8,9].

Wegener's granulomatosis. Wegener's granulomatosis, although not a lymphoma, is discussed here. Oral manifestations are common and may be the first sign of Wegener's granulomatosis [4,10–18]. A painless, progressive swelling of the gingiva in a previously healthy mouth, particularly associated with swollen, inflamed papillae, should arouse suspicion of Wegener's granulomatosis. The gingival enlargement may have a fairly characteristic 'strawberry-like' appearance. Wegener's granulomatosis may also present with oral ulceration, failure of an extraction socket to heal or occasionally swelling of the lip or salivary gland.

Polymorphic reticulosis (syn. lymphomatoid granulomatosis). The most common oral presentation of polymorphic reticulosis is palatal ulceration but there may also occasionally be ulceration elsewhere [17].

Idiopathic midline destructive disease [18]. Downward spread from nasal disease can lead to palatal necrosis and ulceration in idiopathic midline destructive disease. Occasionally the disease presents with delayed healing of an extraction socket [9,17,18].

REFERENCES

1 Baden E, Carter R. Intraoral presentation of American Burkitt's lymphoma after extraction of a mandibular left third molar. *J Oral Maxillofac Surg* 1987; **45**: 689–93.
2 Baden E, Al Saati T, Caverieviere P *et al*. Hodgkin's lymphoma of the oropharyngeal region. *Oral Surg* 1987; **64**: 88–94.
3 Barker GR. Unifocal lymphomas of the oral cavity. *Br J Oral Surg* 1984; **22**: 426–30.
4 Crissman JD, Weiss MA, Gluckman J. Midline granuloma syndrome. A clinicopathologic study of 13 patients. *Am J Surg Pathol* 1982; **6**: 335–8.
5 Eisenbud L, Sciubba JJ, Mir R *et al*. Oral presentations in non-Hodgkins lymphoma: a review of thirty one cases. *Oral Surg* 1983; **56**: 151–6.
6 Ioachim HL, Cooper MC, Hellman GC. Lymphomas in men at high risk for acquired immune deficiency syndrome (AIDS): a study of 21 cases. *Cancer* 1985; **56**: 2831–42.
7 Sirious DA, Miller AS, Harwick RD, Van der Leid EC. Oral manifestations of cutaneous T-cell lymphoma. *Oral Surg* 1993; **75**: 700–5.
8 Nelson JF, Finkelstein MW, Acevedo A *et al*. Midline 'non-healing' granuloma. *Oral Surg* 1984; **58**: 554–60.
9 Tsokos M, Fauci AS, Costa J. Idiopathic midline destructive disease (IMDD). A subgroup of patients with the midline granuloma syndrome. *Am J Clin Pathol* 1982; **77**: 162–7.
10 Abraham-Inpijn L. Oral and otal manifestations as the primary symptoms in Wegener's granulomatosis. *J Head Neck Pathol* 1983; **2**: 20–2.
11 Allen CM, Canisa C, Salewski C, Weiland JE. Wegeners granulomatosis: report of three cases with oral lesions. *J Oral Maxillofac Surg* 1991; **49**: 294–8.
12 Israelson H, Binnie WH, Hurt WC. The hyperplastic gingivitis of Wegener's granulomatosis. *J Periodontol* 1981; **52**: 81–7.
13 Lutcavage GJ, Schaberg SJ, Arendt DA, Malmquist JP. Gingival mass with massive soft-tissue necrosis. *J Oral Maxillofac Surg* 1991; **49**: 1332–8.
14 Parsons E, Seymour RA, MacLeod RI *et al*. Wegener's granulomatosis: distinct gingival lesion. *J Clin Periodontol* 1992; **19**: 64–6.
15 Patten SF, Tomecki KJ. Wegeners granulomatosis: cutaneous and oral mucosal disease. *J Am Acad Dermatol* 1993; **28**: 710–18.
16 Hansen LS, Silverman S, Pons VG *et al*. Limited Wegener's granulomatosis. Report of a case with oral, renal and skin involvement. *Oral Surg* 1985; **60**: 524–30.
17 McDonald TJ, De Remee RA, Weiland LH. Wegener's granulomatosis and polymorphic reticulosis—two diseases or one? Experience with 90 patients. *Arch Otolaryngol* 1981; **107**: 141–6.
18 Fauci AS, Haynes BF, Katz P *et al*. Wegener's granulomatosis: prospective clinical and therapeutic experience with 85 patients for 21 years. *Ann Intern Med* 1983; **98**: 76–85.

Mycosis fungoides

Oral lesions in mycosis fungoides typically are red or white areas on the tongue but are usually late manifestations [1–3].

REFERENCES

1 Barnett ML, Cole RJ. Mycosis fungoides with multiple oral mucosal lesions. *J Periodontol* 1985; **56**: 690–3.
2 Evans GE, Dalziel KL. Mycosis fungoides with oral involvement. *Int J Oral Maxillofac Surg* 1987; **16**: 634–7.
3 Patel SP, Hotterman OA. Mycosis fungoides: an overview. *J Surg Oncol* 1983; **22**: 221–6.

Pseudolymphoma

Rare tumour-like lymphoproliferative infiltrates which lack the malignant potential of lymphomas may be seen intra-orally, notably in the palate [1].

REFERENCE

1 Wright JM, Dunsworth AR. Follicular lymphoid hyperplasia of the hard palate: a benign lymphoproliferative process. *Oral Surg* 1983; **55**: 162–8.

Histiocytoses

The histiocytoses typically produce lytic bone lesions [1,2] but gingival swelling, periodontal destruction with loosening of teeth and mouth ulceration may be seen [3].

REFERENCES

1 Broadbent V, Pritchard J. Histiocytosis X: current controversies. *Arch Dis Child* 1985; **60**: 605–8.
2 Favera BE, McCarthy RC, Mieran GW. Histiocytosis X. *Hum Pathol* 1983; **14**: 663–76.
3 Hartman KS. Histiocytosis X. A review of 114 cases with oral involvement. *Oral Surg* 1980; **49**: 38–54.

Multicentric reticulohistiocytosis

Oral lesions are seen in up to 50% of patients with multicentric reticulohistiocytosis [1]. Lesions are collections of histiocytes which form nodular or granular lesions, particularly in the labial or buccal mucosa. The temporomandibular joint may also be involved as part of the polyarthropathy.

REFERENCE

1 Katz RW, Anderson KF. Multicentric reticulohistiocytosis. *Oral Surg* 1988; **65**: 721–5.

Hypereosinophilic syndrome

Oral erosions affecting buccal, gingival or labial mucosae may be a feature of the hypereosinophilic syndrome [1–3] and herald cardiac involvement [2]. Etoposide therapy may be effective [3].

REFERENCES

1 Aractingi S, Janin A, Zini JM *et al.* Specific mucosal erosions in hypereosinophilic syndrome. *Arch Dermatol* 1996; **132**: 535–541.
2 Leiferman KM, O'Duffy D, Perry HO *et al.* Recurrent incapacitating mucosal ulcerations; a prodrome of the hypereosinophilic syndrome. *Am J Med* 1982; **247**: 1018–20.
3 Smit AJ, van Essen LH, de Vries EG. Successful long-term control of idiopathic hypereosinophilic syndrome with etoposide. *Cancer* 1991; **67**: 2826–7.

Vasculitides

Periarteritis nodosa. Transient submucosal oral nodules may occur singly or in crops along the path of vessels and especially in the tongue. Other mucosal lesions include erythema, papules, haemorrhages or ulceration [1].

REFERENCE

1 Cowpe JG, Hislop WS. Oral presentation of polyarteritis nodosa. *Oral Surg* 1983; **56**: 597–601.

Giant-cell arteritis. Patients may suffer ischaemic pain during mastication, or intermittent claudication of the tongue [1]. Ulceration and necrosis of the tongue or lip have also been observed in a few patients [2,3].

REFERENCES

1 Lamey P-J, Taylor JA, Devine J. Giant cell arteritis: a forgotten diagnosis. *Br Dent J* 1988; **164**: 48–50.
2 Patterson A, Barnard N, Scully C *et al.* Necrosis of the tongue in a patient with intestinal infarction. *Oral Surg* 1992; **74**: 582–6.
3 Scully C, Eveson JW, Barrett AW *et al.* Necrosis of the lip in giant cell arteritis. *J Oral Maxillofac Surg* 1993; **51**: 581–3.

Iatrogenic conditions

Bone-marrow transplantation

Oral complications are common and can be a major cause of morbidity following bone-marrow transplantation. Mucositis, infections, bleeding, xerostomia and loss of taste result from the effects of the underlying disease, chemo- or radiotherapy and GVHD. The ventrum of the tongue, buccal and labial mucosa and gingiva may be affected by ulceration or mucositis [1–6].

Graft-versus-host disease

The oral manifestations of acute GVHD consist of painful mucosal desquamation and ulceration, and/or cheilitis, and the presence of lichenoid plaques or striae. Small, white lesions affect the buccal and lingual mucosa early on, but clear by day 14. Erythema and ulceration are most pronounced at 7–11 days, and may be associated with obvious infection. Candidiasis is common, as is herpes simplex stomatitis (occasionally zoster) and there may be oral purpura, especially in adults [4,7].

The oral lesions in chronic GVHD are coincident with skin lesions, and include generalized mucosal erythema, lichenoid lesions, mainly in the buccal mucosa, and xerostomia. These may be depressed salivary IgA levels in minor gland saliva [8]. Xerostomia is most significant in the first 14 days after transplant and is a consequence of drug treatment, irradiation and/or GVHD.

Lip biopsy is useful in the diagnosis of chronic GVHD and should include both mucosa and underlying minor salivary glands [9]. Histology shows changes similar to those seen in Sjögren's syndrome.

REFERENCES

1 Barrett AP. Oral complications of bone marrow transplantation. *Aust NZ J Med* 1986; **16**: 239–40.
2 Berkowitz RJ, Strandford S, Jones P *et al.* Stomatologic complications of bone marrow transplantation in a pediatric population. *Pediatr Dent* 1987; **9**: 105–10.
3 Dahllof G, Heimdahl A, Modeer T *et al.* Oral mucous membrane lesions in children treated with bone marrow transplantation. *Scand J Dent Res* 1989; **97**: 268–77.
4 Dreizen S, McCredie KB, Dicke KA *et al.* Oral complications of bone marrow transplantation in adults with acute leukaemia. *Postgrad Med* 1979; **66**: 187–93.
5 Seto BG. Oral mucositis in patients undergoing bone-marrow transplantation. *Oral Surg* 1985; **60**: 493–7.
6 Kolbinson DA, Schubert MM, Flourney N *et al.* Early oral changes following bone marrow transplantation. *Oral Surg* 1988; **66**: 130–8.
7 Graham-Brown RAG, Jones JAG, Shaw PV *et al.* A graft-versus-host disease-like syndrome with carcinomatosis. *Br J Dermatol* 1987; **116**: 249–52.
8 Izutsu KT, Menard TW, Schubert MM. Graft versus host disease-related secretory immunoglobulin A deficiency in bone marrow transplant recipients: findings in labial saliva. *Lab Invest* 1985; **52**: 292–7.
9 Sale GE, Shulman HM, Schubert MM. Oral and ophthalmic pathology of graft-versus-host disease in man: predictive value of the lip biopsy. *Hum Pathol* 1981; **12**: 1022–30.

Gastrointestinal diseases

Aphthae in gastrointestinal diseases have been discussed on page 3070. Other types of mouth ulcer are also sometimes found in ulcerative colitis and Crohn's disease.

Ulcerative colitis

Reported oral lesions in ulcerative colitis include aphthae, chronic ulcers and pyostomatitis vegetans. The course of these lesions tends to follow the course of the bowel disease and, although oral lesions may respond to topical therapy (e.g. corticosteroids), systemic treatment is often needed [1–5]. Oral lesions termed pyostomatitis vegetans are deep fissures, pustules and papillary projections. Less than 40 cases have been recorded and most patients have had ulcerative colitis or Crohn's disease [1–6].

Oral lesions are uncommon in pyoderma gangrenosum and are typically painful irregular ulcers with rolled margins and a grey base.

REFERENCES

1 Ballo FS, Camisa C, Allen CM. Pyostomatitis vegetans. *J Am Acad Dermatol* 1989; **21**: 381–7.
2 Basu MK, Asquith P. Oral manifestations of inflammatory bowel disease. *Clin Gastroenterol* 1980; **9**: 307.
3 Chan S, Scully C, Prime SS *et al.* Pyostomatitis vegetans: oral manifestation of ulcerative colitis. *Oral Surg* 1991; **27**: 689–92.
4 Neville B, Laden SA, Smith SE *et al.* Pyostomatitis vegetans. *Am J Dermatopathol* 1985; **7**: 69–77.
5 Thornhill MH, Zakrzewska JM, Gilkes JJH. Pyostomatitis vegetans; report of three cases and review of the literature. *J Oral Pathol Med* 1992; **21**: 128– 33.
6 Van Hale HM, Rogers RS, Zone JJ. Pyostomatitis vegetans: a reactive mucosal marker for inflammatory disease of the gut. *Arch Dermatol* 1985; **121**: 94–8.

Crohn's disease is discussed later (p. 3112).

Dermatological diseases

Several dermatoses can be associated with oral erosions or ulcers; lichen planus (LP) is the most common, pemphigus the most serious.

Lichen planus (Chapter 41)

Oral LP may affect up to 1–2% of the population and is probably about eight times more common than cutaneous LP. The oral mucosa may be involved alone or in association with lesions on skin or other mucosa and oral lesions may precede, accompany or follow lesions elsewhere [1,2]. The association of oral LP with gingival involvement, together with vulvovaginal lesions, has been termed the vulvovaginal–gingival syndrome.

Aetiology. Most oral LP is idiopathic but some lichenoid lesions may be related to dental materials, GVHD, liver disease or drug use (e.g. non-steroidal anti-inflammatory agents). In the UK, oral LP has only weak HLA associations [3], and is only rarely associated with liver disease or immunodeficiency, which have been purported to be related to LP [4]. Chronic liver disease, especially chronic active hepatitis may be associated with erosive LP in persons of southern European extraction [5,6].

Pathology. The pathology is similar to that of cutaneous LP, although sawtooth rete ridges are rarely seen in oral biopsies, and other epithelial changes may be less distinct [2,6].

Clinical features. The common oral lesions of LP are bilateral white lesions in the buccal and/or lingual mucosa [2,7]. They may be reticular, papular or plaque-like (Figs

69.24–69.28). They are often symptomless but may cause soreness. Erosive LP, which frequently affects the dorsum and lateral borders of the tongue or the buccal mucosae on both sides, is uncommon. The erosions are often large, slightly depressed or raised with a yellow slough, and an

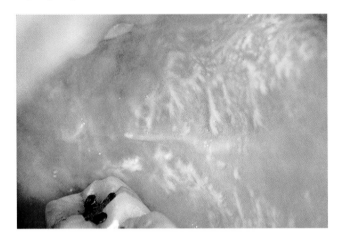

Fig. 69.24 Lichen planus: reticulopapular lesions in the common oral site—the buccal mucosa.

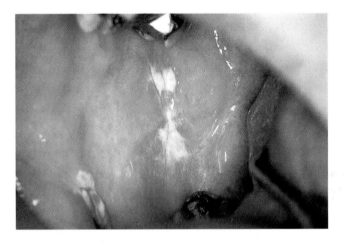

Fig. 69.25 Lichen planus: plaque-like lesions resemble leukoplakia.

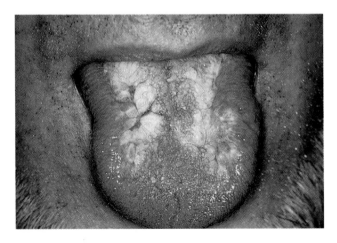

Fig. 69.26 Lichen planus on the tongue.

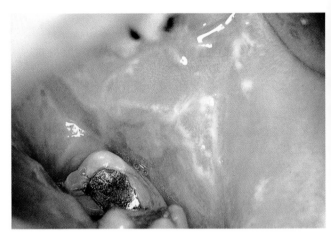

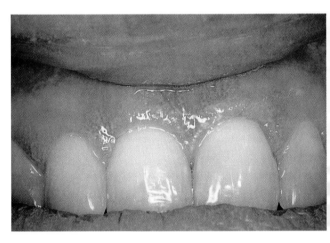

Fig. 69.27 Erosive lichen planus.

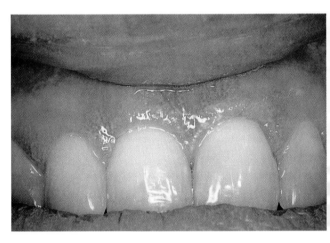

Fig. 69.28 Lichen planus on the gingivae: white and desquamative lesions.

irregular outline (Fig. 69.26), but they are not always as painful as might be imagined. The surrounding mucosa is often erythematous and glazed in appearance, with loss of filiform papillae of the tongue, and there are often pathognomonic whitish striae. LP may also produce a desquamative gingivitis (p. 3108). Candidiasis may complicate oral LP [6].

Prognosis. There appears to be a predisposition for some oral LP, particularly the chronic erosive or atrophic forms, to develop carcinoma—possibly a risk of around 5% over 10 years [6,8,9].

Diagnosis. Biopsy with immunofluorescence is often indicated to exclude keratosis, chronic ulcerative stomatitis with stratified epithelium-specific antinuclear antibodies, lichen sclerosus, lupus erythematosus, malignancy and other disorders.

Management. Consideration should be given to whether dental restorations should be replaced [6,10,11]. Antifungals help control candidiasis that often complicates LP [6].

Topical corticosteroids such as hydrocortisone, triamcinolone, betamethasone, fluocinonide or clobetasol are useful in controlling LP but erosive forms may need controlling with intralesional corticosteroids such as triamcinolone or, occasionally systemic corticosteroids [6,12,13]. Agents such as retinoids and griseofulvin have not been reliably effective [14] or have produced unacceptable adverse effects, but new oral retinoids, temarotene and fenretinide, appear promising [15,16]. Topical cyclosporin (100 mg/ml) swished around the mouth and expectorated has been recommended but has only equivocal value [1,17–19]

In view of the slight risk of premalignancy, especially in erosive LP, patients should be regularly reviewed [20].

REFERENCES

1 Porter SR, Scully C, Eveson JW. The efficacy of topical cyclosporin in the management of desquamative gingivitis due to lichen planus. *Lancet* 1994; **ii**: 753.
2 Scully C, Elkom M. Lichen planus: review and update on pathogenesis. *J Oral Pathol* 1985; **14**: 431–58.
3 Porter K, Klouda P, Scully C *et al.* HLA class I and II antigens in British patients with oral lichen planus. *Oral Surg* 1993; **75**: 176–80.
4 El-Kabir MA, Scully C, Porter SR *et al.* Liver disease and oral lichen planus in English patients. *Clin Exp Dermatol* 1993; **18**: 12–16.
5 Gruppo Italiano Studi Epidemiologica in Dermatologia (GISED). Lichen planus and liver disease: a multicentre case-control study. *Br Med J* 1990; **300**: 227–30.
6 Scully C, Beyli M, Feirrero MC *et al.* Oral lichen planus: a European consensus review of aetiopathogenesis and management. *Eur J Oral Health Sciences* 1997; (in press).
7 Vincent SD, Fotos PG, Baker KA *et al.* Oral lichen planus: the clinical, historical and therapeutic features of 100 cases. *Oral Surg* 1990; **70**: 165–71.
8 Barnard N, Scully C, Eveson JW *et al.* Oral cancer development in oral lichen planus. *J Oral Pathol Med* 1993; **22**: 421–4.
9 Marder MZ, Deesen KC. Transformation of oral lichen planus to squamous cell carcinoma. *J Am Dent Assoc* 1982; **105**: 55–60.
10 Eversole LR, Ringer M. The role of dental restorative metals in the pathogenesis of oral lichen planus. *Oral Surg* 1984; **57**: 383–7.
11 Finne K, Goranson K, Winckler L. Oral lichen planus and contact allergy to mercury. *Int J Oral Surg* 1982; **11**: 236–9.
12 Lozada-Nur F, Miranda C, Maliksi R. Double-blind clinical trial of 0.05% clobetasol propionate ointment in Orabase and 0.05% fluocinonide ointment in Orabase in the treatment of patients with oral vesiculoerosive diseases. *Oral Surg* 1994; **77**: 598–604.
13 Thongprasom K, Lunagjarmekorn L, Sererat T, Taweesap W. Relative efficacy of fluocinolone acetonide compared with triamcinolone acetonide in treatment of oral lichen planus. *J Oral Pathol Med* 1992; **21**: 456–8.
14 Matthews RW, Scully C. Griseofulvin in the treatment of oral lichen planus: adverse drug reactions but little beneficial effect. *Ann Dent* 1992; **L1**: 10–11.
15 Bollag W, Ott F. Treatment of lichen planus with temarotene. *Lancet* 1989; **ii**: 974.
16 Tradati N, Chiesa F, Rossi N *et al.* Successful topical treatment of oral lichen planus and leukoplakias with fenretinide (4HPR). *Cancer Lett* 1994; **76**: 109–11.
17 Eisen D, Ellis CN, Duell EA *et al.* Effect of topical cyclosporin rinse on oral lichen planus: a double-blind analysis. *N Engl J Med* 1990; **323**: 290–4.
18 Sieg P, Von Doarus H, von Zitzewitz V *et al.* Topical cyclosporin in oral lichen planus: a controlled, randomised prospective trial. *Br J Dermatol* 1995; **132**: 790–4.
19 Scully C. Treatment of oral lichen planus. *Lancet* 1990; **336**: 913–14.
20 De Jong WFB, Albrecht M, Banoczy J *et al.* Epithelial dysplasia in oral lichen planus. *Int J Oral Surg* 1984; **13**: 221–5.

Overlap syndromes

Lichen planus pemphigoides. Oral lesions in LP pemphigoides (LPP) may be similar to those of LP or pemphigoid, clinically and histologically [1].

Lichen planus/lichen sclerosus overlap syndrome. This may involve the oral and/or vulval mucosae [2]

REFERENCES

1 Allen CM, Camisa C, Grinwood R. Lichen planus pemphigoides: report of a case with oral lesions. *Oral Surg* 1987; **63**: 184–8.
2 Marren P, Millard P, Chia Y, Wojnarowska F. Mucosal lichen sclerosus/lichen planus overlap syndromes. *Br J Dermatol* 1994; **131**: 118–23.

Pemphigus (Chapter 40)

Oral lesions are the rule in pemphigus vulgaris, but rare in the superficial forms of pemphigus.

Pemphigus vulgaris. The oral mucosa is almost invariably involved in pemphigus vulgaris and oral lesions are commonly the presenting feature (Fig. 69.29). Bullae appear on any part of the oral mucosa including the palate, but so rapidly break that they are rarely seen [1]. Usually, the patient presents with large, painful, irregular and persistent erosions which can sometimes be difficult to differentiate clinically from those of other erosive conditions such as pemphigoid or superficial mucoceles, although intact bullae are more commonly seen in these latter conditions, whereas the Nikolsky sign is more often positive in pemphigus [2]. Rarely in pemphigus vulgaris there can be an acquired macroglossia [3].

Oral smears for cytology are of little practical value. A biopsy of perilesional mucosa should be taken for paraffin sections and immunostaining (Table 69.19) and serum collected for autoantibody titres [4].

Systemic immunosuppression is indicated, typically with corticosteroids and/or azathioprine [5,6]. Mucosal lesions are very recalcitrant, often healing after skin lesions when immunosuppressive therapy is given, and they may

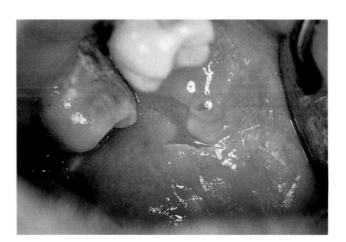

Fig. 69.29 Pemphigus vulgaris: irregular persistent oral erosions.

Table 69.19 Immunostaining in oral mucosal vesiculobullous disorders.

Disease	DIF	Oral mucosal deposits mainly	Pattern of IF	IIF	Autoantibodies against
Pemphigus	+	IgG C3	Epithelial intercellular	+	Epithelial intercellular cement
Mucous membrane pemphigoid	+	C3 IgG	Linear epithelial basement membrane	±	Epithelial basement membrane
Bullous pemphigoid	+	IgG C3	Linear epithelial basement membrane	+	Epithelial basement membrane
Dermatitis herpetiformis	+	IgA C3	Granular epithelial basement membrane	–	Reticulin
Linear IgA disease	+	IgA C3	Linear epithelial basement membrane	–	–
Erythema multiforme	±	C3 IgM	Vessel walls in lamina propria	–	–
Lichen planus†	±	Fibrin* mainly IgM IgG IgA C3	Globular epithelial or lamina propria and in Civatte bodies	–	–
Discoid lupus† erythematosus	+	IgG IgA IgM C3	Granular epithelial basement membrane	±	None, or antinuclear
Angina bullosa haemorrhagica	–	–	–	–	–
Superficial mucoceles	–	–	–	–	–

DIF, direct immunofluorescence (biopsy); IF, immunofluorescence; IIF, indirect immunofluorescence (serology).
* Non-specific deposits. + = present; – = absent. † Rarely vesiculobullous.

persist even though skin lesions are controlled. Topical corticosteroids may then help, or possibly prostaglandin E_2 [7].

REFERENCES

1 Hietanen J. Clinical and cytological features of oral pemphigus. *Acta Odontol Scand* 1982; **40**: 403–14.
2 Laskaris GC, Sklavounou A, Stratigos J. Bullous pemphigoid, cicatricial pemphigoid and pemphigus vulgaris: a comparative clinical survey of 287 cases. *Oral Surg* 1982; **54**: 656–62.
3 Milgraum SS, Kanzler MH, Waldinger TP *et al.* Macroglossia: an unusual presentation of pemphigus vulgaris. *Arch Dermatol* 1985; **121**: 1328–9.
4 Acosta E, Gilkes JJH, Ivanyi L. Relationship between serum autoantibody titres and the clinical activity of pemphigus. *Oral Surg* 1985; **60**: 611–14.
5 Lamey PJ, Rees TD, Binnie WH *et al.* Oral presentation of pemphigus vulgaris and its response to systemic steroid therapy. *Oral Surg* 1992; **74**: 54–7.
6 Mashkilleyson N, Mashkilleyson AL. Mucous membrane manifestations of pemphigus vulgaris. *Acta Derm Venereol (Stockh)* 1988; **68**: 413–21.
7 Morita H, Morisaki S, Kitano Y. Clinical trial of prostaglandin E2 on the oral lesions of pemphigus vulgaris. Br J Dermatol 1995; **132**: 165–6.

Pemphigus vegetans. Oral lesions in pemphigus vegetans are hyperplastic masses which, on the tongue, can give a cerebriform appearance [1,2].

REFERENCES

1 Ahmed AR, Blose DA. Pemphigus vegetans: Neumann type and Hallopeau type. *Int J Dermatol* 1984; **23**: 135–41.
2 Premalatha S, Jayakumar S, Yesudian P *et al.* Cerebriform tongue: a clinical sign in pemphigus vegetans. *Br J Dermatol* 1981; **104**: 587–91.

Paraneoplastic pemphigus. Oral lesions, mainly erosions and ulcers, have been noted in virtually all reported cases, and may be seen in isolation [1].

REFERENCE

1 Bialy-Golan A, Brenner S, Anhalt GJ. Paraneoplastic pemphigus; oral involvement as the sole manifestation. *Acta Derm Venereol (Stockh)* 1996; **76**: 253–4.

IgA pemphigus (syn. intraepidermal neutrophilic IgA dermatosis). Oral lesions, blisters and ulcers have been reported. Dapsone is the therapy of choice [1–3].

REFERENCES

1 Beutner EH, Chorzelski TP, Wilson RM *et al.* IgA pemphigus foliaceus: report of two cases and a review of the literature. *J Am Acad Dermatol* 1989; **20**: 89–97.
2 Borradori L, Saada V, Rybojad M *et al.* Oral intraepidermal IgA pustulosis and Crohn's disease. *Br J Dermatol* 1992; **126**: 383–6.
3 Teraki Y, Amagou N, Hashimoto T. Intracellular IgA dermatosis of childhood. Selective deposition of monomer IgA1 in the intercellular space of the epidermis. *Arch Dermatol* 1991; **127**: 221–4.

Subepithelial autoimmune bullous diseases

A spectrum of subepithelial autoimmune bullous diseases can present with oral blisters and/or erosions, and with immune deposits at the epithelial basement membrane zone. Several distinct groups, and probably several overlap syndromes, exist.

Mucous membrane pemphigoid (Chapter 40). Mucous membrane pemphigoid involves the oral mucosa in more than one-third of cases. The usual lesion, desquamative gingivitis, is characterized by erythematous, glazed, sore gingivae (Fig. 69.30). Bullae are less common, and are seen particularly on the soft palate. They rupture to form erosions [1–4].

The bullae in mucous membrane pemphigoid are subepithelial and tend to persist for longer than those of pemphigus. The bullae may be filled with serous fluid or blood, and then must be differentiated from angina bullosa haemorrhagica (p. 3094), epidermolysis bullosa acquisita and superficial mucoceles (pp. 3086 and 3095) as well as dermatitis herpetiformis and linear IgA disease. Oral lesions may scar but this is not invariable.

A biopsy is required for diagnosis. Serum autoantibodies to epithelial basement membrane may be detected in a few patients (see Table 69.19) but many have immune deposits at the epithelial and mucous gland basement membrane zone [4–10]. A very small minority of patients have an associated internal malignancy which should be excluded.

Topical corticosteroids help if the lesions are restricted to the oral mucosa. Systemic corticosteroids may occasionally be required but tetracyclines with or without nicotinamide may help [3,9]. Dapsone may be useful in the treatment of desquamative gingivitis [9,11].

Bullous pemphigoid. Oral lesions (blisters or ulcers) are rarely seen in bullous pemphigoid.

Vegetating cicatricial pemphigoid (syn. pemphigoid vegetans). A subset of bullous pemphigoid, although clinically indistinguishable from pemphigus vegetans and sometimes producing oral blisters and erosions shows linear deposits of IgG and C3 at the epithelial basement-membrane zone on oral biopsy, but no circulating basement-membrane antibodies [10].

Palate and gingiva have been especially involved in the rare cases thus far described [12,13].

REFERENCES

1 Grattan CEH, Small D, Scully C *et al.* Oral herpes simplex infection in bullous pemphigoid. *Oral Surg* 1986; **61**: 40–3.
2 Manton S, Scully C. Mucous membrane pemphigoid. *Oral Surg* 1988; **66**: 37–40.
3 Silverman S, Gorsky M, Lozada-Nur F *et al.* Oral mucous membrane pemphigoid. *Oral Surg* 1986; **61**: 233–7.
4 Venning VA, Frith PA, Bron AJ *et al.* Mucosal involvement in bullous and cicatricial pemphigoid. A clinical and immunopathological study. *Br J Dermatol* 1988; **118**: 7–15.
5 Fleming MG, Valenzuela R, Bergfeld WF *et al.* Mucous gland basement membrane immunofluorescent in cicatricial pemphigoid. *Arch Dermatol* 1988; **124**: 1407–10.
6 Peng T, Nisengard RJ, Levine MJ. Gingival basement membrane antigens in desquamative lesions of the gingiva. *Oral Surg* 1986; **61**: 584–9.
7 Poskitt L, Wojnarowska F. Minimizing cicatricial pemphigoid orodynia with minocycline. *Br J Dermatol* 1995; **132**: 784–9.
8 Poskitt L, Wojnarowska F. Treatment of cicatricial pemphigoid with tetracycline and nicotinamide. *Clin Exp Dermatol* 1995; **20**: 258–9.
9 Rogers RS, Seehafer JR, Perry H. Treatment of cicatricial (benign mucous membrane) pemphigoid with dapsone. *J Am Acad Dermatol* 1982; **6**: 215–23.
10 Vincent SD, Lilly GE, Baker KA. Clinical, historic and therapeutic features of cicatricial pemphigoid. *Oral Surg* 1993; **76**: 453–9.
11 Matthews RW, Pinkney RC, Scully C. The management of desquamative gingivitis with dapsone. *Ann Dent* 1981; **48**: 41–3.
12 Liu HN, Su WP, Rogers RS *et al.* Clinical variants of pemphigoid. *Int J Dermatol* 1986; **25**: 17–27.
13 Wolf K, Rappersberger K, Steiner A *et al.* Vegetating cicatricial pemphigoid. *Arch Dermatol Res* 1987; **279**: S30–7.

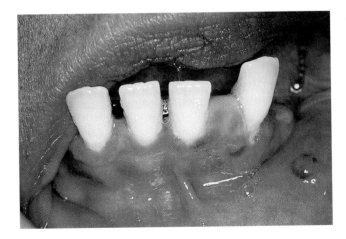

Fig. 69.30 Pemphigoid: vesicles and desquamative gingivitis.

Epidermolysis bullosa acquisita (Chapter 40). Blisters or ulcers may be seen in the oral mucosa in epidermolysis bullosa acquisita (EBA), and biopsy shows IgG and C3 in the sublamina densa zone of the epithelial basement membrane, by immunoelectron microscopy [1,2].

REFERENCES

1 Prost C, Labeille B, Chanssade V *et al.* Immunoelectron microscopy in subepidermal autoimmune bullous diseases: a prospective study of IgG and C3 bound *in vivo* in 32 patients. *J Invest Dermatol* 1987; **89**: 567–73.
2 Rubenstein R, Sterley NB, Fine JD. Childhood epidermolysis bullosa acquisita. *Arch Dermatol* 1987; **123**: 772–6.

Dermatitis herpetiformis and adult linear IgA disease. Oral lesions may occur in dermatitis herpetiformis and in most patients with linear IgA disease. Macules, papules, petechiae, vesicles, bullae and erosions are the usual manifestations [1–8]. These disorders must be differentiated especially from pemphigoid, angina bullosa haemorrhagica and superficial mucoceles.

Salivary IgA antigliadin antibodies may be found but this is not useful diagnostically. Dapsone and sulphapyridine are the most effective therapeutic agents along with a gluten-free diet in dermatitis herpetiformis.

REFERENCES

1 Chan LS, Regezi JA, Cooper KD. Oral manifestations of linear IgA disease. *J Am Acad Dermatol* 1990; **22**: 362–5.
2 Cowan CG, Lamey PJ, Walsh M *et al.* Linear IgA disease (LAD); immunoglobulin deposition in oral and colonic lesions. *J Oral Pathol Med* 1995; **24**: 374–8.
3 Economopoulou P, Laskaris G. Dermatitis herpetiformis: oral lesions as an early manifestation. *Oral Surg* 1986; **62**: 77–80.
4 Hall RP, Waldbauer GV. Characterisation of the mucosal immune response to dietary antigens in patients with dermatitis herpetiformis. *J Invest Dermatol* 1988; **90**: 658–63.
5 Kelly SE, Frith PA, Millard PR *et al.* A clinopathological study of mucosal involvement in linear IgA disease. *Br J Dermatol* 1988; **119**: 161–70.
6 Porter SR, Bain SE, Scully C. Linear IgA disease manifesting as recalcitrant desquamative gingivitis. *Oral Surg* 1992; **74**: 179–82.
7 Porter SR, Scully C, Midda M *et al.* Adult linear IgA disease manifesting as desquamative gingivitis. *Oral Surg* 1990; **70**: 450–3.
8 Wiesenfeld D, Martin A, Scully C *et al.* Oral manifestations in linear IgA disease. *Br Dent J* 1982; **153**: 389–99.

Chronic bullous dermatosis of childhood (Chapter 40). Oral ulceration has been reported [1].

REFERENCE

1 Wojnarowska F, Marsden RA, Bhogal B, Black MM. Chronic bullous disease of childhood, childhood cicatricial pemphigoid and linear IgA disease of adults; a comparative study demonstrating clinical and immunopathological overlap. *J Am Acad Dermatol* 1988; **19**: 792–805.

Toxic epidermal necrolysis (Chapter 40). Oral lesions can be seen in over 95% of patients with toxic epidermal necrolysis (TEN). The blisters and erosions may precede the skin lesions by a day or so and may persist [1–3].

There is no specific therapy [4] but 2% lignocaine and 0.2% aqueous chlorhexidine mouth baths may provide symptomatic relief.

REFERENCES

1 Cohen SG, Glick M, Schaeffer VH. Toxic epidermal necrolysis. *Special Care Dent* 1989; **9**: 6–9.
2 Giallorenzi AF, Goldstein BH. Acute (toxic) epidermal necrolysis: report of a case. *Oral Surg* 1975; **40**: 611–15.
3 Marra LM, Wunderlee RC. Oral presentation of toxic epidermal necrolysis. *J Oral Maxillofac Surg* 1982; **40**: 59–61.
4 Revuz J, Penso D, Roujeau JC. Toxic epidermal necrolysis: clinical findings and prognostic factors in 87 patients. *Arch Dermatol* 1987; **123**: 1160–5.

Erythema multiforme (Chapter 45). In erythema multiforme, the oral mucosa may be involved alone or in association with skin lesions [1–4]. Mucosal lesions begin as erythematous areas which blister and break down to irregular, extensive, painful erosions with extensive surrounding erythema. The labial mucosa is often involved, and a serosanguinous exudate leads to crusting of the swollen lips. A biopsy may be required if the diagnosis is doubtful.

An attempt should be made to identify any precipitating factors. Aciclovir may control herpes simplex-induced erythema multiforme [5].

Oral hygiene should be maintained and, in severe cases, systemic corticosteroids, levamisole or azathioprine may be needed [2,3].

REFERENCES

1 Barrett AW, Scully C, Eveson JW. Erythema multiforme involving the gingiva. *J Periodontol* 1993; **64**: 910–13.
2 Lozada F. Prednisone and azathioprine in the treatment of patients with vesiculoerosive oral diseases. *Oral Surg* 1981; **52**: 257–60.
3 Lozada-Nur F, Gorsky M, Silverman S. Oral erythema multiforme; clinical observations and treatment of 95 patients. *Oral Surg* 1989; **67**: 36–40.
4 Nesbit SP, Gobetti JP. Multiple occurrences of oral erythema multiforme after secondary herpes simplex: report of case and review of literature. *J Am Dent Assoc* 1986; **112**: 348–52.
5 Scully C, Epstein JB, Porter SR. Viruses and chronic diseases of the oral mucosa. *Oral Surg* 1991; **72**: 537–44.

Lichen sclerosus (Chapter 72). Oral lichen sclerosus presents with whitish plaques, papules or a reticular pattern, or erosions—all features of LP [1–4]. Histologically, however, lichen sclerosus has epithelial atrophy with hyperkeratosis, oedema in the papillary corium and the lymphocytic infiltrate is less close to the epithelium than in LP. It has been suggested that mucosal lichen sclerosus is more common than formerly thought and may cause dysplasia [5].

REFERENCES

1 MacLeod RI, Soames JV. Lichen sclerosus et atrophicus of the oral mucosa. *Br J Oral Maxillofac Surg* 1991; **89**: 64–5.
2 Ravits HG, Welsh AL. Lichen sclerosus et atrophicus of the mouth. *Arch Dermatol* 1957; **76**: 56–8.

3 De Araujo VC, Orsini SC, Marcucci G *et al.* Lichen sclerosus et atrophicus. *Oral Surg* 1985; **60**: 655–7.
4 Miller RF. Lichen sclerosus et atrophicus with oral involvement. *Arch Dermatol* 1957; **76**: 43–55.
5 Maren P, Millard P, Chia Y, Wojnarowska F. Mucosal lichen sclerosus/lichen planus overlap syndromes. *Br J Dermatol* 1994; **131**: 118–23.

Chronic ulcerative stomatitis with epithelial antinuclear antibodies. Chronic erosive or ulcerative stomatitis, presenting as desquamative gingivitis with or without lesions on buccal or lingual mucosa and sometimes resembling LP, may be associated with lichenoid histology but stratified, squamous epithelial, antinuclear antibodies. Circulating antibodies are also found. The lesions appear to respond to hydroxychloroquine [1–3].

REFERENCES

1 Jarenko WM, Beutner EH, Kumar V *et al.* Chronic ulcerative stomatitis associated with a specific immunologic marker. *J Am Acad Dermatol* 1990; **22**: 215–20.
2 Beutner EH, Chorzelski TP, Parodi A *et al.* Ten cases of chronic ulcerative stomatitis with stratified epithelium-specific antinuclear antibody. *J Am Acad Dermatol* 1991; **24**: 781–2.
3 Church LF, Schosser RH. Chronic ulcerative stomatitis associated with stratified epithelial specific antinuclear antibody. *Oral Surg* 1992; **73**: 579–82.

Lupus erythematosus (Chapter 58)

Almost half of the patients with systemic lupus erythematosus (SLE) suffer from oral lesions, which begin as red patches which break down to irregular slit-like ulcers which often heal with scarring [1]. Lesions particularly affect the palate. Sjögren's syndrome may occur in SLE. Oral petechiae and herpetic infections are also common. Rarely, dental surgery has been followed by facial swelling [2].

Similar erosions, with a white border, occur in discoid lupus erythematosus (Fig. 69.31). Discoid lupus erythematosus may predispose to oral carcinoma [3]. Oral ulceration has also been described in drug-induced lupus.

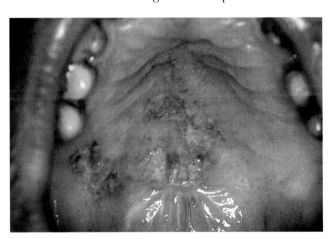

Fig. 69.31 Chronic oral lesions in discoid lupus erythematosus.

Systemic corticosteroids, often with an immunosuppressant, may be required in severe cases.

Other collagen–vascular diseases

Dermatomyositis and mixed connective tissue disease may be associated with non-specific mucosal erosions [4].

Oral involvement in Reiter's syndrome may include red patches or superficial painless mucosal erosions which may resemble erythema migrans (geographical tongue) both clinically and histologically.

REFERENCES

1 Schiodt M. Oral manifestations of lupus erythematosus. *Int J Oral Surg* 1984; **13**: 101–47.
2 Loescher A, Edmondson HD. Lupus erythematosus—a case of facial swelling. *Br J Oral Surg* 1988; **26**: 129–32.
3 Handlers JP, Abrams AM, Aberle AM *et al.* Squamous cell carcinoma of the lip developing in discoid lupus erythematosus. *Oral Surg* 1985; **60**: 382–6.
4 Porter SR, Malamos D, Scully C. Mouth–skin interface: 2. Connective tissue and metabolic disorders. *Update* 1986; **33**: 94–6.

Metabolic disorders

Glucagonoma

Oral ulceration can be a severe manifestation in glucagonoma [1].

REFERENCE

1 Ditty FR, Lang PG. Cutaneous and oral changes as the only manifestations of the glucagonoma syndrome. *South Med J* 1982; **75**: 222–4.

Infective diseases

Oral ulceration is common in some viral infections. It can also occur in several bacterial diseases (notably acute necrotizing gingivitis, tuberculosis and syphilis), but is rare in fungal infections other than the deep mycoses.

Herpes simplex stomatitis

Aetiology. Herpes simplex virus (HSV) infection is a common infection. In general, HSV-1 causes primary herpetic stomatitis (and the secondary infection of recurrent herpes labialis). There are no precise distinctions nowadays, presumably with more frequent orogenital and oroanal sexual practices, and oral infection with HSV-2 is also frequently seen.

With improving socio-economic circumstances and standards of hygiene, a larger number of children are not exposed to HSV and enter adult life without immunity. Cases of primary herpetic stomatitis are, therefore, now seen occasionally in adults, and the manifestations can be severe. HSV is usually transmitted in saliva.

Clinical features. The incubation period is 3–7 days. Many infections with HSV occur in childhood and are subclinical and, where there is disease, it varies greatly in severity. In many it is trivial and passed off as 'teething.'

Primary herpetic stomatitis presents with malaise, anorexia, irritability and fever, anterior cervical lymph nodes which are enlarged and tender, and a diffuse, purple, boggy gingivitis, especially anteriorly, with multiple vesicles followed by round or ovoid ulcers 1–3mm in diameter scattered across the oral mucosa and gingiva (Fig. 69.32) [1–3].

Prognosis. Herpetic stomatitis resolves spontaneously in 7–10 days but HSV remains latent in the trigeminal ganglion. The most obvious sequel is that about one-third of patients are thereafter predisposed to recurrences. HSV is shed intermittently into the saliva.

Diagnosis. The main differential diagnoses are chickenpox and other viral causes of mouth ulcers, and acute leukaemia. A full blood picture, white-cell count and differential, viral studies and a cytological smear (which shows multinucleate giant cells) may therefore be required.

Treatment. Specific antiviral agents are most useful in the very early stages of disease, before most patients present for treatment. In general, antivirals are indicated, especially for immunocompromised patients who may otherwise suffer severe infection. Both oral and intravenous aciclovir appear to be effective.

For most, however, management is supportive with antipyretic analgesics (e.g. paracetamol), sponging with tepid water and a high fluid intake. Analgesics (as elixirs or syrups for children) and, in adults, lignocaine mouthbaths help ease discomfort and 0.2% aqueous chlorhexidine mouthbaths aid resolution.

An antihistamine such as promethazine may help sedate an irritable child.

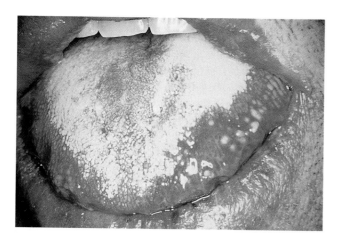

Fig. 69.32 Scattered ulcers and a furred tongue in primary herpetic stomatitis.

Recurrent intraoral herpes simplex infection. Chronic oral herpetic ulcers, often with a raised, white border, and sometimes with a dendritic appearance may occasionally affect apparently healthy individuals, especially at sites of trauma, for example following palatal infiltration of a local anaesthetic. Chronic indolent lesions, usually ulcerative or nodular, may be seen in patients with neutropenia or chronic leukaemia [2,4,5] and, in patients with more severe immunosuppression such as acute leukaemia or HIV infection [1,6,7], more aggressive ulcers may be seen (see Fig. 69.22). Aciclovir may be indicated systemically [8].

REFERENCES

1 Greenberg MS, Cohen SG, Boosz B *et al*. Oral herpes simplex infections in patients with leukaemia. *J Am Dent Assoc* 1987; **114**: 483–6.
2 Grossman ME, Stevens AW, Cohen PR. Herpetic geometric glossitis. *N Engl J Med* 1993; **329**: 1859–60.
3 Scully C. Ulcerative stomatitis gingivitis and rash: a diagnostic dilemma. *Oral Surg* 1985; **59**: 261–3.
4 Barrett AP. Chronic indolent orofacial herpes simplex virus infection in chronic leukaemia. *Oral Surg* 1988; **66**: 387–90.
5 Cohen SG, Greenberg MS. Chronic oral herpes simplex virus infection in immunocompromised patients. *Oral Surg* 1985; **59**: 465–71.
6 Bergmann OJ, Mogensen SC, Ellegaard J. Herpes simplex virus and intraoral ulcers in immunocompromised patients with haematologic malignancies. *Eur J Clin Microbiol Infect Dis* 1990; **9**: 184–90.
7 Scully C. Orofacial herpes simplex virus infections: current concepts in the epidemiology, pathogenesis and treatment, and disorders in which the virus may be implicated. *Oral Surg* 1989; **68**: 701–10.
8 Scully C. Infectious diseases in oral medicine. In: Millard D, Mason DK, eds. *1993 World Workshop on Oral Medicine*. Michigan: University of Michigan, 1995: 16–23.

Chickenpox (Chapter 26)

Chickenpox affects children predominantly and may present with mouth ulcers which resemble those of herpetic stomatitis, but there is no gingivitis [1]. There may be a contact history. Many primary infections with varicella–zoster virus (VZV) are subclinical or produce so few lesions as to pass almost unnoticed. VZV remains latent in sensory ganglia and may be reactivated to produce shingles.

Herpes zoster
SYN. SHINGLES

If shingles affects the maxillary or mandibular divisions of the trigeminal nerve, mouth ulcers are usually seen.

Clinical features. The pain of trigeminal zoster may simulate toothache. Severe pain often precedes, accompanies and follows the rash, and post-herpetic neuralgia may persist for months or years.

The rash is restricted to a dermatome and is unilateral, but sometimes a few chickenpox-type lesions can be found elsewhere. Oral ulcers appear in the distribution of the involved nerve division [2]. There is ulceration of one side of the tongue, floor of mouth, lower labial and buccal mucosa if the mandibular division of the trigeminal nerve is involved. One side of the palate, the upper gingiva and buccal sulcus are involved in maxillary zoster. Rarely, mandibular or maxillary zoster may disturb the formation of developing teeth [3] or cause jaw necrosis [4].

If the geniculate ganglion of the facial nerve is affected, there may be unilateral facial palsy, with vesicles in the ipsilateral ear and ulcers in the soft palate ipsilaterally (*Ramsay–Hunt syndrome*).

Zoster resolves spontaneously but post-herpetic neuralgia can be distressing.

Occasionally there is misdiagnosis of toothache, leading to extraction, the true diagnosis becoming apparent only when the rash appears.

Management. An underlying immune defect, such as acquired immune deficiency syndrome (AIDS) or malignancy should be excluded in zoster.

Treatment is mainly supportive but antivirals such as aciclovir can be useful. Analgesics are indicated in zoster, but the pain may prove refractory to even potent analgesics.

REFERENCES

1 Badger GR. Oral signs of chickenpox (varicella): report of two cases. *ASDC J Dent Child* 1980; **47**: 349–51.
2 Scully C, Samaranayake LP. *Clinical Oral Virology*. Cambridge: Cambridge University Press, 1992.
3 Smith S, Ross JR, Scully C. An unusual oral complication of herpes zoster infection. *Oral Surg* 1984; **57**: 388–9.
4 Wright WE, Davis ML, Geffen DB *et al.* Alveolar bone necrosis and tooth loss: a rare complication associated with herpes zoster infection of the fifth cranial nerve. *Oral Surg* 1983; **56**: 39–46.

Herpangina

Aetiology. Herpangina is caused by Coxsackie viruses. The incubation period is 3–7 days and young children are predominantly affected.

Clinical features. Many infections are subclinical but features of the clinical syndrome include malaise, anorexia, irritability, low fever, slightly enlarged and tender anterior cervical lymph nodes and mouth ulcers, predominantly on the soft palate [1].

Diagnosis. There may be a contact history. It is possible to culture Coxsackie viruses in suckling mice if absolutely necessary.

The main differential diagnosis is primary herpetic stomatitis, but in herpangina there is less fever, no acute gingivitis and ulceration is mainly restricted to the soft palate.

Treatment. The condition is self-limiting, and treatment is supportive only.

REFERENCE

1 Bell EJ, Williams GR, Grist NR *et al.* Enterovirus infections. *Update* 1983; **26**: 967–78.

Hand, foot and mouth disease (Chapter 26)

Aetiology. Hand, foot and mouth disease is caused particularly by Coxsackie A viruses but sometimes by Coxsackie B viruses, or enteroviruses.

Clinical features. The incubation period is 3–10 days and, although young children are predominantly infected, there are occasional outbreaks in adults. Many infections are subclinical but features of the clinical syndrome include:
1 general features—malaise, anorexia, irritability and fever may be present but usually only in severe cases;
2 anterior cervical lymph nodes may occasionally be slightly enlarged and tender;
3 mouth ulcers which are round or ovoid, usually sparse and may affect any site [1–3];
4 rash—painful, sometimes deep-seated vesicles may appear, usually on the hand and / or feet, particularly on digits or at the base of the phalanges.

Hand, foot and mouth disease is self-limiting and only rarely complicated by systemic illness such as encephalitis.

The condition tends to be more severe when it occurs in adults.

Diagnosis and management are as for herpangina.

REFERENCES

1 Conway SP. Coxsackie B2 virus causing simultaneous hand, foot and mouth disease and encephalitis. *J Infect* 1987; **15**: 191.
2 Goh KT, Doraisingham S, Tan JC *et al.* An outbreak of hand, foot and mouth disease in Singapore. *Bull WHO* 1982; **60**: 965–9.
3 Ishimaru Y, Nakano S, Yamaoka K *et al.* Outbreak of hand, foot and mouth disease caused by Enterovirus 71. *Arch Dis Child* 1980; **55**: 583–8.

Infectious mononucleosis (Chapter 26)

Epstein–Barr virus (EBV) is found in pharyngeal epithelium and appears in the saliva of patients with infectious mononucleosis and for several months after clinical recovery. Infection appears to be spread by close oral contact, especially kissing.

Infection is often subclinical. Infectious mononucleosis is protean in its clinical manifestations, which include particularly lymphadenopathy, sore throat, fever, malaise and rashes. In the anginose type (sore-throat type), the throat is sore with soft-palate petechiae and a whitish exudate on oedematous tonsils. There may be non-specific oral ulceration or pericoronitis [1]. The glandular type of infectious mononucleosis is characterized by generalized lymph-node enlargement and splenomegaly; the febrile type by fever.

Similar syndromes may be caused by cytomegalovirus (CMV), human herpesvirus 6 (HHV-6), and by HIV. Characteristic of infectious mononucleosis are large numbers of atypical mononuclear cells in the blood and a wide variety of serological changes, particularly heterophil antibodies which are detectable by the Paul–Bunnell or Monospot tests, usually during the first or second week of illness. Several other antibodies against EBV appear during the course of infectious mononucleosis, but the most frequent is the antibody to viral capsid antigen (VCA), the titre of which reaches a peak at about 4 weeks.

No specific treatment is available, but supportive care should be given. Systemic corticosteroids are required if there is pharyngeal oedema severe enough to hazard the airway.

REFERENCE

1 Scully C, Samaranayake LP. *Clinical Oral Virology.* Cambridge: Cambridge University Press, 1992.

Cytomegalovirus infection

CMV may cause a glandular fever type of syndrome, and rarely causes oral ulceration. Indolent CMV-induced oral ulcers have been described in immunosuppressed patients and in AIDS [1–3].

REFERENCES

1 Epstein JB, Scully C. Cytomegalovirus: a virus of increasing relevance to oral medicine and pathology. *J Oral Pathol Med* 1993; **22**: 348–53.
2 Kanas RJ, Jensen JL, Abrams AM *et al.* Oral mucosal cytomegalovirus as a manifestation of the acquired immune deficiency syndrome. *Oral Surg* 1987; **64**: 183–9.
3 Myerson D, Hackman RC, Nelson JA *et al.* Widespread evidence of histologically occult cytomegalovirus. *Hum Pathol* 1984; **15**: 430–9.

Mucocutaneous lymph-node syndrome (Chapter 26)
SYN. KAWASAKI DISEASE

Mucocutaneous lymph-node syndrome (MLNS) is a disorder of uncertain, but possibly infectious, aetiology. Male children are predominantly affected.

At least one oral feature should be present for the diagnosis of MLNS to be made. The oral and pharyngeal mucosa become generally red and sore and the lips dry and fissured. There may be oral ulceration and a 'strawberry tongue' appearance [1,2].

Cervical lymphadenopathy, conjunctivitis, and fever also occur, followed later by the characteristic desquamation of the skin of the hands and feet.

Early therapy with immunoglobulin is essential to avoid cardiac complications.

REFERENCES

1 Ogden GR, Kerr M. Mucocutaneous lymph node syndrome (Kawasaki disease). *Oral Surg* 1989; **67**: 569–72.
2 Terezhalmy GT. Mucocutaneous lymph node syndrome. *Oral Surg* 1979; **47**: 26–30.

Acute necrotizing (ulcerative) gingivitis and noma

Aetiology. There is no firm evidence of communicability of acute necrotizing gingivitis (ANG), although it may occur in epidemic form, especially in institutions or in the military (trench mouth). Viral respiratory infections, overwork and fatigue, smoking or immune defects may precede the onset of disease, suggesting depression of immunity as a predisposing cause. A similar lesion may be a feature of HIV infection and related diseases.

A mixed, mainly anaerobic, flora (the fusospirochaetal complex), consisting mainly of Fusobacterium nucleatum (*F. fusiformis* or *Bacillus fusiformis*) and *Borrelia vincentii*, is associated with this infection [1,2].

Clinical features. The mouth ulceration is usually restricted to the gingiva, specifically the interdental papillae which appear blunted (Figs 69.33 & 69.34). The history is characteristic with an acute onset of gingival soreness, bleeding and halitosis. ANG occurs especially in the anterior part of the mouth where the affected gingiva are extremely tender to touch and readily bleed on minimal pressure. Occasionally the ulceration extends elsewhere on the gingiva, or onto the adjacent mucosa. There is often enlargement of the cervical lymph nodes and there may be pyrexia and malaise.

Prognosis. Failure to adequately treat ANG may predispose to recurrence and, in malnourished or immunocompromised individuals may lead to noma (cancrum oris) [3–7]. Similar lesions of gangrenous stomatitis are increasingly reported in HIV disease.

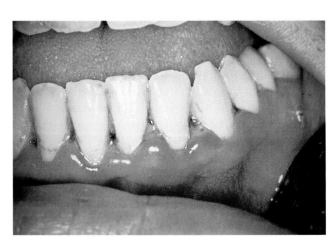

Fig. 69.33 Acute necrotizing gingivitis showing typical ulceration of interdental gingival papillae. This was in human immunodeficiency virus infection.

Secondary syphilis follows after 6–8 weeks, with oral lesions in about one-third of patients [1,3]. These are highly infectious and are usually fairly painless ulcers (mucous patches and snailtrack ulcers).

The most characteristic oral lesion of tertiary syphilis is a localized granuloma (gumma) varying in size from a pinhead to several centimetres affecting particularly the palate, or the tongue. Gummas break down to form deep chronic punched-out ulcers which are not infectious (Fig. 69.35). The most common oral manifestation of tertiary syphilis is, however, a leukoplakia which particularly affects the dorsum of the tongue and has a high potential for malignant change.

Congenital syphilis may, when the permanent teeth erupt, present with dental anomalies such as Hutchinson's teeth (Fig. 69.36). Oral ulcers are rare.

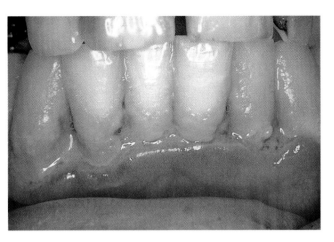

Fig. 69.34 Untreated acute necrotizing gingivitis can lead to extensive gingival ulceration and irreparable damage.

Diagnosis. Diagnosis is mainly from gingival lesions in primary herpetic stomatitis, leukaemias and HIV disease. A bacteriological smear may be helpful.

Treatment. Gentle cleansing with a hydrogen peroxide mouthwash and a soft toothbrush is remarkably effective. Oral metronidazole 200 mg should be given three times daily for 3–7 days to limit the tissue destruction. Penicillin is equally effective. The patient should also be referred for dental advice [1].

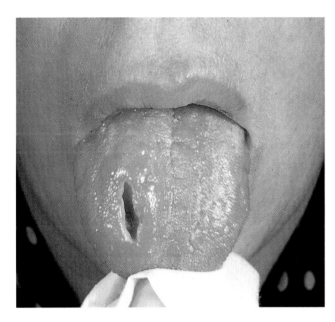

Fig. 69.35 Gumma.

REFERENCES

1 Johnson BD, Engel D. Acute necrotising ulcerative gingivitis: a review of diagnosis, etiology and treatment. *J Periodontol* 1986; **57**: 141–50.
2 Osuji OO. Necrotizing ulcerative gingivitis and cancrum oris (noma) in Ibadan, Nigeria. *J Periodontol* 1990; **61**: 769–72.
3 Enwonwu CO. Infectious oral necrosis (cancrum oris) in Nigerian children. *Community Dent Oral Epidemiol* 1985; **13**: 190–4.
4 Madden N. An interesting case of facial gangrene (from Papua, New Guinea). *Oral Surg* 1985; **59**: 279.
5 Sabiston CB. A review and proposal for the etiology of acute necrotizing gingivitis. *J Clin Periodontol* 1986; **13**: 727–34.
6 Sawyer D, Nwoku AJ. Cancrum oris (noma): past and present. *J Dent Child* 1981; **48**: 138–41.
7 Stassen LFA, Batchelor AGG, Rennie JS *et al.* Cancrum oris in an adult Caucasian female. *Br J Oral Maxillofac Surg* 1989; **27**: 417–22.

Syphilis

Oral ulcers may be seen at any stage but particularly in secondary syphilis [1–3]. In primary syphilis, a primary chancre (hard or Hunterian chancre) may involve the lips, tongue or palate. A small, firm, pink, macule changes to a papule which ulcerates to form a painless, round ulcer with a raised margin and indurated base [4]. Chancres heal spontaneously in 3–8 weeks but are highly infectious and are associated with enlarged, painless regional lymph nodes.

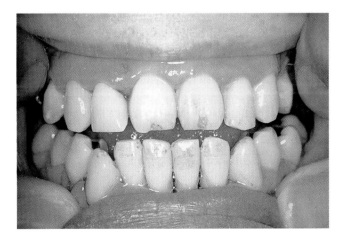

Fig. 69.36 Hutchinson's maxillary central incisors.

Exudate from a suspected oral lesion of syphilis should be examined for treponemes by dark-ground microscopy but, since the diagnosis can be confused by oral commensal treponemes, lesions should first be thoroughly swabbed with a sterile gauze or cotton wool then gently scraped with a sterile spatula; and the scraping examined immediately by dark-ground microscopy. Serology is indicated. Biopsy is not usually indicated, but lesions are characterized by a dense plasma-cell infiltrate.

REFERENCES

1 Manton SL, Eggleston SI, Alexander I *et al.* Oral presentation of secondary syphilis. *Br Dent J* 1986; **160**: 237–8.
2 Samaranayake LP, Scully C. Oral disease and sexual medicine. *Br J Sexual Med* 1988; **15**: 138–43, 174–80.
3 Terezhalmy GT. Oral manifestations of sexually-related diseases. *Ear Nose Throat J* 1983; **62**: 287–96.
4 Cousteau C, Leyder P, Laufer J. Syphilis primaire buccale: un diagnostic parfois difficile. *Rev Stomatol Chir Maxillofac* 1984; **85**: 391–8.

Gonorrhoea

Oral mucosal erythema, sometimes with oedema and ulceration, is occasionally seen in oropharyngeal gonorrhoea. Oropharyngeal asymptomatic carriage of gonococci is more common, in around 4% of those attending clinics for sexually transmitted diseases [1,2].

REFERENCES

1 Brown RT, Lossick JG, Mosure DJ *et al.* Pharyngeal gonorrhoea screening in adolescents: is it necessary? *Pediatrics* 1989; **84**: 623–5.
2 Guinta JL, Fiumara NJ. Facts about gonorrhoea and dentistry. *Oral Surg* 1986; **62**: 529.

Tuberculosis

Oral lesions can develop in pulmonary tuberculosis but are not common. A chronic ulcer, usually of the dorsum of the tongue, is the most common oral presentation but jaw lesions or cervical lymph node involvement may be seen [1–4]. Atypical mycobacteria are not uncommonly involved.

Mycobacterial oral ulcers, particularly caused by *Mycobacterium avium–intracellulare*, have been reported as a complication of AIDS and occasionally in apparently healthy individuals [5]. Cervicofacial infection is occasionally caused by *M. chelonei*, usually in the form of lymph-node abscesses, or occasionally as intraoral swellings [6–9].

REFERENCES

1 Dimitrakopoulos I, Zouloumis L, Lazaridis N *et al.* Primary tuberculosis of the oral cavity. *Oral Surg* 1991; **72**: 712–15.
2 Haddad NM, Zaytoun GM, Hadi U. Tuberculosis of the soft palate: an unusual presentation of oral tuberculosis. *Otol Head Neck Surg* 1987; **97**: 91–9.
3 Michaud M, Blanchette G, Tomich CF. Chronic ulceration of the hard palate: first clinical sign of undiagnosed pulmonary tuberculosis. *Oral Surg* 1984; **57**: 63–7.

4 Waldman RH. Tuberculosis and the atypical mycobacteria. *Otolaryngol Clin North Am* 1982; **15**: 581–96.
5 Morris CA, Grant GH, Everall PH *et al.* Tuberculoid lymphadenitis due to *Mycobacterium chelonei. J Clin Pathol* 1973; **26**: 422–6.
6 Blake GC, Murray JJ, Lee KW. Cervicofacial infection with *Mycobacterium chelonei. Br J Oral Surg* 1976; **13**: 278–81.
7 Boyd BW. Oral infection with associated lymphadenopathy due to *Mycobacterium chelonei. Ala Med* 1984; **54**: 9–10.
8 Pedersen A, Reibel J. Intraoral infection with *Mycobacterium chelonei. Oral Surg* 1989; **67**: 262–5.
9 Volpe F, Schwimmer A, Barr C. Oral manifestations of disseminated Mycobacterium avium-intracellulare in a patient with *AIDS. Oral Surg* 1985; **60**: 567–70.

Epithelioid (bacillary) angiomatosis (Chapter 27)

Oral lesions clinically and to some extent histologically reminiscent of Kaposi's sarcoma have been seen in HIV disease [1–3], sometimes as the first manifestation of HIV infection [3].

REFERENCES

1 Glick M, Cleveland DB. Oral mucosal bacillary epithelioid angiomatosis in a patient with AIDS associated with rapid alveolar bone loss. *J Oral Pathol Med* 1993; **22**: 235–9.
2 Levell NJ, Bewley AP, Chopra S *et al.* Bacillary angiomatosis with cutaneous and oral lesions in an HIV-infected patient from the UK. *Br J Dermatol* 1995; **132**: 113–15.
3 Speight PM, Zakrzewska J, Fletcher CDM. Epithelioid angiomatosis affecting the oral cavity as the first sign of HIV infection. *Br Dent J* 1991; **171**: 367–70.

Fungal infections

Oral fungal infections, apart from candidiasis which rarely causes mouth ulcers in Western societies, are usually seen in the West only in immunocompromised or debilitated patients, including those with AIDS. However, they occasionally may be seen in otherwise healthy persons from the tropics (Table 69.20).

Histoplasmosis. Oral lesions of histoplasmosis are uncommon. They are typically seen in chronic disseminated histoplasmosis, usually as a non-specific lump or ulcer on the tongue, palate, buccal mucosa or gingiva [1–5], sometimes in HIV disease [6,7].

REFERENCES

1 Adekeye EO, Edwards MB, Williams HK. Mandibular African histoplasmosis: imitation of neoplasia or giant cell granuloma. *Oral Surg* 1988; **65**: 81–4.
2 Cobb CM, Shultz RE, Brewer JH *et al.* Chronic pulmonary histoplasmosis with an oral lesion. *Oral Surg* 1989; **67**: 73–6.
3 Goodwin RA, Shapiro JL, Thurman GH *et al.* Disseminated histoplasmosis: clinical and pathologic correlations. *Medicine* 1980; **59**: 93–100.
4 Miller RL, Gould AR, Skolnick JL *et al.* Localised oral histoplasmosis. *Oral Surg* 1982; **53**: 367–74.
5 Scully C, Almeida O. Orofacial manifestations of the systemic mycoses. *J Oral Pathol Med* 1992; **21**: 289–94.
6 Filho FJS, Lopes M, Almeida OPD, Scully C. Mucocutaneous histoplasmosis in AIDS. *Br J Dermatol* 1995; **133**: 472–4.
7 Scully C, Almeida OPD, Sposto MR. Deep mycoses in HIV infection. *Oral Dis* 1997; **3**(Suppl. 1): 200–7.

Table 69.20 Rare orofacial fungal infections.

Infection	Oral manifestations
Aspergillosis	Aspergilloma Rhinocerebral type causes palatal necrosis Disseminated in immunocompromised patients
Blastomycosis	
North American	Oral ulcers, or suppurating granulomas
South American (paracoccidioidomycosis)	Oral ulcers and lymphadenopathy
Coccidioidomycosis	Rarely oral ulcers
Cryptococcosis	Oral ulcers
Histoplasmosis	Lumps or ulcers in mouth
Phycomycosis (mucormycosis, zygomycosis)	Antral involvement with palatal ulceration in immunocompromised patients—especially diabetics
Sporotrichosis	Oral lesions rare

Aspergillosis. Rhinocerebral aspergillosis may ulcerate through to the mouth. This is a rare event, except in the severely immunocompromised [1,2].

REFERENCES

1 Beck-Mannagetta J, Necek D, Grasserbauer M. Solitary aspergillosis of maxillary sinus, a complication of dental treatment. *Lancet* 1983; **ii**: 1260.
2 Schubert MM. Head and neck aspergillosis in patients undergoing bone-marrow transplantation. Cancer 1986; **57**: 1092–6.

Cryptococcus. Cryptococcus neoformans may occasionally produce indolent oral ulcers in immunocomprised patients [1,2].

REFERENCES

1 Glick M, Cohen SG, Cheney RT *et al*. Oral manifestations of disseminated *Cryptococcus neoformans* in a patient with acquired immunodeficiency syndrome. *Oral Surg* 1987; **64**: 454–9.
2 Lynch DP, Naftolin LZ. Oral Cryptococcus neoformans infection in AIDS. *Oral Surg* 1987; **64**: 449–53.

Mucormycosis. Rhinocerebral mucormycosis typically commences in the nasal cavity or paranasal sinuses and invades the palate to produce a black necrotic ulcer, but it might occasionally commence in the palate [1–3]. Most cases are seen in diabetics or in immunocompromised patients. Biopsy and radiography are required for diagnosis. Treatment is surgical debridement together with amphotericin intravenously and/or ketoconazole.

REFERENCES

1 Forteza G, Burgeno M, Martonerll V *et al*. Rhinocerebral mucormycosis. *J Cranio maxillofac Surg* 1988; **16**: 80–4.
2 Hauman CHJ, Raubenheimer EJ. Orofacial mucormycosis. *Oral Surg* 1989; **68**: 624–7.
3 Jones AC, Bentsen TY, Freedman PD. Mucor in the oral cavity. *Oral Surg* 1993; **75**: 455–60.

Blastomycoses. Blastomycoses may produce oral lesions which are typically mulberry-like, ulcerated swellings especially seen on the gingiva and alveolus [1,2].

REFERENCES

1 Almeida OP, Jacks J, Scully C *et al*. Orofacial manifestations of paracoccidioidomycosis (South American blastomycosis). *Oral Surg* 1991; **72**: 430–5.
2 Sposto MR, Scully C, Almeida OPD *et al*. Oral paracoccidioidomycosis: a study of 36 South American patients. *Oral Surg* 1993; **75**: 461–5.

Protozoal infestations

Leishmaniasis is rare in northern Europe and the USA; it is not uncommon, however, in hotter climes and may cause ulcers in the mouth or more commonly on the lips [1–4] particularly in HIV [5–8] or other immunocompromised persons.

REFERENCES

1 Abbas K, El Toumn IA, El Hassan AM. Oral leishmaniasis associated with kala-azar. *Oral Surg* 1992; **73**: 583–4.
2 Baily GG, Pitt MA, Cury A *et al*. Leishmaniasis of the tongue treated with liposomal amphotericin B. *J Infect* 1994; **28**: 327–31.
3 Kerdel-Vegas F. American leishmaniasis. *Int J Dermatol* 1982; **21**: 291–303.
4 Marsden PD, Sampaio RN, Rocha R *et al*. Mucocutaneous leishmaniasis: an unsolved clinical problem. *Trop Doct* 1977; **7**: 7–11.
5 Imhof M, Schofer H, Milbradt R, Lutz T. Mucocutaneous leishmaniasis in a European HIV-positive patient. *Eur J Dermatol* 1995; **5**: 594–6.
6 Michiels JF, Monteil RA, Hofman P *et al*. Oral leishmaniasis and Kaposi's sarcoma in an AIDS patient. *J Oral Pathol Med* 1994; **23**: 45–6.
7 Miralles ES, Nunez M, Hilara *et al*. Mucocutaneous leishmaniasis and HIV. *Dermatology* 1994; **189**: 275–7.
8 Montalban C, Calleja JL, Erice A. Visceral leishmaniasis in patients infected with human immunodeficiency virus. *J Infect* 1990; **21**: 261–70.

Immune defects

Human immunodeficiency virus (Chapter 26) [1–5]

Oral ulceration in patients infected with HIV may be due

to malignant disease (mainly Kaposi's sarcoma or non-Hodgkin's lymphoma) or infection (mainly herpes simplex or zoster) but aphthous-like ulcers are also seen, and there are occasional examples of ulcers due to other neoplasms or infections (other herpesviruses, mycobacteria, histoplasma, cryptococcus and others).

Aphthous-like ulcers in HIV may respond to local treatment or, failing that, 100 mg thalidomide at night for 2 weeks and then 100 mg every fifth day may prove effective [6]. Other mouth ulcers should be treated as appropriate.

REFERENCES

1 Epstein JB, Scully C. HIV infection: clinical features and treatment of thirty-three homosexual men with Kaposi's sarcoma. *Oral Surg* 1991; **71**: 38–41.
2 Porter SR, Scully C. HIV: The surgeon's perspective. 1: Update of pathogenesis, epidemiology, management and risk of nosocomial transmission. *Br J Oral Maxillofac Surg* 1994; **32**: 222–30.
3 Porter SR, Scully C. HIV: The surgeon's perspective. 2: Diagnosis and management of non-malignant oral manifestations. *Br J Oral Maxillofac Surg* 1994; **32**: 231–40.
4 Porter SR, Scully C. HIV: The surgeon's perspective. 3: Diagnosis and management of malignant neoplasms. *Br J Oral Maxillofac Surg* 1994; **32**: 241–7.
5 Scully C, Laskaris G, Pindborg J *et al.* Oral manifestations of HIV infection and their management. *Oral Surg* 1991; **71**: 158–71.
6 Youle M, Clarbour J, Farthing C *et al.* Treatment of resistant aphthous ulceration with thalidomide in patients positive for HIV antibody. *Br Med J* 1989; **298**: 432.

Drug-induced mouth ulcers

A wide range of drugs can occasionally induce mouth ulcers, by a variety of effects. Oral ulcers are regularly produced by cytotoxic agents such as methotrexate [1,2]. Oral use of caustics, or agents such as cocaine can cause erosions or ulcers [3]. Drug-induced ulcers may resemble aphthae or may have features reminiscent of lichenoid or other dermatological disorders. The ulcers usually resolve if the offending drug can be identified and withdrawn.

REFERENCES

1 Berkowitz RJ, Jones P, Barsetti J *et al.* Stomatologic complications of bone marrow transplantation in a pediatric population. *Paediatr Dent* 1987; **9**: 105–10.
2 Oliff A, Bleyer WA, Poplack DG. Methotrexate-induced oral mucositis and salivary methotrexate concentrations. *Cancer Chemother Pharmacol* 1979; **2**: 225–6.
3 Parry J, Porter SR, Scully C *et al.* Mucosal lesions due to oral cocaine use. *Br Dent J* 1996; **180**: 462–4.

Acrodynia

SYN. PINK DISEASE

Oral and perioral ulceration, hypersalivation, gingivitis and early tooth loss are features of acrodynia caused by mercury poisoning, now rarely seen [1].

REFERENCE

1 Dinehart SM, Dillard R, Rainer SS *et al.* Cutaneous manifestations of acrodynia (Pink disease). *Arch Dermatol* 1988; **124**: 107–9.

Radiation-induced mucositis

Radiation of the oral mucosa regularly produces severe mucositis and ulceration, as well as xerostomia and irradiation caries [1].

REFERENCE

1 Singh N, Scully C, Joyston-Bechal S. Oral complications of cancer therapies: prevention and management. *Clin Oncol* 1996; **8**: 15–24.

Disorder of uncertain pathogenesis

Angina bullosa haemorrhagica
SYN. LOCALIZED ORAL PURPURA

This is the term given to a benign, fairly common condition of unknown aetiology that usually presents in the elderly with oral blood blisters. These subepithelial blisters are seen mainly in the soft palate and after a few hours rupture to leave ulcers (Fig. 69.37). The patients appear well otherwise, with no detectable immunological or bleeding disorder [1–3]. Occasional cases are related to the use of corticosteroid inhalers. Only symptomatic care is available.

REFERENCES

1 Hopkins R, Walker DM. Oral blood blisters: angina bullosa haemorrhagica. *Br J Oral Surg* 1985; **23**: 9–16.
2 Stephenson P, Lamey P-J, Scully C *et al.* Angina bullosa haemorrhagica: clinical and laboratory features in 30 patients. *Oral Surg* 1987; **63**: 560–5.
3 Stephenson P, Scully C, Prime SS *et al.* Angina bullosa haemorrhagica: lesional immunostaining and haematological findings. *Br J Oral Surg* 1987; **25**: 488–91.

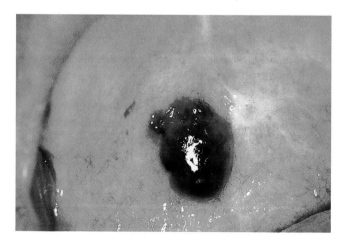

Fig. 69.37 Angina bullosa haemorrhagica: a large blood blister in a typical site on the soft palate. The adjacent whitish lesions are from scarring after a previous biopsy.

Monoclonal plasmacytic ulcerative stomatitis

Ulcerative stomatitis may occasionally appear with a lichenoid rash, related to a plasmacytic infiltrate.

REFERENCES

1 Bowden JR, Scully C, Eveson JW *et al*. Multiple myeloma and bullous lichenoid lesions: an unusual association. *Oral Surg* 1990; **70**: 587–9.
2 Layton SA, Cook JN, Henry JA. Monoclonal plasmacytic ulcerative stomatitis. *Oral Surg* 1993; **75**: 483–7.

Superficial mucoceles

Superficial extravasation mucoceles of the intraoral minor salivary glands in the palate, buccal mucosa or labial mucosa are not uncommon, especially associated with oral lichen planus in middle-aged or elderly women. This is a benign, self-limiting condition that may cause confusion with vesiculobullous disorders [1].

REFERENCE

1 Eveson JW. Superficial mucoceles: pitfall in clinical and microscopic diagnosis. *Oral Surg* 1988; **66**: 318–22.

Eosinophilic ulcer

SYN. TRAUMATIC EOSINOPHILIC GRANULOMA

This is a benign, self-limiting ulcer of unknown aetiology which often affects the tongue and, on biopsy, is characterized by the presence of numerous eosinophils [1–4]. The peripheral blood eosinophil count is normal.

REFERENCES

1 Doyle JL, Geary W, Baden E. Eosinophilic ulcer. *J Oral Maxillofac Surg* 1989; **47**: 349–52.
2 El-Mofty SK, Swanson PE, Wick MR, Miller AS. Eosinophilic ulcer of the oral mucosa: report of 38 new cases with immunohistochemical observations. *Oral Surg* 1993; **75**: 716–22.
3 Elzay RP. Traumatic ulcerative granuloma with stromal eosinophilia (Riga–Fede disease and traumatic eosinophilic granuloma). *Oral Surg* 1983; **55**: 497–506.
4 Sklavounou A, Laskaris G. Eosinophilic ulcer of the oral mucosa. *Oral Surg* 1984; **58**: 431–6.

Necrotizing sialometaplasia

Necrotizing sialometaplasia is an uncommon, benign, self-limiting condition seen predominantly in the posterior hard palate of young adult males, most of whom smoke tobacco [1]. A painless, deep ulcer persists for several weeks before spontaneously healing. Biopsy reveals necrosis and pseudoepitheliomatous changes probably resulting from squamous metaplasia following infarction of minor salivary glands. This benign lesion must be differentiated from malignancy.

REFERENCE

1 Kinney RB, Burton CS, Vollmer RT. Necrotizing sialo-metaplasia: a sheep in wolf's clothing. *Arch Dermatol* 1986; **12**: 208–10.

Mucha–Haberman's disease

Erythematous and ulcerative oral lesions have been reported in pityriasis lichenoides et varioliformis acuta (PLVA; Mucha–Haberman's disease) [1,2].

REFERENCES

1 Burke DP, Adams RM, Arundell FD. Ulceronecrotic Mucha–Haberman's disease. *Arch Dermatol* 1969; **100**: 201–6.
2 McDaniel RK, White JW, Edwards PA. Mucha–Haberman's disease with oral lesions. *Oral Surg* 1982; **53**: 596–601.

Oral soreness

Most oral pain is of local aetiology, usually resulting from odontogenic infections. Neurological, vascular and referred causes are less common, but must also be excluded. Psychogenic pain is all too frequent and this is discussed below.

Chronic soreness may be particularly caused by a deficiency state, geographical tongue, LP or burning mouth syndrome. LP is probably the most common cause of chronic soreness in the buccal mucosae, desquamative gingivitis is the common cause of persistently sore gingiva, and burning mouth syndrome and geographical tongue are the common causes of a sore tongue.

Deficiency glossitis

Aetiology. Deficiency glossitis may be related particularly to deficiency of iron, folate or vitamin B_{12}, and may then be associated with angular stomatitis and/or mouth ulcers. Deficiencies of other B-group vitamins occasionally cause glossitis, usually in chronic alcoholics or in those with malabsorption [1–3].

Pathology. Epithelial atrophy, rarely with some dysplasia, is seen.

Clinical features. In anaemic glossitis the tongue is red, sore and smooth (Fig. 69.38). Occasionally pernicious anaemia can also produce red areas or patterns of red lines.

In many others, the tongue can become sore but appear clinically completely normal and such patients' complaints are liable to be mislabelled as psychogenic.

Diagnosis. A full blood picture and assays of iron, folate and vitamin B_{12} are essential in management, as sore tongue can be the initial symptom of a deficiency and can precede any fall in the haemoglobin level.

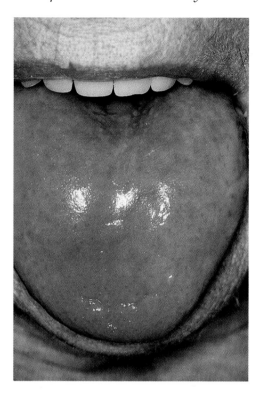

Fig. 69.38 Atrophic glossitis in vitamin B₁₂ deficiency.

Treatment. The cause of the deficiency should be sought before replacement treatment is given.

REFERENCES

1 Drummond JF, White DK, Damin DD. Megaloblastic anaemia with oral lesions: a consequence of gastric bypass surgery. *Oral Surg* 1985; **59**: 149–53.
2 Greenberg MS. Clinical and histologic changes of the oral mucosa in pernicious anaemia. *Oral Surg* 1981; **52**: 38–42.
3 Ramasinghe AW, Warnakulasuriya KAAS, Tennekoon GE *et al*. Oral mucosal changes in iron deficiency anaemia in a Sri Lankan female population. *Oral Surg* 1983; **55**: 29–32.

Burning mouth syndrome

SYN. ORAL DYSAESTHESIA; GLOSSOPYROSIS; GLOSSODYNIA

Burning mouth syndrome most frequently affects middle-aged and elderly females [1–3].

Aetiology. Organic causes of soreness such as candidiasis, diabetes or deficiency states must be excluded but an underlying anxiety about cancer or venereal disease with perhaps excessive tongue activity appears to be the basis for the complaint in most patients (Table 69.21) [2–11]. Contact reactions and pressure urticaria are rare causes [8,12,13].

Clinical features. Although the tongue is most frequently involved, the patient may also occasionally complain of

Table 69.21 Causes of burning mouth.

Local
Candidiasis
Other infections
Geographical tongue
Lichen planus
Oral submucous fibrosis
Dentures

Systemic
Psychogenic
  Cancerophobia
  Depression
  Anxiety states
  Hypochondriasis
Deficiency states
  Pernicious anaemia and other vitamin B deficiencies
  Folate deficiency
  Iron deficiency
Diabetes
Drugs (captopril)

burning lips, gums or palate. This is usually bilateral and often relieved by eating and drinking [1]. In contrast, the pain associated with inflammatory oral lesions is typically made worse by food.

Diagnosis. Oral examination very occasionally reveals an organic cause. Xerostomia should be excluded as this may predispose to candidiasis. Laboratory screening for anaemia, diabetes, a deficiency state or candidiasis should be undertaken.

Management. Reassurance, treatment of any defined underlying organic abnormality and, very occasionally, antidepressants or psychiatric care are indicated and there is some evidence that hormone replacement may help in a few postmenopausal patients [9]. Treatment is often unhelpful, but the condition rarely becomes severe.

REFERENCES

1 Grushka M. Clinical features of burning mouth syndrome. *Oral Surg* 1987; **63**: 30–6.
2 Lamb AB, Lamey PJ, Reeve PE. Burning mouth syndrome: psychological aspects. *Br Dent J* 1988; **165**: 256–60.
3 Van der Waal I. *The Burning Mouth Syndrome*. Copenhagen: Munksgaard, 1990.
4 Browning S, Hislop S, Scully C *et al*. The association between burning mouth syndrome and psychosocial disorders. *Oral Surg* 1987; **64**: 171–4.
5 Feinmann C, Harris M. Psychogenic facial pain. *Br Dent J* 1984; **156**: 165–9, 205–9.
6 Maresky LS, Van der Bijl P, Gird I. Burning mouth syndrome. Evaluation of multiple variables among 85 patients. *Oral Surg* 1993; **75**: 303–7.
7 Rojo L, Silvestre FJ, Bagan JV, de Vincente T. Psychiatric morbidity in burning mouth syndrome. Psychiatric interview versus depression and anxiety scales. *Oral Surg* 1993; **75**: 308–11.
8 Van Joost TH, Van Ulsen J, Van Loon LAJ. Contact allergy to denture materials in the burning mouth syndrome. *Contact Dermatitis* 1988; **18**: 97–9.
9 Wardrop RW, Hailes J, Burger H *et al*. Oral discomfort at menopause. *Oral Surg* 1989; **67**: 535–40.

10 Wray D, Scully C. The sore mouth. *Med Int* 1986; **2**: 1134–8.
11 Zilli C, Brooke RI, Lau CL *et al.* Screening for psychiatric illness in patients with oral dysesthesia by means of the GHQ-28 and the IDA. *Oral Surg* 1989; **67**: 384–9.
12 Dutree-Meulenberg ROGM, Kozel MMA, van Joost TH. Burning mouth syndrome: a possible etiologic role for local contact hypersensitivity. *J Am Acad Dermatol* 1992; **26**: 935–40.
13 Helton J, Storrs F. The burning mouth syndrome: lack of a role for contact urticaria and contact dermatitis. *J Am Acad Dermatol* 1994; **31**: 201–5.

Atypical facial pain

There are several psychogenic types of orofacial pain and, in some population studies, nearly 40% of people have reported frequent headache and facial pain [1–3].

Aetiology. Four main groups of patient appear to suffer from psychogenic pain:
1 normal individuals under extreme stress;
2 those with a personality trait such as hypochondriasis;
3 neurotic, often depressed, persons;
4 psychotic patients.

Clinical features. Atypical facial pain is an ill-defined entity which includes atypical facial pain (or neuralgia), atypical odontalgia and the 'syndrome of oral complaints'. Patients are often middle-aged or elderly females with constant chronic discomfort or pain, often of a dull, boring or burning type. The location of the pain is ill-defined, may cross the midline to involve the other side or may move to another site. The symptoms do not waken the patient from sleep. There are often recent adverse life events such as bereavement or family illness and multiple oral and/or other psychogenic-related complaints, such as headaches, chronic back pains, irritable bowel syndrome or dysmenorrhoea. Over 50% of such patients are depressed or hypochondriacal or have other psychiatric disorders, and some have lost or been separated from parents in childhood [2,3].

Prognosis. Cure is uncommon in most, yet few seem to try or persist in using analgesics. Attempts at relieving the pain by dental treatment are usually unsuccessful and, indeed, may exacerbate the pain. Antidepressants may help (see below).

Diagnosis. There is a total lack of objective signs. Radiographs are advisable but all investigations are usually negative. It is, however, essential to exclude organic disease, for example systemic neoplasms.

Treatment. Some 70% respond to prothiaden, compared with a 50% response to placebo, and those who will respond invariably do so early in treatment [2]. However, many refuse medication or psychiatric help, lack insight and often persist in blaming organic diseases for their pain.

Atypical odontalgia presents with pain indistinguishable from pulpitis or periodontitis but with the absence of detectable pathology [1]. Pain is aggravated by dental intervention. It is probably a variant of atypical facial pain and should be treated similarly.

The syndrome of oral complaints

Multiple pains and other complaints (such as of dry mouth or disturbed taste) may occur simultaneously or sequentially, and relief is rarely found. Patients may bring diaries of their symptoms to emphasize their problem.

REFERENCES

1 Brooke RI. Atypical odontalgia: a report of twenty-two cases. *Oral Surg* 1980; **49**: 196–9.
2 Feinmann C, Harris M. Psychogenic facial pain. *Br Dent J* 1984; **156**: 165–8, 205–8.
3 Remick RA, Blasberg B. Psychiatric aspects of atypical facial pain. *Can Dent Assoc J* 1985; **12**: 913–16.

White lesions

Acquired white lesions in the mouth are usually innocuous keratoses or caused by cheek biting, or chemical burns, but infections, dermatoses (usually LP), neoplastic disorders and other conditions must be excluded (see Table 69.8). Congenital lesions are discussed earlier (p. 3060).

Leukoplakia

The World Health Organization defines leukoplakia as a white patch or plaque on the mucosa that cannot be rubbed off and that is not recognized as a specific disease entity [1]. It therefore implies a diagnosis by exclusion (e.g. exclusion of LP, candidiasis, etc.). The term is also used irrespective of the presence or absence of epithelial dysplasia, although, as discussed below (p. 3099), there is a small premalignant potential to some keratoses.

Leukoplakia is common in adults: around 1% are affected, although some populations show higher prevalences. Most are seen in the 50–70 age group [2–4].

Oral keratoses

Aetiology. The cause of most keratoses is unknown (idiopathic keratoses or leukoplakia) but some are caused by use of tobacco, oral snuff or smokeless tobacco, by chronic irritation or by infective agents or other aetiologies [2,5].

Pathology. Keratoses show, to a varying degree, increased keratin production, change in epithelial thickness and disordered epithelial maturation. Mild dysplasia is not usually regarded as of serious significance. The presence of severe epithelial dysplasia is thought to indicate a considerable risk of malignant development [6].

Clinical features. Keratoses range in size from a few millimetres upwards, and occasionally affect virtually the whole mouth. They most commonly are small, uniformly white, smooth plaques (homogeneous leukoplakia), prevalent in the buccal (cheek) mucosa and usually of low premalignant potential (Fig. 69.39). Up to 90% are of this type.

Less common, but far more serious, are nodular and especially verrucous [7] or speckled leukoplakias (erythroleukoplakia) which consist of white patches or nodules in a red (erythroplakic) area of mucosa (Fig. 69.40). Chronic *Candida* infection is common in speckled leukoplakias and may be associated with an increased risk of malignant change. Candidal leukoplakias are often found at the commissures.

Leukoplakias of the anterior floor of the mouth and undersurface of the tongue (sublingual or floor-of-mouth keratosis) may have a particularly high risk of malignant change (Fig. 69.41). The lesion is more common in women than men and has a typical 'ebbing tide' appearance clinically. Syphilitic leukoplakia, typically found on the dorsum of tongue, may have a high malignant potential.

Paradoxically, malignant change is more likely in non-

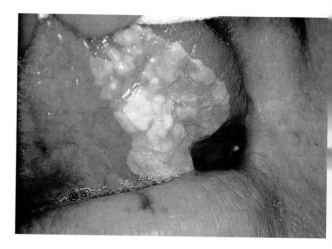

Fig. 69.41 Sublingual keratosis.

smokers than smokers with leukoplakia. Nevertheless, stopping smoking reduces the risk of malignant change in smokers with keratosis.

Trauma occasionally causes benign keratosis, usually at the buccal mucosal occlusal line (Fig. 69.42) or on edentulous ridges when the patient does not wear a denture.

Pipe smoking can lead to a characteristic type of benign keratosis of the palate—stomatitis nicotina (smoker's keratosis; Fig. 69.43). The diffuse palatal keratosis in stomatitis nicotina is covered by red puncta which are the openings of the inflamed palatal salivary glands. Reverse smoking such as is practised in Andhra Pradesh, India, may produce keratosis in the palate, while snuff dipping and the use of smokeless tobacco produces lesions in the vestibule.

The so-called hairy leukoplakia seen in HIV disease and other immunocompromised states is not known to be premalignant (p. 3099)

Most oral leukoplakia is seen without lesions on other mucosae, although rare patients with similar lesions on the genital mucosa have been described.

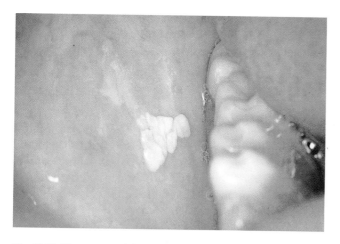

Fig. 69.39 Homogeneous leukoplakia in the buccal mucosa.

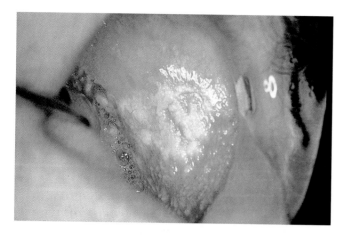

Fig. 69.40 Speckled leukoplakia.

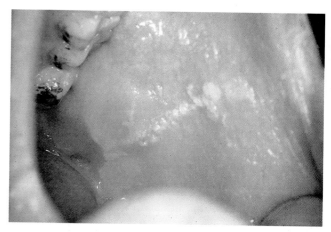

Fig. 69.42 Frictional keratosis and cheek biting (morsicatio buccarum) at the occlusal line.

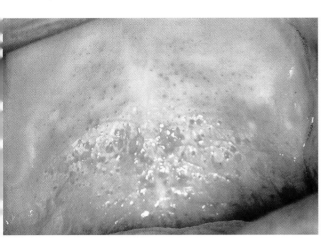

Fig. 69.43 Smoker's keratosis (stomatitis nicotina). The red areas are the orifices of the mucous salivary glands in the palate.

Prognosis. Up to 10% of keratoses seen in some specialist clinics are malignant [4,6,8,9]. Malignant change to carcinoma is most frequent in women older than 50 years and in large lesions. The overall prevalence of malignant change in keratosis is less than 3–6% over 10 years. Sublingual keratoses, speckled leukoplakias and syphilitic leuko-plakias are those most likely to undergo malignant transformation. Up to 30% of these develop into carcinoma. Interestingly, leukoplakias developing in non-smokers have a higher rather than lower risk of malignant change.

There is thus clear evidence of the premalignant potential of some oral leukoplakias, but some leukoplakias (15–30%) regress clinically, not only when supposed aetiological factors have been removed but also sometimes spontaneously.

Diagnosis. It is often difficult to be certain of the precise diagnosis of an oral white patch on clinical examination, as even carcinoma can present as a white lesion. Incisional biopsy should therefore be carried out, selecting for biopsy indurated, red, erosive or ulcerated areas rather than the more obvious whiter areas. Toluidine blue staining may highlight dysplastic areas. Cytology only samples super-ficial squames, overlooks up to 20% of malignancies and is of little diagnostic help.

Candidal leukoplakia, LP, lupus erythematosus and hairy leukoplakia can all be particularly difficult to dif-ferentiate clinically from idiopathic keratosis [10–12].

Treatment. Management of keratoses can be difficult, not least because of the wide extent of some lesions, their frequent admixture with areas of erythroplasia (speckled leukoplakias) and controversy as to the long-term effects of various therapies.

Obvious predisposing factors to be reduced include sharp tooth edges, alcohol consumption, smoking or similar habits (e.g. betel chewing). Some studies have shown regression of leukoplakia in over half of patients who stopped smoking

for 1 year. There may be evidence suggesting syphilis, candidiasis, HIV infection, renal failure or an underlying anaemia in some patients, in which case suitable investi-gations and management should be arranged.

Severely dysplastic and accessible lesions should be excised and the patient should then be reviewed regularly at 3–6 monthly intervals, photographing and rebiopsying if there are changes suggesting malignancy.

Some clinicians advocate removal of mildly or moderately dysplastic lesions but others simply observe as already described.

Topical 0.5% bleomycin in dimethylsulphoxide is being evaluated [13]. Topical or systemic vitamin A derivatives have not been widely used because of their uncertain long-term consequences, although they appear to cause regres-sion of leukoplakia [14].

REFERENCES

1 World Health Organization Collaborating Centre for Oral Precancerous Lesions. Definitions of leucoplakia and related lesions. *Oral Surg* 1978; **45**: 518–39.
2 Axell T, Holmstrup P, Kramer IRH *et al*. International seminar on oral leucoplakia and associated lesions related to tobacco habits. *Community Dent Oral Epidemiol* 1984; **12**: 145–54.
3 Dorey JL, Blasberg B, Conklin RJ *et al*. Oral leucoplakia. *Int J Dermatol* 1984; **23**: 638–42.
4 Shibuya H, Amagasa T, Seto KI *et al*. Leukoplakia-associated mul-tiple carcinomas in patients with tongue carcinoma. *Cancer* 1986; **57**: 843–6.
5 Scully C, Ward-Booth P. Detection and treatment of early cancers of the oral cavity. *Crit Rev Oncol* 1995; **21**: 63–75.
6 Lind PO. Malignant transformation in oral leucoplakia. *Scand J Dent Res* 1987; **95**: 449–55.
7 Hansen LS, Olson JA, Silverman S. Proliferative verrucous leukoplakia. *Oral Surg* 1985; **60**: 285–98.
8 Eveson JW. Oral premalignancy. *Cancer Surv* 1983; **2**: 403–24.
9 Silverman S, Gorsky M, Lozado F. Oral leucoplakia and malignant transformation. *Cancer* 1984; **53**: 563–8.
10 Scully C, Cawson RA. *Colour Aids to Oral Medicine*. Edinburgh: Churchill Livingstone, 1988.
11 Scully C, Flint S, Porter SR. *A Colour Atlas of Oral Medicine*. London: Martin Dunitz, 1996.
12 Shklar G. Oral leucoplakia. *N Engl J Med* 1986; **315**: 1544–5.
13 Malmstrom M, Hietanen J, Sane J *et al*. Topical treatment of oral leucoplakia with bleomycin. *Br J Oral Surg* 1988; **26**: 491–8.
14 Scully C. Oral precancer: preventive and medical approaches to management. *Oral Oncol* 1995; **31B**: 16–26.

Hairy leukoplakia

Aetiology. Hairy leukoplakia (HL) is seen in severe immune defects, especially HIV infection and, occasionally in the apparently immunocompetent [1]. HIV is not found within the genome of epithelial cells in HL and it is more likely that the features are a consequence of an op-portunistic infection with EBV. It is now clear that normal human oral mucosa from HIV-negative individuals may contain latent EBV.

EBV has been shown to be present in HL especially in the upper layers of the epithelium. The oral site of pre-dilection for HL appears to relate to the presence of EBV receptors only on the parakeratinized mucosae such as the lateral margin of the tongue. HL regresses on treatment with antivirals such as aciclovir and ganciclovir but fails to resolve with antifungals, despite the frequent presence of *Candida* species.

Pathology. Histological features of HL include hyperparakeratosis, hyperplasia and ballooning of prickle cells, few or no Langerhans' cells, and only a sparse inflammatory cell infiltrate in the lamina propria.

Clinical features. HL is a white patch, usually seen on the parakeratinized mucosa on the tongue, frequently bilaterally (Fig. 69.44). The lesions are corrugated or have a shaggy or hairy appearance, are mostly symptomless, and, unlike some oral keratoses, have no known premalignant potential [1–5]. The majority of the affected patients who are HIV positive appear eventually to develop AIDS. HL also occurs in HIV-negative persons [6–12].

Diagnosis. Some of the histological features typical of HL, especially the hyperparakeratosis, can be seen in oral white lesions other than HL in HIV-infected persons [13]. Not only are there oral lesions that mimic HL in HIV infection, but lesions similar to HL can be seen in other immunocompromised persons and even in some apparently healthy individuals.

However, most cases can be distinguished from the HL of HIV infection by the absence of EBV DNA on histology and, of course, by examination for HIV serum antibody.

Treatment. HL really needs no treatment but in HIV-infected individuals may occasionally improve spontaneously or with zidovudine. Aciclovir may also prove useful.

Phosphonoformate, and vitamin A acid have produced resolution but are rarely indicated [6].

REFERENCES

1 Schiodt M, Greenspan D, Daniels TE *et al.* Clinical and histologic spectrum of oral hairy leucoplakia. *Oral Surg* 1987; **64**: 716–20.
2 Scully C, Laskaris G, Pindborg J *et al.* Oral manifestations of HIV infection and their management. *Oral Surg* 1991; **71**: 158–66, 167–71.
3 Scully C, Porter SR. Orofacial manifestations in infection with human immunodeficiency viruses (Leading article). *Lancet* 1988; i: 976–7.
4 Scully C, Epstein JB, Porter SR. Oral hairy leucoplakia (Leading article). *Lancet* 1989; ii: 1194.
5 Scully C, McCarthy G. Management of oral health in HIV infection. *Oral Surg* 1992; **73**: 215–25.
6 King GN, Healy CM, Glover T *et al.* Prevalence and risk factors associated with leukoplakia, hairy leukoplakia, erythematous candidiasis and gingival hyperplasia in renal transplant recipients. *Oral Surg* 1994; **78**: 718–21.
7 Euvrard S, Kanitakis J, Puteil-Nobel C *et al.* Pseudo-oral hairy leukoplakia in a renal allograft recipient. *J Am Acad Dermatol* 1994; **30**: 300–3.
8 Itin P, Rufli T, Rudlinger R *et al.* Oral hairy leukoplakia in an HIV-negative renal transplant patient: a marker for immunosuppression? *Dermatologica* 1988; **177**: 126–8.
9 Syrjanen S, Laine P, Happonen R *et al.* Oral hairy leukoplakia is not a specific sign of HIV-infection but related to immunodepression in general. *J Oral Pathol Med* 1989; **18**: 28–31.
10 Greenspan D, Greenspan JS, De Souza YG *et al.* Oral hairy leukoplakia in an HIV-negative renal transplant recipient. *J Oral Pathol Med* 1989; **18**: 32–4.
11 Kanitakis J, Euvrard S, Lefrancois N *et al.* Oral hairy leukopakia in a HIV-negative renal graft recipient. *Br J Dermatol* 1991; **124**: 483–6.
12 Eisenberg E, Krutchkoff D, Yamase H. Incidental oral hairy leukoplakia in immunocompetent persons. *Oral Surg Oral Med Oral Pathol* 1992; **74**: 563–6.
13 Green TL, Greenspan JS, Greenspan D *et al.* Oral lesions mimicking hairy leukoplakia: a diagnostic dilemma. *Oral Surg Oral Med Oral Pathol* 1989; **67**: 422–6.

Cheek biting

SYN. MORSICATIO BUCCARUM

Cheek biting causes a whitish, shredded appearance usually of the buccal or lower labial mucosa at the occlusal line (adjacent to where the teeth meet) (see Fig. 69.42). The habit is most common in tense or anxious individuals who may also show bruxism, mandibular pain dysfunction or other oral features of psychogenic disorders. The lesion is benign but may simulate white-sponge naevus (p. 3060).

Burns

Thermal or chemical burns (due, for example to holding mouthwashes in the mouth or drugs against the buccal mucosa) can cause white sloughing lesions of the mucosa [1].

REFERENCE

1 Bernstein ML. Oral mucosal white lesions associated with excessive use of Listerine mouthwash. *Oral Surg* 1978; **46**: 781.

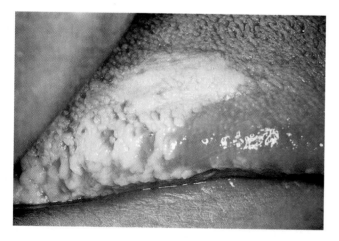

Fig. 69.44 Hairy leukoplakia. Found mainly in human immunodeficiency virus infection, vertical white ridges on the lateral margin of the tongue.

Table 69.22 Intraoral candidiasis.

Types of candidiasis	Usual age at onset	Predisposing factors†
Acute pseudomembranous candidiasis (thrush)*	Any	Local (dry mouth, antimicrobials), General (corticosteroids, leukaemia, human immunodeficiency virus (HIV)
Acute atrophic candidiasis ('antibiotic mouth'; antibiotic sore mouth)	Any	Broad-spectrum antibiotics or corticosteroids
Erythematous candidiasis	Any	HIV especially
Chronic atrophic candidiasis (denture-induced stomatitis)	Adults	Denture-wearing, especially at night
Chronic hyperplastic candidiasis (candidal leukoplakia)*	Usually middle-aged or elderly	Tobacco smoking, denture wearing, immune defect
Median rhomboid glossitis	Third or later decades	Tobacco smoking, denture wearing, HIV
Chronic mucocutaneous candidiasis*	Usually first decade	Often immune defect; rarely endocrinopathy

* White lesions,
† immune defects can predispose to any form.

Candidiasis

Up to 50% of the healthy population harbour *Candida albicans* as an oral commensal. Carriage is more common in cigarette smokers. *Candida* resides particularly on the posterior dorsum of the tongue [1,2].

Infection is likely to result from xerostomia, local disturbances in salivary flora such as occurs during broad-spectrum antimicrobial treatment, or depressed immune responses [1, 3–6]. Of the several clinical presentations of oral candidiasis, only thrush, candidal leukoplakia and chronic mucocutaneous candidiasis present as white lesions: the other types—acute and chronic atrophic candidiasis are red (Table 69.22).

Thrush syn. acute pseudomembranous candidiasis. Healthy neonates, who have yet to develop immunity to *Candida* species, may develop thrush. In other patients, predisposing factors include antibiotic or corticosteroid use, xerostomia and severe T-cell immune defects associated with immunosuppression (e.g. in organ transplantation) or immunodeficiencies such as leukaemia or HIV disease. Oral candidiasis is a common and early feature of HIV infection and may be a portent of developing AIDS [1,2]

The soft, creamy patches of thrush, which resemble milk curds, can be wiped off the oral mucosa with gauze, leaving an area of erythema (Fig. 69.45).

Chronic candidiasis. Long-standing oral candidiasis may produce tough, adherent white patches (chronic hyperplastic candidiasis or candidal leukoplakias) which can have a premalignant potential, and may be indistinguishable from other leukoplakias except by biopsy. Candidal leukoplakias may, however, be speckled. In only a few patients with this type of chronic oral candidiasis can either a local cause or underlying immune defect be identified [2,6]. Chronic mucocutaneous candidiasis syndromes are rare (Chapter 31).

Diagnosis. The diagnosis of oral thrush is usually clinical but it tends to be overdiagnosed by physicians. In contrast, erythematous candidiasis is probably under-diagnosed. In immunosuppressed patients, a Gram-stained smear should be taken to distinguish thrush from the plaques produced by opportunistic bacteria. Hyphae seem to indicate that the *Candida* organisms are acting as pathogens and not simple commensals.

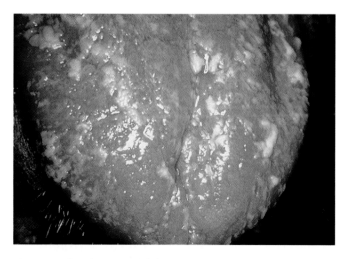

Fig. 69.45 Thrush: scattered white lesions on an erythematous background.

Suspected candidal leukoplakia should be biopsied, both to distinguish it from other non-candidal plaques and also because of possible dyplasia. Although candidal hyphae and a neutrophil infiltrate may be seen on haematoxylin and eosin staining, periodic acid–Schiff (PAS) will demonstrate the purple staining of the hyphae.

Treatment. Acute candidiasis: except in healthy neonates possible predisposing causes should be looked for and treated. Topical polyenes such as nystatin or amphotericin, or imidazoles such as miconazole are often indicated but, in HIV infection, fluconazole may be required.

Chronic hyperplastic candidiasis: the oral lesions of chronic hyper-plastic candidiasis may respond poorly to the polyenes. These cases and some cases of chronic mucocutaneous candidiasis may respond only to fluocytosine, ketoconazole, fluconazole, or itraconazole [3,7–9].

REFERENCES

1 Scully C, El-Kabir M, Samaranayake LP. Candidiasis. In: Millard D, Mason DK, eds. *1993 World Workshop on Oral Medicine.* Michigan: University of Michigan, 1995; 27–51.
2 Smith CB. Candidiasis: pathogenesis, host resistance and predisposing factors. In: Bodey GP, Feinstein V, eds. *Candidiasis.* New York: Raven Press, 1985: 53–72.
3 Burke WA. Use of itraconazole in a patient with chronic mucocutaneous candidiasis. *J Am Acad Dermatol* 1989; **6**: 1309–410.
4 Epstein JB, Truelove EL, Izutzu KT. Oral candidiasis: pathogenesis and host defence. *Rev Infect Dis* 1984; **6**: 96–106.
5 Odds FC. *Candida* infections: an overview. *CRC Crit Rev Microbiol* 1987; **15**: 1–5.
6 Scully C, El-Kabir M, Samaranayake LP. Candida and oral candidiasis. *Crit Rev Oral Biol Med* 1994; **5**: 124–58.
7 Hay RJ, Clayton YM. Fluconazole in the management of patients with chronic mucocutaneous candidiasis. *Br J Dermatol* 1988; **119**: 683–5.
8 Nielson H, Dangaard K, Schiodt M. Chronic mucocutaneous candidiasis: a review. *Tandlaegkbladet* 1985; **89**: 667–73.
9 Porter SR, Scully C. Candidiasis endocrinopathy syndrome. *Oral Surg* 1986; **61**: 573–8.

Koplik's spots (Chapter 26)

White specks may be seen in the buccal mucosa in early measles.

Lichen planus

See Chapter 41.

Psoriasis (Chapter 35)

The oral mucosa is rarely involved in psoriasis with only about 70 cases reported, although there are occasionally white lesions especially in the buccal mucosa, and lesions clinically indistinguishable from geographical tongue (sometimes termed annulus migrans or erythema circinatum) can be seen, with prominent fungiform lingual papillae, particularly in generalized pustular psoriasis [1–8]. These lesions may involve areas other than the tongue. Histologically, spongiform pustules of Kogoj are described.

REFERENCES

1 Heitanen J, Salo OP, Kanerva L *et al.* Study of the oral mucosa in 250 consecutive patients with psoriasis. *Scand J Dent Res* 1984; **92**: 50–4.
2 O'Keefe E, Braverman IM, Cohen T. Annulus migrans; identical lesions in pustular psoriasis, Reiter's syndrome, and geographic tongue. *Arch Dermatol* 1973; **107**: 240–4.
3 Morris LF, Phillips CM, Binnie WH *et al.* Oral lesions in patients with psoriasis; a controlled study. *Cutis* 1992; **49**: 339–44.
4 Pogrel MA, Cram D. Intraoral findings in patients with psoriasis with a special reference to ectopic geographic tongue. *Oral Surg* 1988; **66**: 184–9.
5 Pyle GW, Vitt M, Nieusma G. Oral psoriasis; report of a case. *J Oral Maxillofac Surg* 1994; **52**: 185–7.
6 Sklavounou A, Laskaris G. Oral psoriasis; report of a case and review of the literature. *Dermatologica* 1990; **180**: 157–9.
7 Wagner G, Luckasen J, Goltz R. Mucous membrane involvement in generalised pustular psoriasis. *Arch Dermatol* 1976; **112**: 1010–14.
8 White DK, Leis HJ, Miller AS. Intraoral psoriasis associated with widespread dermal psoriasis. *Oral Surg* 1976; **41**: 174–81.

Pigmented or red lesions

Congenital lesions are described on pages 3059–3068. Localized hyperpigmented lesions are usually amalgam tattoos or naevi, but melanomas and Kaposi's sarcoma must be excluded. Generalized oral mucosal hyperpigmentation is usually racial in origin and only occasionally has a systemic cause such as Addison's disease.

Many oral red lesions are inflammatory in nature, but desquamation (in desquamative gingivitis) is fairly common, and epithelial atrophy is an important cause especially in deficiency glossitis and erythroplasia. Telangiectases are usually red and haemangiomas purplish in colour.

Purpura

Petechiae are usually caused by trauma often from suction, but a bleeding tendency as in infectious mononucleosis, or leukaemias must be excluded (Fig. 69.46). Palatal petechiae may be seen in infectious mononucleosis, HIV infection or rubella. Blood–filled blisters may be seen in localized oral purpura (angina bullosa haemorrhagica) and pemphigoid, and occasionally in amyloidosis. Rarely a purpuric lesion may be seen in pigmented purpuric stomatitis [1].

REFERENCE

1 Scully C, Eveson JW. Pigmented purpuric stomatitis. *Oral Surg* 1992; **74**: 780–2.

Benign migratory glossitis

SYN. LINGUAL ERYTHEMA MIGRANS; GEOGRAPHICAL TONGUE

Definition. A benign, inflammatory condition of the tongue

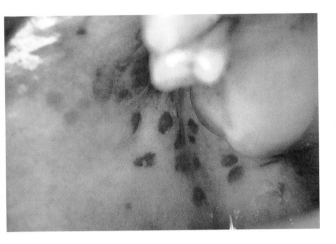

Fig. 69.46 Oral purpura in thrombocytopenia.

with map-like areas of erythema which are not constant.

Lingual erythema migrans is unrelated to cutaneous erythema migrans (Chapter 45).

Aetiology. Unknown, but many patients with a fissured tongue (scrotal tongue) also have lingual erythema migrans. It is a common condition affecting about 1–2% of the population. A positive family history may be obtainable. HLA findings have been equivocal with reports of associations with B15 and DR7 [1].

Some patients with lingual erythema migrans have atopic allergies such as hayfever and a few relate the oral lesions to a particular food, for example cheese, or to stress [2]. Similar oral lesions may be seen in Reiter's syndrome, generalized pustular psoriasis and acrodermatitis continua of Hallopeau. Purported associations with diabetes [3] may be coincidental.

Pathology. There is epithelial thinning at the centre of the lesion with an inflammatory infiltrate mainly of polymorphonuclear leukocytes [4,5].

Clinical features. Geographical tongue may be asymptomatic or cause a sore tongue. Patients of any age may be affected but why the condition sometimes gives rise to symptoms after it has been present asymptomatically for decades is unclear [4,6].

Geographical tongue is characterized by map-like red areas with increased thickness of intervening filiform papillae. Alternatively, there are rounded, sometimes scalloped, reddish areas with a white margin (Figs 69.47 and 69.48). These patterns change from day to day and even within a few hours.

Rarely, other sites, such as the labial or palatal mucosa, are affected. The tongue is usually, but not invariably, affected simultaneously with the other sites [7].

There are no complications and the only differential diagnoses are from psoriasis and larva migrans.

Diagnosis. Clinical examination usually suffices to differentiate the condition from lichen planus, candidiasis or deficiency glossitis.

Treatment. Blood and urine examination may be necessary to exclude anaemia and diabetes. In those with no systemic disorder, no treatment is available except reassurance.

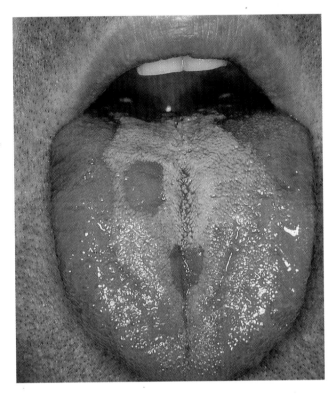

Fig. 69.47 Classical geographical tongue (lingual erythema migrans).

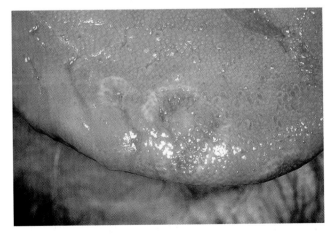

Fig. 69.48 Somewhat less obvious signs of lingual erythema migrans.

REFERENCES

1 Marks R, Tait B. HLA antigens in geographical tongue. *Tissue Antigens* 1980; **15**: 60–2.
2 Marks R, Radden BG. Geographic tongue: a clinicopathological review. *Aust J Dermatol* 1981; **22**: 75–9.
3 Wysocki GP, Daley T. Benign migratory glossitis in patients with juvenile diabetes. *Oral Surg* 1987; **63**: 68–70.
4 Brooks JK, Balciunas BA. Geographic stomatitis: review of the literature and report of five cases *J Am Dent Assoc* 1987; **115**: 421–4.
5 Kullaa-Mikkonen A. Geographic tongue, a scanning electron microscope study. *J Cutan Pathol* 1986; **13**: 154–62.
6 Correll RW, Wescott WB, Jenson JL. Non-painful, erythematous circinate lesions of a protean nature on a fissured tongue. *J Am Dent Assoc* 1984; **109**: 90–1.
7 Luker J, Scully C. Erythema migrans affecting the palate. *Br Dent J* 1983; **155**: 385.

Larva migrans (Chapter 32)

Cutaneous larva migrans is rarely seen in the mouth, where it presents as irregular linear lesions with an inflammatory border [1].

REFERENCE

1 Lopes MA, Zaia AA, Almeida OPD, Scully C. Larva migrans affecting the mouth. *Oral Surg* 1994; **77**: 362–7.

Furred, brown and black hairy tongue

Aetiology and pathology. Children rarely have a furred tongue in health but it may be coated with off-white debris in febrile and other illnesses. Adults, however, not infrequently have a coating on the tongue in health, particularly if they are edentulous, are on a soft, non-abrasive diet, have poor oral hygiene or are fasting. The coating appears more obvious in xerostomic and in ill patients, especially those who cannot maintain oral hygiene. The coating appears to be of epithelial, food and microbial debris; indeed, the tongue is the main oral reservoir of some microorganisms such as *Candida albicans* and some viridans streptococci. The filiform papillae are excessively long and stained by the accumulation of squames and chromogenic microorganisms.

Occasionally, a brown, hairy tongue may be caused by antimicrobial therapy, especially with broad-spectrum drugs such as tetracyclines when it is related to overgrowth of *Candida* species and may respond to withdrawal of the drug. Various medicaments such as chlorhexidine or iron can cause a black or brown superficial staining of the tongue (and teeth).

Clinical features. Black, hairy tongue affects mainly the posterior part of the dorsum of the tongue, especially centrally (Fig. 69.49) [1].

Treatment. Patients with black, hairy tongue may find the condition improves if they increase their standard of oral hygiene, brush the tongue with a toothbrush, use sodium

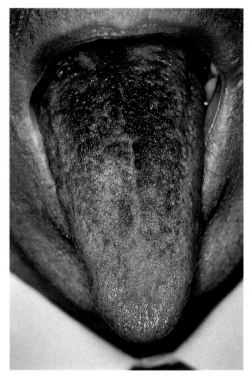

Fig. 69.49 Black, hairy tongue.

bicarbonate mouthwashes or suck a peach stone. Topical tretinoin may be effective [2].

REFERENCES

1 Winer LH. Black hairy tongue. *Arch Dermatol* 1958; **77**: 97–103.
2 Langtry JAA, Carr MM, Steele MC, Ive FA. Topical tretinoin: a new treatment for black hairy tongue (lingua villosa nigra). *Clin Exp Dermatol* 1992; **17**: 163–4.

'Strawberry tongue'

Prominence of the lingual papillae may be seen in scarlet fever, Kawasaki disease and in the Riley–Day syndrome (familial dysautonomia), giving rise to an appearance similar to a strawberry.

Tattoo

Amalgam tattoos are common causes of blue–black pigmentation, usually seen in the mandibular gingiva, or at least close to the teeth (Fig. 69.50), or in the scar of an apicectomy where there has been a retrograde root-filling [1,2]. Radio-opacities may or may not be seen on radiography. Similar lesions can result if for some reason pencil lead or other similar foreign bodies become embedded in the oral tissues [3].

Radiography may help to confirm the diagnosis. Biopsy may be indicated to exclude a naevus or melanoma but otherwise these lesions are innocuous.

Deliberate tattooing is a rare cause of oral pigmentation [4].

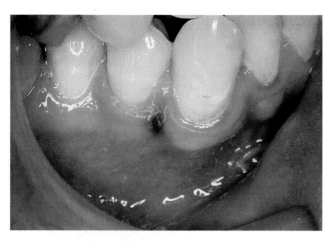

Fig. 69.50 Amalgam tattoo in a common site. This was presumably related to filling of the deciduous predecessor.

REFERENCES

1 Buchner A, Hansen LS. Amalgam pigmentation (amalgam tattoo) of the oral mucosa: a clinicopathological study of 268 cases. *Oral Surg* 1980; **49**: 139–47.
2 Dummett CO. Pertinent considerations in oral pigmentation. *Br Dent J* 1985; **158**: 9–12.
3 Peters E, Gardner DG. A method of distinguishing between amalgam and graphite in tissue. *Oral Surg* 1986; **62**: 73–6.
4 Schawaf M. Gingival tattoo: an unusual gingival pigmentation. *J Oral Med* 1986; **41**: 130–3.

Drug-induced hyperpigmentation

Smoking may cause a greyish brown oral hyperpigmentation because of pigmentary incontinence (Table 69.23).

Table 69.23 Causes of mucosal pigmentation.

Localized
Amalgam tattoo
Ephelis (freckle)
Naevus
Malignant melanoma
Kaposi's sarcoma
Peutz–Jegher's syndrome
Laugier–Hunziker syndrome
Melanotic macules
Complex of myxomas, spotty pigmentation and endocrine
   overactivity

Generalized
Racial
Localized irritation, e.g. smoking
Drugs, e.g. phenothiazines, antimalarials, minocycline,
   contraceptives, mephenytoin
Addison's disease
Nelson's syndrome
Ectopic ACTH (e.g. bronchogenic carcinoma)
Heavy metals
Albright's syndrome
Other rare causes, e.g. haemochromatosis, generalized
   neurofibromatosis, incontinentia pigmenti
Malignant acanthosis nigricans

ACTH, adrenocorticotrophic hormone.

Many of the heavy metals formerly implicated in producing oral hyperpigmentation are not used therapeutically now, although industrial or accidental exposure is still occasionally seen [1]. Purplish gingival discoloration has been rarely reported after exposure to gold salts. Drugs such as antimalarials produce a variety of mucosal colours, ranging from yellow with mepacrine to blue–black with amodiaquine or quinidine. Adrenocorticotrophic hormone (ACTH) therapy may produce brown pigmentation, as may zidovudine, clofazimine, busulphan and some other cytotoxic drugs, oral contraceptives, phenothiazines and some anticonvulsants [2–4].

Minocycline can, in a minority of patients, produce blue–grey gingival pigmentation caused by staining of the underlying bone, and some intrinsic faint bluish grey staining, mainly at the anterior teeth [5,6].

Management. Some drug-induced hyperpigmentation resolves on cessation of exposure to the drug and improved oral hygiene, but resolution can take months or years [6].

REFERENCES

1 Lockhart PB. Gingival pigmentation as the sole presenting sign of chronic lead poisoning in a mentally retarded adult. *Oral Surg* 1981; **52**: 143–9.
2 Axell A, Hedin A. Epidemiologic study of excessive oral melanin pigmentation with special reference to the influence of tobacco habits. *Scand J Dent Res* 1982; **90**: 432–42.
3 Birek C, Main JHP. Two cases of oral pigmentation associated with quinidine therapy. *Oral Surg* 1988; **66**: 59–61.
4 Hertz RS, Beckstead PC, Brown WJ. Epithelial melanosis possibly resulting from the use of oral contraceptives. *J Am Dent Assoc* 1980; **100**: 713–14.
5 Berger RS, Mandel EB, Hayes TJ *et al.* Minocycline staining of the oral cavity. *J Am Acad Dermatol* 1989; **21**: 1300–1.
6 Siller GM, Tod MA, Savage NW. Minocycline-induced oral pigmentation. *J Am Acad Dermatol* 1994; **30**: 350–4.

ACTH-induced hyperpigmentation

Oral hyperpigmentation may be seen in ACTH therapy, Addison's disease, Nelson's syndrome, or ectopic ACTH production (e.g. by bronchogenic carcinoma). The brown or black pigmentation is variable in distribution but is seen typically on the soft palate, buccal mucosa and at sites of trauma [1–4].

REFERENCES

1 Lamey PJ, Carmichael F, Scully C. Oral pigmentation, Addison's disease and results of screening. *Br Dent J* 1985; **158**: 297–305.
2 Merchant HW, Hayes LE, Ellison LT. Soft palate pigmentation in lung disease, including cancer. *Oral Surg* 1976; **41**: 726–33.
3 Moyer GN, Terezhalmy GT, O'Brien JT. Nelson's syndrome: another condition associated with mucocutaneous hyperpigmentation. *J Oral Med* 1982; **1**: 13–17.
4 Scully C. Drug-induced oral mucosal hyperpigmentation. *Prim Dent Care* 1997; **4**: 35–6.

Melanotic macule

Oral melanotic macule is similar to the ephelis and lentigo.

Melanotic macules are usually solitary, discrete, pigmented macules less than 2 cm in diameter, seen especially on the vermilion of the lips, gingiva, buccal mucosa or palate. Most are seen in white adult males and their colour ranges from brown to black [1]. There is melanin in the epithelial basal layer and/or upper lamina propria. Occasionally they are seen along with melanonychia striata (Laugier–Hunziker syndrome) [2,3].

They are benign, but may need excision to exclude melanoma.

Oral mucosal melanotic macule; reactive type

SYN. MELANOACANTHOMA

Melanotic macules occasionally appear suddenly as reactive lesions following trauma. Melanoacanthoma is a misnomer. Most reported cases have been in black people [4]. A hyperpigmented, symptomless macule appears over a course of days or weeks. The course is benign, and some cases resolve spontaneously within 6 months.

Pigment-filled dendritic cells which appear to be melanocytes are found in the stratum malpighii but, in contrast to melanoma, basal layer melanocytes are not increased.

Excision biopsy may be indicated to exclude melanoma.

REFERENCES

1 Buchner A, Hansen LS. Melanotic macule of the oral mucosa. *Oral Surg* 1979; **48**: 244–9.
2 Lamey PJ, Nolan A, Thomson E *et al*. Oral presentation of the Laugier–Hunziker syndrome. *R Dent J* 1991; **171**: 59–60.
3 Laugier P, Hunziker N. Pigmentation melanique lenticulaire essentielle de la muquese jugale et des lèvres. *Arch Belg Dermatol Syphilol* 1970; **26**: 391–9.
4 Horlick HP, Wather RR, Zegarelli DJ *et al*. Mucosal melanotic macule, reactive type. A simulation of melanoma. *J Am Acad Dermatol* 1988; **19**: 786–91.

Melanotic neuroectodermal tumour of infancy

See Chapter 14

Malignant melanoma (Chapter 38)

Oral malignant melanoma is rare. Most patients are over 50 years of age and there is a male preponderance.

Malignant melanoma may arise in apparently normal oral mucosa or in a pre-existent pigmented naevus, most commonly in the palate or maxillary alveolus [1–5]. Metastatic melanoma is rare [4]. Features suggestive of malignancy include a rapid increase in size, change in colour, ulceration, pain, bleeding, the occurrence of satellite pigmented spots or regional lymph-node enlargement. The prognosis is poor unless detected very early [2,3]. Lesions suspected to be malignant melanoma should not be biopsied until the time of definitive surgical excision. The histology may show anaplastic, spindle-shaped or squamoid cells. However, the histology is quite varied and dopa staining may be required to help the diagnosis.

REFERENCES

1 Batsakis JG, Regezi JA, Solomon AR *et al*. The pathology of head and neck tumours: mucosal melanomas. *Head Neck Surg* 1982; **4**: 404–18.
2 Eisen D, Voorhees JJ. Oral melanoma and other pigmented lesions of the oral cavity. *J Am Acad Dermatol* 1991; **24**: 527–37.
3 Hoyt DJ, Jordan T, Fisher SR. Mucosal melanoma of the head and neck. *Arch Otolaryngol Head Neck Surg* 1989; **115**: 1096–9.
4 Patton LL, Brahim JS, Baker AR. Metastatic malignant melanoma of the oral cavity. *Oral Surg* 1994; **78**: 51–6.
5 Rapini RP, Golitz LE, Greer RO *et al*. Primary malignant melanoma of the oral cavity. *Cancer* 1985; **55**: 1543–51.
6 Sooknundun M, Kacker SK, Kapila K *et al*. Oral malignant melanoma (a case report and review of the literature). *J Laryngol Otol* 1986; **100**: 371–5.

Pigmentary incontinence

Melanin pigment ingested by macrophages in the upper lamina propria (pigmentary incontinence) may give rise to hyperpigmentation in lichen planus, especially in dark-skinned people [1].

REFERENCE

1 Cawson RA, Binnie WH, Eveson JW. *Colour Atlas of Oral Disease: Clinical and Pathologic Correlations*. London: Heinemann, 1994: 1515.

Erythroplasia

Erythroplasia is a red, velvety lesion level with, or depressed below, the surrounding mucosa. It is uncommon and affects patients of either sex in their sixth and seventh decades. Some 75–90% of cases prove to be carcinoma or carcinoma-*in-situ* or show severe dysplasia. Erythroplasia usually involves the floor of the mouth, the ventrum of the tongue, or the soft palate (Fig. 69.51) [1–3].

The incidence of malignant change in erythroplasia is 17 times higher than in leukoplakia, and most lesions show dysplasia, carcinoma-*in-situ*, or invasive carcinoma. Areas of erythroplasia should be excised and sent for histological examination.

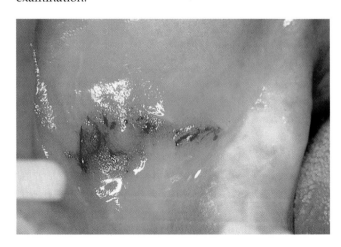

Fig. 69.51 Erythroplasia. (Courtesy of Professor R.A. Cawson, Eastman Dental Institute, London, UK.)

REFERENCES

1 Binnie WH, Rankin KV, Mackenzie IC. Etiology of oral squamous cell carcinoma. *J Oral Pathol* 1983; **12**: 11–29.
2 Eveson JW. Oral premalignancy. *Cancer Surv* 1983; **2**: 403–24.
3 Scully C, Cawson RA. Oral potentially malignant lesions. *J Epidemiol Biostat* 1996; **1**: 3–12.

Denture-induced stomatitis

SYN. DENTURE SORE MOUTH

This common form of mild, chronic, atrophic oral candidiasis occurs only beneath a denture, usually a complete upper denture, and is not often sore despite its name [1,2]. Dentures worn throughout the night, or with a dry mouth, favour development of this infection with *Candida* species. It is not caused by allergy to the denture material but it is not clear why only some denture wearers develop the condition. It is a disease mainly of the middle-aged or elderly and is more prevalent in women than men. Patients appear otherwise healthy.

There is erythema limited to the denture-bearing area (Fig. 69.52), and the stomatitis predisposes to angular stomatitis (Chapter 70). Occasionally, small nodules (papillary hyperplasia) appear in the vault of the palate and initiate a vicious circle since they create an environment that favours growth of *Candida* [2–4].

Dentures should be left out of the mouth at night, in 0.2% aqueous chlorhexidine or 1% hypochlorite (e.g. Milton or Dentural) since the fitting surface is infested with *Candida*. Topical antifungals may be useful to eradicate the mucosal infection [2,5].

REFERENCES

1 Budzt-Jorgensen E. Oral mucosal lesions associated with the wearing of removable dentures. *J Oral Pathol* 1981; **10**: 65–80.
2 Scully C. Chronic atrophic candidiasis. *Lancet* 1986; **ii**: 437–8.
3 Dorey JL, Blasberg B, MacEntee MI *et al*. Oral mucosal disorders in denture wearers. *J Pros Dent* 1985; **53**: 210–13.

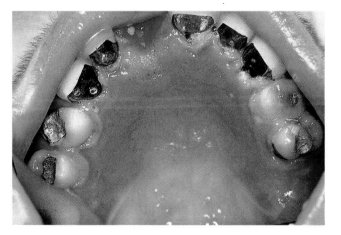

Fig. 69.52 Denture-induced stomatitis, showing diffuse erythema in the denture-bearing area.

4 Samaranyake LP, MacFarlane TW. A retrospective study of patients with recurrent chronic atrophic candidiasis. *Oral Surg* 1981; **52**: 150–3.
5 Walker DM, Stafford DG, Huggett R *et al*. The treatment of denture-induced stomatitis. *Br Dent J* 1981; **151**: 416–19.

Erythematous candidiasis

Oral candidiasis can cause erythema and soreness of the oral mucosa, with or without the more usual thrush.

Median rhomboid glossitis

SYN. CENTRAL PAPILLARY ATROPHY OF THE TONGUE

Aetiology. This red, depapillated, rhomboidal area in the centre line of the dorsum of the tongue, just anterior to the sulcus terminalis, was formerly thought to be caused by persistence of the tuberculum impar. However, it is now thought to be associated with candidiasis [1,2]. Smoking, denture wearing and, occasionally, immune defects, including HIV, predispose to this lesion.

Pathology. Histology shows irregular pseudoepitheliomatous epithelial hyperplasia which may resemble a carcinoma but it is not a malignant condition.

Clinical features. This is typically a red, central lesion of somewhat rhomboidal shape anterior to the sulcus terminalis on the dorsum of the tongue (Fig. 69.53). Occasionally, there is a nodular component. There may also sometimes be a coexistent erythematous candidiasis in the palate [3].

Diagnosis and management. Median rhomboid glossitis is usually diagnosed on clinical grounds, although biopsy may be indicated, since some lesions are nodular and may simulate a neoplasm. It may respond to cessation of smoking and to the use of antifungals.

REFERENCES

1 Touyz LZG, Peters E. Candidal infection of the tongue with non-specific inflammation of the palate. *Oral Surg* 1987; **63**: 304–8.
2 van der Waal I. Candida albicans in median rhomboid glossitis: a post-mortem study. *Int J Oral Maxillofac Surg* 1986; **15**: 322–5.
3 Holmstrup P, Besserman M. Clinical, therapeutic and pathogenic aspects of chronic oral multifocal candidiasis. *Oral Surg* 1984; **56**: 388–95.

Chronic marginal gingivitis

The accumulation of dental bacterial plaque because of inadequate oral hygiene produces non-specific chronic inflammation.

This is an extremely common condition. Over 90% of dentate adults exhibits some degree of gingivitis. It is painless but may manifest with bleeding from the gingival crevice. The gingival margins are red and slightly swollen [1].

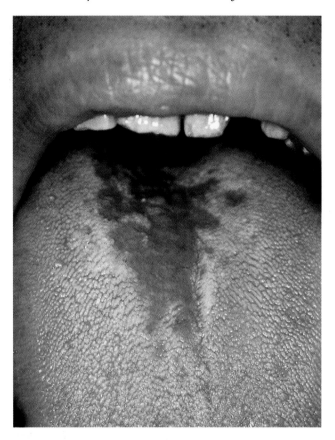

Fig. 69.53 Median rhomboid glossitis.

Dental advice on improved oral hygiene is needed. If untreated it may progress to periodontitis and tooth loss.

REFERENCE

1 Page RC. Gingivitis. *J Clin Periodontol* 1986; **13**: 345–59.

Desquamative gingivitis

In this condition, the labial gingiva are persistently glazed, red and sore but the gingival margins may be spared, differentiating desquamative gingivitis from chronic marginal gingivitis (see Fig. 69.28). Desquamative gingivitis typically affects middle-aged or elderly women and is usually a manifestation of mucous membrane pemphigoid or lichen planus [1–4]. Rarely, it may be seen in pemphigus, dermatitis herpetiformis, linear IgA disease, chronic ulcer-ative stomatitis with epithelial antinuclear antibodies or other dermatoses [4]. This tends to be a chronic recalcitrant condition. The underlying condition should be treated where possible. Improved oral hygiene and use of topical corticosteroids in a nocturnally worn polythene splint may help. Dapsone or topical cyclosporin sometimes may be beneficial in severe cases.

REFERENCES

1 Nisengard RJ, Nieders M. Desquamative lesions of the gingiva. *J Periodontol* 1981; **52**: 500–10.
2 Nisengard RJ, Levine RA. Diagnosis and management of desquamative gingivitis. *Periodontol Insights* 1995; **2**: 4–10.
3 Rees TD. Vesiculo-ulcerative diseases and periodontal practice. *J Periodontol* 1995; **66**: 747–8.
4 Scully C. Oral medicine and periodontal disease. *Periodontol 2000* (in press).

Allergic gingivostomatitis

SYN. ATYPICAL OR PLASMA-CELL
GINGIVOSTOMATITIS

Diffusely red, swollen gingivae with or without oral ulceration may occasionally follow exposure to various allergens and other substances. Such reactions have followed the use of certain chewing gums, confectionery such as mints, and dentifrices [1–7]. More recently, various tartar control dentifrices in which cinnamon, or derivatives such as cinnamaldehyde, are present have been implicated [2]

These lesions resolve on withdrawal of the causal agent and reappear on rechallenge. Biopsy is usually not indicated and is fairly non-specific with epithelial atrophy, oedema and a variable cellular infiltrate in the lamina propria which, in the earlier reported cases due to chewing gum, was often predominantly plasmacytic [1,3,5–7]. Patch testing may be of value in diagnosis.

REFERENCES

1 Kerr DA, McClarchey KD, Regezi JA. Allergic gingivostomatitis (due to gum chewing). *J Periodontol* 1971; **42**: 709–12.
2 Lamey PJ, Lewis MAO, Rees TD *et al.* Sensitivity reaction to the cinnamaldehyde component of toothpaste. *Br Dent J* 1990; **168**: 115–18.
3 Lubow RM, Cooley RL, Hartman KJ *et al.* Plasma cell gingivitis: report of a case. *J Periodontol* 1984; **55**: 234–41.
4 MacLeod FI, Ellis JE. Plasma cell gingivitis related to the use of herbal toothpaste. *Br Dent J* 1989; **166**: 375–6.
5 Owings JR. An atypical gingivostomatitis: a report of four cases. *J Periodontol* 1969; **40**: 538–42.
6 Palmer RM, Eveson JW. Plasma cell gingivitis. *Oral Surg* 1981; **51**: 187–9.
7 Perry HO, Deffnes NF, Sheridan SJ. Atypical gingivostomatitis. *Arch Dermatol* 1973; **107**: 872–8.

Idiopathic plasmacytosis (see also Plasma-cell balanitis, p. 3190)

This term refers to red, velvety gingival lesions associated with a plasmacytic infiltrate. Most cases are restricted to the gingiva (atypical gingivostomatitis, plasmacyte gingivitis, allergic gingivostomatitis) [1] while a few have supraglottic laryngeal lesions [2]. Corticosteroids are the main treatment.

REFERENCES

1 White JW, Olsen KD, Banks PM. Plasma cell orofacial mucositis. *Arch Dermatol* 1986; **122**: 1321–4.
2 Timms M, Sloan P. Association of supraglottic and gingival idiopathic plasmacytosis. *Oral Surg* 1991; **71**: 451–3.

Telangiectasia (Chapter 45)

Oral telangiectases occur mainly in hereditary haemorrhagic telangiectasia, systemic sclerosis, cirrhosis and after radiotherapy.

Kaposi's sarcoma (Chapter 55)

Kaposi's sarcoma (KS) is now seen predominantly as a consequence of HIV infection, mainly in male homosexuals. It appears to be associated with a herpesvirus [1,2]. Up to 50% of male homosexual AIDS patients have developed oral KS but it appears to be declining in frequency and is rare in other HIV-infected patients.

Oral KS is the first presentation of HIV in 20–60% of affected patients, often associated with oral candidiasis. KS affects the hard-palate mucosa in particular (Fig. 69.54). Up to 95% of lesions are seen in the palate, 23% in the gingiva and others on the tongue or buccal mucosa. A red–purple macule is the early lesion, progressing to a purple nodular swelling which may be extensive and ulcerated. Multiple lesions are common [3–6]. Lesions may often be asymptomatic but more than 25% are painful and about 8% bleed. Oral KS is also occasionally seen in other non-HIV immunocompromised patients.

Oral KS may regress occasionally spontaneously, or with zidovudine or systemic vinca alkaloids, etoposide or interferon, but the more usual treatment is local radiotherapy, laser removal or intralesional vinblastine. The latter produces fewer adverse effects than radiotherapy [4,7–9].

REFERENCES

1 Chang Y, Cesarman E, Pessin MS *et al*. Identification of herpesvirus-like DNA sequences in AIDS-associated Kaposi's sarcoma. *Science* 1994; **266**: 1865–9.

2 DiAlberti L, Teo CG, Porter S *et al*. Kaposi's sarcoma herpesvirus in oral Kaposi's sarcoma. *Oral Oncol* 1996; **32B**: 68–9.
3 Epstein JB, Scully C. HIV infection: clinical oral features and management in 33 homosexual males referred with Kaposi's sarcoma. *Oral Surg* 1991; **71**: 38–41.
4 Epstein J, Scully C. Neoplastic disease in the head and neck of patients with AIDS. *Int J Oral Maxillofac Surg* 1992; **2**: 219–26.
5 Ficarra G, Berson AM, Silverman S *et al*. Kaposi's sarcoma of the oral cavity: a study of 134 patients with a review of the pathogenesis, epidemiology, clinical aspects and treatment. *Oral Surg* 1988; **66**: 543–50.
6 Lumerman H, Freedman PD, Kerpel SM *et al*. Oral Kaposi's sarcoma: a clinicopathologic study of 23 homosexual and bisexual men from the New York metropolitan area. *Oral Surg* 1988 **65**: 711–16.
7 Scully C, Porter SR. An ABC of oral health care in HIV infection. *Br Dent J* 1990; **170**: 149–50.
8 Scully C, Spittle M. Malignant tumours of the oral cavity in HIV disease. In: Langdon J, Henk JM, eds. *Malignant Tumours of the Mouth, Jaws and Salivary Glands*. London: Edward Arnold, 1995: 246–57.
9 Porter SR, Scully C, eds. *Oral Health Care for those with HIV Infection and other Special Needs*. Northwood: Science Reviews, 1995: 51–61.

Varicosities

Bluish oral varicosities may often be seen in elderly patients, particularly in the ventrum and lateral margin of the tongue. They are benign and inconsequential.

Loss of elasticity of oral tissues

Fibrosis of oral tissues can follow burns or irradiation. It may also be associated with habits such as the chewing of betel nut (areca), which predisposes to oral submucous fibrosis (see below) and it may be caused by a connective tissue disorder such as scleroderma. Rarely it is occupational (polyvinylchloride workers). Epidermolysis bullosa and mucous membrane pemphigoid may cause scarring and the orofacial region is occasionally involved in multiple idiopathic fibrosis [1].

REFERENCE

1 Lewin IG, Carter JLB, Evans N *et al*. Multiple idiopathic fibrosis presenting as facial pain and trismus. *Br J Oral Surg* 1985; **23**: 135–9.

Oral submucous fibrosis

Aetiology. Oral submucous fibrosis (OSMF) is a chronic disease of the oral mucosa that appears to be caused by exposure to constituents of the areca nut. It is found virtually exclusively in persons from the Indian subcontinent; most of those affected chew areca nut with tobacco, betel leaf and lime [1,2].

Pathology. There is a subepithelial chronic inflammatory reaction with fibrosis extending to the submucosa and muscle. Epithelial changes range from atrophy to keratosis and there may be dysplasia.

Clinical features. OSMF develops insidiously, often initially presenting with oral dysaesthesia and a non-specific vesicular stomatitis [3]. Later there may be symmetrical fibrosis

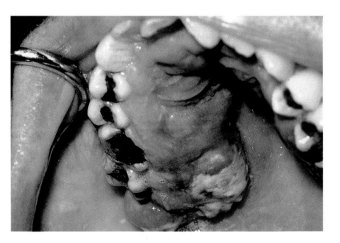

Fig. 69.54 Kaposi's sarcoma in a typical site with a characteristic purplish appearance. (Courtesy of Dr J.B. Epstein, Cancer Control Agency, Vancouver, Canada.)

of the cheeks, lips or palate which may be symptomless and noted only as bands running through the mucosa. This can, however, become so severe that the affected site becomes white and firm, with severe restriction of opening of the mouth.

Oral submucous fibrosis appears to be restricted to the mouth, although many patients are also anaemic. OSMF may predispose to the development of oral carcinoma which occurs in 2–10% of patients over 10 years [4,5].

The diagnosis can be confirmed by biopsy.

Treatment. Management is difficult. Intralesional corticosteroids and jaw exercises may be useful in the early stages, but surgery may be needed to relieve the fibrosis [1,6].

REFERENCES

1 Caniff JP. Mucosal diseases of uncertain etiology: III Oral submucous fibrosis. In: Mackenzie IC, Squier CA, Dabelsteen E, eds. *Oral Mucosal Diseases: Biology, Etiology and Therapy.* Copenhagen: Laegeforeningen Forlag, 1987: 87–91.
2 Caniff JP, Harvey W. The aetiology of oral submucous fibrosis: the stimulation of collagen synthesis by extracts of areca nut. *Int J Oral Surg* 1981; **10**: 163–7.
3 Pindborg JJ, Bhonsle RB, Murti PR *et al.* Incidence and early forms of oral submucous fibrosis. *Oral Surg* 1980; **50**: 40–4.
4 Gupta PC, Bhonsle RB, Murti PR *et al.* An epidemiologic assessment of cancer risk in oral precancerous lesions in India with special reference to nodular leukoplakia. *Cancer* 1989; **63**: 2247–52.
5 Pindborg JJ, Murti PR, Bhonsle RB *et al.* Oral submucous fibrosis as a precancerous condition. *Scand J Dent Res* 1984; **92**: 224–9.
6 Yen DJ. Surgical treatment of submucous fibrosis. *Oral Surg* 1982; **54**: 269–72.

Systemic sclerosis (Chapter 58)

Oral features are common in systemic sclerosis and are generally more obvious in those with diffuse than in localized scleroderma. About 70% of patients have xerostomia, and there is an increase in both caries and periodontal disease. A characteristic finding is of increased width of the periodontal ligament space of all teeth on radiography [1]. There are mandibular erosions in the angle particularly, but also in the condyle, coronoid or digastric regions. Telangiectasia may be seen and most patients have restricted oral opening, with linear wrinkles of the lips [2,3].

REFERENCES

1 Alexandridis C, White SC. Periodontal ligament changes in patients with progressive systemic sclerosis. *Oral Surg* 1984; **58**: 113–18.
2 Masmary Y, Glais R, Pisanty S. Scleroderma: oral manifestations. *Oral Surg* 1981; **52**: 32–7.
3 Wood RE, Lee P. Analysis of the oral manifestations of systemic sclerosis (scleroderma). *Oral Surg* 1988; **65**: 172–8.

Lumps and swellings

Lumps in the mouth range from simple anatomical variants, which can cause the patient considerable concern to lumps caused by inflammatory, cystic (Fig. 69.55), neoplastic and other disorders (Table 69.24).

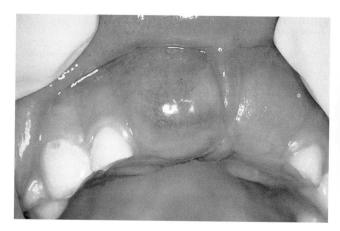

Fig. 69.55 Bluish, fluctuant swelling of an oral cyst, in this case an eruption cyst over an erupting maxillary permanent incisor. (The lesion on the maxillary canine is early dental caries.)

Foliate papillitis

The foliate lingual papillae may become inflamed and swell. Because of their location on the posterolateral tongue this may give undue concern about malignancy. The condition resolves spontaneously.

Torus palatinus and torus mandibularis

Torus palatinus is a developmental benign exostosis sometimes found in the centre of the hard palate. It is a painless non-enlarging, bony, hard lump with a normal overlying mucosa (Fig. 69.56) and a smooth or nodular surface [1,2]. Torus mandibularis is a similar exostosis found lingual to the premolar teeth, usually bilaterally. Tori are common conditions of no consequence, apart from occasionally interfering with denture construction.

The diagnosis is confirmed by radiography. Surgery is rarely indicated.

REFERENCES

1 Eggen S, Natvig B. Relationship between torus mandibularis and number of present teeth. *Scand J Dent Res* 1986; **94**: 233–40.
2 Rezai RF. Torus palatinus, an exostosis of unknown aetiology: review of the literature. *Compend Contin Educ Dent* 1985; **6**: 149–52.

Osteoma mucosae
SYN. OSSEOUS CHORISTOMA

There are rare cases of osteoma of the oral mucosa, usually in the tongue. Most have been in females in the third and fourth decades and have arisen as pedunculated, hard, painless lumps on the dorsum of the tongue immediately posterior to the foramen caecum [1–3]. They may arise from thyroid anlages. Simple excision suffices.

REFERENCES

1 Busuttil A. An osteoma of the tongue. *J Laryngol* 1977; **91**: 259–61.

Table 69.24 Lesions which may cause the complaint of lumps or swellings in the mouth.

Normal anatomical features	Pterygoid hamulus Parotid papillae Foliate or other lingual papillae Unerupted teeth
Developmental	Haemangioma Lymphangioma Maxillary and mandibular tori Hereditary gingival fibromatosis Von Recklinghausen's neurofibromatosis Cysts of developmental origin Odontomes
Inflammatory	Abscess Pyogenic granuloma Oral Crohn's disease Pulse granuloma Sarcoidosis Wegener's granuloma Others
Traumatic	Epulis Fibroepithelial polyp Denture-induced granuloma Mucocele Herniation of buccal fat pad
Infective	Various papillomatous lesions
Cystic	Cysts of odontogenic origin (e.g. dental cysts)
Drug therapy (gingival swelling only)	Oral contraceptive (pill gingivitis) Phenytoin Calcium-channel blockers Cyclosporin
Hormonal	Pubertal gingivitis Pregnancy epulis/gingivitis
Blood dyscrasias	Leukaemia, lymphoma and myeloma
Benign neoplasms	Various
Malignant neoplasms	Primary and secondary
Others	Angioedema Amyloidosis Fibro-osseous diseases Acanthosis nigricans

2 Markaki S, Gearty J, Markakis P. Osteoma of the tongue. *Br J Oral Surg* 1987; **25**: 79–82.
3 Sheridan SM. Osseous choristoma: a report of two cases. *Br J Oral Surg* 1984; **22**: 99–102.

Fibrous nodules

Fibroepithelial polyp

SYN. FIBROUS LUMP

Fibrous lumps are common in the mouth and are seen

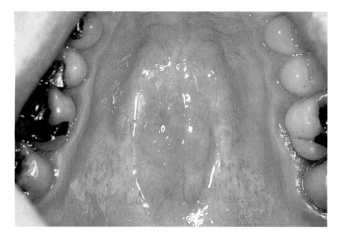

Fig. 69.56 Torus palatinus.

mainly in adults. They appear to be purely reparative in nature. They may attain their full size (which rarely exceeds 2.5 cm diameter) quite rapidly, and then stop growing.

Pathology. A well-keratinized stratified squamous epithelium overlies thick collagenous bundles.

Fibrous lumps should not be confused with the true fibroma, a benign neoplasm derived from fibroblasts, which is rare in the mouth (see below).

Clinical features. The variable inflammatory changes account for the different clinical presentations of fibrous lumps from red, shiny, soft lumps to those which are pale, stippled and firm [1]. Commonly, they are round, pedunculated swellings arising from the marginal or papillary gingiva (epulides), sometimes adjacent to sites of irritation (e.g. a carious cavity). They are usually painless. They may reach quite a large size, but the prognosis is good.

Treatment. Fibrous epulides should be removed down to the periosteum, which should be curetted thoroughly.

Fibroma

The true fibroma, a benign neoplasm of fibroblastic origin, is rare in the oral cavity and many lesions in the past called fibromas were probably fibroepithelial polyps.

Pathology. Histology shows marked proliferation of fibroblasts, with nuclei of uniform shape, size and staining characteristics.

Clinical features. The true fibroma is a continuously enlarging new growth, not necessarily arising at a site of potential trauma. It is a pedunculated growth with a smooth, non-ulcerated, pink surface.

Treatment. Removal should be total, deep and wide.

REFERENCE

1 Lee KW. The fibrous epulis and related lesions. *Periodontics* 1986; **6:** 277–99.

Abscesses

Most intraoral abscesses are odontogenic in origin, as a final consequence of dental caries. Most abscesses discharge in the mouth on the buccal gingiva but occasionally they discharge palatally, lingually, on the chin or submental region (Fig. 69.57), or elsewhere. Very occasionally abscesses follow trauma, a foreign body, or rarely are related to unusual oral infections such as actinomycosis [1], nocardiosis or botryomycosis [2]. Drainage and appropriate antimicrobials are indicated [3]. Dental attention is required; dental abscesses are drained by tooth extraction, incision and drainage, or through the root canal (endodontics).

REFERENCES

1 Brignall ID, Gilhooly M. Actinomycosis of the tongue: a diagnostic dilemma. *Br J Oral Surg* 1989; **27:** 249–53.
2 Small IA, Kobernick S. Botryomycosis of the tongue. *Oral Surg* 1967; **24:** 503–9.
3 Luker J. A case of lingual abscess. *Br Dent J* 1985; **159:** 300.

Pyogenic granuloma (Chapter 55)

Pyogenic granuloma commonly affects the gingiva, the lip or the tongue [1]. In these sites, the lesion should be excised completely. It will readily recur if excision is not adequate.

REFERENCE

1 Vilmann A, Vilmann P, Vilmann H. Pyogenic granuloma: evaluation of oral conditions. *Br J Oral Surg* 1986; **24:** 376–82.

Sarcoidosis

Isolated nodules [1,2] gingival lesions [3], facial or labial

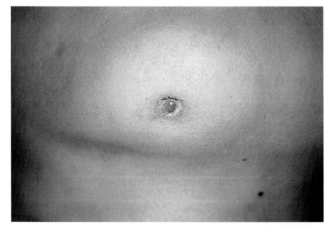

Fig. 69.57 Sinus on chin related to a dental abscess on a mandibular incisor tooth.

swelling [4] and salivary gland involvement are the main oral or perioral lesions of sarcoidosis, but are uncommon. However, even where the mucosa is clinically normal, patients with sarcoidosis may have characteristic changes in palatal or labial salivary gland biopsies [5].

REFERENCES

1 Mendelsohn SS, Field EA, Woolgar J. Sarcoidosis of the tongue. *Clin Exp Dermatol* 1992; **17:** 47–8.
2 Tillman HH, Taylor RG, Carchidi JE. Sarcoidosis of the tongue. *Oral Surg* 1968; **21:** 190–5.
3 Hayter JP, Robertson JM. Sarcoidosis presenting as gingivitis. *Br Med J* 1988; **296:** 1504.
4 Gold RS, Sager E. Oral sarcoidosis: review of the literature. *J Oral Surg* 1976; **34:** 237–44.
5 Van Maarsseveen ACMTH, Van der Waal I, Stam J *et al.* Oral involvement in sarcoidosis. *Int J Oral Surg* 1982; **11:** 21–9.

Oral Crohn's disease
SYN. OROFACIAL GRANULOMATOSIS

Aetiology. Crohn's disease can affect the mouth but some patients appear to develop similar oral lesions because of an adverse reaction to various food additives such as cinnamaldehyde or benzoates [1–11]. The term orofacial granulomatosis is preferred in some centres since it is unclear where in the spectrum of Crohn's disease/sarcoidosis/allergy/infection these lesions (and related conditions such as Melkersson–Rosenthal syndrome and granulomatous cheilitis) lie [8,12–14].

Pathology. Non-caseating granulomas and lymphoedema may be seen but the granulomas tend to be sparse and deep, close to the muscle.

Clinical features. Oral ulcers in classic Crohn's disease may be aphthae due to malabsorption, but may also be due to primary Crohn's disease of the oral mucosa or to coincidental ulceration of other aetiology. Ulcers classically involve the buccal sulcus where they appear as linear ulcers, often with granulomatous masses flanking them.

Mucosal lesions also include thickening and folding of the mucosa to produce a 'cobblestone' type of appearance and mucosal tags. Purple granulomatous enlargements may appear on the gingiva [12]. The lips or face may swell and there may be splitting of the lips and angular stomatitis. Patients may be predisposed to dental caries.

Diagnosis. The oral history is not specific, and investigation of the gastrointestinal tract is mandatory [15,16]. Investigations such as chest radiography, serum angiotensin converting enzyme, gallium scan and a Kveim test may be required to exclude sarcoidosis [9].

Treatment. Elimination diets may be warranted in patients with orofacial granulomatosis if allergy is suspected [11].

Topical or intralesional corticosteroids may effectively control the oral lesions [6] but more frequently systemic corticosteroids, azathioprine or salazopyrine are required. Metronidazole may be of value in some cases [3].

REFERENCES

1 Field EA, Tyldesley WR. Oral Crohn's disease revisited—a 10 year review. *Br J Oral Maxillofac Surg* 1989; **27**: 114–23.
2 Halme L, Meurman JH, Laine P *et al.* Oral findings in patients with active or inactive Crohn's disease. *Oral Surg* 1993; **76**: 175–81.
3 Kano Y, Shiohara T, Yagita A. Treatment of recalcitrant cheilitis granulomatosa with metronidazole. *J Am Acad Dermatol* 1992; **27**: 629–30.
4 Patton DW, Ferguson MM, Forsyth A *et al.* Orofacial granulomatosis: a possible allergic basis. *Br J Oral Maxillofac Surg* 1985; **23**: 235–42.
5 Ronney T. Dental caries prevalence in patients with Crohn's disease. *Oral Surg* 1984; **57**: 623–4.
6 Sakuntabhai A. MacLeod RI, Lawrence CM. Intralesional steroid injection after nerve block anesthesia in the treatment of orofacial granulomatosis. *Arch Dermatol* 1993; **129**: 477–80.
7 Scully C, Cochran KM, Russell RI *et al.* Crohn's disease of the mouth: an indication of intestinal involvement. *Gut* 1982; **23**: 198–201.
8 Scully C, Eveson JW. Orofacial granulomatosis. *Lancet* 1991; **338**: 20–1.
9 Shehade SA, Foulds IS. Granulomatous cheilitis and a positive Kveim test. *Br J Dermatol* 1986; **115**: 619–22.
10 Sundh B, Emilson CG. Salivary and microbial conditions and dental health in patients with Crohn's disease: a 3-year study. *Oral Surg* 1989; **67**: 286–90.
11 Sweatman MC, Tasker R, Warner JO *et al.* Orofacial granulomatosis. Response to elimination diet and provocation by food additives. *Clin Allergy* 1986; **16**: 331–7.
12 Worsaae N, Pindborg JJ. Granulomatous gingival manifestations of Melkersson—Rosenthal syndrome. *Oral Surg* 1980; **49**: 131–8.
13 Worsaae N, Christensen KO, Bondesen S *et al.* Melkersson–Rosenthal syndrome and Crohn's disease. *Br J Oral Surg* 1980; **18**: 254–8.
14 Zimmer WM, Rogers RS, Reeve CM, Sheridan PJ. Orofacial manifestations of Melkersson–Rosenthal syndrome. *Oral Surg* 1992; **74**: 610–19.
15 Wiesenfield DW, Ferguson MM, Mitchell D *et al.* Orofacial granulomatosis: a clinical and pathological analysis. *Q J Med* 1985; **54**: 101–13.
16 Williams AJK, Wray D, Ferguson A. The clinical entity of orofacial Crohn's disease. *Q J Med* 1991; **79**: 451–8.

Pulse granuloma
SYN. LEWAR'S DISEASE

Chronic mandibular periostitis caused by embedded vegetable matter of dietary origin is uncommon but typically presents as a submucosal lump over the lower alveolus. Histology shows amorphous hyaline material and a granulomatous inflammatory reaction [1]. Excision suffices.

REFERENCE

1 Keirby FAR, Soames JV. Periostitis and osteitis associated with hyaline bodies. *Br J Oral Surg* 1985; **23**: 346–50.

Denture-induced hyperplasia
SYN. DENTURE GRANULOMA, EPULIS FISSURATUM

Where a denture flange is overextended and irritates the vestibular mucosa, a linear reparative process may result, eventually producing an elongated fibroepithelial enlargement—denture-induced hyperplasia [1]. The pathology is that of a fibrous lump (p. 3111).

Firm, leaf-like, painless swellings are seen, usually in the buccal or labial vestibule.

A denture-induced granuloma should be excised and examined histologically, if modification of the denture does not induce regression. Rarely, a denture granuloma arises because some other lesion develops beneath a denture and causes the mucosa to be irritated.

REFERENCE

1 Budzt-Jorgensen E. Oral mucosal lesions associated with the wearing of removable dentures. *J Oral Pathol* 1981; **10**: 65–80.

Mucocele

Superficial mucoceles are discussed on page 3095. Deeper mucoceles are more common and are usually seen in the lower labial mucosa where they arise as painless, bluish, cystic fluctuant lesions (Fig. 69.58), usually resulting from the escape of mucus into the lamina propria from a damaged minor salivary gland duct. Care must be taken to exclude a cystic neoplasm particularly in a lesion in the upper lip which might appear to be a mucocele. Excision and cryosurgery are the usual means of treatment.

Buccal fat-pad herniation

Trauma may rarely cause the buccal pad of fat to herniate through the buccinator muscle, producing an intraoral swelling [1]. This usually occurs in males under the age of 4 years. Surgery is indicated.

REFERENCE

1 Fleming P. Traumatic herniation of buccal fat pad: a report of two cases. *J Oral Surg* 1986; **24**: 265–8.

Oral papilloma

Aetiology. These are caused by human papillomaviruses (HPV) [1].

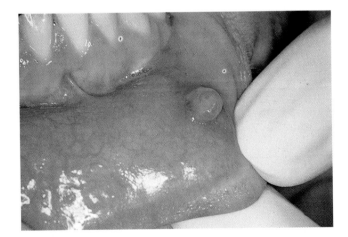

Fig. 69.58 Mucocele in a typical site.

Pathology. Histology includes acanthotic and sometimes hyperkeratotic epithelium with occasional koilocytosis.

Clinical features. Papillomas can appear anywhere in the mouth, but are most common at the junction of the hard and soft palate. The papilloma is a white or pink, cauliflower-like lesion which may resemble a wart. Papillomas of normal colour may be confused with the commoner fibroepithelial polyps, although the latter are commonest at sites of potential trauma.

Prognosis. Unlike some papillomas of the larynx or bowel, oral papillomas remain benign.

Diagnosis. Oral papillomas should be examined histologically to establish a correct diagnosis.

Treatment. Excision must be total, deep and wide enough to include any abnormal cells beyond the zone of the pedicle.

REFERENCE

1 Scully C, Cox MF, Prime SS *et al*. Papillomaviruses: the current status in relation to oral disease. *Oral Surg* 1988; **65**: 526–32.

Warts (Chapter 26)

Common warts (verrucae vulgaris) and venereal warts (condyloma acuminatum) are both caused by papillomaviruses [1–3]. They are rare in the mouth (Fig. 69.59) but are more common in HIV disease. None is known to be premalignant. Most can be removed by excision, cryosurgery or laser.

REFERENCES

1 Green TL, Eversole LP, Leider AS. Oral and labial verruca vulgaris: clinical, histologic and immunohistochemical evaluation. *Oral Surg* 1986; **62**: 410–16.

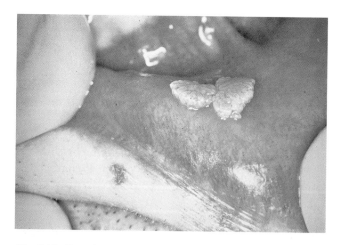

Fig. 69.59 Genital warts on the lower lip in human immunodeficiency virus infection. (There is also a healing herpes simplex lesion on the lip.)

2 Scully C, Cox M, Maitland N *et al*. Papillomaviruses: their current status in relation to oral disease. *Oral Surg* 1988; **65**: 526–32.
3 Scully C, Prime S, Maitland N. Papillomaviruses: their possible role in oral disease. *Oral Surg* 1985; **60**: 166–74.

Focal epithelial hyperplasia
SYN. HECK'S DISEASE

Focal epithelial hyperplasia (FEH) is a rare, benign, familial disorder with no sex predisposition, characterized by multiple, soft, circumscribed, sessile, nodular elevations of the oral mucosa [1,2].

Heck's disease occurs particularly in native Americans and in Inuits in Greenland but has been reported rarely from many other countries. The prevalence in Greenland and Venezuela approaches 35% [1,3,4].

Aetiology. The papillomaviruses HPV-13 and HPV-32 appear to be causal in patients with the genetic predisposition to FEH [5–8].

Pathology. The characteristics of FEH are local epithelial hyperplasia, acanthosis and elongated 'Bronze Age axe' rete ridges, together with a ballooning type of nuclear degeneration. Epithelial cells have a pseudomitotic appearance.

Clinical features. Among native Americans, FEH mainly affects children and usually involves the lower lip, whereas in Eskimos and in white people the lesions are found mainly in the fourth decade and later and often affect the tongue. This is a benign asymptomatic condition, requiring only reassurance.

REFERENCES

1 Axell T, Hammarstrom L, Larsson A. Focal epithelial hyperplasia in Sweden. *Acta Odontol Scand* 1981; **39**: 201–8.
2 Starink TM, Woerdeman MJ. Focal epithelial hyperplasia of the oral mucosa. *Br J Dermatol* 1977; **96**: 375–80.
3 Praetorius-Clausen F, Mogeltoft M, Roed-Petersen B *et al*. Focal epithelial hyperplasia of the oral mucosa in a South-West Greenlandic population. *Scand J Dent J* 1970; **78**: 287–94.
4 Scully C, Cox M, Prime SS *et al*. Papillomaviruses: the current status in relation to oral disease. *Oral Surg* 1988; **65**: 526–32.
5 Beaudenon S, Praetorius F, Kremsdorf D *et al*. A new type of human papillomavirus associated with oral focal epithelial hyperplasia. *J Invest Dermatol* 1987; **88**: 130–5.
6 Garlick JA, Calderon S, Buchner A *et al*. Detection of human papillomavirus in focal epithelial hyperplasia. *J Oral Pathol Med* 1989; **18**: 172–7.
7 Henke RP, Guerin-Reverschon I, Milde-Langosch K *et al*. In situ detection of human papillomavirus types 13 and 32 in focal epithelial hyperplasia of the oral mucosa. *J Oral Pathol Med* 1989; **18**: 419–21.
8 Hernandes-Juaregui P, Eriksonn A, Tamayo-Perez R *et al*. Human papillomavirus type 13 DNA in focal epithelial hyperplasia among Mexicans. *Arch Virol* 1987; **93**: 131–7.

Papillary hyperplasia

Papillary hyperplasia may be seen in the vault of the palate typically in persons with chronic denture-induced stomatitis and occasionally in its absence [1,2]. It may require excision or laser removal.

REFERENCES

1 O'Driscoll PM. Papillary hyperplasia of the palate. *Br Dent J* 1965; **118**: 77–80.
2 Schmitz JF. A clinical study of inflammatory papillary hyperplasia. *J Prosthet Dent* 1964; **14**: 1034–9.

Rhabdomyoma

Rhabdomyomas are rare but most extracardiac rhabdomyomas present in the mouth, typically as lumps in the floor of mouth, tongue or soft palate [1,2]. Most are seen in the sixth decade, predominantly in males. Surgery is effective provided total excision is achieved.

REFERENCES

1 Corio RL, Lewis DM. Intraoral rhabdomyomas. *Oral Surg* 1979; **48**: 525–31.
2 Reid CO, Smith CJ. Rhabdomyoma of the floor of the mouth: a new case and review of recently reported intraoral rhabdomyomas. *Br J Oral Surg* 1985; **23**: 284–91.

Rhabdomyosarcoma

Some 45% of soft-tissue sarcomas in the head and neck region are rhabdomyosarcomas. The most common oral presentation is a progressively enlarging mass: some 20% have enlarged regional lymph nodes [1]. In advanced disease there may be pain, paraesthesia, trismus or loosening of teeth.

The prognosis is poor. Treatment includes cytotoxic chemotherapy, surgery and radiotherapy.

REFERENCE

1 Bras J, Batsakis JG, Luna MA. Rhabdomyosarcoma of the oral soft tissues. *Oral Surg* 1987; **64**: 585–96.

Nodular fasciitis (Chapter 55)

Nodular (pseudosarcomatous) fasciitis affects the head and neck in 20% of cases but rarely involves the mouth [1,2].

REFERENCES

1 Davies HT, Bradley N, Bowerman JE. Oral nodular fasciitis. *Br J Oral Surg* 1989; **27**: 147–51.
2 Kawana T, Yamamoto H, Deguchi A *et al.* Nodular fasciitis of the upper labial fascia. Cytometric and ultrastructural studies. *Int J Oral Surg* 1986; **15**: 464–8.

Verruciform xanthoma

Although verruciform xanthoma was originally described as a distinct oral entity it is now also known occasionally to affect the skin and non-oral mucosae [1]. The aetiology is unknown but may be a reaction to some irritant.

The lesions consist of parakeratotic verruciform epithelium, with large, foamy xanthoma cells containing slightly PAS-positive granules and abundant lipid in the lamina propria between the epithelial pegs [2].

Verruciform xanthoma is usually a solitary, symptomless lesion, typically on the gingiva, with a normal, pale, reddish or keratotic surface [1,2]. Excision is only rarely followed by recurrence.

REFERENCES

1 Neville BW, Weathers DR. Verruciform xanthoma. *Oral Surg* 1980; **49**: 429–34.
2 Nowparast B, Howell FV, Rick GM. Verruciform xanthoma: a clinicopathologic review and report of fifty-four cases. *Oral Surg* 1981; **51**: 619–25.

Lipoma (Chapter 57)

Lipomas are uncommon in the mouth, comprising less than 5% of oral benign tumours [1]. They present as slow-growing, spherical, smooth and soft semifluctuant lumps with a characteristic yellowish colour. Most involve the buccal mucosa or floor of mouth. Occasionally, although benign, they infiltrate. Histology shows adult fat cells gathered into lobules by vascular septa of fibrous connective tissue. Surgery is rarely indicated except for infiltrating lipomas.

REFERENCE

1 Batsakis JG, Regezi JA, Rice DH. The pathology of head and neck tumors: part 8. *Head Neck Surg* 1980; **3**: 145–68.

Myxoma

Myxomas are rare in the oral cavity. They can arise in bone or soft tissue and, although benign, are aggressive and difficult to eradicate because of the tendency to infiltrate normal tissue.

Leiomyoma

This benign tumour of smooth muscle is rare in the oral cavity but usually affects the tongue or palate.

Giant-cell epulis
SYN. PERIPHERAL GIANT-CELL GRANULOMA

Aetiology. The giant-cell epulis probably arises because chronic irritation triggers a reactionary hyperplasia of mucoperiosteum and excessive production of granulation tissue. Giant-cell granulomas are occasionally a feature of hyperparathyroidism.

Pathology. Histology shows many multinucleated giant cells, distributed widely throughout the lesion or gathered into clumps. There is considerable vascularity. Sheets of stromal cells in the younger vascular lesions give way to greater numbers of collagen fibres and well-differentiated fibroblasts in the older lesion. The older lesion may also contain some woven bone. There is no capsule.

***Clinical features*.** The giant-cell epulis characteristically arises interdentally, adjacent to permanent teeth which have had deciduous predecessors [1], i.e. not the permanent molars. Classically, the most notable feature is the deep-red colour, although older lesions tend to be paler.

This is a benign lesion which is cured by excision.

REFERENCE

1 Giansanti JS, Waldron CA. Peripheral giant cell granuloma: review of 720 cases. *J Oral Surg* 1969; **27**: 787–91.

Drug-induced gingival hyperplasia

Gingival hyperplasia is a recognized adverse effect of medication, especially following use of phenytoin, calcium-channel blockers and cyclosporin.

Phenytoin

Phenytoin induces gingival hyperplasia presumably by an effect on fibroblast activity. There is no correlation between the extent of overgrowth and the dose of phenytoin, its serum level, or the age and sex of the patient. Rather, the hyperplasia is aggravated by poor oral hygiene.

***Histology*.** Histology shows marked epithelial thickening with long overgrowths into the connective tissue. Fibroblasts show increased mitotic activity but are not increased in number, and the collagen fibre component is not increased.

***Clinical features*.** Phenytoin can produce a variable degree of gingival enlargement, which characteristically affects the interdental papillae first but which may later involve the marginal and even attached gingiva. The palatal and lingual gingiva are usually involved less than the buccal and labial gingiva [1–4].

The enlargement is characteristically firm, pale and tough, with coarse stippling, but these features may take several years to develop, and earlier lesions may be softer and redder (see Fig. 69.9).

***Treatment*.** The patient's level of plaque control should be improved [5] and a 0.2% aqueous chlorhexidine mouthwash may be helpful. Excision of the enlarged tissue may be indicated, but unfortunately readily recurs, although this is less likely with meticulous oral hygiene, particularly if the phenytoin can be stopped. Folic acid may improve the condition and systemic isotretinoin may be of some value [2].

Calcium-channel blockers

Nifedipine can cause gingival hyperplasia typically affecting the papillae in a similar fashion to phenytoin [3,6]. Several other calcium-channel blockers have a similar effect [7]. Increased numbers of fibroblasts containing strongly sulphated mucopolysaccharides may be demonstrated histochemically. Their cytoplasm contains numerous secretory granules, suggesting an increased production of acid mucopolysaccharides.

Improved oral hygiene may reduce the hyperplasia [8]. Excision of the enlarged tissue may be followed by recurrence, and patients should be warned accordingly. If possible the medication should be changed.

Cyclosporin

Cyclosporin also causes gingival hyperplasia, initially of papillae [3,9]. Only about one-third of patients are affected, more commonly children, and this change may be lessened by meticulous removal of plaque before the drug is introduced.

Other drugs

Hyperplasia has been reported as a reaction to other agents such as tranexamic acid [10].

REFERENCES

1 Hassell TM. Epilepsy and the oral manifestations of phenytoin therapy. In: Myers HM, ed. *Monographs in Oral Science*. Basel: Karger, 1981: 9–12.
2 Norris JF, Cunliffe WJ. Phenytoin-induced gum hypertrophy improved by isotretinoin. *Int J Dermatol* 1987; **26**: 602–3.
3 Slavin J, Taylor J. Cyclosporin, nifedipine and gingival hyperplasia. *Lancet* 1987; **ii**: 739.
4 Stinnett E, Rodu B, Grizzle WE. New developments in understanding phenytoin-induced gingival hyperplasia. *J Am Dent Assoc* 1987; **114**: 814–16.
5 Modeer T, Dahllof G. Development of phenytoin-induced gingival overgrowth in non-institutionalised epileptic children subjected to different plaque control programs. *Acta Odontol Scand* 1987; **45**: 81–5.
6 Shaftic AA, Widdup LL, Abate MA *et al.* Nifedipine-induced gingival hyperplasia. *Drug Intell Clin Pharm* 1986; **20**: 602–5.
7 Steele RM, Schuna AA, Schreiber RT. Calcium antagonist-induced gingival hyperplasia. *Ann Intern Med* 1994; **120**: 663–4.
8 Hancock RH, Swan RH. Nifedipine-induced gingival overgrowth: report of a case treated by controlling plaque. *J Clin Periodontol* 1992; **19**: 12–14.
9 Daley TD, Wysocki GP, Day C. Clinical and pharmacological correlations in cyclosporin-induced gingival hyperplasia. *Oral Surg* 1986; **62**: 417–21.
10 Diamond JP, Chandna A, Williams C *et al.* Tranexamic acid-associated ligneous conjunctivitis with gingival and peritoneal lesions. *Br J Ophthalmol* 1991; **75**: 753–4.

Pregnancy gingivitis and epulis

***Aetiology*.** There can be an exaggerated inflammatory reaction to dental bacterial plaque in pregnancy, presumably mediated by an effect on the immune response. Chronic marginal gingivitis may therefore be aggravated [1,2] and occasionally a pyogenic granuloma (pregnancy epulis) results.

Pathology. Histologically, a pregnancy epulis is a pyogenic granuloma. Despite the vascularity, the immaturity of the vessels may lead to superficial ischaemia and ulceration. Larger lesions are prone to trauma, which may contribute to the ulceration.

Clinical features. Pregnancy gingivitis is characterized by soft, reddish enlargements, usually of the gingival papillae varying from small, smooth enlargements to more extensive, ragged, granular lumps resembling the surface of a strawberry. Changes of pregnancy gingivitis usually appear about the second month of pregnancy, and reach a peak at the eighth month. Poor oral hygiene predisposes to these changes. A similar appearance may occur with oral contraceptives.

Sometimes there is a localized epulis, a pregnancy epulis which, although unsightly, is usually painless. Occasionally it ulcerates or interferes with eating.

Most lesions tend to resolve on parturition.

Treatment. Oral hygiene should be improved. There is one report of a beneficial effect of folic acid on pregnancy gingivitis [3]. An epulis requires excision only if it is being traumatized or is grossly unaesthetic [2].

REFERENCES

1 Amar S, Chung KM, Influence of hormonal variation on the periodontium in women. *Periodontol 2000* 1994; **6**: 79–87.
2 Chiodo GT, Rosenstein DI. Dental treatment during pregnancy: a preventive approach. *J Am Dent Assoc* 1985; **110**: 365–8.
3 Pack ARC, Thomson ME. Effect of topical and systemic folic acid supplementation on gingivitis of pregnancy. *J Clin Periodontol* 1980; **7**: 402–14.

Scurvy (Chapter 59)

Scurvy (vitamin C deficiency) causes gingival swelling, bleeding and oral purpura, but is now rare in the West.

Macroglossia

The tongue may be congenitally enlarged (macroglossia) in Down's syndrome or Beckwith–Wiedemann syndrome or where there is an angioma. It may also enlarge in angioedema, gigantism, acromegaly or amyloidosis.

Angio-oedema (Chapter 47)

Oral swelling may be a feature of angio-oedema. The swelling is of acute onset and is often only mild and transient but there is always the potential for obstruction of the airway. Dental treatment may precipitate an attack in hereditary angio-oedema.

Myeloma and paraproteinaemias

Multiple myeloma very occasionally presents with an intraoral mass or oral bleeding. Bone lesions are more common. Solitary plasmacytomas may also be seen; indeed, some 80% of these rare tumours are found in the head and neck region but typically in the nasal cavity or pharynx rather than in the mouth [1,2].

Waldenstrom's macroglobulinaemia

Oral manifestations in Waldenstrom's macroglobulinaemia include purpura, ulceration and occasional mental nerve anaesthesia [3–5].

REFERENCES

1 Epstein JB, Boss NJS, Stevenson-Moore P. Maxillofacial manifestations of multiple myeloma. *Oral Surg* 1984; **57**: 267–71.
2 Woodruff RK, Whittle JM, Malpas JS. Solitary plasmacytoma. 1. Extramedullary soft tissue plasmacytoma. *Cancer* 1979; **43**: 2340–3.
3 Gamble JW, Driscoll EJ. Oral manifestations of macroglobulinaemia of Waldenstom. *Oral Surg* 1960; **13**: 104–10.
4 Klokkevold PR, Miller DA, Friedlander AH. Mental nerve neuropathy: a symptom of Waldenstrom's macroglobulinaemia. *Oral Surg* 1989; **67**: 689–93.
5 Zulian M, Bellome J, DeBoom GW. Multiple linear ulcers on the dorsum of the tongue in a patient with Waldenstrom's macroglobulinaemia. *J Am Dent Assoc* 1987; **114**: 79–80.

Franklin's disease

SYN. HEAVY-CHAIN DISEASE

Palatal oedema and oral ulceration have been described in a few patients with heavy-chain disease, but the former feature is not as invariable as initially described [1,2].

REFERENCES

1 Kanoch T, Takigawa M, Niwa Y. Cutaneous lesions in heavy chain disease. *Arch Dermatol* 1988; **124**: 1538–40.
2 Seligmann M. Heavy chain diseases. In: IW Delamore, ed. *Multiple Myeloma and Other Paraproteinaemias*. Edinburgh: Churchill Livingstone, 1986: 263–85.

Thrombotic thrombocytopenic purpura

This may present with oral purpura and/or spontaneous gingival haemorrhage [1,2]. Gingival biopsy is a recommended investigation [3,4].

REFERENCES

1 Fox P, Gordon RE, Williams AC. Thrombotic thrombocytopenic purpura: report of a case. *J Oral Surg* 1977; **35**: 921–3.
2 Ridolfi R, Bell W. Thrombotic thrombocytopenic purpura: report of 25 cases and review of the literature. *Medicine* 1981; **60**: 413–28.

3 Goodman A, Ramos P, Petrelli M *et al.* Gingival biopsy in thrombotic thrombocytopenic purpura. *Ann Intern Med* 1978; **89**: 501–4.
4 Nishioka GJ, Chilcoat CC, Aufdenorte TB *et al.* The gingival biopsy in the diagnosis of thrombotic thrombocytopenic purpura. *Oral Surg* 1988; **65**: 580–5.

Amyloidosis (Chapter 59)

In primary amyloidosis the tongue is enlarged and hard. There may also be yellowish submucosal nodules, lumps or petechiae (Fig. 69.60). Rarely, there are similar deposits elsewhere (e.g. in the soft palate), jaw claudication, salivary gland swelling or xerostomia [1–5].

Secondary amyloidoses rarely involves the mouth except in the case of multiple myeloma or haemodialysis-associated amyloid, which may occasionally produce oral nodules [6,7].

Some 10% of patients with oral amyloidosis have amyloid in their submandibular glands.

Solitary intraoral amyloid is rare [8].

Congo red or thioflavine T staining of a biopsy usually confirms the diagnosis, although in extreme cases the deposits are seen on haematoxylin and eosin staining. Treatment is unsatisfactory but the underlying disease, where present, should be treated.

REFERENCES

1 Al-Hashimi I, Drinnan AJ, Uthman AA *et al.* Oral amyloidosis: two unusual case presentations. *Oral Surg* 1987; **63**: 586–91.
2 Babejews A. Occult multiple myeloma associated with amyloid of the tongue. *Br J Oral Maxillofac Surg* 1985; **23**: 298–303.
3 Gertz MA, Kyle RA, Griffing WL *et al.* Jaw claudication in primary systemic amyloidosis. *Medicine* 1986; **65**: 173–9.
4 Salisbury PS, Jacoway JR. Oral amyloidosis: a late complication of multiple myeloma. *Oral Surg* 1983; **56**: 48–50.

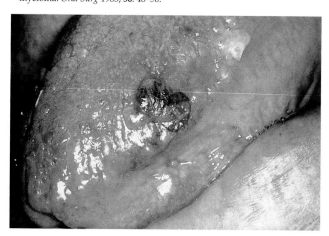

Fig. 69.60 Macroglossia and oral petechiae in amyloidosis.

5 Van der Waal I, Fehmers MCO, Kraal ER. Amyloidosis: its significance in oral surgery. *Oral Surg* 1973; **36**: 469–81.
6 Reinish EI, Raviv M, Srolovitz H, Gornitsky M. Tongue, primary amyloidosis, and multiple myeloma. *Oral Surg* 1994; **77**: 121–5.
7 Guccion JG, Redman RS, Winne CE. Hemodialysis-associated amyloidosis presenting as lingual nodules. *Oral Surg* 1989; **68**: 618–23.
8 Raymond AK, Sneige N, Batsakis JG. Amyloidosis in the upper aerodigestive tracts. *Ann Otol Rhinol Laryngol* 1992; **101**: 794–6.

Acanthosis nigricans (Chapter 34)

Between 30 and 50% of patients with acanthosis nigricans secondary to neoplasia (malignant acanthosis nigricans) have oral lesions, which involve the tongue and lips predominantly. The dorsum and margins of the tongue and the lips are marked by a shaggy appearance, sometimes with non-pigmented, papillomatous growths [1–3].

REFERENCES

1 Mostofi RS, Hayden NP, Soltani K. Oral malignant acanthosis nigricans. *Oral Surg* 1983; **56**: 372–4.
2 Nomachi K, Mori M, Matsuda N. Improvement of oral lesions associated with malignant acanthosis nigricans after treatment of lung cancer. *Oral Surg* 1989; **68**: 74–9.
3 Sedano HO, Gorlin RJ. Acanthosis nigricans. *Oral Surg* 1987; **68**:74–9.

Oral manifestations of systemic diseases

Oral manifestations can occasionally occur in many systemic diseases (Tables 69.25–69.39). Space precludes all but a brief tabular synopsis here. Further details can be found in [1–10].

REFERENCES

1 Jones JH, Mason DK, eds. *Oral Manifestations of Systemic Disease*, 2nd edn. London: Balliére Tindall, 1990.
2 Scully C, Flint S, Porter SR. *Colour Atlas of Oral Diseases*. London: Martin Dunitz, 1996.
3 Millard HD, Mason DK. *1993 World Workshop on Oral Medicine*. Michigan: University of Michigan, 1995.
4 Scully C, Cawson RA. Oral medicine. *Med Int* 1986; **28**: 1129–51.
5 Scully C, Cawson RA. *Medical Problems in Dentistry*, 4th edn. Oxford: Wright, 1998.
6 Scully C, Cawson RA. *Colour Aids to Oral Medicine*. Edinburgh: Churchill Livingstone, 1988.
7 Scully C, Porter SR. Oral medicine. *Med Int* 1990; **76**: 3145–74.
8 Porter SR, Scully C. HIV: the surgeon's perspective. *Br J Oral Maxillofac Surg* 1994; **32**: 222–47 (3 parts).
9 Scully C, Welbury R. *A Colour Atlas of Oral Diseases in Children and Adolescents*. London: Mosby–Wolfe, 1994.
10 Scully C, Samaranayake LP. *Clinical Virology in Oral Medicine and Dentistry*. Cambridge: Cambridge University Press, 1992.

Table 69.25 Endocrine disorders.

Disease	Oral manifestations
Pituitary dwarfism	Microdontia Retarded tooth eruption
Congenital hypothyroidism	Macroglossia Retarded tooth eruption
Congenital hypoparathyroidism	Dental hypoplasia May be chronic candidosis if associated immune defect
Gigantism/acromegaly	Spaced teeth Mandibular prognathism Macroglossia Megadontia (in gigantism)
Hyperparathyroidism	Bone rarefaction Brown tumours
Addison's disease	Mucosal hyperpigmentation
Diabetes mellitus	Periodontal disease Xerostomia Candidiasis Sialosis Lichen planus
Pregnancy	Gingivitis Epulis
Precocious puberty	Accelerated tooth eruption (fibrous dysplasia in Albright's syndrome)

Table 69.26 Liver diseases.

Disease	Oral manifestations
Most liver diseases with jaundice	Bleeding tendency Jaundice
Alcoholic cirrhosis	Bleeding tendency Sialosis
Chronic active hepatitis	Lichen planus
Primary biliary cirrhosis	Sjögren's syndrome Lichen planus

Table 69.27 Psychiatric disease.

Disease	Oral manifestation

Depression, hypochondriasis
and various psychoses
	Various complaints such as dry
	  mouth discharges, pain,
	  disturbed taste and
	  sensation
	Drug reactions
	Often multiple complaints
	Artefactual ulcers

Anxiety states	Cheek biting Bruxism (teeth grinding)
Bulimia	Tooth erosion

Table 69.28 Drug effects.

Tissue	Drug effect	Drugs commonly implicated
Teeth	Discoloration	Tetracyclines Chlorhexidine
	Root anomalies	Phenytoin Cytotoxics
Gingiva	Swelling	Phenytoin Cyclosporin Nifedipine Diltiazem
Salivary glands	Dry mouth	Tricyclic antidepressants Phenothiazines Antihypertensives Lithium
Taste	Disturbed	Metronidazole Penicillamine
Facial movements	Dykinesias	Phenothiazones Metoclopramide
Mucosa	Thrush	Broad-spectrum antimicrobials Corticosteroids Cytotoxic drugs
	Ulcers	Cytotoxic drugs
	Lichenoid lesions	Non-steroidal anti-inflammatory agents
	Erythema multiforme	Barbiturates Sulphonamides

Table 69.29 Gastrointestinal diseases.

Disease	Oral manifestations
Pernicious anaemia	Ulcers Glossitis Angular stomatitis Red lesions
Any cause of malabsorption	Ulcers Glossitis Angular stomatitis
Any cause of regurgitation	Tooth erosions Halitosis
Tylosis	Leukoplakia
Crohn's disease	Facial swelling Mucosal tags Gingival hyperplasia Cobblestoning of mucosa Ulcers Glossitis Angular stomatitis
Coeliac disease	Ulcers Glossitis Angular stomatitis Dental hypoplasia
Peutz–Jegher syndrome (small intestinal polyps)	Melanosis
Chronic pancreatitis	Sialosis (rarely)
Cystic fibrosis	Salivary gland swelling
Gardner's syndrome (familial colonic polyposis)	Osteomas

Table 69.31 Haematological diseases.

Disease	Oral manifestations
Deficiency of the haematinics—iron, folic acid or vitamin B_{12}	Burning mouth sensation Glossitis Ulcers Angular stomatitis
Sickle-cell anaemia	Jaw deformities Osteomyelitis or pain
Thalassaemia major	Jaw deformities
Aplastic anaemia	Ulcers Bleeding tendency
Haemolytic disease of newborn	Tooth pigmentation Enamel defects
Any leukocyte defect	Infections, especially herpetic and candidal Ulcers
Any cause of purpura	Bleeding tendency Purpura
Leukaemia/lymphoma	Infections Ulcers Bleeding tendency and purpura (in leukaemias only) Gingival swelling in myelomonocytic leukaemia
Multiple myeloma	Bone pain Tooth mobility Amyloidosis
Amyloid disease	Enlarged tongue Purpura

Table 69.30 Renal diseases.

Disease	Oral manifestations
Chronic renal failure of any cause	Xerostomia Halitosis/taste disturbance Leukoplakia Dental hypoplasia in children Renal osteodystrophy Bleeding tendency (especially if anticoagulated)
Post-renal transplant (immunosuppressed)	Infections, particularly herpetic and candidal Bleeding tendency if anticoagulated Gingival hyperplasia if on cyclosporin Kaposi's sarcoma (rarely) Hairy leukoplakia (rarely)
Nephrotic syndrome	Dental hypoplasia
Renal rickets (vitamin D resistant)	Delayed tooth eruption Dental hypoplasia (rarely) Enlarged pulp

Table 69.32 Cardiovascular disease.

Disease	Oral manifestations
Any disorder causing right-to-left shunt, e.g. Fallot's tetralogy	Cyanosis Delayed tooth eruption
Angina pectoris	Pain referred to jaw
Hereditary haemorrhagic telangiectasia	Telangiectasis
Giant-cell arteritis (cranial or temporal arteritis)	Tongue pain or necrosis
Polyarteritis nodosa	Ulcers
Any disorder in which anticoagulants are used	Bleeding tendency
Hypertension	Dry mouth and other problems caused by some antihypertensives, e.g. gingival hyperplasia (nifedipine or diltiazem); lichenoid lesions (methyldopa and others)

Table 69.33 Primary and secondary immunodeficiencies.

Disease	Oral manifestations
Severe combined immunodeficiency	Candidiasis Viral infections Ulcers Absent tonsils Recurrent sinusitis
Sex-linked agammaglobulinaemia	Ulcers Recurrent sinusitis Absent tonsils
Common variable immunodeficiency	Recurrent sinusitis Candidiasis
Selective IgA deficiency	Tonsillar hyperplasia Ulcers Viral infections Parotitis
Di George syndrome	Abnormal facies Candidiasis Viral infections Bifid uvula
Ataxia–telangiectasia	Recurrent sinusitis Ulcers Telangiectasia
Wiskott–Aldrich syndrome	Candidiasis Viral infections Purpura
Hereditary angiooedema	Swellings
Chronic benign neutropenia	Ulcers Severe periodontitis
Cyclic neutropenia	Ulcers Severe periodontitis Eczematous lesions of the face
Chronic granulomatous disease	Candidiasis Enamel hypoplasia Acute gingivitis Ulcers
Myeloperoxidase deficiency	Candidiasis
Chediak–Higashi syndrome	Ulcers Periodontitis
Job's syndrome	Abnormal facies
Secondary immune defects	Ulcers Periodontitis Candidiasis Viral infections Malignant neoplasms Hairy leukoplakia

Table 69.34 Metabolic disorders.

Disease	Oral manifestations
Congenital hyperuricaemia (Lesch–Nyhan syndrome)	Self-mutilation
Mucopolysaccharidoses	Spaced teeth Retarded tooth eruption Cystic radiolucencies Temporomandibular joint anomalies Enamel defects Gingival hyperplasia
Niemann–Pick disease	Retarded tooth eruption Loosening of teeth Mucosal pigmentation
Mucolipidoses	Gingival hyperplasia
Hypophosphatasia	Loosening and loss of teeth
Erythropoietic porphyria	Reddish teeth Bullae/erosions Dental hypoplasia
Amyloidosis	Macroglossia Purpura
Vitamin B_{12} or folic acid deficiency	Ulcers Glossitis Angular stomatitis
Scurvy	Gingival swelling Purpura Ulcers
Rickets (vitamin D dependent)	Dental hypoplasia Large pulp chambers Large tooth eruption

Table 69.35 Collagen–vascular diseases.

Disease	Oral manifestations
Any collagen–vascular disease	Sjögren's syndrome
Rheumatoid arthritis	Temporomandibular arthritis Drug reaction (e.g. lichenoid) Ulcers in Felty's syndrome Temporomandibular ankylosis in juvenile arthritides
Lupus erythematosus	White lesions Ulcers
Systemic sclerosis	Stiffness of lips, tongue, etc. Trismus Telangiectasia Mandibular condylar resorption Periodontal ligament widened on X-ray

Table 69.36 Miscellaneous disorders.

Disease	Oral manifestations
Sarcoidosis	Xerostomia Salivary gland swelling Heerfordt syndrome (parotid swelling, lacrimal swelling, facial palsy) Gingival swelling
Behçet's syndrome	Ulcers like aphthae
Sweet's syndrome	Ulcers like aphthae
Reiter's syndrome	Ulcers
Langerhans' cell histiocytosis	Loosening of teeth Jaw radiolucencies
Wegener's granulomatosis	Gingival swellings Ulcers
Kawasaki's disease (mucocutaneous lymph-node syndrome)	Sore tongue Cheilitis
Ellis–van Creveld syndrome (chondroectodermal dysplasia)	Multiple fraena Short roots Hypodontia
Tuberous sclerosis	Enamel defects Gingival fibromatosis

Table 69.37 Other infections.

Disease	Oral manifestations
Syphilis	Chancre Mucous patches Ulcers Gumma Pain from neurosyphilis Leukoplakia Lymph-node enlargement Hutchinson's teeth in congenital syphilis
Gonorrhoea	Pharyngitis (occasionally) Gingivitis (occasionally) Temporomandibular arthritis (rarely)
Tuberculosis (including atypical mycobacteria)	Ulcers (rarely)
Leprosy	Cranial nerve palsies (rarely)
Lyme disease	Facial palsy
Candidiasis	White lesions Red lesions Angular stomatitis
Cryptococcosis	Ulcers
Coccidioidomycosis	Ulcers
Histoplasmosis	Ulcers (especially in immune defects)
Blastomycosis	Ulcers
Mucormycosis Aspergillosis	Antral infections or ulcers (especially in immune defects)

Table 69.38 Viral infections.

Disease	Oral manifestations
Herpes simplex	Ulcers in primary infection Gingivitis in primary infection Vesicles on lips in recurrence (rarely oral ulcers)
Herpes zoster–varicella	Ulcers in chickenpox, or in zoster of maxillary or mandibular divisions of the trigeminal nerve Pain in maxillary or mandibular zoster
Coxsackie and echoviruses	Ulcers in herpangina and hand, foot and mouth disease
Epstein–Barr virus (in infectious mononucleosis)	Sore throat Tonsillar exudate Palatal petechiae Recurrent parotitis (possibly) Hairy leukoplakia
Measles	Koplik's spots
Mumps	Salivary gland swelling
Papillomaviruses	Warts Papillomas Focal epithelial hyperplasia
Human immunodeficiency virus Common	Candidiasis Hairy leukoplakia Gingival and periodontal disease Herpes simplex infection Herpes zoster infection Papillomavirus infection Kaposi's sarcoma Aphthous-like ulcers Xerostomia
Uncommon	Infections Cryptococcus Mycobacteria Histoplasma Cytomegalovirus Others Salivary gland swelling Sjögren's syndrome-like disease Cranial neuropathies Others Fetal AIDS syndrome

Table 69.39 Neurological disorders.

Disease	Oral manifestations
Facial palsy of any cause	Palsy and poor natural cleansing of mouth on same side
Trigeminal neuralgia	Pain
Bulbar palsy	Fasciculation of tongue
Parkinsonism	Drooling Tremor of tongue Dysarthria
Neurosyphilis	Pain (rarely) Dysarthria Tremor of tongue
Cerebral palsy	Spastic tongue Dysarthria Attrition Periodontal disease
Choreoathetosis	Green staining of teeth in kernicterus Hypoplasia of deciduous dentition in congenital rubella
Epilepsy	Trauma to teeth/jaws/mucosa Gingival hyperplasia if taking phenytoin
Down's syndrome	Delayed tooth eruption Macroglossia Scrotal tongue Maxillary hypoplasia Anterior open bite Hypodontia Periodontal disease Cleft lip or palate in some

Chapter 70
The Lips

J.L. BURTON & CRISPIAN SCULLY

Anatomy

The lips extend from the lower end of the nose to the upper end of the chin. They mainly consist of bundles of striated muscle, particularly the *orbicularis oris* muscle, with skin on the external surface and mucous membrane on the inner surface, which has a profusion of minor salivary glands.

The vermilion zone—the transitional zone between the glabrous skin and the mucous membrane—is found only in humans. The vermilion zone contains no hair or sweat glands but contains sebaceous glands (Fordyce spots, see below). The epithelium of the vermilion is distinctive, with a prominent stratum lucidum and a very thin stratum corneum. The dermal papillae there are numerous, with a rich capillary supply, which produces the reddish-pink colour of the lips in white people. Melanocytes are abundant in the basal layer of the vermilion of pigmented skin, but are infrequent in white skin.

The *oral commissures* are the angles where the upper and lower lip meet. The upper lip includes the *philtrum*, a midline depression, extending from the columella of the nose to the superior edge of the vermilion zone [1].

This chapter describes organic lesions affecting the lips: the reader is referred elsewhere for discussion of the lip in neurological and psychiatric disorders.

REFERENCE

1 Zugerman C. The lips: anatomy and differential diagnosis. *Cutis* 1986; **38**: 116–120.

Congenital anomalies

Racial variations

There are considerable racial variations in lip morphology and colour of the vermilion.

Cleft lip

Cleft lip and/or palate are the most common congenital craniofacial abnormalities (Fig. 70.1). Cleft lip occurs in about one per 1000 white-skinned neonates. The prevalence is higher in oriental neonates (about 1.7 per 1000 births) and lower in black neonates (approximately one per 2500 births) and appears reduced if women take multivitamins containing folic acid early in pregnancy [1]. Clefts are often accompanied by impaired facial growth, dental anomalies, speech disorders, poor hearing and psychosocial problems [2]. Clefts can be seen in over 300 different syndromes [3].

Cleft lip is not always complete (i.e. extending into the nostril). A cleft may involve only the upper lip or may

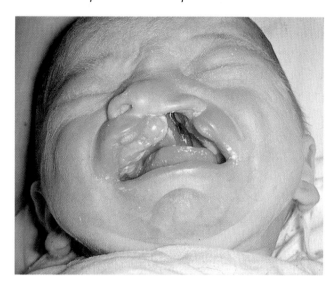

Fig. 70.1 Cleft lip and palate in a baby.

extend to involve the nostril and the hard and soft palates. In about 9% of the cases, the cleft is associated with skin bridges or Simonart's bands.

Isolated cleft lip may be unilateral or bilateral (approximately 20%). When unilateral, the cleft is more common on the left side (about 70%).

Lips are more frequently cleft bilaterally (approximately 25%) when combined with cleft palate. Cleft lip–palate is more common in men. Cleft lip–palate comprises about 50% of the cases, with cleft lip and isolated cleft palate each being about 25%. About 85% of bilateral cleft lips and 70% of unilateral cleft lips are associated with cleft palate. One subgroup have cleft-lip–palate with median facial dysplasia and cerebrofacial malformations [4], others with laryngotracheal oesophageal clefts (Opitz–Firas or G syndrome) or cranial asymmetry (Opitz or B syndrome) [5], others with cardiac defects such as in Shprintzen's syndrome.

Clefts in the middle of the upper lip may be true or false. True median clefts have been described in association with bifid nose and ocular hypertelorism. Other cases of true median labial cleft are associated with polydactyly or other digital anomalies, constituting an autosomal recessive trait called the *orofaciodigital syndrome II*.

Pseudocleft of the middle of the upper lip may occur in *orofaciodigital syndrome I*. A somewhat similar central defect, but of mild degree, is seen in *chondroectodermal dysplasia* (Ellis–van Creveld syndrome). Clefts in the lower lip are rare and usually median but may involve the mandible and sometimes the tongue. Management of cleft lip is discussed elsewhere [6,7].

REFERENCES

1 Shaw GM, Lammer EJ, Wasserman CR *et al*. Risks of orofacial clefts in children born to women using multivitamins containing folic acid periconceptionally. *Lancet* 1995; **346**: 393–6.
2 Habel A, Sell D, Mars M. Management of cleft lip and palate. *Arch Dis Child* 1996; **74**: 360–6.
3 Cohen MM, Bankier A. Syndrome delineation involving orofacial clefting. *Cleft Palate J* 1991; **28**: 119–20.
4 Noordhoff MS, Huang C-S, Lo L-J. Median facial dysplasia in unilateral and bilateral cleft lip and palate: a subgroup of median cerebrofacial malformations. *Plast Reconstr Surg* 1993; **91**: 966–1005.
5 Bershof JF, Guyuron B, Olsen MM. G Syndrome: a review of the literature and a case report. *J Craniomaxillofac Surg* 1992; **20**: 24–7.
6 Kaufman FL. Managing the cleft lip and palate patient. *Pediatr Clin North Am* 1991; **38**: 1127–47.
7 Melnick J. Cleft lip with or without cleft palate. *Can Dent Assoc J* 1986; **14**: 92–8.

Lip pits and sinuses

Dimples are common at the commissures. They are distinguished from *commissural pits* which are distinct definite pits ranging from 1 to 4 mm in diameter and depth [1,2] present from infancy, often showing a familial tendency and probably determined by a dominant gene (Fig. 70.2). Their incidence is from 1 to 20% in various population groups [2,3]; for example, they were found in one series in 12% of white people and 20% of black people [4]. Commissural pits are sometimes associated with aural sinuses or pits. Rarely, they may be infected and present as recurrent or refractory angular cheilitis.

Congenital lip pits or *sinuses* are small, blind fistulae on the vermilion border [5]. They are usually bilateral and symmetrical often just to one side of the philtrum. The pits may be up to 3–4 mm in diameter and up to 2 cm deep. They may communicate with underlying minor salivary glands. They may appear as isolated findings, but are often

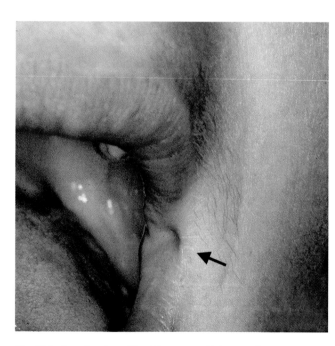

Fig. 70.2 Angular sinus (lip-pit), a congenital anomaly.

(67%) associated with a cleft lip and/or palate—the Van der Woude syndrome [6–9]. This autosomal dominant syndrome [10,11] has a frequency of one in 75 000 to one in 100 000 in white populations (Chapter 12).

Surgical removal may be indicated for cosmetic purposes.

REFERENCES

1 Witkop CJ, Barros L. Oral and genetic studies of Chileans, 1960. I. Oral anomalies. *Am J Phys Anthropol* 1963; **21**: 15–24.
2 Sedano HO. Congenital oral anomalies in Argentinian children. *Comm Dent Oral Epidemiol* 1975; **3**: 61–3.
3 Everett FG, Wescott WB. Commissural lip pits. *Oral Surg Oral Med Oral Pathol* 1961; **14**: 202–9.
4 Baker B. Commissural lip pits. *Oral Surg* 1966; **21**: 56.
5 Watanabe Y, Igaku-Hakushi K, Otake K *et al*. Congenital fistulas of the lower lip. *Oral Surg Oral Med Oral Pathol* 1951; **4**: 709–22.
6 Van der Woude A. Fistula labii inferius congenita and its association with cleft lip and palate. *Am J Hum Gen* 1954; **6**: 244–56.
7 Gordon H, Davis D, Friedberg S. Congenital pits of the lower lip with cleft lip and palate. *S Afr Med J* 1969; **43**: 1275–9.
8 Rintala AE, Lahti AY, Gylling US. Congenital sinuses of the lower lip in connection with cleft lip and palate. *Cleft Palate J* 1970; **7**: 336–46.
9 Tan KL, Wong TT, Ong ES, Chiang SP. Congenital lip pits with cleft lip or palate. *J Singapore Paediatr Soc* 1971; **13**: 75–8.
10 Cervenka J, Gorlin RJ, Anderson VE. The syndrome of pits of the lower lip and cleft lip and/or palate. Genetic considerations. *Am J Hum Genet* 1967; **19**: 416–32.
11 Wang MK, Macomber WB. Congenital deformities of the lips. In: Converse MA, ed. *Reconstructive Plastic Surgery*. WB Saunders, Philadelphia, 1977: 1540–1.

Microstomia

The size of the oral opening has wide individual variability. Some diminution of the oral opening is seen in *craniocarpotarsal dysplasia* ('whistling face syndrome'). Congenital microstomia has also been recorded in association with agnathia or cyclopia hypognathus and occasionally is an isolated phenomenon (see also acquired microstomia, p. 3147).

Double lip

Double lip is a developmental anomaly usually involving the upper lip. A fold of redundant tissue is found on the inner aspect of the involved lip [1]. It is reported to be common among some groups of Africans [2].

Double lip may occur alone or in association with other anomalies. The association with blepharochalasis (laxity of the upper eyelid skin) and sometimes non-toxic thyroid enlargement is known as *Ascher's syndrome* [3] (Chapter 44).

Double lip requires no treatment except for cosmetic purposes.

REFERENCES

1 Beumeir P, Weinberg A, Neuman A *et al*. Congenital double lip: report of five cases and a review of the literature. *Ann Plast Surg* 1992; **28**: 180–2.
2 Sawyer DR, Taiwo EO, Mosadomi A. Oral anomalies in Nigerian children. *Comm Dent Oral Epidemiol* 1984; **3**: 61–3.
3 Halling F, Sandrock D, Merten HA *et al*. Das Ascher Syndrom. *Dtsch Z Mund Kiefer Gesichtschrift* 1991; **15**: 440–4.

Ectopic sebaceous glands

In some people sebaceous glands may be seen as creamy yellow dots (*Fordyce spots*) along the border between the vermilion and the oral mucosa (Chapter 69) (Fig. 70.3). These are not usually evident in infants, but they appear in children after the age of 3 years, increase during puberty and then again in later adult life.

No treatment is indicated though they may be suppressed by isotretinoin [1].

REFERENCE

1 Monk BE. Fordyce spots responding to isotretinoin therapy. *Br J Dermatol* 1993; **129**: 355.

Peutz–Jeghers syndrome

Peutz–Jeghers syndrome is as an autosomal dominant trait characterized by hamartomatous intestinal polyposis and mucocutaneous melanotic pigmentation, especially circumorally [1,2]. Those affected have discrete, brown to bluish black macules mainly around the oral, nasal, and ocular orifices. The lips, especially the lower, have pigmented macules in about 98% of patients (Fig. 70.4). Mucosal and facial hyperpigmentation may also be seen in relatives [3].

Intestinal polyps are found mainly in the small intestine in Peutz–Jeghers syndrome. They rarely undergo

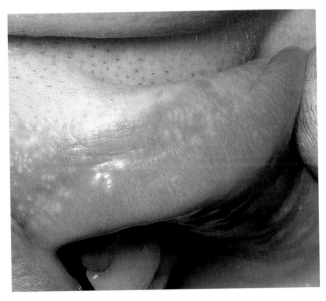

Fig. 70.3 Fordyce spots of the lips. (Courtesy of Addenbrooke's Hospital, Cambridge, UK.)

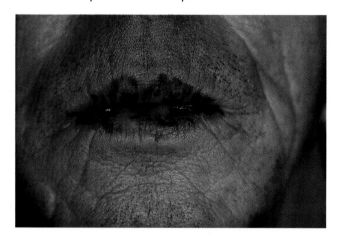

Fig. 70.4 Peutz–Jeghers syndrome.

malignant change but, if they produce intussusception, surgical intervention is required. There is a slightly increased risk of gastrointestinal carcinoma and carcinomas of the pancreas, breast and reproductive organs [4,5] (Chapter 39).

REFERENCES

1 Dummett CO, Barens G. Oromucosal pigmentation: an updated literature review. *J Periodontol* 1971; **42**: 726–36.
2 Wesley RK, Delaney JR, Pensler L. Mucocutaneous melanosis and gastrointestinal polyposis (Peutz–Jeghers syndrome): clinical considerations and report of case. *J Dent Child* 1977; **44**: 131–4.
3 Burdick D, Prior JT. Peutz–Jeghers syndrome: a clinicopathological study of a large family with a 27 year follow-up. *Cancer* 1982; **50**: 2139–46.
4 Buck JL, Harned RK, Lichtenstein JE, Sobin LH. Peutz–Jeghers syndrome. *Radiographics* 1992; **12**: 365–78.
5 Gardiello FM, Welsh SB, Hamilton SR *et al.* Increased risk of cancer in the Peutz–Jeghers syndrome. *N Engl J Med* 1987; **316**: 1511–14.

Laugier–Hunziker–Baran syndrome (Chapter 69)

Laugier–Hunziker syndrome presents with labial, oral mucosal and nail hyperpigmentation. A possible variant of this or Peutz–Jeghers syndrome, has been termed *idiopathic lenticular pigmentation* [1] in which there are oral, labial, perianal and digital hyperpigmented lenticular macules. Similar patients have been reported previously [2,3,4].

REFERENCES

1 Gerbig AW, Hunziker T. Idiopathic lenticular mucocutaneous pigmentation or Laugier–Hunziker syndrome with atypical features. *Arch Dermatol* 1996; **132**: 844–5.
2 Calnan CD. The Peutz–Jegher's syndrome. *Trans St John's Hosp Dermatol Soc* 1960; **44**: 58–64.
3 Bologa EI, Bene M, Pasztor P. Considerations sur la lentiginose eruptive de la face. *Ann Dermatol Syphiligr* 1965; **92**: 277–86.
4 Dupre A, Viraben R. Laugier's disease. *Dermatologica* 1990; **181**: 183–6.

For mucocutaneous pigmented spots and oral myxoma see Chapter 69 and for pseudoxanthoma elasticum see Chapter 44.

Multiple mucosal neuroma syndrome

Familial syndromes of multiple endocrine neoplasia (MEN) occur in at least three separate clinical patterns. The type 2b (also called type 3) MEN syndrome is characterized by medullary carcinoma of the thyroid and phaeochromocytoma, in association with multiple mucosal neuromas and an ab-normal phenotype, a condition inherited as an autosomal dominant, although new cases often arise sporadically. The gene locus is on chromosome 10.

The facial appearance is striking, with thick, slightly everted lips which usually have a slightly bumpy surface due to the multiple neuromas [1,2]. These are actually mucosal and submucosal hamartomatous proliferations of nerve axons, Schwann cells and ganglion cells. Lesions may involve the tongue and commissures but are less frequent on the buccal mucosa, gingivae, palate, pharynx or larynx (Fig. 70.5). The eyelids are thickened, and multiple neuro-mas produce an irregular lumpy appearance.

Ganglioneuromatosis may also occur throughout the gastrointestinal tract, and this may result in constipation or megacolon [3]. Other ocular changes include yellowish masses on the conjunctivae, thickened corneal nerves and keratitis due to decreased tear production [4].

Most patients have an asthenic Marfanoid habitus, with high, arched palate, pectus excavatum, arachnodactyly and kyphoscoliosis, but the lens subluxation and cardiovascular abnormalities of Marfan's syndrome are not present [5–8].

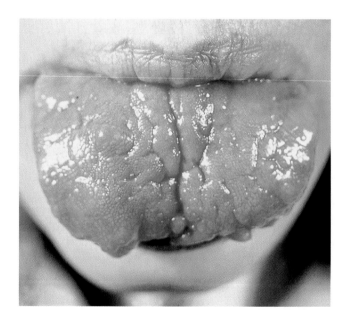

Fig. 70.5 Multiple neuromas of the lips and tongue in a patient with multiple endocrine neoplasia syndrome (type 2). (Courtesy of Dr M. Hartog, Bristol Royal Infirmary, Bristol, UK.)

REFERENCES

1 Brown RS, Colle F, Tashjian AH. The syndrome of multiple endocrine neoplasia and medullary thyroid carcinoma in childhood: importance of recognition of the phenotype. *J Pediatr* 1975; **86**: 77–83.
2 Casino AJ, Sciubba J, Ohri JL *et al.* Oral–facial manifestations of the multiple endocrine neoplasia syndrome. *Oral Surg* 1981; **51**: 516–23.
3 Carney JA, Go VLW, Sizemore GW *et al.* Alimentary tract ganglio-neuromatosis: a major component of the syndrome of multiple endocrine neoplasia. *N Engl J Med* 1976; **295**: 1287–91.
4 Colombo CD, Watson AG. Ophthalmological manifestations of the multiple endocrine neoplasia type 3 syndrome. *Can J Ophthalmol* 1976; **11**: 290–4.
5 Montgomery TB, Mandelstam P, Tachman ML. Multiple endocrine neoplasia type IIB: a description of several patients and review of the literature. *J Clin Hypertens* 1987; **3**: 31–49.
6 Ohishi M, Ishii T, Shiratsychi H, Tashiro H. Mucosal endocrine neoplasia type 3: three cases with mucosal neuromata. *Br J Oral Maxillofac Surg* 1990; **28**: 317–21.
7 Rashid R, Khairi MRA, Dexter RN. Mucosal neuroma, pheochromocytoma and medullary thyroid carcinoma: multiple endocrine neoplasia Type III. *Medicine* 1975; **54**: 89–112.
8 Schimke RN. Multiple endocrine adenomatosis syndromes. *Adv Intern Med* 1976; **21**: 249–65.

Cowden's syndrome (Chapter 12)

Papules may be seen on the lips.

Telangiectasia

Telangiectasia of the lips may be seen in hereditary haemorrhagic telangiectasia [1] (Fig. 70.6) and as an acquired disorder.

REFERENCE

1 Flint SR, Keith O, Scully C. Hereditary haemorrhagic telangiectasia. *Oral Surg Oral Med Oral Pathol* 1988; **66**: 440–4.

Haemangioma

Most haemangiomas of the lip are small and of no consequence [1,2]. Large facial haemangiomas, which can involve the lips, may be associated with Sturge–Weber syndrome (Fig. 70.7) [3] or the Dandy–Walker syndrome, or other posterior cranial fossa malformations [4].

REFERENCES

1 Kaban LB, Mulliken JB. Vascular anomalies of the maxillofacial region. *J Oral Maxillofac Surg* 1986; **44**: 203–13.
2 Stal S *et al.* Haemangioma, lymphangioma and vascular malformations of the head and neck. *Otolaryngol Clin North Am* 1986; **19**: 769–96.
3 Scully C. Orofacial manifestations of the neurodermatoses. *J Dent Child* 1980; **47**: 255–60.
4 Reese V, Frieden IJ, Paller AS. Association of facial hemangiomas with Dandy–Walker and other posterior fossa malformations. *J Pediatr* 1993; **122**: 379–84.

Olmsted's syndrome (Chapter 34)

Mutilating palmoplantar and periorificial keratoderma are the features of this autosomal dominant disorder which sometimes responds to etretinate [1,2].

REFERENCES

1 Lucker GPH, Steijlen PM. The Olmsted syndrome: mutilating palmoplantar and periorificial keratoderma. *J Am Acad Dermatol* 1994; **31**: 508–9.
2 Judge MR, Misch K, Wright P. Palmoplantar and periorificial keratoderma with corneal epithelial dysplasia: a new syndrome. *Br J Dermatol* 1991; **125**: 186–8.

Congenital syphilis

Scars radiating from the vermilion (rhagades) may be seen in congenital syphilis. The small furrows which radiate from the lips in systemic sclerosis can be mistaken for rhagades.

Acquired lip lesions

The prevalence of the commonest lesions of the lips is shown in Table 70.1 [1,2].

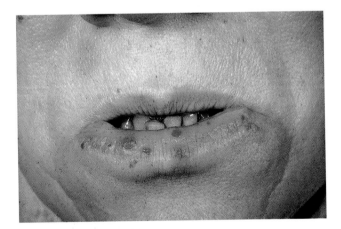

Fig. 70.6 Hereditary haemorrhagic telangiectasia.

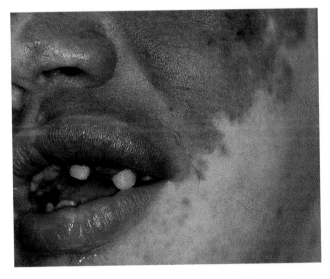

Fig. 70.7 Haemangioma affecting the lip in Sturge–Weber syndrome.

Table 70.1 Prevalence of lip lesions per 1000 population.*

	Men	Women
Leukoplakia	21.8	2.3
Haemangioma	5.2	2.9
Irritation fibroma	3.7	2.6
Herpes labialis	2.4	2.6
Angular cheilitis (stomatitis)	1.8	1.9
Inflammatory ulcer	1.8	1.3
Mucocoele	1.8	1.2

* White Americans over 35 years of age [1].

REFERENCES

1 Bouquot JE. Odd lips: the prevalence of common lip lesions in 23616 white Americans over 35 years of age. *Quintessence Int* 1987; **18**: 277–84,
2 Engel A, Johnson M-L, Haynes SG. Health effects of sunlight exposure in the United States. *Arch Dermatol* 1988; **124**: 72–9.

Leukoplakia (Chapter 69)

Smoking and tobacco-related habits are, with friction, the most common identifiable causes of keratoses but solar keratoses are also seen.

Telangiectasia

Telangiectasia may be seen in Calcinosis, Raynaud's, Esophageal, Sclerodactyly, Telangiectasia (CREST) syndrome [1] (Chapter 58), chronic liver disease, pregnancy and postirradiation.

REFERENCE

1 Veda M, Abe Y, Fujiwara H *et al*. Prominent telangiectasia associated with marked bleeding in CREST syndrome. *J Dermatol* 1993; **20**: 180–4.

Venous lake

SYN. VENOUS VARIX; SENILE HAEMANGIOMA OF LIP

This is a bluish purple, soft swelling, 2–10 mm in diameter, usually seen on the lower lip of an elderly person, due to a venous dilatation (Figure 70.8). The lesion is lined by a single layer of flattened endothelial cells with a thick wall of fibrous tissue. The lesion empties on prolonged pressure [1,2].

A venous lake may be only a trivial cosmetic problem or it can bleed severely after trauma. It can be excised, but careful cryotherapy, electrocautery or treatment with an argon laser [2] can also give good results.

REFERENCES

1 Alcalay J, Sandbank M. The ultrastructure of cutaneous venous lakes. *Int J Dermatol* 1987; **26**: 645–6.

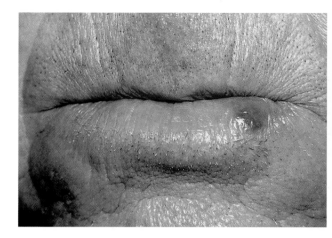

Fig. 70.8 Venous lake of the lip. (Courtesy of Addenbrooke's Hospital, Cambridge, UK.)

2 Neumann RA, Knobler RM. Venous lakes (Bean–Walsh) of the lips—treatment experience with the argon laser and 18 months follow-up. *Clin Exp Dermatol* 1990; **15**: 115–18.

Proliferative vascular lesions

Benign atypical vascular lesions of the lip may exhibit cytological or architectural features that simulate angiosarcoma such that considerable caution is required [1]. The head and neck region is a common location particularly for lobular capillary haemangioma (LCH or pyogenic granuloma) and the lip is a particularly common site for LCH [2] and intravascular papillary endothelial hyperplasia (IPEH, Masson's haemangioma or pseudoangiosarcoma) [3,4]. IPEH is a benign, non-neoplastic, vascular lesion characterized histologically by papillary fronds lined by proliferating endothelium and probably represents an organizing thrombus. Seen mainly in the lip or tongue in females, it may simulate angiosarcoma histologically [5]. Excision suffices.

Vascular lesions such as epithelioid haemangioma, epithelioid haemangioendothelioma, spindle-cell haemangioendothelioma, acquired progressive lymphangioma, or angiosarcoma and Kaposi's sarcoma may also occasionally be seen.

REFERENCES

1 Renshaw AA, Rosai J. Benign atypical vascular lesions of the lip. *Am J Surg Pathol* 1993; **17**: 557–565.
2 Kerr DA. Granuloma pyogenicum. *Oral Surg Oral Med Oral Pathol* 1951; **4**: 158–76.
3 Kuo TT, Sayers CP, Rosai J. Masson's 'Vegetant intravascular hemangioendothelioma': a lesion often mistaken for angiosarcoma. Study of 17 cases located in the skin and soft tissues. *Cancer* 1976; **38**: 1227–36.
4 Mills SE, Cooper PH, Fechner RE. Lobular capillary hemangioma: the underlying lesion of pyogenic granuloma. A study of 73 cases from the oral and nasal mucous membranes. *Am J Surg Pathol* 1980; **4**: 471–9.
5 Tosios K, Koutlas IG, Papanicolaou SI. Intravascular papillary endothelial hyperplasia of the oral soft tissues. *J Oral Maxillofac Surg* 1994; **52**: 1263–8.

Fibrous lumps (Chapter 55)

Fibrous lumps are not uncommon, particularly inside the commissure.

Labial melanotic macule

SYN. SOLITARY LABIAL LENTIGO

The labial melanotic macule is an acquired, small, flat, brown to brown–black, asymptomatic, benign lesion, unchanging in character [1,2]. Melanotic macules may be seen in up to 3% of normal persons, at any age. Most are seen near the midline, on the lower lip vermilion. They are solitary and are more common in young, white women (mean age 30 years) [3,4]. Occasional cases are seen in human immunodeficiency virus (HIV) infection [5].

Clinically, the labial melanotic macule may resemble other lesions such as early melanoma and ephelides, although these tend to fade in winter and darken in summer. Histopathologically, the lip or mucosal epithelium is normal apart from increased pigmentation of the basal layer, accentuated at the tips of rete ridges. There are no naevus cells or elongated rete ridges [3]. The intralesional melanocytes are benign in nature. They can be excised for cosmetic reasons, or hidden by lipstick.

REFERENCES

1 Weathers DR, Corio RL, Crawford BE. The labial melanotic macule. *Oral Surg Oral Med Oral Pathol* 1976; **42**: 192–205.
2 Wescott WB, Correll RW, Friedlander AH. Pigmented macules on the lower lip. *J Am Dent Assoc* 1983; **107**: 100–1.
3 Spann CR, Owen LG, Hodge SJ. The labial melanotic macule. *Arch Dermatol* 1987; **123**: 1029–31.
4 Ho KL, Dervan P, O'Loughlin S, Powell FC. Labial melanotic macule: a clinical, histopathologic and ultrastructural study. *J Am Acad Dermatol* 1993; **28**: 33–9.
5 Ficarra G, Shillitoe EJ, Adler-Storthz K. Oral melanotic macules in patients infected with human immunodeficiency virus. *Oral Surg Oral Med Oral Pathol* 1990; **70**: 748–55.

Cheilitis

SYN. INFLAMMATION OF THE LIPS

Cheilitis may arise as a primary disorder of the vermilion zone, or the inflammation may extend from nearby skin or, less often, from the oral mucosa (Table 70.2).

'Chapping' of the lips

Chapping is a reaction to adverse environmental conditions. It is usually caused by exposure to freezing cold or to hot, dry winds, but acute sunburn can cause very similar changes. The keratin of the vermilion zone loses its plasticity, so that the lips become sore, cracked and scaly. The affected subject tends to lick the lips, or to pick at the scales, which may make the condition worse.

Treatment is by the application of petroleum jelly, and the avoidance of the causative environmental conditions.

Table 70.2 Causes of cheilitis.

Chapping due to cold and wind
Eczematous cheilitis
Contact cheilitis
Drug-induced cheilitis
Infective cheilitis
Angular cheilitis
Ultraviolet irradiation
  Actinic cheilitis
  Actinic prurigo of the lip
Glandular cheilitis
Granulomatous cheilitis
Exfoliative (factitious) cheilitis
Plasma-cell cheilitis
Nutritional cheilitis
Dermatoses
Trauma

Eczematous cheilitis

The lips are often involved secondarily to atopic eczema, but the possibility of contact dermatitis must also be considered (so-called contact cheilitis, see next section).

The treatment of atopic eczema of the lips is with emollients and topical corticosteroids, but the response to hydrocortisone is often poor, and the short-term use of a potent steroid such as fludrocortisone may be required to bring the condition under control.

Contact cheilitis

Definition. Contact cheilitis is an inflammatory reaction of the lips, provoked by the irritant or sensitizing action of chemical agents. A large number of substances have been incriminated, but many cases are caused by lipsticks or lip salves.

Lipsticks. Lipsticks are composed of mineral oils and wax which form the stick, castor oil as a solvent for the dyes, lanolin as an emollient, preservatives, perfumes and colours [1]. The colours may include azo dyes and eosin which is a bromofluorescein derivative. An impurity in the eosin used to be an important sensitizer [2] but eosin is now rarely if ever used in lipstick and lipstick allergy is now uncommon. Other ingredients which are occasionally incriminated include the azo dyes, carmine and oleyl alcohol [3]. Other sensitizers include lanolin, perfumes, azulene, propyl gallate, sesame oil [4], stearates [5], shellac and colophony [6]. Sunscreens applied in the form of a lipstick (e.g. cinnamic aldehyde) can also cause contact cheilitis [7].

Lipsalves and other medicaments. Lipsalves containing lanolin are frequently applied for dryness or chapping. Phenyl salicylate and antibiotics have also been incriminated as a cause of cheilitis [8,9]. Petrolatum chapsticks may cause an unusual form of acne with a single row of large, open comedones along the cutaneous margin of the upper lip [10].

Mouthwashes and dentrifices [11]. Essential oils, such as peppermint, cinnamon, cloves and spearmint and bactericidal agents can cause cheilitis or circumoral dermatitis. Propolis, derived from resin collected by bees, is a well-known sensitizer which has been used in some toothpastes [12,13].

Some patients who brush their teeth frequently with tartar-control dentrifices, which contain pyrophosphate compounds, develop erythema, scaling and fissuring of the perioral area, sometimes with gingivitis or cheilitis. Patch testing to the toothpaste ingredients in 20 patients with this condition was negative and it was postulated that the eruption was a form of irritant contact dermatitis. The oral contents of subjects using tartar control toothpaste became more alkaline than when regular toothpaste was used. Nineteen of the 20 subjects were atopic and presumably had an increased susceptibility to an irritant process [14].

Dental preparations. Mercury and eugenol, both much used in dentistry, may cause cheilitis in the absence of stomatitis. Allergy to epimine-containing materials used for temporary crowns and bridges can cause cheilitis [15]. The subject of allergy to dental preparations has been reviewed elsewhere [16,17].

Foods. Peppermint, carvone, spearmint [18], citrus fruits [19], artichokes [20], nuts [21], pineapple [22], mangoes [23–25], asparagus [26] and cinnamon oil [27,28] are among the food constituents which occasionally cause an allergic cheilitis and dermatitis of the skin around the lips. The oil on the peel of citrus fruits is irritant to the skin, but in addition some sweet oranges contain a weakly phototoxic agent which can cause a reaction in pale-skinned people [29]. Both type I and type IV reactions may occur, and will require different tests.

Miscellaneous objects. Common causes are various objects favoured by obsessional suckers of all ages—metal hair clips, metal pencils, the cobalt paint on blue pencils, etc. [30]. Allergy to nail varnish can also cause cheilitis [31]. The wooden and nickel mouthpieces of musical instruments are a rare cause [32]. Clarinettists' cheilitis due to prolonged playing of reed instruments has also been reported (Fig. 70.9), but this is thought to be due to mechanical factors rather than allergy [33].

The metal mouthpieces of trumpets and other 'brass' instruments can also cause lip problems, including contact dermatitis, lacerations and acne mechanica [34].

Clinical features. Lipstick cheilitis is sometimes confined to the vermilion border but more often extends beyond

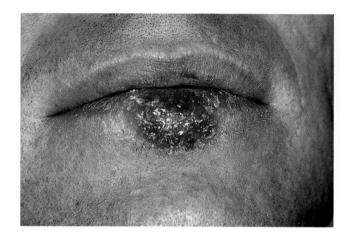

Fig. 70.9 Clarinettists' cheilitis.

it. There may be persistent irritation and scaling or a more acute reaction with oedema and vesiculation. The offending lipstick may have been adopted only recently or may have been in regular use for many years. Exacerbations develop a few hours or over a day after the application. In some cases a lipstick may be well tolerated unless there is also exposure to sunlight.

The other forms a cheilitis vary greatly in their clinical appearance. Those caused by foods commonly also involve the skin around the mouth. If a small, sucked object is responsible, the reaction may be confined to one part of the lips.

Diagnosis. If acute eczematous changes are obviously present, the diagnosis of contact cheilitis presents no difficulty. If the changes are confined to irritation and scaling the various forms of exfoliative cheilitis must be excluded.

If an allergic reaction is suspected, patch tests should be carried out as described in Chapter 20 using the appropriate concentrations of the substances concerned.

Treatment. Topical corticosteroids will give symptomatic relief but the offending substance must be traced and avoided.

REFERENCES

1 Cronin E. *Contact Dermatitis.* Edinburgh: Churchill Livingstone 1980: 141.
2 Calnan CD, Sarkany I. Studies in contact dermatitis II. Lipstick cheilitis. *Trans Rep St John's Hosp Dermatol Soc Lond* 1957; **39**: 28–36.
3 Calnan CD, Sarkany I. Studies in contact dermatitis XII. Sensitivity to oleyl alcohol. *Trans Rep St John's Hosp Dermatol Soc Lond* 1960; **44**: 47–50.
4 Hayakawa R, Matsunaga K, Suzuki M *et al.* Is sesamol present in sesame oil? *Contact Dermatitis* 1987; **17**: 133–5.
5 Hayakawa R, Matsunaga K, Suzuki M *et al.* Lipstick dermatitis due to C$_{18}$ aliphatic compounds. *Contact Dermatitis* 1987; **16**: 215–19.
6 Rademaker M, Kirby JD, White IR. Contact cheilitis to shellac, Lampol 5 and colophony. *Contact Dermatitis* 1987; **15**: 307–8.
7 Maibach HJ. Cheilitis—occult allergy to cinnamic aldehyde. *Contact Dermatitis* 1986; **15**: 106–7.

8 Hindson C. Phenyl salicylate in a lip salve. *Contact Dermatitis* 1980; **6**: 216.

9 Marchand B, Barbier P, Ducombs G *et al.* Allergic contact dermatitis to various salols (phenyl salicylates). A study in man and guinea-pig. *Arch Dermatol Res* 1982; **272**: 61–6.

10 Shelley WB, Shelley ED. Chapstick acne. *Cutis* 1986; **37**: 459–60.

11 Fisher AA. *Contact Dermatitis*, 2nd edn. Philadelphia: Lea & Febiger, 1973: 320.

12 Trevisar G, Kokelj F. Contact dermatitis from propolis; role of gastro-intestinal absorption. *Cantact Dermatitis* 1987; **16**: 48.

13 Young E. Contact dermatitis from sensitivity to propolis. *Contact Dermatitis* 1987; **16**: 49.

14 Beacham BE, Kurgansky D, Gould WM. Circumoral dermatitis and cheilitis caused by tartar control dentifrices. *J Am Acad Dermatol* 1990; **22**: 1029–32.

15 Duxbury AJ, Turner EP, Watts DC. Hypersensitivity to epimine containing dental materials. *Br Dent J* 1979; **147**: 331–3.

16 Kulenkamp D, Hausen BM, Schulz KH. Kontakt Allergie durch neuartige, zahnartzlich verwendete Abdruckmaterialien. *Hautarzt* 1977; **28**: 353–8.

17 Maurice PD, Hopper C, Punnia-Moorthy A *et al.* Allergic contact stomatitis and cheilitis from iodoform used in a dental dressing. *Contact Dermatitis* 1988; **18**: 114–16.

18 Hjorth N, Jervoe P. Allergies to essential oils. *Tandlaegeblader* 1967; **71**: 937.

19 Schur A. Dermatitis venenata: report of a case due to the osage orange. *Arch Dermatol Syphil* 1932; **26**: 312–13.

20 Pindborg JJ. Disorders of the oral cavity and lips. In: Rook AJ, Wilkinson DS, Ebling FJ eds. *Textbook of Dermatology*, 2nd edn. Oxford: Blackwell Scientific Publications, 1972: 1672–1721.

21 Siegal S. Local allergic oedema induced by procaine. *J Allergy* 1958; **29**: 329–35.

22 Polunin J. Pineapple dermatosis. *Br J Dermatol* 1951; **63**: 441–55.

23 Kirby-Smith JL. Mango dermatitis. *Am J Trop Med* 1938; **18**: 373–84.

24 Asai T. About mango-dermatitis. *Jpn J Dermatol Urol* 1939; **46**: 44–5.

25 Brown A, Brown FR. Mango dermatitis. *J Allergy* 1941; **12**: 310–11.

26 Halberg V. Tilfaetden af aspargedermatitis. *Hospitalstid* 1932; **75**: 1235–41.

27 Leifer W. Contact dermatitis due to cinnamon. *Arch Dermatol Syphil* 1951; **64**: 52–5.

28 Miller J. Cheilitis from sensitivity to oil of cinnamon present in bubble gum. *JAMA* 1941; **116**: 131–2.

29 Volden G, Krokan H, Kavli G. Phototoxic and contact toxic reactions of the exocarp of sweet oranges: a common cause of cheilitis? *Contact Dermatitis* 1983; **9**: 201–4.

30 Bruynzeel DP. A child with perioral eczema. *Contact Dermatitis* 1987; **16**: 43.

31 Cronin E. *Contact Dermatitis*. Edinburgh: Churchill Livingstone, 1980: 154.

32 Hausen BM, Bruhn G, Koenig WA. New hydroxyisoflavans as contact sensitizers in cocus wood *Brya ebenus* DC (Fabaceae). *Contact Dermatitis* 1991; **25**: 149–55.

33 Friedman SJ, Connolly SM. Clarinettists' cheilitis. *Cutis* 1986; **38**: 183–4.

34 Bischof RD. Drum and bugle corps: medical issues and problems. *Med Prob Perform Art* 1994; **9**: 131–6.

Drug-induced cheilitis

Haemorrhagic crusting of the lips (Fig. 70.10) is a feature of erythema multiforme (particularly in the Stevens–Johnson syndrome), which is commonly caused by drugs or the herpes simplex virus (Chapter 45), but cheilitis can also occur as an isolated feature of a drug reaction, either as a result of allergy or as a pharmacological effect.

The aromatic retinoids, such as etretinate and isotretinoin, cause dryness and cracking of the lips in most patients. The mechanism of this pharmacological effect is unknown, but is dose related.

Life-threatening anaphylactic reactions have been reported in patients who have applied chlorhexidine gluconate topically to the lips, and in 1984 the Japanese Ministry of Welfare recommended that chlorhexidine should not be used on mucous membranes because of this risk [1].

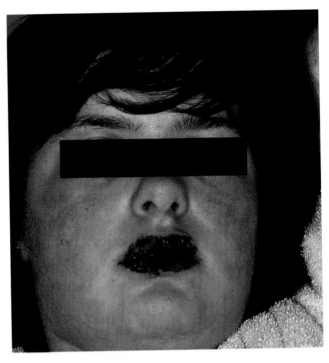

Fig. 70.10 Haemorrhagic crusting of the lips in Stevens–Johnson syndrome.

Nevertheless, chlorhexidine is commonly used as an antiplaque mouthwash in many countries with only rare adverse effects.

Other drugs which can affect the oral mucosa are discussed in Chapter 77.

REFERENCE

1 Okano M, Nomura M, Hata S *et al.* Anaphylactic symptoms due to chlorhexidine gluconate. *Arch Dermatol* 1989; **125**: 50–2.

Infective cheilitis

Viral

Primary oral infection by herpes simplex virus may produce perioral lesions (Fig. 70.11). However, recurrent herpes labialis involving the lip is a very common cause of blisters at the mucocutaneous junction (Fig. 70.12) (Chapter 26). The lesions arise at the mucocutaneous junction as itching papules which progress to vesicles, pustules and then scab. They are unsightly and occasionally become infected with *Staphylococcus* or *Streptococcus*, resulting in impetigo (Fig. 70.13). In immunocompromised persons extensive and persistent lesions may result. In atopic persons the lesions may spread to produce eczema herpeticum (Fig. 70.14). Aciclovir is the standard treatment used as a 5% cream.

Herpes zoster of the maxillary division of the trigeminal nerve affects the upper lip. The lower lip is affected in

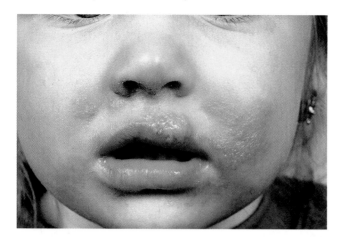

Fig. 70.11 Primary herpetic stomatitis with extraoral lesions.

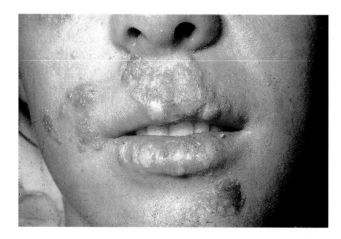

Fig. 70.12 Herpes labialis.

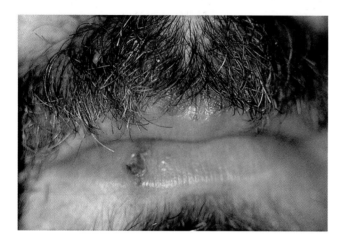

Fig. 70.13 Impetigo.

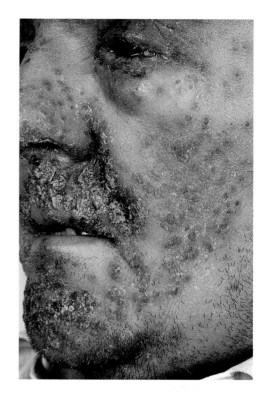

Fig. 70.14 Eczema herpeticum.

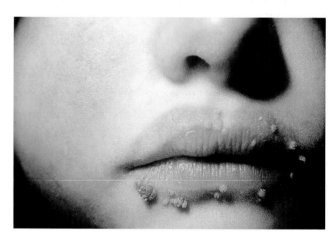

Fig. 70.15 Warts on lips in a boy who was also a lip-sucker.

Bacterial

Dental infection or occasionally a furuncle or carbuncle may cause swelling of the lip. Impetigo may mimic herpes labialis (Chapter 27). Cancrum oris (fusospirochaetal infection) may cause labial and buccal necrosis [8,9].

The lip is the most common extragenital site for a primary syphilitic lesion. Most lip chancres in males tend to occur on the upper lip; in females on the lower lip. In secondary syphilis, moist, flat, papulonodular lesions (condylomata lata) often appear at the mucocutaneous junctions and on mucosal surfaces especially at the com-

mandibular zoster [1]. Various papillomaviruses may cause papillomatous lesions on the lips, especially verruca vulgaris [2–4] (Fig. 70.15). Coxsackie virus (Fig. 70.16), orf [5,6] molluscum contagiosum and vaccinia virus [7] infections of the lips are rare.

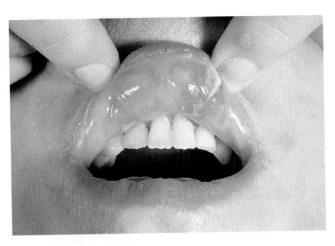

Fig. 70.16 Hand, foot and mouth disease due to Coxsackie virus (note oral and digital lesions).

missures [10]. The tropical treponematoses may present similarly to syphilis.

Rhinoscleroma initially affects the nasal mucosa, but it may spread slowly to the upper lip, producing plaques or nodules with sunken centres. The extreme hardness of the infiltrations is characteristic. The lip can appear to fuse to the alveolar process but the overlying skin and mucosa remain normal.

Protozoal

Cutaneous or mucocutaneous leishmaniasis typically causes swellings on the upper lip with later enlargement and destruction of the lip [11–14] reflecting the three stages of oedema, granulomatous proliferation, and then necrosis.

Fungal

Blastomycosis and paracoccidioidomycosis are uncommon causes of chronic ulceration affecting the lip, producing very similar clinical lesions to leishmaniasis [15].

Others

Red, swollen lips with fissuring and exfoliation are prominent in mucocutaneous lymph-node syndrome (Kawasaki disease).

REFERENCES

1 Smith S, Ross JR, Scully C. An unusual complication of herpes zoster infection. *Oral Surg* 1984; **57**: 388–9.
2 Green TL, Eversole LP, Leider AS. Oral and labial verruca vulgaris: clinical, histological and immunohistochemical evaluation. *Oral Surg Oral Med Oral Pathol* 1986; **62**: 410–16.
3 Scully C, Cox M, Prime S, Maitland N. Papillomaviruses: their current status in relation to oral disease. *Oral Surg Oral Med Oral Pathol* 1988; **65**: 526–32.
4 Scully C, Prime S, Maitland N. Papillomaviruses: their possible role in oral disease. *Oral Surg Oral Med Oral Pathol* 1985; **60**: 166–74.
5 Parnell AG. Ecthyma contagiosum (Orf). *Br J Oral Surg* 1965; **3**: 128–35.
6 Meechan JG, MacLeod RI. Human labial orf: a case report. *Br Dent J* 1992; **173**: 343–4.
7 Scully C. Vaccinia of the lip. *Br Dent J* 1977; **143**: 57–9.
8 Enwonwu CO. Infectious oral necrosis (cancrum oris) in Nigerian children. *Community Dent Oral Epidemiol* 1985; **13**: 190–4.
9 Sawyer D, Nwoku AJ. Cancrum oris (noma): past and present. *J Dent Child* 1981; **48**: 138–41.
10 Manton SL, Eggleston SI, Alexander I, Scully C. Oral presentation of secondary syphilis. *Br Dent J* 1986; **160**: 237–8.
11 Sitheeque MA, Quazi AA, Ahmed GA. A study of cutaneous leishmaniasis involvement of the lips and perioral tissues. *Br J Oral Maxillofac Surg* 1990; **28**: 43–6.
12 Asvesti C, Anastassiadis G, Kolokotronis A, Zographakis I. Oriental sore: a case report. *Oral Surg* 1992; **73**: 56–8.
13 Sanguezą OP, Sanguezą JM, Stiller MJ, Sanguezą P. Mucocutaneous Leishmaniasis: a clinicopathological classification. *J Am Acad Dermatol* 1993; **28**: 927–32.
14 Ramesh V, Mirra RS, Saxena U, Mukherjee A. Post-kala-azar dermal Leishmaniasis: a clinical and therapeutic study. *Int J Dermatol* 1993; **32**: 272–5.
15 Spostos R, Scully C, Almeida OPD *et al.* Oral paracoccidioidomycosis: a study of 36 South American patients. *Oral Surg Oral Med Oral Pathol* 1993; **75**: 461–5.

Angular cheilitis

SYN. ANGULAR STOMATITIS

Definition [1]. Angular cheilitis is an acute or chronic inflammation of the skin and contiguous labial mucous membrane at the angles of the mouth.

Aetiology. Angular cheilitis is a clinical syndrome, in which four main groups of factors are implicated, alone or in combination. Most cases in adults are due to mechanical and/or infective causes but in children nutritional or immune defects are more prominent causes.

Infective agents. These are probably the major cause. In a careful Scandinavian study, either *Candida* or staphylococci were isolated in all patients [2]; none of the patients had iron deficiency or loss of the vertical dimension of occlusion. Other studies have also shown a high incidence of infection with bacteria or yeasts [3,4], although secondary invasion of cheilitis due to atopic eczema is a possibility in some cases.

Oral candidiasis causing cheilitis is particularly common in those wearing dentures (Chapter 31). Permanent cure can be achieved only by eliminating the growth of *Candida* beneath the upper denture [5]. Candidiasis was probably responsible for some of the cases of cheilitis attributed to allergy to denture materials since contamination of denture material by *Candida* may cause false-positive patch-test reactions [6].

Immune deficiency. Angular cheilitis associated with candidiasis resistant to therapy may be an early manifestation of an underlying immunological deficiency.

Diabetes and HIV infection may present with angular stomatitis.

Outbreaks of acute pustular and fissured cheilitis may occur in children, particularly if they are malnourished, and in some cases streptococci or staphylococci have appeared to be causative [7].

Mechanical factors. In the edentulous patient who does not wear a denture or who has inadequate dentures, and also as a normal consequence of the ageing process, the upper lip overhangs the lower at the angles of the mouth, producing an oblique curved fold and keeping a small area of skin constantly macerated. Prognathism may give rise to a similar state of affairs in the young.

The recurrent trauma of dental flossing is a very rare cause of angular cheilitis [8].

Nutritional deficiencies. Nutritional deficiencies, in particular deficiencies of riboflavin, folate, iron and general protein malnutrition, have often been incriminated. Riboflavin deficiency produces smooth, shiny, red lips associated with angular stomatitis, and this combination has been called *cheilosis* [1,9–11]. Crohn's disease or orofacial granulomatosis may be found in some [12].

Other factors. Hypersalivation from any cause may ensure the continued maceration of the angles of the mouth. Cheilitis is common in Down's syndrome, the large tongue and the constant dribbling possibly being contributory factors.

Atopic dermatitis involving the face is often associated with angular cheilitis. The incidence appears also to be increased in seborrhoeic dermatitis but the association with other skin diseases is probably fortuitous.

A rare cause is the presence of sinuses of developmental origin at the angles of the mouth.

Clinical features. All forms of angular cheilitis present as a roughly triangular area of erythema and oedema at one, or more commonly both, angles of the mouth (Fig. 70.17). Linear furrows or fissures radiating from the angle of the mouth (rhagades) are seen in the more severe forms, especially in denture wearers.

Recurrent exudation and crusting are frequent. An eczematous dermatitis may extend some distance onto the cheek or chin as an infective eczematoid reaction (Chapter 17) or as a reaction to topical medicaments.

In atopic dermatitis, especially in children and adolescents, dry scaling and thickening, and sometimes hyperpigmentation, are combined with crusted radial fissures. Licking, as a nervous tic, often perpetuates the changes.

Diagnosis. This is usually obvious. The rhagades which radiate from the angles of the mouth in congenital syphilis are much less inflamed. In all cases in denture wearers,

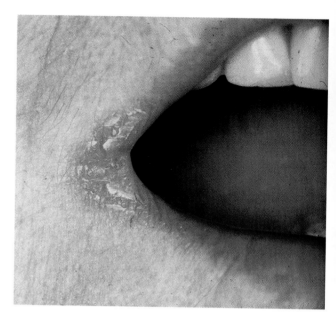

Fig. 70.17 Angular cheilitis.

Candida should be sought not only in the lesions but also beneath the denture.

Treatment. Treatment of angular cheilitis is sometimes difficult and may need to be prolonged. Dentures should be kept out of the mouth at night and stored in a candidacidal solution such as hypochlorite. Denture-induced stomatitis should be treated with an antifungal and new dentures which restore facial contour may help. The skin lesions should be swabbed and staphylococcal infection treated with fusidic acid ointment or cream at least four times daily.

Miconazole may be preferable treatment for candidiasis (cream applied locally, together with the oral gel) as it has some Gram-positive bacteriostatic action but there is a high relapse rate unless treatment is prolonged. Miconazole is absorbed and may potentiate the action of warfarin, phenytoin and the sulphonylureas. Nystatin or amphotericin (as cream or ointment) should therefore be tried first in patients taking these drugs. Fluconazole may be indicated for immuno-compromised patients.

Underlying systemic disease must be sought and treated, and a course of oral iron and vitamin B supplements may be helpful in indolent cases.

In rare intractable cases, surgery or occasionally collagen injections have been advocated to try and restore normal commissural anatomy.

REFERENCES

1 Schoenfeld RJ, Schoenfeld FI. Angular cheilitis. *Cutis* 1977; **19**: 213–16.
2 Ohman SC, Dahlen G, Moller A *et al.* Angular cheilitis—a clinical and microbial study. *J Oral Pathol* 1986; **15**: 213–17.

3 MacFarlane TW, Helnarska SJ. The microbiology of angular cheilitis. *Br Dent J* 1976; **140**: 403.
4 Dahlen G. A retrospective study of microbiologic samples from oral mucosal lesions. *Oral Surg* 1982; **53**: 350–4.
5 Scully C. Chronic atrophic candidosis. *Lancet* 1986; **ii**: 437–8.
6 Salo OP, Hirvonen ML. Yeasts as a cause of false-positive reactions in patch-tests for allergy to dental materials. *Br J Dermatol* 1969; **81**: 338–41.
7 MacFarlane TW, McGill JC, Samaranayake LB. Antibiotic testing and phage typing of *Staphylococcus aureus* isolated from non-hospitalized patients with angular cheilitis. *J Hosp Infect* 1984; **5**: 444–6.
8 Kahana M, Yakalom M, Yakalom R *et al.* Recurrent angular cheilitis caused by dental flossing. *J Am Acad Dermatol* 1986; **15**: 113–14.
9 Murphy NC, Bissada NF. Iron deficiency: an overlooked predisposing factor in angular cheilitis. *J Am Dent Assoc* 1979; **99**: 640–1.
10 Rose JA. Aetiology of angular cheilosis: iron metabolism. *Br Dent J* 1968; **125**: 67–72.
11 Parodi A, Priano L, Rebora A. Chronic zinc deficiency in a patient with psoriasis and alcoholic liver cirrhosis. *Int J Dermatol* 1991; **30**: 45–7.
12 Wiesenfeld D, Ferguson MM, Mitchell DN *et al.* Orofacial granulomatosis; clinical and pathological analysis. *Q J Med* 1985; **213**: 101–13.

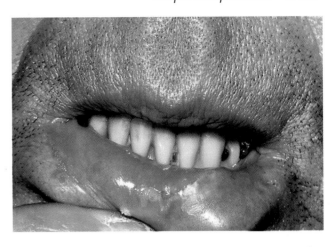

Fig. 70.18 Chronic actinic cheilitis with leukoplakia. (Courtesy of Addenbrooke's Hospital, Cambridge, UK.)

Actinic cheilitis

SYN. ACTINIC KERATOSIS OF LIP;
SOLAR CHEILOSIS

Definition. A premalignant keratosis of the lip caused by exposure to solar irradiation.

Aetioloy. Cheilitis due to acute sunburn is common, and clinically resembles 'chapping'. Actinic cheilitis is most common in hot, dry regions, in outdoor workers and in fair-skinned people (skin types I and II). The vermilion of the lower lip receives a high dose of UV irradiation because it is almost at right angles to the rays of the midday sun and it is poorly protected by keratin and melanocytes. Most actinic cheilitis is seen on the lower lip of fair-skinned men in their fourth to eighth decade of life. Other forms of radiation can cause similar changes including arc welding.

The condition is less common in females, perhaps because of the sunscreen effect of lipstick, and in black people, because of the protective effect of melanin.

Particular care to protect the vermilion of the lips with adequate sunscreens is needed in patients with photo-sensitivity disorders such as xeroderma pigmentosum, and in those whose exposure to UVB is high, such as mountaineers, windsurfers and skiers.

Pathology [1]. The histology shows a flattened or atrophic epithelium, beneath which is a band of inflammatory infiltrate in which plasma cells may predominate. Nuclear atypia and abnormal mitoses may be seen in the more severe cases, and some develop into invasive squamous carcinoma [2]. The collagen generally shows basophilic (elastotic) degeneration [3].

Clinical features (Fig. 70.18). Actinic cheilitis tends to affect the lower lip of adults who have had prolonged exposure to sunlight [4]. In the early stages there may be redness and oedema, but later the lips become dry and scaly. Later still, the epithelium becomes palpably thickened with small, greyish white plaques. Vertical fissuring and crusting may be seen, particularly in cold weather, although sometimes the condition improves during the winter months. At times, vesicles may appear which rupture to form superficial erosions.

Secondary infection may occur and, eventually, warty nodules may form. These tend to vary in size with fluctuation in the degree of oedema and inflammation, but eventually one or more may undergo malignant change, the possibility of which must always be considered when ulceration develops, or there are other suspect features such as:
1 a red and white, blotchy appearance with an indistinct vermilion border;
2 generalized atrophy with focal areas of whitish thickening;
3 persistent flaking and crusting [5].

Diagnosis. It must be remembered that actinic cheilitis may be an early manifestation of a genetic susceptibility to light damage as in xeroderma pigmentosum. Actinic cheilitis can also be part of the syndrome of actinic prurigo [6], which mainly affects native Americans (see below). Other forms of cheilitis must also be considered, including lupus erythematosus and lichen planus of the lips.

Eczematous cheilitis may be induced by contact allergy, or by the photosensitizing action of certain ingredients of lipstick or lip salves. Attacks of herpes simplex may also be induced by sunlight.

Treatment. Treatment of actinic cheilitis is required to relieve symptoms and to prevent development of squamous carcinoma. Three methods give acceptable results.
1 *Topical agents.* For mild cases the application of 5% fluorouracil three times daily for 10 days is suitable. This

produces a brisk erosion, but the lip should heal within 3 weeks [7]. Topical tretinoin [8] or trichloracetic acid [9] may also be effective.

2 *Vermilionectomy (lip shave)* [10]. Under local anaesthesia, the vermilion border is excised with a scalpel and the wound closed by advancing the labial mucosa to the skin. This can be combined with wedge resection if cancer has developed. Postoperative complications are generally more than with laser ablation [11], and include paraesthesiae, lip pruritus and labial scar tension [12].

3 *Laser ablation.* Carbon dioxide laser therapy has been used to vaporize the vermilion with good results and no postoperative paraesthesiae or significant scarring [13–16]. Following treatment, prevention of recurrence by the regular use of a sunscreen lip salve is advisable. Liquid or gel waterproof preparations containing *para*-aminobenzoic acid probably give the best protection [17,18].

REFERENCES

1 Koten JW. Histopathology of actinic cheilitis. *Dermatologica* 1967; **135**: 465–71.
2 Picascia DD, Robinson JK. Actinic cheilitis, a review of the aetiology, differential diagnosis and treatment. *J Am Acad Dermatol* 1987; **17**: 255–64.
3 Schmitt CK. Histologic evaluation of degenerative changes of the lower lip. *J Oral Surg* 1968; **26**: 51–6.
4 Cotaldo E. Solar cheilitis. *J Dermatol Surg Oncol* 1981; **7**: 289–95.
5 La Riviere W, Pickett AB. Clinical criteria in diagnosis of early squamous carcinoma of the lower lip. *J Am Dent Assoc* 1979; **99**: 972–7.
6 Birt AR, Hogg GR. The actinic cheilitis of hereditary polymorphic light eruption. *Arch Dermatol* 1979; **115**: 699–702.
7 Epstein E. Treatment of actinic cheilitis with topical fluorouracil. *Arch Dermatol* 1977; **113**: 906–8.
8 Kligman A. Topical tretinoin: indications, safety and effectiveness. *Cutis* 1987; **39**: 486–8.
9 Turk LL, Winder PR. Carcinomas of the skin and their treatment. *Semin Oncol* 1980; **7**: 376–84.
10 Birt BD. The lip-shave operation for premalignant conditions of the lower lip. *Otolaryngology* 1977; **6**: 407–11.
11 Robinson JK. Actinic cheilitis: a prospective study comparing four treatment methods. *Arch Otolaryngol Head Neck Surg* 1989; **115**: 848–52.
12 Sanchez-Conejo-Mir J, Perez-Bernal AM, Mormo-Jiminez JC *et al.* Follow-up of vermilionectomies. *J Dermatol Surg Oncol* 1986; **12**: 180–4.
13 David LM. Laser vermilion ablation for actinic cheilitis. *J Dermatol Surg Oncol* 1984; **11**: 605–8.
14 Dufresne RG, Garrett AB, Bailin PL, Ratz JL. Carbon dioxide laser treatment of chronic actinic cheilitis. *J Am Acad Dermatol* 1988; **19**: 876–8.
15 Stanley RJ. Actinic cheilitis: treatment with the carbon dioxide laser. *Mayo Clin Proc* 1988; **63**: 230–5.
16 Zelickson BD, Roenigk RK. Actinic cheilitis: treatment with the carbon dioxide laser. *Cancer* 1990; **65**: 1307–11.
17 Lundeen RC, Langlais RP. Sunscreen protection for lip mucosa. A review and update. *J Am Dent Assoc* 1985; **11**: 617–21.
18 Payne TE. An evaluation of actinic blocking agents for the protection of lip mucosa. *J Am Dent Assoc* 1976; **92**: 409–11.

Actinic prurigo

This is a type of familial photodermatitis, which occurs mainly in native Americans living at high altitudes [1,2] especially in Latin America, although a very similar condition has been reported in China [3]. It usually presents in young women as a photosensitive facial rash with pruritic cheilitis affecting the lower lip, and it may be associated with conjunctivitis, eyebrow alopecia and the formation of pterygia.

This type of cheilitis is due to enhanced sensitivity to sunlight and is distinguished from actinic cheilitis, which is due to prolonged and excessive exposure to UV irradiation, by the relative absence of epidermal dysplasia and solar elastosis. There is follicular cheilitis with numerous germinal centres in the lamina propria and a dense perivascular infiltrate composed of plasma cells and lymphocytes, although there may also be many eosinophils [4].

The relationship of actinic prurigo to polymorphous light eruption is uncertain, since pruritic cheilitis is not a prominent feature of the latter disease, although it is almost invariably present in the actinic prurigo of native Americans [5,6].

Treatment with sunscreens, β-carotene, long-term psoralen and UVA (PUVA), and antihistamines has given variable and generally unsatisfactory results. Oral thalidomide may be tried, if it is available and there are no contraindications such as the possibility of pregnancy [7].

REFERENCES

1 Birt AR, Davis RA. Hereditary polymorphic light eruption of American Indians. *Int J Dermatol* 1975; **14**: 105–11.
2 Scheen SR, Connolly SM, Dicken CH. Actinic prurigo. *J Am Acad Dermatol* 1981; **5**: 183–90.
3 Guogi X, Yiming H, Huibao S *et al.* Pruritic cheilitis: six cases. *Oral Surg* 1983; **55**: 359–62.
4 Herrera-Goepfert R, Magana M. Follicular cheilitis. *Am J Dermatopathol* 1995; **17**: 357–361.
5 Calnan CD, Meara RH. Actinic prurigo (Hutchinson's summer prurigo). *Clin Exp Dermatol* 1977; **2**: 365–77.
6 Mounsden T, Kratochvil T, Auclair P *et al.* Actinic prurigo of the lower lip. Review of the literature and report of 5 cases. *Oral Surg Oral Med Oral Pathol* 1988; **65**: 327–32.
7 Londono F. Thalidomide in the treatment of actinic prurigo. *Int J Dermatol* 1973; **12**: 323–8.

Glandular cheilitis

Definition. Glandular cheilitis is characterized by inflammatory changes and swelling of salivary glands in the lips [1–3].

Aetiology. This is an uncommon idiopathic condition which in a few cases has apparently been familial [4]. Although it was originally thought that the condition was due to inflammation of enlarged heterotopic salivary glands, the glands are often normal in size, depth and histology [5]. It is possible that the excessive salivary secretion from minor salivary glands in this condition might be an unusual clinical response to irritation of the lip from some other cause such as actinic damage, repeated licking, etc.

Pathology. In the milder forms there is some fibrosis surrounding the salivary glands, and in the more severe forms there may be a dense chronic inflammatory infiltrate. Only rarely do patients show genuine hyperplasia of the salivary glands or duct ectasia.

Clinical features. The onset is at any age from childhood onwards. In simple glandular cheilitis the lower lip is slightly thickened, and bears numerous pin-head-sized orifices from which mucous saliva can readily be squeezed. The upper lip is rarely involved [6].

In the more severe suppurative form (*Volkmann's cheilitis*) the lip is considerably and permanently enlarged, and subject to episodes of pain, tenderness and increased enlargement. The surface is covered by crusts and scales, beneath which the salivary duct orifices may be discovered. In the most severe forms there may be deep-seated infection with abscess formation, and fistulous tracts.

The condition can evidently be premalignant; in some series 20–30% of cases progress to squamous cancer. This does, of course, support the suggestion that in many cases glandular cheilitis is a consequence of actinic cheilitis [5].

Treatment. Actinic cheilitis, if identified, should be treated appropriately. If the lips are grossly enlarged, excision of an elongated ellipse of tissue may be required, and in other cases shave vermilionectomy may be all that is necessary. Other conditions such as atopic disease or factitial cheilitis would require different treatment.

REFERENCES

1 Rada DC. Cheilitis glandularis. A disorder of ductal ectasia. *J Dermatol Surg Oncol* 1985; **1**: 372–5.
2 Stuller CB, Schaberg SJ, Stokos J. Cheilitis glandularis. *Oral Surg* 1982; **53**: 602–5.
3 Thiele B, Mahrle G, Ippen H. Cheilitis glandularis simplex. *Hautarzt* 1983; **34**: 232–4.
4 Weir TW, Johnson WC. Cheilitis glandularis. *Arch Dermatol* 1971; **103**: 433–7.
5 Swerlick RA, Cooper PH. Cheilitis glandularis: a re-evaluation. *J Am Acad Dermatol* 1984; **10**: 466–72.
6 Winchester L, Scully C, Prime SS, Eveson JW. Cheilitis glandularis: a case affecting the upper lip. *Oral Surg Oral Med Oral Pathol* 1986; **62**: 654–6.

Granulomatous cheilitis
SYN. MIESCHER'S CHEILITIS

Definition. A chronic swelling of the lip due to granulomatous inflammation of unknown cause.

Nomenclature. Melkersson in 1928 [1] described labial oedema in association with recurrent facial palsy. Rosenthal in 1930 emphasized the role of genetic factors and added scrotal tongue to the syndrome. The full syndrome has since been called the *Melkersson–Rosenthal syndrome* [2].

In Miescher's cheilitis the granulomatous changes are confined to the lip, and this is generally regarded as a monosymptomatic form of the Melkersson–Rosenthal syndrome, although the possibility remains that these may be two separate diseases.

Aetiology. The cause is unknown, but there may be a genetic predisposition to the Melkersson–Rosenthal syndrome [3]; siblings have been affected and a scrotal tongue may be present in otherwise normal relatives.

There is no convincing evidence that granulomatous cheilitis is due to an infective agent. Some cases may represent a localized form of sarcoidosis [4] or ectopic Crohn's disease [5,6] or orofacial granulomatosis. There is increasing evidence that some patients with granulomatous cheilitis are predisposed to Crohn's disease [6]. In some cases, granulomatous cheilitis is followed some years later by regional ileitis [7–10]. A few patients react to cobalt [11] or to food additives such as cinnamic aldehyde [12–14], although these reactions are by no means always relevant; for example, in one study only one of nine patients had a relationship between cheilitis and food intake [15].

Pathology. Biopsy of the swollen lip or facial tissues during the early stages of the disease shows only oedema and perivascular lymphocytic infiltration. In some cases of long duration no other changes are seen, but in others the infiltrate becomes more dense and pleomorphic and small focal granulomas are formed, indistinguishable from sarcoidosis or Crohn's disease. Similar changes may be present in cervical lymph nodes [16–19]. In some cases, small granulomas occur in the lymphatic walls [20].

Clinical features. The condition affects the sexes equally. The earliest manifestations usually develop in childhood or adolescence but may be delayed until middle or old age. The earliest cutaneous manifestation is sudden diffuse or nodular swellings [21] involving the upper lip, the lower lip and one or both cheeks in decreasing order of frequency [5,19]. Labial swelling occurs in about 75% and facial swelling in 50% of patients [22]. Less commonly, the forehead, eyelids or one side of the scalp may be involved. The attacks are sometimes accompanied by fever and mild constitutional symptoms, including headache and even visual disturbance. At the first episode the oedema typically subsides completely in hours or days, but after recurrent attacks the swelling may persist, and slowly increases in degree (Fig. 70.19). It gradually becomes firmer and eventually acquires the consistency of firm rubber. After some years, the swelling may very slowly regress.

A fissured or scrotal tongue is seen in 20–40% of cases. It is present from birth in some, which may indicate genetic susceptibility. There may be loss of sense of taste and decreased salivary gland secretion [19].

The regional lymph nodes are enlarged in 50% of cases [3] but not usually very greatly.

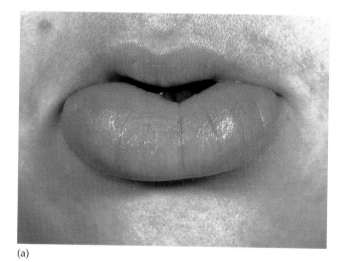

(a)

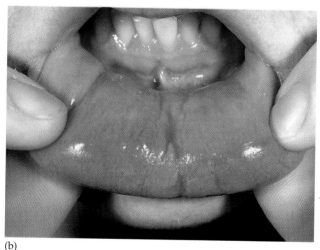

(b)

Fig. 70.19 Granulomatous cheilitis of the lower lip. (Courtesy of Addenbrooke's Hospital, Cambridge, UK.)

Facial palsy of the lower motor neurone type occurs in some 30% of cases. It may precede the attacks of oedema by months or years, but more commonly develops later. Although intermittent at first, the palsy may become permanent. It may be unilateral or bilateral, and partial or complete [19]. Other cranial nerves (the olfactory, auditory, glossopharyngeal and hypoglossal) may occasionally be involved. Involvement of the central nervous system has also been reported, but the significance of the resulting symptoms is easily overlooked as they are very variable, sometimes simulating disseminated sclerosis but often with a poorly defined association of psychotic and neurological features. Autonomic disturbances may occur.

Diagnosis. The essential feature of the syndrome is the granulomatous swelling of lip or face. In the early attacks clinical differentiation from angio-oedema may be impossible in the absence of either scrotal tongue or facial palsy. Persistence of the swelling between attacks should

suggest the diagnosis, which can sometimes be confirmed by biopsy. However, the histological changes are not always conspicuous or specific.

In the established cases, other causes of macrocheilia (Table 70.3) must be excluded. Ascher's syndrome associated with blepharochalasia is likely to cause confusion, although the swelling of the lip is caused by redundant salivary tissue and is present from childhood. Lymphoma is a rare differential diagnosis [23].

Treatment. Reactions to dietary components should be sought and possible antigens avoided. The injection of up to 10 ml triamcinolone (10 mg/l) into the lips after local analgesia may be effective [15,24,25]. The injections may have to be repeated every 4–6 months once a response plateau has been reached. This treatment has also been successfully combined with surgical reduction (cheiloplasty) [26,27]. The injections must be continued periodically after the surgery or there may be an exaggerated recurrence of the condition. Surgery alone is relatively unsuccessful [28].

Systemic corticosteroids are rarely indicated [29]. Not all respond [27,30] and adverse effects may be a problem. Clofazimine appears to help the majority of patients [31,32], in a dose of 100 mg twice daily for 10 days, then twice weekly for 4 months. Metronidazole may also produce resolution in granulomatous cheilitis [33,34].

Table 70.3 Macrocheilia: acute or chronic enlargement of one or both lips.

Acute	Chronic
Traumatic	Developmental
Infective	Familial idiopathic
Pyococcal	Double lip
Anthrax	Ascher's syndrome
Diphtheria	Lymphangioma
Primary syphilis	Haemangioma
Trichophytosis	Neurofibroma
Leishmaniasis	Mucopolysaccharidoses
Herpes simplex	Fucosidosis
Trichiniasis	Coffin–Siris syndrome
Angio-oedema	Acquired
Erythema multiforme	Post-traumatic
Actinic cheilitis	Postinfective
Other forms of cheilitis	on basis of developmental
	lymphatic defect
	Infective
	Tuberculosis
	Leprosy
	Rhinoscleroma
	Leishmaniasis
	Neoplastic
	Melkersson–Rosenthal syndrome
	Cheilitis glandularis
	Sarcoidosis
	Crohn's disease
	Orofacial granulomatosis

Other treatments which have occasionally been helpful include long-term penicillin, erythromycin, sulphasalazine or ketotifen.

REFERENCES

1 Melkersson E. Case of recurrent facial paralysis with angio-neurotic edema. *Hygien* 1928; **90**: 737–41.

2 Wadlington WB, Riley HD, Lowbeer I. The Melkersson–Rosenthal syndrome. *Pediatrics* 1984; **73**: 502–6.

3 Hornstein OP. Melkersson–Rosenthal syndrome: a neuro-mucocutaneous disease of complex origin. *Current Prob in Dermatol* 1973; **5**: 117–56.

4 Shedade SA, Foulds IS. Granulomatous cheilitis and a positive Kveim test. *Br J Dermatol* 1986; **115**: 619–22.

5 Tatnall FM, Dodd HJ, Sarkany I. Crohn's disease with metastatic cutaneous involvement and granulomatous cheilitis. *J R Soc Med* 1987; **80**: 49–50.

6 Kano Y, Shiohara T, Yagita A, Nagashima M. Association between cheilitis granulomatosa and Crohn's disease. *J Am Acad Dermatol* 1993; **28**: 801.

7 Carr D. Granulomatous cheilitis in Crohn's disease. *Br Med J* 1974; **iv**: 636.

8 Talbot T, Jewell L, Schloss E *et al*. Cheilitis antedating Crohn's disease. Case report and literature review. *J Clin Gastroenterol* 1984; **6**: 349–54.

9 Verbov JL. The skin in patients with Crohn's disease and ulcerative colitis. *Trans Rep St John's Hosp Dermatol Soc Lond* 1973; **59**: 30–8.

10 Wiesenfeld D, Ferguson MM, Mitchell DN *et al*. Orofacial granulomatosis: a clinical and pathological analysis. *Q J Med* 1985; **54**: 101–13.

11 Pryce DW, King CM. Orofacial granulomatosis associated with delayed hypersensitivity to cobalt. *Clin Exp Dermatol* 1990; **15**: 384–96.

12 McKenna KE, Walsh MY, Burrows D. The Melkersson–Rosenthal syndrome and food additive hypersensitivity. *Br J Derm* 1994; **131**: 921–2.

13 Patton DW, Ferguson MM, Forsyth A, James J. Orofacial granulomatosis: a possible allergic basis. *Br J Oral Maxillofac Surg* 1985; **23**: 235–42.

14 Sweatman MC, Tasker R, Warner JO *et al*. Orofacial granulomatosis response to elemental diet and provocation by food additives. *Clin Allergy* 1986; **16**: 331–8.

15 Sakuntabhai A, MacLeod RI, Lawrence CM. Intralesional steroid injection after nerve block anaesthesia in the treatment of orofacial granulomatosis. *Arch Dermatol* 1993; **129**: 477–80.

16 Hernandez G, Hernandez F, Lucas M. Miescher's granulomatous cheilitis: literature review. *J Oral Maxillofac Surg* 1986; **44**: 474–8.

17 Kint A, De Brauwere D. Cheilitis granulomatosa und Crohnsche Krankheit. *Hautarzt* 1977; **28**: 319–21.

18 Rhodes EL, Stirling GA. Granulomatous cheilitis. *Arch Dermatol* 1965; **92**: 40–4.

19 Worsaae N, Christensen KC, Schiodt M. Melkersson–Rosenthal syndrome and cheilitis granulomatosa. *Oral Surg* 1982; **54**: 404–13.

20 Nozicka Z. Endovasal granulomatous lymphangitis as a pathogenetic factor in cheilitis granulomatosa. *J Oral Pathol* 1985; **14**: 363–5.

21 Ficarra G, Cicchi P, Amorosi A, Piluso S. Oral Crohn's disease and pyostomatitis vegetans. *Oral Surg Oral Med Oral Pathol* 1993; **75**: 220–4.

22 Zimmer WM, Rogers RS, Reeve CM, Sheridan PJ. Orofacial manifestations of Melkersson–Rosenthal syndrome. *Oral Surg* 1992; **74**: 610–19.

23 Scully C, Eveson JW, Witherow H *et al*. Oral presentation of lymphoma: case report of T-cell lymphoma masquerading as oral Crohn's disease, and review of the literature. *Oral Oncol* 1993; **29B**: 225–30.

24 Cermale D, Serri F. Intralesional injection of triamcinolone in the treatment of cheilitis granulomatosa. *Arch Dermatol* 1963; **72**: 695–6.

25 Williams AJK, Wray D, Ferguson A. The clinical entity of orofacial Crohn's disease. *Q J Med* 1991; **79**: 451–58.

26 Eisenbud L, Hymowitz S, Shapiro R. Cheilitis granulomatosa. *Oral Surg Oral Med Oral Pathol* 1971; **32**: 384–9.

27 Krutchkoff D, James R. Cheilitis granulomatosa: successful treatment with combined local triamcinolone injections and surgery. *Arch Dermatol* 1978; **114**: 1203–6.

28 Scully C, Cochran KM, Russell RI *et al*. Oral Crohn's disease as an indicator of intestinal involvement. *Gut* 1982; **23**: 198–201.

29 Williams PM, Greenberg MS. Management of cheilitis granulomatosa. *Oral Surg* 1991; **72**: 436–9.

30 Allen CM, Camisa C, Hamzeh S, Stephens L. Cheilitis granulomatosa: report of six cases and review of the literature. *J Am Acad Dermatol* 1990; **23**: 444–50.

31 Neuhofer J, Fritsch P. Cheilitis granulomatosa: therapy with clofazimine. *Hautarzt* 1984; **35**: 459–63.

32 Podmore P, Burrows D. Clofazimine—an effective treatment for Melkersson–Rosenthal syndrome or Miescher's cheilitis. *Clin Exp Dermatol* 1986; **11**: 173–8.

33 Kano Y, Shiohara T, Yagita A. Treatment of recalcitrant cheilitis granulomatosa with metronidazole. *J Am Acad Dermatol* 1992; **27**: 629–30.

34 Scully C, Eveson JW. Oral granulomatosis (Leading Article). *Lancet* 1991; **338**: 20–1.

Exfoliative cheilitis

SYN. FACTITIOUS CHEILITIS, *LE TIC DE LÈVRES*

Exfoliative cheilitis is a chronic superficial inflammatory disorder of the vermilion borders of the lips characterized by persistent scaling (Fig. 70.20). The diagnosis is now restricted to those few patients whose lesions cannot be attributed to other causes such as contact sensitization or light (see actinic cheilitis, p. 3197). Many of these cases are now thought to be factitious, owing to repeated lip sucking, chewing or other manipulation of the lips [1,2]. There is no association with dermatological or systemic disease, although rare cases are seen in HIV infection. Some are infected with *Candida* species [3].

Most cases occur in girls or young women, and the majority have a personality disorder [4,5]. The process, which often starts in the middle of the lower lip and spreads to involve the whole of the lower or both lips, consists of scaling and crusting, more or less confined to the vermilion border, and persisting in varying severity for months or years. The patient often complains of irritation or burning, and can be observed frequently biting or sucking the lips. In some cases the condition appears to start with chapping or with atopic eczema, and develops into a habit tic.

In a large Russian series, almost half the cases had associated thyroid disease [6], but this observation has not been confirmed.

Diagnosis. Contact and active cheilitis must be carefully excluded. Chronic exfoliative cheilitis is readily contaminated by *Candida*. In such cases the clinical features are variable and may simulate carcinoma, lichen planus or lupus erythematosus.

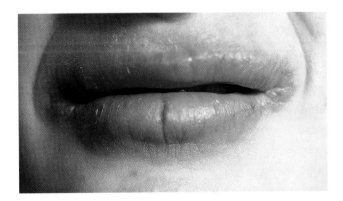

Fig. 70.20 Factitious cheilitis due to repeated lip sucking.

Treatment. Some cases resolve spontaneously [2,7] or with improved oral hygiene [8]. Reassurance and topical corticosteroids may be helpful in some cases [1], but others require psychotherapy or tranquillizers [7,9].

REFERENCES

1 Thomas JR, Greene SL, Dicken CH. Factitious cheilitis. *J Am Acad Dermatol* 1983; **8**: 368–72.
2 Daley TD, Gupta AK. Exfoliative cheilitis. *J Oral Pathol Med* 1995; **24**: 177–9.
3 Reade PC, Rich AM, Hay KD, Radden BG. Cheilo-candidosis—a possible clinical entity. *Br Dent J* 1982; **152**: 305–8.
4 Jeanmougin M, Civatte J, Bertail MA. Cheilites squamo-crouteuses factices. *Ann Dermatol Vénéréol* 1984; **111**: 1007–11.
5 Reade PC, Sim R. Exfoliative cheilitis—a factitious disorder? *Int J Oral Maxillofac Surg* 1986; **15**: 313–17.
6 Kutin SA. Clinical aspects and pathogenesis of exfoliative cheilitis. *Vestn Dermatol Venereol* 1970; **44**: 39–43.
7 Postlethwaite KR, Hendrickse MA. A case of exfoliative cheilitis. *Br Dent J* 1988; **165**: 23.
8 Brooke RI. Exfoliative cheilitis. *Oral Surg* 1978; **45**: 52–5.
9 Crotty CP, Dicken CH. Factitious lip crusting. *Arch Dermatol* 1981; **117**: 338–40.

Plasma-cell cheilitis
SYN. PLASMA-CELL ORIFICIAL MUCOSITIS

Plasma-cell cheilitis is an idiopathic benign inflammatory condition, characterized by dense plasma-cell infiltrates in the lips and other mucosae close to body orifices [1–3]. The condition has been reported (under a wide variety of names) to affect the penis, vulva, lips, buccal mucosa, palate, gingiva, tongue, epiglottis and larynx.

Plasma-cell cheilitis is the counterpart of Zoon's plasma-cell balanitis (Chapter 72). It presents as circumscribed flat or elevated patches of erythema, usually on the lower lip in an elderly person. The cause is unknown, but it responds to the application of powerful topical cortico-steroids such as clobetasol, or to the intradermal injection of triamcinolone [4], or to systemic griseofulvin [5].

A similar lesion, which tends to form a tumorous mass with a hyperkeratotic surface and needs to be differentiated from extramedullary plasmacytoma [6], has been called *plasma-acanthoma* [7,8].

REFERENCES

1 Baughman RD. Plasma cell cheilitis. *Arch Dermatol* 1974; **110**: 725–6.
2 Luders G. Plasmacytosis mucosae: Ein oft verkanntes neues Krankheitsbild. *Munch Med Wschr* 1972; **114**: 8–12.
3 White JW, Olsen KD, Banks PM. Plasma cell orificial mucosis. Report of a case and review of the literature. *Arch Dermatol* 1986; **122**: 1321–4.
4 Jones SK, Kennedy CTC. Response of plasma cell orificial mucositis to topically applied steroids. *Arch Dermatol* 1988; **124**: 1871–2.
5 Tamaki K, Tsukamato K, Ohtake N, Furue M. Treatment of plasma cell cheilitis with griseofulvin. *J Am Acad Dermatol* 1994; **30**: 789–990.
6 Burke WA, Merritt CC, Briggaman RA. Disseminated extramedullary plasmacytomas. *J Am Acad Dermatol* 1986; **14**: 335–9.
7 Ferreira-Marques J. Beitrag zur Kenntnis der Plasmocytosis circumorificialis (Scheuermann) 'Plasmoakanthoma'. *Arch Klin Exp Dermatol* 1962; **215**: 151–64.
8 Ramos E, Silva J. Das Plasmoakanthom. *Hautarzt* 1965; **16**: 7–11.

Nutritional cheilitis

Severe nutritional deficiency, especially pellagra, can cause the vermilion zone to become shiny and cracked, sometimes with eroded areas. Milder degrees of deficiency cause angular cheilitis (p. 3135).

Pyostomatitis vegetans

Erosions and ulcers may be seen in the labial mucosa and on the vermilion in pyostomatitis vegetans—typically seen in ulcerative colitis.

Dermatoses

Lupus erythematosus

Involvement of the vermilion zone is quite common in both discoid and systemic lupus erythematosus [1]. Discoid lupus can be premalignant, and should be treated vigo-rously with topical steroid ointments and sunscreens [2,3]. The cheilitis of systemic lupus erythematosus tends to be more severe, with erosions and haemorrhagic crusts.

Lupus erythematosus can be very difficult to distinguish from lichen planus of the lips, both clinically and by histology (Figs 70.21 & 70.22).

REFERENCES

1 Coulson IH, Marsden RA. Lupus erythematosus cheilitis. *Clin Exp Dermatol* 1986; **11**: 309–13.
2 Martin S, Rosen T, Locker E. Metastatic squamous cancer of lips. Occurrence in Blacks with discoid lupus erythematosus. *Arch Dermatol* 1979; **115**: 1214.
3 Fotos PG, Finkelstein MW. Discoid lupus erythematosus of the lip and face. *J Oral Maxillofac Surg* 1992; **50**: 642–5.

Sarcoidosis (Chapter 60)

Sarcoidosis may cause chronic violaceous lesions on, or swelling of, the lips [1].

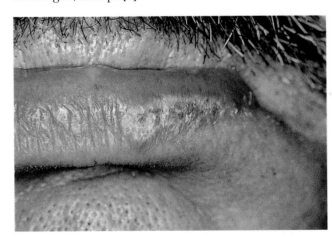

Fig. 70.21 Discoid lupus erythematosus of the lower lip.

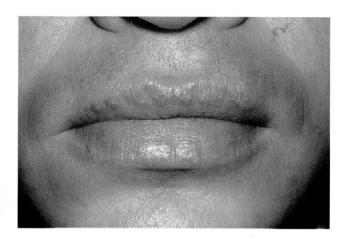

Fig. 70.22 Mild lichen planus of the lips, resembling lupus erythematosus. (Courtesy of Addenbrooke's Hospital, Cambridge, UK.)

REFERENCE

1 James DG. Lupus pernio. *Lupus* 1992; **1**: 129–31.

Lichen planus (Chapter 41)

In most cases of lichen planus of the lips there are characteristic intraoral lesions (Figs 70.22 & 70.23) but some are seen in isolation [1,2].

REFERENCES

1 Itin PH, Schiller P, Gilli L, Buechner SA. Isolated lichen planus of the lip. *Br J Dermatol* 1995; **132**: 1000–2.
2 Allan SJR, Buxton PK. Isolated lichen planus of the lip. *Br J Dermatol* 1996; **135**: 145–6.

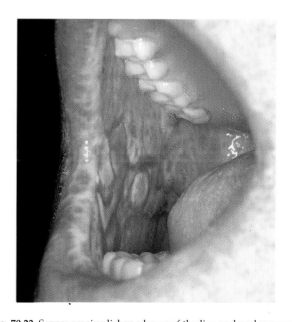

Fig. 70.23 Severe erosive lichen planus of the lips and oral mucosa.

Erythema multiforme (Chapter 45)

Acute labial swelling with a serosanguinous exudate is common in Stevens–Johnson syndrome and is almost pathognomonic [1] (see Fig. 70.10).

REFERENCE

1 Ting HC. Stevens–Johnson syndrome: a review of 34 cases. *Int J Dermatol* 1985; **24**: 587–91.

Focal acantholytic dyskeratosis (Chapter 40)

Focal acantholytic dyskeratosis (FAD) rarely affects the lip as a painful, oozing crusted patch [1].

REFERENCE

1 Ahn SK, Chang SN, Lee SH. Focal acantholytic dyskeratosis on the lip. *Am J Dermatopathol* 1995; **17**: 189–91.

For pemphigus and pemphigoid see Chapter 40.

Traumatic cheilitis

Trauma from habits such as lip licking, use of various musical instruments (see Fig. 70.9) and in some occupations, may cause cheilitis.

Mucous cyst

SYN. MUCOUS RETENTION CYST; RANULA; MUCOCOELE; MYXOID CYST OF LIP

These are usually cystic spaces filled with mucinous material, probably due to traumatic rupture of mucous ducts. They appear as dome-shaped, translucent, whitish blue papules or nodules, typically on the inner surface of the lower lip (Fig. 70.24) [1].

Care should be taken to ensure that the lesion is not a salivary gland tumour with cystic change—especially when dealing with an apparent mucous cyst in the *upper* lip. The cysts can be excised but they also respond well to cryosurgery, using a single freeze–thaw cycle [2].

REFERENCES

1 Lattanand A, Johnson WC. Mucous cyst (mucocele): A clinico-pathologic and histochemical study. *Arch Dermatol* 1970; **101**: 673–8.
2 Bohler-Sommeregger K. Cryosurgical management of myxoid cysts. *J Dermatol Surg Oncol* 1988; **14**: 1405–8.

Lip fissure

A fissure may develop in the lip when a patient, typically a child, is mouth breathing (Fig. 70.25). The aetiology is

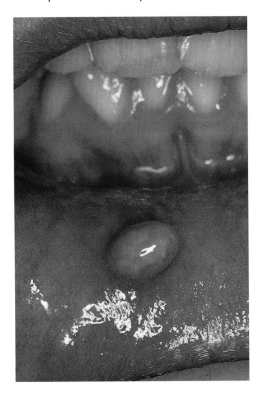

Fig. 70.24 Mucous cyst (ranula) of the lower lip.

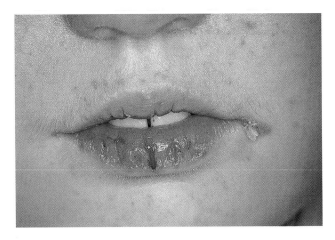

Fig. 70.25 Lip fissure.

obscure, although sun, wind, cold weather and smoking are thought to predispose [1–3]. Contrary to the clinical impression that fissures are seen mainly in the lower lip there is a higher prevalence in the upper lip. A hereditary predisposition for weakness in the first branchial arch fusion seems to exist [1]. Lip fissures are common in Down's syndrome. The lips may also crack in this way if swollen, for example in oral Crohn's disease.

Local applications of silver nitrate, salicylic acid, and antimicrobials seem less effective than excision, preferably with a Z-plasty [1].

REFERENCES

1 Rosenquist B. Median lip fissure: etiology and suggested treatment. *Oral Surg* 1991; **72**: 10–14.
2 Axell T, Skoglund A. Chronic lip fissures. *Int J Oral Surg* 1981; **10**: 354–8.
3 Ecker H. Medial clefts of the lips. *Am J Surg* 1958; **96**: 815.

Injuries

The lips are not infrequently traumatized by a deliberate or accidental blow. The lower lip in particular may be bitten accidentally (as when anaesthetized) [1], or deliberately [2,3] or occasionally in Lesch–Nyhan syndrome [4,5]. Burns may be caused by heat, irradiation, chemicals or electricity.

There are two types of electrical burn: in one the child bites straight through a wire and receives a burn, but the power is cut off; and in the other the child does not bite through the wire but chews on it, receiving several shocks and a number of severe radiating burns. Most children affected are under 4 years of age. Late bleeding from the superficial labial artery is common and thus hospitalization for 21 days is indicated. Long-term treatment is aimed at preventing scarring or contracture of the corner of the mouth.

REFERENCES

1 Gilmour AG, Craven CM, Chustecki AM. Self-mutilation under combined inferior dental block and solvent intoxication. *Br Dent J* 1984; **156**: 438–9.
2 Svirsky JA, Sawyer DR. Dermatitis artefacta of the paraoral region. *Oral Surg Oral Med Oral Pathol* 1987; **64**: 259–63.
3 Lamey PJ, McNab L, Lewis MAO, Gibb R. Orofacial artefactual disease. *Oral Surg Oral Med Oral Pathol* 1994; **77**: 131–4.
4 Scully C. Orofacial manifestations of the Lesch–Nyhan syndrome. *Int J Oral Surg* 1981; **10**: 380–3.
5 LeBlanc J, Epker BN. Lesch–Nyhan syndrome: surgical treatment of a case with lip-chewing. *J Maxillofac Surg* 1981; **9**: 64–7.

Carcinoma

Squamous carcinoma is the commonest malignancy to affect the vermilion zone and, as with squamous carcinoma of the glabrous skin, it is usually due to actinic damage [1]. Like actinic cheilitis it is most common on the lower lip of fair-skinned, outdoor workers in sunny climates, and it is relatively rare in pigmented skin [2–4]. Lip cancer is common in certain population groups in UK, Romania, Hungary, Poland, Spain, Finland, Israel, Canada, USA and in Australia but in most areas reported, the incidence is falling [4–7].

Lip cancer generally occurs in men who are employed in outdoor activities such as farming and fishing [8]. Squamous cancers occur on the lower lip in 89% with 3% on the upper lip and 8% at the commissures [9]. Although sunlight is accepted as the major aetiological factor, some studies have shown a poor correlation between lip-cancer incidence and the rate of annual solar radiation [10]. Other risk factors may include low social class, tobacco smoking,

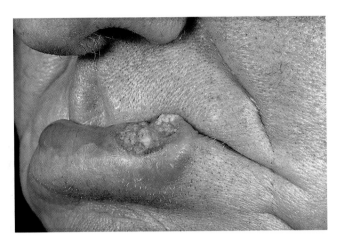

Fig. 70.26 Squamous cell carcinoma.

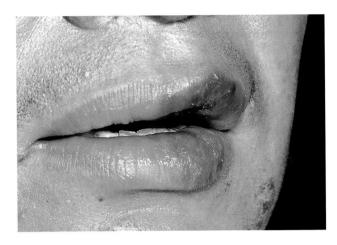

Fig. 70.27 Kaposi's sarcoma of the lips. Courtesy of Dr J. Epstein.

syphilis, poor dentition, infection with herpes simplex virus [3,5,8] and immune suppression [11].

The initial features are a keratinous growth or swelling of the lip (Fig. 70.26), soreness, and ulceration. Most lesions are amenable to surgical excision, with more than 70% surviving for 5 years.

REFERENCES

1 Zitsch RP. Carcinoma of the lip. *Otolaryngol Clin North Am* 1993; **26**: 265–77.
2 Keller AZ. Cellular types, survival, race, nativity, occupations, habits and associated diseases in the pathogenesis of lip cancers. *Am J Epidemiol* 1970; **91**: 486–99.
3 Picascia DD, Robinson JK. Actinic cheilitis: a review. *J Am Acad Dermatol* 1987; **17**: 255–64.
4 Szpak CA, Stone MJ, Frenkel EP. Some observations concerning the demographic and geographic incidence of carcinoma of the lip and buccal cavity. *Cancer* 1977; **40**: 343–8.
5 Keller AZ. The epidemiology of lip, oral and pharyngeal cancers, and the association with selected systemic diseases. *Am J Public Health* 1963; **53**: 1214–28.
6 MacFarlane GJ, Boyle P, Evstifeeva T, Scully C. Epidemiological aspects of lip cancer in Scotland. *Commun Dent Oral Epidemiol* 1993; **21**: 279–82.
7 Scully C, Cawson RA. Potentially malignant oral lesions. *J Epidemiol Biostat* 1996; **1**: 3–12.
8 Pukkala E, Soderholm A-L, Linqvist C. Cancers of the lip and oropharynx in different social and occupational groups in Finland. *Oral Oncol* 1994; **30B**: 209–15.
9 del Regato JA. Cancer of the respiratory system and upper digestive tract. In: del Regato JA, ed. *Ackerman and del Regato's Cancer*, 6th edn. St Louis: CV Mosby, 1985: 248–72.
10 Lindqvist C. Risk factors of lip cancer: a critical evaluation based on epidemiological comparisons. *Am J Public Health* 1979; **69**: 256–60.
11 King GN, Healy C, Glover MT *et al.* Increased prevalence of dysplastic and malignant lip lesions in renal transplant recipients. *N Engl J Med* 1995; **332**: 1052–7.

Other neoplasms

A range of other neoplasms may affect the lip, especially keratoacanthoma (Chapter 36), neoplasms of labial minor salivary glands, lymphomas [1,2], and Kaposi's sarcoma [3] (Fig. 70.27) (Chapter 55) and, rarely, sebaceous adenoma or papillary syringadenoma.

Sebaceous adenoma is a rare benign tumour originating from sebaceous glands, rarely from Fordyce spots, in the elderly. It appears as a well-defined, round, firm lump.

Papillary syringadenoma (syringocystadenoma papilliferum) is a rare benign tumour originating from sweat glands, usually seen at birth or in early life.

Labial salivary glands may show immunoglobulin heavy-chain rearrangement in patients with lymphomas of mucosa-associated lymphoid tissue [1,4].

REFERENCES

1 Morel P, Quiguandon I, Janin A. Involvement of minor salivary glands in gastric lymphomas. *Lancet* 1994; **344**: 139–40.
2 Scully C, Eveson JW, Whitherow H *et al.* Oral presentation of lymphoma: case report of T-cell lymphoma masquerading as oral Crohn's disease, and review of the literature. *Oral Oncol* 1993; **29B**: 225–30.
3 Epstein JB, Scully C. HIV infection: clinical features and treatment of thirty-three homosexual men with Kaposi's sarcoma. *Oral Surg Oral Med Oral Pathol* 1991; **71**: 38–41.
4 Diss TC, Peng H, Wotherspoon AC *et al.* A single neoplastic clone in sequential biopsy specimens from a patient with primary gastric-mucosa-associated lymphoid tissue lymphoma and Sjogren's syndrome. *N Engl J Med* 1993; **329**: 172–5.

Vasculitides

Giant-cell arteritis is a rare cause of ulceration, especially of the upper lip [1,2]. Ulceration of the lips is occasionally a result of leukocytoclastic angiitis.

REFERENCES

1 Pogrel MA. Necrosis of the upper lip from giant cell arteritis. *J Oral Maxillofac Surg* 1985; **43**: 300.
2 Scully C, Eveson JW, Cunningham SJ. Necrosis of the lip in giant cell arteritis: report of a case. *J Oral Maxillofac Surg* 1993; **51**: 581–3.

Lip ulcer due to calibre-persistent artery

A 'calibre-persistent artery' is defined as an artery with a diameter larger than normal near a mucosal or external surface. When such arteries occur in the gut wall (Dieulafay malformation) they may bleed, but in the lip they tend to cause chronic ulceration which can be mistaken for a squamous cancer. The ulcer is attributed to continual pulsation from the large artery running parallel to the surface, although the exact mechanism is obscure [1,2].

Ligation of the artery appears successful [3].

REFERENCES

1 Mike T, Adler P, Endes P. Simulated cancer of lower lip attributed to a 'calibre-persistent artery'. *J Oral Pathol* 1980; **9**: 137–44.
2 Marshall RI, Leppard BJ. Ulceration of the lip associated with a 'calibre-persistent artery'. *Br J Dermatol* 1985; **113**: 757–60.
3 Lovas JGL, Goodday RHB. Clinical diagnosis of calibre-persistent labial artery of the lower lip. *Oral Surg* 1993; **76**: 480–3.

Angio-oedema

Swelling of the lips is a common feature of urticaria and angio-oedema (Chapter 45). It is characterized by the transient nature of the swelling and the lack of scaling and induration (Fig. 70.28).

Reactive perforating collagenosis (Chapter 44)

Crateriform papules of the lower lip have been reported [1].

REFERENCE

1 Trattner A, Lueber A, Sandbank M. Mucosal involvement in reactive perforating collagenosis. *J Am Acad Dermatol* 1991; **25**: 1079–81.

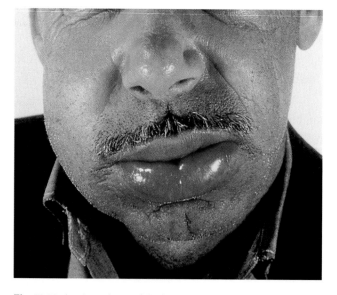

Fig. 70.28 Angio-oedema of the lips.

Hypopigmentation

Vitiligo occasionally involves the lip, usually as an isolated lesion but sometimes associated with vitiligo of the digits and areolae or penis (lip–tip syndrome). It can be easily camouflaged with lipstick.

Body art

Tattooing of the lower lip may occasionally be seen. A tattooed lower lip in a Sudanese woman, for example, signifies that she is married [1]. The Wodaabe people of Nigeria and the Cameroon may tattoo on the skin surface at the angle of the mouth, a practice which has its basis in ritual warding-off of the 'evil eye'. Similar tattoos may be seen on Bedouin women of North Africa. Tattooing of the chin is seen increasingly in Maoris ('Moki') and tattooing inside the lip may now be seen in developed countries. Mathur and Sahoo [2] reported an instance of fatal septicaemia following the placement of tribal tattoo marks at the angle of the mouth in a Nigerian infant.

The practice of piercing oral and facial soft tissues and then placing foreign objects in the defects on a more or less permanent basis is one which has also been largely confined until recently to certain tribal groups in continental Africa and isolated Amazon regions of South America, for example the Suia and Txukahameis tribes of Brazil, but it is now not uncommon in developed countries.

REFERENCES

1 Wilson DF, Grappin G, Miquel JL. Traditional, cultural, and ritual practices involving the teeth and orofacial soft tissues. In: Prabhu SR, Wilson DS, Daftary DK, Johnson NW, eds. *Oral Diseases in the Tropics*. Oxford: Oxford University Press, 1992: 91–124.
2 Mathur DR, Sahoo A. Pseudomonas septicaemia following tribal tattoo marks. *Trop Geogr Med* 1984; **36**: 301–2.

Burning sensation (Chapter 69)

A burning sensation may be seen as part of the burning mouth syndrome [1].

REFERENCE

1 Lamey PJ, Lamb AB. Lip component of the burning mouth syndrome. *Oral Surg Oral Med Oral Pathol* 1994; **78**: 590–3.

Loss of sensation

Labial hypoaesthesia or anaesthesia is often a result of trauma to the mental or inferior alveolar nerves or branches, or other trigeminal nerve branches (Fig. 70.29), or neoplastic involvement of these, but may be caused by diabetes mellitus, connective tissue disease, syphilis,

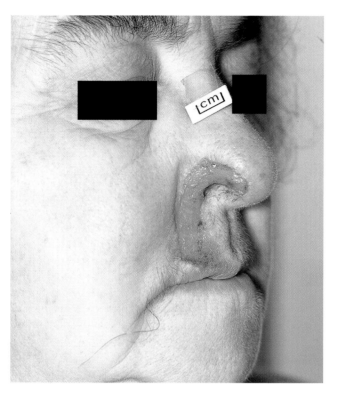

Fig. 70.29 Ulcerative lesion affecting upper lip and nose as a result of trigeminal neuropathy.

amyloidosis, sarcoidosis, sickle-cell disease, vasculitis, demyelinating disease, syringobulbia, or may be idiopathic [1,2].

REFERENCES

1 Burt RK, Sharfman WH, Karp BI, Wilson WH. Mental neuropathy (numb chin syndrome). *Cancer* 1992; **70**: 877–81.
2 Flint SF, Scully C. Isolated trigeminal sensory neuropathy; a heterogeneous group of disorders. *Oral Surg* 1990; **69**: 153–6.

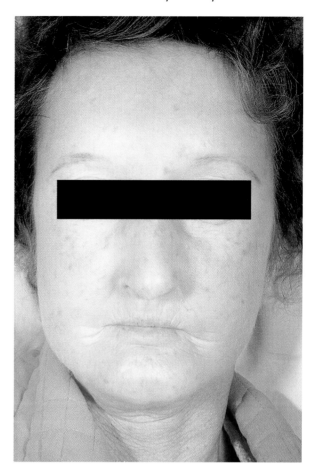

Fig. 70.30 Microstomia and radial lip furrows in systemic sclerosis.

Microstomia

This may occur in systemic sclerosis (Fig. 70.30), lichen myxoedematosus, after burns or after surgery.

For lip augmentation see Chapter 81.

Chapter 71
The Breast

J.L.BURTON

The terms breasts and mammary glands are often accepted as equivalent, but they are not strictly synonymous, because the breasts contain tissues (fat, vessels, nerves, etc.) other than the glandular elements.

In the evolutionary sense, the mammary glands are believed to be related to the apocrine sweat glands, but they show no histological or histochemical similarities [1–3]. In the human embryo, the *'milk lines'* appear at the 7-mm stage as narrow ridges of ectoderm on either side of the midline [4,5], although only two breasts ultimately develop (Fig 71.1).

The skin of the breast does not differ structurally from that of the neighbouring chest wall, but the skin of the nipple and areola is very highly specialized. There are individual and racial variations in the size, shape and colour of the nipple and areola. The periphery of the areola contains hair follicles, and the development of coarse terminal hairs in this site may be a cosmetic problem for some women. The undersurface of the epidermis covering the tip of the nipple resembles that found on tactile surfaces. The nipple is glabrous. Lactiferous ducts, sebaceous glands and apocrine glands open only at its tip. Sensory nerve end organs are also confined to the tip of the nipple. The areola is almost glabrous; there are a few vellus follicles, a few eccrine glands, clusters of large sebaceous glands and the so-called tubercles of Montgomery. These are the ducts of the glands of Montgomery, which are identical in structure with the glands opening at the nipple [3]. The glands of Montgomery are an integral part of the lactiferous apparatus, secreting milk during lactation.

The normal proliferation of the primitive mammary ducts in the girl at puberty is induced by oestrogen but is also dependent on corticosteroids and some somatotrophin [6,7]. These hormones, together with prolactin and progesterone, bring about further proliferation of the lobule–alveolar system during pregnancy. The breasts enlarge during pregnancy, and the veins become prominent. The areolae also enlarge and become darker. This pigmentation decreases after parturition but does not fade completely.

Although most of the more serious diseases of the breast come within the province of the surgeon, the gynaecologist or the endocrinologist, there are some diseases which affect only the breast skin and are wholly the concern of the dermatologist, and others which may involve the skin and present difficult problems in differential diagnosis [8,9].

REFERENCES

1 Giacometti G, Montagna W. The nipple and the areola of the human female breasts. *Anat Rec* 1962; **144**: 191–8.
2 Montagna W. Histology and cytochemistry of human skin: XXXV: The nipple and areola. *Br J Dermatol* 1970; **83**: 2–13.
3 Montagna W, Yun JS. The glands of Montgomery. *Br J Dermatol* 1972; **86**: 126–33.
4 Cowie AT, Tindal JS. *The Physiology of Lactation.* London: Edward Arnold, 1971.
5 Ebling FJG. Differentiation of cells of the skin. In: Goldspink G, ed. *Differentiation and Growth of Cells in Vertebrate Tissues.* London: Chapman and Hall, 1974.
6 Drife JO. Breast development in puberty. *Ann NY Acad Sci* 1986; **464**: 58–65.
7 Rohn RD. Nipple (papilla) development in puberty: longitudinal observations in girls. *Pediatrics* 1987; **79**: 745–7.
8 Haagensen CD. *Disease of the Breast*, 3rd edn. Philadelphia: WB Saunders, 1986.
9 Leis HP. *Diagnosis and Treatment of Breast Lesions.* London: Lewis, 1970.

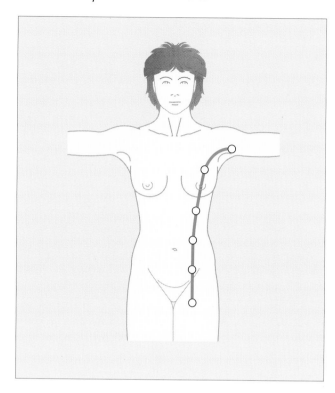

Fig. 71.1 Position of accessory breast tissue along the nipple line ('milk line').

Supernumerary breasts or nipples

Supernumerary (accessory) breasts (polymastia) and the far more common supernumerary nipples (polythelia) usually develop along the course of the embryological milk lines, which run from the anterior axillary folds to the inner thighs (Fig. 71.1). In 10% of cases they occur in other sites [1,2].

Accessory breast tissue may consist of nipple, areola or glandular tissue singly, or in any combination. The condition is very common in women, with an incidence of around 2–4%, although in the majority of cases the accessory nipple is insignificant, appearing as a small brown papule, usually on the chest wall, just below the breast. Much more rarely the condition occurs in men, and in one case a fully developed breast developed on the posterior aspect of the thigh of a male [3]. A familial incidence is sometimes noted [4].

Accessory breasts have been found in association with various rare genodermatoses [5–8], and with a wide variety of other anomalies including unilateral renal agenesis and carcinoma [9–11]. A study of 8000 children in Hungary showed that renal anomalies (mainly obstructive uropathy) were at least 300 times more common in the 1% with supernumerary nipples than in the remainder [12]. This does not seem to be the case, however, in black children [13], and the question of whether to investigate the renal tract in a child with supernumerary nipples and no other obvious anomaly remains contentious [11,14,15].

The Simpson–Golabi–Behmel syndrome is an X-linked condition in which increased pre- and postnatal growth is associated with accessory nipples, coarse facies, polydactyly, midline defects and mild mental retardation [16].

The accessory nipple is usually recognized if the diagnosis is considered, but is often otherwise confused with a pigmented naevus. If functional breast tissue is present, enlargement at puberty or in pregnancy may be embarrassing or painful. Simple excision is advisable, as carcinoma may occur.

REFERENCES

1 Tow SH, Shanmugaratnam K. Supernumerary mammary gland in the vulva. *Br Med J* 1962; **ii**: 1234–6.
2 Shewmake SW, Izumo GT. Supernumerary areolae. *Arch Dermatol* 1977; **113**: 823–5.
3 Camisa C. Accessory breast on the posterior thigh of a man. *J Am Acad Dermatol* 1980; **3**: 467–9.
4 Cellini A, Offidani A. Familial supernumerary nipples and breasts. *Dermatology* 1992; **185**: 56–8.
5 Hay RJ, Wells RS. The syndrome of ankyloblepharon, ectodermal defects and cleft lip and palate. *Br J Dermatol* 1976; **94**: 277–89.
6 Wittebol-Post D, Hennekam RC. Blepharophimosis, ptosis, polythelia and brachydactyly. A new autosomal dominant syndrome? *Clin Dysmorph* 1993; **2**: 346–50.
7 Halper S, Rubenstein D. Aplasia cutis congenita associated with syndactyly and supernumerary nipples; report of a second family. *Pediatr Dermatol* 1991; **8**: 32–4.
8 Bonnekoh B, Wevers A, Spangenberger H *et al*. Keratin pattern of acanthosis nigricans in syndrome-like association with polythelia, polycystic kidneys and syndactyly. *Arch Dermatol* 1993; **129**: 117–82.
9 Varsano IB, Jaber L, Garty B *et al*. Urinary tract abnormalities in children with supernumerary nipples. *Pediatrics* 1984; **73**: 103–5.
10 Mehes K, Pinter A. Minor morphological aberrations in children with isolated urinary tract malformations. *Eur J Pediatr* 1990; **149**: 339–402.
11 Armori M, Filk D, Schlesinger M *et al*. Accessory nipples, any relationship to urinary tract malformation? *Pediatr Dermatol* 1992; **9**: 239–40.
12 Meggyessy V, Mehes K. Association of supernumerary nipples with renal anomalies. *J Pediatr* 1987; **111**: 412–13.
13 Robertson A, Sale P, Sathanarayan MD. Lack of association of supernumerary nipples with renal anomalies in black infants. *J Pediatr* 1986; **109**: 502–3.
14 Hersh J. Association of supernumerary nipples and renal anomalies. *Am J Dis Child* 1988; **142**: 591–2.
15 Mimouni F. Association of supernumerary nipples and renal anomalies. *Am J Dis Child* 1988; **142**: 591–2.
16 Gurrieri F, Cappa M, Neri G. Further delineation of the Simpson–Golabi–Behmel syndrome. *Am J Med Genet* 1993; **46**: 606–7.

Mammary hyperplasia

Excessively large breasts are usually a problem for the plastic surgeon rather than the dermatologist, but there may be a deep groove in the skin of each shoulder, caused by the prolonged pressure from the supportive 'bra strap'. The incidence of submammary intertrigo is increased (Fig. 71.2) and other physical symptoms are common. Women with large breasts may present with aching pain in the neck, back or shoulders, and may develop severe postural abnormalities. Large breasts are less sensitive than small breasts, possibly due to their weight causing chronic traction on the fourth and sixth intercostal nerves [1]. Mammary hyperplasia can also cause psychological disturbances.

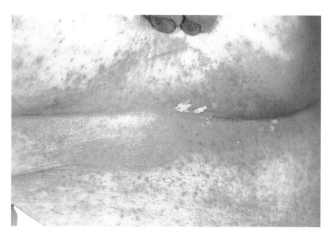

Fig. 71.2 Intertrigo with candidiasis of the submammary skin fold in a woman with large breasts.

Gigantomastia

Gigantomastia is a condition in which the female breasts enlarge progressively until they reach a tremendous size [2,3]. The overlying skin may become inflamed, oedematous and tender, and there may be striae or even severe ulceration [4]. The condition may, or may not, start during pregnancy but the hormone levels are usually normal, and galactorrhoea is not a feature. A suggested cause is increased sensitivity of the breast tissue to normal levels of circulating hormones, but this would not explain why the condition can start for the first time in a second or third pregnancy. Perhaps a more likely possibility is the sudden development of an immune stimulatory globulin, as occurs in Graves' disease.

The condition is occasionally familial [5].

In some cases of Cowden's syndrome, characterized by multiple hamartomas (Chapter 12), fibrocystic disease may lead to massive bilateral hyperplasia of the breasts.

Penicillamine therapy can also cause gigantomastia [6].

Hormone therapy is usually ineffective, but bromocriptine helps some cases [7]. Reduction mammoplasty is usually required, although this decreases breast sensitivity [1].

REFERENCES

1 Slezak S, Dellon A L. Quantitation of sensibility of gynecomastia and alteration following reduction mammoplasty. *Plast Reconstr Surg* 1993; **91**: 1265–7.
2 Gargan TG. Gigantomastia complicating pregnancy. *Plast Reconstr Surg* 1987; **80**: 121–4.
3 Hollingsworth DR, Archer R. Massive virginal breast hypertrophy at puberty. *Am J Dis Child* 1973; **125**: 293.
4 Stavrides S, Hacking A, Tittman A *et al.* Gigantomastia in pregnancy. *Br J Surg* 1987; **74**: 585–6.
5 Kupper D, Dingman D, Broadbent R. Juvenile breast hypertrophy: report of a familial pattern. *Plast Reconstr Surg* 1992; **90**: 303–9.
6 Passas C, Weinstein A. Breast gigantism with penicillamine therapy. *Arthitis Rheum* 1978; **21**: 167–8.
7 Kullander S. Effect of 2 br-alpha-ergocryptin on serum prolactin and clinical

picture in progressive gigantomastia of pregnancy. *Ann Chir Gynecol* 1976; **65**: 227.

Gynaecomastia [1,2]

Gynaecomastia, a benign enlargement of the male breast, may occur as an isolated defect or as a manifestation of a wide range of different pathological states in which it may be a valuable diagnostic sign. The multiplicity of syndromes associated with gynaecomastia reflects the complexity of the hormonal mechanisms concerned in breast enlargement.

Gynaecomastia can be distinguished from fatty enlargement of the breast in obesity (pseudogynaecomastia) by grasping the breast between thumb and forefinger and moving the digits up towards the nipple with the patient supine. In gynaecomastia a rubbery, mobile, disc-like mound will be felt beneath the areola.

The histopathological changes [3] are related to the duration of gynaecomastia and not to its cause. At early stages, there are active proliferating ducts in a vascular fibroblastic stroma. Later, there is progressive fibrosis and hyalinization, and the number of ducts is reduced.

Incidence and aetiology (Table 71.1). Palpable asymptomatic gynaecomastia is common, and can be found in 30–40% of normal men. The incidence of gynaecomastia in boys, and premature thelarche in girls (prepubertal breast development) has increased in recent years in several countries [5–7]. An environmental factor such as the use of hormones in cattle feeds has been postulated as the cause.

Gynaecomastia may result from an imbalance between the stimulatory effect of oestrogens on mammary tissue and the inhibitory effect of androgens. Defective androgen receptors, as found in testicular feminization and related syndromes, may also contribute. The role of prolactin is

Table 71.1 Causes of gynaecomastia [4].

Physiological
  Neonatal
  Adolescent
  Old age
Endocrine disorders
  Hypogonadism, e.g. Klinefelter's
  Excess oestrogen or chorionic gonadotrophin, e.g. from testicular tumour
  Hyperthyroidism
Other diseases
  Starvation, cachexia or refeeding
  Renal haemodialysis
  Liver disease
  Paraplegia
  Erythroderma
Idiopathic (about 25% of cases)
Drugs (see Table 71.2)

less clear, although it may play a part by its indirect effect on gonadal, and possibly adrenal, function. Increased aromatase activity, which increases oestrogen formation in target cells, may also have a role [8].

Physiological gynaecomastia

Gynaecomastia occurs in about 75% of neonates due to circulating oestrogen from the mother. Some enlargement of the breast occurs at puberty in about 60% of normal boys [9]. Serum oestradiol is increased in relation to testosterone in boys with gynaecomastia, and the gynaecomastia regresses as the ratio reverts to normal adult values [10]. The peak incidence is around the age of 14 years, but the onset may be at any age between 10 and 20 years. The degree of enlargement is usually slight, but may be sufficient to cause embarrassment and anxiety. Spontaneous regression usually takes place within a few months, but the enlargement persists for over 2 years in 5% of boys.

Gynaecomastia also occurs in some elderly men as a result of testicular failure [1], and obesity can also produce gynaecomastia by increasing the peripheral aromatization of androgens to oestrogens [8].

Gynaecomastia in endocrine disorders

Gynaecomastia occurs in a very wide range of endocrine disorders. Primary or secondary reduction of testicular androgen production is of special importance. Leprous orchitis may be associated with marked gynaecomastia. Some tumours of the testis are associated with gynaecomastia, notably seminoma, interstitial cell tumour, Sertoli-cell tumour and certain teratomas. The possibility of germ-cell malignancy should be considered even if the testes are normal on palpation [11]. These tumours often produce human chorionic gonadotrophin, which stimulates the normal Leydig cells to secrete excessive amounts of oestradiol [12]. Alpha-fetoprotein and lactic dehydrogenase levels may also be increased. Scrotal ultrasonography may be helpful [11].

Gynaecomastia occurs in most men with Klinefelter's syndrome, and there is an increased risk of breast cancer in this syndrome [13], although other causes of gynaecomastia are not associated with an increased risk of cancer [4].

It has been suggested that partial deficiency of steroid dehydrogenase may be a frequently unrecognized cause of gynaecomastia in otherwise normal males [14].

In other endocrine disorders, gynaecomastia is less common, but may occur in tumours or hyperplasia of the adrenal gland, in pituitary tumours and in hyperthyroidism. It has been reported in association with isolated adrenocorticotrophic hormone (ACTH) deficiency [15]. It is a rare manifestation of bronchial carcinoma.

Gynaecomastia in nutritional, metabolic, renal and hepatic disease

Gynaecomastia may occur during starvation or on resumption of a more adequate diet after prolonged starvation [16]. The endocrine basis of the breast enlargement is inconstant, depending in varying degree on impaired liver function, testicular atrophy and disturbed pituitary function. Gynaecomastia due to human immunodeficiency virus (HIV) infection has been reported [16–18].

In 40–50% of patients receiving maintenance haemodialysis for renal failure, gynaecomastia develops after 2–9 months [19]. It resembles the so-called refeeding gynaecomastia mentioned above.

Impaired liver function in cirrhosis, carcinoma of the liver or haemochromatosis may also be associated with gynaecomastia (Fig. 71.3). Several mechanisms are involved, including decreased testosterone production, excessive oestrogen production from circulating precursors, changes in sex-hormone-binding globulin levels and increased progesterone [20].

The gynaecomastia occasionally observed in patients with mycosis fungoides, extensive erythroderma and other severe widespread and persistent diseases of the skin is presumed to be of nutritional or hepatic origin.

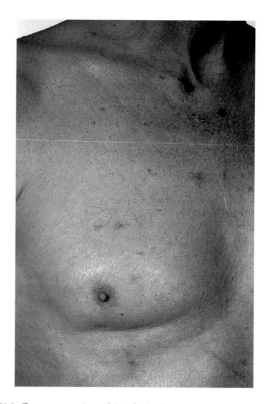

Fig. 71.3 Gynaecomastia and 'spider' telangiectasia in a man with cirrhosis.

Gynaecomastia in diseases of the nervous system

Gynaecomastia may occur in paraplegia as a result of unexplained testicular changes, and is also present in some cases of dystrophia myotonica.

Drug-induced gynaecomastia [17,21–24]

Drugs which can produce gynaecomastia are shown in Table 71.2.

Some of these drugs, such as spironolactone and cimetidine, are antiandrogens, and others, such as isoniazid, may act by the 'refeeding' mechanism. Cytotoxic drugs may damage the testes, but gonadotrophins and oestradiol were also increased in five out of six cases due to cytotoxic drugs [25,26]. Some drugs which act on the central nervous system increase prolactin and thus induce a secondary hypogonadal state. Testosterone might act through its conversion to oestrogens.

Gynaecomastia has been reported in heart failure, but the possible role of drugs as a causative agent was uncertain in some of these cases [27].

Gynaecomastia can also be due to the topical application of oestrogen-containing creams [28].

Table 71.2 Drugs which produce gynaecomastia.

Amiloride
Anabolic steroids
Antiandrogens, e.g. cyproterone acetate
Amiodarone
Amphetamines
Androgens
Busulphan
Captopril
Chorionic gonadotrophin
Cimetidine
Cytotoxic agents
Diazepam
Diethylpropion
Digitalis
Domperidone
Isoniazid
Ketoconazole
Marijuana
Methyldopa
Metoclopramide
Nifedipine
Nitrosoureas
Oestrogens
Penicillamine
Phenothiazines
Phenytoin
Reserpine
Spironolactone
Tricyclic antidepressants
Vincristine

Management of gynaecomastia

Clinical examination may rarely reveal areas of local firmness or irregularity which may suggest the possibility of breast cancer, and this should lead to biopsy or mammography. It should be noted though that gynaecomastia is often asymmetrical, and biopsy is rarely required. Careful examination for other underlying disease and a full drug history are required, particularly if the gynaecomastia is symptomatic, progressive or of recent onset in an adult, but it should be remembered that a large proportion of otherwise normal men have some slight gynaecomastia.

In suitable cases, screening tests may include measurements of serum human chorionic gonadotrophin, plasma testosterone, oestrogen, prolactin and urinary steroid excretion.

For cases with considerable breast discomfort, or if the condition is severe enough to cause embarrassment, treatment with tamoxifen, clomiphene or danazol may be considered [29,30]. Testolactone, an inhibitor of steroid aromatization is safe and effective, but takes 6 months to produce improvement [31].

In extreme cases, reduction mammoplasty or suction lipectomy may be performed by a plastic surgeon [32–34].

REFERENCES

1 Niewohner CB, Nuttal FQ. Gynaecomastia in a hospitalized male population. *Am J Med* 1984; **77**: 633–5.
2 Wheeler CE, Cawley EP, Gray HT *et al.* Occurrence of gynecomastia in conjunction with dermatologic disorders. *Arch Dermatol Syphilol* 1953; **68**: 685–92.
3 Nicolis GL, Modlinger RS, Gabrilove JL. A study of the histopathology of human gynecomastia. *J Clin Endocrinol Metab* 1971; **32**: 173–8.
4 Baunstein GD. Gynecomastia. *N Engl J Med* 1993; **328**: 490–5.
5 Bongiovanni AM. An epidemic of premature thelarche in Puerto Rico. *J Pediatr* 1983; **103**: 245–6.
6 Harlam W, Grillo G. Secondary sex characteristics of boys 12–17 years of age: the US health examination survey. *J Pediatr* 1978; **95**: 293–7.
7 Nizzoli G, Del Corno G, Fara GM *et al.* Gynecomastia and premature thelarche in a schoolchildren population of northern Italy. *Acta Endocrinol* 1986; **279** (Suppl.): 227–31.
8 Bulard J, Mowszowicz I, Schaison G. Increased aromatase activity in pubic skin fibroblasts from patients with isolated gynecomastia. *J Clin Endocrinol Metab* 1987; **64**: 618–23.
9 Nydick M, Bustos J, Dale JH, Jr *et al.* Gynecomastia in adolescent boys. *JAMA* 1961; **178**: 449–54.
10 Mahoney CP. Adolescent gynecomastia. Differential diagnosis and management; a review. *Pediatr Clin North Am* 1990; **37**: 1389–404.
11 Cantwell BM, Richardson PG, Campbell SJ. Gynaecomastia and extragonadal symptoms leading to diagnostic delay in germ-cell tumours in young men. *Postgrad Med J* 1991; **67**: 675–7.
12 Stepanas AV, Samaan NA, Schultz PN *et al.* Endocrine studies in testicular tumour patients with and without gynaecomastia. A report of 45 cases. *Cancer* 1978; **41**: 369–76.
13 Scheike O, Visfeldt J, Petersen B. Male breast cancer. 3: Breast carcinoma in association with Klinefelter syndrome. *Acta Pathol Microbiol Scand* 1973; **81**: 352–8.
14 Cavanah SF, Dons RF. Partial 3 beta hydroxysteroid dehydrogenase deficiency presenting as new-onset gynaecomastia in a eugonadal male. *Metab Clin Exp Med* 1993; **42**: 65–8.
15 Shimatsu A, Suzuki Y, Tanaka S. Gynaecomastia associated with isolated ACTH deficiency. *J Endocrinol Invest* 1987; **10**: 127–9.
16 Smith SR, Chhetri MK, Johanson J. The pituitary–gonadal axis in men with protein-calorie malnutrition. *J Clin Endocrinol Metab* 1975; **41**: 60–9.

17 Antonelli D, Luboshitsky R, Gelbendorf A. Amiodarone-induced gynecomastia. *N Engl J Med* 1986; **315**: 1553.
18 Couderc LJ, Clauvel JP. HIV infection-induced gynecomastia. *Ann Intern Med* 1987; **107**: 257.
19 Freeman RM, Lawton RL, Fearing MO. Gynecomastia; an endocrinologic complication of haemodialysis. *Ann Intern Med* 1968; **69**: 67–72.
20 Farthing MJG, Green JRB, Edwards CRW *et al.* Progesterone, prolactin and gynaecomastia in men with liver disease. *Gut* 1982; **23**: 276–9.
21 Clyne CAC. Unilateral gynaecomastia and nifedipine. *Br Med J* 1986; **292**: 380.
22 Markusse HM, Meyboom RHB. Gynaecomastia associated with captopril. *Br Med J* 1988; **296**: 1262–3.
23 Monson JP, Scott DF. Gynaecomastia induced by phenytoin in men with epilepsy. *Br Med J* 1987; **294**: 612.
24 Tanner LA, Bosco LA. Gynaecomastia association with calcium-channel blocker therapy. *Arch Intern Med* 1988; **148**: 379–80.
25 Trump DL, Pavy MD, Staal S. Gynecomastia in men following antineoplastic therapy. *Arch Intern Med* 1982; **142**: 511–13.
26 Turner AR, Morrish DW, Berry J *et al.* Gynecomastia after cytotoxic therapy for metastatic testicular cancer. *Arch Intern Med* 1982; **142**: 896–7.
27 Murray NP, Daly MJ. Gynecomastia and heart failure—adverse drug reaction or disease process? *J Clin Pharm Ther* 1991; **16**: 275–9.
28 Cimmorra GA. Percutaneous oestrogen induced gynaecomastia. *Br J Plast Surg* 1982; **35**: 209–10.
29 McDermott NT, Hofeldt FD, Kidd GS. Tamoxifen therapy for painful idiopathic gynecomastia. *South Med J* 1990; **83**: 1283–5.
30 Jeffreys DB. Painful gynaecomastia treated with tamoxifen. *Br Med J* 1979; **i**: 111–19.
31 Zachman M, Ejholzer U, Moritano M *et al.* Treatment of pubertal gynaecomastia with testolactone. *Acta Endocrinol* 1986; **279** (Suppl.): 218–26.
32 Courtiss EH. Gynaecomastia: analysis of 159 patients and current recommendations for treatment. *Plast Reconstr Surg* 1987; **79**: 740–53.
33 Rosenberg GJ. Gynaecomastia: suction lipectomy as a contemporary solution. *Plast Reconstr Surg* 1987; **80**: 379–86.
34 Hands LJ, Greenall MJ. Gynaecomastia. *Br J Surg* 1991; **78**: 907–11.

Black galactorrhoea

Galactorrhoea is sometimes caused by drugs such as phenothiazines. In one patient taking perphenazine, the droplets of milk were stained black, due to the concomitant administration of minocycline for acne [1]. The pigment which produces the black discoloration of breast milk in women taking minocycline is thought to be due to an iron chelate of minocycline within macrophages [2].

REFERENCES

1 Basler RSW, Lynch PJ. Black galactorrhea as a consequence of minocycline and phenothiazine therapy. *Arch Dermatol* 1985; **121**: 417–18.
2 Hunt MJ, Salisbury ELC, Grace J, Armati R. Black breast milk due to minocycline therapy. *Br J Dermatol* 1996; **134**: 943–4.

Hypomastia or amastia [1]

Hypomastia is defined as a breast size of 200 ml or less in the adult female. The assessment is made by an instrument such as the volumetric Grossman–Roudner breast-measuring device, which measures the entire breast, including skin, subcutaneous tissue, stroma, parenchyma and areola (available from Cox Uphoff, Santa Barbara, California) [2].

Hypomastia is fairly common in otherwise normal women, in whom it may cause considerable psychological distress. Numerous devices and exercises to enlarge the breasts have been advocated but they act mainly by enlarging the pectoralis major muscle. The breasts usually enlarge during pregnancy, and oral oestrogens, including oral contraceptives, can sometimes be useful. Several augmentation and implantation procedures have been developed over the years, but many of these operations have produced considerable morbidity, ranging from keloids and abscesses to granulomatous induration. The possibility of a unique rheumatological syndrome due to silicone breast implants is discussed below.

In addition to these psychological and surgical problems, small breasts can be associated with *mitral valve prolapse*. In one study approximately 50% of young women with hypomastia had mitral valve prolapse on echocardiography compared with only 6% of control subjects [3]. Identification of these patients is important, because mitral valve prolapse may predispose to bacterial endocarditis, and it can also cause symptomatic arrhythmias [4,5].

Hypomastia is of course a common feature of wasting disease such as tuberculosis and anorexia nervosa, due to loss of fat. It is also a feature of sexual infantilism, particularly the Ullrich–Turner syndrome (Chapter 12) in which amastia may rarely be unilateral [6].

Becker's naevus is occasionally associated with unilateral breast hypoplasia, possibly as a result of enhanced androgen sensitivity [7,8].

Absence or hypoplasia of the breast and nipple may also occur in the *Poland anomaly*, with unilateral absence of the sternocostal part of the pectoralis major muscle, axillary hair loss, ipsilateral syndactyly and dermatoglyphic abnormalities [9].

The AREDYLD syndrome is a form of ectodermal dysplasia, associated with lipoatrophy, diabetes mellitus and amastia [10].

REFERENCES

1 Halkar RK, Abdel-Dayem H, Jahan S. Congenital absence of mammary glands. *Clin Nucl Med* 1985; **10**: 826.
2 Palin WE. Measurement of breast volume. Comparison of techniques. *Plast Reconstr Surg* 1986; **77**: 253–5.
3 Rosenberg CA, Derman G, Grabb WC *et al.* Hypomastia and mitral valve prolapse. Evidence of a linked embryologic and mesenchymal dysplasia. *N Engl J Med* 1983; **309**: 1230–2.
4 Barnet HJM, Boughner DR, Cooper PE. Further evidence relating mitral valve prolapse to cerebral ischaemic events. *N Engl J Med* 1980; **302**: 139–44.
5 Devereux RB. Mitral valve prolapse. *Circulation* 1976; **54**: 3–14.
6 Cohen A, Lavagetto A, Romano C. Ullrich–Turner syndrome with unilateral agenesis of breast, nipple and pectoralis major. *Am J Med Genet* 1992; **44**: 11–12.
7 Formigon M, Alsina MM, Mascaro JM, Rivera F. Becker's naevus and ipsilateral breast hypoplasia. Androgen-receptor study in two patients. *Arch Dermatol* 1992; **128**: 992–3.
8 Moore JA, Schosser RH. Becker's naevus and hypoplasia of the breast and pectoralis major muscles. *Pediatr Dermatol* 1985; **3**: 34–7.
9 David TJ. Nature and etiology of the Poland anomaly. *New Engl J Med* 1972; **287**: 487–9.
10 Breslau-Siderius EJ, Toonstra J, Baart JA *et al.* Ectodermal dysplasia, lipoatrophy, diabetes mellitus and amastia—a second case of the AREDYLD syndrome. *Am J Med Genet* 1992; **44**: 374–7.

Silicone breast implants and autoimmune disease

Silicone gel breast implants, which are supposedly inert, have been widely used to treat hypomastia and amastia (including mastectomy), and approximately 5000 women in the UK receive such implants every year. The short-term side-effects (discomfort, tissue hardening, implant rupture or migration, calcification, abscess and keloid) are well known [1,2]. The most frequent complication is capsular contraction, which becomes more common with increasing duration after the implant. The rate approaches 70% by 4 years after the implantation [3,4]. Affected patients may develop erythema of the chest wall, petechiae and telangiectasia [4].

The possibility has been raised that malignancy or autoimmune connective tissue disease might arise as late sequelae of migration of silicone into the tissues. Silicone has been detected in the surrounding fibrous capsule, with granulomatous reactions [5], and it has also been demonstrated in the liver of women with silicone implants [6].

The safety of silicone implants was initially questioned because of scattered reports of scleroderma and other rheumatological disorders in patients who had received such implants [7]. Antibodies to silicone [8] and antinuclear antibodies [7] were identified in some patients, but their relevance is uncertain.

Because of this concern, the US Food and Drug Administration imposed a moratorium on the use of such implants in January 1992. A legal action against the manufacturers was settled for over four billion US dollars, but the decision to agree to this 'no liability settlement' was apparently taken for financial rather than scientific reasons, because of the escalating costs of potential litigation [9]. The UK Chief Medical Officer concluded in January 1992 that there was no clear evidence to link silicone implants with either cancer or autoimmune disease, and a similar conclusion was reached by an independent advisory committee in Canada [10]. This view was confirmed by an expert advisory group of the UK Department of Health, who reviewed all the available data [9].

The claim [11] that there is an increase in abnormal oesophageal motility among children breastfed by mothers with breast implants, this has been discounted by some experts because of the small numbers of subjects, the lack of adequate controls, and a possible self-selection bias.

However, the controversy continues and it has been argued that the 'silicone implant-associated syndrome', which apparently includes arthralgia, myalgia, sicca complex, paraesthesiae, balance disturbance, night sweats, rashes, and memory loss and fatigue, may represent a disease which is distinct from previously recognized autoimmune connective tissue disorders [3,4,12–16]. It seems clear that further long-term epidemiological studies will be required to resolve this dispute [17].

Many women who have received silicone breast implants produce serum antibodies to a high-molecular-weight antigen which is not a protein but is a complex of synthetic polymers. In a blinded study, women with moderate or severe symptoms of 'rheumatological' disease (fatigue, arthralgia, rash, etc.) were significantly more likely to have these antibodies than asymptomatic women or control women who had not received a breast implant [18].

REFERENCES

1 Ahn CY, Shaw WW. Regional silicone-gel migration in patients with ruptured implants. *Ann Plast Surg* 1994; **33**: 201–8.
2 Holten IW, Barnett RA. Intraductal migration of silicone from intact gel breast prostheses. *Plast Reconstr Surg* 1995; **95**: 563–6.
3 Bridges AJ. Silicone implant controversy continues. *Lancet* 1994; **344**: 1451–2.
4 Solomon G. A clinical and laboratory profile of symptomatic women with silicone breast implants. *Semin Arthritis Rheum* 1994; **24** (Suppl. 1): 29–37.
5 Busch H. Silicone toxicology. *Semin Arthritis Rheum* 1994; **24** (Suppl. 1): 11–17.
6 Pfleiderer B, Garrido L. Migration and accumulation of silicone in the liver of women with silicone gel-filled breast implants. *Magn Reson Med* 1995; **33**: 8–17.
7 Press RI, Peebles CL, Kumagia Y *et al.* Antinuclear autoantibodies in women with silicone breast implants. *Lancet* 1992; **340**: 1304–7.
8 Goldblum RM, Pelley RP, O'Donnell AA *et al.* Antibodies to silicone elastomers and reactions to ventriculo-peritoneal shunts. *Lancet* 1992; **340**: 510–13.
9 Tinkler J, Gott D, Ludgate S. Breast implants; is there an association with connective tissue disease? *Health Trends* 1994; **26**: 25–6.
10 Independent Advisory Committee on Silicone-gel-filled Breast Implants. Summary of the report on silicone-gel-filled breast implants. *Can Med Assoc J* 1992; **147**: 141–6.
11 Levine JJ, Ilowite T. Scleroderma-like oesophageal disease in children breast-fed by mothers with silicone breast implants. *JAMA* 1994; **271**: 213–16.
12 Bridges AJ, Conley C, Wang G *et al.* A clinical and immunologic evaluation of women with silicone breast implants and symptoms of rheumatic disease. *Ann Intern Med* 1993; **118**: 929–36.
13 Vasey FB, Havice DL, Bocanegra TS *et al.* Clinical findings in symptomatic women with silicone breast implants. *Semin Arthritis Rheum* 1994; **24** (Suppl. 1): 22–8.
14 Freundlich B, Altman C, Snadorfi N *et al.* A profile of symptomatic patients with silicone breast implants: a Sjögren's-like syndrome. *Semin Arthritis Rheum* 1994; **24** (Suppl. 1): 44–53.
15 Peters W. Silicone breast implants and autoimmune connective tissue disease. *Ann Plast Surg* 1995; **34**: 103–9.
16 Sanchez-Guerrero J, Schur PH, Sergent JS *et al.* Silicone breast implants and rheumatic disease: clinical, immunologic and epidemiologic studies. *Arthritis Rheum* 1994; **37**: 158–68.
17 Lamm SH. Silicone breast implants and long-term health effects. *J Clin Epidemiol* 1995; **48**: 507–11.
18 Tenenbaum SA, Rice JC, Espinoza LR *et al.* Use of antipolymer antibody assay in recipients of silicone breast implants. *Lancet* 1997; **349**: 449–54.

Rudimentary nipples

Absence or maldevelopment of the nipples may be present as an isolated congenital defect [1], and the association of absent or rudimentary nipples with abnormality of the scalp and pinnae has been reported as an autosomal dominant trait [2,3].

REFERENCES

1 Wilson MG. Absent nipples. *Humangenetik* 1972; **15**: 268–9.

2 Finlay AY, Marks R. An hereditary syndrome of lumpy scalp, odd ears and rudimentary nipples. *Br J Dermatol* 1978; **99**: 423–30.
3 Le Merrer M, Renier D, Briard ML. Scalp defect, nipple absence and ear abnormalities; another case of Finlay syndrome. *Genet Couns* 1991; **2**: 233–6.

Adnexal polyp of neonatal skin

This is a small, usually solitary, tumour which occurs mainly on the areola of the neonate. It is firm and pink but becomes dry and brown and falls off within a few days of birth. Histologically it contains hair follicles, eccrine glands and vestigial sebaceous glands. A survey in Tokyo showed that the condition occurred in 4% of 3257 newborn infants [1].

REFERENCE

1 Hidano A, Kobayishi T. Adnexal polyp of neonatal skin. *Br J Dermatol* 1975; **92**: 659–62.

Inverted nipple

Inverted nipple is common, affecting up to 10% of adult females. The inversion of the nipple may cause psychological distress and an inability to breastfeed. The fault generally lies with short lactiferous ducts, which tether the nipple and prevent it projecting.

Surgical correction is generally unsatisfactory, because although it may provide cosmetic correction, it destroys the breast function [1]. Non-surgical measures include Hoffman's exercises and the use of breast shells, but a controlled trial has cast doubt on their value [2].

Good results have recently been reported with a simple device called the Niplette which exerts chronic negative pressure to suck out the nipple and stretch the subareolar fibres [3]. It consists of a transparent plastic nipple mould with a sealing flange attached to a valve and a syringe port.

REFERENCES

1 Aaiche A. Surgical repair of the inverted nipple. *Ann Plast Surg* 1990; **25**: 457–60.
2 Alexander JM, Grant AM, Campbell MJ. Randomised controlled trials of breast shells and Hoffman's exercises for inverted and non-protractile nipples. *Br Med J* 1992; **304**: 1030–2.
3 McGeorge DD. The Niplette. An instrument for non-surgical correction of inverted nipples. *Br J Plast Surg* 1994; **47**: 46–9.

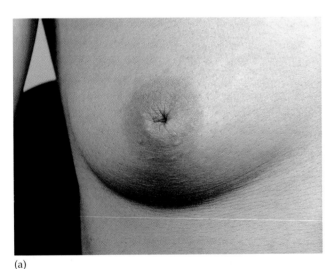

(a)

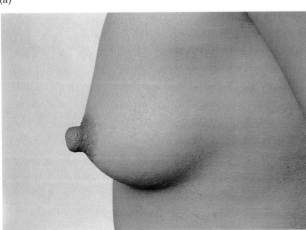

(c)

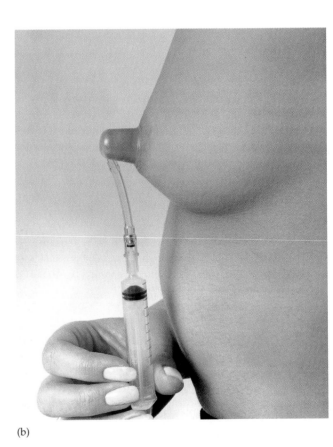

(b)

Fig. 71.4 Inverted nipple (a) before treatment; (b) during application of the Niplette suction device; (c) the nipple after treatment. (Courtesy of the Cannon Rubber Co. Ltd, Lower Road, Glemsford, Suffolk, UK.)

Duct ectasia

The secreting lobules of the breast drain via a branching duct system to the nipple. After the menopause there is a tendency for the major subareolar ducts to dilate and shorten. This may be associated with nipple discharge, nipple retraction or a palpable mass that may be either hard or doughy [1]. The discharge is often 'cheesy', and the nipple retraction is classically slit-like. Surgery may be required in severe cases.

REFERENCE

1 Dixon JM, Mansel RE. Congenital problems and aberrations of normal breast development and involution. *Br Med J* 1994; **309**: 797–800.

Hyperkeratosis of the nipple

This is a rare condition in which the skin of the nipple becomes diffusely thickened and hyperpigmented and covered with filiform or papular warty excrescences. In some cases only the nipple or only the areola is affected. The histology shows acanthosis, hyperkeratosis and papillomatosis [1,2].

Several diseases have been reported to be associated with this condition, although it most frequently develops in women in the second or third decade as an isolated naevoid defect [3,4]. There seems to be a definite association with cutaneous T-cell lymphoma [5,6] (Fig. 71.5), and it has also been seen in some cases of ichthyosis, ichthyosiform erythroderma, acanthosis nigricans, Darier's disease and in men with carcinoma of the prostate treated with oestrogens.

Some cases respond to a keratolytic or to cryotherapy [7], but etretinate is ineffective [8,9].

REFERENCES

1 Schwartz RA. Hyperkeratosis of the nipple and areola. *Arch Dermatol* 1978; **114**: 1844–5.
2 Mehregan AH, Rahbari H. Hyperkeratosis of nipple and areola. *Arch Dermatol* 1977; **113**: 1691–2.
3 Dupré A, Catala D, Christol D. Hyperkératose naevoide des aréoles. Hamartome des aréoles. *Ann Dermatol Vénéréol* 1980; **107**: 305–9.
4 Maycock PM. Hyperkeratosis of the nipples. *Arch Dermatol* 1978; **114**: 1245.
5 Ahn SK, Chung J, Lee WS *et al.* Hyperkeratosis of the nipple and areola simultaneously developing with cutaneous T cell lymphoma. *J Am Acad Dermatol* 1995; **32**: 124–5.
6 Allegue F, Soria AC, Rocamora A *et al.* Hyperkeratosis of the nipple and areola in a patient with cutaneous T cell lymphoma. *Int J Dermatol* 1990; **29**: 519–20.
7 Vestey JP, Bunney MH. Unilateral hyperkeratosis of the nipple: the response to cryotherapy. *Arch Dermatol* 1986; **122**: 1360.
8 Ortonne JP. Naevoid hyperkeratosis of the nipple and areolae mammae. Ineffectiveness of etretinate therapy. *Acta Derm Venereol (Stockh)* 1986; **66**: 175–7.
9 Kuhlman DS, Hodge SJ, Owen LG. Hyperkeratosis of the nipple and areola. *J Am Acad Dermatol* 1985; **13**: 596–8.

Eczema of the nipple

Eczema of the nipple occurs mainly in young women between the ages of 15 and 30 years, and is usually bilateral [1]. It was formerly most common during lactation and was induced by infection and the medicaments applied to combat it, but in the UK it is now seen more often in non-pregnant girls (Fig. 71.6).

Often no cause can be established, particularly in atopic subjects in whom the condition is more frequently found than in non-atopic controls [2]. Contact dermatitis is a possibility, and irregular patches of eczema on the breasts can be due to allergy to nail varnish. Allergy to foam rubber inserts in bra cups can also cause localized eczema. Irritation from friction must also be considered.

Treatment of nipple eczema is with mild topical steroids, but in cases which are resistant to topical steroids, crude coal tar is sometimes helpful.

In every case, the presence of scabies must be carefully excluded. Infection of the nipple and breast ducts with *Candida albicans* can also mimic eczema [3].

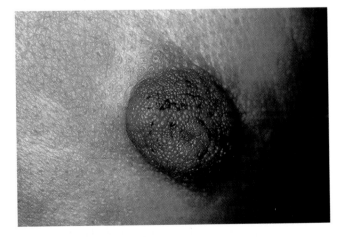

Fig. 71.5 Hyperkeratosis of the nipple in a patient with cutaneous T-cell lymphoma. (Courtesy of Dr S.K. Ahn, Yonsei University, Wonju, Korea.)

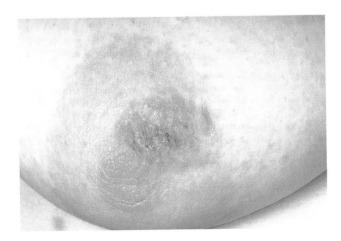

Fig. 71.6 Eczema of the nipple in a young woman.

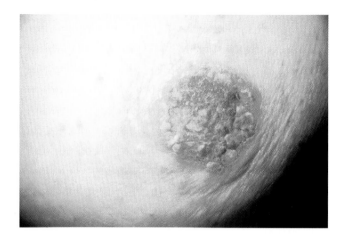

Fig. 71.7 Paget's disease, showing the more clearly defined edge.

The intermittent course, more severe itching, indefinite margin and lack of distortion of the nipple help to distinguish eczema from Paget's disease (Chapter 36, Fig. 71.7). If the diagnosis is at all doubtful, biopsy should be performed, particularly if there has been no response to topical steroids.

REFERENCES

1 Graham DF. Eczema of the nipple. *Trans St John's Hosp Dermatol Soc* 1972; **58**: 98–9.
2 Mevorah B, Frenk E, Wietlisbach V. Minor clinical features of atopic dermatitis. Evaluation of their diagnostic significance. *Dermatologica* 1988; **177**: 360–4.
3 Amir LH. Eczema of the nipple and breast—a case report. *J Hum Lact* 1993; **9**: 173–9.

'Cracked' nipples in lactation

Many women experience discomfort, irritation and fissuring of the nipples early in the puerperium when they are trying to establish breastfeeding. Anatomical features, such as relatively flat nipples, contribute to the development of this problem. Mastitis and deep abscesses may occur due to penetration of the broken skin by pyogenic bacteria. The problem is, in essence, one of friction and irritancy and can be eased considerably by the judicious use of gentle cleansing and emollients such as white soft paraffin. Hydrocortisone cream or 1% chlorhexidine cream can be applied to the fissures, but should be gently sponged off with warm water before breastfeeding.

Jogger's nipples [1]

Long-distance runners of either sex may suffer from irritation of the nipples caused by prolonged friction against a shirt. The problem is more pronounced in women who do not wear a bra, or in men who wear a string vest. The condition is self-healing and can be prevented by the application of tape to the nipples before running.

REFERENCE

1 Levit F. Jogger's nipples. *N Engl J Med* 1977; **297**: 1127.

Nipple rings

Some years ago it became fashionable for various forms of body piercing, including rings through the nipple, to be used by certain male homosexuals and by the punk community, who also pierced ears, eyebrows, nose, lips and genitalia with a variety of rings and other ornaments. This fashion, like that of tattooing, now seems to be spreading into other social groups, particularly in female adolescents. Such nipple rings may cause problems either due to trauma or infection, the development of allergy to the metal, or the development of duct ectasia.

Tassel ornaments suspended from the breasts have of course been popular in some cultures, particularly in the Middle East, for many generations. Some dancers have their nipples pierced to accommodate a ring from which ornaments are suspended and this can cause breast duct ectasia [1,2].

REFERENCES

1 Collins REC. Breast disease associated with tassel dancing. *Br Med J* 1981; **283**: 1660.
2 Healey T. Nipple piercings—unusual artefacts. *Radiology* 1979; **536**: 164–5.

Painful nipples and mastalgia

Painful nipples are common, especially if fissures develop during early lactation, but in other circumstances this symptom can occur as a form of localized mastalgia [1]. The pain tends to be worse in cold weather and the patient can often accurately localize it to the nipple or subareolar area. The condition may be associated with duct ectasia, or periductal mastitis, and the mammogram may show coarse calcification.

It is important that breast cancer should be excluded and if a mass is palpable a surgical opinion is advisable [2].

Women with severe cyclical mastalgia have low plasma levels of the immediate metabolities of gamolenic acid (the essential fatty acid of evening primrose oil) [3]

Breast pain during lactation can be due to colonization of the nipples with *Candida albicans* [4]. The nipple may appear normal, but more often it is red, scaly or cracked, sometimes with a creamy exudate. Risk factors include vaginal candidiasis and the use of broad-spectrum antibiotics. The condition may be misdiagnosed as mastitis, but treatment with bacterial antibiotics will then exacerbate the problem, whereas anti-*Candida* therapy is curative.

Both cyclical and non-cyclical mastalgia often respond to oral medication. Danazol is probably best, followed by bromocryptine and evening primrose oil [5,6]. The last-mentioned has the fewest adverse effects. Some cases will also respond to oral contraceptives, which abolish the mid-cycle increase in breast sensitivity that occurs in most normal women [7]. For severe and refractory cases, tamoxifen may be helpful [8], and excision of a wedge of the areola may also help in difficult cases [1].

Severe nipple pain due to vasospasm can be a feature of Raynaud's phenomenon with the characteristic triphasic (white, blue, red) colour change in the nipple skin. In some cases it can be provoked by breast-feeding [9].

REFERENCES

1 Preece PE, Hughes LE, Mansel RE *et al*. Clinical syndromes of mastalgia. *Lancet* 1976; **ii**: 670–3.
2 Preece PE, Baum M, Mansel RE *et al*. Importance of mastalgia in operable breast cancer. *Br Med J* 1982; **284**: 1299–300.
3 Editorial. Cyclic breast pain—what works and what doesn't. *Drug Ther Bull* 1992; **30**: 1–3.
4 Amir LH, Pakula S. Nipple pain, mastalgia and candidiasis in the lactating breast. *Aust NZ J Obstet Gynaecol* 1991; **31**: 378–80.
5 Gateley CA, Mansel RE. Management of the painful and nodular breast. *Br Med Bull* 1991; **47**: 284–94.
6 Gateley CA, Miers M, Mansel RE, Hughes CE. Drug treatments for mastalgia: seventeen years experience in the Cardiff Mastalgia Clinic. *J R Soc Med* 1992; **85**: 12–15.
7 Robinson JE, Short RV. Changes in breast sensitivity at puberty, during the menstrual cycle and at parturition. *Br Med J* 1977; **i**: 1188–91.
8 Fentiman IS. Tamoxifen and mastalgia. *Drugs* 1986; **32**: 477–80.
9 Lawlor-Smith L, Lawlor-Smith C. Vasospasm of the nipple—a manifestation of Raynaud's phenomenon: case-reports. *Br Med J* 1997; **314**: 644–5.

Erosive adenomatosis of the nipple [1–3]

SYN. BENIGN PAPILLOMATOSIS OF THE NIPPLE;
FLORID PAPILLOMATOSIS OF THE NIPPLE DUCTS;
PAPILLARY ADENOMA OF THE NIPPLE;
SUBAREOLAR DUCT PAPILLOMATOSIS

Definition. A complex benign tumour arising from the lactiferous ducts of the nipple.

Incidence. This is an uncommon tumour, which occurs mainly in middle-aged women, but it can occur at any age, and occasionally in males [4].

Pathology [5–8]. The lesion consists of tubules, with an inner layer of columnar cells and an outer layer of cuboidal myoepithelial cells. The tubules are filled with keratin flakes, and an eosinophilic material, apparently secreted by the columnar cells. The cysts seem to reproduce the terminal portion of the nipple duct system. Within some of the superficial cysts, foreign-body giant cells may be seen. Some degree of intraluminal growth (intraductal papillomatosis) is present in many cases. This ranges from small papillary epithelial tufts to almost complete occlusion of the lumina by solid epithelial plugs, and there may be evidence of apocrine decapitation secretion. The overlying epidermis may show acanthosis and hyperkeratosis.

Clinical features. These are variable. The condition may start with a blood-stained or serous discharge, and the nipple may be enlarged, eroded, crusted or eczematous. There may be a small nodule on the nipple, and the symptoms may be worse in the premenstrual phase. The condition is commonly misdiagnosed as Paget's disease or eczema, and some cases have been mistaken for sweat-gland tumours.

Treatment. Simple excision of the nipple is the treatment of choice.

REFERENCES

1 Brownstein MH, Phelps RG, Magnin PH. Papillary adenoma of the nipple: analysis of 15 new cases. *J Am Acad Dermatol* 1985; **12**: 707–15.
2 Lewis HM, Ovitz ML, Golitz LE. Erosive adenomatosis of the nipple. *Arch Dermatol* 1976; **112**: 1427–8.
3 Bourlond J, Bourlond-Rinert L. Erosive adenomatosis of the nipple. *Dermatology* 1992; **185**: 319–24.
4 Moulin G, Darbon P, Balme B, Frappart L. Erosive adenomatosis of the nipple. Report of 10 cases with immunochemistry. *Ann Dermatol Vénéréol* 1990; **117**: 537–45.
5 Perzin KH, Lattes R. Papillary adenoma of the nipple (florid papillomatosis). A clinico-pathologic study. *Cancer* 1972; **29**: 996–1009.
6 Smith NP, Wilson-Jones E. Erosive adenomatosis of the nipple. *Clin Exp Dermatol* 1977; **2**: 79–84.
7 Diaz NM, Palmer JO, Wick MR. Erosive adenomatosis of the nipple; histology, immunochemistry and differential diagnosis. *Mod Pathol* 1992; **5**: 179–84.
8 Scott P, Kissin MW, Collins C, Webb AJ. Florid papillomatosis of the nipple; a clinico-pathological surgical problem. *Eur J Surg Oncol* 1991; **17**: 211–13.

Circumareolar telangiectasia

White [1] described a 77-year-old man with bilateral patches of perfectly circular telangiectasia centred on the nipple. The condition had been present all his life, with no associated abnormalities. Other associations have rarely been reported with breast telangiectasia [2,3].

REFERENCES

1 White GM, Jeffes EWB. Congenital circumareolar telangiectasia. *Arch Dermatol* 1990; **126**: 1656.
2 Millns JL, Dicken CH. Hereditary acrolabial telangiectasia; a report of blue lips, nails and nipples. *Arch Dermatol* 1979; **75**: 474–8.
3 Schlappner OLA, Shelley WB. Telangiectasia, aphthous stomatitis and hypersplenism. *Arch Dermatol* 1971; **104**: 668.

Mamillary fistula

SYN. PERIAREOLAR ABSCESS

This is a fistula from the areola or periareolar skin into a lactiferous duct [1]. It is a relatively common condition, which affects adult women, and presents as a discharging abscess. There may be a long history of subcutaneous abscesses which are recurrent. This may lead to repeated operations for incision and drainage, and the condition may be mistaken for hidradenitis suppurativa. The condition appears to be due to obstruction of a lactiferous duct, but the literature on the histology is confusing. Some authors have found dilatation and stasis of the major ducts, and others have refuted this [1].

The condition is treated by passing a probe into the opening of the discharging sinus, along the tract of the fistula, and out of the nipple. The track is then laid open, saucerized, and left to heal by granulation. If the excision is not complete the discharging sinus may recur [2]. If the nipple is inverted it may be advisable to correct this defect to prevent recurrence [3].

REFERENCES

1 Lambert ME, Betts CD, Selwood R. Mamillary fistula. *Br J Surg* 1986; **73**: 367–8.
2 Khoola J, Lautsberg L, Yeger Y, Sebbag G. Management of peri-areolar abscess and mamillary fistula. *Surg Gynecol Obstet* 1992; **175**: 306–8.
3 Maier WP, Berger A, Derrick BM. Periareolar abscess in the non-lactating breast. *Am J Surg* 1982; **144**: 359–61.

Breast abscess

This presents, usually in the puerperium, as a red, tender painful swelling in one segment of the breast. It may resolve with the rapid administration of an antistaphylococcal antibiotic but if fever and pain persist, surgical incision and drainage is indicated.

Breast cancer (Fig. 71.8)

This common and important condition lies in the province of the surgeon rather than the dermatologist, but it must be remembered that all physicians have a duty to detect and diagnose early breast cancer, which can sometimes be discovered on routine examination.

A survey in the USA showed that even when women asked specifically for a full physical examination, in 30% the breasts were not examined [1]. Inspection and palpation of the breasts should be included in any full examination,

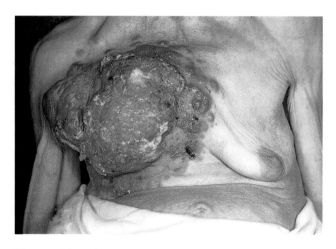

Fig. 71.8 A huge breast cancer with surrounding cutaneous metastases.

although male physicians should explain the necessity for this, and provide a chaperone. The breasts should be inspected with the arms by the side, and then with the arms raised, because in some cases this manoeuvre will demonstrate a visible mass, or a change in contour of the breast, or early retraction or dimpling of the skin caused by fibrosis in a breast cancer. The dermatologist should also remember that redness or oedema of the breast skin can also be due to underlying cancer. Oedema may sometimes occur in the lowest part of the areola or breast when the cancer is central and deep. Breast cancer can also cause flattening, broadening, retraction or inversion of the nipple. It is important that all four quadrants of the breast, including the axillary tail and axillary lymph nodes, should be palpated [1].

The dermatologist should examine the breasts carefully in all patients presenting with skin disease which may be associated with systemic malignancy, for example acanthosis nigricans or dermatomyositis.

The term *peau d'orange* is applied to a circumscribed area of dimpled oedematous or indurated skin resembling the surface of an orange. The finding of peau d'orange should lead to an intensive search for underlying carcinoma. Rarely, it occurs in the absence of any clinically palpable tumour. It has also been reported as a complication of anasarca, nephrotic syndrome and cardiac failure [2].

REFERENCES

1 Haagensen CD. Physician's role in the detection and diagnosis of breast disease. In: Haagensen CD, ed. *Diseases of the Breast*, 3rd edn. Philadelphia: WB. Saunders, 1986: 516–76.
2 McElligott G, Harrington MG. Heart failure and breast enlargement suggesting cancer. *Br Med J* 1986; **292**: 446.

Breast cancer in men

This condition is relatively rare, but it is essential that the diagnosis is not missed, as breast cancer in men has a similar prognosis to that in women, and causes 300 deaths per year in the USA [1]. As in women, the essential feature is a breast mass, but the small amount of breast tissue in the male means that the lesion is more likely to produce nipple inversion, and there is a higher incidence of bloody or serous discharge, and peau d'orange is also more common.

Ninety per cent of breast masses in the male are malignant [2]. Other risk factors include Klinefelter's syndrome [3], a positive family history and a previous prostatic cancer. The disease is commoner in black men and those who have never married [4]. A study of 13 males with breast cancer showed that one had a germ-line mutation affecting the androgen receptor [5].

The risk of developing breast cancer is substantially higher in men who carry the autosomal dominant gene *BRCA2* on chromosome 13q [6]. In one family with this gene there were multiple cases of male breast cancer, but interestingly no increased risk of female breast cancer [7]. Conversely, familial susceptibility to early onset breast and ovarian cancer in women has been linked to the *BRCA1* gene on chromosome 17q, but male breast cancer is rare in families with the *BRCA1* mutation [8].

REFERENCES

1 Nagadowska MM, Fentiman IS. Male breast cancer. *Br J Hosp Med* 1993; **49**: 104–6.
2 Sulyok Z, Koves I. Male breast tumours. *Eur J Surg Oncol* 1993; **19**: 581–6.
3 Scheike O, Visfeldt J, Peterson B. Male breast cancer: breast carcinoma in association with Klinefelter syndrome. *Acta Pathol Microbiol Scand* 1973; **81**: 352–8.
4 Sasco AJ, Lowenfels AB, Pasker de-Jong P. Epidemiology of male breast cancer. A meta-analysis of published case control studies. *Int J Cancer* 1993; **53**: 538–49.
5 Lobacarro JM, Lumbroso S, Belou C. Androgen receptor gene mutation in male breast cancer. *Hum Mol Genet* 1993; **2**: 1799–802.
6 Wooster R, Bignell G, Lancaster J *et al.* Identification of the breast cancer susceptibility gene BRCA2. *Nature* 1995; **378**: 789–91.
7 Thorlacius S, Tryggvadottir L, Olafsdottir GH *et al.* Linkage to BRCA2 region in hereditary male breast cancer. *Lancet* 1995; **346**: 544–5.
8 Stratton MJ, Ford D, Neuhausen S *et al.* Familial male breast cancer is not linked to BRCA1 on chromosome 17q. *Nature Genet* 1994; **7**: 103–7.

Basal cell carcinoma of the nipple [1]

This is a very rare lesion. It can occur in either men or women, usually in old age. It presents as a red eczema-like patch of the nipple or areola and runs a long indolent course. Biopsy is essential to differentiate it from Paget's disease.

REFERENCE

1 Sauven P, Roberts A. Basal cell carcinoma of the nipple. *J R Soc Med* 1983; **76**: 699.

Paget's disease, which is a marker of an underlying breast carcinoma, is discussed in Chapter 36.

Hair sinus of the breast

Hair sinus of the periareolar area of the breast has been observed in women engaged in sheep shearing (roust-abouts' breast) [1] (Fig. 71.9), in canine beauticians who get covered in dog hairs [2] and also in hairdressers. The lesions are similar to the interdigital pilonidal sinuses which occur in barbers [3]. The histology shows a granulomatous reaction. Repeated abscesses and their treatment by lancing may result in inability to breast feed or even lead to women contemplating mastectomy. For such women, there is now a protective brassière on the market, the Baa Bra [4].

The condition should be distinguished from hidradenitis suppurativa, which occasionally affects this area, by the history and by the absence of lesions in the axillae and groins.

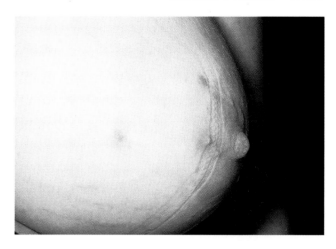

Fig. 71.9 Hair sinuses in a sheep-shearer. (Courtesy of Dr. W. Bowers, Treliske Hospital, Truro, UK.)

REFERENCES

1 Bowers PW. Roustabouts' and barbers' breasts. *Clin Exp Dermatol* 1982; **7**: 445–7.
2 Banerjee A. Pilonidal sinus of the nipple in a canine beautician. *Br Med J* 1985; **291**: 1787.
3 Price SM, Popkin GL. Barbers' interdigital hair sinus. *Arch Dermatol* 1976; **112**: 523.
4 Gardiner G. Roustabouts' breasts. *N Z Med J* 1994; **107**: 494.

Basal cell papillomas

SYN. (SEBORRHOEIC WARTS) (Chapter 36)

These are particularly common in the submammary creases in middle-aged or elderly women, often in association with intertrigo. They are easily removed by cryotherapy or curettage.

Mondor's disease (Fig. 71.10)

SYN. SCLEROSING PERIPHLEBITIS OF THE CHEST WALL

Mondor's disease is usually regarded as an obliterative phlebitis affecting the thoracoepigastric, lateral thoracic or superior epigastric vein. It occurs mainly between the ages of 30 and 60 years and affects women three times as frequently as men. There may be a history of trauma, muscular strain, febrile illness, or of contact dermatitis near the affected vessel. Breast cancer is an occasional cause [3] and mammography is recommended even when no mass is palpable [4,5]. Rarer causes include intravenous drug abuse [6], jellyfish stings [7] and the lupus erythematosus-like syndrome induced by procainamide. However, often no cause is apparent. Rarely the condition is bilateral [8].

There may be some tenderness or discomfort, but there are often no symptoms until the patient discovers a red linear cord running from the lateral margin of the breast, crossing the costal margin and extending to the abdominal wall. The cord is 2–3 mm in diameter and is attached to

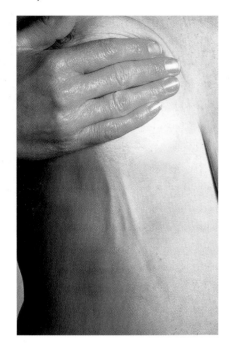

Fig. 71.10 Mondor's disease of the chest wall. (Courtesy of Dr A.Y. Finlay, University Hospital of Wales, Cardiff, UK.)

the skin but not to the deep fascia. It is usually only a few centimetres long, but may extend to 30–40 cm. The symptoms subside in a few weeks and there are no known complications.

REFERENCES

1 Hacker SM. Axillary string phlebitis in pregnancy; a variant of Mondor's disease. *J Am Acad Dermatol* 1994; **30**: 636–8.
2 Bejanga BL. Mondor's disease. Analysis of thirty cases. *J R Coll Surg Edin* 1992; **37**: 322–4.
3 Levi T, Baum M. Mondor's disease as a presenting symptom of breast cancer. *Br J Surg* 1987; **74**: 700.
4 Catania S, Zurrida S, Veronesi P *et al.* Mondor's disease and breast cancer. *Cancer* 1992; **69**: 2267–70.
5 Conant EF, Wilkes AN, Mendelson EB, Feig SA. Superficial thrombophlebitis of the breast. Mammographic findings. *Am J Roentgenol* 1993; **160**: 1201–3.
6 Cooper RA. Mondor's disease secondary to intravenous drug abuse. *Arch Surg* 1990; **125**: 807–8.
7 Ingram DM, Sheiner HJ, Ginsberg A. Mondor's disease of breast resulting from jellyfish sting. *Med J Aust* 1992; **157**: 836–7.
8 Skipworth GB, Morris JB, Goldstein N. Bilateral Mondor's disease. *Arch Dermatol* 1967; **95**: 95–7.

Other conditions which may be confined to the breast

Sunburn is common when the normally covered breasts are exposed, particularly on a beach or a boat.

Vitiligo sometimes shows a striking symmetrical involvement of the breasts.

Morphoea produces characteristic violaceous or ivory-coloured plaques around the areolae.

Bruises and purpura may result from sexual activity such as biting and prolonged sucking.

Psoriasis may also be provoked by the trauma of suckling.

Pityriasis rosea commonly presents with a herald patch on the breast.

Cutaneous larva migrans may occur on the breast when women have lain 'topless' on a tropical beach in the prone position.

Neurofibromas have a predilection for the periareolar skin and may be confined to this region, though café-au-lait spots can then usually be found elsewhere (Fig. 71.11).

Scabies often produces papules around the nipple, which may persist after treatment.

Fox–Fordyce disease (Chapter 43) may produce intensely irritable papules on the areolae.

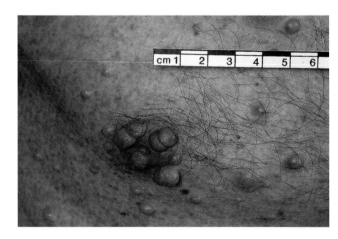

Fig. 71.11 Neurofibromatosis in a male, showing the predilection of this condition for the nipple.

Chapter 72
The Umbilical, Perianal and Genital Regions

F.A.IVE

Introduction

A number of common diseases affect the genitalia and genitocrural folds only incidentally, whereas others present in this region with unusual features. These will be dealt with briefly or by cross-reference to their full description elsewhere. However, there are some conditions which are entirely or predominantly confined to these regions, and these are discussed in more detail.

The chapter is divided into five sections:
1 the umbilicus (included for convenience);
2 the genitocrural region;
3 the perineal and perianal regions;
4 the male genitalia;
5 the female genitalia.

The umbilicus

Although the umbilicus is not strictly part of the genital apparatus, its evolution and connections link it to the pelvic region.

Anatomy and embryology

At birth the umbilical cord contains two arteries and a vein, the rudimentary arachus (allantois) and the vitelline (omphalomesenteric) duct, enveloped in Wharton's jelly. After separation and retraction of the stump, an umbilicus of variable depth is formed. Persistence of the urachal or vitelline ducts at this 'carrefour embryologique' may cause trouble in early or later life. A deeply retracted umbilicus may be the site of infection or foreign bodies.

The umbilicus in the newborn

Haemorrhages may occur from slipped ligatures. The cord normally separates within a week of birth, and the raw surface is epithelialized by day 15. During this time, the umbilicus is prone to infection, especially in maternity hospitals and nurseries. Impetigo (pemphigus neonatorum) or, rarely, more severe bacterial infections, may occur (see below). Talc granulomas are a particular hazard.

The 'absent navel' syndrome has been described as a sign of dystrophic epidermolysis bullosa [1].

Omphalocele

This form of abdominal hernia appears to be more common in African people. In 5 years in Ibadan, 33 cases were seen [2]. The minor form is due to herniation of the umbilical cord; a major form is probably due to a fault of embryonic folding of the fetus.

Developmental errors and congenital anomalies [3]

These are all rare, more common in males, and usually due to failure of obliteration of the omphalomesenteric duct or urachus. They present as fistulae, cysts or polypoid tumours.

Patent urachal duct

The umbilical opening is lined by skin or a pouting mucous membrane. Urine may be seen to escape from it, particularly in the elderly, when an obstruction to micturition exists. The condition is rare.

Persistent vitelline duct and polyp

If a connection with the intestine persists, it may become inflamed or cause a faecal umbilical discharge. More commonly, the remains of the duct give rise to a polyp in later life [4]. This may be accompanied by intermittent bleeding or a more persistent mucoid discharge, sometimes profuse. A symptomless, sterile umbilical discharge should always arouse suspicion. The histopathological features are those of intestinal gastric mucosa. It may be mistaken for a pyogenic granuloma [5].

Periumbilical 'choristia'

Under this title (meaning dysgenetic translocation of tissue) Bellone *et al.* [6] described extending, crusted, erythematous, periumbilical plaques, in which islands of intestinal mucosal cells were found in the epidermis.

Perforating pseudoxanthoma elasticum

This may occur in the umbilicus, and was the only site involved in six obese multiparous American black females [7]. It is only rarely associated with systemic problems [8,9].

Granulomas [5]

The following granulomas may present as such, or with an associated discharge, infection, bleeding or profuse sterile purulent exudate.

Pyogenic granuloma

This is a dull-red, fleshy, polypoid lesion, often pedunculated.

Bleeding readily takes place from trauma. If it occurs early in life, it may be confused with a capillary haemangioma.

Talc granuloma

This lesion, which is probably more frequent than is recognized, occurs in infants and very young children. It is distinguished histologically from a pyogenic granuloma (on which it may supervene) by the doubly refractile talc crystals [10].

Pilonidal sinus

A pilonidal sinus may occur [11].

Ileoumbilical fistula

This may follow laparotomy for Crohn's disease, or may rarely occur spontaneously [12].

Omphalith

In deeply set umbilici, an accumulation of sebum and keratin may lead to the gradual formation of a hard, stone-like mass, which may remain unnoticed for many years until discovered accidentally or revealed by secondary infection or ulceration.

Infections

Infection of the umbilicus in the newborn used to carry a high mortality. It still occurs in some countries. A number of bacterial organisms may be responsible, but staphylococcal, pseudomonal and clostridial species [13] are the most important. Minor forms consist of oozing and crusting, but a spreading oedematous erythema, progressing to gangrene, is of very serious import. Liver abscess, portal vein thrombosis or osteomyelitis can supervene [14]. At any time in later life, but usually after middle age, the umbilicus may be the seat of intertrigo or candidal infection. This is more common in the obese or in those with poor personal hygiene. Genital and perianal warts can occasionally be associated with similar lesions within the umbilicus [15]. Foreign bodies, inserted by children or psychotics, may be overlooked as a cause of purulent infection in a deeply set umbilicus. The periumbilical skin is a common site of schistosomiasis when it affects the skin [16]. Disseminated strongyloidiasis has presented as periumbilical purpura [17].

Eczematous and other conditions

Contact dermatitis is usually due to medicaments. Irritant reactions to soap and quaternary ammonium compounds also occur. The umbilicus is not infrequently involved in bullous and cicatricial pemphigoid, and may be the site of presentation of the latter (Chapter 40).

Periumbilical staining (Cullen's sign) occurs in acute pancreatitis, and occasionally in ruptured ectopic pregnancy or with duodenal ulcer perforation [18].

Umbilical haemorrhage has been described as a complication of cirrhosis following gross ulceration of the umbilical vein [19].

Tumours and implantations

The umbilicus is a site of implantation of endometriomas [20], which may clinically resemble melanomas. A unique case of postoperative endosalpingosis has also been reported [21]. Colonic mucosa was implanted in an infant, after colostomy for Hirschsprung's disease [22]. A single case of carcinoid of the umbilicus has been noted [23]. Paget's disease has also been recorded [24,25]. Skin metastases from neoplasms of the digestive tract occurred in only 3% of 2187 cases [26], but the umbilicus is a characteristic site, especially from cancer of the stomach (Sister Joseph's nodule) (Fig. 72.1) [27], which was the primary source in 33 out of 40 cases [27]. The ovary, uterus and colon are responsible for most of the others [28–30], although the pancreas has also been a rare primary site [31]. A leiomyosarcoma of the small intestinal wall has presented in this way, as has a malignant peritoneal mesothelioma [32,33]. The lesions usually present as firm, irregular nodules, but can occasionally infiltrate diffusely, or ulcerate and produce a foetid discharge. Such metastases were the presenting sign in 18 out of 40 cases, and were a major diagnostic feature in 28 cases [34]. The prognosis is always poor, but not entirely hopeless [35]. Histological identification of the site of the primary tumour may be difficult, and proved possible in only 21 of 85 cases [36,37]. Fine-needle aspiration of the nodule is not particularly helpful in reaching a diagnosis

[37]. Computed tomography (CT) and surgical intervention are obligatory, because it may represent the earliest and only metastasis [30].

Umbilical artery catheterization

Unilateral skin necrosis of the buttock has been reported following indwelling umbilical artery catheterization [38–40], probably due to thrombosis leading to occlusion of the inferior gluteal artery. A similar case was due to misdirection of the tip of the arterial catheter [41]. However, 'spontaneous gangrene' can also occur without catheterization, possibly owing to minor trauma to the umbilicus [38]. Very rarely, the bladder and kidney may also be involved.

REFERENCES

1 Paslin D. People without navels. *Br J Dermatol* 1978; **98**: 584.
2 Nivabueze I, Hekwaba F. Omphalocele: experience in the African tropics. *Postgrad Med J* 1981; **57**: 635–9.
3 Nix TE, Young CJ. Congenital umbilical anomalies. *Arch Dermatol* 1964; **90**: 160–5.
4 Hejazi N. Umbilical polyp: a report of two cases. *Dermatologica* 1975; **150**: 111–15.
5 Laradle De Luna M, Gcioni V, Herrara A *et al.* Umbilical polyps. *Pediatr Dermatol* 1987; **4**: 341–3.
6 Bellone AG, Raimondi L, Gasparini G *et al.* Choristia intestinale périumbilicale en plaques. *Ann Dermatol Vénéréol* 1978; **105**: 601–6.
7 Hicks J, Carpenter CL, Reed RJ. Periumbilical perforating pseudoxanthoma elasticum. *Arch Dermatol* 1979; **115**: 300–3.
8 Goldstein BG, Lesher JL. Periumbilical pseudoxanthoma elasticum with systemic manifestations. *South Med J* 1991; **84**: 788–9.
9 Kim YH, Yoon JS, Lee JH *et al.* Periumbilical pseudoxanthoma elasticum. *Ann Dermatol* 1994; **6**: 49–51.
10 McCallum DJ, Hall GFM. Umbilical granulomata—with particular reference to talc granuloma. *Br J Dermatol* 1970; **83**: 151–6.
11 Eby CS, Jetton RL. Umbilical pilonidal sinus. *Arch Dermatol* 1972; **106**: 893.
12 Reutz TW, Jr, Warden CS, Garcia FJ. Crohn's disease with spontaneous ileoumbilical and ileo-vesical fistulae. *Dig Dis Sci* 1979; **24**: 316–18.
13 Gormley D. Neonatal anaerobic (clostridial) cellulitis and omphalitis. *Arch Dermatol* 1977; **113**: 683–4.
14 Bingham EA, Beare JM. In: Verbov J, ed. *Modern Topics in Paediatric Dermatology*. London: Heinemann, 1979: 43–4.
15 Nathan M. Umbilical warts: a new entity? *Genitourin Med* 1994; **70**: 49–50.
16 Colin M, Loubiere R, Guillaume A *et al.* Les lesions cutanées de bilharziose: a propos de 14 observations. *Ann Dermatol Vénéréol* 1980; **107**: 759–67.
17 Kalb R, Grossman ME. Periumbilical purpura in disseminated strongyloidiasis. *J Am Acad Dermatol* 1986; **256**: 1170–1.
18 Evans DM. Cullen's sign in perforated duodenal ulcer. *Br Med J* 1971; **i**: 154.
19 Douglas JG. Umbilical haemorrhage—an unusual complication of cirrhosis. *Postgrad Med J* 1981; **57**: 461–2.
20 Williams HE, Barsky S, Storino W. Umbilical endometrioma (silent type). *Arch Dermatol* 1976; **112**: 1435–6.
21 Dore N, Landry M, Cadotte M *et al.* Cutaneous endosalpingiosis. *Arch Dermatol* 1980; **116**: 909–12.
22 Peachey RDG. Implantation of colonic mucosa in skin around colostomy. *Br J Dermatol* 1974; **90**: 108.
23 Brody HJ, Stallings WP, Fine RM *et al.* Carcinoid in an umbilical nodule. *Arch Dermatol* 1978; **114**: 570–2.
24 Ueki H, Kohda M. Multilokulärer extramammärer morbus Paget. *Hautarzt* 1979; **30**: 267–70.
25 Remond B, Aractingi S, Blanc F *et al.* Umbilical Paget's disease and prostatic carcinoma. *Br J Dermatol* 1993; **128**: 448–50.
26 Texier L, Geniaux M, Tamisier JM. Métastases cutanées des cancers digestifs. *Ann Dermatol Vénéréol* 1978; **105**: 913–19.
27 Samitz MH. Umbilical metastasis from carcinoma of the stomach. *Arch Dermatol* 1975; **111**: 1478–9.
28 Patel KS, Watkins RM. Recurrent endometrial adenocarcinoma presenting

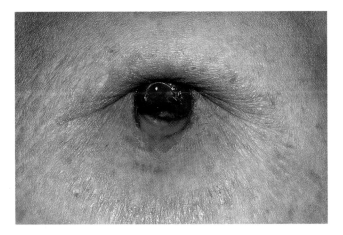

Fig. 72.1 'Sister Joseph's nodule'. (Courtesy of Dr J. Marks, Freeman Hospital, Newcastle-upon-Tyne, UK.)

as an umbilical metastasis. *Br J Clin Pract* 1992; **46**: 69–70.

29 Brustman L, Seltzer V. Sister Joseph's nodule: seven cases of umbilical metastases from gynecologic malignancies. *Gynecol Oncol* 1984; **19**: 155–62.

30 Sharaki M, Abdel-Kader M. Umbilical deposits from internal malignancy (the Sister Joseph's nodule). *Clin Oncol* 1981; **7**: 351–5.

31 Shvili D, Halevy S, Sandbank M. Umbilical metastasis as the presenting sign of pancreatic adenocarcinoma. *Cutis* 1983; **31**: 555–8.

32 Powell FC, Cooper AJ, Massa MC *et al.* Leiomyosarcoma of the small intestine: metastatic to the umbilicus. *Arch Dermatol* 1984; **120**: 402–3.

33 Chen KTK. Malignant mesothelioma presenting as a Sister Joseph's nodule. *Am J Dermatopathol* 1991; **13**: 300–3.

34 Steck WD, Helwig EB. Tumors of the umbilicus. *Cancer* 1965; **18**: 907–15.

35 Chatterjee SN, Bauer HM. Umbilical metastasis from carcinoma of the pancreas. *Arch Dermatol* 1980; **116**: 954–5.

36 Powell FC, Cooper AJ, Massa MC *et al.* Sister Mary Joseph's nodule: a clinical and histologic study. *J Am Acad Dermatol* 1984; **10**: 610–15.

37 Schneider V, Smyczek B. Sister Mary Joseph's nodule. *Acta Cytol* 1990; **34**: 555–8.

38 Bonifazi E, Meneghini C. Perianal gangrene of the buttock: an iatrogenic or spontaneous condition? *J Am Acad Dermatol* 1980; **3**: 596–8.

39 Cutler VE, Stretcher GS. Cutaneous complications of central umbilical artery catheterization. *Arch Dermatol* 1977; **113**: 61–3.

40 Mann PN. Gluteal skin necrosis after umbilical artery catheterisation. *Arch Dis Child* 1980; **55**: 815–17.

41 Rudolph N, Wang HH, Dragutsky D. Gangrene of the buttock: a complication of umbilical artery catheterization. *Pediatrics* 1974; **53**: 106–9.

The genitocrural region

Introduction

This section describes conditions affecting the genitocrural region, irrespective of the sex of the patient. It is a region of the body which is particularly prone to mycotic and pyococcal infections and flexural forms of common dermatoses. Moisture and friction lead to maceration and fissuring. Vegetating reactions are often very resistant to treatment.

Diffuse lymphangiomas or angiomas may cause irregular subcutaneous swellings. Epidermal naevi are not uncommon. Papilliferous moles and skin tags often become large and pedunculated on the inner aspect of the thighs. Dystrophic forms of epidermolysis bullosa may cause separation of the skin during delivery or, if less severe, bullae and erosions at these sites of friction.

Reticulate pigmented anomaly of the flexures (Dowling–Degos) involved the flexures in eight out of 10 patients [1], but may be restricted entirely to the vulval skin [2].

Infestations

Phthiriasis pubis is sometimes overlooked as a cause of pruritus in the female. In the hirsute male, the infestation may be widespread. Oxyuriasis has caused localized urticaria as well as pruritus. Scabies in children is diffuse, and the inguinal glands are often enlarged from secondary infection. Seabather's eruption and 'seaweed dermatitis' affect the bathing trunk area.

Schistosomiasis and amoebiasis cause phagedenic necrosis, fistulae and pseudoelephantiasis, and may also give rise to granulomas and condylomatous masses [3]. Onchocerciasis causes depigmentation, nodules, atrophy, lymphadenopathy and a 'hanging groin', infection and lichenification [4].

Infections

Bacterial or candidal infections complicate eczema, scabies, intertrigo, napkin erythema and many tropical diseases. Vincent's organism, *Pseudomonas aeruginosa* and a wide variety of Gram-negative organisms are commonly found. Giant condylomata acuminata may infiltrate the groin [5].

Gangrenous ecthyma of infants may, very rarely, affect the inguinocrural area, and gangrene has followed operations for inguinal hernia [6].

Erythrasma of the groins

This condition is symptomless and is very often overlooked. Lesions are usually also found in the axillae or toe webs. It may coexist with *Trichophyton rubrum* [7].

Candidiasis

This is extremely common, either as a primary infection, particularly in infants, and in pregnancy and diabetes, or superimposed on other dermatoses. It is a frequent cause of genitocrural pruritus. A glazed, erythematous sheet extends from the genitalia, anus or inguinal folds, and is bordered by a thin, vesicular or slightly macerated edge. Outlying papules rapidly develop small erosions with a collarette edge. In bacterial infections scaling, crusting or oozing are more usual, or folliculitis is present.

Tinea cruris

This condition is much more frequent in males, although females are affected more commonly in hot climates. Spread occurs onto the thighs and pubis. *Epidermophyton floccosum* infections are usually symmetrical or more marked on the side on which the patient 'dresses' (F.A. Ive, personal observation). There is a fine peripheral scaling (eczema marginé of Hebra). Cases have been described in infants [8]. *Trichophyton rubrum* infections are often deceptive or atypical, with irregular or polycyclic margins and extension to the pubis, perianal area and buttocks. When corticosteroids have suppressed scaling and reduced the erythema, the clinical diagnosis may be in doubt. Trichomycosis presents with malodour and discoloured, broken hairs [9], which should be distinguished from those of trichorrhexis nodosa, caused by repeated scratching [10]. Blastomycosis, actinomycosis and other deep fungal infections (Chapter 31) simulate tuberculosis, but are more prone to form fissures, sinuses and vegetating or exuberant granulomatous lesions.

They are distinguished by histological and bacteriological examination.

Among chronic infections, tuberculosis, tertiary syphilis and leishmaniasis are diagnosed by their characteristic features, which are described elsewhere. In tropical countries, tuberculous inguinal lymphadenopathy may be a cause of genitocrural lymphoedema. Amoebiasis involves the groins and perineum by extension from the anus. Hidradenitis suppurativa usually involves the area widely, although localized lesions are sometimes seen.

Venereal diseases

These are fully discussed in Chapters 27 and 30. Granuloma inguinale affects the genitalia only in less than half the cases, causing coalescing nodules, serpiginous ulcers and fungating masses. The buboes and fistulae of lymphogranuloma venereum are characteristic. Vulval (rarely scrotal) lymphoedema and elephantiasis may occur in both diseases.

REFERENCES

1 Wilson Jones E, Grice K. Reticulate pigmented anomaly of the flexures: Dowling–Degos disease, a new genodermatosis. *Arch Dermatol* 1976; **114**: 1150–7.
2 Milde P, Goerz G, Plewig G. Morbus Dowling—Degos mit ausschliesslich genitaler Manifestation. *Hautartz* 1992; **43**: 369–72.
3 Biagi FF, Martuscelli QA. Cutaneous amebiasis in Mexico. *Dermatol Trop* 1963; **2**: 129–36.
4 Nelson GS. 'Hanging groin' and hernia, complications of onchocerciasis. *Trans R Soc Trop Med Hyg* 1958; **52**: 272–5.
5 Eng AM, Morgan NE, Blekys I. Giant condyloma acuminatum. *Cutis* 1979; **24**: 203–6.
6 Audebert C. La gangrene post-operatoire progressive de la peau. *Ann Dermatol Vénéréol* 1981; **108**: 451–5.
7 Schlappner OLA, Rosenblum GA, Rowden G *et al.* Concomitant erythrasma and dermatophytosis of the groin. *Br J Dermatol* 1979; **100**: 147–51.
8 Parry EL, Foshee WS, Hall W *et al.* Diaper dermatophytosis. *Am J Dis Child* 1982; **136**: 273–4.
9 White SW, Smith J. Trichomycosis pubis. *Arch Dermatol* 1979; **115**: 444–5.
10 Chernosky ME, Owen DW. Trichorrhexis nodosa: clinical and investigative studies. *Arch Dermatol* 1966; **94**: 577–85.

Genitocrural dermatitis

The main features in differential diagnosis are as follows.

Contact dermatitis (Chapter 20). This may present suddenly with pruritus, oedema and erythema, or insidiously as a gradual intensification of a pre-existing dermatitis. Sensitization to applied medicaments, contraceptives, or, in men, industrial or other contact agents transferred by hand may be responsible, especially if the scrotum and thighs are also affected.

Constitutional eczema. Infantile napkin erythemas are discussed below and in Chapter 14. The distinction of von Jacquet's eruption from congenital syphilis and from the exuberant plaques and nodules of infantile gluteal granuloma [1,2] is important. Candidiasis may be overlooked as a common cause of genitocrural inflammation, and Langerhans' cell histiocytosis as a rare cause.

In adults, the genitocrural and lower abdominal folds are likely to be involved in any form of seborrhoeic or intertriginous dermatitis. Psoriasis and lichen planus are recognized by their special characteristics, although the diagnosis may be difficult when the former arises in an exclusively flexural distribution. The alternation of flexural seborrhoeic dermatitis and psoriasis may pose diagnostic difficulties.

Acrodermatitis enteropathica and the acquired zinc deficiency syndrome may well be overlooked as causes of genitocrural dermatitis.

Intertrigo

Definition. Intertrigo is a generic name for an inflammatory dermatosis involving the body folds, notably those of the submammary and genitocrural regions.

Pathogenesis. There is no clear distinction between constitutional and infective causes. Physical factors such as obesity, sweating, friction, incontinence and soiling by excreta may cause erythema or fissuring, and render the skin vulnerable to the effect of other agents. Initially, it is marked by soreness or slight itching, and a superficial mild erythema of the opposed surfaces. Secondary infection occurs rapidly, and the condition is then perpetuated as an infective dermatitis. In eczematous subjects this will take on the physical characteristics of eczema; in others, the infection may progress to crusting, pustular or vegetating lesions. The organisms concerned are *Staphylococcus aureus*, rarely the haemolytic streptococcus, *Escherichia coli*, *Proteus* spp. and, occasionally, *Pseudomonas aeruginosa*. In infants, diabetics and the obese, yeasts are often present. Latent diabetes should be borne in mind when the disease is refractory to treatment.

Overtreatment readily induces further irritation or a sensitization dermatitis.

Diagnosis. Candidiasis and contact dermatitis are differentiated by the history, the appearance and miscroscopic examination. The diffuse macerated erythema, often with fissures at the apex of the fold and without a sharply defined edge, distinguishes intertrigo from psoriasis and fungal infections, although scrapings and culture should always be undertaken. Mistakes in diagnosis arise from failure to recognize that two or more aetiological factors may coexist [3]. In India, *Trichosporon* species, which normally cause white piedra trichomycosis, have been implicated in causing cutaneous lesions resembling genitocrural intertrigo [4].

Treatment. In the early stages, the condition can be controlled by avoidance of friction and tight clothing. Driving or sitting for long periods should be avoided. In severe cases, the patient must rest in bed, preferably with groins unclothed and bedclothes lifted by a cradle, the opposed skin surfaces being kept apart with appropriate dressings [5]. Obesity, diabetes and incontinence should receive attention. Wet dressings are often useful initially in acute cases, and may be followed by bland or mild antibacterial creams or lotions. The aniline dyes and magenta paints still have a place in therapy. In general, lotions, paints and powders are more acceptable than creams. Nystatin, hydroxyquinoline and the newer imidazoles can be applied alone or with hydrocortisone.

Bullous and vegetating lesions

Bullous impetigo occurs in childhood, often secondary to scabies. All forms of pemphigus and pemphigoid (especially pemphigus vegetans [6] and pyodermite végétante [7]) affect this region, and juvenile pemphigoid and pemphigoid gestationis affect it selectively and sometimes exclusively. Benign familial pemphigus affected the groins or genitalia in 14 out of 21 patients in one series [8]. It is easily mistaken for intertrigo, especially when a family history is lacking. Secondary infection with herpes simplex has been reported after treatment with retinoids [9]. Seasonal exacerbations over many years should arouse suspicion and compel a biopsy. Subcorneal pustular dermatosis extends outwards from the inguinal folds as flaccid pustules, rapidly rupturing to form gyrate and circinate crusted lesions. Epidermal necrolysis may present as desquamation, sometimes involving the whole region. Severe erythema multiforme involves the genital or anal mucosa in half the cases. Necrolytic migratory erythema also extends in waves from this area [10].

Pemphigus vegetans must be distinguished from vegetating forms of pyoderma, which are not uncommon in the groins, and from blastomycosis and other mycoses, verrucoid forms of tuberculosis, and granuloma inguinale. Careful histological examination and culture are usually essential unless diagnostic lesions are present elsewhere.

Other conditions likely to pose diagnostic problems

Changes in the pattern of pubic hair are dealt with in Chapter 66. Acanthosis nigricans almost invariably affects the groins. Pseudoacanthosis nigricans can present as a macerated intertrigo and secondary infection. These can be distinguished from each other and from lichenification in pigmented skins by a rubber silicone impression technique [11].

Impetigo herpetiformis frequently starts in the groin with small, inflammatory, yellowish green pustules, which rupture to produce scabs and crusts.

Calcinosis involving the upper inner thighs may resemble pseudoxanthoma elasticum [12].

In the 'short-bowel syndrome', kwashiorkor-like changes include an 'enamel paint skin' [13].

REFERENCES

1 Hamado T. Granuloma intertriginosum infantum. *Arch Dermatol* 1975; **111**: 1072–3.
2 Tappeiner J, Pfleger L. Granuloma gluteale infantum. *Hautarzt* 1971; **22**: 383–8.
3 Schlappner OLA, Rosenblum GA, Rowden G et al. Concomitant erythrasma and dermatophytosis of the groin. *Br J Dermatol* 1970; **100**: 147–51.
4 Kamalam A, Senthamilselvi A, Ajuthades K et al. Cutaneous trichosporosis. *Mycopathologia* 1988; **101**: 167–75.
5 Wilkinson DS, ed. *The Nursing and Management of Skin Diseases*, 4th edn. London: Faber, 1977.
6 Winkelmann RK, Su WPD. Pemphigoid vegetans. *Arch Dermatol* 1979; **115**: 446–8.
7 Neuman HAM, Faber WR. Pyodermite vegetante of Hallopeau: immunofluorescence studies performed in an early disease stage. *Arch Dermatol* 1980; **116**: 1169–71.
8 Raaschou-Nielsen W, Reymann F. Familial benign chronic pemphigus. *Acta Derm Venereol (Stockh)* 1959; **39**: 280–91.
9 Stallman D, Schmoeckel C. Morbos Hailey–Hailey mit dissemination und eczema herpeticum unter Etretinat therapie. *Hautartz* 1988; **39**: 454–6.
10 Wilkinson DS. Necrolytic migratory erythema with carcinoma of the pancreas. *Trans St John's Hosp Dermatol Soc* 1973; **59**: 244–50.
11 Sarkany I. A method of studying the microtopography of the skin. *Br J Dermatol* 1962; **74**: 254–9.
12 Cochran RJ, Wilkin JK. An unusual case of calcinosis cutis. *J Am Acad Dermatol* 1983; **8**: 103–6.
13 Smith SR. Skin changes in short bowel syndrome. *Ann Dermatol Vénéréol* 1977; **113**: 657–9.

Pruritus and lichenification

Genitocrural pruritus may be unusually prominent in psoriasis and infective conditions in this area. Lice, *Oxyuris* infestation and diabetes must always be excluded as primary causes. Diffuse or localized pruritus, often severe and spasmodic, occurs with lichen simplex. The psychological mechanisms involved are similar to those discussed in relation to pruritus vulvae and pruritus ani.

Lichenification occurs readily, either as lichen simplex or superimposed on a pre-existing dermatitis. In women, vulval lichenification may spread to involve the thighs and lower abdomen, or the perianal region. In men, the perianal region, scrotum, the root of the penis and pubis are chiefly affected, although a localized area of the inner thigh may be involved alone. Lichenification occurs commonly in atopic patients and in those of an anxious or obsessional nature. The 'giant' form of lichenification described by Pautrier [1] may resemble dermatitis vegetans and be extremely resistant to treatment.

Diagnosis. The appearances are characteristic, even when rubbing is denied. It is important to determine any primary underlying organic cause. To label a disease 'psychosomatic' because an anxious patient has the ability to lichenify a pre-existing organic dermatosis does them a disservice, and delays correct treatment.

Treatment. If no primary cause is evident, and if diabetes and infestations have been excluded, a careful history may disclose relevant psychogenic factors, or a state of extreme tension, anxiety or conflict requiring discussion and reassurance.

Local treatment with corticosteroid applications is supplemented by reassurance, rest and sedation. All factors provoking local itching must, as far as possible, be removed. A short period of complete bed rest, preferably away from home, is often more successful than local therapy.

REFERENCE

1 Pautrier LM. In: Darier J, ed. *Nouvelle Pratique Dermatologique*, Vol. 7. Paris: Masson, 1936: 497.

Diseases particularly affecting infants

These usually involve part or all of the napkin area. They are discussed in this chapter on page 3222 and more fully in Chapter 14.

The perineal and perianal regions

Anatomy and physiology

The central part of the pelvic floor, bounded posteriorly by the coccyx and anococcygeal raphe, and anteriorly by the perineal body and its attachment to the genital organs, encloses one mucocutaneous junction and adjoins another. The natal cleft is deep and firmly fixed to underlying fibrous and fascial tissues, and its sides are steep and closely opposed. Mucous discharges, excreta and moisture are retained easily within it. Proximity to the genital organs and anus give it a special physical and psychological importance.

The perineum is endowed with numerous eccrine sweat glands whose function is retained after lumbar and thoracolumbar sympathectomies. Sweating may be due to an alternative parasympathetic sudomotor pathway from the fourth sacral anterior root. Apocrine glands are present but many are functionless.

A variable number of sebaceous glands are present both in pilosebaceous units and as individual 'free' sebaceous glands at the transitional part of the anal canal.

Developmental anomalies

Gross anomalies will be seen only incidentally by the dermatologist because of skin complications. Minor abnormalities such as haemangiomas, skin tags and papilliferous acanthomas are common on the inner sides of the thighs and infragluteal region. Pigmented, hairy naevi may involve one or both buttocks.

Developmental cysts, fistulae, sinuses and tumours

These are not uncommon, and frequently become infected. They may be mistaken for hidradenitis suppurativa or furuncules. Dermoid cysts occur on or adjacent to the perineal raphe and scrotum. Cloacal sinuses form fistulae from the anus to the adjoining skin; others involve the urethra and perineum.

Chordoma cutis [1]

Chordomas arise from the embryonic precursor of the axial skeleton, the notochord. They can involve the skin of the perineum, sacral area and buttocks by direct extension, recurrence or metastasis. They present as single or multiple, smooth, skin-coloured, non-tender nodules. Sacrococcygeal pain of a persistent nature may precede the diagnosis for years, in a manner that may mimic the presentation of sacral cysts [2], and require scanning procedures to differentiate between them.

Pilonidal cyst and sinus [3]

This common, midline lesion many present as a cyst, often with a pigmented or hairy surface, which ruptures and quickly becomes infected (Fig. 72.2). The sinus usually

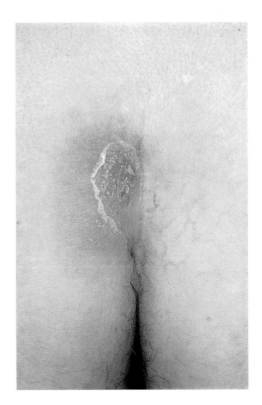

Fig. 72.2 Pilonidal sinus. (Courtesy of Dr D.A. Burns, Leicester Royal Infirmary, UK.)

extends to the sacrum and causes sacrococcygeal fistulae with deep ramifications. This heals if the track is thoroughly cleaned. It may be successfully dealt with on an outpatient basis [4].

Squamous cell carcinomatous change within a pilonidal sinus has been reported occasionally [5].

Because the perineum is at the centre of the anogenital area, it is often involved in conditions primarily involving the perianal skin, groins and scrotum or vulva. These will not be described separately.

Perianal inflammation

The causes of perianal inflammation in infants are dealt with in Chapter 14. In older children, *Oxyuris* infestation causes irritation and excoriations at night. Physical agents, tight underclothes or moisture from discharges are also sources of local inflammation.

Streptococcal perianal disease in children. A number of outbreaks of perianal streptococcal inflammation have been reported from North America. Symptoms include itching, rectal pain and, occasionally, bleeding. Streptococcal sore throats and communal bathing are associated with spread of the disorder [6–8], which may also involve the penis [9], and be associated with outbreaks of guttate psoriasis [10].

In adults, inflammation may result from the coexistence of several factors: haemorrhoids, anal discharge, proctitis, the presence of fissures or the effect of scratching. *Oxyuris* infestation is sometimes postulated but seldom confirmed. Phthiriasis pubis must be excluded. Traumatic lesions are seen in male homosexuals.

Contact dermatitis. This condition results chiefly from antipruritics or antibiotic applications. In 43 suspected cases, neomycin (27%) and 'caine mix' (24%) were the most frequent offenders; quinolines (7%), lanolin (7%) and ethylenediamine (5%) were less common [11].

Fixed drug eruptions may produce striking pigmentation. Lichen planus involving the buttocks and perianal region is extremely irritable, and may become excoriated or hypertrophic. Solitary involvement of the perianal skin may occur (Fig. 72.3). In elderly, debilitated or bed-ridden patients, a persistent patch of erythema on the sacral or ischial region is a sign of impending ulceration.

Five common conditions cause diagnostic difficulties: seborrhoeic dermatitis, psoriasis, contact dermatitis, lichen simplex and mycotic infections. The lesions of seborrhoeic dermatitis are brownish red, with branny or large, greasy scales towards the edge, extending beyond and outside the fold, and involving other areas of the body. Psoriasis has a smooth, glazed surface and a dull-red hue, and is often fissured; other signs of the disease are nearly always present. Contact dermatitis is highly irritable, and has an ill-defined spreading border. When due to a medicament,

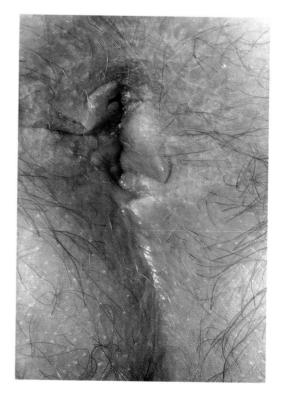

Fig. 72.3 Perianal lichen planus.

the hands may be involved. Gross lichenification simulates psoriasis but is usually unilateral, except when it involves the perianal area. It may occur as a small, intensely irritable area, localized to the edge of the anus in one site, which is indicated exactly by the patient. Mycotic infections are dealt with below. The prior use of topical corticosteroids frequently leads to diagnostic confusion.

Treatment. This should be bland. The strength of added active ingredients should be less than that used elsewhere on the skin. Humidity, natural occlusion of the area and the presence of fissures and excoriations, increase the risk of sensitization. Wet dressings, cool bathing, bland or mildly astringent packs and simple creams are indicated in acute stages. Antibacterials should be chosen with care. Hydroxyquinolines, although reasonably safe, are being displaced by imidazoles. Povidone–iodine cleansing preparations are useful. Psoriasis and lichenification call for more vigorous measures. Tar pastes, dithranol and steroid ointments are tolerated if applied carefully and in an appropriate strength. Prolonged use of strong topical corticosteroids causes a dusky erythema, atrophy or induration. In all cases of perianal and perineal inflammation, the urine should be tested for sugar, and swabs and scrapings examined for organisms. A vaginal or rectal examination is mandatory. Any irregularity of the bowels that causes straining or soiling should be corrected.

Superficial infection of the perianal skin

Although the high temperature and humidity of this area, combined with pressure [12] and friction, encourage colonization by staphylococci, primary pyococcal infections are now uncommon in countries with cultural or acquired habits of cleanliness. The perineal carriage of staphylococci [13] may not cause local lesions in the host, but is especially important in acting as a reservoir from which *Staphylococcus aureus* may be disseminated to other sites or to eczematous lesions elsewhere. In adults, the carriage rate is of the order of 13–22%; in neonates it may be higher. Some persons are better 'dispersers' of staphylococci than others, and the organisms may remain (and even increase) after washing. The risk of dispersion of staphylococci from this site is of obvious importance in hospital operating theatres, where attempts have been made to minimize it by the provision of special clothing [14]. Gram-negative organisms are seldom pathogenic unless the balance of the skin flora is grossly disturbed. *Pseudomonas aeruginosa* may be found in deep ulcers and fissures.

The presence of an infective condition in this area may overlie and disguise a more important lesion of the colon or rectum [15].

Viral infections

In infants, Coxsackie A infections and Kawasaki disease [16] can cause a transient papular or papulovesicular eruption of the perianal area and buttocks. Herpes simplex may occur. Anogenital zoster [17], involving S2–S4, or, less commonly, the ileoinguinal segment of L1–L2, may cause acute cystitis or urinary or faecal retention [18–20]. Vaccinia, usually by indirect transmission [17], is now never seen, but orf still occurs occasionally [21]. Acquired immune deficiency syndrome (AIDS) has presented as anogenital herpes zoster [22]. Cytomegalovirus has been found in perineal ulcers of patients who were immunocompromised from a variety of causes [23].

Condylomata acuminata (Fig. 72.4)

These can be distinguished without difficulty from moist, flat, syphilitic condylomas (Fig. 72.5). Although they occasionally occur in infants and young children, they are normally seen in young adults, and are not always venereal. They may be extraordinarily profuse, extending into the anal canal, especially in homosexuals or in immunodeficient subjects.

The giant condyloma of Buschke–Löwenstein (p. 3185). Only five patients have been reported with lesions in the anal area [24].

Mycotic infections

These are common. Candidiasis causes a bright-red, glazed

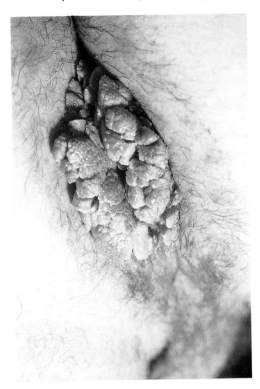

Fig. 72.4 Perianal condylomata acuminata.

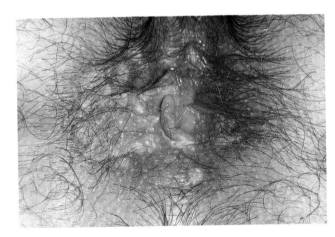

Fig. 72.5 Condylomata lata. (Courtesy of Dr S.C. Gold, St George's Hospital, London, UK.)

area, often with outlying small pustules, and may spread to the groins or natal cleft. Microscopy and culture distinguish it from other fungal infections, and from psoriasis and pyococcal infections. Erythrasma, present also in other sites, was found in 15 of 81 patients examined using Wood's light [25]. All were males. In the author's experience, it is less common. The well-defined, scaly, circinate edge, the spread, and the chronicity of *Trichophyton rubrum* infections offer clues to diagnosis, which is easily verified in the usual way. However, prior treatment with corticosteroids may so disguise the appearance as to trap the unwary. The possibility of fungal infection should therefore be considered in all unusual forms of perianal dermatitis. Histoplasmosis, blastomycosis and other forms of mycotic infection have also been recorded in this area.

REFERENCES

1 Su WPD, Louback JB, Gagne EJ, Scheithauer BW. Cutaneous chordoma: a report of nineteen patients with cutaneous involvement of chordoma. *J Am Acad Dermatol* 1993; **29**: 63–6.
2 Van Kleft E, Van Vyve M. Chronic perineal pain related to meningeal cysts. *Neurosurgery* 1991; **29**: 223–31.
3 Millar DM. Aetiology of post-anal pilonidal disease. *Proc R Soc Med* 1970; **63**: 1263–4.
4 Lord PH, Millar DM. Pilonidal sinus: a simple treatment. *Br J Surg* 1965; **52**: 298–300.
5 Sagi A, Rosenberg L, Grief M *et al.* Squamous cell carcinoma arising in a pilonidal sinus: a case report and review of the literature. *J Dermatol Surg Oncol* 1984; **10**: 210–12.
6 Hirshfeld AJ. Two family outbreaks of cellulitis associated with group A streptococci. *Pediatrics* 1970; **46**: 799–802.
7 Kokx NP, Comstock J, Facklam RR. Streptococcal perianal disease in children. *Pediatrics* 1987; **80**: 659–63.
8 Rehder PA, Eliezer ET, Lane AT. Perianal cellutis. *Arch Dermatol* 1988; **124**: 702–4.
9 Duhra P, Ilchyshyn A. Perianal streptococcal cellulitis with penile involvement. *Br J Dermatol* 1990; **123**: 793–6.
10 Patrizi A, Costa AM, Fiorillo L *et al.* Perianal streptococcal dermatitis associated with guttate psoriasis and/or balanoposthitis: a study of five cases. *Pediatr Dermatol* 1994; **11**: 168–71.
11 Wilkinson JD, Hambly EM, Wilkinson DS. Comparison of patch test results in two adjacent areas in England. *Acta Derm Venereol (Stockh)* 1980; **60**: 245–9.
12 Felman YM, Kikitas JA. Nonvenereal anogenital lesions. *Cutis* 1980; **26**: 347, 351, 354, 357.
13 Noble WC, Somerville DA. In: Rook AJ, ed. *Microbiology of Human Skin*, Vol. 2. *Major Problems in Dermatology*. London: WB Saunders, 1974.
14 Mitchell NJ, Gamble DR. Clothing design for operating room personnel. *Lancet* 1974; **ii**: 1133–6.
15 Grosshans E, Jenn P, Baumann R *et al.* Manifestations anales des maladies du tube digestif. *Ann Dermatol Vénéréol* 1979; **106**: 25–30.
16 Friter BS, Lucky AW. The perineal eruption of Kawasaki syndrome. *Arch Dermatol* 1988; **124**: 1805–10.
17 Bessiere L, Allain D, Meleville J. La vaccine ano-genitale. *Ann Dermatol Vénéréol* 1979; **105**: 339–41.
18 Fungelso PD, Reed WB, Newman SB *et al.* Herpes zoster of the anogenital area affecting urination and defaecation. *Br J Dermatol* 1973; **89**: 285–8.
19 Waugh MA. Herpes zoster of the anogenital area affecting urination and defaecation. *Br J Dermatol* 1974; **90**: 235.
20 Weaver SM, Keelly AP. Herpes zoster as a cause of neurogenic bladder. *Cutis* 1982; **29**: 611–12.
21 Kennedy CTC, Lyell A. Perianal orf. *J Am Acad Dermatol* 1984; **11**: 72–4.
22 Thune P, Andersson T, Skjorten F. AIDS manifesting as anogenital herpes zoster eruption: demonstration of virus-like particles in lymphocytes. *Acta Derm Venereol (Stockh)* 1983; **63**: 540–3.
23 Horn TD, Hood AF. Cytomegalovirus is predictably present in perineal ulcers from immunosuppressed patients. *Arch Dermatol* 1990; **126**: 642–4.
24 Alexander RM, Kaminsky DB. Giant condyloma acuminatum (Buschke–Löwenstein tumour) of the anus. *Dis Colon Rectum* 1979; **22**: 561–5.
25 Bowyer A, McColl I. Erythrasma and pruritus ani. *Acta Derm Venereol (Stockh)* 1971; **51**: 444–7.

Effects of corticosteroids

The prolonged use of potent topical corticosteroids for inflammatory conditions of the groins or perianal area can produce misleading appearances. Tinea incognito [1] is well recognized, but a persistent, deep, livid erythema of the perianal skin may not be regarded as primarily infective. Striae occur readily on the thighs. Multiple perianal comedones followed the application of a topical corticosteroid for 3 years [2]. 'Infantile gluteal granuloma' [3] (Chapter 14), usually affecting infants of 4–6 months, may also occur in incontinent elderly patients [4].

REFERENCES

1 Ive FA, Marks R. Tinea incognito. *Br Med J* 1968; **iii**: 149–52.
2 Oliet EJ, Estes SA. Perianal comedones associated with chronic topical fluorinated steroid use. *J Am Acad Dermatol* 1982; **7**: 405–7.
3 Ortonne JP, Perrot H, Thivolet J. Granulome gluteal infantile (GGI): étude ultrastructurale. *Ann Dermatol Vénéréol* 1980; **107**: 631–4.
4 Maekawa Y, Sakazaki Y, Hayashibara T. Diaper area granuloma of the aged. *Arch Dermatol* 1978; **114**: 382–3.

Danthron erythema [1,2]

This form of irritant contact dermatitis per rectum is due to the use of a laxative containing danthron in situations where there is retention of faeces. It is seen in mentally backward children, in those with Hirschsprung's disease or encopresis, and sometimes in elderly incontinent patients [2–4]. Danthron (1,8-dihydroxyanthroquinone) is reduced in the large bowel to 1,8-dihydroxyanthron, which is the active agent [2]. This is chemically identical to dithranol, and the lesions produced by faecal incontinence are equivalent to dithranol 'burns'.

A bizarre livid erythema in the perianal area, groins, thighs and buttocks, with sharp outlines, corresponds to the area of contact with the faeces. Danthron erythema is easily differentiated from other causes of perianal or inguinocrural lesions.

REFERENCES

1 Bunney MH, Noble IM. Red skin and Dorbanex. *Br Med J* 1974; **ii**: 731.
2 Ippen H. Toxizität und stoffwechsel des cignolins (Wz). *Dermatologica* 1959; **119**: 211–20.
3 Barth JH, Reshad H, Darley CR *et al.* A cutaneous complication of Dorbanex therapy. *Clin Exp Dermatol* 1984; **9**: 95–6.
4 Broholm KA. A controlled trial of a new combined preparation for the treatment of constipation in geriatric patients. *Gerontol Clin (Basel)* 1973; **15**: 25–31.

Hidradenitis suppurativa

Hidradenitis suppurativa (Chapter 27) can give rise to all degrees of inflammation and scarring. Friction and pressure accentuate the inflammatory changes that invade the fat and cause further granulomatous change extending widely over the buttocks and thighs. Persistent perineal sinuses are frequent, and deep lesions cause anal fistulae. In mild cases, only a few isolated lesions are present. Secondary bacterial invasion, often from the gut [1] is an important complicating factor. Seven cases have been associated with an oestrogen–progesterone contraceptive pill [2].

Differential diagnosis. This is not difficult when the condition is well established. The advanced case, with its fluctuant abscesses, burrowing sinuses, epithelial 'bridges', scarring and fibrosis, can scarcely be mistaken for any other disorder. Regional ileitis may cause anal fistulae (see below).

Mild or localized forms are frequently misdiagnosed as furunculosis or 'infected cysts', and confusion occurs with severe acne, developmental fistulae and lymphogranuloma venereum. The relatively painless recurrences in the same or other sites, and oblique sinuses that end in soft, swollen, inflamed nodules are characteristic.

Treatment [3]. Small, localized sinuses may be phenolized successfully, and early lesions may respond to intralesional corticosteroids. However, this treatment may have to be repeated, and recurrent or extensive lesions may require a more radical approach. Marsupialization (as with pilonidal sinuses) [4] and diathermy destruction of the affected tissue have been very successful in some cases, even those involving the scrotum. Treatment with carbon dioxide laser, with secondary intention healing, is very effective [5,6]. The use of Silastic foam dressing may facilitate healing [7]. Otherwise, plastic surgery with complete excision of all the involved skin is required. Long-term antibiotic therapy is often given 'blind', but is seldom of lasting value, although elimination of specific secondary invaders such as *Streptococcus milleri* [1] has given good results. More recently, isotretinoin has been used with mixed results, but is occasionally helpful in difficult cases [8,9]. Antiandrogen therapy has yet to be evaluated.

Lichen sclerosus et atrophicus

The perianal skin is rarely affected alone, but is involved in two-thirds of the cases in which the vulva is affected [10], forming a characteristic 'figure-of-eight' distribution. One case of carcinoma has been reported [11].

REFERENCES

1 Highet AS, Warren RE, Weekes AJ. Bacteriology and antibiotic treatment of perineal suppurative hidradenitis. *Arch Dermatol* 1988; **124**: 1047–51.
2 Stellon AJ, Wakeling M. Hidradenitis suppurativa associated with use of oral contraceptives. *Br Med J* 1989; **298**: 28–9.
3 Mouly MR. A propos des suppurations périnéo-fessieres chroniques et de leur traitement chirurgical. *Bull Soc Fr Dermatol Syphiligr* 1969; **76**: 23–7.
4 Brown SCW, Kazzasi N, Lord PH. Surgical treatment of perineal hidradenitis suppurativa with special reference to recognition of the perianal form. *Br J Surg* 1986; **73**: 978–80.
5 Lapins J, Marcusson JA, Emtestam L. Surgical treatment of chronic hidradenitis suppurativa: CO2 laser stripping—secondary intention technique. *Br J Dermatol* 1994; **131**: 551–6.
6 Finley EM, Ratz JL. Treatment of hidradenitis suppurativa with carbon dioxide laser excision and second-intention healing. *J Am Acad Dermatol* 1996; **34**: 465–9.
7 Morgan WP, Harding KG, Richardson G et al. The use of Silastic foam dressing in the treatment of advanced hidradenitis suppurativa. *Br J Surg* 1980; **67**: 277–80.
8 Brown CF, Gallup DG, Brown VM. Hidradenitis suppurativa of the anogenital region. Response to isotretinoin. *Am J Obstet Gynecol* 1988; **158**: 13–15.
9 Jones DH, Cunliffe W, King K. Hidradenitis suppurativa—lack of success with cis-retinoic acid. *Br J Dermatol* 1982; **107**: 252.
10 Wallace HJ. Lichen sclerosus et atrophicus. *Trans St John's Hosp Dermatol Soc* 1971; **57**: 9–30.
11 Sloan PJM, Goepel J. Lichen sclerosus et atrophicus and perianal carcinoma. *Clin Exp Dermatol* 1981; **6**: 399–402.

Anosacral cutaneous amyloidosis

Fourteen cases of a type of cutaneous amyloidosis have been reported in elderly Japanese people [1,2]. Pigmented macules and glossy hyperkeratotic lesions fan out in lines from the anus. Moderate pruritus was present in eight patients [2]. There are no systemic changes. Amyloid deposits are seen in the upper reticular dermis and around hair follicles. It is thought to represent an ageing process [1].

REFERENCES

1 Yamamoto T, Mukai H. Amyloidosis of the ano-sacral skin. *Jpn J Dermatol* 1981; **91**: 398–443.
2 Yanaghihara M, Fukishima N, Mori S. Anosacral amyloidosis. *Proceedings of 16th Congress on Dermatology*. Tokyo: Tokyo University Press, 1982: 922.

Fissured and ulcerating lesions

Non-specific lesions

Non-specific anal and perianal fissures occurring as a result of chronic constipation in young people may be painless but intensely pruritic. They are usually situated posteriorly. If lateral, a primary lesion in the anal canal should be sought. An oedematous 'sentinel tag' is usually present if the fissure arises in the anus itself. Small erosions and fissures may occur in the sulcus beneath oedematous haemorrhoids or in any area of dermatitis. Proctoscopy is mandatory if the aetiology is in doubt, and especially if the fissure extends to the anal margin or within. Benign fissures are superficial and not indurated, but when persistent they may be painful and cause bleeding, especially in the elderly. Unless they heal quickly under treatment, a biopsy should always be performed to exclude malignancy.

The presence of even a small fissure in an area of dermatitis maintains the pruritus and prolongs the course.

Behçet's disease occasionally presents with multiple shallow ulcers and fissures of the anal margin [1]; psoriasis, lichen simplex and lichen sclerosus et atrophicus may cause splits in the skin folds.

Bacterial perianal infection is commonly seen in leukaemic patients [2].

Anorectal carcinoma may present as an ischiorectal abscess [3–5].

Specific lesions

Syphilis [6]. Anal chancres are often mistaken for fissures; at the anal margin their significance may not be appreciated. Pain on defaecation or at night may be severe, but is often absent. The posterior midline is the site of election. Bilateral lymphadenopathy is extremely rare with other perianal ulcers. Dark-ground examination is useless if lubricants or ointments have been used.

Gonorrhoea. This causes anal inflammation and discharge, or an oedematous perianal dermatitis with multiple fissures and erosions.

Chancroid. This condition can cause extremely painful anal lesions instead of multiple, soft chancres.

Tuberculosis [7] (Chapter 28). This is still seen where tuberculosis is common, but must always be considered, even in western Europe [8]. A primary chancre is exceptional; the accompanying unilateral lymphadenopathy is very suggestive. Indolent, irregular, painful ulcers, fistulae and abscesses may be difficult to distinguish from those accompanying Crohn's disease [4,9]. Lupus vulgaris and verrucous tuberculosis may spread widely over the buttocks and postanal region, or assume a fungating and vegetating appearance.

Langerhans' cell histiocytosis. This condition may cause ulceration in the perianal area [10].

Schistosomiasis (bilharziasis). This condition may present as pruritic papules in the genital, umbilical and perineal regions in countries where it is endemic [11,12]. It is usually preceded by rectal or intestinal symptoms. However, genital lesions simulating viral warts have been seen in holidaymakers returning from fresh-water swimming in Africa [13]. Viable or calcified ova are found in the dermis. The lesions mimic those of subcutaneous tuberculosis.

Ischiorectal abscesses are common in Crohn's disease (see below) but may on occasion herald an underlying anal or rectal carcinoma [3].

Treatment. The patient is often apprehensive, and after a full examination must be reassured that the lesion is benign, when this is so. Small erosions and excoriations frequently heal with treatment for anogenital pruritus. If they are hidden between haemorrhoids or anal tags, protective pastes are helpful. Fissures in psoriasis and seborrhoeic dermatitis are difficult to heal, particularly in the natal cleft. If the underlying disease is satisfactorily controlled, the crack will heal without special attention. Intralesional

corticosteroids may be effective in non-infective inflammatory conditions.

REFERENCES

1 Lockhart-Mummery HE. Non-venereal lesions of the anal region. *Br J Vener Dis* 1963; **39**: 15–17.
2 Carlson GW, Ferguson CM, Amerson JR. Perianal infections in acute leukaemia. *Am Surg* 1988; **54**: 693–5.
3 Drumm J, Donovan IA, Clain A. Unusual presentation of anorectal carcinoma. *Br J Med* 1982; **285**: 1393.
4 McConnell EM. Squamous carcinoma of the anus—a review of 96 cases. *Br J Surg* 1970; **57**: 89–92.
5 Tait WF, Sykes PA. Unusual presentation of anorectal carcinoma. *Br Med J* 1982; **285**: 1742.
6 Samenius B. Primary syphilis of anorectal region. *Proc R Soc Med* 1966; **49**: 629–31.
7 Strescobich D, Donadio R, Aguilar OG *et al.* Fistulas anales de etiología poco frecuente. *Prensa Med Argent* 1969; **56**: 622–3.
8 Lé Bourgeois PC, Poynard T, Modai J *et al.* Ulceration perianale. Ne pas oublier la tuberculose. *Presse Med* 1984; **13**: 2507–9.
9 Morson BC. Histopathology of Crohn's disease. *Proc R Soc Med* 1968; **61**: 79–81.
10 Geniaux B, Lazrak B, Moubid MA. Histiocytoses X. *Bull Soc Fr Dermatol Syphiligr* 1973; **80**: 380–2.
11 Adeyemi-Doru FAB, Osoba OA, Junaid TA. Perigenital cutaneous schistosomiasis. *Br J Vener Dis* 1979; **55**: 446–9.
12 Cohn M, Loubiere R, Guillaume A *et al.* Les lesions cutanées de bilharziose: a propos de 14 observations. *Ann Dermatol Vénéréol* 1980; **107**: 759–67.
13 Goldsmith PC, Leslie TA, Sams V *et al.* Lesions of schistosomiasis mimicking warts on the vulva. *Br Med J* 1993; **307**: 556–7.

Granulomatous, vegetating and stenosing lesions [1,2]

Many banal conditions take on a vegetating appearance in this area, especially in hot, humid climes and in the presence of infection. For these, the term 'dermatitis vegetans' can be used.

Elephantiasis forms of progressive tuberculosis [3] and syphilis are now seldom seen, but deep fungal infections must not be overlooked.

Benign mucosal pemphigoid [4]

This condition (Chapter 40) may affect the groin, perineum and perianal skin, and may cause anal stenosis. The drug clonidine may have been responsible in one case [5]. Pyodermite végétante can be distinguished by the histology and by immunofluorescence studies. Ulcerative colitis may be present [1]. A periorificial form of eosinophilic granuloma may cause ulcerating and vegetating lesions around and within the anal canal.

In the differentiation of these rare, proliferative and granulomatous lesions, repeated biopsies and tissue cultures are usually necessary.

Lymphogranuloma venereum

When unrecognized or undiagnosed, this disease causes

widespread vegetating and scarring lesions of the genito-perineal area. The Frei and complement fixation tests distinguish it from hidradenitis suppurativa.

REFERENCES

1 Forman L. The skin and colon. *Trans St John's Hosp Dermatol Soc* 1966; **52**: 139–62.
2 Goldberg J, Bernstein R. Studies on granuloma inguinale VI. Two cases of perianal granuloma inguinale in male homosexuals. *Br J Vener Dis* 1964; **40**: 137–9.
3 Delacrétaz J, Christeler A. Demonstrations. *Dermatologica* 1969; **139**: 313–19.
4 Lever WF, ed. *Pemphigus and Pemphigoid*. Springfield: Thomas, 1965.
5 Van Joost TH, Faber WR, Manuel HR. Drug-induced anogenital cicatricial pemphigoid. *Br J Dermatol* 1980; **102**: 715–18.

Regional ileitis

SYN. CROHN'S DISEASE

The cutaneous manifestations of Crohn's disease [1–5] are:
1 erythema nodosum;
2 anal and perianal lesions;
3 spreading ulceration of perineum and buttocks after colectomy;
4 skin changes around ileostomies and colostomies;
5 'Sarcoid' type lesions in remote sites;
6 pyoderma gangrenosum;
7 granulomatous cheilitis;
8 epidermolysis bullosa acquisita;
9 non-specific changes due to malabsorption.

Crohn's disease affects any part of the gastrointestinal tract, but particularly the terminal ileum.

A sarcoid-like granulomatous histology is found in about 60% of cases. Anal or perianal lesions occur in a high proportion of all those affected [1,6] and may precede other signs by months or years; therefore they are of considerable diagnostic importance [6] (Fig. 72.6). In one series of 151 consecutive patients, 23 had ulcers and 26 had abscesses or fistulae. In another series [7], 112 out of 329 patients were affected, and in nearly all cases the colon was involved. Suspicion should be aroused whenever the anal margin or perianal skin is the site of pronounced maceration or inflammatory swellings, fistulae or ischiorectal abscesses, multiple ulcers, or florid, 'juicy' skin tags. If there is any doubt about the causation, biopsy of the edge of a lesion and sigmoidoscopy are obligatory.

Perianal manifestations of Crohn's disease in childhood are a major cause of morbidity, but only rarely progress in a destructive manner [8].

Similar, although less extensive, lesions occur, but much less commonly, in ulcerative colitis, and only very rarely in diverticulitis [1]. Syphilis, florid condylomata acuminata [9], anorectal carcinoma presenting with an ischiorectal abscess [10], tuberculosis and amoebiasis must be excluded.

Resection of the affected segment of bowel does not always cure the lesions or prevent their recurrence, especially at ileostomy or colostomy sites.

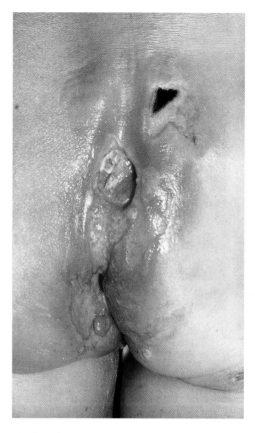

Fig. 72.6 Crohn's disease: perianal lesions. (Courtesy of Dr D.I. McCallum, Inverness, UK.)

Metronidazole given long term in full doses has been reported as helpful in a series of 26 cases [11].

Actinomycosis

Ulcerating and vegetating lesions, often unrecognized and of long duration, have followed trauma in patients with actinomycosis [12]. Correct diagnosis depends on histological confirmation, but the yellow or red grain pus should arouse suspicion [13].

Amoebiasis of the perianal skin [14]

This condition (Chapter 32) is usually associated with bowel infections, but where the disease is endemic, direct inoculation of abraded skin or operation wounds can occur.

Abscesses and fistulae may at first be indolent and symptomless. Ulcers typically extend slowly, with serpiginous outlines, firm cord-like edges and a whitish slough [5]. Sometimes, however, progression is rapid and remorseless, until a phagedenic ulcer completely destroys the perianal and sacral tissues [15]. A black, foul-smelling eschar is surrounded by a violaceous edge resembling pyoderma gangrenosum. The patient is extremely ill. Vegetating or condyloma-like lesions of intermediate severity occur less frequently.

Amoebiasis should be suspected when such a lesion occurs unexpectedly in the course of 'ulcerative colitis' or in a prolonged, mild, undiagnosed colitis. Cases have been described in infants [16]. The diagnosis is made by finding the *Entamoeba* species in a biopsy specimen from the edge of a lesion (which is always secondarily infected) or by examination, while warm, of a fresh high sigmoidoscopy swab. Treatment with metronidazole may be dramatically effective, but in severe cases surgery may also be required.

Granuloma inguinale

The initial rapidly ulcerating papule (Chapter 27) may occur in the perianal region in homosexual males. It is soft, painless and bleeds easily on trauma. It may be hypertrophic, sclerotic or phagedenic. There is normally no regional adenopathy, but a 'pseudobubo' may be present. In the anal canal, the lesion never extends beyond the stratified epithelium and strictures do not occur, but anal stenosis or, rarely, epitheliomatous change can supervene.

REFERENCES

1 Crohn NN, Yarnis H, eds. *Regional Ileitis*, 2nd edn. New York: Grune & Stratton, 1958.
2 Hibbiss JH, Schofield PF. Management of perianal Crohn's disease. *J R Soc Med* 1982; **75**: 414–17.
3 Lockhart-Mummery HE. Non-venereal lesions of the anal region. *Br J Vener Dis* 1963; **39**: 15–17.
4 Rankin GB. National co-operative Crohn's disease study. *Gastroenterology* 1979; **77**: 914–20.
5 Smith JN, Winship DH. Complications and extraintestinal problems in inflammatory bowel disease. *Med Clin North Am* 1980; **64**: 1161–71.
6 Gruwez JA, Christiaens MR, Laquet A. La maladie de Crohn de l'anus. *Acta Endoscopica* 1983; **13**: 285–92.
7 Marks CG, Ritchie JK, Lockhart-Mummery HE. Anal fistulas in Crohn's disease. *Br J Surg* 1981; **68**: 525–7.
8 Markowitz J, Davim F, Aiges H *et al.* Perianal disease in children and adolescents with Crohn's disease. *Gastroenterology* 1984; **86**: 829–33.
9 Thomson JPS, Grace RH. The treatment of perianal and anal condylomata accuminata: a new operative technique. *J R Soc Med* 1978; **71**: 180–5.
10 Tait WF, Sykes PA. Unusual presentation of anorectal carcinoma. *Br Med J* 1982; **285**: 1742.
11 Brandt LJ, Bernstein LH, Boley SJ *et al.* Metronidazole therapy for perianal Crohn's disease. A follow-up study. *Gastroenterology* 1982; **83**: 383–7.
12 Grigoriu D, Delecretaz J. Actinomyocose peri-anale pruritive. *Ann Dermatol Vénéréol* 1981; **108**: 159–61.
13 Millet P, Sonneck J-M, Lanternier G *et al.* Actinomycose perineofessiere et deficit en G6PD. *Ann Dermatol Vénéréol* 1982; **109**: 789–90.
14 Lord PH, Sakellariades P. Perianal skin gangrene due to amoebic infection in a diabetic. *Proc R Soc Med* 1973; **66**: 677–8.
15 Venkataramaiah NR, Reinaerta HHM, Van Roalte JE *et al.* Pseudomalignant cutaneous amoebiasis. *Trop Doct* 1982; **12**: 162–3.
16 Wynne JM. Perineal amoebiasis. *Arch Dis Child* 1980; **55**: 234–6.

Epidermolysis bullosa acquisita and bowel disease [1]

A connection has been recognized between epidermolysis bullosa acquisita and inflammatory bowel disease. There have been several reports of an association with Crohn's disease [2–4].

REFERENCES

1 Ray TL, Levine JB, Weiss W *et al.* Epidermolysis bullosa acquisita and inflammatory bowel disease. *J Am Acad Dermatol* 1982; **6**: 242–52.
2 Chouvet B, Guillet G, Perrot H *et al.* L'epidermolyse bulleuse acquise: association a la maladie de Crohn. Revue generale a propos de deux observations. *Ann Dermatol Vénéréol* 1982; **109**: 53–63.
3 Livden JK, Thunold S, Schsonsby H. Epidermolysis bullosa acquisita and Crohn's disease. *Acta Derm Venereol (Stockh)* 1978; **58**: 241–4.
4 Pegum JS, Wright JT. Epidermolysis bullosa acquisita and Crohn's disease. *Proc R Soc Med* 1973; **66**: 234–5.

Necrotizing and gangrenous lesions

A number of closely associated and overlapping severe gangrenous or necrotizing lesions may affect the anorectal, perineal and scrotal skin and subcutaneous tissues. Although they are often a result of surgery or trauma and thus are primarily of surgical importance, they are mentioned here because of the significance of their early recognition and treatment (see also Chapter 27). These conditions are described under several names [1]:

1 clostridial and non-clostridial [1–3] gangrene;
2 streptococcal cellulitis and myositis;
3 synergistic necrotizing cellulitis;
4 necrotizing fasciitis [4–6];
5 Meleney's progressive bacterial synergistic gangrene [7];
6 synergistic gangrene [8];
7 Fournier's gangrene, etc.

Clinical features [1,5,6]. Although middle-aged and elderly subjects are most often affected, the conditions can follow trauma in young adults, and the prognosis in the latter, given vigorous early treatment, is good [1]. They have also been described in children [9], particularly following circumcision or scalds, but sometimes after a bout of severe diarrhoea [10], or even spontaneously [11]. The infection may present as a primary perirectal abscess in the perineum or on the scrotum or labia. Pain is generally the first symptom, and may be severe. A distinct black spot may appear on the scrotum or labium and is of ominous significance. Tenderness and a dusky erythema extend with extreme rapidity to involve wide areas, and all the perirectal and perineal spaces (hence the terms 'fasciitis' and 'myositis'). Crepitus is an important feature, as is the presence of a dark-brown, turbid fluid without pus. Many patients are diabetic [1,5] or leukaemic; in these, the mortality is much higher than the overall rate of 12–25% [5]. A perianal distribution, old age and delay in treatment also greatly reduce the survival rate.

Bacteriology. Swabs should be taken from the margin of the lesion [8]. An immediate Gram stain will distinguish clostridial infections by the finding of large Gram-positive rods. *Clostridium perfringens* was the most common organism in one series [1], but other clostridia, aerobic and anaerobic streptococci, and *Pseudomonas* species [9] have all been isolated. Anaerobes may easily be missed. A wide variety of secondary organisms are commonly cultured.

Treatment [1]. Early recognition and immediate and aggressive treatment are essential in this devastating condition. Electrolyte and fluid balance must be established, and high-dosage antibiotic therapy started without waiting for the result of culture. This will normally consist of intravenous penicillin (24–30 million units/day [1]) together with a broad-spectrum antibiotic, usually an aminoglycoside or a cephalosporin; this regimen can be modified later.

However, the most important single therapeutic manoeuvre is rapid and extensive debridement of all affected tissue. Other surgical procedures, such as colostomy, may also be necessary. The value of hyperbaric oxygen [12] is disputed, but it should probably be used if available.

REFERENCES

1 Bubrick MP, Hitchcock CR. Necrotizing anorectal and perineal infection. *Surgery* 1979; **86**: 655–62.
2 Bessman AN, Wagner W. Non-clostridial gas gangrene. Report of 48 cases and a review of the literature. *JAMA* 1975; **233**: 958–63.
3 Skiles MS, Covert GK, Fletcher HS. Gas producing clostridial and nonclostridial infections. *Surg Gynecol Obstet* 1978; **147**: 65–7.
4 Fisher JR, Conway MJ, Takeshita RT *et al.* Necrotizing fasciitis: importance of roentgenographic studies for soft tissue gas. *JAMA* 1979; **241**: 803–6.
5 Oh C, Lee C, Jacobson JH. Necrotizing fasciitis of the perineum. *Surgery* 1982; **91**: 49–51.
6 Rosenberg PH, Shuck JM, Tempest BD *et al.* Diagnosis and therapy of necrotizing soft tissue infections of the perineum. *Ann Surg* 1978; **187**: 430–4.
7 Meleney FL. Hemolytic streptococcus gangrene. *Arch Surg* 1924; **9**: 317–64.
8 Flanigan RC, Kursh FD, McDougal WS *et al.* Synergistic gangrene of the scrotum and penis secondary to colorectal disease. *J Urol* 1978; **119**: 369–71.
9 Rabinowitz R, Lewin EB. Gangrene of the genitalia in children with *Pseudomonas* sepsis. *J Urol* 1980; **124**: 431–2.
10 Chuang JH, Wong KS. Necrotising perianal infection in children. *J Pediatr Gastroenterol Nutr* 1990; **10**: 409–12.
11 Boisseau AM, Sarlangue J, Perel Y *et al.* Perineal ecthyma gangrenosum in infancy and early childhood: septicaemic and non-septicaemic forms. *J Am Acad Dermatol* 1992; **27**: 415–18.
12 Schweigel JF, Shim SS. A comparison of the treatment of gas gangrene with and without hyperbaric oxygen. *Surg Gynecol Obstet* 1973; **136**: 969–70.

Pruritus ani

The very common symptom of itching localized to the anus or the nearby perianal skin is seen especially in middle-class, middle-aged white males [1]. It occurs less frequently in females, either alone or with pruritus vulvae. It can be associated with most forms of anal disease and with skin conditions involving the perianal area. The contributory factors are complex and may complement or perpetuate each other.

Anal itching occurs to a variable degree with any inflammatory or eczematous condition of the skin of that area, with anal fissures, whatever their aetiology, and with malignant tumours. Mycotic infection often causes intense pruritus, and diabetes must be excluded in all severe or persistent candidal infections. Threadworm infestations are a well-recognized cause in childhood and occasionally in adults.

Concern here is with anal itching in which there is no obvious primary dermatological cause. Changes secondary to rubbing and scratching are, of course, evident, as may be a contact dermatitis arising from treatment.

Pathogenesis. The common factor linking most forms of pruritus ani is faecal contamination [2,3]. In addition to potential allergens and bacteria, faeces contain endopeptidases of bacterial origin [4,5]. In the presence of pre-existing skin disease, for example seborrhoeic dermatitis or flexural psoriasis, or even in the absence of visible disease, these enzymes are capable of inducing both itching and inflammation [6].

The causes of faecal contamination are as follows (more than one factor may be operative).

Difficulty in cleansing the area. This may be due to the following factors.
1 Simple obesity: poor ventilation and maceration play an additional role.
2 Frequency of defaecation: patients with a colostomy never suffer from perianal itching. Patients with pruritus ani are rarely constipated, although they may sit long at stool owing to faulty training techniques, with resultant prolapse or haemorrhoids and soiling [2,7,8]. Patients frequently admit to two or more motions a day. These are often tense individuals in whom everyday problems induce a profound colonic reflex, resulting in defaecation and soiling.
3 Anatomical factors: it is often noted that the anus is deeply placed. The association of this 'funnel anus' with marked hirsutism causes mechanical problems in the maintenance of hygiene.

Anal leakage. This may be due to the following factors.
1 Local causes such as haemorrhoids, perianal tags or fissures, which interfere with the efficient functions of the anus.
2 Primary anal sphincter dysfunction. Anal canal manometry studies have shown that leakage of infused saline occurs early [9], and in one common group of patients the sphincter relaxes in response to rectal distension in a more rapid and profound manner than in a control group [7]. The arrival of faeces or flatus in the rectum may then regularly result in reflex faecal soiling.

Bacterial contamination. This is frequently a secondary cause, but rarely a primary cause alone. However, cross-infection of staphylococci may occur between the anus and the ears, for example.

Food and drink. The role of ingested metabolites or food chemicals in inducing pruritus ani is still uncertain and virtually unexplored, but anecdotal evidence in individual cases is sometimes compelling [10].

Psychological factors are often involved as causes of pruritus ani, particularly when the itching appears to be out of proportion to the changes observed. However, as Whitlock [11] points out in a careful review, the evidence is unsatisfactory, except perhaps in primary lichen simplex. Psychosexual connotations of suppressed homosexuality certainly do not withstand critical assessment. It is quite understandable, however, that prolonged pruritus ani can lead to tension, irritability or depression, and the treatment of this is an important part of the management of the condition.

Clinical features. These vary somewhat according to the factors responsible, but are all complicated by the effects of rubbing, secondary infection or contact dermatitis.
1 Lichen simplex may be present in a 'pure' form, often localized to a small area at the edge of the anus or slightly away from it. The perception of itch from 'easily alerted' nerve endings is more acute in those of anxious temperament or at times of psychic trauma or fatigue.
2 A more general area of maceration, lichenification and fissuring—the 'mossy bank' anus—may be present. The architecture of the anal margin may be distorted by haemorrhoids, tags, oedema and infection. There is usually a gross degree of discharge [7].
3 Features of acute eczema may be due to secondary infection of possibly minimal seborrhoeic dermatitis or psoriasis, or to contact dermatitis. This should always be suspected when there has been any sudden change of pattern or intensity of a rash. The fingers may also be involved. One of the commonest offenders is the 'caine' group of drugs [12], often self-prescribed.
4 Intense erythema with no obvious features of eczema may occur. This tends to vary in intensity over short periods, and probably represents the pruritic stage of the next group.
5 There may be no visible abnormality at the time of examination. These patients may have noticed erythema at times, or intense itching, and commonly give a story of an intermittent sensation of wet anal margins and slight faecal soiling. It is in this group that dyskinesia of the sphincter appears to be a primary factor.

Diagnosis. A full history, including bowel habits, is essential, and a search for underlying disease must be carried out. A rectal examination will prevent the occasional serious error and will always reassure the patient. Sigmoidoscopy may be indicated if there is marked bowel upset. In the young,

threadworms should be sought with nocturnal 'Sellotape' swabs.

Treatment [2]. Time is well spent in dealing in detail with all aspects of hygiene. Patients should be encouraged to limit evacuation to once daily or less, and to wash and dry the anal area gently with wool or soft toilet tissue afterwards. Underwear should be loose and preferably made of cotton.

Any foods, such as nuts, which provoke the pruritus should be excluded from the diet, and a high-fibre diet should be encouraged if there is any history of constipation or haemorrhoids [13].

When active pathology such as fissures, haemorrhoids or anal spasm are present, surgical help will be needed. Lord's stretch procedure [14] has proved helpful. The long-term results are particularly satisfactory in those patients with strong ultra-low-pressure waves [13]. However, it may not always relieve the pruritus [15]. Simple excision of anal tags is unhelpful in relieving symptoms [16].

Local applications should be mild and soothing. If infection is present or suspected, antibacterials may be combined with mild corticosteroid preparations. Considerable relief from nocturnal itching can be achieved with corticosteroid suppositories. A wick of bandage impregnated with hydrocortisone 1% and silicone 10% inserted in the natal cleft is anti-inflammatory and lubricating. The anal skin is 'quasi-occluded' and is easily damaged by fluorinated corticosteroids. The application of zinc paste with 1–2% phenol is a safe and useful antipruritic and protective application if used both before and after bowel movement, and again at night.

REFERENCES

1 Leiberman DA. Common anorectal disorders. *Ann Intern Med* 1984; **101**: 837–46.
2 Alexander-Williams J. Pruritus ani. *Br Med J* 1983; **287**: 159–60.
3 Kocsard E. Pruritus ani. A symptom of fecal contamination. *Cutis* 1981; **27**: 518.
4 Keele CA. Chemical causes of pain and itch. *Proc R Soc Med* 1957; **50**: 477–84.
5 Shelley WB, Arthur RP. The neurohistology and neurophysiology of the itch sensation in man. *Arch Dermatol* 1957; **76**: 296–323.
6 Andersen PH, Bucher AP, Saeed I *et al.* Faecal enzymes: *in vivo* skin irritation. *Contact Dermatitis* 1994; **30**: 152–8.
7 Eyers AA, Thompson JPS. Pruritus ani: is anal sphincter dysfunction important in aetiology? *Br Med J* 1979; **ii**: 1549–51.
8 Kaufman HD, ed. In: *The Haemorrhoid Syndrome.* Tunbridge Wells: Abacus, 1981: 61.
9 Allan A, Ambrose NS, Silverman S *et al.* Physiological study of pruritus ani. *Br J Surg* 1987; **74**: 576–9.
10 Veren NK, Hattel T, Justesen O *et al.* Dermatoses in coffee drinkers. *Cutis* 1987; **40**: 421–2.
11 Whitlock FA, ed. *Psychophysiological Aspects of Skin Disease.* London: WB Saunders, 1976: 118–21.
12 Wilkinson JD, Hambly EM, Wilkinson DS. Comparison of patch test results in two adjacent areas of England. II. Medicaments. *Acta Derm Venereol (Stockh)* 1980; **60**: 245–9.
13 Hancock BD. In: Kaufman HD, ed. *The Haemorrhoid Syndrome.* Tunbridge Wells: Abacus, 1981: 93–104.

14 Lord PH. Diverse methods of managing haemorrhoids: dilatation. *Dis Colon Rectum* 1973; **16**: 180–92.
15 Ortiza H, Marti J, Jaurieta E *et al.* Lord's procedure: a critical study of its basic principle. *Br J Surg* 1978; **65**: 281–4.
16 Jensen SL. A randomised trial of simple excision of non-specific hypertrophied anal papillae versus expectant management in patients with chronic pruritus ani. *Ann R Coll Surg Engl* 1988; **70**: 348–9.

Chronic perianal pain and the 'perineal syndrome'

A number of names have been given to sensations of pain localized to the anogenital region in the absence of evident organic cause [1,2]. Proctalgia fugax affects young adult males, and occurs chiefly at night in the form of a sudden cramp-like pain, which resolves in a few minutes. 'Coccygodynia', 'descending perineum syndrome' and 'chronic idiopathic anal pain' chiefly affect females. The pain is described as dull and throbbing. In 35 such patients, it was noted that the pain was precipitated by sitting, and that these three conditions differed from proctalgia fugax [1]. Electrophysiological studies gave variable results. There was a high incidence of previous sciatica and damage to the pelvic floor musculature. Treatment was disappointing. Rarely, sacral cysts and even chordoma can present with this symptomatology (see p. 3169).

Such patients will present to surgeons or gynaecologists. However, dermatologists may be confronted by a similar problem in which a patient complains of short-lived episodes of intense burning, which may be accompanied by sweating, limited to the perineum or occasionally the scrotum. Attacks occur without warning, but may be brought about by a full rectum. In one patient, the attacks were severe enough to cause him to stop walking for some minutes. The patients tend to be stressed individuals, as are those with proctalgia fugax [2]. The skin is entirely normal.

The mechanism is unknown. Two patients appeared to have been helped by propantheline, suggesting a cholinergic mechanism [3]. However, the condition may also fall into the group of 'dermatological non-disease' [4], in which the perineum was affected in eight out of 24 patients.

In women, 'vulvodynia' may be comparable (p. 3225). The condition has also been reported in children suffering from intrafamilial stresses [5].

REFERENCES

1 Neill ME, Swash M. Chronic perianal pain: an unsolved problem. *J R Soc Med* 1982; **75**: 96–101.
2 Parks AG, Porter NH, Hardcastle J. The syndrome of descending perineum. *Proc R Soc Med* 1966; **59**: 477–82.
3 Monro PAG, ed. *Sympathectomy*. Oxford: Clarendon Press, 1959: 146.
4 Cotterill JA. A dermatological non-disease—a common and potentially fatal disturbance of cutaneous body image. *Br J Dermatol* 1980; **103** (Suppl. 18): 13.
5 Lask B. Chronic perianal pain. *J R Soc Med* 1982; **75**: 370.

Miscellaneous conditions

Pregnancy, Addison's disease and other pigmentary disorders increase the pre-existing pigmentation. Acanthosis nigricans causes acanthotic and papillomatous lesions in the perineum. The anus is involved in about 5% of cases of Stevens–Johnson syndrome. Leukoplakia is rare, and is usually superimposed on lichen sclerosus et atrophicus.

Anal manifestations of intestinal disease

These have been well documented [1]. Although they are usually non-specific, the particular skin manifestations of tuberculosis, amoebiasis, schistosomiasis and Crohn's disease may lead to diagnosis of the underlying disease by their typical histology.

Anal and perianal lesions in homosexual males [2–4]

These have become of greater significance in view of the increasing prevalence of AIDS [3,5]. Whatever the presentation of the patient, it is important to look for other infective conditions. Painful lesions of the anus in homosexual men are common [6], and may include traumatic lesions and herpes genitalis. Anorectal sepsis, including chronic intersphincteric abscesses, anal fistulae, fissures and ulcerated haemorrhoids were seen more frequently in a group of male homosexuals than in heterosexuals [7]. Cytomegalovirus has been recorded in persistent perineal ulcers in immunosuppressed patients [8]. Epstein–Barr virus DNA has been found recently in epithelial cells from the anal canals of asymptomatic human immunodeficiency virus (HIV)-positive male homosexuals, indicating possible sexual transmissibility [9].

Herpes simplex, gonorrhoea and anal condylomas were commonly associated in a US study on early HIV positivity [10]. Similar findings relate to a central African group with more advanced disease [11]. The importance of primary rectal syphilis has been emphasized [12]. Amoebiasis [13] may be overlooked. Dark-ground examination, and culture and microscopy for ova, should be obligatory [2]. In the absence of organisms, if pus cells are found, a rectal biopsy is indicated. Kaposi's sarcoma of the rectum has been recorded in HIV-positive males [14].

DNA sequences of what appears to be a distinct and newly recognized form of herpesvirus have been found in AIDS-associated Kaposi's sarcoma [15]. An identical agent has been identified in the semen of HIV-positive males [16], indicating a possible sexual mode of transmission, and perhaps explaining the comparative rarity of the disorder in HIV-positive intravenous drug abusers.

Such is the complexity, atypicality and potential severity of infections in homosexual men that all dermatologists to whom they present must not only be aware of the range of such infections, but must either have the facilities for full and accurate identification of pathogens, or refer patients to those who have such facilities.

REFERENCES

1 Grosshans E, Jenn P, Baumann R *et al.* Manifestations anales de maladies du tube digestif. *Ann Dermatol Vénéréol* 1979; **106**: 25–30.
2 Felman YM, Nikitas JA. Sexually transmitted diseases in the male homosexual. *Cutis* 1982; **30**: 706–24.
3 Penneys NS, ed. *Skin Manifestations of AIDS.* London: Martin Dunitz, 1990.
4 Cope R. Mise au point sur les lesions anoperineals et rectales observees au cours du SIDA. *Contracept Fertil Sex* 1994; **22**: 187–94.
5 Matis WL, Triana A, Shapiro R *et al.* Dermatologic findings associated with the human immunodeficiency virus. *J Am Acad Dermatol* 1987; **17**: 746–51.
6 McMillan A, Smith IW. Painful anal ulceration in homosexual men. *Br J Surg* 1984; **71**: 215–16.
7 Carr ND, Mercey D, Slack WW. Non-condylomatous perianal skin disease in homosexual men. *Br J Surg* 1989; **76**: 1064–6.
8 Horn TD, Hood AF. Cytomegalovirus is predictably present in perineal ulcers of immunosuppressed patients. *Arch Dermatol* 1990; **126**: 642–4.
9 Naher H, Lenhard B, Wilms J, Nickel P. Detection of Epstein–Barr virus DNA in anal scrapings from HIV positive homosexual men. *Arch Dermatol Res* 1995; **287**: 608–11.
10 Berger RS, Stoner MF, Hobbs ER *et al.* Cutaneous manifestations of early human immunodeficiency virus exposure. *J Am Acad Dermatol* 1988; **19**: 298–303.
11 Hira SK, Wadhawam D, Kamanga J *et al.* Cutaneous manifestations of human immunodeficiency virus in Lusaka, Zambia. *J Am Acad Dermatol* 1988; **19**: 451–7.
12 Gluckman JB, Kleinman MS, May AG. Primary syphilis of rectum. *NY State J Med* 1974; **74**: 2210–11.
13 Robertson DHH, McMillan A, Young H. Homosexual transmission of amoebiasis. *J R Soc Med* 1982; **75**: 564.
14 Lorenz HP, Wilson W, Leigh B, Schecter WP. Kaposi's sarcoma of the rectum in patients with the Acquired Immune Deficiency Syndrome. *Am J Surg* 1990; **160**: 681–2.
15 Chang Y, Cesarman E, Pessin MS *et al.* Identification of herpes virus-like DNA sequences in AIDS-associated Kaposi's sarcoma. *Science* 1994; **266**: 1865–9.
16 Lin JC, Lin SC, Mar EC *et al.* Is Kaposi's sarcoma-associated herpes virus detectable in semen in HIV infected homosexual men? *Lancet* 1995; **346**: 1601–2.

Premalignant and malignant lesions

The anogenital area is not exposed to solar radiation, the chief cutaneous carcinogen. Treatment of pruritus with such agents as radiotherapy or tar preparations, and the use of radiotherapy for gynaecological malignancy, carry theoretical hazards and can occasionally be incriminated. They do not, however, appear to have influenced greatly the frequency of perineal tumours. Postgranulomatous scarring is an important background to perianal malignancy in areas where venereal granulomas are common, and other scarring processes, such as lichen sclerosus, are a potential hazard. There are a small number of cases where condylomata acuminata precede squamous cell carcinoma of the anal or perianal skin [1,2].

Anal tumours are uncommon, and are mainly squamous cell carcinomas. A variety of tumours may arise on perianal skin. Basal cell carcinoma and malignant melanoma are uncommon, and show no special features requiring comment here; other malignant tumours are rare. In one survey of 71 patients, the female to male ratio was 4:1 [3].

Bowen's disease

Bowen's disease of the perianal skin has no particularly special features. In the recent past, it has been confused with pigmentary multicentric Bowen's disease [4], but this is now by convention called Bowenoid papulosis (p. 3197), and can occur on the genitals as well as the perineum [2,5]. It is regarded as a distinct disorder of uncertain prognosis. True Bowen's disease of the perianal skin varies in its appearance, depending on the degree of moistness of the involved area. It may present as a dry, scaling, erythematous or ulcerating plaque, or be erythematous, moist and velvety, like erythroplasia of Queyrat. A woman with anogenital Bowen's disease has an increased risk of carcinoma *in situ* or invasive malignancy elsewhere in the genital tract [6], and a full gynaecological examination is thus obligatory in such cases [7].

Squamous cell carcinoma

Incidence and aetiology. Fifty-six percent of all anal carcinomas are of the squamous variety [8]. They are slightly more common in women, but seem to be more aggressive in men [9]. In Denmark, the incidence of anal carcinoma has tripled since 1960 to 0.74 cases per 100 000 population. An association with smoking, cervical intraepithelial dysplasia and changing sexual habits has been postulated [10].

Coexistent Crohn's disease has been associated with a 10-fold increase in anal carcinoma [11]. Homosexual males show an increased incidence of the disease, which suggests an association with anal intercourse [12]. An association has been found between verrucous carcinoma of the anus and human papillomavirus (HPV) infection [13].

Clinical features. Symptoms may include bleeding, pain, presence of a mass and change in bowel habit. Examination will reveal a hard mass that may be flat, raised or polypoid [14].

Diagnosis. The commonest tumours of the anal margin are virus warts, which are distinguished by their multiplicity, their lack of induration and ulceration, and their rapid evolution. Rarely these may give rise to anal carcinoma [15]. Syphilitic condylomas are also multiple and not indurated. A syphilitic chancre of the anal margin or canal may be more easily mistaken for carcinoma. Amoebiasis and tuberculosis must also be considered.

Treatment. Surgical excision of the tumour, and of the inguinal lymph nodes when these are involved, is the treatment of choice. For small, well-differentiated tumours, particularly adenocarcinomas, a local excision and repair is ideal. Small squamous and basal cell carcinomas also respond well to irradiation. More extensive lesions require abdominoperineal excision. In all cases, obsessive follow-up is necessary to detect lymph-node metastases before they become fixed. Tumours which are too advanced for surgery may respond to palliative radiotherapy.

Extramammary Paget's disease (Chapter 36)

Seventy-three percent of cases present as pruritus ani [16]. There is disagreement on how often a careful search will reveal an underlying cancer. Two reviews of the literature revealed only a 25% association [3,17]. Despite this, a search for a primary adenocarcinoma of underlying secretory glands should be carried out in perianal Paget's disease. In some cases, the primary tumour is an anorectal, or even more distant, carcinoma [18,19]. The primary tumour and the Paget's cells in the epidermis are usually mucus secreting. In some cases, electron microscopy shows the Paget's cells to be squamous in character, but more recent immunohistochemical and enzyme histochemical methods have demonstrated a close relationship between Paget's cells and sweat-gland epithelial cells [20]. In all cases of perianal Paget's disease, a careful search for a primary tumour must be made [21]. Anorectal carcinomas may arise from rectal mucosa or from the intramuscular glands. In the latter case, the malignant cells may track to the buttock through the ischiorectal fossa, and the Paget's plaque may begin at a distance from the anal margin, rather like an ischiorectal abscess. Topographic studies have shown that the plaque of Paget's disease is much larger than the visible lesion [22]. Any attempt at removal must be radical and histologically controlled [23].

Extensive surgery in conjunction with photodynamic therapy involving infusion of dihaematoporphyrin and an argon pumped dye laser has been effective in curing a patient with previous postoperative recurrences [24].

The pattern of the intramuscular glands and of the wide range of tumours which arise from them ('cloacogenic' carcinoma) resembles genitourinary rather than intestinal endothelium [25]. The carcinoma may spread, either to involve the anorectal mucosa, or through the perianal tissue to produce a chronic fistula *in ano* [26]. It may on occasion mimic a basal cell carcinoma both in clinical and histological appearance [27].

REFERENCES

1 South LM, O'Sullivan JP, Gazet JC. Giant condylomata of Buschke and Löwenstein. *Clin Oncol* 1977; **3**: 107–15.
2 Sturm JT, Christenson CE, Vecker JH *et al.* Squamous cell carcinoma of the anus arising in a giant condyloma acuminatum. *Dis Colon Rectum* 1975; **18**: 147–51.
3 Mohs FE, Blanchard I. Microscopically controlled surgery for extramammary Paget's disease. *Arch Dermatol* 1979; **115**: 706–8.
4 Lloyd KM. Multicentre pigmented Bowen's disease of the groin. *Arch Dermatol* 1970; **101**: 48–51.
5 Wade TR, Kopf AW, Ackerman AB. Bowenoid papulosis of the genitalia. *Arch Dermatol* 1979; **115**: 306–8.
6 Franklin EW, Rutledge FD. Epidemiology of epidermoid carcinoma of the vulva. *Obstet Gynecol* 1972; **39**: 165–72.
7 Reynolds VH, Madden JJ, Franlin JD *et al.* Preservation of anal function after total excision of the anal mucosa for Bowen's disease. *Ann Surg* 1984; **199**: 563–8.
8 Boman B, Moertel CG, O'Connell MJ. Carcinoma of the anal canal. *Cancer* 1984; **54**: 114–25.
9 Serota AI, Weil M, Williams RA. Anal cloacogenic carcinoma. *Arch Surg* 1981; **116**: 456–9.
10 Frisch M, Melbye M, Moller H. Trends in incidence of anal cancer in Denmark. *Br Med J* 1993; **306**: 419–22.
11 Slater G, Greenstein A, Aufses A. Anal carcinoma in patients with Crohn's disease. *Ann Surg* 1984; **199**: 348–50.
12 Cantril ST, Green JP, Schall GL. Primary radiation therapy in the treatment of anal carcinoma. *Radiol Oncol Biol Physiol* 1983; **9**: 1271–8.
13 Chang F, Kosunen O, Kosma VM *et al.* Verrucous carcinoma of the anus containing human papilloma virus type 16 DNA detected by *in situ* hybridisation. *Genitourin Med* 1990; **66**: 342–5.
14 Stearns MW, Urmacher C, Sternberg SS. Cancer of the anal canal. *Curr Probl Cancer* 1980; **4**: 1–44.
15 Goodman P, Halpert RD. Invasive squamous cell carcinoma of the anus arising in condyloma acuminatum: CT demonstration. *Gastrointest Radiol* 1991; **16**: 267–70.
16 Jensen SL, Sjolin KE, Shokouh-Amiri MH. Paget's disease of the anal margin. *Br J Surg* 1988; **75**: 1089–92.
17 Breen JL, Smith CI, Gregori CA. Extramammary Paget's disease. *Clin Obstet Gynecol* 1978; **21**: 1107–15.
18 Fetherston WC, Friedrich EG. The origin and significance of vulvar Paget's disease. *Obstet Gynecol* 1972; **39**: 735–44.
19 Helwig EB, Graham JH. Anogenital (extramammary) Paget's disease: a clinicopathological study. *Cancer* 1963; **16**: 387–403.
20 Hamm H, Vroom TM, Czarnetski BM. Extramammary Paget's cells: further evidence of sweat gland derivation. *J Am Acad Dermatol* 1986; **15**: 1275–81.
21 van der Putte SCK, van Gorp LHM. Adenocarcinoma of the mammary-like glands of the vulva: a unifying concept. *J Cutan Pathol* 1994; **21**: 157–63.
22 Gunn RA, Gallagher S. Vulvar Paget's disease: a topographic study. *Cancer* 1980; **46**: 590–4.
23 Coldiron BM, Goldsmith BA, Robinson JK. Surgical treatment of extramammary Paget's disease. *Cancer* 1991; **67**: 933–8.
24 Petrelli NJ, Cebollero JA, Rodriguez-Bigas M *et al.* Photodynamic therapy in the management of neoplasms of the perianal skin. *Arch Surg* 1992; **127**: 1436–8.
25 Grenvalsky HT, Helwig EB. Carcinoma of the anorectal junction. I. Histological considerations. *Cancer* 1956; **19**: 480–8.
26 Zeinberg VH, Kays S. Anorectal carcinomas of extramucosal origin. *Ann Surg* 1957; **145**: 344–54.
27 Espana A, Redondo P, Idoate MA *et al.* Perianal basal cell carcinoma. *Clin Exp Dermatol* 1992; **17**: 360–2.

The male genitalia

Introduction

The difference between the circumcised and uncircumcised penile skin causes differences in the incidence and appearance of dermatoses of the glans and corona. A long prepuce and poor hygiene predispose to infection and carcinoma, particularly in elderly people. Psoriasis of the exposed glans is easily recognized, but loses its habitual scaling when covered. The deep fold formed by the junction of the prepuce and the penis behind the corona is subject to maceration from epithelial debris and glandular secretion, and is a common site of infection.

Pilosebaceous units are absent on the penis except, sparsely, on the proximal part of the body. On the corona and in its sulcus, modified sebaceous glands—the preputial glands—secrete a fatty substance wrongly believed to be the chief source of smegma, which is mostly derived from desquamating epithelial cells. Free sebaceous (Tyson's) glands open directly onto the surface. Apocrine and eccrine glands are abundant, but there is great variation in the amount of their secretion. The median raphe may be the site of infections, notably gonococcal [1,2].

The rugose and apparently thick skin of the scrotum allows excellent penetration of topical agents. Carcinogens such as soot and tar also penetrate more readily.

The penile and scrotal skin easily become contaminated by urine and urethral discharges; contact with the female genitalia allows cross-infection with sexually transmitted diseases.

The proximity of deep skin folds encourages moisture and maceration. The influence of social customs such as tight clothing and contraceptives add hazards in sophisticated communities. The freedom from photodermatitis is occasionally of diagnostic value.

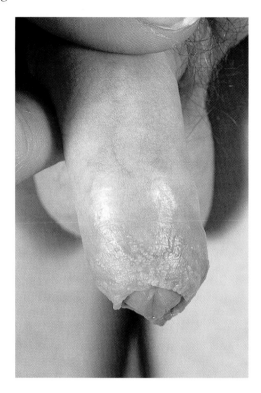

Fig. 72.7 Prominent sebaceous glands on the penis.

REFERENCES

1 Johnson HD, Thin RNT. Disease of the median raphe of the penis. Report of two cases. *Br J Vener Dis* 1972; **49**: 467–8.
2 Sowmini CN, Vijayalakshmi K, Chellamuthiah C *et al*. Infections of the median raphe of the penis: report of three cases. *Br J Vener Dis* 1972; **49**: 469–74.

Developmental and congenital lesions

The more severe embryological and developmental defects will not present to dermatologists. However, they see minor abnormalities affecting the median raphe [1]. Cysts of various types occur here, particularly at the penoscrotal junction or arising from the dysembryonic diverticula of the urethra. These canals may be lined with non-keratinizing clear cells [2]. Occasionally, mixed keratinizing and urethroid epithelia are seen [3]. If they become infected in later life, they are apt to be misdiagnosed [4]. Angiomas, lymphangiomas [5] and lipomas occasionally occur. Unduly profuse or enlarged sebaceous glands of the shaft are often a cause of anxiety to the patient (Fig. 72.7). Ectopic pilosebaceous elements causing naevus comedonicus on the glans have been reported [6]. Syringomas, rare on the genitalia, may present as papular lesions limited to the penis [7]. Nodular hidradenoma (apocrine hidrocystoma) has occurred as a slow-growing tumefaction of the prepuce [8,9]. Multiple calcifying cysts of presumed syringomatous origin have been described [10].

REFERENCES

1 Sowmini CN, Vijayalakshmi K, Chellamuthiah C *et al*. Infections of the median raphe of the penis: report of three cases. *Br J Vener Dis* 1972; **49**: 469–74.
2 Civatte J, Morel P, Bouhanna P. Canal dysembryoplasique de la verge de revelation tardive. *Ann Dermatol Vénéréol* 1982; **109**: 84–5.
3 Claudy AL, Dutoit M, Boucheron S. Epidermal and urethroid penile cyst. *Acta Derm Venereol (Stockh)* 1991; **71**: 61–2.
4 Dupre A, Lassere J, Christol B *et al*. Canaux et kystes dysembryoplasiques du raphe genitoperineal. *Ann Dermatol Vénéréol* 1982; **109**: 81–4.
5 Tsur H, Urson S, Schewach-Millet M. Lymphangioma circumscriptum of the glans penis. *Cutis* 1981; **28**: 642–3.
6 Abdel-A' Al H, Abdel-Azziz AHM. Nevus comedonicus: report of three cases localized on glans penis. *Acta Derm Venereol (Stockh)* 1975; **55**: 78–80.
7 Zalla JA, Perry HO. An unusual case of syringoma. *Arch Dermatol* 1971; **103**: 215–17.
8 Ahmed A, Jones AW. Apocrine cystadenoma. Report of two cases occurring on the prepuce. *Br J Dermatol* 1969; **81**: 899–901.
9 Dé Delanto F, Armijo-Morens M, Martinez FC. Hidradenoma nodulaire (cyst-adenoma apocrine) du penis. *Ann Dermatol Syphiligr* 1973; **100**: 417–22.
10 Katoh N, Okabayashi K, Wakabyashi S *et al*. Dystrophic calcinosis of penis. *J Dermatol* 1993; **20**: 114–17.

Traumatic lesions

The more bizarre forms of self-inflicted or experimental traumatic lesions of the penis rarely present to the dermatologist. However, unusual or unexpected manifestations or artefacts may deceive the unwary. Recurrent or necrotic lesions without evident cause should always be suspect. Ecchymosis may be marked, sometimes tracking back down the median raphe [1]. Traumatic urethral diverticula may be present as soft, compressible, nodulocystic lesions at the site of the penile shaft [2]. They must be distinguished from inclusion cysts, lipomas, lymphangiomas and epithelial tumours. Penile nodules [3] due to the self-insertion of glass beads [4,5] may be mobile and inert, but can cause confusion when associated with other inflammatory penile disorders [6]. Injection of silicone or oil often causes granulomas [5,7]. 'Hair coil strangulation' of the penis owing to the mother's hair encircling the penis (usually after circumcision) [8] causes fistulae or gangrene. Mechanical avulsion has also been noted [9]. Fracture of the penis can occur, with a loud crack, during intercourse. Over 80 cases have been reported in the English literature [10,11].

Zip-fastener and vacuum-cleaner injuries are less common than previously. The role of trauma in penile thrombosis and non-venereal sclerosing lymphangitis is discussed below.

New surgical operations for vascular impotence can involve arterialization of the dorsal vein of the penis producing penile hyperaemia and occasionally ulceration of the glans [12].

'Penile venereal oedema'

This condition occurs within a few hours of intercourse, and affects the shaft and the mucosal surface of the prepuce of circumcised patients. It is attributed to 'non-cooperating partners' with no vaginal secretion. Twenty-five cases were seen in 5 years [13].

REFERENCES

1 Johnson HW, Thin RNT. Disease of the median raphe of the penis. Report of two cases. *Br J Vener Dis* 1972; **49**: 467–8.
2 Maged A. Urethral diverticula in males (with a report of eight cases). *Br J Urol* 1969; **37**: 560–8.
3 Nitidandhaprabhas P. Artificial penile nodules: case reports from Thailand. *Br J Urol* 1975; **47**: 463.
4 Cohen EL, Kim S-W. Subcutaneous artificial penile nodules. *J Urol* 1982; **127**: 135.
5 Datta NS, Kern FB. Silicone granuloma of the penis. *J Urol* 1973; **109**: 840–2.
6 Wolf P, Kerl H. Artificial penile nodules and secondary syphilis. *Genitourin Med* 1991; **67**: 247–9.
7 Stewart RC, Beason ES, Hayes CW. Granulomas of the penis from self-injection with oils. *Plast Reconstr Surg* 1979; **64**: 108–11.
8 Bashir AY, El-Barbary M. Hair coil strangulation of the penis. *J R Coll Surg* 1979; **25**: 47–51.
9 Serrano Ortega S, Sánchez Hurtado G, Dulanto Campos MC *et al.* Avulsion complete de piel de pene. *Actas Dermo Sifilogr* 1980; **71**: 381–2.
10 Davies DM, Mitchell I. Fracture of the penis. *Br J Urol* 1978; **50**: 426.
11 Goh SH, Trapnell JE. Fracture of the penis. *Br J Surg* 1980; **67**: 680–1.
12 Eichmann A, Krahenbuhl A, Hauri D. Post-operative hyperemia of the glans penis with ulcers following revascularization surgery for vascular impotence. *Dermatology* 1992; **184**: 291–3.
13 Canby JP, Wilde H. Penile venereal edema. *N Engl J Med* 1973; **289**: 108.

Penile manifestations of common diseases [1]

Fixed drug eruptions cause recurrent erythematous or bullous lesions. Their rapidity of onset and cyclical pattern are charac-teristic. Other drugs produce severe erythema multiforme-like eruptions of the genital and oral mucosa. Lichen planus

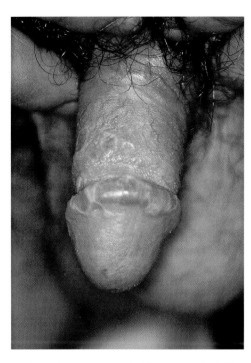

Fig. 72.8 Lichen planus of the penis. (Courtesy of Dr S. Yoganathan, Victoria, Australia.)

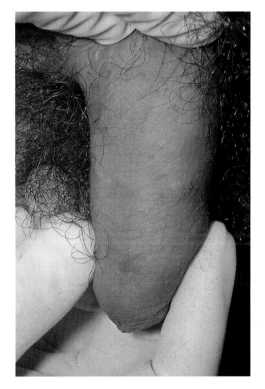

Fig. 72.9 Scabetic papules on the penis. (Courtesy of Dr C. White, Dryburn Hospital, Durham, UK.)

(Fig. 72.8) affects the shaft or glans as multiple, papular, annular or erosive lesions [2], which may even cause phimosis [3]. Lichen nitidus involved the penis in nine out of 43 cases [4]. Psoriasis in the uncircumcised may resemble erythroplasia or plasma cell balanitis. However, confirmatory lesions elsewhere or nail dystrophy are usually present. The tumid pruritic papules of scabies are pathognomonic (Fig. 72.9). They may persist after other lesions have been eradicated.

Granuloma annulare is rare on the penis, and can be confused with annular syphilide [5,6].

The penis is involved in flexural and seborrhoeic forms of eczema, although less markedly than the scrotum and groins. Patches of exudative discoid and lichenoid dermatitis (Chapter 17) may affect the shaft or glans in middle-aged or elderly Jews, and are sometimes the initial presentation.

Overtreatment of common conditions with powerful topical corticosteroids may produce a dusky erythema of the glans and prepuce ('purple penis'), or atrophic striae and increased visibility of blood vessels on the shaft [7].

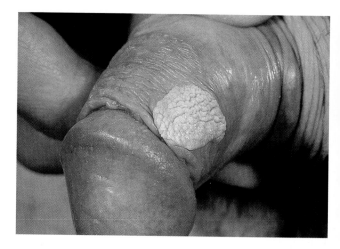

Fig. 72.10 Condyloma acuminatum on the penis.

REFERENCES

1 Coldiron B, Jacobson C. Common penile lesions. *Urol Clin North Am* 1988; **15**: 671–85.
2 Schmitt EC, Pigatto PD, Boneschi V *et al*. Erosiver lichen planus der glans penis. *Hautartz* 1993; **44**: 43–5.
3 Itin P, Hirsbrunner P, Buchner S. Lichen planus: an unusual cause of phimosis. *Acta Dermatologica* 1992; **72**: 41–2.
4 Lapins NA, Willoughby C, Helwig EB. Lichen nitidus. A study of 43 cases. *Cutis* 1978; **21**: 634–7.
5 Hillman RJ, Waldren S, Walker MM *et al*. Granuloma annulare of the penis. *Genitourin Med* 1992; **68**: 47–9.
6 Jain HC, Fischer BK. Annular syphilide mimicking granuloma annulare. *Int J Dermatol* 1988; **27**: 340–1.
7 Stankler L. Striae of the penis. *Br J Dermatol* 1982; **107**: 371–2.

Infective conditions

Early primary syphilis in the prechancre state (Chapter 30), and the erythematous and papular forms of secondary syphilis, although rare, must not be overlooked. Condylomata lata may occur, with fissures and erosions of the coronal sulcus or the free margin of the prepuce, or with papulosquamous lesions of the shaft. The late annular syphilide resembles sarcoidosis or granuloma annulare, and is differentiated only by histology. The presence of a hard penile circumferential fold at the coronal sulcus has been described as a presentation of primary syphilis [1]. Gonococcal lesions may confuse the unwary.

Condylomata acuminata (Chapter 26)

These affect the coronal sulcus (Fig. 72.10), the preputial border and the urethral orifice, sometimes extending within the urethra. They present as soft, velvety, hyperplastic or sessile lesions at sites that are probably determined by microtrauma. The incubation period in 332 patients who developed condylomas after intercourse was 2–3 months [2].

The common classical condylomatous genital warts have been shown to be usually caused by HPV-6, -11 and -16. It is increasingly recognized that cervical intraepithelial neoplasia (CIN) in females is associated with HPV-16, -18, -31, -33 and -35. This group are now regarded as 'high risk' by virtue of their ability to produce dysplastic changes on histological examination [3]. One study has shown that 75% of 25 women were infected by the same type of wart virus as their sexual partner, and that 36% of the group had cervical abnormalities [4].

In men, using colposcopy techniques, subclinical HPV infections of the penis and urethra were discovered in the majority of partners of females both with cervical dysplasia and cervical infection [5–7].

It is recommended that, as in other sexually transmissible disorders, both partners should be examined, and that examination of the male should include the use of acetic acid and some form of magnification technique to identify abnormal sites for biopsy [8]. In a large survey of 478 patients with genital warts attending a special treatment centre, 61% of the women and 32% of the men had another genital infection [9]. The author of the survey stressed the importance of recognizing and dealing with these associated infections, especially *Candida vaginale*, *Neisseria gonorrhoea* and *Trichomonas vaginalis* in order to reduce the moist conditions favourable for wart proliferation.

Despite its toxicity and potential oncogenicity, podophyllin, applied carefully and sparingly, probably remains the first choice of treatment, except in any woman suspected of being pregnant. However, 50% or more patients failed to respond in one trial [10], and only 22% cleared in another [11]. 5-fluorouracil (1% in ethanol) is an alternative [12]. Colchicine has also been used [13]. Purified podophyllotoxin is now available for self-application in males with genital warts. A controlled trial involving 109 males produced an 82%

clearance (versus 13% in controls) after 6 weeks [14]. Cryo-therapy or electrocautery may be required in severe or resistant cases [11]. A technique of cutting off the condylomas to skin level is becoming favoured, as it destroys less normal tissue. Four-fifths of 75 patients treated in this way cleared with one operative procedure, and had little postoperative discomfort [15]. Anal lesions may be concealed, and were the main cause of recurrence. Laser therapy is now an alternative treatment method [16].

Giant condyloma acuminatum

SYN. BUSCHKE–LÖWENSTEIN TUMOUR

This form of condyloma grows relentlessly, and is resistant to topical therapy such as podophyllin. The surface is hard, unlike the exuberant 'cauliflower-like' form of a large condyloma [17]. Although more common in the perianal area or groin [18], it may affect the coronal sulcus, especially in the uncircumcised. Infiltration and penetration of the tumour are characteristic, producing fistulae and sinuses. Histologically, the very acanthotic epithelium forms club-shaped rete ridges. Epidermal cells may show perinuclear halos or hyperchromasia. Viral bodies are not seen, but this may be because the viral material becomes incorporated into the genetic material of the cell [19].

Although metastases are rare, its invasive nature has prompted some workers to regard it as a true carcinoma. Others have compared it with verrucous carcinoma and florid oral papillomatosis [20]. The occurrence of this tumour following renal transplantation emphasizes the importance of ablating all genital warts prior to the introduction of immunosuppressive therapy [21].

Treatment is usually surgical, although aggressive cryo-therapy [11], bleomycin [22] and interferon [23–26] have been used with success.

REFERENCES

1 Goldstein AMB, Fox JN. The hard penile circumferential fold as the presenting finding in primary syphilis: report of six cases. *J Am Acad Dermatol* 1992; **26**: 700–3.
2 Oriel JD. Natural history of genital warts. *Br J Vener Dis* 1971; **47**: 1–13.
3 Lowhagen GB, Bolmstedt A, Ryd W *et al.* The prevalence of 'high risk' HPV types in penile condyloma-like lesions: correlation between HPV type and morphology. *Genitourin Med* 1993; **69**: 87–90.
4 Campion MJ, Singer A, Clarkson PK *et al.* Increased risk of cervical neoplasia in consorts of men with penile condylomata acuminata. *Lancet* 1985; **i**: 943–6.
5 Boon ME, Schneider A, Hogewoning CJA *et al.* Penile studies and heterosexual partners. *Cancer* 1988; **61**: 1652–9.
6 Campion MJ, McCance DJ, Mitchell HS *et al.* Subclinical penile human papilloma virus infection and dysplasia in consorts of women with cervical neoplasia. *Genitourin Med* 1988; **64**: 90–9.
7 Schneider A, Kirchmayr R, De Villers E-M *et al.* Subclinical human papilloma virus infection in male partners of female carriers. *J Urol* 1988; **140**: 1431–4.
8 Sand PK, Bowen LW, Blischke SO *et al.* Evaluation of male consorts of women with genital human papilloma virus infection. *Obstet Gynecol* 1986; **68**: 679–81.

9 Kinghorn GR. Genital warts: incidence of associated genital infections. *Br J Dermatol* 1978; **99**: 405–9.
10 Von Krogh G. Topical treatment of penile condylomata acuminata with podo-phyllin, podophyllotoxin and colchicine: a comparative study. *Acta Derm Venereol (Stockh)* 1978; **58**: 163–8.
11 Simmons PD, Langlet F, Thin RNT. Cryotherapy versus electrocautery in the treatment of genital warts. *Br J Vener Dis* 1981; **57**: 273–4.
12 Von Krogh G. The beneficial effect of 1% 5-fluorouracil in 70% ethanol on therapeutically refractory condylomas in the preputial cavity. *Sex Transm Dis* 1978; **5**: 137–40.
13 Von Krogh G, Ruden A-K. Topical treatment of penile condylomata acumin-ata with colchicine at 48–72 hour intervals. *Acta Derm Venereol (Stockh)* 1980; **60**: 87–9.
14 Beutner KR, Conant MA, Friedman-Kien AE *et al.* Patient applied podofilox for treatment of genital warts. *Lancet* 1989; **i**: 831–4.
15 Thomson JPS, Grace RH. The treatment of perianal and anal condylomata acuminata: a new operative technique. *J R Soc Med* 1978; **71**: 180–5.
16 Bar-Am A, Shilon M, Peyser MR *et al.* Treatment of male genital condyloma-tous lesions by carbon dioxide laser after failure of previous non-laser methods. *J Am Acad Dermatol* 1991; **24**: 87–9.
17 Marshescu S, Braun-Falco O, Konz B. Communications sur les dermatoses précancéreuses. *Bull Soc Fr Dermatol Syphiligr* 1975; **83**: 293–4.
18 Eng AM, Morgan NE, Blekys I. Giant condyloma acuminatum. *Cutis* 1979; **24**: 203–6, 209.
19 Doutre M-S, Beylot C, Bioulac P *et al.* Tumeur de Buschke-Löwenstein: 2 cas feminins. *Ann Dermatol Vénéréol* 1979; **106**: 1031–4.
20 Hughes PSH. Cryosurgery of verrucous carcinoma of the penis (Buschke–Löwenstein tumor). *Cutis* 1979; **24**: 43–5.
21 Domingues JC, Sereijo M, Couto JC *et al.* Buschke–Löwenstein tumour in a renal transplant recipient. *Skin Cancer* 1994; **9**: 27–32.
22 Puissant A, Pringuet R, Noory JY *et al.* Condylome acumine geant (syndrome de Buschke–Löwenstein). Action de la bléomycine. *Bull Soc Fr Dermatol Syphiligr* 1975; **79**: 9–12.
23 Douglas JM, Rogers M, Judson F. The effect of asymptomatic infection with HTLV III on the response of anogenital warts to intralesional treatment with alpha-2 interferon. *J Infect Dis* 1986; **154**: 331–3.
24 Eron LJ, Judson F, Tucker S. Interferon therapy for condylomata acuminata. *N Engl J Med* 1986; **315**: 1059–64.
25 Kirby PK, Kiviat N, Beckman A *et al.* Tolerance and efficacy of recombinant human interferon gamma in the treatment of refractory genital warts. *Am J Med* 1988; **85**: 183–8.
26 Zachariae H, Larsen PM, Sogaard H. Recombinant interferon alpha-2A (Roferon-A) in a case of Buschke–Löwenstein giant condyloma. *Dermatologica* 1988; **177**: 175–9.

Fungal infections

These are rare on the glans, but are documented [1,2]. The lesions, affecting the shaft, were unusual, but the inguinal or pubic areas were also involved in most cases. The incidence may be higher in tropical regions [3]. Pityriasis versicolor is more common, especially if sought using Wood's light [4]. Here also, the infection is more widespread than is at first apparent. Candidal infections are dealt with in the section on balanitis (p. 3188).

Molluscum contagiosum

This condition affects the genital and paragenital areas of infants and young adults. Solitary lesions can be confused with lymphangiomas, and multiple lesions with furuncles. Central umbilication is a characteristic distinguishing feature.

Tuberculosis

This condition was once a common complication of circumcision [5], but is now rare. Orificial tuberculosis occurs as multiple, shallow, crusted ulcers. Papulonecrotic tuberculosis may involve the penis [6]. If successive crops of lesions occur, the eventual scarring leads to a remarkable 'worm-eaten' appearance [7]. A persistent indolent chancriform lesion occurs very rarely at the coronal sulcus, secondary to tuberculosis in the spouse. It lacks the induration of a syphilitic chancre. The inguinal glands enlarge, soften, and sometimes ulcerate. A case of 'anonymous' mycobacterial infection of the glans has been reported [8].

REFERENCES

1 Dekio S, Jidoi J. Tinea of the glans penis. *Dermatologica* 1989; **178**: 112–14.
2 Pillai KG, Singh G, Sharma BM. *Trichophyton rubrum* infection of the penis. *Dermatologica* 1975; **100**: 252–4.
3 Vora NS, Dave JN, Mukhopadyay AK *et al.* Incidence of dermatophytosis of the penis and scrotum. *Indian J Dermatol Venereol Leprol* 1994; **50**: 89–91.
4 Avram A, Rousseiet G, Benazeraf C *et al.* 'Pityriasis versicolor' de la verge. *Bull Soc Fr Dermatol Syphiligr* 1973; **80**: 607–8.
5 Minkin W, Frank SB, Cohen HJ. Penile granuloma. *Arch Dermatol* 1972; **106**: 756.
6 Nishigori C, Taniguchi S, Hayakawa M *et al.* Penis tuberculides: papulonecrotic tuberculides on the glans penis. *Dermatologica* 1986; **172**: 93–7.
7 Jeyakumar W, Ganesh R, Mohanram F *et al.* Papulonecrotic tuberculids of the glans penis: case report. *Genitourin Med* 1988; **64**: 130–2.
8 Schnitzler L, Halligon J, Schubert B *et al.* Quatre cas de 'tuberculose cutanée'. Rôle possible des mycobactéries atypiques. *Bull Soc Fr Dermatol Syphiligr* 1972; **79**: 571–7.

Genital herpes [1–3]

This infection is fully discussed in Chapter 26, and genital infections in the female are dealt with on page 3217. In the UK, most cases are caused by the herpes simplex virus (HSV)-2 strain, although an increasing number are due to HSV-1.

Clinical manifestations. The primary infection usually occurs within a week of sexual exposure (including oral or anal intercourse), but occasionally after a longer interval. Asymptomatic attacks may occur in as many as half the cases [2]. Otherwise, they are usually more severe than recurrent attacks that may follow. The eruption may be preceded by prodromal symptoms, which are often misdiagnosed as influenza [3]. Clustered, tiny papules on an erythematous base develop into vesicles and rapidly break down to form superficial erosions or painful ulcers (Fig. 72.11). The glans, prepuce and fraenum are usually involved; the shaft is rarely involved. The attack lasts 2–3 weeks, but may be complicated by recrudescences [1,4], other infections or viraemic spread. Severe or anomalous forms may cause difficulty in diagnosis, especially in the immunosuppressed patient. Neurological complications include meningeal involvement and sacral radiculitis [5].

Recurrent attacks occur in 30–70% of those affected [3]. These are usually less severe and shorter lived than the

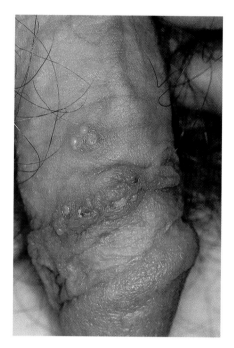

Fig. 72.11 Herpes genitalis.

primary infection. They involve the same or an adjacent area, and may be preceded by prodromal malaise, aching, peculiar pricking sensations or paraesthesiae of the thighs or perineum. Subsequent attacks may involve the buttock [1]. The frequency of attacks varies, but tends to decrease in time. They may be precipitated by trauma, stress and various other events [6]. However minor, they may cause great anxiety and depression in those affected, and must be treated seriously.

Diagnosis. In the early stages, the clustered vesicular eruption is characteristic. However, later stages or anomalous manifestations invite diagnostic errors. The patient must be screened for other coexistent disease, including chancroid and candidiasis. Presence of the virus can be confirmed by electron microscopy, immunofluorescence or tissue culture. It is vital that the correct transport medium is used. The examination of a Papanicolaou-stained slide is less accurate [1]. Neutralizing or complement-fixing antibodies rise to a peak in about 3 weeks, and may be of value in confirming doubtful primary infections.

Treatment [3]. Symptomatic measures include potassium permanganate or similar soaks and mild antibacterial agents, for example colloidal iodine paint.

Oral aciclovir therapy in doses of 200 mg five times per day is superior to topical aciclovir in first-episode genital herpes [7]. Recurrent attacks of herpes will respond well to repeated courses of aciclovir, but intermittent courses appear not to influence the frequency of recurrence. Prophylactic aciclovir in doses of 400 mg twice daily for 5 years has been shown to be safe and effective [8]. Recurrence may occur after cessation of therapy, but viral resistance to aciclovir has not been encountered following long-term prophylaxis [9]. Aciclovir resistance is, however, being reported with increasing frequency in patients with AIDS. An uncontrolled trial of trisodium phosphonoformate (foscarnet) has shown considerable therapeutic benefit [10].

At one time, photoinactivation with neutral red or proflavine was fashionable, but the results were not impressive [11] and the procedure may be carcinogenic [12]. Interferon therapy is unhelpful in genital herpes [13,14].

In all cases, the patient must be counselled about sensible precautions with regard to avoiding intercourse at the time of attacks.

REFERENCES

1 Felman YM, Nikitas JA. Herpes genitalis. *Cutis* 1982; **30**: 442–56.
2 Nahmias AJ *et al.*, eds. In: *The Human Herpesviruses*. New York: Elsevier, 1981.
3 Oates JK. Genital herpes. *Br J Hosp Med* 1983; **29**: 13–22.
4 Jeansson S, Molin L. In: Danielsson D *et al.*, eds. *Proceedings of the Symposium on Genital Infections and their Complications*. Stockholm: Almquist & Wickesell, 1974: 189.
5 Oates JK, Greenhouse PR. Retention of urine in anogenital herpetic infection. *Lancet* 1978; **i**: 691–2.
6 Hill J, Blyth WA. An alternative theory of herpes-simplex recurrence and a possible role for prostaglandins. *Lancet* 1976; **i**: 397–8.
7 Kinghorn GR, Abeywickrame I, Jeavons M *et al.* Efficacy of combined treatment with oral and topical acyclovir in first episode genital herpes. *Genitourin Med* 1986; **62**: 186–8.
8 Goldberg LH, Kaufman R, Kurtz TO *et al.* Longterm suppression of recurrent genital herpes with acyclovir. *Arch Dermatol* 1993; **129**: 582–7.
9 Lehrman SN, Douglas JM, Corey L *et al.* Recurrent genital herpes and suppressive oral acyclovir therapy. *Ann Intern Med* 1986; **104**: 786–90.
10 Erlich KS, Jacobson MA, Koehler JE *et al.* Foscarnet therapy for severe acyclovir resistant herpes simplex virus type-2 infections in patients with acquired immunodeficiency syndrome. *Ann Intern Med* 1989; **110**: 710–13.
11 Kaufman RH, Adam E, Mirkovic RR *et al.* Treatment of genital herpes simplex virus infection with photodynamic inactivation. *Am J Obstet Gynecol* 1978; **132**: 861–9.
12 Berger RS, Papa CM. Photodye herpes therapy—Cassandra confirmed? *JAMA* 1977; **238**: 133–4.
13 Mendelson J, Clecner BYA, Eiley S. Effect of recombinant interferon alpha 2 on clinical course of first episode genital herpes infection and subsequent recurrences. *Genitourin Med* 1986; **62**: 97–101.
14 Shupack J, Stiller M, Davis I *et al.* Topical alpha–interferon ointment with dimethyl sulphoxide in the treatment of recurrent genital herpes. *Dermatology* 1992; **184**: 40–4.

Uncommon and miscellaneous conditions

Several non-venereal diseases affect the penis uniquely or in a distinct fashion. Mention should be made briefly of Fordyce's disease, which simulates lichen planus on the glans; granular cell myoblastoma, which characteristically has the appearance of a truncated dome [1]; neurinoma of the glans [2], and congenital os penis [3]. The term penile horn has been given to a compact tapered keratinous mass arising on areas of acanthosis or condylomas, often after excision. Twenty-five per cent have a dysplastic base, so wide excision is advised [4]. In pellagra, the penile skin may be grossly excoriated. Crohn's disease may very rarely affect the penis as well as the scrotum [5,6].

Pigmentary anomalies

Both vitiligo and occupational leukoderma may involve the scrotum [7]. Wood's light examination may reveal 'hidden' cases. Of 54 patients with occupational vitiligo, the penis or scrotum was affected in 38 [8]. Chemicals in condoms and pessaries have also been incriminated, and hypopigmented macules of the glans have been reported following recurrent gonococcal infection, presumably as a post-inflammatory phenomenon [9].

Acquired hyperpigmented macules of the glans or shaft of the penis are not uncommon [10], and are best regarded as lentigines [11], although in one case atypical histological findings suggested acral lentiginous melanoma [12]. The lesions are generally harmless, but extensive and cosmetically disfiguring pigmentation has been successfully managed by lasers [13]. A relatively recently described paediatric disorder known as the Ruvalcaba–Myhre–Smith syndrome comprises pigmented macules on the glans and penile shaft, associated with macrocephaly, hamartomatous intestinal polyps and a unique lipid storage myopathy [14].

Bullous eruptions (Chapter 40)

Pemphigus vulgaris may develop first on the penis, with

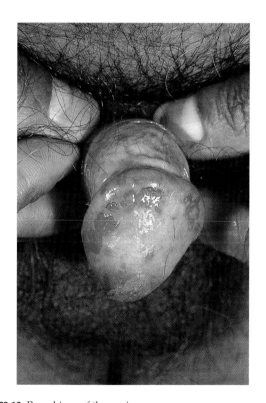

Fig. 72.12 Pemphigus of the penis.

the flaccid bullae rupturing readily to form erosions and crusts (Fig. 72.12). The diagnosis may sometimes be confirmed cytologically by Tzanck smear.

Pemphigus vegetans is exceedingly rare [15].

Pemphigoid. This is more common, and typical lesions will be present elsewhere.

Benign mucosal pemphigoid. This is rare in males, but may involve the corona or glans, in association with ocular and oral lesions. Bullae and irregular cicatrization occur, and the scarring may produce meatal stricture.

Bullous drug reactions, notably fixed drug eruptions, are suggested by acute recurrent lesions and residual pigmentation [16].

Erythema multiforme exudativum. This condition frequently involves the penis. Bullae are common.

Haemorrhagic, thick-roofed bullae may occur in the ivory-white plaques of lichen sclerosus et atrophicus.

Vegetating lesions

Condylomata acuminata become exuberant in the presence of a urethral discharge. An extensive tumour-like form of tuberculosis has been described [17]. Chronic forms of pyoderma are less common than elsewhere on the genitalia, but a fungating and vegetating response to a mixed or fusospirillary infection is seen in the uncircumcised under conditions of poor hygiene or debility. If rapid resolution does not occur with appropriate treatment, a carcinoma must be suspected. Bowen's disease may cause difficulty in diagnosis. Verruciform xanthoma, a condition most often seen in the oral cavity, has been described on the penis [18].

REFERENCES

1 Kern AB, Kaufman JJ, Combes FC. Granular cell myoblastoma: report of a case simulating granuloma inguinale. *Arch Dermatol Syphilol* 1950; **62**: 109–16.
2 Von Parr CA. Solitares neurinom der glans penis. *Dermatologica* 1968; **137**: 150–5.
3 Champion RH, Wegrzyn J. Congenital os penis. *J Urol* 1964; **91**: 663–4.
4 Willsher MK, Daley KJ, Conway JF *et al.* Penile horns. *J Urol* 1984; **132**: 1192–3.
5 Cockburn AG, Krolikowski J, Balogh K *et al.* Crohn's disease of penile and scrotal skin. *Urology* 1980; **15**: 596–8.
6 Slaney G, Muller S, Clay J *et al.* Crohn's disease involving the penis. *Gut* 1986; **27**: 329–33.
7 Moss JR, Stevenson CJ. Incidence of male genital vitiligo: report of a screening programme. *Br J Vener Dis* 1981; **57**: 145–6.
8 James O, Mayes RW, Stevenson CJ. Occupational vitiligo induced by a *p*-tert-butylphenol: a systemic disease? *Lancet* 1977; **ii**: 1217–19.
9 Gaffoor PMA. Hypopigmentation of the glans penis. *Cutis* 1983; **31**: 214.
10 Revuez J, Clerici T. Penile melanosis. *J Am Acad Dermatol* 1989; **20**: 567–70.

11 Kopf AW, Bart RS. Tumor conference 43: penile lentigo. *J Dermatol Surg Oncol* 1982; **8**: 637–9.
12 Leicht S, Youngberg G, Diaz-Miranda C. Atypical pigmented penile macules. *Arch Dermatol* 1988; **124**: 1267–70.
13 Delaney TA, Walker NPJ. Penile melanosis successfully treated with the Q switched ruby laser. *Br J Dermatol* 1994; **130**: 663–4.
14 Gretzula JC, Hevia O, Schachner LS *et al.* Ruvalcaba–Myhre–Smith syndrome. *Pediatr Dermatol* 1988; **5**: 28–32.
15 Castle WN, Wentzell JM, Schwartz BK *et al.* Chronic balanitis due to pemphigus vegetans. *J Urol* 1987; **137**: 289–91.
16 Gaffoor PMA, George WM. Fixed drug eruptions occurring on the male genitals. *Cutis* 1990; **45**: 242–4.
17 Menzel E. Diagnostische gesichtspunkte bei der penistuberkulose. *Z Urol Nephrol* 1966; **59**: 287–91.
18 Ronan SG, Bolano J, Manaligod JR. Verruciform xanthoma of penis. *Urology* 1984; **23**: 600–3.

Balanitis

Definition. Inflammation of the penile skin. Properly, the condition is called 'balanoposthitis', from 'balanitis' referring to inflammation of the glans and 'posthitis' referring to that of the mucous surface of the prepuce. 'Balanitis' is used here to describe acute and chronic forms of inflammation of the glans penis and prepuce resulting from traumatic, irritant or infective causes.

Pathogenesis [1]. There are obvious predisposing factors such as: irritation by smegma, urine, alkalis and external contacts; susceptibility to irritation from clothing, friction and trauma; a long foreskin combined with poor hygiene, and exposure to venereal and vaginal pathogens. Perhaps the most common source of moisture is a failure to dry the glans and prepuce after bathing. Bacteria, yeasts and fusospirillary organisms flourish in the moist, covered preputial sac and saprophytes may become pathogens under conditions of lowered local or general resistance. In humid climates especially, balanitis is far more common in the uncircumcised. A mixed pathogenesis is thus common, and recurrences of seemingly simple infections are often due to continuing non-specific causes of inflammation. In such cases, circumcision may effect a cure.

Irritants and pathogens are normally extraneous in origin, but occasionally derive from infected urine, faeces or perineal foci of infection or carriage. The part played by chlamydiae [2,3] and mycoplasmas [4] has been recorded.

Histopathology. There is no specific histological picture. In infective and superficial erosive forms, the features are those of inflammation, with spongiosis and a more or less intense dermal inflammatory infiltrate. Bacteria, spirochaetes, acid-fast bacilli and other pathogens are found by appropriate methods of examination or staining.

Clinical varieties of balanitis

All morphological forms of acute superficial balanitis may be grouped together, despite aetiological differences.

1 *Traumatic.* Accidental wounds and friction trauma cause erosions, fissures or localized areas of erythema and oedema. Postcoital fraenal erosions are not uncommon. 'Zip fastener' injuries lacerate the prepuce and cause haemorrhage and oedema.

2 *Irritant.* Retained smegma, poor hygiene and retained soap, detergent or inadequate drying may cause an irritant dermatitis. Contact dermatitis affects the shaft rather than the glans, except when medicaments or contraceptives are involved.

3 *Infective.* This is the common cause of balanitis.

Infective forms of balanitis

Erythema of the glans, the coronal sulcus and the inner surface of the prepuce may arise suddenly, with irritation, or develop insidiously and unnoticed by the patient. In a recent study, no specific organism was found in most cases, but 26% of 86 cases grew *Candida* species and 13% group B β-haemolytic *Streptococcus* [5].

In more acute infections, or as a result of treatment, the erythema and oedema extend widely, and phimosis may result. The involved area is red and moist. The edge is usually ill-defined. Maceration and exudation are marked in the uncircumcised. Acute infections are accompanied by offensive, creamy, purulent discharge. Secondary invasion by Vincent's organism and Gram-negative bacteria lead to erosion and ulceration. A great variety of organisms are found on culture: some are obviously pathogenic, and others are doubtfully so. In resistant or recurrent cases the sexual partner should always be examined.

Circinate erosive balanitis. This occurs as an early, short-lived, mucosal presentation of Reiter's disease.

Candidal balanitis [6,7]. *Candida albicans* can be recovered from both the vagina and, less commonly, the coronal sulcus, in the absence of clinical infection. The strains are usually the same in both partners, but it is not always possible to determine whether the source is exogenous, or endogenous from the rectum, anus or mouth. Although candidal balanitis most frequently follows intercourse with an infected partner [8,9], the pathogenicity of the organism also depends upon host factors, of which diabetes is the most important. It should be sought in any severe, persistent or unexplained case, as the balanitis may be a presenting symptom of the disease. In elderly people, it may be associated with cachexia or malignancy.

The distinguishing features include a glazed, non-purulent surface, a slightly scaling edge (in the circumcised) and satellite eroded pustules. The groins may be affected. An acute fulminating oedematous type occurs, although the typical case is mild. Microscopy and culture confirm the diagnosis, and specimens should be taken from both partners, and from the anal as well as the genital areas. It is

wise to examine the blood as well as the urine for sugar. A glucose tolerance test is indicated when there is a family history of diabetes.

An allergic reaction to *Candida* infection in the partner may account for some cases of recurrent balanitis in which burning and erythema of the glans and prepuce occur shortly after intercourse [6,8]. Cultures are negative or non-contributory in the subject, but yeasts are found in the partner.

Recurrent candidal balanitis causes fissuring of the prepuce, fibrosis and sclerosis.

Specific remedies are available for this specific form of balanitis. Both partners, if affected, should be treated concurrently. There is now a large variety of effective anticandidal agents of the polyene or imidazole type. Fluconazole is an oral alternative for severe cases. However, none of these achieves more than a 90% cure rate [6], and it is probable that intestinal or urethral reservoirs—as well as reinfection—contribute to the failure rate in the refractory 10%. The rarity of balanitis in circumcised males is one argument presented in favour of the American custom of neonatal circumcision [10].

Amoebic balanitis [11]. A severe amoebic infection leading to rupture of the prepuce and erosion of the shaft has been reported from New Guinea. *Entamoeba histolytica* was found in direct smears. Emetine or circumcision cured the patients, whose infection was thought to have been contracted through anal intercourse.

Micaceous and keratotic pseudoepitheliomatous balanitis [12]. This is a rare, curious condition in which coronal balanitis gradually takes on a silvery-white appearance, and mica-like crusts and keratotic horny masses form on the glans. There is a loss of elasticity of the prepuce and the general appearance is atrophic.

Histologically, there is extreme hyperkeratosis and pseudoepitheliomatous hyperplasia, with elongation of the rete ridges and acanthosis. It has been regarded as a form of pyodermatitis or a pseudoepitheliomatous response to infection. Another possibility is that it is a variant of lichen sclerosus. It is not considered to be malignant. Circumcision does not cure it. Topical cytotoxic agents have been used [13].

Titanium balanitis [14]. Granules of titanium have been found in skin biopsies from two patients with penile disease. In one case, phimosis and meatal stenosis occurred, but there was no histological suggestion of lichen sclerosus. The source of titanium may have been a topical preparation.

Trichomonal balanitis. This is receiving increasing recognition. It occurs as a superficial or an erosive balanitis in young subjects with trichomoniasis [15] with or without urethritis. It is more common in those with a long pre-puce. Phimosis may occur, but it responds rapidly to metro-nidazole. Occasionally, more severe lesions of chancriform type, or with penile abscesses [16], are seen.

Mycoplasma balanitis [17]. Although not yet widely recog-nized by dermatologists, it has been suggested that a balanitis may accompany mycoplasma urethritis, either as a primary infection or secondary to gonorrhoea. It responds to tetracyclines in high dose.

Chlamydial infections [13]. The D–K serotypes of *Chlamydia trachomatis* are now recognized as the cause of the commonest genital infections in the Western world [1]. L1–L3 serotypes are the cause of lymphogranuloma venereum. The clinical spectrum is still expanding. In the female especially, they may give rise to a variety of clinical diseases—salpingitis, bartholinitis, abacterial urethritis, etc. In the male, by far the most common manifestation is non-gonococcal urethritis, of which over 70000 cases are diagnosed annually in the UK [4]. In homosexual men, it is a cause of proctitis. It is important to be aware of the possibility of this infection in a patient presenting, perhaps, with a non-specific but associated irritant balanitis. The characteristic penile lesions of Reiter's syndrome may also be an indicator of *Chlamydia* infection.

Syphilitic balanitis (Follmann) [18]. This rare condition follows a primary chancre. The glans show a whitish, coalescent surface on an oedematous background. Histo-logically, the multilocular pustules are full of polymorphs, and *Treponema pallidum* is abundant in epidermal scrapings.

Non-specific spirochaetes were associated with penile ulceration in 12% of a South African series. Precise identi-fication of the species was not established, but the micro-scopic appearance suggested that they belonged to the *Borrelia* group [19].

Differential diagnosis. Fixed drug eruptions, contact derma-titis and psoriasis are most likely to cause diagnostic confusion, particularly in the uncircumcised. Aphthae and herpetic lesions are usually characteristic. Porokeratosis of Mibelli is sometimes difficult to distinguish when localized to the penis. Erythroplasia is characterized by its fixed appearance, the impression of thickness on palpation and its velvety surface.

Complications. Venereal disease may become superimposed on a damaged and eroded surface. Treatment may increase the extent of the inflammation if too vigorous, or cause sensitization if prolonged. Phimosis is common. The pecu-liar effect of quaternary ammonium derivatives is dealt with separately (p. 3194).

Necrosis and gangrene may develop in infections complicated by fusospirillary organisms.

All forms of balanitis may become chronic or relapse frequently, especially in elderly people. When this happens, the glans and prepuce gradually undergo sclerotic and fibrotic changes. The final picture is that of an obliterative balanitis.

Carcinoma may complicate long-standing irritative lesions in the uncircumcised.

Treatment. Mild forms of balanitis respond to repeated cool bathing with potassium permanganate or Burow's solution and the application of mild antibacterial creams, with or without weak corticosteroids. Hydroxyquinolines are widely used in the UK, but are conveniently replaced in many cases, even those not due to yeast infections, by the newer imidazoles, for example miconazole, with or without hydrocortisone. Topical gentamicin is sometimes of value. In persistent cases, circumcision may be curative.

REFERENCES

1 Veller Fornasa C, Calabro A, Miglietta A *et al*. Mild balanoposthitis. *Genitourin Med* 1994; **70**: 345–6.
2 Dunlop ENC. Chlamydial genital infection and its complications. *Br J Hosp Med* 1983; **29**: 6–11.
3 Oriel JD, Ridgeway GL, eds. *Current Topics in Infection—Genital Infections by Chlamydia trachomatis*. London: Edward Arnold, 1982.
4 Taylor-Robinson D, McCormack WM. The genital mycoplasmas. II. *N Engl J Med* 1980; **302**: 1063–7.
5 Abdullah AN, Drake SM, Wade AAH *et al*. Balanitis (balanoposthitis) in patients attending a department of genitourinary medicine. *Int J STD AIDS* 1992; **3**: 128–9.
6 Odds FC. Genital candidiasis. *Clin Exp Dermatol* 1982; **7**: 345–54.
7 Winner HL, Hurley R, eds. *Symposium on Candida Infections*. Edinburgh: Churchill Livingstone, 1966.
8 Catterall RD. In: Winner HL, Hurley R, eds. *Symposium on Candida Infections*. Edinburgh: Churchill Livingstone, 1966: 113.
9 Rohatiner JJ. In: Winner HL, Hurley R, eds. *Symposium on Candida Infections*. Edinburgh: Churchill Livingstone, 1966: 118.
10 Fakjian N, Hunter S, Cole GW *et al*. An argument for circumcision. *Arch Dermatol* 1990; **126**: 1046–7.
11 Cooke RA, Rodriguez RB. Amoebic balanitis. *Med J Aust* 1964; **5**: 114–17.
12 Civatte J, Lortat-Jacob E. Balanite pseudo-épithéliomateuse, kératosique et micacée. *Bull Soc Fr Dermatol Syphiligr* 1966; **68**: 164–7.
13 Fleck F, Fleck M, eds. *Organische w. Funktionelle Sexualerkran krungen*. Berlin: Verlag und Gesundheit, 1974.
14 Dundas SAC, Laing RW. Titanium balanitis with phimosis. *Dermatologica* 1988; **176**: 305–7.
15 Michalowski R. Balano-posthites a trichomonas: a propos de 16 observations. *Ann Dermatol Vénéréol* 1981; **108**: 731–8.
16 Duperrat B, Carton F-X. Balanite et abces de la verge à trichomonas. *Bull Soc Fr Dermatol Syphiligr* 1969; **76**: 345.
17 Siboulet A, Catalant F, Deubel M. Balanites et 'mycoplasma'. *Bull Soc Fr Dermatol Syphilol* 1975; **82**: 419–22.
18 Leyjman K, Starzycki Z. Syphilitic balanitis of Follmann developing after the appearance of the primary chancre. A case report. *Br J Vener Dis* 1975; **51**: 138–40.
19 Piot P, Duncan M, van Dyck E *et al*. Ulcerative balanoposthitis associated with non-syphilitic spirochaetal infection. *Genitourin Med* 1986; **62**: 44–6.

Plasma-cell balanitis [1–3]
SYN. ZOON'S BALANITIS, PSEUDO-ERYTHROPLASTIC BALANITIS [4]

Despite the paucity of case reports, this distinctive condition is not excessively rare. Its characteristic features allow ready recognition. It presents in middle-aged or elderly uncircumcised men as one or more indolent circumscribed plaques, almost always on the glans [2], which remain localized indefinitely. The surface is shiny and smooth, reddish brown in colour (Fig. 72.13) and occasionally eroded, in contrast with the velvety appearance of erythroplasia, with which it may be confused. The surface is slightly moist, giving the impression of 'incompletely dried varnish' [4], and is stippled with minute red specks—the 'cayenne pepper' spots. It is important to verify the diagnosis by biopsy.

Histology. Histologically, the changes are also distinctive [2,5]. The epidermis is attenuated, and the horny and granular layers are absent. Individual suprabasal keratinocytes are diamond shaped ('lozenge keratinocytes' [6]). Occasional dyskeratotic cells are seen, but there is no atypia. The intercellular spaces are widened ('watery spongiosis'). The dense, band-like, mixed dermal infiltrate usually contains more than 50% plasma cells, although these are sometimes less numerous [1,6]. Vertically or obliquely orientated vascular proliferation, haemosiderin deposition and free extravasated erythrocytes complete the characteristic pattern.

Variants. Dupre *et al.* [7] have described a variant showing fleshy buds and erosions. A rare vegetating form also occurs. Jonquieres and de Lutzky [4], who also include variants with marked dermal oedema and a predominantly lymphocyte infiltrate, prefer to avoid the name 'plasma cell' for what they consider to be a spectrum of different stages of the same process [8].

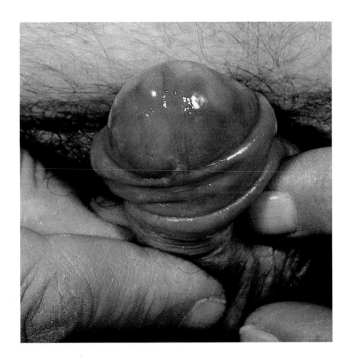

Fig. 72.13 Plasma-cell balanitis.

Aetiology. The aetiology of plasma-cell balanitis remains unclear. It is best regarded as a persistent chronic form of balanitis. Immunological studies [5] in four cases suggested that IgA found in the lesions might be secreted by the infiltrate as a reflection of its mucosal situation. However, in an immunohistochemical study, IgG-producing plasma cells were found to predominate over IgA-positive cells. The plasma-cell reactivity was identical to that found in plasma-cell infiltrates associated with malignant and premalignant skin lesions elsewhere on the body [9].

An IgE-secreting Zoon's balanitis has been described more recently, indicating perhaps that the secretions of the involved plasma cells may be purely fortuitous rather than indicative [10].

Treatment. Topical corticosteroids are not very helpful. Gentamicin may be of benefit. Circumcision is often curative [2,11]. Carbon dioxide laser therapy has its advocates [12].

REFERENCES

1 Bureau Y, Barriere H, Evin Y-P. Les erythroplasies benignes a plasmocytes. *Ann Dermatol Syphiligr* 1962; **89**: 271–84.
2 Souteyrand P, Wong E, MacDonald DM. Zoon's balanitis (balanitis circumscripta plasma cellularis). *Br J Dermatol* 1981; **105**: 195–9.
3 Zoon JJ. Balanoposthite chronique circonscrite benigne a plasmocytes. *Dermatologica* 1952; **105**: 1–7.
4 Jonquieres EDL, De Lutzky FK. Balanitis et vulvites pseudo-erythroplasiques chroniques. *Ann Dermatol Vénéréol* 1980; **107**: 173–80.
5 Dupre A, Bonafe J-L, Castel M. Etude immuno-pathologique de 4 cas de balano-posthite de Zoon. *Ann Dermatol Vénéréol* 1981; **108**: 691–6.
6 Wong E, Souteyrand P, MacDonald DM. Zoon's balanitis (balanitis circumscripta plasma cellularis). *Br J Dermatol* 1981; **105** (Suppl. 19): 28–9 (Abstract).
7 Dupre A, Bonafé JL, Lassere J *et al.* Lésions bourgeonnantes préputiales à plasmocytes: variante anatomo-clinique de la balano-posthite chronique circonscrite bénigne de Zoon. *Bull Soc Fr Dermatol Syphiligr* 1976; **83**: 62–3.
8 Jonquieres EDL. Balanitis pseudoeritroplasicas. *Arch Argent Dermatol* 1971; **21**: 85–95.
9 Toonstra J, Can Wichen DF. Immunohistochemical characterization of plasma cells in Zoon's balanoposthitis and (pre)malignant skin lesions. *Dermatologica* 1986; **172**: 77–81.
10 Nishimura M, Matsuda T, Muto M *et al.* Balanitis of Zoon. *Int J Dermatol* 1990; **29**: 421–3.
11 Ferrandiz C, Ribera M. Zoon's balanitis treated by circumcision. *J Dermatol Surg Oncol* 1984; **10**: 622–5.
12 Baldwin HE, Geronemus RG. The treatment of Zoon's balanitis with the carbon dioxide laser. *J Dermatol Surg Oncol* 1989; **15**: 491–4.

Lichen sclerosus et atrophicus

SYN. BALANITIS XEROTICA OBLITERANS

The old term 'balanitis xerotica obliterans' is probably best discarded because it merely refers to an anatomical situation, similar to 'kraurosis vulvae'. It is still used, however, as a descriptive term by surgeons and others. Most dermatologists believe that almost all cases are due to lichen sclerosus et atrophicus [1,2], although very occasionally other fibrosing or synechial pathological entities such as severe mucosal pemphigoid or very chronic

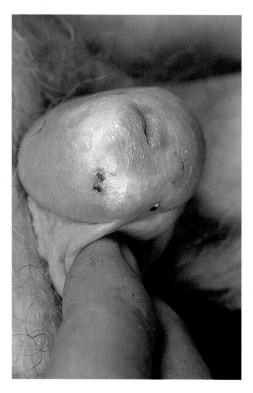

Fig. 72.14 Lichen sclerosus et atrophicus. White plaques and haemorrhagic areas on the glans. (Courtesy of Dr D.A. Burns, Leicester Royal Infirmary, UK.)

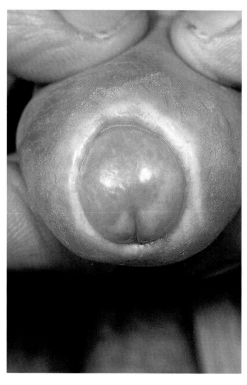

Fig. 72.15 Lichen sclerosus et atrophicus causing phimosis. (Courtesy of Dr D.A. Burns, Leicester Royal Infirmary, UK.)

balanoposthitis may lead to a similar picture. The term 'cicatricial balanitis' is preferable for these other entities.

Definition and aetiology. This is dealt with fully in Chapter 58. Females are affected far more frequently than males [2], although many cases in men are unrecorded or undiagnosed. There is some evidence that the disease has an autoimmune basis. Patients have an increased incidence of autoimmune disorders [3,4]; vitiligo or alopecia areata were or had been present in five out of 25 males in one report [5], and a higher than expected incidence of autoantibodies is found in patients and their relatives [3–5]. However, the results of two studies employing human leukocyte antigen (HLA) typing have been conflicting. In one series of 50 females, HLA-B40 was found to have an increased frequency [6], but in a larger series of 120 patients [7] there was no statistically significant difference from the frequencies found in 8837 random individuals typed in the UK. This suggests that the relationship may not be very strong, at least in males.

Histopathology (Chapter 58). In a biochemical, ultrastructural and immunological study [8], the few elastic fibres present in the superficial dermis were abnormal, and there was a loss of antigenicity of macromolecules in the homogenized zone of collagen. There were no significant biochemical abnormalities. It was not possible to demonstrate a supposed overactivity of elastase.

Clinical features. Although usually a disease of young men, it may occur in childhood and adolescence rather more frequently than is recognized, as its early stages are readily overlooked, and it is not an uncommon cause for circumcision in boys of 5–11 years and above [9,10]. There are three forms of presentation. The patient may recognize typical ivory-white macules or confluent plaques on the glans (Fig. 72.14), or become alarmed at the appearance of a haemorrhagic bulla (often after intercourse), sometimes leading to blood-stained urine if it is situated on the meatus. Alternatively, the condition may be confined to the meatus itself and the adjacent perimeatal mucosa, leading him to present to a surgeon because of difficulty in micturition. The smooth, white appearance of the contracted meatal orifice, and often the surrounding atrophic meatal collar, are distinctive. In other cases, the changes preferentially involve the preputial area, leading to progressive stenosis and eventually phimosis (Fig. 72.15). The shaft is rarely involved.

In Wallace's large series [2], half the patients had been circumcised. The glans was ultimately affected in all; only two cases involved the shaft alone. Meatal lesions were present in half the cases, but meatal strictures were uncommon.

Lesions of lichen sclerosus et atrophicus elsewhere are less frequent than in the female, but should be sought.

Course and prognosis. In most cases the condition appears to reach a certain stage and then 'burn out' and cease to extend further. However, phimosis is common, and is frequently the cause of initial presentation. Meatal strictures may continue to be troublesome over several years. Leukoplakia is less common than in women [11], and was seldom a problem in a series extending over 15 years. Squamous cell carcinoma is rare [11,12], but is highly invasive when it occurs. Rapid early growth may be missed in the uncircumcised [13].

Treatment. Weak topical corticosteroids will usually be sufficient for mild forms not involving the meatus. Powerful corticosteroids are helpful, but should be used for limited periods only [14]. However, meatal involvement may respond to strong corticosteroids inserted by means of a nozzle-headed tube, or to repeated dilatation or meatotomy [15]. Testosterone propionate 1.5% ointment is advocated by some [16]. Leukoplakic areas respond to cryotherapy [17], but careful follow-up is essential. The condition may recur on excised or grafted sites. Circumcision (or a dorsal slit) is advisable when it is impossible to retract the foreskin, as leukoplakic or early neoplastic changes may otherwise be missed [18].

REFERENCES

1 Meyrick Thomas RH, Ridley CM, Black MM. Clinical features and therapy of lichen sclerosus et atrophicus affecting males. *Clin Exp Dermatol* 1987; **12**: 126–8.
2 Wallace HJ. Lichen sclerosus et atrophicus. *Trans St John's Hosp Dermatol Soc* 1971; **57**: 9–30.
3 Goolamali SK, Barnes EN, Irvine WJ *et al.* Organ-specific antibodies in patients with lichen sclerosus. *Br Med J* 1974; **iv**: 78–9.
4 Harrington CI, Dunsmore IR. An investigation into the incidence of autoimmune disorders in patients with lichen sclerosus et atrophicus. *Br J Dermatol* 1981; **104**: 563–6.
5 Meyrick Thomas RH, Ridley CM, Black MM. The association of lichen sclerosus et atrophicus and autoimmune-related disease in males. *Br J Dermatol* 1983; **109**: 661–4.
6 Harrington CI, Gelsthorpe K. The association between lichen sclerosus et atrophicus and HLA-B40. *Br J Dermatol* 1981; **104**: 561–2.
7 Meyrick Thomas RH, Ridley CM, Sherwood F *et al.* The lack of association of lichen sclerosus with HLA-A & B tissue antigens. *Clin Exp Dermatol* 1984; **9**: 290–2.
8 Frances C, Wechsler J, Rouges O. Lichen sclero-atrophique vulvaire (LSAV): étude biochimique, histologique, ultrastructurale et immunologique. *Ann Dermatol Vénéréol* 1981; **108**: 209 (Abstract).
9 Bale PM, Lochhead A, Martin HCO *et al.* Balanitis xerotica obliterans in children. *Pediatr Pathol* 1987; **7**: 617–27.
10 Chalmers RJ, Burton PA, Bennett R *et al.* Lichen sclerosus et atrophicus—a distinctive and common cause of phimosis in boys. *Arch Dermatol* 1984; **120**: 1025–7.
11 Weigand DA. Lichen sclerosus et atrophicus, multiple dysplastic keratoses, and squamous cell carcinoma of the glans penis. *J Dermatol Surg Oncol* 1980; **6**: 45–50.
12 Bart RS, Kopf AW. Tumor conference No 18: squamous cell carcinoma arising in balanitis xerotica. *J Dermatol Surg Oncol* 1978; **4**: 556–8.
13 Schnitzler L, Sayag J, Sayag J *et al.* Epitheliome spino-cellulaire aign de la verge et lichen sclero-atrophique. *Ann Dermatol Vénéréol* 1987; **114**: 979–81.
14 Jorgensen ET, Svensson A. The treatment of phimosis in boys with potent topical steroid (clobetasol propionate 0.05%) cream. *Acta Derm Venereol (Stockh)* 1993; **73**: 55–6.
15 Williams JL, Crawford BH. A method for urethroplasty for urethral strictures. *Br J Urol* 1968; **40**: 712–16.
16 Pasieczny TAH. The treatment of balanitis xerotica obliterans with testosterone propionate ointment. *Acta Derm Venereol (Stockh)* 1977; **57**: 275–7.
17 August PJ, Milward TM. Cryosurgery in the treatment of lichen sclerosus et atrophicus of the vulva. *Br J Dermatol* 1980; **103**: 667–70.
18 Campus GV, Ena P, Seuderi N. Surgical treatment of balanitis xerotica obliterans. *Plast Reconstr Surg* 1984; **73**: 652–7.

Penile ulceration and necrosis

Traumatic lesions

Traumatic ulcers are usually easily recognized, but self-inflicted lesions may be bizarre and unacknowledged. Extravasation of material injected into the dorsal vein by a heroin addict caused local necrosis [1]. Condom catheter drainage systems in paraplegic and geriatric patients may be attached by tapes applied too tightly, causing painless necrosis or gangrene of the glans or shaft [2,3].

Venereal infections

Syphilis must be considered and exluded in any case of penile ulceration, however strongly the possibility is refuted; chancre redux and pseudochancre are rare, but may be overlooked [4]. Chancroid is also a trap for the unwary [5], as it may present in unusual forms—especially in tropical countries—and may coexist with other viral or bacterial infections. Granuloma venereum may also present with ulceration. Multiple erosions with ragged edges result from contamination with *Neisseria gonorrhoeae* [6,7]. Discrete pustules or ulcers may also occur without urethritis. Careful and accurate culture techniques are important in differentiating this group of diseases.

Other infections

Primary tuberculosis [8] may simulate a syphilitic chancre, but lymphadenopathy is more marked. Orificial tuberculous ulcers are multiple, with shallow, ragged edges; bacilli abound. Papulonecrotic tuberculides have involved the penis, and acne scrofulosorum has also been reported [9]. Fusospirillary infections are now uncommon in western Europe. Deep, sloughing, necrotic lesions, and even gangrene, develop with great rapidity. Histoplasmosis and varicella occasionally ulcerate, sometimes deeply. HSV-2 infections have caused necrotic lesions of the glans and shaft [10], and amoebiasis [11] has caused gross tissue loss.

Other causes

Gummas and epitheliomas may ulcerate, especially if neglected. Severe aphthosis sometimes causes quite deep, painful lesions. In Behçet's syndrome, genital ulceration is said to occur in over 90% of cases [12].

Although vasculitis seldom involves the penis, erythema multiforme may produce ulcerative lesions, especially in the Stevens–Johnson form. Curiously, there have also been reports of Wegener's granulomatosis causing penile necrosis [13,14]. Pyoderma gangrenosum may also occur on the penis (Fig. 72.16).

Dequalinium necrosis [15]. An outbreak of 'necrotizing ulcers of the penis' was found to be due to the quaternary ammonium antibacterial agent decamethylene bis(4-aminoquinaldinium). This topical agent was well tolerated on most parts of the body, but caused a necrotic reaction in some subjects in occluded areas. A similar effect has been noted from other quaternary ammonium products [16] and from needles sterilized in these. The antiviral agent foscarnet (phosphono formate) has been implicated in penile ulceration [17].

The treatment of all forms of penile necrosis is determined by initial identification of the cause. In fulminant necrotic or gangrenous lesions, excision of all necrotic tissue may be life-saving. In milder cases, antibacterial dressings and applications may be sufficient. Treatment with dextran polymer particles has been advocated [18].

Penile gangrene

Gangrene of the penis is rare in western Europe. It usually presents to surgeons, but dermatologists may see a few cases. Many cases of penile necrosis, especially those due to trauma, may progress to gangrene. Known predisposing factors are diabetes [19], old age and intravascular coagulation syndromes. Particular causes include varicella in infants, and haemolytic streptococcal, postoperative, malignant and leukaemic diseases. Among rare causes are tuberculosis, syphilis, penile thrombosis, dermatitis artefacta and tourniquet injury [20].

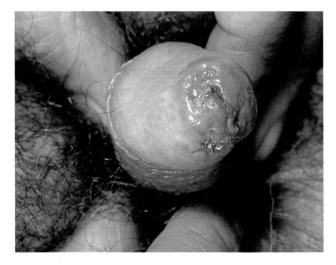

Fig. 72.16 Pyoderma gangrenosum in a patient with severe seronegative arthropathy.

Gangrenous balanitis

SYN. PHAGEDENIC BALANITIS

This condition occurs as an occasional complication of venereal infection and superadded (usually fusospirillary) infection. Operative procedures, such as a dorsal slit, extend the infection.

In the form originally described by Fournier, oedema, blisters and rapidly extending sloughs spread over the penis and scrotum of young men after trivial injury. Severe constitutional symptoms are present, and the condition is sometimes fatal (p. 3199).

Treatment must be immediate and thorough. Complete excision of all the affected area is combined with antibiotic therapy and attention to any underlying disease or venereal infection.

REFERENCES

1 White WB, Barrett S. Penile ulcer in heroin abuse: a case report. *Cutis* 1981; **29**: 62–72.
2 Fauer R, Morrow JW. External urinary devices—use and abuse. *Urology* 1978; **11**: 180–2.
3 Steinhardt J, McRoberts JW. Total distal penile necrosis caused by condom catheter. *JAMA* 1980; **244**: 1238.
4 Evans AJ, Summerly R. Pseudo-chancre redux with negative serology. A case report. *Br J Vener Dis* 1964; **40**: 222–4.
5 McCarley ME, Cruz PD, Sontheimer RD. Chancroid: clinical variants and other findings from an epidemic in Dallas County 1986–87. *J Am Acad Dermatol* 1988; **19**: 330–44.
6 Haim S, Merzbach D. Gonococcal penile ulcer. *Br J Vener Dis* 1970; **46**: 336–7.
7 Landergren G. Gonnorrheal ulcer of the penis: report of a case. *Acta Derm Venereol (Stockh)* 1961; **41**: 320–3.
8 Delzotto A, Christol B, Dezotto L *et al.* Tubercolosi del pene. *Urologica* 1973; **34**: 171–5.
9 Breathnach SM, Black MM. Atypical tuberculide (acne scrofulosorum) secondary to tuberculous lymphadenitis. *Clin Exp Dermatol* 1981; 6: 339–44.
10 Peutherer JF, Smith JW, Robertson DHH. Necrotizing balanitis due to generalized primary infection with herpes simplex virus type 2. *Br J Vener Dis* 1979; **55**: 48–51.
11 Parkash S, Ramakrishnan K, Ananthakrishnan N *et al.* Amoebic ulcer of the penis. *Postgrad Med J* 1982; **58**: 375–7.
12 Haim S, Sobel JD, Friedman-Birnbaum R. Thrombophlebitis. A cardinal symptom of Behçet's syndrome. *Acta Derm Venereol (Stockh)* 1974; **54**: 299–301.
13 Kalis BJ. Case presentations. In: *Proceedings of 16th International Congress on Dermatology.* Tokyo: University of Tokyo Press, 1982: 841.
14 Matsuda O, Mitsukawa S, Ishii N *et al.* A case of Wegener's granulomatosis with necrosis of the penis. *Tohuku J Exp Med* 1976; **118**: 145–51.
15 Coles RB, Wilkinson DS. Necrosis and dequalinium. I. Balanitis. *Trans St John's Hosp Dermatol Soc* 1965; **51**: 46–8.
16 Dupre A, Christol B. Dequalinium necrosis penis. *Bull Soc Fr Dermatol Syphiligr* 1975; **80**: 194–6.
17 Evan LM, Grossmann ME. Forscarnet induced penile ulceration. *J Am Acad Dermatol* 1992; **271**: 124–6.
18 Lassus A, Karvonen J, Juvakoski T. Dextran polymer particles (Debrisan) in the treatment of penile ulcers. *Acta Derm Venereol (Stockh)* 1977; **57**: 361–3.
19 Bour J, Steinhardt G. Penile necrosis in diabetes mellitus and end-stage renal disease. *J Urol* 1984; **132**: 560–2.
20 Thomas AJ, Jr, Timmons JW, Perlwitter AD. Progressive penile amputation. Tourniquet injury secondary to hair. *Urology* 1977; **9**: 42–4.

Granulomatous lesions

Although many infections may develop granulomatous forms, three conditions in particular are properly referred to as granulomas.

Lymphogranuloma venereum (Chapter 27)

This condition is still an important tropical venereal disease, and it became endemic in Finland between 1925 and 1940. Its penile manifestations in 37 patients have been recorded [1]. It may present as lymphangitis, preputial infiltration, or small granulomatous or fistulous lesions. Late complications in the male are unusual; elephantiasis of the penis and scrotum is the most common.

Granuloma inguinale (Chapter 27)

The button-like lesion develops after an incubation period of about 15 days. A painful inguinal adenitis due to secondary infection may be present [2]. Syphilis may coexist [3]. A mutilating and cicatricial form has been described. Streptomycin cured 91% of a series of 122 patients in India, but resistance and side-effects occurred [4]. Tetracyclines in high dose are effective.

Eosinophilic granuloma

This condition is rare in the genital area, and is more common in the perivulval and perianal regions, but it has been described on the penis [5].

Necrobiotic granulomas localized to the penis probably merely represent subcutaneous granuloma annulare [6].

REFERENCES

1 Hopsu-Havu VK, Sonck CE. Infiltrative, ulcerative and fistular lesions of the penis due to lymphogranuloma venereum. *Br J Vener Dis* 1973; **49**: 193–202.
2 Duperrat B, Labouche F. Le granulome vénérien (donovanose) en France. *Ann Dermatol Syphiligr* 1975; **102**: 241–50.
3 Davis CM. Granuloma inguinale: a clinical, histological and ultrastructural study. *JAMA* 1970; **211**: 632–6.
4 Lal S, Nicholas C. Epidemiological and clinical features in 165 cases of granuloma inguinale. *Br J Vener Dis* 1970; **46**: 461.
5 Rousselot M, Privat Y, Bonerandi JJ. Granulome éosinophile du visage. *Bull Soc Fr Dermatol Syphiligr* 1975; **82**: 44–5.
6 Kossard S, Collins AG, Wegman A *et al*. Necrobiotic granulomas localized to the penis: a possible variant of subcutaneous granuloma annulare. *J Cutan Pathol* 1990; **17**: 101–4.

Sclerosing lipogranuloma of penis and scrotum

This name was originally applied to a local reaction to injury of adipose tissue, but it is now felt admissible to narrow the definition to 'a local reactive process following injection of exogenous lipids into the subcutaneous tissues' [1].

Pathogenesis. It follows that the condition should be regarded as factitious [1–3], despite lack of admission by the patient. Paraffin hydrocarbons may be found by infra-red spectrophotometry [1], and severe psychological problems may be present [4].

Histopathology. A hyaline necrosis in the fat lobules and intracellular septa leads to disruption of fat cells and a granulomatous reaction. This is followed by a proliferative phase leading to dense hyaline scar tissue. Ultrastructural studies show a histiocyte-like infiltrate with numerous intracytoplasmic vacuoles [3].

Clinical features. The granuloma affects the shaft of the penis or scrotum. The skin is frequently attached to the tumour, which may become tethered or ulcerated, softening and discharging liquefied adipose tissue. As they evolve, the tumours frequently become cystic, although smaller lesions may fibrose. The condition is intractable.

Treatment. Surgical excision is advocated, although recurrences are usual.

REFERENCES

1 Oertel YC, Johnson FB. Sclerosing lipogranuloma of male genitalia. Review of 23 cases. *Arch Pathol* 1977; **101**: 321–6.
2 Carlson HE. Sclerosing lipogranuloma of the penis and scrotum. *J Urol* 1968; **100**: 656–8.
3 Claudy A, Garcier F, Schmitt D. Sclerosing lipogranuloma of the male genitalia: ultrastructural study. *Br J Dermatol* 1981; **105**: 451–6.
4 Forstorm L, Winkelmann RK. Factitial panniculitis. *Arch Dermatol* 1974; **110**: 747–50.

Pearly penile papules

SYN. HIRSUTOID PAPILLOMAS OF THE PENIS; 'HAIRY' PENIS

Definition and aetiology. Pearly penile papules [1,2] are small, smooth, dome-shaped or hair-like papules involving the penile corona. They appear to be a physiological variant, symptomless and without functional significance. They occur at any age after puberty, but are chiefly detected between the ages of 20 and 50 years. They are unrelated to race, sexual activity or circumcision. An incidence as high as 19% has been reported [3], but this is not in accord with the author's experience.

Histopathology. The lesions consist of a core of normal connective tissue covered by epidermis which is thinned centrally and acanthotic at the periphery [4]. The body of the lesion contains a rich, vascular network surrounded by dense connective tissue and a mild lymphocytic infiltrate. They are best considered as angiofibromas [5].

Clinical features [2,4,6]. The patient complains of 'warts' which are situated on the corona, particularly the anterior

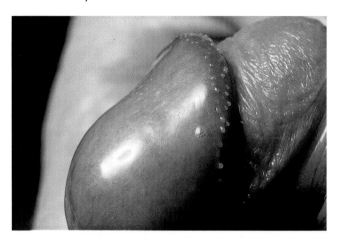

Fig. 72.17 Pearly penile papules. (Courtesy of Dr D.A. Burns, Leicester Royal Infirmary, UK.)

border, in 1–3 irregular rings, partly or completely encircling the glans (Fig. 72.17). The individual papules, which are flesh-coloured, white or red, are 1–3 mm broad and up to 3 mm or more in height. Longer filiform lesions also occur.

Treatment. Reassurance alone is required.

REFERENCES

1 Buschke A. Ueber die Bedeutung de 'papillen' de corona glandis. *Med Klin* 1909; **5**: 1621–3.
2 Tannebaum MH, Becker SW. Papillae of the corona at the glans penis. *J Urol* 1965; **93**: 391–5.
3 Neinstein LS, Goldenring J. Pink pearly papules: an epidemiologic study. *J Pediatr* 1984; **105**: 594–5.
4 Johnson BL, Baxter DL. Pearly penile papules. *Arch Dermatol* 1964; **90**: 166–7.
5 Ackerman AB, Kornberg R. Pearly penile papules: acral angiofibromas. *Arch Dermatol* 1973; **108**: 673–5.
6 Glickman JM, Freeman RG. Pearly penile papules: a statistical study of the incidence. *Arch Dermatol* 1966; **93**: 56–9.

Thrombosis of the penis

Only a few cases of this condition have been described [1,2]. It is said to be more common in black men. The cause is unknown. Of nine cases [3], it followed strenuous intercourse in three and was traumatic in one. Another case has been described with gout [4], and one with thrombophlebitis migrans after resection of the colon for thrombosis of the mesenteric vein [1]. It may also occur in leukaemia and other blood diseases. In granulomatous phlebitis, the veins of the sphincter are affected, but not those of the penis itself [5]. Priapism is the chief sign.

REFERENCES

1 Grossman A, Kaplan HJ, Grossman M *et al.* Thrombosis of the penis: interesting facet of thrombangiitis obliterans. *JAMA* 1965; **192**: 329–31.
2 Leading Article. Priapism. *Br Med J* 1965; **i**: 401–2.
3 Harrow BR, Sloane JA. Thrombophlebitis of superficial penile and scrotal veins. *J Urol* 1963; **89**: 841–2.

4 Aubertin E, Roy A, Fenelon J. On a case of thrombosis of the corpus cavernosum in a patient with gout receiving 3 intravenous injections per week of 50 mg of heparin. *Med Bordeaux* 1960; **137**: 1486–9.
5 Nesbit RM, Hodgson NB. Thromboangiitis obliterans of the spermatic cord. *Trans Am Assoc Genitourin Surg* 1959; **51**: 92–4.

Penile venereal oedema

This uncommon condition [1] accounted for 1.7 per 1000 male visits to a clinic for sexually transmitted diseases [2]. In almost all cases, other venereal diseases were present.

The condition consists of a self-limiting, painless, boggy oedema involving the prepuce and distal penile shaft in sexually active males. There may be some difficulty in separating this condition from non-venereal sclerosing lymphangitis (although this is partly semantic). The two sometimes coexist. They are both related to previous sexual intercourse, and both run a benign course after sexual abstinence. It has been reported in a 2-year-old boy with gonorrhoea [3].

This acute, rapidly developing oedema must be distinguished from angio-oedema and from penoscrotal or penile lymphoedema.

Gonococcal infection at the sites of previous penile prosthetic implants has been recorded as causing acute erythema and oedema of the organ [4].

REFERENCES

1 Wilde H, Canby JP. Penile venereal edema. *Arch Dermatol* 1973; **108**: 263.
2 Wright RA, Judson FN. Penile venereal edema. *JAMA* 1979; **241**: 157–8.
3 Fleisher G, Hodge D, Cromie W. Penile edema in childhood. *Ann Emerg Med* 1980; **9**: 314–15.
4 Nelson R, Gregory JC. Gonococcal infections of penile prostheses. *Urology* 1988; **31**: 391–4.

Non-venereal sclerosing lymphangitis of the penis

SYN. MONDOR'S PHLEBITIS OF THE PENIS [1]

The apparent rarity of this condition is probably misleading [2,3], as it is painless and symptomless. It affects males aged 20–40 years, appearing 24–48 h after intercourse. It appears as single or grouped, doughy, purplish, cord-like lesions arising from or around the coronal sulcus. It may extend to the dorsal lymphatics. Ulceration is rare, and the lesion is self-limiting in a matter of weeks.

Histologically, it has always been believed that the lymphatic vessels were thickened and sclerosed. However, a good case has been made [1] for regarding the early changes as affecting the veins, with occlusion of the lumina by a clot invaded by disintegrating polymorph neutrophils, and granulation tissue in the vein wall, similar to Mondor's phlebitis of the chest wall (Chapter 71).

The aetiology is unknown, but the role of trauma [2–4] is obviously important. Cases have been reported following herpes simplex [5] and coincidental with chlamydial infections [6], gonorrhoea and urethritis [7]. The condition can coexist with and be concealed by penile venereal oedema. It may easily be confused with the hard penile circumferential fold sometimes seen in primary syphilis [8].

REFERENCES

1 Findlay GH, Whiting DA. Mondor's phlebitis of the penis. *Clin Exp Dermatol* 1977; **2**: 65–7.
2 Greenburg RD, Perry TL. Nonvenereal sclerosing lymphangitis of the penis. *Arch Dermatol* 1972; **105**: 728–9.
3 Lassus A, Niemi KM, Valle S-L *et al.* Sclerosing lymphangitis of the penis. *Br J Vener Dis* 1972; **38**: 545–8.
4 Kandil E, Al Kashlan IM. Non-venereal sclerosing lymphangitis of the penis. *Acta Derm Venereol (Stockh)* 1970; **50**: 309–12.
5 Van De Staak WJBM. Non-venereal sclerosing lymphangitis of the penis following herpes progenitalis. *Br J Dermatol* 1977; **96**: 679–80.
6 Kristenssen JK, Scheibel J. Sclerosing lymphangitis of the penis: a possible *Chlamydia* aetiology. *Acta Derm Venereol (Stockh)* 1981; **61**: 455–6.
7 Stolz E, van Kampen WJ. Sklerosierende lymphangitis des penis, der oberlippe und des labium minus. *Hautarzt* 1974; **25**: 231–7.
8 Goldstein AMB, Fox JN. The hard penile circumferential fold as the presenting finding in primary syphilis: report of six cases. *J Am Acad Dermatol* 1992; **26**: 700–3.

Plastic induration of the penis
SYN. PEYRONIE'S DISEASE

This disorder of the penile connective tissue is described in Chapter 44.

Bowenoid papulosis
SYN. MULTIFOCAL INDOLENT PIGMENTED PENILE PAPULES; MULTICENTRIC PIGMENTED BOWEN'S DISEASE

Definition and aetiology. Bowenoid papulosis [1] was first described as a condition affecting the groin by Lloyd [2], but was recognized as an entity by Kopf and co-workers a few years later [3,4]. It consists of indolent, symptomless fleshy papules, which are usually pigmented, involving the genitalia or perigenital areas of both sexes (but chiefly young men). The histological features suggest a preinvasive carcinoma *in situ* but the course is almost certainly benign [5], although one case progressing to true Bowen's disease (in an older man) has been reported [6]. The aetiology is almost certainly viral. DNA sequences closely related to HPV-16 have been found in most cases of Bowenoid papulosis [7,8] of both sexes, but numerous other HPV genotypes have been identified, with types 16, 18 and 33 considered to be the most oncogenic [9]. In females, a higher incidence of abnormal cervical smears is found both in patients and in the partners of men with penile lesions. Most authors [8,10] consider that Bowenoid changes represent a major risk factor in the development of cervical neoplasia, although the observed clinically benign behaviour of the lesions elsewhere on the genitalia remains reassuring [5].

Histopathology. This shows the changes of Bowen's disease, with acanthosis, atypical keratinocytic hyperplasia,

a moderate degree of nuclear dysplasia, and atypical crowded mitotic activity. Pigment is usually prominent in the basal cell layer, and pigment-laden macrophages are present in the dermis. The overall appearance is that of carcinoma *in situ*, although the general pattern of maturation and orderliness has enabled some authors to make a histological distinction from true Bowen's disease [5]. A study based on histomorphological and DNA ploidy analysis favoured the conclusion that bowenoid papulosis was a form of low-grade squamous cell carcinoma *in situ* [11]. Electron microscopy has shown structures resembling viral particles [5,12] within the granular layer. Increased intercellular spaces were found around dysplastic cells which had microvilli protruding from their cytoplasmic membranes. Their nuclei contained dispersed chromatin, with irregular peripheral condensation. Cytoplasmic tonofilaments were short and deranged. Melanocytes were normal in number, but increased numbers of melanosomes were found in basal and squamous cells [5].

Clinical features. The lesions occur in young patients as multiple papules, often grouped, 2–20mm in diameter, with a verrucous or smooth surface, and more commonly on the shaft than the glans (Fig. 72.18). Their colour usually ranges from brown-red to violaceous or black, but they may be rosy [13] or pale. At times they may show a lichenoid or psoriasiform appearance.

Differential diagnosis [14,15]. The lesions may be confused with condylomas, verrucae vulgares (on the shaft), seborrhoeic warts [16], epithelial naevi or lichen planus. The presence of pigmented papules on the penile shaft of a young man should be a pointer to the correct diagnosis.

Treatment. Although bowenoid papules appear to remain benign, cases have not been followed long enough to be certain [5]. Local excision of solitary lesions enables the

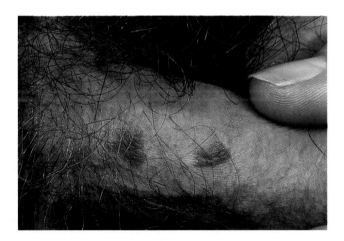

Fig. 72.18 Bowenoid papulosis. (Courtesy of Dr D.A. Burns, Leicester Royal Infirmary, UK.)

diagnosis to be confirmed [8]. Excision, electrocoagulation, electrodesiccation, cryotherapy or 5-fluorouracil have been employed successfully [8,14,15,17]. Subcutaneous injection of interferon-γ, in a regimen of three doses per week of 4×10^6 i.u. for 13 weeks, has been claimed to be effective in some cases [18]. However, close follow-up is essential. Spontaneous regression has occasionally occurred.

REFERENCES

1 Peters MS, Perry HO. Bowenoid papules of the penis. *J Urol* 1981; **126**: 482–4.
2 Lloyd KM. Multicentric pigmented Bowen's disease of the groin. *Arch Dermatol* 1970; **101**: 48–51.
3 Kopf AW, Bart RS. Tumor conference No 11. Multiple bowenoid papules of the penis: a new entity? *J Dermatol Surg Oncol* 1977; **3**: 265–9.
4 Wade TR, Kopf AW, Ackerman B. Bowenoid papulosis of the genitalia. *Arch Dermatol* 1979; **115**: 306–8.
5 Patterson JW, Kas GF, Graham JH *et al.* Bowenoid papulosis. *Cancer* 1986; **57**: 823–36.
6 De Villez RL, Stevens CS. Bowenoid papules of the genitalia. *J Am Acad Dermatol* 1980; **3**: 149–52.
7 Grosshans E, Grossmann L. Bowenoid papulosis. *Arch Dermatol* 1985; **121**: 858–63.
8 Obalek S, Jablonska S, Beaudenon S *et al.* Bowenoid papulosis of the male and female genitalia: risk of cervical neoplasia. *J Am Acad Dermatol* 1986; **14**: 433–44.
9 Schwarz RA, Janniger CK. Bowenoid papulosis. *J Am Acad Dermatol* 1991; **24**: 261–4.
10 Rogozinski TT, Janniger CK. Bowenoid papulosis. *Am Fam Physician* 1988; **38**: 161–4.
11 Böcking A, Chatelain R, Salterberg A *et al.* Bowenoid papulosis: classification as a low grade *in situ* carcinoma of the epidermis on the basis of histomorphologic and DNA ploidy studies. *Ann Quant Cytol Histol* 1989; **11**: 419–25.
12 Kimura S, Hirai A, Harada R *et al.* So-called multicentric pigmented Bowen's disease. *Dermatologica* 1978; **157**: 229–37.
13 Toribio J, Muño MG, Pérez-Oliva N *et al.* Papulosis bowenoide genital. *Actas Dermosifilogr* 1981; **72**: 545–50.
14 Mascaro JM, Torras H, Bou D. Papulosis bowenoide de los genitales. Comentario sobre su significado. *Actas Dermosifilogr* 1980; **71**: 119–28.
15 Taylor DR, Jr, South DA. Bowenoid papulosis: a review. *Cutis* 1981; **27**: 92–8.
16 Friedman SJ, Fox BJ, Albert HL. Seborrhoeic keratoses of the penis. *Urology* 1987; **29**: 204–6.
17 Cutler TC. Bowenoid papulosis of the penis. *Clin Exp Dermatol* 1980; **5**: 97–100.
18 Gross G, Roussaki A, Papendick U. Efficacy of interferons on bowenoid papulosis and other precancerous lesions. *J Invest Dermatol* 1990; **95** (Suppl. 6): 152–7.

Conditions particularly involving the scrotum

Cavernous haemangiomas in infants habitually ulcerate, healing spontaneously after some weeks. Angiokeratoma of Fordyce selectively involves the scrotal skin (Fig. 72.19); the lesions seldom require treatment, although they are easily destroyed by electrodesiccation. The punctate spots of angiokeratoma corporis diffusum are smaller and less hyperkeratotic, and are present elsewhere. Epidermal naevi are distinguished by their usual features. Cutaneous horns, lipomas and even trichofolliculomas [1] occur as occasional or rare curiosities. A pendulous fibroma can be troublesome to the patient. Sebocystomas arise in early life as multiple,

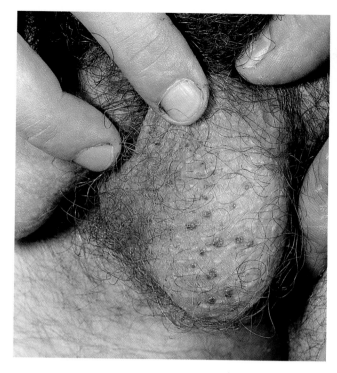

Fig. 72.19 Scrotal angiokeratoma of Fordyce. (Courtesy of Dr D.A. Burns, Leicester Royal Infirmary, UK.)

firm, yellow-white nodules, and must be distinguished from the lesions of idiopathic calcinosis, which sometimes break down and extrude chalky contents.

Acanthosis nigricans, pemphigus vegetans and pyodermite vegetante affect the scrotum; benign familial pemphigus may easily be overlooked as the cause of an erosive dermatitis which is refractory to treatment.

Absorption of topical medicaments is greatly enhanced through the scrotal skin [2]. Corticosteroids should be used sparingly [3]. Hexachlorophane concentrate in baths has caused burns [4]. 5-fluorouracil (Efudix) given to patients for treatment of actinic keratoses of the exposed parts may produce acute dermatitis of an irritant type if used inappropriately on the scrotum [5]. Cysts, sometimes itchy and inflamed, occur in chloracne [6].

Infections and infestations

Condylomata acuminata do not commonly involve the scrotal skin, except in the presence of maceration, infection or discharge.

The scrotum is involved in genitocrural infective dermatitis, when fissuring and superficial ulceration of the penoscrotal junction may be a marked feature. Infection secondary to scabies, pruritus or eczema is occasionally seen. The scrotum is a common site of lichen simplex.

Infestation with *Pthirus pubis* is common in hirsute patients, and scabetic lesions occur, although less frequently than on the penis. Although the scrotum may appear to be spared in fungal infections, it is not infrequently affected [7], but the epidermal reaction is usually poor [8], and may be completely absent in patients treated with cortico-steroids [9].

Schistosomiasis causes fistulae, sinuses, phagedenic ulceration, and pseudoelephantiasis. A chronic papular dermatitis has also been recorded [10]. True elephantiasis, often extraordinary in extent, is caused by *Wuchereria bancrofti*. Calcified nodules may result from encysted worms of either *Wuchereria* or *Onchocerca volvulus* [11].

Erythematous and eczematous conditions

The scrotal skin is frequently involved in seborrhoeic and intertriginous eczema. Eczema confined to the scrotum suggests an exogenous cause, usually industrial. Lichen simplex is most frequent at the scrotoperineal junction, where it is sustained by rubbing through trouser pockets (Fig. 72.20). The pruritus often has a particular 'burning quality' [12].

Scrotal dermatitis and pigmentation, often with scaling and superficial ulceration, formed a characteristic part of an 'oculogenital' syndrome seen in 75% of 8000 American prisoners of war fed on an inadequate diet of rice [13]. Intense burning and itching accompanied the condition, in which conjunctivitis and stomatitis were also present. The patients recovered on a full diet. Riboflavin, and to some extent nicotinic acid, deficiencies have been blamed for a syndrome of scrotal dermatitis, seborrhoeic dermatitis, angular stomatitis and fissuring of the alae nasi. This was reproducible experimentally on a diet low only in riboflavin [14]. However, as these features are seen without any evidence of riboflavin deficiency, it seems possible that other factors such as zinc deficiency (Chapter 59) lead to an increased requirement for the vitamin. The scrotum may be involved in the 'perineal syndrome' (p. 3179).

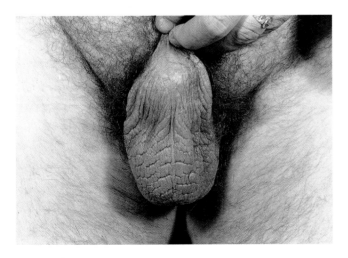

Fig. 72.20 Scrotal lichen simplex.

Increased pigmentation is seen with malabsorption syndromes.

Scrotal gangrene [15,16]

Fournier's 'idiopathic' gangrene carries a high mortality. It develops suddenly and progresses rapidly. Although the patients are often diabetic [15,17,18], the essential cause remains obscure. It has been regarded as a synergistic necrotizing cellulitis, a form of disseminated intravascular coagulation [15,19], or equivalent to necrotizing fasciitis [20]. An immunological deficit, associated with myeloma, was present in one case [21], and may be a contributory factor in others. It has followed vasectomy and lower gut resection. Organisms are not always found, but *Bacteroides fragilis* has sometimes been isolated. Extensive debridement of all affected tissue is essential [22]. In conjunction with supportive measures and aggressive therapy, a 55% survival rate has been achieved [16].

Juvenile gangrenous vasculitis of the scrotum [23]

A less severe form of gangrene, which heals in 15–45 days, is preceded by fever and burning. Polycyclic vasculitic lesions with histological features of angiitis follow. It may be related to aphthosis. Rickettsial infection may also cause scrotal gangrene.

Other conditions

Lymphangiectases may follow filarial infection or be due to lymphangioma circumscriptum. A milky discharge may seep from the scrotum after rupture of the lesions ('weeping scrotum') [24]. Lipogranuloma may involve the scrotum. Crohn's disease does so rarely, and causes boggy oedema and fistulae [25].

Penoscrotal lymphoedema [26] must be distinguished from transitory penile venereal oedema (p. 3196). It occurs as a manifestation of primary hypoplastic lymphatics, or following infection with consequent damage to lymphatic channels. Lymphoedema may also unexpectedly follow local operative procedures.

Acute haemorrhagic oedema (Chapter 14) affects the newborn [27].

Bruised hemiscrotum of the newborn, associated with hard testicular swelling, results from torsion of the spermatic cord and testicular infarction. Uncomplicated neonatal hemiscrotal bruising may result from high venous pressure during difficult deliveries [28].

Macro-orchidism with mental retardation is an important feature of the fragile-X syndrome. Advice from a geneticist should be sought if this disorder is suspected [29].

REFERENCES

1 Nomura M, Hata S. Sebaceous trichofolliculoma on scrotum and penis. *Dermatologica* 1990; **181**: 68–70.

2 Fisher AA. Unique reactions of scrotal skin to topical agents. *Cutis* 1989; **44**: 445–7.

3 Feldman RT, Maibach HI. Regional variation in percutaneous penetration of 14C cortisol in man. *J Invest Dermatol* 1967; **48**: 181–3.

4 Baker H, Ive FA, Lloyd M. Primary irritant dermatitis of the scrotum due to hexachlorophane. *Arch Dermatol* 1969; **99**: 693–6.

5 Shelley WB, Shelley D. Scrotal dermatitis caused by 5-fluorouracil (Efudix). *J Am Acad Dermatol* 1988; **19**: 929–31.

6 Crow KD. Chloracne and its potential clinical implications. *Clin Exp Dermatol* 1981; **6**: 243–57.

7 Dekio S, Li-Mo Q, Kawasaki Y *et al.* Tinea of scrotum. *J Dermatol* 1990; **17**: 448–51.

8 La Touche CJ. Scrotal dermatophytosis. An insufficiently documented aspect of tinea. *Br J Dermatol* 1967; **79**: 339–44.

9 Ive FA, Marks R. Tinea incognito. *Br Med J* 1968; **iii**: 149–52.

10 Walker RR. Chronic papular dermatitis of the scrotum due to *Schistosoma mansoni*. *Arch Dermatol* 1979; **115**: 869–70.

11 Browne SG. Calcinosis circumscripta of the scrotal wall: the aetiological role of *Onchocerca volvulus*. *Br J Dermatol* 1962; **74**: 136–40.

12 Kantor GR. What to do about pruritus scroti. *Postgrad Med* 1990; **88**: 95–102.

13 Jacobs EC. Oculo-oro-genital syndrome: a deficiency disease. *Ann Intern Med* 1951; **35**: 1049–54.

14 Hills OW, Liebert E, Steinberg DL *et al.* Clinical aspects of dietary depletion of riboflavin. *Arch Intern Med* 1951; **87**: 682–93.

15 Feingold DS. Gangrenous and crepitant cellulitis. *J Am Acad Dermatol* 1982; **6**: 289–99.

16 Spirnak JP, Resnick MI, Hampel N *et al.* Fournier's gangrene: report of 20 cases. *J Urol* 1984; **132**: 289–91.

17 Dootson GM, Lott CW, Moisey CU. Fournier's gangrene and diabetes mellitus: survival following surgery. *J R Soc Med* 1982; **75**: 916–17.

18 Katsas AG. Diabetic scrotal gangrene. *J R Soc Med* 1982; **75**: 988.

19 Pande SK, Mewara PC. Fournier's gangrene: a report of 5 cases. *Br J Surg* 1976; **63**: 479–81.

20 Oh C, Lee C, Jacobson JH II. Necrotizing fasciitis of the perineum. *Surgery* 1982; **91**: 49–51.

21 Frier BM, Howie AD. Scrotal gangrene in asymptomatic myeloma. *Br Med J* 1972; **iv**: 26.

22 Pardy B, Eastcott HHG. Diabetic scrotal gangrene. *Proc R Soc Med* 1982; **75**: 829–30.

23 Pinol Aguade J. *XIVe Congress de l'Association des Dermatologistes et Syphiligraphers de Langue Francaise, Geneve, 1973. II Vascularites.* Geneva: Medecine et Hygiene, 1974: 112.

24 Johnson WT. Cutaneous chylous reflux, 'the weeping scrotum'. *Arch Dermatol* 1979; **115**: 464–6.

25 Cockburn AG, Krolikowski J, Bariogh K *et al.* Crohn's disease of penile and scrotal skin. *Urology* 1980; **15**: 596–8.

26 Samsoen M, Deschler JM, Servelle M *et al.* Le lymphoedeme penoscrotal: 2 observations. *Ann Dermatol Vénéréol* 1981; **108**: 541–6.

27 Lambert D, Laurent R, Bouilly D *et al.* Oedeme aigu hemorragique du nourrisson. Donnees immunologiques et ultra structurales. *Ann Dermatol Syphiligr* 1979; **106**: 975–87.

28 Davenport M, Bianchi A, Gough DCS. Idiopathic scrotal haemorrhage in neonates. *Br Med J* 1989; **298**: 1492–3.

29 York Moore DW. New developments in the fragile-X syndrome. *Br Med J* 1992; **305**: 208.

Idiopathic calcinosis of the scrotum [1–4]

Multiple asymptomatic nodules develop in childhood or early adult life [3] as greyish or white, firm nodules scattered in the scrotal skin (Fig. 72.21) In some cases, lesions have been shown to arise in eccrine duct milia [5]. As they increase in size, they may break down to discharge their chalky contents. Some lesions have been shown to arise in epidermal and pilar cysts [6].

Blood calcium and phosphorus levels are normal, in contrast with metastatic calcinosis, which only rarely affects the skin, but which carries a poor prognosis [7]. Histologically, these amorphous deposits may be surrounded by a granulomatous epithelioid cell and foreign-body giant-cell reaction.

True secondary dystrophic calcinosis follows tissue injury, local chronic infection or connective tissue disease. Cases have been reported following onchocerciasis [8].

In most cases, surgical treatment should be limited to the removal of large, discharging lesions. Healing of scrotal skin is often slow. In severe cases, excision and grafting may be necessary [9].

REFERENCES

1 Fisher BK, Dvoretsky I. Idiopathic calcinosis of the scrotum. *Arch Dermatol* 1978; **114**: 957.

2 Moss RL, Shewmake SW. Idiopathic calcinosis of the scrotum. *Int J Dermatol* 1981; **20**: 134–6.

3 Schapiro L, Platt N, Torres-Rodriguez VM. Idiopathic calcinosis of the scrotum. *Arch Dermatol* 1970; **102**: 199.

4 Fuzesi L, Hollweg G, Lagrange W *et al.* Idiopathic calcinosis of the scrotum: scanning electron microscopic study with X-ray microanalysis. *Ultrastructural Pathology* 1991; **15**: 167–73.

5 Dare AJ, Axelsen RA. Scrotal calcinosis: origin from dystrophic calcification of eccrine duct milia. *J Cutan Pathol* 1988; **15**: 142–9.

6 Song DH, Lee KH, Kang WH. Idiopathic calcinosis of the scrotum. *J Am Acad Dermatol* 1988; **19**: 1095–101.

7 Putkonen T, Wangel GA. Renal hyperparathyroidism with metastatic calcification of the skin. *Dermatologica* 1959; **118**: 127–44.

8 Browne SG. Calcinosis circumscripta of the scrotal wall: the aetiological role of *Onchocerca volvulus*. *Br J Dermatol* 1962; **74**: 136–40.

9 Theuvenet WJ, Nolthewus-Puylaert T, Juvaha ZLG *et al.* Massive deformation of the scrotal wall by idiopathic calcinosis of scrotum. *Plast Reconstr Surg* 1984; **74**: 539–43.

Verruciform xanthoma

This condition was first described on scrotal skin in 1981 [1]. It seems to be more common in the Japanese [2]. It may

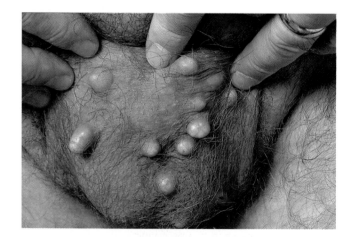

Fig. 72.21 Scrotal calcinosis. (Courtesy of Dr D.A. Burns, Leicester Royal Infirmary, UK.)

also appear in the oral cavity [3] (See Chapter 69). The aetiology and pathogenesis are unknown. Clinically, the lesions are of a red or yellow hue, and may be pedunculated or flat with a granular surface resembling a cauliflower. All reported patients were in good health and normolipaemic. Histologically, all cases showed epidermal acanthosis and papillomatosis, with densely distributed, fat-filled foam cells confined to the superficial papillary dermis [1,4].

No evidence of an infective cause has yet been demonstrated [5].

REFERENCES

1 Shindo Y, Mikoshiba H, Michizuku M *et al*. Two cases of verruciform xanthoma of the scrotum. *Jpn J Clin Dermatol* 1981; **35**: 365–9.
2 Nakamura S, Kanamori S, Nakayama K *et al*. Verruciform xanthoma of the scrotum. *J Dermatol* 1989; **16**: 397–401.
3 Shafer WG. Verruciform xanthoma. *Oral Surg* 1971; **31**: 784–9.
4 Kimura S. Verruciform xanthoma of scrotum. *Arch Dermatol* 1984; **120**: 1378–9.
5 Helm KF, Hopfl RM, Kreider JW *et al*. Verruciform xanthoma in an immunocompromised patient. *J Cutan Pathol* 1993; **20**: 84–6.

Premalignant and malignant lesions of the penis and scrotum

Giant condylomata acuminata [1]

SYN. BUSCHKE–LÖWENSTEIN SYNDROME

This condition occupies an uncertain position on the borderline of malignant disease. These rare but dramatic tumours have many similarities to florid oral papillomatosis of the oral mucosa and epithelioma cuniculatum, in that, although all three conditions have the cytological appearance of a benign condition, they are locally extremely aggressive and tend to recur repeatedly and extensively, even after apparently adequate surgery.

Metastases are rare, but the infiltrative nature of the tumour makes management very difficult [2].

Pathology. The lesion has none of the obvious hallmarks of malignancy. There is extreme acanthosis of the epidermis or mucosa, but little or no cellular atypia or mitotic figures. It has long been suspected that HPV is an aetiological agent, and modern methods of identification of HPV have confirmed the presence of HPV DNA (HPV-6) in these lesions [3,4].

Clinical features. Giant condylomas are found on both the male and female genitalia. Initially, they may appear as no more than a cluster of genital warts, but the lesion expands relentlessly, causing gross local tissue destruction (Fig. 72.22).

Treatment. Because local recurrence is common early and effective therapy is essential. Surgical excision and cryotherapy are effective, but topical wart preparations are not. Even with apparently adequate surgery, the lesion may recur, and in some cases partial penile amputation is necessary.

REFERENCES

1 Schwarz RA. Buschke–Löwenstein tumour: verrucous carcinoma of the penis. *J Am Acad Dermatol* 1990; **23**: 723–7.
2 Grossegger A, Hopfl R, Hussl H *et al*. Buschke–Löwenstein tumour infiltrating pelvic organs. *Br J Dermatol* 1994; **130**: 221–5.
3 Gissmann L, De Villiers EM, Zur Hausen H. Analysis of human genital warts (condylomata acuminata) and other genital tumors for human papillomavirus type 6 DNA. *Int J Cancer* 1982; **29**: 143–6.
4 Zochow KR, Ostrow RS, Bender M *et al*. Detection of human papillomavirus DNA in anogenital neoplasias. *Nature* 1982; **300**: 771–3.

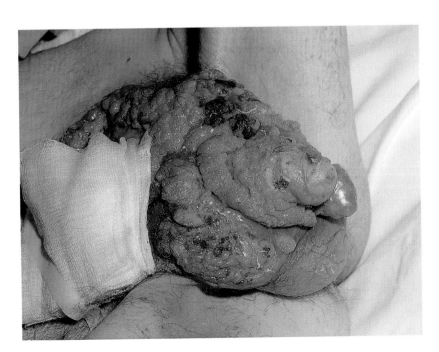

Fig. 72.22 Gross condylomas of Buschke–Löwenstein on the genitalia. Ten years after amputation, this patient is still alive with no recurrence. (Courtesy of Professor R.M. MacKie, Department of Dermatology, Glasgow University, UK.)

Erythroplasia of Queyrat [1,2]

This can be defined as a barely raised, sharply outlined, bright-red, glistening and velvety plaque occurring on mucous membranes, particularly the penis, which is refractory to treatment and eventuates in malignancy [3]. The use of the term should be restricted to an intraepidermal carcinoma, histologically similar to Bowen's disease. Erythroplasia is not associated with Bowen's disease elsewhere, nor with an increase in incidence of internal cancer [4].

Incidence. It is an uncommon condition. On the penis, it does not occur in men circumcised in infancy, and is not confined to elderly people [5]. It has been described on the mucous membranes of the mouth and tongue, and on the vulva. In the last site, British and American authors tend to prefer the designation Bowen's disease rather than erythroplasia.

Pathology. The surface may be denuded of stratum corneum and crusted, or covered by parakeratosis. The epidermis is thickened, particularly in the interpapillary ridges, which may become bulbous and extend quite deeply into the dermis. The other features are similar to those seen in Bowen's disease, with regard to the variety of abnormal cells in the prickle cell layer, large and hyperchromatic nuclei, multinucleate cells, increased mitoses, premature keratinization and disturbance of polarity. The dermis may be infiltrated by inflammatory cells.

Clinical features [3]. The penile lesion is situated on the glans, beginning under the foreskin as a red, glazed, barely raised, well-circumscribed and rather irregularly shaped plaque, which typically has a lacquered appearance. It is soft and supple. Crusting or erosion may occur later. Advanced lesions may spread from the mucous membrane to the skin. Invasive change is indicated by induration, verrucosity or ulceration. Metastasis can occur [6].

Diagnosis. Most of the common inflammatory conditions of the glans of foreskin are less sharply circumscribed and respond to application of a steroid and antimicrobial agent. Biopsy should be performed in cases of doubt.

Treatment. Erythroplasia responds to the local application of antimitotic agents such as 5-fluorouracil cream [7]. Soft X-ray therapy in cumulative doses of between 3200 and 5000 cGy has been helpful in clearing lesions of erythroplasia, but relapse may occur, and long-term follow-up is essential [8]. Alternatively, a radium mould can be used [2]. If there is evidence of invasion the treatment should be that employed for squamous cell carcinoma.

Squamous carcinoma of the penis and scrotum

Incidence and aetiology [9,10]. Squamous carcinomas of the penis and scrotum are caused by differing environmental factors, and they are preventable malignancies. Scrotal cancer, which is commoner in those of lower socio-economic status [11], appears to be caused by contact with mineral oils and tars. It is thus an industrial disease and, with appropriate protective clothing, could be prevented. Men who survive scrotal cancer appear to have a high incidence of other primary malignancies [12]. However, a study of 12 scrotal cancers (nine squamous cell carcinomas and three basal cell carcinomas) suggested that poor hygiene and chronic irritation may also be important [13].

Penile cancer is very rare in the circumcised male [14], and here the association with poor hygiene is well established. Improved hygiene appears to account for the reported falling incidence in Denmark [15]. Unlike scrotal cancer, however, there is no association with socio-economic status. There are studies reporting a high incidence of carcinoma of the cervix in the wives of men with carcinoma of the penis, suggesting a common, probably viral, aetiological factor [16,17]. HPV-16 has been associated with squamous cell carcinoma underlying a penile cutaneous horn [18]. A much increased incidence of squamous cell tumours of both penis and scrotum has been seen in patients with psoriasis who have been exposed to psoralen and UVA (PUVA) [19,20].

There are a few reports [21] of carcinoma of the penis developing as a consequence of lichen sclerosus et atrophicus, and one study reports two such cases in 44 patients with lichen sclerosus et atrophicus [22]. Hypertrophic lichen planus has been associated with penile carcinoma [23].

Clinical features [24,25]. The initial lesion on the penis is almost always within the preputial sac. It may be preceded by erythroplasia, leukoplakia or a warty excrescence, which is frequently misdiagnosed as a wart (Figs. 72.23 & 72.24). Lesions may occasionally be multiple and closely resemble condylomata acuminata [26,27]. The majority of tumours are histologically well-differentiated, and are initially vegetating rather than ulcerative. Despite this, metastases are present in the inguinal glands in about half the cases when first seen [16]. The general characteristics of squamous cell carcinoma are described in Chapter 36.

Diagnosis [28]. Biopsy of any suspicious warty, leukoplakic, reddened or ulcerated area should give a definite diagnosis. A low-grade carcinoma may show only epithelial hyperplasia microscopically for a considerable time before invasion becomes apparent [28].

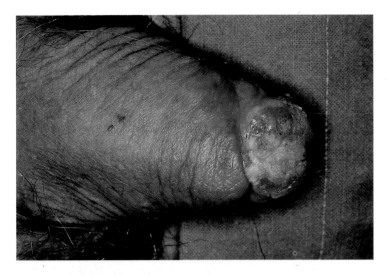

Fig. 72.23 Squamous cell carcinoma of the penis. (Courtesy of Dr W. Taylor, Hartlepool, UK.)

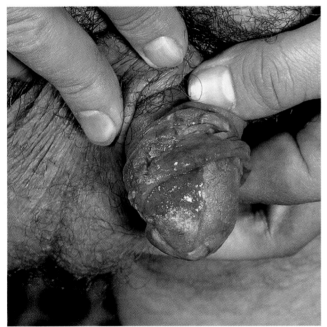

Fig. 72.24 Squamous cell carcinoma of the penis initially mistaken for genital warts.

Treatment. Radiotherapy can be used in cases where the regional nodes are not involved [29], but it is not effective in verrucous cancer [26]. Most authorities recommend partial or complete penile amputation, depending on the extent of the spread, with removal of involved nodes. Mohs' micrographic surgery has been used successfully in one series [4]. Combination chemotherapy can be used in advanced cases.

Other malignant tumours

Extramammary Paget's disease, basal cell carcinoma and malignant melanoma [30] are uncommon on the male genitalia. In a recent report, three out of 24 scrotal basal cell carcinomas had metastasized (a rate of 13%), an incidence that is much higher than the overall rate of less than 0.1% [31]. A variety of connective tissue tumours of the penis have been reported, including malignant haemangioendothelioma, undifferentiated sarcoma and angiosarcoma, dermatofibrosarcoma protuberans [32–35], and leiomyosarcoma.

Secondary metastatic tumours

About 200 cases of secondary metastatic tumours have been reported [36]. The primary sites have been mainly in the bowel and genitourinary tract. Symptoms and signs are variable, but priapism is present in 40% of cases. The presence of a mass, pain and dysuria are common, but acute urinary retention is rare as the urethra is not usually involved.

REFERENCES

1 Dehner LP, Smith BH. Soft tissue tumours of the penis. *Cancer* 1970; **25**: 1431–47.
2 Kaplan C, Kotah A. Erythroplasia of Queyrat (Bowen's disease of the penis). *J Surg Oncol* 1973; **5**: 281–90.
3 Blau S, Hyman AB. Erythroplasia of Queyrat. *Acta Derm Venereol (Stockh)* 1955; **35**: 341–78.
4 Brown MD, Zachary CB, Grekin RC *et al*. Penile tumours: their management by Mohs' micrographic surgery. *J Dermatol Surg Oncol* 1987; **13**: 1163–7.
5 McAninch JW, Moore CA. Precancerous penile lesions in young men. *J Urol* 1970; **104**: 287–90.
6 Avrach WW, Christensen HE. Mestastasizing erythroplasia of Queyrat: report of a case. *Acta Derm Venereol (Stockh)* 1976; **56**: 409–12.
7 Hueser JN, Pugh RP. Erythroplasia of Queyrat treated with topical 5-flourouracil. *J Urol* 1969; **102**: 595–7.
8 Blank AA, Schryder VW. Soft X-ray therapy in Bowen's disease and erythroplasia of Queyrat. *Dermatologica* 1985; **171**: 89–94.
9 Pointon RCS. Carcinoma of the penis. External beam therapy. *Proc R Soc Med* 1975; **68**: 779–81.
10 Schrek R, Lenowitz H. Etiological factors in carcinoma of the penis. *Cancer Res* 1947; **7**: 180–7.
11 Lee WR, Alderson MR, Downes JE. Scrotal cancer in the North-West of England. *Br J Ind Med* 1972; **29**: 188–95.

12 Holmes JG, Kipling MD, Waterhouse JAH. Subsequent malignancies in men with scrotal epithelioma. *Lancet* 1970; **ii**: 214–15.

13 McDonald MW. Carcinoma of scrotum. *Urology* 1982; **19**: 269–74.

14 Melmed EP, Payne JR. Carcinoma of the penis in a Jew circumcised in infancy. *Br J Surg* 1967; **54**: 729–31.

15 Frisch M, Friis S, Kruger-Kjaer S et al. Falling incidence of penis cancer in an uncircumcised population (Denmark 1943–90). *Br Med J* 1995; **311**: 1471.

16 Martinez I. Relationship of squamous cell carcinoma of the cervix uteri to squamous cell carcinoma of the penis among Puerto Rican women married to men with penile carcinoma. *Cancer* 1969; **24**: 777–80.

17 Smith PG, Kinlen LJ, White GC et al. Mortality of wives of men dying with cancer of the penis. *Br J Cancer* 1980; **41**: 422–8.

18 Solivan GA, Smith KJ, James WD. Cutaneous horn of penis: its association with squamous cell carcinoma and HPV 16 infection. *J Am Acad Dermatol* 1990; **23**: 969–72.

19 Stern RS. Members of the Photochemotherapy Follow Up Study. Genital tumors among men with psoriasis exposed to psoralens and ultraviolet A radiation (PUVA) and ultraviolet B radiation. *N Engl J Med* 1990; **322**: 1093–7.

20 de la Brassine, Richert B. Genital squamous cell carcinoma after PUVA therapy. *Dermatology* 1992; **185**: 316–18.

21 Pride HB, Miller OF, Tyler WB. Penile squamous cell carcinoma arising from balanitis xerotica obliterans. *J Am Acad Dermatol* 1993; **29**: 469–73.

22 Bingham JS. Carcinoma of the penis developing in lichen sclerosus et atrophicus. *Br J Vener Dis* 1978; **54**: 350–1.

23 Worheide J, Bonsmann G, Kolde G et al. Plattenepithelkarzinom auf dem Boden eines Lichen ruber hypertrophicus an der Glans penis. *Hautartz* 1991; **42**: 112–15.

24 Hanash KA, Furlow WL, Utz DC et al. Carcinoma of the penis. *J Urol* 1970; **104**: 291–7.

25 Staubitz WJ, Lent MH, Oberkincher OJ. Carcinoma of the penis. *Cancer* 1955; **8**: 371–8.

26 Kraus FT, Perez-Mesa C. Verrucous carcinoma: clinical and pathological study of 105 cases involving oral cavity, larynx and genitalia. *Cancer* 1966; **19**: 26–38.

27 Oranje AP, Brouwer J, Vuzevski VD. Condyloma-like penis carcinoma. *Dermatologica* 1976; **152**: 47–54.

28 Graham JH, Helwig EB, eds. *Tumours of the Skin.* Chicago: Yearbook Medical Publishers, 1964: 209.

29 Hope-Stone H. Carcinoma of the penis. External radiation mould technique. *Proc R Soc Med* 1975; **68**: 777–8.

30 Begun FP, Grossman HB, Dionko AC et al. Malignant melanoma of the penis and male urethra. *J Urol* 1984; **132**: 123–5.

31 Nahass GT, Blauvelt A, Pennys NS. Metastasis from basal cell carcinoma of scrotum. *J Am Acad Dermatol* 1992; **26**: 509–10.

32 Armijo M, Herrera E, De Dulanio F et al. Léiomyosarcome de la verge. Étude ultrastructurale. *Ann Dermatol Vénéréol* 1978; **105**: 267–74.

33 Belaich S, Civatte J, Bonvalet D et al. Dermato-fibrosarcome de Darier–Ferrand de la verge. *Ann Dermatol Vénéréol* 1978; **105**: 331–2.

34 Ghandur-Mnaymneh L, Gonzalez MS. Angiosarcoma of the penis with hepatic angiomas in a patient with low vinyl chloride exposure. *Cancer* 1981; **47**: 1318–24.

35 Isa SS, Almaraz R, McGreen J. Leiomyosarcoma of penis. Case report and review of literature. *Cancer* 1984; **54**: 939–42.

36 Robey EL, Schellhammer PF. Four cases of metastases to the penis and a review of the literature. *J Urol* 1984; **132**: 992–4.

The female genitalia

Introduction

Mention should be made at the outset of three authoritative and excellent accounts of this subject [1–3], which can of necessity be dealt with only briefly below. The reader is referred to these for further information.

REFERENCES

1 Beilby JOW, Ridley CM. Pathology of the vulva. In: Fox H, ed. *Hailes and Taylor's Obstetric and Gynaecological Pathology.* Edinburgh: Churchill Livingstone, 1986.

2 Gardner HL, Kaufman RH, eds. *Benign Diseases of the Vulva and Vagina.* St Louis: Mosby, 1969.

3 Ridley CM, ed. *The Vulva.* London: Churchill Livingstone, 1988.

Anatomy [1–3]

The female external genitalia extend between the pubis and the posterior commissure. The labia majora are equivalent to the scrotum, and the clitoris is the homologue of the penis. The labia majora are endowed with abundant subcutaneous fat and loose connective tissue, allowing considerable oedema to develop in inflammation, with minimal residual damage or scarring. The skin is thick, rugose and hairy on the outer aspect, and smooth and moist on the inner, where it takes on the character of a mucosal surface. Pilosebaceous units and 'free' sebaceous glands are abundant on the labia majora, but only the latter are found on the labia minora (Fig. 72.25). Small mucous glands occur on the skin of the vestibule. Nerve endings are numerous, especially on the clitoris. Apocrine glands, which are twice as abundant as in the male, are found on the mons veneris and labia majora.

Bartholin's glands, homologues of Cowper's glands, are compound, branching, tubular glands which secrete a clear, alkaline mucus into a duct lined deeply by columnar cells and superficially by transitional and then stratified epithelium. They lie between the superficial and deep layers of the urogenital diaphragm, opening by a duct 2cm long at the posterior aspect of the labium minus. The acini are lined by a single layer of columnar or cuboidal cells.

The vagina is lined by stratified squamous epithelium. The cells are stimulated by oestrogen, and mature keratinized cells are shed just before ovulation. The pH in reproductive life is in the region of 3.8–4.2, but is higher at menstruation.

In pregnancy, pigmentation increases, varicosities may develop and the pH falls. At the menopause, vascularity decreases, and the pattern of vessels becomes less regular [4]; the sebaceous glands become less active.

Congenital and developmental conditions

Malformations will not be discussed, as an admirable summary is available [3]. Accessory mammary tissue may become active in pregnancy, and give rise to fibroadenomas [2]. Dermoid cysts at the perineal raphe, and para-urethral cysts, are both rare, but may become infected. Cavernous haemangiomas ulcerate readily, as they do on the scrotum. Angiokeratomas may cause intermittent bleeding, or increase in size in pregnancy. Although rare, all other forms of angiomatous dysplasia, including angiokeratoma corporis diffusum, may occur. Local or general dysplasia of

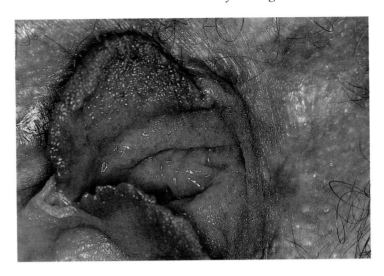

Fig. 72.25 Sebaceous hypertrophy on the labia minora.

the lymphatic system may manifest itself in childhood or young adult life as lymphangiectasia or as recurrent attacks of cellulitis. In adult life, acquired lymphangiomas following radiotherapy for cervical carcinoma may mimic genital wart infection [5]. Perineal, as well as axillary freckling, may occur in neurofibromatosis [6].

Special characteristics of common vulval dermatoses [7]

The normal characteristics of common diseases are modified. The lax tissues of the vulva encourage oedema rather than vesiculation [8]. Psoriasis loses its characteristic scaling; bullous lesions become erosive or vegetating; intertriginous lesions spread from the inguinal or abdominal folds; and secondary infection is common in the obese, middle-aged or elderly patient. Lichenification frequently complicates, and may mask, any pruritic skin lesion.

Urticaria and angio-oedema affecting the vulva give rise to considerable oedema and discomfort, although only rarely to difficulty in micturition [3]. Hereditary angio-oedema, however, may involve the urethra [9]. Dermographism may be confined to the genital and perineal areas [10,11]. Atopic eczema seldom affects the vulva, but lichen simplex is common. Seborrhoeic dermatitis and psoriasis (Fig. 72.26) are easily confused in this area, but other stigmata are usually present. Erythrasma may affect the labia majora, and is often overlooked unless Wood's light examination is carried out.

Fixed drug eruptions, less common now than previously, appear to have a predilection for the genital region. Residual pigmentation must be distinguished from general causes of pigmentation.

Vitiligo commonly involves the vulval area. Cytotoxic drugs may cause loss of pubic as well as scalp hair [2].

Contact dermatitis

The vulva has been shown to be significantly more sus-

ceptible to irritants [12,13]. Irritant contact dermatitis is most commonly seen in overscrupulous women whose enthusiastic use of soap or antiseptics may be combined with a rather guilty conscience [14]. Other culprits may be corrosive chemicals, or deodorant sprays applied too closely. Friction, trauma, moisture or the proximity of infective discharges play a role and are considered below. Allergic contact dermatitis [15] may present as oedema or be mistaken for angio-oedema. It is usually the result of medicaments, especially local anaesthetic and antihistamine creams. Other less common causes are nail varnish,

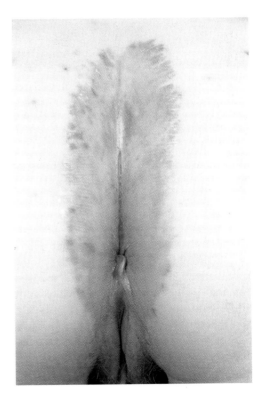

Fig. 72.26 Flexural psoriasis.

perfumes in sprays and sanitary napkins, contraceptives, clothing dyes, etc. A full battery of patch tests may reveal unsuspected sensitivities. This diagnosis should be considered whenever a pruritic vulval dermatosis fails to respond adequately to treatment.

REFERENCES

1 Beilby JOW, Ridley CM. Pathology of the vulva. In: Fox H, ed. *Hailes and Taylor's Obstetric and Gynaecological Pathology*. Edinburgh: Churchill Livingstone, 1986.
2 Gardner HL, Kaufman RH, eds. *Benign Diseases of the Vulva and Vagina*. St Louis: Mosby, 1969.
3 Ridley CM, ed. *The Vulva*. London: Churchill Livingstone, 1988.
4 Ryan TJ. In: *Physiology and Pathophysiology of the Skin*, Vol. 2. London: Academic Press, 1973.
5 Harwood CA, Mortimer PS. Acquired vulval lymphangiomata mimicking genital warts. *Br J Dermatol* 1993; **129**: 334–6.
6 Crowe FW. Axillary freckling as a diagnostic aid in neurofibromatosis. *Ann Intern Med* 1964; **61**: 1142–3.
7 Pincus SH. Vulvar dermatoses and pruritus vulvae. *Dermatol Clin* 1992; **10**: 297–308.
8 Elsner P, Wilhelm D, Maibach HI. Mechanical properties of human forearm and vulvar skin. *Br J Dermatol* 1990; **122**: 607–14.
9 Warin RP, Champion RH. *Urticaria*. London: Saunders, 1974: 114.
10 Sherertz EF. Clinical pearl: symptomatic dermographism as a cause of genital pruritus. *J Am Acad Dermatol* 1994; **31**: 1040–1.
11 Perniciaro C, Bustamenta AS, Guittierrez MM. Two cases of vulvodynia with unusual causes. *Acta Derm Venereol (Stockh)* 1993; **73**: 227–8.
12 Britz MB, Maibach HI. Human cutaneous vulvar reactivity to irritants. *Contact Dermatitis* 1979; **5**: 375–7.
13 Elsner P, Oriba HA, Maibach HI. Vulvar skin physiology: new aspects. *Hautarzt* 1988; **60**: 411–17.
14 Oriba HA, Maibach HI. Vulvar transepidermal water loss decay curves. Effect of occlusion, delipidation and age. *Acta Derm Venereol (Stockh)* 1989; **69**: 461–5.
15 Marren P, Wojnarowska F, Powell S. Allergic contact dermatitis and vulvar dermatoses. *Br J Dermatol* 1992; **126**: 52–6.

Miscellaneous conditions [1–3]

Varicosities of the labial veins may occur unilaterally in association with limb varicosities or appear in pregnancy. Although usually symptomless, they may cause pruritus or discomfort. Phthiriasis, scabies or even insect bites may be an unexpected cause of pruritus.

Vulval oedema accompanies acute infections, and is a feature of Crohn's disease, where it may be associated with lymphangiectasia [4]. Urticaria, angio-oedema and hereditary angio-oedema may involve the vulva, sometimes predominantly, and can occasionally be associated with immediate-type hypersensitivity to seminal plasma [5]. Lymphoedema may be primary or secondary to repeated streptococcal infections [6], lymphogranuloma venereum, granuloma inguinale [7], filariasis, tuberculosis and other chronic infections or neoplasms.

Accidental or purposeful traumatic lesions [1] are seldom seen by dermatologists, and may therefore be overlooked in differential diagnosis.

Darier's disease affecting the vulva produces brownish crusts, which break down and become malodorous; the vagina may be involved [8]. Acanthosis nigricans and seborrhoeic dermatitis may be simulated [3]. Ehlers–Danlos syndrome causes problems during childbirth (Chapter 44). Pseudoxanthoma elasticum also affects the vulva and sometimes the vagina [9].

Non-infective granulomas are uncommon. Midline granuloma has been reported [10]. Eosinophilic granuloma involving the vulval or perianal skin usually affects women aged 15–59 years, presenting as papules, vesicles, pustules, or weeping ulcers, which are often painful or pruritic. Diabetes insipidus is often present [11,12]. Vaginal involvement is rare.

Angiolymphoid hyperplasia with eosinophilia confined to the vulval area has been described [13].

Bullous diseases

Rapidly developing bullae may occur in erythema multiforme. Epidermolysis bullosa may affect the vulva [3], but seldom affects the vagina. In two of six personal cases of pemphigoid gestationis, the vulva was especially affected. Juvenile dermatitis herpetiformis also has a predilection for the genital area [14], as have pemphigus vulgaris and vegetans. The vagina, usually spared in other chronic bullous disease, may be involved, and the cervix has also been affected [15,16]. Familial benign chronic pemphigus of the vulva [17] is easily induced by friction, infection and irritants, and may escape recognition. It may be that the relatively newly described acantholytic and dyskeratotic eruption of the vulva may prove to be a variant of Hailey–Hailey disease [18,19]. Benign mucosal pemphigoid not infrequently involves the vulva, which has also been affected at some stage in all reported cases of necrolytic migratory erythema [20].

Non-scarring pemphigoid of the vagina is rare [21]. One personal case responded well to the intravaginal use of steroid suppositories. Recently, a localized childhood variant has been described [22–24].

Plantar pustulosis has been associated with recurrent sterile pustulosis of the vulva [25].

All secondarily infected chronic bullous diseases may be mistaken for intertrigo.

REFERENCES

1 Beilby JOW, Ridley CM. Pathology of the vulva. In: Fox H, ed. *Hailes and Taylor's Obstetric and Gynaecological Pathology*. Edinburgh: Churchill Livingstone, 1986.
2 Gardner HL, Kaufman RH, eds. *Benign Diseases of the Vulva and Vagina*. St Louis: Mosby, 1969.
3 Ridley CM, ed. *The Vulva*. London: Churchill Livingstone, 1988.
4 Handfield-Jones SE, Prendeville WL, Norman S. Vulval lymphangiectasia. *Genitourin Med* 1989; **65**: 335–7.
5 Chang T-W. Familial allergic seminal vulvovaginitis. *Am J Obstet Gynecol* 1976; **126**: 442–4.
6 Norburn LM, Coles RB. Recurrent erysipelas following vulvectomy. *J Obstet Gynecol* 1960; **67**: 279–80.
7 Sehgal VN, Jain MK, Sharma VK. Pseudo-elephantiasis induced by donovanosis. *Genitourin Med* 1987; **63**: 54–6.

8 Klostermann GF. In: *Handbuch des Speziellen Pathologischen Anatomie und Histologie.* Berlin: Springer-Verlag, 1972.

9 Goodman RM, Smith EW, Paton D *et al.* Pseudoxanthoma elasticum: a clinical and histological study. *Medicine* 1963; **42**: 297–334.

10 Friedmann I. Midline granuloma. *Proc R Soc Med* 1964; **57**: 289–97.

11 Thomas R, Barnhill D, Bibro M *et al.* Histiocytosis X in gynaecology: case presentation and review of literature. *Obstet Gynecol* 1986; **67**: 46–9.

12 Sang YH, Choi IC, Jun JB *et al.* Histiocytosis X with chronic weeping ulcers in the anogenital areas. *Ann Dermatol* 1990; **2**: 128–31.

13 Aguilar A, Embrojo P, Requena L. Angiolymphoid hyperplasia with eosinophilia limited to the vulva. *Clin Exp Dermatol* 1990; **15**: 65–7.

14 Grant PW. Juvenile dermatitis herpetiformis. *Trans St John's Hosp Dermatol Soc* 1968; **54**: 128–36.

15 Friedman D, Haim S, Paldi E. Refractory involvement of cervix uteri in a case of pemphigus vulgaris. *Am J Obstet Gynecol* 1971; **110**: 1023–4.

16 Sagher F, Kekovici B, Romen R. Nikolsky sign on cervix uteri in pemphigus. *Br J Dermatol* 1974; **90**: 407–11.

17 Thiers H, Moulin G, Rochet Y *et al.* Maladie de Hailey–Hailey à localisation vulvaire prédominante: étude génétique et ultra-structurale. *Bull Soc Fr Dermatol Syphiligr* 1975; **75**: 352–5.

18 Cooper PH. Acantholytic dermatoses localised to the vulvocrural area. *J Cutan Pathol* 1989; **16**: 81–4.

19 Van Joost TH, Vuzeuski VD, Tank B *et al.* Benign persistent papular acantholytic and dyskeratotic eruption: a case report and review of the literature. *Br J Dermatol* 1991; **124**: 92–5.

20 Mallinson CN, Bloom SR, Warin AP *et al.* A glucagonoma syndrome. *Lancet* 1974; **ii**: 1–4.

21 Haustein VF. Localized non-scarring bullous pemphigoid of the vagina. *Dermatologica* 1988; **176**: 200–7.

22 Guenther LC, Shum D. Localised childhood vulvar pemphigoid. *J Am Acad Dermatol* 1990; **22**: 762–4.

23 Saad RW, Domloge-Hultsch N, Yancey KB *et al.* Childhood localized vulvar pemphigoid: is it a true variant of bullous pemphigoid? *Arch Dermatol* 1992; **128**: 807–10.

24 Guenther LC, Shum D. Localized childhood vulvar pemphigoid. *J Am Acad Dermatol* 1990; **22**: 762–4.

25 Keefe M, Wakeil RA, Kerr REI. Sweet's syndrome, plantar pustulosis and vulval pustules. *Clin Exp Dermatol* 1988; **13**: 344–6.

Disorders of the sweat glands [1,2]

Fox–Fordyce disease involves the mons pubis and labia, and is extremely pruritic. The pink, follicular papules may be obscured by secondary infection or lichenification. The itching distinguishes this condition from syringomas, but apocrine or miliarial retention cysts [3] may cause difficulty. Rarely, chromhidrosis, trichomycosis and genital white piedra cause discoloration of the pubic hair, and must be distinguished from phthiriasis [4,5].

Hidradenitis suppurativa (Chapter 27)

This condition is less common in this area than it is in the male. The aetiology is obscure. It is not associated with virilization [6]. Seven patients have been described in whom the disorder occurred in association with the use of a combined oestrogen–progestogen contraceptive pill [7]. Secondary inflammation in occluded apocrine glands may be responsible for the signs. Abscesses, sinuses and fistulae develop, often continuously and remorselessly, involving increasingly wider areas as the postinflammatory scarring creates distortion of the tissues. Carcinoma may develop in the affected area [8]. Early lesions are often mistaken for boils, and later ones for lymphogranuloma venereum or Crohn's disease.

Small local lesions respond well to phenolization, cryotherapy, or injections of corticosteroids. More advanced lesions may be helped by appropriate antibiotics, but usually require surgery—either excision and grafting or marsupialization and diathermy; the latter is a technique which has proved very effective in personal cases. Spontaneous regression of activity usually occurs as scarring destroys gland tissue, or with the advent of the menopause.

Tumours of apocrine origin are discussed below.

REFERENCES

1 Beilby JOW, Ridley CM. Pathology of the vulva. In: Fox H, ed. *Hailes and Taylor's Obstetric and Gynaecological Pathology.* Edinburgh: Churchill Livingstone, 1986.

2 Ridley CM, ed. *The Vulva.* London: Churchill Livingstone, 1988.

3 Gardner HL, Kaufman RH, eds. *Benign Diseases of the Vulva and Vagina.* St Louis: Mosby, 1969.

4 Kalter DC, Tschen JA, Cernoch PL *et al.* Genital white piedra; epidemiology, microbiology and therapy. *J Am Acad Dermatol* 1986; **14**: 982–93.

5 White SW, Smith J. Trichomycosis pubis. *Arch Dermatol* 1979; **115**: 444–5.

6 Jemec GBE. The symptomatology of hidradenitis suppurativa in women. *Br J Dermatol* 1988; **119**: 345–50.

7 Stellon AJ, Wakeling M. Hidradenitis suppurativa associated with the use of oral contraceptives. *Br Med J* 1989; **298**: 28–9.

8 Humphrey LJ, Playforth H, Leavell UW, Jr. Squamous cell carcinoma arising in hidradenitis suppurativa. *Arch Dermatol* 1960; **100**: 59–62.

Benign tumours of the vulva [1–4]

These are relatively rare [1]. Melanocytic naevi [5], seborrhoeic warts and especially fibroepithelial polyps, often of considerable size, are not uncommon, although they are usually in the pubic area or genitocrural folds rather than on the vulva itself. They are probably more common in the male on the inner thighs, but form part of the spectrum of 'pseudoacanthosis nigricans' in the middle-aged female, which may act as a marker for insulin resistance [6].

Verruciform xanthomas are rare [7]. Clinically, they mimic the more common benign warty lesions of the vulval area.

Epidermal cysts are seen on the labia majora and in the region of the clitoris. They are especially common in tribal societies which practice female circumcision [8], and may become inflamed, or present because of increasing size. Obstruction of the duct of a Bartholin's gland may occur in the reproductive years, causing a cyst in the posterior part of the labia majora. Marsupialization [1] may be performed if the cyst is troublesome, unless there is suspicion of malignancy, when an excision biopsy is to be preferred. Polypoid lesions of the vulva may rarely represent gross sebaceous gland hyperplasia [9].

Eccrine syringomas are asymptomatic, and occasionally involve the vulva [10], but hidradenoma papilliferum is seen almost exclusively in this region [11,12], especially in the labium majus. It presents as a solitary, firm or soft nodule, up to 4 cm in diameter [3], showing histological features of apocrine-type papillary epithelium, similar to intraduct papillomas of the breast. Over 200 cases had been reported up to 1973 [11]. Rarely, calcified nodules may be found, and these probably represent the female counterpart of idiopathic scrotal calcinosis [13].

Angiokeratoma of the vulva is probably more common than is recognized [14]. The lesions, which are solitary or multiple [15], may cause bleeding in pregnancy. They may correspond to the lesions called 'senile haemangiomas' [1]. They must be distinguished from the more important lesions of angiokeratoma corporis diffusum, which are more widespread.

Numerous types of benign tumours may occasionally occur on the vulva, for example moles, angiomas, capillary naevi and neurofibromas [16,17]. Granular cell myoblastoma [18,19], presenting as flesh-coloured, occasionally pedunculated or ulcerated lesions, is likely to be diagnosed only histologically.

The rare but troublesome leimyoma presents as a solitary, firm, reddish-brown tumour, which may be painful on pressure and with heat or cold. A clitoral leiomyoma associated with a leiomyoma of the oesophagus has been reported [20].

Nodular fasciitis of the vulva is a rare occurrence, but it is important to differentiate it histologically from leiomyosarcoma and malignant fibrous histiocytoma [21].

Lymphocytoma cutis, also a rare lesion in this area, presents as glistening brownish-red nodules, occasionally extending to the urethra and vagina [22].

Endometriosis [1] occasionally occurs on the vulva or in the vagina as a direct implantation. The condition may be becoming more common [3] because of the increased frequency of gynaecological procedures. The lesions are often preceded by uterine curettage, or sometimes occur in episiotomy scars after delivery [23]. They present as firm, bluish nodules, which become tender or bleed during menstruation. The histology is diagnostic.

REFERENCES

1 Beilby JOW, Ridley CM. Pathology of the vulva. In: Fox H, ed. *Hailes and Taylor's Obstetric and Gynaecological Pathology*. Edinburgh: Churchill Livingstone, 1986.
2 Gardner HL, Kaufman RH, eds. *Benign Diseases of the Vulva and Vagina*. St Louis: Mosby, 1969.
3 Ridley CM, ed. *The Vulva*. London: Churchill Livingstone, 1988.
4 Hood AF, Lumadue J. Benign vulval tumours. *Dermatol Clin* 1992; **10**: 371–85.
5 Christensen WN, Friedman KJ, Woodruff JD et al. Histologic characteristics of vulvar nevocellular nevi. *J Cutan Pathol* 1987; **14**: 87–91.
6 Grasinger CC, Wild RA, Parker IJ. Vulvar acanthosis nigricans: a marker of insulin resistance in hirsute women. *Fertil Steril* 1993; **59**: 583–6.
7 De Rosa G, Barra E. Verruciform xanthoma of the vulva: case report. *Genitourin Med* 1989; **65**: 252–4.
8 Onuigbo WIB. Vulval epidermoid cysts in the Igbos of Nigeria. *Arch Dermatol* 1976; **112**: 1405–6.
9 Rocamora A, Santonja C, Vives R et al. Sebaceous gland hyperplasia of the vulva. A case report. *Obstet Gynecol* 1986; **68** (Suppl. 3): 635–55.
10 Panizzon R, Mitsuhashi Y, Schnyder VW. Das Syringom der Vulva. *Hautarzt* 1987; **38**: 607–9.
11 Nielson NC. Hidroadenoma of the vulva. *Acta Obstet Gynecol Scand* 1973; **52**: 387–9.
12 Veraldi S, Schrianchi–Veraldi R, Marini D. Hidradenoma papilliferum of the vulva. *J Dermatol Surg Oncol* 1990; **16**: 674–6.
13 Jameleddine FN, Salmon SM, Shbaklo Z et al. Vulvar calcinosis, the counterpart of idiopathic scrotal calcinosis. *Cutis* 1988; **41**: 273–5.
14 Blair C. Angiokeratoma of the vulva. *Br J Dermatol* 1970; **83**: 409–11.
15 Karlsmark T, Weismann K, Kobayasi T. Ultra-structure of angiokeratoma vulvae. *Acta Derm Venereol (Stockh)* 1988; **68**: 80–2.
16 Schreiber MM. Vulvar von Recklinghausen's disease. *Arch Dermatol* 1963; **88**: 320–1.
17 Lewis FM, Lewis-Jones MS, Toon PG et al. Neurofibromatosis of the vulva *Br J Dermatol* 1992; **127**: 540–1.
18 Gifford RRM, Birch HW. Granular cell myoblastoma of multicentric origin involving the vulva: a case report. *Am J Obstet Gynecol* 1973; **117**: 184–7.
19 Sadler WP, Docherty MB. Malignant myoblastoma vulvae. *Am J Obstet Gynecol* 1951; **61**: 1047–55.
20 Stenchever MA, McDivitt RW, Fisher JA. Leiomyoma of the clitoris. *J Reprod Med* 1973; **10**: 75–6.
21 Li Volsi VA, Brooks JJ. Nodular fasciitis of the vulva. A report of two cases. *Obstet Gynecol* 1987; **69**: 513–16.
22 Matras A. Ein Bertrag zum Lymphocytoma genitale. *Hautarzt* 1964; **15**: 657–61.
23 Paull T, Tedesch L. Perineal endometriosis at the site of episiotomy scar. *Obstet Gynecol* 1972; **40**: 28–34.

Infections of the vulva

Normal flora [1–5]

The skin of the perineal area has a higher pH, temperature and degree of humidity than skin elsewhere, and harbours large numbers of transient and resident organisms, mainly micrococci, diphtheroids and lactobacilli. Only coagulase-positive staphylococci are usually considered pathogenic, but have been found in as many as 67% of normal females [6]. Alpha-haemolytic streptococci were present in 44% of the same series; however, only the β. 240-haemolytic strain, notably of Lancefield groups A and C, are pathogenic. Carriage rates are highest in hospital personnel [7]. Gram-negative bacteria (39%) are usually transient, but may sometimes be pathogenic. Health spa whirlpools appear to encourage the growth of these organisms [8].

Candida albicans is a normal inhabitant of the site. It is asymptomatic in 10% of women, and normally associated with rectal carriage [9]. Its pathogenicity is discussed below.

Colonization in infancy [4]

Although it has been the subject of much study, the method, extent and pattern of neonatal colonization is not accurately defined, and may initially be fortuitous. The significance of the flora in relation to infection in this area is deal with in Chapter 14.

The effect of diabetes

In diabetics whose disease is well-controlled, the flora does not differ significantly from that of normal individuals, but infections, especially candidiasis and erythrasma, are more common, perhaps because of the high skin sugar in diabetic subjects [4]. Necrotizing fasciitis may occur in poorly controlled diabetes [10].

Vaginal flora

Lactobacilli are probably the most common organisms, particularly on the labial mucosa [4]. However, vaginal swabs from preoperative women were sterile in about half the cases [11]. A mixed flora, including coliforms, streptococci and *Bacteroides* species, was found in the remainder, more frequently in the first half of the cycle. The frequency of isolation of *Candida albicans* varies with different groups, and is probably a matter of selection. It is more frequent in pregnancy, due to a reduction in glycogen availability from vaginal epithelium [3]. Its significance is still a matter of controversy. In the pregnant woman, it may well be pathogenic [12], but in the non-pregnant woman the significance is still a matter of opinion [9,13,14].

Bacterial vaginosis is the term used to describe a common clinical entity which results from the interaction between *Gardnerella vaginalis* and anaerobic bacterial overgrowth within the vagina. Although often asymptomatic, it may present as an increase in secretion or malodour. Despite the fact that its incidence is equal in virginal and sexually active groups [15], studies of male sexual partners have revealed a 30% incidence of non-gonococcal urethritis [16]. Suspicions have been raised that this type of abnormal bacterial colonization may in some way be related to prematurity and late miscarriage in pregnant patients [17].

REFERENCES

1 Beilby JOW, Ridley CM. Pathology of the vulva. In: Fox H, ed. *Hailes and Taylor's Obstetric and Gynaecological Pathology*. Edinburgh: Churchill Livingstone, 1986.
2 Gardner HL, Kaufman RH, eds. *Benign Diseases of the Vulva and Vagina*. St Louis: Mosby, 1969.
3 Ridley CM, ed. *The Vulva*. London: Churchill Livingstone, 1988.
4 Noble WC, Somerville DA. In: Rook AJ, ed. *Microbiology of Human Skin*, Vol. 2. *Major Problems in Dermatology*. London: WB Saunders, 1974.
5 Sobel JD. Vulvovaginitis. *Dermatol Clin* 1992; **10**: 339–59.
6 Aly R, Britz MB, Maibach HI. Quantitative microbiology of human vulva. *Br J Dermatol* 1979; **101**: 445–8.
7 Rowan D. Streptococci and the genital tract. *Int J STD AIDS* 1993; **4**: 63–4.
8 Sausker WF, Aeling JL, Fitzpatrick JE et al. *Pseudomonas* folliculitis acquired from a health spa whirlpool. *JAMA* 1978; **239**: 2362–5.
9 Leegard M. Incidence of *Candida albicans* in the vagina of healthy young women. *Acta Obstet Gynecol Scand* 1984; **63**: 85–9.
10 Addison WA, Livengood CH, Hill GB et al. Necrotising fasciitis of vulvar origin in diabetic patients. *Obstet Gynecol* 1984; **63**: 473–9.
11 Neary MP, Allen J, Okubadejo OA et al. Preoperative vaginal bacteria and postoperative infections in gynaecological patients. *Lancet* 1973; **ii**: 1291–4.
12 Carrol CJ, Hurley R, Stanley VC. Criteria for diagnosis of candida vulvovaginitis in pregnant women. *J Obstet Gynaecol* 1973; **80**: 258–63.
13 Hurley R. In: Skinner SA, Carr JG, eds. *Symposium of the Society of Applied Bacteriology*, No. 3. London: Academic Press, 1974.
14 Oriel JD, Partridge BM, Denny MJ et al. Genital yeast infections. *Br Med J* 1972; **iv**: 761–4.
15 Bump RC, Buesching WJ. Bacterial vaginosis in virginal and sexually active

adolescent females: evidence against sexual transmission. *Am J Obstet Gynecol* 1988; **158**: 935–9.
16 Arumainayagam JR, de Silva Y, Shahmanesh M. Anaerobic vaginosis: a study of male sexual partners. *Int J STD AIDS* 1991; **2**: 102–4.
17 Hay PE, Lamont RF, Taylor–Robinson D et al. Abnormal bacterial colonisation of the genital tract and subsequent preterm delivery and late miscarriage. *Br Med J* 1994; **308**: 295–8.

Malacoplakia of the vulva [1]

An unusual granulomatous response to infection—usually by *Escherichia coli*, sometimes *Pseudomonas* species [1] or *Staphylococcus aureus* [2]—has been reported in the vagina [3], on the vulva [4] and the perianal skin [1]. More commonly it involves the urinary or gastrointestinal tract mucosa. The 'soft' plaques may present as an indurated ulcer. Diagnosis is made by searching for and finding Michaelis–Guttmann bodies in the closely packed histiocytes of the infiltrate.

REFERENCES

1 Lewin KJ, Fair WR, Steigbigel RT et al. Clinical and laboratory studies into the pathogenesis of malacoplakia. *J Clin Pathol* 1976; **29**: 354–63.
2 Price HM, Hanrahan JB, Florida RG. Morphogenesis of calcium laden cytoplasmic bodies in malacoplakia of the skin: an electron microscopic study. *Hum Pathol* 1973; **4**: 381–94.
3 Khan AR. Malakoplakia of vagina. *J Ind Med Assoc* 1979; **72**: 254–5.
4 Arul KJ, Emmerson RW. Malacoplakia of the skin. *Clin Exp Dermatol* 1977; **2**: 131–5.

Venereal and 'paravenereal' conditions

For convenience, the main forms of venereal disease as causes of vulvovaginitis will be considered together. The reader is referred to the fuller descriptions of the individual diseases given elsewhere (Chapters 27 and 30).

Syphilis and gonorrhoea must always be thought of in women presenting with vulvovaginitis, particularly as the presentation is not as obvious as in the male.

Gonorrhoea

The incidence is increasing, particularly among younger females. Under poor hygienic conditions, infants may become infected via towels, etc., or during birth. In the female, the signs of infection may be few or absent. Gonococcal vulvitis is rare, but may occur with a mixed discharge. Inflammation involves the urethra, and the paraurethral and Bartholin's glands. The rectum and cervix may also be involved. The rare, soft gonorrhoeal ulcer can occur without urethritis [1]. Several authors [2,3] have stressed the need to take cervical, urethral and rectal swabs if the disease is not to be missed. Repeated cultures may be necessary.

Syphilis

The typical primary chancre is now seldom seen in women.

The posterior commissure or urethral opening are usually affected, but it may occur anywhere from the cervix to the labia majora. Extensive oedema or induration may simulate cellulitis. The lesion must be distinguished from other causes of ulceration.

Condylomata lata are seen in the vulval and anal areas in the secondary stage. The lesions of endemic syphilis resemble condylomas [4], which are also a feature of congenital syphilis. Primary vulval involvement in yaws is rare, but ulcers and crusted nodules may occur on the vulva in the secondary stage.

Chancroid

This is still a relatively rare disease in the UK, but is much more common in tropical regions. An initial ulcerating papule is followed by similar lesions in adjacent and opposing sites. The regional glands enlarge, and may suppurate. Pain, when present, distinguishes the primary lesion from a chancre. Other venereal diseases may coexist and confuse the clinical picture [5].

Granuloma inguinale
SYN. GRANULOMA VENEREUM

This disease of tropical countries is occasionally encountered in immigrants, and in individuals returning from visits to these countries. The lesions occur in any part of the genitocrural area, vagina or cervix. The initial bleb or nodule breaks down to form an ulcer with a rolled edge and crazy-paving appearance [6]. Secondary infection is common, and may lead to constitutional upset [7]. Dissemination can occur. A postinfective thickening of the involved area is not entirely explained by lymphoedema [8]. The diagnosis is made by finding Donovan bodies in smears from biopsy material or the biopsy specimen.

Mycobacterial infections [9] (Chapter 28)

Tuberculosis of the genital tract is rare. A reported prevalence of 3–10% of microscopic tuberculosis of the cervix in patients with pelvic infections [10] seems high for the UK. The primary tuberculous chancre is now extremely rare, most lesions deriving from foci elsewhere. Exogenous infection may be conveyed by sputum or by sexual intercourse. The vulva was involved in three of 26 cases of genital tuberculosis in South Africa [11]. Unilateral Bartholin's gland infection has been reported [12]. Haematogenous spread may involve the vulva. Infection of the endometrium and genital tract may cause a tuberculous vulvovaginitis.

Nodules, ulcers with ragged edges, or fungating masses are seen in this infection. Suppuration and scarring of the regional lymph glands may occur, followed by lymphoedema

of the limb [13]. Smears, histology and culture confirm the diagnosis.

A primary focus of the tuberculous infection must always be sought, and a full course of antituberculous therapy should be given.

Leprosy (Chapter 29)

Vulval lesions are uncommon [14,15]. The pubic hair may be lost [9].

Condylomata acuminata

These affect the mucocutaneous surfaces, and form extensive, vegetating masses which may occlude the vaginal orifice and perianal area, especially in pregnancy or in the presence of a vaginal discharge of coincident venereal infection, which should be treated first. Electrocoagulation may be needed if the infection is voluminous and intravaginal. Secondary syphilis, especially in pregnancy, may cause extensive mucous patches, condylomatous masses, and erythematopapular or psoriasiform lesions, which must be distinguished.

Lymphogranuloma venereum [16]

This condition is rare in women. It is due to a chlamydia of a specific serotype. The initial ulcer, papule or herpetiform lesion occurs in the region of the labia, clitoris, fourchette or in the vagina, when pelvic lymphadenopathy is accompanied by a moderate or severe degree of constitutional upset. The subsequent picture of ulceration, scarring, stricture, lymphoedema and eventually esthiomene completes the sequence of events. The Frei test is positive.

Chlamydia of different serotypes have now been recognized as a frequent cause of cervicitis and Bartholinitis in women, both postgonococcal and non-gonococcal urethritis in men, and conjunctivitis in neonates [17].

REFERENCES

1 Landergren G. Case of gonorrheal ulcer. *Acta Derm Venereol (Stockh)* 1963; **43**: 496.
2 Bhattacharyya MN, Jephcott AE. Diagnosis of gonorrhoea in women. *Br J Vener Dis* 1974; **50**: 109–12.
3 Schroeter AL, Reynolds G. The rectal culture as a test of cure of gonorrhoea in the female. *J Infect Dis* 1972; **125**: 499–503.
4 Wilcox RR, ed. *Textbook of Venereal Diseases and Treponematoses*, 2nd edn. London: Heinemann, 1964.
5 Editorial. Chancroid. *Lancet* 1982; **ii**: 747–8.
6 Gardner HL, Kaufman RH, eds. *Benign Diseases of the Vulva and Vagina*. St Louis: Mosby, 1969.
7 Wilcocks C, Manson-Bahr P, eds. *Manson's Tropical Diseases*, 17th edn. London: Bailliére Tindall, 1972: 645.
8 Douglas CP. Lymphogranuloma venereum and granuloma inguinale of the vulva. *Am J Obstet Gynecol* 1962; **69**: 871–80.
9 Klostermann GF. In: *Handbuch der speziellen pathologischen anatomie und Histologie Weibliche Geschelentsorgave*. Berlin: Springer-Verlag, 1972.

10 Beilby JOW, Ridley CM. Pathology of the vulva. In: Fox H, ed. *Hailes and Taylor's Obstetric and Gynaecological Pathology*. Edinburgh: Churchill Livingstone, 1986.

11 Moore D. Genito-peritoneal tuberculosis—a review of 26 cases. *S Afr Med J* 1954; **28**: 666–70.

12 Schaefer G. Diagnosis and treatment of female genital tuberculosis. *Clin Obstet Gynecol* 1959; **2**: 530–48.

13 Ashworth FL. Tuberculous lymphoedema. *Br Med J* 1974; **iv**: 167.

14 Bonar BE, Rabson AS. Gynaecologic aspects of leprosy. *Obstet Gynecol* 1957; **9**: 33–43.

15 Grabstold DH, Swan L. Genitourinary lesions in leprosy with special reference to the problem of atrophy of the testes. *JAMA* 1952; **149**: 1287–91.

16 Ridley CM, ed. *The Vulva*. London: Churchill Livingstone, 1988.

17 Taylor-Robinson D, Thomas BJ. The role of *Chlamydia trachomatis* in genital tract and associated diseases. *J Clin Pathol* 1980; **33**: 205–33.

Vulvovaginitis

Inflammation of the female external genitalia may result from infective and irritant causes. It is not always possible to separate these. A vaginal discharge can, on occasion, give rise to vulval irritation, and treatment for this may cause a contact dermatitis. Secondary infection of any vulval rash is common, due to the proximity of faeces and urine, and the irresistible desire to scratch. The moisture and warmth engendered by inflammation are conducive to further soreness, irritant dermatitis and scratching. Lichenification is frequent, and may obscure the original cause of the irritation.

Vaginal discharge

This is a common complaint, and is not usually associated with other symptoms. Five conditions account for 95% of all vaginal discharges or infections. A pH higher than 6 is strongly predictive of infection [1].

Mucorrhoea and epithelial discharge

Between 5 and 10% of women complaining of vaginal discharge do not have infection. They have an excess physiological secretion of mucus and vaginal epithelial debris. The discharge is not irritant, it is odourless, and is of a thick, grey-white pasty consistency. Vaginal pH is normal.

'Non-specific vaginitis' [2]

This is the commonest form of vaginitis. The patient complains of excessive, grey, thin discharge, associated with a 'fishy' malodour, which is especially strong immediately after intercourse. Vulval irritation is slight or absent in this group, and symptoms are so few that many women regard their condition as part of the spectrum of normality.

Controversy has surrounded the aetiology, but it is now generally agreed that the disorder is almost invariably associated with infection by a small, aerobic Gram-negative rod known as *Gardnerella vaginalis*, after its discoverer [3]. It would appear that this organism alone is incapable of causing infection, and non-specific vaginitis is now regarded as a complex interrelationship between *Gardnerella* and anaerobic species of bacteria [4], two of which (belonging to a new genus *Mobiluncus*) have been identified only recently [5,6].

Characteristically, the vaginal pH is greater than 5, and the fishy odour of the discharge can be accentuated by the addition of an alkali such as 10% potassium hydroxide (the Whiff test). Treatment with metronidazole 200 mg three times per day for 7 days is effective if the consort is treated at the same time.

Cervicitis

Nearly one-third of women complaining of vaginal discharge do not suffer from vaginal infection. They suffer from a mucopurulent, occasionally blood-stained discharge from infected endocervical mucosa.

The four pathogens most commonly involved are *Neisseria gonorrhoeae*, *Chlamydia trachomatis*, *Trichomonas vaginalis* and herpesvirus hominis.

The discharge from chronic cervicitis is not normally irritating to the vulval skin. Patients' complaints tend to relate either to the discharge itself or to deep pelvic pain and dyspareunia.

Chlamydia trachomatis has been grown from the cervices of 50% of women with mucopurulent cervicitis [7]. It responds to treatment with tetracyclines, and should be regarded as the counterpart of urethritis in males.

Trichomoniasis [8–11]

Infection with *T. vaginalis* is an increasingly infrequent cause of vaginitis and vulvitis in the Western world. As an inhabitant of the female genital tract, the problems of pathogenicity are similar to those of *Candida* species, and depend on a favourable environment for its growth. Infections are rare in children and after the menopause. They are common in poorer social groups.

Trichomonal vaginitis causes a frothy, malodorous, greyish green, watery discharge, and a bright-red or petechiae-studded vaginal mucosa. Although itching is generally less severe than with *Candida* infection, secondary vulvitis occurs from irritation by the discharge [11], which may extend to the genitocrural area. Erythema and swelling of the vestibule and labia minora are often present.

The diagnosis is made by examination of a fresh specimen on a warm slide, or by culture of the discharge. The distress and anxiety caused by this mild but persistent condition has often led to an erroneous diagnosis of 'neurodermatitis', and the dermatologist should be careful to exclude trichomoniasis before making this diagnosis. Coexistent *Candida* infection should also be excluded.

As the male may harbour the infection, and occasionally show signs of it, both partners should receive treatment. Metronidazole (200 mg three times per day for 7 days) is usually successful, but other regimens have their advocates. Relapse is due either to reinfection or to failure to take the tablets. Nimorazole may be more effective if there is a coexistent urinary infection [12].

Candidal vulvovaginitis [8,9,11]

Candida albicans may be present in the vagina of 25% of asymptomatic women as a commensal. Changes in host factors are probably responsible for transition to pathogenicity, and are generally not directly associated with sexual contact. Factors related to cell-mediated immunity are doubtless important, but as yet are ill understood. Pregnancy, diabetes, cystic fibrosis [13], possibly oral antibiotics, the contraceptive pill, immunosuppressive drugs and local tissue damage, for example incontinence rashes and intertrigo, may all favour precipitation of infection. In general, if microscopy reveals the yeast-like (bunch of grapes) form of organisms, the commensal state is most likely, whereas the pseudohyphal (mycelial) form is most often associated with pathogenicity.

Candida infection accounted for one-third of 478 consecutive cases of discharge and pruritus [14]. The vaginitis may be difficult to diagnose clinically unless the skin is involved (Fig. 72.27). The discharge may be slight, the vagina is reddened, and the white, curd-like plaques of thrush may be present. The degree of pruritus varies, but may be considerable. *Candida* may rarely be the cause of the urethral syndrome and cystitis.

The erythema may extend to the inner aspects of the labia and vestibule only. However, when it spreads to the genitocrural region, it classically presents as well-demarcated sheets with a lightly scaling or vesiculopustular edge. Beyond this edge lie grouped or isolated superficial small pustules, which rupture rapidly, leaving a slightly scaly periphery. In such cases, microscopy affords an immediate diagnosis. However, all specimens should be cultured, especially those from the vagina.

In the obese, middle-aged patient, late-onset diabetes should be considered, and appropriate tests carried out.

Candidiasis may coexist with other infections, notably gonorrhoea and trichomonal infection (see above). Alternatively, it may supervene as a secondary invader on other genital dermatoses, especially if predisposing factors are present.

Turolopsis glabrata is very occasionally the cause of a vaginal mycotic infection.

Treatment. The newer imidazole group of drugs (clotrimazole, miconazole and econazole) are now regarded as more reliable than the polyene antibiotics nystatin and amphotericin [15].

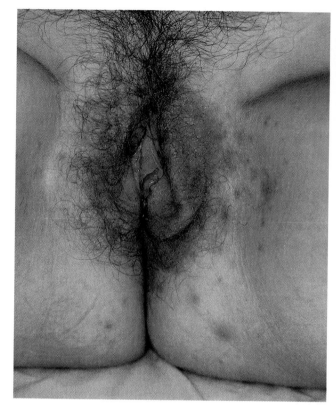

Fig. 72.27 Vulvitis due to *Candida*.

Skin and vaginal therapy must be combined; treatment of the consort is almost mandatory, as 10% were involved in one series [16]. In refractory cases, oral itraconazole or the new triazole, fluconazole, may be helpful in clearing rectal carriage, especially when combined with local therapy.

Other (non-infective) causes of vaginal discharge are less common, and are listed below:
1 atrophic vaginitis;
2 vaginal ulceration;
3 vaginal fistulae;
4 tumours;
5 excessive douching;
6 contraceptive irritation;
7 retained foreign body.

REFERENCES

1 Hanna NF, Taylor-Robinson D, Kalodikki-Karamanoli M *et al.* The relation between vaginal pH and the microbiological status in vaginitis. *Br J Obstet Gynaecol* 1985; **92**: 1267–71.
2 Vontver LA, Eschenbach DA. The role of *Gardnerella vaginalis* in nonspecific vaginitis. *Clin Obstet Gynecol* 1981; **24**: 439–60.
3 Gardner HL. *Haemophilus vaginalis* vaginitis after 25 years. *Am J Obstet Gynecol* 1980; **137**: 385–91.
4 Speigel CA, Amsel R, Eschenbach D *et al.* Anaerobic bacteria in nonspecific vaginitis. *N Engl J Med* 1980; **303**: 601–7.
5 De Boer JM, Plantema FHF. Ultrastructure of the *in situ* adherence of *Mobiluncus* to vaginal epithelial cells. *Can J Microbiol* 1988; **34**: 757–66.
6 Holst E. Reservoir of four organisms associated with bacterial

vaginosis suggests lack of sexual transmission. *J Clin Microbiol* 1990; **28**: 2033–9.

7 Brunham RC, Paavonen J, Stevens CE *et al.* Mucopurulent cervicitis—the ignored counterpart in women of urethritis in men. *N Engl J Med* 1984; **311**: 1–6.

8 Gardner HL, Kaufman RH, eds. *Benign Diseases of the Vulva and Vagina.* St Louis: Mosby, 1969.

9 Ridley CM, ed. *The Vulva.* London: Churchill Livingstone, 1988.

10 Catterall RD. Trichomonal infections of the genital tract. *Med Clin North Am* 1972; **56**: 1203–9.

11 Fleury FJ. Adult vaginitis. *Clin Obstet Gynecol* 1981; **24**: 407–38.

12 Burslem RW. The treatment of trichomonal vaginitis. *Prescribers J* 1973; **13**: 14–16.

13 Saywer SM, Bowes G, Phelan PD. Vulvovaginal candidiasis in young women with cystic fibrosis. *Br J Med* 1994; **308**: 1609.

14 Gray LA, Barnes ML. Vaginitis in women, diagnosis and treatment. *Am J Obstet Gynecol* 1975; **92**: 125–36.

15 Odds FC. Cure and relapse with antifungal therapy. *Proc R Soc Med* 1977; **70** (Suppl. 4): 24–32.

16 Oriel JD, Partridge BM, Denny M *et al.* Genital yeast infections. *Br Med J* 1972; **iv**: 761–4.

Seminal vulvitis

This is a rare condition characterized by vulval oedema, erythema and pruritus following shortly after intercourse [1]. The pruritus is usually confined to the vulval area, but disseminated urticaria may supervene [2]. Most of the patients are atopics who have developed reaginic antibodies to all human seminal plasma. Specific immunotherapy against semen has been successfully employed on occasion [3]. A fixed eruption similar to fixed drug eruption has been reported [4]. One patient was also allergic to her husband's sweat [5]. Other antigens may be transmitted through seminal plasma, and post-coital urticaria in a penicillin-sensitive patient was provoked by penicillin ingested by her consort [6].

Consumption of contaminated marine fish may result in seminal transmission of the toxin to previously unaffected females [7].

Salivary vulvitis [8]

A relatively common and often unrecognized cause of vulval itching is the increasingly common practice of orogenital contact. This may present as vulvitis in the absence of vaginitis. The clinical appearance is non-specific, with generalized erythema and slight oedema of the labia, the introitus and the clitoral and periclitoral tissues.

At other times, a vaginal discharge is associated with the vulvitis, and unusual pathogens such as *Haemophilus* species may be isolated in culture.

In the first group, the likely causation is irritation by digestive enzymes in salivary fluid, whereas the infective group involves the transmission of oral pathogens, which can often be recovered from the mouth of the consort.

Vulval vestibulitis [9–11]; focal vulvitis [12]

The orifices of minor mucous glands are just visible to the naked eye, and are present throughout the vestibule, but are found in greatest density in the posterior fourchette. Patients with chronic dyspareunia and symptoms suggestive of vulvodynia (p. 3225) may show evidence of punctate inflammation and point tenderness on palpation of a gland orifice [13]. Histology shows a variable degree of upper dermal inflammatory infiltrate of mixed cellularity. Residual glands appear histologically normal [14], but clustering of glands exhibiting squamous metaplasia leads to coalescence of ducts and the formation of vestibular epithelial defects. These appear to be characteristic of the condition [14]. Treatment is difficult. The author prefers to try topical rosaniline dyes and intralesional steroids, but therapeutic success has been claimed for laser therapy and surgical excision [15]. Topical aciclovir [16] and transepidermal nerve-stimulator units [17] have their devotees but, as yet, there have not been any controlled therapeutic studies. The title vulvar vestibulitis syndrome is now being used more widely to include the full spectrum of chronic vulvar pain or vulvodynia (see p. 3225).

Plasma-cell vulvitis [9]

This condition is regarded as the analogue of Zoon's balanitis. It is rare, with only 10 case reports in the literature [18]. It is characterized by tender, red, sharply marginated plaques, which can be multiple and situated virtually anywhere within the vulval area [19,20]. Treatment is difficult. The topical combination of an antibiotic with a weak steroid is probably most helpful in affording symptomatic relief. Interferon-α has been used in an atypical case [18].

Circinate vulvovaginitis

This has been recorded in Reiter's disease, as the clinical analogue of the commoner balanitis [21].

Miscellaneous causes of vulvovaginitis [9,17,22]

Infestation with *Enterobius vermicularis* (threadworm) may cause irritation and a secondary vulvovaginitis, especially in children. Occasionally, the worm is found in the vagina itself [23]. Scabies may involve the female genitalia and, like phthiriasis, can lead to secondary infection from scratching. Vulval ulceration may occur in infants with amoebic dysentery [9], and filariasis may cause vulval oedema. Schistosomiasis is considered below.

REFERENCES

1 Chang T. Familial allergic seminal vulvovaginitis. *Am J Obstet Gynecol* 1976; **126**: 442–4.
2 Mathias CGT, Frick OL, Caldwell TM *et al.* Immediate hypersensitivity to seminal fluid and atopic dermatitis. *Arch Dermatol* 1980; **116**: 209–12.
3 Boom BW, van Toorenenbergen AW, Nierop G *et al.* A case of seminal fluid allergy successfully treated with immunotherapy in a one day rush procedure. *J Dermatol* 1991; **18**: 206–10.
4 Best CL, Waters C, Adelman DC. Fixed cutaneous eruption to seminal plasma challenge. *Fertil Steril* 1988; **50**: 532–4.
5 Freeman S. Woman allergic to husband's sweat and semen. *Contact Dermatitis* 1986; **14**: 110–12.
6 Green RL, Green MA. Postcoital urticaria in a penicillin sensitive patient. *JAMA* 1985; **254**: 531.
7 Lange WR, Lipkin KM, Young GC. Can ciguatera be a sexually transmitted disease? *J Clin Toxicol* 1989; **27**: 193–7.
8 Davies BA. Salivary vulvitis. *Obstet Gynecol* 1971; **37**: 238–40.
9 Ridley CM, ed. *The Vulva.* London: Churchill Livingstone, 1988.
10 Friedrich EG. Vulvar vestibulitis syndrome. *J Reprod Med* 1987; **32**: 110–14.
11 McKay M, Frankman O, Horowitz BJ *et al.* Vulvar vestibulitis and vestibular papillomatosis: report of the ISSVD Committee on Vulvodynia. *J Reprod Med* 1991; **36**: 413–15.
12 van der Meijden WI, Blindeman LAJ, Gianotten WA *et al.* Focal vulvitis. *Br J Dermatol* 1994; **131**: 727–8.
13 McKay M. Vulvodynia. *Arch Dermatol* 1989; **125**: 256–62.
14 Pyka RE, Wilkinson EJ, Friedrich EG *et al.* The histopathology of vulvar vestibulitis syndrome. *Int J Gynecol Pathol* 1988; **7**: 249–57.
15 Kaufman RH, Friedrich EG, Jr. The CO$_2$ laser in the treatment of vulvar disease. *Clin Obstet Gynecol* 1985; **28**: 220–9.
16 Friedrich EG. Therapeutic studies in vulvar vestibulitis. *J Reprod Med* 1988; **33**: 514–18.
17 Beilby JOW, Ridley CM. Pathology of the vulva. In: Fox H, ed. *Hailes and Taylor's Obstetric and Gynaecological Pathology.* Edinburgh: Churchill Livingstone, 1986.
18 Movioka S, Nakajima S, Jaguohi H *et al.* Vulvitis circumscripta plasma cellularis treated successfully with interferon alpha. *J Am Acad Dermatol* 1988; **19**: 947–50.
19 Garnier G. Benign plasma-cell erythroplasia. *Br J Dermatol* 1957; **69**: 77–81.
20 Souteyrand P, Wong E, McDonald DM. Zoon's balanitis (balanitis circumscripta plasma cellularis). *Br J Dermatol* 1981; **105**: 195–9.
21 Haake N, Altmeyer P. Circinate vulvo-vaginitis in Reiter's disease. *Hautarzt* 1988; **39**: 748–9.
22 Gardner HL, Kaufman RH, eds. *Benign Diseases of the Vulva and Vagina.* St Louis: Mosby, 1969.
23 Kacker TP. Vulvo-vaginitis in an adult with threadworms in the vagina. *Br J Vener Dis* 1973; **49**: 314–15.

Vulvovaginitis in children [1]

The vaginal mucosa of the child is an excellent bacterial culture medium. It lacks protective factors such as oestrogen stimulation, glycogen and Doderlein lactobacilli, and has a neutral pH. The tissues are thin and easily damaged, and perineal hygiene is frequently poor.

The majority of cases in which a specific cause of infection cannot be discovered respond well to measures designed purely to improve personal cleanliness [2]. Non-specific irritants such as bubble bath solutions may occasionally be responsible, as may pinworm infestation and foreign bodies. *Candida* does not infect the vagina of the pre-pubertal child, although it may induce vulvitis. Gonorrhoea may occur in children, and is becoming a more common cause of vulvovaginitis, especially in more under-privileged parts of North America. Sexual abuse, with or without specific vaginal infection, was a factor in 11% of 54 children with genital problems [2].

REFERENCES

1 Altchek A. Vulvovaginitis, vulvar skin disease, and pelvic inflammatory disease. *J Reprod Med* 1984; **28**: 397–432.
2 Paradise JE, Campos JM, Friedman HM *et al.* Vulvovaginitis and premenarcheal girls; clinical features and diagnostic evaluation. *Pediatrics* 1982; **70**: 193–8.

Corynebacteria [1]

Infection with *Corynebacterium diphtheriae* occurs rarely as a primary genital infection of children [2]; cases in adults have been reported in the past. Where diphtheria is still endemic they may be more common. The typical greyish pseudomembrane is characteristic. Vaginal adhesions may be prevented by local applications to separate the surfaces [3].

Erythrasma (Chapter 27)

This condition, caused by *C. minutissimum*, is rare in the UK before puberty, but may be extensive in tropical areas and in black women, especially in association with diabetes. It was also found in the groins of 18% of mentally subnormal patients [4]. Milder forms are often unnoticed by the patient. Confirmation of the diagnosis is by demonstration of coral-red fluorescence under Wood's light. It responds to oral erythromycin and to topical sodium fusidate, Whitfield's ointment, clotrimazole [5] or miconazole. However, recurrences are common. The vigorous use of an antibacterial soap has been suggested [3].

Trichomycosis (Chapter 27)

This condition is caused by various bacteria, and may be confused with phthiriasis. Careful examination, Wood's light fluorescence and microscopy should prevent diagnostic errors.

Staphylococcal and streptococcal infections

Primary infection with coagulase-positive staphylococci causes impetigo, folliculitis or boils. More chronic forms of pyoderma (lupoid sycosis) are occasionally seen, and are exceedingly difficult to treat; long-term, combined corticosteroid–antibiotic therapy has been fairly successful in personal cases. Secondary infection occurs in any itchy skin disorder, notably scabies, phthiriasis and atopic dermatitis.

An exotoxin associated with phage group 1 staphylococci has been implicated in production of the collapse, fever and morbilliform rash seen in the toxic shock syndrome.

Although the syndrome occurs most commonly in menstruating women who use tampons, the association is not exclusive, and the exotoxin has not as yet been identified [6].

Bartholinitis

Abscesses of Bartholin's gland [7] may be due to pyococcal organisms or to the gonococcus, especially if bilateral [8]. It has been shown [9] that *Chlamydia trachomatis* can be involved in the infection, either alone or in association with gonococci. In another study [7], only 21 of 109 cases were due to staphylococci, whereas 50 were due to *Escherichia coli* and 46 to *Streptococcus faecalis*. The abscess is due to distal blockage of the duct. The patient presents with fever, malaise and a tender swelling arising posterior to the origin of the labium minus. Episodes of bartholinitis often follow intercourse, and recurrent mild attacks may occur until fibrosis supervenes.

Acute streptococcal infections are rare, but erysipelas or cellulitis may follow surgical procedures [10] or destructive and scarring diseases. Persistent lymphoedema usually follows repeated attacks, probably because of progressive damage to an already defective lymphatic system.

Synergistic bacterial gangrene

This severe and rapidly extending disease is due to the synergistic effect of a microaerophilic streptococcus and *Staphylococcus aureus* (Chapter 27).

Gram-negative and anaerobic organisms

The role of Gram-negative enterococci in infections of the vulva and vagina remains doubtful [11,12]. It is unlikely that they are normally pathogenic, although they may play a part in the urethral syndrome of dysuria without significant bacteria. Anaerobic organisms are often found in the normal vagina. Those most commonly isolated include peptostreptococci, peptococci, and *Bacteroides* species.

Women with vaginitis have been reported to have high concentrations of anaerobic organisms [13]. It has been shown [14] that in women with *Gardnerella*-associated 'non-specific vaginitis', peptococci and *Bacteroides* species were isolated more frequently and in higher concentrations that in normal controls. Perhaps the time has come to cease using the term 'non-specific vaginitis'. Combined infections with fusobacteria and *Borrelia vincentii* have been reported in cases of erosive vulvitis in the older literature, but this is now rare. The organisms can be found in very ill patients with necrotic vaginal tissue or retained secretions [2].

Pseudomonas aeruginosa is not a cause of vulvovaginitis [2], but has caused blue staining of napkins in infants [15].

REFERENCES

1 Noble WC, Somerville DA, eds. *Microbiology of Human Skin*. London: WB Saunders, 1974.
2 Beilby JOW, Ridley CM. Pathology of the vulva. In: Fox H, ed. *Hailes and Taylor's Obstetric and Gynaecological Pathology*. Edinburgh: Churchill Livingstone, 1986.
3 Ridley CM, ed. *The Vulva*. London: Churchill Livingstone, 1988.
4 Somerville DA, Seville RH, Cunningham RC *et al.* Erythrasma in a hospital for the mentally subnormal. *Br J Dermatol* 1970; **82**: 355–60.
5 Clayton YM, Connor BL. Comparison of clotrimazole cream, Whitfield's ointment and nystatin ointment for the topical treatment of ringworm infections, pityriasis versicolor, erythrasma and candidiasis. *Br J Dermatol* 1973; **89**: 297–303.
6 Davis JP, Chesney PJ, Wand PJ *et al.* Toxic-shock syndrome: epidemiologic features, recurrence, risk factors, prevention. *N Engl J Med* 1980; **303**: 1429–35.
7 Mayer HGK. Pathogénie et traitement des pretendus abcés et kystes de la glande de Bartholin. *J Gynecol Obstet Biol Reprod* 1972; **1**: 71–6.
8 Gardner HL, Kaufman RH, eds. *Benign Diseases of the Vulva and Vagina*. St Louis: Mosby, 1969.
9 Davies JA, Rees E, Jobson D *et al.* Isolation of *Chlamydia trachomatis* from Bartholin's ducts. *Br J Vener Dis* 1978; **54**: 409–13.
10 Norburn LM, Cole RB. Recurrent erysipelas following vulvectomy. *J Obstet Gynecol* 1960; **67**: 279–80.
11 Bailey RR, Gower PE, Roberts AP *et al.* Urinary tract infection in non-pregnant women. *Lancet* 1973; **ii**: 275–81.
12 Cattell WR, McSherry MA, Northeast A *et al.* Periurethral enterobacterial carriage in pathogenesis of recurrent urinary infection. *Br Med J* 1974; **iv**: 136–9.
13 Levison ME, Trestman I, Quach R *et al.* Quantitative bacteriology of the vagina flora in vaginitis. *Am J Obstet Gynecol* 1979; **133**: 139–44.
14 Speigel CA, Amsel R, Eschenbach D *et al.* Anaerobic bacteria in nonspecific vaginitis. *N Engl J Med* 1980; **303**: 601–7.
15 Thearle MJ, Wise R, Allen JT. Blue nappies (Letter). *Lancet* 1973; **ii**: 499–500.

Fungi

Dermatophyte infections of the genital area are uncommon in women in temperate climates. When present, other sites are also infected. It may be diagnosed easily. Erythrasma is distinguished by its brown colour and lack of scaling edge.

In extensive cases, pityriasis versicolor can involve the genital region.

Viruses [1–3]

Three groups of viruses are important causes of infection in the genital area—the poxviruses, papillomaviruses and herpesviruses. Other viruses seldom give rise to distinctive clinical pictures, although the vulva may be involved in hand, foot and mouth disease, and may ulcerate in infectious mononucleosis. Epstein–Barr virus DNA has been found in association with DNA of HPV in aceto-white vulval lesions. A situation which also pertains in oral hairy leukoplakia [4].

Poxviruses

Accidental autoinoculation of the vulva following smallpox vaccination is not now encountered.

Molluscum contagiosum is becoming very common. Vulval lesions are often seen in childhood and are innocently acquired. In the adult, transmission during sexual intercourse tends to produce pubic lesions more often than infection of the external genitalia. Solitary inflamed lesions are often mistaken for boils, and the eczematous reaction which may surround lesions can be deceptive. The condition is more fully described in Chapter 26.

Papillomaviruses

HPV has still not been propagated in tissue culture. This makes investigation difficult, but DNA hybridization techniques and restriction enzyme analysis have made it clear that numerous strains of HPV exist [5]. Viral DNA extracted from anogenital warts has been shown to contain genome sequences related to HPV-1 and -2. In addition, another distinct species of DNA has been found in some anogenital warts, and designated HPV-6 [6]. Genital HPV infection is stongly associated with cervical neoplasia. HPV genomes have been demonstrated in up to 90% of cervical dysplasias [7]. HPV-16, -18, -13 and -33 are among those most frequently associated with genital cancer, and HPV-16 is regarded as a marker for women who have progressive cervical dysplasia [8].

The incubation period is between 2 and 3 months [9]. It is now generally accepted that nearly all cases are sexually transmitted. The incidence of genital warts has been increasing for several years.

The soft, frond-like, papilliferous lesions are distinctive (Fig. 72.28). When numerous, they become confluent, with a velvety surface. In severe cases, they may cover the inner surfaces of the labia, and extend far into the vagina. Even the bladder and ureter can be involved. Extension to the perineum and perianal area is common, and they may then spread to the rectum. The genitocrural fold is often involved, but not the thighs. In pregnancy, and if an associated vaginal infection is present, condylomas become more profuse.

The only important differential diagnoses are syphilitic condylomas, which are flat, broad-topped and sparse, and carcinoma, which is harder and usually more localized. However, the so-called 'malignant condyloma' and the Buschke–Löwenstein giant condyloma must always be suspected in cases which do not rapidly respond to appropriate treatment. Close supervision and repeated biopsies may be necessary.

All patients should be investigated for other diseases, and any concomitant discharge treated appropriately.

Vulval papillomatosis [3]. Small cutaneous papillae may be seen on the labia minora, within the vestibule (especially around the urethral orifice), and on the posterior aspect of the introitus. These have been described as a normal variant akin to pearly penile papules, and termed 'hirsutes

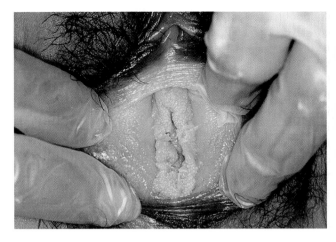

Fig. 72.28 Vulval warts. (Courtesy of Dr A. Robinson, University College Hospital, London, UK.)

papillaris vulvae' [10,11] or, alternatively, 'vestibular papillae' [12] (Fig. 72.29).

There has been concern that these papillae may represent subclinical wart virus infection [13]. Often, they can be more easily seen after application of 3–5% acetic acid solution (aceto-whitening), and may be associated with similar changes within the vagina and on the cervix. There is no evidence that these lesions represent a variant of papillomavirus infection [14–16]. Although many such patients are asymptomatic, a number present with complaints of a persistent burning sensation akin to that which occurs in vulvodynia [17]. It is not yet clear whether ablation of these 'microwarts' produces long-term resolution of this symptomatology.

Condylomata acuminata on the cervix [18] can also be proliferative and show cytological changes of dyskeratosis and koilocytosis [19]. Similar cytological changes can be found in lesions which are flat and white when viewed on

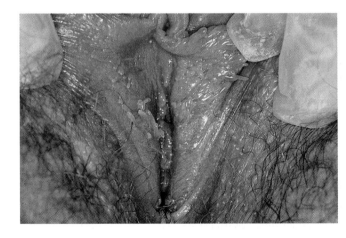

Fig. 72.29 Papilliferous vulva (microwarts). (Courtesy of Dr A. Robinson, University College Hospital, London, UK.)

colposcopy. These are known as flat condylomas, or more correctly as noncondylomatous cervical wart virus infection [20]. It has been concluded that this group of virus-induced lesions can give rise to suspect smears. The biological importance of cervical HPV infection is still being evaluated, but it seems likely that this virus infection is oncogenic [21]. Histological evidence of HPV infection has been found in 91% of 80 women with invasive or preinvasive cervical neoplasia, compared with only 12.5% of controls [22]. Abnormal cervical smears were found 15 times more commonly in women who had previous genital wart infection [9]. It has long been recognized that early sexual activity, promiscuity and low socio-economic status are major risk determinants in cervical cancer [23–25]. It has also been shown that there is a threefold increase in cancer of the penis in the husbands of cervical cancer patients [26]. There is no evidence that HSV-2 is associated with the initiation of cervical neoplasia [27].

Treatment. Podophyllin is the treatment of choice. It is applied in strengths of from 10 to 25%, and the patients are instructed to wash it off 8–24h later. Treatment should be repeated at regular intervals. Podophyllin should not be used in pregnancy because of potential toxicity [28], or for cervical lesions, because of potential carcinogenicity [29]. Diathermy, electrocautery or liquid nitrogen, using a cryoprobe, and carbon dioxide laser [30] are also helpful in difficult cases.

Interferons administered both intralesionally [31] and intramuscularly [32] have been found to be useful in cases of genital wart infection, but varying degrees of systemic upset have been recorded, and the expense of this treatment may limit its usefulness.

Condylomas may regress after delivery [33], but their management in pregnancy poses a problem—particularly if they are florid near the date of delivery. Diathermy destruction of such florid lesions under general anaesthesia may be attempted.

Transmission of warts to newborns via an infected birth canal can give rise to laryngeal papillomatosis, which is very difficult to treat [34], and this has led to the suggestion that all affected mothers should have their infants delivered by caesarean section [35].

Transmission or reinfection from underwear appears to be a possibility, based on evidence from DNA probe analysis, which showed 17% positivity on 74 pairs of used underpants [36].

Herpesviruses [3,37–39]

Both herpes simplex and varicella–zoster viruses affect the vulva. Cytomegalovirus does not, except in immunosuppressed individuals. HSV-2 is mainly responsible for genital infections. The question of antigenic differences is dealt with elsewhere (Chapter 26). HSV-2 infection is usually acquired in early adult life. The virus may then lie dormant or give rise to recurrent infections. As HSV-1 infections are also common, the patient may carry two types of antibody. Neither protects against the other.

Genital herpes [19] due to HSV-2 is now the commonest cause of genital ulceration [37], and was once described as the most important sexually transmitted disease [40].

Many primary and recurrent infections are asymptomatic [41], and recurrences occur in about 50% of those infected [38].

The primary infection is usually more severe or widespread than recurrences. A zosteriform or segmental distribution is not unusual and invites confusion with zoster. The incubation period varies from 2 to 7 days. The grouped vesicles on an inflamed base erode rapidly; deeper ulceration may occur [41]. The vagina, urethra and anal canal may also be involved. Dysuria and retention of urine may occur [42]. The regional lymph nodes are enlarged and tender. Cervicitis is commonly found, if sought [43]. Although systemic effects usually subside in a week, ulceration may persist for 2–6 weeks [44].

Recurrences may occur without coitus, and be precipitated by trauma, fever, local infection, menstruation or stress. Each individual may have her own pattern, for example premenstrual attacks. Prodromal itching and tingling are soon recognized as heralding an attack. These attacks tend to be relatively mild, lasting only 7–10 days, and usually become less frequent with time [40]. It is important to appreciate that this disease is infective even when the patient is asymptomatic, and that viral shedding has been found in asymptomatic women up to 6 months after a clinical attack of genital herpes [45]. In childhood, genital HSV infection, regardless of type, may be an important sign of sexual abuse [46] (p. 3219).

Neurological signs and symptoms have been reported rarely in both primary and recurrent attacks [47]. The diagnosis is usually obvious, although primary attacks may closely resemble zoster. Differentiation from zoster requires viral culture. Primary or secondary syphilis may coexist. Aphthosis, Behçet's syndrome and secondarily infected chancroid may pose difficulties in some cases.

Although transplacental intrauterine infection with HSV is rare [48], the newborn must be protected from contact with the genital tract of mothers with primary HSV infection. Caesarean section is usually performed immediately after rupture of membranes [49]. The risks of infection from mothers with recurrent infection is much lower [50]. The subject of HSV infection is well reviewed by Ridley [3].

Treatment. The use of idoxuridine has now been largely superseded by aciclovir. In severe primary infections, which are often associated with systemic symptoms, many patients require hospitalization.

Intravenous aciclovir, in a dose of 5 mg/kg every 8 h by slow infusion, has been shown to be a safe and effective treatment for the primary attack [51], but does not prevent recurrences.

In less severe cases, or in recurrent attacks, oral aciclovir is preferred. The recommended dose is 200 mg five times daily for 7 days [52]. Topical 5% aciclovir ointment is helpful in speeding healing in mild cases. Gloves should be worn during application to prevent autoinoculation [52]. Recurrent attacks of genital herpes may be treated with oral or topical aciclovir. Long-term suppression of recurrent attacks can be achieved safely by the administration of 400 mg of oral aciclovir twice daily for up to 5 years [53]. No change in viral strain or sensitivity has been found in this or other studies [54,55].

As alternative bland applications, wet dressings or 1% aqueous gentian violet are of help. Steroids should not be used. Topical interferon-β has been used effectively in both labial and genital herpes [56]. Interferon-α2 gel significantly shortens viral shedding in recurrent cases, but is of little therapeutic benefit to the female patient [57].

Varicella–zoster. Varicella only affects the vulva in a random fashion. It may occur in infants by transplacental infection. Zoster may mimic acute primary herpes, but is strictly unilateral and segmental, and is often preceded by pain. Scattered viraemic vesicles are common elsewhere, especially in immunodeficient patients.

Motor involvement leading to bladder and bowel dysfunction is well recognized [58]. When the lesions are sparse, the diagnosis may be difficult. However, a second attack of zoster is unusual [59].

Aciclovir and the more recently introduced famciclovir and valaciclovir are the only effective treatments currently available. Regarding the use of aciclovir in pregnancy, manufacturers advise that animal studies show no evidence of embryotoxic effects, but experience in humans is limited [60]. Famciclovir and valaciclovir are currently contraindicated in pregnancy.

REFERENCES

1 Beilby JOW, Ridley CM. Pathology of the vulva. In: Fox H, ed. *Hailes and Taylor's Obstetric and Gynaecological Pathology*. Edinburgh: Churchill Livingstone, 1986.
2 Gardner HL, Kaufman RH, eds. *Benign Diseases of the Vulva and Vagina*. St Louis: Mosby, 1969.
3 Ridley CM, ed. *The Vulva*. London: Churchill Livingstone, 1988.
4 Voog E, Ricksten A, Lowhagen GB *et al.* Demonstration of Epstein Barr virus DNA in acetowhite lesions of the vulva. *Int J STD AIDS* 1994; **5**: 25–8.
5 Coggin J, zur Hausen H. Workshop on papilloma viruses and cancer. *Cancer Res* 1979; **39**: 545–6.
6 Gissman L, zur Hausen H. Partial characterization of viral DNA from human genital warts (condyloma acuminata). *Int J Cancer* 1979; **25**: 605–9.
7 Gissman L, Schwartz E. Persistence and expression of HPV in genital cancers. *Ciba Foundation Symposium* 1986; **120**: 190–8.
8 Campion MJ, Cuziek J, McCance DJ *et al.* Progressive potential of mild cervical atypia: prospective cytologic, colposcopic and virologic study. *Lancet* 1986; **ii**: 237–40.
9 Mitchell H, Drake M, Medley G. Prospective evaluation of risk of cervical cancer after cytological evidence of human papillomavirus infection. *Lancet* 1986; **i**: 573–5.
10 Altmeyer P, Cliff GN, Holzmann H. Hirsutes papillaris vulvae (pseudokondylome der vulva). *Hautarzt* 1982; **33**: 281–3.
11 Khoda H, Hino Y, Fukuda H. Hirsutoid papillomas of vulva. *J Dermatol* 1986; **13**: 154–6.
12 Friedrich EG, Jr. The vulvar vestibule. *J Reprod Med* 1983; **28**: 773–7.
13 Manoharon V, Somerville JM. Benign squamous papillomatosis—case report. *Genitourin Med* 1987; **63**: 393–5.
14 Moyal-Barracco M, Leibowitch M, Orth G. Vestibular papillae of the vulva. *Arch Dermatol* 1990; **126**: 1594–8.
15 Bergeron C, Ferenczy A, Richart RM *et al.* Micropapillomatosis labialis appears unrelated to human papilloma virus. *Obstet Gynecol* 1990; **76**: 281–5.
16 Fimiani M, Mazzatenta C, Biagioli M *et al.* Vulvar squamous papillomata and human papilloma virus infection. A polymerase chain reaction study. *J Dermatol Res* 1993; **285**: 250–4.
17 Turner MLC, Marinoff SC. Association of human papilloma virus with vulvodynia and the vulvar vestibulitis syndrome. *J Reprod Med* 1988; **33**: 533–7.
18 Meisels A, Fortin R, Roy M. Condylomatous lesions of the cervix. II. Cytological, colposcopic and histopathologic study. *Acta Cytol* 1977; **21**: 379–90.
19 Leading Article. Genital herpes. *Br Med J* 1980; **i**: 1335–6.
20 Laverty CR, Booth N, Hills E *et al.* Noncondylomatous wart virus infection of the postmenopausal cervix. *Pathology* 1978; **10**: 373–8.
21 Tidy JA, Vousden KH, Farrell PJ. Relation between infection with a sub type of HPV 16 and cervical neoplasia. *Lancet* 1989; **i**: 1225–7.
22 Reid R, Stanhope CR, Herschran BR *et al.* Genital warts and cervical cancer. I. Evidence of an association between subclinical papillomavirus infection and cervical malignancy. *Cancer* 1982; **50**: 377–87.
23 Gardner JW, Lyon JL. Low incidence of cervical cancer in Utah. *Gynecol Oncol* 1977; **5**: 68–80.
24 Rotkin ID. A comparison review of key epidemiological studies in cervical cancer related to current searches for transmissible agents. *Cancer Res* 1973; **33**: 1353–67.
25 Thomas DB. An epidemiologic study of carcinoma *in situ* and squamous dysplasia of the uterine cervix. *Am J Epidemiol* 1973; **98**: 10–28.
26 Smith PG, Kinlen LJ, White GC *et al.* Carcinoma of penis and cervix. *Lancet* 1980; **ii**: 417.
27 Francheschi S, Doll R, Gallwey J *et al.* Genital warts and cervical neoplasia: an epidemiological study. *Br J Cancer* 1983; **48**: 621–8.
28 Chamberlain MJ, Reynold AL, Yeoman WB. Toxic effect of podophyllin application in pregnancy. *Br Med J* 1972; **ii**: 391–2.
29 Gueson ET, Liu CT, Emich JP, Jr. Dysplasia following podophyllin treatment of vulvar condyloma acuminata. A case report. *J Reprod Med* 1971; **6**: 159–62.
30 Ferenczy A. Laser therapy in genital condylomata accuminata. *Obstet Gynecol* 1984; **63**: 703–7.
31 Vance JC, Bart BJ, Hansen RC *et al.* Intralesional recombinant alpha-2 interferon for the treatment of patients with condyloma acuminatum or verruca plantaris. *Arch Dermatol* 1986; **122**: 272–7.
32 Week PK, Buddin DA, Whisnant JK. Interferons in the treatment of genital human papillomavirus infections. *Am J Med* 1988; **85** (Suppl. 12A): 159–64.
33 Oriel JD. Natural history of genital warts. *Br J Vener Dis* 1971; **47**: 1–13.
34 Cook TA, Pierre Brunschwig J, Buiel JS *et al.* Laryngeal papilloma: etiologic and therapeutic considerations. *Ann Otol Rhinol Laryngol* 1973; **82**: 649–55.
35 Goldman L. Spread of condyloma acuminata to infants and children. *Arch Dermatol* 1977; **113**: 1294.
36 Bergeron C, Ferenczy A, Richart R. Underwear: contamination by human papillomavirus. *Am J Obstet Gynecol* 1990; **162**: 25–9.
37 Anstey MS. Current concepts of herpes virus infection in woman. *Am J Obstet Gynecol* 1973; **117**: 711–25.
38 Kaufman RH, Faro S. Herpes genitalis: clinical features and treatment. *Clin Obstet Gynaecol* 1985; **28**: 152–63.
39 Lycke E. The pathogenesis of the genital herpes simplex virus infection. *Scand J Infect Dis* 1991; **80** (Suppl. 78): 7–14.
40 Gardner HL. Herpes genitalis: our most important venereal disease. *Am J Obstet Gynecol* 1979; **135**: 553–4.
41 Poste G, Hawkins DF, Thomlinson J. Herpes virus hominis infection of the female genital tract. *Obstet Gynecol* 1972; **40**: 871–90.
42 Ryttor N, Aagaard J, Hertz J. Retention of urine in genital herpetic infection. *Urol Int* 1985; **40**: 22–4.

43 Hutfield DC. Herpes genitalis. *Br J Vener Dis* 1968; **44**: 241–50.
44 Alcheck A. Vulvovaginitis, vulvar skin disease, and pelvic inflammatory disease. *Pediatr Clin North Am* 1981; **28**: 397–435.
45 Adam E, Kaufman RH, Mirkovic RR *et al.* Persistence of virus shedding in asymptomatic women after recovery from herpes genitalis. *Obstet Gynecol* 1979; **54**: 171–3.
46 Kaplan K, Fleisler GR, Paradise JE *et al.* Social relevance of genital herpes simplex in children. *Am J Dis Child* 1984; **138**: 872–4.
47 Leading Article. Herpes simplex encephalitis. *Lancet* 1973; ii: 1426–7.
48 Bendon RW, Perez F, Ray MB. Herpes simplex virus: fetal and decidual infection. *Pediatr Pathol* 1987; **7**: 63–70.
49 Jacob AJ, Epstein J, Madden DC *et al.* Genital herpes infection in pregnant women. *Obstet Gynecol* 1984; **63**: 480–4.
50 Prober OG, Sullender WM, Yasukarra LL. Low risk of herpes simplex virus infections in neonates exposed to the virus at the time of vaginal delivery to mothers with recurrent genital herpes virus infections. *N Engl J Med* 1987; **316**: 240–4.
51 Mindel A, Adler MW, Sutherland S *et al.* Intravenous acyclovir treatment for primary genital herpes. *Lancet* 1982; **i**: 697–703.
52 Lafferty M. Genital herpes: recommendations for comprehensive care. *Postgrad Med* 1988; **83**: 157–65.
53 Goldberg LH, Kaufman TO, Kurtz MA *et al.* Continuous five year treatment of patients with frequently recurring genital herpes simplex virus infection with acyclovir. *J Med Virol Suppl* 1993; **1**: 45–50.
54 Burns WH, Saral R, Santos GW *et al.* Isolation and characterization of resistant herpes simplex virus after acyclovir therapy. *Lancet* 1982; **i**: 421–3.
55 Lehrmann SN, Hill EL, Rooney JF *et al.* Extended acyclovir therapy for herpes genitalis: changes in virus sensitivity and strain variation. *J Antimicrob Chemother* 1986; **18** (Suppl. B): 85–94.
56 Glezerman M, Lunenfield E, Cohen V *et al.* Placebo controlled trial of topical interferon in labial and genital herpes. *Lancet* 1988; **i**: 150–2.
57 Lebwohl M, Sachs S, Conant M *et al.* Recombinant alpha 2 interferon gel treatment of recurrent herpes genitalis. *Antiviral Res* 1992; **17**: 235–43.
58 Fugelso PD, Newman SB, Beamer JE. Herpes zoster of the anogenital area affecting urination and defaecation. *Br J Dermatol* 1973; **89**: 285–8.
59 Juel-Jensen BE. Herpes simplex and zoster. *Br Med J* 1973; **i**: 406–10.
60 *Association of British Pharmaceutical Industry Data Sheet.* London: Datapharm Publications, 1989–90.

Chlamydiae and mycoplasmas [1–4]

Chlamydiae are Gram-negative organisms with many of the features of bacteria, but differ in that they are obligatory intracellular parasites [5].

Different serotypes (D–K) of chlamydiae have been found causing cervicitis in the female partners of men with non-specific and postgonococcal urethritis. The most characteristic picture is a lymphocytic follicular cervicitis [6], most commonly found in the mothers of babies with chlamydia ophthalmia neonatorum [4]. Chlamydiae do not cause vaginitis, but may cause salpingitis and lead to infertility [5].

Specific serotypes of *Chlamydia trachomatis* are responsible for the disease lymphogranuloma venereum.

Lymphogranuloma venereum

Although usually found in tropical areas, a number of cases nevertheless occur in the UK, particularly in men [7]. Transmission is by sexual intercourse or via an alimentary reservoir. The incubation period varies from a few days to a few weeks. The initial papulovesicle, which may quickly ulcerate, occurs at the fourchette or vagina. It is often unnoticed. Lymphadenopathy, often with constitutional

upset, follows this in a week or more. This may be unilateral, and involve the pelvic and perirectal rather than the inguinal glands. These may become fluctuant and discharge, producing ulceration, fistulae and scarring (esthiomene). Strictures and elephantiasis complete the sequence of events. Carcinoma may ultimately supervene.

Rectal lesions present as proctocolitis, followed by rectal stricture, and can be confused with Crohn's disease.

The Frei test is useful in diagnosis, but may give false-negative reactions.

Treatment. This is by full doses of sulphonamides or tetracyclines, often in prolonged or repeated courses.

The mycoplasmas [8]

Mycoplasma hominis and *Ureaplasma urealyticum* (T mycoplasmas) can frequently be isolated from the genital tract. The latter is now best regarded purely as a commensal [9]. *M. hominis* may play a role in *Gardnerella* vaginitis, and both organisms may be responsible for pelvic inflammatory disease, postabortion and postpartum fevers.

REFERENCES

1 Beilby JOW, Ridley CM. Pathology of the vulva. In: Fox H, ed. *Hailes and Taylor's Obstetric and Gynaecological Pathology*. Edinburgh: Churchill Livingstone, 1986.
2 Gardner HL, Kaufman RH, eds. *Benign Diseases of the Vulva and Vagina*. St Louis: Mosby, 1969.
3 Ridley CM, ed. *The Vulva*. London: Churchill Livingstone, 1988.
4 Dunlop EMC. Chlamydial genital infection and its complications. *Br J Hosp Med* 1983; **29**: 6–11.
5 Taylor-Robinson D, Thomas BJ. The role of *Chlamydia trachomatis* in genital tract and associated diseases. *J Clin Pathol* 1980; **33**: 205–33.
6 Hare MJ, Toone E, Taylor-Robinson D *et al.* Follicular cervicitis—colposcopic appearances and association with *Chlamydia trachomatis*. *Br J Obstet Gynaecol* 1981; **88**: 174–80.
7 Willcox RR. In: Morton RS, Harris JRW, eds. *Recent Advances in Sexually Transmitted Diseases*, No. 1. Edinburgh: Churchill Livingstone, 1974.
8 Taylor-Robinson D, McCormack WM. The genital mycoplasmas. *N Engl J Med* 1980; **302**: 1003–10.
9 Wooley PD, Kinghorn GR, Bennet KW *et al.* Significance of *Bacterioides ureolyticus* in the lower genital tract. *Int J STD AIDS*. 1992; **3**: 107–10.

Dermatological manifestations of sexual abuse of children

The diagnosis of childhood sexual abuse [1,2] is of necessity a multidisciplinary exercise. Paediatricians are now familiar with the normal patterns of variation of pre-adolescent genitalia [3], the signs of sexual injury (which may be minimal or absent) and the limitations of the anal dilatation test [2].

Occasionally, the dermatologist is asked to give an opinion on genital skin disease. Lichen sclerosus is the most likely cause of confusion [4,5], but psoriasis, Ehlers–Danlos syndrome and vulvitis of all types may be the subject of enquiry.

The instigation of an investigation into sexual abuse may arise from the discovery of a sexually transmitted disease [6,7]. Bacterial vaginosis alone is not necessarily an indicator of sexual activity [8]. It is advisable that all suspect cases are seen in conjunction with a paediatric specialist.

Gonorrhoea. If gonorrhoea is found, the situation is usually clear cut. With the exception of neonatal infection, and gonococcal eye disease, there is little evidence to support a theory of non-sexual transmission in any age group [9].

Genital warts. These are being increasingly reported as occurring in infants and prepubertal children [10,11]. Papilliferous warts, especially those caused by common genital wart virus types (6 and 11) [12], should be viewed with more suspicion than the hard variety, which may have been transmitted by innocent handling. Neonatal transmission from the birth canal can explain some infections in very young infants [13]. With these exceptions, the presence of papilliferous genital or oral warts in childhood should provoke a suspicion of abuse [14]. It has recently been shown that both genital and skin-type viruses may be found by DNA probe examination of tissue from childhood genital wart infections [15]. The type of papillomavirus present may be helpful in determining the likely mode of transmission, in association with other clinical and social information [16].

Attention has been drawn to a group of children with rather non-specific, but non-viral pseudoverrucous papules and nodules on the perianal skin [17]. Few biopsies were performed, but the authors distinguish this condition from granuloma gluteale infantum, despite clinical similarities [17].

Herpes simplex of the prepubertal genitalia is relatively uncommon [18]. Sexual transmission may be implicated in both HSV-1 and -2 infections. In a review of six cases, sexual abuse was proved in four. In the two innocently acquired cases, HSV-1 infection of the oral cavity immediately preceded the genital signs [19].

Bullous disorders. Localized vulvar pemphigoid is a relatively newly diagnosed condition, and has been misinterpreted as a sign of sexual abuse in childhood [20].

Human immunodeficiency virus. This has rarely been reported as being transmitted by sexual abuse of children [21,22].

REFERENCES

1 American Academy of Dermatology Task Force on Pediatric Dermatology. Genital warts and sexual abuse in children. *J Am Acad Dermatol* 1984; **11**: 529–30.

2 Bamford F, Roberts R. Child sexual abuse. *Br Med J* 1989; **299**: 377–82.

3 Herman-Giddens ME, Frothingham TE. Prepubertal female genitalia: examination for evidence of sexual abuse. *Pediatrics* 1987; **80**: 203–8.

4 Handfield-Jones SE, Hinde FRJ, Kennedy CTC. Lichen sclerosus et atrophicus in children misdiagnosed as sexual abuse. *Br Med J* 1987; **294**: 1404–5.

5 Jenny C, Kirbu P, Furquay D. Genital lichen sclerosus mistaken for child sexual abuse. *Pediatrics* 1989; **83**: 597–9.

6 Dattell BJ, Landers DV, Coulter K *et al.* Isolation of *Chlamydia trachomatis* from sexually abused female adolescents. *Obstet Gynecol* 1988; **72**: 240–2.

7 Herman-Giddens ME, Gutman LT, Berson N. Association of coexisting vaginal infections and multiple abusers in female children with genital warts. *Sex Transm Dis* 1988; **15**: 63–7.

8 Bump RC, Buesching WJ. Bacterial vaginosis in virginal and sexually active adolescent females: evidence against exclusive sexual transmission. *Am J Obstet Gynecol* 1988; **158**: 935–9.

9 Sgroi SM. Pediatric gonorrhoea and child sex abuse: the venereal disease connection. *Sex Transm Dis* 1982; **9**: 154–6.

10 Stumpf P. Increasing occurrence of condylomata acuminata in premenarchal children. *Obstet Gynecol* 1979; **56**: 562–4.

11 Raimer SS. Editorial. Family violence, child abuse and anogenital warts. *Arch Dermatol* 1992; **128**: 842–4.

12 Cohen BA, Honig P, Androphy E. Anogenital warts in children. *Arch Dermatol* 1990; **126**: 1575–80.

13 Sadan O, Koller AB, Adno A *et al.* Massive vulval condylomata acuminata in a 10-month-old child with suspected sexual abuse. *Br J Obstet Gynaecol* 1985; **92**: 1201–3.

14 Seidal J, Zonana J, Trotter E. Condylomata acuminata as a sign of sexual abuse in children. *J Pediatr* 1979; **95**: 553.

15 Fleming KA, Venning V, Evans M. DNA typing of genital warts and diagnosis of sexual abuse of children. *Lancet* 1984; **ii**: 454.

16 Padel AF, Venning VA, Evans MF *et al.* Human papillomavirus in anogenital warts in children: typing by *in situ* hybridisation. *Br Med J* 1990; **300**: 1491–4.

17 Goldberg NS, Esterley NB, Rothman KF *et al.* Perianal pseudoverrucous papules and nodules in children. *Arch Dermatol* 1992; **128**: 240–2.

18 Gardner M, Jones JG. Genital herpes acquired by sexual abuse of children. *J Pediatr* 1984; **104**: 243–4.

19 Kaplan KM, Fleischer GP, Paradise JE *et al.* Social tolerance of genital herpes simplex in children. *Am J Dis Child* 1984; **138**: 872–4.

20 Levine V, Sanchez M, Nestor M. Localised vulvar pemphigoid in a child misdiagnosed as sexual abuse. *Arch Dermatol* 1992; **128**: 804–6.

21 Liedermann BA, Grimm KT. A child with HIV infection. *JAMA* 1986; **256**: 3904.

22 Straka BF, Whitaker DL, Morrison SH *et al.* Cutaneous manifestations of acquired immunodeficiency syndrome in children. *J Am Acad Dermatol* 1988; **18**: 1089–102.

The investigation of vulvovaginitis [1,2]

The previous sections have indicated the complexity of factors involved in vulvovaginitis. Its frequent lack of clear definition, the inexperience of many dermatologists with regard to gynaecological examination procedures, and the frequent high level of anxiety of the patient create an unfavourable milieu in which to work. Moreover, the significance of many of the results obtained from the laboratory remains unknown. Elucidation of the cause of vulvovaginitis in an individual patient requires expertise and time.

A thorough history is essential. The patient should be asked about her initial symptoms and the circumstances under which these occurred, for example the relationship to menstruation, prior illness, change of contraceptive method, use of deodorants, foreign sojourn, etc. Medication— particularly self-medication—may not be fully disclosed by the referring doctor or admitted by the patient. However, 48% of households contain some topical skin preparation [3], and local anaesthetic ointments are freely available. The family history, particularly with reference to diabetes and tuberculosis, should be recorded. The presence of any urinary or intestinal symptoms should be noted. Tactful enquiries should be made about the presence of any symptoms in the sexual partner, about family or marital stresses, and even about sexual technique. Although often irrelevant, these may be a pertinent cause of chronicity or relapse of disease, or may increase the perception of pruritus.

The whole skin should be examined in a good light, with special attention to the mucosae, axillae and submammary areas. Look for dermographism even if no rash is visible [4]. A rash on one hand may be a sign of sensitivity to an applied medicament. Examination of the anogenital region demands good lighting and a comfortable but firm couch or bed, especially for the obese. The vagina and cervix should always be examined in adults, and proctoscopy may be necessary in some cases. The examination of children and young adolescents requires particular gentleness and care. In some cases, a general anaesthetic may be needed [1].

Scrapings from the vaginal wall provide material for hormonal cytology and microbiology; a cervical scrape can be carried out at the same time, and will assuage the undisclosed fears of many patients. Smears for *Trichomonas vaginalis* must be examined fresh on a warm slide. After cleansing with normal saline, light scrapings from the inner aspects of the labia minora allow a similar assessment of the hormonal state in children and virgins [2]. The use of toluidine blue 1%, to detect areas of malignancy [5], is not sufficiently specific to have been accepted for general use in the UK.

The amine-like fish odour of the vaginal discharge in *Gardnerella* vaginitis is very characteristic, and is accentuated by the addition of 10% potassium hydroxide to vaginal secretions on a glass slide. The vaginal pH is high, 5.0–5.5, and a wet mount of a vaginal smear in saline will identify 'clue cells'. These are vaginal epithelial cells with a granular cytoplasmic appearance and indistinct cellular outlines. This indistinct border is caused by the attachment of the small Gram-negative rods to the cell [6].

Bacteriological specimens must be taken in the correct manner, for example moist or transferred to transport medium, and from the appropriate site, for example high vaginal, vulval, and perhaps perianal and nasal. In the presence of an infective condition of any type it is wise to assume that others may coexist [2]. It is often valuable to examine the sexual partner, and to include penile and perianal swabs where appropriate (especially for staphylococci, yeasts and *Trichomonas* species).

A biopsy may be necessary, and the site should be chosen with care.

The urine may have been tested routinely on the first visit, but laboratory examination is necessary to determine infection, and a glucose tolerance test should be performed if diabetes is suspected. Standard serological tests are called for in all cases of suspected venereal or 'paravenereal' disease, and appropriate patch tests whenever contact dermatitis is suspected. The routine testing of all cases of vulvovaginitis of uncertain aetiology can be rewarding.

The reader should consult specialist texts, for example [2], for details of other investigational procedures.

General management [7]. During the period of investigation and diagnostic assessment, some immediate treatment will be required. The more severe cases require rest and sedation; a few may need admission to hospital. All topical irritants and sensitizers should be removed, and cotton, rather than nylon, underwear worn. Soaking underwear in an amphoteric biocide prior to washing has been shown to reduce carriage of candidal yeasts from 85 to 23% [8]. Aqueous cream can be used for cleaning, but in the acute phase, cool 'sitz' baths or wet dressings will give most comfort. All other topical treatment should be bland, but specific agents directed against a likely cause of infection can obviously be used, while the results of culture are awaited. Otherwise, zinc or calamine creams, or a mild steroid/antiseptic cream, are soothing and innocuous.

REFERENCES

1 Capraro VJ, Capraro EJ. Examination of the genital organs in the newborn, the child and the adolescent patient. *Gynecol Pract* 1971; **22**: 169–77.
2 Ridley CM, ed. *The Vulva.* Edinburgh: Churchill Livingstone, 1988.
3 Office of Health Economics. Skin disorders. *Studies in Current Health Problems*, No. 46. London: HMSO, 1973.
4 Shenertz EF. Clinical pearl: symptomatic dermographism as a cause of genital pruritus. *J Am Acad Dermatol* 1994; **31**: 1040–1.
5 Collins CG, Hansen LH, Theriot E. A clinical stain for use in selecting biopsy sites in patients with vulvar disease. *Am J Obstet Gynecol* 1966; **28**: 158.
6 Fleury FJ. Adult vaginitis. *Clin Obstet Gynecol* 1981; **24**: 407–38.
7 Wilkinson DS, ed. *Nursing and Management of Skin Diseases*, 4th edn. London: Faber & Faber, 1977.
8 Rashid S, Collins M, Kennedy RJ. A study of candidosis: the role of fomites. *Genitourin Med* 1991; **67**: 137–42.

Granulomatous lesions [1,2]

Many granulomatous lesions have already been mentioned. All are uncommon in the UK, but much more frequent in tropical regions. In such regions, the initial lesion may not by itself produce a granulomatous picture, but this develops as a result of neglect and secondary infection, and is perhaps accentuated by anaemia and malnutrition. Granulomas may be the end result of superinfections and abscess formation arising from trivial infections [1].

Tuberculosis, which is rare in this site, produces areas of granulation tissue, especially at the fourchette, or scrofuloderma from involvement of the inguinal glands. The warmer body areas are usually not affected by leprosy, and earlier accounts of vulval involvement are open to doubt. Vulvar tertiary syphilis of nodular gummatous form has been reported in the past, and may still occur where the disease is prevalent. Crohn's disease is more likely to involve the perineum, but labial lesions have been described [3–5]. A separate form of vulval granuloma akin to the orofacial lesions seen in Melkersson–Rosenthal syndrome has been described [6,7]. Many protozoal and metazoal diseases can result in granulomatous lesions, often because of secondary infection. Amoebiasis of the vulva may occur in babies with severe amoebic dysentery [8], whereas in the adult lesions of the cervix are more common [9]. Cutaneous leishmaniasis occasionally affects the vulva, and has been seen in the UK [10]. Diagnosis may be difficult if the lesion is of the lupoid type. *Schistosoma* species, especially *S. haematobium*, can cause a chronic warty granulomatous reaction in the genital area, and the warty growths may be indistinguishable from condylomata acuminata [11]. The bladder, urethra, vagina and cervix may also be involved. Rectal mucosal snips, examination of urine and vaginal discharge, and biopsy should confirm the diagnosis. Genital tract cytology is useful in vaginal infections [12].

Cryptococcus neoformans can induce painless ulceration of the vulva in the immunosuppressed patient [13].

Untreated or secondarily infected granuloma inguinale may give rise to a mixed picture of inflammation, lymphoedema, fistula formation and fibrosis. Fistulae and scarring are also the end result of lymphogranuloma venereum, which may be difficult to differentiate from granuloma inguinale.

Hidradenitis suppurativa commonly affects the perigenital areas. It is fully described in Chapter 27. The diagnosis is not usually difficult, especially if the axillae are also involved. However, Crohn's disease, deep fungal infection and lymphogranuloma venereum must be excluded. The deep mycoses may themselves cause granulomas and sinus or fistula formation. Pilonidal sinuses have been recorded on the vulva and clitoris [14,15].

Fat necrosis resulting from corticosteroid injection may cause a painful swelling. Finally, one should remember the possibility of artefactual granuloma production, when the features are bizarre and recurrent. Sclerosing lipogranuloma [16] probably falls into this group. Verruciform xanthoma is a condition which was first described in the mouth [17], but it has also been shown to occur on the genitalia of both sexes [18]. It is rare, and characterized by verrucous epithelial proliferation and xanthoma cells confined to the papillary dermis.

REFERENCES

1 Gardner HL, Kaufman RH, eds. *Benign Diseases of the Vulva and Vagina*. St Louis: Mosby, 1969.
2 Ridley CM, ed. *The Vulva*. London: Churchill Livingstone, 1988.
3 Ansell ID, Hogbin B. Crohn's disease of the vulva. *J Obstet Gynecol* 1973; **80**: 376–8.
4 Laugier MP, Hunziker N, Vidmar B. L'oedeme isolé de la grand levre. Complication cutanée de la maladie de Crohn. *Bull Soc Fr Dermatol Syphiligr* 1971; **78**: 98–100.
5 McCallum DI, Kinmont PDC. Dermatological manifestations of Crohn's disease. *Br J Dermatol* 1968; **80**: 1–8.
6 Hackel H, Hartman AA, Burg G. Vulvitis granulomatosa and anoperineitis granulomatosa. *Dermatologica* 1991; **182**: 128–31.
7 Knopf B, Schaarschmidt H, Wollina U. Monosymptomatisches Melkersson–Rosenthal–Syndrom mit nachfolgender vulvitis und perivulvitis granulomatosa. *Hautarzt* 1992; **43**: 711–13.
8 Rimsza ME, Berg RA. Cutaneous amebiasis. *Pediatrics* 1983; **71**: 595–8.
9 Cohen C. Three cases of amoebiasis of the cervix uteri. *J Obstet Gynecol* 1973; **80**: 476–9.
10 Symmers W St C. Leishmaniasis acquired by contagion: a case of marital infection in Britain. *Lancet* 1960; **i**: 127–32.
11 McKee PH, Wright E, Hutt MSR. Vulval schistosomiasis. *Clin Exp Dermatol* 1983; **8**: 189–94.
12 Berry A. Evidence of gynecologic bilharziasis in cytologic material. *Acta Cytol* 1971; **15**: 482–98.
13 Blocher KS, Weeks JA, Noble RC. Cutaneous cryptococcal infection presenting as vulvar lesion. *Genitourin Med* 1987; **63**: 341–3.
14 Beilby JOW, Ridley CM. Pathology of the vulva. In: Fox H, ed. *Hailes and Taylor's Obstetric and Gynaecological Pathology*. Edinburgh: Churchill Livingstone, 1986.
15 Radman HM, Bhagavan BS. Pilonidal disease of the female genitals. *Am J Obstet Gynecol* 1972; **114**: 271–3.
16 Kempson RL, Sherman AI. Sclerosing lipogranuloma of the vulva. *Am J Obstet Gynecol* 1968; **101**: 854–6.
17 Shafer WB. Verruciform xanthoma. *Oral Surg* 1971; **31**: 784–9.
18 Santa Cruz DJ, Martin SA. Verruciform xanthoma of the vulva. Report of two cases. *Am J Clin Pathol* 1979; **71**: 224–8.

Vulval diseases of infancy

These are seldom confined to the vulva but usually involve part or all of the napkin area.

Napkin rash

Erythematous form. Minor degrees are commonplace, and the dermatologist, in the UK at least, will see only those cases which are severe, unusual or persistent. Newer, more absorbant materials appear to be contributing to a marked decrease in severity [1]. Although it may appear at any age, especially if the child fails to become continent, napkin erythema is a disease of the first few months of life. The erythema, affecting the area in contact with the napkins, and generally sparing the flexures, is characteristic. Superficial erosions and even ulceration occasionally occur. The acute phase gives place to a duller, scaly rash, which may have outlying satellite lesions. When these are micropustular, candidiasis must be suspected.

Some infants appear to be more prone to develop napkin erythema, even when the same standards of care and hygiene apply. Infrequent changings, chafing and friction in association with occlusive pants, inadequate rinsing, fabric softeners and excessively strong concentrations of cleansers or antiseptics may contribute to irritancy, and systemic antibiotic therapy may be a predisposing factor [2].

Frequency of bowel movement, and length of contact of faecal material with the infant's skin, appear to be important factors in both the production and severity of the rash [3]. It is likely that faecal enzymes are primarily responsible for most aspects of napkin erythema. Heat-treated stool, in which all enzymes have been inactivated, does not produce a rash when occluded on the skin of hairless mice [4]. The role of ammonia is becoming clearer. It has been shown that infants with napkin erythema do not produce above-average amounts of ammonia, and that application of ammonia under occlusion to non-traumatized skin does not induce erythema [5]. It has now been shown that the rise in pH resulting from ammonia production by faecal urease increases the activity of faecal proteases and lipases, and that this process can damage skin [4,6]. Urine itself can increase the permeability of occluded skin to irritants of all types, and ammonia can further irritate previously traumatized skin [5,7].

Secondary bacterial infection may occur at any stage. The significance of candidal infection has been disputed. Earlier workers found *Candida* in the skin of less than half affected infants [8].

In its early stages, napkin erythema is characterized by chafing and contact erythema. Some infants may then progress to an intense erythema with a sharp border and satellite pustules. There is a high yield of *Candida* in scrapings from satellite pustules and from the faeces in this group, but recovery rates from the area of intense erythema are lower [9].

In infants with intense erythema only, the rate of recovery of *Candida* will be low, but the rate of rectal carriage is high when compared with controls, and correlates directly with the severity of the rash [3]. It has been shown that *Candida albicans* can activate the alternative complement pathway and produce severe inflammation, which may then suppress further growth of *Candida* and account for its relatively infrequent isolation within the group [9].

Papular forms. Papular forms of napkin rash, which may show central ulceration (Jacquet), are entirely separate from the erythematous form (Fig. 72.30). They are less commonly seen, and are generally a manifestation of parental neglect. Long hours of contact with urine and faeces under occlusion and poor general hygiene characterize this disorder, and it may be that the concept of a prominent role for ammonia in the production of napkin rash originated from consideration of this group [10].

A particular form, the so-called 'gluteal granuloma' [11], has been described, and appears, at least in part, to be associated with prolonged use of potent topical steroids. A number of cases, however, have now been described in incontinent adults in whom steroids were not used [12].

Cytomegalovirus in association with severe napkin rash has been described in an HIV immunosuppressed infant [13].

Treatment. In the papular, necrotic form, parental education,

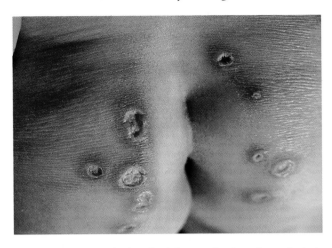

Fig. 72.30 'Nappy rash of neglect': the papulo-ulcerative variant of Jacquet.

supervision and hygiene are usually sufficient to cure the problem. These infants tend not to relapse or suffer problems with oversensitive skins.

There is still controversy with regard to the relative merits of disposable and non-disposable napkins [14,15].

The most effective management of the erythematous forms is total liberation from napkins and, more especially, from occlusive pants. Non-disposable napkins should be washed and rinsed thoroughly; fabric softeners should not be used. The early chafing rashes respond well to zinc creams and even silicone-based barrier creams. Zinc and castor oil cream alone often suffices in mild lesions. In the cases seen by a dermatologist, dermatitic changes are usually prominent, and hydrocortisone in association with either a polyene antibiotic or an imidazole is indicated. The use of Vioform (clioquinol) under occlusive pants is contra-indicated because of the risk of systemic absorption [16]. Soaps should be avoided, and aqueous cream used for washing the area. Relapse is common.

Napkin psoriasis

Occasionally, an eruption in the napkin area presents as a bright-red, glazed, well-demarcated sheet of erythema reminiscent of psoriasis. Secondary lesions may be widely scattered and profuse, often with marked scaling. *Candida* may be found. The appearance is alarming to the mother, but the infant seems little worried by the extensive eruption. There is usually a very satisfactory response to simple topical measures. Over an observation period of 7–15 years some patients subsequently developed psoriasis [17].

Infantile seborrhoeic dermatitis

This unsatisfactory term (Chapter 14) is applied to a dry, scaly eruption involving the skin folds. Vesication does not occur. Secondary infection is common. The cause is unknown, and it may not be same condition as the adult disease of this name. However, a similar association with *Pityrosporum* yeasts has been noted [18]. A generalized form constitutes Leiner's disease.

Contact dermatitis

The effect of napkin-washing materials and antiseptic rinses as a primary cause of rashes in the napkin area has been discussed above. These can certainly cause an irritant dermatitis, especially if the general hygiene is poor and the napkin is left unchanged on skin already damaged by prolonged contact with urine and faeces.

A peculiar, apparently idiosyncratic, glazed, yellowish red scaling confined to the area of a paper napkin liner treated with a very weak solution of quaternary ammonium antiseptic has been observed in four patients (N.J. Bandmann, D.S. Wilkinson, unpublished). It resolved within 48 h when these were left off, and did not recur subsequently. The mechanism is unknown. The necrotic reaction to quaternary ammonium agents [19] is now seldom seen, but may occur unexpectedly and under unusual circumstances [20]. Other causes of contact dermatitis are rare in the infant. Hexachlorophane talc may cause rashes and encephalopathy [21], and anaphylaxis to casein in a soothing application has been reported in a milk-sensitive infant [22].

Other conditions

Dermatophyte infections of the napkin area have been described, especially in warmer climates [23]. Miliaria of the occluded skin is being seen more frequently, especially in neonates. It is due to high ambient temperatures in hospital nurseries associated with the increased insulation effect of newer disposable napkins (F.A. Ive, B. Diffey, unpublished, 1987.)

Acrodermatitis enteropathica is characterized by the poor general condition of the infant, loss of hair, and other typical features. Langerhans' cell histiocytosis should be considered when yellow–brown papules occur with purpura in the napkin region and elsewhere. The diagnosis is confirmed histologically. Kawasaki disease often produces perineal erythema [24]. Haemangiomas of the vulva and napkin area frequently ulcerate and give rise to parental concern, but they heal satisfactorily with the application of a protective antibacterial ointment. Asymptomatic Crohn's disease has presented as unilateral labial hypertrophy in infancy [25].

REFERENCES

1 Longhi F, Carlucci G, Bellucci R *et al*. Diaper dermatitis, a study of contributing factors. *Contact Dermatitis* 1992; **26**: 248–52.
2 Honig PJ, Gribetz B, Leyden JJ. Amoxicillin and diaper dermatitis. *J Am Acad Dermatol* 1988; **19**: 275–9.
3 Jordan WE, Lawson KD, Stewart R *et al*. Diaper dermatitis: frequency and severity among a general infant population. *Pediatr Dermatol* 1986; **3**: 198–207.
4 Buckingham KW, Berg RW. Etiologic factors in diaper dermatitis: the role of faeces. *Pediatr Dermatol* 1986; **3**: 107–12.
5 Leyden JJ, Katz S, Stewart R *et al*. Urinary ammonia and ammonia-producing micro-organisms in infants with and without diaper dermatitis. *Arch Dermatol* 1977; **113**: 1678–80.
6 Berg RW, Buckingham KW, Stewart RL. Etiologic factors in diaper dermatitis: The role of urine. *Pediatr Dermatol* 1986; **3**: 102–6.
7 Berg RW, Milligan MC, Sarbaugh FC. Association of skin wetness and pH with diaper dermatitis. *Pediatr Dermatol* 1994; **11**: 18–20.
8 Dixon PN, Warin RP, English MP. Role of *Candida albicans* infection in napkin rashes. *Br Med J* 1969; **ii**: 23–7.
9 Rebora A, Leyden JJ. Napkin (diaper) dermatitis and gastrointestinal carriage of *Candida albicans*. *Br J Dermatol* 1981; **105**: 551–5.
10 Cooke JV. Dermatitis of the diaper region in infants. *Arch Dermatol Syphilol* 1926; **14**: 539–46.
11 Tappeiner J, Partsch H. Ulceromultilierende neuropathien der unteren extremitaten. *Hautarzt* 1971; **22**: 283–9.
12 Maekawa Y, Sakazaki Y, Hayashibara T. Diaper area granuloma of the aged. *Arch Dermatol* 1978; **114**: 382–3.
13 Thiboutot DM, Beckford A, Mart CR *et al*. Cytomegalovirus diaper dermatitis. *Arch Dermatol* 1991; **127**: 396–8.
14 Campbell RL, Bartlett AV, Sarbargh FC *et al*. Effect of diaper types on diaper dermatitis associated with diarrhoea and antibiotic use in children and day-care centres. *Pediatr Dermatol* 1988; **5**: 83–7.
15 Maleville J, Larregue M, Lardet B *et al*. Dermatitis fessieres du nourisson. *Revue Pediatr* 1982; **18**: 601–10.
16 Stohs SJ, Ezzedeen FW, Anderson K *et al*. Percutaneous absorption of iodochlorhydroxyquinoline in humans. *J Invest Dermatol* 1984; **82**: 195–8.
17 Rasmussen HB, Hagdrup H, Schmidt H. Psoriasiform napkin dermatitis. *Acta Derm Venereol (Stockh)* 1986; **66**: 534–6.
18 Broberg A, Faergemann J. Infantile seborrhoeic dermatitis and *Pityrosporum ovale*. *Br J Dermatol* 1989; **120**: 239–62.
19 Tilsley DI, Wilkinson DS. Necrosis and dequalinium. II. Vulval and extragenital ulceration. *Trans St John's Hosp Dermatol Soc* 1965; **51**: 49–54.
20 August PJ. Cutaneous necrosis due to cetrimide application. *Br Med J* 1975; **i**: 71–6.
21 Larregue M, Laider B, Ramdene P *et al*. Dermite caustique du siege et encephalite secondaires a l'application de talc contaminé par l'hexachlorophene. *Ann Dermatol Vénéréol* 1984; **111**: 789–97.
22 Jarmoc LM, Primack WA. Anaphylaxis to cutaneous exposure to milk protein in a diaper rash ointment. *Clin Pediatr* 1988; **26**: 154–5.
23 Cavanagh RM, Greeson JD. *Trichophyton rubrum*: infection of the diaper area. *Arch Dermatol* 1982; **118**: 446.
24 Friter BS, Lucky AW. The perineal eruption of Kawasaki syndrome. *Arch Dermatol* 1988; **124**: 1805–10.
25 Werlin S, Esterly NB, Oechler H. Crohn's disease presenting as unilateral labial hypertrophy. *J Am Acad Dermatol* 1992; **27**: 893–4.

Vulval pruritus

Vulval pruritus occurs consistently in some dermatoses and inconstantly in others, to an extent which varies with the individual patient. Any itching of a dermatosis involving the vulva may appear disproportionate, especially in anxious or depressed patients. Lichen sclerosus et atrophicus, scabies, phthiriasis, mycotic infections and contact dermatitis are important causes.

Cystitis, proctitis, cervicitis and vaginitis of any type cause itching of variable degree. Anal pruritus, whatever its cause, not infrequently spreads to the vulva. Vulvovaginal candidiasis is a very common cause of pruritus, and trichomonal infections to a lesser extent. Fox–Fordyce disease is accompanied by particularly severe itching.

Infestation with *Enterobius (Oxyuris) vermicularis* is relatively rare in adult women [1].

In 161 patients with pruritus, vulvitis or fungal infections were responsible in 78 and an atrophic or leukoplakic condition in 83 [2]. Paradoxically, dermatologists probably see more cases in which local causes are less obvious.

Vulval neoplasms may also present with pruritus, and the symptoms should never be dismissed lightly. An increase of pruritus in patients with lichen sclerosus et atrophicus (p. 3231) may herald the onset of 'leukoplakia' or a premalignant change.

It has been said [3] that 10% of all gynaecological patients present with pruritus. Local and general causes must first be excluded. Diabetes may present in this way, and the urine should be tested in all cases. In older patients, a glucose tolerance test may be required to detect mild, late-onset diabetes.

Pruritus vulvae is confined to the vulva or perianal area, and does not involve the vagina. However, it may be sufficiently intense to disturb sleep and to affect seriously the mental equilibrium of the patient. In those of a particularly anxious temperament, or when a 'depressive equivalent' is involved, slight degrees of inflammation or infection may give rise to disproportionate itching. The imprecise term 'pruritus vulvae' has been retained to describe those patients in whom there is a complaint of chronic itching without organic cause.

It is important to recognize, however, that short-lived vulval pruritus is not uncommon, and is easily induced by friction, chafing, sweating or the vulval engorgement of pregnancy. In this group there may also be cases of early candidal vulvitis, who have infection and symptoms but no physical signs.

Psychosomatic vulvovaginitis

About 2% of women who present with complaints of vaginal or vulval discomfort defy even the most diligent search for recognizable genital pathology [4]. These patients have usually seen many doctors, and have been treated with a multitude of medicaments. Their complaints may vary from persistent itching, through a spectrum of types of pain, which is often localized and described variously as burning, shooting or gnawing. Dyspareunia is virtually the rule among the group, and it may be that avoidance of intercourse is the 'reward' gained for their very genuine discomfort. It is perhaps to preserve this defence against intercourse that these patients will absolutely resist any suggestion that their symptoms might be psychological in origin, although emotional lability, dependent personality and sexual guilt feelings can often be unmasked on relatively superficial questioning.

The pattern of psychosomatic vulvovaginitis appears to be changing over recent years. Until recently, the common complaint appeared to be itching without organic cause. This is now much less common [5], and in a survey of 900 patients in a combined dermatology/gynaecology clinic, no such patient was seen [6].

Vulvodynia or the vulvar vestibulitis syndrome [7]

Complaints of vulval pain are, however, becoming much more common [8,9]. The term vulvodynia [5,8,10–12] has been applied to a group of symptoms characterized by chronic and often unremitting pain, burning, stinging or rawness of the vulval area. Itching is absent, and careful examination of the involved site should show no sign of either primary disease or secondary damage associated with rubbing or excoriation. Evidence of vulval microwarts or papillomatosis (p. 3216), although probably irrelevant, should be sought and excluded [13]. All adult age groups are involved, and many patients will indicate the precise localization of their symptoms. The disorder can best be described as a dysaesthesia comparable with that seen in glossodynia, the hot scrotum syndrome [14], the chronic perianal pain syndrome [15] or even post-herpetic neuralgia. Topical therapies are usually unhelpful, and the patients and their relatives frequently become resentful and angry. They tend to visit many doctors, and often are driven to try a variety of quack and folk remedies.

Temporary relief of symptoms is seen following injection of local anaesthetic agents, but attempts at long-term nerve blockage by alcohol injection, although helpful in vulvar pruritus, do not influence the burning sensation of vulvodynia [16]. Many patients manifest evidence of endogenous depression [17], and as tricyclic antidepressant therapy is often helpful in other forms of dysaesthesia, its long-term administration in the form of amitriptyline hydrochloride has been tried successfully in doses of 50–75mg daily [8]. Topical therapy with capsaicin has been advocated [18]. Its judicious use combined with topical local anaesthetic has been found helpful in the author's pain clinic (D. Laird, F.A. Ive, unpublished, 1995).

Hallmarks of psychosomatic vulvovaginitis [4]

These are:
1 persistent symptoms of long-standing duration;
2 lack of demonstrable pathology;
3 sexual inactivity as a direct result of symptoms;
4 unsuccessful consultations with many doctors;
5 'allergy' to many common vaginal medicaments;
6 reluctance to accept a psychosomatic causation;
7 emotional lability and dependency.

Lichenification of the vulva (Fig. 72.31)

SYN. LICHEN SIMPLEX; LOCALIZED NEURODERMATITIS

Thickening and hypertrophy of the vulval skin are frequently seen as a result of prolonged rubbing rather than scratching. The initial stimulus to itch may be an underlying seborrhoeic dermatitis, intertrigo, tinea or psoriasis, but in most cases the underlying cause is not evident, and may have been a transient vulvitis or vaginal discharge. Perhaps even more trivial factors such as chafing or sweating may be sufficient to provoke the initial itching sensation. In predisposed individuals the itch–rub cycle supervenes, producing the characteristic picture of lichenification (Chapter 17).

It is important to appreciate that any itching disease of the vulva can become secondarily lichenified; after treatment, all cases must be reviewed in case an underlying 'leukoplakia', Paget's or Bowen's disease has been revealed.

Treatment. Treatment is identical to management of lichenification elsewhere on the body. The patient should be informed of the need to break the rubbing habit. The cutaneous nerves in involved areas appear to work on a hair trigger mechanism, and strenuous efforts should be made to assist the patient by reducing their activation.

In the early stages, topical antibiotics may be prescribed if secondary infection is present. Thereafter, strong topical steroids either applied locally or injected intralesionally are usually needed to provide the prolonged relief from itching necessary to break the rubbing reflex.

Application of strong local steroids should not be prolonged for over 1 month because of risks of local atrophy. Such a length of application is usually unnecessary, however. Soaps and cleansing agents other than aqueous cream should be forbidden.

In severe or extensive cases, Grenz ray therapy in addition to local steroids may be needed to provide the required antipruritic effect. If therapy fails or is only partially effective, a biopsy of the involved area should always be performed.

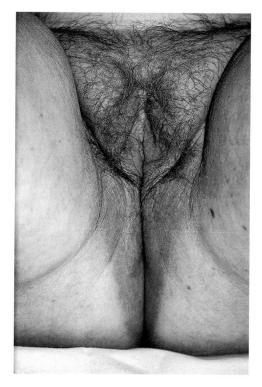

Fig. 72.31 Lichen simplex of the vulva and perineum.

REFERENCES

1 Kacker TP. Vulvovaginitis in an adult with threadworms in the vagina. *Br J Vener Dis* 1973; **49**: 314–15.
2 Mariotti GF. Terapie chirurgiche del plurito vulvare ribeue. *Pubblicita Riv Ital Ginecol* 1964; **48**: 262–82.
3 Jeffcoate TNA, ed. *Principles of Gynaecology*, 3rd edn. London: Butterworths, 1967.
4 Dodson MG, Friedrich EG. Psychosomatic vulvovaginitis. *Obstet Gynecol* 1978; **51** (Suppl. 1): 235–55.
5 Ridley CM, ed. *The Vulva*. London: Churchill Livingstone, 1988.
6 Tovell HMM, Young AW. Classification of vulvar diseases. *Clin Obstet Gynecol* 1978; **21**: 955–61.
7 Marinoff SC, Turner MLC. Vulvar vestibulitis syndrome. *Dermatol Clin* 1992; **10**: 435–44.
8 McKay M. Vulvodynia. *Arch Dermatol* 1989; **125**: 256–62.
9 Goetsch MF. Vulvar vestibulitis and historic features in general gynecologic practice population. *Am J Obstet Gynecol* 1991; **164**: 1609–16.
10 Ridley CM. International Society for the Study of Vulvar Disease (ISSVD). Report of committee on vulvodynia. *J Reprod Med* 1993; **38**: 1–4.
11 Lynch PJ. Vulvodynia. *J Reprod Med* 1986; **31**: 773–80.
12 McKay M. Vulvodynia versus pruritus vulvae. *Clin Obstet Gynecol* 1985; **28**: 123–33.
13 Turner MLC, Marinoff SC. Association of human papilloma virus with vulvodynia and the vulvar vestibulitis syndrome. *J Reprod Med* 1988; **33**: 533–7.
14 Cotterill JA. Dermatological non-disease; a common and potentially fatal disturbance of cutaneous body image. *Br J Dermatol* 1981; **104**: 611–19.
15 Neill ME, Swash M. Chronic perianal pain: an unsolved problem. *J R Soc Med* 1982; **75**: 96–101.
16 Clouser JK, Friedrich EG. A new technique for alcohol injection in the vulva. *J Reprod Med* 1986; **31**: 971–2.
17 Moyal-Burracco M, Consoli S. Brulures vulvaires sans support organique. *Contracept Fert Sex* 1986; **14**: 941–7.
18 Freidrich EG. Therapeutic studies on vulvar vestibulitis. *J Reprod Med* 1988; **33**: 514–18.

Vulval and vaginal bullae and ulcers

Genital ulceration is frequently complicated by secondary infection. Papules and vesicles erode easily on the mucosal surface, so that lesions which do not normally ulcerate may present as ulcers. Vulval and vaginal ulcers may be divided conveniently into acute, chronic and recurrent types.

Acute genital ulceration

The patient presents with an ulcer or discharge and, sometimes, pain and vulval oedema. Alternatively, the ulceration is seen in the course of an acute illness.

Venereal ulcers

These must always be considered first: syphilis, chancroid, gonorrhoea, lymphogranuloma venereum and granuloma inguinale.

The differentiating features are discussed elsewhere. The diagnosis is confirmed by the results of specific bacteriological and serological investigations, which should always be carried out to exclude a double infection. Reiter's syndrome has been associated with ulcerative vulvitis [1].

Non-venereal infective ulcers

Tuberculosis, typhoid, pneumonia and brucellosis. Ulceration occurs rarely in these and other severe acute illnesses. In diphtheria, genital ulcers are seen in children with pharyngeal or nasal infection. The child is ill, and the ulcer is characterized by an adherent greyish membrane, which often extends over much of the swollen, excoriated mucosal surface.

Anaerobic streptococci, *Pseudomonas aeruginosa* and fusospirillary organisms alone or as a superinfection cause rapidly spreading, burrowing ulcers or phagedena and gangrene in the debilitated patient. Herpes simplex, herpes zoster, vaccinia and variola are discussed in Chapter 26.

Hand, foot and mouth disease. Small, rapidly eroding vesicles occasionally occur on the vulva of infants (perhaps more frequently than is reported).

Acute non-infective ulcers

Erythema multiforme. In the severe form (Stevens–Johnson syndrome) the vulva is affected, often severely.

Artefacts. These are rare on the vulva, but may be associated with foreign bodies or trauma from sexual injury [2], and self-induced lesions may deceive the doctor [3].

Ulceration has followed the use of strong quaternary ammonium solutions employed to disinfect a speculum.

Chronic genital ulceration

Any chronic ulcer of the genital mucosa must be considered malignant until proved otherwise. Ulceration occurs particularly on atrophic mucosa or on a patch of leukoplakia. Chronic infective ulcers occur in pyoderma, actinomycosis and other deep mycoses. The late stages of lymphogranuloma venereum cause ulceration and scarring. Vulval ulceration caused by the bite of the brown recluse spider *Loxosceles reclusa* has been reported from the USA [4].

The now outdated term *esthiomene* was applied to chronic ulcerating, vegetating and lymphoedematous lesions of the vulva and perigenital area. Several of the bullous diseases affect the vulva, but only pemphigus vulgaris [5] and

vegetans have a predilection for this area. The flaccid bullae rupture easily to produce erosions. Biopsy (with immunofluorescence studies) will confirm the diagnosis. Juvenile pemphigoid affected the genital area in 36 out of 38 cases [6]. The ruptured vesicles and fissured plaques of benign familial chronic pemphigus may be easily misdiagnosed. Exacerbations may follow friction, infection, irritants and herpes simplex infections [7]. Polydysplastic epidermolysis bullosa affects the mucous membranes more frequently than other types. The mouth and conjunctivae are also likely to be involved.

Cicatricial pemphigoid may produce ulceration and stenosis of the vulva and vagina. Urinary obstruction may be a feature [8,9]. Erosive lichen planus often will be recognizable by its lace-work patterning and accompanying oral lesions. The association of erosions of the vulva, vagina and gingival mucosa has been reported [10,11]. This seriously disabling condition, sometimes referred to as desquamative inflammatory vaginitis [12], may not always be due to lichen planus.

Superficial fissures and ulcers occur in lichen sclerosus, and may also lead to adhesions and urinary obstruction [13].

Recurrent genital ulceration [14]

A multitude of names, often eponymous, disguise a few entities which can be distinguished clinically. The aetiology of many remains unknown.

Recurrent erythema multiforme. The genital area is seldom affected in the usual peripheral type but may be involved when oral lesions are predominant.

Bullous fixed drug eruptions. These are less common (or less commonly recognized) on the vulva than on the penis. With the decline in the use of phenolphthalein, sulphonamides and barbiturates, they are becoming rare, at least in the UK.

Recurrent herpes simplex. This has been discussed earlier.

Recurrent vaginal ulcers. These have been associated with the use of tampons [15].

Aphthosis. This common idiopathic entity may account for some or all cases of: (i) Sutton's ulcer; and (ii) Lipschutz's ulcer (see below).

Behçet's syndrome. For the present, this condition remains distinct from aphthosis because of its other manifestations and differing prognosis (Fig. 72.32).

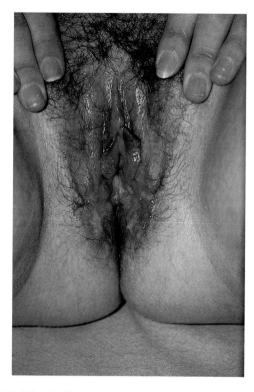

Fig. 72.32 Behçet's disease.

Aphthosis

When aphthae occur on the vulva, the concomitant oral lesions are usually severe. It is important to differentiate between these ulcers and a recurrent herpetic infection [16]. Premenstrual exacerbations are common. The cause is unknown.

The genital lesions are multiple, painful, superficial and yellowish, with a red areola. They affect the labia particularly, and heal quickly.

At present, only symptomatic treatment is available. Topical corticosteroids, or topical tetracyclines, seem to help some patients. Others unaccountably respond to a variety of unproven or experimental forms of treatment, suggesting a high degree of placebo response. Testosterone implants have been recommended in the treatment of females with this condition [17].

Sutton's ulcer (periadenitis mucosa necrotica recurrens). This ulcer is solitary, painful, recurring, and is more common in the mouth [18]. It may be a variant of aphthosis or Behçet's syndrome but normally occurs alone, without any associated abnormalities. Intralesional triamcinolone has been the most effective form of treatment in personal cases.

Lipschutz's ulcer (ulcus vulvae acutum). Lipschutz described three types of ulcer only one of which is now regarded as being a separate entity [19]; the others fall into the pattern of Behçet's syndrome or aphthosis [19]. The remaining form

of ulceration in which lesions are solitary or sparse, is sometimes associated with infection such as typhoid or paratyphoid fever [20]. It is self-limiting, and resolves without treatment. *Bacillus crassus* is no longer regarded as a pathogen in these cases.

Adolescent girls are affected in more than half the cases reported. The lesion is often acute in onset, and may be accompanied by fever. Sparse lesions are surrounded by a reddish areola, and have a firmly adherent membrane, which separates in a few days. The lymphatic glands are usually enlarged, and tests for infectious mononucleosis may be positive [21]. Epstein–Barr virus has been found in such cases [22]. One case was initially misdiagnosed as a high-grade lymphoma [23].

REFERENCES

1 Daunt S O'N, Kotowski KE, O'Reilly AP *et al.* Ulcerative vulvitis in Reiter's syndrome. *Br J Vener Dis* 1982; **58**: 405–7.
2 Wilson KFG. Lower genital tract trauma. *Aust NZ J Obstet Gynecol* 1966; **6**: 291–3.
3 Reich LH, Wehr T. Female genital self-mutilation. *Obstet Gynecol* 1973; **41**: 239–42.
4 Magrina JF, Masterson BJ. *Loxosceles reclusa* spider bite: a consideration in the differential diagnosis of chronic, nonmalignant ulcers of the vulva. *Am J Obstet Gynecol* 1981; **140**: 341–3.
5 Kaufman RH, Watts JM, Gardner HL. Pemphigus vulgaris: genital involvement. Report of two cases. *Obstet Gynecol* 1969; **33**: 264–6.
6 Grant PW. Juvenile dermatitis herpetiformis. *Trans St John's Hosp Dermatol Soc* 1968; **54**: 128–36.
7 Leppard B, Delaney TJ, Sanderson KV. Chronic benign familial pemphigus: induction of lesions by herpesvirus hominis. *Br J Dermatol* 1973; **88**: 609–13.
8 Boyce DC, Valprey JM. Acute ulcerative vulvitis of obscure etiology. *Obstet Gynecol* 1971; **38**: 440–3.
9 McCallum DI. Unusual cause of urinary obstruction. *Br Med J* 1969; **ii**: 637.
10 Pelisse M. The vulvovaginal gingival syndrome. A new form of erosive lichen planus. *Int J Dermatol* 1989; **28**: 381–4.
11 Eisen D. The vulvovaginal–gingival syndrome of lichen planus: the clinical characteristics of 22 patients. *Arch Dermatol* 1994; **130**: 1379–82.
12 Oates JK, Rowen D. Desquamative inflammatory vaginitis. *Genitourin Med* 1990; **66**: 275–9.
13 Damanski M, Barker ME, Sheehan JF. Unusual cause of urinary obstruction. *Br Med J* 1969; **ii**: 385.
14 Ridley CM, ed. *The Vulva*. London: Churchill Livingstone, 1988.
15 Weissberg SM, Dodson MG. Recurrent vaginal and cervical ulcers associated with tampon use. *JAMA* 1983; **250**: 1430–1.
16 Weathers DR, Griffiths JW. Internal ulcerations of recurrent herpes simplex and recurrent aphthae: two distinct clinical entities. *J Am Dent Assoc* 1970; **81**: 81–8.
17 Misra R, Anderson DC. Treatment of recurrent premenstrual orogenital aphthae with implants of low dosage testosterone. *Br Med J* 1989; **299**: 834.
18 Monteleone L. Periadenitis mucosa necrotica recurrens. Report of a case. *Oral Surg Oral Med Oral Pathol* 1967; **23**: 586–91.
19 Berlin C. The pathogenesis of the so-called ulcus vulvae acutum. *Acta Derm Venereol (Stockh)* 1965; **45**: 221–2.
20 Van Joost Th. Casuistische mededelingen. Een zeldzaam geval can een acuut onttaan ulcus vulvae. *Ned Tijdschr Geneeskd* 1971; **115**: 1080–2.
21 Brown ZA, Stenchever MA. Genital ulceration and infectious mononucleosis. *Am J Obstet Gynecol* 1977; **127**: 673–4.
22 Portnoy J, Arontheim GA, Ghibu F *et al.* Recovery of Epstein–Barr virus from genital ulcers. *N Engl J Med* 1984; **311**: 966–8.
23 Eghbali H, Lacut JY, Hoernie B. Genital infectious mononucleosis mimicking high grade non-Hodgkin's lymphoma. *Med Mal Infect* 1989; **19**: 83–6.

The vulval dystrophies

Introduction

The term *vulvar dystrophy* [1] is applied by gynaecologists to describe a group of diseases presenting as white lesions of the vulva. In the past, there has been much confusion over terminology between dermatologists and gynaecologists, and it is hoped that the establishment of a Committee on Terminology of the International Society for the Study of Vulvar Disease (ISSVD) might help to resolve many of the problems of terminology and classification. In 1987, the ISSVD [1] ratified a classification of non-neoplastic disorders of the vulva. It is a necessary compromise between the views of gynaecologists and dermatologists, which, by over simplification and clinical impoverishment, may limit its usefulness to both groups.

Non-neoplastic epithelial disorders of vulval skin and mucosa

These are:
1 Lichen sclerosus;
2 Squamous cell hyperplasia;
3 Other dermatoses.

It is recognized that admixtures of these disorders may occur, and the ISSVD recommends that each component is coded separately. It suggests that squamous cell hyperplasia with atypia is diagnosed as vulval intraepithelial neoplasia (VIN), and coded according to degree of severity (p. 3235). The author's personal preference is a classification [2] based on clinical and histological criteria, which encompasses both benign and malignant disease of the vulva, and which could easily include the VIN schedule.

Reactive and neoplastic disorders of vulval epithelium
(adapted from [2])

1 Benign dermatoses:
 I lichenification;
 II psoriasis;
 III lichen planus;
 IV seborrhoeic dermatitis;
 V eczematous dermatitis (chronic).
2 Vulvar epithelial hyperplasia:
 I without atypia;
 II with atypia (leukoplakia).
3 Lichen sclerosus.
4 Lichen sclerosus with foci of epithelial hyperplasia:
 I without atypia;
 II with atypia (VIN).
5 Squamous cell carcinoma *in situ*/invasive VIN.
6 Paget's disease of the vulva.
7 Plasma-cell vulvitis.

The classification of the ISSVD has, however, finally freed us from the use of such terms as senile genital atrophy and primary vulval atrophy. These terms presumably relate, in major part, to the physiological effects of ageing, and do not represent recognizable disease processes.

Benign dermatoses of the vulva

Lichenification (lichen simplex chronicus) (Chapter 17). The hyperkeratosis is usually ill-defined, and merges into normal skin. Pigmentation is common, even on the normal vulva, and may, on occasion, have to be biopsied to exclude malignant melanoma [3,4]. On the external labia, the diagnosis is not difficult. On the mucosal surface the affected area may be localized, thickened and greyish-white in colour, or more diffuse, with large areas of thickening merging with obvious lichenification of the adjacent skin. Leukoplakia is stark white and more localized.

Psoriasis. The silvery scaling of patches on the outer aspects of the labia is readily recognized. Psoriasis of the vulva is usually of the smooth, 'glazed', flexural type. A rare, severe psoriasiform reaction has been described as part of Reiter's syndrome [5].

Lichen planus [6,7]. The bluish-white papules or delicate, lace-like striae are easily distinguished from the more opaque lesions of leukoplakia, but in the rare absence of lesions elsewhere, a solitary patch of lichen planus may cause diagnostic difficulty and necessitate a biopsy. The vestibule and inner surfaces of the labia minora are most frequently affected (Fig. 72.33). The occurrence of erosions and desquamation of the vaginal epithelium, with or without other signs of more generalized lichen planus, has been included under the generic title *desquamative vaginitis* [8,9]. It can cause vulval and vaginal adhesions, and may account for some cases of chronic atrophic erosive vulval disease. Topical steroid therapy may be of benefit [8]. The author's experience suggests that systemic administration of cyclosporin at doses of about 3mg/kg may be curative in steroid-resistant cases. In long-standing and ulcerative lichen planus, there may be some risk of malignancy [10,11].

Chronic erosive vulvar disease [11] presents many diagnostic problems. Vaginal erosions alone usually suggest either lichen planus or cicatricial pemphigoid. Additional diagnoses of lichen sclerosus [12], intraepithelial neoplasia and focal vulvitis may be considered in cases with solely vulvar involvement.

Seborrhoeic dermatitis. The flexures are usually involved. A combination of erythema, scaling and even crusting may spread over the labia majora.

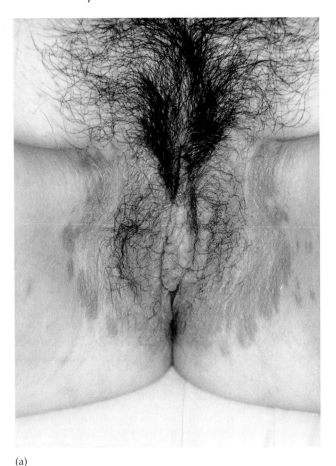

(a)

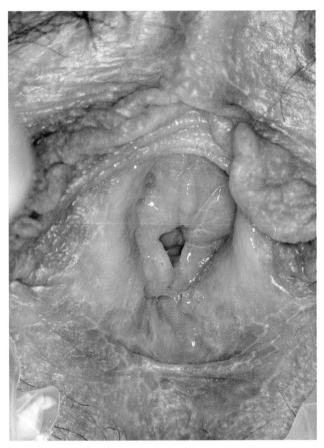

(b)

Fig. 72.33 Lichen planus.

Eczematous dermatitis. This is irritant and allergic eczema of the vulva.

Vulval squamous epithelial hyperplasia

This seems a ponderous term to have imposed upon the profession. Its necessity appears to stem from the fact that many feel unable to accept that 'leukoplakia' means anything more than literally 'white patch'. If it could be accepted that the term leukoplakia represents a combined clinical and histological diagnosis of vulval epithelial hyperplasia with cellular atypia, most of the dermatologist's difficulties would be resolved, and all the above classification would be unnecessary. In the present text the term leukoplakia (as defined above) will continue to be used.

Vulval squamous epithelial hyperplasia without atypia

This term can be limited to such conditions as seborrhoeic warts and epithelial naevi, which might involve any area of the skin, and appear on the vulva largely by chance.

Vulval squamous epithelial hyperplasia with atypia
SYN. LEUKOPLAKIA

This is a diagnosis which cannot be made without histological confirmation, as its clinical appearance can be imitated by such diseases as lichenification, epithelial naevi and lichen planus. The situation is complicated by the fact that a varying degree of lichenification may be superimposed on another disorder. In the presence of a confusing histological picture, it is perfectly legitimate to use a strong topical steroid to clear the lichenification and then rebiopsy the area. Clinically, the condition appears as single or scattered plaques of thickened white skin with rather ill-defined edges extending onto or involving the mucosa. Histologically, it consists of an irregular hyperplastic epithelium with varying degrees of cellular atypicality or loss of polarity. Occasionally, there may be no obvious atypia in the early stages, but careful follow-up and rebiopsy, sometimes after clearing superimposed lichenification with steroids, may then show evidence of increased mitotic activity throughout the epidermal layers, which is the earliest sign of atypia.

Thereafter, there appears to be a progression from slightly atypical hyperplasia to conditions which approximate to intraepithelial carcinoma. It has been reported that more than 55% of cases of carcinoma of the vulva were associated with leukoplakic change elsewhere on the genitalia [13].

The white patches of this disease may appear *de novo*, or as a complication of lichen sclerosus. The factors responsible are unknown; syphilis is not one of them. Suspicion is growing that infectious viral agents (HSV-2 and certain HPV subgroups) may be in part responsible [14–17].

Clinical features and course. Leukoplakia—used in the above context—is usually accompanied by, and may be preceded by, itching, which is sometimes severe. This often indicates its development in the course of lichen sclerosus. Pain and soreness also occur, particularly when it becomes fissured.

It presents as one or more well-demarcated, thickened, stark white or greyish-white patches, which have been likened to white paint that has hardened and cracked. Any part of the vulva, except the vestibule and urethral orifice, may be affected, but especially the clitoris, labia minora and the inner aspects of the labia majora. Fissuring, cracking and ulceration are regarded as poor prognostic signs. When it is widespread, leukoplakia causes stenosis of the vaginal introitus (but not of the urethral meatus).

Leukoplakia is a dynamic process, waxing and waning inexplicably. Different areas in the same patient characteristically vary in extent and appearance within short periods of time, especially in the presence of vulvitis or secondary lichenification.

The course is unpredictable. In some cases, the spread is rapid and extensive. In others, patches show little visible change for years.

Treatment. Excision biopsy is usually indicated, in order to assess the histological picture. However, electrocoagulation or cryotherapy are successful in dealing with lesions which are not frankly neoplastic. Local vulvectomy may be necessary if multiple lesions are present, but should be undertaken only after careful clinical and histological study.

Lichen sclerosus [10,18–21]

This condition is discussed fully in Chapter 58.

Diagnostic features in the genital area. Lichen sclerosus is essentially a disease of women, although it occurs on the penis more commonly than is recognized (p. 3192) [22]. It appears to be less common in Black races, although it has been reported in them [23,24]. The anogenital area was involved in 190 of 200 women affected [10], the vulva alone in 61, and the vulva and perianal area (the 'figure-of-eight' distribution) in 126. The inguinal area was affected in only 25. The average age at presentation ranges from 45 to 54 years, but it may occur in quite young children [23–25]. The presenting symptom is usually pruritus, sometimes soreness, and occasionally dyspareunia, which may be

marked. Vaginitis may precede or accompany any stage of the condition.

The typical appearance of lichen sclerosus, as it affects the skin, is modified in the anogenital region. The ivory-coloured papules with follicular plugging and hyperkeratosis are most likely to be seen at the edge of perianal lesions, and only rarely occur on the vulva. Lesions are present elsewhere on the body in about one-fifth of the patients. Of 41 patients, the skin and the vulva were both affected in 26, the vulva alone in 10 and the skin alone in five [23]. As the disease progresses, sheets of ivory-white (Fig. 72.34a) or light violaceous, atrophic skin show the characteristic 'cigarette-paper' atrophy (Fig. 72.34b). At times, individual papules are absent [10,26], or there is marked hyperkeratosis or a diffuse irregular scaling. Occasionally, the skin feels thick and waxy due to oedema; when this is marked, thick-walled bullae, which are often quite large and haemorrhagic, may form.

On the mucous surfaces the changes are less distinctive. The labia minora and clitoris are affected early, but a general atrophy with marked narrowing of the introitus may follow. The mucosal surface is pale, and may show flecks of haemorrhage, telangiectasia or bulla formation. Fissures, erosions and lichenification may appear in the course of the disease. A statistically significant association with morphoea, and a less certain one with vitiligo, was demonstrated in 380 cases [10]. The possibility that hereditary or familial factors are involved has been suggested by the documentation of 13 familial cases [27], and by its occurrence in monozygotic twins [28]. No relationship appears to exist with parity, age at first intercourse or number of sexual partners [20].

There is a significant increase in the frequency of organ-specific autoantibodies in these patients [29], and a higher incidence of autoimmune disease. However, the only disease which has been shown to have a significant association with lichen sclerosus is pernicious anaemia [18]. In males with lichen sclerosus, an increase in the incidence of autoimmune disease has also been noted [30], but no particular condition was specifically associated. A more recent study of 350 females has confirmed an association with autoimmune disease. Thus, 21% had one or more autoimmune-related disease, 21% had a first-degree relative with autoimmune disease, 42% had at least one raised autoantibody titre and a total of 60% had at least one of these autoimmunological markers [31]. In a separate study, 45% of 76 patients showed abnormal glucose tolerance curves [32].

A significant decrease in certain circulating lymphocyte subsets may be taken as supportive evidence of disordered immunoregulation in some subjects [33].

A statistically significant association of lichen sclerosus with HLA-A29 and -B24 has been claimed [34].

Histopathology. The hallmarks of lichen sclerosus are

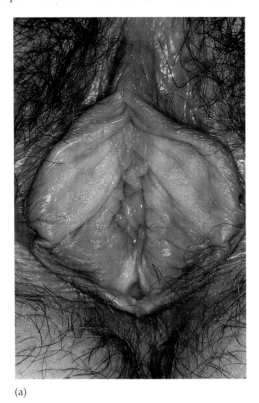

(a)

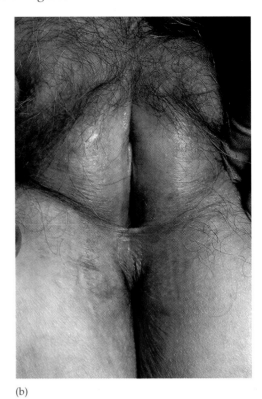

(b)

Fig. 72.34 Lichen sclerosus et atrophicus. (a) An early case. (b) A late case, with loss of the labia minora.

hyperkeratosis, follicular plugging and atrophy of the epidermis and epidermal appendages, associated with a bland oedema of the papillary and superficial dermis, which is delineated on its deeper aspect by a monomorphic lymphocytic infiltrate.

It has been shown that elastic fibres are absent from the superficial dermis in this disease. It is possible that an elastase-type protease is responsible for this degradation of elastic tissue [35].

Small areas of epidermal hypertrophy, which may represent lichenification or leukoplakia, may develop. These areas should be kept under close observation and biopsied regularly [10].

Course and complications. Untreated, the course is progressive, with periods of relative inactivity. Infection, lichenification, erosion and fissuring occur frequently. Contact dermatitis may complicate treatment.

Despite the frequent claims that lichen sclerosus of childhood tends to remit in many cases [10,25,36], recent work has indicated otherwise, and it appears that in most cases the disease persists into adult life [37].

Leukoplakia, often presaged by more intense or persistent itching, eventually occurs in about half the cases [10,38] although at any one time it is found in substantially fewer. A carcinoma supervenes in a proportion of these; exactly how many is difficult to determine. A proportion

of one in six [25] appears too high; a figure of 4.4% of 290 patients [10] is perhaps the minimum for patients under regular observation. The carcinoma always occurs in preexisting leukoplakia. The labia minora and clitoris are particularly affected. Dysuria and urinary tract infections may follow labial fusion.

Treatment. There is no specific therapy. As the danger to the patient lies in the development of leukoplakia and carcinoma, regular observation by an experienced clinician is advisable. Repeated biopsies of suspicious areas may be needed. The first indication of malignancy will usually be the development of hyperplasia and leukoplakia, the treatment of which is discussed below. Vulvectomy should not be undertaken without very careful consideration, but ablation of areas of early premalignancy may be necessary and can be repeated over a period of many years.

The stronger fluorinated corticosteroids, particularly clobetasol propionate (Dermovate), are often very helpful in relieving symptomatology and also in producing clinical improvement. No evidence of atrophy has been found after prolonged application [39]. Intradermal injections of triamcinolone, or cryotherapy, may be helpful for localized areas.

Oral administration of potassium para-aminobenzoate 12 g/day has been recommended as an alternative form of therapy [40]. Numerous reports of open studies of etretinate at a dosage of up to 1 mg/kg body weight are uniformly encouraging [41–43]. Hydroxychloroquine was reported as helpful in one particularly severe case [44].

Differential diagnosis of white vulval patches [19]. A number of conditions of different aetiology and significance give rise to white patches or plaques in the vulval region.

Leukoderma (vitiligo). There should be no difficulty in distinguishing this from the other conditions discussed. Although vitiligo may coexist with lichen sclerosus, the genital region is often involved early in the process.

Infections. Candidal infection causes whitish or yellowish white, curd-like patches, typical of 'thrush'. These are readily removed, and the associated erosions, superficial ulcers and vaginal discharge distinguish them from other white vulval lesions.

Bowen's disease and Paget's disease. These produce raised velvety or indurated lesions which may at times be confused with leukoplakia. A biopsy will enable differentiation of these disorders.

REFERENCES

1 Ridley CM, ed. *The Vulva*. London: Churchill Livingstone, 1988.
2 Sanchez NP, Mihm MC. Reactive and neoplastic epithelial alterations of the vulva. *J Am Acad Dermatol* 1982; **6**: 378–88.
3 Rudolph RI. Vulvar melanosis. *J Am Acad Dermatol* 1990; **23**: 982–4.
4 Carli P, De Giorgi V, Nardini P *et al.* Vulvar melanosis mimicking melanoma: a cause for concern in patients and clinicians. *G Ital Dermatol Venereol* 1994; **129**: 143–6.
5 Edwards L, Hansen RC. Reiter's syndrome of the vulva. *Arch Dermatol* 1992; **128**: 811–14.
6 Edwards L. Vulvar lichen planus. *Arch Dermatol* 1989; **125**: 1677–80.
7 Eisen D. The vulvo-vaginal gingival syndrome: the clinical characteristics of 22 patients. *Arch Dermatol* 1994; **130**: 1379–82.
8 Edwards L, Friedrich EG. Desquamative vaginitis: lichen planus in disguise. *Obstet Gynecol* 1988; **71**: 832–6.
9 Edwards L. Desquamative vulvitis. *Dermatol Clin* 1992; **10**: 325–37.
10 Wallace HJ. Lichen sclerosus et atrophicus. *Trans St John's Hosp Dermatol Soc* 1971; **57**: 9–30.
11 Ridley CM. Chronic erosive vulval disease. *Clin Exp Dermatol* 1990; **15**: 245–52.
12 Marren P, Millard P, Chia Y, Wojnarowska F. Mucosal lichen sclerosus/lichen planus overlap syndromes. *Br J Dermatol* 1994; **131**: 118–23.
13 Way S, ed. *Malignant Disease of the Vulva*. Edinburgh: Churchill Livingstone, 1982.
14 Cabral GA, Marciano-Cabral F, Dry D *et al.* Expression of herpes simplex type 2 antigens in premalignant and malignant human vulvar cells. *Am J Obstet Gynecol* 1982; **143**: 611–19.
15 Darling JR, Chu J, Weiss NA *et al.* The association of condylomata acuminata with squamous cell carcinoma of the vulva. *Br J Cancer* 1984; **50**: 533–5.
16 Kaufman RH, Dressman GR, Burek J *et al.* Herpes virus induced antigens in squamous cell carcinoma *in situ* of the vulva. *N Engl J Med* 1981; **305**: 483–8.
17 Sawchuk WS. Vulvar manifestations of human papillomavirus infection. *Dermatol Clin* 1992; **10**: 405–14.
18 Harrington CI, Dunsmore IR. An investigation into the incidence of autoimmune disorders in patients with lichen sclerosus et atrophicus. *Br J Dermatol* 1981; **104**: 563–6.
19 Ridley CM. Lichen sclerosus. *Dermatol Clin* 1992; **10**: 309–23.
20 Sideri M, Parrazzini F, Rognoni MT. Risk factors for vulvar lichen sclerosus. *Am J Obstet Gynecol* 1989; **161**: 38–42.
21 Wallace HJ, Whimster IW. Vulval atrophy and leukoplakia. *Br J Dermatol* 1951; **63**: 241–57.
22 Chalmers RJG, Burton PA, Bennett R *et al.* Lichen sclerosus et atrophicus—a destructive and common cause of phimosis in boys. *Br J Dermatol* 1982; **107** (Suppl. 22): 29–30.
23 Barclay DL, Macey HB, Jr, Reed RJ. Lichen sclerosus et atrophicus of the vulva in children. A review and report of 5 cases. *Obstet Gynecol* 1966; **27**: 637–42.
24 Chernosky ME, Derbes VJ, Burks JW. Lichen sclerosus et atrophicus in children. *Arch Dermatol* 1957; **75**: 647–52.
25 Dewhirst J. Lichen sclerosus of the vulva in childhood. *Pediatr Adolesc Gynecol* 1983; **1**: 149–62.
26 Surmound D. Lichen sclerosus et atrophicus of the vulva. *Arch Dermatol* 1964; **90**: 143–52.
27 Friedrich EG, MacLaren NK. Genetic aspects of vulvar lichen sclerosus. *Am J Obstet Gynecol* 1984; **150**:161–5.
28 Meyrick Thomas RH, Kennedy CTC. The development of lichen sclerosus et atrophicus in monozygotic twins. *Br J Dermatol* 1986; **114**: 377–9.
29 Goolamali SK, Barnes EW, Irvine WJ *et al.* Organ specific antibodies in patients with lichen sclerosus. *Br Med J* 1974; **iv**: 78–9.
30 Meyrick Thomas RH, Ridley CM, Black MM. The association of lichen sclerosus et atrophicus and autoimmune related disease in males. *Br J Dermatol* 1983; **109**: 661–4.
31 Meyrick Thomas RH, Ridley CM, McGibbon DH *et al.* Lichen sclerosus et atrophicus and autoimmunity. *Br J Dermatol* 1988; **118**: 41–6.
32 Garcia-Bravo B, Sanchez-Pedereno P, Rodriguez-Pichardo A *et al.* Lichen sclerosus et atrophicus. *J Am Acad Dermatol* 1988; **19**: 482–5.
33 Betti R, Lodi A, Marmini A *et al.* T cell peripheral subsets in lichen sclerosus et atrophicus. *Clip Exp Dermatol* 1986; **11**: 569–73.
34 Purcell KG, Spencer LV, Simpson PM *et al.* HLA antigens in lichen sclerosus et atrophicus. *Arch Dermatol* 1990; **126**: 1043–5.
35 Godeau G, Frances C, Hornebeck W *et al.* Isolation and partial characterization of an elastase-type protease in human vulva fibroblasts: its possible involvement in vulvar elastic tissue destruction of patients with lichen sclerosus et atrophicus. *J Invest Dermatol* 1982; **78**: 270–5.
36 Clark JA, Muller SA. Lichen sclerosus et atrophicus in children. A report of 24 cases. *Arch Dermatol* 1967; **95**: 476–82.
37 Ridley CM. Genital lichen sclerosus (lichen sclerosus et atrophicus) in childhood and adolescence. *J R Soc Med* 1993; **86**: 69–75.
38 Nicolau SG, Balus L. Sur la localisation vulvaire du lichen scléroatrophique. *Dermatologica* 1966; **132**: 27–44.
39 Dalziel KL, Millard PR, Wojnarowska F. The treatment of vulval lichen sclerosus with a very potent topical steroid (clobetasol propionate 0.05%) cream. *Br J Dermatol* 1991; **124**: 461–4.
40 Penneys NS. Treatment of lichen sclerosus with potassium paraamino benzoate. *J Am Acad Dermatol* 1984; **10**: 1039–42.
41 Mork NJ, Jensen P, Hoel PS. Vulval lichen sclerosus et atrophicus treated with etretinate (Tigason). *Acta Derm Venereol (Stockh)* 1986; **66**: 363–5.
42 Romppanen V, Rantala I, Lauslahti K *et al.* Light and electron microscopic findings in lichen sclerosus of the vulva during etretinate therapy. *Dermatologica* 1987; **175**: 33–40.
43 Yokota M, Mizuno N. A case of lichen sclerosus et atrophicus of the vulva effectively treated with oral etretinate. *J Dermatol* 1988; **15**: 330–3.
44 Wakelin SH, James MP. Extensive lichen sclerosus et atrophicus with bullae and ulceration—improvement with hydroxychloroquine. *Clin Exp Dermatol* 1994; **19**: 332–4.

Bowenoid papulosis

There have been several reports [1–3] of papular, pigmented, occasionally skin-coloured, or depigmented lesions [4] in the groins and on the genitalia of young adults of both sexes (the youngest reported case is less than 3 years old [5]). When the female is involved, lesions are frequently associated with pregnancy [4].

The clinical appearance of these lesions can vary widely [6]. They have been described variously as verrucous, lichenoid, dry, brown, pigmented or even whitish papules or plaques (Fig. 72.35). The diagnosis is confirmed by biopsy.

These clinically banal, asymptomatic lesions have histological features which are difficult to distinguish from those of Bowen's disease (carcinoma *in situ*) [7]. Cellular uniformity, occasional apparent synchronization of mitoses and absence of pilosebaceous involvement are features peculiar to Bowenoid papulosis [4]. Vesicular changes in epidermal cell chromatin have led to comparison with viral balloon cell changes [8], and lesions have been frequently associated with both HSV-2 [9,10] and condylomata acuminata [7].

As yet the prognosis is unknown. Major surgery is regarded as contraindicated as, so far, only one case of invasive squamous carcinoma has been described [11]. Some cases undergo spontaneous regression [12]. Electrodesiccation or cryotherapy appear to be the treatments of choice, although recurrence has been recorded, and long-term follow-up is required to determine the eventual outcome.

REFERENCES

1 Bhawan J. Multicentric pigmented Bowen's disease: a clinically benign squamous cell carcinoma. *Gynecol Oncol* 1980; **10**: 201–5.
2 Kimura S, Hirai A, Harada R *et al.* So-called multicentric pigmented Bowen's disease. *Dermatologica* 1978; **157**: 229–37.
3 Lloyd KM. Multicentric pigmented Bowen's disease of the groin. *Arch Dermatol* 1970; **101**: 48–51.
4 Ulbright TM, Stehman FB, Roth LM *et al.* Bowenoid dysplasia of the vulva. *Cancer* 1982; **50**: 2910–19.
5 Weitzner JM, Fields KW, Robinson MJ. Pediatric bowenoid papulosis: risks and management. *Pediatr Dermatol* 1989; **6**: 303–5.
6 Bender ME, Katz HI, Posalaky Z. Carcinoma *in situ* of the genitalia. *JAMA* 1980; **243**: 145–7.
7 Wade TR, Kopf AW, Ackerman AB. Bowenoid papulosis of the genitalia. *Arch Dermatol* 1979; **115**: 306–8.
8 Sedel D, Leibowitch M, Pelisse M *et al.* Etats Bowénoides vulvaires de la femme jeune. *Ann Dermatol Vénéréol* 1982; **109**: 811–12.
9 Cabral GA, Marciano-Cabral F, Fry D *et al.* Expression of herpes simplex virus type 2 antigens in premalignant and malignant human vulvar cells. *Am J Obstet Gynecol* 1982; **143**: 611–19.
10 Kaufman RH, Dressman GR, Burek J *et al.* Herpes virus-induced antigens in squamous cell carcinoma *in situ* of the vulva. *N Engl J Med* 1981; **305**: 483–8.
11 Bergeron C, Naghashfar Z, Canaan C *et al.* Human papilloma virus type 16 in an intraepithelial neoplasia (bowenoid papulosis) and co-existent invasive carcinoma of the vulva. *Int J Gynecol Pathol* 1987; **6**: 1–11.
12 Berger BW, Hori Y. Multicentric Bowen's disease of the genitalia: spontaneous regression of lesions. *Arch Dermatol* 1978; **114**: 1698–9.

Premalignant and malignant lesions of the vulva

Premalignant vulvar lesions

A variety of medicosocial factors appear to contribute to the risk of developing carcinoma of the vulva, including smoking, diabetes, low educational status and multiparity [1,2]. A pre-existing viral infection is now regarded as the

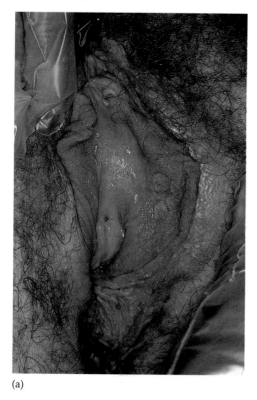

(a)

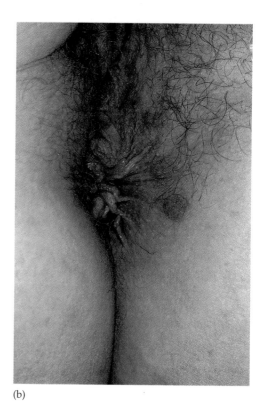

(b)

Fig. 72.35 Bowenoid papulosis. (a) The labia minora in a young adult. (b) Perianal skin in the same patient.

most important specific risk factor. HSV-2 antigens have been found in the genomes of intraepithelial vulval malignancies [3,4]. Previous genital wart infection appears to be similarly relevant. Antigens of HPV-6, -10 and -11 have been identified frequently in low-grade cervical and vulval lesions [5], but a higher risk factor appears to be the presence of HPV-16 and -18, which have been seen in the presence of more advanced lesions [6]. There is speculation that HSV-2 may act as the initiator of cell transformation and that subsequent HPV infection may then promote the development of neoplasia [6].

It is impossible to state definitely how many patients suffering from vulvar epithelial hyperplasia with atypia (leukoplakia) will progress to frank malignancy: one estimate is 10% [7]. Conversely, between 57 and 69% [8] of all squamous cell carcinomas of the vulva show evidence elsewhere on the vulva of hyperplasia and atypia. Progression of true Bowen's disease to vulval carcinoma is probably less frequent, despite its sometimes alarming histological appearance [9].

The true incidence of malignancy developing subsequent to lichen sclerosus et atrophicus is not well established (Fig. 72.36). Wallace's classic work [10] suggested that around 5% of patients progress to vulvar carcinoma, and that those at greatest risk are patients with pruritic ulcerated lesions. There are no reports of malignancy developing after prepubertal lichen sclerosus et atrophicus. Patients with Fanconi's anaemia, one of the chromosome instability syndromes, appear to be prone to both perineal and vulval cancers [11,12].

There is evidence from the West Indies [13,14] that lymphogranuloma venereum and granuloma inguinale increase the likelihood of vulval carcinoma. The patients are younger than those with no evidence of the two diseases, more than half of them show evidence of Bowen's disease of the vulva, and there is a likelihood that the tumour will behave aggressively.

Diagnosis of vulval carcinoma in situ. Careful examination of the whole genital and perianal area is required. Many cases are asymptomatic, and may be found only on routine health checks [15,16]. Overall, 40–60% suffer pruritus [5,7], and others may discover some roughness or irregularity of the skin surface. Magnification ×2 in a good light is essential in examining lesions. Colposcopic examination of the vulva may be helpful, especially when combined with the use of the toluidine blue, a nuclear stain which selectively accentuates subclinically involved zones [17].

Vulval intraepithelial neoplasia [18]

In the belief that the classification of vulval premalignancy into distinct clinical entities is no longer warranted as 'they all behave in the same biological manner', the International

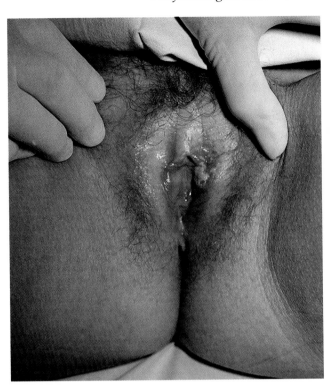

Fig. 72.36 Squamous cell carcinoma arising in lichen sclerosus. (Courtesy of Dr J. McGlone, Dryburn Hospital, Durham, UK.)

Society for the Study of Vulvar Disease (ISSVD) has introduced a classification of vulval intraepithelial neoplasia (VIN). This classification is loosely based on that successfully adopted by pathologists in relation to cervical neoplasia (CIN) [19]:
1 VIN-I (mild atypia);
2 VIN-II (moderate atypia);
3 VIN-III (severe atypia).
The classification lacks any clinical correlates, and includes within it flat condylomas and lesions of bowenoid papulosis, which can spontaneously regress and behave in a very varied 'biological manner'. For this reason, the author will continue to draw clinical distinctions.

Bowen's disease of the vulva [20–22]

Clinical features. Bowen's disease of the vulva clinically differs from bowenoid papulosis, and is best regarded as an analogue of erythroplasia of Queyrat. It is aetiologically related to previous HPV infection, in that 90% of tumours show evidence of viral DNA expression [23], and is characterized by intractable, severe itching. In many cases, there are multiple lesions which are flat, red or pigmented, velvety or granular plaques, with well-demarcated and irregular, occasionally hyperpigmented, margins [24].

A history of bleeding or a palpable mass suggests invasive changes, when examination shows induration, ulceration or a verrucous nodular contour. The anterior vulva, and especially the labia minora, are the main areas involved, in contrast with the rectovaginal involvement following lymphogranuloma venereum in a Jamaican patient [14]. In all patients, lymphatic spread is to the inguinal nodes and thence to the iliac nodes.

Diagnosis. It may be difficult to distinguish clinically between simple lichenification and epithelial hyperplasia with atypia ('leukoplakia', Bowen's disease, and extramammary Paget's disease).

Any vulval lesions which do not respond rapidly to the application or intralesional injection of potent steroids must be biopsied (Fig. 72.37). Any indurated, eroded or ulcerated plaque, nodule or warty lesion, especially in the elderly, is more likely to be squamous cell carcinoma than anything else.

Treatment. Bowen's disease is best treated by complete vulvectomy, with careful histological examination of the specimen to exclude invasive malignancy. This may be an unacceptable procedure to relatively young women, and 5-fluorouracil, which is an effective local treatment, may be used [25]. Cryotherapy has not proved to be helpful [26].

Vulvar malignancy

The American statistical service SEER [1] states that in North America there are 1900 cases annually of vulvar carcinoma. Of these, 82% are squamous cell carcinoma, 5% basal cell carcinoma, 5% adenocarcinoma, 6% melanoma and 1% sarcoma. British statistics reveal that it is the fourth most common tumour of the female genital tract, and comprises 10% of all genital tumours. Sixty per cent of tumours occurred in women over 60 years of age, and over 88% of women were postmenopausal at the onset of the illness. It may develop either *de novo*, or from pre-existing areas of 'leukoplakia' or Bowen's disease [27].

About one-third of patients die within 3 years of diagnosis, despite vigorous therapy [27], and the prognosis is therefore much less favourable than it should be for such an accessible site. A recent large survey in Indiana found a 43% recurrence rate after primary therapy [28]. Earlier diagnosis can greatly improve the prognosis. A survey of cases of early microinvasive carcinoma revealed 100% survival after follow-up for 1–24 years [29].

Clinical features. Any persistent nodule or plaque on the vulva in an older female should be biopsied to exclude vulvar carcinoma. The lesion most commonly presents as an ulcerated nodule, and pre-existing Bowen's disease or leukoplakia should heighten clinical suspicion.

Treatment [27,30]. Until recently, radical surgery such as complete vulvectomy offered the only hope of long-term survival. With earlier presentation and new methods

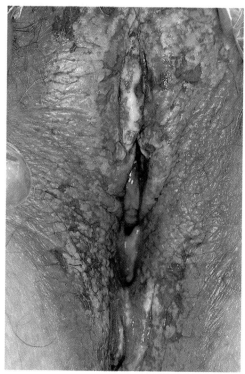

(a)

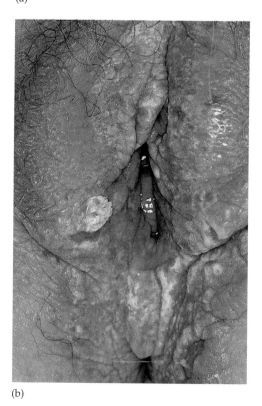

(b)

Fig. 72.37 The potential similarity between benign and dysplastic vulval disease. (a) Benign, cleared by topical steroid therapy. (b) Dysplastic, with squamous cell carcinoma.

of treatment this approach has been somewhat modified, and laser surgery, using the carbon dioxide laser, is now considered a safe and useful method of managing patients with early disease, particularly younger individuals.

Malignant melanoma [31,32]

American figures indicate that 2% of all melanomas in women occur on the vulva [1]. Most lesions begin as superficial spreading melanoma (Fig. 72.38). Nodular growths are slightly less common, and have a worse prognosis [33]. In one series, a 5-year survival of 75% and a median survival of 7.5 years were reported [34]. A recent series, perhaps more realistically, estimated a mortality of 66% over 5 years [35].

Attention has been drawn to an intensely pigmented, asymmetrical, well-demarcated, macular lesion of the vulva, which mimics the clinical appearance of melanoma, but which shows basal layer hyperpigmentation on histological examination and no increase of melanocytes [36].

Basal cell carcinoma

Basal cell carcinoma is rare on the vulva, and usually presents as an itchy tumour of long duration. Local excision is associated with a 20% recurrence rate, and there is a significant association with other primary malignancies [37].

Other rarer vulvar tumours

Secondary tumours and lymphomas are occasionally seen. There are reports of dermatofibrosarcoma [38,39], epithelioid sarcoma [40] and Merkel cell carcinoma [41]

Carcinoma of Bartholin's gland [42] should be suspected when there is a persistent cystic or tender and indurated vulval mass [43]. It can easily be mistaken for an inflammatory process, and it is wise to biopsy all Bartholin gland enlargements. The lesion is an adenocarcinoma and should be treated by radical vulvectomy. Five-year survival is about 30% [44].

Vulvar Paget's disease

Extramammary Paget's disease is fully discussed in Chapter 36. The vulva is the commonest site for this condition.

The lesion is a moist, red, oozing plaque, which is associated with symptoms of burning and pruritus. The majority of lesions are associated with underlying adenocarcinoma of the sweat glands, but cervical [45], urinary tract [46] and rectal carcinoma may also be associated with this condition.

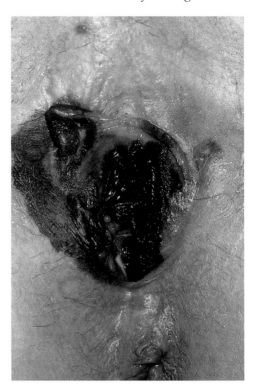

Fig. 72.38 Melanoma of the vulva.

Complete excision of the lesion and removal of the underlying malignancy is the appropriate therapy.

REFERENCES

1 Berg E, Lamp E. High risk factors in gynaecologic cancer. *Cancer* 1981; **48**: 429–41.
2 Newcomb PA, Weiss NS, Darling JR. Incidence of vulvar carcinoma in relation to menstrual, reproductive and medical factors. *J Natl Cancer Inst* 1984; **73**: 391–6.
3 Cabral GA, Marciano-Cabral F, Fry D *et al.* Expression of herpes simplex virus type 2 antigens in premalignant and malignant human vulvar cells. *Am J Obstet Gynecol* 1982; **143**: 611–19.
4 Kaufman RH, Dressman GR, Burek J *et al.* Herpes virus-induced antigens in squamous cell carcinoma *in situ* of the vulva. *N Engl J Med* 1981; **305**: 483–8.
5 Kaufman RH, Gordon A. Squamous cell carcinoma *in situ* of the vulva. *Br J Sex Med* 1986; **13**: 24–7.
6 Zur Hausen H. Human genital cancer: synergism between two virus infections or synergism between a virus infection and initiating events? *Lancet* 1982; **ii**: 1370–2.
7 McAdams AJ, Jr, Kistner RW. The relationship of chronic vulvar disease, leukoplakia and carcinoma *in situ* to carcinoma of the vulva. *Cancer* 1959; **11**: 740–57.
8 Taussig FJ. Cancer of the vulva. An analysis of 155 cases (1911–1940). *Am J Obstet Gynecol* 1940; **40**: 764–79.
9 Ulbright TM, Stehman FB, Roth LM *et al.* Bowenoid dysplasia of the vulva. *Cancer* 1982; **50**: 2910–19.
10 Wallace HJ. Lichen sclerosus et atrophicus. *Trans St John's Hosp Dermatol Soc* 1971; **57**: 9–30.
11 Kennedy AW, Hart WR. Multiple squamous cell carcinomas in Fanconi's anaemia. *Cancer* 1982; **50**: 811–14.
12 Wilkinson EJ, Morgan LS, Friedrich EG. Association of Fanconi's anaemia and squamous cell carcinoma of the lower female genital tract with condylomata acuminata. A report of 2 cases. *J Reprod Med* 1984; **29**: 447–53.

13 Hay DM, Cole FM. Postgranulomatous epidermoid carcinoma of the vulva. *Am J Obstet Gynecol* 1970; **108**: 479–84.

14 Stockhausen BY. Cancer involving the vulva. *West Indian Med J* 1968; **17**: 103–8.

15 Benedet JL, Murphy KJ. Squamous cell carcinoma *in situ* of the vulva. *Gynecol Oncol* 1982; **14**: 213–19.

16 Bernstein J, Kovacs BR, Townsend DE *et al*. Vulvar carcinoma *in situ*. *Obstet Gynecol* 1983; **61**: 304–7.

17 Eliezri YD. The toluidine blue test: an aid in the diagnosis and treatment of early squamous cell carcinomas of mucous membranes. *J Am Acad Dermatol* 1988; **18**: 1339–49.

18 Ridley CM, ed. *The Vulva*. London: Churchill Livingstone, 1988.

19 Wilkinson EJ, Kneale B, Lynch PJ. International Society for the Study of Vulvar Disease: Terminology Committee. *J Reprod Med* 1986; **31**: 973.

20 Bender ME, Katz HI, Posalaky Z. Carcinoma in situ of the genitalia. *JAMA* 1980; **243**: 145–7.

21 Lloyd KM. Multicentric pigmented Bowen's disease of the groin. *Arch Dermatol* 1970; **101**: 48–55.

22 Sedel D, Leibowitch M, Pelisse M *et al*. Etats Bowénoides vulvaires de la femme jeune. *Ann Dermatol Vénéréol* 1982; **109**: 811–12.

23 Zur Hausen H. Human papilloma viruses in the pathogenesis of anogenital cancer. *Virology* 1991; **184**: 9–13.

24 Abell MR, Gosling JRG. Intraepithelial and infiltrative carcinoma of vulva: Bowen's type. *Cancer* 1961; **14**: 318–29.

25 Woodruff JD, Julian C, Puray T *et al*. The contemporary challenge of carcinoma *in situ* of the vulva. *Am J Obstet Gynecol* 1973; **115**: 677–86.

26 Marren P, Dawber R, Wojnarowska F *et al*. Failure of cryosurgery to eradicate vulval intraepithelial neoplasia: a pilot study. *J Eur Acad Dermatol Venereol* 1993; **2**: 247–52.

27 Way S, ed. *Malignant Disease of the Vulva*. Edinburgh: Churchill Livingstone, 1982.

28 Tilmans AS, Sutton GP, Look KY. Recurrent squamous carcinoma of the vulva. *Am J Obstet Gynecol* 1992; **167**: 1383–9.

29 Kunschner A, Kanbour AI, David B. Early vulvar carcinoma. *Am J Obstet Gynecol* 1978; **132**: 599–606.

30 Morley GW. Cancer of the vulva: a review. *Cancer* 1981; **48**: 597–601.

31 Edington PT, Monaghan J. Malignant melanoma of the vulva and vagina. *Br J Obstet Gynaecol* 1980; **87**: 422–4.

32 Bradgate MG, Rollason TP, McConkey CC, Powell J. Malignant melanoma of the vulva: a clinicopathological study of 50 women. *Br J Obstet Gynaecol* 1990; **97**: 124–33.

33 Itala J, Di Paola GR, Tueda NG. Melanoma of the vulva. The experience of Buenos Aires University. *J Reprod Med* 1986; **31**: 836–8.

34 Beller V, Demopoulos RI, Beckman EM. Vulval melanocarcinoma. *J Reprod Med* 1986; **31**: 315–19.

35 Sutherland C, Chmiel JS, Henson DE, Winchester DP. Patient characteristics, methods of diagnosis, and treatment of mucous membrane melanoma in the USA. *J Am Coll Surg* 1994; **179**: 561–72.

36 Carli P, De Giorgi V, Nardini P, Gonnelli F. Vulval melanosis mimicking malignant melanoma: a cause for concern for patients and clinicians. *G Ital Dermatol Venereol* 1994; **129**: 143–6.

37 Palladino VS, Duffy JL, Bures GJ. Basal cell carcinoma of the vulva. *Cancer* 1969; **24**: 460–70.

38 Agress R, Figge DC, Taimimi H *et al*. Dermatofibrosarcoma of the vulva. *Gynecol Oncol* 1983; **16**: 288–91.

39 Soltan MH. Dermatofibrosarcoma protuberans of the vulva: case report. *Br J Obstet Gynaecol* 1981; **88**: 203–5.

40 Ulbright TM, Brokaw SA, Stehman FB *et al*. Epithelioid sarcoma of vulva. *Cancer* 1983; **52**: 1462–9.

41 Bottles K, Lacey CG, Goldberg J *et al*. Merkel cell carcinoma of the vulva. *Obstet Gynecol* 1984; **63** (Suppl.): 61–3.

42 Lurmann K. Das primare karzinom der Bartholinschen Druse. *Zentralbl Gynakol* 1974; **96**: 1044–7.

43 Dodson MG, O'Leary JA, Avorette HE. Primary carcinoma of Bartholin's gland. *Obstet Gynecol* 1970; **35**: 578–84.

44 Noumoff JS, Farber M. Tumours of the vulva. *Int J Dermatol* 1986; **25**: 552–63.

45 McKee PH, Hertogs KT. Endocervical adenocarcinoma and vulval Paget's disease: a significant association. *Br J Dermatol* 1980; **103**: 443–8.

46 Powell FC, Bjornsson J, Doyle JA *et al*. Genital Paget's disease and urinary tract malignancy. *J Am Acad Dermatol* 1985; **13**: 84–90.

Chapter 73
Racial Influences on Skin Disease

D.J.GAWKRODGER

Definition and classification of race

The concept of race was first developed in the 18th century as an arbitary classification to help understand evolution and human variation [1]. The division of our species *Homo sapiens* into 'races' is to some extent artificial given that the species shows a continuous variability of characteristics and all humans are apparently derived from common ancestors (see Chapter 2). However, there are obviously differences between groups of humans which, in the present context, have an influence on the appearance and susceptibility to disease. The classification into racial groups therefore allows an examination of the genetic and environmental influences on human morphology and on disease.

Definitions

Many definitions are unsatisfactory. A race has been defined as 'a group united by heredity' or 'a major segment of a species' or 'a breeding population' [2]. It can also be regarded as 'one of the divisions of humankind as differentiated by physical characteristics' [1].

Scientifically, race is a matter of genetic variation. A definition that takes this into account is that of Boyd, who defined race as 'a population which differs significantly from other populations in regard to the frequency of one or more of the genes it possesses' [3]. Even this gives considerable latitude to defining quite a small subgroup as a 'race'.

Ethnicity

Another concept to consider is that of ethnicity. This is different from race but equally difficult to define. Ethnicity can be regarded as a 'people or tribe' and implies shared origins or social background, shared cultural traditions that are maintained between generations and, often, a common language or religion [1,4,5]. One or more of these things leads to a sense of identity as a group.

Racial origins

Little is known about how the races originally differentiated and why they assumed their own characteristics. Conventional theory outlines that a change in gene frequency can occur due to mixture (with other races), mutation, natural selection and genetic drift (i.e. the accidental loss of a gene from the communal pool) [6]. It is assumed that some differences, such as skin pigmentation, are an adaptation to environmental conditions, although often it is still unclear as to exactly what advantage is conferred. Migrations of populations over the last few thousand years have meant that in certain places there has long been an admixture of genes. For example, many invaders who have swept over Europe in the last 2000 years, including Romans, Celts, Slavs and Moors, have left a genetic legacy behind them. In view of this it is difficult to accept the concept of a 'pure' race. Isolated groups such as the Australian aborigines, who are thought to have migrated from the South Pacific Islands, may not have had much intermixture of genes from other races until recent times.

No racial group is characterized by a completely distinctive genetic make-up [7]. There is considerable genetic variation within racial groups and sharing of genetic characteristics between them.

Classification of races

In the past, classifications have relied on various physical characteristics such as stature, cephalic index, nasal index, prognathism, capacity of the skull, hair texture, hairiness, skin colour, hair and eye colour, and other special traits such as the epicanthic fold of the eyelid (a Mongoloid feature) or steatopygia (a heavy deposit of fat in the buttocks, seen in Bushmen and Hottentot women) [8]. A satisfactory classification must take most of these factors into account. There are three main divisions, namely, Mongoloid, black African and Caucasoid, which account for over 90% of the world's population [8]. The remaining groups, grouped together by Coon [9] as the Australoid and Capoid races, occupy a doubtful position as they frequently show some features of the other races. These main races broadly show a geographical grouping. Within each 'geographical' race it is possible to define 'local' races and so on. A convenient division of the geographical races, albeit with some reservations, is as follows [8–10].
1 Australoid: Australian aborigines, Melanesians, Papuans and Negritos.
2 Capoid: Bushmen and Hottentots.
3 Caucasoids: Europeans, peoples of the Mediterranean, Middle East and most of the Indian subcontinent, and the Ainu of Japan.
4 Mongoloids: peoples of East Asia, Indonesia and Polynesia, native Americans and Eskimos.
5 Negroids: black people and pygmies of Africa.

REFERENCES

1 Senior PA, Bhopal R. Ethnicity as a variable in epidemiological research. *Br Med J* 1994; **309**: 327–30.
2 Garn SM. *Human Races*. Springfield: Thomas, 1961.
3 Boyd WC. *Genetics and the Races of Man*. Oxford: Basil Blackwell, 1950.
4 Marmot MG. General approaches to migrant studies: the relation between disease, social class and ethnic origin. In: Cruickshank JK, Beevers DG, eds. *Ethnic Factors in Health and Disease*. London: Wright, 1989: 12–17.
5 Bhopal RS, Phillimore P, Kohli HS. Inappropriate use of the term 'Asian': an obstacle to ethnicity and health research. *J Public Health Med* 1991; **13**: 244–6.
6 Rife DC. Race and heredity. In: Kuttner RE, ed. *Race and Modern Science*. New York: Social Science Press, 1967: 141–68.
7 Cooper R. A note to the biological concept of race and its application in epidemiological research. *Am Heart J* 1984; **108**: 715–23.
8 Kroeber AL. *Anthropology: Biology and Race*. New York: Harcourt Brace and World, 1963.
9 Coon CS. *The Living Races of Man*. New York: AA Knopf, 1965.
10 Baker JR. *Race*. London: Oxford University Press, 1974.

Characteristics and variations between racial groups

There is a considerable overlap of features between the racial groups; for example, not all black Africans have tightly curled hair and not all Caucasoids have a lightly pigmented skin. Some characteristics may show considerable variation within a race, for example head shape for Caucasoids is very variable, but other features are much more constant, for example straight, black hair is almost universal in Mongoloids.

Australoids. Australian aborigines show some black African features such as black skin, a broad nose and prognathism, but their hirsutism, full beards and wavy hair are more Caucasoid. In addition they have heavy eyebrow ridges [1,2,3].

Capoids. Bushmen and Hottentots show mainly black African characteristics but some of their features are possibly Caucasoid (e.g. thin lips) or Mongoloid (e.g. a type of epicanthic fold) [1,4,5].

Caucasoids. There are at least four Caucasoid sub-races extending from Europe, the Mediterranean and North Africa across to the Indian subcontinent. All show wavy hair and abundant facial and body hair. The skin colour is fair to brown and the nose is usually narrow. The Ainu of Japan are classified as Caucasoids, mainly because of their heavy body hair, curly scalp and beard hair and European-like facial features [1,4,5].

Mongoloids. This group extends through the extremes of climatic conditions, from the extreme north (Eskimos) to the equator (Malaysian types) and includes the Chinese and the native Americans in North and South America. Body hair is scanty and scalp hair is straight and black [2,3].

Negroids. Originally confined to Africa. The main characteristics are dark pigmentation, tightly curled hair and a broad nose [4,5].

Jews. Jews, on the whole, are not a race but a cultural community. They usually approximate genetically to the community in which they live [2,5]. However, certain genes are more frequent in certain Jewish communities than in the surrounding population.

The black people of North America are regarded by some

as a local race [6]. A study of blood groups in American blacks has revealed the following admixture of Caucasoid genes: in Oakland (California) 22%, in Detroit 26%, in New York 19%, in Charleston 4% [3]. Some also may have native American genes [4]. Many of the studies on dermatology in 'Negroids' have been done on black Americans and hence may not be strictly applicable for all black Africans.

There is now a tendency in the USA and elsewhere for individuals with any degree of black African descent to adopt the term 'black'. This has come about because of a new consciousness by this group of a shared identity. In some places the term 'black' has been more widely used and may be implied to include some darkly skinned Caucasoids such as Mediterranean or Indian people [7]. Quite often, the description 'Afro-Caribbean' is used and, in North America, recently there has been a tendency to use 'African American'. The term 'black African' will therefore often be used to avoid any confusion about which group is being referred to. The terms Australoid, Mongoloid and Caucasoid will also be used to describe racial groups.

REFERENCES

1 Baker JR. *Race*. London: Oxford University Press, 1974.
2 Dunn LC. *Heredity and Evolution in Human Populations*. Cambridge, MA: Harvard University Press, 1959.
3 Reed TE. Caucasian genes in American negroes. *Science* 1969; **165**: 762–8.
4 Coon CS. *The Living Races of Man*. New York: AA Knopf, 1965.
5 Kroeber AL. *Anthropology: Biology and Race*. New York: Harcourt Brace and World, 1963.
6 Cobb WM. Physical anthropology of the American Negro. *Am J Phys Anthropol* 1942; **29**: 113–223.
7 Banton M. *The Idea of Race*. Cambridge: Tavistock Publications, 1977.

Ethnic groups

Some groups of humans do not fit easily into a race, for example pygmies, but ethnicity creates a new category for each group [1,2]. Ethnicity is a social phenomenon with imprecise and fluid boundaries. It is often used, incorrectly, as interchangeable with race [3]. Broad ethnic divisions, for instance into Asian or Afro-Caribbean, may have limited value due to the great diversity of cultural and other variations within the groups. Nonetheless, because of the association with social and cultural factors, ethnicity often has a bearing on disease.

A current recommendation is that, in describing disease or characteristics in a racial or ethnic group, the most precise description possible is given for that group [4]. This will be followed when appropriate but, where it seems desirable to look at racial characteristics more generally, the broad racial groupings will be applied.

REFERENCES

1 Cooper R. A note on the biological concept of race and its application in epidemiological research. *Am Heart J* 1984; **108**: 715–23.
2 Senior PA, Bhopal R. Ethnicity as a variable in epidemiological research. *Br Med J* 1994; **309**: 327–30.
3 Sheldon TA, Parker H. Race and ethnicity in health research. *J Public Health Med* 1992; **14**: 104–10.
4 McKenzie K, Crowcroft NS. Describing race, ethnicity, and culture in medical research. *Br Med J* 1996; **312**: 1054.

Racial variations in the structure and function of the skin

The degree of pigmentation is one of the most obvious and immediate factors in distinguishing the main geographical races. Other differences in the structure and function of the skin are less obvious and not so well studied but are of some importance.

Pigmentation

Variation

Skin colour depends largely on the content and distribution of melanin in the epidermis. In Caucasoids, the constitutive skin colour (i.e. the amount of melanin pigmentation in the absence of sun exposure) is darkest on the upper thigh and lightest on the lumbar area, whereas in black Africans the abdomen is darkest, although the lumbar area is also the lightest [1]. Males are normally darker than females. In general, the geographical distribution of the intensity of racial pigmentation correlates with the areas of greatest sun exposure, although there are anomalies such as the Tasmanian Australoids who were dark although they lived in a temperate latitude, and native Americans (Mongoloids) who have a similar pigmentation across the whole continent of North America.

Melanosomes

The density of melanocytes differs between various parts of the body [2] and is similar in most races, although melanocytes may be more numerous in the Australian aborigine [3]. There are differences in the size, distribution and shape of melanosomes. In Caucasoids the melanosomes are small and aggregated in groups of three or more within a membrane in the keratinocyte [4] and are broken up by lysosomal enzymes before reaching the stratum corneum [5]. In black Africans and Australoids the melanosomes are larger, distributed singly within keratinocytes, and persist up to the stratum corneum.

Inheritance

Skin colour is continuously variable and its inheritance is complex. Three or four genes seem to be involved in the colour differences between Caucasoids and black Africans [6], whereas only one gene is thought to be important in Australian aborigines [7].

3242 Chapter 73: Racial Influences on Skin Disease

Physiological effects of skin pigmentation

The minimal erythema dose in black African skin is about 33 times that for Caucasoid [4]. Obviously a pigmented skin protects against sunlight and particularly against sunburn and skin cancer. However, it seems doubtful that protection against skin cancer conveys an evolutionary advantage, as under 'natural' conditions survival is unlikely to be affected. According to Wasserman [8,9] racial pigmentation is a secondary phenomenon, related to resistance to infection. The disadvantages of a pigmented skin are increased heat absorption and reduced vitamin D synthesis. Black Africans absorb 30% more heat than Caucasoids, although this is partially offset by more efficient sweating [10,11].

REFERENCES

1 Selmanowitz VJ, Krivo JM. Pigmentary demarcation lines. *Br J Dermatol* 1975; **93**: 371–7.
2 Szabo G. Quantitative histological investigations on the melanocyte system of the human epidermis. In: Gordon M, ed. *Pigment Cell Biology*. New York: Academic Press, 1959: 99–125.
3 Mitchell RE. The skin of the Australian aborigine: a light and electron-microscopical study. *Aust J Dermatol* 1968; **9**: 314–28.
4 Olson RL, Gaylor J, Everett MA. Skin color, melanin and erythema. *Arch Dermatol* 1973; **108**: 541–4.
5 Hori Y, Toda K, Pathak MA. A fine structure study of the human epidermal melanosome complex and its acid phosphate activity. *J Ultrastruct Res* 1968; **25**: 109–20.
6 Harrison GA. Differences in human pigmentation, measurement, geographic variation and causes. *J Invest Dermatol* 1973; **60**: 418–26.
7 Gates RR. The genetics of the Australian aborigines. *Acta Genet Med* 1960; **9**: 7–50.
8 Wasserman HP. Melanokinetics and the biological significance of melanin. *Br J Dermatol* 1970; **82**: 530–4.
9 Wasserman HP. *Ethnic Pigmentation*. Amsterdam: Excerpta Medica, 1974.
10 Blum HF. Physiological effects of sunlight on man. *Physiol Rev* 1945; **25**: 483–530.
11 Blum HF. Does the melanin pigment of human skin have adaptive value? *Q Rev Biol* 1961; **36**: 50–63.

Hair

Variations in hair depend on a wide range of genetically controlled factors both between and within races [1]. Hair form is inherited separately from skin colour, and of the two is the more dominant.

Hair forms

Hair form depends on the three-dimensional structure of the hair shaft. There are broadly four hair types—straight, wavy, helical and spiral [2,3]. Helical forms coil with a constant diameter. Spiral forms coil with a decreasing diameter outwards: the extreme of this is 'peppercorn' hair which is tightly curled and shows multiple kinks [4]. Hair that is elliptical in cross-section is curly whereas round hair is straight.

Mongoloid hair is usually straight, circular in diameter, and with the largest diameter of all the races. The hair in black Africans and Capoids tends to be short, helical or spiral, flattened or elliptical in cross-section, and midway between the Mongoloid and Caucasoid in thickness. Spiral hair is produced by hair follicles that are curved and upwardly convex towards the epidermis. Black African hair tends to be drier and more brittle than the hair of other races, probably due in part to its intrinsic properties [5].

In Caucasoids the hair is variable and may be straight, wavy, or helical and round or oval in cross-section. It tends to be the thinnest in diameter of all the races. Despite these variations for scalp hair, beard, pubic and eyelash hair is elliptical in all races. The morphology and chemical composition of hair is similar in all races [6].

Hair colour

Mongoloids, black Africans, Capoids and Australoids have hair that is predominantly black although it may be red in colour. Caucasoid hair is widely variable: in northern Europe it tends to be blond, in southern and eastern Europe it is commonly black [7]. However, blond hair may be found in North Africa and the Middle East, and is even seen in some Australoids. Greying of the hair starts on average in the third decade in Caucasoids, and in the fourth decade in black Africans. Caucasoids show more balding over the vertex than do black Africans [8].

Body hair

Caucasoids have earlier and greater axillary and beard growth than Mongoloids [9] and more extensive male secondary sexual hair. In general, Mongoloids have less body hair than Caucasoids, with Negroids and Capoids occupying an intermediate position.

Selective advantage of hair forms

Any evolutionary advantage conferred by the different hair forms is unclear. Short, curly hair facilitates evaporation of sweat but thick wavy hair provides a greater degree of physical protection.

REFERENCES

1 Baden HP. Chemistry, structure and function of hair. In: Baden HP, ed. *Symposium on Alopecia*. New York: HP Publishing, 1987: 3–10.
2 Steggerda M, Seibert HC. Size and shape of head hairs from 6 racial groups. *J Hered* 1942; **32**: 315–18.
3 Vernall DG. Study of the size and shape of hair from 4 races of man. *Am J Phys Anthropol* 1961; **19**: 345–50.
4 Hrdy D. Quantitative hair form variation in 7 populations. *Am J Phys Anthropol* 1973; **39**: 7–17.
5 Halder RM. Hair and scalp disorders in blacks. *Cutis* 1983; **32**: 378–80.
6 Hrdy D, Baden HP. Biochemical variations of hair keratins in man and non-human primates. *Am J Phys Anthropol* 1973; **39**: 19–24.
7 Sunderland E. Hair colour variation in the United Kingdom. *Ann Hum Genet* 1955; **20**: 312–13.

8 Setty LR. Hair patterns of the scalp in white and negro males. *Am J Phys Anthropol* 1970; **33**: 49–55.
9 Hamilton JB. Age, sex and genetic factors in the regulation of hair growth in man; a comparison of Caucasian and Japanese populations. In: Montagna W, Ellis RA, eds. *The Biology of Hair Growth*. New York: Academic Press, 1958: 399–433.

Sweat glands

Eccrine glands

There is little or no difference in the sweating ability of black Africans as compared to Caucasoids [1]. A study in the Bantu did show a greater number of sweat glands per unit area than in European Caucasoids [2], but such changes are now thought to be due to adaption to climatic factors [3]. Increased sweating is known to be accompanied by hypertrophy of the sweat glands [4]. Indeed, in Australoids, sweat glands were noted to be larger but not more numerous than in Caucasoids [1].

Keratosis punctata, a hyperkeratosis of the acrosyringeal orifice seen on the palmar creases, is found in 1–2% of black Africans and in less than 0.1% of Latin Americans, but it is not seen in European or Middle Eastern Caucasoids [5].

Apocrine glands

An early paper mentions that apocrine glands are more numerous in black African skin than in Caucasoid skin [6], but the variation in the distribution of apocrine glands between individuals is so great [7] that it is difficult to place much emphasis on this report.

REFERENCES

1 Green LMA. The distribution of eccrine sweat glands of Australian aborigines. *Aust J Dermatol* 1971; **12**: 143–8.
2 Glaser S. Sweat glands in Negro and European. *Am J Phys Anthropol* 1934; **18**: 371–6.
3 Kawahata A, Sakamoto H. Some observations on sweating of the Aino. *Jpn J Physiol* 1951; **2**: 166–9.
4 Warter G, Diolombi G. Sweat gland tumours in Niger. *Ann Dermatol Vénéréol* 1989; **116**: 621–7.
5 Pierard-Franchimont C, Pierard GE, Melotte P et al. Keratosis punctata of the palmar creases. *Ann Soc Belg Med Trop* 1989; **69**: 257–61.
6 Homma H. On apocrine sweat glands in white and negro men and women. *Bull Johns Hopkins Hosp* 1926; **38**: 365–71.
7 Woollard HH. The cutaneous glands of man. *J Anat* 1930; **64**: 415–21.

Sebaceous glands

Black African skin showed no consistent difference in sebaceous gland activity as compared with Caucasoid skin [1]. There have been no substantial studies on the comparative number of sebaceous glands in the different races.

REFERENCE

1 Pochi PE, Strauss JS. Sebaceous gland activity in black skin. *Dermatol Clin* 1988; **6**: 349–51.

The epidermis

Comparative studies have been performed on black African and Caucasoid epidermis. The stratum corneum in both has an equal thickness although in black skin there are more cell layers and it requires more tape strips to remove it than Caucasoid stratum corneum [1]. The stratum corneum in black subjects seems to show greater intracellular cohesion than in Caucasoids. It has a higher lipid content [2] and an increased electrical resistance [3]. There is no difference in corneocyte surface area between Caucasoids, Mongoloids and black Africans, but desquamation was up to 2.5 times greater from black skin, compared with the other two races [4]. Recently, it has been found that quantities of cerumides in the stratum corneum are lower in black Africans than in Caucasoids [5]. The composition of ear wax (cerumen) varies between different races: in black Africans and Caucasoids, it is honey-coloured, wet and sticky, in Mongoloids, it is grey, dry and brittle [6].

Not surprisingly, black African epidermis is more effective at blocking the transmission of ultraviolet radiation, transmitting only 7.4% of UVB as compared to 29.4% for Caucasoid epidermis [7]. Black African skin shows a higher transepidermal water loss than Caucasoid [8]; this is thought to be due to differences in thermo regulation and in the stratum corneum lipids. Some substances do not penetrate black skin as well as Caucasoid, but this is not universally the case [9].

REFERENCES

1 Weigand DA, Haygood C, Gaylor JR. Cell layers and density of Negro and Caucasian stratum corneum. *J Invest Dermatol* 1974; **62**: 563–8.
2 Rienertson RP, Wheatley VR. Studies on the chemical composition of human epidermal lipids. *J Invest Dermatol* 1959; **32**: 49–59.
3 Johnson LC, Corah NL. Racial differences in skin resistance. *Science* 1963; **139**: 766–7.
4 Corcuff P, Lotte C, Rougier A, Maibach HI. Racial differences in corneocytes. *Acta Derm Venereol (Stockh)* 1991; **71**: 146–8.
5 Sugino K, Imokawa G, Maibach HI. Ethnic difference of stratum corneum lipid in relation to stratum corneum function. *J Invest Dermatol* 1993; **100**: 597–9.
6 Hanger HC, Mulley GP. Cerumen: its fascination and clinical importance. *J R Soc Med* 1992; **85**: 346–9.
7 Kaidbey KH, Agin PP, Sayre RM et al. Photoprotection by melanin—a comparison of black and caucasian skin. *J Am Acad Dermatol* 1979; **1**: 249–60.
8 Wilson D, Berardesca E, Maibach HI. In vitro transepidermal water loss: differences between black and white human skin. *Br J Dermatol* 1988; **119**: 647–52.
9 Wedig JH, Maibach HI. Percutaneous penetration of dipyrithione in man: effect of skin color (race). *J Am Acad Dermatol* 1981; **5**: 433–8.

The dermis

Black African skin may be slightly more extensible than Caucasoid [1], although the difference is small. The vasodilatory response after exposure to nicotinate is reduced in black Africans compared with Caucasoids, and hyperaemia after vasoconstrictive stimuli may be different [1,2].

3244 *Chapter 73: Racial Influences on Skin Disease*

REFERENCES

1 Berardesca E. Racial differences in skin function. *Acta Derm Venereol (Stockh)* 1994; **185**(Suppl.): 44–6.
2 Berardesca E, de Rigal J, Leveque JL, Maibach HI. *In vivo* biophysical characterization of skin physiological differences in races. *Dermatologica* 1991; **182**: 89–93.

Peripheral vascular responses to cold

Eskimos (Mongoloids) are able to maintain a higher hand blood flow than Caucasoids under identically cold conditions [1]. At –12°C the finger temperature in black Africans fell more rapidly (and the metabolic rate rose less rapidly) than in Caucasoids under similar conditions [2]. The extent to which these observations represent physiological adaptions, rather than significant inter-racial differences, is not known.

REFERENCES

1 Brown GM, Page J. Effect of chronic exposure to cold on temperature and blood flow of hand. *J Appl Physiol* 1952; **5**: 221–7.
2 Rennie DW, Adams T. Comparative thermoregulatory responses of negroes and white persons to acute cold stress. *J Appl Physiol* 1957; **11**: 201–4.

Common diseases that show racially dependent variations

Many dermatoses manifest themselves similarly in the different races but not infrequently, due to differences in pigmentation, hair or other factors, the appearance of a disorder varies depending on the racial constitution of the individual. It is not intended here to provide a comprehensive list of every possible racially-influenced dermatosis but rather to select the most important differences, especially for the commonest conditions.

Dermatoses that in white Caucasoid skin appear red or brown appear black, grey or purple in pigmented skin. Furthermore, any pigmentation may mask an erythematous reaction. Inflammation in pigmented skin may provoke reactions of a hyperpigmentary or hypopigmentary nature that persist after the initiating eruption has faded [1]. These pigmentary reactions may be of greater concern to the patient than the eruption itself and are often the reason why medical help is sought. Pigmented skin may have an inherent tendency to show reaction patterns that are different from those seen in white Caucasoid skin. For example, follicular, papular and annular patterns are seen more frequently in Afro-Caribbean skin than in Caucasoid [1].

There are few data on the frequency with which people of different races attend a dermatologist. In an office-based study in the USA, patients classified as 'white' or 'Asian or Pacific Islander' attended a dermatologist proportionally more than 'black' people or 'native Americans or Eskimos', but this may well have been because of economic or social reasons [2].

REFERENCES

1 McLaurin CI. Unusual patterns of common dermatoses in blacks. *Cutis* 1983; **32**: 352–60.
2 Fletcher AB, Feldman SR, Bradham DD. Office-based physician services provided by dermatologists in the United States in 1990. *J Invest Dermatol* 1994; **102**: 93–7.

Acne

The prevalence of acne seems to be similar in both North American black Africans and Caucasoids [1], although it may be more severe in the latter [2]. However, acne is less common in the Mongoloid Japanese [3]. In pigmented skin, acne lesions may become hyperpigmented (Fig. 73.1).

'Pomade' acne is seen in certain Afro-Caribbean groups due to the custom of anointing the scalp hair with pomades, oils and creams. Up to 70% of long-term users of pomades suffer from this complication [4]. It may be seen in children as well as adults. There is some evidence that black Africans react to comedogenic substances in a different way from Caucasoids. Kaidbey and Kligman studied the comedogenic effects of coal tar in Caucasoids and black Africans and found that, whereas Caucasoids

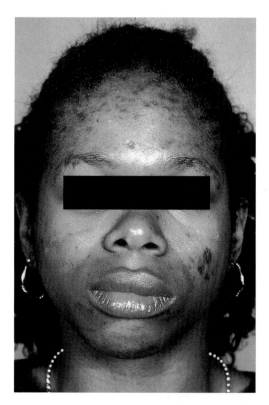

Fig. 73.1 Pigmentation associated with acne. (Courtesy of Dr A.G. Messenger, Royal Hallamshire Hospital, Sheffield, UK.)

produced an inflammatory response with papules and pustules, black Africans did not usually show this but rather developed small comedones [5].

REFERENCES

1 Pochi PE, Strauss JS. Sebaceous gland activity in black skin. *Dermatol Clin* 1988; **6**: 349–51.
2 Wilkins JW, Jr, Voorhees JJ. Prevalence of nodulocystic acne in white and negro males. *Arch Dermatol* 1970; **102**: 631–4.
3 Hamilton JB, Terada H, Mestler GE. Greater tendency to acne in white Americans than Japanese populations. *J Clin Endocrinol* 1964; **24**: 267–72.
4 Verhagen AR. Pomade acne in black skin. *Arch Dermatol* 1974; **110**: 465.
5 Kaidbey KH, Kligman AM. A human model of coal tar acne. *Arch Dermatol* 1974; **109**: 212–15.

Atopic eczema

The inheritance of atopic eczema is 'polygenic'. It is a disease that is seen worldwide and in all races. Comparative figures are not generally available. There was an impression in the UK that atopic eczema may be more common in Caucasoids from the Indian subcontinent [1], but a subsequent cohort study has not confirmed this [2]. It may be that over-representation of Asian children with atopic eczema in dermatology clinics results from a lower level of familiarity with the disease in this community. In another study, from London, UK, it was suggested that atopic eczema is more prevalent in 'black Caribbean' children than in other ethnic groups including Asians [3]. In India, it is suggested that atopic eczema is not as severe as in Western countries [4].

In black Africans, there is a tendency towards the development of follicular lesions in atopic eczema, and a micropapular follicular form of lichenification resembling lichen nitidus is common [1,5,6]. The follicular eruption may predate the onset of other features of the disease [5,6]. Flexural involvement may be less common than in other races, but the severity of the eczema seems to be no different [3].

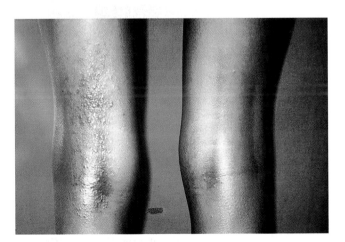

Fig. 73.2 Hyperpigmentation associated with atopic eczema.

Lichenification is seen in all races but is particularly pronounced in Mongoloids. Postinflammatory hyperpigmentation is a problem in black skin (Fig. 73.2).

REFERENCES

1 Graham-Brown RAC, Berth-Jones J, Dure-Smith B *et al*. Dermatologic problems for immigrant communities in a Western environment. *Int J Dermatol* 1990; **29**: 94–101.
2 Berth-Jones J, George S, Graham-Brown RAC. A birth cohort study on prevalence of atopic dermatitis. *Br J Dermatol* 1994; **131** (Suppl. 44): 24–5.
3 Williams HC, Pembroke AC, Fordyke H *et al*. London-born black Caribbean children are at increased risk of atopic dermatitis. *J Am Acad Dermatol* 1995; **32**: 212–17.
4 Kanwar AJ, Dhar S. Severity of atopic dermatitis in India. *Br J Dermatol* 1994; **131**: 733–4.
5 McLaurin CI. Unusual patterns of common dermatoses in blacks. *Cutis* 1983; **32**: 352–60.
6 Rosen T, Martin S. *Atlas of Black Dermatology*. Boston: Little, Brown and Co., 1981.

Contact dermatitis

Studies using irritants suggest that black African skin is less susceptible to irritants than Caucasoid skin [1,2], although the difference is not detectable when the stratum corneum has been removed.

There is little evidence that there is any racial predisposition for the development of allergic contact dermatitis. A study by the North American Contact Dermatitis Group found no racial differences, although the numbers were such that the results were only applicable to black Africans and Caucasoids [3]. Others have confirmed these findings [4,5]. A study from Singapore of contact sensitivity to topical medicaments showed no differences between Chinese, Malays and Indians [6].

However, certain patterns of contact dermatitis are recognized in specific groups due to the use of traditional or ethnic preparations. Indian women may develop an allergic contact dermatitis to materials in 'Bindi', a pigment applied as a paste or powder to the central forehead for religious and social reasons [7].

Some reported differences in the prevalence of contact allergy to certain allergens are likely to represent a difference in exposure. The equal sex incidence of nickel allergy in Nigeria [8], distinct from the female preponderance in most Western countries [9], is probably due to the equal popularity of the wearing of jewellery by both men and women in Nigeria. Clinically, contact dermatitis appears different in black skin as compared with Caucasoid. In the latter, acute contact dermatitis produces vesiculation and exudation, whereas in black skin, lichenification and disordered pigmentation are more common. Hyperpigmentation occurs after contact with mild irritants [10] and certain chemicals, for example phenolic detergents [11], cause hypopigmentation.

REFERENCES

1 Marshall EK, Lynch V, Smith HV. On dichlorethylsulphide (mustard gas) II. Variation in susceptibility of the skin to dichlorethylsulphide. *J Pharmacol Exp Ther* 1919; **12**: 291–301.
2 Weigand DA, Gaylor JR. Irritant reaction in negro and caucasian skin. *South Med J* 1974; **67**: 548–51.
3 Rudner J, Clendenning WE, Epstein E *et al.* Epidemiology of contact dermatitis in North America 1972. *Arch Dermatol* 1973; **108**: 537–40.
4 Fisher AA. Contact dermatitis in black patients. *Cutis* 1977; **20**: 308–9.
5 Kligman AM, Epstein W. Updating the maximization test for identifying contact allergens. *Contact Dermatitis* 1975; **1**: 231–9.
6 Goh CL. Contact sensitivity to topical medicaments. *Int J Dermatol* 1989; **28**: 25–8.
7 Kumar AS, Pandhi RK, Bhutani LK. Bindi dermatoses. *Int J Dermatol* 1986; **25**: 434–5.
8 Olumide YM. Contact dermatitis in Nigeria. *Contact Dermatitis* 1975; **12**: 241–6.
9 Gawkrodger DJ, Vestey JP, Wong WK *et al.* Contact clinic survey of nickel-sensitive subjects. *Contact Derm* 1986; **14**: 165–9.
10 Berardesca E, Maibach HI. Contact dermatitis in blacks. *Dermatol Clin* 1988; **6**: 363–8.
11 Fisher AA. Vitiligo due to contactants. *Cutis* 1976; **17**: 431–7.

Kaposi's sarcoma

The appearance of the lesions of acquired immune deficiency syndrome (AIDS)-related Kaposi's sarcoma can show variation between the different races. In black Africans, lesions may vary from being slightly hyperpigmented to being a deep purple in colour [1]. The classical form of Kaposi's sarcoma is commonest in mid-European Caucasoids of Jewish lineage, and occurs 10 times more frequently in males than in females [2]. Another, more rapidly progressive form, affects black Africans in central Africa [3].

REFERENCES

1 Penneys NS. AIDS in black patients. *Dermatol Clin* 1988; **6**: 435–42.
2 Friedman-Birnbaum R, Weltfriend S, Katz I. Kaposi's sarcoma: retrospective study of 67 cases with the classical form. *Dermatologica* 1990; **180**: 13–17.
3 Oluwasanmi JO, Williams AO, Alli AF. Superficial cancer in Nigeria. *Br J Cancer* 1969; **23**: 714–28.

Keloid formation

Keloids occur in all races but are more common in black Africans and Mongoloids than in Caucasoids. The exact incidence ratio for black Africans over Caucasoids varies from twice to 19 times according to the study consulted [1]. In Malaysia, Chinese are more prone to keloids than Indians or Malays [2]. In Hawaii, keloids are five times more common in the Japanese and three times more frequent in the Chinese, than in Caucasoids [3]. Keloids can occur anywhere on the body but have a predilection for the shoulders, ears, upper back and anterior chest (Fig. 73.3). They usually follow trauma to the skin but can arise spontaneously. In black Africans they may develop in areas of scarification.

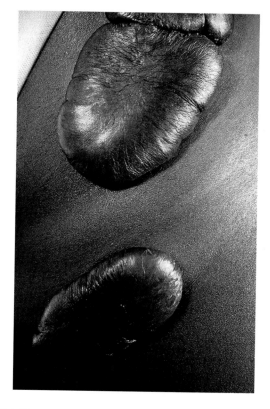

Fig. 73.3 Huge spontaneous keloids in an African. (Courtesy of Professor J.L. Burton, Bristol Royal Infirmary, Bristol, UK.)

REFERENCES

1 Kelly AP. Keloids. *Dermatol Clin* 1988; **6**: 413–24.
2 Alhady SM, Sivanantharajah K. Keloids in various races: a review of 175 cases. *Plast Reconstr Surg* 1969; **44**: 564–6.
3 Arnold HL Jr, Grauer FH. Keloids: etiology and management by excision and intensive prophylactic radiation. *Arch Dermatol* 1959; **80**: 772–7.

Lichen planus

Lichen planus is a worldwide problem and occurs in all races. In Singapore, lichen planus was proportionally more common in Indians and less common in Chinese and Malays than would be expected, given the composition of the local population [1]. There are no other studies to suggest a racial predisposition although the appearances may differ between races. In darkly pigmented patients, papules of lichen planus typically are purple in colour (Fig. 73.4). Oral lesions are said to be uncommon in black Africans but frequent in Caucasoids, while the hypertrophic variant, and possibly the erosive type, are more often seen in black Africans [2]. In black Africans, postinflammatory hyperpigmentation may be prolonged [3]. In Asian Caucasoids, itching is often not prominent and hyperpigmentation is a more common presentation [4]. Histologically, Asian Caucasoids show less inflammation and basal cell degeneration than black Africans or European Caucasoids [4].

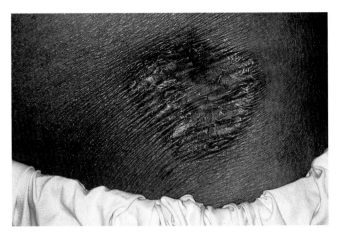

Fig. 73.4 Hyperpigmented lichen planus.

REFERENCES

1 Vijayasingham SM, Lim KB, Yeoh KH *et al.* Lichen planus: a study of 72 cases in Singapore. *Ann Acad Med Singapore* 1988; **17**: 541–4.
2 Rosen T, Martin S. *Atlas of Black Dermatology.* Boston: Little, Brown and Co., 1981.
3 McLaurin CI. Unusual patterns of common dermatoses in blacks. *Cutis* 1983; **32**: 352–60.
4 Fallowfield ME, Harwood C, Cook MG, Marsden RA. Lichen planus in Asians? *Br J Dermatol* 1993; **129** (Suppl. 42): 59.

Lichen simplex chronicus

Lichenification is particularly readily induced in Mongoloid and black African skin (Fig. 73.5). Lichen simplex chronicus may affect the neck, forearms and lower legs, and be associated with hyperpigmentation [1]. A common variant is lichen simplex chronicus of the scrotum in elderly black African males.

REFERENCE

1 Rosen T, Martin S. *Atlas of Black Dermatology.* Boston: Little, Brown and Co., 1981.

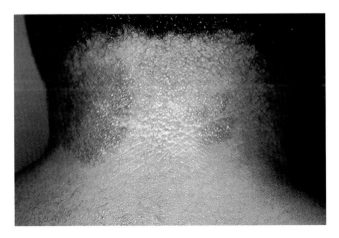

Fig. 73.5 Hyperpigmented lichen simplex chronicus.

Lupus erythematosus

It used to be said that lupus erythematosus was uncommon in black Africans but this is no longer believed to be the case. Indeed, the black populations of North America and North Africa seem to develop severe forms of the disease [1]. In New Zealand systemic lupus erythematosus was found to be three times as common in Mongoloids as in Caucasoids [2].

Lupus erythematosus is closely associated with certain genetic and human leukocyte antigen (HLA) markers. North American and European Caucasoids with systemic lupus erythematosus show an increased frequency of a C4A, CYP21A gene deletion, often in association with the HLA-B8, -DR3, C4A*Q0 extended haplotype [3]. In African Americans, a large C4A, CYP21A gene deletion, particularly associated with HLA-B44, -DR2, and -DR3 alleles, is a strong genetic risk factor for the development of systemic lupus erythematosus [3]. Complete or partial deficiency of C4A allele has also been identified as a genetic determinant of systemic lupus erythematosus in Chinese and Japanese Mongoloids [4]. West Indian and, to a lesser extent, North African, black people have a more severe form of systemic lupus erythematosus than European Caucasoids, mainly due to a higher prevalence of renal disease [1]. The mortality from systemic lupus erythematosus in African Americans is higher than in Caucasoids [5]. Discoid lupus erythematosus also seems to have a nearly similar incidence in all races. In those with a dark skin, the face, scalp and, commonly, the lower lip, tend to be affected. Hypopigmentation and gross scarring may result.

REFERENCES

1 Gioud-Paquet M, Chamot AM, Bourgeois P *et al.* Différences symptomatiques et pronostiques selon la communauté éthnique dans le lupus érythemateux systemique. Etude contrôlee sur 3 populations. *Presse Med* 1988; **17**: 103–6.
2 Hart HH, Grigor RR, Caughey DE. Ethnic differences in the prevalence of systemic lupus erythematosus. *Ann Rheum Dis* 1983; **42**: 529–32.
3 Olsen ML, Goldstein R, Arnett FC *et al.* C4A gene deletion and HLA associations in black Americans with systemic lupus erythematosus. *Immunogenetics* 1989; **30**: 27–33.
4 Dunkley H, Gatenby PA, Hawkins B *et al.* Deficiency of C4A is a genetic determinant of systemic lupus erythematosus in three ethnic groups. *J Immunogenet* 1987; **14**: 209–18.
5 Reveille JD, Bartolucci A, Alarcon GS. Prognosis in systemic lupus erythematosus. Negative impact of increasing age at onset, black race, and thrombocytopenia, as well as causes of death. *Arthritis Rheum* 1990; **33**: 37–48.

Melanocytic naevi

Caucasoids have more melanocytic naevi than other races. Black Africans have the fewest naevi with Mongoloids occupying an intermediate position [1]. Caucasoid children had a median total number of 17 naevi, compared with 2.5 in non-Caucasoids [1]. Young Caucasoid adults had a median of 61 naevi, compared with 16 for non-Caucasoids [1]. A study of schoolchildren in Queensland, Australia, confirmed these findings but found an even higher prevalence of naevi [2]. Children less than 12 years old had a mean of 28 naevi, with boys having significantly more than girls, and those with a pale skin and light-coloured hair having the highest prevalence [2]. Non-Caucasoid heritage has a protective effect for naevus development independent of pigmentary characteristics [2].

REFERENCES

1 Rampen FH, de Wit PE. Racial differences in mole proneness. *Acta Derm Venereol (Stockh)* 1989; **69**: 234–6.
2 Green A, Siskind V, Hansen ME *et al*. Melanocytic nevi in school-children in Queensland. *J Am Acad Dermatol* 1989; **20**: 1054–60.

Palmoplantar keratodermas (Chapter 34)

Some palmoplantar keratodermas are said to be seen more often in black Africans than in other races [1]. One example is keratosis punctata of the palmar creases [2], in which small crateriform pits are visible on the palmar creases (Fig. 73.6). *Focal acral hyperkeratosis* is a type of papular keratoderma, dominantly inherited in familial cases, that occurs almost exclusively in black Africans [3]. It is characterized by oval or polygonal papules, which may show central pigmented pits, situated on the borders of the palms and soles.

REFERENCES

1 Shrank AB, Harman RRH. The incidence of skin disease in a Nigerian teaching hospital dermatological clinic. *Br J Dermatol* 1966; **78**: 235–41.
2 Penas PF, Rois-Buceta L, Sanchez-Perez J *et al*. Keratosis punctata of the palmar creases: case report and prevalence study in caucasians. *Dermatology* 1994; **188**: 200–2.
3 Lucker GPH, van der Kerkhof PCM, Steijlen PM. The hereditary palmoplantar keratoses: an updated review and classification. *Br J Dermatol* 1994; **131**: 1–14.

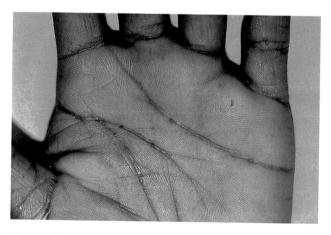

Fig. 73.6 Keratosis punctata of the palmar creases with hyperpigmentation. (Courtesy of Dr D.J. Barker, Bradford Royal Infirmary, Bradford, UK.)

Photodermatoses

Racial pigmentation protects from some of the immediate and long-term adverse effects of sunlight. However, even a pigmented skin may be sunburnt, although it may be difficult to see the erythema because of the pigmentation [1]. Conditions such as polymorphic light eruption occur in all races but some have a particular presentation depending on the race of the individual. In black Africans or Australoids, for example, an actinic cheilitis (or discoid lupus erythematosus) may affect the lower lip, which may not be protected by the same amount of pigment as on other sites of the body.

One photodermatosis that seems to have a racial predilection is actinic prurigo of native Americans [2], although it may be a form of polymorphic light eruption [3] (Chapter 25). It may present as a lower lip cheilitis, but also produces a conjunctivitis, pterygium and eyebrow alopecia [2]. Actinic prurigo has a female/male ratio of 3:1 and usually has an onset in the first two decades of life [4]. Those with an early onset tend to have cheilitis and may improve; those with a later onset have a milder disease which may be more persistent [4].

REFERENCES

1 Willis I. Photosensitivity reactions in black skin. *Dermatol Clin* 1988; **6**: 369–75.
2 Mounsdon T, Kratochvil F, Auclair P *et al*. Actinic prurigo of the lower lip. Review of the literature and report of five cases. *Oral Surg Oral Med Oral Pathol* 1988; **65**: 327–32.
3 Fletcher DC, Romanchuk KG, Lane PR. Conjunctivitis and pterygium associated with the American Indian type of polymorphous light eruption. *Can J Ophthalmol* 1988; **23**: 30–3.
4 Lane PR, Hogan DJ, Martel MJ *et al*. Actinic prurigo: clinical features and prognosis. *J Am Acad Dermatol* 1992; **26**: 683–92.

Pityriasis rosea

In black Africans, this eruption shows several unusual features. It shows an 'inverse' pattern, with lesions on the face, neck, extremities and lower abdomen, rather than on the trunk as is usual [1]. In addition, it may be papular, may affect the palms and soles, and shows a brown–grey or even purple pigmentation [2,3]. The recurrence rate seems to be higher in black Africans than in other races [4] and the hyperpigmentation which may follow can persist for some months.

REFERENCES

1 McLaurin CI. Unusual patterns of common dermatoses in blacks. *Cutis* 1983; **32**: 352–60.
2 Hendricks AA, Lohr JA. Pityriasis in infancy. *Arch Dermatol* 1979; **115**: 896–7.
3 Jacyk WK. Pityriasis rosea in Nigerians. *Int J Dermatol* 1980; **19**: 397–9.
4 Chuang TY, Illstrup DM, Perry HO *et al*. Pityriasis rosea in Rochester, Minnesota, 1969 to 1978. *J Am Acad Dermatol* 1982; **7**: 80–9.

Postinflammatory pigmentary changes

Pigmented skin shows more of a pigmentary reaction following trauma or inflammation than non-pigmented or lightly pigmented skin. In black Africans it is also not uncommon to see secondary hypopigmentation after eczema, pityriasis alba, sarcoidosis, leprosy, herpes zoster, pityriasis versicolor or other common eruptions [1,2]. It may also follow cryotherapy and the topical use or intralesional injection of corticosteroids. Table 73.1 lists causes of hypopigmentation in a pigmented skin [1–3]. Sometimes unusual patterns of pigmentation are found; for example, black Africans with systemic sclerosis may develop a mottled and vitiligo-like hypopigmentation [3] (Chapter 58). Complete or patchy 'leopard skin' depigmentation may be seen with onchocerciasis (Fig. 73.7). On the other hand, some dermatoses result in hyperpigmentation, and it is not unusual to find both hyper- and hypopigmentation coexisting in the same individual.

Hyperpigmentation may occur in black African skin with acne, eczema, sarcoidosis, psoriasis, mycosis fungoides, lichen planus, fixed drug eruption and lupus erythematosus, and frequently is seen when the skin is lichenified, as in chronic eczema [2]. Hyperpigmentation, particularly of the face, may also be acquired due to exposure to a variety of agents. These include exogenous ochronosis from hydroquinone-containing skin-bleaching creams, and mercury deposition from skin-lightening creams containing mercury, and also from exposure to photosensitizing drugs and herbal potions [4].

REFERENCES

1 Olumide YM, Odunowo BD, Odiase AO. Depigmentation in black African patients. *Int J Dermatol* 1990; **29**: 166–74.
2 McLaurin CI. Unusual patterns of common dermatoses in blacks. *Cutis* 1983; **32**: 352–60.
3 Kenney JA, Jr. Pigmentary disorders in black skin. *Clin Dermatol* 1989; **7**: 1–10.
4 Olumide YM, Odunowo BD, Odiase AO. Regional dermatoses in the African. Part 1. Facial hypermelanosis. *Int J Dermatol* 1991; **30**: 186–9.

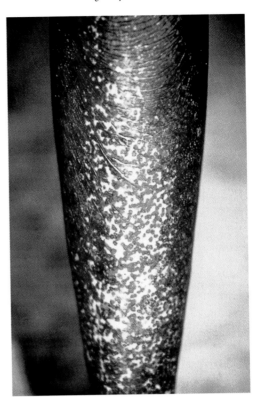

Fig. 73.7 Onchocerciasis showing 'leopard skin' depigmentation. (Courtesy of Dr M.E. Murdoch, St Thomas' Hospital, London, UK.)

Psoriasis

The genetic basis for psoriasis is well established although not well understood. It is relatively common in European Caucasoids (prevalence about 2%), although within the Caucasoid group it is said to vary, being more common in Parsees than in Hindus or Moslems [1]. A high prevalence is reported in East Africans [2] and a low prevalence in West Africans [3–5], which may explain the low prevalence

Table 73.1 Causes of hypopigmentation in a pigmented skin.

Division	Disorders
Congenital or genetic	Albinism, piebaldness
Infections	Leprosy, onchocerciasis, pinta, pityriasis vesicolor, herpes zoster
Papulosquamous disorders	Pityriasis alba, pityriasis rosea, pityriasis lichenoides chronica, psoriasis, seborrhoeic dermatitis
Physical or chemical agents	Burns, cryotherapy, ammoniated mercury, hydroquinone products, fluorinated corticosteroids
Postinflammatory	Discoid lupus erythematosus, systemic sclerosis, sarcoidosis, some eczematous eruptions
Miscellaneous	Vitiligo, idiopathic guttate hypomelanosis

in African Americans. Psoriasis is almost unknown in the Mongoloid native Americans [3] and Eskimos [6], and in Australian aborigines [7]. It is rare in the Japanese (Mongoloid), although the prevalence in the latter is increasing [8]. The prevalence in Mongoloids in Hong Kong, mainland China and Japan was estimated to be 0.3% [9].

In black skin, psoriatic plaques may appear violaceous or bluish black due to pigmentary incontinence. Grey, silvery scales may be seen. Postinflammatory hyperpigmentation may be left after clearing of the lesions [10]. This may be a persistent cosmetic disability.

REFERENCES

1 Gans O. Some observations on the pathogenesis of psoriasis. *Arch Dermatol* 1952; **66**: 598–611.
2 Verhagen AR, Koten JW. Psoriasis in Kenya. *Arch Dermatol* 1967; **96**: 39–41.
3 Kerdel-Vegas F. The challenge of tropical dermatology. *Trans St Johns Hosp Dermatol Soc* 1973; **59**: 1–9.
4 Lomholt G. Psoriasis in Uganda: a comparative study with other parts of Africa. In: Farber EM, Cox AJ, eds. *Psoriasis. Proceedings of the First International Symposium.* Stanford: Stanford University Press, 1971: 41.
5 Obasi OE. Psoriasis vulgaris in the Guinea Savannah region of Nigeria. *Int J Dermatol* 1986; **25**: 181–3.
6 Horrobin DF. Low prevalence of coronary heart disease, psoriasis, asthma and rheumatoid arthritis in Eskimos: are they caused by high dietary intake of eicosapentaenoic acid, a genetic variation of essential fatty acid metabolism or both? *Med Hypotheses* 1987; **22**: 421–8.
7 Green AC. Australian aborigines and psoriasis. *Aust J Dermatol* 1984; **25**: 18–24.
8 Yasudo T, Ishikawa E, Mori S. Psoriasis in the Japanese. In: Farber EM, Cox AJ, eds. *Psoriasis. Proceedings of the First International Symposium.* Stanford: Stanford University Press, 1971: 25–34.
9 Yip SY. The prevalence of psoriasis in the mongoloid race. *J Am Acad Dermatol* 1984; **10**: 965–8.
10 Rosen T, Martin S. *Atlas of Black Dermatology.* Boston: Little, Brown and Co., 1981.

Sarcoidosis

In the USA, sarcoidosis is 10 times more common in African Americans than in Caucasoids [1]. Skin signs are seen in between one-tenth and one-third of patients with sarcoidosis [2]. Erythema nodosum is the commonest non-specific lesion of sarcoidosis, but is much more frequent in Caucasoids than in black Africans [3,4]. In Africans, the commonest sarcoidal skin lesions are flesh-coloured or slightly hypopigmented papules which tend to occur around the nose, mouth and occiput [2]. Hypopigmented macules, violaceous plaques (often on the face or arms) and subcutaneous nodules are also seen. Ulceration may occur. Lupus pernio is apparently infrequent in black Africans [2].

In contrast to the American experience, sarcoidosis was said to be uncommon in West Africans but this may not be the case [5]. It has a very low reported prevalence in the Far East.

REFERENCES

1 Abeles H, Robins AB, Chaves AD. Sarcoidosis in New York City. *Am Rev Respir Dis* 1961; **84**: 120–1.
2 Minus HR, Grimes PE. Cutaneous manifestations of sarcoidosis in blacks. *Cutis* 1983; **32**: 361–8.
3 Caruthers B, Day TB, Minus HR *et al.* Sarcoidosis: a comparison of cutaneous manifestations with chest radiographic changes. *J Natl Med Assoc* 1975; **67**: 364–7.
4 James DG. Dermatological aspects of sarcoidosis. *Q J Med* 1959; **28**: 108–24.
5 Alabi GO, George AO. Cutaneous sarcoidosis and tribal scarifications in West Africa. *Int J Dermatol* 1989; **28**: 29–31.

Skin cancer

Most forms of skin malignancy and sun-induced degenerative change are more common in North European Caucasoids than in other racial groups. Black Africans have the lowest incidence (1/70 that of Caucasoids) of non-melanoma skin cancer [1], with Mongoloids occupying an intermediate position. In black people, squamous cell carcinoma is the commonest tumour [2], as opposed to basal cell carcinoma in Caucasoids. Scarring, for example from burns or discoid lupus erythematosus, is a predisposing factor in squamous cell carcinoma in Africans [3]. The prognosis in black Africans in the USA is generally worse than in Caucasoids because of later presentation or more aggressive disease [4].

Malignant melanoma is 10 times more common in North American 'European' Caucasoids than in African Americans, with an incidence in New Mexican Hispanic Caucasoids and Puerto Rico Hispanic Caucasoids of 3.7 and 1.6 times that of African Americans [5]. Puerto Rico Hispanics have more admixture of African genes than Hispanics from New Mexico. In black Africans malignant melanoma mostly affects the soles or palms [2]. Presentation may be delayed. Malignant melanoma of the sole of the foot, in North America, has a similar incidence in black people as in Caucasoids [6]. In the Mongoloid Japanese the acral lentiginous type of malignant melanomas makes up a large proportion of cases and the incidence at this site is similar to that for Caucasoids in other sites [7].

Japanese residents in Hawaii had a rate for non-melanoma skin cancer that was 88 times higher than that reported in Japan [8]. This higher rate was attributed to increased sun exposure, and possibly to arsenic exposure.

REFERENCES

1 Scotto J, Fraumeni JF, Jr. Skin-cancer other than melanoma. In: Scottenfeld D, Fraumeni JF, Jr, eds. *Cancer Epidemiology and Prevention.* Philadelphia: WB Saunders, 1982; 996–1011.
2 Halder RM, Bang KM. Skin cancer in blacks in the United States. *Dermatol Clin* 1988; **6**: 397–405.
3 Mora RG, Perniciaro C. Cancer of the skin in blacks: a review of 163 patients with cutaneous squamous cell carcinoma. *J Am Acad Dermatol* 1981; **5**: 535–43.
4 Halder RM, Bridgeman-Shah S. Skin cancer in African Americans. *Cancer* 1995; **75**: 667–73.

5 Bergfelt L, Newell GR, Sider JG *et al.* Incidence and anatomical distribution of cutaneous melanoma among United States Hispanics. *J Surg Oncol* 1989; **40**: 222–6.

6 Stevens NG, Liff JM, Weiss NS. Plantar melanoma: is the incidence of melanoma of the sole of the foot really higher in blacks than in whites? *Int J Cancer* 1990; **45**: 691–3.

7 Elwood JM. Epidemiology and control of melanoma in white populations and in Japan. *J Invest Dermatol* 1989; **92**: 214S–21S.

8 Leong GK, Stone JL, Farmer ER *et al.* Nonmelanoma skin cancer in Japanese residents of Kauai, Hawaii. *J Am Acad Dermatol* 1987; **17**: 233–8.

Syphilis

The primary chancre is similar in Caucasoids and black Africans but the manifestations of secondary syphilis can be different. In Caucasoids, macular lesions are common but in black Africans, follicular and papular forms are more frequent and may be hyperpigmented [1]. Annular secondary syphilis is almost unique to Negroids [2], corymbose forms (a central lesion with surrounding small satellites) are also seen [1]. Palmoplantar lesions in black Africans may be keratotic. The non-venereal treponematoses yaws, pinta and bejel are endemic in certain parts of the world. No racial predilection exists, although the appearances may be modified in different races.

REFERENCES

1 Rosen T, Martin S. *Atlas of Black Dermatology.* Boston: Little, Brown and Co., 1981.

2 McLaurin CI. Annular facial dermatoses in blacks. *Cutis* 1983; **32**: 369–70.

Vitiligo

Vitiligo has the same incidence in all races [1] but its manifestations are much more significant in those with a dark skin than in lightly pigmented individuals (Fig. 73.8). In Afro-Caribbeans, vitiligo may show a 'trichrome' pattern, with hypopigmented as well as depigmented areas.

REFERENCE

1 Kenney JA. Vitiligo. *Dermatol Clin* 1988; **6**: 425–34.

Diseases with a distinct racial or ethnic predisposition

Hair disorders

Dissecting folliculitis (Chapter 66)
SYN. DISSECTING CELLULITIS; PERIFOLLICULITIS CAPITIS ABSCEDENS ET SUFFODIENS

This is an uncommon, chronic, progressive and suppurative scalp disorder that almost exclusively affects Afro-Caribbean males. Painful, boggy, sterile abscesses form on the scalp (Fig. 73.9) and are connected by sinus tracts [1]. As the disease progresses, scarring and alopecia are seen, and keloids may form [2]. The cause is unknown. Treatment has been difficult in the past as intralesional steroids and systemic antibiotics provide only partial relief, but it is now known that isotretinoin is effective in this condition, although it needs to be continued for 4 months after clinical control is achieved to prevent relapse [3]. Resistant cases may require surgical excision and grafting [4]. Dissecting folliculitis may be associated with acne conglobata and

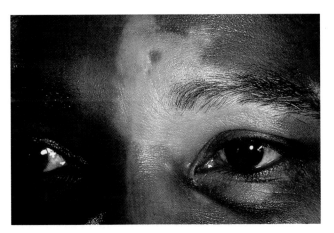

Fig. 73.8 Vitiligo. (Courtesy of Dr A.G. Messenger, Royal Hallamshire Hospital, Sheffield, UK.)

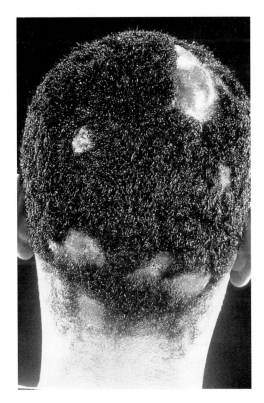

Fig. 73.9 Dissecting cellulitis of the scalp. (Courtesy of Dr H.C. Williams, Queen's Medical Centre, Nottingham, UK.)

hidradenitis suppurativa, to form the so-called 'follicular occlusion' triad, in which abnormal follicular keratinization and occlusion occur [5].

REFERENCES

1 Halder RM. Hair and scalp disorders in blacks. *Cutis* 1983; **32**: 378–80.
2 Scott DA. Disorders of the hair and scalp in blacks. *Dermatol Clin* 1988; **6**: 387–95.
3 Scerri L, Williams HC, Speight EL, Allen BR. Dissecting cellulitis of the scalp: response to isotretinoin. *Br J Dermatol* 1995; **133** (Suppl. 45): 41.
4 Dellon AL, Orlando JC. Perifolliculitis capitis: surgical treatment for the resistant case. *Ann Plast Surg* 1982; **9**: 254–9.
5 Baden HP. *Diseases of the Hair and Nails.* Chicago: Year Book Medical Publishing, 1987.

Folliculitis keloidalis (Chapter 27)

SYN. ACNE KELOIDALIS NUCHAE

This condition is seen almost exclusively in black Africans; males being mostly affected [1]. Firm, discrete, follicular and perifollicular papules develop, usually on the nape of the neck, but often extending into the occipital scalp or beyond (Fig. 73.10). Complications include pustule formation, hypertrophic scars, keloids and alopecia [2]. The aetiology is unknown but probably related to the curved shape of the hair follicle. Treatment includes intralesional steroid injection, and topical and systemic antibiotics [1].

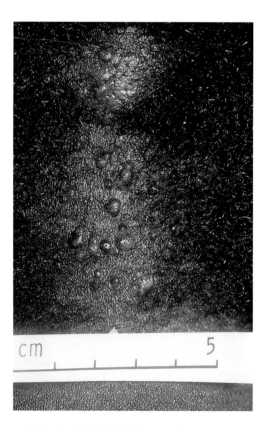

Fig. 73.10 Folliculitis keloidalis. (Courtesy of Dr A.G. Messenger, Royal Hallamshire Hospital, Sheffield, UK.)

REFERENCES

1 Halder RM. Hair and scalp disorders in blacks. *Cutis* 1983; **32**: 378–80.
2 Rosen T, Martin S. *Atlas of Black Dermatology.* Boston: Little, Brown and Co., 1981.

Hot-comb alopecia (Chapter 66)

Hot combing is a method of straightening curly black hair, although it has to a large extent been replaced by chemical methods [1]. Oil is applied to the hair and acts as a lubricant and heat conductor. A metal comb, heated from 150 to 260°C, is applied to the hair, re-arranging the hydrogen and disulphide bonds and straightening the hair [2]. The hot comb and oil may break the hair and a traction alopecia may also result. Repeated contact of the hot oil with the scalp can produce a scarring alopecia [3]. Recent evidence suggests that hot combing may not be the reason for the hair loss, which is usually seen in young adult women, and that the histological end-result, follicular degeneration, may have some other cause [4].

Hair-shaft breakage may also be seen with the inappropriate use of chemical relaxers and straighteners [1]. A scarring alopecia may also be seen, again in young women, following the use of hair-straightening chemicals [5].

REFERENCES

1 Scott DA. Disorders of the hair and scalp in blacks. *Dermatol Clin* 1988; **6**: 387–95.
2 Halder RM. Hair and scalp disorders in blacks. *Cutis* 1983; **32**: 378–80.
3 LoPresti P, Papa CM, Kligman AM. Hot comb alopecia. *Arch Dermatol* 1968; **98**: 234–8.
4 Sperling LC, Sau P. The follicular degeneration syndrome in black patients: 'hot comb alopecia' revisited and revised. *Arch Dermatol* 1992; **128**: 68–74.
5 Nicholson AG, Harland CC, Ball RH *et al.* Chemically induced cosmetic alopecia. *Br J Dermatol* 1993; **128**: 537–41.

Pseudofolliculitis barbae (Chapter 23)

This is a disorder common in black African males who shave and is related to the curved hair follicles found in such individuals [1]. Once shaved, the cut hair retracts beneath the skin surface into the curved follicle and grows in a circular direction. The sharpened hair end either penetrates the wall of the follicle causing a foreign-body reaction or grows out of the follicle but re-enters the skin and penetrates the dermis, again setting up an inflammatory reaction [1]. Perifollicular papules and pustules develop and scarring may result (Fig. 73.11). The beard area is usually affected but pseudofolliculitis may involve any site that is shaved, including the pubic area and the scalp [2]. Recommended treatment is to grow a beard, use electric clippers, depilatory creams or a manual razor, sometimes with topical or systemic antibiotics [3].

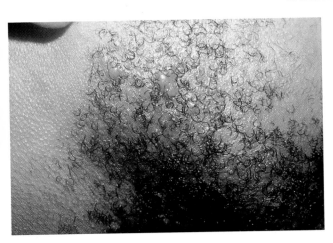

Fig. 73.11 Pseudofolliculitis barbae. (Courtesy of Dr C. St J. O'Doherty, Queen Elizabeth II Hospital, Welwyn Garden City, London, UK.)

REFERENCES

1 Scott DA. Disorders of the hair and scalp in blacks. *Dermatol Clin* 1988; **6**: 387–95.
2 Smith JD, Odom RB. Pseudofolliculitis capitis. *Arch Dermatol* 1977; **113**: 328–9.
3 Brown LA. Pathogenesis and treatment of pseudofolliculitis barbae. *Cutis* 1983; **32**: 373–5.

Traction alopecia (Chapter 66)

Traction alopecia (Fig. 73.12) is mainly seen in black Africans because of the practices of plaiting or tightly braiding the hair into multiple braids (corn rowing), although it is not entirely confined to this group [1]. It may also follow the use of tight rollers or 'picking out' the hair with a hard comb to create the 'Afro' hairstyle [2]. Hairs are loosened from their follicles and inflammation and atrophy may result. The distribution depends on the pattern of braiding but often involves the temporal regions. Treatment consists of persuading the patient to discontinue the offending practice. In long-standing cases alopecia may be permanent.

REFERENCES

1 Scott DA. Disorders of the hair and scalp in blacks. *Dermatol Clin* 1988; **6**: 387–95.
2 Halder RM. Hair and scalp disorders in blacks. *Cutis* 1983; **32**: 378–80.

Variations of normal pigmentation

Futcher's or Voigt's lines

These are sharply demarcated bilateral lines of pigmentation (Fig. 73.13) that are seen at the anterolateral junction usually of the upper arms, where there is a transition from extensor to flexor surface and from darker to lighter

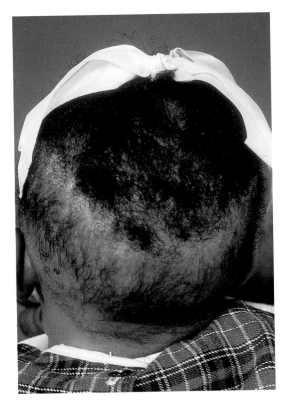

Fig. 73.12 Traction alopecia. (Courtesy of Dr A.G. Messenger, Royal Hallamshire Hospital, Sheffield, UK.)

pigmentation [1]. The lines correspond to a dermatome [2]. A second hyperpigmented line may occur on the posteromedial part of the lower aspect of the limbs [3]. The presence of Futcher's lines is proportional to the degree of pigmentation of the individual; they are present in 25% of black Africans [3]. Overall about 75% of black people have at least one line hypo- or hyperpigmented [3]. These lines may be seen to a lesser extent in other races.

REFERENCES

1 Henderson AL. Skin variations in blacks. *Cutis* 1983; **32**: 376–7.
2 Futcher PH. A peculiarity of pigmentation of the upper arms of negroes. *Science* 1938; **88**: 570–1.
3 McLaurin CI. Cutaneous reaction patterns in blacks. *Dermatol Clin* 1988; **6**: 353–62.

Hyperpigmentation of the palms and soles

Discrete, ill-defined or mottled macular pigmentation is frequently seen on the palms and soles (Fig. 73.14) of African patients, especially those with a darker skin colour [1].

REFERENCE

1 Chapel TA, Taylor RM, Pinkus H. Volar melanotic macules. *Int J Dermatol* 1979; **18**: 222–5.

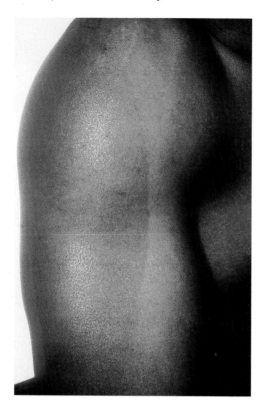

Fig. 73.13 Futcher's lines. (Courtesy of the late Dr R.R.M. Harman, Bristol Royal Infirmary, Bristol, UK.)

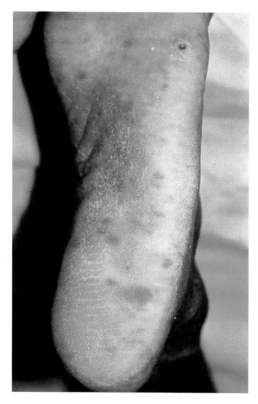

Fig. 73.14 Mottled macular pigmentation on the soles. (Courtesy of Dr D.J. Barker, Bradford Royal Infirmary, Bradford, UK.)

Midline hypopigmentation

This appears as a line or band of hypopigmentation, or as discrete oval macules, on the anterior chest and mid-sternal area. Lesions sometimes extend down to the abdomen or up to the neck, where lines of hypopigmentation may radiate out to the clavicles [1,2]. It is commonly seen in black African males but may occur in other races.

REFERENCES

1 Selmanowitz V, Krivo JM. Hypopigmented markings in negroes. *Int J Dermatol* 1973; **12**: 229–35.
2 Weary PE, Behlen CH. Unusual familial hypopigmentary anomaly. *Arch Dermatol* 1965; **92**: 54–5.

Mongolian spot (Chapter 39)
SYN. CONGENITAL DERMAL MELANOCYTOSIS

Mongolian spot refers to a slatey brown or blue–grey macular pigmentation observed at birth or in the neonatal period (Fig. 73.15). It is present in 100% of Mongoloid babies [1], between 70 and 96% of black Africans, and in up to 10% of Caucasoids [2,3]. The pigmentation is usually faint, round or oval in shape, and ranges in size from a few millimetres to greater than 10 cm in diameter. Mongolian spots are normally located over the sacral area, but the buttocks, flank or shoulders may be involved. Occasionally multiple or extensive lesions are seen. The pigmentation generally reaches its peak at 2 years and fades by the age of 6 or 7 years.

REFERENCES

1 Leung AK. Mongolian spots in Chinese children. *Int J Dermatol* 1988; **27**: 106–8.
2 Cordova A. The Mongolian spot: a study of ethnic differences and a literature review. *Clin Pediatr* 1981; **20**: 714–19.

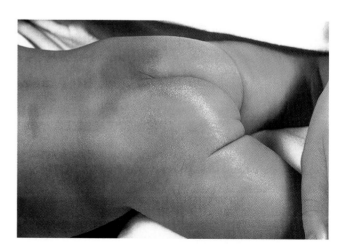

Fig. 73.15 Mongolian spot. (Courtesy of Professor S.S. Bleehen, Royal Hallamshire Hospital, Sheffield, UK.)

3 Osburn K, Schosser RH, Everett MA. Congenital pigmented and vascular lesions in newborn infants. *J Am Acad Dermatol* 1987; **16**: 788–92.

Nail pigmentation

Longitudinal bands of brown or black pigmentation may be seen (Fig. 73.16), and occur with a higher frequency on the thumb and index fingernails [1,2]. They are present in more than 50% of all black Africans, are more common in those with heavy pigmentation, and increase with advancing age.

REFERENCES

1 Leyden JJ, Spott D, Goldschmidt H. Diffuse and banded melanin pigmentation in nails. *Arch Dermatol* 1972; **105**: 548–50.
2 Monash S. Normal pigmentation in the nails of the negro. *Arch Dermatol* 1932; **25**: 876–81.

Oral pigmentation

Oral macular pigmentation is seen in black Africans. It most often affects the gingivae but may also involve the hard palate, buccal mucosa and tongue [1].

REFERENCE

1 Dummett CO, Sakumura JS, Barens G. The relationship of facial skin complexion to oral mucosal pigmentation and tooth color. *J Prosthet Dent* 1980; **4**: 392–6.

Pigmentary disorders

Acanthosis nigricans (Chapter 34)

In some Mongoloid native American tribes, acanthosis nigricans is very common [1]. It may indicate a high risk of diabetes mellitus.

REFERENCE

1 Stuart CA, Smith MM, Gilkison CR *et al.* Acanthosis nigricans among Native Americans: an indicator of high diabetes risk. *Am J Public Health* 1994; **84**: 1839–42.

Dermatosis papulosa nigra (Chapter 34)

This condition is characterized by hyperpigmented, smooth-surfaced, round or filiform papules usually on the face (Fig. 73.17), but sometimes on the neck or upper trunk [1,2]. The papules measure 1–5 mm in diameter. It is most common in black Africans, affecting up to three-quarters of adults — the majority being women — but is occasionally found in Caucasoids and Mongoloids [1]. The cause is unknown.

REFERENCES

1 Grimes PE, Arora S, Minus HR *et al.* Dermatosis papulosa nigra. *Cutis* 1983; **32**: 385–92.
2 Hairston N, Reed R, Derbes V. Dermatosis papulosa nigra. *Arch Dermatol* 1964; **89**: 655–8.

Naevus of Ota (Chapter 38)

Macular pigmentation, due to dermal melanocytes, is seen adjacent to the eye and also involves the sclera (Fig. 73.18). The pigmentation in naevus of Ota is variable and may be blue, slatey blue or brown. The naevus is usually unilateral and affects the eyelid, maxillary and zygomatic areas, regions that are innervated by the first and second branches of the trigeminal nerve [1]. It is most common in Mongoloids but may occur in other racial groups. The prevalence in the Japanese is 0.4–0.8% [2]. Over 80% of cases appear in women. About two-thirds of patients have ocular involvement, commonly of the sclera but also of the cornea, conjunctiva and retina [1]. Malignant melanoma

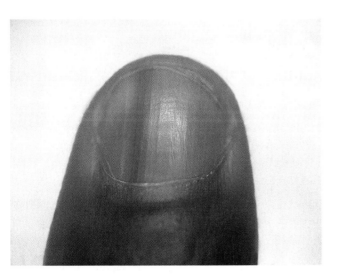

Fig. 73.16 Nail pigmentation.

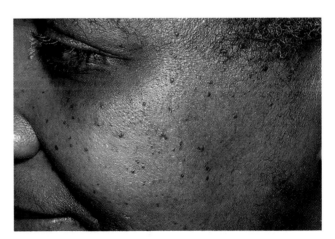

Fig. 73.17 Dermatosis papulosa nigra.

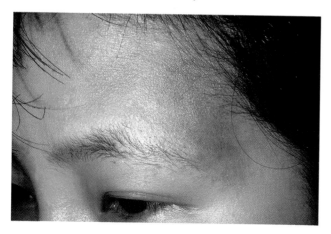

Fig. 73.18 Naevus of Ota.

may develop in the naevus of Ota, more frequently in Caucasoid than Mongoloid patients [3].

REFERENCES

1 Kopf AW, Weidman AI. Nevus of Ota. *Arch Dermatol* 1962; **85**: 195–208.
2 Jimbow M, Jimbow K. Pigmentary disorders in oriental skin. *Clin Dermatol* 1989; **7**: 11–27.
3 Jay B. Malignant melanoma of the orbit in a case of oculodermal melanocytosis (naevus of Ota). *Br J Ophthal* 1965; **49**: 359–63.

Naevus of Ito (Chapter 38)

This is a variant of the naevus of Ota, and is characterized by macular pigmentation involving the shoulder, supraclavicular area, sides of the neck and upper arm—the areas supplied by the posterior supraclavicular and lateral brachial nerves [1,2]. It is more common in the Japanese and may occur alone or associated with a naevus of Ota.

REFERENCES

1 Ito M. Studies on melanin: nevus fusco-caeruleus acromiodeltoideus. *Tohoku J Exp Med* 1954; **60**: 10.
2 Mishima Y, Mevorah B. Nevus Ota and nevus Ito in American negroes. *J Invest Dermatol* 1961; **36**: 133–54.

Other conditions

Ainhum (Chapter 44)

Ainhum is characterized by the development of a constricting band around a digit (often the fifth toe) which may progress to spontaneous amputation of the digit [1]. It is generally found in black inhabitants of tropical countries but has been described in African Americans [2].

The trauma and infection associated with walking barefoot may stimulate fibrosis. Pseudo-ainhum occurs in all races as a feature of mutilating keratoderma.

REFERENCES

1 Browne S. Ainhum: a clinical and etiological study of 83 cases. *Ann Trop Med Parasitol* 1961; **55**: 314–20.
2 Hucherson DC. Ainhum (dactylolysis spontanea): review of 10 cases. *Ann Surg* 1950; **132**: 312–14.

Cutaneous amyloidosis (Chapter 59)

Both the lichenoid type and the macular type are more common in Mongoloid subjects but may be seen in any racial group [1–3]. Lichen amyloidosus consists of discrete, firm papules which often involve the lower leg, extensor aspect of the arms and lower back. The pigmented macular variant commonly affects the scapular region and shows a rippled pattern of pigmentation.

REFERENCES

1 Black MM, Wilson-Jones E. Macular amyloidosis. A study of 21 cases with special reference to the role of the epidermis and its histogenesis. *Br J Dermatol* 1971; **84**: 199–209.
2 Tay CH, DaCosta JL. Lichen amyloidosus. Clinical study of 40 cases. *Br J Dermatol* 1970; **82**: 129–36.
3 Looi LM. Primary localised cutaneous amyloidosis in Malaysians. *Aust J Dermatol* 1991; **32**: 39–44.

Disseminate and recurrent infundibulofolliculitis (Chapter 27)

This is a type of follicular eczema mainly seen in black Africans [1,2]. Pruritic, follicle-based papules are present on the neck, trunk or limbs. Juxtaclavicular beaded lines are a somewhat similar condition. They consist of asymptomatic parallel rows of skin-coloured papules on the neck and overlying the clavicles [1]. They are also seen in Caucasoids.

REFERENCES

1 McLaurin CI. Cutaneous reaction patterns in blacks. *Dermatol Clin* 1988; **6**: 353–62.
2 Rosen T, Martin S. *Atlas of Black Dermatology*. Boston: Little, Brown and Co., 1981.

Facial Afro-Caribbean childhood eruption

In facial Afro-Caribbean childhood eruption (FACE), monomorphic flesh-coloured or hypopigmented papules are seen on the face, particularly around the mouth (Fig. 73.19), eyelids and ears, in Afro-Caribbean children [1,2]. The eruption persists for several months but resolves spontaneously without scarring. The cause is unknown.

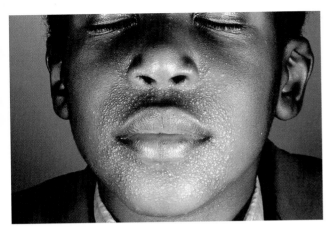

Fig. 73.19 Facial Afro-Caribbean childhood eruption. (Courtesy of Dr H.C. Williams, Queen's Medical Centre, Nottingham, UK.)

REFERENCES

1 Marten RH, Presbury DGC, Adamson JE *et al.* An unusual papular and acneiform facial eruption in the negro child. *Br J Dermatol* 1976; **91**: 435–8.
2 Williams HC, Ashworth J, Pembroke AC *et al.* FACE—facial Afro-Caribbean childhood eruption. *Clin Exp Dermatol* 1990; **15**: 163–6.

Hamartoma moniliformis (Chapter 15)

An asymptomatic disorder of small, discrete, flesh-coloured papules seen over the face and neck [1]. Histology reveals an increase in collagen and elastic fibres, capillary endothelial hyperplasia and proliferation of dermal nerves. The condition was first recognized in mentally retarded black children [1], but may occur in Caucasoid children and in mentally normal children.

REFERENCE

1 Butterworth T, Graham JH. Linear papular ectodermal–mesodermal hamartoma (hamartoma moniliformis). *Arch Dermatol* 1970; **101**: 191–205.

Infantile acropustulosis (Chapter 14)

Crops of small, intensely itchy papules appear between 2 and 10 months of age. The papules evolve into pustules and are mostly found on the palms, soles, wrists and ankles [1,2]. Lesions clear within 3 weeks but recur until the disease resolves spontaneously at the age of about 2 or 3 years. It occurs predominantly in black African infants and the cause is unknown.

REFERENCES

1 Jarratt M, Ramsdell W. Infantile acropustulosis. *Arch Dermatol* 1979; **115**: 834–6.
2 Kahn G, Rywlin AM. Acropustulosis of infancy. *Arch Dermatol* 1979; **115**: 831–3.

Mudi-chood

A papulosquamous eruption, known as mudi-chood, is seen in young Caucasoid women in India on the nape of the neck and upper back. It seems to be due to the effects of oils applied to the hair [1]. The early lesions are follicular pustules, although later, flat-topped brownish black papules, with a keratinous rim, are seen (Fig. 73.20). Histologically, there is parakeratosis and acanthosis [2]. Reducing the use of oils or cutting the hair shorter results in cure.

REFERENCES

1 Gharpuray MB, Kulkarni V, Tolat S. Mudi-chood: an unusual tropical dermatosis. *Int J Dermatol* 1992; **31**: 396–7.
2 Sugathan P, Balaraman Nair M. Mudi-chood: a new dermatosis. In: Marshall J, ed. *Essays on Tropical Dermatology*, Vol. 2. Amsterdam: Exerpta Medica, 1972: 183.

Papular eruption in black males

Described in young African American males, this monomorphic eruption consists of pruritic dermal papules with a predilection for the trunk, upper arms and postauricular area [1]. The condition may be persistent and resistant to treatment. The cause is not known.

REFERENCE

1 Rosen T, Algra RJ. Papular eruption in black men. *Arch Dermatol* 1980; **116**: 416–18.

Papuloerythroderma of Ofuji (Chapter 17)

The unusual eruption, characterized by solid papules coalescing into erythroderma with sparing of the body

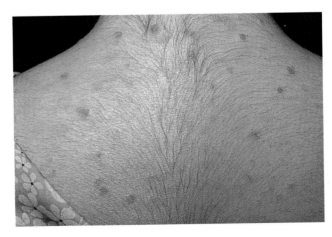

Fig. 73.20 Mudi-chood. (Courtesy of Dr P. Sugathan, Baby Memorial Hospital, Calicut, India.)

folds, was first described in elderly Mongoloid Japanese men but has since also been reported in Caucasoids [1]. The cause is unknown.

REFERENCE

1 Nazzari G, Crovato F, Nigro A. Papuloerythroderma (Ofuji): two additional cases and a review of the literature. *J Am Acad Dermatol* 1992; **26**: 499–501.

Pityriasis rotunda (Chapter 34)

An eruption of discrete, large, scaly, oval or round plaques on the trunk, mostly reported in Mongoloid or black African individuals [1,2]. It is a type of acquired ichthyosis and in some cases is associated with serious disease such as tuberculosis, leprosy, cirrhosis or underlying malignancy.

REFERENCES

1 Rubin MG, Mathes B. Pityriasis rotunda: two cases in black Americans. *J Am Acad Dermatol* 1986; **14**: 74–8.
2 Grimalt R, Gelmetti C, Brusasco A *et al*. Pityriasis rotunda: report of a familial occurrence and review of the literature. *J Am Acad Dermatol* 1994; **31**: 866–71.

Sickle-cell disease (Chapter 50)

Sickle-cell disease occurs in black African races. The main cutaneous findings are the hand–foot syndrome and leg ulceration. The hand–foot syndrome is the most common and often the initial manifestation of the disease in children and consists of painful, non-pitting oedema of the hands and feet, caused by infarction of the small bones [1]. Ischaemic leg ulcers are, overall, the most frequent skin complication of sickle-cell disease, but are rare under the age of 15 years [2].

REFERENCES

1 Stevens MC, Padwick M, Serjeant GR. Observations on the natural history of dactylitis in homozygous sickle cell disease. *Clin Pediatr* 1981; **20**: 311–17.
2 Morgan AG. Proteinuria and leg ulcers in homozygous sickle cell disease. *J Trop Med Hyg* 1982; **85**: 205–8.

Transient neonatal pustular melanosis (Chapter 14)

A transient eruption of sterile vesicles and pustules, with surrounding erythema, which is present at birth. The vesicles rupture easily and leave pigmented macules that fade within the first few weeks of life [1,2]. It affects 4.4% of black Africans and 0.2% of Caucasoid neonates and tends to involve the face, neck, lower back and shins.

REFERENCES

1 Barr RJ, Globerman LM, Werber FA. Transient neonatal pustular melanosis. *Int J Dermatol* 1979; **18**: 636–8.
2 Ramamurthy RS, Reveri M, Esterly NB *et al*. Transient neonatal pustular melanosis. *J Pediatr* 1976; **88**: 831–5.

Vascular naevi (Chapter 15)

Vascular birthmarks, such as the naevus flammeus, usually seen on the neck (the 'stork mark') or sometimes on the forehead or eyelids, or the port-wine stain naevus, are more common in Caucasoids than in black Africans or, to a lesser extent, in Mongoloids [1]. Naevus flammeus is seen in 30% of Caucasoid newborns and in 22% of black newborns [1]. Port-wine stain naevi are found in 1% of Caucasoid infants but are rarer in other races [1].

REFERENCE

1 Osburn K, Schosser RH, Everett MA. Congenital pigmented and vascular lesions in newborn infants. *J Am Acad Dermatol* 1987; **16**: 788–92.

Chapter 74
The Ages of Man and their Dermatoses

R.A.C. GRAHAM-BROWN

Introduction

Human life is a continuum, but within the continuum there are several identifiable phases, which we (the present and previous authors and editors) have called, after Shakespeare, 'The Ages of Man' [1]. We all begin by passing through a period of development to the point of 'maturity', which is then followed by a process of intrinsic ageing leading inexorably to senescence. During these ages, alterations take place in the structure and function of the skin, and there are important differences in the range, presentation, prognosis and treatment of skin disorders at various points in life. Indeed, some of the physiological events that accompany puberty, pregnancy, the menopause and old age can, of themselves, be sufficient reason for the patient to seek specialist dermatological advice.

This chapter aims to provide an overview of these stages in the life of the skin. The dermatological problems of the neonatal period and infancy have been dealt with elsewhere (Chapter 14). This section, therefore, will deal principally with the skin and skin disorders of puberty, the menstrual cycle, pregnancy, childbirth and the puerperium, the menopause, and old age.

REFERENCE

1 Shakespeare W. *As You Like It* II. vii. 139.

Birth to puberty

Somatic growth

Growth, defined as an increase in size, occurs in most tissues, including the reproductive system. In particular, the changes in the skeleton, which can be monitored radiologically, and in the visible teeth, have been used as indices of maturity [1].

Between birth and maturity the skeleton and body keep in step with increases in weight of 20–25-fold, whereas the somatic muscles increase by 30–40-fold, and the nervous system by less than five-fold. The surface area of the skin increases seven-fold. In the first year after birth the body length increases by about 50% to around 75 cm, and another 12–13 cm are added in the second year. Subsequently, growth remains steady at 6 cm/year until the spurt associated with puberty. Weight follows a similar pattern.

Postnatal growth is dependent on growth hormone, or somatotrophin, secreted by the anterior pituitary, although other hormonal interactions may also be involved [2,3]. Human growth hormone is a protein with 191 amino acids. It exerts an effect on a number of tissues which include the viscera and bone. In particular, it affects stature by stimulating proliferation of cartilage cells at the epiphyseal plates, an action which ceases once the epiphyses of the long bones have fused. Growth hormone also antagonizes the actions of insulin, possibly by reducing the binding of insulin at its target sites, or by interacting with a second-messenger system.

Some of the effects of growth hormone are indirect, in the sense that they are mediated through the production of polypeptide growth factors in the target tissue. The most important of these, which effects the uptake of sulphate into cartilage, is somatomedin C, initially called 'sulphation factor' but now known to be identical with insulin-like growth factor 1 (IGF-1) and closely similar to IGF-2. Somatomedins have also been shown to stimulate incorporation of [^{14}C] leucine into glycosaminoglycans in cartilage and of [^{14}C] proline into collagen.

The secretion of growth hormone from the pituitary is mediated by the interaction between hypothalamic growth hormone-releasing hormone and somatostatin. Negative feedback by both somatomedin C and growth hormone itself may also be involved. The basal concentration of growth hormone in the plasma is below 1 mIU/l, but it can reach peaks of up to 60 times this amount in adolescence. Bursts of secretion occur every 1–2 h during sleep, but can also be produced by physiological and psychological stresses.

Excessive secretion before puberty gives rise to gigantism, but once the epiphyses of the long bones have fused, it results in thickening of the bones and enlargement of the hands and feet, known as acromegaly. Acromegalics have, on average, abnormally high sebum secretion.

Deficiency of growth hormone, either in isolation or as a component of general hypopituitarism, is one cause of short stature. In a number of other syndromes dwarfism is associated with cutaneous manifestations.

REFERENCES

1 Sinclair D. *Human Growth after Birth*, 5th edn. Oxford: Oxford University Press, 1989.
2 O'Riordan JLO, Malan PG, Gould RP, eds. *Essentials of Endocrinology*, 2nd edn. Oxford: Blackwell Scientific Publications, 1988.
3 Underwood LE, Van Wyk JJ. Normal and aberrant growth. In: Wilson JD, Foster DW, eds. *Textbook of Endocrinology*. Philadelphia: WB Saunders, 1985: 155–205.

Sexual development

The period between infancy and puberty that we call childhood is, in relation to sexual development, a hiatus in hormonally controlled events that have already been initiated in the fetus. While the dermatological problems of the neonatal period are so distinctive and of such practical importance as to merit a separate chapter, an understanding of the hormonal status of the fetus and the neonate, and of the cutaneous implications, is an essential starting point for a journey through 'the Ages of Man'.

Males become differentiated from females by their possession of a Y chromosome which causes the indifferent gonads to become testes [1,2]. The fetal testes secrete a factor known as anti-Müllerian hormone, which induces regression of the Müllerian ducts between the seventh and eighth weeks of gestation, and testosterone, which causes virilization of the Wolffian duct to form most of the male system. Conversion of the testosterone to 5 α-dihydrotestosterone (Chapter 4) is necessary for the development of the prostate, from the urinogenital sinus, and of the external genitalia. In the latter trimesters the testicles descend to their position in the scrotum in response to gonadotrophin from the fetal pituitary, in addition to testosterone.

In females, where the testicular secretions are lacking, the Müllerian ducts persist and give rise to the reproductive tract.

The fetal testis continues to secrete testosterone even after birth [3]. At 50 days of age the level of plasma testosterone (250 ng/100 ml) is more than seven times that in the umbilical cord (35 ng/100 ml), and is thus unlikely to be of maternal origin. It falls to the low level of childhood by about 6 months.

In males, this production of testosterone appears to be reflected by the activity of the sebaceous glands, which become functional by 17 weeks of gestation. The glands are large at birth; and the skin surface lipid is high, around 400 g/cm^2, remaining so for about 3 months [4,5]. A level of about 100 g/cm^2 is maintained throughout childhood.

The neonatal skin-surface lipid is, however, equally high in females, and the same explanation cannot be applied. In fact, the hormonal pattern is also different; the maximum plasma testosterone occurs immediately after birth, and falls within days [3]. Furthermore, in both females and males the pattern of dehydroepiandrosterone very closely follows that of the casual sebum levels [6]. For these reasons, it seems possible that the production of sebum in the neonatal period, and the occurrence of acne [7–9], may be related to adrenal activity.

Sebaceous activity starts to increase again towards the end of childhood, in advance of other signs of approaching puberty [10,11]. Dramatic changes take place between the ages of 8 and 9 years, in both males and females [12], and it seems possible that these are related to an increase in output of adrenal androgens. Comedones start to increase around this period [13].

REFERENCES

1 Grumbach MM, Conte FA. Disorders of sexual differentiation. In: Wilson JD, Foster DW, eds. *Textbook of Endocrinology*. Philadelphia: WB Saunders, 1985: 312–401.
2 O'Riordan JLH, Malan PG, Gould RP, eds. *Essentials of Endocrinology*. Oxford: Blackwell Scientific Publications, 1988.
3 Forest MG, Cathiard AM, Bertrand JA. Evidence of testicular activity in early infancy. *J Clin Endocrinol Metab* 1973; **37**: 148–51.
4 Agache P, Blanc D, Barrand C *et al.* Sebum levels during the first year of life. *Br J Dermatol* 1980; **103**: 643–9.
5 Emanuel SV. Quantitative determination of the sebaceous gland's function, with particular mention of the method employed. *Acta Derm Venereol (Stockh)* 1936; **17**: 444.
6 de Peretti D, Forest MG. Unconjugated DHEA plasma levels in normal subjects from birth to adolescence in humans: the use of a sensitive radio immuno-assay. *J Clin Endocrinol Metab* 1976; **43**: 982–91.
7 Bessone L. Acne infantum. Parte I. *Chron Dermatol* 1971; **2**: 3–20.
8 Bessone L. Acne infantum. Parte II. *Chron Dermatol* 1971; **2**: 643–96.

9 Bessone L. Acne infantum. Parte III. *Chron Dermatol* 1972; **3**: 75–99.

10 Constans S, Makki S, Petiot F *et al.* Sebaceous levels from 6 to 15 years: comparison with pubertal events. *J Invest Dermatol* 1985; **84**: 454–5.

11 Pochi PE, Strauss JS, Downing DT. Age-related changes in sebaceous gland activity. *J Invest Dermatol* 1979; **73**: 108–11.

12 Ramasastry P, Downing DT, Pochi PE *et al.* Chemical composition of human skin surface lipids from birth to puberty. *J Invest Dermatol* 1970; **54**: 139–44.

13 Burton JL, Cunliffe WJ, Stafford I *et al.* The prevalence of acne vulgaris in adolescence. *Br J Dermatol* 1971; **85**: 119–26.

The skin in childhood

The skin, along with other organ systems, undergoes some degree of maturation during the hiatus of childhood, before the resumption of sexual development at puberty and the transition to adulthood. The skin disorders seen in children in part reflect these physiological changes, but many of the most troublesome cutaneous problems result from intrinsic genetic abnormalities conditioned by environmental influences. A good example is atopic dermatitis (Chapter 18). The influence of the environment changes, of course, as the child becomes more mobile and travels further and further afield.

School years bring exposure to a wide variety of infections and contagions, such as measles, chickenpox, impetigo, warts, molluscum contagiosum, scabies and head lice. There is also a gradual increase in contact with potential irritants at school during lessons, in sporting activities such as swimming and team games, and in hobbies. The wearing of jewellery and cosmetics, and exposure to sensitizers such as rubber chemicals in footwear and preservatives in medicaments, bring a further range of dermatological problems in the form of allergic contact dermatitis, which is not as rare before puberty as is often suggested [1]. One disorder that seems to have a definite predilection for the prepubertal period in girls is lichen sclerosus et atrophicus [2], which may improve and disappear as puberty approaches, although this is not always the case [3]. In boys, the same pathological changes are frequently found in prepuces removed to relieve phimosis [4].

There has also been an increasing awareness in recent years that both girls and boys may present to the dermatologist with symptoms and signs which indicate sexual abuse [5]. Vulval or perianal soreness and inflammation for which no other cause can be found should be considered suspicious, as should the presence of anogenital warts [6], although some are innocently acquired. Proof of sexual abuse is always a difficult matter unless there has been disclosure or confession from within the family unit. Furthermore, the social and legal implications of formal investigations for the child and its family are enormous. Inquiries must therefore be undertaken with care, although there is a well-established framework in many countries to deal with the problem, generally involving paediatricians, social workers and police [5]. It is also important to note that the changes associated with lichen sclerosus and Crohn's disease in childhood can be mistaken, by non-dermatologists, for evidence of sexual abuse [2].

Table 74.1 Disorders in which short stature may occur with cutaneous changes.

Often severe	Moderate
Rothmund–Thomson syndrome	Turner's syndrome
Bloom's syndrome	Hypohidrotic ectodermal
Cockayne's syndrome	dysplasia
Bird-headed dwarfism	Marinesco–Sjögren syndrome
Progeria	Xeroderma pigmentosum
Cornelia de Lange syndrome	Trichorhinophalangeal
Cartilage–hair hypoplasia	syndrome
Conradi's disease	Focal dermal hypoplasia
Polydysplastic epidermolysis	Werner's syndrome
bullosa	Darier's disease
Ataxia–telangiectasia	Atopic dermatitis
Leprechaunism	
GAPO	
Short stature, alopecia and	
macular degeneration	

GAPO, growth retardation, alopecia, pseudo-anodontia, optic atrophy

Syndromes of short stature

There are several disorders in which abnormal or delayed growth and development are accompanied by cutaneous changes. Some lead to short stature (a term preferred to 'dwarfism'), which is a common feature of chromosomal abnormalities. In others, delayed sexual development (infantilism) is also present, and this will be discussed briefly in relation to premature and delayed puberty. It is important to note that due allowance must be made for parental height in assessing possible delayed growth in a child [7].

Some of the more important of the disorders in which skin changes accompany short stature are listed in Table 74.1.

Furthermore, it is well known that severe skin disease of any kind in childhood may have a considerable impact on general physical development. Atopic dermatitis is a good example, short stature being very common in severely affected individuals, at least until puberty [8], although the assessment of this may be complicated by systemic or topical steroid therapy.

REFERENCES

1 Balato N, Lembo G, Patruno C *et al.* Patch-testing in children. *Contact Dermatitis* 1989; **20**: 305–7.

2 Ridley CM. Lichen sclerosus et atrophicus. *Semin Dermatol* 1989; **8**: 54–63.

3 Holder JE, Berth-Jones J, Graham-Brown RAC. Lichen sclerosus et atrophicus presenting in childhood: a follow-up study. *Br J Dermatol* 1994; **131** (Suppl 44): 50.

4 Bale PM, Lochhead A, Martin HCO *et al.* Balanitis xerotica obliterans in children. *Pediatr Pathol* 1987; **7**: 617–27.

5 Berth-Jones J, Graham-Brown RAC. Childhood sexual abuse—a dermatological perspective. *Clin Exp Dermatol* 1990; **15**: 321–30.

6 Hanson RM, Glasson M, McCrossin I *et al.* Anogenital warts in childhood. *Child Abuse Neglect* 1989; **13**: 225–33.

7 Tanner JM, Goldstein H, Whitehouse RH. Standards for children's height at ages 2–9 years allowing for height of parents. *Arch Dis Child* 1970; **45**: 755–62.

8 Verbov J. Atopic and other dermatitis. In: *Essential Paediatric Dermatology.* Bristol: Clinical Press, 1988: 29–46.

Puberty and adolescence

Hormonal events and cutaneous changes

Puberty is the period over which the secondary sexual characters gradually become manifest as the reproductive system develops to full capacity and there is rapid somatic growth [1–3]. The term adolescence embraces these events, but is also used in a wider sense to include the phase of psychological and social adjustment to the physical changes. Thus, depending on the society, adolescence may be prolonged well beyond the completion of puberty.

The onset of puberty in the male is heralded by an increase in testicular volume which results from the appearance of a lumen in each seminiferous tubule and an increase in the size and number of the Leydig cells which produce testosterone. This hormone is responsible for secondary changes such as enlargement of the penis and larynx, growth of pubic hair, axillary hair and beard, and also for a rise in sebum excretion and increased axillary sweating. Slight growth of the pubic hair, probably provoked by androgens from the adrenal, may be one of the earliest visible signs of impending puberty, but it proceeds slowly and does not even reach the pattern of the adult female until around the age of 15 years. Facial hair only starts to appear about 2 years later. A full account of the patterns of hair development is given in Chapter 66.

In 95% of white British boys studied by Tanner [4–6] the genitalia started to enlarge at between 9.5 and 13.5 years (mean 11.6±0.9 years of age), and functional maturity, indicated by ability to ejaculate, was achieved between the ages of 13 and 17 (mean 14.9±1.1) years. The adolescent growth spurt, when the average gain in height reached a peak of 10 cm/year, a velocity of growth similar to that at the age of 2 years, usually occurred between 12.5 and 15 years (mean 14.1±0.9), i.e. about 3 years after the first signs of genital enlargement.

In girls, one of the first signs of puberty is the onset of breast development (thelarche), indicated by the elevation of the breast and papilla to form a small mound known as the breast bud [5,7]. This usually occurs at between 8 and 13 years of age, with an average at 11, but the breasts continue to enlarge for about 2 more years. Growth of the breasts is provoked by the secretion of oestrogens by the ovary; the further development of the secretory alveoli during pregnancy requires the action of progesterone as well. Pubic hair also starts to develop early (Chapter 66). The most obvious feature of puberty, namely first menstruation or menarche, occurs at an average age of 13 years, but within an age range of 10–16.5 years. The early menstrual cycles do not usually involve ovulation, so full reproductive function is generally delayed for a further year or two. The growth spurt, with a peak height gain of 8 cm/year occurs between 10.5 and 13 years of age in white British girls [7]. This is about 2 years earlier than in boys. It is also noteworthy that rapid somatic growth precedes the major events of sexual maturation in girls but accompanies or succeeds them in boys.

The pubertal growth spurt appears, in both sexes, to be dependent on androgenic steroids as well as on growth hormone. Boys with growth hormone deficiency respond less well to testosterone than do normal subjects, not only in relation to acceleration of growth but also for development of the secondary sexual characteristics [8,9].

Gonadal function in both sexes is initiated by two gonadotrophic hormones of the pituitary, namely follicle-stimulating hormone (FSH) and luteinizing hormone (LH). In the male, initiation of spermatogenesis requires both hormones, but secretion of testosterone by the Leydig cells needs only LH. It may be noted that, when the earliest sign of puberty in the female is the appearance of pubic hair, this probably results from stimulation by androgens from the adrenal cortex, so-called adrenarche, and is thus dependent on an output of hypophyseal adrenocorticotrophic hormone (ACTH).

Levels of serum FSH and LH rise in both sexes between the ages of 6 and 17 years [10]. As puberty develops, LH is released in pulses, at first only at night but later also during the day [11,12]. The secretion of both gonadotrophins from the pituitary is controlled by a single releasing hormone, gonadotrophin releasing hormone (GnRH), a decapeptide produced in the hypothalamus. This is influenced by negative feedback of the gonadotrophins, steroid hormones and a peptide called inhibin, which is produced by the gonads [13].

The important question, therefore, is: what initiates the pulsatile release of GnRH to invoke the onset of puberty? [14,15]. Animal studies show that the central component of the neuroendocrine mechanism which governs gonadal function is fully mature by birth [14]. Pulsatile GnRH release occurs during infancy, but there is then a hiatus in GnRH release between infancy and puberty [16]. The mechanisms which control this juvenile quiescence and eventual pubertal reawakening remain uncertain.

It has long been assumed that the initiation of puberty depends on the achievement of a particular body size or composition, suggesting the existence of a central growth tracking device or 'somatometer', rather than chronological age [14,17]. It is not understood how the central nervous system detects such changes in somatic development. The metabolites or hormones which are used by the brain as signals of metabolic maturity have yet to be identified. One suggestion is that developing bone produces a peptide which enters the circulation and imposes the prepubertal hiatus. This would explain the congruence of puberty with bone age rather than with chronological age. It is, for example, known that in children with constitutional delay of growth and puberty or with isolated growth hormone deficiency, sexual maturity is chronologically delayed but occurs at normal skeletal age [14].

It is also unclear whether season influences the timing of puberty, as it does for the majority of species which live in changing habitats (see [18] for a review). An annual rhythm in human reproductive success exists in most societies, but it has long been controversial whether this is related to biological or sociological factors [19]. Marked seasonal effects on the timing of puberty have been noted in the female rhesus monkey [20], and, in common with most mammals in temperate latitudes, it is the changing photoperiod which is used to time puberty [18]. Studies in sheep and various species of hamster establish unequivocally that the daily pattern of melatonin secretion from the pineal gland provides an endocrine measure of day length, and mediates its effect on reproductive function. Melatonin is secreted during the hours of darkness, and provides an accurate measure of the length of night. Melatonin is not directly pro- or antigonadotrophic it solely provides a seasonal cue. Humans show a clear daily rhythm of melatonin secretion [21], so the question arises whether it plays a role in triggering puberty. Tumours of the pineal gland have been associated with both precocious and delayed puberty [22,23], although there is no experimental evidence that abnormal melatonin secretion causes reproductive malfunction in such cases. The amplitude of the nocturnal rise in melatonin secretion declines over the period of childhood, and has led to a hypothesis that puberty results from a decrease in melatonin secretion [24]. This view is not supported by animal studies. In both the rhesus monkey and sheep, for example, puberty occurs in the autumn, when the periods of melatonin secretion are actually increasing [18,20]. It may be noted that the initial increase in LH secretion in the pubertal human first occurs at night, when melatonin secretion is high, rather than during the day when melatonin secretion is basal [25]. It seems likely that, although the human has retained a melatonin secretory system, the seasonal information that it conveys, at least, has become disregarded in the course of evolution.

Social cues may also play a part in the induction of gonadal activity, as demonstrated in many mammalian species. For example, introduction of a ram can induce an increase in LH pulse frequency and ovulation in both the seasonally anoestrus and prepubertal sheep, and this appears to be effected through a pheromonal mechanism [16,26]. The demonstration that extracts of male axillary secretions can affect the menstrual cycle when applied to the female upper lip [27] suggests that similar cues may play a role in humans.

REFERENCES

1 Falkner F, Tanner JM, eds. *Human Growth*, Vols 1,2,3. New York: Plenum Press, 1986.
2 Sinclair D. *Human Growth after Birth*, 5th edn. Oxford: Oxford University Press, 1989.
3 Underwood LE, Van Wyk JJ. Normal and aberrant growth. In: Wilson JD, Farber DW, eds. *Williams' Textbook of Endocrinology*, 7th edn. Philadelphia: WB Saunders, 1985: 155–205.
4 Marshall WA, Tanner JM. Variations in the pattern of pubertal changes in boys. *Arch Dis Child* 1970; **45**: 13–23.
5 Tanner JM. *Growth at Adolescence*. Oxford: Blackwell Scientific Publications, 1962.
6 Tanner JM, Whitehouse RH. Clinical longitudinal standards for height, weight, height velocity, weight velocity and stages of puberty. *Arch Dis Child* 1976; **51**: 170–9.
7 Marshall WA, Tanner JM. Variations in pattern of pubertal changes in girls. *Arch Dis Child* 1969; **44**: 291–303.
8 Tanner JM, Whitehouse RH. The pattern of growth in children with growth hormone deficiency before, during and after treatment. In: Pecile A, Müller EE, eds. *Growth and Growth Hormone*. Amsterdam: Excerpta Medica, 1972: 429–51.
9 Zachmann M, Aynsley-Green A, Prader A. Interrelations of the effects of growth hormone and testosterone in hypopituitarism. In: Pecile A, Müller EE, eds. *Growth Hormone and Related Peptides*. Amsterdam: Excerpta Medica, 1976: 286–96.
10 Faiman C, Winter JSD. Gonadotrophins and sex hormone patterns in puberty: clinical data. In: Grumbach MM, Grave GD, Mayer FE, eds. *Control of the Onset of Puberty*. New York: John Wiley & Sons, 1974: 33–5.
11 Plant TM. Puberty in primates. In: Knobil E, Neill JD, Ewing LL *et al*, eds. *The Physiology of Reproduction*. New York: Raven Press, 1988: 1763–88.
12 Wu FCW, Borrow SM, Nicol K *et al*. Ontogeny of pulsatile gonadotrophin secretion and pituitary responsiveness in male puberty in man: a mixed longitudinal and cross-sectional study. *J Endocrinol* 1989; **123**: 347–59.
13 O'Riordan JLH, Malan PG, Gould RP. *Essentials of Endocrinology*. Oxford: Blackwell Scientific Publications, 1988.
14 Plant TM, Fraser MO, Medhamurthy R *et al*. Somatogenic control of GnRH neuronal synchronization during development in primates: a speculation. In: Delemarre-van de Waal HA, Plant TM, van Rees GP *et al.*, eds. *Control of the Onset of Puberty*, Vol. III. Amsterdam: Excerpta Medica, 1989: 111–21.
15 Terasawa E, Claypool LE, Gore AC *et al*. The timing of the onset of puberty in the female rhesus monkey. In: Delemarre-van de Waal HA, Plant TM, van Rees GP *et al.*, eds. *Control of the Onset of Puberty*, Vol. III. Amsterdam: Excerpta Medica, 1989: 123–36.
16 Foster DL, Ebling FJP, Ryan KD *et al*. Mechanisms timing puberty: a comparative approach. In: Delemarre-van de Waal HA, Plant TM, van Rees GP *et al.*, eds. *Control of the Onset of Puberty*, Vol III. Amsterdam: Excerpta Medica, 1989: 227–45.
17 Frisch RE. Body fat, puberty and fertility. *Biol Rev* 1984; **59**: 161–88.
18 Ebling FJP, Foster DL. Pineal melatonin rhythms and the timing of puberty in mammals. *Experientia* 1989; **45**: 946–54.
19 Roenneberg T, Aschoff J. Annual rhythm of human reproduction: I. Biology, Sociology or both? *J Biol Rhythm* 1990; **5**: 195–216.
20 Wilson ME, Gordon TP. Season determines timing of first ovulation in outdoor-housed rhesus monkeys. *J Reprod Fertil* 1989; **85**: 583–91.
21 Arendt J. Melatonin and the human circadian system. In: Miles A, Philbrick DRS, Thompson C, eds. *Melatonin, Clinical Perspectives*. Oxford: Oxford University Press, 1988: 43–61.
22 Reichlin S. Neuroendocrinology. In: Williams RH, ed. *Textbook of Endocrinology*. Philadelphia: WB Saunders, 1981: 492–567.
23 Weinberger LM, Grant FC. Precocious puberty and tumors of the hypothalamus. *Arch Intern Med* 1941; **67**: 762–92.
24 Waldhauser F, Weizsenbacher G, Tatzer E *et al*. Alterations in nocturnal serum melatonin levels with growth and aging. *J Clin Endocrinol Metab* 1988; **66**: 648–52.
25 Fevre M, Segel T, Marks JM *et al*. LH and melatonin secretion patterns in pubertal boys. *J Clin Endocrinol Metab* 1979; **47**: 1383–6.
26 Ebling FJP, Foster DL. Seasonal breeding—a model for puberty? In: Delemarre-van de Waal HA, Plant TM, van Rees GP *et al.*, eds. *Control of the Onset of Puberty*, Vol III. Amsterdam: Excerpta Medica, 1989: 253–64.
27 Cutler WB, Preti G, Krieger A *et al*. Human axillary secretions influence women's menstrual cycles: the role of donor extract from men. *Horm Behav* 1986; **20**: 463–73.

Dermatoses of puberty and adolescence

Adolescence is a difficult period for most people. It is a time when the whole emphasis of relationships is supposed to change from the herd bond of the 'gang' to the pair bond of courtship and sexual involvement, but this does not happen all at once or completely. Most of us retain a need for the approbation of our peers throughout life, as well as a desire to develop a close one-to-one relationship. The tensions involved in this are at their most acute during adolescence and, for this reason, many skin diseases, which first presented during childhood, only begin to exert their most damaging influences after the onset of puberty. Adolescence is a bad time to have skin disease, especially on the face or on the extremities.

The physiological changes which occur in the skin during puberty and adolescence also have several effects, and may result in sufficient distress to cause the individual to seek medical advice. There are several examples of this: the increase in sebum production often results in unacceptably greasy hair, on which many hours and much money is expended; teenagers often present with secondary sexual hair which they perceive to be abnormal, largely as a result of the pressure exerted by the media; young men become anguished when male-pattern balding begins in the teenage years; members of both sexes become disturbed by the onset of 'body odour'.

It has been pointed out that the pressures of coping with a maturing skin are particularly acute for a girl who is persuaded by advertisers that she should have plenty of hair on her head, but none on her face, under her arms or on her legs. Her skin should be free from grease, spots and wrinkles and, moreover, should be odourless [1]. Puberty makes this ideal image virtually impossible to achieve. Several disorders cause special problems or make their first appearance in adolescence. The classic example is acne vulgaris but there are several others (Table 74.2).

Teenagers may present with a variety of skin disorders in which self-inflicted injury is an important component (Fig. 74.1), varying from mild excoriated acne to severe habitual mutilation. The mental state of these individuals ranges from simple, mild anxiety to gross personality disorder, psychotic disturbance and instability. Extreme forms of deliberate self-harm almost invariably begin in adolescence, but most continue for many years [2].

Table 74.2 Disorders which present in or cause particular problems during adolescence.

Acne vulgaris
Acne excoriée and neurotic excoriation
Self-mutilation and dermatitis artefacta
Seborrhoeic dermatitis
Pityriasis versicolor
Hyperhidrosis
Axillary bromhidrosis (body odour)
Hidradenitis suppurativa
Fox–Fordyce disease
Polymorphic light eruption
Epidermolysis bullosa simplex (Weber–Cockayne syndrome)
Psoriasis
Atopic dermatitis

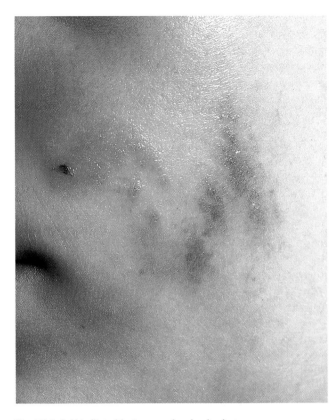

Fig. 74.1 Self-inflicted lesions on the cheek of a teenager.

Seborrhoeic dermatitis is generally seen only from adolescence onwards, as is pityriasis versicolor in temperate climates. An explanation for this may lie in the alterations in sebum that appear to occur at puberty [3], especially if it is accepted that yeast organisms play a role in seborrhoeic dermatitis (Chapter 17). This alteration in sebum is also said to be responsible for the virtual disappearance of scalp ringworm after puberty.

Teenagers may seek help for a number of different axillary problems. Severe eccrine hyperhidrosis can be a very distressing complaint, but usually responds well to treatment (Chapter 43), as does axillary odour (bromhidrosis). More difficult to deal with are abnormalities of the apocrine glands (hidradenitis and Fox–Fordyce disease).

Polymorphic light eruption often presents for the first time in adolescence, and can ruin summer holidays. So does psoriasis [4]; 25% of 5600 patients with psoriasis dated the onset of their disease to between the ages of 10 and 20 years [5]. The impact of the appearance of psoriasis on a teenager should not be underestimated. The patient will be told that psoriasis is probably genetic, that it is likely to continue to be a lifelong problem, and that there is no satisfactory cure. All this has to be assimilated during a period of increasing awareness of the importance of being attractive.

Atopic dermatitis can also be a major problem for the teenager and his or her family. It may present for the first time in adolescence, but this is rare. More commonly, children do not grow out of it as they have been led to believe, or atopic dermatitis may disappear during childhood only to reappear in adolescence. In this situation the skin changes and pruritus are often severe, and usually have already affected the enjoyment of childhood. The adolescent is then quite abruptly faced with the prospect of the skin problem continuing for an apparently indefinite period into adult life. Many, if not all, affected teenagers become increasingly depressed and frustrated, and a sense of hopelessness can descend on the whole family. Many patients completely lose faith in orthodox medicine and seek advice from homeopaths, herbalists, naturopaths and others. A truly sympathetic and holistic approach is therefore required if the dermatologist is to retain the confidence of his or her young patient and the latter's relatives through this difficult period. Good communications need to be cultivated and maintained. Professional counselling facilities can be very helpful, but are often neglected or not available.

Another troublesome aspect of atopic dermatitis in adolescence is that there is a greater tendency to develop involvement of the hands (and feet) as the years go by. This can lead to real difficulties in choosing a suitable occupation (see below). Furthermore, treatment parameters usually differ in adolescents and adults from those in childhood atopic dermatitis [6]. In particular, the information and support needs are different and, in practical therapeutic terms, steroid-sparing strategies may become more important.

Some congenital and genetic diseases, such as tuberous sclerosis and neurofibromatosis may actually progress during the teenage years, causing increasing physical and cosmetic disability. Others (e.g. ichthyotic disorders, pigmentary anomalies and port-wine stains), even though largely static, may exert a greater effect because of the social and psychological tensions of adolescence.

However, some disorders improve at puberty. For example, atopic dermatitis clears in many individuals, and autosomal dominant ichthyosis tends to improve.

Skin disease and career

Young people with skin disease are often not aware that they may be at a major disadvantage in pursuing some occupations.

The armed forces medically examine all recruits, and are unlikely to accept anyone with psoriasis, significant atopic dermatitis or bad acne. It is, therefore, preferable for acne to be eradicated before, rather than after, application.

Psoriasis and eczema of the hands can cause trouble for those hoping to work in catering. Although they may be accepted by colleges to study, sufferers often find it difficult to obtain subsequent employment.

Hand dermatitis among hairdressers is a far greater problem in those with active atopic dermatitis and in those who have been troubled in the past than in non-sufferers [7]. A teenager with atopic dermatitis may work in a hair salon for months or even years suffering with hand dermatitis before eventually giving up. The same applies to nursing, where many committed individuals are rejected at the occupational health screen because of eczema. The reasons given include the exposure to irritants that the skin will inevitably have during a nurse's normal duties, and the increased risk of acquiring hepatitis and acquired immune deficiency syndrome (AIDS) through broken skin.

Any teenager with a chronic skin disease, especially of the hands, should therefore be made aware of the potential difficulties that he or she may face in the choice of a future occupation. It is better that a change be made early on than after working hard to achieve a set of educational and vocational goals which are unobtainable.

REFERENCES

1 Cotterill JA. Infantile cutaneous ideas. *Br J Dermatol* 1987; **117** (Suppl. 32): 22–3.
2 Favazza AR, Conterio K. Female habitual self-mutilators. *Acta Psychiatr Scand* 1989; **79**: 283–9.
3 Stewart ME, Steele WA, Downing DT. Changes in the relative amounts of endogenous and exogenous fatty acids in sebaceous lipids during early adolescence. *J Invest Dermatol* 1989; **92**: 371–8.
4 Ingram JT. The significance and management of psoriasis. *Br Med J* 1954; **ii**: 823–8.
5 Farber EM, Nall LM. The natural history of psoriasis in 5600 patients. *Dermatologica* 1974; **148**: 1–18.
6 Graham-Brown RAC. Managing adults with atopic dermatitis. *Dermatol Clin* 1996; **124**: 531–7.
7 Cronin E. Hairdresser. *Contact Dermatitis*. Edinburgh: Churchill Livingstone, 1980: 134–9.

Premature and delayed puberty and hypogonadism

The dermatologist will occasionally see patients with abnormally early or delayed puberty, or with various hypogonadal syndromes. The appearance or non-appearance of sexual hair, or the onset of acne lesions in late childhood are the usual reasons for such referrals. Premature and delayed puberty are matters for endocrinological investigations, but the dermatologist should at least be aware of the range of diagnostic possibilities.

Premature puberty

Signs of puberty before the age of 10 years are generally held to be abnormal. This may be due to an early onset of complete (or true) puberty, in which the changes are triggered by early activation of the normal hypothalamo-pituitary–gonadal axis. In some instances, early signs of puberty are due to false (or pseudo-) puberty, in which sex hormone secretion is independent of the normal control mechanisms. Partial or incomplete puberty is also recognized, and there are two forms: thelarche (isolated breast development), and pubarche (isolated development of pubic and axillary hair). The former may be unilateral and be confused with tumours. It is not clear what causes isolated breast enlargement, although tissue hypersensitivity to oestrogen has been suggested (Chapter 71). Pubarche is often associated with adrenal androgen secretion, and this may be a priming phenomenon in the early phases of normal pubertal development [1]. Indeed, the very early, isolated appearance of sexual hair may presage a true early puberty, and the distinction can be a very fine one. Table 74.3 gives a clinical classification of early puberty.

Most instances of premature, complete puberty are constitutional. Although this may be sporadic, there is often a strong family history. Indeed, it seems likely that many families never present at all, accepting that it is quite normal for them. This is particularly true for girls, in whom approximately 80% of premature puberty is thought to be constitutional [2]. There is no difference in the order of events, but mental and emotional development may lag behind the physical changes. In boys, where the event is rarer, there is more often an underlying pathological condition [2].

The investigation of complete premature puberty is obviously a complex process, especially if a neurogenic origin is suspected, but the dermatologist should always look for other features of the specific syndromes listed in Table 74.3: McCune–Albright syndrome, neurofibromatosis, tuberous sclerosis and Silver's syndrome (short stature, craniofacial disproportion and clinodactyly [3]), as well as hypothyroidism.

Table 74.3 Classification of premature puberty. (From Rayner [2].)

Complete (true)	False (pseudopuberty)
Constitutional	Adrenal lesions
Sporadic	Congenital adrenal
Familial	hyperplasia
Cerebral/neurogenic	Tumours
Tumours	Cushing's syndrome/
Development defects	hyperplasia
CNS infections	Ovarian tumours
CNS trauma	Testicular tumours
McCune–Albright	Iatrogenic (sex hormones)
syndrome	
Neurofibromatosis	*Extrapituitary gonadotrophin-*
Tuberous sclerosis	*secreting tumours*
Silver's syndrome	Teratoma
Hypothyroidism	Chorionepithelioma
Pineal lesions	Hepatoblastoma

Incomplete
Premature thelarche,
  pubarche

CNS, central nervous system.

REFERENCES

1 Ducharme JR, Forest MG, De Peretti E *et al*. Plasma adrenal and gonadal sex steroids in human pubertal development. *J Clin Endocrinol Metab* 1976; **42**: 468–76.
2 Rayner PHW. Early puberty. In: Brook CGD, ed. *Clinical Paediatric Endocrinology*. Oxford: Blackwell Scientific Publications, 1981: 224–39.
3 Silver HK. Asymmetry, short stature, and variations in sexual development: a syndrome of congenital malformations. *Am J Dis Child* 1964; **107**: 495–515.

Delayed puberty and hypogonadism

Puberty can be considered delayed if there is no sign of sexual development by the age of 15 years in boys and 14 years in girls [1]. There are a number of important causes, listed in Table 74.4. Constitutional delay accounts for at least 50% of male cases, and is much more common than in girls [1].

As with premature puberty, pubertal delay requires endocrinological investigation. However, a dermatologist can make a useful contribution if the patient presents first in the skin clinic. For example, examination may reveal the obesity, short stature and mental retardation of the Prader–

Table 74.4 Causes of delayed puberty. (From Chaussain [1], Kulin [2] and Santen and Kulin [3].)

Constitutional delay
Hypogonadotrophism
  Isolated gonadotrophin deficiency
    Hypogonadotrophic eunuchoidism (Kallmann's syndrome)
  Multiple hormonal deficiency states
    Idiopathic
    Tumours
    Langerhans' cell histiocytosis
    Tuberculosis
    Sarcoidosis
    Vascular disease
    Haemochromatosis
  Hyperprolactinaemia
  Specific syndromes with hypogonadotrophism
    Prader–Willi
    Laurence–Moon–Biedl
    Multiple lentigines
    Rud's
    Cerebellar ataxia
  Systemic disease
    Chronic renal failure
    Congenital heart disease
    Cystic fibrosis
    Thalassaemia major
    Diabetes mellitus
    Hypothyroidism
    Gluten intolerance
    Anorexia nervosa
  Excessive exercise
Hypergonadotrophic hypogonadism
  Klinefelter's syndrome
  Ullrich–Turner's syndrome
  Dystrophia myotonica
  Trisomy 21 (Down's syndrome)
  17β-Hydroxylase deficiency
  Androgen insensitivity (testicular feminization syndrome)
  Surgical accidents (e.g. during herniorraphy)
  Testicular torsion
  Anorchia and bilateral cryptorchidism
  Irradiation and cytotoxic drugs
  Orchitis (e.g. mumps)
  Polycystic ovarian disease

Willi syndrome, the polydactyly of the Laurence–Moon–Biedl syndrome, or the increased height and gynaecomastia of Klinefelter's syndrome.

Many extraneous factors can also affect the onset of puberty. For example, malnutrition and extreme forms of exercise, such as long-distance running and ballet training, may delay markedly onset of puberty, probably by interfering with hypothalamic triggering mechanisms [4,5].

REFERENCES

1 Chaussain J-L. Late puberty. In: Brook CGD, ed. *Clinical Paediatric Endocrinology.* Oxford: Blackwell Scientific Publications, 1981: 240–7.
2 Kulin HE. Disorders of sexual maturation: delayed adolescence and precocious puberty. In: De Groot LJ, ed. *Endocrinology*, 2nd edn. Philadelphia: WB Saunders, 1989: 1873–99.
3 Santen RJ, Kulin HE. Evaluation of delayed puberty and hypogonadism. In: Santen RJ, Swerdloff RS, eds. *Male Reproductive Dysfunction.* New York: Marcel Dekker, 1986: 145–89.
4 MacConnie SE, Barkan A, Lampman RM *et al.* Decreased hypothalamic gonadotrophin releasing hormone secretion in male marathon runners. *N Engl J Med* 1986; **315**: 411–17.
5 Warren PW. Effects of undernutrition on reproductive function in the human. *Endocrinol Rev* 1983; **4**: 363–77.

The menstrual cycle

Hormonal influences [1,2]

The menstrual cycle involves changes in the genital tract which are brought about by two hormones from the ovary. At the start of each cycle, after menstruation is completed, the repair and proliferation of the endometrium and the synthesis of receptors for progesterone and oestradiol within its cells is effected by the rising secretion of oestradiol. Following ovulation and the formation of the corpus luteum, the rise in progesterone causes the endometrium to double in thickness and the tubular glands to become tortuous and sacculated. The maintenance of this secretory phase is dependent on both oestradiol and progesterone, and the breakdown of the endometrium which causes menstrual bleeding is a consequence of the withdrawal of these hormones. The cyclic hormonal changes also affect the vaginal epithelium, which can be monitored through desquamated cells in vaginal smears, the consistency and pH of the cervical mucus, and several features of the skin.

Synthesis of oestrogens in the ovary first involves the production of the androgens, androstenedione and testosterone, in the theca interna cells of the follicle, and then their aromatization to oestrone and oestradiol in the granulosa cells. These processes are stimulated by LH from the pituitary, but the increased production of oestradiol between the eighth and 10th days of the cycle is also dependent on FSH in the sense that this is responsible for the development of numbers of primary follicles in the early follicular phase, which increases the number of granulosa cells.

Ovulation in the middle of the cycle is associated with surges in both LH and, to a lesser extent, FSH. The surge in LH lasts for about 36 h, and is affected by pulsatile output of GnRH from the hypothalamus. It appears that feedback by oestradiol is responsible. In the early follicular phase, oestradiol acts to inhibit secretion of gonadotrophin, but, as the follicle ripens, a threshold is exceeded which switches the feedback from negative to positive.

REFERENCES

1 O'Riordan JLH, Malan PG, Gould RP, eds. *Essentials of Endocrinology.* Oxford: Blackwell Scientific Publications, 1988.
2 Ross GT. Disorders of the ovary and female reproductive tract. In: Wilson JD, Foster DW, eds. *Textbook of Endocrinology.* Philadelphia: WB Saunders, 1985: 206–58.

Cutaneous changes

Many women notice changes in their skin and hair during the course of the monthly cycle. For example, 70% of Scottish women reported a few acne papules during the premenstrual phase of their cycle, and a significant number of others experienced textural variations. Some found the skin and hair greasier (35%), others drier (16%) [1], despite the fact that sebum production has not reliably been shown to alter significantly. Pre-existing skin disorders, other than acne, may also undergo premenstrual exacerbation; examples are psoriasis, rosacea, atopic dermatitis, lupus erythematosus, anogenital pruritus, recurrent aphthae and herpes simplex [2,3].

Some women experience premenstrual flushing identical in quality to that associated with the menopause. In one study of 120 women with classical features of the so-called premenstrual syndrome, 72% were observed to have such flushing episodes [4]. This phenomenon may be related in part to the general increase in cutaneous vascularity during the second half of the menstrual cycle [5], but detailed investigation of one of these women revealed that each flush (recorded using skin resistance and finger temperature) coincided with a measurable pulse of LH. Identical findings are reported in menopausal flushes (p. 3277), suggesting a common pathogenesis.

Other cutaneous disturbances described in the 'premenstrual syndrome', include minor, non-specific abnormalities and recurrent boils. Premenstrual oedema has also been described, most commonly of the feet and ankles, but occasionally involving the hands and even the face. In rare individuals this may be very marked.

Autoimmune progesterone dermatitis (Fig. 74.2)

There are also patients in whom the regular appearance of skin changes in the premenstrual period is associated with evidence of hypersensitivity to progesterone. This has generally been established by skin testing, deliberate challenge with progesterone, or the presence of antibodies [6], and the term autoimmune progesterone dermatitis has been coined for this syndrome. The cutaneous lesions vary, and may resemble

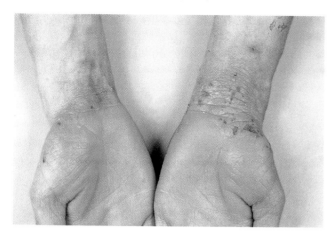

Fig. 74.2 Autoimmune progesterone dermatitis. (Courtesy of Dr J.D. Wilkinson, High Wycombe, UK)

eczema, particularly the pompholyx type, urticaria, erythema multiforme [7] or dermatitis herpetiformis [8]. Many patients develop the eruption after receiving exogenous synthetic progesterone preparations.

Treatment of autoimmune progesterone dermatitis can be difficult. Most patients are unresponsive to topical steroids and antihistamines, but some respond to oestrogen or tamoxifen therapy [6]. One resistant patient required bilateral oophorectomy [8].

REFERENCES

1 Sutherland H. Stewart I. A critical analysis of the premenstrual syndrome. *Lancet* 1965; **i**: 1180–3.
2 Anderson RH. Autoimmune progesterone dermatitis. *Cutis* 1984; **33**: 490–1.
3 Dalton K. Premenstrual tension: an overview. In: Friedmann RC, ed. *Behavior and the Menstrual Cycle*. New York: Marcel Dekker, 1982: 217–42.
4 Casper RF, Graves GR, Reid RL. Objective measurement of hot flushes associated with the premenstrual syndrome. *Fertil Steril* 1987; **47**: 341–4.
5 Edwards EA, Duntley SQ. Cutaneous vascular changes in women in reference to the menstrual cycle and ovariectomy. *Am J Obstet Gynecol* 1949; **57**: 501–9.
6 Stephens CJM, Wojnarowska FT, Wilkinson JD. Autoimmune progesterone dermatitis responding to tamoxifen. *Br J Dermatol* 1989; **121**: 135–7.
7 Wojnarowska FT, Greaves MW, Peachey RGD *et al*. Progesterone-induced erythema multiforme. *J R Soc Med* 1985; **78**: 407–8.
8 Shelley WB, Purcel R, Spount S. Autoimmune progesterone dermatitis. *JAMA* 1964; **190**: 35–8.

Pregnancy, childbirth and the puerperium

Pregnancy, childbirth and the puerperium are associated with profound physiological endocrine upheavals. Many of the consequent cutaneous changes should be considered normal, although not every woman is happy to accept them in this light. The physiological events of pregnancy and its resolution may also modify a number of concomitant dermatoses and tumours, and there are also some pathological skin conditions which are virtually pregnancy-specific.

Endocrine background [1–3]

Pregnancy is characterized by the advent of a new endocrine organ (the placenta). The endocrine changes of pregnancy start soon after the fertilized ovum becomes implanted in the endometrium, when the developing trophoblast begins to secrete chorionic gonadotrophin. This, in turn, stimulates production of oestrogen and progesterone by the corpus luteum. The increase in the concentration of these steroids suppresses the production of FSH by the pituitary and thus prevents further ovulation. At about the ninth week of pregnancy the fetoplacental unit becomes able to synthesize both pregnenolone and progesterone. Pregnenolone crosses to the fetus and is converted to dehydroepiandrosterone by the developing fetal adrenal. This, in turn, is returned to the placenta to be aromatized to oestriol. From the 12th week onwards the fetoplacental unit provides increasing amounts of oestriol and progesterone, and the corpus luteum of pregnancy regresses.

The placenta also produces lactogen (hPL) in quantities as great as 1g/day by late pregnancy. This hormone has some somatotrophic as well as lactogenic properties. A human chorionic thyrotrophin (hCT), structurally different from pituitary thyroid-stimulating hormone (TSH), has also been isolated, and there is evidence that the placenta produces an adrenocorticotrophic hormone (ACTH)-like substance, an LH-releasing hormone and a thyrotrophin-releasing hormone.

Placental hormones, by a variety of interactions, induce physiological adaptations to pregnancy including, for example, a considerable increase in blood volume. The thyroid enlarges and takes up more iodine. The pituitary also enlarges and increases its output of ACTH, prolactin and gonadotrophins. Circulating cortisol rises, due mainly to a decrease in its rate of clearance combined with an increase in cortisol-binding globulin.

The breasts enlarge during pregnancy, most noticeably towards term. In the early phases of the first pregnancy there is a rapid growth and branching of the terminal portions of glandular tissue, together with an increase in the vascularity of the breast as a whole. Later, true acini appear for the first time, and alveolar secretion begins during the second trimester. In the last weeks there is considerable parenchymal cell enlargement and distension of the alveoli with colostrum [3].

The state of pregnancy is terminated, at least in part, by an alteration in the balance of the antagonistic actions of oestrogen and progesterone. This is probably 'fine-tuned' by the fetal pituitary–adrenal axis and its effect on oestrogen production [2]. Thus, abnormalities of the fetal brain, such as anencephaly, may lead to abnormally early or late onset of parturition. The tendency of labour to be delayed in mothers bearing children with X-linked ichthyosis is due to a reduction in the processing of hormones by the placental enzyme steroidal sulphatase (Chapter 34).

After birth, the mother's hormonal status changes yet

again. Levels of prolactin rise steadily towards the end of pregnancy, and at childbirth the apparently inhibitory effect of the fetoplacental steroid hormones is suddenly lost, leaving prolactin acting unopposed. This initiates lactation [3].

REFERENCES

1 Casey ML, Macdonald PC, Simpson ER. Endocrinological changes of pregnancy. In: Wilson JD, Foster DW, eds. *Williams' Textbook of Endocrinology*, 7th edn. Philadelphia: WB Saunders, 1985: 422–37.
2 Buster JE, Simon JA. Placental hormones, hormonal preparation for and control of parturition, and hormonal diagnosis of pregnancy. In: De Groot LJ, ed. *Endocrinology*, 2nd edn. Philadelphia: WB Saunders, 1989: 2043–73.
3 Friesen HG, Cowden EA. Lactation and galactorrhoea. In: De Groot LJ, ed. *Endocrinology*, 2nd edn. Philadelphia: WB Saunders, 1989: 2074–86.

Physiological skin changes related to pregnancy

Pigmentation (Chapter 39)

Most women notice a generalized increase in skin pigmentation during pregnancy, and the change is more marked in dark-haired women than in fair-haired women. Areas that are already pigmented become darker, in particular the nipples, areolae, genital areas and the midline of the abdominal wall. In consequence, the 'linea alba' ('white line') may become brown. The pigmentation usually fades after delivery, but seldom to its previous level. Many women also notice an increase in the size, activity and number of melanocytic naevi.

In about 70% of women, especially those of dark complexion, chloasmal pigmentation also develops during the second half of pregnancy. Its intensity is not necessarily proportional to that of the general melanosis. Irregular, sharply marginated areas of pigmentation develop in a roughly symmetrical pattern either on the forehead and temples, or on the central part of the face, or both. It usually fades completely after parturition, but may persist.

Similar changes occur in other species. The pigmentary changes of pregnancy have been induced experimentally in non-pregnant guinea-pigs by the injection of small doses of oestrogen and progesterone [1]. The extent to which human pigmentary changes are due to these steroids or to melanocyte-stimulating hormones derived from pro-opiomelanocortin (Chapter 39) is uncertain [2–4].

Hair and nail changes

Many women maintain that hair growth on the scalp is more vigorous during pregnancy. In the latter part, the proportion of follicles in anagen rises, but a compensatory decrease after parturition associated with shedding of hairs may result in noticeable postpartum alopecia [5,6]. Spontaneous recovery is usual. Mild frontoparietal recession may also occur [7].

Minor degrees of hypertrichosis are not uncommon. Hirsutism, accompanied by acne and, in severe cases, by other evidence of virilization, occurs rarely, usually during the second half of pregnancy. It may result from an androgen-secreting tumour, luteoma, lutein cysts or polycystic ovary disease [8,9]. All cases should be thoroughly investigated. A female fetus may be masculinized. In the absence of a tumour which can be eradicated, the problem tends to recur in subsequent pregnancies. Hirsutism may regress between pregnancies, but this is not always complete.

Pregnant women often report brittleness of the nail plate, and some develop distal onycholysis, similar to that seen occasionally in thyrotoxicosis [7].

Eccrine, apocrine and sebaceous gland activity

Eccrine activity may be noticeably increased during pregnancy [7], although palmar sweating diminishes [10]. This may be responsible for the recognized increased frequency of miliaria. It is often said that apocrine gland activity is reduced during pregnancy, but the evidence is conflicting. Hurley and Shelley [11] were unable to find any increase in apocrine sweating immediately postpartum, but they pointed out that Fox–Fordyce disease usually improves in pregnancy, which suggests that apocrine activity has been reduced.

Although there is considerable individual variation, the rate of sebum excretion tends to increase during pregnancy and return to normal after delivery [12].

The rise in sebum excretion during the last trimester of pregnancy, at a time when oestrogens, which suppress sebum secretion, are being produced in large quantities, suggests that a powerful sebotrophic stimulus is released. The sebum excretion rate in women with twins or triplets is no greater than the rate in women with a single fetus, suggesting that the sebotrophic factor comes from the pituitary rather than the placenta [13]. Sebum excretion does not fall in women who are lactating [14], and suckling presumably promotes secretion of pituitary factors, such as prolactin, which either stimulate sebaceous glands directly or enhance their response to androgens.

REFERENCES

1 Snell RS, Bischitz PG. The effect of large doses of estrogen and progesterone on melanin pigmentation. *J Invest Dermatol* 1960; **35**: 73–82.
2 Dahlberg BCG. Melanocyte stimulating substances in the urine of pregnant women. *Acta Endocrinol* 1961; **60** (Suppl.): 1–51.
3 McGuinness BW. Melanocyte stimulating hormone: a clinical and laboratory study. In: The pigment cell—molecular, biological and clinical aspects (Part II). *Ann NY Acad Sci* 1963 **100**: 640–57.
4 Thody AJ, Plummer NA, Burton JL *et al.* Plasma β-melanocyte stimulating hormone levels in pregnancy. *J Obstet Gynaecol Br Comm* 1974; **81**: 875–7.
5 Lynfield YL. Effect of pregnancy on the human hair cycle. *J Invest Dermatol* 1960; **35**: 323–7.
6 Pecoraro V, Barman JM, Astore I. The normal trichogram of pregnant women. In: Montagna W, Dobson RL, eds. *Advances in Biology of Skin*, Vol. IX. *Hair Growth*. Oxford: Pergamon, 1969: 203–20.

7 Winton GB, Lewis CW. Dermatoses of pregnancy. *J Am Acad Dermatol* 1982; **6**: 977–8.

8 Fayez JA, Bunch TR, Miller GL. Virilization in pregnancy associated with polycystic ovary disease. *Obstet Gynecol* 1974; **44**: 511–21.

9 Judd HL, Benirschke K, De Vane G *et al*. Maternal virilization developing during a twin pregnancy. *N Engl J Med* 1973; **288**: 118–22.

10 MacKinnon PCB, MacKinnon IL. Palmar sweating in pregnancy. *J Obstet Gynaecol Br Emp* 1955; **62**: 298–9.

11 Hurley HL, Shelley WB. *The Human Apocrine Gland in Health and Disease*. Springfield: Thomas 1960: 65–6.

12 Burton JL, Cunliffe WJ, Millar DG *et al*. Effect of pregnancy on sebum excretion. *Br Med J* 1970; **ii**: 769–71.

13 Burton JL, Shuster S, Cartlidge M. The sebotrophic effect of pregnancy. *Acta Derm Venereol (Stockh)* 1975; **55**: 11–13.

14 Burton JL, Shuster S, Cartlidge M *et al*. Lactation, sebum excretion and melanocyte-stimulating hormone. *Nature* 1973; **243**: 349–50.

Vascular changes

The vascular changes of pregnancy do not differ qualitatively from those in hyperthyroidism or cirrhosis. All are thought to be due to the sustained high levels of circulating oestrogen. Vascular 'spiders' (Chapter 45) are very common in white women but less so in black women [1]. They usually disappear postpartum. Palmar erythema is also common, affecting at least 70% of white women, and 30% of black women [2]. In some, it takes the form of a diffuse, pink mottling of the whole palm, whereas in others the changes are confined to the thenar and hypothenar eminences [3]. Palmar erythema and vascular spiders commonly occur together.

Less commonly, pregnant women develop small haeman-

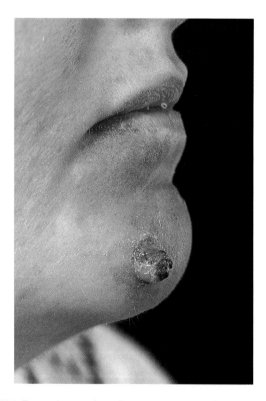

Fig. 74.3 Pyogenic granuloma in a port-wine stain during pregnancy. This woman had similar lesions in three successive pregnancies.

giomas [4,5]. These usually affect the head and neck (Fig. 74.3), and occur in approximately 5% of pregnancies [4].

Varicose veins of the legs and haemorrhoids are frequent complications of pregnancy. A rarer, but more serious, event is the development of deep-vein thrombosis, which can lead to permanent damage to the leg veins and, occasionally, death from pulmonary embolism. Many pregnant women also develop non-pitting oedema of the face, eyelids, feet and hands. The swelling is usually most pronounced in the early morning and disappears during the course of the day. There is no known treatment, but it is important to recognize and differentiate the condition from cardiac, renal or pre-eclamptic oedema.

Gingivitis and pregnancy 'epulis'

Approximately 80% of pregnant women develop some gingival oedema and redness [6]. This can become painful and ulcerative, especially if oral hygiene is poor. In about 2% the gingival changes are associated with the appearance of a small, vascular lesion similar to a pyogenic granuloma, known as a pregnancy epulis or granuloma gravidarum. This may bleed profusely on contact. These phenomena, like palmar erythema and vascular spiders, are probably due to the general increase in vascularity associated with high oestrogen levels.

In most women, gum changes resolve after parturition. Vitamin C has been used to try to improve the symptomatology.

REFERENCES

1 Winton GB, Lewis CW. Dermatoses of pregnancy. *J Am Acad Dermatol* 1982; **6**: 977–98.

2 Cummings K, Derbes VJ. Dermatoses associated with pregnancy. *Cutis* 1967; **3**: 120–5.

3 Black MM, Mayou SC. Skin diseases in pregnancy. In: de Swiet M, ed. *Medical Disorders in Obstetric Practice*, 2nd edn. Oxford: Blackwell Scientific Publications, 1989: 808–29.

4 Hellreich PD. The skin changes of pregnancy. *Cutis* 1974; **13**: 82–6.

5 Letterman G, Schuster M. Cutaneous haemangiomas of the face in pregnancy. *Plast Reconstr Surg* 1962; **29**: 293–300.

6 Hilming F. Gingivitis gravidarum. Studies on clinic and on etiology with special reference to the influence of vitamin C. *Oral Surg Oral Med Oral Pathol* 1952; **5**: 734–51.

Dermatoses modified by pregnancy

Some dermatoses worsen during pregnancy, some improve, and many are unpredictable.

Table 74.5 gives a list of those dermatoses and tumours which are commonly modified by pregnancy and the puerperium. The details of most of these are discussed elsewhere in this book. However, some specific points should be noted here.

Infections and immunity in pregnancy

Cell-mediated immunity is depressed during normal

Table 74.5 Dermatoses and tumours modified by pregnancy.

Infections
Candidiasis
Trichomoniasis
Condylomata acuminata
Pityrosporum folliculitis
Herpes simplex
Herpes varicella/zoster
Leprosy

Autoimmune disorders
Lupus erythematosus
Dermatomyositis/polymyositis
Pemphigus
Systemic sclerosis

Metabolic disorders
Porphyria cutanea tarda
Acrodermatitis enteropathica

Disorders of connective tissue
Ehlers–Danlos syndrome
Pseudoxanthoma elasticum

Tumours
Bowenoid papulosis
Langerhans' cell histiocytosis
Mycosis fungoides
Malignant melanoma
Neurofibromatosis

Miscellaneous
Atopic dermatitis
Erythema multiforme
Erythrokeratoderma variabilis
Psoriasis (and 'impetigo herpetiformis')
Acne
Hidradenitis suppurativa
Fox–Fordyce disease

pregnancy [1], which probably accounts for the increased frequency and severity of certain infections such as candidiasis. Condylomata acuminata, too, can be exacerbated, growing very rapidly and occasionally obstructing the birth canal. *Candida*, genital warts and herpes simplex can be transmitted to the baby during childbirth. In babies of very low birth weight, candidiasis and herpes simplex can be life-threatening [2]. In view of the known oncogenic potential of some strains, there is a debate about whether mothers infected with human papillomavirus should routinely be offered caesarean section, as generally practised for active herpes simplex infection. However, there is doubt whether this practice prevents neonatal infection [3] either by herpesvirus or by genital warts [4]. Bowenoid papulosis (Chapter 72), a condition closely linked with wart virus infection, may appear for the first time, or deteriorate during pregnancy [5].

Podophyllin should never be used in the treatment of warts during pregnancy because of potential maternal and fetal toxicity, and physical treatments are preferable [6].

The immune alterations of pregnancy, childbirth and the puerperium have an adverse effect on leprosy in more than one-third of patients [7]. Leprosy reactional states are more common, and the decline in immune reactivity may also lead to an increase in drug resistance [7]. Furthermore, there are specific problems with some antileprosy drugs: thalidomide cannot be used because of its teratogenicity, and clofazimine has been associated with unexplained fetal deaths [8].

Autoimmune disorders

The outcome of most pregnancies in women with systemic lupus erythematosus is undoubtedly better than was once thought, although a few develop renal damage, and disease exacerbation may be severe enough to cause death [6]. Lupus in the mother may affect the baby (neonatal lupus) (Chapter 14). Cutaneous lupus does not appear to be affected by pregnancy [9].

Most women with systemic sclerosis do not experience major problems, and some appear to improve [10]. Occasionally, however, there is severe, progressive deterioration of renal function, with hypertension and pre-eclampsia. This may lead to fetal loss or even maternal death [11].

Dermatomyositis and polymyositis are generally unaffected by pregnancy, but some patients may deteriorate.

Metabolic disease

There is no consensus about the effects of pregnancy on porphyria cutanea tarda. Some women experience few problems, and Marks suggested that endogenous oestrogen might be less harmful than exogenous compounds because of the complete absence of deterioration of the porphyria during one normal pregnancy [12]. However, some cases do show clinical and biochemical deterioration, and on one occasion this was shown to be parallel to the physiological rise in oestrogen [13]. Acrodermatitis enteropathica is said always to deteriorate in pregnancy [14].

Disorders of connective tissue

Women with Ehlers–Danlos syndrome types I and IV often have major problems, including bleeding, wound dehiscence and uterine lacerations [6] (Chapter 44). They should probably be counselled to avoid pregnancy altogether. Some patients with pseudoxanthoma elasticum have suffered major gastrointestinal bleeds necessitating blood transfusion [15].

Tumours

The relationship between malignant melanoma and pregnancy (and, indeed, exogenous oestrogens) has been discussed for many years [6]. One large series suggests that melanoma developing during pregnancy carries a slightly worse prognosis, but that pregnancy following excision of a tumour does not affect prognosis [16]. Epidemiological studies from the USA have failed to show significant associations between melanoma and reproductive and other hormonal factors in women [17]. Neurofibromas may grow during pregnancy, or appear for the first time. Rupture of major blood vessels in neurofibromatosis has also been reported [18,19], and hypertension is a common complication. Pregnancy may exacerbate mycosis fungoides [20] and the eosinophilic granuloma form of Langerhans' cell histiocytosis [21].

Miscellaneous dermatoses

Atopic dermatitis often improves in pregnancy, but this is unpredictable; in some patients it is exacerbated. Breast feeding is often a problem for those suffering from atopic dermatitis because of nipple eczema, and the puerperium may herald a deterioration in hand eczema because of exposure to irritants.

Pregnancy may trigger erythema multiforme, and vaginal stenosis has been described in severe Stevens–Johnson syndrome occurring in pregnancy [22].

Marked deterioration in erythrokeratoderma variabilis occurred during pregnancy in two related women [23].

The effects of pregnancy on psoriasis are variable, although often consistent in the same individual. A rare occurrence is the sudden eruption of acute pustular psoriasis. This used to be considered as a distinct entity called *impetigo herpetiformis*, but this term is probably best discarded.

Acne may improve, but is occasionally exacerbated during pregnancy. This can cause management problems, because a number of antiacne drugs are contraindicated in pregnancy.

Hidradenitis suppurativa and Fox–Fordyce disease often improve considerably, and it is generally presumed that this is due to a reduction in apocrine gland activity.

REFERENCES

1 Weinberg ED. Pregnancy-associated depression of cell-mediated immunity. *Rev Infect Dis* 1984; **5**: 814–31.
2 Chapel TA, Gagliardi C, Nichols W. Congenital cutaneous candidiasis. *J Am Acad Dermatol* 1982; **6**: 926–8.
3 Prober CG, Sullender WM, Yasukawa LL *et al.* Low risk of herpes simplex virus infections in neonates exposed to the virus at the time of vaginal delivery to mothers with recurrent genital herpes simplex virus infections. *N Engl J Med* 1989; **314**: 240–4.
4 Chuang TY. Condylomata acuminata (genital warts). *J Am Acad Dermatol* 1987; **16**: 376–84.
5 Patterson JW, Kao GF, Graham JH *et al.* Bowenoid papulosis: a clinicopathologic study with ultrastructural observations. *Cancer* 1986; **57**: 823–36.
6 Winton GB. Skin diseases aggravated by pregnancy. *J Am Acad Dermatol* 1989; **20**: 1–13.
7 Duncan ME, Pearson JMH, Ridley DS *et al.* Pregnancy and leprosy: the consequences of alterations of cell-mediated and humoral immunity during pregnancy and lactation. *Lepr Rev* 1982; **55**: 129–42.
8 Farb H, West DP, Pedvis-Leftick A. Clofazimine in pregnancy complicated by leprosy. *Obstet Gynecol* 1982; **59**: 122–3.
9 Yell JA, Burge SM. The effect of hormonal changes on cutaneous disease in lupus erythematosus. *Br J Dermatol* 1993; **129**: 18–22.
10 Johnson TR, Banner EA, Winkelmann RK. Scleroderma and pregnancy. *Obstet Gynecol* 1964; **23**: 467–9.
11 Karlen JR, Cook WA. Renal scleroderma and pregnancy. *Obstet Gynecol* 1974; **44**: 349–54.
12 Marks R. Porphyria cutanea tarda. *Arch Dermatol* 1982; **118**: 452.
13 Lamon JM, Frykholm BC. Pregnancy and porphyria cutanea tarda. *Genet Clin Johns Hopkins Hosp* 1979; **145**: 235–7.
14 Bronson DM, Barsky R, Barsky S. Acrodermatitis enteropathica: recognition at long last during a recurrence in pregnancy. *J Am Acad Dermatol* 1983; **9**: 140–4.
15 Lao TT, Walters BNJ, de Swiet M. Pseudoxanthoma elasticum and pregnancy: two case reports. *Br J Obstet Gynaecol* 1984; **91**: 1049–50.
16 MacKie RM, Bufalino R, Sutherland C. The effect of pregnancy on melanoma prognosis. *Br J Dermatol* 1990; **123** (Suppl. 37): 40.
17 Holly EA, Cress RD, Ahn DK. Cutaneous melanoma in women. III. Reproductive factors and oral contraceptive use. *Am J Epidemiol* 1995; **141**: 943–50.
18 Brade DB, Bolan JC. Neurofibromatosis and spontaneous hemothorax in pregnancy: two case reports. *Obstet Gynecol* 1984; **63** (Suppl.): 35–8.
19 Tapp E, Hickling RS. Renal artery rupture in a pregnant woman with neurofibromatosis. *J Pathol* 1969; **97**: 398–402.
20 Vonderheid EC, Dellatore DL, van Scott EJ. Prolonged remission of tumor-stage mycosis fungoides by topical immunotherapy. *Arch Dermatol* 1981; **117**: 586–9.
21 Growdon WA, Cline M, Tesler A *et al.* Adverse effects of pregnancy on multifocal eosinophilic granuloma. *Obstet Gynecol* 1986; **67** (Suppl.): 2–6.
22 Graham-Brown RAC, Cochrane GW, Swinhoe JR *et al.* Vaginal stenosis due to bullous erythema multiforme (Stevens–Johnson syndrome). *Br J Obstet Gynaecol* 1981; **88**: 1156–7.
23 Gewirtzman GB, Winkler NW, Dobson RL. Erythrokeratoderma variabilis, a family study. *Arch Dermatol* 1978; **114**: 112–14.

AIDS and pregnancy

AIDS is a worldwide problem, and there have now been many pregnancies in women infected by human immunodeficiency virus (HIV). The infection has often only become apparent after birth when the children developed AIDS, although it appears that pregnancy may accelerate the development of AIDS symptoms [1,2]. If opportunistic infections, such as *Pneumocystis* pneumonia or listeriosis, develop in a pregnant woman with AIDS, the outcome is generally fatal [3,4]. This contrasts with the more usual 70% recovery rate in non-pregnant AIDS patients and suggests that the immune suppression of pregnancy may be additive to that of HIV infection. Kaposi's sarcoma has also been reported in AIDS in pregnancy [5]. The effects of maternal HIV infection on the child can be devastating [6].

REFERENCES

1 Minkoff H, Nanda D, Menez R *et al.* Pregnancies resulting in infants with acquired immunodeficiency syndrome or AIDS-related complex. *Obstet Gynecol* 1987; **69**: 285–7.
2 Minkoff H, Nanda D, Menez R *et al.* Pregnancies resulting in infants with acquired immunodeficiency syndrome or AIDS-related complex: follow-up of mothers, children, and subsequently born siblings. *Obstet Gynecol* 1987; **69**: 288–91.
3 Minkoff H, de Regt RH, Landesman S *et al. Pneumocystis carinii* pneumonia associated with acquired immunodeficiency syndrome in pregnancy: a report of three maternal deaths. *Obstet Gynecol* 1986; **67**: 284–7.
4 Wetli CV, Roldan ED, Fujaco RM. Listeriosis as a cause of maternal death: an obstetric complication of acquired immunodeficiency syndrome (AIDS). *Am J Obstet Gynecol* 1983; **147**: 7–9.
5 Rawlinson KF, Zubrow AB, Harris MA *et al.* Disseminated Kaposi's sarcoma in pregnancy: a manifestation of acquired immune deficiency syndrome. *Obstet Gynecol* 1984; **63** (Suppl.): 2–6.
6 Winton GB. Skin disease aggravated by pregnancy. *J Am Acad Dermatol* 1989; **20**: 1–13.

The dermatoses of pregnancy

Irritation, rashes and other skin changes are common in pregnancy. The possibility that the patient has an unrelated skin condition such as scabies must not be overlooked. There are, however, several skin changes which appear to be specifically related to pregnancy and the puerperium, distinct from physiological events, and not due to exacerbation of a pre-existing condition.

Pruritus gravidarum

Itching in pregnancy is dealt with here because it is uncertain whether it is an extension of the physiological changes, or a specific dermatosis [1–3].

As many of one-fifth of pregnant women experience some itching [4]. In most, this can be attributed to some identifiable skin disorder such as scabies, eczema, urticaria, a drug eruption or one of the specific, pregnancy-related, inflammatory dermatoses discussed below. However, there is also a small group of women who experience intense pruritus without evident primary cutaneous changes, and it is to these patients that the term pruritus gravidarum is applied.

It is generally considered that pruritus gravidarum is a mild variant of recurrent cholestasis of pregnancy, and occurs in 0.02–2.4% of pregnancies [5]. The itching usually begins in the third trimester and is often localized to the abdomen, although it may also be very widespread. The patient may be mildly icteric. Liver–function tests are occasionally abnormal, with a raised alkaline phosphatase [2].

It is probable that the irritation results from abnormal hepatic excretion of bile acids induced by endogenous oestrogen and progesterone, both of which have been shown to affect the handling of bile acids [6,7].

The itching usually subsides rapidly after childbirth, but may persist for some weeks into the puerperium. It may also recur with subsequent pregnancies, and the use of oral contraceptive pills. Recurrent attacks increase the liability to cholelithiasis [4].

Striae

Striae distensae (striae gravidarum) are a common and striking feature of most pregnancies. They are dealt with fully in Chapter 44.

Skin tags

SYN. MOLLUSCUM FIBROSUM GRAVIDARUM

Multiple tags often appear in the second half of pregnancy. These are most common on the face, the side of the neck, in the axillae and under the breasts. The histological features are those of ordinary skin tags [8]. They are usually small, but may reach 5 mm in size. They generally regress in the puerperium, and it has been suggested that they are probably due to hormonal factors [2].

'Cracked' and sore nipples

Many women experience discomfort, irritation and fissuring of the nipples, especially early in the puerperium as they are trying to establish breastfeeding. Anatomical features, such as relatively flat nipples, contribute to the development of this problem. Mastitis and deep abscesses may occur due to penetration of the broken skin by pyogenic bacteria. The problem is, in essence, one of friction and irritation, and can be eased considerably by the judicious use of gentle cleansing and emollients.

Inflammatory dermatoses specific to pregnancy

Classification. The older literature is confusing. Dermatoses considered distinct by some authors are lumped together by others. Holmes and Black [9] have suggested a rationalization of the terminology, and have proposed a classification which seems the most logical for practical use (Table 74.6), even though alternatives are still employed. Ackerman and colleagues wish to go further. They argue [10] that there really are only two dermatoses in this category: pruritic urticarial papules and plaques of pregnancy (PUPPP) and pemphigoid gestationis. However, I shall briefly discuss some of the other dermatoses that have been reported as being pregnancy-associated, drawing attention to those descriptions that appear to be at least clinically distinct from PUPPP or pemphigoid gestationis, and reviewing whether others are really distinct entities or not.

Pemphigoid (herpes) gestationis [11,12]

This rare and highly characteristic disorder affects approximately one in 150 000 pregnancies and is considered in detail in Chapter 40. The disease usually appears in the second or third trimester, and presents with an intensely itchy urticarial or vesiculobullous eruption. Immunofluorescence reveals a linear band of IgG at the basement-membrane zone, identical to that seen in bullous pemphigoid. Recent studies involving tissue typing have supported earlier suggestions of a genetic predisposition [13].

Polymorphic eruption of pregnancy

SYN. PRURITIC URTICARIAL PAPULES AND PLAQUES OF PREGNANCY

In addition to the above designations, these skin changes have been known as toxaemic rash of pregnancy [14], toxic erythema of pregnancy [15] and 'late-onset' prurigo of

Table 74.6 Specific dermatoses of pregnancy. (From Shornick [12].)

Pemphigoid (herpes) gestationis
Polymorphic eruption of pregnancy
Prurigo of pregnancy
Pruritic folliculitis of pregnancy

pregnancy [16]. It is probable also that some patients with this condition have been recorded in the literature as prurigo gestationis (see below), erythema multiforme and pemphigoid (herpes) gestationis.

If there is agreement that all these disorders are one and the same, there is still no consensus on which name to use. In the UK, as proposed by Holmes and Black [9,11], the term polymorphic eruption of pregnancy is favoured. Elsewhere, the lengthy descriptive phrase 'pruritic urticarial papules and plaques of pregnancy' or 'PUPPP', as suggested by Lawley *et al.* [17], still finds favour.

Incidence. Polymorphic eruption of pregnancy occurs in approximately one in 240 pregnancies [2]. The eruption begins in the third trimester, usually of a first pregnancy, but is occasionally delayed until a few days postpartum. It rarely recurs in subsequent pregnancies [11,17,18], but when it does it is often less severe [2].

Aetiology. The cause remains obscure, although the condition has been related to abnormal weight gains in the mother and the newborn, and to twin pregnancy [19]. As the disorder occurs predominantly in primigravidae in the third trimester, it has been postulated that excessive abdominal distension may act as a trigger for the skin changes.

Pathology [11,16,17]. The histology of this condition is non-specific, and there are many similarities with the early, prebullous phase of pemphigoid gestationis. Most biopsies show epidermal and upper dermal oedema, with a perivascular infiltrate of lymphocytes and histiocytes. There may be a striking number of eosinophils (as there may be in pemphigoid gestationis). Spongiotic vesicles are also seen, and there may be patchy parakeratosis.

Immunofluorescence is uniformly negative, even by immunoelectron microscopy, and this provides the best means of distinguishing this disorder from pemphigoid gestationis, should there be any diagnostic doubt [20].

Clinical features [11,16,17]. The patient usually complains of intense itching. The skin lesions closely resemble the very early stage of pemphigoid gestationis. The eruption consists predominantly of urticated papules and plaques. Less commonly, vesicles, target lesions and polycyclic erythematous areas are seen.

The most striking feature, however, is the distribution of the lesions. They usually begin, and predominate, on the abdomen, often closely following the lines of the striae, where present (Fig. 74.4). The umbilicus is frequently spared. Lesions often also appear on the upper arms and thighs.

Despite the outdated term toxaemic rash of pregnancy, there is no suggestion that polymorphic eruption has any adverse effect on the outcome of the pregnancy. Indeed, the babies tend to be larger than normal [19].

Treatment. Some patients improve with topical calamine or steroids and systemic sedative antihistamines. Most women are relieved to learn that the condition is not serious, that all should be well with them and their baby, and that the rash will disappear at or soon after childbirth.

Prurigo of pregnancy [16]

SYN. EARLY-ONSET PRURIGO OF PREGNANCY; PRURIGO GESTATIONIS OF BESNIER

The main differences between this disorder and polymorphic eruption of pregnancy are that it begins earlier—usually between 25 and 30 weeks' gestation—and that there are no urticated lesions. It occurs in one in 300 pregnancies.

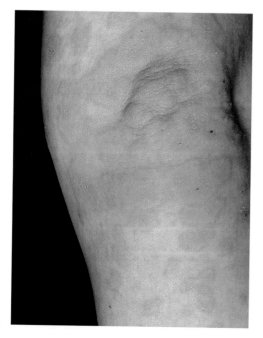

(a)

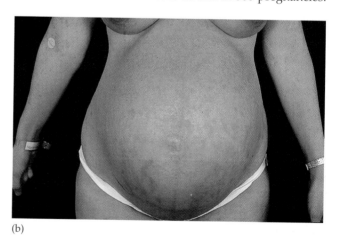

(b)

Fig. 74.4 Typical lesions of polymorphic eruption of pregnancy: (a) on the arm, and (b) on the abdomen. (Courtesy of Dr D.A. Burns, Leicester Royal Infirmary, UK).

Clinically, there are multiple excoriated papules over the abdomen and on the extensor surfaces of the limbs. Histology reveals acanthosis and parakeratosis, with perivascular lymphocytic infiltration around upper dermal vessels. Immunofluorescence is negative. The lesions tend to persist throughout pregnancy, and may continue well into the puerperium, although the pruritic element often settles shortly after delivery [2]. As with polymorphic eruption of pregnancy, the mother and fetus are unaffected, but prurigo of pregnancy may recur in successive pregnancies, which can cause significant distress to the pregnant woman.

Only symptomatic treatment is available, and this is often rather unsatisfactory.

Pruritic folliculitis of pregnancy [21]

This disorder begins in the second or third trimester, and usually resolves within 2 weeks of delivery. The eruption consists of masses of itchy, red, follicular papules. It strongly resembles steroid-induced acne. Histology reveals a nonspecific folliculitis. Immunofluorescence is negative. There is no adverse effect on mother or baby.

Less well-defined dermatoses

Papular dermatitis of pregnancy

Considerable controversy surrounds this entity. It was first described by Spangler and coworkers in 1962, who reported a widespread papular eruption, which they estimated to occur only once in every 2400 pregnancies [22]. In the original description, the rash consisted of widespread, 3–5 mm, intensely itchy papules with a smaller, central crust. There were several laboratory abnormalities, including markedly raised urinary chorionic gonadotrophin levels and low urinary oestriol. Of most significance was the observation that there appeared to be a 30% fetal mortality with this eruption. However, there have been no other convincing reports, and a recent review of 85 patients found no evidence of increased fetal loss [23]. The confusion may have arisen because Spangler and coworkers included fetal deaths in pregnancies unaffected by a rash, and spontaneous abortions without qualifying these by gestational age [2].

It is now generally accepted that the changes reported as papular dermatitis of pregnancy are probably those of pregnancy prurigo, and that the fetal loss in Spangler's series was overestimated.

Autoimmune progesterone dermatitis of pregnancy

There is a single case report of a patient who developed an odd, acneiform rash on the extremities and buttocks in two successive pregnancies [24]. There was an associated arthritis and a positive skin-test reaction to progesterone. The author used the term autoimmune progesterone dermatitis to describe this phenomenon, thereby leading to confusion with the condition of the same name which is not pregnancy associated (see above). However, the clinical features of the two disorders are quite distinct.

Prurigo annularis

Two reported cases [7] had annular, scaly lesions which persisted for years postpartum. Whether it really had anything to do with the pregnancy must be in doubt.

REFERENCES

1 Anonymous. Itching in pregnancy. *Br Med J* 1975; **3**: 608.
2 Black MM, Mayou SC. Skin diseases in pregnancy. In: de Swiet M, ed. *Medical Disorder in Obstetric Practice*, 2nd edn. Oxford: Blackwell Scientific Publications, 1989: 808–29.
3 Winton GB, Lewis CW. Dermatoses of pregnancy. *J Am Acad Dermatol* 1982; **6**: 977–98.
4 Furhoff WR. Itching in pregnancy. A 15-year follow-up study. *Acta Med Scand* 1974; **196**: 403–10.
5 Alcalay J, Wolf JE. Pruritic urticarial papules and plaques of pregnancy: the enigma and the confusion. *J Am Acad Dermatol* 1988; **19**: 1115–16.
6 Holzbach RT. Jaundice in pregnancy. *Am J Med* 1976; **61**: 367–76.
7 Sasseville D, Wilkinson RD, Schnader JY. Dermatoses of pregnancy. *Int J Dermatol* 1981; **20**: 223–41.
8 Cummings K, Derbes VJ. Dermatoses associated with pregnancy. *Cutis* 1967; **3**: 120–5.
9 Holmes RC, Black MM. The specific dermatoses of pregnancy. *J Am Acad Dermatol* 1983; **8**: 405–12.
10 Ackerman AB, Cavegn BM, Robinson MJ, Abad-Casintahan MF. *Ackerman's Resolving Quandaries in Dermatology, Pathology and Dermatopathology.* Baltimore: Williams and Wilkins, 1995: 219–21.
11 Holmes RC, Black MM. The specific dermatoses of pregnancy: a reappraisal with special emphasis on a proposed simplified clinical classification. *Clin Exp Dermatol* 1982; **7**: 65–73.
12 Shornick JK. Herpes gestationis. *J Am Acad Dermatol* 1987; **17**: 539–56.
13 Shornick JK, Jenkins RD, Artlett CM *et al.* Class II MHC typing in pemphigoid gestationis. *Clin Exp Dermatol* 1995; **20**: 123–6.
14 Bourne G. Toxaemic rash of pregnancy. *Proc R Soc Med* 1962; **55**: 462–4.
15 Holmes RC, Black MM, Dann J *et al.* A comparative study of toxic erythema of pregnancy and herpes gestationis. *Br J Dermatol* 1982; **106**: 499–510.
16 Nurse DS. Prurigo of pregnancy. *Australas J Dermatol* 1968; **9**: 258–67.
17 Lawley TJ, Hertz KC, Wade TR *et al.* Pruritic urticarial papules and plaques of pregnancy. *JAMA* 1979; **241**: 1696–9.
18 Yancey KB, Hall RP, Lawley TJ. Pruritic urticarial papules and plaques of pregnancy. *J Am Acad Dermatol* 1984; **10**: 473–80.
19 Cohen LM, Capeless EL, Krusinski PA *et al.* Pruritic urticarial papules and plaques of pregnancy and its relationship to maternal–fetal weight gain and twin pregnancy. *Arch Dermatol* 1989; **125**: 1534–6.
20 Jurecka W, Holmes RC, Black MM *et al.* An immunoelectron microscopy study of the relationship between herpes gestationis and polymorphic eruption of pregnancy. *Br J Dermatol* 1983; **108**: 147–51.
21 Zoberman E, Farmer ER. Pruritic folliculitis of pregnancy. *Arch Dermatol* 1981; **117**: 20–2.
22 Spangler AS, Reddy W, Bardiwal WA *et al.* Papular dermatitis of pregnancy. *JAMA* 1962; **181**: 577–81.
23 Vaughan Jones SA, Bhogal BS, Black MM. A prospective study of the specific dermatoses of pregnancy in 85 pregnant women including hormone profiles and effects on pregnancy outcome. *Br J Dermatol* 1996; **135** (Suppl. 47): 18.
24 Bierman SM. Autoimmune progesterone dermatitis. *Arch Dermatol* 1973; **107**: 896–901.

The menopause

Hormonal and physiological changes

Strictly speaking, the menopause is a fixed, single point in a woman's life: it is her last menstrual period [1–4]. The surrounding years, or climacteric, are a time of change and readjustment to the new phase which the menopause brings. Literally, climacteric means a step up the ladder. It is a crucial phase for a woman, preparing her for the years to come which, in modern societies at least, may now represent as much as one-third of her life [5].

The age of menopause has been the subject of much study, and some of the data have been criticized because of flaws in its collection and interpretation [6]. However, menopause occurs between the ages of 45 and 55 years in 65–70% of women, and the median age in most Western populations is around 50 years. The onset appears to occur a little earlier in developing countries than in Western societies [6], a fact which may be related to nutritional status, as there is also a relationship between body weight and menopausal age [7]. True premature menopause before the age of 40 occurs in less than 1% of women [8], but can follow surgery, irradiation, viral infections (especially mumps), accompany various enzymatic and hormonal defects, or be associated with a number of systemic disorders, such as Addison's disease, rheumatoid arthritis, diabetes or myasthenia gravis [1].

During the reproductive years, oestrogen is produced mainly by ovarian follicles, but at the menopause there are very few follicles left, the ovaries become atrophic, and the levels of ovary-derived oestrogen fall. There may be intermittent bursts of oestrogen in the immediate post-menopausal period due to residual follicular activity, but ultimately the level of plasma oestradiol falls to less than 20 pg/l for the rest of the woman's life [6]. The ratio of oestradiol to oestrone changes, with oestrone becoming the more abundant hormone [9]. After the menopause, most oestrogens are derived from the direct peripheral conversion to oestrone of androstenedione, which has been produced by the adrenals. Some oestrone may arise through the alternative pathway via testosterone and oestradiol [6]. The pituitary–gonadal feedback loop is virtually absent, and levels of gonadotrophins are elevated in consequence.

These hormonal changes are reflected in a number of physiological changes [1]. Breast glandular tissue decreases, and fibrous tissue increases. The body of the uterus becomes smaller and its muscles are partly replaced by fibrous tissue, and the endometrium regresses and becomes atrophic. However, it still retains the capacity to respond to exogenous hormones. The vagina becomes shorter and narrower, and the vaginal epithelium atrophies. The pH of the vagina rises, and infections become more frequent. The external genitalia atrophy, with a loss of vulval subcutaneous fat, and thinning of the vulval epithelium. Pubic hair diminishes.

The epithelium of the lower urinary tract also atrophies and this, together with the increased tendency to prolapse, increases the frequency of urinary tract infections. There is a loss of elasticity in the pelvic supporting ligaments, contributing to prolapse.

There are no structural cutaneous changes that are specifically associated with the menopause, but there are oestrogen receptors in the skin, suggesting that the skin is a target organ for oestrogen and that its withdrawal may be important [10]. It is interesting that there is a far greater concentration of oestrogen receptors in facial skin than in skin on the breasts or thigh. It is possible that some of the changes seen after the menopause, such as dryness, epidermal thinning and loss of dermal elasticity, may result, in part, from lower circulating oestrogen levels. Certainly, administration of oestrogen to castrated animals leads to thickening of the dermis and decreased breakdown of collagen. Oestrogen given to postmenopausal women also increases dermal thickness [11], and in preliminary studies has been shown to improve skin elasticity and deformability [12]. The application of topical oestrogens to the face in menopausal women has also been reported to improve various parameters, including reduction in the depth of wrinkles [13]. However, the picture is not as clear-cut with regard to the epidermis. Animal work has suggested a biphasic response, with initial thickening and later thinning [14], whereas human studies have produced conflicting results [11]. Hormone-replacement therapy (HRT) may increase the skin's water-holding capacity [15].

REFERENCES

1 Barbo DM. The physiology of the menopause. *The Postmenopausal Woman. Med Clin North Am* 1987; **71**: 11–22.
2 Hammond CB. Menopause—an American view. In: Campbell S, ed. *The Management of the Menopause and Post-Menopausal Years*. London: MTP Press, 1976: 405–21.
3 London DR, Shaw RW. Gynaecological endocrinology. In: O'Riordan JLH, ed. *Recent Advances in Endocrinology and Metabolism*. Edinburgh: Churchill Livingstone, 1981: 91–110.
4 Ross GT. Disorders of the ovary and female reproductive tract. In: Wilson JD, Foster DW, eds. *Williams' Textbook of Endocrinology*, 7th edn. Philadelphia: WB Saunders, 1981: 206–58.
5 Brenner S, Politi Y. Dermatologic diseases and problems of women throughout the life cycle. *Int J Dermatol* 1995; **34**: 369–79.
6 Gosden RG. *Biology of Menopause*. London: Academic Press, 1985: 1–15.
7 Sherman BM, Wallace RB, Bean JA et al. Relationship of body weight to menarchal and menopausal age: implications for breast cancer risk. *J Clin Endocrinol Metab* 1979; **52**: 488–93.
8 Coulam CB, Anderson SC, Annegan JF. Incidence of primary ovarian failure. *Obstet Gynecol* 1986; **67**: 604–6.
9 Baird DT. Synthesis and secretion of steroid hormones by the ovary *in vivo*. In: Zuckerman L, Weir JB, eds. *The Ovary*, vol 3, 2nd edn. New York: Academic Press, 1977: 305–57.
10 Hasselquist M, Goldberg N, Schreter A et al. Isolation and characterisation of the estrogen receptors in human skin. *J Clin Endocrinol Metab* 1980; **50**: 76–82.
11 Marks R, Shahrad F. Skin changes at the time of the climacteric. *Clin Obstet Gynecol* 1977; **4**: 207–26.
12 Pierard GE, Letawae C, Dowlatti A et al. Effect of hormone replacement therapy for menopause on the mechanical properties of skin. *J Am Geriatr Soc* 1995; **43**: 662–5.
13 Schmidt JB, Binder M, Macheiner W et al. Treatment of skin ageing symptoms in perimenopausal females with estrogen compounds. A pilot study. *Maturitas* 1994; **20**: 25–30.
14 Ebling FJ. Some effects of oestrogen on epidermis. *J Endocrinol* 1953; **9**: 31–2.
15 Pierard-Franchimont C, Letawe C, Goffin V et al. Skin water-holding capacity and transdermal estrogen therapy for menopause: a pilot study. *Maturitas* 1995; **22**: 151–4.

Skin disorders of the menopause

Atrophic vulvovaginitis

It has been known for many years that the atrophic changes in the female external genitalia described above respond, at least partially, to topical oestrogens [1].

Menopausal flushing

The most consistent and distressing complaint associated with the menopause is flushing [2]. This is usually described as a sudden feeling of intense heat in the face, neck and chest, often accompanied by discomfort and sweating. Although the intensity and duration vary, it typically lasts 3–5min. Visible changes occur in about 50% of women, and generally consist of a blotchy erythema on the face, neck, upper chest and breasts. Some women also develop palpitations, throbbing in the head and neck, headaches, waves of nausea and anxiety attacks. Sleep disturbance is not uncommon [3]. It is possible to measure several physiological changes during hot flushes, including increased temperature, pulse rate and respiratory rate [4,5].

Flushes are associated with pulsatile release of LH [6], presumably due to low circulating oestrogen levels and failure of the normal feedback mechanisms. However, flushing can occur after hypophysectomy [7], and so LH itself cannot be responsible for the observed vasomotor instability. One suggested mechanism involves alteration of hypothalamic catecholamine levels, and a failure of normal central thermoregulatory centres through LH-releasing hormone neurones [2]. However, flushes similar to those seen in the menopause can be induced by an enkephalin analogue. This is blocked by naloxone infusions [8], and it seems likely that menopausal hot flushes may also be mediated by an opiate-dependent central mechanism [9].

The consensus is that oestrogen therapy is the most effective treatment for symptomatic hot flushes [2], although not all authorities have always agreed [5]. A non-hormonal alternative, when oestrogens are contraindicated, is a mixture of ergotamine, belladonna alkaloids and phenobarbitone [2].

Keratoderma climactericum

This term has been used to describe the appearance of hard skin on the palms and soles, especially around the heels. Although originally reported as a specific association with the menopause [10], the same changes are seen in men and women at other ages, many of whom are obese. It may, therefore, be a non-specific effect. There has been a report of a therapeutic response to systemic retinoids [11].

Lichen sclerosus et atrophicus

This disorder is considered in detail in Chapter 72 but is mentioned here because of its apparent frequent onset at or around the menopause, and because of the significant symptomatology it may cause.

Complications of HRT

The increasing use of HRT, largely to prevent osteoporosis and cardiovascular disease, has revealed a number of problems associated with this treatment. There is an ongoing debate regarding the relationship between HRT and cancers of the breast and genital tract, but this is beyond the scope of this chapter. However, HRT may be responsible for a number of cutaneous problems, which should at least receive a mention here.

Oestrogen therapy may trigger or exacerbate amongst others: chloasma (melasma); spider angiomas; darkening of naevi; the skin changes of porphyria cutanea tarda; acanthosis nigricans [12,13]. Many clinicians also report encountering urticarial or eczematous dermatoses which appear in patients on HRT and subside on cessation of treatment. Allergic reactions have been reported to the transdermal patches frequently used as delivery systems for HRT. These may be to the adhesives or to the oestrogens themselves [14].

REFERENCES

1 Artner J, Gitsch E. Über lokalwirkungen von Östriol. *Gerburtshilfe Frauenheilk* 1959; **19**: 812–19.
2 Barbo DM. The physiology of the menopause. In: *The Postmenopausal Woman. Med Clin North Am* 1987; **71**: 11–22.
3 Erlick Y, Tataryn IV, Meldrum DR *et al.* Association of waking episodes with menopausal hot flushes. *JAMA* 1981; **245**: 1741–4.
4 Molnar GW. Body temperatures during menopausal hot flushes. *J Appl Physiol* 1975; **38**: 499–503.
5 Mulley G, Mitchell JRA. Menopausal flushing: does oestrogen therapy make sense? *Lancet* 1976; **i**: 1397–8.
6 Ravnikar V, Elkind-Hirsch K, Schiff I *et al.* Vasomotor flushes and the release of peripheral immunoreactive luteinizing hormone releasing hormone in postmenopausal women. *Fertil Steril* 1985; **41**: 881–7.
7 Mulley G, Mitchell JRA, Tattersall RB. Hot flushes after hypophysectomy. *Br Med J* 1977; **2**: 1062.
8 Stubbs WA, Delitala G, Jones A *et al.* Hormonal and metabolic responses to an enkephalin analogue in normal man. *Lancet* 1978; **ii**: 1225–7.
9 Casper RF, Yen SSC. Neuroendocrinology of 3 menopausal flushes: an hypothesis of flush mechanism. *Clin Endocrinol* 1985; **22**: 293–312.
10 Haxthausen H. Keratoderma climactericum. *Br J Dermatol* 1934; **46**: 161–7.
11 Deschamps P, Leory D, Pedailles S *et al.* Keratoderma climactericum (Haxthausen's disease). Clinical signs, laboratory findings and response to etretinate in 10 patients. *Dermatologica* 1986; **172**: 259–62.
12 Graham-Brown RAC. Dermatologic problems of the menopause. *Clin Dermatol* 1997; **15**: 143–5.
13 Banuchi SR, Cohen L, Lorincz AL *et al.* Acanthosis nigricans following diethylstilboestrol therapy. *Arch Dermatol* 1974; **109**: 544–6.
14 Angelini G. Topical drugs. In: Rycroft RJG, Menné T, Frosch PJ, eds. *Textbook of Contact Dermatitis*, 2nd edn. Berlin: Springer-Verlag; 1995: 493.

Old age

Introduction

Senescence in the skin is a gradual process which ultimately results in the appearances and functional differences that we associate with old age. However, by no means all of these changes are purely intrinsic. The skin is particularly vulnerable to the 'ageing' effects of a number of environmental insults, especially UV radiation, and in women there are additional hormonal changes at the menopause (p. 3276). These factors are superimposed on the background changes of intrinsic senescence, and care needs to be exercised in interpreting which are most important in determining any particular aspect of the appearance and function of the skin in an elderly person. There have, however, been increasing efforts to disengage the roles of these intertwined and contemporaneous processes.

Biology of ageing

Ageing is the decline in the power of self-maintenance, the increase in susceptibility to disease, and the growing probability of death as age advances. Ultimate senescence is as much a biological necessity as initial survival; evolutionary progress has occurred because animals are programmed for both. In the words of Macfarlane Burnet [1], 'The two basic evolutionary needs of all species of higher animal are survival to reproductive age, and death when survival offers no reproductive advantages to the species.'

Modern theories of ageing fall into two categories which, philosophically speaking, start from opposite poles. The first views ageing as an ordered process delicately programmed by the genes [2], the second suggests that ageing is caused by the progressive retention and amplification of errors in the replication of genetic information in the somatic cells [1]. From the practical viewpoint, both types of theory emphasize the intrinsic inevitability of the process.

If the ageing of most of the bodily organs has, however reluctantly, to be accepted, the ageing of the facial skin appears to be a matter of widespread concern. The reason is that the skin plays a major part in our social and sexual interactions; the concern is not so much to do with physiological functions, which may remain adequate in old age, but about continuing effectiveness, particularly of the facial skin, in communication. To display sexuality or assert social status it is necessary to have skin and hair which look, feel and smell attractive.

The ageing of skin has so far been studied for social and commercial reasons in affluent white populations. Some of these subjects are ill adapted for the environments they now occupy or the lifestyles they endure or enjoy. It must not therefore be assumed that the data obtained will necessarily apply to skin with greater pigmentation, especially that of Mongoloid and Negroid populations.

The most obvious signs of an ageing skin are atrophy, laxity, wrinkling, sagging, dryness, yellowness, a multiplicity of pigmented and other blemishes, and sparse grey hair. Some of these stigmata clearly have genetic components, and some are mimicked by heritable disorders. The abnormal texture

of the dermis in cutis laxa makes young children look old; in progeria, on the other hand, the connective tissue remains evenly dense, although the epidermis shows mottled pigmentation [3].

Intrinsic changes of ageing fall into two categories: those which appear to be engendered within the tissues themselves, and those which are the result of alterations, including hormonal, caused by senile changes in other organs. An example of the former is the greying of hair, and of the latter, the lowering of sebaceous gland activity consequent upon reduction of androgen secretion.

Into a third category must be put changes which are mainly the result of environmental factors. These may be overriding; for example, it has been stated that on exposed skin more than 90% of age-associated cosmetic problems are caused by UV radiation [4].

REFERENCES

1 Burnet M. *Intrinsic Mutagenesis: a Genetic Approach to Ageing.* Lancaster: MTP Press, 1974.
2 Bergsma D, Harrison DE. *Genetic Effects on Aging.* New York: Alan R Liss, 1978.
3 Lapiere CM. The ageing dermis: the main cause of the appearance of old skin. *Br J Dermatol* 1990; **122** (Suppl. 35): 5–11.
4 Leyden JJ. Clinical features of ageing skin. *Br J Dermatol* 1990; **122** (Suppl. 35): 1–3.

The ageing skin

Dermis

It cannot be doubted that wrinkling of senescent skin is almost entirely the result of changes in the dermis. The debatable questions concern the nature of these changes and the extent to which they are intrinsic or environmentally caused [1,2].

The dermis diminishes in bulk, and in absolute terms the collagen per unit area of unexposed skin decreases with age [3]. There also appears to be a steady decrease in the number and size of mast cells and fibroblasts [2]. While it is often assumed that the lax skin of the aged is due to lack of water, there is evidence that, on the contrary, water content increases between the fourth and ninth decades [4].

Gross morphological changes, especially in the collagen and elastin fibres, have been revealed by electron and light microscopy. Their relationship to molecular changes as determined by physical and chemical methods requires interpretation. Moreover, it has long been clear that such changes are largely the result of exposure to solar radiation [5].

In the dermis of young adults the collagen bundles are well organized. They form a rhomboid network with the individual bundles lying at angles to one another. Intertwined among the collagen bundles lie single branching elastic fibres, apparently aligned haphazardly, in planes parallel with the surface at all levels beneath the dermo-epidermal junction. The network of collagen bundles, although composed of inextensible fibres, is itself extensible as the bundles rotate relative to one another to form parallel alignments. It seems likely that the return of the network to its unstretched state is brought about by the interwoven elastic fibres [6]. Thus, in cutis laxa, an uncommon disorder in which the skin hangs in folds, the elastic fibres appear to be reduced in number and degenerate (Chapter 44).

The various descriptions of changes in ageing based on histological staining techniques are often confusing. In general, it appears that the collagen bundles become fragmented and disorientated, and elastin fibres become progressively reduced [7]. However, in senile skin from exposed areas there may, paradoxically, be a striking increase in fibres which take up elastin stains in actinic elastosis (Chapter 44).

Elastic fibres gradually disintegrate with age, even in protected skin, and after the age of 70 years most fibres appear abnormal [8–10]. Similar changes can be produced in protected buttock skin within hours by incubating it with pancreatic elastase and bovine chymotrypsin [8].

Epidermis

Many differences between a senile and young epidermis have been described, but a consistent interpretation of the ageing process has proved difficult. In part, this is because the epidermis varies from site to site. Young skin from the back [11], like that from the scalp and axilla [12], has deep and complex rete ridges, whereas that of the face [12] has a fairly flat dermo-epidermal junction. It is widely agreed that in areas where the junction is corrugated in youth, it becomes flattened in the aged [12–17].

Similarly, there are differences in epidermal thickness, even in young skin. On the face or on the dorsum of the hand, for example, it is considerably greater than on the arms, legs or trunk [12]. In many areas the whole epidermis becomes thinner with age, and the cells become less evenly aligned on the basement membrane and less regular in size, shape and staining properties [12,16–19].

The question of whether these changes result from alterations in the rate of cell replication has also engendered controversy, largely because of differing methods of study [20]. However, there is now some consensus that the cell turnover rate is halved between the third and seventh decades of life [18,21,22], notwithstanding an earlier finding that the frequency of mitoses in abdominal skin increases from childhood until the fifth decade and then levels out [23]. The evidence that the rate of epidermal repair and wound healing declines with age [24] is consonant with the view that epidermopoeisis is decreased.

The permeability of the skin also changes with age, although some of the data are contradictory [25]. According to Christophers and Kligman [13], the capacity of the isolated horny layer *in vitro* to restrict water loss does not differ between young adults and persons over 70 years of age, but the aged skin is decidedly more permeable to chemical substances. However, *in vivo*, they found that the percutaneous absorption of testosterone appeared to be reduced in old age. A possible explanation is that, although substances enter aged skin more easily than young skin, they are removed more slowly into the circulation because of changes in the dermal matrix and reduction in the vasculature [4]. The response to blistering agents, such as 50% ammonium hydroxide, is initially quicker in old than in young subjects, but the formation of the full blister takes longer [26].

These physiological differences must be largely related to changes in the stratum corneum, yet neither its thickness nor the number of cell layers seem to vary with age, at least on the back [13]. However, Marks [27] showed that the surface area of individual corneocytes from non-exposed areas of the arms, thighs and lower abdomen increases with age, and suggested that this might reflect an increased transit time [28].

A change in the nature of the corneocytes is also indicated by the tendency of the senescent epidermal surface, especially that of the lower legs, to become dry, flaky and sometimes itchy. Apart from reduced function of the skin glands, the water-binding capacity of the stratum corneum appears to be reduced [29].

Pigmentation

The most obvious senile change in white skin is irregularity of pigmentation. Yellow or brown macules, known as 'liver spots', develop on the backs of the hands and exposed parts of the face in more than 50% of persons over 45 years of age. Very rarely such *senile lentigines* develop into *lentigo maligna* which is a precancerous condition, although it progresses very slowly [30].

The senile lentigo consists of a localized proliferation of melanocytes at the dermo-epidermal junction [31]. In general, however, the number of dopa-positive melanocytes in both exposed and unexposed skin decreases in old age, although their size increases. Their reaction to dopa becomes variable, and some no longer donate pigment [30,32,33].

Even heavily pigmented skin darkens. A study of 578 adult natives of New Guinea revealed that pigmentation increased with age in skin exposed to the sun, but not in axillary skin, and that males darkened more than females [34].

Greying of hair

Greying usually becomes evident around the age of 50 years, by which time about half the population has about 50% grey or white body hairs and an even greater proportion has some depigmented scalp hair [35].

The bulbs of grey or white hairs show various abnormalities, but it is uncertain which are critical. In general, the bulbs appear to lack, or be deficient in, tyrosinase, the enzyme necessary for the first stages of melanin synthesis [36]. Structurally, the follicles of grey hairs still have melanocytes placed normally over the dermal papilla, but the cytoplasm may contain large vacuoles and the melanosomes may be only lightly melanized [30]. The follicles of fully white hairs may completely lack melanocytes. However, among grey or white hairs, there may be a few normal bulbs producing dark hairs.

An unexplained fact is that at all ages from their appearance on the chest in males, and probably elsewhere, grey hairs tend to be thicker and longer than pigmented ones [35].

Premature greying of hair, even before the age of 20 years, is a feature of several hereditary syndromes, and is also associated with a number of disorders induced by organ-specific antibodies. A survey of the age prevalence of normal greying of hair in men [37] showed that it fitted a simple mathematical model of ageing consonant with the view that the condition is 'autoaggressive' or 'autoimmune' in character and arises from somatic gene mutations.

Hair follicles [38]

Changes in the hair follicles vary greatly between sites. For example, it can be widely observed that hair becomes sparse on the vertex while it is still luxuriant on the occiput, and that greying usually starts at the temples.

In the scalp, the density of hair follicles steadily decreases with age, more rapidly in bald than in non-bald persons [39]. The overall capacity of the follicles to produce long hairs is progressively reduced, at least on the vertex, and especially in males. This cannot be accounted for by any diminution in the rate of growth, which remains substantially unchanged [40]. It must, therefore, result from a shortening of the duration of anagen. This is reflected by the gradual rise in the proportion of follicles in telogen, both in non-bald subjects [41] and in persons with pattern alopecia, where it becomes evident in advance of visible baldness [42].

Scalp hair also becomes finer, especially in persons with visible alopecia. In a group of 58 white women with diffuse alopecia, 13 of whom were clinically hypothyroid, there was a gradual reduction in mean diameter which appeared to be an exaggeration of a trend also found in normal subjects [43]. The diameters showed a wide range, with a single peak around 0.08 mm in normal persons, but two peaks at 0.04 and 0.06 mm, respectively, in patients with alopecia, suggesting that not all the follicles behave identically.

The weight of beard grown per day reaches a peak in the fourth decade, and starts to decrease slightly in the seventh decade [44]. As the density of the hairs remains constant, the decrease in weight must be accounted for by a reduction

in the rate of growth, in diameter, or in both. Evidence that the linear growth of beard hair is correlated solely with levels of 5 α-dihydrotestosterone (DHT) in the plasma, not with testosterone, whereas hair density is significantly correlated solely with testosterone, not with DHT [45], suggests that the age changes may result not so much from reduced production of testosterone as by lessened peripheral metabolism.

Chest hairs, which are also androgen-dependent, reach a maximum in number, breadth and length around the fifth decade, and then start to diminish markedly [35].

Axillary hair reaches a peak in mass and in rate of production towards the end of the third decade in males and females alike, and this is followed by a rapid decline, somewhat more severe in females [44,46]. Pubic hair appears to follow a similar pattern.

If most of the changes with ageing involve reductions in the amount of hair, this is not true of all sites. In the male the eyebrows may become more bushy, and visible hairs develop around the external auditory meati. In the female, hirsutism may occur as a result of endocrine changes associated with the menopause (p. 3276).

Sebaceous and apocrine glands

Sebum production is at its greatest in early adulthood, and lessens in old age. A view that it remains unchanged until past the age of 70 years in men, but falls after the menopause in women, has not been entirely sustained [47,48].

Measurements of the sustainable rate of wax ester secretion after depletion of the sebum reservoir by absorption with bentonite clay suggest that sebum secretion declines steadily through each decade by about 23% in men and 32% in women [49]. The fatty acid composition also changes [50].

The predominant belief is that, in spite of their decreased output, the sebaceous glands increase in size because turnover of cells is slower in senility [51,52]. However, in one study in 14 women the glands appeared to become smaller, and the sebocytes flatter, with age [53].

The axillary apocrine glands also regress with age and produce less odour [12].

Eccrine glands

Spontaneous sweating on the finger tips declines in old age, due to a combination of a reduction in the number of glands [54] and of the output per gland [55]. On the forearm, the response to adrenalin has been shown to be reduced by ageing equally in men and women, suggesting an intrinsic deterioration of the glands, an interpretation supported by histological evidence. In contrast, the effect of age on the response to mecholyl is much greater in the male than in the female, suggesting that ageing affects cholinergic sweating indirectly through the hormonal balance in the blood [55]. Such a hypothesis is borne out by the evidence that the maximum rate of cholinergic sweating is much greater in adult males than in females or in juveniles, and is thus probably androgen-dependent [56].

Nail growth

The rate of linear nail growth increases until well into the third decade. From about the age of 25 years it starts to decrease. Until the age of 70 years nail growth is greater in men than in women, but thereafter the situation appears to be reversed [57].

Nerves and sensation

Age often decreases sensory perception and increases the threshold for pain [26,58]. There is evidence for progressive disorganization or loss of some sense organs; for example, the density of Meissner corpuscles in the little finger falls from over 30/mm^2 in young adults to about 12 by the age of 70 years [59].

Langerhans' cells and immune functions

Langerhans' cells become considerably reduced in number in elderly people, even in light-protected areas [60,61]. T-cells, similarly, are reduced in percentage and absolute number, and lose their responsiveness to specific antigens [4,62]. The number of B-cells does not seem to be affected by age, but their dysfunction is reflected by increased auto-antibody formation and serum levels of IgA and IgG [62–65]. Elderly skin appears to have a much reduced capacity to produce cytokines such as epidermal cell thymocyte-activating factor [31], and interleukin 2 (IL-2) [66]. However, the production of some cytokines (e.g. IL-4) increases with age [66]. The decreased intensity of delayed hypersensitivity reactions [67], the increased risk of photocarcinogenesis, and the greater susceptibility to chronic skin infections are some of consequences of the ageing of the immune system [21].

REFERENCES

1 Ebling FJG. Physiological background to skin ageing. *Int J Cosmet Sci* 1982; **4**: 103–10.
2 Kligman AM, Lavker RM. Cutaneous aging: the differences between intrinsic aging. *J Cutan Ageing, Cosmetol Dermatol* 1988; **1**: 5–12.
3 Shuster S, Bottoms E. Senile degeneration of skin collagen. *Clin Sci* 1963; **25**: 487–91.
4 Kligman AM. Perspectives and problems in cutaneous gerontology. *J Invest Dermatol* 1979; **73**: 39–46.
5 Knox JM, Cockerell EG, Freeman RG. Etiological factors and premature aging. *JAMA* 1962; **179**: 630–6.
6 Hall DA. *The Ageing of Connective Tissue*. New York: Academic Press, 1976.
7 Boisson H, Pieraggi MT, Julian M et al. In: Robert L, Robert B, eds. *Frontiers of Matrix Biology*, Vol. 1. *Ageing of Connective Tissue, Skin*. Basel: Karger, 1973: 190.
8 Braverman IM, Fonferko E. Studies in cutaneous aging: 1 The elastic fibre network. *J Invest Dermatol* 1982; **78**: 434–43.
9 Stadler R, Orfanos CE. Reifung und Alterung der elastischen Fasern: Electronenmikroskopische Studien in verschiedenen Altersperioden. *Arch Dermatol Res* 1978; **262**: 97.
10 Tsuji T, Hamada T. Age-related changes in human dermal elastic fibres. *Br J Dermatol* 1981; **105**: 57–63.
11 Eller JJ, Eller WD. Oestrogenic ointments. Cutaneous effects of topical applications of natural oestrogens with report of three hundred and twenty-one biopsies. *Arch Dermatol Syphilol* 1949; **59**: 449–64.
12 Montagna W. Morphology of the aging skin: the cutaneous appendages. In: Montagna W, ed. *Advances in Biology of Skin*, Vol. VI. *Aging*. Oxford: Pergamon Press, 1965: 1–16.
13 Christophers E, Kligman AM. Percutaneous absorption in aged skin. In: Montagna W, ed. *Advances in Biology of Skin*. Vol. IV. *Aging*. Oxford: Pergamon Press, 1965: 163–76.
14 Hill WR, Montgomery H. Regional changes and changes caused by age in the normal skin. *J Invest Dermatol* 1940; **3**: 321–45.
15 Lavker RM, Zheng P, Dong G. Morphology of aged skin. *Dermatol Clin* 1986; **4**: 379–84.
16 Montagna W, Carlisle K. Structural changes in aging human skin. *J Invest Dermatol* 1979; **73**: 47–53.
17 Montagna W, Carlisle K. Structural changes in ageing skin. *Br J Dermatol* 1990; **122**: (Suppl. 35): 61–70.
18 Gilchrest BA. *Skin and Ageing Processes*. Boca Raton: CRC Press, 1984.
19 Lavker RM. Structural alterations in exposed and unexposed aged skin. *J Invest Dermatol* 1979; **73**: 59–66.
20 Epstein WL, Maibach HT. Cell renewal in the human epidermis. *Arch Dermatol* 1965; **92**: 462–8.
21 Cerimele D, Celleno L, Serri F. Physiological changes in ageing skin. *Br J Dermatol* 1990; **122** (Suppl. 35): 13–20.
22 Grove GL, Kligman AM. Age-associated changes in human epidermal cell renewal. *J Gerontol* 1983; **38**: 137–42.
23 Thuringer JM, Katzberg AA. The effect of age on mitosis in the human epidermis. *J Invest Dermatol* 1959; **33**: 35–9.
24 Goodson WH III, Hunt TK. Wound healing and aging. *J Invest Dermatol* 1979; **73**: 88–91.
25 Roskos KV, Guy RH, Maibach H. Percutaneous absorption in the aged. In: Gilchrest BA, ed. *Dermatologic Clinics: The Aging Skin*. Philadelphia: WB Saunders, 1986: 455–65.
26 Grove GL, Duncan S, Kligman AM. Effect of ageing on the blistering of human skin with ammonium hydroxide. *Br J Dermatol* 1982; **107**: 393–400.
27 Marks R. Measurement of biological ageing in human epidermis. *Br J Dermatol* 1981; **104**: 627–33.
28 Baker H, Blair CP. Cell replacement in the human stratum corneum in old age. *Br J Dermatol* 1968; **80**: 367–72.
29 Raab WP. The skin surface and stratum corneum. *Br J Dermatol* 1990; **122** (Suppl. 35): 37–41.
30 Fitzpatrick TB, Szabo G, Mitchell RE. Age changes in the human melanocyte system. In: Montagna W, ed. *Advances in Biology of Skin*, Vol. VI, *Aging*. Oxford: Pergamon Press, 1965: 35–50.
31 Cawley EP, Curtis AC. Lentigo senilis. *Arch Dermatol Syphilol* 1950; **62**: 635–41.
32 Gilchrest BA, Blog FB, Szabo G. Effect of aging and chronic sun exposure on melanocytes in human skin. *J Invest Dermatol* 1979; **73**: 141–3.
33 Ortonne JP. Pigmentary changes in the ageing skin. *Br J Dermatol* 1990; **122** (Suppl. 35): 21–8.
34 Walsh RJ. Variation in the melanin content of the skin of New Guinea natives at different ages. *J Invest Dermatol* 1964; **42**: 261–5.
35 Hamilton JB, Terada H, Mestler GE et al. I: Coarse sternal hairs, a male secondary sex character that can be measured quantitatively: the influence of sex, age and genetic factors. II: Other sex-differing characters: relationship to age, to one another, and to values for coarse sternal hairs. In: Montagna W, Dobson RL, eds. *Advances of Biology of Skin*, Vol. IX. *Hair Growth*. Oxford: Pergamon Press, 1969: 129–51.
36 Fitzpatrick TB, Brunet P, Kukita A. The nature of hair pigment. In: Montagna W, Ellis RA, eds. *The Biology of Hair Growth*. New York: Academic Press, 1958: 255–303.
37 Burch PRJ, Murray JJ, Jackson D. The age-prevalence of arcus senilis, greying of hair, and baldness. Etiological considerations. *J Gerontol* 1971; **26**: 364–72.
38 Ebling FJG. Age changes in the cutaneous appendages. *J Appl Cosmetol* 1985; **3**: 243–56.
39 Giacometti L. The anatomy of the human scalp. In: Montagna W, ed. *Advances in Biology of Skin*. Vol VI. *Aging*. Oxford: Pergamon Press, 1965: 97–120.
40 Barman JM, Astore I, Pecoraro V. The normal trichogram of people over 50 years but apparently not bald. In: Montagna W, Dobson RL, eds. *Advances*

in *Biology of Skin*. Vol. IX. *Hair Growth*. Oxford: Pergamon Press, 1969: 211–20.

41 Pecoraro V, Astore I, Barman JM. The pre-natal and post-natal hair cycles in man. In: Baccaredda-Boy A, Moretti G, Frey JR, eds. *Biopathology of Pattern Alopecia, Proceedings of the International Symposium*, Rapallo, Italy, July 1967. Basel: Karger, 1968: 29–38.

42 Braun-Falco O, Christophers E. Hair root pattern in male pattern alopecia. In: Baccaredda-Boy A, Moretti G, Frey JR, eds. *Biopathology of Pattern Alopecia*. Basel: Karger, 1968: 141–5.

43 Jackson D, Church RE, Ebling FJ. Hair diameter in female baldness. *Br J Dermatol* 1972; **87**: 361–7.

44 Hamilton JB. Age, sex and genetic factors in the regulation of hair growth in man: a comparison of Caucasian and Japanese populations. In: Montagna W, Ellis RA, eds. *The Biology of Hair Growth*. New York: Academic Press, 1958: 399–433.

45 Farthing MJG, Mattei AM, Edwards CRW *et al*. Relationship between plasma testosterone and dihydrotestosterone concentrations and male facial hair growth. *Br J Dermatol* 1982; **107**: 559–67.

46 Pecoraro V, Astore I, Barman JM. Growth rate and hair density of the human axilla. A comparative study of normal males and females and pregnant and post-partum females. *J Invest Dermatol* 1971; **56**: 362–5.

47 Pochi PE, Strauss JS. The effect of aging on the activity of the sebaceous gland in man. In: Montagna W, ed. *Advances in Biology of Skin*. Vol. VI, *Aging*. Oxford: Pergamon Press, 121–7.

48 Pochi PE, Strauss JS, Downing DT. Age-related changes in sebaceous gland activity. *J Invest Dermatol* 1979; **73**: 108–11.

49 Jacobsen E, Billings JK, Frantz RA *et al*. Age-related changes in sebaceous wax ester secretion rates in men and women. *J Invest Dermatol* 1985; **85**: 483–5.

50 Yamamoto A, Serizawa S, Ito M *et al*. Effect of aging on sebaceous gland activity and on the fatty acid composition of wax esters. *J Invest Dermatol* 1987; **89**: 507–12.

51 Kumar P, Barton SP, Marks R. Tissue measurements in senile sebaceous gland hyperplasia. *Br J Dermatol* 1988; **118**: 397–402.

52 Plewig G, Kligman AM. Proliferative activity of the sebaceous glands of the aged. *J Invest Dermatol* 1978; **70**: 314–17.

53 Ito N, Mashiko T, Sato Y. Morphological changes of sebaceous glands with ageing in human females; computer graphic analysis and ultrastructural study. *J Invest Dermatol* 1988; **90**: 570.

54 Oberste-Lehn H. Effects of aging on the papillary body of the hair follicles and on the eccrine sweat glands. In: Montagna W, ed. *Advances in Biology of Skin*. Vol. VI. *Aging*. Oxford: Pergamon Press, 1965: 17–34.

55 Silver AF, Montagna W, Karacan I. The effect of age on human eccrine sweating. In: Montagna W, ed. *Advances in Biology of Skin*. Vol. IV. *Aging*. Oxford: Pergamon Press, 1965; 129–50.

56 Rees J, Shuster S. Pubertal induction of sweat gland activity. *Clin Sci* 1980; **60**: 689–92.

57 Orentreich N, Markofsky J, Vogelman JH. The effect of aging on the rate of linear nail growth. *J Invest Dermatol* 1979; **73**: 126–30.

58 Schludermann E, Zubeck JP. Effect of age on pain sensibility. *Percept Motor Skills Res Exchange* 1962; **14**: 295–301.

59 Winkelmann RK. Nerve changes in aging skin. In: Montagna W, ed. *Advances in Biology of Skin*. Vol. IV. *Aging*. Oxford: Pergamon Press, 1965: 51–61.

60 Gilchrest BA, Murphy G, Soter NA. Effect of chronologic aging and ultraviolet irradiation on Langerhans cells in human epidermis. *J Invest Dermatol* 1982; **79**: 85–8.

61 Thiers H, Maize JC, Spicer SS *et al*. The effect of aging and chronic sun exposure on human Langerhans cell population. *J Invest Dermatol* 1984; **82**: 223–6.

62 Makinodan T. Immunodeficiencies of ageing. In: Doria G, Eshkol A, eds. *The Immune System: Functions and Therapy of Dysfunction*. New York: Academic Press, 1980: 55–63.

63 Diaz-Jouanen E, Strickland RG, Williams RC Jr. Studies of human lymphocytes in the newborn and the aged. *Am J Med* 1975; **58**: 620–8.

64 Kay MMB, Makinodan T. Immunobiology of aging: evaluation of current status. *Clin Immunol Immunopathol* 1976; **6**: 394–413.

65 Reddy MM, Goh K. B- and T-lymphocytes in man. IV: Circulating B-, T-, and null lymphocytes in aging population. *J Gerontol* 1979; **34**: 5–8.

66 Ben-Yahuda A, Weksler ME. Host resistance and the immune system. *Clin Geriatr Med* 1992; **8**: 701–11.

67 Walford DS, Willkens RF, Decker JL. Impaired delayed hypersensitivity in an aging population: association with antinuclear reactivity and rheumatoid factor. *JAMA* 1968; **203**: 831–5.

Skin disease in old age

The demography of most nations is changing. Higher standards of housing, hygiene and nutrition, together with improvements in health-care services have meant that the average lifespan has increased considerably over the last century. Added to this, many couples are now limiting their families to two or three children at most. Virtually every Western society is therefore experiencing an increase in the average age of its population. The provision of health care for elderly people is consequently becoming more and more important, and disease of the skin is no exception to this [1]. Elderly patients present in dermatology clinics and consulting rooms with a wide variety of skin problems; a few are more or less specific to old age, but most are familiar skin disorders whose clinical expression, physical and emotional consequences, and management may be altered by the age of the patient and the problems that increasing age bring with it.

The reasons an individual seeks advice for skin changes in old age may be as much influenced by personality and social conditioning as by the absolute severity of the problem. Although some societies are still said to view the outward signs of age, such as wrinkles and grey hair, as marks of distinction, it is clear that in much of the world, 'Westernization' is resulting in an increasing degree of social stigmatization associated with looking old. Furthermore, it has been recognized for a long time that, contrary to the popular belief of the young, elderly people are often anxious to look attractive [2].

Thus, particularly in rich and highly developed societies, there is an increasing reluctance to accept the physiological consequences of old age and the effects of environmental exposure. A myth has begun to develop that these ageing changes are abnormal, and many older people with plentiful spare time and financial resources have become obsessed with the pursuit of an eternally youthful appearance (Fig. 74.5). One reason for this is that the pharmaceutical and cosmetic industries have invested heavily in the promotion of the concept that 'young is beautiful'. A great deal of money is being, and will continue to be, devoted to the study of compounds which may arrest or reverse the visible effects of ageing. Some are claiming success, most notably with retinoic acid for wrinkles. Such research is also increasingly gaining credence in mainstream medical circles, and dermatologists are becoming more and more involved in this area of practice.

However, the majority of people accept (albeit increasingly reluctantly) that ageing is a natural process, and only seek medical advice when skin changes are particularly troublesome or severe, or develop earlier than might otherwise have been expected.

Skin changes of sufficient severity to warrant medical attention in elderly patients may result from the interplay of several different factors:

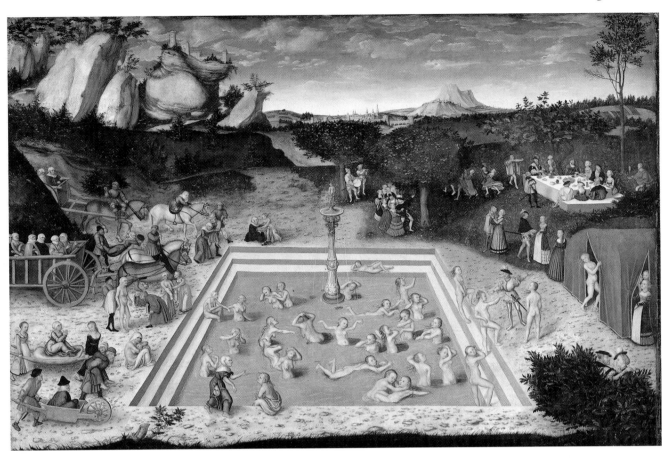

Fig. 74.5 *Der Jungbrunnen*. Lucas Cranach the Elder painted this picture of the Fountain of Youth in 1546, when he was 72 years of age. On the left, a succession of aged and decrepid women are brought to the fountain by an interesting variety of primitive transport. As they move through the basin they are transformed into lovely young maidens. The eternal desire for and, indeed, the possible advantages of rejuvenation are wonderfully expressed. (Courtesy of Staatliche Museen zu Berlin, Gemäldegalerie, Berlin, Germany.)

1 the alterations in structure and function of the ageing skin;

2 the cumulative effects of exposure to a variety of environmental insults, especially UV radiation;

3 the cutaneous consequences of ageing or age-related disease in other organ systems;

4 changes in the environment—decreasing occupational exposure, increasing leisure exposure to potential irritants and sensitizers;

5 social circumstances, with poor nutrition, home care and mobility often contributing to the expression, perpetuation and failure to resolve of skin problems;

6 physiological problems, such as dementia, increasing rigidity of attitude and refusal to accept advice;

7 increasing physical frailty, resulting in a relative incapacity to carry out tasks correctly.

Of particular practical importance are the latter three problems, which are frequently ignored. For example, an elderly patient may be too proud to point out that physical incapacity prevents the twice-daily application of a cream, or may deliberately refuse or forget to relate relevant facts about the home situation. The onus is very much on the dermatologist to consider these factors when dealing with skin disease in the elderly patient.

The incidence of skin problems in old age

It is hard to estimate the true frequency of skin disease in the population as a whole, let alone specifically in older age groups. One problem is that the line between that which is physiological and the 'truly' pathological becomes increasingly difficult to draw with advancing years. Another is that studies of skin problems in the elderly have used different types of population and diagnostic groupings which are not directly comparable (Table 74.7). It is probably better, therefore, to think of skin problems rather than just skin disease in this age group.

However, it is clear that skin problems are common in elderly people. The general scale of this can be gauged from the findings of a large American study, in which dermatological examination of 20 000 non-institutionalized US citizens revealed that 40% of those aged between 65 and 74 years had some significant dermatological problem [3]. 'Significant',

Table 74.7 Studies on the incidence of skin disease in elderly people.

Reference	No. of patients	Population studied
Droller, 1955 [5]	476	Random; at home
Young, 1958 [8]	330	Ambulatory outpatients from skin clinic; chosen 'at random'
Epstein, 1962 [9]	687	US private practice
Tindall and Smith, 1963 [6]	163	Volunteers; at home; black and white people
Verbov, 1975 [12]	170	Mainly outpatients; some inpatients
Weisman et al. (1980) [7]	584	Residents of old peoples' homes
Beauregard and Gilchrest, 1987 [4]	68	Volunteers: housing projects, geriatric home visits, medical centre employees
McFadden and Hande, 1987 [10]	257	Dermatology outpatients

in this context, was defined as requiring, in the view of the examining doctor, a dermatological opinion. Smaller studies on elderly individuals selected randomly and not from skin clinics give much the same impression [4–7]. For example, of 68 volunteers aged between 50 and 91 years, living in Boston, USA, two-thirds of the entire group and 83% of those aged over 80 years complained of skin problems of some kind [4]. In a European study, 77.4% of a population of 584 elderly residents of a municipal old peoples' home in Denmark were found to have a skin problem [7].

Many of the skin problems which are found most commonly on random examination of elderly people are not those for which elderly patients necessarily seek attention from specialist or non-specialist doctors. Although eczemas, pruritus, easy bruising and dryness (under various headings) are certainly seen in skin clinics, tumours, both benign and malignant, tend to figure more prominently than inflammatory problems [8–12].

REFERENCES

1 Gilchrest BA. Demography of skin disease in the elderly. In: *Skin and Aging Processes*. Boca Raton: CRC Press, 1984: 1.
2 Kligman AM, Graham JA. The psychology of appearance in the elderly. *Dermatol Clin* 1986; **4**: 501–7.
3 Johnson M-LT. Skin conditions and related need for medical care among persons 1–74 years. United States. 1971–1974. *Vital Health Statistics*: Series 11, Data from the National Health Survey; no 212, DHEW Publication no. (PHS) 79–1660. Hyattsville, ML: US Department of Health, Education and Welfare, 1978.
4 Beauregard S, Gilchrest BA. A survey of skin problems and skin care regimens in the elderly. *Arch Dermatol* 1987; **123**: 1638–43.
5 Droller H. Dermatologic findings in a random sample of old persons. *Geriatrics* 1955; **10**: 421–4.
6 Tindall JP, Smith JG. Skin lesions of the aged and their association with internal changes. *JAMA* 1963; **186**: 1039–42.
7 Weisman K, Krakauer R, Wanscher B. Prevalence of skin disease in old age. *Acta Derm Venereol (Stockh)* 1980; **60**: 352–3.
8 Young AW. Dermatologic complaints presented by 330 geriatric patients. *Geriatrics* 1958; **13**: 428–34.
9 Epstein NN. The aging skin. Part 1: Some problems of the aging skin with particular reference to environmental factors. In: Rees RB, ed. *Dermatoses due to Environmental and Physical Factors*. Springfield: Thomas, 1962: 28–38.
10 McFadden N, Hande K-H. A survey of elderly new patients at a dermatology outpatient clinic. *Acta Derm Venereol (Stockh)* 1987; **69**: 260–2.
11 Stern RS, Johnson M-L, DeLozier J. Utilization of physician services for dermatologic complaints. *Arch Dermatol* 1977; **113**: 1062–6.
12 Verbov J. Skin problems in the older patient. *Practitioner* 1975; **215**: 612–22.

Specific skin problems in old age

Most of the skin disorders which are particularly troublesome in the elderly patient are described elsewhere in this book. However, one or two points should be emphasized about certain specific disorders.

Wrinkles and elastosis

These changes, together with greying of the hair, are most readily associated with an aged appearance. The different clinical forms of wrinkles, and the clinical syndromes associated with elastosis, are described in Chapter 44, and the histological changes of the ageing dermis are discussed above. Plastic surgeons and dermatologists are becoming increasingly involved in their management. Chemical peels, collagen implants and face-lift operations are in wide use, and topical retinoids are currently being evaluated in the treatment and prevention of wrinkling [1–3].

Pruritus

Itching in old age can be so severe that it ruins quality of life completely [4]. The itch may be localized or generalized; and may or may not be accompanied by skin changes. It is crucial to examine an itchy elderly person carefully for primary cutaneous disease: in one study, 142 of 162 elderly patients had an identifiable cause for their itching (including xerosis), leaving only 20 to whom the term senile pruritus was applicable [5]. Diagnoses which are particularly easy to miss are scabies (often due to the inadequate examination facilities in residential homes for the elderly) and bullous pemphigoid, which often begins with a non-specific, or even no, rash [6]. Non-specific skin changes in anogenital itch may also conceal important diagnoses: candidiasis in undiagnosed diabetes; lichen sclerosus et atrophicus, the classical signs of which may easily be obscured by secondary excoriation and inflammation.

If a primary skin disorder has been ruled out, it is important to investigate any elderly patient with generalized itching for systemic causes: renal disease, cholestasis (especially chronic liver disease), thyroid disease, anaemia or cancer.

The relationship between carcinomas and pruritus in the elderly patient is controversial, but there is no doubt that lymphomas, leukaemias and other myelodysplastic disorders may present in this way [7]. The frequency with which a systemic cause is found varies, but is high enough to justify a routine search [4], and a useful algorithm for this has been provided by Champion [8].

When all these causes have been excluded, there remains a small core of elderly patients with intractable pruritus. In some, the itching is accompanied by xeroderma, but in others the skin feels relatively normal to the touch. The management of such patients is extremely difficult, and is often totally unsatisfactory for all concerned. The topical use of emollients, soothing preparations such as menthol in calamine, and potent topical steroids may be helpful. However, many of those with the worst pruritus are quite unable to manage topical therapy by themselves, and it is necessary to resort to relatively sedative systemic drugs, such as phenothiazine-type antihistamines. These, too, have their drawbacks, not the least of which is the development of confusion and disorientation.

Senile xerosis and asteatotic eczema

SYN. ECZEMA CRAQUELÉ

The ageing skin often feels 'dry' to the touch, although the reason for this is not clear. As mentioned above, water loss is not increased in aged skin [9], but the water content of the epidermis appears to be somewhat reduced [10]. It has been suggested that xerosis reflects minor abnormalities in epidermal maturation [7].

The dryness is often worse in the winter, a fact that has given rise to many of the alternative names used for these changes: winter eczema, prurigo or pruritus hiemalis. The changes are often most pronounced on the legs. In some patients, the surface texture of the skin assumes a cracked appearance resembling crazy paving. This is known as asteatotic eczema or eczema craquelé (Fig. 74.6). Frequent washing is certainly a causative factor in susceptible individuals [11], and central heating may also play a role by reducing atmospheric humidity. Perhaps it is not surprising that this problem is commonly seen in geriatric inpatients.

The use of emollients to reduce requirements for soaps and detergents will improve xerosis in most patients and, because high water temperatures appears to increase the tendency to irritant reactions [12], so will reducing the bath temperature. Moisturizing preparations in the bath are generally held to be effective [4], but bath oils can make the bath very slippery, which has its own risks in the elderly and frail patient.

Eczema

The aged may suffer from any of the clinical types of eczema. Atopic dermatitis, for example, occasionally continues into

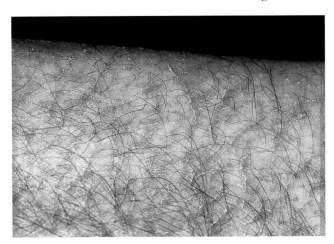

Fig. 74.6 Eczema craquelé.

old age or even appears for the first time. However, certain patterns such as asteatotic eczema are more common and more troublesome in elderly subjects.

Seborrhoeic dermatitis may be more common in the elderly infirm and in those confined to bed [13]. In the aged patient, especially the obese, a flexural pattern is often encountered, which may mimic intertrigo and flexural psoriasis.

Some elderly patients present for the first time with a discoid or nummular eczema, and most patients with Sulzberger–Garbe disease (generally considered to be a variant of discoid eczema) are elderly.

Gravitational eczema is much commoner in the elderly patient (Chapter 17), and may be complicated by contact sensitivity.

Contact dermatitis of irritant or allergic origin is generally considered to be less common in elderly people, partly because of decreased occupational exposure [14]. This may also reflect the decline in immune reactivity that occurs with age [15] and the fact that irritant responses to some substances are reduced in intensity [16]. However, patch test positivity remains quite common, presumably from exposure earlier in life. Allergic contact dermatitis remains a significant problem in elderly people, especially due to local medicaments, such as aminoglycosides, lanolin, parabens, antihistamines and anaesthetics. Other sensitizers which continue to cause trouble in old age include rubber in gloves and shoes, plastics in hearing aids and spectacle frames, plants, and hair dyes [14].

Marked secondary lichenification and chronic lichen simplex are also often seen in older patients.

Bullous disorders

Pemphigoid (Chapter 40) is much more frequent in the elderly than in other age groups. Old age modifies the management of all blistering diseases because of unwanted effects of drugs, or because of physical and social circumstances. For example, steroids precipitate glucose intolerance more often in the elderly, and sulphapyridine or sulphamethoxy-pyridazine may be better first-line drugs than dapsone for dermatitis herpetiformis because of the tendency for dapsone to cause haemolysis [17]. Drug regimens need to be kept simple, and written down where necessary.

Psoriasis

There is a distinct peak of onset of psoriasis in later life which is not as clearly associated with a family history as in patients whose disease begins earlier. This is reflected in different human leukocyte antigen (HLA) associations [18].

Psoriasis causes increased problems in the elderly patient. Disease of lesser extent and severity may be relatively more disabling in old age than in youth, and the systemic effects of widespread, or acute pustular, psoriasis are less well tolerated than in younger individuals. Flexural psoriasis is a particular problem in the elderly patient [19], but other patterns are also seen. Eruptive guttate disease, however, is rare in old age.

Treatment can be difficult. The patient may be unable to apply topical therapies, and there may be problems in travelling to and from the hospital for outpatient dithranol, or in standing for psoralen and UVA (PUVA) therapy. One solution is the use of systemic therapy, especially methotrexate. There is less reason for concern over long-term toxicity in the elderly patient, relatively small doses may keep the patient comfortable (perhaps because of diminished renal clearance), and the drug is generally well tolerated.

Leg ulcers (Chapter 50)

Leg ulcers are a major problem. Most are due to venous hypertension, but arterial disease becomes increasingly important with advancing years. Poor wound healing in elderly people [20], perhaps associated with other illnesses and poor nutrition, may also play a role in the perpetuation of some ulcers.

In managing chronic leg ulcers in the elderly patient it is important to take an overview of the whole situation. Strenuous efforts to heal a stable ulcer in someone who is coping independently at home may be inappropriate in some cases if long-stay inpatient treatment will be required.

Decubitus ulcers [21]
See Chapter 23.

Herpes zoster and post-herpetic neuralgia [22]

Shingles is much commoner in old age, the relative incidence rising from 4/1000/year at age 55 years to 10/1000/year at age 90 years. It has been estimated that 25% of people over the age of 65 develop shingles at some time, and that all who have had chickenpox would do so were they to live to 100 years old. Post-herpetic neuralgia is also much commoner in elderly people. About 50% of patients over the age of 60 years experience pain, and the incidence rises to as many as 75% of the over-70s.

Skin tumours

Most skin tumours are commoner in elderly people: benign, such as seborrhoeic keratoses, senile lentigines and skin tags; dysplastic, such as actinic keratoses; and cancers, especially basal and squamous cell carcinomas. Lentigo maligna is seen predominantly in the elderly, and the highest age-specific incidence rates for invasive malignant melanoma are also in those over 60 [23]. There is also an association between increasing age and decreasing 5-year survival in malignant melanoma [24]. It is not clear why this should be, but elderly patients seem to present with thicker lesions [24,25], and recent evidence suggests that the proportion of nodular melanomas may rise with increasing age [25]. The tendency to wait longer before presenting for treatment also extends to other tumours, and lesions such as that shown in Fig. 74.7 are essentially restricted to elderly people.

Infections with ectoparasites

Outbreaks of scabies in residential homes for the elderly are not uncommon, and are usually attributable to one individual with a heavy infection, verging on Norwegian or crusted scabies. Clothing lice (Chapter 33) are, in the UK, almost exclusively seen in elderly vagrants.

REFERENCES

1 Ellis CN, Weiss JS, Hamilton TA *et al*. Sustained improvement with prolonged topical tretinoin (retinoic acid) for photoaged skin. *J Am Acad Dermatol* 1990; **23**: 629–37.

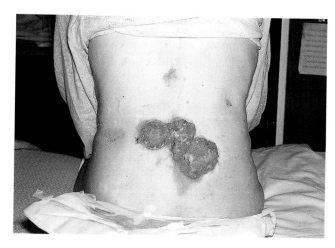

Fig. 74.7 A large, neglected basal cell carcinoma on the back of an elderly lady.

2 Kligman AM, Grove GL, Hirose R *et al.* Topical tretinoin to photoaged skin. *J Am Acad Dermatol* 1986; **15**: 836–59.

3 Marks R, Lever L. Studies on the effects of topical retinoic acid on photoageing. *Br J Dermatol* 1990; **122** (Suppl. 35): 93–5.

4 Graham-Brown RAC, Monk BE. Pruritus and xerosis. In: Monk BE, Graham-Brown RAC, Sarkany I, eds. *Skin Disorders in the Elderly*. Oxford: Blackwell Scientific Publications, 1988: 133–46.

5 Young AW. The diagnosis of pruritus in the elderly. *J Am Geriatr Soc* 1967; **15**: 750–8.

6 Barker DJ. Generalised pruritus as the presenting feature of bullous pemphigoid. *Br J Dermatol* 1986; **109**: 237–9.

7 Gilchrest BA. Pathologic processes associated with aging. In: *Skin and Aging Processes*. Boca Raton: CRC Press, 1984: 37–56.

8 Champion RH. Generalised pruritus. *Br Med J* 1984; **289**: 751–3.

9 Kligman AM. Perspectives and problems in cutaneous gerontology. *J Invest Dermatol* 1979; **73**: 39–46.

10 Potts RO, Buras EM, Chrisman DA. Changes with age in the moisture content of human skin. *J Invest Dermatol* 1984; **82**: 97–100.

11 Graham-Brown RAC. Soaps and detergents in the elderly. *Clin Dermatol* 1996; **14**: 85–7.

12 Lazar AP, Lazar P. Dry skin, water and lubrication. *Dermatol Clin* 1991; **9**: 45–51.

13 Tager A, Berlin C, Scen RJ. Seborrhoeic dermatitis in acute cardiac disease. *Br J Dermatol* 1964; **76**: 367–9.

14 Monk BE, Graham-Brown RAC. Eczema. In: Monk BE, Graham-Brown RAC, Sarkany I, eds. *Skin Disorders in the Elderly*. Oxford: Blackwell Scientific Publications, 1988: 147–57.

15 Bach J-F. Immunosenescence. *Triangle* 1986; **25**: 25–31.

16 Bettley FR, Donoghue E. The irritant effect of soap on normal skin. *Br J Dermatol* 1960; **72**: 67–76.

17 Leonard JN. Dermatitis herpetiformis, bullous pemphigoid, cicatricial pemphigoid and linear IgA disease. In: Fry L, ed. *Skin Problems in the Elderly*. Edinburgh: Churchill Livingstone, 1985: 182–201.

18 Henseler T, Christophers E. Psoriasis of early and late onset: characterization of two types of psoriasis vulgaris. *J Am Acad Dermatol* 1985; **13**: 450–6.

19 Marks R. *Skin Disease in Old Age*. London: Martin Dunitz, 1987: 49–63.

20 Eaglstein WH. Wound healing and aging. *Dermatol Clin* 1986; **4**: 481–4.

21 Bliss MR, Silvers JR. Pressure sores. In: Monk BE, Graham-Brown RAC, Sarkany I, eds. *Skin Disorders in the Elderly*. Oxford: Blackwell Scientific Publications, 1988: 97–112.

22 Peto TEA, Juel-Jensen BE. Varicella zoster virus disease. In: Monk BE, Graham-Brown RAC, Sarkany I, eds. *Skin Disorders in the Elderly*. Oxford: Blackwell Scientific Publications, 1988: 80–96.

23 Elwood JM, Lee JAH. Recent data on the epidemiology of malignant melanoma. *Semin Oncol* 1975; **2**: 149–54.

24 Morris BT, Sober AJ. Cutaneous malignant melanoma in the older patient. *Dermatol Clin* 1986; **4**: 473–80.

25 Keefe M, White JE, Perkins P. Nodular melanomas in the over-50 age group: the next target for health education. *Br J Dermatol* 1990; **123** (Suppl. 37): 59.

Chapter 75
General Aspects of Treatment

J.A.COTTERILL & A.P.WARIN

General principles

The general principles for the treatment of skin diseases are essentially the same as for other branches of medicine. There are, however, important aspects and details peculiar to dermatology that readily escape the non-specialist, attention to which may make so much difference to the success or otherwise of therapy. In particular, topical therapy in many situations may be in danger of being relegated to an unimportant role. Patients may decry local applications. During history taking, many patients say they have had no treatment, 'only a few ointments'. They may also be unaware of the potential harm that can be done by topical therapy, whether self-administered or iatrogenic. Careful nursing and instruction of the patient on how to use any remedy can be much more important than in other branches of medicine.

Although dermatologists have available to them many more agents of proven beneficial pharmacological activity than were available to their predecessors, they still have to persuade, console and counsel and must convince many patients that no specific key is available for their particular problem.

Thus, the most central aspect of dermatological management is the consultation, which often demands great skill in communication techniques.

The dermatological consultation

The various manoeuvres employed by patients and doctors in the consultation 'gamesmanship' have been described [1].

The individual dermatologist will, however, develop his or her own preferred technique of consultation as he or she matures in the specialty over the years. Thus, there are those dermatologists who like to see their patients completely naked so that they can be sure they are missing no other dermatological pathology. However, seeing a patient initially entirely naked may lead to a considerable loss of valuable data. The patient's dress provides psychosocial information, and the gait of the patient as he or she walks into the consulting room can give some useful information. In particular, the depressed patient often has a characteristic 'droop', whilst the anxious patient is moving in all directions at the same time, typically sitting on the edge of the chair. The depressed patient may be slow in all his or her responses to questions. An anxious person may continuously twirl a ring on a finger, and the quivering lips or the moistening of an eye in response to a question may indicate important stress-provoking factors. The language employed by the patient in describing the symptoms is also important. Whilst light eruptions such as porphyria may produce a burning sensation in the skin, very few other skin conditions do this and symptoms described emotively in this way may indicate that functional factors are important in pathogenesis. The patient who brings in an enormous bag of medicaments, all of which have done 'nothing at all' to help, may also indicate a psychological or psychiatric aspect to the case. A 'hollow' history and the 'belle indifference' of the classical patient with dermatitis artefacta can be appreciated only by taking a good history. Little matchboxes and plastic bags containing detritus are very characteristic of patients with delusions of parasitosis.

What do patients want?

Patients consult dermatologists because they want help with their skin problems. Patients require not only information and medical treatment, but also explanation, understanding and emotional support [2]. Whilst patients may hold elaborate, and sometimes sophisticated, theories about their own skin problems, most patients need to know the answers to three basic questions: 'Why me?', 'Why now?' and 'Why this particular illness?' [2]. Moreover, patients can be divided into two groups. There are those who search and demand more information about their problems (monitors) and those who deliberately avoid information, especially if it has negative connotations (blunters) and so patients who complain about lack of information may paradoxically be the most well-informed [3]. Above all, the patient values a doctor who listens, although not all doctors may yet have learned to hear what their patients are saying [4].

Eye contact is vital if meaningful data are to be gathered from the patient [5]. Doctors with a mechanistic inter-rogative style who offer no eye contact usually turn off any meaningful verbal communication from the patient.

Body image, self-esteem and the leper complex

An individual's body image is largely cutaneous, so skin disease affecting any part of the body surface may produce considerable depression in body image, self-esteem, confidence and secondary depression [6]. This is particularly true where skin disease affects areas such as the scalp, hair, face, hands and genital area. The stigma of skin disease can readily produce a 'leper complex' in the individual patient, which compels the patient to withdraw from society and physical contact with other human beings [7,8]. It is vital, therefore, that the dermatologist provides reassurance by touching the patient at some stage during the consultation.

REFERENCES

1 Cotterill JA. Dermatological games. *Br J Dermatol* 1981; **105**: 311–20.
2 Armstrong D. What do patients want? Someone who will hear their questions. *Br Med J* 1991; **303**: 261–2.
3 Miller SM, Brody DS, Summerton JS. Strategies of coping with threat: implications for Health. *J Pers Soc Psychol* 1988; **54**: 142–8.
4 Smith C, Armstrong D. Comparisons of criteria derived by governments for evaluating general practitioner services. *Br Med J* 1989; **299**: 494–6.
5 Davenport S, Goldberg D, Millar T. How psychiatric disorders are missed during medical consultations. *Lancet* 1987; **i**: 439–41.
6 Hardy GE, Cotterill JA. A study of depression and obsessionality in dysmorphophobic and psoriatic patients. *Br J Psychiatry* 1982; **140**: 19–22.
7 Ginsburg IA, Link BG. Feelings of stigmatization in patients with psoriasis. *J Am Acad Dermatol* 1989; **20**: 53–63.
8 MacKenna RMB. Psychiatric factors in cutaneous disease. *Lancet* 1944; **ii**: 679–81.

Timing

A dermatosis is rarely a static event. The effect of the patient's actions and attitudes, the frequent development of anxiety or depression and the daily variations in the internal and external milieu require frequent reappraisal and adjustment of treatment. Topical corticosteroids should be reduced in strength as the disease recedes.

The timing of a return to work often involves a difficult decision; even the return of a patient from hospital to his or her environment may be misjudged. In either case, a relapse may cause the patient to lose confidence. In all dermatological therapy, Napoleon's dictum may be remembered with advantage: 'la puissance ne consiste pas à frapper fort ou à frapper souvent, mais à frapper juste'.

Failure to appreciate the natural history of disease has been responsible for much unnecessary therapy, and for a wrong assessment of therapeutic needs. For instance, in alopecia areata, specific therapy is lacking, and the average duration is unaffected by empirical measures. Infantile eczema tends to improve with time and nummular eczema 'burns itself out' in months or years. In these diseases, the patient is ill-served by measures that can only alter the immediate situation without an additional planned campaign to sustain him or her over this prolonged period. A diminishing concentration of topical corticosteroids, measures designed to distract attention from the disease and manoeuvres designed to help morale are necessary parts of the whole treatment. In diseases with a short-lived but hectic course, such as erythema multiforme exudativum, oral steroids, if given at all, should be 'tailed off' once the expected peak of the disease is past. In chronic diseases, such as psoriasis, systemic sclerosis, lichen sclerosus of the vulva, ichthyosiform erythroderma or dermatitis herpetiformis, therapy should be on the lines of a siege operation or, sometimes, as a deliberately planned retreat in which the disease is contained and held in check. It is a wise precaution to hold a therapeutic reserve whenever possible, for periods of exceptional activity of the disease process.

Compliance

It is too easily assumed that the patient will take or has taken the medicines prescribed. A thrice-daily routine is difficult, especially for those who travel to work. This has encouraged drug manufacturers to attempt to find once-daily substitutes, for example for antibiotics. The reasons for non-compliance cannot easily be evaluated [1–3], but levels of anxiety, degree of motivation and the patient's attitude to the doctor and the disease, and that of others in his or her social environment, are important factors.

In poorer countries, the cost of treatment and, in developed countries, more complex socio-economic issues may determine the degree to which treatment is continued as long as is necessary [2].

Side-effects

Because of the public's greater awareness of drugs, bolstered by exuberant presentation by the media, any doctor is put in a difficult position. The patient needs basic information [4,5]. If the doctor does not explain possible major side-effects, he or she is guilty of neglect; if the doctor over-stresses these, he or she will invite non-compliance. If too many of the minor possible side-effects are included, the doctor will invite a psychological reaction. The doctor must assess the patient's common sense and exert his or her own. Care must be taken with those with compromised hepatic or renal function, and the elderly, who easily become confused about dosage; various aids to overcome this problem have been devised [6].

REFERENCES

1 Evans L, Spelman M. The problem of non-compliance with drug therapy. *Drugs* 1983; **25**: 63–76.
2 Goodman LJ, Swartwout JE. Socioeconomic issues in dermatology. *J Am Acad Dermatol* 1981; **5**: 711–20.
3 Witowski JA. Compliance: the dermatological patient. *Br J Dermatol* 1988; **27**: 608–11.
4 Editorial. What should we tell patients about their medicines? *Drug Ther Bull* 1981; **19**: 73–4.
5 Hermann F, Herxheimer A, Lionel NDW. Package inserts for prescribed medicines: what minimum information do patients need? *Br Med J* 1978; **ii**: 1132–5.
6 Atkinson L, Gibson I, Andrews J. An investigation into the ability of elderly patients continuing to take prescribed drugs after discharge from hospital and recommendations concerning improving the situation. *Gerontology* 1978; **24**: 225–34.

Therapy

General management

Explanation

Like all doctors, but perhaps more than most, dermatologists must achieve rapid rapport with their patients and be seen either to assuage the symptoms and signs of visible disease or to bring the patient—and the relatives or parents—to accept chronicity or irreversible changes. Dermatology has been called an 'applied intuitive art': if so, an easy understanding must be achieved between the artist and sitter. Allowance must be made for symptoms of anxiety—aggression, lack of faith, mistrust. If necessary, the dermatologist must gradually overcome these to become therapeutic in the clinical situation.

Patients nowadays demand and deserve a far fuller explanation of their disease than was formerly either possible or even considered desirable. No longer is it appropriate to give a learned diagnosis, a prescription and little else.

Patients may be well-informed or misinformed, but they are informed. Recourse to the Book of Proverbs or Job is not received with the understanding it used to command. It is never easy to explain autoimmune diseases or the aetiology of atopic dermatitis in easily comprehensible terms. The intelligence of the patient must be gauged; a suitable metaphor or simile is often apt. In any case, the patient's questions must be answered. In seeking clues to the causation of conditions such as contact dermatitis or chronic urticaria, one should always listen attentively to the patient's explanation. He or she may well be wrong, but occasionally the patient is right, however unexpected the answer.

Nevertheless, his or her account of the onset and course of the disease may have become distorted by time or for medicolegal reasons and can never be believed in cases of dermatitis artefacta. The patient's memory (or suppression of memory) of drug or topical medicaments given is usually defective, especially if self-administered.

Avoidance of aggravating factors

General advice that might be considered common sense to the dermatologist may be quite unfamiliar to some patients. Such advice includes care with environmental temperature and, at times, humidity. Advice should be given on appropriate clothing, which should not be too constricting, too hot or too harsh. Irritants and sensitizers should be avoided where possible. Many patients retain the belief that skin disease is a manifestation of dirt or germs to be expunged with vigour and exorcized with soap and water or worse. Care should indeed be taken with soap, but it is seldom necessary to proscribe bathing. It is surprising how often patients will be applying inappropriate household germicides, and in totally inappropriate concentrations. Advice to stop scratching usually causes more frustration and alienation unless something is done to help the sensation of itching.

Regimen

Rest and relaxation can play a major part in treating many dermatoses. With others, there are positive benefits in remaining at work or at school. Decisions, including economic ones, are often neatly balanced, but the patient will often require positive guidance on how much activity is to be encouraged.

The arguments for and against admission to hospital clearly depend on so many variables other than the purely medical ones. The last 30 years have seen a great reduction in beds for dermatology patients in many countries. The reasons include better treatments, which do away with the need for admission, improved facilities for home nursing, and better transport to outpatient facilities. The dramatic rises in cost of maintaining patients in hospital, whether at the expense of themselves or of their health services, also militate against admission.

No firm guidelines can be laid down about which particular diseases need to be treated on an inpatient basis. These will vary from culture to culture and even from town to town. No doubt many diseases might benefit from time in hospital but this may not be feasible. Sometimes, a short stay before complete remission has been achieved will allow the acute crisis to be averted, allow patients to be taught how to manage themselves, and also build up a better relationship between patient, doctors and nurses.

Recent years have seen the emergence of dermatological intensive care units for the management of such acute, life-threatening emergencies as toxic epidermal necrolysis, pemphigus and erythroderma. These have been pioneered at Creteil, France [1,2] and have pointed the way forward to improving what can be a poor prognosis.

Quite often, the need for hospitalization is avoided if the patient is given precise instructions how to do at home almost everything that might have been done in hospital.

Diet

The value of dietary regimens in the treatment of most skin diseases has not been proven. Some exceptions to this rule are discussed below, but even these are not universally accepted. There has been a renewed interest in this subject in recent years in western Europe and the USA, stimulated in part by the media and in part by a general trend towards reduced dependence on drugs and a return to a belief in 'simplistic' medicine. Sensible advice on diet, aimed chiefly at the obese or those overweight for their age and height, plays an obvious part in the treatment of conditions such as intertrigo and gravitational eczema or leg ulceration.

The effects of malnutrition due to starvation, unfortunately still prevalent in many parts of the world, need no underlining, but malnutrition may also occur in any patient with anorexia nervosa or carcinomatosis (especially carcinoma of the throat or oesophagus). Bowel-shortening operations, total parenteral nutrition and precolectomy dietary regimens have led to selective deficiencies, for example of essential fatty acids [3,4] or zinc [5], but these are now usually recognized and corrected.

Even in advanced industrial communities, quite marked malnutrition is seen in elderly people living alone, in whom financial stringency, apathy, boredom, dementia or immobility lead to a diet deficient in folic or ascorbic acid or even in protein itself. Chronic alcoholics may suffer from avitaminosis or from general malnutrition. A growing group of 'food faddists' (and a smaller group of those believing themselves to suffer from 'total allergy') may also become deprived of essential vitamin or protein requirements. Although the dermatologists in Europe and the USA do not generally need to concern themselves with vitamin therapy, elderly alcoholics or misguided patients

are still admitted to dermatological wards with scurvy or gross vitamin B complex deficiency, both of which may be unrecognized.

Whenever there is doubt, it is simpler and cheaper to give ascorbic acid than to attempt to measure serum levels: a gradual return to a full and balanced diet may, in the apathetic, require sip-feeds with protein-containing supplements and possibly added vitamins. Intramuscular high-potency vitamin supplements are of value, especially in alcoholics. Nasal drip feeding is sometimes indicated.

Food metabolites and toxins

Technical advances in recent years have greatly extended our knowledge of foods and their metabolites. It has been suggested [6] that some food peptides can act as exogenous 'hormones'. Such 'exorphens', for example those derived from milk or wheat protein, have an opiate-like activity, which will be lacking in patients on a gluten-free diet. The importance of trace elements such as zinc is now fully established, but there is increasing interest in plant-derived toxins and 'microtoxins' [7], such as protease inhibitors, haemagglutinins, goitrogens, cyanogens, glossypol, etc. Fortunately, cooking destroys many of these, but they are not without importance in poorer countries, where the diet may be heavily biased towards one-plant products. The toxic oil syndrome resulted in multisystem organ damage, including the skin, from an unknown toxin present in rapeseed oil, denatured with aniline, used for cooking [8]. The eosinophilia–myalgia syndrome, another multisystem disorder, associated with tryptophan therapy, may also be due to a toxic contaminant of this amino-acid drug [9] (Chapter 77).

Special dietary regimens

These are obligatory in some genetic conditions and in some diseases of metabolic origin, useful in the control of a few important dermatological conditions, and of disputed value in some others.

Genetic conditions. Phenylketonuria and Refsum's disease are well-known examples; the control of tyrosinaemia II is a more recent one [10].

Metabolic disease. Diabetes is, of course, the best-known example. Hypercholesterolaemic xanthomatosis benefits from a strict limitation of dietary cholesterol. Patients with carotenaemia should avoid carotenoids.

Special diets in other diseases. Claims made for special diets in a number of common diseases such as psoriasis and acne have not been convincing, although there was some reduction of pain and frequency of aphthous ulcers in patients on a gluten-free diet [11]; this requires further investigation. Fish oil may be helpful in some patients with psoriasis, particularly with regard to reducing pruritus and inflammation to some extent [12].

Although a fasting diet gave some temporary benefits to patients with atopic eczema, rosacea and palmoplantar pustulosis [13], change to a vegetarian diet caused regression. The authors of this study believed that the improvement during fasting might be related to neutrophil leukocyte turnover, as reflected by the serum concentration of lactoferrin.

Atopic eczema [14,15] (Chapter 18). There has been a revival of interest in dietary factors in this disease in recent years, particularly on the part of allergists. The radioallergosorbent test (RAST) and the scratch-chamber technique [16] have given this interest further stimulus, although the difficulty of relating the results of these tests to the history has not been completely resolved [17]. The subject is extremely complicated and still under intensive investigation. The role of evening primrose oil in the management of atopic eczema is also controversial [18], as is the use of Chinese herbal remedies (see Chapter 76).

Chronic urticaria. The extent of food allergens in the causation of chronic urticaria (Chapter 47) is still disputed. In the management of a condition that is so tedious and prolonged, it is always worthwhile considering carefully planned exclusion diets.

Intolerance to food dyes and preservatives is responsible for a modest proportion of cases of chronic urticaria [19–22]. If the history, supplemented by a diary, fails to incriminate the cause, a diet free from these agents [17,20] may be used as a diagnostic manoeuvre. Intolerance to other drugs or foodstuffs may coexist—a complicating factor in assessment. Yeasts, another possible cause [13], are present in bread, sausage, wine, beer, Marmite and yeast tablets [17]. Other responsible chemical substances or constituents include salicylates [19], sulphur dioxide, quinine, menthol and possibly food flavourings.

Dermatitis herpetiformis [16,23,24]. Despite initial doubt, withdrawal of dietary gluten appears to be of definite benefit in patients with this disease. Of 42 patients treated with a gluten-free diet, 71% were able to discontinue drugs after a mean period of 29 months, although a reduction in dose became possible after a mean period of 8 months. Only five of 30 patients on a normal diet (14%) were able to do so [16]. However, the improvement in the skin condition and the intestinal intraepithelial lymphocyte count were closely related to the strictness with which the diet was carried out.

There are data to suggest that elemental iodine may also exacerbate this condition [25].

A dietician's advice is invaluable, as is the advice and encouragement given by belonging to the Coeliac Society.

Very rarely, it may be necessary to include a milk-free diet [23,26].

Drug regimens. Patients taking monoamine oxidase inhibitors must avoid foods containing amines. Corticosteroids are catabolic and extra milk and protein (and possibly anabolic steroids) may be needed in elderly patients on long-term treatment.

REFERENCES

1 Revuz J, Roujeau JC, Guillaume JC. Treatment of toxic epidermal necrolysis, Creteil's experience. *Arch Dermatol* 1987; **123**: 1156–8, 1160–5.
2 Roujeau JC, Revuz J. Intensive care in dermatology. In: Champion RH, Pye RJ, eds. *Recent Advances in Dermatology*, Vol. 8. Edinburgh: Churchill Livingstone, 1990: 85–99.
3 Prottey C, Hartop PJ, Press M. Correction of the cutaneous manifestations of essential fatty acid deficiency in man by application of sunflower-seed oil to the skin. *J Invest Dermatol* 1975; **64**: 228–34.
4 Riella MC, Broviac JW, Wells M et al. Essential fatty acid deficiency in human adults during total parenteral nutrition. *Ann Intern Med* 1975; **83**: 786–9.
5 Weismann K, Hjorth N, Fischer A. Zinc depletion syndrome with acrodermatitis during long-term intravenous feeding. *Clin Exp Dermatol* 1976; **1**: 237–42.
6 Morley JE. Food peptides: a new class of hormones? *JAMA* 1982; **247**: 2379–80.
7 Liener IE. *Toxic Constituents of Plant Foodstuffs*, 2nd edn. New York: Academic Press, 1980.
8 Tabuenca JM. Toxic–allergic syndrome caused by rapeseed oil denatured with aniline. *Lancet* 1981; **ii**: 567–8.
9 Acheson D. *L-Tryptophan and Eosinophilia–Myalgia Syndrome in the USA.* London: Department of Health, 1989: PL/CMO(89)11.
10 Machino H, Miki Y, Kawatsu T et al. Successful dietary control of tyrosinemia II. *J Am Acad Dermatol* 1983; **9**: 533–9.
11 Walker DM, Dolby AE, Mead J et al. Effect of gluten-free diet on recurrent aphthous ulceration. *Br J Dermatol* 1980; **103**: 111.
12 Bittiner SB, Tucker WFG, Cartwright I et al. A double-blind randomised placebo-controlled trial of fish oil in psoriasis. *Lancet* 1988; **i**: 378–80.
13 Lithell H, Bruce A, Gustafsson IB et al. A fasting and vegetarian diet treatment trial on chronic inflammatory disorders. *Acta Derm Venereol (Stockh)* 1983; **63**: 397–403.
14 Atherton DJ, Sewell M, Soothill JF et al. A double-blind controlled crossover trial of an antigen-avoidance diet in atopic eczema. *Lancet* 1978; **i**: 401–3.
15 Hanifin JM, Rajka G. Diagnostic features of atopic dermatitis. *Acta Derm Venereol Suppl (Stockh)* 1980; **92**: 44–7.
16 Fry L, Leonard JN, Swain F et al. Long-term follow-up of dermatitis herpetiformis with and without dietary gluten withdrawal. *Br J Dermatol* 1982; **107**: 631–40.
17 August PJ. *Proceedings of the First Food Allergy Workshop.* Oxford: Medical Education Services, 1980: 76–81.
18 Editorial. Gamolenic acid in atopic eczema: EPOGAM. *Drug Ther Bull* 1990; **28**: 69–70.
19 Doeglas HMG. Reactions to aspirin and food additives in patients with chronic urticaria, including the physical urticarias. *Br J Dermatol* 1975; **93**: 135–44.
20 Michaelsson G, Juhlin L. Urticaria induced by preservatives and dye additives in food and drugs. *Br J Dermatol* 1973; **88**: 525–32.
21 Rudski E, Czubalski K, Grzywa ZI. Detection of urticaria with food additives intolerance by means of diet. *Dermatologica* 1980; **161**: 57–62.
22 Warin RP, Smith RJ. Challenge test battery in chronic urticaria. *Br J Dermatol* 1976; **94**: 401–6.
23 Fry L. The treatment of dermatitis herpetiformis. *Clin Exp Dermatol* 1982; **7**: 633–42.
24 Katz SI, Hall RP III, Lawley TJ et al. Dermatitis herpetiformis. The skin and the gut. *Ann Intern Med* 1980; **93**: 857–74.
25 Alexander JO. *Dermatitis Herpetiformis.* London: WB Saunders, 1975: 313–21.
26 Engquist A, Pock-Steen OCL. Dermatitis herpetiformis and milk-free diet. *Lancet* 1971; **ii**: 438–9.

Gene therapy

Gene therapy is relevant to the skin in two ways. Firstly, the skin keratinocytes or fibroblasts can be transfected with a known gene in order to correct a metabolic disease. Secondly, genetic diseases of the skin could be corrected by inserting genes into keratinocytes or fibroblasts, but only those areas of skin most severely affected would benefit. For example, in recessive epidermolysis bullosa, inserting a normal type VII collagen gene into keratinocytes might be useful in selected severely affected areas. In order for such gene transfer to have a long-lasting effect, the transfected gene must be placed into stem cells of the skin or else the cells will be quickly lost and the effect therefore lost too. This presents a major problem for treatment of genetic skin diseases. Some early experiments are of interest. Malignant melanoma was treated by an infusion of tumour infiltrating lymphocytes manipulated to excrete large amounts of tumour necrosis factor [1]. Steroid sulphatase deficiency has been corrected by gene transfer into cultured keratinocytes from patients with X-linked ichthyosis [2]. Animal models already exist where keratinocytes are used to secrete factors, for example human growth hormone and factor IX, into the circulation.

Possible epidermal diseases that might be appropriately treated by gene therapy include epidermolytic hyperkeratosis, various forms of epidermolysis bullosa and xeroderma pigmentosum.

There is a long way to go before gene therapy becomes relevant to clinical practice, but it has great potential and is an exciting area of research [3].

REFERENCES

1 Rosenberg SA. TNF/TIL Human gene therapy. Clinical Protocol. *Hum Gene Ther* 1990; **1**: 443–62.
2 Jensen TG, Jensen UB, Ibsen HH *et al.* Correction of steroid sulphatase deficiency by gene transfer into basal cells of tissue cultured epidermis from patients with recessive x-linked ichthyosis. *Exp Cell Res* 1993; **209**: 392–7.
3 Moss C, Savin J. *Dermatology and the New Genetics*. Oxford: Blackwell Science, 1995.

Systemic drug therapy

Drug therapy may be specific, empirical or placebo in its effect. Dermatology has suffered more than most specialties from an abundance of empirics and placebos. It has not been shown that dermatological patients respond more to placebos than others, but the presence of an obvious and visible disease and the anxiety that this engenders endow all forms of treatment with an aura of suggestibility that often confuses the judgement of the patient and physician alike. The past records of dermatological therapy give abundant evidence of the 'wish to believe'. The results of 'double-blind' trials have destroyed the edifice of this belief.

Drugs should not be despised if they help the patient, but they should never be regarded as pharmacologically active without unequivocal evidence of their effectiveness. There must be no confusion in the dermatologist's mind. At his or her command there are a few specific remedies, a number of empirical ones and many placebos. The first are accepted because their action is known. The second are effective in 'double-blind' trials, although their mode of action remains unknown. The third are effective in a manner that bears no relation to the pharmacology of the drug or the pathogenesis of the disease; often, the physician endows them with his or her personality. It is important to be acquainted with the concept of the doctor as a drug and that problems may arise, as with any drug, with overdose, underdose or idiosyncratic reactions [1].

The placebo [2–5]

The placebo ('I shall please') has long been a cause of dissension among doctors and of benefit to patients. Those who extolled its virtues were accused of deceit and those who did not were led into errors of judgement on the effects of the drug they were prescribing. Trials of new therapeutic agents are still often poorly controlled, and neglect of the placebo effect [2] has led to unwarranted optimism. Too little attention has been given to the response of itching to inert drugs, despite the excellent early classical studies on the subject [6]. Any relationship between a physician and a patient creates a situation in which the placebo response may occur; the degree depends upon the personality and optimism of the physician or of the patient, the setting or nature of the communication [5], fatigue and concentration. Every prescription written may have a placebo effect in the signature. The physical and emotional act of giving and receiving creates a psychological bond. Primitive modes of religious or magical therapy leaned heavily on hieratical manipulation of the placebo situation. The occurrence of adverse effects—including rashes—in the course of placebo therapy (so-called nocebo effect) is well attested in clinical trials of many agents. Even true addiction and dependence have occurred. Every drug is also a placebo and every placebo exerts some drug-like effects. In one trial, 14% of 69 patients were found to react consistently with placebo responses [7]; an additional 55% were inconsistent reactors. Variations in the placebo response to tablets of different colours—green is best for anxiety—have been demonstrated [8]. Minor aberrations of normal physiological function may occur for many placebo effects. When an inert preparation was given to three groups with widely differing advice about the nature of the drug, those who believed it to resemble amphetamines were found to have a significantly raised pulse rate [4].

It is now accepted that the efficacy of a new drug or local preparation must be shown to be statistically and consistently superior to a matched 'dummy'. Regrettably, this is not always clear in published reports.

The placebo response in dermatology

The less effective any existing treatment, the more likely are any favourable effects to be of placebo type. Lichen planus, alopecia areata and chronic urticaria have been 'cured' in the past with many different preparations, which have not been shown to be pharmacologically effective in these diseases. But the patient has been sustained through the natural course by receiving a potion or a lotion that at least sustains the faith and the hope and, at most, is free from potential toxicity. The placebo effect is also apparent in the control of insomnia and pruritus, and extends to physical methods of treatment, notably acupuncture (p. 3300).

Preparations. Placebos must be harmless. Many drugs that are *not* harmless are really only being given as placebos. Lactose tablets are commonly given but even this substance is not totally harmless. Aspirin should be avoided. Carefully worded instructions may reinforce a placebo effect [6], as may an unusual size or shape of tablet.

No official placebo is included in the British National Formulary, but many manufacturers will supply inert preparations matched to their own products.

In general, physicians should be aware that the effect of a drug they are prescribing may be a placebo effect. On the other hand, it has been cogently argued that a placebo works better if the physician also believes in it!

Ethics. Most but not all physicians would agree that the administration of a placebo as a therapeutic measure is justifiable if no known effective treatment exists. In any case, it is less likely to harm the patient than a poorly tested or a powerful 'new' drug of uncertain value. In some cases, the deliberate use of a placebo initially may be valuable in ensuring rapport with a patient who claims to be prone to all the side-effects known for all drugs taken; and to assess the placebo response reactions. It also gains time for the anxious patient to accept a prolonged or incurable condition while a situation of rapport is being built up. This presupposes, of course, that no widely accepted active agent is available that is likely to be more beneficial.

In all cases, particularly in drug trials, the overriding consideration must always be the benefit to the patient. The doctor is always in a particularly authoritative position and must not abuse this authority. The patient's fully informed consent (with a witness) must always be obtained if a 'controlled' trial is embarked on. It is doubtful whether the use of 'dummy' preparations is ever justified in children, even with the parents' consent.

It is very important that none of us loses sight of the fact that we should not do harm to the patient, especially in an experimental situation. The so-called experiment where a mother aged 80 years was injected with malignant melanoma cells from her 50-year-old daughter, which led to the mother's most unpleasant death from metastatic malignant melanoma, must never be repeated [9]. It is essential that any proposed research is vetted by a well-qualified ethical committee before any projects are undertaken.

REFERENCES

1 Balint M, ed. *The Doctor, His Patient and the Illness*. London: Pitman Medical, 1975: 5.
2 Benson H, Epstein MD. The placebo effect. A neglected asset in the care of patients. *JAMA* 1975; **232**: 1225–6.
3 Brodeur DW. The effects of stimulant and tranquillizer placebos on healthy subjects in a real-life situation. *Psychopharmacology* 1965; **7**: 444–52.
4 Editorial. The clinical use of placebos. *Drug Ther Bull* 1965; **3**: 58–60.
5 Lasagna L, Mosteller F, von Felsinger JM *et al*. A study of the placebo response. *Am J Med* 1954; **16**: 770–9.
6 Beecher HK. Pruritus: comparison of the antipruritic effect of morphine and papaverine in experimental and pathological itch in man. In: *Measurement of Subjective Responses. Quantitative Effects of Drugs*. New York: Oxford University Press, 1959: 389–98.
7 Lasagna L. Some explored and unexplored psychological variables in therapeutics. *Proc R Soc Med* 1962; **55**: 773–6.
8 Shapira K, McClelland HA, Griffiths NR *et al*. Study on the effects of tablet colour in the treatment of anxiety states. *Br Med J* 1970; **ii**: 446–9.
9 Papworth M, ed. *Human Guinea Pigs*. Middlesex: Penguin Books, 1967: 156–7.

Antihistamines

These are discussed in Chapter 76. In the hands of many non-dermatologists, the sight of a rash evokes a reflex desire to prescribe antihistamines. These drugs are, of course, no panacea. If they are to be prescribed, there should be some thought whether they are being used for their ability to antagonize other mediators such as acetylcholine (usually considered as a side-effect), or for a central effect. Otherwise, their use must be considered as placebo, albeit usually a harmless placebo. The advent of new 'non-sedating' antihistamines, said not to cross the blood–brain barrier, makes it important not to thoughtlessly prescribe the newest antihistamine for the management of all types of pruritus (Chapters 16 & 76). Every general practitioner should have a working knowledge of short-acting, long-acting, sedative and non-sedative types.

Psychopharmacological agents

In recent years, there has been a marked trend, in the UK at least, away from reliance on these drugs or willingness to take them on the part of the patient. Even the conservative dermatologist, who may feel on occasions that the short-term administration of sedatives or hypnotics would be of help in reducing itching or restoring normal sleep patterns, may encounter unexpected resistance by the patient. Unfortunately, reasonable alternatives—discussion, the encouragement of the development of relaxation or autosuggestive techniques—are time consuming and seldom carried out by busy practitioners. Thus, anxiety may intensify until the acute 'emergency' situation, so well known to dermatologists, develops. In such cases, rest, adequate sleep and some form of sedation become imperative and may be obtained only by removal of the patient from his or her environment to hospital.

Two situations in which the rational use of psycho-pharmacological agents may be necessary are anxiety and depression. Many agents are available for the treatment of these conditions, and national and individual differences in prescribing are widespread. One drug often replaces another for reasons of improved efficacy. The dermatologist is best advised to choose two or three, preferably having short- or medium-term and more prolonged effects, and to use them appropriately.

Anxiety

Environmental sources of anxiety and tension have increased in modern industrialized life. Anxiety, not always recognized or acknowledged by the patient, may be an essential driving force in some individuals ('trait' anxiety) [1]; only when this increases, as a result of extra stresses or the presence of disease, may it become marked ('state' anxiety). Then, the symptoms themselves, for example the intensity of pruritus, may become part of a general stress response characterized by emotional overarousal [2].

Whilst the benzodiazepines [2–4] are the safest and most effective anxiolytics at present in use, there is now considerable literature on habituation and addiction to this group of drugs [5,6]. A large number are available: the main difference lies in their different plasma half-lives [2]. They are equally effective for treating both anxiety and insomnia, although the causes of the latter should be examined before recourse to drug therapy [7]. They are widely used, especially by older females in the lower socio-economic groups [8]. Diazepam and chlordiazepoxide are the best known. Nitrazepam, used as a hypnotic, has a half-life of about 30 h and may thus accumulate on repeated use. A single dose of diazepam is frequently given to allay apprehension in young children before minor operative procedures [9,10]. When appropriate, a suitable analgesic should be given before the diazepam [11]. The intravenous use of benzodiazepines carries a risk of thrombosis or ischaemia [12,13]. This drug should be diluted with blood and given slowly [12] and resuscitation facilities should be to hand. The benzodiazepines have no antidepressive effect and may, in fact, enhance depression. The side-effects are those of any drug affecting the central nervous system, including oversedation [14]. Effects of alcohol are potentiated [15]. Because of their addictive and habituating

properties, many dermatologists are now reluctant to use this group of drugs, particularly in the long term. Their use in adequate doses in the short term to prevent nocturnal pruritus and give the patient a good night's sleep can be justified. However, conventional doses of sedative antihistamines such as hydroxyzine may be equally effective and not accompanied by the risk of addiction or habituation.

Depressive states

Depression is common in dermatological patients and may present in many different guises. It is unusual for the patient to say 'I am depressed'. However, the condition is so common in dermatological patients that the attending dermatologist should always ask him- or herself 'is this particular patient depressed or not?'.

Depression with suicidal ideation is common, both in patients with psoriasis [16] and Darier's disease [17], and any extensive skin disease, particularly if it affects important body image areas, such as the face, may produce a very severe reactive depression. It is known that patients with chronic urticaria and generalized pruritus are more likely to be depressed than controls [18], and acne scarring, particularly in males, may produce severe reactive depression and even suicide [19]. Dermatological patients may become significantly depressed when they are treated with corticosteroids orally or parenterally, and depressed dermatological patients are twice as likely to be admitted to hospital, and to remain as inpatients twice as long as non-depressed dermatological patients [20]. The commonest psychiatric disease present in patients with dermatological delusional disease and with body dysmorphic disorder (dermatological non-disease), in particular, is depression [21].

Finally, dermatological patients who go to litigation are more likely to be depressed than their non-litigious peers [22]. The treatment of depression, therefore, is of vital importance in dermatological practice. If accompanied by anxiety, the depressive element may be marked. The distinction between the two is not always easily made, but may become apparent if a patient fails to respond to anxiolytics. Whilst tricyclic antidepressants such as amitriptyline in adequate dosage are effective in anxious and depressed patients, they also have some sedative properties and are not particularly helpful in patients with pure primary anxiety [2].

Doxepin is both a potent antidepressant and has very marked antihistamine activity. This antidepressant is useful in the itchy, depressed, elderly patient and in some patients with neurodermatitis [23].

The new generation of selective serotonin reuptake inhibitors have a particular place in the management of depression. This group of drugs is effective in a significant proportion of dysmorphophobic patients and also has a place in the management of obsessive–compulsive disorder. It should be noted, however, that the dose to achieve therapeutic success in these conditions is much higher than that normally required for depression alone (see Chapter 64).

Other drugs in use [4]

Butyrophenone derivations such as haloperidol are also used for anxiety, depression and alcohol withdrawal symptoms. Chloral hydrate (0.3–2 g) should not be despised as a hypnotic, particularly in children. The unpleasant taste of paraldehyde has limited its oral use, but it is an effective and quick-acting hypnotic, especially for hypomanic states, given by intramuscular injection (5–10 ml). Beta-adrenoceptor antagonists ('β-blockers') have not found much place in dermatology, although symptoms mediated by the β-division of the sympathetic nervous system have been helped by propranolol [24]. A number of side-effects have been reported [25]. Pimozide has a special place in the management of patients with delusions of parasitosis [26].

Topical therapy

The dictum 'primum non nocere', has a special significance in relation to the vulnerability of damaged skin, often with an impaired barrier function, to develop either sensitivity or irritant reactions to local applications that the same patient might find harmless at other times. There is a particular temptation to be overzealous in treatment when faced with a disease that fails to react to initial therapy. Visual evidence of failure is particularly hard to accept with equanimity. Full details of topical therapy are given in Chapter 78.

EMLA cream (a eutectic mixture of 5% lignocaine and prilocaine) is particularly useful as a local anaesthetic cream in children to try and ensure pain-free venepuncture and may also be used to try and minimize distress during curettage of lesions of molluscum contagiosum or in removing genital warts. Its use may ensure that the injection of keloids in children causes minimal distress, and it has a place in anaesthetizing the skin in children with port-wine stains during laser therapy. The cream is best applied under occlusion 1–4 h before the planned procedure [27]. A recently introduced amethocaine-containing gel has been claimed to be more effective than the EMLA local anaesthetic in patients with port-wine stains [28].

Cosmetic camouflage

Cosmetic camouflage is very useful in the management of a wide range of dermatological problems ranging from scarring to vitiligo, and vascular anomalies such as port-wine stains. In the UK, the Red Cross offers a voluntary service and in some hospitals the occupational therapists are trained to do this work.

REFERENCES

1 Spielberger CD. Anxiety as an emotional state. In: Spielberger CD, ed. *Anxiety. Current Trends in Theory and Research*, Vol. 1. New York: Academic Press, 1972: 23–49.
2 Lader M, Peturrson H. Rational use of anxiolytic/sedative drugs. *Drugs* 1983; **25**: 514–28.
3 Committee on the Review of Medicines. Systemic review on the benzodiazepines. Guidelines for data sheets on diazepam, chlordiazepoxide, medazepam, clorazepate, lorazepam, oxazepam, temazepam, triazolam, nitrazepam, and flurazepam. *Br Med J* 1980; **280**: 910–12.
4 Garattini S, Mussini E, Randall LO, eds. *The Benzodiazepines*. New York: Raven Press, 1973.
5 Marks J, ed. *The Benzodiazepines. Use, Overuse, Misuse, Abuse*. Lancaster: MTP Press, 1978.
6 Petursson H, Lader MH. Withdrawal from long-term benzodiazepine treatment. *Br Med J* 1981; **283**: 643–5.
7 Editorial. Temazepam for insomnia? *Drug Ther Bull* 1978; **16**: 21–2.
8 Lader M. Benzodiazepines—the opium of the masses? *Neuroscience* 1978; **3**: 159–65.
9 Gordon NY, Turner DJ. Oral paediatric premedication. A comparative trial of either phenobarbitone, trimeprazine or diazepam with hyoscine, prior to guillotine tonsillectomy. *Br J Anaesth* 1968; **41**: 136–42.
10 Haq IU, Dundee JW. Studies of drugs given before anaesthesia. XVI: Oral diazepam and trimeprazine for adenotonsillectomy. *Br J Anaesth* 1968; **40**: 972–8.
11 Editorial. Sedation for minor procedures. *Drug Ther Bull* 1976; **14**: 19–20.
12 Driscoll EJ, Gelfman SS, Sweet JB *et al*. Thrombophlebitis after intravenous use of anesthesia and sedation: its incidence and natural history. *J Oral Surg* 1979; **37**: 809–15.
13 Editorial. Coronary artery bypass. *Drug Ther Bull* 1981; **19**: 9–11.
14 Edwards JG. Adverse effects of antianxiety drugs. *Drugs* 1981; **22**: 495–514.
15 Linnoila M, Mattila MJ, Kitchell BS. Drug interactions with alcohol. *Drugs* 1979; **18**: 299–311.
16 Gupta MA, Schork NJ, Gupta AK *et al*. Suicidal ideation in psoriasis. *Int J Dermatol* 1993; **32**: 188–90.
17 Denicoff KD, Lehman ZA, Rubinow DR *et al*. Suicidal ideation in Darier's disease. *J Am Acad Dermatol* 1990; **22**: 196–8.
18 Sheehan-Dare R, Cotterill JA. Anxiety and depression in patients with chronic urticaria and generalised pruritus. *Br J Dermatol* 1990; **123**: 769–74.
19 Cotterill JA, Cunliffe WJ. Suicide in dermatological patients. *Br J Dermatol* 1997 (Accepted for publication).
20 Pulimood S, Rajagopalan B, Rajagopalan M *et al*. Psychiatric morbidity among dermatology in-patients. *Natl Med J India* 1996; **9**: 208–10.
21 Hardy G, Cotterill JA. A study of depression and obsessionality in dysmorphophobic and psoriatic patients. *Br J Psychiatry* 1982; **140**: 19–22.
22 Cotterill JA. Why do patients sue? Paper presented at the Vth Congress of the European Academy of Dermatology and Venereology, October 1996.
23 Koo JYM. The treatment of chronic cutaneous sensory syndrome with psychotropic medications. *Proceedings of the Second International Congress on Dermatology and Psychiatry*, Leeds, 1989.
24 Tyrer P. Use of beta-blocking drugs in psychiatry and neurology. *Drugs* 1980; **20**: 300–8.
25 Clerens A, Guilmot-Bruneau MM, Defresne C *et al*. Revue: a propos des beta-bloquants en dermatologie. *Dermatologica* 1981; **163**: 5–11.
26 Koblenzer CS, ed. *Psychocutaneous Disease*. New York: Grune & Stratton, 1987: 20.
27 Clarke S, Radford M. Topical anaesthesia for venepuncture. *Arch Dis Child* 1986; **61**: 1132–5.
28 Armstrong DKB, Handley J, Allen GE. Effect of percutaneous local anaesthesia on pain caused by pulsed dye laser treatment of port wine stains. *Br J Dermatol* 1996; **135** (Suppl. 47): 14.

Dressings

The type of dressing to be used for covering the skin during topical treatment requires careful consideration. Wet dressings lower the temperature of the treated area, occluded dressings increase it. The purpose of a dressing is to keep the agent used in close apposition to the skin and, normally, to allow the free evaporation of sweat. It should prevent or minimize friction, chafing and damage from rubbing and scratching, and be comfortable for the patient. It should enable the patient, whenever possible, to carry on with normal life while retaining in place the applications used, without undue soiling or staining of clothing.

Cool, light dressings should be used for covering wet dressings or creams in acute eczematous conditions; cotton gloves should be worn at night to keep ointments and pastes in place. In particular circumstances, paste bandages covered with tubular gauze may be applied for several days at a time in chronic eczema, and polyethylene occlusive dressings may be used to increase penetration of corticosteroids.

When wet dressings are applied, several layers of linen soaked in the solution are kept constantly dampened by removing the outer layers and soaking them in a fresh solution. Such dressings can be kept in place with a loose outer covering if the patient is at rest in bed. Otherwise tubular gauze is useful. Pastes may be applied on strips of linen and laid over the affected area, but are best applied directly to the skin and covered with a stockinette of firm tubular gauze or elasticated tubular net.

In any raw or exuding lesions, plain paraffin gauze or non-adherent gauze is preferable and can be removed without discomfort. This in turn may be covered with ordinary gauze, linen or other dressings as appropriate.

Tubular gauze

By ingenious techniques of folding and cutting, this closely woven, fine, tubular gauze provides a covering in the shape of sandals, stockings, helmets, vests, etc. An experienced nurse can very rapidly cover the whole surface of the body and the dressings will stay in place for 12–24 h. A 'suit' of Tubegauze may be worn as underclothing beneath ordinary clothes. Oozing of pastes through the gauze is prevented by dusting with an inert powder. Surgical stockinette, which is thicker, is also widely used for the same purpose.

Elasticated tubular net

This type of bandage is increasingly used in a wide variety of situations. It has the advantage of simplicity, adaptability and easy removal. It is relatively long lasting and can be washed without significant loss of elasticity.

Occlusive dressings

Initial enthusiasm for polyethylene occlusion over topical corticosteroids has been tempered by a recognition of its limitations and adverse effects. However, used judiciously, it remains a very valuable technique. A piece or tube of polyethylene, particularly of the self-clinging film type, is secured over the treated area and left in place for 8 h or longer. In psoriasis, for which it was originally chiefly used, the immediate results are good, but relapse occurs rapidly after its use is discontinued. Its main value in this disease is as a preliminary short-term treatment before passing on to other therapy. Certain side-effects should be noted. The rustling is aesthetically disturbing to some patients or their spouses and a disagreeable odour accompanies prolonged occlusion. Folliculitis may occur especially on hairy limbs. The risk can be reduced by restricting the occlusion to 10–12 h a day, by thorough cleansing before application, by the concomitant use of antibacterial bath additives or emulsions, or by steroid–antibacterial preparations. It is best to avoid occlusion over antiseptics for prolonged spells as contact dermatitis to antiseptics is likely to occur. In hospital wards, there is the added risk of contamination by *Pseudomonas aeruginosa* [1]. Absorption of corticosteroids may occur to a significant degree under widespread occlusion. In extensive psoriasis, the danger of approaching a significant systemic dose is evident. Local atrophy is sometimes reversible after several months, but if advanced, will be permanent.

Occlusive therapy remains of value in the treatment of chronic eczematous or psoriatic conditions of the hands, feet and scalp, where polyethylene gloves, bags or contrived helmets are used overnight.

Leg dressings

Crepe or elastic net bandaging may be used over applications. Old pyjama trousers or long underpants are of value underneath ordinary trousers to prevent staining of the clothes. Tubular elastic bandages, or elastic webbing bandages, give more support. In the application of compressive leg bandaging, pressure must be carefully and evenly applied from the base of the toes to below the knees. Selective pressure, with or without foam pads or slats of paste bandage, may be concentrated at the blow-out site in the form of a pad. In general, the mistake is to exert too little, rather than too much, pressure. The technique can be learnt only by experience. Pressure bandaging is dealt with in more detail in Chapter 50.

Four-layer compression for venous ulcers

A multilayer bandaging system for venous leg ulcers where the ankle/brachial arterial Doppler index is 0.8 or greater has been reported to heal 69% of ulcers at 12 weeks and 83% at 24 weeks [2]. A further study of 514 venous leg ulcers, all with ankle/brachial Doppler index of 0.8 or greater, showed healing rates of 14% at 12 weeks and 57% at 24 weeks with a prediction of 80% healing at 2 years [3].

The four layers include a cotton-wool layer, a crepe layer, an elastic layer of Elset and finally a layer of Coban. Correctly applied, this four-layer system achieves a pressure of 40 mmHg at the ankle and the system stays in place for a week before changing.

As an alternative to the described four-layer system, there are now two high-compression elastic bandages available in the UK (Setopress and Tensopress), which can either be used on their own or, possibly more appropriately, by the application of a cotton-wool layer underneath, followed by crepe and then Setopress or Tensopress replacing the Elset and Coban layers of the four-layer system described above.

Leg-ulcer dressings

These are discussed in more detail in Chapter 50. Non-adhesive gauzes are pleasant for the patient, but abundant exudate may spread beneath them. Hydrocolloid and alginate dressings are very useful and usually deliver a clean, epithelializing surface. These dressings can be left on for up to a week, although they may need changing more often if the wounds weep excessively. In messy ulcers, an alternative dressing used in polyurethane foam dressing sheets and these are especially useful, as they are hydrophilic and non-adhesive. Proteolytic enzymes [4] hydrolyse collagen fibres. They are applied after cleaning the ulcer and removing any loose debris. They are useful only on patients admitted to hospital and are used to help to loosen firm eschar or debris and should only be used for up to a week at a time. They will certainly prevent new epithelium being formed, and so it is important to discontinue such agents once the wound has been debrided.

Small dextranomer beads provide an ingenious way of drawing up exudates and their contents, thus removing bacteria and degradation products to the surface [5,6]. They do often appear to produce a clean, dry ulcer bed, but the drying effect may occasionally cause some pain. More specialized leg-ulcer and wound dressings are considered in Chapter 50.

Felt, Sorbo and plastic foam

These can be used to supplement pressure or to protect areas vulnerable to trauma or friction. Foam pads to localize pressure over intercommunicating veins are more effective if extended some way up the saphenous vein and beneath the malleolus. The cotton-wool layer of the four-layer system is particularly helpful in this regard and can be used to pad out difficult areas such as prominent malleoli.

Compression stockings

While plain paraffin gauze (tulle gras) or non-adherent gauze dressings fulfil most needs, there is a place for the short-term use of medicated dressings in open infected lesions. Several varieties are now available but should be used with discretion over leg ulcers, where the risk of sensitization is high [7].

Medicated paste bandages

Of the several types available, the zinc paste, coal-tar paste and iodohydroxyquinoline bandages are most frequently used. They should be cut or folded frequently and moulded to the skin while being applied, avoiding constriction at the bends of the knees and elbows. They are useful in atopic dermatitis, discoid and other forms of chronic eczema, lichen simplex, hypertrophic lichen planus, prurigo, artefacts and gravitational eczema and ulceration. They are covered by any conventional form of dressing appropriate to the site. Corticosteroids can be applied beneath these, if required.

Wet-wrap dressings

Wet-wrap dressings are especially useful in children with severe atopic eczema. They are usually applied overnight but in severe cases can be applied throughout the day. The child is bathed with emollients added; the child's skin is then covered in an emollient cream, and on areas of eczema a mildly potent or moderately potent topical corticosteroid is applied. Damp tubular gauze is applied and, in severe, cases, a complete suit to cover the limbs and body is made. On the outside, a dry layer of tubegauze is applied and the dressings are left on either overnight or for a 24-h period.

Corticosteroid-impregnated tapes

An acrylic-backed adhesive tape impregnated with flurandrenolone, $4 \mu g/cm^2$, offers a cosmetically attractive and simple form of occlusive dressing (Cordran, Haelan tape) for lichen simplex, hypertrophic lichen planus, hyperkeratotic palmar eczema, local patches of lupus erythematosus and some cases of localized palmoplantar pustulosis.

Colostomy dressings

These usually come to the notice of dermatologists only if sensitization or irritant dermatitis has developed. It is usual for any reaction from colostomy dressings to be of contact irritant type rather than contact allergic.

Allergic contact dermatitis

Patients with ulcers or eczema of the leg appear to be particularly prone to develop sensitization reactions to parabens, antibiotics, antiseptics, lanolin and topical corticosteroids. This may limit the choice of dressings used. They may also become sensitized to rubber chemicals in elasticated supports: this imposes a considerable restriction in the choice of supporting devices used to control oedema. Keep all topical treatments simple and as far as possible free from potential allergens. It is important, therefore, to avoid as far as possible antiseptics, topical antibiotics and products containing lanolin in particular.

REFERENCES

1 Noble WC, Savin JA. Steroid cream contaminated with Pseudomonas aeruginosa. *Lancet* 1966; **i**: 347–9.
2 Moffat CJ, Franks PJ, Oldridge M *et al*. Community clinic for leg ulcers and impact on healing. *Br Med J* 1992; **305**: 1389–92.
3 Thompson B, Powell, Warin AP. Healing rates of venous leg ulcers in the community using the 'Charing Cross' 4-layer system. *Br J Dermatol* 1995; **133** (Suppl. 45): 32.
4 Niermann MM. Treatment of dermal and decubitus ulcers. *Drugs* 1978; **15**: 226–30.
5 Frank DH, Robson MC, Heggars JP. Evaluation of Debrisan as a treatment of leg ulcers. *Ann Plast Surg* 1979; **3**: 395–400.
6 Jacobson S, Rothman U, Arturson G *et al*. A new principle for the cleansing of infected wounds. *Scand J Plast Reconstr Surg* 1976; **10**: 65–72.
7 Wilkinson JD, Hambly EM, Wilkinson DS. Comparison of patch test results in two adjacent areas of England. II Medicaments. *Acta Derm Venereol (Stockh)* 1980; **60**: 245–9.

Physical measures

Physiotherapy

The role of physiotherapists has assumed increased importance in recent years. Their duties have extended far from the massage and simple forms of heat and light therapy of the past. They have become valuable members of a team devoted to a wide range of physiotherapeutic manoeuvres and to rehabilitation in the widest context.

In dermatology, the physiotherapist is probably not sufficiently invited to participate in the overall management of the patient with chronic or disabling diseases. Rehabilitation is discussed below, but techniques of relaxation are of benefit to many tense patients with irritable or vasolabile skin disease. Muscular relaxation is a key that opens the door to emotional relaxation, but it requires some experience and training to use the key effectively. Relaxation techniques [1] are a valuable adjunct to drug therapy and may even supplant it. Massage and re-education in limb movement are of great practical value in patients with constricting scars and deforming linear scleroderma, for which we have so little to offer. The influence of communal participation of physiotherapeutic activities, in which warmth, touch and encouragement combine to create an ambience conducive to relaxation and to a feeling of positive activity, should not be underestimated.

Massage [2] is valuable in the treatment of lymphoedema (Chapter 51) and in rosacea.

Some physiotherapists have expertise in the management of venous leg ulceration and can participate in treatment from an early stage through the period of healing and rehabilitation.

Tap water iontophoresis is performed by many physiotherapy departments and is particularly useful in patients with hyperhidrosis of the hands, feet and axillae [3].

Other modes of physical medicine, such as short-wave diathermy, play a small part in dermatological management.

Ultrasound has found a secure place in the treatment of soft-tissue disease and injury [4,5] and may occasionally be of adjuvant value in conditions such as scleroderma [6], panniculitis and other dermatological conditions affecting deeper tissues.

Phototherapy, often performed by physiotherapists, is discussed in Chapter 35.

Acupuncture

The empirical basis on which this technique rested for so long has been dramatically changed by the discovery of the endorphins, and recent work has indicated that the response to acupuncture can be mediated centrally by endorphins and enkephalins [7]. It has been shown that acupuncture can reduce the effect of histamine-induced itch and flare in healthy subjects [8]. The acupuncture points described in ancient Chinese medical literature correspond to some of the so-called trigger points described in Western medicine, and are said to represent areas of low electrical resistance.

Low-dose helium neon laser light and other types of lasers directed at acupuncture points have been claimed to be effective in a wide variety of conditions, but no valid double-blind clinical trials have been carried out. Anecdotally, post-herpetic neuralgia and atopic dermatitis seem to be helped in some patients by acupuncture, but it is difficult to assess the results of treatment. However, there are few risks as long as the needles are properly sterilized.

Biofeedback techniques

These involve the induction of a learned response aimed at controlling or modifying vascular responses [9] or inappropriate bodily responses to various centrally mediated stimuli. They may reduce emotional intensification of erythema and have been used to control flushing, for patients with dyshidrosis whose disease flared with stress [10] and in patients with atopic dermatitis [11]. Thirty-three patients with eczema were trained to decrease or increase electrical conductivity of the skin. Those who were trained to decrease skin conductance showed clinical improvement, while the controls who were trained in the opposite direction did not. The positive response was accompanied by a significant decrease in measured conductance and anxiety [12]. Eleven of 14 patients with chronic hyperhidrosis improved following biofeedback training. The most important aspect of the treatment was thought to be relaxation [13]. However, there is considerable individual variability in responses [1], and the main value may lie in anxiety reduction [14] and in the active involvement of the patient in self-help. It has been suggested that the techniques may be the 'ultimate placebo' [15] and their place in dermatology may remain limited by the time and patience required. Nevertheless, further developments in these methods may prove rewarding in specific dermatological situations, given a highly motivated and suitable subject.

Behaviour therapy

The use of behaviour therapy in dermatology was well summarized by Bar and Kuypers, who described four main therapeutic approaches [16].

Systemic desensitization is employed mainly in neurotic disorders where anxiety is the main clinical feature. An attempt is made to induce inhibition of anxiety following repeated exposures to weak anxiety-raising stimuli, after which progressively stronger stimuli are introduced. This type of behaviour therapy has limited application in dermatological practice.

In aversion therapy, patients with persistent behaviour disorders such as compulsive scratching or pathological hair pulling can be treated. The patient is given an unpleasant stimulus, for example a mild electric shock, whenever the unadaptive habit is demonstrated or displayed.

Operant techniques can be used to modify compulsive habits, and awards are given to reinforce good behaviour and bad behaviour is either punished or ignored. In children, a token may be given after a period of good (non-scratching) behaviour as part of a so-called token economy system.

Assertive training is employed in patients who are afraid of expressing their emotions and also experience extreme social fear. This technique is said to be most useful in patients with facial erythema or erythrophobia and also has a place in the treatment of patients with hyperhidrosis.

An operant technique was used successfully to modify the scratching behaviour in a patient with long-standing severe dermatitis, which had defied all traditional therapy [17]. As soon as the patient was observed scratching he was asked to fold his arms and think of something pleasant. Normal social attention was then withheld as a mild punishment. This man improved. The technique of habit reversal has an important place in the management of both adults and children with atopic eczema [18–20]. The patients were taught situation awareness so that they could recognize situations that made them itch. The patients were also instructed either to grasp an object or to keep the hands firmly on the itching area and pinch it if necessary but not scratch it. A strong correlation was demonstrated between a reduction in scratching and an improvement in skin status [19,20].

REFERENCES

1 Volow MR, Erwin CW, Cipolat AL. Biofeedback control of skin potential level. *Biofeedback Self Regul* 1979; **4**: 133–43.
2 Foldi M, Casley-Smith JR. *Lymphangiology*. Stüttgart: Schattauer, 1983: 677.
3 Abel E, Morgan K. The treatment of idiopathic hyperhidrosis by glycopyrronium bromide and tap water iontophoresis. *Br J Dermatol* 1974; **91**: 87–91.
4 Dyson M, Suckling J. Stimulation of tissue repair by ultrasound. A survey of the mechanisms involved. *Physiotherapy* 1978; **64**: 105–8.
5 Dyson M, Franks C, Suckling J. Stimulation of healing of varicose ulcers by ultrasound. *Ultrasonics* 1976; **14**: 232–6.
6 Rudolph RI, Leyden JJ. Physiatrics for deforming linear scleroderma. *Arch Dermatol* 1976; **112**: 995–7.
7 Mayer DJ, Price DD, Rafil A. Antagonism of acupuncture analgesia in man by the narcotic antagonist naloxone. *Brain Res* 1977; **121**: 368–72.
8 Belgrade MJ, Solomon LM, Lichter EA. The effect of acupuncture on experimentally-induced itch. *Acta Derm Venerol (Stockh)* 1984; **64**: 129–33.
9 Friar LR, Beatty J. Migraine: management by trained control of vasoconstriction. *J Consult Clin Psychol* 1976; **44**: 46–53.
10 Koldys KW, Meyer RP. Biofeedback training in the therapy of dyshidrosis. *Cutis* 1979; **24**: 219–21.
11 Haynes SN, Wilson CC, Jaffe PG, Britton BT. Biofeedback treatment of atopic dermatitis. Controlled case studies of eight cases. *Biofeedback Self Regul* 1979; **4**: 195–209.
12 Miller RM, Coger RW. Skin conductance conditioning with dyshidrotic eczema patients. *Br J Dermatol* 1986; **115**: 435–40.
13 Duller P, Doyle Gentry W. Use of biofeedback in treating chronic hyperhidrosis: a preliminary report. *Br J Dermatol* 1980; **103**: 143–6.
14 Green EE, Green AM, Walters ED. Biofeedback training for anxiety tension reduction. *Ann NY Acad Sci* 1974; **233**: 157–61.
15 Stroebel CF, Glueck BC. Biofeedback treatment in medicine and psychiatry: an ultimate placebo? In: Birk L, ed. *Biofeedback: Behavioural Medicine*. New York, Grune & Stratton, 1973: 19–33.
16 Bar LHJ, Kuypers BRM. Behaviour therapy in dermatological practice. *Br J Dermatol* 1973; **88**: 591–8.
17 Cataldo MF, Varni JW, Russo DC, Estes SA. Behaviour therapy techniques in treatment of exfoliative dermatitis. *Arch Dermatol* 1980; **116**: 919–22.
18 Bridgett C, Noren P, Staughton R. *Atopic Skin Disease. A Manual for Practitioners*. Petersfield: Wrightson Biomedical Publishing, 1996: 43–7.
19 Melin L, Frederiksen T, Noren P et al. Behavioural treatment of scratching in patients with atopic dermatitis. *Br J Dermatol* 1986; **115**: 467–74.
20 Bridrett C, Moréy P, Staughton R. *Atopic Skin Disease: A Manual for Practitioners*. Petersfield: Wrightson Biomedical Publishing, 1996: 43–7.

Heliotherapy and actinotherapy [1–5]

The use of artificial UV radiation in dermatological therapy was pioneered by Finsen at the turn of the century, but its study has received a great stimulus in recent decades with the advent of psoralen and UVA (PUVA) therapy, the increasing popular demand for a 'healthy' tan and with the increasing realization of the potential harm from any form of UV radiation. Artificial sources of UV radiation are unable to simulate natural sunlight precisely, but they can in theory emit wavelengths that are appropriate for a particular purpose.

The types of UV lamp available will not be discussed in detail. PUVA is discussed in Chapter 35. The carbon arc lamp is now little used. The main source of UV radiation is the mercury vapour lamp, the radiation emitted depending on the pressure within the lamp, the phosphors coating the tube and other variables, which help to provide a more continuous spectrum like that of sunlight. The Kromayer lamp was designed mainly for contact therapy. It emits considerable amounts of shorter UV radiation and is not now used very much for therapeutic purposes. Alpine sunlamps and Theraktin lamps are examples of mercury vapour lamps that have been available for many years. A comparison of Phillips TL-12 and Sylvaner UV6 and UV21 tubes showed them to be equivalent in effect [4]. The xenon lamp [6] emits a more continuous spectrum, which makes it valuable for experimental and testing purposes but expense limits its therapeutic use. UV lamps provide a much more powerful source of UV radiation than natural sunlight, although a properly designed therapeutic course of UV radiation may give an amount of radiation comparable with that from a fortnight's sunny holiday.

Dermatological uses

Where natural sunlight is lacking [7] actinotherapy may be simulated with the Alpine sunlamp or with banks of fluorescent UVB lamps. The role of UVB in the treatment of psoriasis is traditional and has been disputed but now seems to be gaining favour again (Chapter 35). In particular, narrow-band UVB has a useful role in the management of psoriasis [8], difficult and severe atopic eczema [9], polymorphic light eruption [10], and other photodermatoses [11]. Acne vulgaris may be helped by exposure to UVB but the effect is less dramatic than that of natural sun. However, it must be remembered that there are data to suggest that UV radiation is comedogenic, and acne aestivalis is a distinct clinical entity [12]. Chilblains and erythrocyanosis have been treated with doses of four or more minimal erythema doses of UVB, repeated three or more times (Chapter 25). In some clinics, very short-wave (bactericidal) doses of UV radiation, given conveniently by the contact Kromayer lamp, are used for leg ulcers. The dose must be many times that of the minimal erythema dose [1].

Phototherapy is used also to treat neonatal icterus and may be helpful in controlling the pruritus of primary biliary cirrhosis [13] and uraemia [14], and even the intensive pruritus of acquired immune deficiency syndrome (AIDS) [15]. Traditionally, it has been used empirically to speed

resolution (or perhaps disguise the lesions) of pityriasis lichenoides chronica. Carefully graded exposure to natural sunlight, UVB, UVA or PUVA can also be used to cause increased pigmentation and tanning for the treatment or prophylaxis of light-sensitive dermatoses, especially polymorphic light eruption.

The influence of UV radiation on the immune system is important [2,16].

Sunbeds [17,18]

These have achieved a considerable popularity in recent years. Some sun beds and sun-tan parlours provide UVB. In England, many now emit mainly or entirely UVA. As UVA is biologically very much less active than UVB, small traces of UVB in a light source can be very significant. UVA is much less effective in producing a durable tan, but may achieve some [19–21]. There is little evidence that this does much towards positive health, and it probably potentiates the harmful effects of UVB, especially the photo-ageing effects. Patients with any form of light sensitivity, and those on photosensitizing drugs or in contact with topical photosensitizers, must take special care.

REFERENCES

1 Diffey BL. *Ultraviolet Radiation in Medicine. Medical Physics Handbooks II.* Bristol: Adam Hilger, 1982.
2 Editorial. Skin photobiology. *Lancet* 1983; **i**: 566–8.
3 Magnus IA, ed. *Dermatological Photobiology.* Oxford: Blackwell Scientific Publications, 1976.
4 Schothorst AA, Boer J, Suurmond D *et al.* Application of controlled high dose rates in UV-B phototherapy for psoriasis. *Br J Dermatol* 1984; **110**: 81–7.
5 Wadsworth H, Chanmugam APP. *Electrophysical Agents in Physiotherapy.* Australia: Science Press, 1980.
6 Berger DS. Specification and design of solar ultraviolet simulators. *J Invest Dermatol* 1969; **53**: 192–9.
7 Diffey BL, Larko O, Swanbeck G. UV-B doses received during different outdoor activities and UV-B treatment of psoriasis. *Br J Dermatol* 1982; **106**: 33–41.
8 Green C, Lakshmipathi T, Johnson BE *et al.* A comparison of the efficacy and relapse rates of narrow-band UVB (TL-01) monotherapy, vs. etretinate (re-TL-01), vs. etretinate-PUVA (re-PUVA) in the treatment of psoriasis patients. *Br J Dermatol* 1992; **127**: 5–9.
9 George SA, Bilsland DJ, Johnson BE *et al.* Narrow-band (TL-01) air conditioned phototherapy for chronic severe adult atopic dermatitis. *Br J Dermatol* 1993; **128**: 49–56.
10 Blisland D, George SA, Gibbs NK *et al.* The comparison of narrow-band phototherapy (TL-01) and photo-chemotherapy (PUVA) in the management of polymorphic light eruption. *Br J Dermatol* 1993; **129**: 708–12.
11 Collins P, Ferguson J. Narrow-band UVB (TL-01) phototherapy: an effective preventive treatment for the photodermatoses. *Br J Dermatol* 1995; **132**: 956–63.
12 Hjorth M, Sjolin KE, Sylvest B *et al.* Acne aestivalis—Mallorca acne. *Acta Derm Venereol (Stockh)* 1972; **52**: 61–4.
13 Hanid MA, Levi AJ. Phototherapy for pruritus in primary biliary cirrhosis. *Lancet* 1980; **ii**: 530.
14 Gilchrest BA, Rowe JW, Brown RS *et al.* Relief of uremic pruritus with ultraviolet phototherapy. *N Engl J Med* 1977; **297**: 136–8.
15 Gorin I, Lessana-Leibowitch M, Fortier P *et al.* Successful treatment of the pruritus of human immunodeficiency virus infection and acquired immunodeficiency syndrome with psoralens plus UV-A therapy. *J Am Acad Dermatol* 1989; **20**: 511–13.
16 Fox IJ, Perry LL, Sy M-S *et al.* The influence of ultraviolet light irradiation on the immune system. *Clin J Immunol Immunopathol* 1980; **17**: 141–55.

17 Epstein JH. Suntan salons and the American skin. *South Med J* 1981; **74**: 837–40.
18 Hawk JLM. Sunbeds. *Br Med J* 1982; **286**: 329.
19 Kaidbey KH, Kligman AM. Photopigmentation with trioxsalen. *Arch Dermatol* 1974; **109**: 674–7.
20 Kaidbey KH, Kligman AM. Sunburn protection by longwave ultraviolet radiation-induced pigmentation. *Arch Dermatol* 1978; **114**: 46–8.
21 Langner A, Kligman AM. Tanning without sunburn with aminobenzoic acid-type sunscreen. *Arch Dermatol* 1972; **106**: 338–43.

Hypothermia and hyperthermia

Cooling of the scalp to 25° with ice turban packs or chemical coolants has been used to prevent or reduce hair loss during the critical period after administration of chemotherapeutic drugs [1]. Cooling of port-wine stains prior to treatment with the argon laser has also been tried to improve the efficacy of laser therapy and also to minimize scarring [2].

Resulting from the demonstration of the potential of hyperthermia as an antitumour agent [3,4], there have been occasional reports of its value in treating deep mycoses [5], leishmaniasis and myobacterial infections. Some similarity between the kinetics of tumour cells and psoriasis cells has prompted its use in the form of ultrasound in this disease [6]. Chemically generated heat in exothermic bags was used in 22 psoriatics in comparison with Goeckerman's regime [7], with apparent success and without side-effects. This convenient form of therapy requires further study.

REFERENCES

1 Guy R, Shah S, Parker H *et al*. Scalp cooling by thermocirculator. *Lancet* 1982; i: 937–8.
2 Gilchrest BA, Rosen S, Noe JM. Chilling port wine stains improves response to argon laser. *Plast Reconstr Surg* 1982; **69**: 278–83.
3 Cavaliere R, Ciocatto EC, Giovanella BC *et al*. Selective heat sensitivity of cancer cells. Biochemical and clinical studies. *Cancer* 1967; **20**: 1351–81.
4 Suit HD, Shwayder M. Hyperthermia: potential as an anti-tumor agent. *Cancer* 1974; **34**: 122–9.
5 Tagami H, Ohi M, Aoshima T *et al*. Topical heat therapy for cutaneous chromomycosis. *Arch Dermatol* 1979; **115**: 740–1.
6 Orenberg EK, Deneau DG, Farber EM. Response of chronic psoriatic plaques to localized heating induced by ultrasound. *Arch Dermatol* 1980; **116**: 893–7.
7 Urabe H, Nishitani K, Konda H. Hyperthermia in the treatment of psoriasis. *Arch Dermatol* 1981; **117**: 770–4.

Hypnotherapy

See Chapter 64.

Abreactive therapy

This technique, used widely after World War II to treat diseases thought to be tension related, appeared to be of value at the time [1,2]. However, it has been little used in recent years [3].

REFERENCES

1 Shorvon HJ, Rook AJ, Wilkinson DS. Psychological treatment in skin disorders with special reference to abreactive techniques. *Br Med J* 1950; ii: 1300–4.
2 Slater E, Roth M, eds. *Clinical Psychiatry*. London: Ballière, 1969.
3 Whitlock FA. Psychophysiological aspects of skin disease. In: Rook AJ, ed. *Major Problems in Dermatology*, Vol. 8. London: WB Saunders, 1976: 226–7.

Climatotherapy [1]

A calm and restful environment is of value in the treatment of disease in which emotional factors play a part, even a secondary one. When this environment includes constant sunshine, particularly at the seaside [2], conditions such as acne and psoriasis will usually benefit. In high altitude sanitoria, a reduction in air-borne allergens can be expected to help some atopic patients. Psoriatics have benefited greatly by visits to the Dead Sea [3] and other specialized centres in Europe (Chapter 35). It is difficult for those of us who do not have the advantages of these retreats to assess realistically the specific claims made for them in relation to alterations in enzymes, vitamin levels [1,4] and cutaneous reactivity [5], but the psychological benefits appear to be long lasting.

REFERENCES

1 Purschel W, Pahl O, Knust T. Fluvographische Untersuchungen bei Psoriasis Vulgaris wahrend Klimatherapie/Nordsee. *Zeitschr Hautkrankheit* 1980; **55**: 193–209.
2 Molin L. Climate therapy for Swedish psoriatics on Hvar, Yugoslavia. *Acta Derm Venereol (Stockh)* 1972; **52**: 155–60.
3 Avrach WW, Niordsen AM. Psoriasisbehandling ved det d'ode Hav. *Ugeskrift Laeger* 1974; **136**: 2687–90.
4 Zlatkov NB, Babushkina N, Stransky L. Influence of helio- and thalasso-therapy on the vitamin A and beta-carotene levels in psoriasis. *Dermatol Monatsschr* 1976; **162**: 746–9.
5 Purschel W. Dermatologische Klimatherapie an der Nordsee. Klinisch-analytische Untersuchungen am konstitutionellen Ekzematoid mit/ohne/Asthma bronchiale und/oder Rhinitis atopica. *Dermatologica* 1973; **146** (Suppl. 1): 1–98.

Homeopathy [1]

Homeopathy is a system of therapy originated by Samuel Hahnemann in the latter part of the 18th century. Central to the theory of homeopathy is the thesis that those agents that produce symptoms of any given disease will, in a much smaller dosage, cure that disease. Others have described homeopathy as a harnessing of an energy unknown to orthodox science.

Proponents of homeopathy state that there are three essential processes in the preparation of remedies, namely dilution, succussion and trituration. By dilutating the drug, the toxicity of the original product disappears and during succussion and trituration some supposed mechanical energy is imparted to the remedy, imprinting the pharmacological message of the original drug upon the molecules in the diluent. From the practical point of view there seems no doubt that many patients are happy to consult with homeopathic practitioners, and most of these consultations do no harm unless a patient is advised to stop their oral or topical steroids suddenly. There is no doubt that homeopathic practitioners spend a great deal of time with the patient and some patients undoubtedly benefit from this enhanced level of communication which they are unlikely to find in a busy National Health Service clinic.

Despite two centuries of work, there are very few controlled clinical trials that allow homeopathy to be assessed [1].

In a study of alternative medicine, utilized by patients with atopic dermatitis and psoriasis, it was found that over 50% of patients with atopic eczema and over 40% of patients with psoriasis reported previous or current use of one or more forms of alternative medicine, and homeopathy, health-food preparations and herbal remedies were used most. The use was related to disease duration and disease severity and inefficiency of therapy prescribed by physicians as judged by the patients. The author concluded that the use of alternative medicine is commonplace and should be of concern to dermatologists [2].

REFERENCES

1 Cotterill JA. Alternative medicine and dermatology. In: Champion RH, ed. *Recent Advances in Dermatology*, No. 7. Edinburgh: Churchill Livingstone, 1986: 257–8.
2 Jenssen P. Use of alternative medicine by patients with atopic dermatitis and psoriasis. *Acta Derm Venereol (Stockh)* 1990; **70**: 421–4.

Occupational therapy and rehabilitation

A person conditioned to an active life does not take kindly to bed rest. Patients with skin diseases should be encouraged to become mobile as soon as their state allows it. Those with venous leg ulcers should not be kept in bed for long periods (although periodic elevation of the leg is important), but should have active and passive leg exercises to reduce the risk of thrombosis, foot drop and atrophy of the leg muscles. They should be encouraged to walk for increasing periods, rather than sitting, in order to re-educate their leg movements. The elderly patient with exfoliative dermatitis or pemphigus should be stimulated to pass his or her time without boredom, which passes imperceptibly in the aged into depression and despondency. In the alien milieu of a hospital ward, the elderly patient quickly deteriorates mentally and physically. Subsequent discharge or rehabilitation may then be extremely difficult. Occupational therapy should not only engage manual skill but also satisfy the emotional and intellectual needs of the patient of any age.

Patient self-help groups [1]

Increasingly, patients want to know more about their skin disease and its treatment. It is not always possible to meet all the patient's needs in an outpatient appointment, and, moreover, there is a limit to how much a patient can take in at one outpatient visit. This is where the self-help groups are increasingly important. The concept of self-help is that patients 'own' their own disease and find out more about their disease for themselves and are not just passively reliant on doctors and nurses for information and help. Such groups generate information, emotional support and advice. Patients can meet others with similar skin diseases and so realize that they are not alone. Patient self-help groups usually raise funds to support their activities, which will include research grants. They also lobby Members of Parliament to ensure that the needs of skin patients are heard and met. Pressure is often put on the purchasing Health Authority and the provider units to improve their service and to increase the amount of money spent on dermatology. Lastly, such groups attempt to diminish the stigma of skin disease that still exists in the community. The role of the patients' self-help group in dermatology is increasingly important to patients with skin disease and their general practitioners, dermatologists and nurses alike.

REFERENCE

1 Funnell C. Importance of patients' self-help groups—a British perspective. *Retinoids Today Tomorrow* 1995; **41**: 6–8.

Disability from skin diseases and quality of life

Skin diseases do not often kill, but they can make life a misery. Too often skin diseases are dismissed by the general public and even by doctors as being trivial. Several centres have addressed disability from skin diseases and quality of life (QOL) and have looked mainly at effects of acne, eczema, psoriasis and leg ulcers.

Disability was studied in patients with acne, psoriasis or eczema attending a hospital clinic, and 64% of patients said their skin disease affected their work. Eighty per cent of patients expressed some subjective psychological effects, mostly anxiety, lack of confidence, depression or embarrassment [1].

An eczema disability index (EDI) has been developed [2] and used in conjunction with a general health questionnaire—the sickness impact profile (UK SIP). The EDI and the UK SIP were used to assess the effect of a course of cyclosporin treatment on the lives of patients with atopic dermatitis. A major improvement was found in QOL and disability after 8 weeks of cyclosporin treatment [3]. In children, it has been shown that atopic eczema has a major impact on QOL [4].

It has been recognized for many years that psoriasis affects patients' lives. In one study [5], 84% of patients with psoriasis expressed difficulties in establishing social contacts and relationships and stated it was the worst aspect of their psoriasis, although soreness and irritation were also important.

The psoriasis disability index (PDI) was developed to assess the degree to which psoriasis impaired QOL. A significant decrease in PDI was found after a spell of inpatient treatment [6]. The same workers have also studied the level of disability of patients with severe psoriasis [7]. The mean PDI was 38.2% and most patients felt it would be worse to have diabetes, asthma or bronchitis. However, 49% would be prepared to spend 2–3 h each day on treatment if it kept their skin clear of psoriasis. Ninety-eight per cent of patients would prefer a cure to a gift of £1000. Seventy-one per cent would pay £1000 for a cure and 38% would pay £10 000 for a cure. There was a good correlation between PDI score and the amount a patient had indicated they would pay for a cure.

Patients with leg ulcers have been studied, and 81% of patients have mobility problems related to their ulcer. For younger patients, leg ulcers cause loss of work and earnings. There was a strong correlation between time spent on their ulcer and feelings of anger and resentment [8]. A dermatology life quality index (DLQI) has been developed as a simple tool to use in routine clinical management of many skin diseases [9]. This index has shown that atopic eczema, psoriasis and generalized pruritus have greater impact on QOL than acne, basal cell epithelioma or viral wart. The DLQI for 100 healthy volunteers was 1.6%. For dermatology patients the score was 24.2%.

All these studies have helped to describe the level of disability, both physical and psychological, that patients with skin disease experience. The measurement of disability and QOL is important in assessing individual patients, but it is also important in winning resources for the better provision of services for patients with skin disease.

REFERENCES

1 Jowett S, Ryan T. Skin disease and handicap: an analysis of the impact of skin conditions. *Soc Sci Med* 1985; **20**: 425–9.
2 Eun HC, Finlay AY. Measurement of atopic dermatitis disability. *Ann Dermatol* 1990; **2**: 9–12.
3 Salek MS, Finlay AY, Luscombe DK *et al.* Cyclosporin greatly improves the quality of life of adults with severe atopic dermatitis. A randomised double blind placebo controlled trial. *Br J Dermatol* 1993; **129**: 422–30.
4 Lewis-Jones MS, Finlay AY. The children's dermatology life quality index (C.D.L.Q.I.). Initial validation and practical use. *Br J Dermatol* 1995; **132**: 942–9.
5 Jobling RG. Psoriasis—a preliminary questionnaire study of sufferers' subjective experience. *Clin Exp Dermatol* 1976; **1**: 233–6.
6 Finlay AY, Kelly SE. Psoriasis—an index of disability. *Clin Exp Dermatol* 1987; **12**: 8–11.
7 Finlay AY, Coles EC. The effect of severe psoriasis on the quality of life of 369 patients. *Br J Dermatol* 1995; **132**: 236–44.
8 Philips TE, Stanton B, Provan BA *et al.* A study of the impact of leg ulcers on the quality of life. Financial, social and psychological implications. *J Am Acad Dermatol* 1994; **31**: 49–53.
9 Finlay AY, Khan GK. Dermatology life quality index (D.L.Q.I.). A simple practical measure for routine clinical use. *Clin Exp Dermatol* 1994; **19**: 210–16.

Some specific groups for whom problems of readjustment and rehabilitation may be important are outlined below.

Children with infantile atopic eczema. The main need is for dialogue with the parents and sustained contact to help relieve the inevitable tensions and emotional stresses that the condition imposes on them. Special problems arise in children where hospital admission is required. This is best dealt with in children's units. Joint management with nursing staff trained for the special requirements of sick children and expertise in basic dermatological therapy is invaluable. The parents should be encouraged to participate in the ward activity and will gain confidence in helping in the management of the problem.

The young adult atopic eczema patient. The problems here are often those of personality and environmental stresses rather than of working conditions. Apparent resolution in the protected environment of a hospital ward does not always survive exposure to the harsher emotional stresses of outside life. However, a temporary withdrawal from an adverse environment is usually helpful. It is important that the dermatologist discusses with both the patient and his or her family possible future employment. For instance, the youngster with severe hand eczema is unlikely to be able to nurse or become a hairdresser, or be able to follow a successful career in catering or engineering involving the continued exposure to coolant oils. Early counselling about future work prospects can prevent a lot of misery later on.

The older child. Children with disabling or disfiguring diseases demand special attention towards adjustment to the various epochs of their life relationships with other children, the first school, and the passage through puberty. Play and companionship in the early years mark the transition from maternal social relationships. Disfigurement or disease is always a source of childish cruelty and integration into the social group requires much skilled help from nursing staff and mother figures. The transition to school and pressure of examinations call for guidance and careful management. The difficulties of a spastic child or a deaf and mute child are evident enough to arouse sympathy. The emotionally volatile, scratching atopic or the obviously disfigured child receives less sympathy and attention, although his or her needs are as great.

The young manual worker. There will be much anxiety about the manual worker's future working capacity. After all relevant investigations have been carried out, the work possibilities should be assessed. With the patient's consent, contact with his or her firm's medical officer and general practitioner should be routine, and the results of patch tests, etc. should be conveyed with an interpretation that is relevant to the occupation. To a worker, persistent hand eczema may mean the difference between a livelihood or disablement. Anxieties may not be readily revealed and may require patience to uncover. Re-education in working procedure, an explanation of irritant (or allergic) dermatitis and attention to the causes of persistence and relapse should be part of the normal procedure of treatment. After suffering a severe attack of dermatitis, a patient is likely to be suspicious of any agent to be handled on return to work, but he or she should be encouraged to persist at work during the first critical weeks in which non-specific factors may temporarily exacerbate the condition. The patient should be seen at intervals for at least 3 months after return to work. The employers should be willing to grant time to attend hospital for this purpose.

Medicolegal aspects of dermatology [1]

A recent survey among members of the British Association of Dermatologists indicated that a significant proportion of dermatologists in the UK were concerned about the possibility of being sued, and an even greater percentage had altered their practice because of this concern [2].

There are several measures that minimize the possibility of litigation, and good and effective communication between the dermatologist and the patient is the most important. Moreover, continuing effective communication is necessary after the patient has been seen, especially if there has been dermatological surgery, so that if there are any problems these can be dealt with rapidly and effectively. There is nothing more frustrating for the patient than to find the dermatologist elusive, and resulting patient anger can initiate speedy legal retribution. It is important that not only the dermatologist but also all associated staff adopt an open and easy policy as far as communication with patients is concerned.

A second necessary line of defence against possible litigation involves making adequate and comprehensive case notes. This is particularly important as far as pigmented lesions are concerned, where it is prudent to record the variability or otherwise of the shape, the size and degree of pigmentation of the lesion. There has been a recent increase in litigation involving patients with malignant melanoma, not only over allegations about failure to make an accurate diagnosis, but also in regard to possible delay in seeing the patient after referral by the general practitioner. It is good practice for the dermatologist to see all the referral letters from the primary care physician so an informed assessment of urgency can be made. Even so, the vast numbers of anxious patients referred on account of recent change in pigmented lesions,

the majority of which turn out to be absolutely benign, makes running an effective dermatological service very difficult. Particular difficulties arise when the general practitioner does not label the referral letter 'Urgent' and the patient subsequently turns out to have a malignant melanoma. In this instance, the information given by the general practitioner in the referral letter may or may not be sufficient to allocate an urgent appointment.

Dissatisfaction with scars after lesion removal is another potential area of litigation. It is good practice to explain that spread scars are the almost universal accompaniment of excision of lesions on the back and legs and the development of not only hypertrophic scarring but also keloid scarring should be emphasized, particularly in keloid-prone areas such as presternal skin and over the deltoid area. Comprehensive notes recording that a full discussion has taken place about the future cosmetic appearance of the scar, including possible diagrams of how a lesion will be excised, are both very helpful in rebutting potential litigation.

Consultant dermatologists have a responsibility to train others, and faulty technique using liquid nitrogen is a relatively common cause of litigation against general practitioners. Skin necrosis, and even peripheral neuropathy, are the commonest causes for litigation following inappropriate liquid nitrogen treatment.

Skin and subcutaneous atrophy following injections of triamcinolone in inappropriate sites, such as the arm, or too superficially, or at the same site in the buttock are also relatively common causes of cosmetic litigation as far as the general practitioner dermatologist is concerned.

It is very important that colleagues refrain from making disparaging remarks about other colleagues in front of patients. It is also important not to use emotive words, such as 'dermatitis' to, for example, an engineering worker, who may equate this diagnosis immediately with a diagnosis of industrial dermatitis, and, therefore, financial compensation.

One other potential pitfall for the dermatologist is the side-effects from the use, not only of oral, but also of topical, steroids. Skin atrophy, striae, depression of the pituitary–adrenal axis and avascular necrosis of the femoral neck are particular examples. Avascular necrosis of the femoral neck is more common in alcoholic individuals and special care should be exercised, not only using oral steroids, but also topical steroids, in such patients [3]. It should be remembered, however, that avascular necrosis of the femoral neck has also been described in patients receiving physiological corticosteroid replacement therapy [4]. Patients on long-term oral steroid therapy should be advised about prophylaxis for osteoporosis [5].

Particular care needs to be exercised to avoid prescribing drugs that have previously caused an allergic reaction in a particular patient [1]. Although the resulting medical problem may not be severe, there is always a chance of a much more severe allergic reaction leading to the development of potentially fatal toxic epidermal necrolysis.

Avoidance of drug interactions is also important, particularly where potent drugs, such as methotrexate, cyclosporin, warfarin and corticosteroids are concerned. A recent study of 790 claims against general practitioners has shown that the largest proportion (25%) were related to errors in prescribing, monitoring or administering medicine [6].

Careful systems of work are vital to prevent burning of normal skin during the use of various forms of ultraviolet light, including PUVA therapy and topical dithranol (anthralin) treatment. Management changes in the British National Health Service, attempting to achieve a skill mix, have led to relatively inexperienced nurses being given the task of dithranol or UV therapy. Hospital managers should be told about the possible disastrous consequences of such a policy in dermatological patients, where nursing treatment expertise, built up over many years, is vital to ensure best results. Care also needs to be exercised in the topical treatment of ulcers, where the prescription of topical agents containing neomycin have led to the development of deafness [7].

Why do patients go to litigation? [8]

There are four main reasons why people sue their doctors and the decision to take legal action is not only determined by the original 'injury', but also by insensitive handling and poor communication after the original incident. The patient seeks explanations when things go wrong and these explanations are often considered inadequate by patients who sue their doctors. The four main reasons that emerged from a recent analysis of 227 patients and relatives were, firstly, a concern with standards of care. Both patients and relatives wanted to prevent similar incidents in future. Secondly, there is a need for an explanation to know how the injury happened and why. Thirdly, there was a belief that the doctor or hospital involved should have to account and apologize for their actions. Lastly, financial compensation for pain and suffering was a significant factor. Moreover, the patients and their relatives all expressed a desire for greater honesty and assurances that lessons had been learned from their experiences [8].

Litigation and patients with psychiatric problems [9]

Whilst patients may quite correctly seek financial compensation for errors made by their dermatologist, it is possible that some patients are more likely to go to litigation than others.

In a recent study involving nearly 100 patients, suing either their doctors or their employers, and seen for medicolegal purposes, a very significant past or present history of psychiatric disturbance was found in almost 70% of the litigants [9]. The commonest psychiatric disease present was depression, but anxiety, alcoholism and personality disorder were all represented. The medicolegal patient may also be trying to deceive both the dermatologist and the court. In this series there were two patients with artefact dermatitis and one with dermatitis simulata.

It is easy to miss a diagnosis of depression in dermatological patients and it is thought that perhaps 50% of depressed patients in medical practice go unrecognized [10]. The depressed patient with dysmorphophobia is particularly likely to be angry, and this anger can be directed at the dermatologist or doctor, but, more commonly, internally, resulting ultimately in suicide [11].

Dysmorphophobic patients tend to haunt dermatologists, and particularly those who are undertaking cosmetic procedures, such as laser treatment and skin resurfacing. Even though the results of treatment are good, the patient may remain dissatisfied. Before any cosmetic procedures are undertaken in a depressed patient, it is very important to make sure that communication between the patient and the doctor is optimum. Photography before and after any procedure is also important, so that there is some objective measure of the outcome. Preoperative assessment by a psychiatrist may be indicated in patients with long-standing or gross psychiatric psychopathology.

Preparing a medicolegal report [1]

The data necessary to prepare a medical report on a patient seen with possible occupational dermatosis are described in Chapter 22.

Dermatologists may be asked by solicitors to prepare medicolegal reports. The commonest request is to prepare a report about alleged industrial dermatitis. Less often, a report on the dermatological consequences of an accident, either on the road, in the factory or, for instance, following a badly performed perm, may be sought. Thirdly, there may be a request to prepare a medical report, either on behalf of a litigant or a dermatologist involved in a medical negligence case.

It should be noted that the report has to be based on a complete and detailed enquiry of the relevant events, and a conventional medical history is not sufficient [1].

It should be remembered that the medical report may eventually go before a judge in court and it is humiliating for an expert witness to be questioned by a barrister about numerous spelling and grammatical errors. It is important that the dermatologist does not become biased on one side or the other. The expert witness has a duty to the court, and the medical report should be formulated to help the court. Solicitors may try and manipulate individual reports, asking the dermatologist to omit certain sentences and add others. As a generalization, this type of pressure should be resisted. Although the solicitor may wish you to amend the report for a tactical reason, the best guideline to follow is that the report should not be changed to such an extent that the writer can no longer agree with the content [12].

In a civil case involving, for instance, a claim for compensation for industrial dermatitis, the test of whether there is a causal relationship between exposure to coolant oil and the development of subsequent dermatitis depends on balance of probabilities. If, on balance of probabilities, there is more than a 50% chance that an individual's skin problem was caused, for instance, by coolant oil, that is sufficient for the claimant to establish the case. In contrast, in a criminal matter, the burden of proof has to be beyond all reasonable doubt, i.e. 99% or above certainty. In a medical negligence case, the solicitor may seek a report dealing mainly with diagnosis, causation and prognosis and seek a separate report dealing with liability and negligence.

The essence of negligence is that there has been a breach of a duty of care resulting in damage, and in medical cases this occurs in a context of diagnosis and/or treatment. There are four essential components, and all four must be present and proven before the patient can succeed in the action against the doctor [13].

1 The doctor must have had a duty of care to the plaintiff.
2 There must have been a breach of that duty.
3 The plaintiff must have suffered damage.
4 The damage must be a consequence of a breach of duty of care.

The Bolam test is often used to determine whether there has been a breach of duty of care. In this particular case the judge stated that 'a doctor is not guilty of negligence if he has acted in accordance with the practice accepted as proper by a responsible body of medical men skilled in that particular art'. This Bolam principle remains vital and central to how a doctor's professional behaviour is to be judged by other doctors, and not by lawyers, politicians or administrators.

It should be noted that in exercising reasonable care, there may be an act of either commission or omission and each of these categories could lay the dermatologist open to litigation if harm has occurred. Moreover, a distinction must be made between an error of clinical judgement and negligence.

It is reassuring that the medical defence organizations in the UK still regard dermatology as a low-risk specialty, with few and relatively low-cost claims. On the other hand, plastic and reconstructive surgery involves a higher risk, as does cosmetic practice, especially when not carried out by consultant dermatologists or plastic surgeons.

It is important to remember that if something has gone wrong with patient care, a full and frank explanation with as little delay as possible will do much to diffuse the anger, upset and resentment that the patient feels and ultimately may reduce the risk that the patient will go to litigation [8]. There is a need for an explanation of how the injury has happened and why [8]. The doctor adopting this open type of approach could find him- or herself in direct conflict with the 'never admit anything' insurance type of mentality and it is important that Trust managers in the UK National Health Service, for instance, do not put pressure on their medical practitioners to adopt this approach. A prompt explanation is vital, as any delay would be seen as an attempt at cover up.

Consent [14]

Any treatment that entails the physical touching of a competent adult patient without consent constitutes the tort of battery. Consent provides a defence that makes the touching lawful. From the legal profession's point of view it is important to establish whether a competent adult patient consented to treatment or not and a requirement to obtain consent is imposed by law. In English law, once a patient has been informed in broad terms of the nature of the intended procedure and gives consent, the consent is valid, although there may be difficulties in deciding what constitutes the nature of the treatment or procedure and information in broad terms. It is very important to continue to review the information given to patients before obtaining consent. The use of information leaflets and documentation for the patient to read about treatment or surgical procedures is very helpful in this regard [15].

The court appearance

Fortunately, less than 1% of cases, where a medical report has been requested, ever threatens to reach court, and in the majority of these cases a settlement is often reached out of court before the scheduled hearing. Should your appearance be necessary as an expert witness in court, it is important to follow several rules, but usually the expert witness drifts into this type of work without any training. Good preparation before the scheduled hearing is important and the original clinical notes, taken when preparing the medical report, can also be very useful. It is important to take the attitude that you are there to help the court, rather than to take one side or the other. Speak clearly and slowly enough to allow the judge to make notes. Do not fidget and do keep your evidence simple [16]. Take your time, when you need to, before answering the barrister's questions. When you are unclear as to what the barrister is asking, you may politely ask if the question might be rephrased. Emotionally, it may be difficult to switch from the role of a caring medical practitioner to an adversarial court system. Do not try and cross swords with an aggressive barrister, and address your comments at the judge, or jury if present. Remember, you are perfectly at liberty to ask for a short break if you have been in the witness box for some time and are getting tired.

REFERENCES

1 Sanderson KV. Dermatology. In: Jackson JP, ed. *A Practical Guide to Medicine and the Law*. London: Springer-Verlag, 1991: 96–114.
2 Cotterill JA. A survey of members of the BAD on the perceived threat of litigation. (Submitted for publication, 1997)
3 Cunliffe WJ, Burton JL, Holti G, Wright V. Hazards of steroid therapy in hepatic failure. *Br J Dermatol* 1975; **93**: 183–5.
4 Williams PL, Corbett M. Avascular necrosis of bone complicating corticosteroid replacement therapy. *Ann Rheum Dis* 1983; **42**: 276–9.
5 Walsh LJ, Wong CA, Pingle M, Tattersfield AE. Use of oral corticosteroids in the community and the prevention of secondary osteoporosis: a cross sectional study. *Br Med J* 1996; **313**: 344–6.
6 Green S, Goodwin H, Moss J. *Problems in General Practice*. Medication, errors: claims for negligence against GP members 1996. Data published by the Medical Defence Union Risk Management Team.
7 Editorial. Deafness after topical neomycin. *Br Med J* 1969; **4**: 181–2.
8 Vincent C, Young M, Phillips A. Why do people sue doctors? A study of patients and relatives taking legal action. *Lancet* 1994; **343**: 1609–13.
9 Cotterill JA. Why do patients sue? Paper presented at the European Academy of Dermatology and Venereology, Lisbon, Portugal, October 1996.
10 Mayou R, Hawton K. Psychiatric disorder in the general hospital. *Br J Psychiatry* 1986; **149**: 172–190.
11 Cotterill JA, Cunliffe WJ. Suicide in dermatological patients. *Br J Dermatol* 1997 (Accepted for publication).
12 Cummin J. In: Leadbetter S, ed. *The Civil Perspective in Limitations of Expert Evidence*. London: Royal College of Physicians and RC of Pathologists, 1996: 11–18.
13 Knight B. The legal basis of medical negligence. In: Jackson JP, ed. *A Practical Guide to Medicine and the Law*. London: Springer-Verlag, 1991: 278–88.
14 Palmer RN. Consent and confidentiality. In: Jackson JP, ed. *A Practical Guide to Medicine and the Law*. London: Springer-Verlag, 1991: 19–41.
15 Shah M, Lewis FM. Cutaneous surgery: preoperative information on what the patient expects. *J Eur Ac Dermatol Venereol* 1996; **7**: 86–7.
16 Stephens M. The criminal legal perspective. In: Leadbetter S, ed. *Limitations of Expert Evidence*. London: Royal College of Physicians and Royal College of Pathologists, 1996: 3–10.

Emergency treatment of anaphylaxis [1–3]

Anaphylaxis is often unpredictable and may occur as the result of the introduction of an antigen parenterally into a sensitized person, or it may occur after the ingestion of foods or drugs, or even after topical application to the skin. Anaphylaxis is often thought to be associated with an atopic predisposition but non-atopic persons seem equally liable to develop such reactions after parenteral injection or insect stings. The severity of anaphylaxis is determined by the sensitivity of the individual, as well as by the dose and rate of absorption. Reactions can develop with alarming speed, the more severe reactions usually occurring within 1–5 min, although they may be delayed for 1–2 h or longer. Death can occur almost instantaneously. Skin testing in atopic subjects or in those suspected of being acutely sensitive should be carried out with great discretion, starting with a weak strength and usually using the prick test technique initially. An emergency tray containing the following items must always be at hand: adrenaline (epinephrine) 1:1000 (1 mg/ml) in individual phials; injectable antihistamine, for example chlorpheniramine; hydrocortisone for intravenous or intramuscular injection. Most hospitals maintain prepacked boxes containing an anaesthetic airway, tourniquet, instruments for cutting down on veins, and other materials needed for acute resuscitation. Oxygen and suction apparatus should be available. A salbutamol inhaler is useful for asthmatic symptoms. At the onset of anaphylactic shock, the patient should be lying flat, and the airway secured if they are unconscious. A tourniquet above the site of injection may prevent further rapid absorption of the antigen. The first medication to be given if the attack is of any considerable severity is an injection of adrenaline (epinephrine) 1:1000. At first, 0.25–0.5 ml can be injected into and around the site of injection of the antigen to slow absorption. A further 0.25–0.5 ml can be injected subcutaneously, intramuscularly for more severe reactions or even intravenously for catastrophic reactions. Intravenous adrenaline is not without its own hazards. Care must be taken with repeated subcutaneous injections. If the patient is very shocked, absorption may be very slow, but as the circulation is restored there may be a sudden overdosage. After the initial injection of adrenaline, or in mild cases to replace it, an injection of an antihistamine intravenously or intramuscularly can be given. Injections of corticosteroids do little for the immediate effects of an IgE-mediated reaction, but they do help in preventing the effects of secondary mediators and lessen delayed relapses. Oxygen is often required. Laryngeal obstruction may require intubation or even a tracheostomy. Where rapid relief of symptoms is not achieved, an emergency call for those skilled in intensive care rapidly becomes appropriate. Intravenous infusion of plasma expanders may be needed if there is hypovolaemic shock.

The management of anaphylaxis in a hospital setting, when preparations are in hand in case such reactions develop, does not present much difficulty. Two situations need special attention. First, the patient already known to be at risk of anaphylaxis from allergens that cannot always be avoided should carry with them an adrenaline syringe for injection and should understand how it should be used. A demonstration should be arranged. The patient should also wear a bracelet or necklace carrying details of their allergies. Adrenaline taken by inhalation can help in the management of minor episodes of anaphylaxis but is no substitute for injections in more severe cases. Second, anaphylactic shock is often badly managed in hospital casualty departments; often only antihistamines and hydrocortisone are given and adrenaline is delayed or even not given at all [4]. The most important drug is adrenaline (epinephrine) given quickly subcutaneously in mild episodes and intramuscularly if severe. Volume replacement of patients in anaphylactic cardiogenic shock is important.

Adrenaline (epinephrine) dosage in anaphylaxis

Adults: 0.5 ml of 1:1000 solution i/m.
Children: 0.01 ml of 1:1000 solution/kg i/m.

REFERENCES

1 Bochner BS, Lichtenstein LM. Anaphylaxis. *N Engl J Med* 1991; **324**: 1785–90.
2 *British National Formulary*, No. 29. London: British Medical Association and the Pharmaceutical Society of Great Britain, 1995.
3 Youlten LJF. Drug induced anaphylaxis. *Clin Exp Allergy* 1989; **19**: 233–5.
4 Fisher M. The treatment of acute anaphylaxis. *Br Med J* 1995; **311**: 731–3.

Chapter 76
Systemic Therapy

R.J.HAY, M.W.GREAVES & A.P.WARIN

Systemic corticosteroid therapy

Sex hormones and related compounds

Antihistamines

Other antiallergic drugs

Systemic non-steroidal anti-inflammatory therapy

Interferons

Essential fatty acids

Retinoids

Immunosuppressive and cytotoxic drugs

Alkylating agents
Antimetabolites
Cyclosporin

PUVA

Photodynamic therapy

Photopheresis

Plasmapheresis

Gold

Chelating agents

Antibiotics and antibacterial agents

Antifungal drugs

Antiviral drugs

Antiparasitic agents

Drugs to improve the peripheral circulation

Miscellaneous drugs used in special ways in dermatology
Antimalarials
Dapsone, sulphapyridine
Clofazimine
Sulphasalazine
Thalidomide
Colchicine
Traditional Chinese herbal medicine for atopic eczema

Transdermal delivery systems

Introduction

Topical therapy is the most logical way to treat many skin diseases, with a minimal risk of systemic toxicity. However, there are many drugs where an adequate effect can be achieved only by the systemic route. Some of these drugs, for example antibiotics, are used in specific ways by dermatologists. A brief survey of some of the more important drugs or those used in special ways in dermatology will be given here, with no attempt to describe the pharmacology in detail. Other drugs are described elsewhere in these volumes.

The important subject of drug reactions and interactions is referred to in Chapter 77. The particular problems of prescribing for special groups, such as children, pregnant women, lactating women and elderly people are dealt with in some detail in the British National Formulary [1] (and other national formularies), as are the difficulties in prescribing for patients with liver failure, renal failure and diseases affecting other organs. Where there is any doubt the advice of a clinical pharmacologist, a pharmacist or the drug manufacturer should be sought or information obtained from such reference works as Martindale [2] and Goodman and Gilman [3]. The *ABPI Data Sheet Compendium*

[4] is also valuable. The dosage for children is often calculated roughly on the basis of age, but should more accurately be based on body weight or, even better, body surface [1].

REFERENCES

1 *British National Formulary*, No 31. London: British Medical Association and the Pharmaceutical Society of Great Britain, 1996
2 Reynolds JEF. *Martindale. The Extra Pharmacopoeia*, 30th, edn. London: Pharmaceutical Trade Press, 1993.
3 Gilman AG, Goodman LS, Rall TW. *Goodman and Gilman's The Pharmacological Basis of Therapeutics*, 8th edn. New York: Pergamon, 1990.
4 Association of British Pharmaceutical Industry. *ABPI Data Sheet Compendium*. London: Datapharm, 1996–7.

Systemic corticosteroid therapy

Corticosteroids, first introduced into dermatology by Marion Sulzberger [1], owe at least part of their mode of action to inhibition of phospholipase A_2 (PLA_2). This membrane enzyme causes transformation of membrane phospholipids to a variety of pro-inflammatory lipids including the prostaglandins, the leukotrienes and platelet-activating factor. Corticosteroids do not inhibit this enzyme directly;

they do so by evoking formation of a cell-membrane protein called lipocortin [2]. A number of chronic inflammatory disorders are associated with circulating autoantibodies against lipocortin [3], which may explain the steroid resistance of these conditions [4]. However, lipocortin does not explain all the anti-inflammatory actions of corticosteroids in skin, and other proposed mechanisms include a cytostatic action, a 'stabilizing' action on lysosomal membranes, and suppression of cytokine expression.

Indications

Since skin lesions are accessible the topical route is preferable where corticosteroid treatment is indicated since the risk of potentially harmful exposure of internal tissues and organs to the corticosteroid is reduced. Systemic corticosteroid treatment is therefore only indicated in special circumstances. These include the following.
1 Acute, self-limited, steroid-sensitive disorders, for example acute contact allergic dermatitis where the offending allergen is evident. In these circumstances a 1 week course of oral prednisone in reducing dosage may be sufficient.
2 Acute anaphylactic reactions, for example following a bee or wasp sting or a drug to which the patient is sensitized. Hydrocortisone should be given intravenously in a dosage of 100 mg, after prior administration of adrenaline 0.5 mg s.c., and chlorpheniramine 4 mg i. m. (adult doses).
3 Acute autoimmune connective tissue diseases and generalized immunological vascular disorders, for example systemic lupus erythematosus, dermatomyositis, polyarteritis nodosa, giant-cell arteritis, Wegener's granulomatosis.
4 Chronic, disabling immunological bullous diseases, for example pemphigus vulgaris, pemphigoid.
5 Acute generalized exfoliative dermatitis, for example due to a severe drug reaction.
6 A number of miscellaneous disorders including severe lichen planus, pyoderma gangrenosum, and sarcoidosis, in which there is evidence of cardiac, renal, ocular or extensive pulmonary or cutaneous involvement.
7 Although systemic steroids are often used, the value of such treatment is unproven in erythema multiforme (Stevens–Johnson syndrome), toxic epidermal necrolysis, chronic urticaria and cutaneous T-cell lymphoma.

Pharmacological considerations

Corticosteroids are anti-inflammatory, immunosuppressive, antiproliferative and vasoconstrictive. The pharmacokinetics and special characteristics of the multiple individual preparations available will not be considered here but some general principles are to be stated.

Prednisone and prednisolone

Like cortisone and hydrocortisone, prednisone and pred-nisolone differ chemically only in the presence of an hydroxy group instead of a keto group at C11. The biological properties are similar but prednisone has to be metabolically transformed in the liver to the 11β-hydroxy derivative to acquire biological potency and hence prednisone should not be given to patients with liver disease. Both drugs possess four times the glucocorticoid potency and relatively less mineralocorticoid (salt-retaining) activity than hydrocortisone and cortisone.

Route of administration

Intramuscular

The intramuscular route, especially for triamcinolone, is popular in the USA for systemic steroid administration for short-term (less than 4 weeks) treatment. Triamcinolone does not differ significantly from prednisolone in its actions on a short-term basis, although in the long term it possesses greater mineralocorticoid activity. In the longer term, intramuscular steroids, especially in depot formulation, can cause marked hypothalamo-pituitary–adrenal suppression and severe local atrophic changes although the latter partially remit after a year or more. In the event of untoward steroid-induced complications, the drugs cannot be withdrawn promptly.

Intravenous

The intravenous route is useful in emergency treatment of acute anaphylaxis and in the pre- and postoperative cover of patients who have previously been receiving systemic steroid treatment for 4 weeks or more. A suitable regimen is 25 mg hydrocortisone preoperatively at the time of induction of anaesthesia, 100 mg during the operation and 100 mg on the first postoperative day—all doses being intravenous.

Thereafter the patient can be maintained on oral therapy as required. In fact, hypotensive crises attributable to adrenal insufficiency are extremely rare in patients withdrawn from glucocorticoid therapy and subsequently undergoing surgery without supplemental corticosteroid cover [5].

Pulsed steroid therapy

This is usually administered as doses of 1 g of methylprednisolone given intravenously over several hours using an intravenous line. The dose can be repeated daily for up to 5 days. It may be indicated in patients with severe bullous dermatoses, especially pemphigus vulgaris. It is a potentially hazardous procedure, and thromboembolism, cardiac arrest and steroid psychosis are occasional complications.

Oral steroids

Route of administration and dosage. Oral steroids may be taken in a single daily dose or using an alternate-day regimen.

Single daily dose. Short-term systemic steroid therapy is best given as a single daily dose. Prednisone and prednisolone have minimal mineralocorticoid activity and have a sufficiently prolonged action to ensure the sustained effectiveness of a single daily dose. The single dose should be given first thing in the morning. This is because the maximum rate of adrenocortical cortisol secretion occurs early in the morning and therefore less pituitary–adrenal suppression occurs at this time, whilst therapeutic efficacy is maintained [6].

Alternate-day dosage. Prolonged therapy may be instituted using an alternate-day dose regimen (twice the daily dose on alternate days with no steroid treatment on the other days) [7]. Conversion from a daily to an alternate-day regime should be carried out gradually rather than abruptly, for example by progressive diminution of the dose on even-numbered days while building up the dose on odd-numbered days. In order to prevent alternate-day relapses it may be necessary to maintain a small dose on the even-numbered day. Institution of an alternate-day systemic steroid regimen reduces, but does not prevent, steroid toxicity. Posterior subcapsular cataracts and osteoporosis may remain problems [8,9]. Alternate-day systemic steroid therapy is not always as effective as daily treatment when given in equivalent doses.

Systemic steroid toxicity

A comprehensive account of the range of unwanted side-effects consequent upon systemic steroid therapy is beyond the scope of this text. The reviews by Storrs [10] and Gallant and Kenny [11] are recommended. However, a number of points are worth emphasizing here.

The approximate physiological daily cortisol secretion by the adrenal cortex is 20 mg daily for an average adult (prednisone equivalent 5 mg daily). Short courses of prednisolone, for example up to 30 mg daily for less than 2 weeks, although suppressing pituitary–adrenal function, do not require tapering because recovery is rapid. However, for patients with a longer history of oral steroid treatment, gradual reduction of dosage prior to discontinuation is important because abrupt reduction may lead to the 'steroid-withdrawal' syndrome, which resembles the clinical features of adrenocortical insufficiency. Random plasma-cortisol determination may be within normal limits and stimulation tests of pituitary and adrenal function may also be normal [12].

Tests of pituitary–adrenal function

Baseline plasma-cortisol levels and study of diurnal variation of plasma cortisol are crude estimates of hypothalamo-pituitary–adrenal integrity. The adrenocorticotrophic hormone (ACTH)-stimulation test measures adrenal but not hypothalamo-pituitary integrity. The metyrapone test is based upon inhibition of an enzyme involved in synthesis of a cortisol precursor (2-deoxycortisol) resulting in reduction in cortisol levels and a consequent increase in ACTH. The cortisol precursors are measured in the urine and the resultant values give an indication of hypothalamo-pituitary–adrenal integrity. Stress tests including insulin-induced hypoglycaemia measure the integrity of the whole hypothalamo-pituitary–adrenal system, and are best carried out with the assistance of a specialized unit.

Systemic corticosteroids and pregnancy

Although there is little concrete evidence that systemic corticosteroids are harmful in pregnancy it is prudent to avoid their use whenever possible, as there have been sporadic reports of the association of their use with still-birth, spontaneous abortion and cleft palate [13].

Systemic corticosteroids and cataracts

Posterior subcapsular cataracts are a recognized complication of systemic corticosteroid therapy. Screening by slit-lamp examination on patients in whom prolonged treatment with systemic corticosteroids is contemplated may help to obviate medicolegal consequences [8].

ACTH or tetracosactrin

Although these agents are not corticosteroids they provoke increased secretion of endogenous adrenal corticoids and will therefore be considered here. There is little or no evidence to support the use of ACTH or tetracosactrin in place of systemic steroids. Their anti-inflammatory actions depend entirely upon increased hydrocortisone production by the adrenal cortex. They also suffer from the disadvantage that they stimulate adrenal androgen as well as hydrocortisone production and cause more salt and water retention than prednisolone [14]. Maximum response of adult adrenals is no more than 100 mg of cortisol daily. ACTH and tetracosactrin have to be given by injection and can cause anaphylactic reactions. There is no sound evidence for the often asserted view that these drugs are associated with less growth retardation in children than with oral corticosteroids. The only arguable advantage of ACTH or tetracosactrin therapy is a reduced likelihood of pituitary–adrenal suppression [2] and this view has been challenged [14]. Certainly overall, and dose for dose, manifestations of steroid toxicity are at least as frequent as in oral corticosteroid treatment.

REFERENCES

1 Sulzberger MB, Witten VH. The effect of topically applied compound E in selected dermatoses. *J Invest Dermatol* 1952; **19**: 101–2.
2 Flower RJ. Background and discovery of lipocortins. *Agents Actions* 1986; **17**: 255–62.
3 Hirata F, Del Carmine R, Nelson CA *et al.* Presence of autoantibody for phospholipase inhibitory protein lipomodulin in patients with rheumatic diseases. *Proc Natl Acad Sci USA* 1981; **78**: 3190–4.
4 Rivers JK, Podgorski MR, Goulding NJ *et al.* The presence of autoantibody to recombinant lipocortin-I in patients with psoriasis and psoriatic arthritis. *Br J Dermatol* 1990; **123**: 569–72.
5 Kehlet H, Binder C. Adrenocortical function and clinical course during and after surgery in unsupplemented glucocorticoid treated patients. *Br J Anaesthesiol* 1973; **45**: 1043–8.
6 Nugent CA, Ward J, MacDiamid WD *et al.* Glucocorticoid toxicity: single versus divided daily doses of prednisolone. *J Chron Dis* 1965; **18**: 323–32.
7 Reichling GH, Kligman AM. Alternate-day corticosteroid therapy. *Arch Dermatol* 1961; **83**: 980–3.
8 Castrow FF. Atopic cataracts versus steroid cataracts. *J Am Acad Dermatol* 1981; **5**: 64–6.
9 MacGregor RR, Sheagren JN, Lipsett MB *et al.* Alternate day prednisone therapy. Evaluation of delayed hypersensitivity responses, control of disease and steroid side effects. *N Engl J Med* 1969; **280**: 1427–31.
10 Storrs FJ. Use and abuse of systemic corticosteroid therapy. *J Am Acad Dermatol* 1979; **1**: 95–105.
11 Gallant C, Kenny P. Oral glucocorticoids and their complications. *J Am Acad Dermatol* 1986; **14**: 161–77.
12 Amatruda TT, Hollingsworth DR, D'Esopo G *et al.* A study of the mechanism of the steroid withdrawal syndrome. Evidence for integrity of the hypothalamic–pituitary–adrenal system. *J Clin Endocrinol* 1960; **20**: 339–54.
13 Reinisch JM, Simon NG, Karow WG *et al.* Prenatal exposure to prednisolone in humans and animals retards uterine growth. *Science* 1978; **202**: 436–8.
14 Hirschmann JV. Some principles of systemic glucocorticoid therapy. *Clin Exp Dermatol* 1986; **11**: 27–33.
15 Axelrod L. Glucocorticoid therapy. *Medicine* 1976; **55**: 39–65.

Sex hormones and related compounds

Androgens

Testosterone is the most potent androgen and is currently only used for replacement therapy although it has been used to treat hereditary angio-oedema [1]. Although many derivatives of testosterone have been developed with a pronounced anabolic action (the 'anabolic steroids'), they nevertheless retain significant and often troublesome virilizing activity.

Anabolic steroids

Danazol (100–600 mg daily). Danazol is a synthetic steroid derived from ethisterone. It has a high affinity for androgen receptors, and although itself a weak androgen, it has marked antiandrogenic activity. It also inhibits gonadal steroid production and reduces secretion of follicle-stimulating hormone (FSH) and luteinizing hormone (LH) by the pituitary. It increases the hepatic synthesis of a number of proteins including complement C1 esterase

inhibitor and antitrypsin [2,3]. It is of great value in hereditary angio-oedema due to C1 esterase inhibitor deficiency. It causes enhanced production by the liver of functional C1 esterase inhibitor, but its beneficial effect is probably due to more complex actions [4]. It can also be used to treat more severely affected patients with cholinergic urticaria who are unresponsive to antihistamines [5], probably due to its ability to enhance hepatic synthesis of antitrypsin, and can be used to inhibit ovulation in autoimmune progesterone dermatitis. Apart from its troublesome virilizing actions it may cause hepatotoxicity, and liver function tests should be carried out before, and at monthly intervals during, treatment.

Stanazolol (2.5–10 mg daily). Stanazolol is also a potent anabolic steroid with mild virilizing activity. It is just as effective as danazol in hereditary angio-oedema and with similar side-effects, but considerably cheaper. Additionally, it has marked fibrinolytic properties, and has been used successfully to prevent progression of lipodermatosclerosis [6]. Its side-effects are similar to those of danazol.

Antiandrogens [7]

Cyproterone acetate. Cyproterone is a potent antiandrogen which competes with androgens at receptor sites. In low doses (2 mg daily), usually in combination with ethinyl oestradiol, it can be used for treatment of acne in females [8]. It can also be used to treat hirsutes and other signs of virilization in females. Liver toxicity is an occasional problem and the drug is contraindicated in pregnancy. Spironolactone and flutamide are also potent anti-androgens but are unlicensed for the above indications.

Oestrogens

Ethinyl oestradiol (10–35 μg daily). Ethinyl oestradiol is valuable replacement therapy in the treatment of postmenopausal symptoms including hot flushes, vaginitis and vaginal atrophy [9]. Plasma levels of FSH and LH which are elevated in postmenopausal females are useful guides to dosage. Ethinyl oestradiol should be avoided in patients with a history of breast cancer, liver or thromboembolic disease.

Antioestrogens

Tamoxifen (20 mg daily). Tamoxifen is an antioestrogenic drug which acts at receptor sites to block oestrogen binding. It therefore inhibits ovulation in fertile women. It may be useful in the treatment of progesterone dermatitis or progesterone erythema multiforme [10] as an alternative to oophorectomy [11]. Side-effects are those associated with the menopause, together with abnormal vaginal bleeding. Bone density may be affected in the course of long-term treatment.

REFERENCES

1 Spaulding WB. Methyl testosterone therapy for hereditary episodic edema (hereditary angioneurotic edema). *Ann Intern Med* 1960; **53**: 739–45.
2 Gadek JE, Fulmer JD, Gelfand JA *et al.* Danazol-induced augmentation of serum α-antitrypsin levels in individuals with marked deficiency of this antiprotease. *J Clin Invest* 1980; **66**: 82–7.
3 Gelfand JA, Sherins RJ, Alling DW, Frank MM. Treatment of hereditary angioedema with danazol. Reversal of clinical and biochemical abnormalities. *N Engl J Med* 1976; **295**: 1444–8.
4 Warin AP, Greaves MW, Gatecliff M *et al.* Treatment of hereditary angioedema by low dose attenuated androgens: disassociation of clinical response from levels of C1 esterase inhibitor and C4. *Br J Dermatol* 1980; **103**: 405–9.
5 Wong E, Eftekhari N, Greaves MW, Milford Ward A. Beneficial effects of danazol on symptoms and laboratory changes in cholinergic urticaria. *Br J Dermatol* 1987; **116**: 553–6.
6 Burnand K, Clemenson G, Morland M *et al.* Venous lipodermatosclerosis: treatment by fibrinolytic enhancement and elastic compression. *Br Med J* 1980; **280**: 7–11.
7 Thomson DS. Pharmacology of antiandrogens in the skin. In: Greaves MW, Shuster S, eds. *Pharmacology of the skin.* II. Berlin: Springer-Verlag, 1990: 483–93.
8 Hansted B, Reymann F. Cyproterone acetate in the treatment of acne vulgaris in adult females. *Dermatologica* 1982; **164**: 117–26.
9 Tzingouris VA, Aksu MF, Greenblatt RB. Estriol in the management of the menopause. *JAMA* 1978; **239**: 1638–41.
10 Wojnarowska F, Greaves MW, Peachey RDG *et al.* Progesterone induced erythema multiforme. *J R Soc Med* 1985; **78**: 407–8.
11 Mayou SC, Charles Holmes R, Kenney A, Black MM. A premenstrual urticarial eruption treated with bilateral oophorectomy and hysterectomy. *Clin Exp Dermatol* 1988; **13**: 114–16.

Antihistamines

Historical note

The first effective and safe antihistamine, neoantergan, was based upon a molecule '2786 RP' discovered by Parisian investigators, Bovet and Walthert in 1944 [1]. This antihistamine, known as anthisan or mepyramine maleate, was one of a series of diamethylamino-*n*-propyl phenothiazine compounds. Soon afterwards in the USA, diphenhydramine (Benadryl) was launched and found to be effective by O'Leary and Farber [2] in 35 patients with chronic urticaria. In the UK, definition of the actions and potential role of the first generation antihistamines was pioneered by Warin and colleagues [3,4] in urticaria.

It had long been recognized that not all of the actions of histamine, notably that of stimulation of gastric acid secretion, could be blocked by antihistamines. This puzzle was unravelled by Black [5] who described a subset of histamine receptors designated H_2 which led to the development of the first clinically useful H_2 antihistamine, cimetidine, subsequently to be found effective in the management of chronic urticaria [6]. The later discovery of a third subset of histamine auto receptors, H_3, [7], has as yet, not generated any clinically useful applications in dermatology. However, the new class of H_1 antihistamines including terfenadine, in which troublesome sedative side-effects of the classical antihistamines are minimalized by substitutions on the basic imidazole ring, thus preventing the drug from crossing the blood–brain barrier, has been the biggest recent milestone in the long history of antihistamines [8].

Histamine receptors

Four classes of histamine receptors are presently recognized (Table 76.1). The discovery of H_2 receptors [5], alluded to above, was followed by demonstration of expression of H_1 and H_2 receptors in human skin. Histamine-induced vasodilatation and wealing are mediated by both classes of receptor, whereas itching is only served by H_1 receptors [9–11]. H_3 receptors are responsible for the ability of histamine in some tissues to regulate, by inhibitory feedback, its own biosynthesis and release. H_3 receptors, which also regulate transmitter release at autonomic nerve terminals, have not been convincingly shown to be represented in skin. On the other hand, the recently described intracellular (H_{ic}) histamine receptors which are responsible for the ability of histamine to promote cell and tissue growth (e.g. in embryonic tissue and wound healing) [12] are probably

Table 76.1 Histamine receptors.

Receptors	Main action relevant to skin	Expression in skin	Antagonist
H_1	Vasodilatation Vasopermeability Itch	Yes	Chlorpheniramine Terfenadine
H_2	Vasodilatation Vasopermeability	Yes	Cimetidine Ranitidine
H_3	Regulation of histamine Neurotransmitter release	?	Thioperamide*
H_{ic}	Intracellular messenger for promotion of cell growth	?	DPPE*

DPPE, N_1N-diethyl-2-[4-(phenyl methyl) phenoxy] ethanamine HCl.
* Experimental antagonists.

expressed in skin although this has not yet been specifically demonstrated.

Other actions of antihistamines

Most H_1 antihistamines also express anticholinergic activity, resulting in the well-known side-effects of the earlier 'classical' antihistamines which include dryness of the mouth, blurring of vision and constipation. Drowsiness is also a feature of many early antihistamines. Available evidence suggests that histamine plays a role in the maintenance of the waking state which may go some way towards explaining the sedative actions of some H_1 antihistamines. Many H_1 antagonists also prevent release of mediators from activated mast cells although in most cases only in a higher concentration than that achieved clinically. This response does not involve H_1 receptors [13]. Two H_1 antagonists, ketotifen and cetirizine, deserve mention as they have been claimed to be potent inhibitors of release of mast-cell products [14–16]. However, no evidence of reduced urinary excretion of histamine or its metabolites was detected in patients with mastocytosis treated by the H_1 antihistamine, ketotifen [15]. Cetirizine has also been claimed to possess selective inhibitory activity against eosinophil-rich dermatoses [16,17] but the clinical relevance of this action is unclear.

H_1 antihistamines (Table 76.2)

These are conveniently classified as first- and second-generation H_1 antihistamines. The first-generation drugs, although potent, are accompanied by troublesome atropine-like side-effects, and also cause drowsiness [18] which may be useful or disadvantageous, depending upon the clinical context.

First-generation H_1 antihistamines

These are exemplified by chlorpheniramine (an alkylamine), diphenhydramine (an aminoalkyl ether) and hydroxyzine, (a piperazine). Plasma half-lives of these drugs are variable

Table 76.2 Pharmacokinetic and pharmacodynamic activity of representative first- and second-generation antihistamines [8,34].

H_1 antagonist	T_{max} (h)	Half-life (h)	Weal suppression duration (h)
Chlorpheniramine	2.8	27.9	24
Hydroxyzine	2.1	20.0	24
Diphenhydramine	1.7	9.2	12–24
Terfenadine	1.0	17	12–24
Astemizole	3.0	9.5 days	Variable
Loratadine	1.0	7.8–11.0	12–24
Cetirizine	0.9	7.4	24

T_{max}, time of maximum plasma concentration.

(chlorpheniramine about 24 h; hydroxyzine 20 h; diphenhydramine 9 h), although peak plasma concentrations are reached in about 2 h. Protein binding is almost total, and metabolism occurs via the hepatic microsomal cytochrome P-450 system. Thus, the half life of certain H_1 antihistamines may be prolonged by patients receiving microsomal oxygenase inhibitors such as ketoconazole, erythromycin, doxepin or cimetidine.

The principal actions of H_1 antihistamines are on vasodilatation and increased vascular permeability, thus reducing the redness, weal and axon reflex flare reactions in acute urticaria, and suppressing the associated itching. The clinical effects of these H_1 antihistamines usually persist longer than measurable plasma levels would suggest, because of persistence of tissue levels or because of active metabolites. Once-daily administration is therefore adequate. In urticaria, first-generation H_1 antagonists reduce the size, duration and frequency of weals and greatly alleviate the itching. Although more often a nuisance, the sedative effects of first generation H_1 antihistamines have been claimed to be highly beneficial in suppressing itching in some patients with atopic eczema [19]. They are enhanced by other sedative drugs, especially alcohol. Other side-effects of these antihistamines include tachycardia, with prolongation of the QT interval on the electrocardiogram and other arrythmias as well as psychological disturbances.

Second-generation H_1 antihistamines [8]

These are exemplified by terfenadine astemizole, loratadine and cetirizine, none of which produces sedation significantly greater than that caused by an otherwise identical placebo, provided recommended dosage is used. The absorption and metabolism of second-generation H_1 antihistamines resembles that of the first generation described above. The plasma half-lives of terfenadine, astemizole and cetirizine are listed in Table 76.2. These drugs in recommended dosages do not significantly cross the blood–brain barrier, thus accounting for their minimally sedating characteristics. Terfenadine is almost completely devoid of histamine H_2 or cholinergic receptor blockade. Given in doses of 60 mg twice daily or 120 mg once daily it is effective in the treatment of chronic urticaria [20]. Drugs which inhibit hepatic metabolism via the cytochrome P-450 system (ketoconazole, itraconazole, erythromycin, other macrolide antibiotics, cimetidine and doxepin) should not be given concurrently with terfenadine since they may promote adverse effects of terfenadine including cardiac arrhythmias, the best recognized of which is torsades de pointes (ventricular tachycardia) [21–23]. Thirty-three cases of cardiac arrythmias including 14 deaths attributed to terfenadine have been reported to the UK Committee on Safety of Medicines. Terfenadine is also contraindicated in patients with liver or heart disease. Patients developing torsades de pointes should be treated as for astemizole-induced ventricular tachycardia (see below). Terfenadine may cause rashes which occasionally (and paradoxically) include urticaria [24]. Recently fexofenadine, the major active metabolite of terfenadine, has been licensed in the UK as an alternative to terfenadine. Terfenadine has been withdrawn in several European countries at the time of writing (1997).

Astemizole also undergoes first-pass metabolism via the liver cytochrome P-450 system but its half-life together with its active metabolite dimethylastemizole is prolonged at 9.5 days [8]. It binds with greater avidity to H_1-receptor sites than any other H_1 antihistamine, evidence of histamine weal suppression being evident 4 weeks or more after discontinuation [25], but it has not been shown to be teratogenic. Like terfenadine, it must not be coadministered with macrolide antibiotics, imidazole antifungals or doxepin, because of the risk of cardiac arrhythmia. Patients developing torsades de pointes should be treated by withdrawal of the drug, intravenous magnesium sulphate and isoprenaline, temporary cardiac pacing and if necessary direct current cardioversion [26]. Patients with a pre-existing QT interval prolongation are especially at risk [26]. Other side-effects of astemizole include increase in appetite and excessive weight gain [8].

Loratadine is a potent minimal sedation antihistamine which is also substantially free of anticholinergic side-effects. Loratadine is not metabolized through the liver cytochrome P-450 enzyme system to any great extent and is therefore believed free of cardiac arrhythmic complications. It inhibits evoked release of leukotrienes from human lung *in vitro* but is less active in suppressing histamine release [27]. How relevant these 'antiallergic' properties are to its therapeutic action is unclear.

Like loratadine, cetirizine which is an active metabolite of hydroxyzine is only minimally metabolized via the liver and therefore can be administered safely with macrolide antibiotics, imidazole antifungals and doxepin. In recommended dosage it has minimal sedative and anticholinergic actions. As mentioned previously [16,17] cetirizine is claimed to be effective in diseases involving heavy eosinophil infiltration. It has been proposed, on this basis, that cetirizine is especially valuable in patients with the common physical urticaria, delayed pressure urticaria [28], although adequate confirmation of this claim is lacking.

H_1-antihistamine therapy in childhood

The second-generation, low-sedation antihistamines are probably safer in children than the older, 'classical' antihistamines; liquid formulations of astemizole, cetirizine, loratadine and terfenadine are available in the UK. Overdose of the first-generation antihistamines may cause severe toxicity including hyperpyrexia and convulsions in children.

H_1-antihistamine therapy in pregnancy

No antihistamines administered systemically should be deemed safe in the first trimester of pregnancy. However, of the available H_1 antihistamines, chlorpheniramine [29] and tripelennamine [30] have shown little or no evidence of teratogenicity experimentally and are probably the least risky to use.

Development of tolerance during H_1-antihistamine therapy

Although tolerance of the first-generation H_1 antihistamines was reported soon after their introduction into medical practice [31], little or no information is available on the molecular basis of this phenomenon [32]. Suppression of wealing due to mast-cell activation and to histamine progressively dwindled in response to single doses of 75 mg hydroxyzine given daily for 3 weeks; no tolerance was demonstrated in response to chlorpheniramine 16 mg daily in the same study [33]. Interestingly, this study showed that hydroxyzine, but not chlorpheniramine caused tolerance not only to itself but to several other first-generation antihistamines.

H_2 antihistamines

Cimetidine

The presence of H_2 receptors expressed on human skin blood vessels [9,10] prompted exploration of the value of H_2 antihistamines, coadministered with H_1 antihistamines, in the treatment of chronic urticaria. The object was to achieve an H_1 antihistamine-sparing effect, thus mitigating unwanted first-generation H_1 antihistamine side-effects including drowsiness and atropine-like side-effects. This strategy proved modestly successful [6,35–37]. However, the subsequent availability of the second-generation, low-sedation antihistamines has undermined the need for an H_1-antihistamine-sparing regimen. Since ranitidine, unlike cimetidine, is not metabolized via the liver cytochrome P-450 system, it should probably be used in preference to cimetidine if H_2 antihistamine therapy is instituted.

REFERENCES

1 Bovet D, Walthert F. Structure chemique et activité pharmacodynamique des antihistaminiques de synthese. *Ann Pharma Fr* 1944, Suppl. 4.

2 O'Leary PA, Faber EM. Benadryl in the treatment of urticaria. *Proc Staff Meet Mayo Clin* 1945; **20**: 429–32.

3 Bain WA, Broadbent JL, Warin RP. Comparison of anthisan (mepyramine maleate) and phenengan as histamine antagonists. *Lancet* 1949; **ii**: 47–52.

4 Bain WD, Hellier FF, Warin RP. Some aspects of the action of histamine antagonists. *Lancet* 1948; **ii**: 964–6.

5 Black JW, Duncan WA, Durrant CJ *et al*. Definition and antagonism of histamine H_2 receptors. *Nature* 1972; **236**: 385–90.

6 Commens CA, Greaves MW. Cimetidine in chronic idiopathic urticaria: a randomised double blind study. *Br J Dermatol* 1978; **99**: 675–9.

7 Arrang JM, Garbarg M, Schwartz JC. Autoinhibition of brain histamine release mediated by a novel (H₃) class of histamine receptor. *Nature* 1983; **302**: 832–7.

8 Simons FER. Recent advances in H₁ antagonist treatment. *J Allergy Clin Immunol* 1990; **86**: 995–9.

9 Marks R, Greaves MW. Vascular reactions to histamine and compound 48/80 in human skin: suppression by a histamine H₂ receptor blocking agent. *Br J Clin Pharmacol* 1977; **4**: 367–9.

10 Robertson I, Greaves MW. Responses of human skin blood vessels to synthetic histamine analogues. *Br J Clin Pharmacol* 1978; **5**: 319–22.

11 Davies MG, Greaves MW. Sensory responses of human skin to synthetic histamine analogues and histamine. *Br J Clin Pharmacol* 1980; **9**: 461–5.

12 Brandes LJ, LaBella FS, Glavin GB et al. Histamine as an intracellular messenger. *Biochem Pharmacol* 1990; **40**: 1677–81.

13 Rimmer SJ, Church MK. The pharmacology and mechanism of action of histamine H₁ antagonists. *Clin Exp Allergy* 1990; **20** (Suppl. 2): 3–17.

14 Huston DP, Bressler RB, Kaliner M et al. Prevention of mast cell degranulation by Ketotifen in patients with physical urticarias. *Ann Intern Med* 1986; **104**: 507–10.

15 Mallet AI, Norris P, Rendell NB et al. The effect of disodium cromoglycate and ketotifen on the excretion of histamine and N-methylimidazole acetic acid in urine of patients with mastocytosis. *Br J Clin Pharmacol* 1989; **27**: 88–91.

16 Charlesworth EN, Kagey-Sobotka A, Norman PS, Lichtenstein LM. Effect of cetirizine on mast cell mediator release and cellular traffic during the cutaneous late phase reaction. *J Allergy Clin Immunol* 1989; **83**: 905–12.

17 Leprevost C, Capron M, De Vos C et al. Inhibition of eosinophil chemotaxis by a new anti allergic compound (cetirizine). *Int Arch. Allergy Appl Immunol* 1988; **87**: 9–13.

18 Monti JM. Involvement of histamine in the control of the waking state. *Life Sci* 1993; **53**: 1331–8.

19 Krause L, Shuster S. Mechanism of action of antipruritic drugs. *Br Med J* 1983; **287**: 1199–200.

20 Grant JA, Bernstein DI, Buckley CE et al. Double blind comparison of terfenadine, chlorpheniramine and placebo in the treatment of chronic idiopathic urticaria. *J Allergy Clin Immunol* 1988; **81**: 574–9.

21 MacConnell TJ, Stanners AJ. Torsades de pointes complicating treatment with terfenadine. *Br Med J* 1991; **302**: 1469.

22 Honig PK, Woosley RL, Zamani K et al. Changes in the pharmacokinetics and electrocardiographic pharmacodynamics of terfenadine with concomitant administration of erythromycin. *Clin Pharmacol Ther* 1992; **52**: 231–8.

23 Rao KA, Adlakha A, Verman-Ansil B et al. Torsades de pointes ventricular tachycardia associated with overdose of astemizole. *Mayo Clin Proc* 1994; **69**: 589–93.

24 Stricker BHCH, Van Dijke CPH, Isaacs AI, Lindquist M. Skin reactions to terfenadine. *Br Med J* 1986; **293**: 536.

25 Kailasam V, Matthews KP. Controlled clinical assessment of astemizole in the treatment of chronic idiopathic urticaria and angioedema. *J Am Acad Dermatol* 1987; **16**: 797–804.

26 Broadhurst P, Nathan AW. Cardiac arrest in a young woman with the long QT syndrome and concomitant astemizole ingestion. *Br Heart J* 1993; **70**: 469–70.

27 Temple DM, McClusky M. Loratidine, an antihistamine, blocks antigen and ionophore-induced leukotriene release from human lung *in vitro*. *Prostaglandins* 1988; **35**: 549–54.

28 Kontou-Fili K, Maniatakou G, Demaka P et al. Therapeutic effects of cetirizine in delayed pressure urticaria: Clinicopathologic findings. *J Am Acad Dermatol* 1991; **24**: 1090–3.

29 Pratt WR. Allergic diseases in pregnancy and breast feeding. *Ann Allergy* 1981; **47**: 355.

30 Schatz M, Hoffman CP, Zeiger RS et al. The course and management of asthma and allergic diseases during pregnancy. In: Middleton E, Reed CE, Ellis EE et al., eds. *Allergy Principles and Practice*; Vol. 2, 4th edn. St Louis: Mosby Year Book, 1993: 1301–42.

31 Wyngaarden JB, Seevers MH. The toxic effects of antihistamine drugs. *JAMA* 1951; **145**: 277–82.

32 Monash S. Development of refractory condition of skin towards antihistaminic drugs after antihistamine therapy as determined by histamine iontophoresis. *J Invest Dermatol* 1950; **15**: 1.

33 Long WF, Taylor RJ, Wagner CJ et al. Skin test suppression by antihistamines and the development of subsensitivity. *J Allergy Clin Immunol* 1985; **76**: 113–17.

34 Simons FER, Simons KJ. The pharmacology and use of H₁ receptor-antagonist drugs. *N Engl J Med* 1994; **330**: 1663–70.

35 Breathnach SM, Allen R, Milford Ward A, Greaves MW. Symptomatic dermographism: natural history, clinical features, laboratory investigations and response to therapy. *Clin Exp Dermatol* 1983; **8**: 463–76.

36 Kaur S, Greaves MW, Eftekhari N. Factitious urticaria (dermographism) treatment by cimetidine and chlorpheniramine in a randomised double blind study. *Br J Dermatol* 1981; **104**: 185–90.

37 Bleehen SS, Thomas SE, Greaves MW et al. Cimetidine and chlorpheniramine in the treatment of chronic idiopathic urticaria: a multicentre randomised double blind study. *Br J Dermatol* 1987; **117**: 81–8.

Other antiallergic drugs

The only antiallergic agent of dermatological relevance is sodium cromoglycate. Although ineffective in suppressing mast-cell activation in the skin [1] it inhibits release of histamine and other mast-cell-derived mediators from mast cells of lung, conjunctiva, nose and gastrointestinal tracts. It therefore has no proven role in the skin. However, it does ameliorate the diarrhoea associated with mastocytosis [2].

REFERENCES

1 Pearce CA, Greaves MW, Plummer VM, Yamamoto S. Effect of disodium cromoglycate on antigen-evoked histamine release from human skin. *Clin Exp Immunol* 1974; **17**: 437–40.

2 Soter NA, Austen KF, Wasserman SI. Oral disodium cromoglycate in the treatment of systemic mastocytosis. *N Engl J Med* 1979; **301**: 465–9.

Systemic non-steroidal anti-inflammatory therapy

Non-steroidal anti-inflammatory drugs (NSAID) are defined as substituted phenolic or benzene-ring compounds which owe their pharmacological actions mainly to inhibition of the enzyme cyclo-oxygenase (COX) (prostaglandin synthetase). This enzyme complex was shown by Vane in 1971 to transform arachidonic acid into prostaglandins [1]. However, NSAID undoubtedly influence other pro-inflammatory molecular pathways.

Transformation of arachidonic acid and the mode of action of NSAID

There are two forms of COX: a constitutive enzyme (COX-1) and an induced enzyme (COX-2) (Fig. 76.1). NSAID act mainly by inhibition of COX-2 [2]. In contrast, inhibition of COX-1 by NSAID probably accounts for some of their unwanted side-effects including gastric ulceration.

Arachidonic acid is also transformed via the lipoxygenase pathways (5-lipoxygenase; 12-lipoxygenase) to form a group of strongly pro-inflammatory hydroxy fatty acids of which the best known is leukotriene B₄ (LTB₄) (Fig. 76.2) [3]. Because of the proposed role of the leukotrienes and other hydroxy fatty-acid products of arachidonic acid

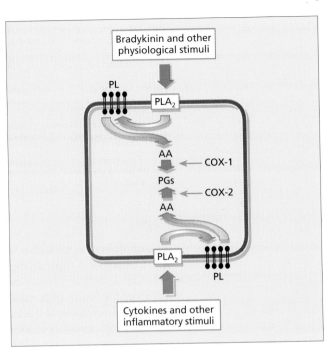

Fig. 76.1 Transformation of arachidonic acid to prostaglandins by cyclooxygenases (COX) 1 and 2.

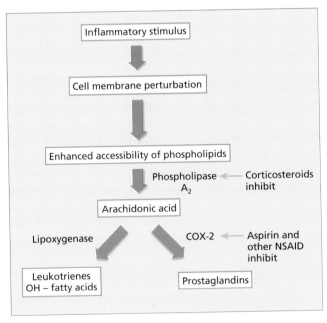

Fig. 76.2 Generation of eicosanoids from cell membrane lipids in the inflammatory response. Arachidonic acid, released from cell membrane phospholipid by the action of phospholipase A_2 is further transformed by COX-2 to prostaglandin, and by lipoxygenase to leukotrienes and related fatty acids.

in the pathogenesis of psoriasis [4] and other inflammatory dermatoses [5], several generally unsuccessful attempts have been made to develop selective lipoxygenase-

inhibiting NSAID for clinical dermatological use [6]. These compounds have generally proved ineffective, toxic or both.

Acetyl salicylic acid (aspirin) is the archetypal NSAID and has been shown to owe its anti-inflammatory action to inhibition of COX-2 [1]. Its role in the management of skin diseases is limited. Administration of aspirin has been shown to suppress ultraviolet erythema in humans [8]. Furthermore, Roberts and colleagues have proposed that aspirin be co-administered with H_1 and H_2 anti-histamines in the management of the diarrhoea of systemic mastocytosis, which is believed to be mainly due to over production of prostaglandin D2 by the increased population of mast cells in the involved tissues [9]. Although originally proposed to be antipruritic, aspirin administration probably does not allay the itching of atopic eczema [10].

The early phase of UVB-induced erythema is due at least in part to release of vasoactive prostaglandins [11]. Oral administration of indomethacin has been demonstrated to reduce the erythema and concurrently suppress the increased tissue levels of cyclo-oxygenase products in the UVB-irradiated skin [12]. Proposed clinical indications for oral indomethacin include cutaneous vasculitis [13] and erythema nodosum [14] although these indications have not yet been confirmed by placebo-controlled, double-blind trials. The value of oral indomethacin in the management of psoriatic arthritis is well established, although there are unconfirmed reports that oral indomethacin may exacerbate the skin lesions of psoriasis [15]. That there has been little or no success in the development of clinically useful lipoxygenase inhibitors for use in the skin has already been alluded to [6].

Adverse reactions to systemic NSAID are unfortunately common place. Reactions occur most frequently in response to piroxicam, sulindac, meclofenamate, tolmetin and phenylbutazone [16]. The best known and probably the most severe include Stevens–Johnson syndrome and toxic epidermal necrolysis. Photosensitivity is very common especially with piroxicam, but the underlying mechanisms, which involve phototoxicity in many instances, are unknown [17].

REFERENCES

1 Vane JR. Inhibition of prostaglandin synthesis as a mechanism of action for aspirin-like drugs. *Nature New Biol* 1971; **231**: 232–5.
2 Mitchell JA, Larkin S, Williams TJ. Cyclooxygenase-2 regulation and relevance in inflammation. *Biochem Pharmacol* 1995; **50**: 1535–42.
3 Samuelsson B, Hammarstrom S. Nomenclature for leukotrienes. *Prostaglandins* 1980; **19**: 645–8.
4 Brain S, Camp RDR, Dowd P *et al*. The release of leukotriene B4-like material in biologically active amounts from the lesional skin of patients with psoriasis. *J Invest Dermatol* 1984; **83**: 70–3.
5 Barr RM, Brain S, Camp RD *et al*. Levels of arachidonic acid and its metabolites in human allergic and irritant contact dermatitis. *Br J Dermatol* 1984; **111**: 23–8.
6 Barr RM, Black AK, Dowd PM *et al*. The *in vitro* 5-lipoxygenase and cyclo-

oxygenase inhibitor L-652, 343 does not inhibit 5-lipoxygenase *in vivo* in human skin. *Br J Clin Pharmacol* 1988; **25**: 23–6.

7 Vane JR, Botting RM. Formation by the endothelium of prostacyclin, nitric oxide and endothelin. *J Lipid Mediat* 1993; **6**: 395–404.

8 Miller WS, Ruderman FR, Smith JG, Jr. Aspirin and ultraviolet light-induced erythema in man. *Arch Dermatol* 1967; **95**: 357–8.

9 Roberts LJ, Sweetman BJ, Lewis RA *et al*. Increased production of prostaglandin D2 in patients with systemic mastocytosis. *N Engl J Med* 1980; **303**: 1400–4.

10 Daly BM, Shuster S. Effect of aspirin on pruritus. *Br Med J* 1986; **293**: 907.

11 Black AK, Fincham N, Greaves MW, Hensby CN. Time course changes in levels of arachidonic acid and prostaglandin D2, E2 and F2 in human skin following ultraviolet B irradiation. *Br J Pharmacol* 1980; **10**: 453–7.

12 Kobza Black A, Greaves MW, Hensby CN *et al*. Effects of indomethacin on prostaglandins E$_2$ F$_{2\alpha}$ and arachidonic acid in human skin 24h after UV-B and UV-C irradiation. *Br J Clin Pharmacol* 1978; **6**: 261–6.

13 Millns JL, Randle HW, Solley GO, Dicken CH. The therapeutic response of urticaria vasculitis to indomethacin. *J Am Acad Dermatol* 1980; **3**: 349–55.

14 Callen JP. Erythema nodosum. In: Provost T, Farmer ER, eds *Current Therapy in Dermatology, 1985–1986*. Dekker and CV Mosby Co., 158–160.

15 Katayama H, Kawada A. Exacerbation of psoriasis induced by indomethacin. *J Dermatol (Tokyo)* 1981; **8**: 323–7.

16 Bigby M, Stern R. Cutaneous reactions to non-steroidal anti inflammatory drugs. *J Am Acad Dermatol* 1985; **12**: 866–76.

17 Kaidbey KH, Mitchell FN. Photosensitising potential of certain non-steroidal anti-inflammatory agents. *Arch Dermatol* 1989; **125**: 783–6.

Interferons

Interferons are naturally occurring antiviral cytokines now available for therapeutic use through recombinant DNA technology. This group of compounds exhibits antiviral, cytostatic and immunomodulatory properties and has therefore found application in both malignant and inflammatory dermatoses. Three types of interferon are available: interferon-α (IFN-α), IFN-β and IFN-γ. Unfortunately, side-effects are common, including influenza-like symptoms with fever, hepatotoxicity and leukopenia; and this has limited clinical usage of these interferons.

Kaposi's sarcoma

Because of its antiviral, antiangiogenic and tumouristatic properties, interferon ought to be an ideal treatment for acquired immune deficiency syndrome (AIDS)-related Kaposi's sarcoma. There have been numerous reports of remissions induced by IFN-α; invariably at the cost of troublesome side-effects. In earlier studies [1], high doses did induce remissions especially in patients without associated opportunistic infections [2]. Subsequent studies suggested that better results were obtained in the presence of sustained CD4 T-lymphocyte counts [3]. There is some evidence of synergism between IFN-α and zidovudine [4,5]. Coadministration of granulocyte/macrophage colony-stimulating factor (GM-CSF) with IFN-α has been shown to limit the bone-marrow-suppressant side-effects of the latter [6]. IFN-γ is ineffective in Kaposi's sarcoma.

Other skin malignancy

There has been much interest in the treatment of metastatic melanoma with IFN-α either alone or in combination with a vaccine. Alone it brings about significant, albeit temporary, remission in 20% of patients [7]. Alternatively, IFN-α has been administered subsequent to melanoma lysate vaccine, leading to a higher response rate than IFN-α or melanoma lysate vaccine given alone [1]. IFN-α treatment is probably worth considering in these patients. IFN-α is also a treatment option in Sézary syndrome. One study involving six patients [9] led to a complete remission in two and a partial remission in one. Combination treatment with IFN-α and other antitumour measures needs to be explored in the Sézary syndrome.

Atopic eczema

Recombinant IFN-γ has been administered on a double-blind, placebo-controlled basis to atopic dermatitis patients with demonstrably superior effect compared with placebo control [10]. The rationale for IFN-γ treatment is based upon the findings of high serum IgE levels, predominant type 2 helper T cell (Th2) cells producing interleukin 4 (IL-4) and IL-5 coupled with low production of IFN-γ by Th1 cells in atopic subjects. Administration of IFN-γ, according to this scheme, results in isotype switching away from IgE production, due to inhibition of growth of IL-4 and IL-5-producing Th2 cells [11]. About one-half of the IFN-γ treated patients, but only about one-quarter of the placebo-treated patients, experienced significant clinical improvement [10]. There was no reduction in serum IgE in the IFN-γ-treated group but the blood eosinophil count fell in these patients. Side-effects including leukopenia were frequent in the actively treated patients. IFN-γ treatment has yet to establish itself as a useful sole or adjunctive treatment for atopic eczema.

REFERENCES

1 Krown SE, Real FX, Cunningham RS *et al*. Preliminary observations on the effect of recombinant leucocyte alpha interferon in homosexual men with Kaposi's sarcoma. *N Engl J Med* 1983; **308**: 1071–6.

2 Groopman JE, Gottlieb MS, Goodman J *et al*. Recombinant alpha$_2$-interferon therapy for Kaposi's sarcoma associated with the acquired immune deficiency syndrome. Clinical response and prognostic parameters. *Ann Intern Med* 1984; **100**: 671–6.

3 Lane HC, Feinberg J, Kovaks JA *et al*. Anti retroviral effects of interferon-α in AIDS-associated Kaposi's sarcoma. *Lancet* 1988; **ii**: 1218–22.

4 Stadler R, Bratzke B, Schaart F, Orfanos CE. Long term combined r INF-alpha-2α and zidovudine therapy for HIV-associated Kaposi's sarcoma. Clinical consequences and side effects. *J Invest Dermatol* 1990; **95**: 170S–5S.

5 Podzamczer D, Bolao F, Clotet B *et al*. Low dose interferon-alpha combined with zidovudine in patients with AIDS associated Kaposi's sarcoma. *J Intern Med* 1993; **233**: 247–53.

6 Scadden DT, Bering HA, Levine JD *et al*. Granulocyte monocyte colony-stimulating factor mitigates neutropenia of combined interferon-alpha and zidovudine treatment of acquired immunodeficiency syndrome-associated Kaposi's Sarcoma. *J Clin Oncol* 1991; **9**: 802–8.

7 Kirkwood JM, Strawderman MH, Ernstoff MS *et al.* Interferon alpha-2β adjuvant therapy of high risk resected cutaneous melanoma: the eastern cooperative group trial EST 1684. *J Clin Oncol* 1996; **14**: 7–17.

8 Mitchell MS. Immunotherapy of melanoma. Epidemiology and clinical manifestations. *J Invest Dermatol Symposium Proc* 1996; **1**: 215–18.

9 Olsen EA, Rosen ST, Vollmer RT *et al.* Interferon alpha-2a in the treatment of cutaneous T cell lymphoma. *J Am Acad Dermatol* 1989; **20**: 395–407.

10 Hanifin JM, Schneider LC, Leung DYM *et al.* Recombinant interferon gamma therapy for atopic dermatitis. *J Am Acad Dermatol* 1993; **28**: 189–97.

11 Gajewski TF, Fitch FW. Anti proliferative effect of IFN-γ inhibits proliferation of TH_2 but not TH_1 murine helper T lymphocyte clones. *J Immunol* 1988; **140**: 4245–52.

Essential fatty acids

Essential fatty acids are simply defined as those which cannot be synthesized by humans. The major essential fatty acids found in humans are the ω-6 fatty acids linoleic acid and its products, γ-linolenic acid and arachidonic acid, precursors of important mediators of inflammation, the eicosanoids. Arachidonic acid is synthesized from linoleic acid in the liver. Although vertebrates cannot synthesize linoleic acid *de novo*, plants can synthesize both linoleic and γ-linolenic acids, important constituents of evening primrose oil. Skin, unlike liver, is devoid of δ-5 desaturase and cannot convert γ-linolenic acid to arachidonic acid directly. Thus, arachidonic acid found in skin is not directly dietary in origin.

Deficiency of essential fatty acids in the diet of humans leads to a scaly dermatitis and impaired skin-barrier function associated with reduced tissue levels of linoleic and arachidonic acid and increased levels of an abnormal fatty acid 5, 8, 11 (ω-9) eicosatrienoic acid. This syndrome is found in patients following bowel resection and prolonged parenteral nutrition [1,2] and can be rectified by topical application of eicosanoids [3] or linoleic acid from sunflower-seed oil [4]. In the latter instance, skin levels of fatty acids were not reported but presumably any correction of cutaneous arachidonic acid deficiency would have been dependent upon systemic absorption. Other cutaneous manifestations of essential fatty acid deficiency include hypopigmentation of hair and alopecia [1,2]. Studies in essential fatty acid-deficient mice suggest that linoleic acid but not arachidonic acid is pivotal in the maintenance of efficient barrier function in the skin [5].

Linoleic acid and γ-linoleic acid in atopic dermatitis

Current interest in essential fatty acids in atopic dermatitis originates in an observation by Hansen [6] that patients with this disorder had elevated serum levels of linoleic acid but reduced levels of its δ-6-desaturase products, γ-linoleic acid and dihomo-γ-linolenic acid. Subsequent plasma analyses [7] have supported these findings and extended them to show that plasma of atopic dermatitis patients is also depleted of arachidonic acid, a δ-desaturase product

of dihomo-γ-linolenic acid. The results were compatible with a proposed defect of δ-6-desaturase in atopic dermatitis and it has been further speculated that insufficiency of these essential fatty acids might bring about prostaglandin-2-series deficiency and even explain some of the abnormalities of immune function which are a recognized feature of this disorder. These findings were followed by a number of reports suggesting that oral replacement therapy using oil from the seed of evening primrose caused clinical improvement in the skin of patients with atopic dermatitis [8] and that the improvement correlated with increased plasma levels of dihomo-γ-linolenic acid. The value of evening primrose oil remains a controversial issue. A meta-analysis of nine trials suggested that this treatment is of significant value in atopic eczema [9]. However, puzzlingly, a large placebo-controlled study which reported negative results [10] was omitted from the meta-analysis. The British National Formulary (1997) states that: 'the evidence in favour of a useful therapeutic effect (in atopic eczema) is poor'.

Eicosapentaenoic acid and related fatty acids

These polyunsaturated fatty acids possess a longer chain length than linoleic acid and more double bonds, and are found in large quantities in fish oils, in which eicosapentaenoic acid (EPA) and docosahexaenoic acid predominate. There are fundamental differences between the lipoxygenase metabolites of EPA and of arachidonic acid. The lipoxygenase metabolite of EPA is LTB_5 which is much less potent as a mediator of leukocyte chemotaxis than LTB_4 which has been proposed as a major polymorphonuclear chemoattractant mediator in psoriasis [11]. Attempts have been made to modify the severity of psoriasis by long-term administration of diet supplemented by fish oil [12] which caused rapid incorporation of EPA and docosahexaenoic acid into neutrophils and epidermis, the majority of patients showing clinical improvement. Subsequent experience [13] suggests that EPA dietary supplementation, which by itself causes only marginal improvement of psoriasis, may enhance the efficacy of co-administered conventional psoriatic therapy. The most frequently prescribed dietary source of fish oil is MAX-EPA, a concentrated fish oil product. The daily intake is 60–75 g flavoured with fruit juice and containing 180 mg EPA and 120 mg docosahexaenoic acid per gram of oil. Double-blind, controlled trials are impractical owing to the persistent fishy odour emanating from users of this product.

EPA has also been proposed as a supplementary treatment for patients receiving cyclosporin treatment for psoriasis and other dermatoses due to its supposed protective action on renal function [14].

REFERENCES

1 Press M, Kikuchi H, Shimoyama T *et al*. Diagnosis and treatment of essential fatty acid deficiency in man. *Br Med J* 1974; **1**: 247–50.
2 Skolnik P, Eaglstein WH, Ziboh VA. Human essential fatty acid deficiency. *Arch Dermatol* 1977; **113**: 939–41.
3 Ziboh VA, Hsia SL. Effects of prostaglandin E on rat skin. Inhibition of sterol ester biosynthesis and clearing of scaly lesions in essential fatty acid deficiency. *J Lipid Res* 1972; **13**: 458–67.
4 Press M, Hartop PJ, Prottey C. Correction of essential fatty acid deficiency in man by the cutaneous application of sunflower seed oil. *Lancet* 1974; **i**: 597–9.
5 Elias PM, Brown BE, Ziboh VA. The permeability barrier in essential fatty acid deficiency; evidence for a direct role for linoleic acid in barrier function. *J Invest Dermatol* 1980; **74**: 230–3.
6 Hansen AE. Serum lipid changes and therapeutic effects of various oils in infantile eczema. *Proc Soc Exp Biol Med* 1933; **31**: 160–1.
7 Manku MS, Horrobin DF, Morse NL *et al*. Essential fatty acids in the plasma phospholipids of patients with atopic eczema. *Br J Dermatol* 1984; **110**: 643–8.
8 Lovell CR, Burton JL, Horrobin DF. Treatment of atopic eczema with evening primrose oil. *Lancet* 1981; **i**: 278.
9 Morse PF, Horrobin DF, Manku MS *et al*. Meta-analysis of placebo controlled studies of the efficacy of Epogam in the treatment of atopic eczema. Relationship between plasma essential fatty acid changes and clinical response. *Br J Dermatol* 1989; **121**: 75–90.
10 Bamford JTM, Gibson RW, Penier CM. Atopic eczema unresponsive to evening primrose oil (linoleic and γ-linolenic acids). *J Am Acad Dermatol* 1985; **13**: 959–65.
11 Brain SD, Camp RDR, Greaves MW. Psoriasis and leucotriene B$_4$. *Lancet* 1982; **ii**: 762–3.
12 Ziboh VA, Cohen KA, Ellis CN *et al*. Effects of dietary supplementation of fish oil on neutrophil and epidermal fatty acids. *Arch Dermatol* 1986; **122**: 1277–82.
13 Maurice PDL, Allen BR, Barkley ASJ *et al*. The effects of dietary supplementation with fish oil in patients with psoriasis. *Br J Dermatol* 1987; **117**: 599–606.
14 Elzinga L, Kelley VE, Houghton DC *et al*. Modification of experimental nephrotoxicity with fish oil as the vehicle for cyclosporine. *Transplantation* 1987; **43**: 271–5.

Retinoids

This class of compounds covers both the synthetic and the natural forms of vitamin A (the term vitamin A includes the preformed vitamin A alcohol, retinol, its aldehyde, retinal, and its acid, *trans*-retinoic acid, as well as the provitamin, β-carotene). Chemical manipulation of retinol has led to numerous new compounds which are less toxic than the parent molecule.

The mode of action of the retinoids has not been completely elucidated but they have profound effects on differentiation, cell growth and immune response. They are used especially in dermatology but also have a role or a potential role in cancer prevention and perhaps cancer therapy.

Effect on differentiation

It has been known for many years that vitamin A deficiency results in epithelial squamous metaplasia and that vitamin supplements reverse this effect. Retinoids have now been shown to reduce differentiation in a number of cell types, for example mouse teratocarcinoma and

human myeloid leukaemia cells, and to cause regression of bronchial metaplasia in heavy smokers [1]. Epidermis undergoes profound changes and shows hypergranulosis and hyperplasia with decreased numbers of tonofilaments and desmosomes and widening of intracellular spaces [2]. The effect on desmosomes appears to contribute to the keratolytic effect of retinoids in hyperkeratotic disorders.

Effect on carcinogenesis [2,3]

In models of carcinogenesis the induction of the enzyme ornithine decarboxylase occurs during transformation [4]. The enzyme induction is inhibited by retinoids and this inhibition has been used to test the anticarcinogenic effect of new retinoids.

Tumour growth [3]

The growth of a number of human tumour-cell lines, for example melanoma, seems to be inhibited by retinoids but the response may be variable. Retinoids have not yet established themselves as of major importance in cancer treatment. High concentrations of retinoids cause cytotoxicity through membrane labilization, although at lower doses membrane stabilization may occur.

Receptors

There are specific retinol and retinoic acid receptors. The activity of retinoids is mediated through these in a similar manner to steroid hormones. There are at least three retinoic acid receptors, all of which belong to the family of steroid–thyroid–vitamin D receptors. The receptors have a more significant effect on differentiation [5] than on the inhibition of tumour growth.

Cell surface effects

Retinoids affect transformed cell surfaces and lead to loss of anchorage-independent growth, cell adhesiveness and density-dependent growth [6]. It is not clear whether these effects are exerted directly by the retinoid involvement in glycosyl transfer reactions or through changes in gene expression.

Immunostimulation

In animal models retinoids may act as an adjuvant and stimulate antibody formation to antigens that were previously not immunogenic [7,8]. In addition, retinoids may stimulate cell-mediated cytotoxicity.

Neutrophil migration

The migration of neutrophils is reduced by retinoids both

in experimental models of inflammation [9] and in patients with acne [10]. The mode of action is unknown.

Skin flora

Retinoids do not seem to have an appreciable direct action on the skin flora.

Ageing

The effects of retinoids on the ageing process, particularly the ageing skin, are complex. The emphasis is currently on topical therapy.

Isotretinoin (13-*cis*-retinoic acid)

Isotretinoin has been shown to be very effective in the treatment of severe, recalcitrant cystic acne unresponsive to antibacterial agents and to be superior to etretinate. Dose ranges have varied considerably from 0.1 to 2.0 mg/kg/day, but the most widely used regimen at present is 1.0 mg/kg/day as a 16-week course. This produces prolonged remission in the majority of patients (Chapter 42). Topical isotretinoin also appears to suppress acne [11].

In a long-term study of up to 10 years (mean 9 years) post-isotretinoin, 85% clinical improvement has resulted from a 4-month course and 69% of patients were still free of acne. Twenty-three per cent required a second course the relapse occurring within 3 years in 96% of patients [12]. The need for a second course of isotretinoin is more likely if low-dose regimens are used (0.1 mg/kg and 0.5 mg/kg). The most effective dose commensurate with side-effects is 1 mg/kg/day for 4 months [13]. In addition to acne, isotretinoin has been used in the treatment of Gram-negative folliculitis, rosacea and, rather less successfully, hidradenitis suppurativa and steatocystoma multiplex.

In acne the major therapeutic effect seems to be a profound reduction in sebaceous gland size and activity. There are reductions in bacterial flora, but it is likely that these changes are secondary to the reduction in sebum secretion. The anti-inflammatory and desquamating effects of retinoids may also play a beneficial role.

A wide range of disorders of keratinization have been found to be responsive to isotretinoin. In Europe this group of disorders is now usually treated with acitretin.

Etretinate

This retinoid has now been superceded by acitretin, which is the hydrolysis product and active metabolite of etretinate [14]. The major disadvantage of etretinate is its binding to body fat for up to 2 years after a course has been completed. Etretinate is 50 times more lipophilic than acitretin [15]. The elimination half-life of etretinate is over 100 days, whereas acitretin is 2 days [16,17].

Acitretin

In most respects, this drug resembles the parent compound. It is less bound to fat than etretinate, and it had been hoped that the time interval, after stopping the drug and before pregnancy was advised, might be shortened. However, it has been shown in some patients that there is reverse metabolism to etretinate and therefore the same restriction of 2 years is advised between the end of a course and pregnancy being advised [18]. The efficacy of acitretin is very similar to etretinate and in general is used in slightly lower doses. Acitretin is effective in various forms of psoriasis although in plaque psoriasis the results are often disappointing [19,20]. The efficacy can be improved by adding UVA, photochemotherapy (psoralen and UVA (PUVA)) or UVB phototherapy [19] (Chapter 35).

Acitretin is effective in pustular psoriasis, both palmoplantar or generalized (Von Zumbusch) [21,22], also in erythrodermic psoriasis.

In many skin conditions, reports have been confined to etretinate prior to the development of acitretin. Most clinicians would agree that the effects are similar with slightly lower doses of acitretin being required. The following disorders of keratinization are often responsive to retinoids: epidermolytic hyperkeratosis, keratoderma, X-linked ichthyosis, ichthyosis vulgaris, erythrokeratoderma variabilis, pityriasis rubra pilaris, discoid lupus erythematosus and lichen planus, Darier's disease, lamellar ichthyosis and non-bullous ichthyosiform erythroderma. Long-term treatment is required as worthwhile remissions following cessation of treatment have not been reported. Toxicity therefore may prove to be a problem in these patients.

A range of skin tumours may sometimes clear with retinoids. These include solar keratoses, keratoacanthoma, epidermodysplasia verruciformis, basal cell epithelioma and leukoplakia. However, these preparations may be of particular value in the prevention of tumours in those patients with high-risk disorders such as xeroderma pigmentosum, porokeratosis of Mibelli, familial self-healing squamous epithelioma of the skin and in those transplantation patients with extensive sunlight-damaged skin.

A number of side-effects are common to all the retinoids. These appear to be dose related and are largely cutaneous. They include cheilitis, conjunctivitis, dryness of mucous membranes and epistaxis, desquamation of hands and feet, pruritus, myalgia, arthralgia, lethargy and alopecia [23–25]. Intracranial hypertension may occur and is a reason not to combine isotretinoin with tetracyclines. Likewise, it is better to avoid supplementary therapy with vitamin A in patients on synthetic retinoids. Retinoids also appear to increase the hepatotoxicity of methotrexate.

Patients may develop abnormal liver enzyme levels during therapy with retinoids. Not all values have returned to normal on cessation of the drug [26].

Increase in very low density lipoprotein (VLDL) cholesterol and reduction in high-density lipoprotein (HDL) cholesterol have been reported with retinoid therapy. Many patients receiving isotretinoin have been reported with elevated serum VLDL triglyceride in the absence of a preceding hyperlipoproteinaemia. These levels have returned to normal on cessation of treatment, but all patients should be screened for hyperlipoproteinaemia prior to treatment with any retinoid.

An ossification disorder resembling idiopathic skeletal hyperostosis has been reported in patients receiving long-term retinoids. These drugs should only be given to younger children when there are good indications [27–29].

Teratogenicity

Retinoids are known to be teratogenic. Maternal ingestion of retinoids early in pregnancy can lead to fetal abnormalities [30] and the infants seem to have a characteristic appearance [31,32].

It is important that women are not pregnant prior to starting treatment. Effective contraception is mandatory during and after a course of treatment. Isotretinoin has a short half-life and therefore contraceptive measures need to be taken for only 1 month after cessation of treatment, but etretinate has a long half-life. The makers recommend that conception should not occur for 2 years after cessation of acitretin therapy. It is preferable to check blood levels at that time to confirm that no drug is detectable, even though it is recognized that only a minority of patients back-metabolize acitretin to etretinate. Males can safely father children even when they are taking the drug.

REFERENCES

1 Gouveia J, Mathé G, Hercent T *et al.* Degree of bronchial metaplasia in heavy smokers and its regression after treatment with a retinoid. *Lancet* 1982; **i:** 710–12.
2 Elias PM, Williams ML. Retinoids, cancer, and the skin. *Arch Dermatol* 1981; **117:** 160–80.
3 Editorial. Retinoids and control of cutaneous malignancy. *Lancet* 1988; **ii:** 545–6.
4 Boutwell RK. Retinoids and inhibition of ornithine decarboxylase activity. *J Am Acad Dermatol* 1982; **6** (Suppl.): 796–800.
5 Jetten AM, Jetten MER. Possible role of retinoic acid binding protein in retinoid stimulation of embryonal carcinoma cell differentiation. *Nature* 1979; **278:** 180–2.
6 Dron LD, Blalock JE, Gifford GE. Retinoic acid and the restoration of anchorage dependent growth to transformed mammalian cells. *Exp Cell Res* 1978; **117:** 15–22.
7 Dresser DW. Adjuvancity of vitamin A. *Nature* 1968; **217:** 527–9.
8 Sporn MB, Roberts AB, Goodman DS, eds. *The Retinoids*, Vols 1 and 2. Orlando: Academic Press, 1984.
9 Dubertret L, Lebreton C, Touraine R. Inhibition of neutrophil migration by etretinate and its main metabolite. *Br J Dermatol* 1982; **107:** 681–5.
10 Norris DA, Tonnesen MG, Lee LA *et al.* 13-cis-retinoic acid has major anti-inflammatory activity *in vivo. Clin Res* 1983; **31:** 593 (Abstract).
11 Chalker DK, Lesher JL, Graham-Smith J *et al.* Efficacy of topical isotretinoin 0.05% gel in acne vulgaris; results of a multicenter, double blind investigation. *J Am Acad Dermatol* 1987; **17:** 251–4.

12 Layton AM, Knaggs H, Taylor J *et al.* Isotretinoin for acne vulgaris—10 years later: safe and effective treatment. *Br J Dermatol* 1993; **129:** 292–6.
13 Stainforth JM, Layton AM, Taylor JP *et al.* Isotretinoin for the treatment of acne vulgaris; which factors may predict the need for more than one course? *Br J Dermatol* 1993; **129:** 297–301.
14 Paravicini U: On the metabolism and pharmacokinetics of an oral aromatic retinoid. *Ann NY Acad Sci* 1981; **359:** 55–67.
15 Brindley C: An overview of recent clinical pharmacokinetic studies with acitretin (Ro 10-1670 etretin). *Dermatologica* 1989; **178:** 179–87.
16 Larsen FG, Jacobsen P, Larsen CG, *et al.* Pharmacokinetics of etretin and etretinate during long-term treatment of psoriasis patients. *Pharmacol Toxicol* 1988; **62:** 159–65.
17 Parvicini U, Camenzind M, Gower M *et al.* Multiple dose pharmacokinetics of Ro 10-1670, the main metabolite of etretinate (Tigason). In: Saurat JH, ed. *Retinoids: New Trends in Research and Therapy*, Basel: Karger, 1985: 289–92.
18 Weigand UW, Jenson BK. Pharmacokinetics of acitretin in humans. In: Saurat JH, ed. *Retinoids: 10 years On.* Basel: Karger, 1991: 192–203.
19 Geiger JM, Czarnetzki BM. Acitretin (RO 10-1670, etretin); Overall evaluation of clinical studies. *Dermatologica* 1988; **176:** 182–90.
20 White SI, Marks JM, Shuster S. Etretinate in pustular psoriasis of palms and soles. *Br J Dermatol* 1985; **113:** 581–5.
21 Kingston T, Matt L, Lowe N. Etretin therapy for severe psoriasis. *Arch Dermatol* 1987; **123:** 55–8.
22 Wolska H, Jablonska S, Bounameaux Y. Etretinate in severe psoriasis. *J Am Acad Dermatol* 1983; **9:** 883–9.
23 Orfanos CE, Ehlert R, Gollmick K. The retinoids: a review of their clinical pharmacology and therapeutic use. *Drugs* 1987; **34:** 459.
24 Strauss JS. Retinoids and acne. *J Am Acad Dermatol* 1982; **6:** 546.
25 Ward A, Brogden RN, Heel RC *et al.* Isotretinoin. A review of its pharmacological properties and therapeutic efficacy in acne and other skin disorders. *Drugs* 1984; **28:** 6–37.
26 Thune P, Mark NJ. A case of centrolobular toxic necrosis of the liver due to aromatic retinoid-tigason (Ro 10-935). *Dermatologica* 1980; **160:** 405–8.
27 Carey BM, Parker GJS, Cunliffe WJ *et al.* Skeletal toxicity with isotretinoin therapy; a clinico-radiological evaluation. *Br J Dermatol* 1988; **119:** 609–14.
28 Pittsley RA, Yoder FW. Retinoid hyperostosis. Skeletal toxicity associated with long-term administration of 13-cis-retinoic acid for refractory ichthyosis. *N Engl J Med* 1983; **308:** 1012–14.
29 Wilson DJ, Kay V, Charig M *et al.* Skeletal hyperostosis and extraosseous calcification in patients receiving long-term etretinate (Tigason). *Br J Dermatol* 1988; **119:** 597–607.
30 Rosa FW. Teratogenicity of isotretinoin. *Lancet* 1983; **ii:** 513.
31 Benke EP. The isotretinoin teratogen syndrome. *JAMA* 1984; **251:** 3267–9.
32 Cruz E de la, Sun S, Van Guanichyakorn K *et al.* Multiple congenital malformations associated with maternal isotretinoin therapy. *Pediatrics* 1984; **74:** 428–30.

Immunosuppressive and cytotoxic drugs

These drugs, which have been primarily developed for use in oncology, must be approached with great caution when they become part of a dermatologist's armamentarium; it is essential that the treatment is not more disabling than the disease. An understanding of the clinical pharmacology of these drugs and their possible side-effects is required for the proper management of patients [1]. Brief details are given below of those drugs that may be of value in dermatological practice. A more complete review can be found in [2].

Alkylating agents

The effect of these drugs is dependent on proliferation and

is expressed only when cells enter the S phase. Alkylation of DNA by these drugs leads to impaired replication.

Cyclophosphamide [3]

Dose: 1–3 mg/kg body weight daily in two or three divided doses. Cyclophosphamide is inactive *in vitro* but is metabolized to an active antimitotic agent which also has profound immunosuppressive activity. It has been successfully used together with corticosteroids in the treatment of pemphigus and pemphigoid, Wegener's granulomatosis, systemic lupus erythematosus, polymyositis, mycosis fungoides and histiocytosis X.

Chlorambucil

Dose: 0.1–0.2 mg/kg/day in one or two doses. Chlorambucil is slow acting and rather less toxic than cyclophosphamide. It has been successfully used in the treatment of mycosis fungoides, Behçet's disease, lupus erythematosus, Wegener's granulomatosis, steroid-resistant sarcoidosis and in combination with prednisone for Sézary syndrome. Benefit has been reported in lichen myxoedematosus [4], granuloma annulare [5] and as a steroid-sparing agent for patients with recalcitrant dermatomysitis [6].

Mustine injection

This is the original nitrogen mustard. It may be used topically in mycosis fungoides (Chapter 56); one method of desensitization for topical therapy involves intravenous injection of gradually increasing doses [7].

Dacarbazine injection (DTIC)

Doses 2–4.5 mg/kg i.v. daily for 10 days. This is an imidazole derivative whose mode of action is unknown. It is used particularly for the treatment of metastatic malignant melanoma [2] (Chapter 38).

REFERENCES

1 Calabresi P, Parks RE, Jr. Antiproliferate agents and drugs used for immunosuppression. In: Gilman AG, Goodman LS, Rall TW *et al.*, eds. *Goodman and Gilman's The Pharmacological Basis of Therapeutics*, 7th edn. New York: Macmillan, 1985: 1247–306.
2 Ho VC, Zloty DM. Immunosuppressive agents in dermatology (Review). *Dermatol Clin* 1993; **11**: 73–85.
3 Razzaque Ahmed A, Honibal SM. Cyclophosphamide (cytoxan). A review on relevant pharmacology and clinical uses. *J Am Acad Dermatol* 1984; **11**: 1115–26.
4 Wieder JM, Barton KL, Baron JM *et al.* Lichen myxedematosus treated with chlorambucil. *J Dermatol Surg Oncol* 1993; **19**: 475–6.
5 Winkelmann RK, Stevens JC. Successful treatment response of granuloma annulare and carpal tunnel syndrome to chlorambucil. *Mayo Clin Proc* 1994; **69**: 1163–5.
6 Sinoway PA, Callen JP. Chlorambucil. An effective corticosteroid-sparing agent for patients with recalcitrant dermatomyositis. *Arthritis Rheum*, 1993; **36**: 319–24.
7 Van Scott EJ, Kalmanson JD. Complete remissions of mycosis fungoides lymphoma induced by topical nitrogen mustard (HN2). Control of delayed hypersensitivity to HN2 by desensitization and by induction of specific immunologic tolerance. *Cancer* 1973; **32**: 18–30.

Antimetabolites

Methotrexate

This folic acid antagonist binds to dihydrofolate reductase and prevents the production of tetrahydrofolic acid, the active coenzyme form of folic acid. It is cell-cycle specific, acting in the S phase, and is also a powerful immunosuppressant, but with little anti-inflammatory activity.

Low doses are well absorbed from the gastrointestinal tract. The majority of the drug is excreted unchanged in the urine within 24 h. Care should therefore be taken in the elderly and in other circumstances where there is renal impairment.

For its use in psoriasis see Chapter 35. It has also been employed in a wide variety of other diseases, including Reiter's disease, pityriasis rubra pilaris, ichthyosiform erythroderma, sarcoidosis and keratoacanthoma. It is effective in pemphigus vulgaris and foliaceus, bullous pemphigoid and corticosteroid-resistant dermatomyositis. Leucovorin (folinic acid) is a potent antidote in methotrexate overdose [1].

The side-effects of methotrexate on the blood are easily monitored. Rather more difficult to monitor is the hepatoxicity that can develop after many years of methotrexate treatment and may not be detected by liver-function tests. The measurement of serum amino-terminal propeptide of type III procollagen and the use of dynamic hepatic scintigraphy do show some promise, but to date there is no substitute for regular liver biopsies, performed during the first 3 months of treatment and subsequently after each 1.5 g of methotrexate [2,3].

Azathioprine

Dose: 1.5–3.0 mg/kg/day. It is converted in the body to mercaptopurine, an inhibitor of purine synthesis and an immunosuppressive; in addition, it has powerful anti-inflammatory properties. It appears to be inferior to methotrexate in the treatment of psoriasis but may be useful for psoriatic arthritis. Azathioprine is of value in producing steroid sparing in pemphigus vulgaris, pemphigoid, systemic lupus erythematosus, dermatomyositis, Wegener's granulomatosis, chronic actinic dermatitis and perhaps pityriasis rubra pilaris and intractable eczema in adults.

Myelosuppression is a relatively common side-effect of azathioprine and can come on very quickly and certainly between regular blood monitoring. It can be severe. It is now known that thiopurine methyltransferase (TPMT) is a major enzyme involved in the metabolism of azathioprine. TPMT activity is determined by an allelic polymorphism for either high or low enzymic activity. Homozygotes for low-activity allele are known to be at high risk for myelosuppression. Homozygotes for the high-activity allele may be inadequately immunosuppressed with conventional empirical doses of azathioprine [4,5].

Azathioprine-induced shock in dermatology patients has only been reported rarely but can be life threatening [6].

Bleomycin

This is a polypeptide antibiotic given parenterally which has no immunosuppressive action and its toxicity is confined to the skin (pigmentation, inflammatory lesions especially on the palms and fingers) [7] and lungs. It is effective against squamous cell carcinoma of the skin and elsewhere and in inducing remission in mycosis fungoides and other lymphomas. It has been used intralesionally for the treatment of intractable virus warts [8,9].

Hydroxyurea

Dose: 500 mg two or three times daily. Hydroxyurea blocks pyrimidine synthesis: it causes much more short-term marrow suppression than methotrexate, necessitating frequent blood counts. However, it is less effective than methotrexate and has little effect on psoriatic arthropathy. A combination of hydroxyurea with retinoids has been reported to be particularly effective [10]. Hydroxyurea is easy to administer, relatively inexpensive and has few contraindications or side-effects. Leukopenia can develop and the blood needs regular monitoring. Hydroxyurea does have a place in those patients who cannot take other drugs because of systemic disorders such as hyperlipidaemia, mild renal impairment, cardiopulmonary disease and mild liver disease [11].

Melphalan

This is used mainly in the treatment of myelomatosis and polycythaemia. Other indications include scleromyxoedema.

Adverse effects

These are considered in some detail in Chapters 35 and 77. Most of these agents have certain unwanted effects in common, as would be expected from their antimitotic action upon rapidly dividing cells. Thus, all of them except bleomycin cause bone-marrow depression. This is usually manifest as leukopenia or thrombocytopenia; megaloblastic anaemia occurs with hydroxyurea and rarely with methotrexate.

Mucosal irritation occurs, with the production of nausea, vomiting and ulceration; gastrointestinal side-effects are uncommon with hydroxyurea and azathioprine. Methotrexate has a higher incidence of such effects and is also hepatotoxic, although less so when given in intermittent weekly dosage. It is especially important to keep the alcohol intake as low as possible to prevent methotrexate-induced hepatotoxicity. A diffuse anagen alopecia is very common with cyclophosphamide but is much less frequent with other agents.

The reproductive system is also affected. All these agents can cause azoospermia and anovulation; they are all potential teratogens. It is therefore mandatory to institute effective contraceptive measures. Sterile haemorrhagic cystitis occurs in up to 10% of patients on cyclophosphamide and may even be fatal. The immunosuppressive action gives rise to an increased liability to infection. Virus infection such as measles, varicella and herpes simplex may become generalized and the patient may become seriously ill. Bacterial, fungal and yeast infections may also disseminate with fatal results. There is an increased incidence of non-Hodgkin's lymphoma and cutaneous squamous-cell carcinoma in patients with renal transplants receiving immunosuppression (corticosteroids, azathioprine, cyclophosphamide, cyclosporin or chlorambucil). Other immunosuppressants are less strongly associated with the promotion of malignancy.

Bleomycin appears to cause no immunosuppression but it does produce significant and unique adverse reactions in the skin and lungs. When the total dose exceeds 150 mg, many patients develop a variety of cutaneous manifestations including infiltrated plaques, nodules and bands on the hands with gangrene of the fingertips and hyperpigmentation on the trunk. Up to 10% develop progressive pulmonary fibrosis which may be reversible with high-dose steroid therapy if detected early.

REFERENCES

1 Bertino JR, Levitt M, McCullough JL *et al.* New approaches to chemotherapy with folate antagonists: use of leucovorin 'rescue' and enzymic folate depletion. *Ann N Y Acad Sci* 1971; **186**: 486–95.
2 van Dooren-Greebe RJ, Kuijpers ALA, Buijs WCA *et al.* Value of dynamic hepatic scintigraphy and serum aminoterminal propeptide of type III procollagen for early detection of methotrexate-induced hepatic damage in psoriasis patients. *Br J Dermatol* 1996; **134**: 481–7.
3 Roenigk HH, Auerbach R, Maibach HI *et al.* Methotrexate and psoriasis. Revised guidelines. *J Am Acad Dermatol* 1988; **19**: 145–6.
4 Snow JL, Gibson LE. The role of genetic variation in thiopurine methyl-transferase activity and the efficacy and/or side effects of azathioprine therapy in dermatologic patients. *Arch Dermatol* 1995; **131**: 193–7.
5 Anstey A. Azathioprine in dermatology; a review in the light of advances in the understanding of methylation pharmacokinetics. *J R Soc Med* 1995; **88**: 155–60.
6 Jones JJ, Ashworth J. Azathioprine induced shock in dermatology patients. *J Am Acad Dermatol* 1993; **29**: 795–6.
7 Cohen IS, Mosher MB, O'Keefe EJ *et al.* Cutaneous toxicity of bleomycin therapy. *Arch Dermatol* 1973; **107**: 553–5.
8 Shumack PH, Haddock MJ. Bleomycin: an effective treatment for warts. *Aust J Dermatol* 1979; **20**: 41–2.

9 James MP, Collier PM, Aherne W *et al.* Histologic, pharmacologic, and immunocytochemical effects of injection of bleomycin into viral warts. *J Am Acad Dermatol* 1993; **28**: 933–7.

10 Wright S, Baker H, Warin AP. Treatment of psoriasis with a combination of etretinate and hydroxyurea. *J Dermatol Treat* 1990; **1**: 211–14.

11 Wolverton SE. Hydroxyurea therapy (Review). *J Am Acad Dermatol* 1991; **25**: 518–24.

Cyclosporin [1]

This drug was isolated and purified in 1972 from a soil fungus found in Norway. Its main use until recently has been as an immunosuppressant in patients having kidney, liver, heart, bone-marrow or other transplants. It has increasing uses in dermatology, but its use demands careful attention to detail. It is a cyclic polypeptide made up of 11 amino acids. The main mode of action is on helper T cells whose cell cycle is blocked in G0 or early G1 and whose production of various lymphokines, notably IL-2, is inhibited. It may also have some direct effect on DNA synthesis and proliferation of keratinocytes [2]. Apart from its use in transplant patients, cyclosporin has been used to treat a wide range of general medical diseases in which T cells contribute—rheumatoid arthritis, systemic lupus erythematosus, polymyositis and dermatomyositis, uveitis, thyrotoxicosis, diabetes, biliary cirrhosis, various nephropathies, colitis, Crohn's disease and others. Dermatological uses [3–5] include notably psoriasis [6], pustular psoriasis [7] and psoriatic arthritis. Cyclosporin is particularly effective in widespread plaque psoriasis. Treatment at low doses (3–5 mg/kg/day) for 1–3 months will produce substantial improvement in over 60% of patients [8]. Most patients relapse once cyclosporin is discontinued.

The other main use of cyclosporin in skin diseases is atopic dermatitis. It is a very effective treatment [9], but relapse occurs within a few weeks of discontinuing the drug, although at 1 year later and still off the drug, the eczema was only about 50% of the severity before cyclosporin treatment was started [10]. Cyclosporin has also been reported to benefit patients with chronic dermatitis of the hands [11].

Cyclosporin is also used for pemphigus, pemphigoid, mycosis fungoides and Sézary syndrome. There are also reports of benefit of cyclosporin in dermatomyositis [12] and pyoderma gangrenosum [13].

Absorption of the drug from the gut is variable, often about 30%, although a new formulation of cyclosporin is now available which has a better absorption and is now replacing the original product. Excretion is mainly via the liver but again the rate is variable. Appropriate control therefore may demand assessment of blood levels of the drug, although for practical purposes with the smaller doses usually used in dermatology monitoring renal function by serum creatinine estimations and blood pressure may suffice.

Cyclosporin has little toxicity on the bone marrow or liver but does have a considerable and largely reversible toxicity on the kidney [14].

Short-term (mean 2.4 months) cyclosporin at a dose of 5 mg/kg/day was associated with a significant but small and reversible increase in blood pressure, but only a transient, mild reduction in glomerular filtration rate, (GFR) which did not reach significance [15]. Renal function and biopsy findings have been studied in patients who have taken cyclosporin continuously for 5 years (average 3.3 mg/kg/day). Six of eight patients who had renal biopsies showed tubular atrophy and arteriolar hyalinosis, four had increase in interstitium and two showed increased instance of glomerular obsolescence. Renal function was assessed by GFR and serum creatinine. Both a fall in the GFR and a rise in serum creatinine correlated with the severity of the cyclosporin nephrotoxicity seen on biopsy [16]. Other side-effects include nausea and vomiting, hypertension, hypertrichosis, tremor, hyperkalaemia. Long-term toxicity may include an increased tendency for lymphomas. There are notable interactions with ketoconazole, erythromycin and other drugs which increase blood levels; with rifampicin and hydantoinates, which decrease blood levels; and with non-steroidal anti-inflammatory drugs which seem to increase the nephrotoxicity without changing the blood levels.

REFERENCES

1 Kahan BD. Cyclosporine. *N Engl J Med* 1989; **321**: 1725–38.

2 Furue M, Gaspari AH, Katz SI, Effect of cyclosporin A on epidermal cells. II. Cyclosporin A inhibits proliferation of normal and transformed keratinocytes. *J Invest Dermatol* 1988; **90**: 796–800.

3 Biren CA, Barr RJ. Dermatologic application of cyclosporine. *Arch Dermatol* 1986; **122**: 1028–32.

4 Gupta AK, Brown MD, Ellis CN *et al.* Cyclosporine in dermatology. *J Am Acad Dermatol* 1989; **21**: 1245–56.

5 Page EH, Wexler DM, Guenther LC. Cyclosporin A. *J Am Acad Dermatol* 1986; **14**: 785–91.

6 Bos JD, Mevinharde MMHM, Van Joost T *et al.* Use of cyclosporin in psoriasis. *Lancet* 1989; **ii**: 1500–2.

7 Reitamo S, Erkko P, Remitz A *et al.* Cyclosporine in the treatment of palmoplantar pustulosis. *Arch Dermatol* 1993; **129**: 1273–79.

8 Ellis CN, Fradin MS, Messana JM *et al.* Cyclosporine for plaque-type psoriasis; results of a multidose, double-blind trial. *N Engl J Med* 1991; **324**: 277–84.

9 Van Joost TH, Heule F, Korstanje M *et al.* Cyclosporin in atopic dermatitis; a multicentre placebo-controlled study. *Br J Dermatol* 1994; **130**: 634–40.

10 Granlund H, Erkko P, Sinisalo M *et al.* Cyslosporin in atopic dermatitis; time to relapse and effect of intermittent therapy. *Br J Dermatol* 1995; **132**: 106–12.

11 Reitamo S, Granlund H. Cyclosporin A in the treatment of chronic dermatitis of the hands. *Br J Dermatol* 1994; **130**: 75–8.

12 Kavanagh GM, Ross JS, Black MM. Dermatomyositis treated with cyclosporin. *J R Soc Med* 1991; **184**: 306.

13 de Hijas C, del-Rio E, Gorospe MA *et al.* Large peristomal pyoderma gangrenosum successfully treated with cyclosporine and corticosteroids. *J Am Acad Dermatol* 1993; **29**: 1034–5.

14 Editorial. Cyclosporin hypertension. *Lancet* 1988; **ii**: 1234.

15 Brown AL, Wilkinson R, Thomas TH *et al.* The effect of short-term low-dose cyclosporin on renal function and blood pressure in patients with psoriasis. *Br J Dermatol* 1993; **128**: 550–5.

16 Powles AV, Cook T, Hulme B *et al*. Renal function and biopsy findings after 5 years' treatment with low-dose cyclosporin for psoriasis. *Br J Dermatol* 1993; **128**: 159–65.

PUVA [1]

Photochemotherapy with 8-methoxypsoralen followed by UVA radiation for psoriasis is considered in detail in Chapter 35. If necessary, 5-methoxypsoralen can be substituted, especially if a patient is nauseated by 8-methoxypsoralen.

PUVA is also of value in mycosis fungoides (MF) (Chapter 56) [2]. Seventy-three patients with MF were treated with PUVA, which produced clinical and histological clearance in a very high proportion of patients with pretumour-stage MF. The response of patients with tumours was less satisfactory, such patients requiring, in addition, radiotherapy.

PUVA may be used in selected children with severe atopic eczema [3]. Fifty-three children (mean age 11.2 years) had twice-weekly PUVA; 39 (74%) of them achieved a clear or nearly clear skin. The mean duration of treatment to remission was 37 weeks with mean cumulative UVA dose of 1118 J/cm. This relatively high UVA exposure is of concern. However, 22 children remain in remission a year after discontinuing PUVA.

PUVA has been described to be of benefit in a whole range of dermatological conditions. Some of the reports involve large numbers of patients and others only single-case reports. For an excellent review of the uses of PUVA in conditions other than psoriasis, including hand eczema, nodular prurigo, vitiligo, the various photodermatoses, granuloma annulare, lichen planus, lyphomatoid papulosis, urticaria, aquagenic pruritus, urticaria pigmentosa, idiopathic pruritus and many other conditions, refer to [4].

The main concern about PUVA is the long-term risk of skin cancer. The risk of melanoma does not appear to be increased, but the risk of non-melanoma skin cancer certainly is, and long-term PUVA substantially increases the risk of squamous cell carcinoma (SCC). After less than 15 years, 25% of patients exposed to 300 or more treatments of PUVA have had at least one SCC and most of these have had multiple tumours [5]. There is a specially high risk of SCC of the male genitalia [6]. Skin cancers or premalignant lesions have been reported to occur in half of high-dose PUVA patients (greater than 2000 J/cm) [7].

These findings have led to a recommendation that PUVA patients should not receive more than 1000 J/cm or greater than 150 treatments in a lifetime unless there are strong indications otherwise [8]. The male genitalia should be protected while receiving PUVA treatment.

REFERENCES

1 Moseley H, Ferguson J. Photochemotherapy: a reappraisal of its use in dermatology. *Drugs* 1989; **38**: 822–37.
2 Briffa DV, Warin AP, Harrington CI *et al*. Photochemotherapy in mycosis fungoides—a study of 73 patients. *Lancet* 1980; **ii**: 49–53.
3 Sheenan MP, Atherton DJ, Norris P *et al*. Oral psoralen photochemotherapy in severe childhood atopic eczema: an update. *Br J Dermatol* 1993; **129**: 431–6.
4 Honig B, Morison WL, Karp D. Photochemotherapy beyond psoriasis. *J Am Acad Dermatol* 1994; **31**: 775–90.
5 Stern RS, Laird N. The carcinogenic risk of treatments for severe psoriasis. *Cancer* 1994; **73**: 2759–64.
6 Stern RS. Genital tumours among men with psoriasis exposed to psoralens and ultraviolet A radiation (Puva) and ultraviolet B radiation. *N Engl J Med* 1990; **322**: 1093–7.
7 Lever LR, Farr PM. Skin cancers or premalignant lesions occur in half of high-dose Puva patients. *Br J Dermatol* 1994; **131**: 215–19.
8 British Photodermatology Group. British Photodermatology Group guidelines for PUVA. *Br J Dermatol* 1994; **130**: 246–55.

Photodynamic therapy

Photodynamic therapy (PDT) is based on an elegantly conceived principle. The sensitizer (usually a haemato-porphyrin derivative) can be given by intravenous injection and the tumour exposed to the appropriate wavelength of visible light. It has been shown that the tumour destruction in PDT is the result of both direct tumour-cell inactivation and indirect effects such as blood-vessel occlusion [1].

PDT using intravenous treatment is limited by the general cutaneous photosensitivity that can last up to 2 months. Alternatively, topical sensitization using δ-amino laevulinic acid (ALA) can be used, and so avoiding the generalized photosensitivity problem. This technique has been used successfully for the PDT of basal cell carcinoma (BCC) and various other cutaneous neoplasms [2,3].

In a further study, a laser light source was substituted, thereby avoiding the risks of hyperthermic effects in addition to the desired photodynamic ones [4]. Eighty BCCs, 10 Bowen's lesions and four lesions of cutaneous T-cell lymphoma were treated. All the superficial BCCs and 64% of the nodular lesions responded completely to a single treatment. The others responded to a second treatment. Bowen's lesions responded completely in 90% of cases to a single treatment, and two of four T-cell lymphomas responded completely. Follow-up was from 6 to 14 months.

PDT is not yet used widely but it is likely to have a role for patients with multiple skin cancers and for patients with diffuse lesions who might otherwise require Mohs margin controlled excision, especially for recurrent tumours. It is a safe and relatively simple and effective treatment.

REFERENCES

1 Henderson BW, Dougherty TJ. How does photodynamic therapy work? *Photochem Photobiol* 1992; **55**: 145–57.

2 Kennedy JC, Pottier RH, Pross DC. Photodynamic therapy with endogenous protoporphyrin IX: basic principles and present clinical experience. *J Photochem Photobiol B* 1990; **6**: 143–8.
3 Wolf P, Rieger E, Kerl H. Topical photodynamic therapy with endogenous porphyrins after application of 5-aminolevulinic acid. *J Am Acad Dermatol* 1993; **28**: 17–21.
4 Svanberg K, Andersson T, Killander D *et al*. Photodynamic therapy of non-melanoma malignant tumours of the skin using topical amino levulinic acid sensitization and laser irradiation. *Br J Dermatol* 1994; **130**: 743–51.

Photopheresis

Edelson [1] pioneered the use of photopheresis (extracorporeal photochemotherapy, ECP) in the treatment of cutaneous T-cell lymphoma (CTCL). The patient takes 8-methoxypsoralen orally (0.6 mg/kg) and 2 hours later the patient's blood is centrifuged in an extracorporeal system and the lymphocyte-enriched fraction is exposed to UVA. Transient activation of the psoralens results and subsequent DNA cross-linking. Altered cells of the malignant clone are then returned to the patient. The exact mechanism of action is not fully understood but it is thought that the patient's immune system is stimulated to destroy the already altered or damaged malignant T lymphocytes. Patients with Sézary syndrome demonstrate the most significant response. In the initial study by Edelson *et al*. [2] of 29 erythrodermic patients, six had a complete remission, another six had a 50% improvement but five had no change or got worse. The remaining patients had variable improvement. In a follow-up study of the same patients [3], four of the six who showed complete response remained in complete remission. Other patients continued on treatment with variable response. It is evident that only a minority of patients have a complete response but many more patients will gain some worthwhile improvement.

Another study looked at the effect of ECP in the 'red man' or 'pre-Sézary syndrome' [4]. Six of seven patients treated lost all signs of their erythroderma.

Systemic sclerosis treated with ECP showed promising results [5]. Seventy-nine patients were studied in a control trial. Sixty-eight percent of patients receiving ECP showed a significant response while 32% who received D-penicillamine treatment responded. Ten per cent of the ECP group and 32% of the D-penicillamine group deteriorated over the 6 months of treatment.

ECP has been reported to be of benefit in graft versus host disease [6]. It has been reported to be successful in eight out of nine episodes of acute rejection after cardiac transplantation [7] and in five of six episodes of rejection after lung transplantation [8].

ECP seems to have some interesting and important immunomodulating effects, some of which are becoming clinically important.

REFERENCES

1 Edelson RL. Cutaneous T cell lymphoma: mycosis fungoides, Sézary syndrome and other variants. *J Am Acad Dermatol* 1980; **2**: 89–106.
2 Edelson RL, Berger CL, Gasparro FP *et al*. Treatment of cutaneous T-cell lymphoma by extracorporeal photochemotherapy. *N Engl J Med* 1987; **316**: 297–303.
3 Heald P, Rook A, Perez M *et al*. Treatment of erythrodermic cutaneous T-cell lymphoma with extracorporeal photochemotherapy. *J Am Acad Dermatol* 1992; **27**: 427–33.
4 Zachariae H, Bjerring, Brodthagen *et al*. Photopheresis in the Red Man or Pre Sézary Syndrome. *Dermatology* 1995; **190**: 132–5.
5 Rook AH, Freundlich B, Jegasothy BV *et al*. Treatment of systemic sclerosis with extracorporeal photochemotherapy. *Arch Dermatol* 1992; **128**: 337–46.
6 Owsianowski M, Gollnick H, Siegert W *et al*. Successful treatment of chronic graft-versus-host disease with extracorporeal photopheresis. *Bone Marrow Transplant* 1994; **14**: 845–8.
7 Costanzonordin MR, Hubbell EA, O'Sullivan EJ *et al*. Photopheresis versus corticosteroids in the therapy of heart transplant rejection; preliminary clinical report. *Circulation* 1992; **86**: 242–50.
8 Slovis B, James L, Lloyd E *et al*. Photopheresis for chronic rejection of lung allografts. *N Engl J Med* 1995; **332**: 962.

Plasmapheresis

Plasmapheresis (plasma exchange) has been used for many years in patients with severe systemic lupus erythematosus in whom high-dose corticosteroids and immunosuppressants were not controlling their disease [1,2]. However, the evidence that it is effective when added to immunosuppression treatment with prednisolone and cyclosporin treatment in severe lupus nephritis is lacking [3]. It can also be life saving in Goodpasture's syndrome [4]. It is used in myaesthenia gravis, Waldenstom's macroglobulinaemia, cryoglobuminaemia, thrombotic thrombocytopenic purpura and Guillain–Barré syndrome. Plasmapheresis is occasionally used in acute polymyositis or dermatomyositis, but in a controlled trial involving 39 patients, it was shown to be no more effective than sham apheresis [5]. Plasmapheresis has been shown to be effective in a series of eight patients with pemphigus, in whom the treatment was added to their glucocorticoid and immunosuppressive therapy, which had not been controlling their disease [6]. Bullous pemphigoid seems to be less successfully treated by plasmapheresis. In a study involving 100 patients, it was found that neither azathioprine nor plasmapheresis was effective as an adjuvant to corticosteroid [7]. Solar urticaria has been reported to respond to plasmapheresis when added to photochemotherapy (PUVA) which had not been effective on its own [8].

REFERENCES

1 Euler HH, Schroeder JO, Harten P *et al*. Treatment-free remission in severe systemic lupus erythematosus following synchronization of plasmapheresis with subsequent pulse cyclosphosphamide. *Arthritis Rheum* 1994; **37**: 1784–94.
2 Erickson RW, Franklin WA, Emlen W. Treatment of hemorrhagic lupus

pneumonitis with plasmapheresis (Review). *Semin Arthritis Rheum* 1994; **24**: 114–23.

3 Lewis EJ, Hunsicker LG, Lan SP *et al*. A control trial of plasmapheresis therapy in severe lupus nephritis. *N Engl Med* 1992; **326**: 1371–9.

4 Shumak KH, Rock GA. Therapeutic plasma exchange. *N Engl J Med* 1984; **310**: 762–71.

5 Miller RW, Leitman SF, Cronin ME *et al*. Controlled trial of plasma exchange and leukapheresis in polymyositis and dermatomyositis. *N Engl J Med* 1992; **326**: 1380–4.

6 Sondergaard K, Carstens J, Jorgensen J *et al*. The steroid-sparing effect of long-term plasmapheresis in pemphigus. *Acta Derm Venereol (Stockh)* 1995; **75**: 150–2.

7 Guillaume JC, Vaillant L, Bernard P *et al*. Controlled trial of azathioprine and plasma exchange in addition to prednisolone in the treatment of bullous pemphigoid. *Arch Dermatol* 1993; **129**: 49–53.

8 Hudson-Peacock MJ, Farr PM, Diffey BL *et al*. Combined treatment of solar urticaria with plasmapheresis and PUVA. *Br J Dermatol* 1993; **128**: 440–2.

Gold (sodium aurothiomalate)

Dose: 10 mg i.m. as a test dose, followed by 50 mg at weekly intervals. Although this regimen was devised for treatment of rheumatoid arthritis it has been successfully used in the treatment of pemphigus [1]. If there has been no improvement by the time the total dose reaches 1 g, treatment should be stopped. If improvement does occur, the frequency of the injections is reduced every 2–3 weeks. Renal, hepatic and marrow damage must be looked for and rashes are common. Auranofin is an oral preparation of gold, rather less effective than the parenteral preparation. Its main advantage is that its tissue half-life is much less than with injectible gold. Dose: 3–6 mg daily, increasing to 9 mg daily after 3–6 months. It has also been used in discoid lupus erythematosus.

REFERENCE

1 Penneys NS, Eaglstein WH, Frost P. Management of pemphigus with gold compounds. *Arch Dermatol* 1976; **112**: 185–7.

Chelating agents

Chelating agents are available which form complexes with a number of heavy metals. They are only occasionally of use in dermatology.

d-Penicillamine [1]

This is a degradation product of penicillin and chelates copper, mercury, zinc and lead. It is used for Wilson's disease, lead poisoning, cystinuria and rheumatoid arthritis [1,2]. Its dermatological interest lies in its ability to cause a variety of diseases, including systemic lupus erythematosus-like syndrome, pemphigus-like bullous eruptions, lichenoid and other eruptions and elastosis perforans [3–5]. It is of possible benefit in scleroderma [6].

Desferrioxamine

This is used in the treatment of various iron-storage diseases. In general, acute iron overload seems to respond much more satisfactorily. However, it is logical to use it in porphyria cutanea tarda as long as iron overload is present, although its value has yet to be proved (Chapter 59).

REFERENCES

1 Editorial. d-Penicillamine in rheumatoid arthritis. *Lancet* 1975; **i**: 1123–5.

2 Multicentre Trial Group. Controlled trial of D-penicillamine in severe rheumatoid arthritis. *Lancet* 1973; **i**: 275–80.

3 Hewitt J, Benveniste M, Lessana-Leibowitch M. Pemphigus induced by d-penicillamine: an experimental pemphigus. *Br J Dermatol* 1975; **93** (Suppl. 11): 12.

4 Levy RS, Fisher M, Alter JN. Penicillamine: review and cutaneous manifestations. *J Am Acad Dermatol* 1983; **8**: 548–58.

5 Tan SG, Rowell NR. Pemphigus-like syndrome induced by d-penicillamine. *Br J Dermatol* 1976; **95**: 99–100.

6 Jayson MIV, Lovell C, Black CM *et al*. Penicillamine therapy in systemic sclerosis. *Proc R Soc Med* 1977; **70** (Suppl. 3): 82–8.

Antibiotics and antibacterial agents

Antibiotics were originally substances synthesized by microorganisms which were toxic to other microorganisms at high dilution. The term is now more widely applied to any drug with therapeutic activity against living organisms, particularly bacteria. Antifungals and antivirals are drugs with activity against fungi and viruses, respectively.

Many antibiotics are now synthetic or semisynthetic. They are usually divided into bacteriostatic and bactericidal groups, although the distinction is not complete; erythromycin, for example, may be either bactericidal or bacteriostatic depending on the nature of the infecting organism and the drug concentration achieved.

In clinical use, antibiotics are divided into those with a narrow spectrum of activity and those broad-spectrum drugs which act against Gram-positive and Gram-negative organisms. In the laboratory, antibiotics can be divided into five main groups:

1 antibiotics which interfere with bacterial cell synthesis, for example the penicillins, cephalosporins and glycopeptide antimicrobials such as vancomycin and teichoplanin;

2 antibiotics affecting bacterial cell-membrane permeability, for example the polymyxins;

3 antibiotics which inhibit bacterial protein biosynthesis, for example the tetracyclines, aminoglycosides, macrolides, lincosamides and chloramphenicol;

4 antibiotics which affect bacterial nucleic acid metabolism, for example the rifamycins and quinolones;

5 *para*-aminobenzoic acid (PABA) antagonists such as the sulphonamides.

Drug resistance

Bacterial resistance can emerge in three ways. When all sensitive bacteria have been eradicated, any remaining inherently resistant bacteria are free to multiply; this is the commonest form of resistance. Less frequently, bacteria may acquire resistance to a drug to which they were initially sensitive. The third form, which is cause for concern, is transferable drug resistance. Here, extra-chromosomal genetic information affecting the expression of resistance contained in a plasmid or a transposable section of chromosomal DNA can be transferred from one bacterium, which may be non-pathogenic, to another previously susceptible bacterium. This often takes place in the bowel or skin and may involve a variety of different organisms. Information on multiple drug resistance can be transferred with a single plasmid.

The mechanisms of drug resistance are variable and include changes in permeability of the cell membrane or antibiotic efflux, alterations in ribosomes, altered cell-wall precursors or target enzymes and the emergence of auxotrophs which have different growth substrates.

Sulphonamides

These antibacterial drugs were introduced into clinical practice in the 1930s, but the frequency of resistance combined with adverse events have limited their use. The combination of a sulphonamide (sulphamethoxazole) with trimethoprim, known as cotrimoxazole, however, is still used in dermatology although less frequently than previously.

Sulphonamides are derivatives of *para*-amino-benzenesulphonamide: many have been synthesized but only a few are of clinical significance. They act by inhibiting the bacterial enzyme dihydrofolic acid synthetase which converts PABA to dihydrofolic acid. Mammalian cells and resistant bacteria do not synthesize folic acid and are unaffected.

Sulphonamides are bacteriostatic and are inhibited by pus. Most are well absorbed orally. They are distributed through all body tissues, metabolized in the liver and excreted mainly by the kidneys. With the exception of some sulphonamides such as sulphadimidine, crystalluria is a potential risk unless adequate fluid intake is ensured.

Adverse effects. Although the frequency of serious adverse events is low, sulphonamides can cause a number of serious problems. Besides crystalluria, they may rarely cause blood dyscrasias such as acute haemolytic anaemia (particularly in patients with glucose-6-phosphate dehydrogenase deficiency), fever, serum sickness and a large variety of skin reactions including erythema nodosum and erythema multiforme. Potentially fatal cases of the severe form of erythema multiforme have followed the use of long-acting sulphonamides [1]. Because of the relatively high incidence of this reaction, the long-acting sulphonamides are little used.

Uses. There are now very few situations where they are drugs of first choice. They are of value in lymphogranuloma venereum, chancroid, nocardiosis and toxoplasmosis (combined with pyrimethamine). Sulphapyridine is now used only as an alternative to dapsone in dermatitis herpetiformis and allied conditions.

Sulphadimidine

Dose: 3g initially, then up to 6g daily in divided doses. For urinary tract infections, two-thirds of these doses are given.

Sulphapyridine

Dose: 0.5–1.5g daily as an alternative to dapsone in dermatitis herpetiformis.

Silver sulphadiazine

This has a role as a topical non-absorbable antimicrobial with a broad spectrum.

REFERENCE

1 Baker H. Drug reactions IV. Erythema multiforme gravis and long acting sulphonamides. *Br J Dermatol* 1968; **80**: 844–6.

Trimethoprim [1]

Trimethoprim is a synthetic antimicrobial agent in its own right. It is a potent inhibitor of bacterial dihydrofolic acid reductase which converts dihydrofolic acid to tetra-hydrofolic acid but has many thousand times less effect on the comparable mammalian enzyme. Trimethoprim is very well absorbed orally, distributed widely through most body tissues and is excreted almost completely by the kidney. Although available as a separate drug, it has been used mainly in combination with sulphamethoxazole in the proportions 1 to 5 as cotrimoxazole. This is a logical mix as these drugs inhibit successive stages in bacterial folate metabolism and it is not surprising that their combined effect is synergistic. Both drugs used singly are bacteriostatic but cotrimoxazole appears to be bactericidal.

Cotrimoxazole Tablets BP

These contain sulphamethoxazole 400mg and trimethoprim 80mg. The dose is two tablets twice daily. Double strength cotrimoxazole (960mg) is also available. It is effective against a wide range of Gram-positive and Gram-negative bacteria as well as *Nocardia* and is in general well tolerated. It is best avoided in pregnancy, however, and in infants under 6 weeks and therefore in lactating mothers feeding young babies. Adverse reactions are similar to those seen with sulphonamides. Typical skin reactions may occur in up to 8% of patients and this has limited its use for relatively benign conditions such as acne. Impairment of red-cell folate utilization may occur particularly in the elderly and supplements of folinic acid may be necessary [1]. Rarer side-effects include renal impairment and hepatic reactions.

Cotrimoxazole may be used for urinary tract and respiratory infections but, in infections affecting the skin, is of value in chancroid, atypical mycobacterial infections [2] and mycetoma. Cotrimoxazole has potential value in the treatment of *Pneumocystis* infections particularly in AIDS patients in whom, unfortunately, there is a high frequency of adverse reactions.

REFERENCES

1 Kucer SA, Bennett NMcK. *The Use of Antibiotics*, 3rd edn. London: Heinemann, 1979.
2 Barrow GI, Hewitt M. Skin infection with *Mycobacterium marinum* from a tropical fish tank. *Br Med J* 1971; **ii**: 505–6.

Penicillins

The basic structure of a penicillin consists of a thiazolidine ring, a β-lactam ring and a variable side chain. The starting point for the semisynthetic penicillins, of which there are now many, is 6-aminopenicillamic acid. It is convenient to divide the penicillins into five main groups according to their antibacterial properties and consequent clinical usage:
1 penicillinase-sensitive penicillins (natural penicillins), for example benzyl penicillin (penicillin G), and phenoxymethyl penicillin (penicillin V);
2 penicillinase-resistant penicillins, for example methicillin, flucloxacillin;
3 amino penicillins, which are broad-spectrum penicillins (vulnerable to penicillinase), for example ampicillin, amoxycillin.
By combining clavulanic acid, a potent β-lactamase inhibitor, with amoxycillin (Augmentin) the spectrum of activity has been broadened to cover penicillin-resistant staphylococci:
4 carboxy penicillins, for example carbenicillin;
5 other penicillins, which include extended-spectrum penicillins for example piperacillin, aminopenicillins and penicillins which are stable against Gram-negative lactamases, for example temocillin.

Toxicity. The penicillins as a whole are remarkably nontoxic to humans [1]. The main problems with their use are hypersensitivity reactions which are not uncommon:

an incidence between 1 and 10% is usually accepted [2], and it appears that administration of these drugs by the oral route is associated with a lower frequency of adverse reactions than the intravenous route [3]. These reactions range from skin rashes to vasculitis to anaphylaxis. Cross-reactivity in this allergy is usual.

Penicillinase-sensitive penicillins (penicillin)

Penicillin is the drug of choice against *Streptococcus pyogenes* group A, *Treponema pallidum* and *Bacillus anthracis* as well as in yaws, actinomycosis and diphtheria. Notwithstanding the emergence of resistant strains of the organism, it remains an important drug against gonorrhoea. In most serious infections, penicillin is given by injection as benzyl penicillin but treatment may be continued with oral penicillin V and this drug also has a role in prophylaxis against streptococcal cellulitis in patients with lymphoedema.

Benzyl penicillin injection BP (penicillin G). Dose: 300 mg (0.5 mega units) four times daily up to 1.8 g (3 mega-units) daily. If higher blood levels are required, probenecid may be given to block renal tubular excretion of penicillin. Long-acting injectable preparations are available.

Phenoxymethyl penicillin (penicillin V). Dose: 250–500 mg orally every 6 h.

Penicillinase-resistant penicillins

For practical purposes this means cloxacillin or flucloxacillin, which are resistant to staphylococcal β-lactamase and are drugs of choice against penicillin-resistant staphylococci [4]. Flucloxacillin is somewhat less effective against other Gram-positive infections. Adequate levels are achieved by the oral route but parenteral administration is preferred in serious infections.

Flucloxacillin. Dose: 250–500 mg every 6 h and at least 30 min before food.

Amino penicillins

Ampicillin is commonly used, having a spectrum of activity against Gram-positive and -negative bacteria. It is acid stable and therefore absorbed orally but is not resistant to penicillinase. It is little used in dermatology but is important as a cause of drug rashes. These occur in about 5–10% of all patients treated but in a majority of those with infectious mononucleosis, cytomegalovirus infections or lymphatic leukaemia [2]. The typical morbilliform rash is thought to be toxic in nature and unrelated to true penicillin hypersensitivity. Amoxycillin is almost identical, is twice as well absorbed as ampicillin but is more expensive. It should probably only replace ampicillin in the patient known to be susceptible to antibiotic-induced diarrhoea [5]. Where an even broader spectrum is needed, perhaps in the treatment of heavily infected leg ulcers with surrounding cellulitis, amoxicillin with clavulanic acid (Augmentin) is worth consideration [6,7]. Its role in dermatology is, however, to be a limited one.

Ampicillin. Dose: 250 mg to 1 g every 6 h and at least 30 min before a meal.

Amoxycillin capsules. Dose: 250–500 mg every 8 h.

Amoxycillin 250 mg and clavulanic acid (Augmentin) tablets. Dose: 1–2 tablets every 8 h.

Other penicillins

Carbenicillin, ticarcillin, and azlocillin must all be given by injection or infusion and have little place in dermatology.

REFERENCES

1 Garrod LP, Lambert HP, O'Grady F. *Antibiotics and Chemotherapy* 5th edn. Edinburgh: Churchill Livingstone, 1981.
2 Beeley L. Allergy to penicillin. *Br Med J* 1984; **228**: 511–12.
3 Saxon A. Immediate hypersensitivity reactions to β-lactam antibiotics. *Rev Infect Dis* 1983; **5** (Suppl. 2): 368–73.
4 Neu HC. Antistaphylococcal penicillins. *Med Clin North Am* 1982; **66**: 51–66.
5 Dyas A, Wise R. Ampicillin and alternatives. *Br Med J* 1983; **286**: 583–5.
6 Anonymous. Augmentin—nice idea, but more trials please. *Drug Ther Bull* 1982; **20**: 21–4.
7 Rolinson GN, Watson A, eds. Augmentin clavulanate—potentiated amoxycillin. Proceedings of First Symposium. Amsterdam: *Excerpta Medica*, 1980.

Cephalosporins [1,2]

The cephalosporins are derivatives of 7-amino-cephalosporamic acid and are similar in structure and properties to the penicillins. They are bactericidal, acting on peptidoglycans in bacterial cell walls, and have wide spectra of activity encompassing Gram-negative organisms and staphylococci—penicillin-resistant staphylococci are generally susceptible but the degree of effectiveness varies between cephalosporins. Many are given parenterally but some orally effective ones are available, for example cephalexin, cefaclor. They are all excreted by the kidney but unlike penicillin may cause tubular damage. Their main role is perhaps as alternative therapy in penicillin hypersensitivity but this is not without risk as some 8–10% of all penicillin-allergic patients react to cephalosporins. Apart from this they have little dermatological use.

REFERENCES

1 Anonymous. Cephalosporins. Now and tomorrow. *Drug Ther Bull* 1982; **20**: 85–8.

2 Donowitz GR, Mandell GL. β-Lactam antibiotics. *N Engl J Med* 1988; **318**: 490–500.

Quinolones [1]

The chief quinolone antibiotics are more correctly classified as 4-quinolones. Their mode of action is via inhibition of DNA synthesis. Their spectrum of activity is broad and generally includes both Gram–positive and -negative bacteria. The principal quinolone in wide use is ciprofloxacin; others include norfloxacin and ofloxacin. This can be given orally in doses of 750 mg twice daily for soft-tissue infections [2]. Ciprofloxacin is active *in vitro* against a wide range of bacteria from *Escherichia coli* to *Yersinia enterocolitica*. It is also active against staphylococci and streptococci as well as *Mycobacterium tuberculosis*, although atypical mycobacteria are generally less sensitive. In dermatology, ciprofloxacin is best reserved for severe infections such as those occurring in the immunocompromised patient.

REFERENCES

1 Gentry LO. Review of quinolones in treatment of infections of the skin and skin structure. *J Antimicrob Chemother* 1991; **28** (Suppl C): 97–110.
2 Fass RJ. Treatment of skin and soft tissue infections with oral ciprofloxacin. *J Antimicrob Chemother* 1986; **18** (Suppl.): 153–7.

Tetracyclines

These are orally effective broad-spectrum antibiotics with relatively low toxicity. The original three tetracyclines were chlortetracycline, oxytetracycline and tetracycline. Later derivatives include demethylchlortetracycline, methacycline, doxycycline and minocycline (the last three being synthetic). They act by inhibition of protein synthesis through ribosomal binding. With the exception of minocycline they all have similar spectra of activity differing, however, in their absorption, distribution and excretion.

Both streptococci and staphylococci may be resistant to tetracyclines, although the incidence of staphylococcal resistance is less than previously and such strains are sensitive to minocycline [1]. However, as much more effective agents are available for these organisms the tetracyclines are generally not used in these infections.

The tetracyclines are bacteriostatic against many Gram-positive and Gram-negative bacteria and are also active against rickettsiae, *Mycoplasma, Chlamydia*, which cause lymphogranuloma venerum, psittacosis and trachoma, as well as amoebae.

Absorption of some tetracyclines is impaired by simultaneously taking milk, aluminium, calcium or magnesium salts or iron preparations due to chelation. However, food does not interfere with the absorption of doxycycline or minocycline. All tetracyclines are concentrated in the liver and excreted into the bile, whence they enter an enterohepatic circulation. Urinary excretion is significant and renal failure may be exacerbated by all except doxycycline [2].

Side-effects [3–5]. A variety of rashes has been described (Chapter 77), including phototoxicity especially shown by demethylchlortetracycline [6]. Glossitis, cheilitis and persistent pruritus ani may occur. Gastrointestinal disturbances are dose dependent [7] and are much more common with daily doses of 2 g or more, which are rarely used in dermatology. Nausea and vomiting are direct irritant effects; diarrhoea may be the result of superinfection, resistant staphylococci being especially dangerous. Minocycline can cause vertigo and hyperpigmentation. The latter is usually slate grey and can affect the skin, nails and sclerae [8]. Tetracyclines are deposited in growing teeth and bones [9] and their use should be avoided in pregnancy, during lactation and in childhood. Rarely, there may be diffuse fatty degeneration of the liver. An uncommon dermatological problem is the development of Gram-negative folliculitis after tetracycline therapy of acne [10,11].

Dermatological uses. Apart from the infections mentioned above, tetracyclines are rarely drugs of first choice. The exception, of course, is the treatment of acne vulgaris [12,13] (Chapter 42) and rosacea (Chapter 46).

Tetracycline, chlortetracycline, oxytetracycline

Daily dosages range from 500 mg (for acne) up to 3 g.

Doxycycline, minocycline

Daily dosages, 100–200 mg. Doxycycline is the ordinary tetracycline of choice in patients with renal impairment. Minocycline is usually effective against staphylococci resistant to other tetracyclines and is used increasingly as a first line treatment of acne (50 mg twice daily).

Preparations are also available as syrups, and injections for intramuscular, intravenous or intralesional use. Tetracycline resistance has been reported in *Propionibacterium acnes* and caution should be exercised over the use of repeated courses of these antibiotics.

REFERENCES

1 Finland M. Commentary. Twenty-fifth anniversary of the discovery of aureomycin: the place of the tetracyclines in antimicrobial chemotherapy. *Clin Pharmacol Ther* 1974; **15**: 3–8.
2 Ribush N, Morgan T. Tetracyclines and renal failure. *Med J Aust* 1972; **i**: 53–5.
3 Ad Hoc Committee Report. Systemic antibiotics for treatment of acne vulgaris. *Arch Dermatol* 1975; **111**: 1630–6.
4 Clendenning WE. Complications of tetracycline therapy. *Arch Dermatol* 1965; **91**: 628–32.
5 Kunin CM. The tetracyclines. *Pediatr Clin North Am* 1968; **15**: 43–55.
6 Falk MS. Light sensitivity due to demethylchlortetracycline. Report of four cases. *JAMA* 1960; **172**: 1156–7.
7 Garrod LP, Lambert HP, O'Grady F. *Tetracyclines. Antibiotics and Chemotherapy*, 5th edn. Edinburgh: Churchill Livingstone 1981: 169–82.
8 Angeloni VL, Salasche SJ, Ortiz R. Nail, skin and scleral pigmentation induced by minocycline. *Cutis* 1987; **40**: 229–33.
9 Macaulay JC, Leistyna JA. Preliminary observations on the prenatal administration of demethylchlortetracycline. *Pediatrics* 1964; **34**: 423–4.
10 Fulton JE, McGinley K, Leyden J *et al*. Gram-negative folliculitis in acne vulgaris. *Arch Dermatol* 1968; **98**: 349–53.
11 Leyden JL, Marples RR, Mills OH *et al*. Gram-negative folliculitis—complication of antibiotic therapy in acne vulgaris. *Br J Dermatol* 1973; **88**: 533–8.
12 Fry L, Ramsay CA. Tetracycline in acne vulgaris. Clinical evaluation and sebum production. *Br J Dermatol* 1966; **78**: 653–60.
13 Smith EL, Mortimer PR. Tetracycline in acne vulgaris. *Br J Dermatol* 1967; **79**: 78–84.

Macrolides

The main macrolide antibiotics are erythromycin and its derivatives azithromycin and clarithromycin. They work by binding to ribosomes and inhibiting protein synthesis.

Erythromycin [1]

Dose 1–2 g daily in divided doses. This is the most widely used member of the macrolide group of antibiotics. It is active mainly against Gram-positive organisms such as staphylococci and streptococci. Staphylococci may rapidly develop resistance, especially in hospital, where in some studies as many as 50% of strains may be resistant; streptococci are also occasionally resistant.

Side-effects include an allergic cholestatic hepatitis which occurs only with erythromycin estolate. Otherwise gastrointestinal problems such as dyspepsia and diarrhoea are not uncommon. Erythromycin is an extremely useful drug for the outpatient treatment of staphylococcal or streptococcal pyodermas, especially in the penicillin-allergic patient. It may also be used for atypical mycobacterial infections. Particular dermatological uses are for erythrasma and acne; it may safely be given in renal failure as less than 5% is excreted in the urine.

Azithromycin and clarithromycin [2]

These are newer macrolide agents with a somewhat different spectrum of activity than erythromycin and longer half life. At present they are little used in dermatology although they show promise as treatment for atypical mycobacterial infections.

REFERENCES

1 Washington JA, Wilson WR. Erythromycin. A microbial and clinical perspective after 30 years of clinical use. 1. *Mayo Clin Proc* 1984; **60**: 189–203.

2 Piscitelli SC, Danziger LH, Rodvold KA. Clarithromycin and azithromycin. *Clin Pharm* 1992; **11**: 137–52.

Aminoglycosides

This group includes streptomycin (see below), neomycin, gentamicin, amikacin and tobramycin. They are little used in dermatological practice, their chief use being against Gram-negative infections. They inhibit protein synthesis; bacteria may rapidly become resistant, and cross-resistance occurs within the group. Normally there is almost no absorption by mouth. They are ototoxic and, to a lesser degree, nephrotoxic.

Dermatological uses. These are few. Streptomycin is still used in some countries for tuberculosis, is effective in tularaemia and some forms of actinomycetoma and can be used as an alternative to tetracyclines in granuloma venereum. The topical use of neomycin is discussed in Chapter 78.

Gentamicin [1]

This is still the most widely used of the aminoglycosides [2]. Although it has a broad spectrum of activity, its use should be restricted to the treatment of serious Gram-negative infections, especially those due to *Pseudomonas aeruginosa* [3,4]. It has a synergistic effect with carbenicillin against *Pseudomonas* and other Gram-negative organisms. It should not be used in pregnancy and should be controlled by measurements of its plasma concentration.

REFERENCES

1 Second International Conference of Gentamicin. An aminoglycoside antibiotic. *J Infect Dis* 1971; **124** (Suppl.).
2 Sande MA, Mandell GL. Antimicrobial agents. The aminoglycosides. In: Gilman AG, Goodman LS, Rall TW, Murad F, eds. *Goodman and Gilman's The Pharmacological Basis of Therapeutics*, 7th edn. New York: Macmillan 1985: 1150–69.
3 Bulger RJ, Sidell S, Kirby WMM. Laboratory and clinical studies of gentamicin. A new broad spectrum antibiotic. *Ann Intern Med* 1963; **59**: 593–604.
4 Jao RL, Jackson GG. Gentamicin sulfate. New antibiotic against Gram-negative bacilli. *JAMA* 1964; **189**: 817–22.

Spectinomycin

This is an aminocyclitol antibiotic derived from a streptomycete species and is related to the aminoglycosides. Its use in dermatology is limited but it is very effective in the management of gonorrhoea as a single intramuscular injection [1].

REFERENCE

1 Holloway WJ. Spectinomycin. *Med Clin North Am* 1982; **66**: 169–84.

Lincosamides

Lincomycin and its derivative clindamycin (which ought to be used in preference to lincomycin) act against Gram-positive cocci including some penicillin-resistant staphylococci. They are highly active against *Bacteroides* infections and penetrate well into bone.

Side effects. Diarrhoea may occur in up to 20% of cases; pseudomembranous colitis may supervene and may last for weeks after the drug has been withdrawn [1,2]. There have been a number of deaths from this complication: one severe case has been reported in a patient treated for acne.

Clindamycin

This is an effective alternative drug for the treatment of acne [3]; however, in view of its known toxicity, it is now rarely used systemically for this condition. It is useful in a 1% formulation for the topical treatment of mild to moderate acne.

REFERENCES

1 Tedesco FJ, Barton RW, Alpers DH. Clindamycin associated colitis. A prospective study. *Ann Intern Med* 1974; **81**: 429–33.
2 Viteri AL, Howard PH, Dyck WP. The spectrum of lincomycin–clindamycin colitis. *Gastroenterology* 1974; **66**: 1137–44.
3 Christian GL, Krueger GG. Clindamycin vs placebo as adjunctive therapy in moderately severe acne. *Arch Dermatol* 1975; **111**: 997–1000.

Chloramphenicol

This would be a useful drug for a number of infections were it not for bone-marrow aplasia which occurs in one in 40 000 courses of treatment [1]. This has been known for 25 years, and yet a survey of 576 cases of blood dyscrasia due to chloramphenicol concluded that in most cases there had been no indication to justify its use. Nevertheless, it remains an alternative treatment for typhoid fever and *Haemophilus influenzae* meningitis.

REFERENCE

1 Polak BCP, Wesseling H, Schut D *et al.* Blood dyscrasias attributed to chloramphenicol. A review of 576 published and unpublished cases. *Acta Med Scand* 1972; **192**: 409–14.

Rifamycins

See page 3337.

Polymyxins

Polymyxin B and polymyxin E (Colistin) are relatively toxic drugs which are not absorbed from the gastrointestinal tract. Their use for Gram-negative infections has been largely superceded by gentamicin and ciprofloxacin. Polymyxin B is used topically.

Glycopeptide antibiotics

The two main examples of this group are vancomycin and teichoplanin. They act by inhibition of peptidoglycan polymer formation in bacterial cell walls. Vancomycin is chiefly used for the treatment of serious staphylococcal infections such as septicaemia as well as other life-threatening conditions such as pseudomembranous colitis. It has no obvious use in skin disease [1].

REFERENCE

1 Wise RI, Kory M, eds. Reassessments of vancomycin—a potentially useful antibiotic. *Rev Infect Dis* 1981; **3** (Suppl.): 199–300.

Fusidic acid [1]

This is produced by a strain of *Fusidium coccineum* and has the basic structure of a steroid, although it shows little in the way of metabolic effects. It is a very safe drug, primarily used for staphylococcal infections, although it is also active against other Gram-positive bacteria and the Gram-negative cocci. Nearly all strains of staphylococci are outstandingly sensitive to fucidin but there may be a few resistant mutants which can multiply rapidly. However, concomitant administration of penicillin can be used to kill any resistant mutants as they emerge. It is available for oral use, as an injection and for topical application. It is a useful drug for staphylococcal osteomyelitis, in particular, and its indiscriminate prescription for minor infections should be discouraged for fear of encouraging resistant strains.

REFERENCE

1 Verbist L. The antimicrobial activity of fusidic acid. *J Antimicrob Chemother* 1990; **25** (Suppl. B): 1–5.

Metronidazole [1,2]

Metronidazole is a synthetic agent active against protozoa and anaerobic bacteria. It is particularly useful in trichomoniasis, amoebiasis and giardiasis and has proved extremely valuable against *Bacteroides* and *Helicobacter* species [2]. For the dermatologist it has a limited role in the treatment of tetracycline-failed rosacea [3]. Metronidazole is well absorbed by the oral or rectal route and it may be applied topically. It may also be given intravenously. It is available as 200 and 400 mg tablets, the usual adult dose by mouth being 200 mg twice daily for rosacea, 200 mg every 8 h for *trichomonas* infections, 400 mg

every 8 h for anaerobic bacterial infections and 800 mg every 8 h for amoebiasis. The suppositories contain 500 mg and in anaerobic infections are prescribed in the adult dose of 1 g every 8 h at first, dropping to 1 g every 12 h. Topical formulations are available for the treatment of rosacea. The fate and mode of excretion of metronidazole are not fully understood [4]; it is generally regarded as safe in hepatic and renal disease. There is no evidence that it is a human teratogen, and it may be given to lactating mothers, although it causes darkening of milk and may give it a bitter taste. In normal doses and for short periods it is generally a remarkably safe drug but minor gastro-intestinal side-effects such as nausea, an unpleasant taste in the mouth and black, hairy tongue are not uncommon. Vomiting, abdominal pain and diarrhoea may follow. Darkening of urine, headache and drowsiness also occur, and leukopenia may be noted. Much less common adverse reactions are peripheral neuropathy, particularly associated with prolonged treatment, and central nervous system effects (dizziness, ataxia and fits) from high dosage. Fears that metronidazole might be a carcinogen are not to date supported by factual evidence. The only important interaction is with alcohol which produces a disulphiram-like reaction in some patients.

REFERENCES

1 Phillips I, Collier J, eds. *Metronidazole*. London: Royal Society of Medicine International Congress and Symposium Series, No. 18, 1979.
2 Rosenblatt JE, Edson RS. Metronidazole. *Mayo Clin Proc* 1983; **53**: 154–62.
3 Saihan EM, Burton JL. A double-blind trial of metronidazole versus oxytetracycline therapy for rosacea. *Br J Dermatol* 1980; **102**: 443–5.
4 Somogyi AA, Kong CE, Gurr FW *et al*. Metronidazole pharmacokinetics in patients with acute renal failure. *J Antimicrob Chemother* 1984; **13**: 183–9.

Antituberculous drugs (Chapter 28)

The important first-line drugs for the treatment of *Mycobacterium tuberculosis* infections are isoniazid, rifampicin, ethambutol and, in some cases, streptomycin [1,2]. In the initial period of treatment, usually 60 days or until sensitivities are available, three of these drugs are used concurrently. For the continuation phase of therapy two drugs to which the organism is sensitive are sufficient for cure without the occurrence of resistant strains (for details see Chapter 28).

Second-line drugs such as pyrazinamide, ethionamide, cycloserine, *para*-aminosalicyclic acid or thiacetazone may be required where drug resistance or adverse reactions preclude the use of more than one of the four first-line agents.

The emergence of multidrug-resistant strains of *Mycobacterium tuberculosis* (MDR-TB) is a major potential threat [3], particularly as they may affect AIDS patients who expectorate large numbers of bacilli.

Isoniazid

This is a synthetic, orally absorbed bactericidal agent usually given in a dose of 300 mg/day to adults (5–10 mg/kg every 24 h). It is excreted mainly by the kidney after acetylation and further metabolism. It can be used in pregnancy [4] but during lactation should be supplemented with pyridoxin because of the theoretical risk of toxic side-effects (see below). In severe renal failure the adult dosage should be reduced to 200 mg/day. Adverse reactions may be divided into toxic and allergic. Toxic reactions are more common in slow acetylators and include most commonly peripheral neuropathy but also convulsions, mental disturbances and a pellagra-like rash [5]. They are usually reversible on cessation of therapy. Pyridoxine 10 mg/day given prophylactically will reduce the incidence of these problems where high doses are used. The main allergic reactions are rashes, agranulocytosis and hepatitis, this last being apparently more common in patients with pre-existing liver disease [6].

Rifampicin

This is a synthetically modified antibiotic of the rifamycin group, bactericidal and very effective against *M. tuberculosis*, many atypical myobacteria and Gram-positive cocci. It is also useful in leprosy. To counter the emergence of resistant strains it is always used in combination with other antimicrobials.

Rifampicin is well absorbed orally and is available as 150 mg capsules and a 100 mg/5 ml mixture. In adults it is usual to prescribe 450–600 mg daily as a single dose before breakfast (10 mg/kg/day). Excretion is predominantly in the bile and so hepatic impairment is an indication for avoidance or at least lower dosage. In pregnancy, rifampicin is best avoided but where it has been used the incidence of abnormalities noted at birth has not been excessively high—4.3% compared with 1.8% in tuberculous controls [7]. If used in late pregnancy it may cause haemorrhagic problems in neonates. Rifampicin is generally regarded as a relatively non-toxic antituberculous drug but many different adverse reactions have been described: mild gastrointestinal disturbances, rashes—particularly flushing [8,9]. Transient impairment of liver function as revealed by elevation of transaminase levels is common but need not usually interrupt therapy. Orange–red discolouration of urine, saliva and sweat may be noticed. Thrombocytopenia, however, is an uncommon side-effect which must not be ignored. Three other serious adverse reactions are a flu-like illness, a syndrome of dyspnoea, wheezing and hypotension and the occurrence of renal failure, all of which are characteristically associated with intermittent or irregular medication [10]. Drug interactions occur with warfarin (diminished anticoagulant effect), oral contraceptives (possibly) and corticosteroids (diminished steroid effect).

Other rifamycins. Rifabutin has particular activity against *M. avium–intracellulare* in addition to *M. tuberculosis*. It is used, for instance, as prophylaxis in patients with low CD4 counts.

Streptomycin

This is an aminoglycoside antibiotic used mainly in the treatment of tuberculosis. It must be administered parenterally and is commonly given in a dose of 500–1000 mg/day by intramuscular injection. Lower doses are preferred in patients over 40 [11]. Excretion is by the kidney so that dosage should be reduced in renal impairment. Dose reduction is also important in the premature infant. Of the important side-effects the most common is vertigo which is especially troublesome in elderly people. Deafness may also develop and both these eighth-nerve effects are dose related [12]. These two adverse reactions provide a strong contraindication to the use of streptomycin in pregnancy and lactation as the infant may be affected, and in patients with pre-existing vestibular or auditory impairment. Allergic reactions include skin eruptions from the trivial to exfoliative dermatitis, eosinophilia and drug fever. Contact sensitization to streptomycin is a well-recognized hazard among nurses, justifying precautions to avoid skin contamination, for example by wearing gloves. Because streptomycin is a neuromuscular blocking agent it may increase the effects of suxamethonium and other similar drugs and should be used only with extreme caution in myasthenia gravis.

Ethambutol

This is a synthetic agent effective only against *M. tuberculosis* and some atypical mycobacteria. It is orally absorbed and is available on its own as 100 and 400 mg tablets and in combination with isoniazid in a variety of strengths. The usual initial dose is 15 mg/kg/day in adults and 25 mg/kg/day in children, reducing later in that age group to 15 mg/kg/day. It may also be used as intermittent treatment in a dose of 45–50 mg/kg twice weekly. Excretion is mainly via the kidney necessitating reduction of dosage in renal impairment. Optic (retrobulbar) neuritis with diminished visual acuity and red–green colour blindness slowly reversible on cessation of therapy was a relatively common side-effect of higher-dose schedules but should be rare with currently recommended levels [13,14]. It seems to be more effective to train patients to check their own vision regularly when on this drug than to rely on periodic ophthalmic examinations. Ethambutol may also, although rarely, cause peripheral neuropathy and renal damage, and may precipitate attacks of gout. It appears not to be a teratogen in humans and is not contraindicated during lactation.

Para-aminosalicylic acid

This drug is much less active than the above drugs but has a role in preventing the emergence of resistant strains of *M. tuberculosis*. It is given in the large dose 10–20 g/day and unfortunately is associated with a high incidence of minor but unpleasant side effects [15]—gastrointestinal symptoms occur in nearly all patients. Allergic reactions with rashes and fever are common and there seems to be either cross-hypersensitivity with streptomycin or potentiation of streptomycin allergy. Although once a valued drug in triple therapy, its use is now largely restricted to poorer countries where its low cost is a major consideration.

Other antituberculous drugs [2]

A number of other antituberculous drugs are available and may be required if resistance or hypersensitivity reactions preclude the use of standard treatment. They include pyrazinamide, capreomycin, ethionamide and cycloserine, Pyrazinamide is bactericidal and low-priced.

REFERENCES

1 Garrod LP, Lambert HP, O'Grady F. Tuberculosis and leprosy. *Antibiotics and Chemotherapy*, 5th edn. Edinburgh: Churchill Livingstone, 1981: 398–418.
2 Kucers A, Bennett NMcK. Drugs mainly for tuberculosis. In: *The Use of Antibiotics*, 3rd edn. London: Heinemann, 1979: 799–862.
3 Frieden TR, Sterling T, Pablos-Mendez A *et al*. The emergence of drug-resistant tuberculosis in New York City. *N Engl J Med* 1993; **328**: 521–6.
4 Ludford J, Doster B, Woolpert SF. Effect of isoniazid on reproduction. *Am Rev Respir Dis* 1973; **108**: 1170–4.
5 Horne NW. Side effects of isoniazid. *Practitioner* 1972; **208**: 263–4.
6 Girling DJ. The hepatic toxicity of antituberculosis regimens containing isoniazid, rifampicin and pyrazinamide. *Tubercle* 1978; **59**: 13–32.
7 Steen JSM, Stainton-Ellis DM. Rifampicin in pregnancy. *Lancet* 1977; ii: 604–5.
8 Girling DJ. Adverse reactions to rifampicin in antituberculous regimens. *J Antimicrob Chemother* 1977; **3**: 115–32.
9 Girling DJ, Hitze KL. Adverse reactions to rifampicin. *Bull WHO* 1979; **57**: 45–9.
10 Flynn CT, Rainford DJ, Hope E. Acute renal failure and rifampicin: danger of unsuspected intermittent dosage. *Br Med J* 1974; ii: 482.
11 Line DH, Poole GW, Waterworth PM. Serum streptomycin levels and dizziness. *Tubercle* 1970; **51**: 76–81.
12 Ballantyne J. Iatrogenic deafness. *J Laryngol Otol* 1970; **84**: 967–1000.
13 Clarke GEM, Cuthbert J, Cuthbert RJ *et al*. Isoniazid plus ethambutol in the initial treatment of pulmonary tuberculosis. *Br J Dis Chest* 1972; **66**: 272–5.
14 Lees AW, Allan GW, Smith J *et al*. Toxicity for rifampicin plus isoniazid and rifampicin plus ethambutol therapy. *Tubercle* 1971; **52**: 182–90.
15 Russouw JE, Saunders SJ. Hepatic complications of antituberculous chemotherapy. *Q J Med* 1975; **44**: 1–16.

Antileprosy agents

Sulphones

The sulphones were the first effective compounds used for the treatment of leprosy. The principle agent is 4, 4-diaminodiphenyl sulphone (dapsone). The sulphones are related to the sulphonamides, and probably act in the same way. *Mycobacterium leprae* is usually extremely sensitive [1] but may become resistant. The sulphones are bacteriostatic, not bactericidal.

Dapsone. This drug is orally absorbed and is available in the form of 50 and 100 mg tablets. The usual adult dose in leprosy is 50–100 mg/day. It is excreted mainly in the urine [2]. Some degree of haemolysis is an extremely common adverse reaction [3,4]. In pregnancy and lactation there is clearly a risk of haemolysis and Met-haemoglobinaemia in the baby but the presence of dapsone in breast milk may have prophylactic value against leprosy [5]. Resistance to dapsone is known to occur in about 20% of patients who receive the drug for the treatment of leprosy as a single agent. With the use of multiple-drug regimens this complication is thought to be much rarer. Leprosy apart, dapsone is a well-established means of suppressing the cutaneous lesions of dermatitis herpetiformis [6] and several other diseases. Most dermatologists are more familiar with the use of the drug in this way and further details are described on page 3345.

Clofazimine (Lamprene) [7,8]

This oral synthetic drug is a phenazine dye. The usual dose is 100 mg three times a week or 100 mg daily in combination with rifampicin if sulphone resistance has occurred [9]. It has an anti-inflammatory effect which may prevent erythema nodosum from developing. For lepra reactions 300 mg/day is recommended. Clofazimine has a very long half-life: 70 days or more. It accumulates in the tissues and is slowly excreted in urine, sweat, sebum and milk.

The main side-effect is the emergence of red–brown to black discoloration of skin and conjunctivae but urine and sputum become red, too, and breast milk may be discoloured. Mild gastrointestinal reactions may occur and ichthyosiform rashes [10]. In general clofazimine is a well-tolerated drug which may be prescribed in pregnancy and during lactation. In renal and hepatic impairment biochemical tests of function are recommended from time to time but the drug may be used. Clofazimine may be valuable in treating pyoderma gangrenosum [11] and perhaps also in discoid lupus erythematosus.

Rifampicin

This drug has been discussed previously (under antituberculosis therapy). It seems to be bactericidal for *M. leprae* in very low dosage and acts much more rapidly than dapsone, rendering the patient non-contagious in a few days or weeks [12]. It does not shorten the total duration of treatment, which should be continued with dapsone.

Thiambutosine

This is a diphenylthiourea, useful as a second-line drug when dapsone cannot be used. Resistance may develop, especially after 1 year of treatment.

REFERENCES

1 Shepard CC, Levy L, Fasal P. The sensitivity to dapsone (DDS) of *Mycobacterium leprae* from patients with and without previous treatment. *Am J Trop Med Hyg* 1969; **18**: 258–63.
2 Alexander JO'D, Young E, McFadyen T *et al.* Absorption and excretion of 35S dapsone in dermatitis herpetiformis. *Br J Dermatol* 1970; **83**: 620–31.
3 Anonymous. Adverse reactions to dapsone. *Lancet* 1981; **ii**: 184–5.
4 Cream JJ, Scott GL. Anaemia in dermatitis herpetiformis. The role of dapsone-induced haemolysis and malabsorption. *Br J Dermatol* 1970; **82**: 333–42.
5 Forrest JM. Drugs in pregnancy and lactation. *Med J Aust* 1976; **ii**: 138–41.
6 Fry L, Walkden V, Wojnarowska F *et al.* A comparison of IgA positive and IgA negative dapsone responsive dermatoses. *Br J Dermatol* 1980; **102**: 371–82.
7 Levy L. Pharmacological studies of clofazimine. *Am J Trop Med Hyg* 1974; **23**: 1097–109.
8 Rodriguez JN, Albalos RM, Reich CV *et al.* Effects of the administration of B663 (Lamprene R, clofazimine) on three groups of lepromatous and borderline cases of leprosy. *Int J Leprosy* 1974; **42**: 276–88.
9 Yawalker SJ, Vischer W. Lamprene (clofazimine) in leprosy. *Leprosy Rev* 1979; **50**: 135–44.
10 Michaelsson G, Molin L, Ohman S *et al.* Clofazimine. A new agent for the treatment of pyoderma gangrenosum. *Arch Dermatol* 1976; **112**: 344–9.
11 Kark EC, Davis BR, Pomeranz JR. Pyoderma gangrenosum treated with clofazimine. Report of three cases. *J Am Acad Dermatol* 1981; **4**: 152–9.
12 Browne SG. The drug treatment of leprosy. *Practitioner* 1975; **215**: 493–500.

Antifungal drugs [1–3]

The drugs available for systemic use against fungal diseases are few in number. There are three main families of antifungals: the polyenes (amphotericin B); the azoles, which include the imidazoles (e.g. ketoconazole, miconazole) and the triazoles (fluconazole and itraconazole); and the allylamines. There is also a miscellaneous group of drugs such as griseofulvin, tolnaftate and flucytosine. Most antifungals work through damage to or inhibition of the fungal cell membrane. The main exceptions are the pyrimidine analogue, flucytosine, which affects RNA and DNA synthesis and potassium iodide, which probably affects phagocytic function.

Polyenes [4]

Nystatin [4]

Nystatin was the first polyene antibiotic discovered and is still valuable today as a topical anti-*Candida* agent. It is not absorbed from the gut in significant amounts.

Amphotericin B [1,4]

This is a polyene antibiotic derived from *Streptomyces nodosus*. It has a very wide range of activity against *Candida* spp. and almost all deep fungal pathogens. Resistance is rare. Absorption from the gut is negligible and so, as with nystatin, tablets and lozenges are for practical purposes topical therapy for the mouth or prophylaxis. For systemic use amphotericin B must be given by slow intravenous infusion in 5% dextrose. This solution is unstable; it should be used promptly and other drugs should not be added, except heparin or hydrocortisone. The definitive adult dose range is normally in the range of 0.4–1 mg/kg/day but toxicity is minimized if there is a build up from a very low dose (1 mg) on the first day, to full dosage by days 3–5. In the seriously ill patient a more rapid build-up to full dosage over 24–48 h is necessary.

The fate of amphotericin in the body is not fully understood [5]. Only small amounts appear in urine; much is probably bound to sterol-containing membranes. Adverse reactions are common, initially: fever, rigors, hypotension, nausea, vomiting, tinnitus and bronchospasm. Phlebitis at the site of infusion is also frequent. Hypokalaemia and hypochromic anaemia may occur and, rarely, liver-function abnormalities. Nephrotoxicity is of great importance; renal clearance may be decreased and tubular damage may develop. These are particularly a problem of extended treatment but are potentially reversible. If renal impairment is severe, therapy must therefore be interrupted and should be restarted at a lower dosage.

Amphotericin B is used principally for systemic mycoses such as candidosis, aspergillosis, mucormycosis and cryptococcosis as well as the endemic respiratory infections such as histoplasmosis.

Lipid-associated amphotericins

Recently, three new formulations of lipid-associated amphotericin B—a liposomal formulation (AmBisome), a colloidal dispersion (ABCD) and a lipid complex (ABLC)—have been developed. They can be used at much higher dosage (mean 3–5 mg/day) without nephrotoxicity [6].

Flucytosine [7]

This is a synthetic cytosine analogue which is converted to 5-fluorouracil in the body. It is effective against yeasts, including *Candida* spp., *Cryptococcus neoformans* and many of the fungi involved in chromoblastomycosis. It is orally absorbed but may be given intravenously too. The tablets contain 500 mg, the usual adult dose being 150 mg/kg/day. Lower doses are necessary in renal failure. It is important to monitor serum levels, aiming to achieve 40–60 mg/l and to avoid toxic levels—above 120 mg/l. Because resistance, both primary and secondary, is well recognized, sensitivity testing initially and at intervals is strongly recommended. It is rarely used on its own. In cryptococcal meningitis in the non-AIDS patient, flucytosine and amphotericin B are given in combination. They appear to be more effective as a combination than amphotericin B on its own and the daily dose of the latter can be reduced to 0.4–0.6 mg/kg.

The main side-effects are nausea, vomiting, diarrhoea and rashes, but thrombocytopenia and neutropenia may also occur.

Azoles

Miconazole

This is a commonly used topical imidazole, poorly absorbed by the oral route. It may be administered intravenously by slow infusion three times in 24 h, the usual adult dose being 1.8–3 g/day. Side-effects are not particularly common. They include pruritus, rashes, fever, faintness and venous thrombosis at the infusion site. Anorexia, nausea, vomiting and diarrhoea occur and anaphylaxis is a rare but genuine problem. It is seldom used now except in infections due to *Scedosporium apiospermum* [8].

Ketoconazole [9,10]

Ketoconazole is a broad-spectrum imidazole which is available in different topical formulations from cream to shampoo or as an oral agent. The drug is well absorbed after oral administration, although lower levels are seen in patients who are neutropenic. It is effective in chronic mucocutaneous candidosis and widespread dermatophytosis. It can also be used topically for pityriasis versicolor. It also appears to be effective in mycetoma infections caused by *Madurella mycetomatis* but not in sporotrichosis. Certain systemic mycoses such as paracoccidioidomycosis and those with soft-tissue lesions are the most sensitive [10].

Adverse events are not common but include headache, vomiting and giddiness as well as nausea. It also leads to blockade of androgen biosynthesis by interference with cytochrome P-450 at high dosage [11]. This results in symptoms such as gynaecomastia in men and menstrual irregularities in women. In addition, it causes asymptomatic changes in liver function and overt hepatitis on occasions [12]. The true frequency of the latter is estimated to be about one in 10 000 but it may be more common in patients receiving treatment for nail disease. It is more common also in those with a prior history of liver disease. While this is a comparatively uncommon complaint it is sufficient to limit the use of the drug in superficial fungal disease. Also, much of its function has been assumed by the development of itraconazole and fluconazole (see below). Drug resistance is also seen rarely [13].

Itraconazole [14]

Itraconazole is a triazole antifungal drug which is avidly

bound in tissue, including skin. Its serum levels are generally low after a 100–200-mg dose. It is given orally and has a broad spectrum of action against the main fungal pathogens. It is effective in dermatophytosis, candidosis and *Malassezia* infections. Originally used in doses of 100 mg daily it is now often given at 200 mg or 400 mg. At higher doses it is possible to use shorter courses such as 400 mg daily for 1 week in tinea corporis. Because it is retained for very long periods in the nail it is used in pulses of 400 mg daily for 1 week per month for 3–4 months [15].

In vaginal candidosis it is given as a single day's treatment of 600 mg and it produces responses in oropharyngeal candidiasis in doses of 100–200 mg daily. For recalcitrant pityriasis versicolor a total dose of 1000 mg is necessary. Other infections responding to itraconazole include sporotrichosis, chromomycosis, paracoccidioidomycosis and histoplasmosis [14]. It has also been reported to be effective in cryptococcal meningitis, particularly as a long-term suppressive therapy of human immunodeficiency virus (HIV)-positive patients. Itraconazole is unusual amongst azoles in producing responses against aspergillosis.

Although itraconazole may occasionally cause nausea and headache, more serious adverse reactions, such as hepatic reactions and anaphylaxis, are extremely rare.

A new formulation of itraconazole in cyclodextrin has recently become available. This oral solution is much better absorbed in AIDS patients.

Fluconazole [16]

Fluconazole is also a triazole antifungal which is well absorbed after oral administration. It may also be given intravenously. Unusually for an azole it is mainly excreted via the kidney. It is active against a range of fungal pathogens.

The principle uses of fluconazole in dermatology are in the treatment of oropharyngeal and vaginal candidosis [17]. In the latter disease, it is effective in a single dose of 150 mg; with oropharyngeal infections, treatment responses are rapid, often within 3 days of starting therapy with 50–100 mg daily [18]. For dermatophytosis it has been found that weekly doses of 150 mg may be effective after 2–3 weeks and a similar weekly pulse has been used for onychomycosis. In systemic mycoses it is used in the management of cryptococcosis either as primary therapy or long-term suppression and in systemic candidosis [19].

Few adverse effects apart from nausea and dyspepsia have been attributed to fluconazole. The dose of the drug has to be reduced in patients with renal impairment.

Certain fungi such as *Candida krusei*, *C. glabrata* and some strains of *C. albicans* may be primarily resistant to fluconazole and secondary resistance may develop in immunocompromised patients [16].

Allylamines

Terbinafine [20]

Terbinafine is a fungicidal allylamine antifungal, similar to naftifine. It works by the inhibition of squalene epoxidation in the synthesis of the ergosterol in the fungal cell membrane [21]. The accumulation of squalene in the cell is thought to contribute to its *in vitro* fungicidal activity. It may be given orally or topically in a dose of 125 mg twice daily. Its chief use is in dermatophytosis, where it is highly effective even in patients with chronic infections of the hands and feet. In onychomycosis it is given in doses of 250 mg daily for 6 weeks for fingernails and 12 weeks for toe nails [22]. It is less active when given orally in superficial candidosis and pityriasis versicolor. In dermatophytosis there is a particularly low relapse rate with this drug. Recently, it has been shown to be active in a range of other deep fungal infections from sporotrichosis to chromoblastomycosis.

There are few side-effects apart from the occasional episode of gastrointestinal discomfort. Loss of taste may occur but is reversible. Skin rashes have also been reported. Hepatic reactions are extremely rare.

Griseofulvin [23]

Griseofulvin is derived from a number of *Penicillium* species. It is a fungistatic drug whose principal activity is directed against dermatophytes. Its mode of action is via the inhibition of the formation of intracellular microtubules.

The usual human dose is 10 mg/kg daily in tablet or, in children, solution form. Treatment duration varies between 2 and 4 weeks for tinea corporis to over 1 year for onychomycosis. The success rate even after 1 year of treatment for toenail infections is less than 30–40%.

Drug interaction with phenobarbitone and coumarin anticoagulants occur. Side effects include headaches and nausea but serious reactions are extremely rare. There are a few reports of apparent precipitation or exacerbation of systemic lupus erythematosus and porphyrias by griseofulvin.

Potassium iodide [2]

In the form of a saturated aqueous solution (100 g in 100 ml water) this is the preferred treatment for lymphocutaneous sporotrichosis and subcutaneous zygomycosis (basidiobolomycosis). It is administered orally starting with 0.6 ml three times a day and gradually increasing until a level of four or five times the dose is attained in an adult. The mode of action is obscure. Progress must be expected to be slow and treatment should be continued until 4 weeks after apparent cure. Iodides are best avoided in pregnancy because of the risk of goitre and hypothyroidism in the infant. Adverse reactions include iododerma, salivary and lacrimal gland swelling and hypersecretion, and gastrointestinal disturbances, as well as anxiety, depression and hypothyroidism.

REFERENCES

1 Bennett JE. Chemotherapy of systemic mycoses. *N Engl J Med* 1974; **290**: 30–2.
2 Roberts DT. The current status of systemic antifungal agents. *Br J Dermatol* 1982; **106**: 597–602.
3 Speller DCE, ed. *Antifungal Chemotherapy*. Chichester: John Wiley and Sons, 1980.
4 Medoff G, Kobayashi GA. The polyenes In: Speller DCE, ed. *Antifungal Chemotherapy*. Chichester: John Wiley and Sons, 1980: 3–33.
5 Atkinson AJ, Bennett JE. Amphotericin B pharmacokinetics in humans. *Antimicrob Agents Chemother* 1978; **13**: 271–6.
6 Janknegt R, de Marie S, Bakker-Woudenberg AJM *et al*. Liposomal and lipid formulations of amphotericin B. *Clin Pharmacokinet* 1991; **23**: 279–91.
7 Bennett JE. Flucytosine. *Ann Intern Med* 1977; **86**: 319–22.
8 Lutwick LI, Rytel MW, Yanez JP *et al*. Deep infections of Petriellidium boydii treated with miconazole. *JAMA* 1979 **241**: 272–3.
9 Cox FW, Stiller RL, South DA *et al*. Oral ketoconazole for dermatophyte infections. *J Am Acad Dermatol* 1982; **6**: 455–62.
10 Jones HE. *Ketoconazole Today*. Manchester: Adis Press, 1987.
11 Stern RS. Ketoconazole; assessing the risks. *J Am Acad Dermatol* 1982; **6**: 544.
12 Heinberg JK, Svejgaard E. Toxic hepatitis during ketoconazole treatment. *Br Med J* 1981; **283**: 825–6.
13 Ryley JF, Wilson RG, Barrett-Bee KJ. Azole resistance in Candida albicans. *Sabouraudia* 1984; **22**: 53–63.
14 Grant SM, Clissold SP. Itraconazole. *Drugs* 1989; **37**: 310–44.
15 Hay RJ, ed. *Itraconazole*. Manchester, Adis Press, 1994.
16 Powderly WB, Van't Wout JW, eds. *Fluconazole*. York: Marius Press, 1992.
17 Brammer KW. Treatment of vaginal candidiasis with a single oral dose of fluconazole. *Eur J Clin Microbiol Infect Dis* 1988; **7**: 364–7.
18 Dupont B, Drouhet E. Fluconazole in the management of oropharyngeal candidosis in a predominantly HIV antibody positive group of patients. *J Med Vet Mycol* 1988; **26**: 67–71.
19 Stern JJ, Hartman BJ, Sharkey P *et al*. Oral fluconazole therapy for patients with acquired immunodeficiency syndrome and cryptococcosis—experience with 22 patients. *Am J Med* 1988; **85**: 477–80.
20 Jones TC, Villars VV. Terbinafine. In: Ryley J, ed. *Chemotherapy of Fungal Diseases*. Berlin: Springer–Verlag, 1990: 455–82.
21 Ryder NS, Meith H. Allylamine antifungal drugs In: Borgers M, Hay R, Rinaldi MG, eds. *Current Topics in Medical Mycology*, Vol. 4 New York: Springer-Verlag, 1992: 158–88.
22 Van der Schroeff JG, Cirkel PKS, Crijns MB *et al*. A randomised treatment duration-finding-study of terbinafine in onychomycosis. *Br J Dermatol* 1992; **126** (Suppl. 39): 36–9.
23 Davies RR. Griseofulvin. In: Speller DCE, ed. *Antifungal Chemotherapy*. Chichester: John Wiley and Sons, 1980: 149–82.

Antiviral drugs

With the spread of HIV infection, considerable efforts have now been expended in searching for new antiviral drugs. Despite this there are still few effective antiviral agents [1]. Because there are fewer steps involved in the assembly of viruses, and these are inextricably associated with human metabolic and other cellular functions, the ratio between antiviral activity and host toxicity is often a narrow one.

Other approaches to treatment have involved the use of interferons which have proved to be of limited value in most viral infections apart from some genital papillomavirus infections and many of the available preparations are associated with dose limiting side-effects when given intravenously.

Drug resistance will occur with antivirals but often it involves a modification of the viral genome which may, in turn, affect viral pathogenetic mechanisms. This alteration in viruses may affect their capacity to cause disease except in severely immunocompromised patients such as those with AIDS.

Vidarabine (adenosine arabinoside, ARA-A)

This purine nucleoside acts by inhibiting viral DNA synthesis. It has effects mainly against the herpes group of viruses and appears to be effective in early cases of herpes simplex encephalitis and in varicella–zoster infections of immunocompromised subjects. However, its use has largely been superceded by aciclovir. At a dose of 10 mg/kg/day i.v. it causes mainly mild gastrointestinal side-effects and in 5% of subjects rashes. CNS and haematological side-effects have also been reported [2]. A 3% ointment has an established place in the topical treatment of herpes simplex keratoconjunctivitis.

Idoxuridine

This synthetic nucleoside is effective against DNA viruses, particularly the herpes group. Its use is now restricted to topical application because of severe bone-marrow and hepatic toxicity when given intravenously. It has been used in 5–40% concentration in DMSO to shorten the duration of clinical symptoms in herpes zoster infections. It can also be used in herpes keratitis but is less effective in genital herpes simplex infections [3].

Aciclovir [4–7]

This antiviral agent works by inhibition of DNA synthesis. Its mode of action involves activation by thymidine kinase and subsequent inhibition of viral polymerase. Resistance to aciclovir has been recorded sometimes, following alterations to or deficiency of thymidine kinase. This has been associated with lack of response to therapy [8,9]. This is a very active agent against herpes viruses. In serious infections it has been used intravenously but it is also available as 200-mg tablets, as an ophthalmic ointment and as a cream [5]. Unfortunately, it has no effect on the latent phase of either herpes simplex or zoster and is apparently ineffective in clinical practice against other viruses. The intravenous dose for serious systemic herpes simplex infections is 5 mg/kg every 8 h by slow infusion (over 1 h). In herpes zoster 10 mg/kg every 8 h is advised. Orally, 200 mg every 4 h (five times a day) is effective and remarkably safe treatment for severe vulvovaginal herpes simplex [10], for example.

Studies with aciclovir have shown that it is possible to suppress recurrences of herpes simplex by intermittent administration over a long period. This has given rise to concerns over the risk of drug resistance and this approach is really only indicated in a few patients with incapacitating recurrent attacks of infection [11].

Aciclovir is less effective against herpes zoster unless given in greater doses for example 10 mg/kg i.v. 8 hourly [12]. It is therefore mainly used for treatment of varicella–zoster infection in immunocompromised patients.

The main route of excretion is renal [13]. Side-effects include elevation of blood urea and creatinine which may rarely progress to acute renal failure. In patients with established renal impairment lower doses are indicated. Although animal and human evidence shows no teratogenic activity, as aciclovir is a relatively new drug it is best avoided in pregnancy. There is currently no information about drug levels in human milk when given during lactation.

New drugs related to aciclovir

These include ganciclovir, famciclovir and penciclovir [14].

Famciclovir is well absorbed after oral administration. It is used at doses of 250–500 mg up to three times daily. At these doses it appears to be as effective as the higher dose regimen of intravenous aciclovir and is well tolerated. There is also a lower frequency of post-herpetic neuralgia after its use.

Penciclovir is a promising treatment for severe herpes simplex infections and because of its pharmacokinetic properties is given less frequently than aciclovir.

Ganciclovir [15] is another deoxyguanosine analogue which can be used in the treatment or prophylaxis of cytomegalovirus (CMV) infections. It is also active against other herpes viruses. Its use is generally reserved for CMV infections in severely immunocompromised patients when it is given in starting doses of 5 mg/kg/12 hours i.v. It can also be used as long-term suppressive therapy to prevent relapse. However, there is a high frequency of nephrotoxicity as well as metabolic disturbances such as hypokalaemia or hypocalcaemia.

Zidovudine (AZT, Retrovir) [16]

AZT has been developed as a drug for the treatment of human retrovirus infections. Its principal site of action is the inhibition of virus-RNA-dependent DNA polymerase (reverse transcriptase) [17]. AZT is given by oral route and the normal dose is 250–500 mg daily; variations to this regimen and drug combinations are under assessment. The use of AZT in patients with AIDS or symptomatic

HIV infections has been found to result in higher levels of circulating CD4 lymphocytes and, in some studies, a decrease in mortality over the short term. Treated patients are still infectious and the therapy does not cure the infection. It is currently used to treat HIV patients with CD4 counts lower than $500/mm^3$ [18]. It has been suggested that AZT may benefit some skin complications of AIDS such as psoriasis. Administration of AZT to infected women in the second and third trimesters of pregnancy significantly reduces the risk of neonatal infection [19].

The main toxic side-effects of zidovudine are neutropenia and anaemia which occur in the majority of patients, particularly at higher doses. This is a particular problem in advanced disease. Other side-effects include headache, myalgia and nausea. Progressive nail pigmentation has been described in black patients [20]. Resistance to AZT occurs regularly with long-term use, although its clinical significance is less clear.

Other antiretroviral agents

These include zalcitabine (DDC) a dideoxynucleotide analogue and stavudine which is a thymidine analogue. Both have been used for treatment of patients with very low CD4 counts or where there is AZT resistance. Zalcitabine causes a painful neuropathy. Pancreatitis, rashes, ulceration and hepatitis have been described. Stavudine also causes a painful neuropathy.

Foscarnet phosphonoformate [21]

Foscarnet is a pyrophosphate analogue that inhibits herpes virus polymerase. It is active against most herpes viruses including CMV. It also inhibits reverse transcriptase and has activity *in vitro* against HIV, particularly in combination with AZT. It is given intravenously in severe herpes simplex and CMV infections or topically. It is an alternative drug for severe aciclovir resistant herpes simplex infections and for this indication the usual initial treatment is 40 mg/kg every 8 hours. Adverse effects include renal tubular damage, malaise, nausea and headache. Tremor and hallucination may occur at high doses.

REFERENCES

1 Hirsch MS, Swartz MN. Antiviral agents. *N Engl J Med* 1980; **302**: 903–7, 949–53.
2 Whitley RJ, Spruance S, Hayden F. Vidarabine therapy of mucocutaneous herpes simplex virus infection in the immunocompromised host. *J Infect Dis* 1984; **149**: 1–8.
3 Silvestri DL, Corey L, Holmes KK. Ineffectiveness of topical idoxuridine in dimethyl sulfoxide for therapy of genital herpes. *JAMA* 1982; **248**: 953–9.
4 Elion GB. The biochemistry and mechanisms of action of acyclovir. *J Antimicrob Chemother* 1983; **12**: (Suppl. B): 9–17.
5 Fiddian AP, Yeo JM, Clark AE. Treatment of herpes labialis. *J Infect* 1983; **6**: (Suppl. 1): 41–7.
6 King DH, Galasso G, eds. Symposium on acyclovir. *Am J Med* 1982; **73** (Suppl. 1).
7 Field HJ, Phillips I, eds. Acyclovir. Based on the Second International Acyclovir Symposium. *J Antimicrob Chemother* 1983; **12** (Suppl. B): 1–11.
8 Field HJ, Larder BA, Darby G. Isolation and characterization of acyclovir resistant strains of herpes simplex virus. *Am J Med* 1982; **73** (Suppl. 1): 369–71.
9 Dekker C, Ellis MN, Hunter G et al. Virus resistance in clinical practice. *J Antimicrob Chemother* 1983; **12** (Suppl. B): 137–52.
10 Bryson YJ. Current status and prospects for oral acyclovir treatment of first episode and recurrent genital herpes simplex virus. *J Antimicrob Chemother* 1983; **12** (Suppl. B): 61–9.
11 Thomas RHM, Dodd HJ, Yeo JM et al. Oral acyclovir in the suppression of recurrent non-genital herpes simplex virus infection. *Br J Dermatol* 1985; **113**: 731–5.
12 Huff JC, Bean B, Balfour HH et al. Therapy of herpes zoster with oral acyclovir. *Am J Med* 1988; **85** (Suppl. 2A): 84–9.
13 De Miranda P, Blum MR. Pharmacokinetics of acyclovir after intravenous and oral administration. *J Antimicrob Chemother* 1983; **12** (Suppl. B): 27–37.
14 Vere Hodge RA. Review antiviral portraits series. Number 3. Famciclovir and penciclovir. *Antiviral Chem Chemother* 1993; **4**: 67–84.
15 Laskin OL, Cederberg DM, Mills J et al. Ganciclovir for the treatment and suppression of serious infections caused by cytomegalovirus. *Am J Med* 1987; **83**: 201–7.
16 Hirsch MS. AIDS commentary—azidothymidine. *J Infect Dis* 1988; **157**: 427–31.
17 Yaschoan R, Broder S. Development of antiretroviral therapy for the acquired immunodeficiency syndrome and related disorders. *N Engl J Med* 1988; **316**: 557–64.
18 McLeod GX, Hammer SM. Zidovudine: five years later. *Ann Intern Med* 1992; **117**: 487–501.
19 Graham NMH, Zeger SL, Park LP et al. The effects on survival of early treatment of human immunodeficiency virus infection. *N Engl J Med* 1992; **326**: 1037–42.
20 Furth PA, Kazakis AM. Nail pigmentation changes associated with azidothymidine (zidovudine). *Ann Intern Med* 1988; **107**: 350.
21 Oleg B, Behrmetz S, Eriksson B. Clinical use of foscarnet (phosphonoformate). In: De Clerq E, ed. *Clinical Use of Antiviral Drugs*. Amsterdam: Martinus Nijhoff Publishing 1991: 223–40.

Antiparasitic agents

Drugs that are used to treat parasitic infections which affect the skin include antibacterial agents such as metronidazole and cotrimoxazole as well as those with specific activity against parasites. This section will largely be concerned with the latter group.

Drugs used to treat roundworms

The benzimidazoles. Mebendazole and albendazole are the best known of these compounds. Mebendazole or methyl 5-benzoylbenzimidazole-2 carbamate is a synthetic drug which is active against diverse species such as *Ascaris*, *Enterobius* and *Trichuris* [1]. It is also active against the adult forms of *Trichinella spiralis* and some filariae such as *Loa loa*. It works through blocking the assembly of microtubules. It is poorly absorbed from the gastrointestinal tract. Adverse events are not common and are mainly seen at high doses. The more common but trivial side-effects are abdominal pain and diarrhoea.

Albendazole or methyl 5-*n*-propoxythio-2-benzimidazole carbamate has broad-spectrum activity for parasites from *Ascaris* to *Trichuris* [2,3]. Albendazole is absorbed after oral administration but this is enhanced in the presence of a fatty meal. Once again it is well tolerated and abdominal pain and diarrhoea are the main side-effects. Liver and bone-marrow toxicity occur only at high doses.

Thiabendazole is less used than previously. It is well absorbed and is active against a range of nematodes as well as some fungi. However side effects such as nausea and vomiting are common.

Diethyl carbamazine

Diethyl carbamazine (DEC) is discussed in Chapter 32. It is a piperazine derivative used in the treatment of microfilariae [4]. It rapidly kills these microorganisms, an event which leads to considerable inflammation which can cause damage in the eye and skin. It acts by affecting microfilarial muscle activity and affects their membranes leading to increased host killing capacity. In onchocerciasis it can cause severe itching, oedema, erythema and hypotension, the DEC reaction. The dose is usually built up from an initial 50 mg dose depending on the infection.

Ivermectin

This is a macrocyclic lactone which is used for intestinal parasites in animals and for the management of onchocerciasis [5–7]. It is also effective against *Sarcoptes scabiei*. Its advantage in onchocerciasis is that it is microfilaricidal but does not lead to severe inflammatory responses. Ivermectin blocks neuromuscular transmission in helminths. Ivermectin is well absorbed after oral administration. Side-effects are not common but include fever, itching and headache. A mild DEC-like reaction may occur in some patients. Its usual dose is 150 μg/kg orally, repeated when necessary every 6–12 months.

Pentavalent antimony

The main variants used for the treatment of leishmaniasis are sodium stibogluconate and meglumine antimoniate. Neither is orally active and both have to be given parenterally (intramuscularly or intravenously) [8]. There is a slow elimination phase which may give rise to toxicity at high dosage. Common adverse events include abdominal pain, nausea and headache [9]. Other effects are renal impairment, pancreatitis and alterations in electrocardiogram (ECG) and cardiac arrhythmias. In particular the QT interval may be prolonged.

REFERENCES

1 Keystone JS, Murdoch JK. Mebendazole. *Ann Intern Med* 1979; **91**: 582–6.
2 Jones SK, Reynolds NJ, Oliwiecki S *et al*. Oral albendazole for the treatment of cutaneous larva migrans. *Br J Dermatol* 1990; **122**: 99–101.
3 Pugh RNH, Teesdale CH, Burnham GM. Albendazole in children with hookworm infection. *Ann Trop Med Parasitol* 1986; **80**: 565–7.
4 Hawking F. Diethyl carbamazine and new compounds for the treatment of filariasis. *Adv Pharmacol Chemother* 1979; **16**: 129–94.
5 Taylor HR. Recent developments in the treatment of onchocerciasis. *Bull WHO* 1984; **62**: 509–15.
6 Collins RC, Gonzalez-Peralta C, Castro J *et al*. Ivermectin: Reduction in prevalence and infection intensity of *Onchocerca volvulus* following biannual treatments in five Guatemalan communities. *Am J Trop Med Hyg* 1992; **47**: 156–69.
7 Pacque M, Greene BM, Munoz B *et al*. Ivermectin therapy: a 5 year follow up. *J Infect Dis* 1991; **164**: 1035–6.
8 Navin TR, Arana BA, Arana FA *et al*. Placebo-controlled clinical trial of sodium stibogluconate (pentostam) versus ketoconazole for treating cutaneous leishmaniasis in Guatemala. *J Infect Dis* 1992; **165**: 528–34.
9 Ballou WR, McClain JB, Gordon DM *et al*. Safety and efficacy of high dose stibogluconate therapy for American cutaneous leishmaniasis. *Lancet* 1987; **2**: 13–16.

Drugs to improve the peripheral circulation

Raynaud's phenomenon and perniosis are the principal dermatological indications for systemic vasodilator therapy. Raynaud's phenomenon occurs in a primary, usually mild form unassociated with systemic disease, or secondary to underlying connective tissue disease or less commonly a hyperviscosity disorder or cervical rib. It can also be caused by administration of drugs with a vasoconstrictor action and rarely can be occupational.

The use of calcium-channel blocking agents has revolutionized the management of Raynaud's phenomenon. Nifedipine is the treatment of choice [1]. It acts by inhibiting contraction of smooth-muscle cells by reducing the cellular uptake of calcium, a process fundamental to vasospasm; it also reduces platelet aggregability. Modified release nifedipine 20-60 mg daily is usually effective. Diltiazem is also useful but verapamil less so. Side-effects include flushing, headaches and peripheral oedema. The response of primary Raynaud's phenomenon is usually more impressive than that secondary to connective tissue disease. Use of calcium-channel antagonists can occasionally precipitate erythromelalgia [2].

Severe Raynaud's phenomenon (see Chapter 24) especially that secondary to systemic sclerosis and other connective tissue diseases, is more difficult to treat and may be poorly responsive to nifedipine. For these patients intravenous prostacyclin or one of its stable analogues may be necessary [3]. Prostacyclin inhibits platelet aggregability, increases red-cell deformability, and decreases blood viscosity. For reasons which are poorly understood, it causes sustained clinical benefit, a single low-dose infusion (0.5 ng/kg/min) often causing clinical remission for several weeks [4]. Side-effects include flushing, headaches and hypotension. Other systemically administered drugs reported to be useful include ketanserin [5], a serotonin antagonist and dazoxiben, a thromboxane synthetase inhibitor [6]. Alpha-adrenergic-blocking agents, for example thymoxamine, a non-selective α-adrenoceptor blocker, in dosage 40 mg three times daily or prazosin, a selective α-adrenergic-blocking agent, in dosage 0.5–1.0 mg three times daily may suffice in mild cases. Recently, the use of intravenous calcitonin gene-related peptide (CGRP) has been recommended for severe Raynaud's phenomenon [7]. CGRP, which was given in dosage 0.6 µg/min for 3 h/day on 5 consecutive days, causes flushing, diarrhoea, headache and hypotension.

Perniosis also responds well to calcium-channel antagonists. A double-blind, cross-over, placebo-controlled study of nifedipine in 10 patients [8] showed a convincing response in the nifedipine phase of the trial. The dosage and side-effects of nifedipine, which is the drug of choice for perniosis, are as for Raynaud's phenomenon.

Other drugs reported to improve the peripheral circulation include oxpentifylline, fibrinolytic agents including stanazolol and low-molecular-weight dextran infusion. However, adequate evidence of efficacy is lacking in these instances.

REFERENCES

1 Smith CD, McKendry RJR. Controlled trial of nifedipine in the treatment of Raynaud's phenomenon. *Lancet* 1982; **ii**: 1299–301.
2 Drenth JPH, Michiels JJ, Van Joost T, Vuzeuski VD. Verapamil induced secondary erythermalgia. *Br J Dermatol* 1992; **127**: 292–4.
3 Dowd PM, Martin MFR, Cook ED *et al*. Treatment of Raynaud's phenomenon by intravenous infusion of prostacyclin (PG12). *Br J Dermatol* 1982; **106**: 81–9.
4 Torby HI, Madhok R, Capell HA *et al*. A double blind randomised multicentre comparison of two doses of intravenous iloprost in the treatment of Raynaud's phenomenon secondary to connective tissue diseases. *Ann Rheum Dis* 1991; **50**: 800–4.
5 Roald OK, Seem E. Treatment of Raynaud's phenomenon with ketanserin in patients with connective tissue disorders. *Br Med J* 1984; **289**: 577–9.
6 Tindell H, Tooke JE, Menys VC *et al*. Effect of dazoxiben, a thromboxane synthebase inhibitor on skin blood flow following cold challenge in patients with Raynaud's phenomenon. *Eur J Clin Invest* 1985; **15**: 20–3.
7 Bunker CB, Reavley C, O'Shaungmessy DJ, Dowd PM. Calcitonin gene related peptide in treatment of severe peripheral vascular insufficiency in Raynaud's Phenomenon. *Lancet* 1993; **342**: 80–3.
8 Dowd PM, Rustin MHA, Lanigan S. Nifedipine in the treatment of chilblains. *Br Med J* 1986; **293**: 923–4.

Miscellaneous drugs used in special ways in dermatology

Antimalarials

A variety of drugs have been used in the treatment of malaria. However, for over 35 years it has been well known that several of these drugs may have other useful properties in the management of skin diseases [1,2]. There are several diseases where there is an undoubted beneficial effect—discoid and systemic lupus erythematosus, polymorphic light eruption and solar urticaria (Chapters 58 and 25). They are of some value in rheumatology, where there is a resurgence of their use, as well as their more obvious application in diseases caused by some protozoa. Their use in sarcoidosis and porphyria cutanea tarda is discussed elsewhere (Chapters 59 and 60).

The mode of action of antimalarials is complex and their usage is largely on empirical grounds. They can interfere with many biological processes. They bind to DNA, stabilize membranes, inhibit hydrolytic enzymes, interfere with prostaglandin synthesis and block chemotaxis [1,2].

The major problem with chloroquine is the retinopathy and potential blindness [3,4]. There are considerable problems in defining the criteria for the diagnosis of retinopathy and the estimate that 3–5% of patients who receive the drug may develop this complication is almost certainly too high. A number of questions remain unanswered. It is generally agreed that the risk to the retina of giving chloroquine sulphate 250 mg daily for 3 months is virtually negligible, although the drug is cumulative to some extent from one year to another. It has long been thought that it is the total cumulative dose that determines the retinal toxicity. It has recently been suggested that it is the daily dose that counts and that 4 mg/kg choroquine daily is likely to be safe [5].

Because of the potential retinopathy with chloroquine, hydroxychloroquine or mepacrine are the two antimalarial drugs now used. Hydroxychloroquine is more effective than mepacrine but is said to have some ocular toxicity albeit less than with chloroquine. It is likely that in the doses used by dermatologists (up to 400 mg/day) the risk of ocular toxicity is negligible. In many hospitals the ophthalmologists will not agree to screen or monitor patients as they think the risk is so small, but if hydroxychloroquine is continued for more than a few months it would seem prudent to obtain ophthalmological screening, which should also be sought before starting treatment. Mepacrine lacks ocular toxicity, and is often an effective drug, especially in discoid lupus erythematosus and Hutchinson's chilblain lupus. In effective doses (200 mg/day) it usually causes the skin to turn yellow and occasionally produces lichenoid reactions. Ocular toxicity of antimalarials as used in dermatology is well reviewed by Cox *et al.* [6].

REFERENCES

1 Isaacson D, Elgart M, Turner ML. Anti-malarials in dermatology. *Int J Dermatol* 1982; **21**: 379–95.
2 Koranda FC. Antimalarials. *J Am Acad Dermatol* 1981; **4**: 650–5.
3 Olansky AJ. Antimalarials and ophthalmologic safety. *J Am Acad Dermatol* 1982; **6**: 19–23.
4 Portnoy JZ, Callen JP. Ophthalmologic aspects of chloroquine and hydroxychloroquine therapy. *Int J Dermatol* 1983; **22**: 273–8.
5 Ochsendorf FR, Runne U. Chloroquin-Retinopathie: Vermeidbar durch Beachtung der maximalen Tagesdosis. *Hautarzt* 1988; **39**: 341–2.
6 Cox NH, Paterson WD. Ocular toxicity of antimalarials in dermatology; a survey of current practice. *Br J Dermatol* 1994; **131**: 878–22.

Dapsone, sulphapyridine [1–6]

Dapsone (DDS) first came into medicine as an antibacterial agent but was found to be less effective and more toxic than sulphonamides. Likewise, its activity against tuberculosis was disappointing. Nevertheless, it has been the mainstay in the treatment of leprosy for many years (Chapter 29). It also has some action against malaria and other parasites.

However, it has also proved a very valuable drug in the management of a wide range of mainly uncommon dermatoses. Its mode of action is not fully understood. Although many of the diseases found empirically to respond to this drug have in common the involvement of either polymorphs or immune complexes, the metabolic action of dapsone cannot yet be explained simply in these terms. The diseases for which dapsone is particularly effective are dermatitis herpetiformis and erythema elevatum diutinum. Other diseases also favourably but not invariably influenced include other bullous diseases (pemphigoid, mucous membrane pemphigoid, linear IgA disease, chronic bullous disease of childhood, bullous eruption of systemic lupus erythematosus, subcorneal pustular dermatosis), pyoderma gangrenosum, rheumatoid arthritis and collagen diseases, relapsing polychondritis, acne conglobata, leukocytoclastic vasculitis and granuloma faciale.

Toxicity is a considerable problem with dapsone but overall the drug has probably fewer long-term side-effects than do corticosteroids or sulphapyridine. The main toxic side-effect is haemolysis which is not usually dependent on glucose-6-phosphate dehydrogenase deficiency, although that enzyme defect may compound the problem. Some haemolysis is almost invariably found on therapeutic doses. Methaemoglobinaemia is also common and is responsible for the bluish lips etc., commonly seen in patients on this drug. A level of 3% methaemoglobinaemia is often unnoticed, 12% may be acceptable, but 20% usually not. Regular blood checks of haemoglobin and reticulocytes but also including white cells and platelets should therefore be undertaken in all patients for the first few months after starting dapsone. Dapsone has several other but less common side-effects, including agranulocytosis, peripheral neuropathy, drug rashes, renal damage, hypoalbuminaemia, cholestasis, psychoses and reversible male infertility. A dose of 100 mg daily is often used as a starting dose. Many patients with dermatitis herpetiformis can be controlled on very much less. Some diseases can only be controlled by larger doses, but the incidence of side-effects then rises very sharply and most dermatologists prefer not to exceed a dose of 100–150 mg daily. It is possible to reduce dapsone-dependent methaemoglobinaemia by the concomitant administration of cimetidine (400 mg three times daily) [7]. A useful review of the use and side-effects of dapsone was published by Stern [8].

Other drugs which share some of the useful assets of dapsone include sulphapyridine and, to a lesser extent, sulphamethoxypyridazine. Others are less commonly used [3]. Sulphapyridine is in general less effective than dapsone

and, in doses which are effective, tends to cause more side-effects, especially marrow suppression, although not haemolysis. The usual dose is 0.5 g twice or three times daily.

Clofazimine

This antileprotic drug has also been used especially in pyoderma gangrenosum and in lupus erythematosus and Sweet's disease.

REFERENCES

1 Bernstein JE, Lorincz AL. Sulfonamides and sulphones in dermatologic therapy. *Int J Dermatol* 1981; **20**: 81–8.
2 Katz SI. Sulfoxone (Diasone) in the treatment of dermatitis herpetiformis. *Arch Dermatol* 1982; **118**: 809–12.
3 Lang PG, Jr, Stenson WF, Lobos E. Sulfones and Sulfonamides in dermatology today. *J Am Acad Dermatol* 1979; **1**: 479–92.
4 Samsoen M, Bousquet F, Basset A. Les sulfones-indications en dehors des maladies infectieuses. *Ann Dermatol Vénéréol* 1981; **108**: 911–20.
5 Wozel G. The story of sulfones in tropical medicine and dermatology. *Int J Dermatol* 1989; **28**: 17–21.
6 Wozel G, Barth J. Current aspects of modes of action of dapsone. *Int J Dermatol* 1988; **27**: 547–52.
7 Coleman MD, Scott AK, Breckenridge AM *et al*. The use of Cimetidine as a selective inhibitor of Dapsone N hydroxylation in man. *Br J Clin Pharmacol* 1990; **30**: 761–7.
8 Stern RS. Systemic Dapsone. *Arch Dermatol* 1993; **129**: 301.

Sulphasalazine

This drug is best known for its activity in inflammatory bowel disease and rheumatoid arthritis with their associated skin problems. The mode of action is uncertain [1,2]. It is not very well absorbed from the gut and does have side-effects. Among other activities it may be a 5-lipoxygenase inhibitor. It has been found to be of some value in pustular psoriasis, arthropathic psoriasis and psoriasis vulgaris [1–5]. Its use in other conditions such as dermatitis herpetiformis, scleroderma and acne [6] has been recommended but is less well established. Sulphasalazine has been reported to be useful in metastatic cutaneous Crohn's disease [7,8].

REFERENCES

1 Farr M, Kitas GD, Waterhouse L *et al*. Treatment of psoriatic arthritis with sulfasalazine: a one year open study. *Clin Rheumatol* 1988; **7**: 372.
2 Stenson WG, Lobos E. Sulfasalazine inhibits the synthesis of chemotactic lipids by neutrophils. *J Clin Invest* 1982; **69**: 494–7.
3 Gupta AK, Ellis CN, Siegel MT *et al*. Sulfasalazine: a potential psoriasis therapy. *J Am Acad Dermatol* 1989; **20**: 797–800.
4 Gupta AK, Ellis CN, Siegel MT *et al*. Sulfasalazine improves psoriasis: a double blind analysis. *Arch Dermatol* 1990; **126**: 487–93.
5 Newman ED, Perruquet JL, Harrington TM. Sulfsalazine therapy in psoriatic arthritis; clinical and immunologic response. *J Rheumatol* 1997; **18**: 1379–82.
6 Schoch EP, McCuiston CH. Effect of salicylazosulfapyridine (azulfidine) on pustular acne and certain other dermatoses. *J Invest Dermatol* 1955; **25**: 123–6.
7 Peltz S, Vetsey JP, Ferguson A *et al*. Disseminated metastatic cutaneous Crohn's disease. *Clin Exp Dermatol* 1993; **18**: 55–9.

8 Kolansky G, Kimbrough-Green C, Dubin HV. Metastatic Crohn's disease of the face. *Arch Dermatol* 1993; **129**: 1348–9.

Thalidomide

Thalidomide is an interesting drug whose name is linked with the causation of severe birth defects so that its use is very restricted and it must never be given to pregnant women. It also has other toxic side-effects, notably causing peripheral neuropathy [1–3], so that the manufacturers advise against its use. It can be helpful in severe leprosy reactions (Chapter 29). It can also be helpful in some, but by no means all, patients with nodular prurigo [4], lupus erythematosus [5,6], light-sensitive dermatoses, aphthosis [7], Behçet's disease, Weber–Christian disease, pyoderma gangrenosum, sarcoid, graft-versus-host disease and adult Langerhans' cell histiocytosis [8], although other treatments are to be preferred. It is a drug whose use must always be kept under the strictest control and it must be used only by patients who are able to understand the problems. It is important to check regularly for peripheral neuropathy. Guidelines for the clinical use and dispensing of thalidomide have been drawn up by Judge *et al.* [9].

REFERENCES

1 Aronson IK, Yu R, West DP *et al.* Thalidomide-induced peripheral neuropathy. *Arch Dermatol* 1984; **120**: 1466–70.
2 Clemmensen OJ, Olsen PZ, Andersen KE. Thalidomide neurotoxicity. *Arch Dermatol* 1984; **120**: 338–41.
3 Wulff CH, Asboe-Hansen G, Brodthagen H. Development of polyneuropathy during thalidomide therapy. *Br J Dermatol* 1985; **112**: 475–80.
4 Johnke H, Zachariae H. Thalidomide treatment of prurigo nodularis (Danish). *Ugeskrift for Laeger* 1993; **155**: 3028–30.
5 Holm AL, Bowers KE, McMeekin TO, Gaspari AA. Chronic cutaneous lupus erythematosus treated with thalidomide. *Arch Dermatol* 1993; **129**: 1548–50.
6 Knop J, Bonsmann G, Happle R *et al.* Thalidomide in the treatment of sixty cases of chronic discoid lupus erythematosus. *Br J Dermatol* 1983; **108**: 461–6.
7 Bowers PW, Powell RJ. Effect of thalidomide on orogenital ulceration. *Br Med J* 1983; **287**: 799–800.
8 Thomas L, Ducros B, Secchi T *et al.* Sussessful treatment of adult's Langerhans cell histiocytosis with Thalidomide. *Arch Dermatol* 1993; **129**: 1261.
9 Judge MR, Kobza-Black A, Hawk JL. Guidelines for the clinical use and dispensing of thalidomide. *Postgraduate Med J* 1995; **71**: 123.

Colchicine [1,2]

Colchicine has been used in the treatment of gout for many centuries and is still a valuable remedy. It is also of use in familial Mediterranean fever and has been advocated for cirrhosis. It has an antimitotic action (for which it is sometimes used topically) but its useful effects in skin diseases probably depend more on its suppression of various aspects of polymorph activity, notably chemotaxis. This confers on it an anti-inflammatory effect. It may also inhibit histamine release from mast cells. Its use is somewhat restricted by its side-effects, especially those on the gastrointestinal tract, but the bone marrow and kidney may also be affected. It should be avoided in pregnancy.

It is not therefore a first-line drug but can prove of value in Behçet's disease [3], chronic bullous dermatosis of childhood (linear IgA disease) [4], pustular psoriasis [5], relapsing polychondritis [6], leukocytoclastic vasculitis, urticarial vasculitis [7], epidermolysis bullosa acquisita [8] and Sweet's syndrome—all diseases in which polymorphs are presumed to play a role. A common dose is 0.5–1 mg by mouth daily, although larger doses are used by rheumatologists.

REFERENCES

1 Malkinson FD. Colchicine. New uses of an old, old drug. *Arch Dermatol* 1982; **118**: 453–7.
2 Aram H. Colchicine in dermatologic therapy. *Int J Dermatol* 1983; **22**: 566–9.
3 deBois MH, Geelhoed-Duvijvestijn PH, Westdt ML. Behcet's syndrome treated with colchicine. *Netherlands J Med* 1991; **38**: 175–6.
4 Zeharia A, Hodak E, Mukamel M *et al.* Sussessful treatment of chronic bullous dermatosis of childhood with colchicine. *J Am Acad Dermatol* 1994; **30**: 660–1.
5 Takigawa M, Miyachi Y, Uehara M *et al.* Treatment of pustulosis palmaris et plantaris with oral doses of colchicine. *Arch Dermatol* 1982; **118**: 458–602.
6 Askari AD. Colchicine for treatment of relapsing polychondritis. *J Am Acad Dermatol* 1984; **10**: 506–10.
7 Asherson RA, Buchanan N, Kenwright S *et al.* The normocomplementemic urticarial vasculitis syndrome—report of a case and response to colchicine. *Clin Exp Dermatol* 1991; **16**: 424–7.
8 Megahed M, Scharffetter-Kochanek K. Epidermolysis bullosa acquisita—successful treatment with colchicine. *Arch Dermatol Res* 1994; **286**: 35–46.

Traditional Chinese herbal medicine for atopic eczema

The treatment involves taking a 'tea' prepared from a decoction of plant materials. Usually 10 or so plant materials are included. Trials have also been performed using a tablet form of treatment. No product licence is yet available for the use of Chinese herbal medicine in eczema. Trials have, however, shown a beneficial response in children [1] and adults [2] with atopic eczema. Even when treatment is effective and continued, it often wears off after 6–12 months. Relapses occur once treatment is stopped. Of concern are the reports of hepatotoxicity associated with Chinese herbal remedies [3–6]. While Chinese herbs cannot yet be recommended for the routine treatment of children with atopic eczema, they did help about half the children who took part in the Great Ormond Street Hospital Trial [7]. The risk of hepatic side-effects requires further study.

REFERENCES

1 Sheehan MP, Atherton DJ. A controlled trial of traditional Chinese medical plants in widespread non-exudative atopic eczema. *Br J Dermatol* 1992; **126**: 179–84.
2 Sheehan MP, Rustin MHA, Atherton DJ *et al.* Efficacy of traditional Chinese herbal therapy in adult atopic dermatitis. *Lancet* 1992; **340**: 13–17.
3 Davies EG, Pollock I, Steele HM. Chinese herbs for eczema. *Lancet* 1990; **336**: 177.
4 Graham-Brown R. Toxicity of Chinese herbal remedies. *Lancet* 1992; **340**: 673.

5 Perharic-Walton L, Murray V. Toxicity of Chinese herbal remedies. *Lancet* 1992; **340**: 673.

6 Mostefa-Cara N, Pauwels A, Pinus E *et al*. Fatal hepatitis after herbal tea. *Lancet* 1992; **340**: 674.

7 Sheehan MP, Atherton DJ. One year follow up of children treated with Chinese medicinal herbs for atopic eczema. *Br J Dermatol* 1994; **130**: 488–93.

Transdermal delivery systems

The blood is the target for penetration in transdermal delivery systems. There are two major routes for drug penetration through skin: the stratum corneum and shunts via hair follicles and eccrine sweat gland ducts [1].

With drugs metabolized in the liver achievement of therapeutic blood levels is enhanced by transdermal delivery because of avoidance of the 'first pass' effect inherent in oral administration. Thus, transdermally delivered drugs show reduced differences in 'peak' and 'trough' blood levels, and a different profile of metabolites [2]. Efficiency of transdermal delivery is greater with lipid-soluble drugs. Additional advantages include ability to use short half-life drugs, better patient compliance, reduced dosage frequency, avoidance of unpredictable intestinal absorption and gastric irritation, and fewer complications.

Recent examples of drugs marketed in a transdermal form include scopolamine, clonidine, nitroglycerine, oestradiol and nicotine. Within the transdermal 'patch', the drug, which may be formulated in a liquid, solid, ointment or cream form, behaves as a reservoir. The blood levels are proportional to the active surface area of the 'patch', and drug delivery occurs over a period of 1–7 days. Skin irritation and sensitization are significant difficulties with transdermal delivery systems, which contain several sources of problems besides the drug itself including the adhesive, vehicle penetration enhancers and polymers. More advanced transdermal delivery systems are now available which should enable continuous or pulsed delivery of new drugs including genetically engineered products [3].

REFERENCES

1 Scheuplein RJ, Blank IH. Permeability of the skin. *Physiol Rev* 1971; **51**: 702–47.

2 Powers MS. Pharmacokinetics and pharmacodynamics of transdermal dosage forms of 17b-oestradiol: comparison with conventional oral oestrogen used for hormone replacement. *Am J Obstet Gynecol* 1985; **152**: 1099–106.

3 Flynn GL, Stewart BS. Percutaneous drug penetration: choosing candidates for transdermal development. *Drug Dev Res* 1988; **13**: 169–185.

Chapter 77
Drug Reactions

S.M.BREATHNACH

Introduction [1–4]

A drug may be defined as a chemical substance, or combination of substances, administered for the investigation, prevention or treatment of diseases or symptoms, real or imagined. The distinction between drugs and 'other chemicals' is not always easily made, as chemicals of very diverse structure are increasingly added to foods and beverages as dyes, flavours or preservatives. Such chemicals may cause harmful side-effects. Moreover, chemicals used in agriculture or in veterinary medicine may contaminate human food. In addition, with the advent of therapeutic agents that may be useful for improving the appearance, as with minoxidil for androgenetic alopecia and tretinoin for photo-aged skin, the distinction between drugs and cosmetics has become blurred [5].

An adverse drug reaction may be defined as an unde-

sirable clinical manifestation resulting from administration of a particular drug; this includes reactions due to overdose, predictable side-effects and unanticipated adverse manifestations. Adverse drug reactions may be said to be the inevitable price we pay for the benefits of modern drug therapy [6]. They are costly both in terms of the human illness caused and in economic terms, and can undermine the doctor–patient relationship. Sometimes, reactions result from human error [7]. In one study, 0.9% of 530 medication errors resulted in adverse drug reactions [8]; these usually involve errors at the ordering stage, but may also occur at the administration stage [9]. In hospitals, medication errors occur at a rate of about one per patient per day; dispensing errors made by pharmacy staff range from 0.87 to 2.9% [10]. Approximately one in 2000 of all deaths for which there were records of Coroner's Inquests in one district were related to drugs; of these, 20% were due to errors

[11]. Confusion may occur between drugs with similar spelling of their brand names [12,13]. It has been proposed that licensing authorities should exercise more control over the naming of new proprietary formulations, that non-proprietary and new proprietary names should be internationalized, and that doctors should issue printed prescriptions if possible [14]. The average extra length of stay for patients with an adverse drug event in one study in the USA was 1.9 days, and the average extra cost of hospitalization was $1939 [15]. In another study, at a university-affiliated hospital, the mean cost of an adverse drug reaction or medication error varied from $95 for additional laboratory tests to $2640 for intensive care; the estimated total cost for the medication-related problems reported in 1994 was almost $1.5 million [16]. Drug reactions, principally to corticosteroids and methotrexate, accounted for 32% of claims and 26% of dollar losses in dermatology malpractice suits in the USA from 1963 to 1973 inclusive [17]. Medication side-effects, most frequently to corticosteroids, antibiotics and chemotherapeutic agents, represented 26% of lawsuits in a study of dermatology residency programmes in the USA between 1964 and 1988 [18]. If legal consequences are to be avoided, consistent care is needed at every stage from drug manufacture to administration [19].

It is in everyone's interests to minimize the chances of their occurrence, and to this end government regulatory bodies and the pharmaceutical industry collaborate to ensure adequate screening of new products. In addition to extensive *in vitro* and animal testing, prolonged and strictly controlled clinical trials are essential. Even so, hazards cannot be completely eliminated, for a serious reaction of low incidence may not be suspected until a very large number of patients have been treated with a new drug. Premarketing clinical trials conducted before a new drug is licensed will not identify adverse reactions occurring in less than 0.1–1% of patients, or those occurring only after prolonged administration, or with a long latency period, or only in susceptible patients, or when the drug is combined with some other factor, such as another drug [20,21].

Another problem is that only a very small fraction of all adverse reactions are ever reported to monitoring agencies, and first warning is still often given by anecdotal reports published in medical journals [22,23]. Many of these reports are subsequently validated but a substantial proportion of poorly documented reports are not [23,24]. In an analysis of 5737 articles from 80 countries between 1972 and 1979, only half the reports contained enough information for the calculation of the frequency of a particular reaction [24]. The usefulness of anecdotal case reports has again been called into question [25]. Since incorrect reports may have serious legal and other consequences, a heavy responsibility rests with medical editors; a chance association or coincidental reaction should not be allowed to enter the literature. Criteria for assessment of potential drug reactions have been promulgated: these include recurrence on challenge, existence of a pharmacological basis for the reactions, the occurrence of immediate acute or local reactions at the time of administration, of previously known reactions with a new route of administration, or of repeated rare reactions, and the presence of immunological abnormalities [23,26]. In the assessment of an unrecorded new reaction the existence of similar but unpublished reports to the manufacturers or to the Committee on Safety of Medicines is of particular importance.

REFERENCES

1 Bork K. *Cutaneous Side Effects of Drugs.* Philadelphia: WB Saunders, 1988.
2 Breathnach SM, Hintner H. *Adverse Drug Reactions and the Skin.* Oxford: Blackwell Scientific Publications, 1992.
3 Zürcher L, Krebs A. *Cutaneous Drug Reactions.* Basel: Karger, 1992.
4 Litt JZ, Pawlak WA, Jr. *Drug Eruption Reference Manual.* New York: Parthenon, 1997.
5 Lavrijsen APM, Vermeer BJ. Cosmetics and drugs. Is there a need for a third group: cosmeceutics? *Br J Dermatol* 1991; **124**: 503–4.
6 Nolan L, O'Malley K. Adverse drug reactions in the elderly. *Br J Hosp Med* 1989; **41**: 446–57.
7 Wright D, Mackenzie SJ, Buchan I *et al.* Critical events in the intensive therapy unit. *Lancet* 1991; **338**: 676–8.
8 Bates DW, Boyle DL, Vander Vliet MB *et al.* Relationship between medication errors and adverse drug events. *J Gen Intern Med* 1995; **10**: 199–205.
9 Bates DW, Cullen DJ, Laird N *et al.* Incidence of adverse drug events and potential adverse drug events. Implications for prevention. ADE Prevention Study Group. *JAMA* 1995; **274**: 29–34.
10 Allan EL, Barker KN. Fundamentals of medication error research. *Am J Hosp Pharm* 1990; **47**: 555–71.
11 Ferner RE, Whittington RM. Coroner's cases of death due to errors in prescribing or giving medicines or to adverse drug reactions: Birmingham 1986–1991. *J R Soc Med* 1994; **87**: 145–8.
12 Fine SN, Eisdorfer RM, Miskovitz PF, Jacobson IM. Losec or Lasix? *N Engl J Med* 1990; **322**: 1674.
13 Faber J, Azzugnuni M, Di Romana S, Vanhaeverbeek M. Fatal confusion between 'Losec' and 'Lasix'. *Lancet* 1991; **337**: 1286–7.
14 Aronson JK. Confusion over similar drug names. Problems and solutions. *Drug Saf* 1995; **12**: 55–60.
15 Evans RS, Classen DC, Stevens LE *et al.* Using a hospital information system to assess the effects of adverse drug events. *Proc Ann Symp Comp Appl Med Care* 1993: 161–5.
16 Schneider PJ, Gift MG, Lee YP *et al.* Cost of medication-related problems at a university hospital. *Am J Health System Pharm* 1995; **52**: 2415–18.
17 Altman J. Survey of malpractice claims in dermatology. *Arch Dermatol* 1975; **111**: 641–4.
18 Hollabaugh ES, Wagner RF, Jr, Weedon VW, Smith EB. Patient personal injury litigation against dermatology residency programs in the United States, 1964–1988. *Arch Dermatol* 1990; **126**: 618–22.
19 Day AT. Adverse drug reactions and medical negligence. *Adverse Drug Reaction Bull* 1995; **172**: 651–4.
20 Bruinsma W. Drug monitoring in dermatology. *Int J Dermatol* 1986; **25**: 166–7.
21 Committee of Management, Prescribers' Journal. Adverse Drug Reactions. *Prescr J* 1991; **31**: 1–3.
22 Leading Article. Crying wolf on drug safety. *Br Med J* 1982; **284**: 219–20.
23 Venning GR. Validity of anecdotal reports of suspected adverse drug reactions: the problem of false alarms. *Br Med J* 1982; **284**: 249–52.
24 Venulet J, Blattner R, von Bülow J, Berneker GC. How good are articles on adverse drug reactions? *Br Med J* 1982; **284**: 252–4.
25 Stern RS, Chan H-L. Usefulness of case report literature in determining drugs responsible for toxic epidermal necrolysis. *J Am Acad Dermatol* 1989; **21**: 317–22.
26 Stern RS, Wintroub BU. Adverse drug reactions: reporting and evaluating cutaneous reactions. *Adv Dermatol* 1987; **2**: 3–18.

Incidence of drug reactions [1,2]

Data collection

It is difficult to obtain reliable information on the incidence of drug reactions, despite attempts at monitoring by government and the pharmaceutical industry. One problem is the lack of standardized coding for drug reactions [3]. Moreover, the information that is available must be interpreted with considerable care, because data will be biased, depending on the method of collection [1,2]. Thus, data on medical inpatients, especially from acute care facilities, may indicate a relatively high incidence, since these patients are generally sicker and receive more intensive drug treatment. By contrast, spontaneous reporting may underestimate the true incidence. National schemes for collating reported adverse drug reactions exist in many countries, and the World Health Organisation's Adverse Reaction Collaborating Centre, in Uppsala, provides a very large database [2]. The UK's 'yellow card' reporting scheme solicits adverse drug reaction reports from doctors, dentists, Her Majesty's coroners, and drug manufacturers; the wide availability of reporting forms is important in encouraging reporting [2]. 'Pharmacovigilence' in France, which involves reporting to regional centres, and most other national schemes, also rely entirely on spontaneous reporting [4,5]. Institution of an adverse drug reaction reporting project in Rhode Island in the USA increased the rate of reporting of such reactions more than 17-fold over a 2-year period [6]. The quality of adverse-event reporting to the United States Food and Drug Administration improved following introduction of the MedWatch scheme [7]. Specialty-based systems for spontaneous reporting of adverse drug reactions (e.g. the Adverse Drug Reaction Reporting System of the American Academy of Dermatology [8] and the Gruppo Italiano Studi Epidemiologici in Dermatologia [9]) have also been introduced. In the UK, the speciality-based Cutaneous Reactions Database established at the Institute of Dermatology in 1988 was unfortunately closed in 1990 because of a meagre response [10]. Inherent difficulties with spontaneous reporting are that reactions associated with newly marketed drugs, those of unusual morphology, and reactions starting soon after initiation of therapy are more likely to be notified; at best only a crude estimate of true incidence is provided [11–13]. All national spontaneous reporting systems are compromised by under-reporting [2]; in the UK, surveys suggest that rarely more than 10% of serious reactions are notified to the Committee on Safety of Medicines [14,15]. A survey of 44 000 patients receiving one or other of seven new drugs suggested that under-reporting by the spontaneous system may be as high as 98% when compared with information collected by the more objective 'event monitoring' system [4]. Heavy prescribing by a minority of doctors immediately following licensing may place patients at unnecessary risk, and affects safety monitoring of new drugs: the 10% of doctors who prescribed most heavily accounted for 42% of total prescribing in a survey of 28 402 general practitioners asked to supply postmarketing data on 27 new drugs dispensed in England between September 1984 and June 1991, but returned proportionately far fewer questionnaires [16]. Reasons for under-reporting include lack of time, lack of report forms and the misconception that absolute confidence in the diagnosis of an adverse reaction was important [17]; workload may affect reporting [18]. Another factor is the perceived deterrent to reporting adverse drug reactions caused by fear of involvement in litigation [19]; reporting of errors should be free of recrimination [20]. The offer of a small fee increased the rate of reporting in one hospital study almost 50-fold [21].

Pharmacoepidemiology, the epidemiological assessment of adverse drug effects, and pharmacovigilance, the process of identifying and responding to safety issues about marketed drugs, necessitate making use of information from clinical trials, spontaneous reporting systems, specialty-based reporting systems, case reports, prescription monitoring, case series, cohort studies, case–control studies, population-based registries using computerized material, and special surveillance programmes (e.g. the Boston Collaborative Drug Surveillance Program, in the United States) [22–24].

REFERENCES

1 Breathnach SM, Hintner H. *Adverse Drug Reactions and the Skin*. Oxford: Blackwell Scientific Publications, 1992.
2 Rawlins MD, Breckenridge AM, Wood SM. National adverse drug reaction reporting—a silver jubilee. *Adverse Drug React Bull* 1989; **138**: 516–19.
3 Bonnetblanc JM, Roujeau JC, Benichou C. Standardized coding is needed for reports of adverse drug reactions. *Br Med J* 1996; **312**: 776–7.
4 Fletcher AP. Spontaneous adverse drug reaction reporting vs event monitoring: a comparison. *J R Soc Med* 1991; **84**: 341–4.
5 Moore N, Paux G, Begaud B *et al*. Adverse drug reaction monitoring: doing it the French way. *Lancet* 1985; **ii**: 1056–8.
6 Scott HD, Thacher-Renshaw A, Rosenbaum SE *et al*. Physician reporting of adverse drug reactions. Results of the Rhode Island Adverse Drug Reaction Reporting Project. *JAMA* 1990; **263**: 1785–8.
7 Piazza-Hepp TD, Kennedy DL. Reporting of adverse events to MedWatch. *Am J Health Syst Pharm* 1995; **52**: 1436–9.
8 Stern RS, Bigby M. An expanded profile of cutaneous reactions to nonsteroid anti-inflammatory drugs. Reports to a specialty-based system for spontaneous reporting of adverse reactions to drugs. *JAMA* 1984; **252**: 1433–7.
9 Gruppo Italiano Studi Epidemiologici in Dermatologia. Spontaneous monitoring of adverse reactions to drugs by Italian dermatologists; a pilot study. *Dermatologica* 1991; **182**: 12–17.
10 Kobza Black A, Greaves MM. Cutaneous reactions database closure. *Br J Dermatol* 1990; **123**: 277.
11 Griffin JP, Weber JCP. Voluntary systems of adverse reaction reporting—Part I. *Adverse Drug React Acute Poisoning Rev* 1985; **4**: 213–30.
12 Griffin JP, Weber JCP. Voluntary systems of adverse reaction reporting—Part II. *Adverse Drug React Acute Poisoning Rev* 1986; **5**: 23–55.
13 Griffin JP, Weber JCP. Voluntary systems of adverse reaction reporting—Part III. *Adverse Drug React Acute Poisoning Rev* 1989; **8**: 203–15.
14 Rawlins MD. Spontaneous reporting of adverse drug reactions I: The data. *Br J Clin Pharmacol* 1988; **26**: 1–5.
15 Bem JL, Mann RD, Rawlins MD. Review of yellow cards 1986 and 1987. *Br Med J* 1988; **296**: 1319.

16 Inman W, Pearce G. Prescriber profile and post-marketing surveillance. *Lancet* 1993; **342**: 658–61.

17 Belton KJ, Lewis SC, Payne S *et al.* Attitudinal survey of adverse drug reaction reporting by medical practitioners in the United Kingdom. *Br J Clin Pharmacol* 1995; **39**: 223–6.

18 Bateman DN, Sanders GL, Rawlins MD. Attitudes to adverse drug reaction reporting in the Northern Region. *Br J Clin Pharmacol* 1992; **34**: 421–6.

19 Kaufman MB, Stoukides CA, Campbell NA. Physicians' liability for adverse drug reactions. *South Med J* 1994; **87**: 780–4.

20 Upton DR, Cousins DH. Avoiding drug errors. Reporting of errors should be free of recrimination. *Br Med J* 1995; **311**: 1367.

21 Feely J, Moriarty S, O'Connor P. Stimulating reporting of adverse drug reactions by using a fee. *Br Med J* 1990; **300**: 22–3.

22 Stern RS, Wintroub BU. Adverse drug reactions: reporting and evaluating cutaneous reactions. *Adv Dermatol* 1987; **2**: 3–18.

23 Stern RS. Epidemiologic assessment of adverse drug effects. *Semin Dermatol* 1989; **8**: 136–40.

24 Rawlins MD. Pharmacovigilance: paradise lost, regained or postponed? *J R Coll Physicians Lond* 1995; **29**: 41–5.

General incidence of adverse drug reactions

The incidence of adverse drug reactions varies from 6 [1] to 30% [2], with at least 90 million courses of drug treatment given yearly in the US [3]. The reported percentage of patients who develop an adverse drug reaction during hospitalization varies markedly in different studies from 1.5 to 44%, although in most studies the incidence is about 10–20% [4]. About 3–8% of hospital admissions are a consequence of adverse drug reactions [5–7]. A survey of 30 195 randomly selected hospital records in 51 hospitals in the state of New York found that 19% of adverse events caused by medical treatment were the result of drug complications; the most frequently implicated classes of drug responsible were antibiotics, antitumour agents and anticoagulants [8]. 18% of adverse drug reactions were caused by negligence, and allergic/cutaneous complications constituted 14% of all drug-related complications. Less information is available about the incidence among outpatients. It has been estimated that about one in 40 consultations in general practice is the result of adverse drug reactions [9], and eventually 41% of patients develop a reaction [10]. In one multicentre general practice study in the UK, the percentage of consultations involving an adverse drug reaction increased from 0.6% for patients aged 0–20 years to 2.7% for patients aged over 50 years [11]; in another study, 2.5% of consultations were the result of iatrogenic illness [12]. Fatal reactions to drugs are more common than is generally realized. It was previously estimated that penicillin caused 300 deaths each year in the USA alone [13]. Anaphylactic reactions to penicillin were reported in 1968 to occur in about 0.015%, and fatal reactions in up to 0.002% (i.e. one per 50 000), of treatment courses [14]. These figures may be somewhat less today, with use of newer β-lactam antibiotics. The risk of fatal aplastic anaemia with chloramphenicol therapy was reported as at least one in 60 000 [15], and the risk of a fatal outcome from treatment with monoamine oxidase inhibitors may be of the same order. It has been estimated

that the incidence of fatality as a result of a drug reaction among inpatients is between 0.1 and 0.3% [16,17].

REFERENCES

1 DeSwarte RD. Drug allergy—Problems and strategies. *J Allergy Clin Immunol* 1984; **74**: 209–21.

2 Jick H. Adverse drug reactions: the magnitude of the problem. *J Allergy Clin Immunol* 1984; **74**: 555–7.

3 Goldstein RA. Foreword. Symposium proceedings on drug allergy: prevention, diagnosis, treatment. *J Allergy Clin Immunol* 1984; **74**: 549–50.

4 Breathnach SM, Hintner H. *Adverse Drug Reactions and the Skin.* Oxford: Blackwell Scientific Publications, 1992.

5 McKenney JM, Harrison WL. Drug-related hospital admissions. *Am J Hosp Pharm* 1976; **33**: 792–5.

6 Levy M, Kewitz H, Altwein W *et al.* Hospital admissions due to adverse drug reactions: a comparative study from Jerusalem and Berlin. *Eur J Clin Pharmacol* 1980; **17**: 25–31.

7 Black AJ, Somers K. Drug-related illness resulting in hospital admission. *J R Coll Phys Lond* 1984; **18**: 40–1.

8 Leape LL, Brennan TA, Laird N *et al.* The nature of adverse events in hospitalized patients. Results of the Harvard Medical Practice Study II. *N Engl J Med* 1991; **324**: 377–84.

9 Kellaway GSM, McCrae E. Intensive monitoring of adverse drug effects in patients discharged from acute medical wards. *NZ Med J* 1973; **78**: 525–8.

10 Martys CR. Adverse reactions to drugs in general practice. *Br Med J* 1979; **ii**: 1194–7.

11 Lumley LE, Walker SR, Hall CG *et al.* The under-reporting of adverse drug reactions seen in general practice. *Pharm Med* 1986; **1**: 205–12.

12 Mulroy R. Iatrogenic disease in general practice: its incidence and effects. *Br Med J* 1973; **ii**: 407–10.

13 Parker CW. Allergic reactions in man. *Pharmacol Rev* 1983; **34**: 85–104.

14 Idsøe O, Guthe T, Willcox RR, De Weck AL. Nature and extent of penicillin side reactions, with particular reference to fatalities from anaphylactic shock. *Bull WHO* 1968; **38**: 159–88.

15 Witts LJ. Adverse reactions to drugs. *Br Med J* 1965; **ii**: 1081–6.

16 Davies DM, ed. *Textbook of Adverse Drug Reactions*, 3rd edn. Oxford: Oxford University Press, 1985: 1–11.

17 Caranasos GJ, May FE, Stewart RB, Cluff LE. Drug-associated deaths of medical inpatients. *Arch Intern Med* 1976; **136**: 872–5.

Risk of adverse drug reactions among different patient groups

Certain patient groups are at increased risk of developing an adverse drug reaction. Women are more likely than men to develop adverse drug reactions [1]. The incidence of such reactions increases with the number of drugs taken both in hospital inpatients [2–4] and outpatients [5,6]. Although data are somewhat conflicting [7], the burden of evidence suggests that the incidence of adverse reactions increases with patient age [1,8]. While those over 65 years of age comprise only 12% of the population in the US, 33% of all drugs are prescribed for this age group, and the elderly have a significantly higher incidence of adverse drug reactions, related to decreased organ reserve capacity, altered pharmacokinetics and pharmacodynamics, and polypharmacy [9]. Similarly, in the UK the elderly are dispensed twice as many prescriptions as the national average [10]. Adverse drug reactions contribute to the need for hospitalization in 10–17% of elderly inpatients [11–13]. Inappropriate medication is a major cause of adverse drug reactions in elderly patients; 27% of elderly patients on medication admitted to a teaching hospital experienced adverse drug reactions, of which almost 50% were due to drugs with absolute contraindications and/or that were unnecessary [14]. Adverse drug reactions occur in between 6 and 17% of children admitted to specialist paediatric hospitals [15].

Patients with Sjögren's syndrome (SS) have also been reported to have a high frequency of drug allergy. In a different series, drug allergy has been reported in 43% of SS patients, compared with 9% of patients with systemic lupus erythematosus (LE) without SS [16], 62% of SS patients [17], and 41% of rheumatoid arthritis patients with SS, compared with 17% of those without SS [18]. Antibiotic allergy is increased in LE [19].

REFERENCES

1 Davies DM, ed. *Textbook of Adverse Drug Reactions*, 3rd edn. Oxford: Oxford University Press, 1985: 1–11.
2 Vakil BJ, Kulkarni RD, Chabria NL *et al*. Intense surveillance of adverse drug reactions. An analysis of 338 patients. *J Clin Pharmacol* 1975; **15**: 435–41.
3 May FE, Stewart RB, Cluff LE. Drug interactions and multiple drug administration. *Clin Pharmacol Ther* 1977; **22**: 322–8.
4 Steel K, Gertman PM, Crescenzi C, Anderson J. Iatrogenic illness on a general medical service at a university hospital. *N Engl J Med* 1981; **304**: 638–42.
5 Kellaway GSM, McCrae E. Intensive monitoring of adverse drug effects in patients discharged from acute medical wards. *NZ Med J* 1973; **78**: 525–8.
6 Hutchinson TA, Flegel KM, Kramer MS *et al*. Frequency, severity, and risk factors for adverse reactions in adult outpatients: a prospective study. *J Chronic Dis* 1986; **39**: 533–42.
7 Gurwitz JH, Avorn J. The ambiguous relation between aging and adverse drug reactions. *Ann Intern Med* 1991; **114**: 956–66.
8 Nolan L, O'Malley K. Adverse drug reactions in the elderly. *Br J Hosp Med* 1989; **41**: 446–57.
9 Sloan RW. Principles of drug therapy in geriatric patients. *Am Fam Physician* 1992; **45**: 2709–18.
10 Black D, Denham MJ, Acheson RM *et al*. Medication for the elderly. A report of the Royal College of Physicians. *J R Coll Physicians Lond* 1984; **18**: 7–17.
11 Col N, Fanale JE, Kronholm P. The role of medication noncompliance and adverse drug reactions in hospitalizations of the elderly. *Arch Intern Med* 1990; **150**: 841–5.
12 Levy M, Kewitz H, Altwein W *et al*. Hospital admissions due to adverse drug reactions: a comparative study from Jerusalem and Berlin. *Eur J Clin Pharmacol* 1980; **17**: 25–31.
13 Williamson J, Chopin JM. Adverse reactions to prescribed drugs in the elderly: a multicentre investigation. *Age Ageing* 1980; **9**: 73–80.
14 Lindley CM, Tully MP, Paramsothy V, Tallis RC. Inappropriate medication is a major cause of adverse drug reactions in elderly patients. *Age Ageing* 1992; **21**: 294–300.
15 Rylance G, Armstron D. Adverse drug events in children. *Adv Drug React Bull* 1997; **184**: 689–702.
16 Katz J, Marmary Y, Livneh A, Danon Y. Drug allergy in Sjögren's syndrome. *Lancet* 1991; **337**: 239.
17 Bloch KJ, Buchanan WW, Wohl MJ, Bunim JJ. Sjögrens's syndrome: a clinical, pathological and serological study of 62 cases. *Medicine* 1965; **44**: 187–231.
18 Williams BO, Onge RAST, Young A *et al*. Penicillin allergy in rheumatoid arthritis with special reference to Sjögren's syndrome. *Ann Rheum Dis* 1969; **28**: 607–11.
19 Petri M, Allbritton J. Antibiotic allergy in systemic lupus erythematosus: a case-control study. *J Rheumatol* 1992; **19**: 265–9.

Acquired immunodeficiency syndrome

Patients with the acquired immunodeficiency syndrome (AIDS) appear to be at increased risk for adverse drug reactions [1–5], especially from sulphonamides including co-trimoxazole (trimethoprim–sulphamethoxazole) [6–10], other sulphur congeners, for example dapsone [11], pentamidine, antituberculosis regimens containing thiacetazone [12,13] or isoniazid and rifampicin, amoxicillin–clavulanate [14,15], clindamycin, pyrimethamine [16] and thalidomide. Human immunodeficiency virus (HIV)-positive individuals have been postulated to have a systemic glutathione deficiency, resulting in a decreased capacity to scavenge reactive hydroxylamine derivatives of sulphonamides, although this has been disputed (see pharmacogenetic mechanisms of drug reactions, below). Patients with AIDS are more likely to have particularly severe reactions, ranging from erythema multiforme to toxic epidermal necrolysis (TEN) (especially with sulphonamides, clindamycin, phenobarbital and chlormezanone) [17,18], and to demonstrate multiple cutaneous drug reactions [3].

REFERENCES

1 Coopman SA, Stern RS. Cutaneous drug reactions in human immunodeficiency virus infection. *Arch Dermatol* 1991; **127**: 714–17.
2 Bayard PJ, Berger TG, Jacobson MA. Drug hypersensitivity reactions and human immunodeficiency virus disease. *J Acquir Immune Defic Syndr* 1992; **5**: 1237–57.
3 Carr A, Tindall B, Penny R, Cooper DA. Patterns of multiple-drug hypersensitivities in HIV-infected patients. *AIDS* 1993; **7**: 1532–3.
4 Sadick NS, McNutt NS. Cutaneous hypersensitivity reactions in patients with AIDS. *Int J Dermatol* 1993; **32**: 621–7.
5 Coopman SA, Johnson RA, Platt R, Stern RS. Cutaneous disease and drug reactions in HIV infection. *N Engl J Med* 1993; **328**: 1670–4.
6 Kletzel M, Beck S, Elser J *et al*. Trimethoprim–sulfamethoxazole oral desensitization in hemophiliacs infected with human immunodeficiency virus with a history of hypersensitivity reactions. *Am J Dis Child* 1991; **145**: 1428–9.
7 Carr A, Swanson C, Penny R, Cooper DA. Clinical and laboratory markers of hypersensitivity to trimethoprim-sulfamethoxazole in patients with *Pneumocystis carinii* pneumonia and AIDS. *J Infect Dis* 1993; **167**: 180–5.
8 Mathelier-Fusade P, Leynadier F. Intolerance aux sulfamides chez les sujets infectés par le VIH. Origine toxique et allergique. *Presse Med* 1993; **22**: 1363–5.
9 Chanock SJ, Luginbuhl LM, McIntosh K, Lipshultz SE. Life-threatening reaction to trimethoprim/sulfamethoxazole in pediatric human immunodeficiency virus infection. *Pediatrics* 1994; **93**: 519–21.
10 Roudier C, Caumes E, Rogeaux O *et al*. Adverse cutaneous reactions to trimethoprim–sulfamethoxazole in patients with the acquired immunodeficiency syndrome and *Pneumocystis carinii* pneumonia. *Arch Dermatol* 1994; **130**: 1383–6.
11 Jorde UP, Horowitz HW, Wormser GP. Utility of dapsone for prophylaxis of *Pneumocystis carinii* pneumonia in trimethoprim-sulfamethoxazole-intolerant, HIV-infected individuals. *AIDS* 1993; **7**: 355–9.
12 Nunn P, Kibuga D, Gathua S *et al*. Cutaneous hypersensitivity reactions due to thiacetazone in HIV-1 seropositive patients treated for tuberculosis. *Lancet* 1991; **337**: 627–30.
13 Pozniak AL, MacLeod GA, Mahari M *et al*. The influence of HIV status on single and multiple drug reactions to antituberculous therapy in Africa. *AIDS* 1992; **6**: 809–14.
14 Battegay M, Opravil M, Wütrich B, Lüthy R. Rash with amoxycillin-clavulanate therapy in HIV-infected patients. *Lancet* 1989; **ii**: 1100.
15 Paparello SF, Davis CE, Malone JL. Cutaneous reactions to amoxicillin-clavulanate among Haitians. *AIDS* 1994; **8**: 276–7.
16 Piketty C, Weiss L, Picard-Dahan C *et al*. Toxidermies à la pyrimethamine chez les patients infectés par le virus de l'immunodeficience acquise. *Presse Med* 1995; **24**: 1710.
17 Porteous DM, Berger TG. Severe cutaneous drug reactions (Stevens–Johnson

syndrome and toxic epidermal necrolysis) in human immunodeficiency virus infection. *Arch Dermatol* 1991; **127**: 740–1.

18 Saiag P, Caumes E, Chosidow O *et al.* Drug-induced toxic epidermal necrolysis (Lyell syndrome) in patients infected with the human immunodeficiency virus. *J Am Acad Dermatol* 1992; **26**: 567–74.

Drug reaction frequency in relation to types of medication

The incidence of reactions to a particular drug must obviously be related to the quantity prescribed [1]. Nearly one in every 10 prescriptions in the USA in 1981 contained either hydrochlorothiazide or codeine [2]. One in every five prescriptions was for a diuretic or other cardiovascular drug; analgesics and antiarthritics constituted 13%; anti-infectives 13%; and sedatives and other psychotropics 11% of prescriptions. Of the 10 drugs most frequently reported by the yellow-card system to the UK Committee on Safety of Medicines in the first 6 months of 1986, seven were non-steroidal anti-inflammatory drugs (NSAIDs) (accounting for 74% of serious adverse reactions); the remaining drugs were the angiotensin-converting enzyme (ACE) inhibitors enalapril and captopril (accounting for 19% of serious reactions) and co-trimoxazole (accounting for 7% of serious adverse reactions) [3]. In another study, anti-inflammatory agents were the drugs responsible for almost 50% of the reactions necessitating admission to a general medical ward; most of the drug-related admissions to the hospital as a whole were caused by digoxin, phenytoin, tranquillizers, antihypertensives, cardiac depressants and antineoplastic agents [4]. Adverse drug reactions accounted for 8% of 1999 consecutive admissions to medical wards in yet another study [5]; the drugs most frequently involved were antirheumatics and analgesics (27%), cardiovascular drugs (23%), psychotropic drugs (14%), antidiabetics (12%), antibiotics (7%) and corticosteroids (5%). Nitrofurantoin and insulin were associated with admission rates of 617 and 182 per million daily doses, compared with 10 for diuretics and seven for benzodiazepines. Adverse drug reactions were responsible for the admission of 2% of 5227 consecutive patients to the University Hospital Centre in Zagreb [6]; drugs incriminated included acetylsalicylic acid (aspirin) (38%), other NSAIDs (23%), cardiovascular agents (20%) and antimicrobials (3%). In a study of cutaneous drug eruptions among children and adolescents in north India, antibiotics were responsible for most eruptions, followed by antiepileptics; cotrimoxazole was the commonest antibacterial culprit, followed by penicillin and its semisynthetic derivatives, and then sulphonamides, and antiepileptics were the most frequently incriminated drugs in erythema multiforme, Stevens–Johnson syndrome and TEN [7].

REFERENCES

1 Committee on Safety of Medicines. CSM Update: Non-steroidal anti-inflammatory drugs and serious gastrointestinal reactions—2. *Br Med J* 1986; **292**: 1190–1.

2 Baum C, Kennedy DL, Forbes MB, Jones JK. Drug use in the United States in 1981. *JAMA* 1984; **251**: 1293–7.

3 Mann RD. The yellow card data: the nature and scale of the adverse drug reactions problem. In: Mann RD, ed. *Adverse Drug Reactions*. Carnforth: Parthenon, 1987: 5–66.

4 Black AJ, Somers K. Drug-related illness resulting in hospital admission. *J R Coll Phys Lond* 1984; **18**: 40–1.

5 Hallas J, Gram LF, Grodum E *et al.* Drug related admissions to medical wards: a population based survey. *Br J Clin Pharmacol* 1992; **33**: 61–8.

6 Huic M, Mucolic V, Vrhovac B *et al.* Adverse drug reactions resulting in hospital admission. *Int J Clin Pharmacol Ther* 1994; **32**: 675–82.

7 Sharma VK, Dhar S. Clinical pattern of cutaneous drug eruption among children and adolescents in north India. *Pediatr Dermatol* 1995; **12**: 178–83.

Incidence of drug eruptions

Drug eruptions are probably the most frequent of all manifestations of drug sensitivity, although their incidence is difficult to determine. The baseline rate of rash development, reflecting a variety of different causes, was similar for 36 recently marketed drugs in the UK at around one per 1000 patients per month from the second to the sixth month of one study; however, the rate for rash in the first month after prescription varied substantially from 0.9 to 6.4 per 1000 patients per month, and was highest for diltiazem [1]. Most estimates of the incidence of drug eruptions are inaccurate, because many mild and transitory eruptions are not recorded, and because skin disorders are sometimes falsely attributed to drugs. There have been several studies of the incidence of drug eruptions [1–7]. The reaction rate has been reported as about 2% [4,7]. A survey [6] of adverse cutaneous drug reactions in inpatients found one-third were fixed drug reactions, one-third exanthematous and 20% were urticaria or angio-oedema; the high frequency of fixed drug reactions reflects the fact that the patients under study had been admitted to hospital. Antimicrobial agents were most frequently incriminated (42%), then antipyretic/anti-inflammatory analgesics (27%), with drugs acting on the central nervous system accounting for 10% of reactions. A few drugs gave specific reactions (e.g phenazone salicylate caused a fixed eruption, while penicillin and salicylates caused urticaria); however, most were capable of causing several types of eruption. Exanthematous eruptions, urticaria and generalized pruritus were the commonest reactions in another large series [7]. The average patient had received eight different medications, which contributed considerably to the difficulties in identifying the causative drugs. Antibiotics, blood products and inhaled mucolytics together caused 75% of the eruptions; amoxicillin (51 cases/1000 exposed), trimethoprim–sulphamethoxazole (33 cases/1000 exposed) and ampicillin (33 cases/1000 exposed) caused the most reactions. Desensitizing vaccines, muscle relaxants, intravenous anaesthetics and radiological contrast media were the most frequent causes of anaphylaxis or anaphylactoid reactions reported to the UK Committee on Safety of Medicines in 1986/1987 [8]. The chairman of the Committee accordingly advised in 1986 that desensitizing vaccines only be given where full cardiorespiratory resuscitation facilities are available. Quinidine, cimetidine, phenylbutazone, hydrochlorothiazide (especially in combination with amiloride) and frusemide have also been frequently implicated in drug eruptions [9,10]. In the US and in the UK, antibiotics, hypnotics and tranquillizers are the most frequent offenders; on a reaction per dose basis, penicillin, warfarin and imipramine are the three drugs most frequently incriminated [11]. The prevalence of a history of penicillin allergy in the US population has been estimated to be between 5 and 10% [12]. An international study of 1790 patients from 11 countries documented the frequency of allergic reactions to long-term benzathine penicillin prophylaxis for rheumatic fever at 3.2%; anaphylaxis occurred in 0.2% (1.2/10 000 injections), and the fatality rate was 0.05% (0.31/10 000 injections) [13]. Reactions to sulphonamides may affect up to 5% of those treated [14]. Cutaneous reactions to common drugs such as digoxin, antacids, paracetamol (acetaminophen), nitroglycerine, spironolactone, meperidine, aminophylline, propranolol, prednisone, salbutamol and diazepam are very rare [9].

Epidemiological data suggest that a relatively small number of drugs are responsible most often for the most serious reactions [15]. Even where the eruption is apparently the only manifestation, death can result from exfoliative dermatitis, erythema multiforme or epidermal necrolysis. The incidence of TEN has been estimated at 1.2 cases per million per year in France based on nationwide surveillance between 1981 and 1985 inclusive [16]. Another study, based on the data of the Group Health Cooperative of Puget Sound, Seattle, Washington (which covers about 260 000 individuals), investigated hospitalized patients from 1972 to 1986 inclusive. The incidence of erythema multiforme, Stevens–Johnson syndrome and TEN was estimated at 1.8 cases per million person-years for patients aged between 20 and 64 years; the incidence for patients aged less than 20 years, and 65 years or greater, increased to 7 and 9 cases per million person-years, respectively [17]. The incidence of TEN was estimated at 0.5 per million per year. Reaction rates per 100 000 exposed individuals were as follows: phenobarbital 20, nitrofurantoin 7, co-trimoxazole and ampicillin 3 and amoxicillin 2. An Italian study estimated the incidence of TEN at about 1.2 cases per million per year [18]. A study based on computerized Medicaid billing data for 1980 to 1984 from the states of Michigan, Minnesota and Florida reported an incidence of Stevens–Johnson syndrome of 7.1, 2.6 and 6.8 per million per year, respectively; penicillins, especially aminopenicillins, were most frequently

implicated [19]. In West Germany, the overall annual risk of TEN and of Stevens–Johnson syndrome was estimated over the years 1981 through 1985 as 0.93 and 1.1 per million, respectively; drugs most frequently implicated were antibiotics (sulphonamides and β-lactam agents), and analgesics and non-steroidal anti-inflammatory agents [20]. In this study, it was possible to attribute the cause of the TEN to a drug in 88% of cases. Another study estimated the incidence for West Germany and Berlin for Stevens–Johnson syndrome and TEN as up to 1.89 per million inhabitants per year [21]. An ongoing international case–control study of TEN and Stevens–Johnson syndrome in relation to the use of drugs is being carried out, based on data collection in France, Italy, Germany and Portugal [22]. The incidence of TEN (cases/million/year) has been reported to be 2.7 times higher, and the fatality twice as high (51% compared with 25%), in the elderly compared with younger adults; the same drugs (NSAIDs, antibacterials and anticonvulsants) are incriminated in both groups [23].

REFERENCES

1 Kubota K, Kubota N, Pearce GL *et al.* Signalling drug-induced rash with 36 drugs recently marketed in the United Kingdom and studied by Prescription-Event Monitoring. *Int J Clin Pharmacol Ther* 1995; **33**: 219–25.
2 Kaplan AP. Drug-induced skin disease. *J Allergy Clin Immunol* 1984; **74**: 573–9.
3 Kauppinen K. Cutaneous reactions to drugs. With special reference to severe mucocutaneous bullous eruptions and sulphonamides. *Acta Derm Venereol (Stockh)* 1972; Suppl. **68**: 1–89.
4 Arndt KA, Jick H. Rates of cutaneous reactions to drugs. A report from the Boston Collaborative Drug Surveillance Program. *JAMA* 1976; **235**: 918–22.
5 Kauppinen K, Stubb S. Drug eruptions: Causative agents and clinical types. A series of inpatients during a 10-year period. *Acta Derm Venereol (Stockh)* 1984; **64**: 320–4.
6 Alanko K, Stubb S, Kauppinen K. Cutaneous drug reactions: clinical types and causative agents. A five year survey of in-patients (1981–1985). *Acta Derm Venereol (Stockh)* 1989; **69**: 223–6.
7 Bigby M, Jick S, Jick H, Arndt K. Drug-induced cutaneous reactions. A report from the Boston Collaborative Drug Surveillance Program on 15 438 consecutive inpatients, 1975 to 1982. *JAMA* 1986; **256**: 3358–63.
8 Bem JL, Mann RD, Rawlins MD. Review of yellow cards 1986 and 1987. *Br Med J* 1988; **296**: 1319.
9 Kalish RS. Drug eruptions: a review of clinical and immunological features. *Adv Dermatol* 1991; **6**: 221–37.
10 Thestrup-Pedersen K. Adverse reactions in the skin from antihypertensive drugs. *Dan Med Bull* 1987; **34**: 3–5.
11 Davies DM, ed. *Textbook of Adverse Drug Reactions*, 3rd edn. Oxford: Oxford University Press, 1985: 1–11.
12 Green CR, Rosenblum A. Report of the Penicillin Study Group—American Academy of Allergy. *J Allergy Clin Immunol* 1971; **48**: 331–43.
13 International rheumatic fever study group. Allergic reactions to long-term benzathine penicillin prophylaxis for rheumatic fever. *Lancet* 1991; **337**: 1308–10.
14 Anonymous. Hypersensitivity to sulphonamides—A clue? (Editorial). *Lancet* 1986; **ii**: 958–9.
15 Stern RS, Steinberg LA. Epidemiology of adverse cutaneous reactions to drugs. *Dermatol Clin* 1995; **13**: 681–8.
16 Roujeau J-C, Guillaume J-C, Fabre J-D *et al.* Toxic epidermal necrolysis (Lyell syndrome). Incidence and drug etiology in France, 1981–1985. *Arch Dermatol* 1990; **126**: 37–42.
17 Chan H-L, Stern RS, Arndt KA *et al.* The incidence of erythema multiforme, Stevens–Johnson syndrome, and toxic epidermal necrolysis. A population-based study with particular reference to reactions caused by drugs among outpatients. *Arch Dermatol* 1990; **126**: 43–7.

18 Naldi L, Locati F, Marchesi L, Cainelli T. Incidence of toxic epidermal necrolysis in Italy. *Arch Dermatol* 1990; **126**: 1103–4.

19 Strom BL, Carson JL, Halpern AC *et al*. A population-based study of Stevens–Johnson syndrome. Incidence and antecedent drug exposures. *Arch Dermatol* 1991; **127**: 831–8.

20 Schöpf E, Stühmer A, Rzany B *et al*. Toxic epidermal necrolysis and Stevens–Johnson syndrome. An epidemiologic study from West Germany. *Arch Dermatol* 1991; **127**: 839–42.

21 Rzany B, Mockenhaupt M, Baur S *et al*. Epidemiology of erythema exudativum multiforme majus, Stevens–Johnson syndrome, and toxic epidermal necrolysis in Germany (1990–1992): structure and results of a population-based registry. *J Clin Epidemiol* 1996; **49**: 769–73.

22 Kaufman DW. Epidemiologic approaches to the study of toxic epidermal necrolysis. *J Invest Dermatol* 1994; **102**: 31S–33S.

23 Bastuji-Garin S, Zahedi M, Guillaume JC, Roujeau JC. Toxic epidermal necrolysis (Lyell syndrome) in 77 elderly patients. *Age Ageing* 1993; **22**: 450–6.

Classification and mechanisms of drug reactions [1–11]

Drug reactions may arise as a result of immunological allergy directed against the drug itself, a reactive metabolite or some contaminant of the drug or, more commonly, by non-immunological mechanisms, such as pseudoallergic reactions caused by non-immune mediated degranulation of mast cells and basophils. Autoimmune reactions, in which the drug elicits an immune reaction to autologous structures, may also occur. Drug reactions may be predictable (type A) or unpredictable (type B) (Table 77.1). About 80% of drug reactions are predictable, usually dose related, a function of the known pharmacological actions of the drug and occur in otherwise normal individuals.

Table 77.1 Classification of adverse drug reactions.

1 *Non-immunological*
Predictable
    Overdosage
    Side-effects
    Cumulation
    Delayed toxicity
    Facultative effects
    Drug interactions
    Metabolic alterations
    Teratogenicity
    Non-immunological activation of effector pathways
    Exacerbation of disease
    Drug-induced chromosomal damage
Unpredictable
    Intolerance
    Idiosyncrasy

2 *Immunological (unpredictable)*
IgE-dependent drug reactions
Immune complex-dependent drug reactions
Cytotoxic drug-induced reactions
Cell-mediated reactions

3 *Miscellaneous*
Jarisch–Herxheimer reactions
Infectious mononucleosis–ampicillin reaction

Side-effects are unavoidable at the regular prescribed dose. Unpredictable reactions are dose independent, not related to the pharmacological action of the drug and may have a basis in pharmacogenetic variation in drug bioactivation and drug or metabolite detoxification or clearance. Intolerance refers to an expected drug reaction occurring at a lower dose, while idiosyncratic and hypersensitivity reactions are qualitatively abnormal unexpected responses. Type C reactions include those associated with prolonged therapy (e.g. analgesic nephropathy), and type D consists of delayed reactions (e.g. carcinogenesis and teratogenicity). The skin has a limited repertoire of morphological reaction patterns in response to a wide variety of stimuli, and it is therefore often impossible to identify an offending drug, or the pathological mechanism involved, on the basis of clinical appearances alone. We therefore remain relatively ignorant about the mechanisms underlying many clinical drug eruptions.

REFERENCES

1 Rawlins MD, Thompson JW. Mechanisms of adverse drug reactions. In: Davies DM, ed. *Textbook of Adverse Drug Reactions*, 3rd edn. Oxford: Oxford University Press, 1985: 12–38.

2 Wintroub BU, Stern R. Cutaneous drug reactions: pathogenesis and clinical classification. *J Am Acad Dermatol* 1985; **13**: 833–45.

3 Stern RS, Wintroub BU, Arndt KA. Drug reactions. *J Am Acad Dermatol* 1986; **15**: 1282–8.

4 Breathnach SM, Hintner H. *Adverse Drug Reactions and the Skin*. Oxford: Blackwell Scientific Publications, 1992.

5 Weiss ME. Drug allergy. *Med Clinics N Am* 1992; **76**: 857–82.

6 Gibaldi M. Adverse drug effect-reactive metabolites and idiosyncratic drug reactions: Part I. *Ann Pharmacother* 1992; **26**: 416–21.

7 Anderson JA. Allergic reactions to drugs and biological agents. *JAMA* 1992; **268**: 2844–57.

8 Pichler WJ. Medikamentenallergien. *Therapeut Umschau* 1994; **51**: 55–60.

9 Rieder MJ. Mechanisms of unpredictable adverse drug reactions. *Drug Saf* 1994; **11**: 196–212.

10 Breathnach SM. Mechanisms of drug eruptions: Part I. *Australas J Dermatol* 1995; **36**: 121–7.

11 Bonnetblanc JM, Vaillant L, Wolkenstein P. Facteurs predisposants des reactions cutanées aux medicaments. *Ann Dermatol Vénéréol* 1995; **122**: 484–6.

Non-immunological drug reactions

Overdosage

The manifestations are a predictable exaggeration of the desired pharmacological actions of the drug, and are directly related to the total amount of drug in the body. Overdosage may be absolute, as a result of a prescribing or dispensing error, or of deliberate excess intake by the patient. It may also occur despite standard dosage due to varying individual rates of absorption, metabolism or excretion (see below). An inappropriately large dose may be given to an infant or very old person or to one with renal impairment. Drug interaction (see below) may also cause drug overdosage.

Side-effects

These include unwanted or toxic effects, which are not separable from the desired pharmacological action of the drug. Examples are the drowsiness induced by antihistamines; the atropine-like anticholinergic properties of some phenothiazines, many antihistamines, and tricyclic antidepressants; and the anagen alopecia caused by cytotoxic drugs.

Cumulative toxicity

Prolonged exposure may lead to cumulative toxicity. Accumulation of drugs in the skin may lead to colour disturbance, either as a result of deposition within phagocytic cells or mucous membranes (e.g. with prolonged administration of gold, silver, bismuth or mercury), or due to binding of the drug or a metabolite to a skin component (e.g. with high-dose chlorpromazine therapy).

Delayed toxicity

Examples are the keratoses and skin tumours that appear many years after inorganic arsenic, and the delayed hepatotoxicity associated with methotrexate therapy.

Facultative effects

These include the consequences of drug-induced alterations in skin or mucous membrane flora. Antibiotics that destroy Gram-positive bacteria may allow the multiplication of resistant Gram-negative species. Broad-spectrum antibiotics, corticosteroids and immunosuppressive drugs may promote multiplication of *Candida albicans* and favour its transition from saphrophytism to pathogenicity. Corticosteroids promote the spread of tinea and erythrasma. Antibiotics such as clindamycin and tetracycline may be associated with pseudomembranous enterocolitis following bowel superinfection with *Clostridium difficile*.

Drug interactions

Interactions between two or more drugs administered simultaneously may occur before entry into the body in an intravenous drip, in the intestine, in the blood and/or at tissue receptor sites, or indirectly by acceleration or slowing in the rate of drug metabolism or excretion. It should be remembered that adverse consequences of drug interactions may occur not only on introduction of a drug, but also on removal of a drug that causes acceleration of drug metabolism, since this may result in effective overdosage of the remaining drug. The subject of drug interactions has been extensively reviewed [1]. Combinations of drugs with potential adverse interactions continue to be prescribed [2].

Intestinal drug interactions. Examples are that phenobarbitone inhibits absorption of griseofulvin [1], antacids inhibit absorption of tetracycline [3] and tetracycline may decrease absorption of the oral contraceptive [4]. Whether the latter is of real significance is a matter of debate [5].

Displacement from carrier or receptor sites. Most drugs are reversibly bound to carrier proteins in plasma or extracellular fluid; bound drug acts as a reservoir, preventing excessive fluctuation in the level of the active unbound fraction. Displacement from a carrier protein augments drug activity, while displacement from a receptor site diminishes it. Many acidic drugs such as salicylates, coumarins, sulphonamides and phenylbutazone are bound to plasma albumin, and compete for binding sites. Thus, a sulphonamide may displace tolbutamide from albumin leading to hypoglycaemia; or aspirin, sulphonamides, clofibrate or phenylbutazone may displace warfarin from albumin, causing bleeding and ecchymoses. Similarly, sulphonamides and aspirin may increase methotrexate toxicity. Ciprofloxacin increases plasma levels of theophylline.

Enzyme stimulation or inhibition. A drug may either stimulate or inhibit metabolic enzymes important to its own degradation or that of another agent, with significant clinical consequences. Thus, some drugs induce synthesis of drug-metabolizing enzymes in liver microsomes. The liver microsomal hydroxylating system (which mediates metabolism of phenytoin and debrisoquine) is based on cytochrome P-450, and appears to be a family of enzymes capable of acting on different substrates including barbiturates, fatty acids and endogenous steroids. The cytochrome P-450-dependent system also catalyses deamination (e.g. amphetamine), dealkylation (e.g. morphine, azathioprine), sulphoxidation (e.g. chlorpromazine, phenylbutazone), desulphuration (thiopentone) and dehalogenation (e.g. halogenated anaesthetics). This lack of specificity accounts for the ability of an inducing agent to stimulate metabolism of many other drugs, and of one drug to inhibit metabolism of a structurally unrelated drug. Antibiotics, if administered over a period (e.g. rifampicin for tuberculosis), can be enzyme inducers. Barbiturates stimulate metabolism of griseofulvin, phenytoin and coumarin anticoagulants, and griseofulvin induces increased metabolism of coumarins. Similarly, rifampicin, phenytoin and carbamazepine increase the metabolism of cyclosporin A [6]. Drugs causing enzyme inhibition include chloramphenicol, cimetidine, monoamine oxidase inhibitors, *p*-aminosalicylic acid, pethidine and morphine. Dicoumarol, chloramphenicol and phenylbutazone inhibit metabolic inactivation of tolbutamide. Allopurinol inhibits metabolism of azathioprine and mercaptopurine by xanthine oxidase. Cimetidine inhibits liver enzymes and decreases hepatic blood flow, therefore potentiating the action of some β-blockers (propranolol) and benzodiazepines, carbamazepine, warfarin, morphine, phenytoin and theophylline. Ketoconazole may potentiate oral anticoagulants [7] and erythromycin may potentiate carbamazepine [8]; both may potentiate cyclosporin. Nifedipine and cyclosporin are both metabolized by the same cytochrome P-450 enzyme, P-450 cpn; cyclosporin potentiates the action of nifedipine, phenytoin and to a lesser extent valproate by decreasing P-450 cpn availability by competitive inhibition [9].

Altered drug excretion. Examples are the well-known probenecid-induced reduction in the renal excretion of penicillin, and aspirin-induced reduction in renal clearance of methotrexate.

REFERENCES

1 Griffin JP, D'Arcy PF, Speirs CJ. *A Manual of Adverse Drug Interactions*, 4th edn. London: Wright (Butterworth), 1988.
2 Beers MH, Storrie MS, Lee G. Potential adverse drug interactions in the emergency room. An issue in the quality of care. *Ann Intern Med* 1990; **112**: 61–4.
3 Garty M, Hurwitz A. Effect of cimetidine and antacids on gastrointestinal absorption of tetracycline. *Clin Pharmacol Ther* 1980; **28**: 203–7.
4 Bacon JF, Shenfield GM. Pregnancy attributable to interaction between tetracycline and oral contraceptives. *Br Med J* 1980; **280**: 293.
5 Fleischer AB, Resnick SD. The effect of antibiotics on the efficacy of oral contraceptives. *Arch Dermatol* 1989; **125**: 1562–4.
6 Schofield OMV, Camp RDR, Levene GM. Cyclosporin A in psoriasis: interaction with carbamazepine. *Br J Dermatol* 1990; **122**: 425–6.
7 Smith AG. Potentiation of oral anticoagulants by ketoconazole. *Br Med J* 1984; **288**: 188–9.
8 Wroblewski BA, Singer WD, Whyte J. Carbamazepine-erythromycin interaction: Case studies and clinical significance. *JAMA* 1986; **255**: 1165–7.
9 McFadden JP, Pontin JE, Powles AV et al. Cyclosporin decreases nifedipine metabolism. *Br Med J* 1989; **299**: 1224.

Metabolic changes

Drugs may induce cutaneous changes by their effects on nutritional or metabolic status. Thus, drugs such as phenytoin that interfere with folate absorption or metabolism increase the risk of aphthous stomatitis, and isotretinoin may cause xanthomas by elevation of very-low-density lipoproteins (VLDL) [1].

REFERENCE

1 Dicken CH. Eruptive xanthomas associated with isotretinoin (13-*cis*-retinoic acid). *Arch Dermatol* 1980; **116**: 951–2.

Teratogenicity and other effects on the fetus [1–6]

The advent of isotretinoin has focused the attention of dermatologists considerably on the problem of teratogenicity in general [5]. The fetus is particularly at risk from drug-induced developmental malformations during the period of organogenesis, which lasts from about the third to the 10th week of gestation. Thalidomide, retinoids and cytotoxic drugs are proven teratogens. Heavy alcohol intake, which produces the 'fetal alcohol syndrome'; smoking; anticonvulsants (especially phenytoin and trimethadione); warfarin and antiplatelet drugs; inhalational anaesthetics; lithium; quinine; ACE inhibitors; misoprostol; certain antimicrobials, for example trimethoprim, pyramethamine, aminoglycosides, 4-quinolones and itraconazole; and cocaine are probably teratogenic. High-dose corticosteroids have been linked to cleft palate. A major correlation has been found between the incidence of glucocorticoid-induced cleft palate and the chromosome 8 segment identified by *N*-acetyl transferase in mice [7]. 6-aminonicotinamide-induced cleft palate and phenytoin-induced cleft lip with or without cleft palate are also influenced by this genetic region but not as strongly. Sex hormones, psychotropic drugs, benzodiazepines, tetracycline, rifampicin, penicillamine and the folate antagonist pyrimethamine are possibly teratogenic and should be avoided in the first trimester of pregnancy. Chlorpheniramine appears safe to use. The potential adverse effects on the fetus and on the breastfed infant of a number of drugs not infrequently used by the dermatologist have been reviewed [4].

Drugs may also cause fetal damage later in pregnancy. Warfarin may cause haemorrhage, and phenytoin near to term produces a coagulation defect in the neonate, which is correctable by vitamin K. Antithyroid drugs and iodides may cause neonatal goitre and hypothyroidism. Fetal adrenal atrophy may follow high-dose maternal corticosteroid therapy. The non-steroidal anti-inflammatory drugs have various ill effects, although aspirin has been advocated in pregnancy for the prevention of fetal growth retardation. Tetracyclines are deposited in developing bones and cause discoloration and enamel hypoplasia of teeth [8]. Aminoglycoside antibiotics are ototoxic, and chloroquine has caused a neonatal chorioretinitis. Androgens and progestogens may virilize the fetus. Stilboestrol administered from early pregnancy for several months has been associated with female and male genital tract abnormalities, and carcinoma of the vagina 20 years later in the offspring.

REFERENCES

1 Ellis C, Fidler J. Drugs in pregnancy: adverse reactions. *Br J Hosp Med* 1982; **28**: 575–84.
2 Kalter H, Warkany J. Congenital malformations: Etiologic factors and their role in prevention. *N Engl J Med* 1983; **308**: 424–31, 491–7.
3 Ashton CH. Disorders of the fetus and infant. In: Davis DM, ed. *Textbook of Adverse Drug Reactions*, 3rd edn. Oxford: Oxford University Press, 1985: 77–127.
4 Stockton DL, Paller AS. Drug administration to the pregnant or lactating woman: a reference guide for dermatologists. *J Am Acad Dermatol* 1990; **23**: 87–103.
5 Mitchell AA. Teratogens and the dermatologist. New knowledge, responsibilities, and opportunities. *Arch Dermatol* 1991; **127**: 399–401.
6 Ferner RE. Teratogenic drugs—an update. *Adverse Drug Reaction Bull* 1993; **161**: 607–10.

7 Karolyi J, Erickson RP, Liu S, Killewald L. Major effects on teratogen-induced facial clefting in mice determined by a single genetic region. *Genetics* 1990; **126**: 201–5.
8 Witkop CJ, Wolf RO. Hypoplasia and intrinsic staining of enamel following tetracycline therapy. *JAMA* 1963; **185**: 1008–11.

Effects on spermatogenesis

Most chemotherapeutic agents potentially damage sperm; conception should also be avoided after griseofulvin for 3 months. A number of drugs cause oligospermia [1], which may come to light only as a result of infertility investigations; oestrogens, androgens, cyproterone acetate, cytotoxic drugs, including methotrexate given for psoriasis [2], colchicine, most monoamine oxidase inhibitors, keto-conazole and sulphasalazine have all been incriminated. The synthetic retinoids isotretinoin and etretinate do not seem to affect the numbers of sperm [3,4].

REFERENCES

1 Drife JO. Drugs and sperm. *Br Med J* 1982; **284**: 844–5.
2 Sussman A, Leonard J. Psoriasis, methotrexate, and oligospermia. *Arch Dermatol* 1980; **116**: 215–17.
3 Schill W-B, Wagner A, Nikolowski JM, Plewig G. Aromatic retinoid and 13-cis- retinoic acid: spermatological investigations. In: Orfanos CE, Braun-Falco O, Farber EM *et al.*, eds. *Retinoids, Advances in Basic Research and Therapy.* Berlin: Springer-Verlag, 1981: 389–95.
4 Töröck L, Kása M. Spermatological and endocrinological examinations connected with isotretinoin treatment. In: Saurat JH, ed. *Retinoids: New Trends in Research and Therapy.* Basel: Karger, 1985: 407–10.

Non-immunological activation of effector pathways (anaphylactoid reactions)

Certain drugs, such as opiates, codeine, amphetamine, polymyxin B, *d*-tubocurarine, atropine, hydralazine, pentamidine, quinine and radiocontrast media, may release mast-cell mediators directly to produce urticaria or angio-oedema [1–6]. Some drugs, such as radiocontrast media, may activate complement by an antibody-independent method [7]. Anaphylactic-like responses to cyclo-oxygenase inhibitors such as aspirin and other non-steroidal anti-inflammatory agents may lead to amplified mast-cell degranulation and enhanced biosynthesis of lipoxygenase products of arachidonic acid, which cause vasodilatation and oedema [8,9]. ACE inhibitors, which cause or exacerbate angio-oedema, may potentiate bradykinin activity; they have been reported to enhance bradykinin-induced cutaneous wheals in normal individuals [10,11].

REFERENCES

1 Schoenfeld MR. Acute allergic reactions to morphine, codeine, meperidine hydrochloride and opium alkaloids. *NY State J Med* 1960; **60**: 2591–3.
2 Comroe JH, Dripps RD. Histamine-like action of curare and tubocurarine injected intracutaneously and intra-arterially in man. *Anesthesiology* 1946; **7**: 260–2.

3 Greenberger PA. Contrast media reactions. *J Allergy Clin Immunol* 1984; **74**: 600–5.
4 Assem ESK, Bray K, Dawson P. The release of histamine from human basophils by radiological contrast agents. *Br J Radiol* 1983; **56**: 647–52.
5 Rice MC, Lieberman P, Siegle RL, Mason J. *In vitro* histamine release induced by radiocontrast media and various chemical analogs in reactor and control subjects. *J Allergy Clin Immunol* 1983; **72**: 180–6.
6 Watkins J. Markers and mechanisms of anaphylactoid reactions. *Monogr Allergy* 1992; **30**: 108–29.
7 Arroyave CM, Bhatt KN, Crown NR. Activation of the alternative pathway of the complement system by radiographic contrast media. *J Immunol* 1976; **117**: 1866–9.
8 Stevenson DD, Lewis RA. Proposed mechanisms of aspirin sensitivity reactions. *J Allergy Clin Immunol* 1987; **80**: 788–90.
9 Morassut P, Yang W, Karsh J. Aspirin intolerance. *Semin Arthr Rheum* 1989; **19**: 22–30.
10 Wood SM, Mann RD, Rawlins MD. Angio-oedema and urticaria associated with angiotensin converting enzyme inhibitors. *Br Med J* 1987; **294**: 91–2.
11 Ferner RE. Effects of intradermal bradykinin after inhibition of angiotensin converting enzyme. *Br Med J* 1987; **294**: 1119–20.

Exacerbation of disease

Examples of adverse drug effects on pre-existing skin conditions include: lithium exacerbation of acne and psoriasis, β-blocker induction of a psoriasiform dermatitis [1] and corticosteroid withdrawal resulting in exacerbation of psoriasis; cimetidine, penicillin or sulphonamide exacerbation of LE; and vasodilator exacerbation of rosacea. Sometimes, a drug may unmask a latent condition, as when barbiturates precipitate symptoms of porphyria.

REFERENCE

1 Abel EA, Dicicco LM, Orenberg EK *et al.* Drugs in exacerbation of psoriasis. *J Am Acad Dermatol* 1986; **15**: 1007–22.

Intolerance

The characteristic effects of the drug are produced to an exaggerated extent by an abnormally small dose. This may simply represent an extreme within normal biological variation. Alternatively, the intolerance may be contributed to by delayed metabolism or excretion due to impaired hepatic or renal function, or by genetic variation in the rate of drug metabolism (see below).

Idiosyncrasy

This term describes an uncharacteristic response, not predictable from animal experiments, and not mediated by an immunological mechanism. The cause is often unknown, but genetic variation in metabolic pathways may be involved. Such genetic abnormalities include: glucose-6-phosphate dehydrogenase (G6PD) deficiency, hereditary met-haemoglobinaemia, porphyria, glucocorticoid glaucoma and malignant hyperthermia of anaesthesia, all of which are characterized by unusual pharmacological responses to various drugs.

Pharmacogenetic mechanisms and genetic influences underlying intolerance and idiosyncratic reactions [1–3]

The pharmacokinetics of drugs, including their absorption, plasma protein binding, distribution, metabolism and elimination, may be influenced by genetic factors. Oxidation, hydrolysis and acetylation are the three metabolic pathways most subject to genetic influence. Genetic factors also influence pharmacodynamics, i.e. tissue or organ responsiveness. Thus genetic variations in all these areas may underlie both intolerance and idiosyncrasy. Variation in the regulation and expression of the human cytochrome P-450 enzyme system may play a key role in both interindividual variation in sensitivity to drug toxicity and tissue-specific damage [4]. Pharmacogenetic variability probably underlies reactions such as TEN. It has been proposed that most patients who have a severe adverse cutaneous drug reaction have an abnormal metabolism of the offending drug [5].

Examples of genetically mediated intolerance include pupil size responses to phenylephrine and parasympatholytics and the very rare dominantly inherited familial resistance to coumarin anticoagulants, the result of mutation in the receptor for vitamin K and anticoagulants. Low red cell G6PD levels, inherited as a sex-linked dominant, are common in black people, certain Levantine peoples and Philippinos, and result in a chronic deficit of reduced glutathione sulphydryl (SH) groups. Affected individuals are at risk of acute haemolysis on exposure to antimalarials, sulphonamides, dapsone, nitrofurantoin, phenacetin, aspirin and chloramphenicol, all of which may oxidize the few reduced SH groups in older red cells. Genetic variation in thiopurine methyltransferase activity may be linked to the side-effects of azathioprine therapy, as homozygotes for the low activity allele are at risk of myelosuppression, while homozygotes for high activity are inadequately immunosuppressed with conventional doses of azthioprine [6]. Increased susceptibility to aminoglycoside-induced deafness in two Japanese pedigrees was associated with a particular mitochondrial DNA polymorphism [7].

REFERENCES

1 Rawlins MD, Thompson JW. Mechanisms of adverse drug reactions. In: Davies DM, ed. *Textbook of Adverse Drug Reactions*, 3rd edn. Oxford: Oxford University Press, 1985: 12–38.
2 Shear NH, Bhimji S. Pharmacogenetics and cutaneous drug reactions. *Semin Dermatol* 1989; **8**: 219–26.
3 Lennard MS, Tucker GT, Woods HF. Inborn 'errors' of drug metabolism. Pharmacokinetic and clinical implications. *Clin Pharmacokinet* 1990; **19**: 257–63.
4 Park BK, Pirmohamed M, Kitteringham NR. The role of cytochrome P450 enzymes in hepatic and extrahepatic human drug toxicity. *Pharmacol Ther* 1995; **68**: 385–424.
5 Chosidow O, Bourgault L, Roujeau JC. Drug rashes. What are the targets of cell-mediated cytotoxicity? *Arch Dermatol* 1994; **130**: 627–9.
6 Snow JL, Gibson LE. The role of genetic variation in thiopurine methyl-
transferase activity and the efficacy and/or side effects of azathioprine therapy in dermatologic patients. *Arch Dermatol* 1995; **131**: 193–7.
7 Hutchin T, Haworth I, Higashi K et al. A molecular basis for human hypersensitivity to aminoglycoside antibiotics. *Nucleic Acids Res* 1993; **21**: 4174–9.

Oxidation. Anticonvulsants, many hypnotics, tricyclic antidepressants, anticoagulants and various anti-inflammatory and anxiolytic agents are eliminated by oxidation. For many drugs, oxidation rates vary as a continuous spectrum within the population. Genetic differences in metabolism of sulphonamides may underlie idiosyncratic toxicity [1–6]. Oxidative metabolism of sulphonamides by cytochrome P-450 enzymes and *N*-acetylation yields a reactive hydroxylamine intermediate [7], which is inactivated by glutathione conjugation. The hydroxylamine metabolite is toxic to lymphocytes, and the lymphocyte toxicity is markedly increased in patients with a history of hypersensitivity or with glutathione synthetase deficiency. HIV-positive individuals have been reported in some studies to have a systemic glutathione deficiency, resulting in a decreased capacity to scavenge hydroxylamine derivatives of sulphonamides, which may partially explain the increased frequency of sulphonamide reactions [8–10]. However, other studies have not been able to confirm intracellular glutathione deficiency in peripheral blood cells of HIV-infected patients [11,12].

Phenytoin, phenobarbital and carbamazepine are oxidized by the cytochrome P-450 enzyme system into potentially reactive arene-oxide intermediates; liver microsomal epoxide hydrolase (mEH) converts such reactive intermediates to non-toxic dihydrodiols [13–16]. Phenytoin hypersensitivity syndrome appears to be associated with an inherited deficiency of epoxide hydrolase, which is primarily responsible for detoxifying the toxic arene-oxide intermediate [13–15]. Activated phenytoin was shown to be toxic to lymphocytes from patients with phenytoin reactions and, to a lesser degree, to lymphocytes from their parents [15]. However, a genetic defect altering the structure and function of the mEH protein was thought unlikely to be responsible for predisposing patients to anticonvulsant adverse reactions in another study [16].

Increased toxic effects of culprit drug-reactive metabolites, generated by a microsomal oxidation system, were found toward lymphoid cells in patients with TEN (13 each with sulphonamide and anticonvulsant reactions) and in first-degree relatives, while oxygen free radical and/or aldehyde detoxification pathways were normal [17].

Impaired metabolism of phenacetin and phenformin, inherited as a result of genetic polymorphism in liver microsomal oxidation, may result in adverse reactions [18,19]. The induction of liver enzymes responsible for drug oxidation may itself be under genetic control [20]. There is a fourfold increase in toxicity with penicillamine in patients with rheumatoid arthritis with a genetically determined poor capacity to sulphoxidate the structurally related mucolytic agent, carbocysteine [21].

REFERENCES

1 Shear NH, Spielberg SP. *In vitro* evaluation of a toxic metabolite of sulfadiazide. *Can J Physiol Pharmacol* 1985; **63**: 1370–2.
2 Shear NH, Spielberg SP. An *in vitro* lymphocytotoxicity assay for studying adverse reactions to sulphonamides. *Br J Dermatol* 1985; **113**: 112–13.
3 Shear N, Spielberg S, Grant D *et al*. Differences in metabolism of sulfonamides predisposing to idiosyncratic toxicity. *Ann Intern Med* 1986; **105**: 179–84.
4 Anonymous. Hypersensitivity to sulphonamides—A clue? (Editorial). *Lancet* 1986; **ii**: 958–9.
5 Rieder MJ, Uetrecht J, Shear NH *et al*. Synthesis and *in vitro* toxicity of hydroxylamine metabolites of sulphonamides. *J Pharmacol Exp Ther* 1988; **244**: 724–8.
6 Rieder MJ, Uetrecht J, Shear NH *et al*. Diagnosis of sulfonamide hypersensitivity reactions by in-vitro 'rechallenge' with hydroxylamine metabolites. *Ann Intern Med* 1989; **110**: 286–9.
7 Meekins CV, Sullivan TJ, Gruchalla RS. Immunochemical analysis of sulfonamide drug allergy: identification of sulfamethoxazole-substituted human serum proteins. *J Allergy Clin Immunol* 1994; **94**: 1017–24.
8 Buhl R, Jaffe HA, Holroyd KJ *et al*. Systemic glutathione deficiency in symptom-free HIV-seropositive individuals. *Lancet* 1989; **334**: 1294–8.
9 van der Ven AJAM, Koopmans PP, Vree TB, van der Meer JWM. Adverse reactions to co-trimoxazole in HIV infection. *Lancet* 1991; **338**: 431–3.
10 Koopmans PP, van der Ven AJ, Vree TB, van der Meer JWM. Pathogenesis of hypersensitivity reactions to drugs in patients with HIV infection: allergic or toxic? *AIDS* 1995; **9**: 217–22.
11 Aukrust P, Svardal AM, Muller F *et al*. Increased levels of oxidized glutathione in CD4+ lymphocytes associated with disturbed intracellular redox balance in human immunodeficiency type 1 infection. *Blood* 1995; **86**: 258–67.
12 Pirmohamed M, Williams D, Tingle MD *et al*. Intracellular glutathione in the peripheral blood cells of HIV-infected patients: failure to show a deficiency. *AIDS* 1996; **10**: 501–7.
13 Shear NH, Spielberg SP. Anticonvulsant hypersensitivity syndrome. *In vitro* assessment of risk. *J Clin Invest* 1988; **82**: 1826–32.
14 Spielberg SP, Gordon GB, Blake DA *et al*. Predisposition to phenytoin hepatotoxicity assessed *in vitro*. *N Engl J Med* 1981; **305**: 722–7.
15 Spielberg SP. *In vitro* assessment of pharmacogenetic susceptibility to toxic drug metabolites in humans. *Fed Proc* 1984; **43**: 2308–13.
16 Gaedigk A, Spielberg SP, Grant DM. Characterization of the microsomal epoxide hydrolase gene in patients with anticonvulsant adverse drug reactions. *Pharmacogenetics* 1994; **4**: 142–53.
17 Wolkenstein P, Charue D, Laurent P *et al*. Metabolic predisposition to cutaneous adverse drug reactions. Role in toxic epidermal necrolysis caused by sulfonamides and anticonvulsants. *Arch Dermatol* 1995; **131**: 544–51.
18 Shahidi NT. Acetophenetidin sensitivity. *Am J Dis Child* 1967; **113**: 81–2.
19 Eichelbaum M. Defective oxidation of drugs: pharmacokinetic and therapeutic implications. *Clin Pharmacokin* 1982; **7**: 1–22.
20 Vessell ES, Passananti T, Greene FE, Page JG. Genetic control of drug levels and of the induction of drug-metabolizing enzymes in man: individual variability in the extent of allopurinol and nortryptiline inhibition of drug metabolism. *Ann NY Acad Sci* 1971; **179**: 752–3.
21 Dasgupta B. Adverse reactions profile: 2. Penicillamine. *Prescribers' J* 1991; **31**: 72–7.

Hydrolysis. Genetic influence on drug hydrolysis is well illustrated in the case of suxamethonium, which normally results in only very brief neuromuscular blockade due to rapid hydrolysis by plasma pseudocholinesterase. Genetically determined atypical cholinesterases cannot hydrolyse the drug, leading to prolonged apnoea in affected individuals; conversely, dominantly inherited resistance to suxamethonium, mediated by a highly active cholinesterase, has been reported.

Acetylation. Isoniazid, many sulphonamides, hydralazine, dapsone, procainamide, etc. are inactivated by conversion to acetyl conjugates. Acetylation rates vary greatly, with a bimodal frequency distribution, and there is marked ethnic variation. Rapid inactivation is dominantly inherited, and is commonest amongst Eskimos and Japanese and least common amongst certain Mediterranean Jews. The LE-like syndrome due to procainamide may occur more in fast acetylators, implying that a conjugate and not the parent compound is responsible [1]. Slow acetylators, in whom higher and more persistent drug levels occur, are more liable to develop adverse reactions to isoniazid (pellagra-like syndrome and peripheral neuritis), dapsone (haemolysis) [2] and hydralazine (LE-like syndrome) [3,4]. A slow acetylation phenotype is a risk factor for hypersensitivity to trimethoprim–sulphamethoxazole in HIV-infected subjects [5,6], and for sulphonamide-induced TEN and Stevens–Johnson syndrome independent of HIV infection [7,8].

REFERENCES

1 Davies DM, Beedie MA, Rawlins MD. Antinuclear antibodies during procainamide treatment and drug acetylation. *Br Med J* 1975; **iii**: 682–4.
2 Ellard GA, Gammon PT, Savin LA, Tan RSH. Dapsone acetylation in dermatitis herpetiformis. *Br J Dermatol* 1974; **90**: 441–4.
3 Perry HM JR, Sakamoto A, Tan EM. Relationship of acetylating enzyme to hydralazine toxicity. *J Lab Clin Med* 1967; **70**: 1020–1.
4 Russell GI, Bing RF, Jones JA *et al*. Hydralazine sensitivity: clinical features, autoantibody changes and HLA-DR phenotype. *Q J Med* 1987; **65**: 845–52.
5 Carr A, Gross AS, Hoskins JM *et al*. Acetylation phenotype and cutaneous hypersensitivity to trimethoprim–sulphamethoxazole in HIV-infected patients. *AIDS* 1994; **8**: 333–7.
6 Delomenie C, Grant DM, Mathelier-Fusade P *et al*. N-acetylation genotype and risk of severe reactions to sulphonamides in AIDS patients. *Br J Clin Pharmacol* 1994; **38**: 581–2.
7 Wolkenstein P, Carriere V, Charue D *et al*. A slow acetylator genotype is a risk factor for sulphonamide-induced toxic epidermal necrolysis and Stevens–Johnson syndrome. *Pharmacogenetics* 1995; **5**: 255–8.
8 Dietrich A, Kawakubo Y, Rzany B *et al*. Low N-acetylating capacity in patients with Stevens–Johnson syndrome and toxic epidermal necrolysis. *Exp Dermatol* 1995; **4**: 313–16.

Influence of human leukocyte antigen (HLA)-types. An association between HLA types and susceptibility to drug eruptions has been reported on several occasions, particularly in relation to gold (HLA-DRw3, HLA-DR5 and HLA-B8) and penicillamine toxicity [1–6]. Penicillamine toxicity is associated with HLA phenotypes as follows [1]: HLA-DR3 and -B8 are associated with renal toxicity, -DR3, -B7 and -DR2 with haematological toxicity, -A1 and -DR4 with thrombocytopenia, and cutaneous adverse reactions are linked to HLA-DRW6. DR1/DR4 heterozygosity, or the DR5 subtypes DRB1* 1102 or DRB1*1201, were found in 61% of patients with intolerance to tiopronin given for rheumatoid arthritis [7].

A positive association with AW33 and B17/BW58 haplotypes, and a negative association with the A2 haplotype, has been reported in southern Chinese patients with drug eruptions after exposure to allopurinol [8]. Aspirin-sensitive asthma is associated with HLA-DQw2 [9]. HLA-linkage associations with certain bullous disorders have been reported [10,11]. Hydralazine-induced LE is commonest in female patients with the HLA-DRw4 haplotype [12,13]. The above findings indicate that there may be genetic predisposition to develop certain drug eruptions.

REFERENCES

1 Dasgupta B. Adverse reactions profile: 2. Penicillamine. *Prescribers' J* 1991; **31**: 72–7.
2 Wooley PH, Griffin J, Payani GS *et al*. HLA-DR antigens and toxic reaction to sodium aurothiomalate and D-penicillamine in patients with rheumatoid arthritis. *N Engl J Med* 1980; **303**: 300–2.
3 Latts JR, Antel JP, Levinson DJ *et al*. Histocompatibility antigens and gold toxicity: a preliminary report. *J Clin Pharmacol* 1980; **20**: 206–9.
4 Bardin T, Dryll A, Debeyre N *et al*. HLA system and side effects of gold salts and D-penicillamine treatment of rheumatoid arthritis. *Ann Rheum Dis* 1982; **41**: 599–601.
5 Emery P, Panayi GS, Huston G *et al*. D penicillamine induced toxicity in rheumatoid arthritis: the role of sulphoxidation status and HLA-DR3. *J Rheumatol* 1984; **11**: 626–32.
6 Rodriguez-Perez M, Gonzalez-Dominguez J, Mataran L *et al*. Association of HLA-DR5 with mucocutaneous lesions in patients with rheumatoid arthritis receiving gold sodium thiomalate. *J Rheumatol* 1994; **21**: 41–3.
7 Ju LY, Paolozzi L, Delecoeuillerie G *et al*. A possible linkage of HLA-DRB haplotypes with tiopronin intolerance in rheumatoid arthritis. *Clin Exp Rheumatol* 1994; **12**: 249–54.
8 Chan SH, Tan T. HLA and allopurinol drug eruption. *Dermatologica* 1989; **179**: 32–3.
9 Mullarkey MF, Thomas PS, Hansen JA *et al*. Association of aspirin-sensitive asthma with HLA-DQw2. *Am Rev Respir Dis* 1986; **133**: 261–3.
10 Roujeau J-C, Bracq C, Huyn NT *et al*. HLA phenotypes and bullous cutaneous reactions to drugs. *Tissue Antigens* 1986; **28**: 251–4.
11 Mobini N, Ahmed AR. Immunogenetics of drug-induced bullous diseases. *Clin Dermatol* 1993; **11**: 449–60.
12 Batchelor JR, Welsh KI, Mansilla Tinoco R *et al*. Hydralazine-induced systemic lupus erythematosus: influence of HLA-DR and sex on susceptibility. *Lancet* 1980; **i**: 1107–9.
13 Russell GI, Bing RF, Jones JA *et al*. Hydralazine sensitivity: clinical features, autoantibody changes and HLA-DR phenotype. *Q J Med* 1987; **65**: 845–52.

Drug-induced chromosomal damage [1–3]

This may be studied by examining the chromosomes of patients or animals exposed to drugs, or *in vitro* by the addition of drugs to cell cultures; substances capable of inducing chromosomal damage are termed clastogens. Effects may be dose related, but *in vitro* results may not be representative of the *in vivo* situation. Antimitotic and antibiotic agents have been the most studied, but psychotropics, anticonvulsants, hallucinogens, immuno-suppressants and oral contraceptives have also been investigated and shown to cause, in varying degree, chromosomal damage. Damage ranges from staining variations through 'gaps' in staining, chromosome breaks, gross aberrations such as deletions, fragments, translocations, inversions, etc. to polyploidy. Such damage may be stable and retained over a succession of cell divisions, or transient.

REFERENCES

1 Shaw MW. Human chromosome damage by chemical agents. *Ann Rev Med* 1970; **21**: 409–32.
2 Bender MA, Griggs HG, Bedford JS. Mechanisms of chromosomal aberration production. III, Chemicals and ionizing radiation. *Mutat Res* 1974; **23**: 197–212.
3 Rawlins MD, Thompson JW. Mechanisms of adverse drug reactions. In: Davies DM, ed. *Textbook of Adverse Drug Reactions*, 3rd edn. Oxford: Oxford University Press, 1985; 12–38.

Miscellaneous

Jarisch–Herxheimer reaction

This is the focal exacerbation of lesions of infective origin when potent antimicrobial therapy is initiated, and is classically observed in the treatment of early syphilis with penicillin; it may also occur 3 days after starting griseofulvin therapy, during therapy with diethyl-carbamazine for onchocerciasis and thiabendazole for strongyloidiasis, and with penicillin or minocycline for erythema chronic migrans due to *Borrelia burgdorferi* infection [1]. The reaction has been attributed to sudden release of pharmacologically and/or immunologically active substances from killed microorganisms or damaged tissues. There is, however, little evidence that it is an allergic reaction [2]. Clinically there may be fever, rigors, lymphadenopathy, arthralgia, and transient macular urticarial eruptions; a vesicular eruption has also been described [3].

REFERENCES

1 Weber K. Jarisch–Herxheimer-Reaktion bei Erythema-migrans-Krankheit. *Hautarzt* 1984; **35**: 588–90.
2 Skog E, Gudjónsson H. On the allergic origin of the Jarisch–Herxheimer reaction. *Acta Derm Venereol (Stockh)* 1966; **46**: 136–43.
3 Rosen T, Rubin H, Ellner K *et al*. Vesicular Jarisch–Herxheimer reaction. *Arch Dermatol* 1989; **125**: 77–81.

Infectious mononucleosis-ampicillin reaction. Ampicillin almost always causes a severe morbilliform eruption when given to a patient with infectious mononucleosis or lymphatic leukaemia (see later). The reaction occurs much less frequently with amoxycillin. The exact mechanism responsible is not known.

Immunological drug reactions

Allergic hypersensitivity reactions result from immunological sensitization to a drug, by previous exposure to that drug or to a chemically related cross-reacting substance [1–7]. Although drugs frequently elicit an immune response, clinically evident hypersensitivity reactions are manifest only in a small proportion of exposed individuals. Thus, using highly sensitive passive haemagglutination assays, IgM class antibodies to the penicilloyl group (the major hapten determinant derived from penicillin) are detectable in almost 100% of normal individuals, even in the absence of a history of penicillin therapy; 40% of patients receiving more than 2g of penicillin for more than 10 days develop IgG class antibodies [8]. Macromolecular drugs such as protein or peptide hormones, insulin or dextran are antigenic in their own right. By contrast, most drugs are small organic molecules with a molecular mass of less than 1kDa; conjugation of free drug as a hapten with a macromolecular carrier is then required to initiate an immune response. Fortunately, many drugs have only a limited capacity to form covalent bonds with tissue proteins. Clinical sensitization may also result from allergy to reactive drug metabolites as haptens, or to minor contaminants.

Clinical features distinguishing allergic from non-allergic drug reactions. Prior exposure before sensitization should have been without adverse effect. If there has been no previous exposure, there should be a latent period of several days of uneventful therapy before the reaction supervenes, during which primary sensitization occurs. Thereafter, reactions may develop within minutes (or even seconds) and certainly within 24h. Allergic reactions do not resemble the pharmacological action of the drug, may follow exposure to doses far below the therapeutic level and are reproducible on readministration (if judged safe).

Factors concerned in the development of hypersensitivity. The route of administration of a drug may affect its immunogenicity and the nature of any allergy. Topical drug exposure is more likely to result in sensitization than oral administration, and favours development of contact dermatitis; thus, poison ivy is a potent contact sensitizer, but oral ingestion may promote tolerance. Anaphylaxis is more likely to be associated with intravenous drug administration. However, anaphylaxis may sometimes occur as fast after oral penicillin administration [9]. Whether allergy develops or not may also depend on the antigenic load in terms of degree of drug exposure, and individual genetic variation in drug absorption and metabolism. Thus, as stated above, an LE-like syndrome with antinuclear antibody formation following hydralazine therapy occurs more frequently in slow acetylators of the drug [10]. Hydralazine-related systemic LE is 10 times more frequent in HLA-DR4-positive patients than in the population at large, and is commoner in females. Allergic drug reactions are less common in childhood and possibly in the aged; in the latter, this may be related to impaired immunological responsiveness. Immunosuppression may increase the risk by inhibiting the regulatory function of suppressor T cells [11]. Environmental factors may also affect susceptibility to drug hypersensitivity, as for example the well recognized increase in ampicillin-induced morbilliform eruptions associated with infectious mononucleosis, and photo-allergic reactions to drugs such as thiazide diuretics or phenothiazines.

The duration of hypersensitivity. The duration of allergic sensitivity is unpredictable. Although there is a general tendency for immunological responses to a drug to fall off with time, provided the patient is not re-exposed to the drug or a related substance, this can never be relied on; where necessary, safe confirmatory procedures (if available) should be carried out.

REFERENCES

1 de Weck AL. Pathophysiologic mechanisms of allergic and pseudo-allergic reactions to foods, food additives and drugs. *Ann Allergy* 1984; **53**: 583–6.
2 Wintroub BU, Stern R. Cutaneous drug reactions: pathogenesis and clinical classification. *J Am Acad Dermatol* 1985; **13**: 833–45.
3 Rawlins MD, Thompson JW. Mechanisms of adverse drug reactions. In: Davies DM, ed. *Textbook of Adverse Drug Reactions*, 3rd edn. Oxford: Oxford University Press, 1985; 12–38.
4 De Swarte RD. Drug allergy: An overview. *Clin Rev Allergy* 1986; **4**: 143–69.
5 Stern RS, Wintroub BU, Arndt KA. Drug reactions. *J Am Acad Dermatol* 1986; **15**: 1282–8.
6 Blaiss MS, de Shazo RD. Drug allergy. *Pediatr Clin North Am* 1988; **35**: 1131–47.
7 Kalish RS. Drug eruptions: a review of clinical and immunological features. *Adv Dermatol* 1991; **6**: 221–37.
8 Weiss ME, Adkinson NF. Immediate hypersensitivity reactions to penicillin and related antibiotics. *Clin Allergy* 1988; **18**: 515–40.
9 Simmonds J, Hodges S, Nicol F, Barnett D. Anaphylaxis after oral penicillin. *Br Med J* 1978; **ii**: 1404.
10 Perry HM, Jr, Sakamoto A, Tan EM. Relationship of acetylating enzyme to hydralazine toxicity. *J Lab Clin Med* 1967; **70**: 1020–1.
11 Lakin JD, Grace WR, Sell KW. IgE antipolymyxin B antibody formation in a T-cell depleted bone marrow transplant patient. *J Allergy Clin Immunol* 1975; **56**: 94–103.

Drug eruptions may occur as a result of a variety of different immunological mechanisms as described below (see also Chapter 10).

IgE-dependent (type I) drug reactions: urticaria and anaphylaxis [1]

In vivo cross-linkage by polyvalent drug–protein conjugates of two or more specific IgE molecules, fixed to sensitized tissue mast cells or circulating basophil leukocytes, triggers the cell to release a variety of chemical mediators including histamine, peptides such as eosinophil chemotactic factor of anaphylaxis, lipids such as leukotriene C_4 or prostaglandin D_2, and a variety of pro-inflammatory cytokines [2]. These in turn have effects on a variety of target tissues including skin, respiratory, gastrointestinal and/or cardiovascular systems. Eosinophil degranulation may also result in release of pro-inflammatory mediators [3]. Dilatation and increased permeability of small blood vessels with resultant oedema and hypotension, contraction of bronchiolar smooth muscle and excessive mucus secretion, and chemotaxis of inflammatory cells, including polymorphs and eosinophils, occurs. Clinically, this may produce pruritus, urticaria, bronchospasm, laryngeal oedema and in severe cases anaphylactic shock with hypotension and possible death. Immediate reactions occur within minutes of drug administration; accelerated reactions may occur within hours or days, and are generally urticarial but may involve laryngeal oedema. Penicillins are the commonest cause of IgE-dependent drug eruptions.

REFERENCES

1 Champion RH, Greaves MW, Kobza Black A, eds. *The Urticarias*. Edinburgh: Churchill Livingstone, 1985.
2 Schwartz LB. Mast cells and their role in urticaria. *J Am Acad Dermatol* 1991; **25**: 190–204.
3 Leiferman KM. A current perspective on the role of eosinophils in dermatologic diseases. *J Am Acad Dermatol* 1991; **24**: 1101–12.

Antibody-mediated (type II) drug reactions

Binding of antibody to cells may lead to cell damage following complement-mediated cytolysis. The classical example of immune complex formation between a drug (as hapten) bound to the surface of a cell (in this case, platelets) and IgG-class antibody, with subsequent complement fixation, was the purpura caused by apronalide (Sedormid). A further example is the thrombocytopenic purpura that may result from antibodies to quinidine–platelet conjugates [1,2]. A number of drugs including penicillin, quinine and sulphonamides may rarely produce a haemolytic anaemia by this method. Methyldopa very occasionally induces a haemolytic anaemia mediated by autoantibodies directed against red-cell antigens.

REFERENCES

1 Christie DJ, Weber RW, Mullen PC *et al.* Structural features of the quinidine and quinine molecules necessary for binding of drug-induced antibodies to human platelets. *J Lab Clin Med* 1984; **104**: 730–40.
2 Gary M, Ilfeld D, Kelton JG. Correlation of a quinidine-induced platelet-specific antibody with development of thrombocytopenia. *Am J Med* 1985; **79**: 253–5.

Immune complex-dependent (type III) drug reactions

Urticaria and anaphylaxis. Immune complexes may activate the complement cascade, with resultant formation of anaphylatoxins such as the complement protein fragments C3a and C5a, which trigger release of mediators from mast cells and basophils directly, resulting in urticaria or anaphylaxis.

Serum sickness. Serum sickness-like reactions and other immune complex-mediated conditions necessitate a drug antigen to persist in the circulation for long enough for antibody, largely of IgG or IgM class, to be synthesized and to combine with it to form circulating antibody–antigen immune complexes. They therefore develop about 6 days or more after drug administration. Serum sickness occurs when antibody combines with antigen in antigen excess, leading to slow removal of persistent complexes by the mononuclear phagocyte system. It was usually seen in the context of serum therapy with large doses of heterologous antibody, as with horse antiserum for the treatment of diphtheria. It has been reported more recently with antilymphocyte globulin therapy [1]. Clinical manifestations of serum sickness include fever, arthritis, nephritis, neuritis, oedema, and an urticarial or papular rash.

Vasculitis [2–4]. Drug-induced immune complexes play a part in the pathogenesis of cutaneous necrotizing vasculitis. Deposition of immune complexes on vascular endothelium results in activation of the complement cascade, with generation of the anaphylatoxins C3a and C5a, which have chemotactic properties. Vasoactive amines and pro-inflammatory cytokines are released from basophils and mast cells, with resultant increased vascular permeability and attraction of neutrophil polymorphonuclear cells. Immune complex interaction with platelets via their Fc receptors causes platelet aggregation and microthrombus formation. Release by neutrophils of lysosomal enzymes contributes further to local inflammation. These events lead to the histological appearance of leukocytoclastic vasculitis. Deposition of immunoglobulins and complement in and around blood vessel walls is detectable by direct immunofluorescence staining of skin biopsies. Hydralazine and the hydroxylamine metabolite of procainamide bind to complement component C4 and inhibits its function; this may impair clearance of immune complexes, and predispose to development of an LE syndrome [4].

The Arthus reaction. The Arthus reaction is a localized form of immune complex vasculitis. Intradermal or subcutaneous injection of antigen such as a vaccine into a sensitized individual with circulating precipitating antibodies, usually of IgG_1 class, leads to local immune complex formation and the cascade of events described above. Clinically, there is erythema and oedema, haemorrhage, and occasionally necrosis at the injection site, which reaches a peak at 4–10h, and then gradually wanes.

REFERENCES

1 Lawley TJ, Bielory L, Gascon P *et al.* A prospective clinical and immunologic analysis of patients with serum sickness. *N Engl J Med* 1984; **311**: 1407–13.
2 Mackel SE, Jordon RE. Leukocytoclastic vasculitis. A cutaneous expression of immune complex disease. *Arch Dermatol* 1983; **118**: 296–301.
3 Sams WM. Hypersensitivity angiitis. *J Invest Dermatol* 1989; **93**: 78S–81S.
4 Sim E. Drug-induced immune complex disease. *Complement Inflamm* 1989; **6**: 119–26.

Cell-mediated reactions (type IV reactions)

The role of delayed type cell-mediated immune reactions in contact drug hypersensitivity, as to penicillin [1], is well established, but the importance of such mechanisms involving specific effector lymphocytes in other varieties of cutaneous drug allergy is uncertain. It is nevertheless thought that a number of drug reactions, including erythema multiforme, TEN, lichenoid reactions, LE-like reactions and some morbilliform reactions, involve T-lymphocyte responses to altered self. It has been proposed that viruses may non-specifically stimulate cytotoxicity in general, which spills over to affect target cells altered by drug antigen [2]. The involvement of the skin immune system (Chapter 10) in cell-mediated drug eruptions, and graft-versus-host disease as a model for cutaneous drug eruptions, have been reviewed [3,4].

There is increasing evidence for a role for T cells and cell-mediated immunity in some drug eruptions. Sulphamethoxazole-reactive lymphocytes can be detected in peripheral blood of patients with drug-induced eruptions, at a frequency of 1/172000, within the range of the frequency of urushiol-reactive T cells found in patients with urushiol (poison ivy) dermatitis [5]. Patients with acute drug allergy to carbamazepine, phenytoin, sulphamethoxazole, allopurinol or paracetamol had activated drug-specific CD4+ or CD8+ T cells in the circulation [6]. CD8+ T cells predominate in the epidermis in drug-induced maculopapular and bullous eruptions and patch-test reactions to β-lactam antibiotics. β-Lactam-specific peripheral and epidermal T lymphocytes from bullous exanthems are predominantly T-cell receptor αβ+, CD8+, CD4–, display a Th1-like cytokine pattern, proliferate in an antigen- and major histocompatibility complex (MHC)-specific manner and are cytotoxic against epidermal keratinocytes in lectin-induced cytotoxicity assays [7–9]. By contrast, T-cell lines from patients with penicillin-induced urticarial exanthems are predominantly T-cell receptor αβ+, CD4+, CD8–, with a Th2-like cytokine pattern. Proliferation of CD8+ dermal T cells, from a sulphamethoxazole-induced bullous exanthem, to sulphamethoxazole was significantly increased in the presence of liver microsomes, suggesting that microsomal enzymes, such as the cytochrome P-450 system, generate highly reactive metabolites, which are the nominal antigens for T-cell activation [9,10]. The expression of the intercellular adhesion molecule 1 (CAM-1) by target keratinocytes plays an important role in the cytotoxicity of epidermal T cells in bullous drug eruptions [11]. Penicillin G may stimulate T cells directly by binding to MHC molecules on the cell surface. Alternatively, it may bind to soluble proteins like human serum albumin, which require processing for presentation in an immunogenic form. These different modes of presentation, which elicit a variety of immunological reactivities, may explain the heterogeneity of clinical pictures seen in penicillin allergy [12]. Morbilliform drug hypersensitivity reactions in HIV-infected subjects showed spongiosis, hydropic generation of the basal layer, Civatte bodies, an epidermal lymphocytic infiltrate, and perivascular lymphocytes and macrophages [13]. Immunohistochemistry demonstrated CD8+, HLA-DR+ T lymphocytes, marked depletion of epidermal Langerhans' cells and strong keratinocyte interleukin 6 (IL-6), IL-1β tumour necrosis factor-α (TNF-α) and, to a lesser degree, interferon-γ (IFN-γ) expression.

REFERENCES

1 Stejskal VDM, Forsbeck M, Olin R. Side chain-specific lymphocyte responses in workers with occupational allergy induced by penicillins. *Int Arch Allergy Appl Immunol* 1987; **82**: 461–4.
2 Chosidow O, Bourgault L, Roujeau JC. Drug rashes. What are the targets of cell-mediated cytotoxicity? *Arch Dermatol* 1994; **130**: 627–9.
3 Breathnach SM, Hintner H. *Adverse Drug Reactions and the Skin*. Oxford: Blackwell Scientific Publications, 1992.
4 Breathnach SM. Mechanisms of drug eruptions: Part I. *Australas J Dermatol* 1995; **36**: 121–7.
5 Kalish RS, LaPorte A, Wood JA, Johnson KL. Sulfonamide-reactive lymphocytes detected at very low frequency in the peripheral blood of patients with drug-induced eruptions. *J Allergy Clin Immunol* 1994; **94**: 465–72.
6 Mauri-Hellweg D, Bettens F, Mauri D. Activation of drug-specific CD4+ and CD8+ T cells in individuals allergic to sulfonamides, phenytoin, and carbamazepine. *J Immunol* 1995; **155**: 462–72.
7 Hertl M, Geisel J, Boecker C, Merk HF. Selective generation of CD8+ T-cell clones from the peripheral blood of patients with cutaneous reactions to beta-lactam antibiotics. *Br J Dermatol* 1993; **128**: 619–26.
8 Hertl M, Bohlen H, Jugert F et al. Predominance of epidermal CD8+ T lymphocytes in bullous cutaneous reactions caused by β-lactam antibiotics. *J Invest Dermatol* 1993; **101**: 794–9.
9 Hertl M, Merk HF. Lymphocyte activation in cutaneous drug reactions. *J Invest Dermatol* 1995; **105** (Suppl.): S95–8.
10 Hertl M, Jugert F, Merk HF. CD8+ dermal T cells from a sulphamethoxazole-induced bullous exanthem proliferate in response to drug-modified liver microsomes. *Br J Dermatol* 1995; **132**: 215–20.
11 Hertl M, Rönnau A, Bohlen H et al. The cytotoxicity of epidermal T lymphocytes in bullous drug reactions is strongly but not completely abrogated by inhibition of ICAM-1 on target cells. *Arch Dermatol Res* 1993; **285**: 63 (Abstract).
12 Brander C, Mauri-Hellweg D, Bettens F et al. Heterogeneous T cell responses to beta-lactam-modified self-structures are observed in penicillin-allergic individuals. *J Immunol* 1995; **155**: 2670–8.
13 Carr A, Vasak E, Munro V et al. Immunohistological assessment of cutaneous drug hypersensitivity in patients with HIV infection. *Clin Exp Immunol* 1994; **97**: 260–5.

Erythema multiforme/Stevens–Johnson syndrome. Herpes simplex genome has been identified in the lesions of herpes-induced erythema multiforme [1], and by extrapolation, drug hapten-specific T cells could be involved in the pathogenesis of drug-induced erythema multiforme and Stevens–Johnson syndrome. Peripheral blood mononuclear cells obtained from a patient with carbamazepine-induced erythema multiforme at the time of disease showed increased binding to ICAM-1+ heterologous keratinocytes, and to autologous keratinocytes *in vitro*, which could be inhibited completely by antibodies to lymphocyte function-associated antigen-1 (LFA-1), the ligand for ICAM-1 [2]. Autoantibodies against desmosomal plaque proteins desmoplakin I and II were found in seven of 10 patients with erythema multiforme major, associated with suprabasal acantholysis [3].

REFERENCES

1 Brice SL, Krzemien D, Weston WL *et al.* Detection of herpes simplex virus DNA in cutaneous lesions of erythema multiforme. *J Invest Dermatol* 1989; **93**: 183–7.
2 Bruynzeel I, van der Raaij EMH, Boorsma DM *et al.* Increased adherence to keratinocytes of peripheral blood mononuclear leucocytes of a patient with drug-induced erythema multiforme. *Br J Dermatol* 1993; **129** 45–9.
3 Foedinger D, Sterizcky B, Elbe A *et al.* Autoantibodies against desmoplakin I and II define a subset of patients with erythema multiforme major. *J Invest Dermatol* 1996; **106**: 1012–16.

Toxic epidermal necrolysis [1–6]. CD4+ T cells predominate in the upper dermis, while epidermal CD8+ T cells and macrophages are variable and Langerhans' cells virtually disappear. Keratinocytes express HLA-DR and ICAM-1, and there is endothelial cell ICAM-1, vascular cell adhesion molecule 1 (VCAM-1) and E-selectin expression. Prominent involvement of the monocyte–macrophage lineage, including factor XIIIa+ HLA-DR+ dendrocytes and CD68+ Mac 387+ macrophages before, during and after epidermal necrosis was reported in one study [6], with dense labelling of the epidermis for TNF-α. Thus, cytokines released by activated mononuclear cells and keratinocytes may contribute to local cell death in TEN. Keratinocytes from TEN patients have been reported to undergo extensive apoptosis [7], perhaps as a result of lymphocyte activation with apoptosis occurring via the *Fas* (a membrane receptor expressed after exposure to IFN-γ with a ligand on the lymphocyte surface) or perforin-granzyme routes [8,9]. In a patient with carbamazepine-induced TEN, lymphocytes were more susceptible to cytotoxic killing by liver microsome-induced carbamazepine intermediates than by the parent drug [10].

REFERENCES

1 Merot Y, Gravallese E, Guillén FJ, Murphy GF. Lymphocyte subsets and Langerhans' cells in toxic epidermal necrolysis. Report of a case. *Arch Dermatol* 1986; **122**: 455–8.
2 Villada G, Roujeau J-C, Cordonnier C *et al.* Toxic epidermal necrolysis after bone marrow transplantation: Study of nine cases. *J Am Acad Dermatol* 1990; **23**: 870–5.
3 Miyauchi H, Hosokawa H, Akaeda T *et al.* T-cell subsets in drug-induced toxic epidermal necrolysis. Possible pathogenic mechanism induced by CD8-positive T cells. *Arch Dermatol* 1991; **127**: 851–5.
4 Villada G, Roujeau JC, Clerici T *et al.* Immunopathology of toxic epidermal necrolysis: keratinocytes, HLA-DR expression, Langerhans cells, and mononuclear cells: an immunopathologic study of five cases. *Arch Dermatol* 1992; **128**: 50–3.
5 Correia O, Delgado L, Ramos JP *et al.* Cutaneous T-cell recruitment in toxic epidermal necrolysis: further evidence of CD8+ lymphocyte involvement. *Arch Dermatol* 1993; **129**: 466–8.
6 Paquet P, Nikkels A, Arrese JE *et al.* Macrophages and tumor necrosis factor α in toxic epidermal necrolysis. *Arch Dermatol* 1994; **130**: 605–8.
7 Paul C, Wolkenstein P, Adle H *et al.* Apoptosis as a mechanism of keratinocyte death in toxic epidermal necrolysis. *Br J Dermatol* 1996; **134**: 710–14.
8 Sayama K, Yonehara S, Watanabe Y, Miki Y. Expression of *Fas* antigen on keratinocytes *in vivo* and induction of apoptosis in cultured keratinocytes. *J Invest Dermatol* 1994; **103**: 330–4.
9 Chu JL, Ramos P, Rosendorff A *et al.* Massive upregulation of the *Fas* ligand in *lpr* and *gld* mice: implications for *Fas* regulation and the graft-versus-host-disease-like wasting syndrome. *J Exp Med* 1995; **181**: 393–8.
10 Friedmann PS, Strickland I, Pirmohamed M, Park BK. Investigation of mechanisms in toxic epidermal necrolysis induced by carbamazepine. *Arch Dermatol* 1994; **130**: 598–604.

Lichenoid drug eruptions. The mechanisms underlying lichenoid drug eruptions are essentially unknown, but they may develop as a result of autoreactive cytotoxic T-cell clones directed against a drug/class II MHC antigen complex, such that keratinocytes and Langerhans' cells are viewed by the immune system as 'non-self'. Cloned murine autoreactive T cells produce a lichenoid reaction in recipient animals following injection [1]. The presence of epidermotropic T cells correlates with that of class II MHC (HLA-DR) expressing keratinocytes and Langerhans' cells in lichenoid eruptions [2].

REFERENCES

1 Shiohara T. The lichenoid tissue reaction. An immunological perspective. *Am J Dermatopathol* 1988; **10**: 252–6.
2 Shiohara T, Moriya N, Tanaka Y *et al.* Immunopathological study of lichenoid skin diseases: correlation between HLA-DR-positive keratinocytes or Langerhans cells and epidermotropic T cells. *J Am Acad Dermatol* 1988; **18**: 67–74.

Lupus erythematosus (LE)-like syndrome induced by drugs. Drug-induced LE, with production of antihistone antibodies, may result from interaction between the drug and nuclear material to produce a drug-nucleoprotein complex that is immunogenic. Alternatively, drugs may alter immunoregulation in such a way that autoantibody production is favoured; procainamide and hydralazine modulate lymphocyte function directly and induce autoreactivity. Thus, drugs may cause a systemic LE-like condition by a mechanism analogous to that in immunostimulatory graft-versus-host disease [1]. Hydralazine, isoniazid, and the hydroxylamine metabolites of procainamide and practolol, may also predispose to the development of an LE-like syndrome by inhibiting binding of C4 and in turn of C3 to immune complexes, thus preventing complement-mediated clearance of immune complexes by solubilization and opsonization [2].

REFERENCES

1 Gleichman E, Pals ST, Rolinck AG *et al.* Graft-versus-host reactions: clues to the etiopathogenesis of a spectrum of immunological diseases. *Immunol Today* 1984; **5**: 324–32.
2 Sim E. Drug-induced immune complex disease. *Complement Inflamm* 1989; **6**: 119–26.

Drug-induced pemphigus. Immunoprecipitation studies have shown that patients with drug-induced pemphigus foliaceus and pemphigus vulgaris often have circulating autoantibodies with the same antigenic specificity at a molecular level as autoantibodies from patients with idiopathic pemphigus [1]. Binding of an active thiol group in a drug to the pemphigus antigen complex might result in autoantibody production, or culprit drugs may result in immune dysregulation. In addition, drugs with thiol groups in their molecule, such as penicillamine, captopril and thiopronine, and piroxicam can cause acantholysis directly *in vitro* in the absence of autoantibody [2].

REFERENCES

1 Korman NJ, Eyre RW, Stanley JR. Drug-induced pemphigus: autoanti-bodies directed against the pemphigus antigen complexes are present in penicillamine and captopril-induced pemphigus. *J Invest Dermatol* 1991; **96**: 273–6.
2 Ruocco V, Pisani M, de Angelis E, Lombardi ML. Biochemical acantholysis provoked by thiol drugs. *Arch Dermatol* 1990; **126**: 965–6.

Fixed drug eruptions. Graft autotransplantation investigations carried out in the 1930s demonstrated cutaneous memory in involved skin in fixed drug eruption [1]. Serum factors from patients with fixed drug eruption have been reported to cause inflammation on injection into a previously involved site, but not into normal skin [2], and to induce lymphocyte blast transformation [3,4]. However, cell-mediated rather than humoral immunity is thought to play the major role in the development of lesions in this condition.

Lesional skin contains increased numbers of both helper and suppressor T lymphocytes [5–8], and T suppressor/cytotoxic T cells may be seen adjacent to necrotic keratinocytes in the epidermis [6]. T cells may persist within lesional skin and contribute to immunological memory [7,9]; CD8+ suppressor/cytotoxic T cells were present in suprabasal epidermis in involved skin 3 weeks after challenge [5]. T cells from lesional epidermis in two patients with fixed drug eruption utilized a very limited range of Vα and Vβ genes compared with peripheral blood T cells, indicating some expansion or preferential migration of T cells recognizing a restricted set of antigens [10]. Keratinocytes in lesional skin express ICAM-1 [11], which is involved in interaction between keratinocytes and lymphocytes, HLA-DR [6] and the chemotactic protein IP-10 [8], findings that suggest a role for cytokines in the evolution of the histological changes [8,11]. ICAM-1 was noted to be induced on endothelium and keratinocytes 1.5 h after drug challenge, and there was increased reactivity in lesional skin *in vitro* to TNF-α and IFN-γ, as well as to the causative drug [12]; drug-induced, TNF-α-dependent keratinocyte ICAM-1 expression in lesional skin may provide a localized initiating stimulus for epidermal T-cell activation. Early release of histamine from mast cells or basophils has been reported in fixed drug eruption, based on suction blister fluid levels [13]. Significantly higher frequencies of HLA-B22 and -Cwl antigens were found in

36 patients with fixed drug eruption, and familial cases occur, suggesting a genetic predisposition [14].

REFERENCES

1 Korkij W, Soltani K. Fixed drug eruption. A brief review. *Arch Dermatol* 1984; **120**: 520–4.
2 Wyatt E, Greaves M, Søndergaard J. Fixed drug eruption (phenolphthalein). *Arch Dermatol* 1972; **106**: 671–3.
3 Gimenez-Camarasa JM, Garcia-Calderon P, De Moragas JM. Lymphocyte transformation test in fixed drug eruption. *N Engl J Med* 1975; **292**: 819–21.
4 Suzuki S, Asai Y, Toshio H *et al.* Drug-induced lymphocyte transformation in peripheral lymphocytes from patients with drug eruption. *Dermatologica* 1978; **157**: 146–53.
5 Hindsén M, Christensen OB, Gruic V, Löfberg H. Fixed drug eruption: an immunohistochemical investigation of the acute and healing phase. *Br J Dermatol* 1987; **116**: 351–6.
6 Murphy GF, Guillén FJ, Flynn TC. Cytotoxic T lymphocytes and phenotypically abnormal epidermal dendritic cells in fixed cutaneous eruption. *Hum Pathol* 1985; **16**: 1264–71.
7 Visa K, Käyhkö K, Stubb S, Reitamo S. Immunocompetent cells of fixed drug eruption. *Acta Derm Venereol (Stockh)* 1987; **67**: 30–5.
8 Smoller BR, Luster AD, Krane JF *et al.* Fixed drug eruptions: evidence for a cytokine-mediated process. *J Cutan Pathol* 1991; **18**: 13–19.
9 Scheper RJ, Von Blomberg M, Boerrigter GH *et al.* Induction of immunological memory in the skin. Role of local T cell retention. *Clin Exp Immunol* 1983; **51**: 141–8.
10 Komatsu T, Moriya N, Shiohara T. T cell receptor (TCR) repertoire and function of human epidermal T cells: restricted TCR V alpha-V beta genes are utilized by T cells residing in the lesional epidermis in fixed drug eruption. *Clin Exp Immunol* 1996; **104**: 343–50.
11 Shiohara T, Nickoloff BJ, Sagawa Y *et al.* Fixed drug eruption. Expression of epidermal keratinocyte intercellular adhesion molecule-1 (ICAM-1). *Arch Dermatol* 1989; **125**: 1371–6.
12 Teraki Y, Moriya N, Shiohara T. Drug-induced expression of intercellular adhesion molecule-1 on lesional keratinocytes in fixed drug eruption. *Am J Pathol* 1994; **145**: 550–60.
13 Alanko K, Stubb S, Salo OP, Reitamo S. Suction blister fluid histamine in fixed drug eruption. *Acta Derm Venereol (Stockh)* 1992; **72**: 89–91.
14 Pellicano R, Ciavarella G, Lomuto M, Di Giorgio G. Genetic susceptibility to fixed drug eruption: evidence for a link with HLA-B22. *J Am Acad Dermatol* 1994; **30**: 52–4.

Histopathology of drug reactions [1]

In most patterns of reaction to drugs, the histological changes are no more distinctive than are the clinical features. For example, urticaria, erythema multiforme, TEN and exfoliative dermatitis provoked by drugs cannot be differentiated from the same reactions resulting from other causes. Graft-versus-host reaction-type drug eruptions in the acute phase show a predominance of epidermal CD8+ T cells, reduced epidermal OKT6+ Langerhans' cells, and increased keratinocyte expression of HLA-DR and ICAM-1 [2]. By contrast, Langerhans' cells from lesional maculopapular drug eruptions reportedly increased in number by 66% and displayed more intense staining and more prominent dendrites in one study [3].

The histological changes in the vegetating iododermas and bromodermas, in certain lichenoid eruptions, and in fixed drug eruptions are not pathognomonic, but are sufficiently characteristic to be of importance in differential diagnosis. The histology of a number of other drug eruptions has been reviewed [4]. Amiodarone-induced hyperpigmentation shows a lymphocytic dermatitis and yellowish-brown granules within several cell types; the drug or a metabolite composes at least a portion of the deposits. Clofazimine-induced hyperpigmentation involves accumulation of a ceroid lipofuscin within lipid-laden macrophages. The cutaneous eruption of lymphocyte recovery after chemotherapeutic agents is a maculopapular eruption with a non-specific superficial perivascular dermatitis. Chemotherapy-induced acral erythema reveals a non-specific interface dermatitis. Specific reactions occur with etoposide (starburst cells) and busulphan (large, atypical keratinocytes), while other chemotherapeutic agents may involve sweat glands: neutrophilic eccrine hidradenitis is characterized by neutrophil infiltration and by necrosis; syringosquamous metaplasia involves squamous metaplasia of the sweat duct. Drug-induced generalized pustular toxic erythema is characterized by subcorneal pustules and occasional eosinophils. Cephalosporins may produce a syndrome clinically and histologically like pemphigus, and naproxen produces one like porphyria cutanea tarda. The photosensitive dermatitis associated with quinine and piroxicam is histologically a non-specific spongiotic dermatitis. A lichenoid giant-cell dermatitis may be caused by methyldopa or chlorothiazide, while phenytoin and carbamazepine dermatitis histologically imitates mycosis fungoides.

Bromodermas and iododermas

In bromoderma, verrucous pseudoepitheliomatous hyperplasia is associated with abscesses containing neutrophils and eosinophils in the epidermis, and a dense dermal infiltrate initially consisting mainly of neutrophils and eosinophils, and later containing many lymphocytes, plasma cells and histiocytes. The abundant dilated blood vessels may show endothelial proliferation. In iododermas, ulceration is more marked, but there is usually less epithelial hyperplasia. Both conditions must be differentiated from blastomycosis and coccidiomycosis, and from pemphigus vegetans.

Fixed eruptions

In the acute stage, the epidermal changes may be indistinguishable from erythema multiforme, with loss of cell outlines and necrosis of the lower epidermis. In less acute lesions, the epidermis may show little abnormality but the dermis is oedematous and there is a conspicuous perivascular lymphocytic infiltrate. Later, there is increased melanin in the epidermis and within melanophages in the dermis.

Lichenoid eruptions

The changes may be non-specific or may resemble

idiopathic lichen planus, although the cellular infiltrate tends to be more pleomorphic and less dense, and the presence of focal parakeratosis, focal interruption of the granular layer, and cytoid bodies in the cornified and granular layers suggest a drug cause [5]. Later, there may be scarring with destruction of the sweat glands.

REFERENCES

1 Elder D, Elenitsas R, Jaworsky C, Johnson B, Jr, eds. *Lever's Histopathology of the Skin*, 8th edn. Philadelphia: JB Lippincott, 1997.
2 Osawa J, Kitamura K, Saito S *et al.* Immunohistochemical study of graft-versus-host reaction (GVHR)-type drug eruptions. *J Dermatol* 1994; **21**: 25–30.
3 Dascalu DI, Kletter Y, Baratz M, Brenner S. Langerhans' cell distribution in drug eruption. *Acta Derm Venereol (Stockh)* 1992; **72**: 175–7.
4 Fitzpatrick JE. New histopathologic findings in drug eruptions. *Dermatol Clin* 1992; **10**: 19–36.
5 Van den Haute V, Antoine JL, Lachapelle JM. Histopathological discriminant criteria between lichenoid drug eruption and idiopathic lichen planus: retrospective study on selected samples. *Dermatologica* 1989; **179**: 10–13.

Types of clinical reaction [1–13]

The mucocutaneous reactions that may result from adverse drug reactions have been the subject of extensive reviews, to which the reader is referred for further information. The following section details a number of different drug-induced reaction patterns; see also the discussion of adverse effects of individual drugs (p. 3397). It is unfortunate that, while certain drugs are commonly associated with a specific reaction, most drugs are capable of causing several different types of eruption.

REFERENCES

1 Davies DM, ed. *Textbook of Adverse Drug Reactions*, 3rd edn. Oxford: Oxford University Press, 1985.
2 Stern RS, Wintroub BU. Adverse drug reactions: reporting and evaluating cutaneous reactions. *Adv Dermatol* 1987; **2**: 3–18.
3 Seymour RA, Walton JG. *Adverse Drug Reactions in Dentistry*. Oxford: Oxford University Press, 1988.
4 Bork K. *Cutaneous Side Effects of Drugs*. Philadelphia: WB Saunders, 1988.
5 Dukes MNG, ed. *Meylers Side Effects of Drugs*, 11th edn. Amsterdam: Elsevier, 1988.
6 Alanko K, Stubbs S, Kauppinen K. Cutaneous drug reactions: clinical types and causative agents. A five year survey of in-patients (1981–1985). *Acta Derm Venereol (Stockh)* 1989; **69**: 223–6.
7 Shear NH, ed. Adverse reactions to drugs. *Semin Dermatol* 1989; **8**: 135–226.
8 Kalish RS. Drug eruptions: a review of clinical and immunological features. *Adv Dermatol* 1991; **6**: 221–37.
9 Pavan-Langston D, Dunkel EC. *Handbook of Ocular Drug Therapy and Ocular Side Effects of Systemic Drugs*. Boston: Little, Brown and Company, 1991.
10 Breathnach SM, Hintner H. *Adverse Drug Reactions and the Skin*. Oxford: Blackwell Scientific Publications, 1992.
11 Zürcher L, Krebs A. *Cutaneous Drug Reactions*. Basel: Karger, 1992.
12 Bruinsma WA. *A Guide to Drug Eruptions: File of Side Effects in Dermatology*, 6th edn. Oosthuizen, The Netherlands: File of Medicines, 1996.
13 Litt JZ, Pawlak WA, Jr. *Drug Eruption Reference Manual*. New York: Parthenon, 1997.

Exanthematic (maculopapular) reactions

These are the most frequent of all cutaneous reactions to

drugs, and can occur after almost any drug at any time up to 3 (but usually 2) weeks after administration; they may be accompanied by fever, pruritus and eosinophilia. It is not possible to identify the offending drug by the nature of the eruption. The clinical features are variable; the lesions may be scarlatiniform, rubelliform or mobilliform, or may consist of a profuse eruption of small papules showing no close resemblance to any infective exanthem (Fig. 77.1). Less common are eruptions with large macules, polycylic and gyrate erythema, reticular eruptions and sheet-like erythema. The distribution is also variable, but it is generally symmetrical. The trunk and extremities are usually involved, and not uncommonly intertriginous areas may be favoured, but the face may be spared. Palmar and plantar lesions may occur, and sometimes the eruption is generalized. Purpuric lesions, especially on the legs, and erosive stomatitis may develop. There may be relative sparing of pressure areas. If the administration of the drug is continued, an exfoliative dermatitis may develop, although occasionally the eruption subsides despite continuation of the medication.

Table 77.2 Drugs causing exanthematic reactions.

Most common	Less common
Ampicillin and penicillin	Cephalosporins
Phenylbutazone and other pyrazolones	Barbiturates
Sulphonamides	Thiazides
Phenytoin	Naproxen
Carbamazepine	Isoniazid
Gold	Phenothiazines
Gentamicin	Quinidine
	Meprobamate
	Atropine

Morbilliform drug eruptions usually, but not always, recur on rechallenge. It is useful, in differentiating exanthematic drug eruptions from viral exanthemata, to remember that viral rashes may start on the face and progress to involve the trunk, and are more often accompanied by conjunctivitis, lymphadenopathy and fever. Maculopapular drug eruptions usually fade with desquamation, sometimes with postinflammatory hyperpigmentation. Commoner causes are listed in Table 77.2.

Purpura

A purpuric element to a drug eruption is not uncommon, but primarily purpuric drug-induced rashes also occur. Many drugs may interfere with platelet aggregation [1], but with the exception of aspirin, this does not usually result in bleeding. A number of drugs have been implicated in the development of drug-induced purpura [2–4]. Several mechanisms may be involved. These include altered coagulation after anticoagulants or some cephalosporins, allergic and non-allergic thrombocytopenia, altered platelet function (as after valproic acid) or vascular causes, including steroid-induced fragility and loss of support. Cytotoxic drug therapy may result in non-allergic purpura due to bone-marrow depression, with a platelet count of less than $30\,000/mm^3$. Bleomycin may induce thrombocytopenia by causing endothelial damage and consequent platelet aggregation [5]. A large number of drugs has been reported to cause allergic thrombocytopenia [2–4]. Heparin may cause purpura with overdosage or due to an allergic thrombocytopenia [6]. The classical example of complement-mediated destruction of platelets, following immune-complex formation between a drug (as hapten) bound to the platelet surface, and IgG class antibody, was the purpura caused by apronalide (Sedormid). Quinine, quinidine [7,8] and chlorothiazide may also cause allergic purpura. Tissue plasminogen activator (alteplase) has been associated with painful purpura [9]. A purpuric vasculitislike rash followed secondary spread of a contact dermatitis to balsam of Peru [10].

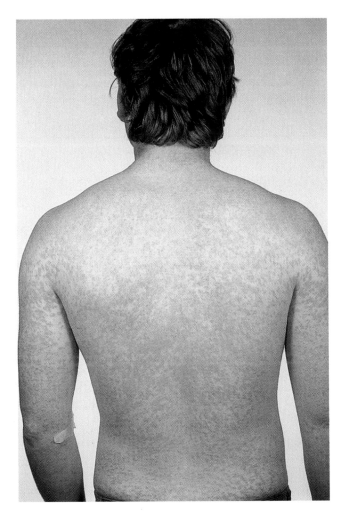

Fig. 77.1 Maculopapular erythema caused by ampicillin.

Capillaritis (pigmented purpuric eruption) may be due to aspirin, carbromal or more rarely to thiamine or meprobamate [11–14], carbamazepine, and phenacetin; it may be due to formation of antibody to a drug/capillary endothelial cell complex [12]. Chronic pigmented purpura is recorded with thiamine propyldisulphide and chlordiazepoxide [13] and aminoglutethimide [15]. NSAIDs, diuretics, meprobamate and ampicillin were the commonest drug cause of pigmented purpuric eruptions in one study [16].

REFERENCES

1 George JN, Shattil SJ. The clinical importance of acquired abnormalities of platelet function. *N Engl J Med* 1991; **324**: 27–39.
2 Miescher PA, Graf J. Drug-induced thrombocytopenia. *Clin Haematol* 1980; **9**: 505–19.
3 Moss RA. Drug-induced immune thrombocytopenia. *Am J Haematol* 1980; **9**: 439–46.
4 Bork K. *Cutaneous Side Effects of Drugs*. Philadelphia: WB Saunders, 1988.
5 Hilgard P, Hossfeld DK. Transient bleomycin-induced thrombocytopenia. A clinical study. *Eur J Cancer* 1978; **14**: 1261–4.
6 Babcock RB, Dumper CW, Scharfman WB. Heparin-induced thrombocytopenia. *N Engl J Med* 1976; **295**: 237–41.
7 Christie DJ, Weber RW, Mullen PC *et al.* Structural features of the quinidine and quinine molecules necessary for binding of drug-induced antibodies to human platelets. *J Lab Clin Med* 1984; **104**: 730–40.
8 Gary M, Ilfeld D, Kelton JG. Correlation of a quinidine-induced platelet-specific antibody with development of thrombocytopenia. *Am J Med* 1985; **79**: 253–5.
9 DeTrana C, Hurwitz RM. Painful purpura: an adverse effect to a thrombolysin. *Arch Dermatol* 1990; **126**: 690–1.
10 Bruynzeel DP, van den Hoogenband HM, Koedijk F. Purpuric vasculitis-like eruption in a patient sensitive to balsam of Peru. *Contact Dermatitis* 1984; **11**: 207–9.
11 Peterson WC, Manick KP. Purpuric eruptions associated with use of carbromal and meprobamate. *Arch Dermatol* 1967; **95**: 40–2.
12 Carmel WJ, Dannenberg T. Nonthrombocytopenic purpura due to Miltown (2-Methyl-2-n-propyl-1,3-propanediol dicarbamate). *N Engl J Med* 1956; **255**: 7701.
13 Nishioka K, Katayama I, Masuzawa M *et al.* Drug-induced chronic pigmented purpura. *J Dermatol (Tokyo)* 1989; **16**: 220–2.
14 Abeck D, Gross GE, Kuwert C *et al.* Acetaminophen-induced progressive pigmentary purpura (Schamberg's disease). *J Am Acad Dermatol* 1992; **27**: 123–4.
15 Stratakis CA, Chrousos GP. Capillaritis (purpura simplex) associated with use of aminoglutethimide in Cushing's syndrome. *Am J Hosp Pharm* 1994; **51**: 2589–91.
16 Pang BK, Su D, Ratnam KV. Drug-induced purpura simplex: clinical and histological characteristics. *Ann Academy Med (Sing)* 1993; **22**: 870–2.

Annular erythema

Erythema annulare centrifugum has been reported in association with chloroquine and hydroxychloroquine [1], oestrogens, cimetidine [2], penicillin, salicylates, and piroxicam, as well as with hydrochlorothiazide [3], spironolactone [4] thiacetazone [5] and the phenothiazine levomepromazine [6]. Annular erythema has occurred with vitamin K [7].

REFERENCES

1 Ashurst PJ. Erythema annulare centrifugum due to hydroxychloroquine sulfate and chloroquine sulfate. *Arch Dermatol* 1967; **95**: 37–9.
2 Merrett AC, Marks R, Dudley FJ. Cimetidine-induced erythema annulare centrifugum: no cross-sensitivity with ranitidine. *Br Med J* 1981: **283**: 698.
3 Goette DK, Beatrice E. Erythema annulare centrifugum caused by hydrochlorothiazide-induced interstitial nephritis. *Int J Dermatol* 1988; **27**: 129–30.
4 Carsuzaa F, Pierre C, Dubegny M. Érythème annulaire centrifuge a l'aldactone. *Ann Dermatol Vénéréol* 1987; **114**: 375–6.
5 Ramesh V. Eruption resembling erythema annulare centrifugum. *Australas J Dermatol* 1987; **28**: 44.
6 Blazejak T, Hölzle E. Phenothiazin-induziertes Pseudolymphom. *Hautarzt* 1990; **41**: 161–3.
7 Kay MH, Duvic M. Reactive annular erythema after intramuscular vitamin K. *Cutis* 1986; **37**: 445–8.

Pityriasis rosea-like reactions

The best known drug cause of a pityriasiform rash is gold therapy [1], but several other drugs have been implicated, including metronidazole [2], captopril [3], isotretinoin [4] and omeprazole [5] and are listed in Table 77.3.

Table 77.3 Drugs causing pityriasis rosea-like drug reactions.

Arsenicals	Captopril
Bismuth	Griseofulvin
Gold	Isotretinoin
Barbiturates	Metronidazole
β-Blockers	Pyribenzamine
Clonidine	Methoxypromazine
	Omeprazole

REFERENCES

1 Wile UJ, Courville CJ. Pityriasis rosea-like dermatitis following gold therapy: report of two cases. *Arch Dermatol* 1940; **42**: 1105–12.
2 Maize JC, Tomecki J. Pityriasis rosea-like drug eruption secondary to metronidazole. *Arch Dermatol* 1977; **113**: 1457–8.
3 Wilkin JK, Kirkendall WM. Pityriasis rosea-like rash from captopril. *Arch Dermatol* 1982; **118**: 186–7.
4 Helfman RJ, Brickman M, Fahey J. Isotretinoin dermatitis simulating acute pityriasis rosea. *Cutis* 1984; **33**: 297–300.
5 Buckley C. Pityriasis rosea-like eruption in a patient receiving omeprazole. *Br J Dermatol* 1996; **135**: 660–1.

Psoriasiform eruptions

See Chapter 35 and Table 77.4.

Exfoliative dermatitis

Exfoliative dermatitis is one of the most dangerous patterns of cutaneous reaction to drugs [1–5]. It may follow exanthematic eruptions or may develop, as in some reactions to arsenicals and the heavy metals, as erythema and exudation in the flexures, rapidly generalizing. The eruption may start several weeks after initiation of the

Table 77.4 Drugs reported to exacerbate psoriasis.

Antimalarials
β-Blockers
Lithium salts
Non-steroidal anti-inflammatory drugs
  Ibuprofen
  Indomethacin (but see text)
  Meclofenamate sodium
  Pyrazolon derivatives (phenylbutazone, oxyphenbutazone)
Miscellaneous
  Captopril
  Chlorthalidone
  Cimetidine
  Clonidine
  Gemfibrozil
  Interferon
  Methlydopa
  Penicillamine
  Penicillin
  Terfenadine
  Trazodone

Table 77.5 Drugs causing erythroderma and exfoliative dermatitis.

Allopurinol	Hydantoins
p-Amino salicylic acid	Isoniazid
Ampicillin	Lithium
Barbiturates	Nitrofurantoin
Captopril	d-Penicillamine
Carbamazepine	Penicillin
Cefoxitin	Phenylbutazone
Chloroquine	Quinidine
Chlorpromazine	Streptomycin
Cimetidine	Sulphonamides
Diltiazem	Sulphonylureas
Gold	Thiacetazone
Griseofulvin	

therapy. An eczematous dermatitis in patients previously sensitized by contact may also become universal.

The main drugs implicated are listed in Table 77.5. In one large series, sulphonamides, antimalarials and penicillin were most frequently implicated [1]. In another series from India [3], the commonest associated drugs were isoniazid (20%), thiacetazone (15%), topical tar (15%), and a variety of homeopathic medicines (20%), with phenylbutazone, streptomycin and sulphadiazine each accounting for 5% of cases. Phenytoin is a well-recognized cause [6]. Recently incriminated drugs have included captopril, cefoxitin, cimetidine and ampicillin.

REFERENCES

1 Nicolis GD, Helwig EB. Exfoliative dermatitis. A clinicopathologic study of 135 cases. *Arch Dermatol* 1973; **108**: 788–97.
2 Hasan T, Jansén DT. Erythroderma: a follow-up of fifty cases. *J Am Acad Dermatol* 1983; **8**: 836–4.
3 Sehgal VN, Srivastava G. Exfoliative dermatitis. A prospective study of 80 patients. *Dermatologica* 1986; **173**: 278–84.
4 Sage T, Faure M. Conduite à tenir devant les érythrodermies de l'adulte. *Ann Dermatol Vénéréol* 1989; **116**: 747–52.
5 Irvine C. 'Skin failure'—a real entity: discussion paper. *J R Soc Med* 1991; **84**: 412–13.
6 Danno K, Kume M, Ohta M *et al.* Erythroderma with generalized lymphadenopathy induced by phenytoin. *J Dermatol (Tokyo)* 1989; **16**: 392–6.

Anaphylaxis and anaphylactoid reactions

This systemic reaction, which usually develops within minutes to hours (the vast majority within the first hour), is often severe and may be fatal [1–3]. Fatal drug-induced anaphylactic shock was estimated at 0.3 cases per million inhabitants per year, based on notifications to the Danish Committee on Adverse Drug Reactions and to the Central Death Register during the period 1968–90 [3]. The most frequent causes were contrast media for X-ray examinations, antibiotics and extracts of allergens. In less severe cases, there may be premonitory dizziness or faintness, skin tingling and reddening of the bulbar conjunctiva, followed by urticaria, angio-oedema, broncho-spasm, abdominal pain and vasomotor collapse. It usually develops on second exposure to a drug, but may develop during the first treatment if this lasts sufficiently long for sensitization to occur. Anaphylaxis is unlikely to occur with a drug taken continuously for several months; by contrast, intermittent administration may predispose to anaphylaxis [1]. It is commoner after parenteral than oral drug administration. Beta-blockers enhance anaphylactic reactions caused by other allergens, and may make resuscitation more difficult [4].

The principal drug causes are shown in Table 77.6. Antibiotics (especially penicillin) and radiocontrast media are the most common known causes of anaphylactic events [2]; the incidence of such reactions is for each about one in 5000 exposures [5,6], of which less than 10% are fatal [2]. The risk for recurrent anaphylactic reactions is 10–20% for penicillins [5] and 20–40% for radiocontrast media [7].

Anaphylactoid reactions are those that clinically resemble an immediate immune response but in which the mechanism is undetermined. Some drugs and agents, such as mannitol and radiographic contrast media, can stimulate mediator release by an as yet unknown direct mechanism independent of IgE or complement. Anaphylactoid reactions may be produced by non-steroidal analgesics and anti-inflammatory reagents [8,9], including aspirin and other salicylates, indomethacin, phenylbutazone, propyphenazone, metimazol and tolmetin [10], as well as by radiographic contrast media, δ-tubocurarine, benzoic acid preservatives [11], tartrazine dyes, sulphite preservatives [12] and ciprofloxacin [13].

Animal sera	Dextrans
Vaccines containing egg protein	Mannitol
Desensitizing agents including pollen vaccines	Sorbitol complexes
Antibiotics	Enzymes
Penicillins	Trypsin
Cephalosporins	Streptokinase
Aminoglycosides	Chymopapain
Tetracyclines	Steroids
Sulphonamides	Progesterone
Antifungal agents	Hydrocortisone
Fluconazole	Polypeptide hormones
Ketoconazole	Insulin
Blood products	Corticotrophin
Angiotensin converting enzyme inhibitors	Vasopressin
Radiographic contrast media	Food and drug additives
Non-steroidal anti-inflammatory drugs (NSAIDs)	Benzoates
Salicylates	Sulphites
Other NSAIDs (e.g. Phenylbutazone, aminopyrine,	Tartrazine dyes
propyphenazone, metamizol, tolmetin)	Hydantoins
Narcotic analgesics	Hydralazine
Anaesthetic agents	Quinidine
Local and general	Anticancer drugs
Muscle relaxants	Vitamins
Suxamethonium	Protamine
Curare	

Table 77.6 Drugs causing urticaria or anaphylaxis.

REFERENCES

1 Sussman GL, Dolovich J. Prevention of anaphylaxis. *Semin Dermatol* 1989; **8**: 158–65.

2 Bochner BS, Lichtenstein LM. Anaphylaxis. *N Engl J Med* 1991; **324**: 1785–90.

3 Lenler-Petersen P, Hansen D, Andersen M *et al.* Drug-related fatal anaphylactic shock in Denmark 1968–1990. A study based on notifications to the Committee on Adverse Drug Reactions. *J Clin Epidemiol* 1995; **48**: 1185–8.

4 Toogood JH. Risk of anaphylaxis in patients receiving beta-blocker drugs. *J Allergy Clin Immunol* 1988; **81**: 1–5.

5 Weiss ME, Adkinson NF. Immediate hypersensitivity reactions to penicillin and related antibiotics. *Clin Allergy* 1988; **18**: 515–40.

6 Ansell G, Tweedie MCK, West DR *et al.* The current status of reactions to intravenous contrast media. *Invest Radiol* 1980; **15** (Suppl. 6): S32–9.

7 Greenberger P, Patterson R, Kelly J *et al.* Administration of radiographic contrast media in high-risk patients. *Invest Radiol* 1980; **15** (Suppl. 6): S40–3.

8 Antépara I, Martín-Gil D, Dominguez MA, Oehling A. Adverse drug reactions produced by analgesic drugs. *Allergol Immunopathol* 1981; **9**: 545–54.

9 Stevenson DD. Diagnosis, prevention and treatment of adverse reactions to aspirin (ASA) and nonsteroidal anti-inflammatory drugs (NSAID). *J Allergy Clin Immunol* 1984; **74**: 617–22.

10 Rossi AC, Knapp DE. Tolmetin-induced anaphylactoid reactions. *N Engl J Med* 1982; **307**: 499–500.

11 Michils A, Vandermoten G, Duchateau J, Yernault J-C. Anaphylaxis with sodium benzoate. *Lancet* 1991; **337**: 1424–5.

12 Twarog FJ, Leung DYM. Anaphylaxis to a component of isoetharine (sodium bisulfite). *JAMA* 1982; **248**: 2030–1.

13 Davis H, McGoodwin E, Reed TG. Anaphylactoid reactions reported after treatment with ciprofloxin. *Ann Intern Med* 1989; **111**: 1041–3.

Urticaria

Urticaria (Chapter 47) is, after an exanthematous eruption, the second most common type of drug reaction (Fig. 77.2). Urticaria usually occurs within 36 h of drug administration;

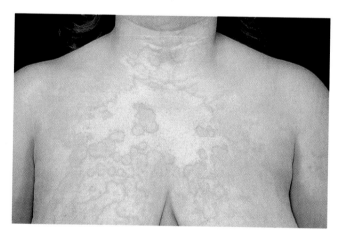

Fig. 77.2 Urticaria induced by acetylsalicylic acid. (Courtesy of St John's Institute of Dermatology, London, UK.)

on rechallenge, lesions may develop within minutes. Angio-oedema, involving oedema of the deep dermis or subcutaneous and submucosal areas, is more rarely seen than urticaria as an adverse drug reaction, and occurs in less than 1% of patients receiving the particular drug.

The commoner drug causes of urticaria/angio-oedema are listed in Table 77.6. The frequency of urticaria/angio-oedema or anaphylactic responses to aspirin and other NSAIDs is about 1% in an outpatient population and is familial [1]. Aspirin (salicylates) may also aggravate chronic urticaria [2]. In addition, an unsuspected agent, for example the yellow dye tartrazine, may really be responsible for an urticaria attributed to aspirin or another drug. The analgesic codeine is also a cause of urticaria [3]. Penicillin is a very well documented cause of acute urticaria, but the role of this drug in chronic urticaria is controversial [4]. Urticaria develops in about 1% of patients receiving blood transfusions [5]. There have been numerous papers on the potential role of food and drug additives [6–14], including preservatives such as benzoic acid, butylated hydroxyanisole (BHA), butylated hydroxytoluene (BHT), sulphites and rarely aspartame, as well as tartrazine dyes, in the development of chronic urticaria. However, a recent study suggested that common food additives are seldom if ever of significance in urticaria [15]. Urticaria may follow alcohol consumption [16].

Certain drugs, such as opiates, codeine, amphetamine, polymyxin B, δ-tubocurarine, atropine, hydralazine, pentamidine, quinine and radiocontrast media, may release mast-cell mediators directly. Cyclo-oxygenase inhibitors, such as aspirin and indomethacin, and ACE inhibitors, such as captopril and enalapril, may cause urticaria or angio-oedema by pharmacological mechanisms. ACE inhibitors may cause increased frequency, intensity and duration of bouts of idiopathic angio-oedema during long-term use [17,18].

REFERENCES

1 Settipane GA, Pudupakkam RK. Aspirin intolerance. III. Subtypes, familial occurrence and cross reactivity with tartrazine. *J Allergy Clin Immunol* 1975; **56**: 215–21.
2 Settipane RA, Constantine HP, Settipane GA. Aspirin intolerance and recurrent urticaria in normal adults and children. Epidemiology and review. *Allergy* 1980; **35**: 149–54.
3 De Groot AC, Conemans J. Allergic urticarial rash from oral codeine. *Contact Dermatitis* 1986; **14**: 209–14.
4 Boonk WJ, Van Ketel WG. The role of penicillin in the pathogenesis of chronic urticaria. *Br J Dermatol* 1982; **106**: 183–90.
5 Shulman IA. Adverse reactions to blood transfusion. *Texas Med* 1990; **85**: 35–42.
6 Simon RA. Adverse reactions to drug additives. *J Allergy Clin Immunol* 1984; **74**: 623–30.
7 Hannuksela M, Lahti A. Peroral challenge tests with food additives in urticaria and atopic dermatitis. *Int J Dermatol* 1986; **25**: 178–80.
8 Supramaniam G, Warner JO. Artificial food additives intolerance in patients with angioedema and urticaria. *Lancet* 1986; **ii**: 907–9.
9 Juhlin L. Additives and chronic urticaria. *Ann Allergy* 1987; **59**: 119–23.
10 Goodman DL, McDonnell JT, Nelson HS *et al.* Chronic urticaria exacerbated by the antioxidant food preservatives, butylated hydroxyanisole (BHA) and butylated hydroxytoluene (BHT). *J Allergy Clin Immunol* 1990; **86**: 570–5.
11 Settipane GA. Adverse reactions to sulfites in drugs and foods. *J Am Acad Dermatol* 1984; **10**: 1077–80.
12 Kulczycki A, Jr. Aspartame-induced urticaria. *Ann Intern Med* 1986; **104**: 207–8.
13 Neuman I, Elian R, Nahum H *et al.* The danger of 'yellow dyes' (tartrazine) to allergic subjects. *J Allergy* 1972; **50**: 92–8.
14 Miller K. Sensitivity to tartrazine. *Br Med J* 1982; **285**: 1597–8.
15 Hannuksela M, Lahti A. Peroral challenge tests with food additives in urticaria and atopic dermatitis. *Int J Dermatol* 1986; **25**: 178–80.
16 Ormerod AD, Holt PJA. Acute urticaria due to alcohol. *Br J Dermatol* 1983; **108**: 723–4.
17 Chin HL. Severe angioedema after long-term use of an angiotensin-converting enzyme inhibitor. *Ann Intern Med* 1990; **112**: 312.
18 Kozel MMA, Mekkes JR, Bos JD. Increased frequency and severity of angio-oedema related to long-term therapy with angiotensin-converting enzyme inhibitor in two patients. *Clin Exp Dermatol* 1995; **20**: 60–1.

Serum sickness

Serum sickness, a type III immune complex-mediated reaction, may occur between 5 days and 3 weeks after initial exposure [1–5], and in its complete form combines fever, urticaria, angio-oedema, joint pain and swelling, lymphadenopathy, and occasionally nephritis or endocarditis, with eosinophilia. In minor forms of serum sickness, fever, urticaria and transitory joint tenderness may be the only manifestations.

Drugs implicated include heterologous serum [1,2], immune globulin (as treatment for Kawasaki syndrome) [6], aspirin, antibiotics [7,8], including penicillin [3,7], amoxicillin [7], flucloxacillin [7], cefaclor [9–14], cefprozil [15], piperacillin [16], ciprofloxacin [17], cefatrazine [18], co-trimoxazole [7], triacetyloldendomycin [7], streptomycin, sulphonamides, sulphasalazine [19], thiouracils, intravenous streptokinase [20,21], *N*-acetylcysteine [22] and staphylococcal protein A immunomodulation [23]. Fifteen per cent of 32 women in an *in vitro* fertilization (IVF) programme developed serum sickness 8–12 days after oocyte retrieval by echographic puncture, when a medium containing bovine serum was employed for rinsing follicles [24]. Patients had specific IgG antibodies against, and positive intradermal skin testing to, bovine serum albumin. A characteristic serpiginous, erythematous and purpuric eruption developed on the hands and feet at the borders of palmar and plantar skin in a series of patients treated with intravenous infusions of horse antithymocyte globulin for bone-marrow failure [1,2]. Circulating immune complexes, low serum C4 and C3 levels, and elevated plasma C3a anaphylatoxin levels, were found. Direct immunofluorescence revealed the presence of immunoreactants including IgM, C3, IgE, and IgA in the walls of dermal blood vessels.

REFERENCES

1 Lawley TJ, Bielory L, Gascon P *et al.* A prospective clinical and immunologic analysis of patients with serum sickness. *N Engl J Med* 1984; **311**: 1407–13.
2 Bielory L, Yancey KB, Young NS *et al.* Cutaneous manifestations of serum sickness in patients receiving antithymocyte globulin. *J Am Acad Dermatol* 1985; **13**: 411–17.
3 Erffmeyer JE. Serum sickness. *Ann Allergy* 1986; **56**: 105–9.
4 Lin RY. Serum sickness syndrome. *Am Fam Physician* 1986; **33**: 157–62.
5 Virella G. Hypersensitivity reactions. *Immunol Ser* 1993; **58**: 329–41.
6 Comenzo RL, Malachowski ME, Meissner HC *et al.* Immune hemolysis, disseminated intravascular coagulation, and serum sickness after large doses of immune globulin given intravenously for Kawasaki disease. *J Pediatr* 1992; **120**: 926–8.
7 Martin J, Abbott G. Serum sickness-like illness and antimicrobials in children. *NZ Med J* 1995; **108**: 123–4.
8 Smith JM. Serum sickness-like reactions with antibiotics. *NZ Med J* 1995; **108**: 258.
9 Hebert AA, Sigman ES, Levy ML. Serum sickness-like reactions from cefaclor in children. *J Am Acad Dermatol* 1992; **25**: 805–8.

10 Stricker BH, Tijssen JG. Serum sickness-like reactions to cefaclor. *J Clin Epidemiol* 1992; **45**: 1177–84.

11 Vial T, Pont J, Pham E *et al.* Cefaclor-associated serum sickness-like disease: eight cases and review of the literature. *Ann Pharmacother* 1992; **26**: 910–14.

12 Parra FM, Igea JM, Martin JA *et al.* Serum sickness-like syndrome associated with cefaclor therapy. *Allergy* 1992; **47**: 439–40.

13 Kearns GL, Wheeler JG, Childress SH, Letzig LG. Serum sickness-like reactions to cefaclor: role of hepatic metabolism and individual susceptibility. *J Pediatr* 1994; **125**: 805–11.

14 Grammer LC. Cefaclor serum sickness. *JAMA* 1996; **275**: 1152–3.

15 Lowery N, Kearns GL, Young RA, Wheeler JG. Serum sickness-like reactions associated with cefprozil therapy. *J Pediatr* 1994; **125**: 325–8.

16 Rye PJ, Roberts G, Staugas RE, Martin AJ. Coagulopathy with piperacillin administration in cystic fibrosis: two case reports. *J Paediatr Child Health* 1994; **30**: 278–9.

17 Guharoy SR. Serum sickness secondary to ciprofloxacin use. *Vet Hum Toxicol* 1994; **36**: 540–1.

18 Plantin P, Milochau P, Dubois D. Maladie serique medicamenteuse apres prise de cefatrizine. Premier cas reporté. *Presse Med* 1992; **21**: 1915.

19 Brooks H, Taylor HG, Nichol FE. The three week sulphasalazine syndrome. *Clin Rheumatol* 1992; **11**: 566–8.

20 Patel A, Prussick R, Buchanan WW, Sauder DN. Serum sickness-like illness and leukocytoclastic vasculitis after intravenous streptokinase. *J Am Acad Dermatol* 1991; **24**: 652–3.

21 Clesham GJ, Terry HJ, Jalihal S, Toghill PJ. Serum sickness and purpura following intravenous streptokinase. *J R Soc Med* 1992; **85**: 638–9.

22 Mohammed S, Jamal AZ, Robison LR. Serum sickness-like illness associated with N-acetylcysteine therapy. *Ann Pharmacother* 1994; **28**: 285.

23 Smith RE, Gottschall JL, Pisciotta AV. Life-threatening reaction to staphylococcal protein A immunomodulation. *J Clin Apheresis* 1992; **7**: 4–5.

24 Morales C, Braso JV, Pellicer A *et al.* Serum sickness due to bovine serum albumin sensitization during in vitro fertilization. *J Invest Allergol Clin Immunol* 1994; **4**: 246–9.

Erythema multiforme

Erythema multiforme (Chapter 45) is a very well-recognized pattern of adverse cutaneous drug reaction [1–7], although in a prospective study of cases of erythema multiforme, only 10% were drug related [2]. In another study, antecedent medication use, especially cephalosporins, was recorded in 59% of erythema multiforme patients and 68% of Stevens–Johnson syndrome patients [3]. Clinically, macular, papular or urticarial lesions, as well as the classical iris or 'target lesions', are distributed preferentially on the distal extremities. Lesions may involve the palms or trunk, as well as the oral and genital mucous membranes.

Drugs implicated (Table 77.7) include sulphonamides and co-trimoxazole, barbiturates, pyrazolone derivatives

Table 77.7 Drugs causing erythema multiforme or Stevens–Johnson syndrome.

Antibiotics
Sulphonamides
   Trimethoprim–sulphamethoxazole
   Sulfadoxine–pyrimethamine
Sulphones
Penicillins and ampicillin
Cephalosporins
   Ceftazidime
Quinolones
Rifampicin
Tetracyclines
Erythromycin
Thiacetazone

Antifungal or antiyeast preparations
Griseofulvin
Terbinafine
Nystatin

Non-steroidal anti-inflammatory drugs
Salicylates
Fenbrufen
Ibuprofen
Sulindac
Paracetamol (acetaminophen)
Pyrazolone derivatives
   Antipyrine
   Phenylbutazone
   Phenazone

Metals
Arsenic
Bromides
Mercury
Gold
Iodides

Anticonvulsants
Barbiturates
Carbamazepine
Hydantoin derivatives
Lamotrigine
Trimethadione

Antihypertensives
Frusemide
Hydralazine
Minoxidil
Thiazide diuretics

Drugs acting on the central nervous system
Danazol
Lithium
Mianserin
Phenothiazines
Trazodone

Miscellaneous
Allopurinol
Chlorpropamide
Codeine
Cyclophosphamide
Methaqualone
Nitrogen mustard
Pentazocine
Phenolphthalein
Progesterone
Topical agents: see text
Vaccination

(phenylbutazone), phenolphthalein, rifampicin, penicillins, hydantoin derivatives, carbamazepine, phenothiazines, chlorpropamide, thiazide diuretics, and sulphones. Recent reports have incriminated phenazone, minoxidil, fenbrufen, mianserin, sulindac, methaqualone, ceftazidime [8], trazodone [9], progesterone [10], lithium [11], ampicillin [12], danazol [13], intradural prednisolone acetate [14], indapamide and sertraline [15], allopurinol [16], suramin [17] and terbinafine [18]. Erythema multiforme may follow vaccination.

A large number of topical medications may induce erythema multiforme-like eruptions [19], including: balsam of Peru, chloramphenicol, econazole, ethylenediamine, furazolidone, mafenide acetate cream used to treat burns, the muscle relaxant mephensin, neomycin, nifuroxime, promethazine, scopolamine, sulphonamides, ophthalmic anticholinergic preparations (scopolamine hydrobromide and tropicamide drops), vitamin E, the antimycotic agent pyrrolnitrin, as well as proflavine, budesonide [20], topical nitrogen mustard [21], sesquiterpene lactones in herbal medicine [22], bufexamac [23] and phenylbutazone [24]. In addition, contact with a number of environmental substances may induce erythema-multiforme-like reactions [25], including nickel, formaldehyde, trichloroethylene, phenyl sulfone derivative, the insecticide methyl parathion, nitrogen mustard, epoxy compounds and trinitrotoluene.

REFERENCES

1 Kauppinen K. Cutaneous reactions to drugs. With special reference to severe mucocutaneous bullous eruptions and sulphonamides. *Acta Derm Venereol (Stockh)* 1972; **52** (Suppl. 68): 1–89.

2 Huff JC, Weston WL, Tonnesen MG. Erythema multiforme: a critical review of characteristics, diagnostic criteria, and causes. *J Am Acad Dermatol* 1983; **8**: 763–75.

3 Stewart MG, Duncan NO, III, Franklin DJ *et al*. Head and neck manifestations of erythema multiforme in children. *Otolaryngol Head Neck Surg* 1994; **111**: 236–42.

4 Gebel K, Hornstein OP. Drug-induced oral erythema multiforme. Results of a long-term retrospective study. *Dermatologica* 1984; **168**: 35–40.

5 Nethercott JR, Choi BC. Erythema multiforme (Stevens–Johnson syndrome)—chart review of 123 hospitalized patients. *Dermatologica* 1985; **171**: 383–96.

6 Fabbri P, Panconesi E. Erythema multiforme ('minus' and 'maius') and drug intake. *Clin Dermatol* 1993; **11**: 479–89.

7 Rzany B, Hering O, Mockenhaupt M *et al*. Histopathological and epidemiological characteristics of patients with erythema exudativum multiforme major, Stevens–Johnson syndrome and toxic epidermal necrolysis. *Br J Dermatol* 1996; **135**: 6–11.

8 Pierce TH, Vig SJ, Ingram PM. Ceftazidime in the treatment of lower respiratory tract infection. *J Antimicrob Chemother* 1983; **12** (Suppl. A): 21–5.

9 Ford HE, Jenike MA. Erythema multiforme associated with trazadone therapy. *J Clin Psychiatry* 1985; **46**: 294–5.

10 Wojnarowska F, Greaves MW, Peachey RDG *et al*. Progesterone-induced erythema multiforme. *J R Soc Med* 1985; **78**: 407–8.

11 Balldin J, Berggren U, Heijer A, Mobacken H. Erythema multiforme caused by lithium. *J Am Acad Dermatol* 1991; **24**: 1015–16.

12 Garty BZ, Offer I, Livni E, Danon YL. Erythema multiforme and hypersensitivity myocarditis caused by ampicillin. *Ann Pharmacother* 1994; **28**: 730–1.

13 Reynolds NJ, Sansom JE. Erythema multiforme during danazol therapy. *Clin Exp Dermatol* 1992; **17**: 140.

14 Lavabre C, Chevalier X, Larget-Piet B. Erythema multiforme after intradural injection of prednisolone acetate. *Br J Rheumatol* 1992; **31**: 717–18.

15 Gales BJ, Gales MA. Erythema multiforme and angioedema with indapamide and sertraline (Letter). *Am J Hosp Pharm* 1994; **51**: 118–19.

16 Kumar A, Edward N, White MI *et al*. Allopurinol, erythema multiforme, and renal insufficiency. *Br Med J* 1996; **312**: 173–4.

17 Katz SK, Medenica MM, Kobayashi K *et al*. Erythema multiforme induced by suramin. *J Am Acad Dermatol* 1995; **32**: 292–3.

18 Todd P, Halpern S, Munro DD. Oral terbinafine and erythema multiforme. *Clin Exp Dermatol* 1995; **20**: 247–8.

19 Fisher AA. Erythema multiforme-like eruptions due to topical medications: Part II. *Cutis* 1986; **37**: 158–61.

20 Stingeni L, Caraffini S, Assalve D *et al*. Erythema multiforme-like contact dermatitis from budesonide. *Contact Dermatitis* 1996; **34**: 154–5.

21 Newman JM, Rindler JM, Bergfeld WF. Stevens–Johnson syndrome associated with topical nitrogen mustard therapy. *J Am Acad Dermatol* 1997; **36**: 112–14.

22 Mateo MP, Velasco M, Miquel FJ, de la Cuadra J. Erythema multiforme-like eruption following allergic contact dermatitis from sesquiterpene lactones in herbal medicine. *Contact Dermatitis* 1995; **33**: 449–50.

23 Koch P, Bahmer FA. Erythema multiforme-like, urticarial papular and plaque eruptions from bufexamac: report of 4 cases. *Contact Dermatitis* 1994; **31**: 97–101.

24 Kerre S, Busschots A, Dooms-Goossens A. Erythema multiforme-like contact dermatitis due to phenylbutazone. *Contact Dermatitis* 1995; **33**: 213–14.

25 Fisher AA. Erythema multiforme-like eruptions due to topical miscellaneous compounds: Part III. *Cutis* 1986; **37**: 262–4.

Stevens–Johnson syndrome [1–9]

This comprises fever, malaise, myalgia, arthralgia, and extensive erythema multiforme of the trunk, with occasional skin blisters and erosions covering less than 10% of the body's surface area. Abnormalities of liver function may be present. Stevens–Johnson syndrome should be differentiated from TEN, in which typically sheet-like erosions involve more than 30% of the body surface with widespread purpuric macules or flat, atypical target lesions, and in which there is severe involvement of conjunctival, corneal, irideal, buccal, labial and genital mucous membranes [8,9]. There may be significant differences between countries in the clinical classification of severe cutaneous reactions, indicating the need for precise definitions [10]. The mean time from first drug administration to onset of Stevens–Johnson syndrome or TEN was 7 ± 6 days (range, 1–28 days) in one study [11]. A longer incubation period was observed with thiacetazone (10 ± 6 days), phenytoin (12 ± 9 days), and carbamazepine (11 ± 3 days).

Drugs potentially causing Stevens–Johnson syndrome are listed in Table 77.7. A retrospective study from Malaysia reported that the most common causes of Stevens–Johnson syndrome were sulphonamides, tetracycline and the penicillin derivatives [12]. In the USA, NSAIDs were reported to be an important cause [13]. Severe Stevens–Johnson-like reactions have been described resulting from sulphonamides with or without trimethoprim [14–16] and following malaria prophylaxis with Fansidar (pyrimethamine and sulphadoxine) [17,18]. Patients with AIDS are at an increased risk of developing severe Stevens–Johnson reactions to co-trimoxazole and thiacetazone [19–

21]. Re-exposure to drugs suspected of causing a reaction has resulted in fatality and should not be carried out for diagnostic purposes [1]. The culprit drugs in a study from Thailand included the following: antibiotics (penicillin, sulphonamides, tetracycline, erythromycin); anticonvulsants (phenytoin, carbamazepine, barbiturates); antitubercular drugs (thiacetazone); analgesics (acetylsalicylic acid, fenbufen); sulphonylurea; and allopurinol. The total mortality rate was 14%: 5% for Stevens–Johnson-syndrome, and 40% for TEN [11]. Data from surveillance networks in France, Germany, Italy and Portugal on 245 people hospitalized because of Stevens–Johnson syndrome or TEN [22] indicate that for drugs usually used for short periods, relative risks were increased as follows: trimethoprim–sulphamethoxazole and other sulphonamide antibiotics 172, chlormezanone 62, aminopenicillins 6.7, quinolones 10 and cephalosporins 14, and for paracetamol (acetaminophen) 0.6 in France but 9.3 in the other countries. For drugs used for months or years, the increased risk was largely in the first 2 months, and was as follows: carbamazepine 90, phenobarbital 45, phenytoin 53, valproic acid 25, oxicam NSAIDs 72, allopurinol 52 and corticosteroids 54. For many drugs, including thiazide diuretics and oral hypoglycaemic agents, there was no significant increase in risk. The excess risk did not exceed five cases per million users per week for any of the drugs. Other drugs implicated in Stevens–Johnson syndrome include ciprofloxacin [23], terbinafine [24], nystatin [25] and cyclophosphamide [26].

REFERENCES

1 Bianchine JR, Macaraeg PVJ, Lasagna L et al. Drugs as etiologic factors in the Stevens–Johnson syndrome. *Am J Med* 1968; **44**: 390–405.
2 Kauppinen K. Cutaneous reactions to drugs. With special reference to severe mucocutaneous bullous eruptions and sulphonamides. *Acta Derm Venereol (Stockh)* 1972; **52** (Suppl. 68): 1–89.
3 Böttiger LE, Strandberg I, Westerholm B. Drug-induced febrile mucocutaneous syndrome. With a survey of the literature. *Acta Med Scand* 1975; **198**: 229–33.
4 Ruiz-Maldonado R. Acute disseminated epidermal necrosis types 1, 2, and 3: Study of sixty cases. *J Am Acad Dermatol* 1985; **13**: 623–35.
5 Nethercott JR, Choi BC. Erythema multiforme (Stevens–Johnson syndrome)—chart review of 123 hospitalized patients. *Dermatologica* 1985; **171**: 383–96.
6 Ting HC, Adam BA. Stevens–Johnson syndrome, a review of 34 cases. *Int J Dermatol* 1985; **24**: 587–91.
7 Assier H, Bastuji-Garin S, Revuz J, Roujeau JC. Erythema multiforme with mucous membrane involvement and Stevens–Johnson syndrome are clinically different disorders with distinct causes. *Arch Dermatol* 1995; **131**: 539–43.
8 Bastuji-Garin S, Rzany B, Stern RS et al. Clinical classification of cases of toxic epidermal necrolysis, Stevens–Johnson syndrome, and erythema multiforme. *Arch Dermatol* 1993; **129**: 92–6.
9 Roujeau JC. The spectrum of Stevens–Johnson syndrome and toxic epidermal necrolysis: a clinical classification. *J Invest Dermatol* 1994; **102**: 28S–30S.
10 Stern RS, Albengres E, Carlson J et al. An international comparison of case definition of severe adverse cutaneous reactions to medicines. *Drug Saf* 1993; **8**: 69–77.
11 Leenutaphong V, Sivayathorn A, Suthipinittharm P, Sunthonpalin P. Stevens–Johnson syndrome and toxic epidermal necrolysis in Thailand. *Int J Dermatol* 1993; **32**: 428–31.
12 Gebel K, Hornstein OP. Drug-induced oral erythema multiforme. Results of a long-term retrospective study. *Dermatologica* 1984; **168**: 35–40.
13 Stern R, Bigby M. An expanded profile of cutaneous reactions to nonsteroidal anti-inflammatory drugs. *JAMA* 1984; **252**: 1433–7.
14 Carrol OM, Bryan PA, Robinson RJ. Stevens–Johnson-syndrome associated with long-acting sulfonamides. *JAMA* 1966; **195**: 691–3.
15 Azinge NO, Garrick GA. Stevens–Johnson syndrome (erythema multiforme) following ingestion of trimethoprim-sulfamethoxazole on two separate occasions in the same person. A case report. *J Allergy Clin Immunol* 1978; **62**: 125–6.
16 Aberer W, Stingl G, Wolff K. Stevens–Johnson-Syndrom und toxische epidermale Nekrolyse nach Sulfonamideinahme. *Hautarzt* 1982; **33**: 484–90.
17 Hornstein OP, Ruprecht KW. Fansidar-induced Stevens–Johnson syndrome. *N Engl J Med* 1982; **307**: 1529–30.
18 Miller KD, Lobel HO, Satriale RF et al. Severe cutaneous reactions among American travelers using pyrimethamine-sulfadoxine (Fansidar) for malaria prophylaxis. *Am J Trop Med Hyg* 1986; **35**: 451–8.
19 De Raeve L, Song M, Van Maldergem L. Adverse cutaneous drug reactions in AIDS. *Br J Dermatol* 1988; **119**: 521–3.
20 Porteous DM, Berger TG. Severe cutaneous drug reactions (Stevens–Johnson syndrome and toxic epidermal necrolysis) in human immunodeficiency virus infection. *Arch Dermatol* 1991; **127**: 740–1.
21 van der Ven AJAM, Koopmans PP, Vree TB, van der Meer JWM. Adverse reactions to co-trimoxazole in HIV infection. *Lancet* 1991; **338**: 431–3.
22 Roujeau JC, Kelly JP, Naldi L et al. Medication use and the risk of Stevens–Johnson syndrome or toxic epidermal necrolysis. *N Engl J Med* 1995; **333**: 1600–7.
23 Bhatia RS. Stevens Johnson syndrome following a single dose of ciprofloxacin. *J Assoc Phys India* 1994; **42**: 344.
24 Rzany B, Mockenhaupt M, Gehring W, Schöpf E. Stevens–Johnson syndrome after terbinafine therapy. *J Am Acad Dermatol* 1994; **30**: 509.
25 Assier-Bonnet HJ, Aractingi S, Cadranel J et al. Stevens–Johnson syndrome induced by cyclophosphamide: report of two cases. *Br J Dermatol* 1996; **135**: 864–5.
26 Garty B-Z. Stevens–Johnson syndrome associated with nystatin treatment. *Arch Dermatol* 1991; **127**: 741–2.

Toxic epidermal necrolysis

There is a degree of overlap between Stevens–Johnson syndrome and TEN; Stevens–Johnson syndrome may evolve into TEN, and several drugs can produce both entities [1–13]. Clinically, the condition presents within a few hours or days of medicament administration with an initial 'burning' morbilliform eruption accompanied by systemic flu-like symptoms. There is rapid progression to areas of confluent erythema, often starting in the axillae and groins, followed by blistering and widespread exfoliation, especially on pressure areas. Blisters on the palms tend to remain intact. Mucous membranes (particularly the buccal and less commonly the genital, nasal and ophthalmic ones) are often involved. Nail shedding may occur. Pigmentary changes and a sicca syndrome are frequent sequelae. Healing occurs by re-epithelialization; most patients completely heal their skin lesions in about 3–4 weeks, but mucosal lesions take longer. Ocular complications occur in 40–50% of survivors and include conjunctivitis, pseudomembrane formation, photophobia, ectropion, entropion with trichiasis, synblepharon and corneal vascularization, corneal opacities, and corneal ulceration and scarring. Blindness may result. There is an appreciable mortality of the order of 20–30% [13,14]. Patients with AIDS have a dramatically increased incidence of TEN; 14 of 80 consecutive cases of TEN patients were HIV infected, and 15 cases of AIDS-associated TEN occurred in the Paris area over a study period, compared with the expected 0.04 cases [15]. Sulphonamides (sulpha-diazine, trimethoprim–sulphamethoxazole, sulphadoxine), clindamycin, phenobarbital, chlormezanone were impli-cated [15], as were sulphadiazine and pyrimethamine/clindamycin [16].

A large number of different drugs have been implicated, but the commonest triggers (Table 77.8) include anti-epileptic drugs (phenytoin, barbiturates, carbamazepine and lamotrigine [17,18]), sulphonamides, ampicillin and other β-lactam antibiotics [19], allopurinol, NSAIDs (especially pyrazolon derivatives, e.g. phenylbutazone, and oxicam derivatives) [20] and pentamidine. The absolute incidence of phenytoin-induced TEN is very low, with nine cases reported in the USA over the past decade, compared with 2 million Americans who take phenytoin [8]. Similarly, four of 232 390 patients on trimethoprim–sulfamethoxazole developed erythema multiforme or Stevens–Johnson syndrome, while only one of 196 397 prescribed cephalexin developed TEN [21]. Other antibiotics, antifungals and antiprotozoal drugs incriminated include ciprofloxacin [22,23], vancomycin [24], thiacetazone [25], fluconazole [26], terbinafine [27,28], griseofulvin [29,30] and fansidar [31]. Miscellaneous causes include fluoxetine [32], methotrexate [33], IL-2 [34], etretinate [35], omeprazole [36], ranitidine [37] and famotidine [38]. Immunization with diphtheria–pertussis–tetanus (DPT), measles, poliomyelitis, smallpox and influenza vaccines has been recorded as a cause of TEN [8]. A single case of fatal TEN following the second exposure to diatrizoate solution for excretory pyelography has been documented [39].

In France, a recent survey showed two main classes of drug were most often responsible: antibacterial agents (especially sulphonamides); NSAIDs including oxyphenabutazone, and fenbufen; and phenytoin [40]. The incidence of erythema multiforme, Stevens–Johnson syndrome and TEN in a United States series with the following drugs were reported as follows: phenobarbital 20, nitrofurantoin 7, cotrimoxazole and ampicillin each 3, and amoxicillin 2, per 100 000 exposed patients [41]. In India by contrast, one-third of cases are the result of drugs used for the treatment of tuberculosis, especially thiacetazone and isoniazid [42]. Review of the English language literature from 1966 to 1987 suggested that allopurinol, NSAIDs, phenytoin and the sulphonamide antibiotics were most frequently responsible [43]. A recent study from the USA reported that penicillins, especially aminopenicillins, were most frequently implicated [44]. In West Germany, drugs most frequently implicated were antibiotics (sulphonamides and β-lactam agents) and analgesics and NSAIDs [45].

Identification of the responsible drug is often difficult, because patients frequently take more than one medication. A helpful guideline is that most drugs that cause TEN have been first given between 1 and 3 weeks previously. However, phenytoin-induced TEN may occur any time between 2 and 8 weeks after initiation of therapy. Unfortunately, there is no reliable test to confirm the aetiological role of a given drug in an individual case.

Table 77.8 Drugs causing toxic epidermal necrolysis.

Antibiotics	*Anticonvulsants*
Sulphonamides	Barbiturates
Penicillins	Carbamazepine
Amoxicillin	Lamotrigine
Ampicillin	Phenytoin
Ethambutol	
Isoniazid	*Antifungal agents*
Streptomycin	Griseofulvin
Tetracycline	Terbinafine
Thiacetazone	
	Gastrointestinal drugs
Non-steroidal anti-inflammatory drugs	Famotidine
Pyrazolon-derivatives	Omeprazole
Phenylbutazone	Ranitidine
Oxyphenabutazone	
Oxicam-derivatives	*Miscellaneous*
Isoxicam	Allopurinol
Fenbufen	Chlorpromazine
Salicylates	Dapsone
	Gold
	Nitrofurantoin
	Pentamidine
	Tolbutamide
	Vaccination

REFERENCES

1 Heng MCY. Drug-induced toxic epidermal necrolysis. *Br J Dermatol* 1985; **113**: 597–60.
2 Fabrizio PJ, McCloshey WW, Jeffrey LP. Drugs causing toxic epidermal necrolysis. *Drug Intell Clin Pharmacol* 1985; **19**: 733–5.
3 Guillaume J-C, Roujeau J-C, Penso D et al. The culprit drugs in 87 cases of toxic epidermal necrolysis (Lyell's syndrome). *Arch Dermatol* 1987; **123**: 1166–70.
4 Revuz J, Penso D, Roujeau J-C et al. Toxic epidermal necrolysis. Clinical findings and prognosis factors in 87 patients. *Arch Dermatol* 1987; **123**: 1160–5.
5 De Felice GP, Caroli R, Auteliano A. Long-term complications of toxic epidermal necrolysis (Lyell's disease): clinical and histopathologic study. *Ophthalmologica* 1987; **195**: 1–6.
6 Ruiz-Maldonado R. Acute disseminated epidermal necrosis types 1, 2 and 3: study of 60 cases. *J Am Acad Dermatol* 1985; **13**: 623–35.
7 Roujeau J-C, Chosidow O, Saiag P, Guillaume J-C. Toxic epidermal necrolysis (Lyell syndrome). *J Am Acad Dermatol* 1990; **23**: 1039–58.
8 Avakian R, Flowers FP, Araujo OE, Ramos-Caro FA. Toxic epidermal necrolysis: a review. *J Am Acad Dermatol* 1991; **25**: 69–79.
9 Parsons JM. Toxic epidermal necrolysis. *Int J Dermatol* 1992; **31**: 749–68.
10 Paquet P. Les medicaments responsables de necrolyse epidermique toxique (syndrome de Lyell). *Thérapie* 1993; **48**: 133–9.
11 Lyell A. Drug-induced toxic epidermal necrolysis. I. An overview. *Clin Dermatol* 1993; **11**: 491–2.
12 Roujeau JC. Drug-induced toxic epidermal necrolysis. II. Current aspects. *Clin Dermatol* 1993; **11**: 493–500.
13 Roujeau JC, Stern RS. Severe adverse cutaneous reactions to drugs. *N Engl J Med* 1994; **331**: 1272–85.
14 Kelly JP, Auquier A, Rzany B et al. An international collaborative case-control study of severe cutaneous adverse reactions (SCAR). Design and methods. *J Clin Epidemiol* 1995; **48**: 1099–108.
15 Saiag P, Caumes E, Chosidow O et al. Drug-induced toxic epidermal necrolysis

(Lyell syndrome) in patients infected with the human immunodeficiency virus. *J Am Acad Dermatol* 1992; **26**: 567–74.

16 Caumes E, Bocquet H, Guermonprez G *et al.* Adverse cutaneous reactions to pyrimethamine/sulfadiazine and pyrimethamine/clindamycin in patients with AIDS and toxoplasmic encephalitis. *Clin Infect Dis* 1995; **21**: 656–8.

17 Creamer JD, Whittaker SJ, Kerr-Muir M, Smith NP. Phenytoin-induced toxic epidermal necrolysis: a case report. *Clin Exp Dermatol* 1996; **21**: 116–20.

18 Sterker M, Berrouschot J, Schneider D. Fatal course of toxic epidermal necrolysis under treatment with lamotrigine. *Int J Clin Pharmacol Ther* 1995; **33**: 595–7.

19 Romano A, Di Fonso M, Pocobelli D *et al.* Two cases of toxic epidermal necrolysis caused by delayed hypersensitivity to beta-lactam antibiotics. *J Invest Allergol Clin Immunol* 1993; **3**: 53–5.

20 Stratigos JD, Bartsokas SK, Capetanakis J. Further experiences of toxic epidermal necrolysis incriminating allopurinol, pyrazolone, and derivatives. *Br J Dermatol* 1972; **86**: 564–7.

21 Jick H, Derby LE. A large population-based follow-up study of trimethoprim-sulfamethoxazole, trimethoprim, and cephalexin for uncommon serious drug toxicity. *Pharmacotherapy* 1995; **15**: 428–32.

22 Tham TCK, Allen G, Hayes D *et al.* Possible association between toxic epidermal necrolysis and ciprofloxacin. *Lancet* 1991; **338**: 522.

23 Moshfeghi M, Mandler HD. Ciprofloxacin-induced toxic epidermal necrolysis. *Ann Pharmacother* 1993; **27**: 467–9.

24 Vidal C, Gonzalez Quintela A, Fuente R. Toxic epidermal necrolysis due to vancomycin. *Ann Allergy* 1992; **68**: 345–7.

25 Ipuge YA, Rieder HL, Enarson DA. Adverse cutaneous reactions to thiacetazone for tuberculosis treatment in Tanzania. *Lancet* 1995; **346**: 657–60.

26 Azon-Masoliver A, Vilaplana J. Fluconazole-induced toxic epidermal necrolysis in a patient with human immunodeficiency virus infection. *Dermatology* 1993; **187**: 268–9.

27 Carstens J, Wendelboe P, Sogaard H, Thestrup-Pedersen K. Toxic epidermal necrolysis and erythema multiforme following therapy with terbinafine. *Acta Derm Venereol (Stockh)* 1994; **74** 391–2.

28 White SI, Bowen-Jones D. Toxic epidermal necrolysis induced by terbinafine in a patient on long-term antiepileptics. *Br J Dermatol* 1996; **134**: 188–9.

29 Taylor B, Duffill M. Toxic epidermal necrolysis from griseofulvin. *J Am Acad Dermatol* 1988; **19**: 565–7.

30 Mion G, Verdon G, Le Gulluche Y *et al.* Fatal toxic epidermal necrolysis after griseofulvin. *Lancet* 1989; **2**: 1331.

31 Sturchler D, Mittelholzer ML, Kerr L. How frequent are notified severe cutaneous adverse reactions to Fansidar? *Drug Saf* 1993; **8**: 60–8.

32 Bodokh I, Lacour JP, Rosenthal E *et al.* Syndrome de Lyell ou necrolyse epidermique toxique et syndrome de Stevens–Johnson après traitement par fluoxetine. *Thérapie* 1992; **47**: 441.

33 Collins P, Rogers S. The efficacy of methotrexate in psoriasis—a review of 40 cases. *Clin Exp Dermatol* 1992; **17**: 257–60.

34 Wiener JS, Tucker JA, Jr, Walther PJ. Interleukin-2-induced dermatotoxicity resembling toxic epidermal necrolysis. *South Med J* 1992; **85**: 656–9.

35 McIvor A. Fatal toxic epidermal necrolysis associated with etretinate (Letter). *Br Med J* 1992; **304**: 548.

36 Cox NH. Acute disseminated epidermal necrosis due to omeprazole. *Lancet* 1992; **340**: 857.

37 Miralles ES, Nunez M, del Olmo N, Ledo A. Ranitidine-related toxic epidermal necrolysis in a patient with idiopathic thrombocytopenic purpura. *J Am Acad Dermatol* 1995; **32**: 133–4.

38 Brunner M, Vardarman E, Goldermann R *et al.* Toxic epidermal necrolysis (Lyell syndrome) following famotidine administration. *Br J Dermatol* 1995; **133**: 814–15.

39 Kaftori JK, Abraham Z, Gilhar A. Toxic epidermal necrolysis after excretory pyelography. Immunologic-mediated contrast medium reaction? *Int J Dermatol* 1988; **27**: 346–7.

40 Roujeau J-C, Guillaume J-C, Fabre J-D *et al.* Toxic epidermal necrolysis (Lyell syndrome). Incidence and drug etiology in France, 1981–1985. *Arch Dermatol* 1990; **126**: 37–42.

41 Chan H-L, Stern RS, Arndt KA *et al.* The incidence of erythema multiforme, Stevens–Johnson syndrome, and toxic epidermal necrolysis. A population-based study with particular reference to reactions caused by drugs among outpatients. *Arch Dermatol* 1990; **126**: 43–7.

42 Nanda A, Kaur S. Drug-induced toxic epidermal necrolysis in developing countries. *Arch Dermatol* 1990; **126**: 125.

43 Stern RS, Chan H-L. Usefulness of case report literature in determining drugs responsible for toxic epidermal necrolysis. *J Am Acad Dermatol* 1989; **21**: 317–22.

44 Strom BL, Carson JL, Halpern AC *et al.* A population-based study of Stevens–Johnson syndrome. Incidence and antecedent drug exposures. *Arch Dermatol* 1991; **127**: 831–8.

45 Schöpf E, Stühmer A, Rzany B *et al.* Toxic epidermal necrolysis and Stevens–Johnson syndrome. An epidemiologic study from West Germany. *Arch Dermatol* 1991; **127**: 839–42.

Fixed eruptions [1–5]

Fixed eruptions characteristically recur in the same site or sites each time the drug is administered; with each exposure, however, the number of involved sites may increase. Usually, just one drug is involved, although independent lesions from more than one drug have been described [6]. Cross-sensitivity to related drugs may occur, such as between phenylbutazone and oxyphenbutazone and between tetracycline type drugs. There may be a refractory period after the occurrence of a fixed eruption.

Acute lesions usually develop 30 min to 8 h after drug administration as sharply marginated, round or oval itchy plaques of erythema and oedema becoming dusky violaceous or brown, and sometimes vesicular or bullous (Fig. 77.3). The eruption may initially be morbilliform, scarlatiniform or erythema multiforme-like; urticarial, nodular or eczematous lesions are less common. Lesions are sometimes solitary at first, but with repeated attacks new lesions usually appear and existing lesions may increase in size. A multifocal bullous fixed drug eruption due to mefenamic acid resembled erythema multiforme [7]. Occasionally, involvement is so extensive as to mimic toxic epidermal necrolysis [8,9].

Lesions are commoner on the limbs than on the trunk; the hands and feet, genitalia and perianal areas are favoured sites. Perioral and periorbital lesions may occur.

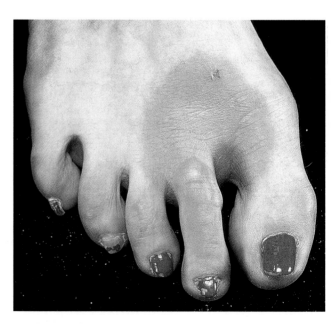

Fig. 77.3 Bullous fixed drug eruption with hyperpigmentation. (Courtesy of St John's Institute of Dermatology, London, UK.)

Genital [10] and oral mucous membranes [11] may be involved in association with skin lesions, or alone. In the case of isolated male genital fixed drug eruption (often affecting only the glans penis), the drugs most commonly implicated in one series were: co-trimoxazole (trimethoprim–sulphamethoxazole), tetracycline and ampicillin [10], and with oral fixed drug eruption, co-trimoxazole, oxyphenbutazone and tetracycline were the most common causative drugs [11]. Pigmentation of the tongue may occur as a form of fixed drug eruption in heroin addicts [12]. As healing occurs, crusting and scaling are followed by pigmentation, which may be very persistent and occasionally extensive, especially in pigmented individuals; pigmentation may be all that is visible between attacks. Non-pigmenting fixed reactions have been reported in association with the sympathomimetic agents pseudoephidrine and tetrahydrozoline hydrochloride, diflunisal, thiopental, piroxicam, the radiopaque contrast medium iothalamate, and arsphenamine [13,14].

The number of drugs capable of producing fixed eruptions is very large [9]. However, most fixed drug reactions are due to one or other of the substances listed in Table 77.9. Earlier series incriminated particularly analgesics, sulphonamides and tetracyclines. In a report from Finland, phenazones caused most eruptions, with barbiturates, sulphonamides, tetracyclines and carbamazepine causing fewer reactions [15]. A series from India reported that acetylsalicylic acid was the drug most commonly implicated in children [16]. A drug-specific clinical pattern in fixed drug eruptions based on a study of 113 patients has been reported as follows [17]. Trimethoprim–sulphamethoxazole caused the maximum incidence (36.3%), followed by tetracycline (15.9%), pyrazolones (14.2%), sulphadiazine (12.4%), dipyrine (9.3%), paracetamol (acetaminophen) (7.9%), aspirin (1.7%), thiacetazone (0.88%) and levamisole (0.88%). Sulphonamides, including trimethoprim–sulphamethoxazole, induced lesions on the lips, trunk and limbs, with only minimal involvement of mucosae. Tetracycline caused lesions only on the glans penis. Pyrazolones affected mainly the lips and mucosae, with a few lesions of the trunk and limbs. Dipyrine, aspirin, and paracetamol (acetaminophen) caused lesions of the trunk and limbs, sparing the lips, genitalia and mucosae. Levamisole caused associated constitutional disturbances with extensive skin lesions, as did thiacetazone [17]. Paracetamol (acetaminophen) is a rare cause of fixed drug eruption [18]; other drugs implicated have included codeine [19], ciprofloxacin [20], terbinafine [21] and dimenhydrinate [22]. Familial occurrence of fixed drug eruption has occurred occasionally [23,24].

REFERENCES

1 Korkij W, Soltani K. Fixed drug eruption. A brief review. *Arch Dermatol* 1984; **120**: 520–4.
2 Kauppinen K, Stubb S. Fixed eruptions: causative drugs and challenge tests. *Br J Dermatol* 1985; **112**: 575–8.
3 Sehgal VN, Gangwani OP. Fixed drug eruption. Current concepts. *Int J Dermatol* 1987; **26**: 67–74.

Table 77.9 Drugs causing fixed eruptions.

Antibacterial substances	Nonsteroidal anti-inflammatory agents
Sulphonamides (co-trimoxazole)	Aspirin (acetylsalicylic acid)
Tetracyclines	Oxyphenbutazone
Penicillin	Phenazone (antipyrine)
Ampicillin	Metimazole
Amoxicillin	Paracetamol (acetaminophen)
Erythromycin	Ibuprofen
Trimethoprim	Various non-proprietory analgesic combinations
Nystatin	Phenolphthalein and related compounds
Griseofulvin	Miscellaneous
Dapsone	Codeine
Arsenicals	Hydralazine
Mercury salts	Oleoresins
p-Amino-salicylic acid	Sympathomimetics
Thiacetazone	Sympatholytics
Quinine	Parasympatholytics
Metronidazole	Hyoscine butylbromide
Clioquinol	Magnesium hydroxide
Barbiturates and other tranquillizers	Magnesium trisilicate
Barbiturate derivatives	Anthralin
Opium alkaloids	Chlorthiazone
Chloral hydrate	Chlorphenesin carbamate
Benzodiazepines	Food substitutes and flavours
Chlordiazepoxide	
Anticonvulsants	
Dextromethorphan	

4 Kanwar AJ, Bharija SC, Singh M, Belhaj MS. Ninety-eight fixed drug eruptions with provocation tests. *Dermatologica* 1988; **177**: 274–9.

5 Sehgal VN, Gangwani OP. Fixed drug eruptions: A study of epidemiological, clinical and diagnostic aspects of 89 cases from India. *J Dermatol (Tokyo)* 1988; **15**: 50–4.

6 Kivity S. Fixed drug eruption to multiple drugs: clinical and laboratory investigation. *Int J Dermatol* 1991; **30**: 149–51.

7 Sowden JM, Smith AG. Multifocal fixed drug eruption mimicking erythema multiforme. *Clin Exp Dermatol* 1990; **15**: 387–8.

8 Saiag P, Cordoliani F, Roujeau JC et al. Érytheme pigmenté fixe bulleux disséminé simulant un syndrome de Lyell. *Ann Dermatol Vénéréol* 1987; **114**: 1440–2.

9 Baird BJ, De Villez RL. Widespread bullous fixed drug eruption mimicking toxic epidermal necrolysis. *Int J Dermatol* 1988; **27**: 170–4.

10 Gaffoor PMA, George WM. Fixed drug eruptions occurring on the male genitals. *Cutis* 1990; **45**: 242–4.

11 Jain VK, Dixit VB, Archana. Fixed drug eruption of the oral mucous membrane. *Ann Dent* 1991; **50**: 9–11.

12 Westerhof W, Wolters EC, Brookbakker JTW et al. Pigmented lesions of the tongue in heroin addicts—fixed drug eruption. *Br J Dermatol* 1983; **109**: 605–10.

13 Alanko K, Kanerva L, Mohell-Talolahti B et al. Nonpigmented fixed drug eruption from pseudoephedrine. *J Am Acad Dermatol* 1996; **35**: 647–8.

14 Krivda SJ, Benson PM. Nonpigmenting fixed drug eruption. *J Am Acad Dermatol* 1994; **31**: 291–2.

15 Stubb S, Alanko K, Reitamo S. Fixed drug eruptions: 77 cases from 1981 to 1985. *Br J Dermatol* 1989; **120**: 583.

16 Kanwar AJ, Bharija SC, Belhaj MS. Fixed drug eruptions in children: a series of 23 cases with provocative tests. *Dermatologica* 1986; **172**: 315–18.

17 Thankappan TP, Zachariah J. Drug-specific clinical pattern in fixed drug eruptions. *Int J Dermatol* 1991; **30**: 867–70.

18 Zemtsov A, Yanase DJ, Boyd AS, Shehata B. Fixed drug eruption to Tylenol: report of two cases and review of the literature. *Cutis* 1992; **50**: 281–2.

19 Gonzalo-Garijo MA, Revenga-Arranz F. Fixed drug eruption due to codeine. *Br J Dermatol* 1996; **135**: 498–9.

20 Dhar S, Sharma VK. Fixed drug eruption due to ciprofloxacin. *Br J Dermatol* 1996; **134**: 56–8.

21 Munn SE, Russell Jones R. Terbinafine and fixed drug eruption. *Br J Dermatol* 1995; **133** 815–16.

22 Gonzalo-Garijo MA, Revenga-Arranz F. Fixed drug eruption due to dimenhydrinate. *Br J Dermatol* 1996; **135**: 661–2.

23 Pellicano R, Silvestris A, Iannantuono M et al. Familial occurrence of fixed drug eruptions. *Acta Derm Venereol (Stockh)* 1992; **72**: 292–3.

24 Hatzis J, Noutsis K, Hatzidakis E et al. Fixed drug eruption in a mother and her son. *Cutis* 1992; **50**: 50–2.

Lichenoid eruptions

Lichenoid eruptions and lichen planus are discussed in Chapter 41. Lichenoid drug eruptions tend to be extensive, and may develop weeks or months after initiation of therapy; they may progress to an exfoliative dermatitis [1,2]. Lesions may be rather more psoriasiform than in idiopathic lichen planus, and oral involvement is rare. Hyperpigmentation, alopecia, and skin atrophy with anhidrosis due to sweat-gland atrophy, may develop. Resolution of the skin eruption may be slow after cessation of therapy, on average from 1 to 4 months, but up to 24 months with gold [2].

Some of the drugs that induce this pattern of reaction are listed in Table 77.10 [2]. Photodistributed lichenoid lesions may be seen with quinine, quinidine, thiazide diuretics (Fig. 77.4), frusemide, diazoxide, tetracyclines, ethambutol, chlorpromazine, carbamazepine, 5-fluorouracil and pyritinol [2]. Unlike idiopathic lichen planus, the lichenoid eruption following quinacrine (mepacrine) may

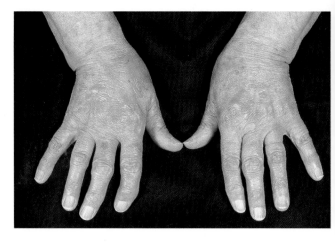

Fig. 77.4 Lichenoid photosensitivity eruption caused by thiazide diuretic. (Courtesy of A. Ive, Dryburn Hospital, Durham, UK.)

undergo malignant change [3]. Lichenoid eruptions may also result from contact dermatitis in photographic workers who handle certain colour film developers containing *p*-phenylenediamines [4,5]. Either eczematous or lichenoid eruptions may be produced; even when lesions are lichenoid clinically and histologically, patch tests are eczematous [5]. Other inducers of contact lichenoid eruptions include dental restorative materials, musk ambrette, nickel, aminoglycoside antibiotics and gold. Oral involvement may be caused by NSAIDs, gold salts, penicillamine, sulphonylureas, ACE inhibitors, methyldopa, allopurinol, ketoconazole, cyanamide and dental restorative materials [2]. Lichen planus pemphigoides occurs after captopril and cinnarizine; bullous lesions with labetalol and tiopronin; lichen planus pigmentosus with gold; exfoliative dermatitis with nifedipine; and ulcerative lesions with hydroxyurea, methyldopa, propranolol and lithium carbonate.

Histologically, changes may be non-specific or may resemble idiopathic lichen planus, although the cellular infiltrate tends to be more pleomorphic and less dense, and the presence of focal parakeratosis, focal interruption of the granular layer, and cytoid bodies in the cornified and granular layers suggest a drug cause [6]. The histopathology of photodistributed, as opposed to non-photodistributed lichenoid drug eruptions has been shown to be often indistinguishable from that of idiopathic lichen planus [7].

REFERENCES

1 Almeyda J, Levantine A. Drug reactions XVI. Lichenoid drug eruptions. *Br J Dermatol* 1971; **85**: 604–7.

2 Halevy S, Shai A. Lichenoid drug eruptions. *J Am Acad Dermatol* 1993; **29**: 249–55.

3 Bauer F. Quinacrine hydrochloride drug eruption (tropical lichenoid dermatitis). Its early and late sequelae and its malignant potential. A review. *J Am Acad Dermatol* 1981; **4**: 239–48.

4 Buckley WR. Lichenoid eruptions following contact dermatitis. *Arch Dermatol* 1958; **78**: 454–7.

Table 77.10 Drugs causing lichenoid eruptions.

Gold salts	Antitubercular drugs
Antimalarials	Ethambutol
Mepacrine (quinacrine, atebrin)	Isoniazid
Chloroquine	p-Aminosalicylic acid
Quinine	Streptomycin
Quinidine	Cycloserine
Pyrimethamine	Antifungal drugs
Penicillamine	Ketoconazole
Diuretics	Chemotherapeutic agents
Thiazides	Hydroxyurea
Frusemide	5-fluorouracil
Spironolactone	Heavy metals
Diazoxide	Mercurials
Antihypertensive agents	Arsenicals
β-Blockers	Bismuth
ACE inhibitors	Miscellaneous
Captopril	Tetracyclines
Enalapril	Carbamazepine
Methyldopa	Phenytoin
Calcium channel blockers:	Procainamide
Nifedipine	Allopurinol
Cinnarizine	Iodides and radiocontrast media
Flunarizine	Tiopronin (mercaptopropionylglycine)
Phenothiazine derivatives	Pyritinol
Metopromazine	Cyanamide
Levomepromazine	Dapsone
Chlorpromazine	Amiphenazole
Sulphonylurea hypoglycaemic agents	Levamisole
Chlorpropamide	Nandrolone furylpropionate
Tolazamide	
Non-steroidal antiinflammatory drugs	
Phenylbutazone	
Suphasalazine and mesalazine	

ACE, angiotensin-converting enzyme.

5 Fry L. Skin disease from colour developers. *Br J Dermatol* 1965; **77**: 456–61.

6 Van den Haute V, Antoine JL, Lachapelle JM. Histopathological discriminant criteria between lichenoid drug eruption and idiopathic lichen planus: retrospective study on selected samples. *Dermatologica* 1989; **179**: 10–13.

7 West AJ, Berger TG, LeBoit PE. A comparative histopathologic study of photodistributed and nonphotodistributed lichenoid drug eruptions. *J Am Acad Dermatol* 1990; **23**: 689–93.

Photosensitivity

Drug–light reactions, which cause eruptions on exposed areas, with sparing of upper eyelids, submental and retro-auricular areas, may be phototoxic or photo-allergic; these cannot always be distinguished clinically, and some drugs may produce cutaneous involvement by both mechanisms [1–5]. The main drugs implicated in photosensitivity reactions are listed in Table 77.11.

REFERENCES

1 Johnson BE, Ferguson J. Drug and chemical photosensitivity. *Semin Dermatol* 1990; **9**: 39–46.

2 Elmets CA. Cutaneous phototoxicity. In: Lim HW, Soter NA, eds. *Clinical Photomedicine*. New York: Marcel Dekker, 1993: 207–26.

3 Deleo VA. Photoallergy. In: Lim HW, Soter NA, eds. *Clinical Photomedicine* New York: Marcel Dekker, 1993: 227–39.

4 Gould JW, Mercurion MG, Elmets CA. Cutaneous photosensitivity diseases induced by exogenous agents. *J Am Acad Dermatol* 1995; **33**: 551–73.

5 González E, González S. Drug photosensitivity, idiopathic photodermatoses, and sunscreens. *J Am Acad Dermatol* 1996; **35**: 871–5.

Phototoxic reactions

Phototoxic reactions are commoner than photoallergic ones, and can be produced in almost all individuals given a high enough dose of drug and sufficient light irradiation. They occur within 5–20 h of the first exposure, and resemble exaggerated sunburn. Erythema, oedema, blistering, weeping, desquamation and residual hyperpigmentation occur on exposed areas; there may be photo-onycholysis. The following are well-recognized causes of phototoxicity: tetracyclines [1–4], especially demeclocycline, less frequently doxycycline, oxytetracycline, and tetracycline, and rarely minocycline and methacycline; other antibacterials including sulphonamides and fluoroquinolones [4]; phenothiazines, especially chlorpromazine, promethazine

Table 77.11 Drugs causing photosensitivity.

Frequent	*Less frequent: systemic*
Amiodarone	Ampicillin
Phenothiazines	Antidepressants: tricyclic
Chlorpromazine	Imipramine
Promethazine	Protriptyline
Psoralens	Antidepressants: MAOI
Sulphonamides	Phenelzine
Co-trimoxazole	Antifungal agents
Tetracyclines	Griseofulvin
Demeclocycline	Ketoconazole
Thiazides	β-Blockers
Non-steroidal anti-inflammatory drugs	Carbamazepine
Azapropazone	Cimetidine
Piroxicam	Cytotoxic agents
Carprofen	Dacarbazine
Tiaprofenic acid	Fluorouracil
Benoxaprofen (withdrawn)	Mitomycin
Nalidixic acid	Vinblastine
Coal tar	Diazepam
	Frusemide
Less frequent: topical	Methyldopa
Antihistamines	Oral contraceptives
Local anaesthetics	Quinine
Benzydamine	Quinidine
Hydrocortisone	Sulphonylureas
Sunscreens	Chlorpropamide
PABA	Tolbutamide
Benzophenone	Retinoids
Halogenated salicylanilides	Isotretinoin
	Etretinate
	Triamterene

PABA, *p*-aminobenzoic acid; MAOI, monoamine oxidase inhibitors.

and less commonly thioridazine; frusemide [5] and nalidixic acid [4,6], both of which produce a pseudo-porphyria syndrome, with blistering of the exposed areas; NSAIDs including ibuprofen [7], piroxicam [8–11], carprofen and tiaprofenic acid [12]; psoralens; amiodarone (which causes photosensitivity in over 50% of cases) [13]; certain anticancer drugs [14] including dacarbazine [14,15], 5-fluorouracil, mitomycin and vinblastine; coal tar and its derivatives; fibric acid derivatives including bezafibrate and fenofibrate [16,17]; and the non-steroid anti-androgen flutamide given for prostatic carcinoma [18].

REFERENCES

1 Cullen SI, Catalano PM, Helfmann RS. Tetracycline sun sensitivity. *Arch Dermatol* 1966; **93**: 77.
2 Frost P, Weinstein GP, Gomez EC. Phototoxic potential of minocycline and doxycycline. *Arch Dermatol* 1972; **105**: 681–3.
3 Layton AM, Cunliffe WJ. Phototoxic eruptions due to doxycycline—a dose-related phenomenon. *Clin Exp Dermatol* 1993; **18**: 425–7.
4 Wainwright NJ, Collins P, Ferguson J. Photosensitivity associated with antibacterial agents. *Drug Saf* 1993; **9**: 437–40.
5 Burry JN, Lawrence JR. Phototoxic blisters from high frusemide dosage. *Br J Dermatol* 1976; **94**: 495–9.

6 Ramsay CA, Obreshkova E. Photosensitivity from nalidixic acid. *Br J Dermatol* 1974; **91**: 523–8.
7 Bergner T, Przybilla B. Photosensitisation caused by ibuprofen. *J Am Acad Dermatol* 1992; **26**: 114–16.
8 Stern RS. Phototoxic reactions to piroxicam and other nonsteroidal antiinflammatory agents. *N Engl J Med* 1983; **309**: 186–7.
9 Serrano G, Bonillo J, Aliaga A et al. Piroxicam-induced photosensitivity. *In vivo* and *in vitro* studies of its photosensitizing potential. *J Am Acad Dermatol* 1984; **11**: 113–20.
10 Figueiredo A, Fontes Ribeiro CA, Conçalo S et al. Piroxicam-induced photosensitivity. *Contact Dermatitis* 1987; **17**: 73–9.
11 Serrano G, Fortea JM, Latasa JM. Oxicam-induced photosensitivity. Patch and photopatch testing studies with tenoxicam and piroxicam photoproducts in normal subjects and in piroxicam–droxicam photosensitive patients. *J Am Acad Dermatol* 1992; **26**: 545–8.
12 Przybilla B, Ring J, Galosi A, Dorn M. Photopatch test reactions to tiaprofenic acid. *Contact Dermatitis* 1984; **1**: 55–6.
13 Ferguson J, Addo HA, Jones S et al. A study of cutaneous photosensitivity induced by amiodarone. *Br J Dermatol* 1985; **113**: 537–49.
14 Kerker BJ, Hood AF. Chemotherapy-induced cutaneous reactions. *Semin Dermatol* 1989; **8**: 173–81.
15 Bonifazi E, Angelini G, Meneghini CL. Adverse photoreaction to dacarbazine (DITC). *Contact Dermatitis* 1981; **7**: 161.
16 Leenutaphong V, Manuskiatti W. Fenofibrate-induced photosensitivity. *J Am Acad Dermatol* 1996; **35**: 775–7.
17 Serrano G, Fortea JM, Latasa JM et al. Photosensitivity induced by fibric acid derivatives and its relation to photocontact dermatitis to ketoprofen. *J Am Acad Dermatol* 1992; **27**: 204–8.
18 Fujimoto M, Kikuchi K, Imakado S, Furue M. Photosensitive dermatitis induced by flutamide. *Br J Dermatol* 1996; **135**: 496–7.

Photo-allergic reactions

Photo-allergic reactions require a latent period during which sensitization occurs, and usually appear within 24 h of re-exposure to drug and light in a sensitized individual; unlike phototoxic reactions, they may spread beyond irradiated areas. Most systemic drugs causing photo-allergy also cause phototoxicity. There may be cross-reactivity with chemically related substances.

Photo-allergic reactions may occur as a result of local photocontact dermatitis to a topical photo-allergen. Photocontact dermatitis is a relatively common cause of photosensitivity, accounting for 9% of cases in a multicentre study [1]. Topical photo-allergens include antihistamines, chlorpromazine, local anaesthetics, benzydamine, hydro-cortisone, desoximetasone and sunscreens containing *p*-aminobenzoic acid (PABA) and its derivatives. Contact and photo-allergy to benzophenones in PABA-free sunscreens may be commoner than is realized [2]. Halogenated salicylanilides, previously used as a disinfectant in soaps, and related compounds also cause a photocontact dermatitis.

Photo-allergic reactions may in addition occur as a result of systemically administered drugs [3], such as phenothiazines (chlorpromazine, promethazine), sulpho-namides, aromatic sulphonamides such as thiazide diuretics [4,5] and oral hypoglycaemic agents (chlorpropamide and tolbutamide), griseofulvin [6] and quinidine [7,8]. Quinidine-induced photo-eruptions may be either eczema-tous or lichenoid; a persistent livedo reticularis-like eruption may be seen in severe cases of quinidine photosensitivity.

Enalapril has caused a photosensitive lichenoid eruption [9]. Tricyclic antidepressants may cause allergy as well as photosensitivity [10]. NSAIDs, disinfectants, sunscreens, phenothiazines and fragrances caused photo-allergic reactions most often in a 5-year survey by the German, Austrian and Swiss photopatch-test group [11].

REFERENCES

1 Wennersten G, Thune P, Brodthagen H *et al.* The Scandinavian multicenter photopatch study. Preliminary results. *Contact Dermatitis* 1984; **10**: 305–9.
2 Knobler E, Almeida L, Ruxkowski AM *et al.* Photoallergy to benzophenone. *Arch Dermatol* 1989; **125**: 801–4.
3 Giudici PA, Maguire HC. Experimental photoallergy to systemic drugs. *J Invest Dermatol* 1985; **85**: 207–11.
4 Robinson HN, Morison WL, Hood AF. Thiazide diuretic therapy and chronic photosensitivity. *Arch Dermatol* 1985; **121**: 522–4.
5 Addo HA, Ferguson J, Frain-Bell W. Thiazide-induced photosensitivity: a study of 33 subjects. *Br J Dermatol* 1987; **116**: 749–60.
6 Kojima T, Hasegawa T, Ishida H *et al.* Griseofulvin-induced photodermatitis. Report of six cases. *J Dermatol (Tokyo)* 1988; **15**: 76–82.
7 Bruce S, Wolf JE, Jr. Quinidine-induced photosensitive livedo reticularis-like eruption. *J Am Acad Dermatol* 1985; **12**: 332–6.
8 Schurer NY, Holzle E, Plewig G, Lehmann P. Photosensitivity induced by quinidine sulfate: experimental reproduction of skin lesions. *Photodermatol Photoimmunol Photomed* 1992; **9**: 78–82.
9 Kanwar AJ, Dhar S, Ghosh S. Photosensitive lichenoid eruption due to enalapril. *Dermatology* 1993; **187**: 80.
10 Ljunggren B, Bojs G. A case of photosensitivity and contact allergy to systemic tricyclic drugs, with unusual features. *Contact Dermatitis* 1991; **24**: 259–65.
11 Hölzle E, Neumann N, Hausen B *et al.* Photopatch testing: the 5-year experience of the German, Austrian and Swiss photopatch test group. *J Am Acad Dermatol* 1991; **25**: 59–68.

Porphyria and pseudoporphyria

A number of drugs may precipitate porphyria cutanea tarda with resultant photosensitivity, or cause a pseudo-porphyria syndrome with bulla formation. The reader is referred to Chapter 59.

Photorecall reactions

A curious photorecall-like eruption occurred, restricted to an area of sunburn sustained 1 month previously, in a patient treated with cefazolin and gentamicin [1]. A recurrent cutaneous reaction localized to the site of pelvic radiotherapy for adenocarcinoma of the prostate followed sun exposure in one patient [2]. Methotrexate is associated with severe reactivation of sunburn [3,4].

REFERENCES

1 Flax SH, Uhle P. Photo recall-like phenomenon following the use of cefazolin and gentamicin sulfate. *Cutis* 1990; **46**: 59–61.
2 Del Guidice SM, Gerstley JK. Sunlight-induced radiation recall. *Int J Dermatol* 1988; **27**: 415–16.
3 Mallory SB, Berry DH. Severe reactivation of sunburn following methotrexate use. *Pediatrics* 1986; **78**: 514–15.

4 Westwick TJ, Sherertz EF, McCarley D, Flowers FP. Delayed reactivation of sunburn by methotrexate: sparing of chronically sun-exposed skin. *Cutis* 1987; **39**: 49–51.

Photo-onycholysis

Photo-onycholysis may be caused by tetracycline, PUVA therapy, and the fluoroquinolone antibiotics pefloxacine and ofloxacine.

Pigmentation reactions

Hyperpigmentation (Table 77.12)

Drug-induced alteration in skin colour [1–3] may result from increased (or more rarely decreased) melanin synthesis, increased lipofuscin synthesis, cutaneous deposition of drug-related material, or most commonly as a result of postinflammatory hyperpigmentation (e.g. fixed drug eruption). Oral contraceptives may induce chloasma [4]. Other drugs implicated in cutaneous hyperpigmentation include minocycline [5,6], antimalarials [7,8], chlorpromazine [9,10], imipramine [11] and desimipramine [12], amiodarone [13], carotene, and heavy metals. Long-term (more than 4 months) antimalarial therapy may result in brownish or blue–black pigmentation, especially on the shin, face, and hard palate or subungually. Yellowish discoloration may occur with mepacrine (quinacrine) or amodiaquin. Long-term high-dose phenothiazine (especially chlorpromazine) therapy results in a blue–grey or brownish pigmentation of sun-exposed areas, the result of a photo-toxic reaction, with pigment deposits in the lens and cornea [10]. The cancer chemotherapeutic agents may be associated with pigmentation as follows [14]. Skin pigmentation may be caused by bleomycin, busulphan, topical carmustine, cyclophosphamide, daunorubicin, fluorouracil, hydroxyurea, topical mechlorethamine, methotrexate, mithramycin, mitomycin and thiotepa. Busulphan and doxorubicin cause mucous membrane pigmentation. Nail

Table 77.12 Drugs causing pigmentation.

Oral contraceptives	Chemotherapeutic agents
Minocycline	Miscellaneous
Antimalarials	Amiodarone
Chloroquine	Carotene
Hydroxychloroquine	Clofazimine
Mepacrine	Pefloxacin
Antidepressants	Sulphasalazine
Chlorpromazine	
Imipramine	
Heavy metals	
Gold	
Lead	
Silver	

pigmentation may result from bleomycin, cyclophosphamide, daunorubicin, doxorubicin and fluorouracil. Methotrexate may induce pigmentation of the hair, and cyclophosphamide of teeth. Sulphasalazine has caused reversible hyperpigmentation [15], and pefloxacin blue–black pigmentation of the legs [16].

Gold may cause blue–grey pigmentation in light exposed areas (*chrysiasis*) [17,18] and silver may cause a similar discoloration (*argyria*) [19]. Lead poisoning can cause a blue–black line at the gingival margin and grey discoloration of the skin. Clofazimine produces red–brown discoloration of exposed skin and the conjunctivae, together with red sweat, urine and faeces [20]. Slate-grey to blue–black pigmentation may occur after long-term topical application of hydroquinone, causing ochronosis [21].

Hypopigmentation

Topical thiotepa has produced periorbital leukoderma [22]. Hypopigmentation has occurred as a result of occupational exposure to monobenzyl ether of hydroquinone, *p*-tertiary-butyl catechol, *p*-tertiary-butyl phenol, *p*-tertiary-amylphenol, monomethyl ether of hydroquinone, and hydroquinone [23]. In addition, hypopigmentation may result from phenolic detergent germicides [24], and following use of diphencyprone for alopecia areata [25,26]. Depigmentation of the skin and hair occurred after a phenobarbital-induced eruption [27]. Photoleukomelanodermatitis occurred due to afloqualone for cervical spondylosis; photopatch and oral challenge tests were positive [28].

REFERENCES

1 Levantine A, Almeyda J. Drug reactions: XXII. Drug induced changes in pigmentation. *Br J Dermatol* 1973; **89**: 105–12.
2 Granstein RD, Sober AJ. Drug- and heavy metal-induced hyperpigmentation. *J Am Acad Dermatol* 1981; **5**: 1–18.
3 Ferguson J, Frain-Bell W. Pigmentary disorders and systemic drug therapy. *Clin Dermatol* 1989; **7**: 44–54.
4 Smith AG, Shuster S, Thody AJ *et al*. Chloasma, oral contraceptives, and plasma immunoreactive beta-melanocyte-stimulating hormone. *J Invest Dermatol* 1977; **68**: 169–70.
5 Dwyer CM, Cuddihy AM, Kerr RE *et al*. Skin pigmentation due to minocycline treatment of facial dermatoses. *Br J Dermatol* 1993; **129**: 158–62.
6 Pepine M, Flowers FP, Ramos-Caro FA. Extensive cutaneous hyperpigmentation caused by minocycline. *J Am Acad Dermatol* 1993; **28**: 292–5.
7 Tuffanelli D, Abraham RK, Dubois EJ. Pigmentation from antimalarial therapy. Its possible relationship to the ocular lesions. *Arch Dermatol* 1963; **88**: 419–26.
8 Leigh IM, Kennedy CTC, Ramsey JD, Henderson WJ. Mepacrine pigmentation in systemic lupus erythematosus. New data from an ultrastructural, biochemical and analytical electron microscope investigation. *Br J Dermatol* 1979; **101**: 147–53.
9 Benning TL, McCormack KM, Ingram P *et al*. Microprobe analysis of chlorpromazine pigmentation. *Arch Dermatol* 1988; **124**: 1541–4.
10 Wolf ME, Richer S, Berk MA, Mosnaim AD. Cutaneous and ocular changes associated with the use of chlorpromazine. *Int J Clin Pharmacol Ther Toxicol* 1993; **31**: 365–7.
11 Hashimoto K, Joselow SA, Tye MJ. Imipramine hyperpigmentation: A slate-gray discoloration caused by long-term imipramine administration. *J Am Acad Dermatol* 1991; **25**: 357–61.
12 Steele TE, Ashby J. Desipramine-related slate-gray skin pigmentation. *J Clin Psychopharmacol* 1993; **13**: 76–7.
13 Zachary CB, Slater DN, Holt DW *et al*. The pathogenesis of amiodarone-induced pigmentation and photosensitivity. *Br J Dermatol* 1984; **110**: 451–6.
14 Kerber BJ, Hood AF. Chemotherapy-induced cutaneous reactions. *Semin Dermatol* 1989; **8**: 173–81.
15 Gabazza EC, Taguchi O, Yamakami T *et al*. Pulmonary infiltrates and skin pigmentation associated with sulfasalazine. *Am J Gastroenterol* 1992; **87**: 1654–7.
16 Le Cleach L, Chosidow O, Peytavin G *et al*. Blue–black pigmentation of the legs associated with pefloxacin therapy. *Arch Dermatol* 1995; **131**: 856–7.
17 Leonard PA, Moatamed F, Ward JR *et al*. Chrysiasis: the role of sun exposure in dermal hyperpigmentation secondary to gold therapy. *J Rheumatol* 1986; **13**: 58–64.
18 Smith RW, Leppard B, Barnett NL *et al*. Chrysiasis revisited: a clinical and pathological study. *Br J Dermatol* 1995; **133**: 671–8.
19 Gherardi R, Brochard P, Chamak B *et al*. Human generalized argyria. *Arch Pathol Lab Med* 1984; **108**: 181–2.
20 Thomsen K, Rothenborg HW. Clofazimine in the treatment of pyoderma gangrenosum. *Arch Dermatol* 1979; **115**: 851–2.
21 Williams H. Skin lightening creams containing hydroquinone. The case for a temporary ban. *Br Med J* 1992; **305**: 903–4.
22 Harben DJ, Cooper PH, Rodman OG. Thiotepa-induced leukoderma. *Arch Dermatol* 1979; **115**: 973–4.
23 Stevenson CJ. Occupational vitiligo: clinical and epidemiological aspects. *Br J Dermatol* 1981; **105** (Suppl. 21): 51–6.
24 Kahn G. Depigmentation caused by phenolic detergent germicides. *Arch Dermatol* 1970; **102**: 177–87.
25 Hatzis J, Gourgiotou K, Tosca A *et al*. Vitiligo as a reaction to topical treatment with diphencyprone. *Dermatologica* 1988; **177**: 146–8.
26 Henderson CA, Ilchyshyn A. Vitiligo complicating diphencyprone sensitization therapy for alopecia universalis. *Br J Dermatol* 1995; **133**: 496–7.
27 Mion N, Fusade T, Mathelier-Fusade P *et al*. Depigmentation cutaneophanerienne consecutive a une toxidermie au phenobarbital. *Ann Dermatol Vénéréol* 1992; **119**: 927–9.
28 Ishikawa T, Kamide R, Niimura M. Photoleukomelanodermatitis (Kobori) induced by afloqualone. *J Dermatol* 1994; **21**: 430–3.

Acneiform and pustular eruptions

The term acneiform is applied to eruptions that resemble acne vulgaris [1,2] (Chapter 42). Lesions are papulopustular but comedones are usually absent. Adrenocorticotrophic hormone (ACTH), corticosteroids [3], as with dexamethasone in neurosurgical patients, anabolic steroids for bodybuilding [4], androgens (in females), oral contraceptives, iodides and bromides may produce acneiform eruptions. Isoniazid may induce acne, especially in slow inactivators of the drug [5]. Other drugs implicated in the production of acneiform rashes include dantrolene [6], danazol [7], quinidine [8], lithium [9,10] and azathioprine [11].

In addition, pustular reactions (toxic pustuloderma, acute generalized exanthematous pustulosis) have been reported in association with a number of drugs [12]. The main differential diagnosis of a generalized pustular drug eruption is pustular psoriasis [13]. Two histological patterns may be seen; either a toxic pustuloderma with spongiform intraepidermal pustules, papillary oedema and a mixed upper dermal perivascular inflammatory infiltrate; or a leukocytoclastic vasculitis with neutrophil collections both below and within the epidermis, suggesting passive neutrophil elimination via the overlying epidermis [14,15]. The presence of eosinophils in the inflammatory infiltrate is a helpful pointer to a drug cause [13]. A responsible drug was found in 87% of a series of 63 patients with acute generalized exanthematous pustulosis; antibiotics were implicated as the causative agent in 80% of individuals [15]. The latter included particularly ampicillin, amoxicillin, spiramycin, erythromycin and cyclins. Hypersensitivity to mercury was also recorded as a precipitating cause. Pustulosis developed within 24 hours of drug administration. It often started on the face or in flexural areas, rapidly became disseminated with fever, and settled spontaneously with desquamation. Facial oedema, purpura, vesicles, blisters and erythema multiforme-like lesions were also seen; transient renal failure was noted in 32% of cases. Acute generalized exanthematic pustulosis is usually due to penicillins or macrolides [16,17]. There have been individual reports of pustular drug reactions with ampicillin (which may be localized [18]), amoxycillin (with or without clavulanic acid) [19], propicillin [20], imipinem [21], cephalosporins (cephalexin and cephadrine) [22,23], co-trimoxazole [24], doxycycline [25], chloramphenicol succinate, norfloxacin [26], ofloxacin [27], streptomycin sulphate [28], isoniazid, salazosulphapyridine/salazopyrine [29,30], pyrimethamine, piperazine ethionamate, frusemide, nitrazepam, itraconazole [31], diltiazem [32,33], captopril [34] and enalapril [35], acetylsalicylic acid [36], naproxen [37], allopurinol [38], the mucolytic agent eprazinone [39], hydroxychloroquine [40] and chlorpromazine [41]. Cases of generalized pustulation in association with the anticonvulsant hypersensitivity syndrome caused by phenytoin [42] and carbamazepine [43] have been recorded. Acne rosacea was temporally associated with daily high-dose B vitamin supplement therapy in one patient [44], and eosinophilic pustular folliculitis (Ofuji's disease) developed in association with use of the cerebral activator indeloxazine hydrochloride [45]. Patch testing with the culprit drug may be positive in patients with acute generalized exanthematous pustulosis [46].

REFERENCES

1 Hitch JM. Acneform eruptions induced by drugs and chemicals. *JAMA* 1967; **200**: 879–80.
2 Bedane C, Souyri N. Les acnés induites. *Ann Dermatol Vénéréol* 1990; **117**: 53–8.
3 Hurwitz RM. Steroid acne. *J Am Acad Dermatol* 1989; **21**: 1179–81.
4 Merkle T, Landthaler M, Braun-Falco O. Acne-conglobata-artige Exazerbation einer Acne vulgaris nach Einnahme von Anabolika und Vitamin-B-Komplex-haltigen Präparaten. *Hautarzt* 1990; **41**: 280–2.
5 Cohen LK, George W, Smith R. Isoniazid-induced acne and pellagra. Occurrence in slow inactivators of isoniazid. *Arch Dermatol* 1974; **109**: 377–81.
6 Pembroke AC, Saxena SR, Kataria M, Zilkha KD. Acne induced by dantrolene. *Br J Dermatol* 1981; **104**: 465–8.
7 Greenberg RD. Acne vulgaris associated with antigonadotrophic (Danazol) therapy. *Cutis* 1979; **24**: 431–2.
8 Burkhart CG. Quinidine-induced acne. *Arch Dermatol* 1981; **117**: 603–4.
9 Heng MCY. Cutaneous manifestations of lithium toxicity. *Br J Dermatol* 1982; **106**: 107–9.
10 Kanzaki T. Acneiform eruption induced by lithium carbonate. *J Dermatol* 1991; **18**: 481–3.
11 Schmoeckel C, von Liebe V. Akneiformes Exanthem durch Azathioprin. *Hautarzt* 1983; **34**: 413–15.
12 Webster GF. Pustular drug reactions. *Clin Dermatol* 1993; **11**: 541–3.
13 Spencer JM, Silvers DN, Grossman ME. Pustular eruption after drug exposure: is it pustular psoriasis or a pustular drug eruption? *Br J Dermatol* 1994; **130**: 514–19.
14 Burrows NP, Russell Jones RR. Pustular drug eruptions: a histopathological spectrum. *Histopathology* 1993; **22**: 569–73.
15 Roujeau J-C. Bioulac-Sage P, Bourseau C *et al.* Acute generalized exanthematous pustulosis. Analysis of 63 cases. *Arch Dermatol* 1991; **127**: 1333–8.
16 Manders SM, Heymann WR. Acute generalized exanthemic pustulosis. *Cutis* 1994; **54**: 194–6.
17 Trevisi P, Patrizi A, Neri I, Farina P. Toxic pustuloderma associated with azithromycin. *Clin Exp Dermatol* 1994; **19**: 280–1.
18 Jay S, Kang J, Watcher MA *et al.* Localized pustular skin eruption. Localized pustular drug eruption secondary to ampicillin. *Arch Dermatol* 1994; **130**: 787, 790.
19 Armster H, Schwarz T. Arzneimittelreaktion auf Amoxicillin unter dem Bild eines toxischen Pustuloderms. *Hautarzt* 1991; **42**: 713–16.
20 Gebhardt M, Lustig A, Bocker T, Wollina U. Acute generalized exanthematous pustulosis (AGEP): manifestation of drug allergy to propicillin. *Contact Dermatitis* 1995; **33**: 204–5.
21 Escallier F, Dalac S, Foucher JL *et al.* Pustulose exanthématique aiguë généralisée imputabilité a l'imipéneme (Tienam®). *Ann Dermatol Vénéréol* 1989; **116**: 407–9.
22 Kalb RE, Grossman ME. Pustular eruption following administration of cephadrine. *Cutis* 1986; **38**: 58–60.
23 Jackson H, Vion B, Levy PM. Generalized eruptive pustular drug rash due to cephalexin. *Dermatologica* 1988; **177**: 292–4.
24 MacDonald KJS, Green CM, Kenicer KJA. Pustular dermatosis induced by co-trimoxazole. *Br Med J* 1986; **293**: 1279–80.
25 Trueb RM, Burg G. Acute generalized exanthematous pustulosis due to doxycycline. *Dermatology* 1993; **186**: 75–8.
26 Shelley ED, Shelley WB. The subcorneal pustular eruption: an example induced by norfloxacin. *Cutis* 1988; **42**: 24–7.
27 Tsuda S, Kato K, Karashima T *et al.* Toxic pustuloderma induced by ofloxacin. *Acta Derm Venereol (Stockh)* 1993; **73**: 382–4.
28 Kushimoto H, Aoki T. Toxic erythema with generalized follicular pustules caused by streptomycin. *Arch Dermatol* 1981; **117**: 444–5.
29 Marce S, Schaeverbeke T, Bannwarth B *et al.* Pustulose exanthematique aigue generalisee apres prise de sulfasalazine. *Presse Med* 1993; **22**: 271.
30 Gallais V, Grange F, De Bandt M *et al.* Toxidermie a la salazosulfapyridine. Erythrodermie pustuleuse et syndrome pseudolymphomateux: 2 observations. *Ann Dermatol Vénéréol* 1994; **121**: 11–14.
31 Heymann WR, Manders SM. Itraconazole-induced acute generalised exanthematic pustulosis. *J Am Acad Dermatol* 1996; **33**: 130–1.
32 Lambert DG, Dalac S, Beer F *et al.* Acute generalized exanthematous pustular dermatitis induced by diltiazem. *Br J Dermatol* 1988; **118**: 308–9.
33 Janier M, Gerault MH, Carlotti A *et al.* Acute generalized exanthematous pustulosis due to diltiazem. *Br J Dermatol* 1993; **129**: 354–5.
34 Carroll J, Thaler M, Grossman E *et al.* Generalized pustular eruption associated with converting enzyme inhibitor therapy. *Cutis* 1995; **56**: 276–8.
35 Ferguson JE, Chalmers RJ. Enalapril-induced toxic pustuloderma. *Clin Exp Dermatol* 1996; **21**: 54–5.
36 Ballmer-Weber BK, Widmer M, Burg G. Acetylsalicylsaure-induzierte generalisierte Pustulose. *Schweiz Med Wochenschr* 1993; **123**: 542–6.
37 Grattan CEH. Generalized pustular drug rash due to naproxen. *Dermatologica* 1989; **179**: 57–8.
38 Boffa MJ, Chalmers RJ. Allopurinol-induced toxic pustuloderma. *Br J Dermatol* 1994; **131**: 447.
39 Faber M, Maucher OM, Stengel R, Goerttler E. Epraxinonenexanthem mit subkornealer Pustelbildung. *Hautarzt* 1984; **35**: 200–3.
40 Lotem M, Ingber A, Segal R, Sandbank M. Generalized pustular drug rash induced by hydroxychloroquine. *Acta Derm Venereol (Stockh)* 1990; **70**: 250–1.
41 Burrows NP, Ratnavel RC, Norris PG. Pustular eruptions after chlorpromazine. *Br Med J* 1994; **309**: 97.

42 Kleier RS, Breneman DL, Boiko S. Generalized pustulation as a manifestation of the anticonvulsant hypersensitivity syndrome. *Arch Dermatol* 1991; **127**: 1361–4.

43 Commens CA, Fischer GO. Toxic pustuloderma following carbamazepine therapy. *Arch Dermatol* 1988; **124**: 178–9.

44 Sherertz EF. Acneiform eruption due to 'megadose' vitamins B6 and B12. *Cutis* 1991; **48**: 119–20.

45 Kimura K, Ezoe K, Yokozeki H *et al.* A case of eosinophilic pustular folliculitis (Ofuji's disease) induced by patch and challenge tests with indeloxazine hydrochloride. *J Dermatol* 1996; **23**: 479–83.

46 Moreau A, Dompmartin A, Castel B *et al.* Drug-induced acute generalized exanthematous pustulosis with positive patch tests. *Int J Dermatol* 1995; **34**: 263–6.

Eczematous eruptions

Allergic contact dermatitis is discussed in Chapter 20. This section concerns the entity termed 'systemic contact-type dermatitis medicamentosa' [1–5] (Table 77.13). A patient initially sensitized to a drug by way of allergic contact dermatitis may develop an eczematous reaction when the same, or a chemically related substance, is subsequently administered systemically. The eruption tends to be symmetrical, and may involve first, or most severely, the site(s) of the original dermatitis, before becoming generalized. Patients with a contact allergy to ethylene-diamine may develop urticaria or systemic eczema following injection of aminophylline preparations containing ethylenediamine as a solubilizer for theophylline [6,7]. Patients with contact allergy to parabens may develop systemic eczema on medication with a drug containing parabens as a preservative [8]. Similarly, sensitized patients may develop eczema following oral ingestion of neomycin or hydroxyquinolines [9]. Diabetic patients sensitized by topical preparations containing *p*-amino compounds, such as *p*-phenylenediamine hair dyes, *p*-aminobenzoic acid sunscreens and certain local anaesthetic agents (e.g. benzocaine), may develop a systemic contact dermatitis with the hypoglycaemic agents tolbutamide or chlorpropamide. Sulphonylureas may also induce eczematous eruptions in sulphanilamide-sensitive patients as a result of cross-reactivity. Phenothiazines can produce allergic contact dermatitis, photo-allergic reactions and eczematous contact-type dermatitis, and may cross-react with certain antihistamines. Tetraethylthiuram disulphide (Antabuse) for the management of alcoholism can cause eczematous reactions in patients sensitized to thiurams via rubber gloves. 'Systemic contact-type dermatitis' reactions have also been described with [4]: acetylsalicylic acid, codeine [10], phenobarbital, pseudoephedrine hydrochloride and norephedrine hydrochloride [11], ephedrine [12], erythromycin [13], isoniazid [14], dimethyl sulphoxide, hydroxyquinone, nystatin, subcutaneous hydromorphone given for cancer pain [15], amlexanox [16], enoxolone [17], vitamin B_1, vitamin C, parabens, butylated hydroxyanisole, hydroxytoluene and tea-tree oil [18]. Allergic eczematous reactions to endogenous or exogenous systemic corticosteroids

Table 77.13 Systemic drugs that can reactivate allergic contact eczema to chemically related topical medicaments. From Fisher [1].

Systemic drug	Topical medicament
Ethylenediamine antihistamines Aminophylline Piperazine	Aminophylline suppositories and ethylenediamine hydrochloride
Organic and inorganic mercury compounds	Ammoniated mercury
Tincture of Benzoin inhalation	Balsam of Peru
Procaine Acetohexamide *p*-Amino salicylic acid Azo dyes in foods and drugs Chlorothiazide Chlorpropamide Tolbutamide	Benzocaine (*p*-amino compound) and glyceryl *p*-aminobenzoic acid sunscreens
Chloral hydrate	Chlorobutanol
Iodochlorhydroxyquinoline	Halogenated hydroxyquinoline creams (Vioform)
Iodides, iodinated organic compounds, radiographic contrast media	Iodine
Streptomycin, kanamycin, paromycin, gentamicin	Neomycin sulphate
Nitroglycerine tablets	Nitroglycerine ointment
Disulfiram (Antabuse)	Thiuram (rubber chemical)

have been documented in patients who are patch-test positive to topical corticosteroids [19].

The term 'baboon syndrome' denotes a characteristic pattern of systemic allergic contact dermatitis, provoked by ampicillin, amoxicillin, nickel, heparin and mercury, in which there is diffuse erythema of the buttocks, upper inner thighs and axillae [20–22]. Patch tests are commonly positive and usually vesicular, although histology of the eruption itself may show leukocytoclastic vasculitis; oral challenge with the suspected antigen may be required to substantiate the diagnosis. Antabuse (disulfiram) therapy of a nickel-sensitive alcoholic patient may induce this syndrome, as this drug leads to an initial acute increase in the blood nickel concentration [20]. Cases have been described from Japan under the name 'mercury exanthem' following inhalation of mercury vapour from crushed thermometers in patients with a history of mercury allergy.

The term 'endogenic contact eczema' [23] refers to the occurrence of an eczematous contact drug reaction following primary sensitization by oral therapy, as in the case of a patient with a drug-related exanthem who later develops localized dermatitis due to topical therapy. Thus, eczematous eruptions may develop following therapy with penicillin [24], methyldopa, allopurinol, indomethacin, sulphonamides, gold therapy, quinine, chloramphenicol, clonidine or bleomycin [25]. The alkylating agent mitomycin C administered intravesically for carcinoma of the bladder has been associated with an eczematous eruption, particularly on the face, palms and soles in some patients; these may have positive patch tests to the drug [26,27].

Some of the more important causes of eczematous drug reactions are listed in Table 77.13. Sensitivity to the suspected drug may be confirmed by subsequent patch testing, when the skin reaction has settled.

REFERENCES

1 Fisher AA. *Contact Dermatitis*. Philadelphia: Lea and Febiger, 1986.
2 Rycroft RJG, Menné T, Frosch PJ, Benezra CM, eds. *Textbook of Contact Dermatitis*. Berlin: Springer-Verlag, 1992.
3 Cronin E. Contact Dermatitis XVII. Reactions to contact allergens given orally or systemically. *Br J Dermatol* 1972; **86**: 104–7.
4 Menné T, Veien NK, Maibach HI. Systemic contact-type dermatitis due to drugs. *Semin Dermatol* 1989; **8**: 144–8.
5 Aquilina C, Sayag J. Eczéma par réactogenes internes. *Ann Dermatol Vénéréol* 1989; **116**: 753–65.
6 Berman BA, Ross RN. Ethylenediamine: systemic eczematous contact-type dermatitis. *Cutis* 1983; **31**: 594–8.
7 Hardy C, Schofield O, George CF. Allergy to aminophylline. *Br Med J* 1983; **286**: 2051–2.
8 Aeling JL, Nuss DD. Systemic eczematous 'contact-type' dermatitis medicamentosa caused by parabens. *Arch Dermatol* 1974; **110**: 640.
9 Ekelund E-G, Möller H. Oral provocation in eczematous contact allergy to neomycin and hydroxy-quinolines. *Acta Derm Venereol (Stockh)* 1969; **49**: 422–6.
10 Rodriguez F, Fernandez L, Garcia-Abujeta JL *et al.* Generalized dermatitis due to codeine. *Contact Dermatitis* 1995; **32**: 120.
11 Tomb RR, Lepoittevin JP, Espinassouze F *et al.* Systemic contact dermatitis from pseudoephedrine. *Contact Dermatitis* 1991; **24**: 86–8.
12 Villas Martinez F, Badas AJ, Garmendia Goitia JF, Aguirre I. Generalized dermatitis due to oral ephedrine. *Contact Dermatitis* 1993; **29**: 215–16.
13 Fernandez Redondo V, Casas L, Taboada M, Toribio J. Systemic contact dermatitis from erythromycin. *Contact Dermatitis* 1994; **30**: 311.
14 Meseguer J, Sastre A, Malek T, Salvador MD. Systemic contact dermatitis from isoniazid. *Contact Dermatitis* 1993; **28**: 110–1.
15 de Cuyper C, Goeteyn M. Systemic contact dermatitis from subcutaneous hydromorphone. *Contact Dermatitis* 1992; **27**: 220–3.
16 Hayakawa R, Ogino Y, Aris K, Matsunaga K. Systemic contact dermatitis due to amlexanox. *Contact Dermatitis* 1992; **27**: 122–3.
17 Villas Martinez F, Joral Badas A, Garmendia Goitia JF, Aguirre I. Sensitization to oral enoxolone. *Contact Dermatitis* 1994; **30**: 124.
18 de Groot AC, Weyland JW. Systemic contact dermatitis from tea tree oil. *Contact Dermatitis* 1992; **27**: 279–80.
19 Lauerma AI, Reitamo S, Maibach HI. Systemic hydrocortisone/cortisol induces allergic skin reactions in presensitized subjects. *J Am Acad Dermatol* 1991; **24**: 182–5.
20 Andersen KE, Hjorth N, Menné T. The baboon syndrome: systemically-induced allergic contact dermatitis. *Contact Dermatitis* 1984; **10**: 97–100.
21 Herfs H, Schirren CG, Przybilla B, Plewig G. Das 'Baboon-Syndrom'. Eine besondere Manifestation einer hamatogenen Kontaktreaktion. *Hautarzt* 1993; **44**: 466–9.
22 Duve S, Worret W, Hofmann H. The baboon syndrome: a manifestation of haematogenous contact-type dermatitis. *Acta Derm Venereol (Stockh)* 1994; **74**: 480–1.
23 Pirilä V. Endogenic contact eczema. *Allerg Asthma* 1970; **16**: 15–19.
24 Girard JP. Recurrent angioneurotic oedema and contact dermatitis due to penicillin. *Contact Dermatitis* 1978; **4**: 309.
25 Lincke-Plewig H. Bleomycin-Exantheme. *Hautarzt* 1980; **31**: 616–18.
26 Colver GB, Inglis JA, McVittie E *et al.* Dermatitis due to intravesical mitomycin C: a delayed-type hypersensitivity reaction? *Br J Dermatol* 1990; **122**: 217–24.
27 De Groot AC, Conemans JMH. Systemic allergic contact dermatitis from intravesical instillation of the antitumor antibiotic mitomycin C. *Contact Dermatitis* 1991; **24**: 201–9.

Bullous eruptions

Bullous drug eruptions encompass many different clinical reactions and pathomechanisms [1,2]. Isolated blisters, often located preferentially on the extremities, may be caused by a wide variety of chemically distinct drugs. Fixed drug eruptions, erythema multiforme and drug-induced vasculitis may have a bullous component, and drug-induced TEN is associated with widespread blistering; these are reviewed elsewhere in this chapter. The specific drug-induced entities of porphyria and pseudoporphyria, bullous pemphigoid, pemphigus and linear IgA disease are discussed here.

Bullous eruption in drug overdosage

Bullae, often at pressure areas, may be seen in patients comatose after overdosage with barbiturates (Fig. 77.5), methadone, meprobamate, imipramine, nitrazepam or glutethimide [1–5].

REFERENCES

1 Bork K. *Cutaneous Side Effects of Drugs*. Philadelphia: WB Saunders, 1988.
2 Breathnach SM, Hintner H. *Adverse Drug Reactions and the Skin*. Oxford: Blackwell Scientific Publications, 1992.

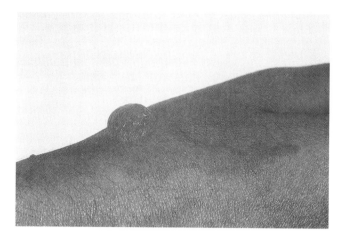

Fig. 77.5 Bullous eruption in barbiturate overdose. (Courtesy of Charing Cross Hospital, London, UK.)

3 Brehmer-Andersson E, Pedersen NB. Sweat gland necrosis and bullous skin changes in acute drug intoxication. *Acta Derm Venereol (Stockh)* 1969; **49**: 157–62.
4 Mandy S, Ackerman AB. Characteristic traumatic skin lesions in drug-induced coma. *JAMA* 1970; **213**: 253–6.
5 Herschtal D, Robinson MJ. Blisters of the skin in coma induced by amitriptyline and chlorazepate dipotassium. Report of a case with underlying sweat gland necrosis. *Arch Dermatol* 1979; **115**: 499.

Drug-induced porphyria

Porphyria is discussed in Chapter 59. Drugs reported to exacerbate the acute hepatic porphyrias are listed in Table 77.14; these either cause excess destruction of haem, or else inhibit haem synthesis [1–3].

Pseudoporphyria

Pseudoporphyria, in which porphyria-like blistering of exposed areas on the extremities occurs in the absence of abnormal porphyrin metabolism, may be caused by high-dose frusemide [4], naproxen [5,6] and other NSAIDs [7,8],

Table 77.14 Drugs that are unsafe to use in patients with acute intermittent porphyria, porphyria cutanea tarda or variegate porphyria.

Aminoglutethimide	Meprobamate
Barbiturates	Novobiocin
Carbamazepine	Oestrogens
Carbromal	Primadone
Chlorpropamide	Progestagens
Danazol	Pyrazolone derivatives
Diclofenac	Rifampicin
Diphenylhydantoin (phenytoin)	Sulphonamides
Ergot preparations	Tolbutamide
Glutethimide	Trimethadione
Griseofulvin	Valproic acid

combined carisoprodol and aspirin [9], nalidixic acid [10], tetracyclines [11] and sulphonylurea drugs. Phototoxic mechanisms have been implicated in some cases. A similar syndrome has been reported in a patient taking very large doses of pyridoxine (vitamin B_6) [12].

REFERENCES

1 Targovnick SE, Targovnik JH. Cutaneous drug reactions in porphyrias. *Clin Dermatol* 1986; **4**: 111–17.
2 Köstler E, Seebacher C, Riedel H, Kemmer C. Therapeutische und pathogenetische Aspekte der Porphyria cutanea tarda. *Hautarzt* 1986; **37**: 210–16.
3 Ayala F, Santoianni P. Drug-induced cutaneous porphyria. *Clin Dermatol* 1993; **11**: 535–9.
4 Burry JN, Lawrence JR. Phototoxic blisters from high frusemide dosage. *Br J Dermatol* 1976; **94**: 495–9.
5 Judd LE, Henderson DW, Hill DC. Naproxen-induced pseudoporphyria: a clinical and ultrastructural study. *Arch Dermatol* 1986; **122**: 451–4.
6 Lang BA, Finlayson LA. Naproxen-induced pseudoporphyria in patients with juvenile rheumatoid arthritis. *J Pediatr* 1994; **124**: 639–42.
7 Stern RS. Phototoxic reactions to piroxicam and other nonsteroidal anti-inflammatory agents. *N Engl J Med* 1983; **309**: 186–7.
8 Taylor BJ, Duffill MB. Pseudoporphyria from nonsteroidal anti-inflammatory drugs. *NZ Med J* 1987; **100**: 322–3.
9 Hazen PG. Pseudoporphyria in a patient receiving carisoprodol/aspirin therapy. *J Am Acad Dermatol* 1994; **31**: 500.
10 Keane JT, Pearson RW, Malkinson FD. Nalidixic acid-induced photosensitivity in mice: a model for pseudoporphyria. *J Invest Dermatol* 1984; **82**: 210–13.
11 Hawk JLM. Skin changes resembling hepatic cutaneous porphyria induced by oxytetracycline photosensitization. *Clin Exp Dermatol* 1980; **5**: 321–5.
12 Baer R, Stilman RA. Cutaneous skin changes probably due to pyridoxine abuse. *J Am Acad Dermatol* 1984; **10**: 527–8.

Drug-induced bullous pemphigoid

Idiopathic bullous pemphigoid is discussed in Chapter 40. In drug-induced bullous pemphigoid, patients tend to be younger; tissue-bound and circulating anti-basement-membrane zone IgG antibodies may be absent, or additional antibodies such as intercellular or antiepidermal cytoplasmic antibodies may be detected. Some cases of drug-induced bullous pemphigoid are short-lived, whereas others become chronic. Drug-induced bullous or cicatricial pemphigoid have been reported with a number of medications [1–4], especially with frusemide [5,6], but also with penicillamine [7–9], the penicillamine analogue tiobutarit [10], penicillin [11] and its derivatives [12], sulphasalazine, salicylazo-sulphapyridine, phenacetin [13], enalapril [14], novoscabin, topical fluorouracil, and PUVA therapy [15]. In the case of enalapril-induced bullous pemphigoid, the IgG antibody was directed against the 230-kDa bullous pemphigoid antigen [14]. Cicatricial pemphigoid has been described in association with penicillamine [9] and clonidine [16]. An association with vaccination for influenza and with tetanus toxoid and induction of bullous pemphigoid has been noted rarely [17–19].

REFERENCES

1 Ahmed AR, Newcomer VD. Drug-induced bullous pemphigoid. *Clin Dermatol* 1987; **5**: 8–10.
2 Ruocco V, Sacerdoti G. Pemphigus and bullous pemphigoid due to drugs. *Int J Dermatol* 1991; **30**: 307–12.
3 Fellner MJ. Drug-induced bullous pemphigoid. *Clin Dermatol* 1993; **11**: 515–20.
4 Van Joost T, Van't Veen AJ. Drug-induced cicatricial pemphigoid and acquired epidermolysis bullosa. *Clin Dermatol* 1993; **11**: 521–7.
5 Fellner MJ, Katz JM. Occurrence of bullous pemphigoid after furosemide therapy. *Arch Dermatol* 1976; **112**: 75–7.
6 Castel T, Gratacos R, Castro J *et al.* Bullous pemphigoid induced by furosemide. *Clin Exp Dermatol* 1981; **6**: 635–8.
7 Brown MD, Dubin HV. Penicillamine-induced bullous pemphigoid-like eruption. *Arch Dermatol* 1987; **123**: 1119–20.
8 Rasmussen HB, Jepsen LV, Brandrup F. Penicillamine-induced bullous pemphigoid with pemphigus-like antibodies. *J Cutan Pathol* 1989; **16**: 154–7.
9 Bialy-Golan A, Brenner S. Penicillamine-induced bullous dermatoses. *J Am Acad Dermatol* 1996; **35**: 732–42.
10 Yamaguchi R, Oryu F, Hidano A. A case of bullous pemphigoid induced by tiobutarit (D-penicillamine analogue). *J Dermatol (Tokyo)* 1989; **16**: 308–11.
11 Alcalay J, David M, Ingber A *et al.* Bullous pemphigoid mimicking bullous erythema multiforme: an untoward side effect of penicillins. *J Am Acad Dermatol* 1988; **18**: 345–9.
12 Hodak E, Ben-Shetrit A, Ingber A, Sandbank M. Bullous pemphigoid: an adverse effect of ampicillin. *Clin Exp Dermatol* 1990; **15**: 50–2.
13 Kashihara M, Danno K, Miyachi Y *et al.* Bullous pemphigoid-like lesions induced by phenacetin: report of a case and an immunopathologic study. *Arch Dermatol* 1984; **120**: 1196–9.
14 Pazderka Smith E, Taylor TB, Meyer LJ, Zone JJ. Antigen identification in drug-induced bullous pemphigoid. *J Am Acad Dermatol* 1993; **29**: 879–82.
15 Abel EA, Bennett A. Bullous pemphigoid. Occurrence in psoriasis treated with psoralens plus long-wave ultraviolet radiation. *Arch Dermatol* 1979; **115**: 988–9.
16 Van Joost T, Faber WR, Manuel HR. Drug-induced anogenital cicatricial pemphigoid. *Br J Dermatol* 1980; **102**: 715–18.
17 Bodokh I, Lacour JP, Bourdet JF *et al.* Réactivation de pemphigoïde bulleuse après vaccination antigrippale. *Thérapie* 1994; **49**: 154.
18 Venning VA, Wojnarowska F. Induced bullous pemphigoid. *Br J Dermatol* 1995; **132**: 831–2.
19 Fournier B, Descamps V, Bouscarat F *et al.* Bullous pemphigoid induced by vaccination. *Br J Dermatol* 1996; **135**: 153–4.

Drug-induced pemphigus

The variants of idiopathic pemphigus are discussed in Chapter 40. A number of drugs have been implicated in drug-induced pemphigus (Table 77.15) [1,2], usually of foliaceus type, but the erythematosus, herpetiformis and urticaria-like forms also occur; drug-induced pemphigus vulgaris is rare. Most patients with drug-induced pemphigus have tissue-bound and/or low-titre circulating autoantibodies with the same antigenic specificity at a molecular level as autoantibodies from patients with the corresponding subtype of idiopathic pemphigus [3,4]; however, in the case of penicillamine-induced pemphigus, 10% do not have tissue-bound, and more than 30% do not have circulating, autoantibodies. About 80% of cases are caused by drugs associated with a thiol group in the molecule, especially penicillamine [5–7], but also the structurally related ACE inhibitors captopril [8–10] and ramipril [11], gold sodium thiomalate, drugs with disulphide bonds such as pyritinol [12], S-thiopyridoxine, thiopronine, which is chemically related to penicillamine

Table 77.15 Drugs implicated in the development of pemphigus.

Thiol drugs	Non-thiol drugs
Penicillamine	*Antibiotics*
Captopril, Ramipril	Penicillin and derivatives
Gold sodium thiomalate	Rifampicin
Pyritinol	Cephalexin
Thiamazole	Cefadroxil
Thiopronine	Ceftazidine
Mercapto-propionylglycine	
	Pyrazolone derivatives
	Aminophenazone
	Aminopyrine
	Azapropazone
	Oxyphenylbutazone
	Phenylbutazone
	Miscellaneous
	Glibenclamide
	Hydantoin
	Levodopa
	Lysine acetylsalicylate
	Nifedipine
	Phenobarbital
	Piroxicam
	Progesterone
	Propranolol
	Interferon-β and interleukin 2
	Heroin

and used as an alternative therapy in penicillamine intolerance [4,13], and mercapto-propionylglycine [14], as well as those with a sulphur-containing ring that may undergo metabolic change to the thiol form, such as piroxicam [15]. Penicillin [16,17] and its derivatives ampicillin [17], procaine penicillin and amoxycillin, may also cause pemphigus. Other drugs that cause pemphigus may contain an active amide group [18].

Rifampicin [19], cephalexin [20], cefadroxil, ceftazidime [21], pyrazolone derivatives [22], propranolol, propranolol-meprobamate [23], optalidon, pentachlorophenol, phenobarbital [24], nifedipine [25], phosphamide, hydantoin, combinations of indomethacin and aspirin [26], glibenclamide [27], as well as heroin [28], have all been established as rare causes of pemphigus-like reaction. Fatal pemphigus vulgaris has been recorded after IFN-β and IL-2 therapy for lymphoma [29].

REFERENCES

1 Brenner S, Wolf R, Ruocco V. Drug-induced pemphigus. I. A survey. *Clin Dermatol* 1993; **11**: 501–5.
2 Ruocco V, De Angelis E, Lombardi ML. Drug-induced pemphigus. II. Pathomechanisms and experimental investigations. *Clin Dermatol* 1993; **11**: 507–13.
3 Korman NJ, Eyre RW, Stanley JR. Drug-induced pemphigus: autoantibodies directed against the pemphigus antigen complexes are present in penicillamine and captopril-induced pemphigus. *J Invest Dermatol* 1991; **96**: 273–6.

4 Verdier-Sevrain S, Joly P, Thomine E *et al.* Thiopronine-induced herpetiform pemphigus: report of a case studied by immunoelectron microscopy and immunoblot analysis. *Br J Dermatol* 1994; **130**: 238–40.

5 Zillikens D, Zentner A, Burger M *et al.* Pemphigus foliaceus durch Penicillamin. *Hautarzt* 1993; **44**: 167–71.

6 Jones E, Sobkowski WW, Murray SJ, Walsh NMG. Concurrent pemphigus and myasthenia gravis as manifestations of penicillamine toxicity. *J Am Acad Dermatol* 1993; **28**: 655–6.

7 Bialy-Golan A, Brenner S. Penicillamine-induced bullous dermatoses. *J Am Acad Dermatol* 1996; **35**: 732–42.

8 Clement M. Captopril-induced eruptions. *Arch Dermatol* 1981; **117**: 525–6.

9 Katz RA, Hood AF, Anhalt GJ. Pemphigus-like eruption from captopril. *Arch Dermatol* 1987; **123**: 20–1.

10 Kaplan RP, Potter TS, Fox JN. Drug-induced pemphigus related to angiotensin-converting enzyme inhibitors. *J Am Acad Dermatol* 1992; **26**: 364–6.

11 Vignes S, Paul C, Flageul B, Dubertret L. Ramipril-induced superficial pemphigus. *Br J Dermatol* 1996; **135**: 657–8.

12 Civatte J, Duterque M, Blanchet P *et al.* Deux cas de pemphigus superficiel induit par le pyritinol. *Ann Dermatol Vénéréol* 1978; **105**: 573–7.

13 Alinovi A, Benoldi D, Manganelli P. Pemphigus erythematosus induced by thiopronin. *Acta Derm Venereol (Stockh)* 1982; **62**: 452–4.

14 Lucky PA, Skovby F, Thier SO. Pemphigus foliaceaus and proteinuria induced by α-mercaptopropionylglycine. *J Am Acad Dermatol* 1983; **8**: 667–72.

15 Martin RL, McSweeny GW, Schneider J. Fatal pemphigus vulgaris in a patient taking piroxicam. *N Engl J Med* 1983; **309**: 795–6.

16 Duhra PL, Foulds IS. Penicillin-induced pemphigus vulgaris. *Br J Dermatol* 1988; **118**: 307.

17 Fellner MJ, Mark AS. Penicillin- and ampicillin-induced pemphigus vulgaris. *Int J Dermatol* 1980; **19**: 392–3.

18 Wolf R, Brenner S. An active amide group in the molecule of drugs that induce pemphigus: a casual or causal relationship? *Dermatology* 1994; **189**: 1–4.

19 Lee CW, Lim JH, Kang HJ. Pemphigus foliaceus induced by rifampicin. *Br J Dermatol* 1984; **111**: 619–22.

20 Wolf R, Dechner E, Ophir J, Brenner S. Cephalexin. A nonthiol drug that may induce pemphigus vulgaris. *Int J Dermatol* 1991; **30**: 213–15.

21 Pellicano R, Iannantuono M, Lomuto M. Pemphigus erythematosus induced by ceftazidime. *Int J Dermatol* 1993; **32**: 675–6.

22 Chorzelski TP, Jablonska S, Blaszczyk M. Autoantibodies in pemphigus. *Acta Derm Venereol (Stockh)* 1966; **46**: 26.

23 Goddard W, Lambert D, Gavanou J, Chapius JL. Pemphigus acquit apres traitement par l'association propranolol-meprobamate. *Ann Dermatol Vénéréol* 1980; **107**: 1213–16.

24 Dourmishev AL, Rahman MA. Phenobarbital-induced pemphigus vulgaris. *Dermatologica* 1986; **173**: 256–8.

25 Kim SC, Won JH, Ahn SK. Pemphigus foliaceus induced by nifedipine. *Acta Derm Venereol (Stockh)* 1993; **73**: 210–11.

26 DeMento FJ, Grover RW. Acantholytic herpetiform dermatitis. *Arch Dermatol* 1973; **107**: 883–7.

27 Fellner MJ, Winiger J. Pemphigus erythematosus and heroin addiction. *Int J Dermatol* 1978; **17**: 308–11.

28 Paterson AJ, Lamey PJ, Lewis MA *et al.* Pemphigus vulgaris precipitated by glibenclamide therapy. *J Oral Pathol Med* 1993; **22**: 92–5.

29 Ramseur WL, Richards F, Duggan DB. A case of fatal pemphigus vulgaris in association with beta interferon and interleukin-2 therapy. *Cancer* 1989; **63**: 2005–7.

Linear IgA disease

Idiopathic linear IgA disease is discussed in Chapter 40. The drugs implicated as a cause of this condition have been reviewed [1–3], and include vancomycin especially [1–6], but also amiodarone, ampicillin, captopril, cefamandole, diclophenac, glibenclamide, IFN-γ, iodine, lithium, penicillin G [7], phenytoin and somatostatin. Most patients lack circulating antibodies to the basement membrane; resolution of the rash follows discontinuation of medication.

REFERENCES

1 Collier PM, Wojnarowska F. Drug-induced linear immunoglobulin A disease. *Clin Dermatol* 1993; **11**: 529–33.

2 Kuechle ML, Stegemeir E, Maynard B *et al.* Drug-induced linear IgA bullous dermatosis: Report of six cases and review of the literature. *J Am Acad Dermatol* 1994; **30**: 187–92.

3 Geissmann C, Beylot-Barry M, Doutre MS, Beylot C. Drug-induced linear IgA bullous dermatosis. *J Am Acad Dermatol* 1995; **32**: 296.

4 Carpenter S, Berg D, Sidhu-Malik N *et al.* Vancomycin-associated linear IgA dermatosis. A report of three cases. *J Am Acad Dermatol* 1992; **26**: 45–8.

5 Piketty C, Meeus F, Nochy D *et al.* Linear IgA dermatosis related to vancomycin. *Br J Dermatol* 1994; **130**: 130–1.

6 Whitworth JM, Thomas I, Peltz S *et al.* Vancomycin-induced linear IgA bullous dermatosis (LABD). *J Am Acad Dermatol* 1996; **34**: 890–1.

7 Combemale P, Gavaud C, Cozzani E *et al.* Dermatose a IgA lineaire (DIAL) induite par penicilline G. *Ann Dermatol Vénéréol* 1993; **120**: 847–8.

Vasculitis

Drug-induced cutaneous necrotizing vasculitis [1–3] may also involve internal organs, including the heart, liver and kidneys, with fatal results. The patterns of polyarteritis nodosa, Henoch–Schönlein vasculitis and hypocomplementaemic vasculitis are not seen commonly with drugs. Drugs that have been implicated are listed in Table 77.16. These include ampicillin, sulphonamides, frusemide (furosemiole) [4], thiazide diuretics, phenylbutazone and other NSAIDs, quinidine, amiodarone [5], hydralazine [6], enalapril [7], propylthioruacil [8,9], mefloquine [10], cimetidine [11], coumadin [12,13], anticonvulsants including phenytoin and in isolated cases carbamazepine and trimethadione [14,15], zidovudine [16], fluoxetine [17], didanosine [18], piperazine [19], centrally acting appetite suppressants [20], hyposensitization therapy [21,22], bacillus

Table 77.16 Drugs recorded as inducing vasculitis.

Additives	Levamisole
Allopurinol	Maprotiline
Aminosalicylic acid	Mefloquine
Amiodarone	Methotrexate
Amphetamine	Penicillin
Ampicillin	Phenacetin
Aspirin	Phenothiazines
Arsenic	Phenylbutazone
Captopril	Phenytoin
Carbamazepine	Piperazine
Cimetidine	Procainamide
Coumadin	Propylthiouracil
Didanosine	Quinidine
Enalapril	Radiocontrast media
Erythromycin	Streptomycin
Ethacrynic acid	Sulphonamides
Fluoroquinolone antibiotics	Trazodone
Fluoxetine	Tetracycline
Frusemide	Thiazides
Griseofulvin	Trimethadione
Guanethidine	Vaccination
Hydralazine	Zidovudine
Iodides	

Calmette–Guérin (BCG) vaccination (which may cause a papulonecrotic type of vasculitis) [23], radiographic contrast media [24], food and drug additives including dye excipients such as tartrazine (FD&C yellow No. 5), ponceau, sodium benzoate, 4-hydroxybenzoic acid [25,26], vitamin B$_6$ [27] and the use of a nicotine patch [28]. Leukocytoclastic vasculitis and necrotizing angiitis have also been documented in drug abusers [29–31].

REFERENCES

1 Mullick FG, McAllister HA, Jr, Wagner BM, Fenoglio JJ, Jr. Drug-related vasculitis. Clinicopathologic correlations in 30 patients. *Hum Pathol* 1979; **10**: 313–25.

2 Mackel SE, Jordon RE. Leukocytoclastic vasculitis. A cutaneous expression of immune complex disease. *Arch Dermatol* 1983; **118**: 296–301.

3 Sanchez NP, Van Hale HM, Su WPD. Clinical and histopathologic spectrum of necrotizing vasculitis. Report of findings in 101 cases. *Arch Dermatol* 1985; **121**: 220–4.

4 Hendricks WM, Ader RS. Furosemide-induced cutaneous necrotizing vasculitis. *Arch Dermatol* 1977; **113**: 375–6.

5 Staubli M, Zimmerman A, Bircher J. Amiodarone-induced vasculitis and polyserositis. *Postgrad Med J* 1985; **61**: 245–7.

6 Peacock A, Weatherall D. Hydralazine-induced necrotizing vasculitis. *Br Med J* 1981; **282**: 1121–2.

7 Carrington PR, Sanusi ID, Zahradka S, Winder PR. Enalapril-associated erythema and vasculitis. *Cutis* 1993; **51**: 121–3.

8 Vasily DB, Tyler WB. Propylthiouracil-induced cutaneous vasculitis. Case presentation and review of literature. *JAMA* 1980; **243**: 458–61.

9 Gammeltoft M, Kristensen JK. Propylthio-uracil-induced cutaneous vasculitis. *Acta Derm Venereol (Stockh)* 1982; **62**: 171–3.

10 Scerri L, Pace JL. Mefloquine-associated cutaneous vasculitis. *Int J Dermatol* 1993; **32**: 517–18.

11 Mitchell GG, Magnusson AR, Weiler JM. Cimetidine-induced cutaneous vasculitis. *Am J Med* 1983; **75**: 875–6.

12 Tanay A, Yust I, Brenner S et al. Dermal vasculitis due to coumadin hypersensitivity. *Dermatologica* 1982; **165**: 178–85.

13 Tamir A, Wolf R, Brenner S. Leukocytoclastic vasculitis: another coumarin-induced hemorrhagic reaction. *Acta Derm Venereol (Stockh)* 1994; **74**: 138–9.

14 Drory VE, Korczyn AD. Hypersensitivity vasculitis and systemic lupus erythematosus induced by anticonvulsants. *Clin Neuropharmacol* 1993; **16**: 19–29.

15 Kaneko K, Igarashi J, Suzuki Y et al. Carbamazepine-induced thrombocytopenia and leucopenia complicated by Henoch-Schonlein purpura symptoms. *Eur J Pediatr* 1993; **152**: 769–70.

16 Torres RA, Lin RY, Lee M, Barr MR. Zidovudine-induced leukocytoclastic vasculitis. *Arch Intern Med* 1992; **152**: 850–1.

17 Roger D, Rolle F, Mausset J et al. Urticarial vasculitis induced by fluoxetine. *Dermatology* 1995; **191**: 164.

18 Herranz P, Fernandez-Diaz ML, de Lucas R et al. Cutaneous vasculitis associated with didanosine. *Lancet* 1994; **344**: 680.

19 Balzan M, Cacciottolo JM. Hypersensitivity vasculitis associated with piperazine therapy. *Br J Dermatol* 1994; **131**: 133–4.

20 Papadavid E, Yu RC, Tay A, Chu AC. Urticarial vasculitis induced by centrally acting appetite suppressants. *Br J Dermatol* 1996; **134**: 990–1.

21 Phanuphak P, Kohler PF. Onset of polyarteritis nodosa during allergic hyposensitisation treatment. *Am J Med* 1980; **68**: 479–85.

22 Merk H, Kober ML. Vasculitis nach spezifischer Hyposensibilisierung. *Z Hautkr* 1982; **57**: 1682–5.

23 Lübbe D. Vasculitis allergica vom papulonekrotischen Typ nach BCG-Impfung. *Dermatol Mschr* 1982; **168**: 186–92.

24 Kerdel FA, Fraker DL, Haynes HA. Necrotizing vasculitis from radiographic contrast media. *J Am Acad Dermatol* 1984; **10**: 25–9.

25 Michäelsson G, Petterson L, Juhlin L. Purpura caused by food and drug additives. *Arch Dermatol* 1974; **109**: 49–52.

26 Lowry MD, Hudson CF, Callen JP. Leukocytoclastic vasculitis caused by drug additives. *J Am Acad Dermatol* 1994; **30**: 854–5.

27 Ruzicka T, Ring J, Braun-Falco O. Vasculitis allergica durch vitamin B$_6$. *Hautarzt* 1984; **35**: 197–9.

28 Van der Klauw MM, Van Hillo B, Van den Berg WH et al. Vasculitis attributed to the nicotine patch (Nicotinell). *Br J Dermatol* 1996; **34**: 361–4.

29 Citron BP, Halpen M, McCarron M et al. Necrotizing angiitis associated with drug abuse. *N Engl J Med* 1970; **283**: 1003–11.

30 Lignelli GJ, Bucheit WA. Angiitis in drug abusers. *N Engl J Med* 1971; **284**: 112–13.

31 Gendelman H, Linzer M, Barland P et al. Leukocytoclastic vasculitis in an intravenous heroin abuser. *NY State J Med* 1983; **83**: 984–6.

LE-like syndrome

A reaction resembling idiopathic LE has been reported in association with a large variety of drugs [1–6], although only about 5% of cases of systemic LE are drug induced. Cutaneous manifestations are in general rare: 18% and 26%, respectively, of patients with procainamide- and hydralazine-induced LE had skin changes in one series [6]. Photosensitivity may be prominent; some patients develop discoid LE lesions; urticarial or erythema multiforme-like lesions may also be seen. Constitutional symptoms may be present, and there may be evidence of Raynaud's disease, arthritis or polyserositis. Renal involvement is rare, as is central nervous system involvement. The condition usually, but not always, resolves after discontinuation of the drug. Abnormal laboratory findings include the presence of LE cells, and of antinuclear antibodies directed against ribonucleoprotein, single-stranded DNA, and especially against histones [7,8]. Antibodies against native double-stranded DNA are rarely found in drug-induced LE, and complement levels are normal; deposition of immunoreactants in uninvolved skin is rare. Patients with drug-induced LE may have the lupus anticoagulant [9,10].

A partial list of drugs reported to induce a systemic LE-like syndrome or exacerbate idiopathic LE is given in Table 77.17. Drugs most commonly implicated in inducing LE include especially hydralazine [11,12] and procainamide [13,14], and less commonly β-blockers, methyldopa [15,16],

Table 77.17 Drugs inducing lupus erythematosus-like syndromes.

Allopurinol	Nitrofurantoin
Aminoglutethimide	Oral contraceptives
p-Aminosalicylic acid	Penicillin
β-Blockers	Penicillamine
Captopril	Phenothiazine
Carbamazepine	Phenylbutazone
Chlorpromazine	Primidone
Clonidine	Procainamide
Co-trimoxazole	Thiazide diuretics
Ethosuximide	Thiouracils
Gold salts	Quinidine
Griseofulvin	Streptomycin
Hydantoins	Sulphasalazine
Hydralazine	Sulphonamides
Ibuprofen	Tetracycline
Isoniazid	Thionamide
Lithium	Trimethadione
Methyldopa	Valproate
Methysergide	

isoniazid, most anticonvulsants in clinical use including phenytoin, carbamazepine, ethosuximide, trimethadione, primidone and valproate (but not phenobarbital or benzodiazepines) [17], and quinidine [18,19]. LE following penicillamine therapy [20,21], and subacute LE with positive Ro/SS-A antibodies in association with thiazide diuretics such as hydrochlorothiazide [22–27], have also been reported. A gyrate subacute LE has been described in association with captopril [28], and a lupus-like syndrome with 2-mercaptopropionylglycine [29]. The oral contraceptive induced LE lesions on the palms and feet of a patient [30]. In addition, a number of drugs may exacerbate a pre-existing systemic LE, such as griseofulvin, β-blockers, sulphonamides [31], testosterone and oestrogens.

REFERENCES

1 Reidenberg MM. The chemical induction of systemic lupus erythematosus and lupus-like illnesses. *Arthritis Rheum* 1981; **24**: 1004–9.
2 Harmon CE, Portnova JP. Drug-induced lupus: clinical and serological studies. *Clin Rheum Dis* 1982; **8**: 121–35.
3 Stratton MA. Drug-induced systemic lupus erythematosus. *Clin Pharm* 1985; **4**: 657–63.
4 Totoritis MC, Rubin RL. Drug-induced lupus. Genetic, clinical, and laboratory features. *Postgrad Med* 1985; **78**: 149–52.
5 Moureaux P. Les formes cutanées du lupus. *Allerg Immunol* 1995; **27**: 196–9.
6 Dubois EL. Serologic abnormalities in spontaneous and drug-induced systemic lupus erythematosus. *J Rheumatol* 1975; **2**: 204–14.
7 Hobbs RN, Clayton AL, Bernstein RM. Antibodies to the five histones and poly(adenosine diphosphate-ribose) in drug-induced lupus: implications for pathogenesis. *Ann Rheum Dis* 1987; **46**: 408–16.
8 Totoritis MC, Tan EM, McNally EM *et al.* Association of antibody to histone complex H2A-H2B with symptomatic procainamide-induced lupus. *N Engl J Med* 1988; **318**: 1431–6.
9 Bell WR, Boss GR, Wolfson JS. Circulating anticoagulant in the procainamide-induced lupus syndrome. *Arch Intern Med* 1977; **137**: 1471–3.
10 Canoso RT, Sise HS. Chlorpromazine-induced lupus anticoagulant and associated immunologic abnormalities. *Am J Hematol* 1982; **13**: 121–9.
11 Mansilla Tinoco R, Harland SJ, Ryan PJ *et al.* Hydralazine, antinuclear antibodies, and the lupus syndrome. *Br Med J* 1982; **284**: 936–9.
12 Russell GI, Bing RF, Jones JA *et al.* Hydralazine sensitivity: clinical features, autoantibody changes and HLA-DR phenotype. *Q J Med* 1987; **65**: 845–52.
13 Dubois EL. Procainamide induction of a systemic lupus erythematosus-like syndrome. Presentation of six cases, review of the literature, and analysis and follow up of reported cases. *Medicine* 1969; **48**: 217–28.
14 Blomgren SE, Condemi JJ, Vaughan JH. Procainamide-induced lupus erythematosus. Clinical and laboratory observations. *Am J Med* 1972; **52**: 338–48.
15 Harrington TM, Davis DE. Systemic lupus-like syndrome induced by methyldopa therapy. *Chest* 1981; **79**: 696–7.
16 Dupont A, Six R. Lupus-like syndrome induced by methyldopa. *Br Med J* 1982; **285**: 693–4.
17 Drory VE, Korczyn AD. Hypersensitivity vasculitis and systemic lupus erythematosus induced by anticonvulsants. *Clin Neuropharmacol* 1993; **16**: 19–29.
18 McCormack GD, Barth WF. Quinidine induced lupus syndrome. *Semin Arthritis Rheum* 1985; **15**: 73–9.
19 Cohen MG, Kevat S, Prowse MV *et al.* Two distinct quinidine-induced rheumatic syndromes. *Ann Intern Med* 1988; **108**: 369–71.
20 Chalmers A, Thompson D, Stein HE *et al.* Systemic lupus erythematosus during penicillamine therapy for rheumatoid arthritis. *Ann Intern Med* 1982; **97**: 659–63.
21 Condon C, Phelan M, Lyons JF. Penicillamine-induced type II bullous systemic lupus erythematosus. *Br J Dermatol* 1997; **136**: 474–5.
22 Reed BR, Huff JC, Jones SK *et al.* Subacute cutaneous lupus erythematosus associated with hydrochlorothiazide therapy. *Ann Intern Med* 1985; **103**: 49–51.
23 Berbis P, Vernay-Vaisse C, Privat Y. Lupus cutané subaigu observé au cours d'un traitement par diurétiques thiazidiques. *Ann Dermatol Vénéréol* 1986; **113**: 1245–8.
24 Darken M, McBurney EI. Subacute cutaneous lupus erythematosus-like drug eruption due to combination diuretic hydrochlorothiazide and triamterene. *J Am Acad Dermatol* 1988; **18**: 38–42.
25 Wollenberg A, Meurer M. Thiazid-Diuretika-induzierter subakut-kutaner Lupus erythematodes. *Hautarzt* 1991; **42**: 709–12.
26 Goodrich AL, Kohn SR. Hydrochlorothiazide-induced lupus erythematosus: A new variant? *J Am Acad Dermatol* 1993; **28**: 1001–2.
27 Brown CW, Jr, Deng JS. Thiazide diuretics induce cutaneous lupus-like adverse reaction. *J Toxicol Clin Toxicol* 1995; **33**: 729–33.
28 Patri P, Nigro A, Rebora A. Lupus erythematosus-like eruption from captopril. *Acta Derm Venereol (Stockh)* 1985; **65**: 447–8.
29 Katayama I, Nishioka K. Lupus like syndrome induced by 2-mercaptopropionylglycine. *J Dermatol (Tokyo)* 1986; **13**: 151–3.
30 Furukawa F, Tachibana T, Imamura S, Tamura T. Oral contraceptive-induced lupus erythematosus in a Japanese woman. *J Dermatol (Tokyo)* 1991; **18**: 56–8.
31 Petri M, Allbritton J. Antibiotic allergy in systemic lupus erythematosus: a case-control study. *J Rheumatol* 1992; **19**: 265–9.

Dermatomyositis reactions

Dermatomyositis has been reported to be precipitated by a variety of drugs, including penicillamine [1–3], NSAIDs (niflumic acid and diclofenac) [4], carbamazepine [5] and vaccination, as with BCG [6]. Acral skin lesions simulating chronic dermatomyositis have been reported during long-term hydroxyurea therapy [7]. Allergy to benzalkonium chloride has caused a dermatomyositis-like reaction [8].

REFERENCES

1 Simpson NB, Golding JR. Dermatomyositis induced by penicillamine. *Acta Derm Venereol (Stockh)* 1979; **59**: 543–4.
2 Wojnorowska F. Dermatomyositis induced by penicillamine. *J R Soc Med* 1980; **73**: 884–6.
3 Carroll GC, Will RK, Peter JB *et al.* Penicillamine induced polymyositis and dermatomyositis. *J Rheumatol* 1987; **14**: 995–1001.
4 Grob JJ, Collet AM, Bonerandi JJ. Dermatomyositis-like syndrome induced by nonsteroidal anti-inflammatory agents. *Dermatologica* 1989; **178**: 58–9.
5 Simpson JR. 'Collagen disease' due to carbamazepine (Tegretol). *Br Med J* 1966; **ii**: 1434.
6 Kass E, Staume S, Mellbye OJ *et al.* Dermatomyositis associated with BCG vaccination. *Scand J Rheumatol* 1979; **8**: 187–91.
7 Richard M, Truchetet F, Friedel *et al.* Skin lesions simulating chronic dermatomyositis during long-term hydroxyurea therapy. *J Am Acad Dermatol* 1989; **21**: 797–9.
8 Cox NH. Allergy to benzalkonium chloride simulating dermatomyositis. *Contact Dermatitis* 1994; **31**: 50.

Scleroderma-like reactions

Penicillamine [1,2], bleomycin [3,4], bromocryptine [5], vitamin K (phytomenadione) [6,7], sodium valproate [8] and 5-hydroxytryptophan combined with carbidopa [9,10] (see also the eosinophilia–myalgia syndrome below) have all been implicated in either localized or generalized morphea-like, or systemic sclerosis-like, reactions. Eosinophilic fasciitis has been associated with tryptophan ingestion in some cases [11], as well as with phenytoin [12].

REFERENCES

1 Bernstein RM, Hall MA, Gostelow BE. Morphea-like reaction to D-penicillamine therapy. *Ann Rheum Dis* 1981; **40**: 42–4.
2 Miyagawa S, Yoshioka A, Hatoko M *et al.* Systemic sclerosis-like lesions during long-term penicillamine therapy for Wilson's disease. *Br J Dermatol* 1987; **116**: 95–100.
3 Finch WR, Rodnan GP, Buckingham RB *et al.* Bleomycin-induced scleroderma. *J Rheumatol* 1980; **7**: 651–9.
4 Snauwaert J, Degreef H. Bleomycin-induced Raynaud's phenomenon and acral sclerosis. *Dermatologica* 1984; **169**: 172–4.
5 Leshin B, Piette WW, Caplin RM. Morphea after bromocriptine therapy. *Int J Dermatol* 1989; **28**: 177–9.
6 Brunskill NJ, Berth-Jones J, Graham-Brown RAC. Pseudosclerodermatous reaction to phytomenadione injection (Texier's syndrome). *Clin Exp Dermatol* 1988; **13**: 276–8.
7 Pujol RM, Puig L, Moreno A *et al.* Pseudoscleroderma secondary to phytonadione (vitamin K1) injections. *Cutis* 1989; **43**: 365–8.
8 Goihman-Yahr M, Leal G, Essenfeld-Yahr E. Generalized morphea: a side effect of valproate sodium? *Arch Dermatol* 1980; **116**: 621.
9 Chamson A, Périer C, Frey J. Syndrome sclérodermiforme et poïkilodermique observé au cours d'un traitement par carbidopa et 5-hydroxytryptophanne. Culture de fibroblastes avec analyse biochimique du métabolisme du collagene. *Ann Dermatol Vénéréol* 1986; **113**: 71.
10 Joly P, Lampert A, Thomine E, Lauret P. Development of pseudo-bullous morphea and scleroderma-like illness during therapy with L-5-hydroxytryptophan and carbidopa. *J Am Acad Dermatol* 1991; **25**: 332–3.
11 Gordon ML, Lebwohl MG, Phelps RG *et al.* Eosinophilic fasciitis associated with tryptophan ingestion. A manifestation of eosinophilia-myalgia syndrome. *Arch Dermatol* 1991; **127**: 217–20.
12 Buchanan RR, Gordon DA, Muckle TJ *et al.* The eosinophilic fasciitis syndrome after phenytoin (Dilantin) therapy. *J Rheumatol* 1980; **7**: 733–6.

Chemical and industrial causes of scleroderma-like reactions [1]

Scleroderma-like changes formed part of the clinical spectrum of the Spanish toxic oil syndrome, which resulted from contamination of rapeseed cooking oil with acetanilide [2]. Scleroderma-like changes have been induced by industrial exposure to vinyl chloride [3], epoxy resins [1,4], organic solvents [5] including perchlorethylene [6], trichlorethylene and trichlorethane [7], and in coal miners due to silica exposure [8,9].

REFERENCES

1 Ishikawa O, Warita S, Tamura A, Miyachi Y. Occupational scleroderma. A 17-year follow-up study. *Br J Dermatol* 1995; **133**: 786–9.
2 Rush PJ, Bell MJ, Fam AG. Toxic oil syndrome (Spanish oil disease) and chemically induced scleroderma-like conditions. *J Rheumatol* 1984; **11**: 262–4.
3 Harris DK, Adams WGF. Acroosteolysis occurring in men engaged in the polymerisation of vinyl chloride. *Br Med J* 1967; **3**: 712–24.
4 Yamakage A, Ishikawa H, Saito Y, Hattori A. Occupational scleroderma-like disorders occurring in men engaged in the polymerization of epoxy resins. *Dermatologica* 1980; **161**: 33–44.
5 Yamakage A, Ishikawa H. Generalized morphea-like scleroderma occurring in people exposed to organic solvents. *Dermatologica* 1982; **165**: 186–93.
6 Sparrow GP. A connective tissue disease similar to vinyl chloride disease in a patient exposed to perchlorethylene. *Clin Exp Dermatol* 1977; **2**: 17–22.
7 Flindt-Hansen H, Isager H. Scleroderma after occupational exposure to tricholorethylene and trichlorethane. *Acta Derm Venereol (Stockh)* 1987; **67**: 263–4.
8 Rodnan GP, Benedek TG, Medsger TA, Jr, Cammarata RJ. The association of progressive systemic sclerosis (scleroderma) with coalminers' pneumoconiosis and other forms of silicosis. *Ann Intern Med* 1967; **66**: 323–4.
9 Rustin MHA, Bull HA, Ziegler V *et al.* Silica-associated systemic sclerosis is clinically, serologically and immunologically indistinguishable from idiopathic systemic sclerosis. *Br J Dermatol* 1990; **123**: 725–34.

Eosinophilia–myalgia syndrome

Ingestion of tryptophan, taken as a mild antidepressant, a 'natural hypnotic', or by athletes to increase pain tolerance, was associated with the eosinophilia–myalgia syndrome [1–4], characterized by eosinophilia, myalgia, arthralgia, limb swelling, fever, weakness and fatigue, respiratory complaints, pulmonary hypertension, arrhythmias, ascending polyneuropathy and a variety of cutaneous manifestations. The latter included diffuse morbilliform erythema, urticaria, angio-oedema, dermatographism, livedo reticularis, alopecia and papular mucinosis. Some patients developed chronic muscle weakness, with diffuse scleroderma-like or fasciitis-like skin changes. The eosinophilia–myalgia syndrome is now thought to have been caused by a contaminant of L-tryptophan following a change in the manufacturing process between October 1988 and June 1989 [5,6].

REFERENCES

1 Kaufman LD, Seidman RJ, Phillips ME, Gruber BL. Cutaneous manifestations of the L-tryptophan-associated eosinophilia–myalgia syndrome: a spectrum of sclerodermatous skin disease. *J Am Acad Dermatol* 1990; **23**: 1063–9.
2 Reinauer S, Plewig G. Das Eosinophilie-Myalgie Syndrom. *Hautarzt* 1991; **42**: 137–9.
3 Gordon ML, Lebwohl MG, Phelps RG *et al.* Eosinophilic fasciitis associated with tryptophan ingestion. A manifestation of eosinophilia–myalgia syndrome. *Arch Dermatol* 1991; **127**: 217–20.
4 Connolly SM, Quimby SR, Griffing WL, Winkelmann RK. Scleroderma and L-tryptophan: A possible explanation of the eosinophilia-myalgia syndrome. *J Am Acad Dermatol* 1991; **23**: 451–7.
5 Slutsker L, Hoesly FC, Miller LM *et al.* Eosinophilia–myalgia syndrome associated with exposure to tryptophan from a single manufacturer. *JAMA* 1990; **264**: 213–17.
6 Mayeno AN, Lin F, Foote CS *et al.* Characterization of 'peak E', a novel amino acid associated with eosinophilia–myalgia syndrome. *Science* 1990; **250**: 1707–8.

Erythema nodosum [1]

Sulphonamides, other antibiotics [2], a variety of analgesics, antipyretics and anti-infectious agents, as well as the contraceptive pill [2–5] and treatment of haematological disorders with granulocyte colony-stimulating factor [6] or all-*trans*-retinoic acid [7] have all been implicated in the aetiology of erythema nodosum. Erythema nodosum leprosum was induced by prolonged recombinant IFN-γ (in 60% of patients within 7 months) [8] and by co-trimoxazole [9].

REFERENCES

1 Bork K. *Cutaneous Side Effects of Drugs.* Philadelphia: WB Saunders, 1988.

2 Puavilai S, Sakuntabhai A, Sriprachaya-Anunt S *et al*. Etiology of erythema nodosum. *J Med Assoc Thailand* 1995; **78**: 72–5.

3 Posternal F, Orusco MMM, Laugier P. Eythème noueux et contraceptifs oraux. *Bull Dermatol* 1974; **81**: 642–5.

4 Bombardieri S, Di Munno O, Di Punzio C, Pasero G. Erythema nodosum associated with pregnancy and oral contraceptives. *Br Med J* 1977; **i**: 1509–10.

5 Muller-Ladner U, Kaufmann R, Adler G, Scherbaum WA. Rezidivierendes Erythema nodosum nach Einnahme eines niedrig dosierten oralen Antikonzeptivums. *Mediz Klin* 1994; **89**: 100–2.

6 Nomiyama J, Shinohara K, Inoue H. Erythema nodosum caused by the administration of granulocyte colony-stimulating factor in a patient with refractory anemia. *Am J Hematol* 1994; **47**: 333.

7 Hakimian D, Tallman MS, Zugerman C, Caro WA. Erythema nodosum associated with all-*trans*-retinoic acid in the treatment of acute promyelocytic leukemia. *Leukemia* 1993; **7**: 758–9.

8 Sampaio EP, Moreira AL, Sarno EN *et al*. Prolonged treatment with recombinant interferon-gamma induces erythema nodosum leprosum in lepromatous leprosy patients. *J Exp Med* 1992; **175**: 1729–37.

9 Nishioka S de A, Goulart IM, Burgarelli MK *et al*. Necrotizing erythema nodosum leprosum triggered by cotrimoxazole? *Int J Lepr Mycobact Dis* 1994; **62**: 296–7.

Pseudolymphomatous eruptions: anticonvulsant hypersensitivity syndrome

A number of drugs may produce a reaction pattern that simulates a lymphoma [1–5]. The pseudolymphoma syndrome associated with anticonvulsant drugs comprises fever, a generalized rash and lymphadenopathy, with variable hepatosplenomegaly, abnormal liver function, arthralgia, eosinophilia and blood dyscrasias. Phenytoin especially, but also phenobarbital and carbamazepine, mephytoin and trimethadione have been implicated [6–9]. Cutaneous lesions in patients with reactions to phenytoin or carbamazepine may show histological features of mycosis fungoides; cutaneous lesions resembling those of mycosis fungoides in the absence of fever have been reported with phenytoin and carbamazepine. Phenobarbital has produced a hypersensitivity syndrome resembling Langerhans' cell histiocytosis [10].

Other drugs have been associated with mycosis fungoides-like drug eruptions, including allopurinol, antidepressants (e.g. fluoxetine [11,12] and amitriptyline [12]), phenothiazines [13], thioridazine, benzodiazepines, antihistamines [4], β-blockers (e.g. atenolol [14]), ACE inhibitors [15], calcium-channel blockers, salazosulphapyridine [16], lipid-lowering agents, mexiletine, cyclosporine, d-penicillamine and amiloride hydrochloride with hydrochlorothiazide. A generalized cutaneous B-cell pseudolymphoma was induced by neuroleptics [17].

The pseudolymphoma syndrome usually responds to drug withdrawal, although not for many months in some cases [5]; failure to recognize this syndrome has resulted in use of antitumour therapy, sometimes with fatal outcome. Occasionally, a true lymphoma may develop. Cutaneous T-cell lymphoma and the Sézary syndrome have been reported in association with silicone breast implants [18,19].

REFERENCES

1 Kardaun SH, Scheffer E, Vermeer BJ. Drug-induced pseudolymphomatous skin reactions. *Br J Dermatol* 1988; **118**: 545–52.

2 Sigal M, Pulik M. Pseudo-lymphomes medicamenteux a expression cutanée predominante. *Ann Dermatol Vénéréol* 1993; **120**: 175–80.

3 Handfield-Jones SE, Jenkins RE, Whittaker SJ *et al*. The anticonvulsant hypersensitivity syndrome. *Br J Dermatol* 1993; **129**: 175–7.

4 Magro CM, Crowson AN. Drugs with antihistaminic properties as a cause of atypical cutaneous lymphoid hyperplasia. *J Am Acad Dermatol* 1995; **32**: 419–28.

5 Magro CM, Crowson AN. Drug-induced immune dysregulation as a cause of atypical cutaneous lymphoid infiltrates: a hypothesis. *Hum Pathol* 1996; **27**: 125–32.

6 Wolf R, Kahane E, Sandbank M. Mycosis fungoides-like lesions associated with phenytoin therapy. *Arch Dermatol* 1985; **121**: 1181–2.

7 Rijlaarsdam U, Scheffer E, Meijer CJLM *et al*. Mycosis fungoides-like lesions associated with phenytoin and carbamazepine therapy. *J Am Acad Dermatol* 1991; **24**: 216–20.

8 Shuttleworth D, Graham-Brown RAC, Williams AJ *et al*. Pseudo-lymphoma associated with carbamazepine. *Clin Exp Dermatol* 1984; **9**: 421–3.

9 Welykyj S, Gradini R, Nakao J, Massa M. Carbamazepine-induced eruption histologically mimicking mycosis fungoides. *J Cutan Pathol* 1990; **17**: 111–16.

10 Nagata T, Kawamura N, Motoyama T *et al*. A case of hypersensitivity syndrome resembling Langerhans cell histiocytosis during phenobarbital prophylaxis for convulsion. *Jpn J Clin Oncol* 1992; **22**: 421–7.

11 Gordon KB, Guitart J, Kuzel T *et al*. Pseudo-mycosis fungoides in a patient taking clonazepam and fluoxetine. *J Am Acad Dermatol* 1996; **34**: 304–6.

12 Crowson AN, Magro CM. Antidepressant therapy. A possible cause of atypical cutaneous lymphoid hyperplasia. *Arch Dermatol* 1995; **131**: 925–9.

13 Blazejak T, Hölzle E. Phenothiazin-induziertes Pseudolymphom. *Hautarzt* 1990; **41**: 161–3.

14 Henderson CA, Shamy HK. Atenolol-induced pseudolymphoma. *Clin Exp Dermatol* 1990; **15**: 119–20.

15 Furness PN, Goodfield MJ, MacLennan KA *et al*. Severe cutaneous reactions to captopril and enalapril: histological study and comparison with early mycosis fungoides. *J Clin Pathol* 1986; **39**: 902–7.

16 Gallais V, Grange F, De Bandt M *et al*. Toxidermie a la salazosulfapyridine. Erythrodermie pustuleuse et syndrome pseudolymphomateux: 2 observations. *Ann Dermatol Vénéréol* 1994; **121**: 11–14.

17 Luelmo Aguilar J, Mieras Barcelo C, Martin-Urda MT *et al*. Generalized cutaneous B-cell pseudolymphoma induced by neuroleptics. *Arch Dermatol* 1992; **128**: 121–3.

18 Duvic M, Moore D, Menter A, Vonderheid EC. Cutaneous T-cell lymphoma in association with silicone breast implants. *J Am Acad Dermatol* 1995; **32**: 939–42.

19 Sena E, Ledo A. Sézary syndrome in association with silicone breast implant. *J Am Acad Dermatol* 1995; **33**: 1060–1.

Acanthosis nigricans-like and ichthyosiform eruptions

See Chapter 34.

Hair changes (see also Chapter 66)

Drug-induced alopecia

A considerable number of drugs have been reported to cause hair loss [1–5]; the most important causes are listed in Table 77.18. Cytotoxic drugs may cause alopecia by either anagen or telogen effluvium. Chemotherapeutic agents implicated in the production of alopecia include amsacrine, bleomycin, cyclophosphamide, cytarabine, dactinomycin, daunorubicin, doxorubicin, etoposide, fluorouracil, methotrexate and the nitrosureas [2]. Telogen alopecia has been caused by anticoagulants (heparin and

Table 77.18 Drugs causing alopecia.

Anticoagulants	Retinoids
Coumarins	Acitretin
Dextran	Etretinate
Heparin	Isotretinoin
Heparinoids	Miscellaneous
Anticonvulsants	Albendazole
Carbamazepine	Allopurinol
Valproic acid	Amphetamine
Cytotoxic agents	Antithyroid drugs
Drugs acting on the CNS	Bromocriptine
Amitriptyline	Captopril
Doxepin	Cholestyramine
Haloperidol	Cimetidine
Lithium	Dixyrazine
Hypocholesterolemic agents	Gentamicin
Clofibrate	Gold
Nicotinic acid	Ibuprofen
Triparanol	Levodopa
Antithyroid drugs	Metoprolol
Carbimazole	Oral contraceptives
Thiouracils	Propranolol
	Trimethadione

Table 77.19 Drugs causing hypertrichosis.

Androgens	Penicillamine
Corticosteroids	Phenytoin
Cyclosporin A	Psoralens
Diazoxide	Streptomycin
Minoxidil	

coumarin anticoagulants), thyreostatic drugs (carbimazole and thiouracils), levodopa, propranolol, albendazole and oral contraceptives. Retinoids cause alopecia by disrupting keratinization. Hydantoins may cause scalp alopecia and hypertrichosis elsewhere, and retinoids and clofibrate may cause alopecia by interfering with keratinization. Temporary hair loss has been described after 5-aminosalicylic acid enemas [6] and bromocriptine [7], and danazol has induced generalized alopecia [8]. Certain β-blockers have caused increased hair loss [9–11] as have dixyrazine [12] and ibuprofen [13].

Drug-induced hypertrichosis

The hirsutism induced in women by corticosteroids, androgens and certain progestogens is well recognized. Other drugs that may cause hypertrichosis are listed in Table 77.19 [3,4]. Up to 50% of children treated with diazoxide, and up to 40% of patients on cyclosporin A, develop hirsutism. Zidovudine has caused excessive growth of eyelashes [14].

REFERENCES

1 Brodin MB. Drug-related alopecia. *Dermatol Clin* 1987; **5**: 571–9.

2 Kerber BJ, Hood AF. Chemotherapy-induced cutaneous reactions. *Semin Dermatol* 1989; **8**: 173–81.
3 Rook A, Dawber R. *Diseases of the Hair and Scalp*, 2nd edn. Blackwell Scientific Publications: Oxford, 1990.
4 Merk HF. Drugs affecting hair growth. In: Orfanos CE, Happle R, eds. *Hair and Hair Diseases*. Springer-Verlag: Berlin, 1990: 601–9.
5 Pillans PI, Woods DJ. Drug-associated alopecia. *Int J Dermatol* 1995; **34**: 149–58.
6 Kutty PK, Raman KRK, Hawken K, Barrowman JA. Hair loss and 5-aminosalicylic acid enemas. *Ann Intern Med* 1982; **97**: 785–6.
7 Blum I, Leiba S. Increased hair loss as a side effect of bromocriptine treatment. *N Engl J Med* 1980; **303**: 1418.
8 Duff P, Mayer AR. Generalized alopecia: an unusual complication of danazol therapy. *Am J Obstet Gynecol* 1981; **141**: 349–50.
9 England JR, England JD. Alopecia and propranolol therapy. *Aust Fam Physician* 1982; **11**: 225–6.
10 Graeber CW, Lapkin RA. Metoprolol and alopecia. *Cutis* 1981; **28**: 633–4.
11 Fraunfelder FT, Meyer SM, Menacker SJ. Alopecia possibly secondary to topical ophthalmic β-blockers. *JAMA* 1990; **263**: 1493–4.
12 Poulsen J. Hair loss, depigmentation of hair, ichthyosis, and blepharo-conjunctivitis produced by dixyrazine. *Acta Derm Venereol (Stockh)* 1981; **61**: 85–8.
13 Meyer HC. Alopecia associated with ibuprofen. *JAMA* 1979; **242**: 142.
14 Klutman NE, Hinthorn DR. Excessive growth of eyelashes in a patient with AIDS being treated with zidovudine. *N Engl J Med* 1991; **324**: 1896.

Drug-induced hair discoloration (see Chapter 66)

Drug-induced change in hair colour usually occurring 3–12 months after the onset of treatment is a rare but well-recognized phenomenon [1,2]. Darkening of hair has occurred during treatment with verapamil [3], tamoxifen [4], carbidopa [5] and *p*-aminobenzoic acid. Etretinate has caused both darkening as well as lightening, curling and kinking of hair [6]. Greying of hair has been reported with chloroquine and mephenesin [7]. Chloroquine depigmentation is reversible and occurs only in red- or blonde-haired individuals; both IFN-α [8] and chloroquine are capable of arresting phaeomelanin synthesis.

REFERENCES

1 Rook A. Some chemical influences on hair growth and pigmentation. *Br J Dermatol* 1965; **77**: 115–29.
2 Bublin JG, Thompson DF. Drug-induced hair colour changes. *Clin Pharmacol Ther* 1992; **17**: 297–302.
3 Read GM. Verapamil and hair colour change. *Lancet* 1991; **338**: 1520.
4 Hampson JP, Donnelly A, Lewisones MS, Pye JK. Tamoxifen induced hair colour change. *Br J Dermatol* 1995; **132**: 483–4.
5 Reynolds NJ, Crossley J, Ferguson I, Peachey RDG. Darkening of white hair in Parkinson's disease. *Clin Exp Dermatol* 1989; **14**: 317–18.
6 Vesper JL, Fenske A. Hair darkening and new growth associated with etretinate therapy. *J Am Acad Dermatol* 1996; **34**: 860.
7 Spillane JD. Brunette to blonde. Depigmentation of hair during treatment with oral mephenesin. *Br Med J* 1963; **i**: 997–8.
8 Fleming CJ, MacKie RM. Alpha interferon-induced hair discolouration. *Br J Dermatol* 1996; **135**: 337–8.

Nail changes

Drug-induced nail abnormalities have been the subject of several reviews [1–7] (see Chapter 65). Heavy metals may induce changes as follows: arsenic causes transverse, broad, white lines (Mee's lines), silver causes blue discoloration of the lunulae, gold results in thin and brittle nails with longitudinal streaking, yellow–brown discoloration and onycholysis, and lead produces partial leukonychia. D-penicillamine therapy is associated with the yellow-nail syndrome and nail dystrophy. Cytotoxic agents may produce transverse or longitudinal pigmentation, splinter haemorrhages, Beau's lines, leukonychia, Mee's lines, onycholysis, shortening of lunulae, pallor, atrophy, nail shedding and slow growth; acute paronychia has occurred with methotrexate. Beta-blockers may induce a psoriasiform nail dystrophy with onycholysis and subungual hyperkeratosis. Thiazide diuretics may result in onycholysis. Discoloration or pigmentation occurs with antimalarials (blue–brown discoloration), lithium (golden discoloration), phenolphthalein (dark-blue discoloration), phenothiazines (blue–black or purple pigmentation), phenytoin (pigmentation), psoralens and tetracyclines (yellow pigmentation). Oral contraceptives may induce photo-onycholysis and onycholysis, and are associated with an increased growth rate and reduced splitting and fragility. By contrast, heparin reduces nail growth and causes transverse banding and subungual haematomas. Retinoids cause thinning and increased fragility, onychoschizia, onycholysis, temporary nail shedding, onychomadesis, ingrowing nails, periungual granulation tissue and paronychia.

Onycholysis

Drugs causing onycholysis [6,7] and photo-onycholysis, are listed in Table 77.20.

REFERENCES

1 Daniel CR, III, Scher RK. Nail changes secondary to systemic drugs or ingestants. *J Am Acad Dermatol* 1984; **10**: 250–8.
2 Fenton DA, Nail changes due to drugs. In: Samman PD, Fenton DA. *The Nails in Disease*, 4th edn. London: Heinemann, 1986: 121–5.
3 Fenton DA, Wilkinson JD. The nail in systemic diseases and drug-induced changes. In: Baran R, Dawber RPR, eds. *Diseases of the Nails and their Management*. Blackwell Scientific Publications: Oxford, 1984: 205–65.
4 Daniel CR, III, Scher RK. Nail changes secondary to systemic drugs or ingestants. In: Scher RK, Daniel CR, III, eds. *Nails: Therapy, Diagnosis, Surgery*. Philadelphia: WB Saunders, 1990: 192–201.
5 Zaias N. *The Nail in Health and Disease*, 2nd edn. East Norwalk, Connecticut: Appleton Lange, 1990.
6 Baran R, Juhlin L. Drug-induced photo-onycholysis. Three subtypes identified in a study of 15 cases. *J Am Acad Dermatol* 1987; **17**: 1012–16.
7 Daniel CR. Onycholysis: an overview. *Semin Dermatol* 1991; **10**: 34–40.

Oral conditions (see also Chapter 69)

Adverse drug reactions affecting the mouth have been extensively reviewed [1–3]. Disturbance of taste has been reported with a wide variety of drugs [4], including captopril, griseofulvin and metronidazole.

Xerostomia

Dryness of the mouth (xerostomia) may result from anticholinergic side-effects of drugs. Xerostomia has been recorded in association with antidepressants, tranquillizers, anti-Parkinsonian drugs, antihypertensives and gastrointestinal antispasmodics (Table 77.21). Parotitis with salivary sialadenitis has been reported in up to 15% of patients taking phenylbutazone, and may be associated with fever and a rash [5]. A similar syndrome may occur with repeated administration of iodinated contrast media [6] and with nitrofurantoin [7].

REFERENCES

1 Zelickson BD, Rogers RS, III. Drug reactions involving the mouth. *Clin Dermatol* 1986; **4**: 98–109.
2 Korstanje MJ. Drug-induced mouth disorders. *Clin Exp Dermatol* 1995; **20**: 10–18.
3 Parks ET. Lesions associated with drug reactions. *Dermatol Clin* 1996; **14**: 327–37.
4 Griffin JP. Drug-induced disorders of taste. *Adv Drug React Toxicol Rev* 1992; **11**: 229–39.
5 Speed BR, Spelman DW. Sialadenitis and systemic reactions associated with phenylbutazone. *Aust NZ J Med* 1982; **12**: 261–4.
6 Chohen JC, Roxe DM, Said R et al. Iodide mumps after repeated exposure to iodinated contrast media. *Lancet* 1980; i: 762–3.

Table 77.20 Drugs causing onycholysis.

Antibiotics	Miscellaneous
Cephaloridine	Acridine
Cloxacillin	Captopril
Chloramphenicol	Norethindrone and mestranol
Chlortetracycline	Practolol (now discontinued)
Demethylchlortetracycline	Psoralens
Doxycycline,	Phenothiazines
Fluoroquinolones	Retinoids
Minocycline	Sulpha-related drugs
Tetracycline hydrochloride	Thiazides
Chemotherapeutic agents	*Photo-onycholysis*
Adriamycin	Oral contraceptives
Bleomycin	Psoralens
5-fluorouracil	Fluoroquinolones
Mitozantrone	Tetracyclines

Table 77.21 Drugs associated with xerostomia.

Antidepressants	Minor tranquillizers
Tricyclic	Diazepam
Amitriptyline	Chordiazepoxide
Doxepin	Hydroxyzine
Imipramine	Anti-Parkinsonian drugs
Monoamine oxidase inhibitors	Antihypertensives (ganglion blockers)
Isocarboxazid	
Phenelzine	Gastrointestinal antispasmodics
Psychotropic agents	Atropine
Chlorpromazine	Propantheline bromide
Thioridazine	Phenobarbital
Haloperidol	
Prochlorperazine	

7 Meyboom RH, van Gent A, Zinkstok DJ. Nitrofurantoin-induced parotitis. *Br Med J* 1982; **285**: 1049.

Stomatitis

Type I immediate hypersensitivity and type IV delayed hypersensitivity reactions may be involved in allergic stomatitis [1]. The allergic stomatitides may present with clinical appearances that mimic classic oral vesiculobullous and ulcerative lesions. Stomatitis may form a part of drug-induced lichenoid reactions, fixed drug reactions or erythema multiforme, but may also arise separately from these conditions as a side-effect of a number of drugs (Table 77.22). Chemotherapeutic agents causing stomatitis or buccal ulceration include [2] actinomycin D, adriamycin, amsacrine, bleomycin, busulfan, chlorambucil, cyclophosphamide, dactinomycin, daunorubicin, doxorubicin, fluorouracil, IL-2, mercaptopurine, methotrexate, mithramycin, mitomycin, nitrosureas, procarbazine and vincristine. Penicillamine may induce stomatitis or ulceration as part of drug-induced pemphigus [3] or a lichenoid drug eruption. Gold therapy is another well-recognized cause of stomatitis [4–6]. Allergic reactions to dental materials and therapy may cause stomatitis. Positive patch tests to mercuric chloride were seen in 42%, and to copper sulphate in 16%, of patients with oral mucosal lesions associated with amalgam restorations, compared with 9% of controls, in one series [7]. It has been postulated that mercury released from dental amalgams can cause hypersensitivity/toxic reactions resulting in lichen planus lesions, and may play a major role in the pathogenesis of gingivitis, periodontitis and periodontal disease [8]. Mercuric chloride caused statistically significant increased IFN-γ release, but not proliferation, in lymphocyte cultures from patients with hypersensitivity to amalgam restorations [9].

REFERENCES

1 Jainkittivong A, Langlais RP. Allergic stomatitis. *Semin Dermatol* 1994; **13**: 91–101.
2 Kerker BJ, Hood AF. Chemotherapy-induced cutaneous reactions. *Semin Dermatol* 1989; **8**: 173–81.

Table 77.22 Drugs causing stomatitis or buccal ulceration.

Chemotherapeutic agents	Antihypertensive agents
Antirheumatic drugs	Captopril
Gold	Hydralazine
Naproxen	Methyldopa (rare)
Indomethacin	Miscellaneous
Penicillamine	Chlorpromazine
Zomepirac	Valproic acid
Antidepressants	
Amitriptyline	
Doxepin	
Imipramine	

3 Hay KD, Muller HK, Rade PC. D-penicillamine-induced mucocutaneous lesions with features of pemphigus. *Oral Surg* 1978; **45**: 385–95.
4 Glenert U. Drug stomatitis due to gold therapy. *Oral Surg* 1984; **58**: 52–6.
5 Gall H. Allergien auf zahnärztliche Werkstoffe und Dentalpharmaka. *Hautarzt* 1983; **34**: 326–31.
6 Wiesenfeld D, Ferguson MM, Forsyth A *et al.* Allergy to dental gold. *Oral Surg* 1984; **57**: 158–60.
7 Nordlind K, Liden S. Patch test reactions to metal salts in patients with oral mucosal lesions associated with amalgam restorations. *Contact Dermatitis* 1992; **27**: 157–60.
8 Swartzendruber DE. The possible relationship between mercury from dental amalgam and diseases. I: Effects within the oral cavity. *Med Hypoth* 1993; **41**: 31–4.
9 Nordlind K, Liden S. In vitro lymphocyte reactivity to heavy metal salts in the diagnosis of oral mucosal hypersensitivity to amalgam restorations. *Br J Dermatol* 1993; **128**: 38–41.

Hyperpigmentation

Hyperpigmentation of the buccal mucosa may occur with chemotherapeutic agents [1]. Oestrogen is associated with gingival hypermelanosis [2]. Amalgam tattoos with localized hyperpigmentation of the buccal mucosa result from implantation of amalgam in soft tissues, especially of the gingival or alveolar mucosa [3].

Reactions caused by antibacterial, antifungal and immunosuppressive therapy

Systemic antibiotics or immunosuppressive medication [4], and corticosteroids administered by aerosol [5], may lead to development of candidiasis of the buccal mucosa. Black, hairy tongue may be associated with broad-spectrum antibiotic therapy and with griseofulvin treatment.

Gingival hyperplasia

Gingival hyperplasia may be caused by phenytoin [6], nifedipine [7], diltiazem [8] felodipine, verapamil and cyclosporin A [9].

REFERENCES

1 Krutchik AN, Buzdar AU. Pigmentation of the tongue and mucous membranes associated with cancer chemotherapy. *South Med J* 1979; **72**: 1615–16.
2 Hertz RS, Beckstead PC, Brown WJ. Epithelial melanosis of the gingiva possibly resulting from the use of oral contraceptives. *J Am Dent Assoc* 1980; **100**: 713–14.
3 Buchner A, Hansen LS. Amalgam pigmentation (amalgam tattoo) of the oral mucosa: a clinicopathologic study of 268 cases. *Oral Surg* 1980; **49**: 139–47.
4 Torack RM. Fungus infections associated with antibiotic and steroid therapy. *Am J Med* 1957; **22**: 872–82.
5 Chervinsky P, Petraco AJ. Incidence of oral candidiasis during therapy with triamcinolone acetonide aerosol. *Ann Allergy* 1979; **43**: 80–3.
6 Hassell TM, Page RC, Narayanan AS, Cooper CG. Diphenylhydantoin (dilantin) gingival hyperplasia: drug induced abnormality of connective tissue. *Proc Natl Acad Sci USA* 1976; **73**: 2909–12.
7 Benini PL, Crosti C, Sala F *et al.* Gingival hyperplasia by nifedipine. Report of a case. *Acta Derm Venereol (Stockh)* 1985; **65**: 362–5.

8 Giustiniani S, Robustelli della Cuna F, Marieni M. Hyperplastic gingivitis during diltiazem therapy. *Int J Cardiol* 1987; **15**: 247–9.
9 Frosch PJ, Ruder H, Stiefel A *et al*. Gingivahyperplasie und Seropapeln unter Cyclosporinbehandlung. *Hautarzt* 1988; **39**: 611–16.

Important or widely prescribed drugs

Antibacterial agents

Beta-lactam antibiotics

Inaccurate antibiotic allergy histories are frequently documented in the medical record by hospital doctors [1]. Reactions to β-lactam antibiotics may be immediate, accelerated or delayed [2–5]. Non-immediate reactions to penicillins are a reproducible phenomenon, suggesting that a specific mechanism is responsible [6]. In one study, 39% of 74 subjects with a cutaneous reaction to a penicillin derivative had a non-immediate reaction, in 93% to an amino penicillin (10.3% ampicillin, 82.7% amoxicillin). There was a positive delayed direct challenge, and a delayed skin-test response in 65% of cases, and a lymphomonocytic infiltrate on skin biopsy [6]. Cross-reactivity exists between several members of this group of antibiotics, but restricted sensitivity to a single penicillin derivative also occurs [7]. As a group, penicillins had a higher frequency of allergic reactions than cephalosporins, in a study of patients with cystic fibrosis treated with parenteral β-lactam antibiotics [8].

REFERENCES

1 Absy M, Glatt AE. Antibiotic allergy: inaccurate history taking in a teaching hospital. *South Med J* 1994; **87**: 805–7.
2 Vega JM, Blanca M, Garcia JJ *et al*. Immediate allergic reactions to amoxicillin. *Allergy* 1994; **49**: 317–22.
3 Warrington RJ, Silviu-Dan F, Magro C. Accelerated cell-mediated immune reactions in penicillin allergy. *J Allergy Clin Immunol* 1993; **92**: 626–8.
4 Ortiz-Frutos FJ, Quintana I, Soto T *et al*. Delayed hypersensitivity to penicillin. *Allergy* 1996; **51**: 134–5.
5 Lopez Serrano C, Villas F, Cabanas R, Contreras J. Delayed hypersensitivity to beta-lactams. *J Invest Allergol Clin Immunol* 1994; **4**: 315–19.
6 Terrados S, Blanca M, Garcia J *et al*. Nonimmediate reactions to betalactams: prevalence and role of the different penicillins. *Allergy* 1995; **50**: 563–7.
7 Blanca M, Vega JM, Garcia J *et al*. New aspects of allergic reactions to betalactams: crossreactions and unique specificities. *Clin Exp Allergy* 1994; **24**: 407–15.
8 Pleasants RA, Walker TR, Samuelson WM. Allergic reactions to parenteral beta-lactam antibiotics in patients with cystic fibrosis. *Chest* 1994; **106**: 1124–8.

Penicillin

Toxic reactions to penicillin are extremely rare and usually only follow massive doses, but can occur with normal doses in patients with renal impairment; encephalopathy with epilepsy may result from binding of the β-lactam ring to γ-aminobutyric acid receptors [1]. By contrast, immunological reactions are common [2–4]; allergy to penicillin has been reported in up to 10% of patients treated [5]. All forms of penicillin, including the semi-synthetic penicillins, are potentially cross-allergenic; in general, allergic reactions to semisynthetic compounds are commoner than to natural penicillins. All four types of immunological reaction may occur: urticaria and anaphylactic shock (type 1), haemolytic anaemia or agranulocytosis (type 2), allergic vasculitis or serum sickness-like reaction (type 3) and allergic contact dematitis [6] (type 4). Immediate reactions occur within 1 h, and take the form of urticaria, laryngeal oedema, bronchospasm and/or anaphylactic shock. So-called accelerated reactions with the same clinical features develop 1–72 h later. Reactions occurring more than 72 h after exposure are termed late reactions; these include maculopapular rashes with scarlatiniform and morbilliform exanthemata, urticaria, serum sickness, erythema multiforme, haemolytic anaemia, thrombocytopenia, and neutropenia. Fever is the commonest reaction.

The antigenic structures responsible for penicillin allergy include a 'major determinant', the penicilloyl group formed by spontaneous hydrolysis of penicillin (penicilloyl polylysine is used for skin testing) and additional antigenic compounds to which benzyl penicillin is metabolized, termed 'minor determinants' [3]. Most immediate-type anaphylactic hypersensitivity reactions are mediated by IgE antibodies to minor antigenic determinants, whereas accelerated reactions are usually the result of IgE antibodies directed against the major antigenic determinant [3,7].

For information on skin testing for penicillin, see page 3510.

Anaphylactic reactions to penicillin reportedly occur in about 0.015% of treatment courses; fatal reactions occurred in between 0.0015 and 0.002% (i.e. one in 50–100 000) of treatment courses [8]. Young and middle-aged adults aged 20–49 years are at most risk [9]. Atopy does not augment the risk of a reaction to β-lactam antibiotics, but may increase the risk of any reaction being severe [3]. Anaphylaxis is commoner after parenteral administration, and is very rare, but has been recorded, after oral ingestion [9]. Maculopapular reactions occur in about 2% of treatment courses [3]; where there is a history of a prior penicillin reaction, the risk of a subsequent reaction increases to about 10% [10]. A fair proportion (33% in one study) of children may lose their skin-test reactivity within a year [11]. In practice, when penicillin is given to children said to be allergic to penicillin, very few experience an adverse reaction [7]. In adults, the rate of disappearance of penicillin-specific IgE is highly variable, from 10 days to indefinite persistence [3]. For a group of penicillin-allergic patients, the time lapsed since a previous reaction is inversely related to the risk of a further IgE-mediated reaction [10]. In one study, 80–90% of patients were skin-test positive 2 months after an acute allergic reaction, but less than 20% were skin-test positive 10 years later [12]. Nevertheless, patients with a prior history of an IgE-dependent reaction remain at risk of recurrence, even though IgE antibodies become undetectable by skin testing [13]. Most serious and fatal allergic reactions to β-lactam antibiotics occur in individuals who have never had a prior allergic reaction; a negative history should therefore not induce a false sense of security [3]. Continuous prophylactic treatment is associated with a very low incidence of reactions [14].

Activation of allergy in a sensitized individual may require only minute amounts of the drug as from contaminated syringes, dental root-canal fillings, viral vaccines, contaminated milk or meat products, and contamination of transfused blood [15]. Urticaria and wheezing occurred in the penicillin-sensitive spouse of a man receiving parenteral mezlocillin, and was postulated to have arisen as a result of seminal fluid transmission of penicillin [16]. Hypersensitivity reactions have occurred after intrauterine placement, in penicillin-sensitive patients, of spermatozoa or embryos exposed to penicillin *in vitro* [17].

Penicillin has been reported to cause erythema multiforme [18], vesicular and bullous eruptions, exfoliative dermatitis [19], vascular purpura or fixed eruptions, postinflammatory elastolysis (cutis laxa), which was generalized and eventually fatal in one case [20], and a very few cases of pemphigus vulgaris [21,22], pemphigoid [23] and pustular psoriasis [24]. It has been proposed that penicillin may have a role in chronic 'idiopathic' urticaria [25].

Cloxacillin and flucloxacillin

Cloxacillins cross-react with penicillins, but unlike ampicillin do not produce distinctive eruptions. Flucloxacillin rarely elicits primary penicillin hypersensitivity. In one case report, parenteral cloxacillin was tolerated, but oral administration caused progressive generalized erythema with pruritus, facial angio-oedema and tachycardia [27]. Flucloxacillin has been implicated as a cause of cholestatic jaundice; this complication is rare, and the risk is greater in elderly patients and those receiving therapy for more than 2 weeks [27].

REFERENCES

1 Barrons RW, Murray KM, Richey RM. Populations at risk for penicillin-induced seizures. *Ann Pharmacother* 1992; **26**: 26–9.
2 Erffmeyer JE. Penicillin allergy. *Clin Rev Allergy* 1986; **4**: 171–88.
3 Weiss ME, Adkinson NF. Immediate hypersensitivity reactions to penicillin and related antibiotics. *Clin Allergy* 1988; **18**: 515–40.
4 Weber EA, Knight A. Testing for allergy to antibiotics. *Semin Dermatol* 1989; **8**: 204–12.
5 Van Arsdael PP. The risk of penicillin reactions. *Ann Intern Med* 1968; **69**: 1071.
6 Stejskal VDM, Forsbeck M, Olin R. Side chain-specific lymphocyte responses in workers with occupational allergy induced by penicillins. *Int Arch Allergy Appl Immunol* 1987; **82**: 461–4.
7 Anonymous. Penicillin allergy in childhood. *Lancet* 1989; **i**: 420.
8 Idsøe O, Guthe T, Willcox RR, de Weck AL. Nature and extent of penicillin side reactions, with particular reference to fatalities from anaphylactic shock. *Bull WHO* 1968; **38**: 159–88.
9 Simmonds J, Hodges S, Nicol F, Barnett D. Anaphylaxis after oral penicillin. *Br Med J* 1978; **ii**: 1404.
10 Sogn DD. Penicillin allergy. *J Allergy Clin Immunol* 1984; **74**: 589–93.
11 Chandra RK, Joglekar SA, Tomas E. Penicillin allergy: anti-penicillin IgE antibodies and immediate hypersensitivity skin reactions employing major and minor determinants of penicillin. *Arch Dis Child* 1980; **55**: 857–60.
12 Sullivan TJ, Wedner JH, Shatz GS *et al.* Skin testing to detect penicillin allergy. *J Allergy Clin Immunol* 1981; **68**: 171–80.
13 Adkinson NF, Jr. Risk factors for drug allergy. *J Allergy Clin Immunol* 1984; **74**: 567–72.
14 Wood HF, Simpson R, Feinstein AR *et al.* Rheumatic fever in children and adolescents. A long-term epidemiologic study of subsequent prophylaxis, streptococcal infections, and clinical sequelae. I. Description of the investigative techniques and the population studied. *Ann Intern Med* 1964; **60** (Suppl. 5): 6–17.
15 Michel J, Sharon R. Non-haemolytic adverse reaction after transfusion of a blood unit containing penicillin. *Br Med J* 1980; **i**: 152–3.
16 Burks JH, Fliegalman R, Sokalski SJ. An unforeseen complication of home parenteral antibiotic therapy. *Arch Intern Med* 1989; **149**: 1603–4.
17 Smith YR, Hurd WW, Menge AC *et al.* Allergic reactions to penicillin during in vitro fertilization and intrauterine insemination. *Fertil Steril* 1992; **58**: 847–9.
18 Staretz LR, DeBoom GW. Multiple oral and skin lesions occurring after treatment with penicillin. *J Am Dent Assoc* 1990; **121**: 436–7.
19 Levine BB. Skin rashes with penicillin therapy: current management. *N Engl J Med* 1972; **286**: 42–3.
20 Kerl H, Burg G, Hashimoto K. Fatal, penicillin-induced, generalized, postinflammatory elastolysis (cutis laxa). *Am J Dermatopathol* 1983; **5**: 267–76.
21 Duhra PL, Foulds IS. Penicillin-induced pemphigus vulgaris. *Br J Dermatol* 1988; **118**: 307.
22 Fellner MJ, Mark AS. Penicillin- and ampicillin-induced pemphigus vulgaris. *Int J Dermatol* 1980; **19**: 392–3.
23 Alcalay J, David M, Ingber A *et al.* Bullous pemphigoid mimicking bullous erythema multiforme: an untoward side effect of penicillins. *J Am Acad Dermatol* 1988; **18**: 345–9.
24 Katz M, Seidenbaum M, Weinrauch L. Penicillin-induced generalized pustular psoriasis. *J Am Acad Dermatol* 1988; **17**: 918–20.
25 Boonk WJ, Van Ketel WG. The role of penicillin in the pathogenesis of chronic urticaria. *Br J Dermatol* 1982; **106**: 183–90.
26 Torres MJ, Blanca M, Fernandez J *et al.* Selective allergic reaction to oral cloxacillin. *Clin Exp Allergy* 1996; **26**: 108–11.
27 Fairley CK, McNeil JJ, Desmond P *et al.* Risk factors for development of flucloxacillin-associated jaundice. *Br Med J* 1993; **306**: 233–5.

Ampicillin

A morbilliform rash, with onset on the extremities, becoming generalized, occurs in 5–10% of patients treated with ampicillin, and usually develops 7–12 days after onset of therapy. This time interval suggests an allergic mechanism, but the rash disappears spontaneously even if ampicillin is continued, and may not develop on re-exposure [1]. Skin tests are generally negative. An urticarial reaction, present in about 1.5% of patients, indicates the presence of type I IgE-mediated general penicillin allergy [2,3]. Administration of ampicillin when a patient has infectious mononucleosis leads to florid morbilliform and sometimes purpuric eruptions in up to 100% of patients [4,5]. Cutaneous reactions to ampicillin are increased in cytomegalovirus infection [6], in chronic lymphatic leukaemia [7], with allopurinol administered concomitantly [8] or in renal insufficiency. Ampicillin has been reported to cause a fixed drug eruption [9], erythema multiforme and Stevens–Johnson syndrome [10,11], TEN [12], Henoch–Schönlein purpura [13], serum sickness [14] and pemphigus vulgaris [15] in individual cases. Administration of ampicillin to a patient with a history of psoriasis resulted in erythroderma on two separate occasions [16]. A recurrent localized pustular skin eruption developed on the cheeks with ampicillin in one case [17].

Delayed intradermal skin tests and patch tests, indicating delayed hypersensitivity, were positive in about half of 60 subjects with maculopapular reactions to the aminopenicillins ampicillin and amoxicillin [18]; in another study, hypersensitivity to an antigenic determinant in the side-chain structure was suggested, as intradermal and patch tests were positive to ampicillin but there was good tolerance to benzylpenicillin [19]. Re-exposure of patients to ampicillins and other penicillins is contraindicated after urticarial reactions; anaphylactic reactions to ampicillin have been recorded. The risk is far less after morbilliform rashes but is not negligible.

REFERENCES

1 Adcock BB, Rodman DP. Ampicillin-specific rashes. *Arch Family Med* 1996; **5**: 301–4.

2 Bass JW, Crowley DM, Steele RW *et al*. Adverse effects of orally administered ampicillin. *J Pediatr* 1973; **83**: 106–8.

3 Leading Article. Ampicillin rashes. *Br Med J* 1975; **ii**: 708–9.

4 Weiss ME, Adkinson NF. Immediate hypersensitivity reactions to penicillin and related antibiotics. *Clin Allergy* 1988; **18**: 515–40.

5 Pullen H, Wright N, Murdoch J McC. Hypersensitivity reactions to antibacterial drugs in infectious mononucleosis. *Lancet* 1967; **ii**: 1176–8.

6 Klemola E. Hypersensitivity reactions to ampicillin in cytomegalovirus mononucleosis. *Scand J Infect Dis* 1970; **2**: 29.

7 Cameron SJ, Richmond J. Ampicillin hypersensitivity in lymphatic leukaemia. *Scot Med J* 1972; **16**: 425–7.

8 Jick H, Slone D, Shapiro S *et al*. Excess of ampicillin rashes associated with allopurinol or hyperuricemia. A report from the Boston Collaborative Drug Surveillance Program, Boston University Medical Center. *N Engl J Med* 1972; **286**: 505–7.

9 Arndt KA, Parrish J. Ampicillin rashes. *Arch Dermatol* 1973; **107**: 74.

10 Gupta HL, Dheman R. Ampicillin-induced Stevens–Johnson syndrome. *J Indian Med Assoc* 1979; **72**: 188–9.

11 Garty BZ, Offer I, Livni E, Danon YL. Erythema multiforme and hypersensitivity myocarditis caused by ampicillin. *Ann Pharmacother* 1994; **28**: 730–1.

12 Tagami H, Tatsuta K, Iwatski K, Yamada M. Delayed hypersensitivity in ampicillin-induced toxic epidermal necrolysis. *Arch Dermatol* 1983; **119**: 910–13.

13 Beeching NJ, Gruer LD, Findlay CD, Geddes AM. A case of Henoch–Schönlein purpura syndrome following oral ampicillin. *J Antimicrob Chemother* 1982; **10**: 479–82.

14 Caldwell JR, Cliff LE. Adverse reactions to antimicrobial agents. *JAMA* 1974; **230**: 77–80.

15 Fellner MJ, Mark AS. Penicillin- and ampicillin-induced pemphigus vulgaris. *Int J Dermatol* 1980; **19**: 392–3.

16 Saito S, Ikezawa Z. Psoriasiform intradermal test reaction to ABPC in a patient with psoriasis and ABPC allergy. *J Dermatol (Tokyo)* 1990; **17**: 677–83.

17 Lim JT, Ng SK. An unusual drug eruption to ampicillin. *Cutis* 1995; **56**: 163–4.

18 Romano A, Di Fonso M, Papa G *et al*. Evaluation of adverse cutaneous reactions to aminopenicillins with emphasis on those manifested by maculopapular rashes. *Allergy* 1995; **50**: 113–18.

19 Lopez Serrano C, Villas F, Cabanas R, Contreras J. Delayed hypersensitivity to beta-lactams. *J Invest Allergol Clin Immunol* 1994; **4**: 315–19.

Amoxicillin

Cutaneous eruptions including urticaria, morbilliform, or maculopapular rashes occur in between 1 and 2% of treatment courses with amoxicillin [1–3]. Immediate allergy (anaphylaxis or urticaria/angio-oedema) to amoxicillin has occurred in patients with good tolerance of benzylpenicillin, aztreonam and ceftazidime [4,5]. However, amoxicillin has been reported to cross-react with penicillin on first exposure [6]. Amoxicillin caused an unusual intertriginous eruption in two patients [7]. Serum sickness has been reported with amoxicillin in children [8]. Amoxicillin has caused a fixed eruption [9], and a curious, recurrent, localized, pustular eruption [10]. This drug has also been implicated in the development of an acute generalized exanthematous pustulosis [11]. There may be an increased frequency of rash with amoxicillin and clavulanate therapy in HIV-positive patients [12]. Amoxicillin, like clavulanic acid and flucloxacillin, may cause a cholestatic hepatitis [13]. This occurs at a frequency of one in 6000 adults when the drug is combined with clavulinic acid (co-amoxiclav) [14].

Methicillin

Methicillin caused reappearance of a recently faded ampicillin rash in a patient with glandular fever [15].

REFERENCES

1 Wise PJ, Neu HC. Experience with amoxicillin: an overall summary of clinical trials in the United States. *J Infect Dis* 1974; **129** (Suppl.): S266–7.

2 Levine LR. Quantitative comparison of adverse reactions to cefaclor versus amoxicillin in a surveillance study. *Pediatr Infect Dis* 1985; **4**: 358–61.

3 Bigby M, Jick S, Jick H, Arndt K. Drug-induced cutaneous reactions. A report from the Boston Collaborative Drug Surveillance Program on 15 438 consecutive inpatients, 1975 to 1982. *JAMA* 1986; **256**: 3358–63.

4 Vega JM, Blanca M, Garcia JJ *et al*. Immediate allergic reactions to amoxicillin. *Allergy* 1994; **49**: 317–22.

5 Martin JA, Igea JM, Fraj J *et al*. Allergy to amoxicillin in patients who tolerated benzylpenicillin, aztreonam, and ceftazidime. *Clin Infect Dis* 1992; **14**: 592–3.

6 Fellner MJ. Amoxicillin cross reacts with penicillin on first exposure. *Int J Dermatol* 1993; **32**: 308–9.

7 Wolf R, Brenner S, Krakowski A. Intertriginous drug eruption. *Acta Derm Venereol (Stockh)* 1992; **72**: 441–2.

8 Chopra R, Roberts J, Warrington RJ. Severe delayed-onset hypersensitivity reactions to amoxicillin in children. *Can Med Assoc J* 1989; **140**: 921–3.

9 Chowdhury FH. Fixed genital drug eruption. *Practical Med* 1982; **226**: 1450.

10 Shuttleworth D. A localized, recurrent pustular eruption following amoxycillin administration. *Clin Exp Dermatol* 1989; **14**: 367–8.

11 Roujeau J-C, Bioulac-Sage P, Bourseau C *et al*. Acute generalized exanthematous pustulosis. Analysis of 63 cases. *Arch Dermatol* 1991; **127**: 1333–8.

12 Battegay M, Opravil M, Wütrich B, Lüthy R. Rash with amoxycillin-clavulanate therapy in HIV-infected patients. *Lancet* 1989; **ii**: 1100.

13 Anonymous. Drug-induced cholestatic hepatitis from common antibiotics. *Med J Aust* 1992; **157**: 531.

14 Anonymous. Revised indications for co-amoxiclav (Augmentin). *Curr Probl Pharmacovig* 1997; **23**: 8.

15 Fields DA. Methicillin rash in infectious mononucleosis. *West J Med* 1981; **133**: 521.

Cephalosporins [1]

In general, cephalosporins are fairly well tolerated [1–3], adverse reactions ranging from 1 to 10% [1]; parenteral administration may cause minor adverse reactions, including thrombophlebitis and pain. The most common adverse effects are allergic reactions, occurring in 1–3% [2] of patients; haematological toxicity occurs in less than 1% of patients. Anaphylaxis is rare (less than 0.02%) [1]. Other reactions include localized gastrointestinal disturbances, hepatotoxicity, nephrotoxicity and mild central nervous system effects. Cephalosporin reactions are minimally, if at all, increased in patients with histories of penicillin allergy [1]. Postmarketing studies of second- and third-generation cephalosporins showed no increase in allergic reactions in patients with a history of penicillin allergy. Cephalosporin antibiotics are safe in penicillin-allergic patients and penicillin skin tests do not identify potential reactors [1]. Isolated independent hypersensitivity to individual cephaplosporins, such as cefazolin [4,5], cefonicid [6] and cefuroxime [7] with good tolerance to other β-lactam antibiotics has been described.

Hypersensitivity reactions include various exanthemata and contact urticaria [8]; cases of anaphylaxis to cefaclor [9], and of fatal anaphylactic shock related to cephalothin [10] have been reported. Vulvovaginitis and pruritus ani are not uncommon. Delayed reactions have been reported with cefonicid [6] and cefuroxime [11]. Serum sickness reactions occur [12–13], especially with cefaclor. Exfoliative dermatitis has been attributed to cefoxitin [14]. Disulfuram-like reactions to alcohol have been described with newer members of this group. Pustular reactions have been documented with cephadrine, cephalexin and cephazolin [15–17]. Ceftazidime has been implicated in the development of erythema multiforme [18]. Cephalosporins [19] including cephalexin [20] have been reported to cause TEN, and cephalexin has precipitated pemphigus vulgaris [21]. Cephazolin has caused an unusual fixed drug eruption [22]. A curious photo recall-like phenomenon followed the use of cephazolin and gentamicin sulphate, in that the eruption was restricted to an area of sunburn sustained 1 month previously [23].

REFERENCES

1 Anne S, Reisman RE. Risk of administering cephalosporin antibiotics to patients with histories of penicillin allergy. *Ann Allergy Asthma Immunol* 1995; **74**: 167–70.

2 Thompson JW, Jacobs RF. Adverse effects of newer cephalosporins. An update. *Drug Saf* 1993; **9**: 132–42.

3 Matsuno K, Kunihiro E, Yamatoya O *et al.* Surveillance of adverse reactions due to ciprofloxacin in Japan. *Drugs* 1995; **49** (Suppl. 2): 495–6.

4 Igea JM, Fraj J, Davila I *et al.* Allergy to cefazolin: study of *in vivo* cross reactivity with other betalactams. *Ann Allergy* 1992; **68**: 515–19.

5 Warrington RJ, McPhillips S. Independent anaphylaxis to cefazolin without allergy to other beta-lactam antibiotics. *J Allergy Clin Immunol* 1996; **98**: 460–2.

6 Martin JA, Alonso MD, Lazaro M *et al.* Delayed allergic reaction to cefonicid. *Ann Allergy* 1994; **72**: 341–2.

7 Marcos Bravo C, Luna Ortiz I, Gonzalez Vazquez R. Hypersensitivity to cefuroxime with good tolerance to other betalactams. *Allergy* 1995; **50**: 359–61.

8 Tuft L. Contact urticaria from cephalosporins. *Arch Dermatol* 1975; **111**: 1609.

9 Nishioka K, Katayama I, Kobayashi Y, Takijiri C. Anaphylaxis due to cefaclor hypersensitivity. *J Dermatol (Tokyo)* 1986; **13**: 226–7.

10 Spruell FG, Minette LJ, Sturner WQ. Two surgical deaths associated with cephalothin. *JAMA* 1974; **229**: 440–1.

11 Romano A, Pietrantonio F, Di Fonso M, Venuti A. Delayed hypersensitivity to cefuroxime. *Contact Dermatitis* 1992; **27**: 270–1.

12 Kearns GL, Wheeler JG, Childress SH, Letzig LG. Serum sickness-like reactions to cefaclor: role of hepatic metabolism and individual susceptibility. *J Pediatr* 1994; **125**: 805–11.

13 Grammer LC. Cefaclor serum sickness. *JAMA* 1996; **275**: 1152–3.

14 Kannangara DW, Smith B, Cohen K. Exfoliative dermatitis during cefoxitin therapy. *Arch Intern Med* 1982; **142**: 1031–2.

15 Kalb R, Grossman ME. Pustular eruption following administration of cephadrine. *Cutis* 1986; **38**: 58–60.

16 Jackson H, Vion B, Levy PM. Generalized eruptive pustular drug rash due to cephalexin. *Dermatologica* 1988; **177**: 292–4.

17 Fayol J, Bernard P, Bonnetblanc JM. Pustular eruption following the administration cefazolin: a second case report. *J Am Acad Dermatol* 1988; **19**: 571.

18 Pierce TH, Vig SJ, Ingram PM. Ceftazidime in the treatment of lower respiratory tract infection. *J Antimicrob Chemother* 1983; **12** (Suppl. A): 21–5.

19 Nichter LS, Harman DM, Bryant CA *et al.* Cephalosporin-induced toxic epidermal necrolysis. *J Burn Care Rehabil* 1983; **4**: 358–60.

20 Hogan DJ, Rooney ME. Toxic epidermal necrolysis due to cephalexin. *J Am Acad Dermatol* 1987; **17**: 852.

21 Wolf R, Dechner E, Ophir J, Brenner S. Cephalexin. A non-thiol drug that may induce pemphigus vulgaris. *Int J Dermatol* 1991; **30**: 213–15.

22 Sigal-Nahum M, Konqui A, Gauliet A, Sigal S. Linear fixed drug eruption. *Br J Dermatol* 1988; **118**: 849–51.

23 Flax SH, Uhle P. Photo recall-like phenomenon following the use of cefazolin and gentamicin sulfate. *Cutis* 1990; **46**: 59–61.

Monobactams

Monobactams (e.g. aztreonam) show weak cross-reactivity with IgE antibodies to penicillin [1,2], but immediate hypersensitivity on first exposure to aztreonam in penicillin-allergic patients has been recorded [3,4]. In general, aztreonam is well tolerated in high-risk patients allergic to other β-lactam antibiotics, but there is a 20% sensitization rate following exposure [5]. However, aztreonam and the monobactams can be safely given to penicillin-allergic patients [6]. Generalized urticaria to aztreonam but good tolerance of the other β-lactams has been recorded [7].

Carbapenems

Cross-reactivity and allergic reactions to imipenem occur in patients known to be allergic to penicillin [8]. Carbapenems should be avoided in patients with penicillin allergy [6]. Imipenem combined with cilastatin, a non-antibiotic enzyme inhibitor which prevents breakdown of imipenem to nephrotoxic metabolites, may cause phlebitis or pain at the site of infusion [9]. Imipenem has been associated with a pustular eruption [10], and imipenem–cilastatin with palmoplantar pruritus during infusion in a child with AIDS [11].

REFERENCES

1 Adkinson NF, Saxon A, Spence MR, Swabb EA. Cross-allergenicity and immunogenicity of aztreonam. *Rev Infect Dis* 1985; **7** (Suppl. 4): S613–21.
2 Saxon A, Hassner A, Swabb EA *et al.* Lack of cross-reactivity between aztreonam, a monobactam antibiotic, and penicillin-allergic subjects. *J Infect Dis* 1984; **149**: 16.
3 Hantson P, de Coninck B, Horn JL, Mahieu P. Immediate hypersensitivity to aztreonam and imipenem. *Br Med J* 1991; **302**: 294–5.
4 Alvarez JS, Del Castillo JAS, Garcia IS, Ortiz MJA. Immediate hypersensitivity to aztreonam. *Lancet* 1990; **335**: 1094.
5 Moss RB. Sensitization to aztreonam and cross-reactivity with other beta-lactam antibiotics in high-risk patients with cystic fibrosis. *J Allergy Clin Immunol* 1991; **87**: 78–88.
6 Kishiyama JL, Adelman DC. The cross-reactivity and immunology of beta-lactam antibiotics. *Drug Saf* 1994; **10**: 318–27.
7 de la Fuente Prieto R, Armentia Medina A, Sanchez Palla P *et al.* Urticaria caused by sensitization to aztreonam. *Allergy* 1993; **48**: 634–6.
8 Saxon A, Adelman DC, Patel A *et al.* Imipenem cross-reactivity with penicillin in humans. *J Allergy Clin Immunol* 1988; **82**: 213–17.
9 Anon. Imipenem + cilastatin—a new type of antibiotic. *Drug Ther Bull* 1991; **29**: 43–4.
10 Escallier F, Dalac S, Foucher JL *et al.* Pustulose exanthématique aiguë généralisée: imputabilité a l'imipéneme (Tienam®). *Ann Dermatol Vénéréol* 1989; **116**: 407–9.
11 Machado ARL, Silva CLO, Galvão NAM. Unusual reaction to imipenem-cilastatin in a child with the acquired immunodeficiency syndrome. *J Allergy Clin Immunol* 1991; **87**: 754.

Tetracyclines

Many of the side-effects are common to all drugs within the group, and cross-sensitivity occurs [1]. Nausea, vomiting and diarrhoea are well-recognized dose-related effects. Oral or vaginal candidiasis may occur as a result of overgrowth of commensals. Resumption of therapy does not necessarily lead to recurrence of the vaginitis [2].

Photosensitivity

All tetracyclines, but especially demethylchlortetracycline, may cause phototosensitive eruptions [1,3–6], which clinically resemble exaggerated sunburn, sometimes with blistering. Phototoxicity is thought to be involved, in that high serum levels predispose to its occurrence. Reactions to both UVA and UVB have been reported. High concentrations of tetracycline are found in sun-damaged skin [3]. Symptoms may persist for months [1]. Photo-onycholysis may develop in finger- and (if exposed) toenails; the thumb (normally less exposed) may be spared [7,8]. Tetracycline therapy is best avoided if there is a prospect of considerable sun exposure. Porphyria cutanea tarda-like changes may develop after chronic sun exposure

[6,9]. A photosensitive lichenoid rash has been attributed to demethylchlortetracycline [10].

REFERENCES

1 Wright AL, Colver GB. Tetracyclines—how safe are they? *Clin Exp Dermatol* 1988; **13**: 57–61.
2 Hall JH, Lupton ES. Tetracycline therapy for acne: incidence of vaginitis. *Cutis* 1977; **20**: 97–8.
3 Blank H, Cullen SI, Catalano PM. Photosensitivity studies with demethylchlortetracycline and doxycycline. *Arch Dermatol* 1968; **97**: 1–2.
4 Frost P, Weinstein GP, Gomez EC. Phototoxic potential of minocycline and doxycycline. *Arch Dermatol* 1972; **105**: 681–3.
5 Kaidbey KH, Kligman AM. Identification of systemic phototoxic drugs by human intradermal assay. *J Invest Dermatol* 1978; **70**: 272–4.
6 Hawk JLM. Skin changes resembling hepatic cutaneous porphyria induced by oxytetracycline photosensitization. *Clin Exp Dermatol* 1980; **5**: 321–5.
7 Baker H. Photo-onycholysis caused by tetracyclines. *Br Med J* 1977; **ii**: 519–20.
8 Kestel JL, Jr. Photo-onycholysis from minocycline. Side effects of minocycline therapy. *Cutis* 1981; **28**: 53–4.
9 Epstein JH, Tuffanelli DL, Seibert JS, Epstein WL. Porphyria-like cutaneous changes induced by tetracycline hydrochloride photosensitization. *Arch Dermatol* 1976; **112**: 661–6.
10 Jones HE, Lewis CW, Reisner JE. Photosensitive lichenoid eruption associated with demeclocycline. *Arch Dermatol* 1972; **106**: 58–63.

Pigmentation

Methacycline is a rare cause [1]. Long-term minocycline therapy for acne may result in pigmentation. While this is generally held to be a rare event, it may occur in about 1.4% of patients [2–5]. The average time for the development of pigmentary changes was 5 months, and onset of this complication did not seem to be related to cumulative dosage of the drug [3]. Minocycline-induced pigmentation resolves after treatment with the Q-switched ruby laser [6]. Facial hyperpigmentation was reported in two sisters on long-term minocycline therapy, who were also being treated with Dianette (cyproterone acetate and ethinyl-oestradiol); it was suggested that pigmentation occurred either as a result of a genetic alteration in the metabolic handling of the drug, or due to accentuation by the concomitant therapy [7]. Other drugs, including amitryptyline [2], phenothiazines, and 13-*cis*-retinoic acid, have been implicated in the accentuation of minocycline-related hyperpigmentation.

Three types of pigmentation are described with minocycline and may occur in combination or isolation [3]. A focal type with well-demarcated blue–black macules is seen in areas of previous inflammation or scarring, especially in relation to acne scars. Minocycline has been associated with postinflammatory hyperpigmentation in women who have undergone sclerotherapy [8]. Macular or more diffuse hyperpigmentation may appear distant from acne sites, especially on the extensor surface of the lower legs, forearms and on sun-exposed areas. These two types resolve on cessation of therapy, with a mean time to resolution of 12 months [3]. A more persistent diffuse brown–grey change may develop, especially in sun-exposed areas [5]. The oral cavity and lips may be involved [9,10]. Conjunctival pigmentation may occur with tetracyclines [11,12] and scleral pigmentation with minocycline [13,14]. Minocycline can cause nail pigmentation and longitudinal melanonychia [5,13–16], and tetracycline may produce yellow discoloration of the nail [17]. Cutaneous osteomas presenting as blue skin nodules that fluoresce yellow under UV light may rarely develop in patients on treatment with tetracycline [18] or minocycline [19] for acne. Black galactorrhea occurred in a patient taking both minocycline and phenothiazines [20].

Pigmentation may also involve, bones, teeth, thyroid, aorta and endocardium [16,21]. Histological and electron-microscopic studies have demonstrated increased melanin, haemosiderin and either minocycline or a metabolite in the skin [22–24]; pigment may be seen in dermal histiocytes and eccrine myoepithelial cells [23]. Minocycline is metabolized to form a brown–black degradation product [25].

REFERENCES

1 Möller H, Rausing A. Methacycline pigmentation: a five-year follow-up. *Acta Derm Venereol (Stockh)* 1980; **60**: 495–501.
2 Basler RSW, Goetz CS. Synergism of minocycline and amitryptyline in cutaneous hyperpigmentation. *J Am Acad Dermatol* 1985; **12**: 577.
3 Layton AM, Cunliffe WJ. Minocycline induced pigmentation in the treatment of acne—a review and personal observations. *J Dermatol Treat* 1989; **1**: 9–12.
4 Dwyer CM, Cuddihy AM, Kerr RE *et al*. Skin pigmentation due to minocycline treatment of facial dermatoses. *Br J Dermatol* 1993; **129**: 158–62.
5 Pepine M, Flower FP, Ramos-Caro FA. Extensive cutaneous hyperpigmentation caused by minocycline. *J Am Acad Dermatol* 1993; **28**: 292–5.
6 Collins P, Cotterill JA. Minocycline-induced pigmentation resolves after treatment with the Q-switched ruby laser. *Br J Dermatol* 1996; **135**: 317–19.
7 Eedy DJ, Burrows D. Minocycline-induced pigmentation occurring in two sisters. *Clin Exp Dermatol* 1991; **16**: 55–7.
8 Leffell DJ. Minocycline hydrochloride hyperpigmentation complicating treatment of venous ectasia of the extremities. *J Am Acad Dermatol* 1991; **24**: 501–2.
9 Siller GM, Tod MA, Savage NW. Minocycline-induced oral pigmentation. *J Am Acad Dermatol* 1994; **30**: 350–4.
10 Chu P, Van SL, Yen TS, Berger TG. Minocycline hyperpigmentation localized to the lips: an unusual fixed drug reaction? *J Am Acad Dermatol* 1994; **30**: 802–3.
11 Brothers DM, Hidayat AA. Conjunctival pigmentation associated with tetracycline medication. *Ophthalmology* 1981; **88**: 1212–15.
12 Messmer E, Font RL, Sheldon G, Murphy D. Pigmented conjunctival cysts following tetracycline/minocycline therapy. Histochemical and electron microscopic observations. *Ophthalmology* 1983; **90**: 1462–8.
13 Angeloni VL, Salasche SJ, Ortiz R. Nail, skin, and scleral pigmentation induced by minocycline. *Cutis* 1988; **42**: 229–33.
14 Sabroe RA, Archer CB, Harlow D *et al*. Minocycline-induced discolouration of the sclerae. *Br J Dermatol* 1996; **135**: 314–16.
15 Mallon E, Dawber RPR. Longitudinal melanonychia induced by minocycline. *Br J Dermatol* 1995; **130**: 794–5.
16 Wolfe ID, Reichmister J. Minocycline hyperpigmentation: skin, tooth, nail, and bone involvement. *Cutis* 1984; **33**: 475–8.
17 Hendricks AA. Yellow lunulae with fluorescence after tetracycline therapy. *Arch Dermatol* 1980; **116**: 438–40.
18 Walter JF, Macknet KD. Pigmentation of osteoma cutis caused by tetracycline. *Arch Dermatol* 1979; **115**: 1087–8.
19 Moritz DL, Elewski B. Pigmented postacne osteoma cutis in a patient treated with minocycline: Report and review of the literature. *J Am Acad Dermatol* 1991; **24**: 851–3.
20 Basler RSW, Lynch PJ. Black galactorrhea as a complication of minocycline and phenothiazine therapy. *Arch Dermatol* 1985; **121**: 417–18.
21 Butler JM, Marks R, Sutherland R. Cutaneous and cardiac valvular pigmentation with minocycline. *Clin Exp Dermatol* 1985; **10**: 432–7.
22 Sato S, Murphy GF, Bernard JD *et al*. Ultrastructural and x-ray microanalytical observations on minocycline-related hyperpigmentation of the skin. *J Invest Dermatol* 1981; **77**: 264–71.
23 Argenyi ZB, Finelli L, Bergfeld WF *et al*. Minocycline-related cutaneous hyperpigmentation as demonstrated by light microscopy, electron microscopy and x-ray energy spectroscopy. *J Cutan Pathol* 1987; **14**: 176–80.
24 Okada N, Moriya K, Nishida K *et al*. Skin pigmentation associated with minocycline therapy. *Br J Dermatol* 1989; **121**: 247–54.
25 Nelis HJCF, DeLeenheer AP. Metabolism of minocycline in humans. *Drug Metab Disposition* 1982; **10**: 142–6.

Other cutaneous side-effects

Allergic reactions are far less common than with penicillin. Morbilliform, urticarial, erythema multiforme-like and bullous eruptions [1,2], exfoliative dermatitis and erythema nodosum [3] have been reported, as well as a recurrent follicular acneiform eruption in one patient [4]. Minocycline has caused eosinophilic cellulitis and pustular folliculitis with eosinophilia [5]. Gram-negative folliculitis of the face is uncommon but well recognized; *Proteus* may be responsible, and the condition responds to ampicillin [6]. Tetracyclines are a well known cause of fixed drug eruptions [7–9], and minocycline [10] and doxycycline [11] have caused Stevens-Johnson syndrome. TEN has been recorded [12]. It has been suggested that tetracyclines may exacerbate psoriasis [13,14]. An eruption resembling Sweet's syndrome has occurred with minocycline [15,16]. Pruritus at the site of active acne has been recorded within 2–6 weeks of starting oral tetracyclines (oxytetracycline, doxycycline or minocycline) [17].

REFERENCES

1 Shelley WB, Heaton CL. Minocycline sensitivity. *JAMA* 1973; **224**: 125–6.
2 Fawcett IW, Pepys J. Allergy to a tetracycline preparation—a case report. *Clin Allergy* 1976; **6**: 301–4.
3 Bridges AJ, Graziano FM, Calhoun W, Reizner GT. Hyperpigmentation, neutrophilic alveolitis, and erythema nodosum resulting from minocycline. *J Am Acad Dermatol* 1990; **22**: 959–62.
4 Bean SF. Acneiform eruption from tetracycline. *Br J Dermatol* 1971; **85**: 585–6.
5 Kaufmann D, Pichler W, Beer JH. Severe episode of high fever with rash, lymphadenopathy, neutropenia, and eosinophilia after minocycline therapy for acne. *Arch Intern Med* 1994; **154**: 1983–4.
6 Leyden JJ, Marples RR, Mills OH, Jr, Kligman AM. Gram-negative folliculitis—a complication of antibiotic therapy in acne vulgaris. *Br J Dermatol* 1973; **88**: 533–8.
7 Jolly HW, Sherman II, Jr, Carpenter CL *et al*. Fixed drug eruptions due to tetracyclines. *Arch Dermatol* 1978; **114**: 1484–5.
8 Fiumara NJ, Yaqub M. Pigmented penile lesions (fixed drug eruptions) associated with tetracycline therapy for sexually transmitted diseases. *Sex Transm Dis* 1980; **8**: 23–5.
9 Chan HL, Wong SN, Lo FL. Tetracycline-induced fixed drug eruptions; influence of dose and structure of tetracyclines. *J Am Acad Dermatol* 1985; **13**: 302–3.
10 Shoji A, Someda Y, Hamada T. Stevens–Johnson syndrome due to minocycline therapy. *Arch Dermatol* 1987; **123**: 18–20.

11 Curley RK, Verbov JL. Stevens–Johnson syndrome due to tetracyclines—a case report (doxycycline) and review of the literature. *Clin Exp Dermatol* 1987; **12**: 124–5.

12 Tatnall FM, Dodd HJ, Sarkany I. Elevated serum amylase in a case of toxic epidermal necrolysis. *Br J Dermatol* 1985; **113**: 629–30.

13 Tsankov M, Botev-Zlatkov M, Lazarova AZ *et al*. Psoriasis and drugs: influence of tetracyclines on the course of psoriasis. *J Am Acad Dermatol* 1988; **19**: 629–32.

14 Bergner T, Przybilla B. Psoriasis and tetracyclines. *J Am Acad Dermatol* 1990; **23**: 770.

15 Mensing H, Kowalzick L. Acute febrile neutrophilic dermatosis (Sweet's syndrome) caused by minocycline. *Dermatologica* 1991; **182**: 43–6.

16 Thibault MJ, Billick RC, Srolovitz H. Minocycline-induced Sweet's syndrome. *J Am Acad Dermatol* 1992; **27**: 801–4.

17 Yee KC, Cunliffe WJ. Itching in acne—an unusual complication of therapy. *Dermatology* 1994; **189**: 117–19.

Gastrointestinal absorption and drug interactions

Absorption of tetracyclines is reduced when taken with meals, especially those containing calcium or iron, such as milk, or drugs such as iron or antacids [1]. The decrease in serum levels following a test meal has been reported as follows: oxytetracycline 50% [1], minocycline 13% [1] and doxycline 20% [2]. Oxytetracycline may have a hypoglycaemic effect in insulin-dependent diabetics [3], and tetracyclines can potentiate the action of warfarin by depressing prothrombin activity, and elevate serum levels of lithium given simultaneously [4].

REFERENCES

1 Leyden JJ. Absorption of minocycline HCl and tetracycline hydrochloride. Effect of food, milk and iron. *J Am Acad Dermatol* 1985; **12**: 308–12.

2 Welling PG, Koch PA, Lau CC, Craig WA. Bioavailability of tetracycline and doxycycline in fasted and nonfasted subjects. *Antimicrob Agents Chemother* 1977; **11**: 462–9.

3 Miller JB. Hypoglycaemic effect of oxytetracycline. *Br Med J* 1966; **2**: 1007.

4 McGennis AJ. Lithium carbonate and tetracycline interaction. *Br Med J* 1978; i: 1183.

Systemic side-effects of tetracyclines

Long-term use of tetracycline for acne may rarely result in benign intracranial hypertension [1,2]. As retinoids may potentiate this effect, it is safest not to use them in combination with tetracycline therapy for acne. Oesophageal ulceration has been described in a number of patients [3]. With the exception of doxycycline and minocycline, tetracyclines may exacerbate renal failure. Combination therapy with tetracyclines and nephrotoxic drugs such as gentamicin or diuretics should be avoided [4]. Deteriorated tetracyclines have caused a nephropathy accompanied by an exanthematic eruption. Patients should be warned not to use outdated or poorly stored tetracycline, because degraded tetracycline can cause a Fanconi-type syndrome comprising renal tubular acidosis and proteinuria [5,6] and lactic acidosis [7]. Dose-related vestibular disturbance has been reported with minocycline [8].

A severe, self-limiting eruption associated with acute hepatic failure, fatal in one instance, has been reported in two patients after a few weeks of routine therapy with minocycline for acne [9]. Minocycline has been reported to cause other serious, albeit rare, adverse events, including a serum sickness-like reaction, and a hypersensitivity syndrome reaction [10,11]. Serum sickness-like reactions occur at about 15 days, while the hypersensitivity syndrome develops at about 23 days [11]. Reversible pulmonary infiltration with eosinophilic or neutrophilic alveolitis has been rarely described in association with tetracycline [12] and especially minocycline therapy [13–15]. There have been isolated case reports linking tetracycline with systemic LE [16]. A drug-induced systemic LE-like syndrome occurs rarely with minocycline [17–20] on average 2 years after the start of therapy [11]. Hepatitis, sometimes with the histological features of chronic active hepatitis, has been fatal [19], and may be associated with polyarthralgia and positive antinuclear antibodies, but negative or only weakly positive anti-DNA antibodies; patients usually recover within 3 months of drug cessation [19]. For this reason, it has been suggested that the use of minocycline in acne should be restricted to patients unresponsive to other tetracyclines [19,20].

REFERENCES

1 Walters BNJ, Gubbay SS. Tetracycline and benign intracranial hypertension: report of five cases. *Br Med J* 1979; **282**: 19–20.

2 Pearson MG, Littlewood SM, Bowden AN. Tetracycline and benign intracranial hypertension. *Br Med J* 1981; **282**: 568–9.

3 Channer KS, Hollanders D. Tetracycline-induced oesophageal ulceration. *Br Med J* 1981; **282**: 1359–60.

4 Wright AL, Colver GB. Tetracyclines—how safe are they? *Clin Exp Dermatol* 1988; **13**: 57–61.

5 Moser RH. Bibliographies on diseases: medical progress. Reactions to tetracyclines. *Clin Pharmacol Ther* 1966; **7**; 117–31.

6 Frimpter GW, Timpanelli AE, Eisenmenger WJ *et al*. Reversible 'Fanconi syndrome' caused by degraded tetracycline. *JAMA* 1963; **184**: 111–13.

7 Montoliu J, Carrera M, Darnell A *et al*. Lactic acidosis and Fanconi's syndrome due to degraded tetracycline. *Br Med J* 1981; **281**: 1576–7.

8 Allen JC. Minocycline. *Ann Intern Med* 1976; **85**: 482–7.

9 Davies MG, Kersey PJW. Acute hepatitis and exfoliative dermatitis associated with minocycline. *Br Med J* 1989; **298**: 1523–4.

10 Kaufmann D, Pichler W, Beer JH. Severe episode of high fever with rash, lymphadenopathy, neutropenia, and eosinophilia after minocycline therapy for acne. *Arch Intern Med* 1994; **154**: 1983–4.

11 Knowles SR, Shapiro L, Shear NH. Serious adverse reactions induced by minocycline. Report of 13 patients and review of the literature. *Arch Dermatol* 1996; **132**: 934–9.

12 Ho D, Tashkin DP, Bein ME, Sharma O. Pulmonary infiltrates with eosinophilia associated with tetracycline. *Chest* 1979; **76**: 33–5.

13 Bando T, Fujimura M, Noda Y *et al*. Minocycline-induced pneumonitis with bilateral hilar lymphadenopathy and pleural effusion. *Intern Med* 1994; **33**: 177–9.

14 Sitbon O, Bidel N, Dussopt C *et al*. Minocycline and pulmonary eosinophilia. A report on eight patients. *Arch Intern Med* 1994; **154**: 1633–40.

15 Dykhuizen RS, Zaidi AM, Godden DJ *et al*. Minocycline and pulmonary eosinophilia. *Br Med J* 1995; **310**: 1520–1.

16 Domz CA, Minamara DH, Hozapfel HF. Tetracycline provocation in lupus erythematosus. *Ann Intern Med* 1959; **50**: 1217.

17 Byrne PAC, Williams BD, Pritchard MH. Minocycline-related lupus. *Br J Rheumatol* 1994; **33**: 674–6.

18 Gordon PM, White MI, Herriot R *et al.* Minocyline-associated lupus erythematosus. *Br J Dermatol* 1995; **132**: 120–1.

19 Gough A, Chapman S, Wagstaff K *et al.* Minocycline-induced autoimmune hepatitis and systemic lupus erythematosus-like syndrome. *Br Med J* 1996; **312**: 169–72.

20 Ferner RE, Moss C. Minocycline for acne. First line antibacterial treatment of acne should be with tetracycline or oxytetracycline. *Br Med J* 1996; **312**: 138.

Effects on the fetus and on teeth

There is little evidence that tetracycline is teratogenic [1]. There is an isolated case report of congenital abnormalities in a child whose mother took clomocycline for acne [2]. Yellow discoloration of the teeth due to tetracycline exposure during mineralization of the deciduous or permanent teeth is well known [3–5]. A yellow–brown fluorescent discoloration is formed as a result of a complex with calcium orthophosphate. Tetracyclines should not be given to pregnant women or children under the age of 12 years. Tetracyclines are excreted in breast milk, but chelation with calcium decreases their absorption, so that tooth discoloration is probably prevented [1].

Tetracycline may be deposited up to late adolescence in calcifying teeth such as the molars, but as these are not normally visible this is not a problem [5]. Minocycline may rarely stain the teeth of adults [6–8].

REFERENCES

1 Wright AL, Colver GB. Tetracyclines—how safe are they? *Clin Exp Dermatol* 1988; **13**: 57–61.

2 Corcoran R, Castles JM. Tetracycline for acne vulgaris and possible teratogenesis. *Br Med J* 1977; **ii**: 807–8.

3 Conchie JM, Munroe JD, Anderson DO. The incidence of staining of permanent teeth by the tetracyclines. *Can Med Ass J* 1970; **103**: 351–6.

4 Moffitt JM, Cooley RO, Olsen NH, Hefferren JJ. Prediction of tetracycline-induced tooth discolouration. *J Am Dental Assoc* 1974; **88**: 547–52.

5 Grossman ER. Tetracycline and staining of the teeth. *JAMA* 1986; **225**: 2442.

6 Poliak SC, DiGiovanna JJ, Gross EG *et al.* Minocycline-associated tooth discoloration in young adults. *JAMA* 1985; **254**: 2930–2.

7 Rosen T, Hoffmann TJ. Minocycline-induced discoloration of the permanent teeth. *J Am Acad Dermatol* 1989; **21**: 569.

8 Berger RS, Mandel EN, Hayes TJ, Grimwood RR. Minocycline staining of the oral cavity. *J Am Acad Dermatol* 1989; **21**: 1300–1.

Tetracyclines and the contraceptive pill

Tetracyclines have been reported to interfere with the action of the contraceptive pill [1,2], and it is standard practice to inform female patients of this and to suggest use of an additional or alternative method of contraception while on medication. However, there is controversy as to whether there is really a significant risk of interaction [3–5].

REFERENCES

1 Bacon JF, Shenfield GM. Pregnancy attributable to interaction between tetracycline and oral contraceptives. *Br Med J* 1980; **280**: 293.

2 Hughes BR, Cunliffe WJ. Interactions between the oral contraceptive pill and antibiotics. *Br J Dermatol* 1990; **122**: 717–18.

3 Fleischer AB, Jr, Resnick SD. The effect of antibiotics on the efficacy of oral contraceptives. *Arch Dermatol* 1989; **125**: 1562–4.

4 Orme ML'E, Back DJ. Interactions between oral contraceptive steroids and broad-spectrum antibiotics. *Clin Exp Dermatol* 1986; **11**: 327–31.

5 De Groot AC, Eshuis H, Stricker BHC. Oral contraceptives and antibiotics in acne. *Br J Dermatol* 1991; **124**: 212.

Sulphonamides and trimethoprim

Reactions occur in 1–5% of those exposed [1–5]. They are commoner in patients with AIDS [6–8], and slow acetylators are at greater risk [9]. Type I reactions (urticaria and anaphylaxis) are rare but recorded. Phototoxic and photo-allergic eruptions occur [10,11]. Morbilliform and rubelliform rashes are seen, and erythema multiforme, Stevens–Johnson syndrome and TEN [12–17], erythema nodosum [1], generalized exfoliative dermatitis [1,18,19] and fixed eruptions [20] are all well known. In addition, an LE-like syndrome and allergic vasculitis [21] are documented. Agranulocytosis or haemolytic anaemia is occasionally precipitated.

REFERENCES

1 Koch-Weser J, Sidel VW, Dexter M *et al.* Adverse reactions to sulfisoxazole, sulfamethoxazole, and nitrofurantoin. Manifestations and specific reaction rates during 2,118 courses of therapy. *Arch Intern Med* 1971; **128**: 399–404.

2 Kauppinen K, Stubb S. Drug eruptions: Causative agents and clinical types. A series of inpatients during a 10-year period. *Acta Derm Venereol (Stockh)* 1984; **64**: 320–4.

3 Bigby M, Jick S, Jick H, Arndt K. Drug-induced cutaneous reactions. A report from the Boston Collaborative Drug Surveillance Program on 15438 consecutive inpatients, 1975 to 1982. *JAMA* 1986; **256**: 3358–63.

4 Anon. Hypersensitivity to sulphonamides—a clue? (Editorial). *Lancet* 1986; **ii**: 958–9.

5 Rieder MJ, Uetrecht J, Shear NH *et al.* Diagnosis of sulfonamide hypersensitivity reactions by *in-vitro* 'rechallenge' with hydroxylamine metabolites. *Ann Intern Med* 1989; **110**: 286–9.

6 De Raeve L, Song M, Van Maldergem L. Adverse cutaneous drug reactions in AIDS. *Br J Dermatol* 1988; **119**: 521–3.

7 van der Ven AJAM, Koopmans PP, Vree TB, van der Meer JWM. Adverse reactions to co-trimoxazole in HIV infection. *Lancet* 1991; **338**: 431–3.

8 Roudier C, Caumes E, Rogeaux O *et al.* Adverse cutaneous reactions to trimethoprim–sulfamethoxazole in patients with the acquired immunodeficiency syndrome and *Pneumocystis carinii* pneumonia. *Arch Dermatol* 1994; **130**: 1383–6.

9 Carr A, Gross AS, Hoskins JM *et al.* Acetylation phenotype and cutaneous hypersensitivity to trimethoprim–sulphamethoxazole in HIV-infected patients. *AIDS* 1994; **8**: 333–7.

10 Epstein JH. Photoallergy. A review. *Arch Dermatol* 1972; **106**: 741–8.

11 Hawk JLM. Photosensitizing agents used in the United Kingdom. *Clin Exp Dermatol* 1984; **9**: 300–2.

12 Kauppinen K. Cutaneous reactions to drugs. With special reference to severe mucocutaneous bullous eruptions and sulphonamides. *Acta Derm Venereol (Stockh)* 1972; **52** (Suppl. 68): 1–89.

13 Jick H, Derby LE. A large population-based follow-up study of trimethoprim-sulfamethoxazole, trimethoprim, and cephalexin for uncommon serious drug toxicity. *Pharmacotherapeutics* 1995; **15**: 428–32.

14 Carrol OM, Bryan PA, Robinson RJ. Stevens–Johnson-syndrome associated with long-acting sulfonamides. *JAMA* 1966; **195**: 691–3.

15 Aberer W, Stingl G, Wolff K. Stevens–Johnson-Syndrom und toxische epidermale Nekrolyse nach Sulfonamideinahme. *Hautarzt* 1982; **33**: 484–90.

16 Chan H-L, Stern RS, Arndt KA *et al.* The incidence of erythema multiforme,

Stevens–Johnson syndrome, and toxic epidermal necrolysis. A population-based study with particular reference to reactions caused by drugs among outpatients. *Arch Dermatol* 1990; **126**: 43–7.

17 Schöpf E, Stühmer A, Rzany B *et al*. Toxic epidermal necrolysis and Stevens–Johnson syndrome. An epidemiologic study from West Germany. *Arch Dermatol* 1991; **127**: 839–42.

18 Nicolis GD, Helwig EB. Exfoliative dermatitis. A clinicopathologic study of 135 cases. *Arch Dermatol* 1973; **108**: 788–97.

19 Sehgal VN, Srivastava G. Exfoliative dermatitis. A prospective study of 80 patients. *Dermatologica* 1986; **173**: 278–84.

20 Sehgal VN, Gangwani OP. Fixed drug eruption. Current concepts. *Int J Dermatol* 1987; **26**: 67–74.

21 Lehr D. Sulfonamide vasculitis. *J Clin Pharmacol* 1972; **2**: 181–9.

Sulphasalazine

Rashes occur in 1–5% of patients, and may be widespread as part of a hypersensitivity syndrome with hepatitis and encephalopathy [1–5], but desensitization is possible [6]. Blood disorders attributable to sulphasalazine occur at a rate of three per 1000 users [7]. An autoimmune syndrome has been described [8]. Photosensitivity [9] and a fixed eruption [10] have been documented. TEN, erythroid hypoplasia and agranulocytosis have been reported [11]. Bronchiolitis obliterans and alveolitis are well-recognized complications, and acute hypersensitivity pneumonia is recorded. LE, including cerebral LE, may be induced [12]. Reversible oligospermia may occur [13], and reversible hair loss has been attributed to use of this drug in enemas [14]. Many of the above adverse effects are attributable to the carrier molecule, sulphapyridine, which delivers 5-aminosalicylic acid, the component of sulphasalazine active in ulcerative colitis, to its site of action in the colon; patients who are slow acetylators may be especially prone to side-effects [15]. Urticaria, and possibly the renal toxicity, are due to the 5-aminosalicylic acid component [16].

Mesalazine (5-aminosalicylic acid)

Fever, erythematous skin eruption and lung involvement [17] and fever, diarrhoea, exfoliative dermatitis, marked atypical lymphocytosis, and severe hepatotoxicity [18] have been described in patients with a previous history of sulphasalazine hypersensitivity. Additional cutaneous hypersensitivity reactions including vasculitis [19], a Kawasaki-like syndrome [20], and an LE-like syndrome [21] have been documented. This drug may cause renal damage, and is associated with blood dyscrasia [22] including fatal bone-marrow suppression and thrombocytopaenia [23].

Olsalazine

This drug, which consists of a dimer of two molecules of 5-aminosalicylic acid linked by an azo bond, dispenses with the unwanted effects of sulphapyridine. Nonetheless, up to one in five patients experience diarrhoea, rash, nausea and abdominal pain severe enough to stop treatment with the drug [16].

Sulphamethoxypyridazine

Obliterative bronchiolitis and alveolitis have been documented in a patient with linear IgA disease of adults [24].

REFERENCES

1 Leroux JL, Ghezail M, Chertok P, Blotman F. Hypersensitivity reaction to sulfasalazine: skin rash, fever, hepatitis and activated lymphocytes. *Clin Exp Rheumatol* 1992; **10**: 427.

2 Gran JT, Myklebust G. Toxicity of sulphasalazine in rheumatoid arthritis. Possible protective effect of rheumatoid factors and corticosteroids. *Scand J Rheumatol* 1993; **22**: 229–32.

3 Gabay C, De Bandt M, Palazzo E. Sulphasalazine-related life-threatening side effects: is N-acetylcysteine of therapeutic value? *Clin Exp Rheumatol* 1993; **11**: 417–20.

4 Schoonjans R, Mast A, Van Den Abeele G *et al*. Sulfasalazine-associated encephalopathy in a patient with Crohn's disease. *Am J Gastroenterol* 1993; **88**: 1416–20.

5 Rubin R. Sulfasalazine-induced fulminant hepatic failure and necrotizing pancreatitis. *Am J Gastroenterol* 1994; **89**: 789–91.

6 Koski JM. Desensitization to sulphasalazine in patients with arthritis. *Clin Exp Rheumatol* 1993; **11**: 169–70.

7 Jick H, Myers MW, Dean AD. The risk of sulfasalazine- and mesalazine-associated blood disorders. *Pharmacotherapeutics* 1995; **15**: 176–81.

8 Vyse T, So AK. Sulphasalazine-induced autoimmune syndrome. *Br J Rheumatol* 1992; **31**: 115–16.

9 Watkinson G. Sulfasalazine: a review of 40 years' experience. *Drugs* 1986; **32**: 1–11.

10 Kanwar AJ, Singh M, Yunus M, Belhaj MS. Fixed eruption to sulphasalazine. *Dermatologica* 1987; **174**: 104.

11 Maddocks JL, Slater DN. Toxic epidermal necrolysis, agranulocytosis and erythroid hypoplasia associated with sulphasalazine. *J R Soc Med* 1980; **73**: 587–8.

12 Rafferty P, Young AC, Haeny MR. Sulphasalazine-induced cerebral lupus erythematosus. *Postgrad Med J* 1982; **58**: 98–9.

13 Drife JO. Drugs and sperm. *Br Med J* 1982; **84**: 844–5.

14 Kutty PK, Raman KRK, Hawken K, Barrowman JA. Hair loss and 5-aminosalicylic acid enemas. *Ann Intern Med* 1982; **97**: 785–6.

15 Das KM, Eastwood MA, McManus JPA, Sircus W. Adverse reactions during salicylazosulfapyridine therapy and the relation with drug metabolism and acetylator phenotype. *N Engl J Med* 1973; **289**: 491–5.

16 Anonymous. Olsalazine—a further choice in ulcerative colitis. *Drug Ther Bull* 1990; **28**: 57–8.

17 Hautekeete ML, Bourgeois N, Potvin P *et al*. Hypersensitivity with hepatotoxicity to mesalazine after hypersensitivity to sulfasalazine. *Gastroenterology* 1992; **103**: 1925–7.

18 Aparicio J, Carnicer F, Girona E, Gmez A. Cutaneous hypersensitivity reaction to mesalazine. *Am J Gastroenterol* 1996; **91**: 620–1.

19 Lim AG, Hine KR. Fever, vasculitic rash, arthritis, pericarditis, and pericardial effusion after mesalazine. *Br Med J* 1994; **308**: 113.

20 Waanders H, Thompson J. Kawasaki-like syndrome after treatment with mesalazine. *Am J Gastroenterol* 1991; **86**: 219–21.

21 Dent MT, Ganatpathy S, Holdworth CD, Channer KC. Mesalazine-induced lupus-like syndrome. *Br Med J* 1992; **305**: 159.

22 Anonymous. Blood dyscrasias and mesalazine. *Curr Probl Pharmacovig* 1995; **21**: 5.

23 Daneshmend TK. Mesalazine-associated thrombocytopenia. *Lancet* 1991; **337**: 1297–8.

24 Godfrey KM, Wojnarowska F, Friedland JS. Obliterative bronchiolitis and alveolitis associated with sulphamethoxypyridazine (Lederkyn) therapy for linear IgA disease of adults. *Br J Dermatol* 1990; **123**: 125–31.

Sulfadoxine

This sulphonamide is used in malaria prophylaxis in

combination with pyrimethamine. The risk of reactions seems to be very low, but drug fever, TEN and photodermatitis have been recorded [1]. Stevens–Johnson syndrome may occur with Fansidar (pyrimethamine and sulphadoxine) for malaria prophylaxis [1–4] or with sulphadoxine alone [5]. TEN has occurred with Fansidar in an AIDS patient [6].

REFERENCES

1 Koch-Weser J, Hodel C, Leimer R, Styk S. Adverse reactions to pyrimethamine/sulfadoxine. *Lancet* 1982; **ii**: 1459.
2 Hornstein OP, Ruprecht KW. Fansidar-induced Stevens–Johnson syndrome. *N Engl J Med* 1982; **307**: 1529–30.
3 Miller KD, Lobel HO, Satriale RF *et al*. Severe cutaneous reactions among American travelers using pyrimethamine–sulfadoxine (Fansidar) for malaria prophylaxis. *Am J Trop Med Hyg* 1986; **35**: 451–8.
4 Ortel B, Sivayathorn A, Hönigsmann H. An unusual combination of phototoxicity and Stevens–Johnson syndrome due to antimalarial therapy. *Dermatologica* 1989; **178**: 39–42.
5 Hernborg A. Stevens–Johnson syndrome after mass prophylaxis with sulfadoxine for cholera in Mozambique. *Lancet* 1985; **i**: 1072–3.
6 Raviglione MC, Dinan WA, Pablos-Mendez A *et al*. Fatal toxic epidermal necrolysis during prophylaxis with pyrimethamine and sulfadoxine in a human immunodeficiency virus-infected person. *Arch Intern Med* 1988; **148**: 2863–5.

Trimethoprim–sulphamethoxazole (co-trimoxazole)

The general incidence and patterns of reactions to this mixture of sulphamethoxazole and trimethoprim are about the same as for sulphonamides in general; cutaneous reactions are seen in 3.3% of patients [1–3]. Severe cutaneous reactions of all types occur in about one per 100 000 users of the drug [2,3]. In view of these severe reactions, the drug is now indicated primarily for *Pneumocystis carinii* pneumonia, and for acute exacerbations of chronic bronchitis and urinary tract infections, and otitis media in children, only where there is good reason to prefer this combination [4]. There is a greatly increased incidence of reactions in patients with AIDS [5–13]. In one study, 18 of 38 patients with AIDS and *P. carinii* pneumonia treated with trimethoprim–sulfamethoxazole developed cutaneous reactions within a median of 11 days. It is sometimes possible to continue treatment through a hypersensitivity reaction, as reported for 67% of cases in the above study [14]. Adjuvant corticosteroids reduce the incidence of adverse cutaneous reactions to co-trimoxazole in patients with AIDS who are treated for hypoxaemic *P. carinii* pneumonia, but the incidence of mucocutaneous herpes simplex virus infection is higher [15]. If it is deemed essential to continue the drug, desensitization can be attempted [16,17].

Fixed eruptions occur [18–22], and may be due to the sulphonamide or trimethoprim components; a widespread fixed eruption mimicking TEN has been documented in one case [23]. Pustular reactions [24] and Sweet's syndrome [25] have been documented. Severe reactions have included erythema multiforme or Stevens–Johnson syndrome [26,27], which has been fatal [27], TEN in AIDS patients [5,11,12], cutaneous vasculitis [28] and fatal agranulocytosis [29]. One patient developed a rapidly progressive subepidermal bullous eruption within hours of intravenous trimethoprim–sulphamethoxazole [30].

REFERENCES

1 Jick J. Adverse reactions to trimethoprim–sulphamethoxazole in hospitalized patients. *Rev Infect Dis* 1982; **4**: 426–8.
2 Lawson DH, Paice BJ. Adverse reactions to trimethoprim–sulfamethoxasole. *Rev Infect Dis* 1982; **4**: 429–33.
3 Huisman MV, Buller HR, TenCate JW. Co-trimoxasole toxicity. *Lancet* 1984; **ii**: 1152.
4 Anonymous. Revised indications for co-trimoxazole (Septrin, Bactrim, various generic preparations). *Curr Probl Pharmacovig* 1995; **21**: 5.
5 Coopman SA, Johnson RA, Platt R, Stern RS. Cutaneous disease and drug reactions in HIV infection. *N Engl J Med* 1993; **328**: 1670–4.
6 Mitsuyasu R, Groopman J, Volberding P. Cutaneous reaction to trimethoprim–sulfamethoxazole in patients with AIDS and Kaposi's sarcoma. *N Engl J Med* 1983; **308**: 1535–6.
7 Gordin FM, Simon GL, Wofsy CB *et al*. Adverse reactions to trimethoprim sulfamethoxazole in patients with the acquired immune deficiency syndrome. *Ann Intern Med* 1984; **100**: 495–9.
8 Cohn DL, Penley KA, Judson FN *et al*. The acquired immunodeficiency syndrome and a trimethoprim–sulfamethoxazole-adverse reaction. *Ann Intern Med* 1984; **100**: 311.
9 Kovacs JA, Hiemenz JW, Macher AM *et al*. *Pneumocystis carinii* pneumonia: a comparison between patients with the acquired immunodeficiency syndrome and patients with other immunodeficiencies. *Ann Intern Med* 1984; **100**: 663–71.
10 De Raeve L, Song M, Van Maldergem L. Adverse cutaneous drug reactions in AIDS. *Br J Dermatol* 1988; **119**: 521–3.
11 Arnold P, Guglielmo J, Hollander H. Severe hypersensitivity reaction upon rechallenge with trimethoprim–sulfamethoxazole in a patient with AIDS. *Drug Intell Clin Pharmacol* 1988; **22**: 43–4.
12 Coopman SA, Stern RS. Cutaneous drug reactions in human immunodeficiency virus infection. *Arch Dermatol* 1991; **127**; 714–17.
13 Chanock SJ, Luginbuhl LM, McIntosh K, Lipshultz SE. Life-threatening reaction to trimethoprim/sulfamethoxazole in pediatric human immunodeficiency virus infection. *Pediatrics* 1994; **93**: 519–21.
14 Roudier C, Caumes E, Rogeaux O *et al*. Adverse cutaneous reactions to trimethoprim–sulfamethoxazole in patients with the acquired immunodeficiency syndrome and *Pneumocystis carinii* pneumonia. *Arch Dermatol* 1994; **130**: 1383–6.
15 Caumes E, Roudier C, Rogeaux O *et al*. Effect of corticosteroids on the incidence of adverse cutaneous reactions to trimethoprim–sulfamethoxazole during treatment of AIDS-associated *Pneumocystis carinii* pneumonia. *Clin Infect Dis* 1994; **18**: 319–23.
16 Kletzel M, Beck S, Elser J *et al*. Trimethoprim–sulfamethoxazole oral desensitization in hemophiliacs infected with human immunodeficiency virus with a history of hypersensitivity reactions. *Am J Dis Child* 1991; **145**: 1428–9.
17 Carr A, Penny R, Cooper DA. Efficacy and safety of rechallenge with low-dose trimethoprim–sulphamethoxazole in previously hypersensitive HIV-infected patients. *AIDS* 1993; **7**: 65–71.
18 Talbot MD. Fixed genital drug reaction. *Practitioner* 1980; **224**: 823–4.
19 Varsano I, Amir Y. Fixed drug eruption due to co-trimoxazole. *Dermatologica* 1989; **178**: 232.
20 Van Voorhees A, Stenn KS. Histological phases of bactrim-induced fixed drug eruption. The report of one case. *Am J Dermatopathol* 1987; **9**: 528–32.
21 Bharija SC, Belhaj MS. Fixed drug eruption due to cotrimoxazole. *Australas J Dermatol* 1989; **30**: 43–4.
22 Lim JT, Chan HL. Fixed drug eruptions due to co-trimoxazole. *Ann Acad Med Sing* 1992; **21**: 408–10.
23 Baird BJ, De Villez RL. Widespread bullous fixed drug eruption mimicking toxic epidermal necrolysis. *Int J Dermatol* 1988; **27**: 170–4.
24 MacDonald KJS, Green CM, Kenicer KJA. Pustular dermatosis induced by co-trimoxazole. *Br Med J* 1986; **293**: 1279–80.

25 Walker DC, Cohen PR. Trimethoprim–sulfamethoxazole-associated acute febrile neutrophilic dermatosis: case report and review of drug-induced Sweet's syndrome. *J Am Acad Dermatol* 1996; **34**: 918–23.
26 Azinge NO, Garrick GA. Stevens–Johnson syndrome (erythema multiforme) following ingestion of trimethoprim-sulfamethoxazole on two separate occasions in the same person. A case report. *J Allergy Clin Immunol* 1978; **62**: 125–6.
27 Beck MH, Portnoy B. Severe erythema multiforme complicated by fatal gastro-intestinal involvement following co-trimoxasole therapy. *Clin Exp Dermatol* 1979; **4**: 201–4.
28 Wåhlin A, Rosman N. Skin manifestations with vasculitis due to co-trimoxazole. *Lancet* 1976; **ii**: 1415.
29 Lawson DH, Henry DA, Jick H. Fatal agranulocytosis attributed to co-trimoxazole therapy. *Br Med J* 1976; **ii**: 316.
30 Roholt NS, Lapiere JC, Traczyk T *et al.* A nonscarring sublamina densa bullous drug eruption. *J Am Acad Dermatol* 1995; **32**: 367–71.

Trimethoprim

Used alone, this substance causes less reaction than sulphonamides; fixed eruption has been proven [1–3]. Two patients experienced life-threatening immediate reactions and one patient developed generalized urticaria following oral trimethoprim–sulphamethoxazole; prick tests and oral challenge tests were positive with trimethoprim, but not to sulphamethoxazole [4].

REFERENCES

1 Kanwar AJ, Bharija SC, Singh M, Belhaj MS. Fixed drug eruption to trimethoprim. *Dermatologica* 1986; **172**: 230–1.
2 Hughes BR, Holt PJA, Marks R. Trimethoprim associated fixed drug eruption. *Br J Dermatol* 1987; **116**: 241–2.
3 Lim JT, Chan HL. Fixed drug eruptions due to co-trimoxazole. *Ann Acad Med Sing* 1992; **21**: 408–10.
4 Alonso MD, Marcos C, Davila I *et al.* Hypersensitivity to trimethoprim. *Allergy* 1992; **47**: 340–2.

Aminoglycosides

Gentamicin, tobramycin, streptomycin and kanamycin cross-react and are all potentially ototoxic and nephrotoxic. Exanthematic eruptions are common with streptomycin, developing in 5% or more of patients. Continued treatment may lead to generalized exfoliative dermatitis with these drugs [1] in a minority, but in a proportion of patients the rash subsides and treatment can be continued. Fever and eosinophilia may be associated with the reactions. Urticaria [2], maculopapular rashes, drug fever and eosinophilia are well recognized with this group of drugs. Skin necrosis following subcutaneous injection of aminoglycoside antibiotics (gentamycin, sisomycin and netilmicin) has been reported in elderly females with a history of thrombosis being treated with heparin anticoagulant therapy [3–5]. The reaction has also occurred following intramuscular sisomycin in a patient with defective fibrinolysis and abnormal neutrophil function [6]. A toxic erythema with generalized follicular pustulosis has been documented with streptomycin [7]. Deafness has rarely followed topical therapy with neomycin, including administration of aerosol preparations in the treatment of extensive burns. An anaphylactic reaction due to streptomycin occurred during *in vitro* fertilization immediately after embryo transfer [8].

REFERENCES

1 Karp S, Bakris G, Cooney A *et al.* Exfoliative dermatitis secondary to tobramycin sulfate. *Cutis* 1991; **47**: 331–2.
2 Schretlen-Doherty JS, Troutman WG. Tobramycin-induced hypersensitivity reaction. *Ann Pharmacother* 1995; **29**: 704–6.
3 Taillandier J, Manigaud G, Fixy P, Dumont D. Nécroses cutanées induites par la gentamicine sous-cutanée. *Presse Med* 1984; **13**: 1574–5.
4 Duterque M, Hubert Asso AM, Corrard A. Lésions nécrotiques par injections sous cutanées de gentamicine et de sisomicine. *Ann Dermatol Vénéréol* 1985; **112**: 707–8.
5 Bernard P, Paris M, Cantanzano G, Bonnetblanc JM. Vascularite cutanée localisée induite par la Nétilmicine. *Presse Med* 1987; **16**: 915–16.
6 Grob JJ, Mege JL, Follano J *et al.* Skin necrosis after injection of aminoglycosides. Arthus reaction, local toxicity, thrombotic process or pathergy? *Dermatologica* 1990; **181**: 258–62.
7 Kushimoto H, Aoki T. Toxic erythema with generalized follicular pustules caused by streptomycin. *Arch Dermatol* 1981; **117**: 444–5.
8 Abeck D, Kuwert C, Segnini-Torres M *et al.* Streptomycin-induced anaphylactic reaction during *in vitro* fertilization (IVF). *Allergy* 1994; **49**: 388–9.

Macrolide antibiotics

Macrolides account for 10–15% of the worldwide oral antibiotic market, with severe adverse reactions being rare [1]. Gastrointestinal reactions occur in 15–20% of patients on erythromycins and in 5% or fewer patients treated with some recently developed macrolide derivatives that seldom or never induce endogenous release of motilin, such as roxithromycin, clarithromycin, dirithromycin, azithromycin and rikamycin. Except for troleandomycin and some erythromycins administered at high dose and for long periods of time, the hepatotoxic potential of macrolides is low. Transient deafness and allergic reactions to macrolide antibacterials are highly unusual and are more common with the erythromycins than with the recently developed 14-, 15- and 16-membered macrolides.

Erythromycin

This is one of the most innocuous antibiotics in current use. Cholestasis caused by the estolate ester is the only potentially serious side-effect. Hypersensitivity skin reactions are rare but when they occur skin tests may be positive [2,3]. Erythema multiforme, Stevens–Johnson syndrome, toxic pustuloderma [4], systemic contact dermatitis [5] and vasculitis have all been recorded.

Azithromycin

This drug has caused toxic pustuloderma [6].

Spiramycin

Rashes, usually transient erythema, may occur in up to 1% of cases. Spiramycin, given for toxoplasmosis in pregnancy, was associated in one case with an erythematous maculopapular pruritic eruption with eosinophilia and raised γ-glutamyl transpeptidase [7]. The drug has caused an allergic vasculitis [8].

REFERENCES

1 Periti P, Mazzei T, Mini E, Novelli A. Adverse effects of macrolide antibacterials. *Drug Saf* 1993; **9**: 346–64.
2 Van Ketel WG. Immediate and delayed-type allergy to erythromycin. *Contact Dermatitis* 1976; **2**: 363–4.
3 Shirin H, Schapiro JM, Arber N *et al.* Erythromycin base-induced rash and liver function disturbances. *Ann Pharmacother* 1992; **26**: 1522–23.
4 Roujeau J-C, Bioulac-Sage P, Bourseau C *et al.* Acute generalized exanthematous pustulosis. Analysis of 63 cases. *Arch Dermatol* 1991; **127**: 1333–8.
5 Fernandez Redondo V, Casas L, Taboada M, Toribio J. Systemic contact dermatitis from erythromycin. *Contact Dermatitis* 1994; **30**: 311.
6 Trevisi P, Patrizi A, Neri I, Farina P. Toxic pustuloderma associated with azithromycin. *Clin Exp Dermatol* 1994; **19**: 280–1.
7 Ostlere LS, Langtry JAA, Staughton RCD. Allergy to spiramycin during prophlyactic treatment of fetal toxoplasmosis. *Br Med J* 1991; **302**: 970.
8 Galland MC, Rodor F, Jouglard J. Spiramycin allergic vasculitis: first report. *Therapie* 1987; **42**: 227–9.

Clindamycin and lincomycin

These antibiotics have become particularly associated with a potentially lethal pseudomembranous colitis due to superinfection with *Clostridium difficile* [1–3]. Vancomycin or metronidazole are the treatments of choice for this complication. Hypersensitivity skin reactions are rare with lincomycin but common with clindamycin, occurring in up to 10% of patients. Erythema multiforme and anaphylaxis are very rare [4].

REFERENCES

1 Dantzig PI. The safety of long-term clindamycin therapy for acne. *Arch Dermatol* 1976; **112**: 53–4.
2 Tan SG, Cunliffe WJ. The unwanted effects of clindamycin in acne. *Br J Dermatol* 1976; **94**: 313–15.
3 Leading Article. Antibiotic-associated colitis: a progress report. *Br Med J* 1978; **i**: 669–71.
4 Lochmann O, Kohout P, Vymola F. Anaphylactic shock following the administration of clindamycin. *J Hyg Epidemiol Microbiol Immunol* 1977; **21**: 441–7.

Miscellaneous antibiotics

Chloramphenicol

Although contact dermatitis from topical application is common, hypersensitivity skin reactions to oral therapy are rare. Macular, papular and urticarial eruptions are reported [1]. Pruritus may be prominent. Erythema multiforme and TEN [2] occur rarely. There is a risk of aplastic anaemia [3] and death has exceptionally followed the use of eye drops [4].

REFERENCES

1 Unsdek HE, Curtiss WP, Neill EJ. Skin eruption due to chloramphenicol (Chloromycetin®). *Arch Dermatol Syphilol* 1951; **64**: 217.
2 Mathe P, Aubert L, Labouche F *et al.* Syndrome de Lyell. Etiologie médicamenteuse: rôle probable de chloramphénicol. *J Méd Bordeaux* 1965; **42**: 1367–76.
3 Hargraves MM, Mills SD, Heck FJ. Aplastic anemia associated with the administration of chloramphenicol. *JAMA* 1952; **149**: 1293–300.
4 Fraunfelder FT, Bagby GC. Ocular chloramphenicol and aplastic anemia. *N Engl J Med* 1983; **308**: 1536.

Fusidic acid

Topical use can lead to contact dermatitis but hypersensitivity reactions to oral or parenteral use are very rare; jaundice has accompanied intravenous use. Acanthosis nigricans-like lesions have been reported after local application [1].

REFERENCE

1 Teknetzis A, Lefaki I, Joannides D, Minas A. Acanthosis nigricans-like lesions after local application of fusidic acid. *J Am Acad Dermatol* 1993; **28**: 501–2.

Metronidazole and tinidazole

Metronidazole. Pruritus, fixed eruptions and generalized erythema [1–3] are rare. A pityriasis rosea-like eruption has been described [4]. A reversible peripheral neuropathy may complicate prolonged therapy.

Tinidazole. A fixed eruption with cross-reactivity with metronidazole has been reported [5,6].

REFERENCES

1 Naik RPC, Singh G. Fixed drug eruption due to metronidazole. *Dermatologica* 1977; **155**: 59–60.
2 Shelley WB, Shelley ED. Fixed drug eruption due to metronidazole. *Cutis* 1987; **39**: 393–4.
3 Knowles S, Choudhury T, Shear NH. Metronidazole hypersensitivity. *Ann Pharmacother* 1994; **28**: 325–6.
4 Maize JC, Tomecki KJ. Pityriasis rosea-like drug eruption secondary to metronidazole. *Arch Dermatol* 1977; **113**: 1457–8.
5 Kanwar AJ, Sharma R, Rajagopalan M, Kaur S. Fixed drug eruption due to tinidazole with cross-reactivity with metronidazole. *Dermatologica* 1990; **181**: 277.
6 Mishra D, Mobashir M, Zaheer MS. Fixed drug eruption and cross-reactivity between tinidazole and metronidazole. *Int J Dermatol* 1990; **29**: 740.

Nitrofurantoin

Pruritus, morbilliform rashes and urticaria may be seen occasionally. Erythema multiforme, erythema nodosum [1], exfoliative dermatitis, and an LE-like syndrome [2] are documented. Acute or chronic pulmonary reactions may accompany these skin manifestations, and may lead to pulmonary fibrosis [3]. Polyneuritis is a dose-dependent toxic reaction. Hepatitis, cholestatic jaundice and marrow suppression may occur rarely. Abnormal immuno-electrophoretic patterns may be induced [4].

REFERENCES

1 Chisholm JC, Hepner M. Nitrofurantoin induced erythema nodosum. *J Natl Med Assoc* 1981; **73**: 59–61.
2 Selross O, Edgren J. Lupus-like syndrome associated with pulmonary reaction to nitrofurantoin. *Acta Med Scand* 1975; **197**: 125–9.
3 Rantala H, Kirvelä O, Anttolainen I. Nitrofurantoin lung in a child. *Lancet* 1979; **ii**: 799–80.
4 Teppo AM, Haltia K, Wager O. Immunoelectrophoretic 'tailing' of albumin line due to albumin-IgG antibody complexes: a side effect of nitrofurantoin treatment? *Scand J Immunol* 1976; **5**: 249–61.

Quinolones

These compounds are related to nalidixic acid; central nervous system toxicity, upper gastrointestinal tract reactions and phototoxicity have been recorded [1–7]. Cross-reactivity occurs [8]. Gastrointestinal side-effects occur in up to 6% of patients. Hypersensitivity reactions involving the skin have been reported in 0.5–2% of patients, and in up to 2.4% of patients receiving cinoxacin; they most frequently manifest themselves as rash or pruritus. Fever, urticaria, angio-oedema and anaphylactoid reactions are rare. Anaphylactic or anaphylactoid reactions have been documented with cinoxacin [9], ciprofloxacin (1.2 per 100 000 prescriptions) [10,11] and pipemidic acid [12]. Fixed drug eruption due to pipemidic acid is recorded [13]. Norfloxacin [14] and ofloxacin [15] have caused a pustular eruption. Ciprofloxacin [16,17], pefloxacin, fleroxacin [18] and enoxacin [19] have been associated with photosensitivity. Pefloxacine and ofloxacine have caused photo-onycholysis [20]. Hypersensitivity leukocytoclastic vasculitis has been reported with both ofloxacin and ciprofloxacin [21,22] and serum sickness with ciprofloxacin [23]. Intravenous administration of ciprofloxacin through small veins at the dorsum of the hands may be associated with local reactions at the site of infusion [24]. Stevens–Johnson syndrome or TEN have been described with quinolones [25] including ciprofloxacin [26].

Nalidixic acid. Cutaneous reactions are common, occurring in up to 5% of patients; various hypersensitivity reactions are seen, including exfoliative dermatitis. Phototoxicity is now well recognized [27–31]. A bullous photodermatitis may occur, usually on the hands or feet; chronic scarring and increased skin fragility may mimic porphyria cutanea tarda. Long-wave UV light is responsible [30]. An LE-like syndrome has been reported [32], as well as transient alopecia.

REFERENCES

1 Christ W, Lehnert T, Ulbrich B. Specific toxicologic aspects of the quinolones. *Rev Infect Dis* 1988; **10** (Suppl. 1): S141–6.
2 Wolfson JS, Hooper DC. Fluoroquinolone antimicrobial agents. *Clin Microbiol Rev* 1989; **2**: 378–424.
3 Hooper DC, Wolfson JS. Fluoroquinolone antimicrobial agents. *N Engl J Med* 1991; **324**: 384–94.
4 Sisca TS, Heel RC, Romankiewicz JA. Cinoxacin: a review of its pharmacological properties and therapeutic efficacy in the treatment of urinary tract infections. *Drugs* 1983; **25**: 544–69.
5 Campoli-Richards DM, Monck JP, Price A *et al.* Ciprofloxacin. A review of its antibacterial activity, pharmacokinetic properties and therapeutic use. *Drugs* 1988; **35**: 373–447.
6 Norrby SR, Lietman PS. Safety and tolerability of fluoroquinolones. *Drugs* 1993; **45** (Suppl.) **3**: 59–64.
7 Matsuno K, Kunihiro E, Yamatoya O *et al.* Surveillance of adverse reactions due to ciprofloxacin in Japan. *Drugs* 1995; **49** (Suppl. 2): 495–6.
8 Davila I, Diez ML, Quirce S *et al.* Cross-reactivity between quinolones. Report of three cases. *Allergy* 1993; **48**: 388–90.
9 Stricker BHC, Slagboom G, Demaeseneer R *et al.* Anaphylactic reactions to cinoxacin. *Br Med J* 1988; **297**: 1434–5.
10 Davis H, McGoodwin E, Reed TG. Anaphylactoid reactions reported after treatment with ciprofloxacin. *Ann Intern Med* 1989; **111**: 1041–3.
11 Deamer RL, Prichard JG, Loman GJ. Hypersensitivity and anaphylactoid reactions to ciprofloxacin. *Ann Pharmacother* 1992; **26**: 1081–4.
12 Gerber D. Anaphylaxis caused by pipemidic acid. *S Afr Med J* 1985; **67**: 999.
13 Miyagawa S, Yamashina Y, Hirota S, Shirai T. Fixed drug eruption due to pipemidic acid. *J Dermatol (Tokyo)* 1991; **18**: 59–60.
14 Shelley ED, Shelley WB. The subcorneal pustular drug eruption: an example induced by norfloxacin. *Cutis* 1988; **42**: 24–7.
15 Tsuda S, Kato K, Karashima T *et al.* Toxic pustuloderma induced by ofloxacin. *Ann Dermatol Vénéréol* 1993; **73**: 382–4.
16 Nederost ST, Dijkstra JWE, Handel DW. Drug-induced photosensitivity reaction. *Arch Dermatol* 1989; **125**: 433–4.
17 Ferguson J, Johnson BE. Ciprofloxacin-induced photosensitivity: *in vitro* and *in vivo* studies. *Br J Dermatol* 1990; **123**: 9–20.
18 Bowie WR, Willetts V, Jewesson PJ. Adverse reactions in a dose-ranging study with a new long-acting fluoroquinolone, fleroxacin. *Antimicrob Agents Chemother* 1989; **33**: 1778–82.
19 Izu R, Gardeazabal J, Gonzalez M *et al.* Enoxacin-induced photosensitivity: study of two cases. *Photodermatol Photoimmunol Photomed* 1992; **9**: 86–8.
20 Baran R, Brun P. Photo-onycholysis induced by the fluoroquinolones pefloxacine and ofloxacine. Report on 2 cases. *Dermatologica* 1986; **173**: 185–8.
21 Huminer C, Cohen JD, Majafla R, Dux S. Hypersensitivity vasculitis due to ofloxacin. *Br Med J* 1989; **299**: 303.
22 Choc U, Rothschield BM, Laitman L. Ciprofloxacin-induced vasculitis. *N Engl J Med* 1989; **320**: 257–8.
23 Guharoy SR. Serum sickness secondary to ciprofloxacin use. *Vet Hum Toxicol* 1994; **36**: 540–1.
24 Thorsteinsson SB, Bergan T, Johannesson G *et al.* Tolerance of ciprofloxacin at injection site, systemic safety and effect on electroencephalogram. *Chemotherapy* 1987; **33**: 448–51.
25 Roujeau JC, Kelly JP, Naldi L *et al.* Medication use and the risk of Stevens–Johnson syndrome or toxic epidermal necrolysis. *N Engl J Med* 1995; **333**: 1600–7.
26 Tham TCK, Allen G, Hayes D *et al.* Possible association between toxic epidermal necrolysis and ciprofloxacin. *Lancet* 1991; **338**: 522.
27 Baes H. Photosensitivity caused by nalidixic acid. *Dermatologica* 1968; **136**: 61–4.
28 Birkett DA, Garretts M, Stevenson CJ. Phototoxic bullous eruptions due to nalidixic acid. *Br J Dermatol* 1969; **81**: 342–4.
29 Ramsay CA, Obreshkova E. Photosensitivity from nalidixic acid. *Br J Dermatol* 1974; **91**: 523–8.
30 Rosén K, Swanbeck G. Phototoxic reactions from some common drugs provoked by a high-intensity UVA lamp. *Acta Derm Venereol (Stockh)* 1982; **62**: 246–8.
31 Nederost ST, Dijkstra JWE, Handel DW. Drug-induced photosensitivity reaction. *Arch Dermatol* 1989; **125**: 433–4.
32 Rubinstein A. LE-like disease caused by nalidixic acid. *N Engl J Med* 1979; **301**: 1288.

Synergistins

An eczematous-like drug eruption is recorded after oral antibiotic synergistins, pristinamycin and virginiamycin, following contact sensitization with topical virginiamycin [1].

REFERENCE

1 Michel M, Dompmartin A, Szczurko C *et al*. Eczematous-like drug eruption induced by synergistins. *Contact Dermatitis* 1996; **34**: 86–7.

Vancomycin

Allergic skin reactions are not uncommon, occurring in up to 5% of patients. Rapid intravenous infusion of vancomycin can cause a histamine-induced anaphylactoid reaction characterized by flushing, a maculopapular eruption of the neck, face, trunk and extremities, the so-called 'red man syndrome', prolonged hypotension, and in rare cases cardiac arrest [1–3]. Desensitization has been successfully achieved in patients with vancomycin hypersensitivity [4–6]. TEN has occurred [7]. Vancomycin has been reported to have induced linear IgA bullous dermatosis [8–11].

REFERENCES

1 Pau AK, Khakoo R. Red-neck syndrome with slow infusion of vancomycin. *N Engl J Med* 1985; **313**: 756–7.
2 Valero R, Gomar C, Fita G *et al*. Adverse reactions to vancomycin prophylaxis in cardiac surgery. *J Cardiothor Vasc Anes* 1991; **5**: 574–6.
3 Killian AD, Sahai JV, Memish ZA. Red man syndrome after oral vancomycin. *Ann Intern Med* 1991; **115**: 410–31.
4 Lin RY. Desensitization in the management of vancomycin hypersensitivity. *Arch Intern Med* 1990; **150**: 2197–8.
5 Anne S, Middleton E, Jr, Reisman RE. Vancomycin anaphylaxis and successful desensitization. *Ann Allergy* 1994; **73**: 402–4.
6 Wong JT, Ripple RE, MacLean JA *et al*. Vancomycin hypersensitivity: synergism with narcotics and 'desensitization' by a rapid continuous intravenous protocol. *J Allergy Clin Immunol* 1994; **94**: 189–94.
7 Vidal C, Gonzalez Quintela A, Fuente R. Toxic epidermal necrolysis due to vancomycin. *Ann Allergy* 1992; **68**: 345–7.
8 Baden LA, Apovian C, Imber MJ, Dover JS. Vancomycin-induced linear IgA bullous dermatosis. *Arch Dermatol* 1988; **124**: 1186–8.
9 Carpenter S, Berg D, Sidhu-Malik N *et al*. Vancomycin-associated linear IgA dermatosis. A report of three cases. *J Am Acad Dermatol* 1992; **26**: 45–8.
10 Piketty C, Meeus F, Nochy D *et al*. Linear IgA dermatosis related to vancomycin. *Br J Dermatol* 1994; **130**: 130–1.
11 Whitworth JM, Thomas I, Peltz S *et al*. Vancomycin-induced linear IgA bullous dermatosis (LABD). *J Am Acad Dermatol* 1996; **34**: 890–1.

Topical antibiotics

The side-effects of topical antibiotics have been reviewed [1]. Allergic contact dermatitis is rare with topical clindamycin, erythromycin and tetracycline, polymyxin B, gentamicin, and mupirocin, but is more frequent with neomycin.

Bacitracin

Anaphylaxis due to bacitracin allergy has followed topical application of this antibiotic [2–5]. The patients had had multiple prior exposures and previous local reactions of pruritus, urticaria or possible allergic contact dermatitis. Two patients with anaphylactic reactions to Polyfax ointment, containing polymixin B and bacitracin, have been reported; one had previously documented positive patch tests to Polyfax, and the other had clinical intolerance to the preparation [5]. Another patient developed anaphylaxis to a similar proprietary mixture (Polysporin) [6]. Intracutaneous injection of bacitracin in sensitive individuals induces histamine release with large weal-and-flare reactions [7].

Chloramphenicol

Urticaria and angio-oedema have been described with topical use [8]. Fatal aplastic anemia has followed the use of eye drops containing this antibiotic [9].

Sulphonamides

Erythema multiforme and Stevens–Johnson syndrome have been reported from topical preparations [10,11].

REFERENCES

1 Hirschmann JV. Topical antibiotics in dermatology. *Arch Dermatol* 1988; **124**: 1691–700.
2 Roupe G, Strannegård Ö. Anaphylactic shock elicited by topical administration of bacitracin. *Arch Dermatol* 1969; **100**: 450–2.
3 Shechter JF, Wilkinson RD, Del Carpio J. Anaphylaxis following the use of bacitracin ointment: report of a case and review of the literature. *Arch Dermatol* 1984; **120**: 909–11.
4 Katz BE, Fisher AA. Bacitracin: a unique topical antibiotic sensitiser. *J Am Acad Dermatol* 1987; **17**: 1016–24.
5 Eedy DJ, McMillan JC, Bingham EA. Anaphylactic reactions to topical antibiotic combinations. *Postgrad Med J* 1990; **66**: 858–9.
6 Knowles SR, Shear NH. Anaphylaxis from bacitracin and polymyxin B (Polysporin) ointment. *Int J Dermatol* 1995; **34**: 572–3.
7 Bjorkner B, Moller H. Bacitracin: a cutaneous allergen and histamine releaser. *Acta Derm Venereol (Stockh)* 1973; **53**: 487–91.
8 Schewach-Millet M, Shapiro D. Urticaria and angioedema due to topically applied chloramphenicol ointment. *Arch Dermatol* 1985; **121**: 587.
9 Fraunfelder FT, Bagby GC. Ocular chloramphenicol and aplastic anemia. *N Engl J Med* 1983; **308**: 1536.
10 Genvert GI, Cohen EJ, Donnenfeld ED, Blecher MH. Erythema multiforme after use of topical sulfacetamide. *Am J Ophthalmol* 1985; **99**: 465–8.
11 Gottschalk HR, Stone OJ. Stevens–Johnson syndrome from ophthalmic sulphonamide. *Arch Dermatol* 1976; **112**: 513–14.

Antituberculous drugs

Severe cutaneous reactions, such as Stevens–Johnson syndrome and TEN, and multiple drug reactions to antituberculous drugs, including thiacetazone, streptomycin and isoniazid, occur more often in HIV-positive patients [1–5]. The World Health Organisation has advised against use of thiacetazone in tuberculosis patients with known, or suspected, HIV infection in view of the severe cutaneous hypersensitivity [3–5]. The following drugs are reported to cause contact dermatitis: isoniazid, rifampicin, ethambutol, *p*-aminosalicylic acid, streptomycin, and kanamycin [6]. The incidence of other reactions to individual drugs is difficult to assess because several drugs are usually used in combination.

Cycloserine

A lichenoid drug eruption with positive patch tests and resolution 4 months after withdrawal was reported [7].

Ethambutol

Hypersensitivity reactions are very rare. Side-effects are largely confined to visual disturbances, with loss of acuity, colour blindness and restricted visual fields; these are usually reversible if the drug is stopped promptly. Patients should have ophthalmic assessments prior to and during therapy. Lichenoid reactions occur and may be restricted to light-exposed sites [8,9].

Ethionamide

Eczema, chiefly affecting the forehead, acneiform eruptions, butterfly eruptions on the face, stomatitis, alopecia and purpura have been reported.

Isoniazid

Allergic skin reactions occur in fewer than 1% of patients. An acneiform eruption, usually occurring in slow inactivators of the drug, is well recognized [10,11]. Urticaria, purpura, and an LE-like syndrome [12,13] have been reported. Rarely, a pellagra-like syndrome has been induced in malnourished patients, due to metabolic antagonism of nicotinic acid with resultant pyridoxine deficiency [10,14]. Exfoliative dermatitis [15] and Stevens–Johnson syndrome [2] have been reported.

Rifampicin

Cutaneous hypersensitivity reactions are very uncommon. There have been isolated reports of bullous erythema multiforme, TEN [16] and pemphigus [17,18]; existing pemphigus may also be exacerbated [19]. Altered liver function, usually transient, and thrombocytopenic purpura may occur. Rifampicin has precipitated porphyria cutanea tarda [20]. It induces liver enzymes and may thus reduce the effectiveness of a number of drugs including oral contraceptives.

Streptomycin

See aminoglycosides above.

Thiacetazone

Severe cutaneous hypersensitivity reactions have been reported, including maculopapular rashes, which progress to mucosal involvement with constitutional symptoms, Stevens–Johnson syndrome, and TEN, especially in HIV-seropositive patients [2,3,5,21,22]. Cutaneous hypersensitivity reactions have been reported in 20% of HIV-seropositive patients, compared with 1% of HIV-seronegative patients who receive the drug as part treatment for tuberculosis [22]. Figurate erythematous eruptions resembling erythema annulare centrifugum may occur [23].

REFERENCES

1 Pozniak AL, MacLeod GA, Mahari M *et al*. The influence of HIV status on single and multiple drug reactions to antituberculous therapy in Africa. *AIDS* 1992; **6**: 809–14.
2 Dukes CS, Sugarman J, Cegielski JP, Lallinger GJ, Mwakyusa DH. Severe cutaneous hypersensitivity reactions during treatment of tuberculosis in patients with HIV infection in Tanzania. *Trop Geograph Med* 1992; **44**: 308–11.
3 Chintu C, Luo C, Bhat G *et al*. Cutaneous hypersensitivity reactions due to thiacetazone in the treatment of tuberculosis in Zambian children infected with HIV-I. *Arch Dis Child* 1993; **68**: 665–8.
4 Nunn P, Porter J, Winstanley P. Thiacetazone—avoid like poison or use with care? *Trans R Soc Trop Med Hyg* 1993; **87**: 578–82.
5 Kelly P, Buve A, Foster SD *et al*. Cutaneous reactions to thiacetazone in Zambia—implications for tuberculosis treatment strategies. *Trans R Soc Trop Med Hyg* 1994; **88**: 113–15.
6 Holdiness MR. Contact dermatitis to antituberculous drugs. *Contact Dermatitis* 1986; **15**: 282–8.
7 Shim JH, Kim TY, Kim HO, Kim CW. Cycloserine-induced lichenoid drug eruption. *Dermatology* 1995; **191**: 142–4.
8 Frentz G, Wadskov S, Kssis V. Ethambutol-induced lichenoid eruption. *Acta Derm Venereol (Stockh)* 1981; **61**: 89–91.
9 Grossman ME, Warren K, Mady A, Satra KH. Lichenoid eruption associated with ethambutol. *J Am Acad Dermatol* 1995; **33**: 675–6.
10 Cohen LK, George W, Smith R. Isoniazid-induced acne and pellagra. Occurrence in slow acetylators of isoniazid. *Arch Dermatol* 1974; **109**: 377–81.
11 Oliwiecki S, Burton JL. Severe acne due to isoniazid. *Clin Exp Dermatol* 1988; **13**: 283–4.
12 Grunwald M, David M, Feuerman EJ. Appearance of lupus erythematosus in a patient with lichen planus treated by isoniazid. *Dermatologica* 1982; **165**: 172–7.
13 Sim E, Gill EW, Sim RB. Drugs that induce systemic lupus erythematosus inhibit complement C4. *Lancet* 1984; **ii**: 422–4.
14 Schmutz JL, Cuny JF, Trechot P *et al*. Les érythèmes pellagroïdes médicamenteux. Une observation d'érythème pellagroïde secondaire a l'isoniazide. *Ann Dermatol Vénéréol* 1987; **114**: 569–76.
15 Rosin MA, King LE, Jr. Isoniazid-induced exfoliative dermatitis. *South Med J* 1982; **75**: 81.
16 Okano M, Kitano Y, Igarashi T. Toxic epidermal necrolysis due to rifampicin. *J Am Acad Dermatol* 1987; **17**: 303–4.
17 Gange RW, Rhodes EL, Edwards CO, Powell MEA. Pemphigus induced by rifampicin. *Br J Dermatol* 1976; **95**: 445–8.
18 Lee CW, Lim JH, Kang HJ. Pemphigus foliaceus induced by rifampicin. *Br J Dermatol* 1984; **111**: 619–22.
19 Miyagawa S, Yamanashi Y, Okuchi T *et al*. Exacerbation of pemphigus by rifampicin. *Br J Dermatol* 1986; **114**: 729–32.

20 Millar JW. Rifampicin-induced porphyria cutanea tarda. *Br J Dis Chest* 1980; **74**: 405–8.

21 Fegan D, Glennon J. Cutaneous sensitivity to thiacetazone. *Lancet* 1991; **337**: 1036.

22 Nunn P, Kibuga D, Gathua S *et al*. Cutaneous hypersensitivity reactions due to thiacetazone in HIV-1 seropositive patients treated for tuberculosis. *Lancet* 1991; **337**: 627–30.

23 Ramesh V. Eruption resembling erythema annulare centrifugum. *Australas J Dermatol* 1987; **28**: 44.

Antileprotic drugs

Clofazimine

This drug regularly causes a reversible, dose-dependent, brown–orange pigmentation of the skin [1–3]. Biopsy specimens from two lepromatous leprosy patients on long-term clofazimine therapy revealed ceroid–lipofuscin pigment as well as clofazimine inside macrophage phagolysosomes [3]. Reddish-blue pigmentation occurred in scarred areas of LE in one patient [4]. Xeroderma, pruritus, phototoxicity, acne and non-specific rashes are described [2]. Gastrointestinal symptoms may occur early due to direct irritation of the gut and are quickly reversible; ulcerative enteritis may occur after 9–14 months of treatment. After high-dose, prolonged therapy, persistent diarrhoea, abdominal pain and weight loss, associated with deposition of crystalline clofazimine in the small intestinal submucosa and mesenteric lymph nodes, may occur [5,6]. Splenic infarction has been associated with this syndrome [7,8].

REFERENCES

1 Thomsen K, Rothenborg HW. Clofazimine in the treatment of pyoderma gangrenosum. *Arch Dermatol* 1979; **115**: 851–2.

2 Yawalker SJ, Vischer W. Lamprene (clofazimine) in leprosy. Basic information. *Lepr Rev* 1979; **50**: 135–44.

3 Job CK, Yoder L, Jacobson RR, Hastings RC. Skin pigmentation from clofazimine therapy in leprosy patients: a reappraisal. *J Am Acad Dermatol* 1990; **23**: 236–41.

4 Kossard S, Doherty E, McColl I, Ryman W. Autofluorescence of clofazimine in discoid lupus erythematosus. *J Am Acad Dermatol* 1987; **17**: 867–71.

5 Harvey RF, Harman RRM, Black C *et al*. Abdominal pain and malabsorption due to tissue deposition of clofazimine (Lamprene) crystals. *Br J Dermatol* 1977; **97** (Suppl. 15): 19.

6 Venencie PY, Cortez A, Orieux G *et al*. Clofazimine enteropathy. *J Am Acad Dermatol* 1986; **15**: 290–1.

7 Jopling WAH. Complications of treatment with clofazimine (Lamprene: B.663). *Lepr Rev* 1976; **47**: 1–3.

8 McDougal AC, Horsfall WR, Hede JE, Chaplin AJ. Splenic infarction and tissue accumulation of crystals associated with the use of clofazimine (Lamprene: B.663) in the treatment of pyoderma gangrenosum. *Br J Dermatol* 1980; **102**: 227–30.

Dapsone

Fixed eruptions occur in 3% of West Africans being treated for leprosy. Erythema multiforme [1] and exfoliative dermatitis [2] have been described during leprosy treatment. Another uncommon side-effect is a hypersensitivity reaction (dapsone or sulphone syndrome) within the first month or so, with fever, a widespread erythematous eruption studded with pustules, exfoliative dermatitis, hepatitis, lymphadenopathy and anaemia [3–9]. In Vanuatu, 24% of 37 patients treated with daily dapsone 100 mg, clofazimine, and monthly rifampicin and clofazimine for leprosy over 4 years, developed the dapsone syndrome, with a fatality rate of 11% [10]. The increase in reactions may have related to a high starting dose of dapsone, possibly enhanced by the combination with clofazimine and rifampicin and a genetic susceptibility of the Melanesian population.

Red-cell life is always shortened, but clinical haemolytic anaemia is uncommon; patients with low red-cell glucose-6-phosphate dehydrogenase levels [11], and slow acetylators [12] are at a special risk of developing this complication. Methaemoglobinaemia and Heinz-body formation are seen [13]. Agranulocytosis is rare but well recognized and may occur in the first weeks of therapy [14–16]. For patients receiving the drug for dermatitis herpetiformis, this side-effect occurred at a median dosage of 100 mg/day and a median duration of therapy of 7 weeks [15]. The total risk was one case per 3000 patient-years of exposure to the drug; however, agranulocytosis was estimated to occur in one in 240 to one in 425 new patients receiving dapsone for dermatitis herpetiformis [15]. Agranulocytosis occurred in approximately one in 10 000 to one in 20 000 US soldiers receiving dapsone for malarial prophylaxis [17]. Elderly patients do not tolerate dapsone well, and sulphaphyridine or sulphamethoxypyridazine (the latter obtainable on a named patient basis from Lederle Laboratories) is to be preferred for IgA-related diseases. A fatal haematological reaction developed in a Burmese boy during induction of treatment for lepromatous leprosy [18].

Severe but usually reversible hypoalbuminaemia due to failure of albumin production [19,20] or an atypical nephrotic syndrome, may occur. Rarely, dapsone causes a peripheral neuropathy, usually purely motor or mixed sensorimotor and usually recovering within a year [21–24], and optic atrophy [24]. Permanent retinal damage has followed overdosage [25]. Headaches [26], and occasionally a psychosis [27], may be precipitated.

REFERENCES

1 Dutta RK. Erythema multiforme bullosum due to dapsone. *Lepr India* 1980; **52**: 306–9.

2 Browne SG. Antileprosy drugs. *Br Med J* 1971; **iv**: 558–9.

3 Tomecki KJ, Catalano CJ. Dapsone hypersensitivity: the sulfone syndrome revisited. *Arch Dermatol* 1981; **117**: 38–9.

4 Mohle-Boetani J, Akula SK, Holodniy M *et al*. The sulfone syndrome in a patient receiving dapsone prophylaxis for *Pneumocystis carinii* pneumonia. *West J Med* 1992; **156**: 303–6.

5 Barnard GF, Scharf MJ, Dagher RK. Sulfone syndrome in a patient receiving steroids for pemphigus. *Am J Gastroenterol* 1994; **89**: 2057–9.

6 Saito S, Ikezawa Z, Miyamoto H, Kim S. A case of the 'dapsone syndrome.' *Clin Exp Dermatol* 1994; **19**: 152–6.

7 Chalasani P, Baffoe-Bonnie H, Jurado RL. Dapsone therapy causing sulfone syndrome and lethal hepatic failure in an HIV-infected patient. *South Med J* 1994; **87**: 145–6.

8 Bocquet H, Bourgault-Villada I, Delfau-Larue MH *et al.* Syndrome d'hypersensibilite a la dapsone. Clone T circulant transitoire. *Ann Dermatol Vénéréol* 1995; **122**: 514–16.

9 Prussick R, Shear NH. Dapsone hypersensitivity syndrome. *J Am Acad Dermatol* 1996; **35**: 346–9.

10 Reeve PA, Ala J, Hall JJ. Dapsone syndrome in Vanuatu: a high incidence during multidrug treatment (MDT) of leprosy. *J Trop Med Hyg* 1992; **95**: 266–70.

11 Beutler E. Glucose-6-Phosphate dehydrogenase deficiency. *Lancet* 1991; **324**: 169–74.

12 Ellard GA, Gammon PT, Savin LA, Tan RSH. Dapsone acetylation in dermatitis herpetiformis. *Br J Dermatol* 1974; **90**: 441–4.

13 Wagner A, Marosi C, Binder M *et al.* Fatal poisoning due to dapsone in a patient with grossly elevated methaemoglobin levels. *Br J Dermatol* 1995; **133**: 816–17.

14 Potter MN, Yates P, Slade R, Kennedy CTC. Agranulocytosis caused by dapsone therapy for granuloma annulare. *J Am Acad Dermatol* 1989; **20**: 87–8.

15 Hörnstein P, Keisu M, Wiholm B-E. The incidence of agranulocytosis during treatment of dermatitis herpetiformis with dapsone as reported in Sweden, 1972 through 1988. *Arch Dermatol* 1990; **126**: 919–22.

16 Cockburn EM, Wood SM, Waller PC, Bleehen SS. Dapsone-induced agranulocytosis: spontaneous reporting data. *Br J Dermatol* 1993; **128**: 702–3.

17 Ognibene AJ. Agranulocytosis due to dapsone. *Ann Intern Med* 1970; **75**: 521–4.

18 Frey HM, Gershon AA, Borkowsky W, Bullock WE. Fatal reaction to dapsone during treatment of leprosy. *Ann Intern Med* 1981; **94**: 777–9.

19 Kingham JG, Swain P, Swarbrick ET *et al.* Dapsone and severe hypoalbuminaemia: a report of two cases. *Lancet* 1979; **ii**: 662–4.

20 Cowan RE, Wright JT. Dapsone and severe hypoalbuminaemia in dermatitis herpetiformis. *Br J Dermatol* 1981; **104**: 201–4.

21 Waldinger TP, Siegle RJ, Weber W *et al.* Dapsone-induced peripheral neuropathy. Case report and review. *Arch Dermatol* 1984; **120**: 356–9.

22 Ahrens EM, Meckler RJ, Callen JP. Dapsone-induced peripheral neuropathy. *Int J Dermatol* 1986; **25**: 314–16.

23 Rhodes LE, Coleman MD, Lewis-Jones MS. Dapsone-induced motor peripheral neuropathy in pemphigus foliaceus. *Clin Exp Dermatol* 1995; **20**: 155–6.

24 Homeida M, Babikr A, Daneshmend TK. Dapsone-induced optic atrophy and motor neuropathy. *Br Med J* 1980; **281**: 1180.

25 Kenner DJ, Holt K, Agnello R, Chester GH. Permanent retinal damage following massive dapsone overdose. *Br J Ophthalmol* 1980; **64**: 741–4.

26 Guillet G, Krausz I, Guillet Guillet MH, Carlhant D. Survenue de cephalées en cours de traitement par dapsone. *Ann Dermatol Vénéréol* 1992; **119**: 46.

27 Fine J-D, Katz SI, Donahue MJ, Hendricks AA. Psychiatric reaction to dapsone and sulfapyridine. *J Am Acad Dermatol* 1983; **9**: 274–5.

Thalidomide

Teratogenicity (phocomelia), gastric intolerance, drowsiness, neuropsychiatric upset and a sensory peripheral neuropathy developing after several months have been reported [1]. A dermatitis associated with eosinophilia develops in a few cases of erythema nodosum leprosum treated with thalidomide over several years [2]. Hypersensitivity reactions characterized by fever, tachycardia, and an extensive erythematous macular eruption developed on rechallenge in a number of patients with HIV infection treated with thalidomide for severe aphthous oropharyngeal ulceration [3]. In addition, brittle fingernails, exfoliative erythroderma [4], face or limb oedema, pruritus, red palms and xerostomia have been described [5].

REFERENCES

1 Revuz J. Actualité du thalidomide. *Ann Dermatol Vénéréol* 1990; **117**: 313–21.

2 Waters MFR. An internally controlled double blind trial of thalidomide in severe erythema nodosum leprosum. *Lepr Rev* 1971; **42**: 26–42.

3 Williams I, Weller IVD, Malin A *et al.* Thalidomide hypersensitivity in AIDS. *Lancet* 1991; **337**: 436–7.

4 Bielsa I, Teixido J, Ribera M, Ferrandiz C. Erythroderma due to thalidomide: report of two cases. *Dermatology* 1994; **189**: 179–81.

5 Tseng S, Pak G, Washenik K *et al.* Rediscovering thalidomide: a review of its mechanism of action, side effects, and potential uses. *J Am Acad Dermatol* 1996; **35**: 969–79.

Antifungal drugs

Dermatological aspects of antifungal drugs have been reviewed [1–3]. Rashes occur as follows: itraconazole in 1.1% of cases, with pruritus in 0.7%, and the drug is teratogenic; fluconazole in 1.8% of cases, and exfoliative dermatitis is recorded; terbinafine in 2.7% of cases, including erythema, urticaria, eczema, pruritus, and isolated Stevens–Johnson syndrome and TEN [3].

REFERENCES

1 Lesher JL, Smith JG, Jr. Antifungal agents in dermatology. *J Am Acad Dermatol* 1987; **17**: 383–94.

2 Gupta AK, Sauder DN, Shear NH. Antifungal agents: an overview. Part I. *J Am Acad Dermatol* 1994; **30**: 677–98.

3 Gupta AK, Sauder DN, Shear NH. Antifungal agents: an overview. Part II. *J Am Acad Dermatol* 1994; **30**: 911–33.

Amphotericin

Skin reactions are rare. The 'grey syndrome', characterized by ashen colour, acral cyanosis and prostration may occur as an immediate reaction to infusion. Allergic reactions occur to liposomal amphotericin [1,2].

Fluconazole

Angio-oedema has occurred [3]. An anaphylactic reaction occurred in a patient who had previously received ketoconazole and metronidazole, suggesting cross-sensitization [4], and Stevens–Johnson syndrome has been reported in a patient with AIDS [5]. Thrombocytopenia is described [6].

Flucytosine

Transitory macular and urticarial rashes have been seen. A toxic erythema occurred in a patient [7]. Anaphylaxis has been reported in a patient with AIDS [8]. Bone-marrow depression can occur.

REFERENCES

1 Tollemar J, Ringden O, Andersson S *et al.* Randomized double-blind study of liposomal amphotericin B (Ambisome) prophylaxis of invasive fungal

infections in bone marrow transplant recipients. *Bone Marrow Transplant* 1993; **12**: 577–82.

2 Ringden O, Andstrom E, Remberger M *et al*. Allergic reactions and other rare side-effecs of liposomal amphotericin. *Lancet* 1994; **344**: 1156–7.

3 Abbott M, Hughes DL, Patel R, Kinghorn GR. Angio-oedema after fluconazole. *Lancet* 1991; **338**: 633.

4 Neuhaus G, Pavic N, Pletscher M. Anaphylactic reaction after oral fluconazole. *Br Med J* 1991; **302**: 1341.

5 Gussenhoven MJE, Haak A, Peereboom-Wynia JDR, van't Wout JW. Stevens–Johnson syndrome after fluconazole. *Lancet* 1991; **338**: 120.

6 Mercurio MG, Elewski BE. Thrombocytopenia caused by fluconazole therapy. *J Am Acad Dermatol* 1996; **32**: 525–6.

7 Thyss A, Viens P, Ticchioni M *et al*. Toxicodermieau cours d'un traitement par 5 fluorocytosine. *Ann Dermatol Vénéréol* 1987; **114**: 1131–2.

8 Kotani S, Hirose S, Niiya K *et al*. Anaphylaxis to flucytosine in a patient with AIDS. *JAMA* 1988; **260**: 3275–6.

Griseofulvin

Reactions to griseofulvin are uncommon and usually mild; headaches and gastrointestinal disturbances are the most frequent. Morbilliform, erythematous or, rarely, haemorrhagic eruptions are occasionally seen [1,2]. Photodermatitis [3,4] with sensitivity to wavelengths above 320nm is by no means rare; clinically, these are mainly eczematous, although pellagra-like changes may be seen [4]. The reaction is thought to be photoallergic and photopatch tests are positive in some cases; there may be photocross-reactivity with penicillin [4]. Histology may be non-specific; direct immunofluorescence showed immunoglobulin and complement at the dermo-epidermal junction and around papillary blood vessels in one series [4]. Urticaria and a fixed drug eruption [5,6], cold urticaria [7], severe angio-oedema [8], erythema multiforme [9], serum sickness [10], exfoliative dermatitis [11] and TEN [12,13] are recorded. Exacerbation of LE has been reported [14–18], with fatality in one case [17]. Patients with anti-SSA/Ro and SSB/La antibodies may be at an increased risk of developing a drug eruption [18,19]. Temporary granulocytopenia has been reported, and proteinuria may occur. Hepatitis and a morbilliform eruption are recorded [20]. Griseofulvin may interfere with the action of anticoagulants and the contraceptive pill [21], and should be avoided in pregnancy as potentially teratogenic; men should avoid conception for 6 months after taking the drug.

REFERENCES

1 Faergemann J, Maibach H. Griseofulvin and ketoconazole in dermatology. *Semin Dermatol* 1983; **2**: 262–9.

2 Von Pöhler H, Michalski H. Allergisches Exanthem nach Griseofulvin. *Dermatol Monatschr* 1972; **58**: 383–90.

3 Jarratt M. Drug photosensitization. *Int J Dermatol* 1976; **15**: 317–23.

4 Kojima T, Hasegawa T, Ishida H *et al*. Griseofulvin-induced photodermatitis. Report of six cases. *J Dermatol (Tokyo)* 1988; **15**: 76–82.

5 Feinstein A, Sofer E, Trau H, Schewach-Millet M. Urticaria and fixed drug eruption in a patient treated with griseofulvin. *J Am Acad Dermatol* 1984; **10**: 915–17.

6 Savage J. Fixed drug eruption to griseofulvin. *Br J Dermatol* 1977; **97**: 107–8.

7 Chang T. Cold urticaria and photosensitivity due to griseofulvin. *JAMA* 1965; **193**: 848–50.

8 Goldblatt S. Severe reaction to griseofulvin: sensitivity investigation. *Arch Dermatol* 1961; **83**: 936–7.

9 Rustin NHA, Bunker CB, Dowd P, Robinson TWE. Erythema multiforme due to griseofulvin. *Br J Dermatol* 1989; **120**: 455–8.

10 Prazak G, Ferguson JS, Comer JE, McNeil BS. Treatment of tinea pedis with griseofulvin. *Arch Dermatol* 1960; **81**: 821–6.

11 Reaves LE, III. Exfoliative dermatitis occurring in a patient treated with griseofulvin. *J Am Geriatr Soc* 1964; **12**: 889–92.

12 Taylor B, Duffill M. Toxic epidermal necrolysis from griseofulvin. *J Am Acad Dermatol* 1988; **19**: 565–7.

13 Mion G, Verdon G, Le Gulluche Y *et al*. Fatal toxic epidermal necrolysis after griseofulvin. *Lancet* 1989; **2**: 1331.

14 Alexander S. Lupus erythematosus in two patients after griseofulvin treatment of *Trichophyton rubrum* infection. *Br J Dermatol* 1962; **74**: 72–4.

15 Anderson WA, Torre D. Griseofulvin and lupus erythematosus. *J Med Soc NJ* 1966; **63**: 161–2.

16 Watsky MS, Linfield YL. Lupus erythematosus exacerbated by griseofulvin. *Cutis* 1976; **17**: 361–3.

17 Madhok R, Zoma A, Capell H. Fatal exacerbation of systemic lupus erythematosus after treatment with griseofulvin. *Br Med J* 1985; **291**: 249–50.

18 Miyagawa S, Okuchi T, Shiomi Y, Sakamoto K. Subacute cutaneous lupus erythematosus lesions precipitated by griseofulvin. *J Am Acad Dermatol* 1989; **21**: 343–6.

19 Miyagawa S, Sakamoto K. Adverse reactions to griseofulvin in patients with circulating anti-SSA/Ro and SSB/La autoantibodies. *Am J Med* 1989; **87**: 100–2.

20 Gaudin JL, Bancel B, Vial T, Bel A. Hepatite aigue cytolytique et eruption morbiliforme imputables à la prise de griseofulvin. *Gastroenterol Clin Biol* 1993; **17**: 145–6.

21 Coté J. Interaction of griseofulvin and oral contraceptives. *J Am Acad Dermatol* 1990; **22**: 124–5.

Ketoconazole

Pruritus and gastrointestinal upset are the most frequent side-effects [1]. Urticaria and angio-oedema are recorded [2]. Severe anaphylaxis has been observed in two patients, one of whom had previously reacted to topical miconazole [3]. Other adverse reactions include exfoliative erythroderma [4]. The drug may block testosterone synthesis, causing dose-dependent lowering of serum testosterone and resultant oligospermia, impotence, decreased libido and gynaecomastia in some men [5–7]. It also blocks the cortisol response to ACTH, and may lead to adrenal insufficiency [7–9]. Hypothyroidism has been documented [10]. The most serious side-effect is idiosyncratic hepatitis, which occurs in about one in 10000 patients, and which may lead to fulminant and potentially fatal hepatic necrosis [11–17]. Trichoptilosis has resulted from misuse of ketoconazole 2% shampoo [18].

REFERENCES

1 Faergemann J, Maibach H. Griseofulvin and ketoconazole in dermatology. *Semin Dermatol* 1983; **2**: 262–9.

2 Gonzalez-Delgado P, Florido-Lopez F, Saenz de San Pedro B *et al*. Hypersensitivity to ketoconazole. *Ann Allergy* 1994; **73**: 326–8.

3 Van Dijke CPH, Veerman FR, Haverkamp HC. Anaphylactic reactions to ketoconazole. *Br Med J* 1983; **287**: 1673.

4 Rand R, Sober AJ, Olmstead PM. Ketoconazole therapy and exfoliative erythroderma. *Arch Dermatol* 1983; **119**: 97–8.

5 Graybill JR, Drutz DJ. Ketoconazole: a major innovation for treatment of fungal disease. *Ann Intern Med* 1980; **93**: 921–3.

6 Moncada B, Baranda L. Ketoconazole and gynecomastia. *J Am Acad Dermatol* 1982; **7**: 557–8.
7 Pont A, Graybill JR, Craven PC *et al.* High-dose ketoconazole therapy and adrenal and testicular function in humans. *Arch Intern Med* 1984; **144**: 2150–3.
8 Pont A, Williams P, Loose D *et al.* Ketoconazole blocks adrenal steroid synthesis. *Ann Intern Med* 1982; **97**: 370–2.
9 Sonino N. The use of ketoconazole as an inhibitor of steroid production. *N Engl J Med* 1987; **317**: 812–18.
10 Kitching NH. Hypothyroidism after treatment with ketoconazole. *Br Med J* 1986; **293**: 993–4.
11 Horsburgh CR, Jr, Kirkpatrick CJ, Teutsch CB. Ketoconazole and the liver. *Lancet* 1982; **i**: 860.
12 Stern RS. Ketoconazole: assessing its risks. *J Am Acad Dermatol* 1982; **6**: 544.
13 Rollman O, Lööf L. Hepatic toxicity of ketoconazole. *Br J Dermatol* 1983; **108**: 376–8.
14 Duarte PA, Chow CC, Simmons F, Ruskin J. Fatal hepatitis associated with ketoconazole therapy. *Arch Intern Med* 1984; **144**: 1069–70.
15 Lewis J, Zimmerman HJ, Benson GD, Ishak KG. Hepatic injury associated with ketoconazole therapy: analysis of 33 cases. *Gastroenterology* 1984; **86**: 503–13.
16 Lake-Bakaar G, Scheuer PJ, Sherlock S. Hepatic reactions associated with ketoconazole in the United Kingdom. *Br Med J* 1987; **294**: 419–22.
17 Knight TE, Shikuma CY, Knight J. Ketoconazole-induced fulminant hepatitis necessitating liver transplantation. *J Am Acad Dermatol* 1991; **25**: 398–400.
18 Aljabre SH. Trichoptilosis caused by misuse of ketoconazole 2% shampoo. *Int J Dermatol* 1993; **32**: 150–1.

Nystatin

A fixed drug eruption has been reported [1], as has Stevens–Johnson syndrome in an isolated case [2].

REFERENCES

1 Pareek SS. Nystatin-induced fixed eruption. *Br J Dermatol* 1980; **103**: 679–80.
2 Garty B-Z. Stevens–Johnson syndrome associated with nystatin treatment. *Arch Dermatol* 1991; **127**: 741–2.

Terbinafine

This drug is well tolerated with few side-effects [1]. Idiosyncratic hepatitis has been reported [2]; up to September 1992, seven cases of hepatobiliary disorders of varying severity had been reported to the UK Committee on Safety of Medicines. Neutropenia and pancytopenia are recorded [3]. A severe erythema annulare centrifugum-like psoriatic drug eruption [4], erythema multiforme and Stevens–Johnson syndrome [5,6], and TEN [7] have all been reported.

REFERENCES

1 Villars V, Jones TC. Present status of the efficacy and tolerability of terbinafine (Lamisil) used systemically in the treatment of dermatomycoses of skin and nails. *J Dermatol Treat* 1990; **1** (Suppl. 2): 33–8.
2 Lowe G, Green C, Jennings P. Hepatitis associated with terbinafine treatment. *Br Med J* 1993; **306**: 248.
3 Kovacs MJ, Alshammari S, Guenther L, Bourcier M. Neutropenia and pancytopenia associated with oral terbinafine. *J Am Acad Dermatol* 1994; **31**: 806.
4 Wach F, Stolz W, Hein R, Landthaler M. Severe erythema anulare centrifugum-like psoriatic drug eruption induced by terbinafine. *Arch Dermatol* 1995; **131**: 960–1.
5 McGregor JM, Rustin MHA. Terbinafine and erythema multiforme. *Br J Dermatol* 1994; **131**: 587–8.
6 Todd P, Halpern S, Munro DD. Oral terbinafine and erythema multiforme. *Clin Exp Dermatol* 1995; **20**: 247–8.
7 White SI, Bowen-Jones D. Toxic epidermal necrolysis induced by terbinafine in a patient on long-term anti-epileptics. *Br J Dermatol* 1996; **134**: 188–9.

Antiviral agents

Aciclovir

In general, there are very few side-effects [1]. Intravenous use may cause inflammation and phlebitis. A nephropathy may develop with intravenous use, especially in patients with renal failure, due to renal precipitation of the drug; the dose should be reduced in patients with impaired renal function. An encephalopathy may occur. Peripheral oedema has been reported very rarely [2,3], as has a vesicular eruption [4].

REFERENCES

1 Arndt KA. Adverse reactions to acyclovir: topical, oral, and intravenous. *J Am Acad Dermatol* 1988; **18**: 188–90.
2 Hisler BM, Daneshvar SA, Aronson PJ, Hashimoto K. Peripheral edema and oral acyclovir. *J Am Acad Dermatol* 1988; **18**: 1142–3.
3 Medina S, Torrelo A, España A, Ledo A. Edema and oral acyclovir. *Int J Dermatol* 1991; **30**: 305–6.
4 Buck ML, Vittone SB, Zaglul HF. Vesicular eruptions following acyclovir administration. *Ann Pharmacother* 1993; **27**: 1458–9.

Azidothymidine (zidovudine)

This drug, used in the management of AIDS, may cause gastrointestinal upset and marrow suppression (with serious anaemia in 32% and leukopenia in 37%), myalgia, headache and insomnia [1–4]. Such side-effects have been reported in health-care workers treated with zidovudine for attempted prophylaxis of HIV infection following accidental needlestick injury [5,6]. Zidovudine-related thrombocytopenia resulted in ecchymoses around Kaposi's sarcoma lesions in a patient with AIDS, simulating rapid intracutaneous spread of neoplasm [7]. Vaginal tumours have been documented in rodents. Diffuse pigmentation, as well as isolated hyperpigmented spots on the palms, soles and fingers, and pigmentation of the fingernails and buccal mucosa have been described [8–13]. Postural hypotension has been recorded [14]. Hypertrichosis of the eyelids has occurred [15]. A possible link with neutrophilic eccrine hidradenitis has been postulated in HIV-infected patients [16]. Hypersensitivity reactions from rash to anaphylaxis have been documented [17,18]. Other reported cutaneous reactions including acne, pruritus, urticaria and leukocytoclastic vasculitis [19].

REFERENCES

1 Gill PS, Rarick M, Brynes RK *et al.* Azidothymidine associated with bone marrow failure in AIDS. *Ann Intern Med* 1987; **107**: 502–5.

2 Richman DD, Fiscal MA, Grieco MH *et al*. The toxicity of azidothymidine (AZT) in the treatment of patients with AIDS or AIDS-related complex: a double blind, placebo-controlled trial. *N Engl J Med* 1987; **317**: 192–7.
3 Gelmon K, Montaner JS, Fanning M *et al*. Nature, time course and dose dependence of zidovudine-related side-effects: results from the Multicenter Canadian Azidothymidine Trial. *AIDS* 1989; **3**: 555–61.
4 Moore RD, Creagh-Kirk T, Keruly J *et al*. Long-term safety and efficacy of zidovudine in patients with advanced human immunodeficiency virus infection. *Arch Intern Med* 1991; **151**: 981–6.
5 Centers for Disease Control. Public health service statement on management of occupational exposure to human immunodeficiency virus, including considerations regarding zidovudine post-exposure use. *MMWR* 1990; **39**: 1–14.
6 Jeffries DJ. Zidovudine after occupational exposure to HIV. Hospitals should be able to give it within an hour. *Br Med J* 1991; **302**: 1349–51.
7 Barnett JH, Gilson E. Zidovudine-related thrombocytopenia simulating rapid growth of Kaposi's sarcoma. *Arch Dermatol* 1991; **127**: 1068–9.
8 Azon-Masoliver A, Mallolas J, Gatell J, Castel T. Zidovudine-induced nail pigmentation. *Arch Dermatol* 1988; **124**: 1570–1.
9 Fisher CA, McPoland PR. Azidothymidine-induced nail pigmentation. *Cutis* 1989; **43**: 552–4.
10 Bendick C, Rasokat H, Steigleder GK. Azidothymidine-induced hyper-pigmentation of skin and nails. *Arch Dermatol* 1989; **125**: 1285–6.
11 Greenberg RG, Berger TG. Nail and mucocutaneous hyperpigmentation with azidothymidine therapy. *J Am Acad Dermatol* 1990; **22**: 327–30.
12 Grau-Massanes M, Millan F, Febrer MI *et al*. Pigmented nail bands and mucocutaneous pigmentation in HIV-positive patients treated with zidovudine. *J Am Acad Dermatol* 1990; **22**: 687–8.
13 Tadini G, D'Orso M, Cusini M *et al*. Oral mucosa pigmentation: a new side effect of azidothymidine therapy in patients with acquired immunodeficiency syndrome. *Arch Dermatol* 1991; **127**: 267–8.
14 Loke RHT, Murray-Lyon IM, Carter GD. Postural hypotension related to zidovudine in a patient infected with HIV. *Br Med J* 1990; **300**: 163–4.
15 Klutman NE, Hinthorn DR. Excessive growth of eyelashes in a patient with AIDS being treated with zidovudine. *N Engl J Med* 1991; **324**: 1896.
16 Smith KJ, Skelton HG, III, James WD *et al*. Neutrophilic eccrine hidradenitis in HIV-infected patients. *J Am Acad Dermatol* 1990; **23**: 945–7.
17 Carr A, Penny R, Cooper DA. Allergy and desensitization to zidovudine in patients with acquired immunodeficiency syndrome (AIDS). *J Allergy Clin Immunol* 1993; **91**: 683–5.
18 Wassef M, Keiser P. Hypersensitivity of zidovudine: report of a case of anaphylaxis and review of the literature. *Clin Infect Dis* 1995; **20**: 1387–9.
19 Torres RA, Lin RY, Lee M, Barr MR. Zidovudine-induced leukocytoclastic vasculitis. *Arch Intern Med* 1992; **152**: 850–1.

Dideoxycytidine

A maculopapular reaction with oral ulceration developed in 70% of patients treated with this new anti-AIDS agent, but resolved spontaneously in those who continued on therapy [1].

REFERENCE

1 McNeely MC, Yarchoan R, Broder S, Lawley TJ. Dermatologic complications associated with administration of 2′,3′-dideoxycytidine in patients with human immunodeficiency virus infection. *J Am Acad Dermatol* 1989; **21**: 1213–17.

Foscarnet

A generalized cutaneous rash has been reported with use of this drug in AIDS [1]. Genital ulceration, both of the penis [2,3] and vulva [4], are documented. In one study [2], 15% of 60 patients treated with intravenous foscarnet developed penile ulceration [2].

REFERENCES

1 Green ST, Nathwani D, Goldberg DJ *et al*. Generalised cutaneous rash associated with foscarnet usage in AIDS. *J Infect* 1990; **21**: 227–8.
2 Katlama C, Dohin E, Caumes E *et al*. Foscarnet induction therapy for cytomegalovirus retinitis in AIDS: comparison of twice-daily and three-times-daily regimens. *J Acquir Immune Defic Syndr* 1992; **5** (Suppl. 1): S18–24.
3 Evans LM, Grossman ME. Foscarnet-induced penile ulcer. *J Am Acad Dermatol* 1992; **27**: 124–6.
4 Caumes E, Gatineau M, Bricaire F *et al*. Foscarnet-induced vulvar erosion. *J Am Acad Dermatol* 1993; **28**: 799.

Idoxuridine

Severe alopecia and loss of nails followed parenteral use [1].

REFERENCE

1 Nolan DC, Carruthers MM, Lerner AM. *Herpesvirus hominis* encephalitis in Michigan: report of thirteen cases, including six treated with idoxuridine. *N Engl J Med* 1970; **282**: 10–13.

Protease inhibitors

Saquinivir causes rashes, and indinavir causes taste disturbance and dry skin [1].

REFERENCE

1 Anonymous. Safety issues with anti-HIV drugs. *Curr Probl Pharmacovig* 1997; **23**: 5.

Antimalarials [1–3]

Pruritus, lichenoid eruptions, exfoliative dermatitis, pigment changes, bleaching of hair, alopecia, photosensitivity with exacerbation of psoriasis and porphyria cutanea tarda, retinopathy, and corneal opacities have all been reported.

REFERENCES

1 Ribrioux A. Antipaludéens de synthese et peau. *Ann Dermatol Vénéréol* 1990; **117**: 975–90.
2 Ochsendorf FR, Runne U. Chloroquin und Hydroxychloroquin: Nebenwirkungsprofil wichtiger Therapeutika. *Hautarzt* 1991; **42**: 140–6.
3 Ziering CL, Rabinowitz LG, Esterly NB. Antimalarials for children: Indications, toxicities, and guidelines. *J Am Acad Dermatol* 1993; **28**: 764–70.

Chloroquine and hydroxychloroquine

Pruritus is common in Africans on acute or prolonged treatment, but rare in Europeans [1–4]. Pigmentary changes develop in about 25% of patients receiving any of the antimalarials for more than 4 months [5–8]; chloroquine binds to melanin [8]. Blackish-purple patches on the shins are often seen, and brown–grey pigmentation may appear in light-exposed skin [7]. The nailbeds may be pigmented diffusely or in transverse bands, and the hard palate is diffusely pigmented. By contrast, red–blonde (but not dark) hair may be bleached [9].

Photosensitivity may be seen [10]; in addition, certain types of porphyria may be provoked [11]. Effects on psoriasis are unpredictable, but precipitation of severe psoriasis has long been recognized [12–17], including erythroderma [17]. However, 88% of a series of 50 psoriatics who were treated with standard doses of chloroquine noted no change in their psoriasis [18]. Lichenoid eruptions are uncommon, and erythema annulare centrifugum is rare [19]. TEN with oral involvement has been documented. A pustular eruption with hydroxychloroquine has been reported [20]. Toxic psychosis has been described with hydroxychloroquine [21]. All antimalarials are potentially teratogenic.

Chloroquine and hydroxychloroquine may cause serious ophthalmic side-effects [22,23]. Corneal deposits occur in 95% of patients on long-term therapy, but of these 95% are asymptomatic [24]. A potentially irreversible retinopathy leading to blindness may develop in 0.5–2% of cases [25,26]. The retinal changes may progress after the drug is stopped. Use of less than 250 mg (or 4 mg/kg) daily of chloroquine, with pretreatment and 6-monthly ophthalmological assessment, using an Amsler grid, is recommended. Malarial prophylaxis with two tablets weekly is said not to carry an appreciable risk.

REFERENCES

1 Spencer HC, Poulter NR, Lury JD, Poulter CJ. Chloroquine-associated pruritus in a European. *Br Med J* 1982; **285**: 1703–4.
2 Salako LA. Toxicity and side-effects of antimalarials in Africa: a critical review. *Bull WHO* 1984; **62** (Suppl.): 63–8.
3 Mnyika KS, Kihamia CM. Chloroquine-induced pruritus: its impact on chloroquine utilization in malaria control in Dar es Salaam. *J Trop Med Hyg* 1991; **94**: 27–31.
4 Ezeamuzie IC, Igbigbi PS, Ambakederemo AW *et al.* Halofantrine-induced pruritus amongst subjects who itch to chloroquine. *J Trop Med Hyg* 1991; **94**: 184–8.
5 Dall JLC, Keane JA. Disturbances of pigmentation with chloroquine. *Br Med J* 1959; **i**: 1387–9.
6 Tuffanelli D, Abraham RK, Dubois EJ. Pigmentation from antimalarial therapy; its possible relationship to the ocular lesions. *Arch Dermatol* 1963; **88**: 419–26.
7 Levy H. Chloroquine-induced pigmentation. Case reports. *S Afr Med J* 1982; **2**: 735–7.
8 Sams WM, Epstein JH. The affinity of melanin for chloroquine. *J Invest Dermatol* 1965; **45**: 482–8.
9 Dupré A, Ortonne J-P, Viraben R, Arfeux F. Chloroquine-induced hypopigmentation of hair and freckles. Association with congenital renal failure. *Arch Dermatol* 1985; **121**: 1164–6.
10 Van Weelden H, Boling HH, Baart de la Faille H, Van Der Leun JC. Photosensitivity caused by chloroquine. *Arch Dermatol* 1982; **118**: 290.
11 Davis MJ, Vander Ploeg DE. Acute porphyria and coproporphyrinuria following chloroquine therapy: a report of two cases. *Arch Dermatol* 1957; **75**: 796–800.
12 O'Quinn SE, Kennedy CB, Naylor LZ. Psoriasis, ultraviolet light and chloroquine. *Arch Dermatol* 1964; **90**: 211–16.
13 Baker H. The influence of chloroquine and related drugs on psoriasis and keratoderma blenorrhagicum. *Br J Dermatol* 1966; **78**: 161–6.
14 Abel EA, Dicicco LM, Orenberg EK *et al.* Drugs in exacerbation of psoriasis. *J Am Acad Dermatol* 1986; **15**: 1007–22.
15 Nicolas J-F, Mauduit G, Haond J *et al.* Psoriasis grave induit par la chloroquine (nivaquine). *Ann Dermatol Vénéréol* 1988; **115**: 289–93.
16 Luzar MJ. Hydroxychloroquine in psoriatic arthropathy: exacerbation of psoriatic skin lesions. *J Rheumatol* 1982; **9**: 462–4.
17 Slagel GA, James WD. Plaquenil-induced erythroderma. *J Am Acad Dermatol* 1985; **12**: 857–62.
18 Katugampola G, Katugampola S. Chloroquine and psoriasis. *Int J Dermatol* 1990; **29**: 153–4.
19 Ashurst PJ. Erythema annulare centrifugum. Due to hydroxychloroquine sulfate and chloroquine sulfate. *Arch Dermatol* 1967; **95**: 37–9.
20 Lotem M, Ingber A, Segal R, Sandbank M. Generalized pustular drug rash induced by hydroxychloroquine. *Acta Derm Venereol (Stockh)* 1990; **70**: 250–1.
21 Ward WQ, Walter-Ryan WG, Shehi GM. Toxic psychosis: a complication of antimalarial therapy. *J Am Acad Dermatol* 1985; **12**: 863–5.
22 Olansky AJ. Antimalarials and ophthalmologic safety. *J Am Acad Dermatol* 1982; **6**: 19–23.
23 Portnoy JZ, Callen JP. Ophthalmologic aspects of chloroquine and hydroxychloroquine safety. *Int J Dermatol* 1983; **22**: 273–8.
24 Easterbrook M. Ocular side effects and safety of antimalarial agents. *Am J Med* 1988; **85**: 23–9.
25 Marks JS. Chloroquine retinopathy: is there a safe daily dose? *Ann Rheum Dis* 1982; **41**: 52–8.
26 Easterbrook M. Dose relationships in patients with early chloroquine retinopathy. *J Rheumatol* 1987; **14**: 472–5.

Mefloquine

Dizziness, nausea, erythema, and neurological disturbance are documented. Stevens–Johnson syndrome [1] and exfoliative dermatitis [2] have been recorded.

REFERENCES

1 Ven Den Enden E, Van Gompel A, Colebunders R, Van Den Ende J. Mefloquine-induced Stevens–Johnson syndrome. *Lancet* 1991; **337**: 683.
2 Martin GJ, Malone JL, Ross EV. Exfoliative dermatitis during malarial prophylaxis with mefloquine. *Clin Infect Dis* 1993; **16**: 341–2.

Mepacrine (atabrine, quinacrine)

This drug constantly causes yellow staining of the skin, which may involve the conjunctiva and may mimic jaundice [1]. Lichenoid eruptions are well known. Large numbers of military personnel given mepacrine for malaria prophylaxis in the Second World War developed a tropical lichenoid dermatitis, which was quickly followed by anhidrosis, cutaneous atrophy, alopecia, nail changes, altered pigmentation and keratoderma [2,3]. A few patients developed localized bluish-black hyperpigmentation confined to the palate, face, pretibial area and nailbeds after prolonged administration of more than a year. Years later, lichenoid nodules, scaly red plaques, atrophic lesions on the soles, erosions and leukoplakia of the tongue, and fungating warty growths appeared [3,4]. Progression to squamous cell carcinoma, especially on the palm, has occurred. Ocular toxicity is much less than with chloroquine.

REFERENCES

1 Leigh JM, Kennedy CTC, Ramsey JD, Henderson WJ. Mepacrine pigmentation in systemic lupus erythematosus. *Br J Dermatol* 1979; **101**: 147–53.
2 Bauer F. Late sequelae of atabrine dermatitis: a new premalignant entity. *Aust J Dermatol* 1978; **19**: 9–12.
3 Bauer F. Quinacrine hydrochloride drug eruption (tropical lichenoid dermatitis). Its early and late sequelae and its malignant potential. A review. *J Am Acad Dermatol* 1981; **4**: 239–48.
4 Callaway JL. Late sequelae of quinacrine dermatitis, a new premalignant entity. *J Am Acad Dermatol* 1979; **1**: 456.

Pyrimethamine

This folate antagonist can cause agranulocytosis even in very low dosage, especially when combined with dapsone [1]. A lichenoid eruption has been reported [2], as has photosensitivity. The reported rate for all serious reactions to pyrimethamine–sulphadoxine (Fansidar) in one study was 1 : 2100 prescriptions, and for cutaneous reactions including Stevens–Johnson syndrome was 1 : 4900, with a fatality rate of 1 : 11 100 [3]. In another study [4], severe cutaneous adverse reactions, including erythema multiforme, Stevens–Johnson syndrome and TEN, to Fansidar were estimated at 1.1 (0.9–1.3) per million. Similar rates for severe reactions to pyrimethamine–dapsone (Maloprim) were 1 : 9100 prescriptions, and for blood dyscrasias 1 : 20 000, with a fatality rate of 1 : 75 000. For developing countries with mainly single dose use, the risk was estimated at 0.1 per million, compared with mainly prophylactic use in Europe and North America at a risk of 10 and 36 per million, respectively. Prophylactic use thus had a 40 times higher risk than single dose therapeutic use [4]. Reactions to pyrimethamine are more common in patients with HIV infection [5]. Epidermal necrolysis, angio-oedema, bullous disorders and serious hepatic disorders also occurred. Because few serious reactions have been recorded with chloroquine and proguanil, it has been recommended that use of compound antimalarials should be restricted [3].

REFERENCES

1 Friman G, Nyström-Rosander C, Jonsell G *et al.* Agranulocytosis associated with malaria prophylaxis with Maloprim. *Br Med J* 1983; **286**: 1244–5.
2 Cutler TP. Lichen planus caused by pyrimethamine. *Clin Exp Dermatol* 1980; **5**: 253–6.
3 Phillips-Howard PA, West LJ. Serious adverse drug reactions to pyrimethamine–sulphadoxine, pyrimethamine–dapsone and to amodiaquine in Britain. *J R Soc Med* 1990; **83**: 82–5.
4 Sturchler D, Mittelholzer ML, Kerr L. How frequent are notified severe cutaneous adverse reactions to Fansidar? *Drug Saf* 1993; **8**: 160–8.
5 Piketty C, Weiss L, Picard-Dahan C *et al.* Toxidermies a la pyrimethamine chez les patients infectés par le virus de l'immunodeficience acquise. *Presse Med* 1995; **24**: 1710.

Quinine

Purpura due to quinine may or may not be thrombo-cytopenic [1,2]. Erythematous, urticarial, photo-allergic [3–5], bullous and fixed eruptions are recorded. Lichenoid eruptions are rare. If contact allergic sensitivity is already present, eczematous reactions may occur, as in 'systemic contact-type eczema' [6]. Splinter haemorrhages, and a maculopapular and a photosensitive papulonecrotic eruption, due to a lymphocytic vasculitis, has been recorded in one case [7].

REFERENCES

1 Belkin GA. Cocktail purpura. An unusual case of quinine sensitivity. *Ann Intern Med* 1967; **66**: 583–6.
2 Helmly RB, Bergin JJ, Shulman NR. Quinine-induced purpura: observation on antibody titers. *Arch Intern Med* 1967; **20**: 59–62.
3 Ljunggren B, Sjövall P. Systemic quinine photosensitivity. *Arch Dermatol* 1986; **122**: 909–11.
4 Ferguson J, Addo HA, Johnson BE *et al.* Quinine induced photosensitivity: clinical and experimental studies. *Br J Dermatol* 1987; **117**: 631–40.
5 Diffey BL, Farr PM, Adams SJ. The action spectrum in quinine photosensitivity. *Br J Dermatol* 1988; **118**: 679–85.
6 Calnan CD, Caron GA. Quinine sensitivity. *Br Med J* 1961; **ii**: 1750–2.
7 Harland CC, Millard LG. Another quirk of quinine. *Br Med J* 1991; **302**: 295.

Antihelminthics

Amocarzine (CGP 6140)

This macro- and microfilaricidal drug used for the therapy of onchocerciasis may be associated with dizziness and pruritus with or without a rash [1].

Benzimidazole compounds

These are used both for the therapy of intestinal helminthiasis and also for hydatid disease; fever, gastrointestinal upset, reversible neutropenia and transient abnormalities in liver function are reported. Telogen effluvium has been documented with both albendazole [2,3] and mebendazole.

Ivermectin

Fever, rash, pruritus, local swelling and tender regional lymphadenopathy are documented [4]. The incidence of moderate adverse reactions including pruritus, localized rash and fever was 4% in a study of patients with onchocerciasis from Ecuador [5], and increased itching and/or rash occurred in 8% of cases in another study [6]. Patients with reactive onchodermatitis (*sowda*) may have severe pruritus and limb swelling with ivermectin [7]. A 3-year placebo-controlled, double-blind trial involving 7148 patients given ivermectin annually for onchocerciasis by mass distribution identified musculosketetal pains, oedema of the face or extremities, itching and papular rash as adverse reactions; bullous skin lesions that did not recur developed in five persons [8].

Levamisole

Prolonged use at high dosage as an immunostimulant is associated with type I reactions with itching, pruritus and urticaria. Lichenoid [9] and non-specific [10] rashes, leukocytoclastic vasculitis with a reticular livedo pattern due to circulating immune complexes [11] and cutaneous necrotizing vasculitis [12] have been reported.

Niridazole

Urticaria and a pellagra-like dermatitis have been described.

Piperazine

Occupational dermatitis has been caused [13]. Previous contact sensitization induced by ethylenediamine has led to severe cross-reactions on subsequent oral administration of piperazine, including generalized exfoliative dermatitis [14].

Tetrachlorethylene

This drug has caused TEN.

Thiabendazole

An unusual body odour is well known after the administration of this drug. Skin reactions, consisting of urticaria or maculopapular rashes, are infrequent and usually mild and transient. Erythema multiforme [15] and TEN [16] have been reported.

REFERENCES

1 Poltera AA, Zea-Flores G, Guderian R *et al*. Onchocercacidal effects of amocarzine (CGP 6140) in Latin America. *Lancet* 1991; **337**: 583–4.
2 Karawifa MA, Yasawi MI, Mohamed AE. Hair loss as a complication of albendazole therapy. *Saudi Med J* 1988; **9**: 530.
3 Garcia-Muret MP, Sitjas D, Tuneu L, de Moragas JM. Telogen effluvium associated with albendazole therapy. *Int J Dermatol* 1990; **29**: 669–70.
4 Bryan RT, Stokes SL, Spencer HC. Expatriates treated with ivermectin. *Lancet* 1991; **337**: 304.
5 Guderian RH, Beck BJ, Proano S, Jr, Mackenzie CD. Onchocerciasis in Ecuador, 1980–86: epidemiological evaluation of the disease in the Esmerldas province. *Eur J Epidemiol* 1989; **5**: 294–302.
6 Whitworth JAG, Maude GH, Luty AJF. Expatriates treated with ivermectin. *Lancet* 1991; **337**: 625–6.
7 Guderian RH, Anselmi M, Sempertegui R, Cooper PJ. Adverse reactions to ivermectin in reactive onchodermatitis. *Lancet* 1991; **337**: 188.
8 Burnham GM. Adverse reactions to ivermectin treatment for onchocerciasis. Results of a placebo-controlled, double-blind trial in Malawi. *Trans R Soc Trop Med Hyg* 1993; **87**: 313–17.
9 Kirby JD, Black MM, McGibbon D. Levamisole-induced lichenoid eruptions. *J R Soc Med* 1980; **73**: 208–11.
10 Parkinson DR, Cano PO, Jerry LM *et al*. Complications of cancer immunotherapy with levamisole. *Lancet* 1977; **ii**: 1129–32.
11 Macfarlane DG, Bacon PA. Levamisole-induced vasculitis due to circulating immune complexes. *Br Med J* 1978; **i**: 407–8.
12 Scheinberg MA, Bezera JBG, Almeida LA, Silveira LA. Cutaneous necrotising vasculitis induced by levamisole. *Br Med J* 1978; **i**: 408.
13 Calnan CD. Occupational piperazine dermatitis. *Contact Dermatitis* 1975; **1**: 126.
14 Burry JN. Ethylenediamine sensitivity with a systemic reaction to piperazine treatment. *Contact Dermatitis* 1978; **4**: 380.
15 Humphreys F, Cox NH. Thiabendazole-induced erythema multiforme with lesions around melanocytic naevi. *Br J Dermatol* 1988; **118**: 855–6.
16 Robinson HM, Samorodin CS. Thiabendazole-induced toxic epidermal necrolysis. *Arch Dermatol* 1976; **112**: 1757–60.

Drugs for *Pneumocystis*

Pentamidine

This drug is increasingly being used in the treatment and prophylaxis of *Pneumocystis carinii* pneumonia in patients with AIDS. Urticaria including contact urticaria [1], or maculopapular eruption proceeding to erythroderma, has been reported with nebulized therapy [2,3]. TEN may occur with systemic therapy [4,5].

REFERENCES

1 Belsito DV. Contact urticaria from pentamidine isethionate. *Contact Dermatitis* 1993; **29**: 158–9.
2 Leen CLS, Mandal BK. Rash due to nebulised pentamidine. *Lancet* 1988; **ii**: 1250–1.
3 Berger TG, Tappero JW, Leoung GS, Jacobson MA. Aerosolized pentamidine and cutaneous eruptions. *Ann Intern Med* 1989; **110**: 1035–6.
4 Wang JJ, Freeman AI, Gaeta JF, Sinks LF. Unusual complications of pentamidine in the treatment of *Pneumocystis carinii* pneumonia. *J Pediatr* 1970; **77**: 311–14.
5 Walzer PD, Perl DP, Krogstadt DJ *et al*. *Pneumocystis carinii* pneumonia in the United States: Epidemiologic, diagnostic and clinical features. *Ann Intern Med* 1974; **80**: 83–93.

Non-steroidal anti-inflammatory drugs

Acetylsalicylic acid and related compounds

Aspirin

Reactions to aspirin [1–4] occur in 0.3% of normal subjects [2,4]. These are usually sporadic, but occasionally more than one family member may be affected, and an HLA-linkage has been reported [5]. Urticaria or angio-oedema is the commonest reaction [1]. Two types of specific IgE antibody were found in sera from aspirin-sensitive patients with salicyloyl and *O*-methylsalicyloyl disks using radioallergosorbent tests (RAST), favouring an IgE-dependent mechanism [6]. Chronic idiopathic urticaria is often aggravated by aspirin [7,8]; this exacerbation probably has a non-allergic basis. It has been estimated that patients with chronic urticaria or angio-oedema have a risk of up to 30% of developing a flare in the condition following administration of aspirin or a NSAID [3]. The reaction is dose dependent and is greater when the urticaria is in an active phase. Aspirin may render the skin of such patients more reactive to histamine [5]. The syndrome of nasal polyposis, bronchial asthma and aspirin intolerance is well known [4,9]; up to 40% of patients with nasal polyps, and 4% of patients with asthma, may develop bronchoconstriction on exposure to aspirin, but only 2% develop urticaria [4]. Anaphylactoid responses may occur [3]; these may involve abnormalities of platelet function [10]. Cross-sensitivity between aspirin and tartrazine is now thought to be rare [3]. Oral desensitization is feasible if essential, and may be maintained by daily aspirin intake [3].

Other reported reactions include purpura, scarlatiniform erythema, erythema multiforme, fixed eruption and a lichenoid eruption (which recurred on challenge) [11], but all are rare [1]. Neonatal petechiae may result from aspirin therapy of the mother [12]. Aspirin has been reported to provoke generalized pustular psoriasis [13]. Oral ulceration may follow prolonged chewing of aspirin [14], and at the site of an insoluble aspirin tablet placed at the side of an aching tooth.

Nephropathy, marrow depression and gastric haemorrhage are well-recognized hazards. The elderly are at an increased risk of developing such complications [15]. The drug may interfere with renal clearance, for example of methotrexate. Aspirin is safe to administer to patients with glucose-6-phosphate deficiency [16].

REFERENCES

1 Baker H, Moore-Robinson M. Drug reactions. IX. Cutaneous responses to aspirin and its derivatives. *Br J Dermatol* 1970; **82**: 319–21.
2 Settipane RA, Constantine HP, Settipane GA. Aspirin intolerance and recurrent urticaria in normal adults and children. Epidemiology and review. *Allergy* 1980; **35**: 149–54.
3 Stevenson DD. Diagnosis, prevention and treatment of adverse reactions to aspirin and nonsteroidal anti-inflammatory drugs. *J Allergy Clin Immunol* 1984; **74**: 617–22.
4 Morassut P, Yang W, Karsh J. Aspirin intolerance. *Semin Arthritis Rheum* 1989; **19**: 22–30.
5 Mullarkey MF, Thomas PS, Hansen JA *et al*. Association of aspirin-sensitive asthma with HLA-DQw2. *Am Rev Respir Dis* 1986; **133**: 261–3.
6 Daxun Z, Becker WM, Schulz KH, Schlaak M. Sensitivity to aspirin: a new serological diagnostic method. *J Invest Allergol Clin Immunol* 1993; **3**: 72–8.
7 Champion RH, Roberts SOB, Carpenter RG, Roger JH. Urticaria and angio-oedema. A review of 554 patients. *Br J Dermatol* 1969; **81**: 588–97.
8 Doeglas HMG. Reactions to aspirin and food additives in patients with chronic urticaria, including the physical urticarias. *Br J Dermatol* 1975; **93**: 135–44.
9 Samter M, Beers RF. Intolerance to aspirin. Clinical studies and consideration of its pathogenesis. *Ann Intern Med* 1968; **68**: 975–83.
10 Wüthrich B. Azetylsalizylsäure-Pseudoallergie: eine Anomalie der Thrombozyten-Funktion? *Hautarzt* 1988; **39**: 631–4.
11 Bharija SC, Belhaj MS. Acetylsalicylic acid may induce a lichenoid eruption. *Dermatologica* 1988; **177**: 19.
12 Stuart MJ, Gross SJ, Elrad H, Graeber JE. Effects of acetylsalicylic-acid ingestion on maternal and neonatal hemostasis. *N Engl J Med* 1982; **307**: 909–12.
13 Shelley WB. Birch pollen and aspirin psoriasis. *JAMA* 1964; **189**: 985–8.
14 Claman HN. Mouth ulcers associated with prolonged chewing of gum containing aspirin. *JAMA* 1967; **202**: 651–2.
15 Karsh J. Adverse reactions and interactions with aspirin. Considerations in the treatment of the elderly patient. *Drug Saf* 1990; **5**: 317–27.
16 Beutler E. Glucose-6-Phosphate dehydrogenase deficiency. *Lancet* 1991; **324**: 169–74.

Diflunisal

Various cutaneous reactions have been reported in up to 5% of patients, including pruritus, urticaria, exanthemata, Stevens–Johnson syndrome, erythroderma [1] and a lichenoid photoreactive rash [2]. A non-pigmenting fixed drug eruption has been documented [3].

REFERENCES

1 Chan L, Winearls C, Oliver D *et al*. Acute interstitial nephritis and erythroderma associated with diflunisal. *Br Med J* 1980; **280**: 84–5.
2 Street ML, Winkelmann RK. Lichenoid photoreactive epidermal necrosis with diflunisal. *J Am Acad Dermatol* 1989; **20**: 850–1.
3 Roetzheim RG, Herold AH, Van Durme DJ. Nonpigmenting fixed drug eruption caused by diflunisal. *J Am Acad Dermatol* 1991; **24**: 1021–22.

Paracetamol (acetaminophen)

This drug is a major metabolite of phenacetin, and has largely replaced it. Allergic reactions are very rare, considering that it has been estimated that more than 1.4 billion tablets are sold per annum in the UK [1,2]. Urticaria [3], anaphylaxis, a widespread maculopapular eruption, fixed eruption [2,4–7], exfoliative dermatitis [8] and delayed hypersensitivity reactions [9] have been seen.

REFERENCES

1 Stricker BHC, Meyboom RHB, Lindquist M. Acute hypersensitivity reactions to paracetamol. *Br Med J* 1985; **291**: 938–9.
2 Thomas RH, Munro DD. Fixed drug eruption due to paracetamol. *Br J Dermatol* 1986; **115**: 357–9.
3 Cole FOA. Urticaria from paracetamol. *Clin Exp Dermatol* 1985; **10**: 404.
4 Guin JD, Haynie LS, Jackson D, Baker GF. Wandering fixed drug eruption: a mucocutaneous reaction to acetaminophen. *J Am Acad Dermatol* 1987; **3**: 399–402.
5 Guin JD, Baker GF. Chronic fixed drug eruption caused by acetaminophen. *Cutis* 1988; **41**: 106–8.
6 Valsecchi R. Fixed drug eruption to paracetamol. *Dermatologica* 1989; **179**: 51–8.
7 Duhra P, Porter DI. Paracetamol-induced fixed drug eruption with positive immunofluorescence findings. *Clin Exp Dermatol* 1990; **15**: 293–5.
8 Girdhar A, Bagga AK, Girdhar BF. Exfoliative dermatitis due to paracetamol. *Indian J Dermatol Venereol Lepr* 1984; **50**: 162–3.
9 Ibanez MD, Alonso E, Munoz MC *et al*. Delayed hypersensitivity reaction to paracetamol (acetaminophen). *Allergy* 1996; **51**: 121–3.

Phenacetin

Capillaritis, vasculitis, and a bullous pemphigoid-like eruption [1] have been documented.

Salicylamide

Use of teething jellies containing this substance has resulted in severe urticaria in infants [2].

REFERENCES

1 Kashihara M, Danno K, Miyachi Y *et al*. Bullous pemphigoid-like lesions induced by phenacetin. Report of a case and an immunopathologic study. *Arch Dermatol* 1984; **120**: 1196–9.
2 Bentley-Phillips B. Infantile urticaria caused by salicylamide teething powder. *Br J Dermatol* 1968; **80**: 341.

Other NSAIDs

Dermatological aspects of the NSAIDs have been extensively reviewed [1–13]. All of these drugs inhibit the enzyme cyclo-oxygenase, and decrease the production of prostaglandins and thromboxanes [6]. NSAIDs represent about 5% of all prescriptions in the UK [5] and USA [2]; nearly one in seven Americans were treated with a NSAID in 1984, and in 1986 100 million prescriptions for these drugs were written in the USA [14]. NSAIDs accounted for 25% of all suspected adverse drug reactions reported to the UK Committee on Safety of Medicines in 1986 [5,15]. Reactions to NSAIDs occur in about one in 50 000 administrations; NSAIDs should be avoided in patients known to be intolerant of aspirin [6]. In a large series, allergic or pseudoallergic reactions were observed in 0.2% of patients exposed to minor analgesics (including aspirin and pyrazolones, mainly metamizole, propyphenazone) and in 0.8% of patients exposed to NSAIDs (including the pyrazolone oxyphenbutazone); most reactions were cutaneous, mainly maculopapular exanthemata, urticaria and angio-oedema [10]. Piroxicam, meclofenamate sodium, sulindac, and zomepirac sodium had the highest reaction rates relative to the number of new prescriptions in the US [1,2]. In contrast, naproxen, fenoprofen, ibuprofen and indomethacin all had low rates of reaction; ibuprofen is available as a non-prescription drug in the US and the UK. In another study of 2747 patients with rheumatoid arthritis, toxicity index scores computed from symptoms, laboratory abnormalities and hospitalizations attributed to NSAID therapy indicated that indomethacin, tolmetin sodium and meclofenamate sodium were the most toxic, and buffered aspirin, salsalate and ibuprofen the least toxic [16].

Cutaneous adverse reactions to NSAIDs were, in order of frequency in one study [11], urticaria/angio-oedema, fixed eruptions, exanthemata, erythema multiforme and Stevens–Johnson syndrome. Drug exanthemata and urticaria occur in 0.2–9% of patients treated with NSAIDs [2,6]. Drug exanthemata develop in 1% of patients on phenylbutazone, and 0.3% of patients on indomethacin [6]; they are most frequently associated with diflunisal, sulindac, meclofenamate sodium, piroxicam and phenylbutazone. All of the NSAIDs, but particularly aspirin and tolmetin, may cause urticaria and anaphylactoid reactions, especially in a patient with a history of aspirin-induced urticaria. Pyrazolone NSAIDs, feprazone, nimesulide, piroxicam and flurbiprofen cause fixed drug eruptions. While all NSAIDs may precipitate exfoliative erythroderma, this is commonest with phenylbutazone [6]. All of the NSAIDs, but particularly phenylbutazone, piroxicam, fenbufen and sulindac, may cause Stevens–Johnson syndrome or TEN [6]. Oral lichenoid lesions have also been recorded with NSAIDs [17]. Psoriasis has been reported anecdotally to be exacerbated by indomethacin and meclofenamate sodium, but there is no definitive evidence that NSAIDs consistently exacerbate psoriasis [5]. Contact dermatitis induced by topical NSAIDs is rare but increasing; ketoprofen and bufexamac are major contact allergens [13]. Children on NSAIDs were 2.4 times as likely to have shallow facial scars, as described in drug-induced pseudoporphyria, in one study; this relative risk was increased to 6 with naproxen [18].

Most of the NSAIDs causing photosensitivity are phenylpropionic acid derivatives: carprofen, ketoprofen, tiaprofenic acid, naproxen and nabumetone [19–24]. NSAIDs that cause photosensitivity absorb UV radiation at longer than 310 nm, resulting in the generation of singlet oxygen molecules, which damage cell membranes [12]. The cutaneous photosensitivity appears to be elicited by a phototoxic mechanism [19–21,24]. The phototoxic reactions with NSAIDs are immediate, consisting of itching, burning, erythema and at higher fluences wealing; this contrasts with the delayed reactions associated with psoralens and tetracyclines, which produce abnormal delayed erythema or exaggerated sunburn. Propionic acid derivatives may also precipitate photo-urticaria by mast-cell degranulation [23]. Piroxicam, an enolic acid derivative structurally unrelated to phenylpropionic acid, is the most frequently cited non-phenylpropionic acid NSAID to cause photosensitivity [20,21,25]; phototoxicity to the parent drug has not been elicited in volunteers or experimental animals, although a phototoxic metabolite has been identified *in vitro*. Indomethacin, sulindac [26], meclofenamate sodium and phenylbutazone have all been associated with photosensitivity [2]. NSAIDs may cause pseudoporphyria changes [27].

Apart from the cutaneous complications, NSAIDs may cause a variety of adverse effects [14,28–30], including gastrointestinal bleeding, intestinal perforations and acute deterioration in renal function with interstitial nephritis [28]; the elderly and patients with impaired renal function or receiving concomitant diuretic therapy are most at risk. NSAIDs may inhibit platelet aggregation and increase bleeding times [29]. Aplastic anaemia is a recognized complication, and has occurred in the same individual with two different NSAIDs (sulindac and fenbufen) [31]. Hepatic syndromes [30], pneumonitis (naproxen, ibuprofen, fenoprofen and sulindac can elicit pulmonary infiltrates with eosinophilia [32]) and neurological problems, such as headache, aseptic meningitis and dizziness, are recorded [14]. Niflumic acid and diclofenac both precipitated a dermatomyositis-like syndrome in a patient [33]. The potential for adverse interactions between NSAIDs and other drugs is considerable [14].

REFERENCES

1 Stern RS, Bigby M. An expanded profile of cutaneous reactions to nonsteroid anti-inflammatory drugs. Reports to a specialty-based system for spontaneous reporting of adverse reactions to drugs. *JAMA* 1984; **252**: 1433–7.

2 Bigby M, Stern R. Cutaneous reactions to non-steroidal anti-inflammatory drugs. A review. *J Am Acad Dermatol* 1985; **12**: 866–76.

3 O'Brien WM, Bagby GF. Rare reactions to nonsteroidal anti-inflammatory drugs. *J Rheumatol* 1985; **12**: 13–20.

4 Roujeau JC. Clinical aspects of skin reactions to NSAIDs. *Scand J Rheumatol* 1987; **65** (Suppl.): 131–4.

5 Greaves MW. Pharmacology and significance of nonsteroidal anti-inflammatory drugs in the treatment of skin diseases. *J Am Acad Dermatol* 1987; **16**: 751–64.

6 Bigby M. Nonsteroidal anti-inflammatory drug reactions. *Semin Dermatol* 1989; **8**: 182–6.

7 Arnaud A. Allergy and intolerance to nonsteroidal anti-inflammatory agents. *Clin Rev Allergy Immunol* 1995; **13**: 245–51.

8 Van Arsdel PP, Jr. Pseudoallergic reactions to nonsteroidal anti-inflammatory drugs. *JAMA* 1991; **266**: 3343–4.

9 Bottoni A, Criscuolo D. Cutaneous adverse reactions following the administration of nonsteroidal antiinflammatory drugs and antibiotics: an Italian survey. *Int J Clin Pharmacol Ther Toxicol* 1992; **30**: 257–9.

10 Oberholzer B, Hoigne R, Hartmann K *et al*. Die Haufigkeit von unerwunschten Arzneimittelwirkungen nach Symptomen und Syndrome. Aus den Erfahrungen des CHDM und der SANZ. Als Beispiel: die allergischen und pseudoallergischen Reaktionen unter leichten Analgetika und NSAIDs. *Therapeut Umschau* 1993; **50**: 13–19.

11 Anonymous. Cutaneous reactions to analgesic-antipyretics and nonsteroidal anti-inflammatory drugs. Analysis of reports to the spontaneous reporting system of the Gruppo Italiano Studi Epidemiologici in Dermatologia. *Dermatology* 1993; **186**: 164–9.

12 Figueras A, Capella D, Castel JM, Laorte JR. Spontaneous reporting of adverse drug reactions to non-steroidal anti-inflammatory drugs. A report from the Spanish System of Pharmacovigilance, including an early analysis of topical and enteric-coated formulations. *Eur J Clin Pharmacol* 1994; **47**: 297–303.

13 Gebhardt M, Wollina U. Kutane Nebenwirkungen nichtsteroidaler Antiphlogistika (NSAID). *Zeitschr Rheumatol* 1995; **54**: 405–12.

14 Brooks PM, Day RO. Nonsteroidal antiinflammatory drugs—differences and similarities. *N Engl J Med* 1991; **324**: 1716–25.

15 Committee on Safety of Medicines. Nonsteroidal anti-inflammatory drugs and serious gastrointestinal adverse reaction—1. *Br Med J* 1986; **292**: 614.

16 Fries JF, Williams CA, Bloch DA. The relative toxicity of nonsteroidal antiinflammatory drugs. *Arthritis Rheum* 1991; **34**: 1353–60.

17 Hamburger J, Potts AJC. Non-steroidal anti-inflammatory drugs and oral lichenoid reactions. *Br Med J* 1983; **287**: 1258.

18 Wallace CA, Farrow D, Sherry DD. Increased risk of facial scars in children taking nonsteroidal antiinflammatory drugs. *J Pediatr* 1994; **125**: 819–22.

19 Ljunggren B. Propionic acid-derived nonsteroidal anti-inflammatory drugs are phototoxic *in vitro*. *Photodermatology* 1985; **2**: 3–9.

20 Stern RS. Phototoxic reactions to piroxicam and other nonsteroidal antiinflammatory agents. *N Engl J Med* 1983; **309**: 186–7.

21 Diffey BL, Daymond TJ, Fairgreaves H. Phototoxic reactions to piroxicam, naproxen and tiaprofenic acid. *Br J Rheumatol* 1983; **22**: 239–42.

22 Przybilla B, Ring J, Schwab U *et al*. Photosensibilisierende Eigenschaften nichtsteroidaler Antirheumatika im Photopatch-Test. *Hautarzt* 1987; **38**: 18–25.

23 Kaidbey KH, Mitchell FN. Photosensitizing potential of certain nonsteroidal anti-inflammatory agents. *Arch Dermatol* 1989; **125**: 783–6.

24 Kochevar IE. Phototoxicity of nonsteroidal inflammatory drugs. Coincidence or specific mechanism? *Arch Dermatol* 1989; **125**: 824–6.

25 Serrano G, Bonillo J, Aliaga A *et al*. Piroxicam-induced photosensitivity and contact sensitivity to thiosalicylic acid. *J Am Acad Dermatol* 1990; **23**: 479–83.

26 Jeanmougin M, Manciet J-R, Duterque M *et al*. Photosensibilisation au sulindac. *Ann Dermatol Vénéréol* 1987; **114**: 1400–1.

27 Taylor BJ, Duffill MB. Pseudoporphyria from nonsteroidal anti-inflammatory drugs. *NZ Med J* 1987; **100**: 322–3.

28 Clive DM, Stoff JS. Renal syndromes associated with nonsteroidal anti-inflammatory drugs. *N Engl J Med* 1984; **310**: 563–72.

29 Ekenny GN. Potential renal, haematological and allergic adverse effects associated with nonsteroidal anti-inflammatory drugs. *Drugs* 1992; **44** (Suppl. 5): 31–7.

30 Carson JL, Willett LR. Toxicity of nonsteroidal anti-inflammatory drugs. An overview of the epidemiological evidence. *Drugs* 1993; **46** (Suppl. 1): 243–8.

31 Andrews R, Russell N. Aplastic anaemia associated with a non-steroidal anti-inflammatory drug: relapse after exposure to another such drug. *Br Med J* 1990; **301**: 38.

32 Goodwin SD, Glenny RW. Nonsteroidal anti-inflammatory drug-associated pulmonary infiltrates with eosinophilia. Review of the literature and Food and Drug Administration Adverse Drug Reaction reports. *Arch Intern Med* 1992; **152**: 1521–4.

33 Grob JJ, Collet AM, Bonerandi JJ. Dermatomyositis-like syndrome induced by nonsteroidal anti-inflammatory agents. *Dermatologica* 1989; **178**: 58–9.

Proprionic acid derivatives

Carprofen. This drug causes photosensitivity [1].

Fenbufen. Morbilliform and erythematous rashes, erythema multiforme [2], Stevens–Johnson syndrome and allergic vasculitis have been recorded rarely. Fenbufen has caused exfoliative dermatitis, haemolytic anaemia and hepatitis [3], and was the drug implicated most commonly in adverse reactions reported to the UK Committee on Safety of Medicines in 1986 and 1987. A florid erythematous rash with pulmonary eosinophilia has been described in four cases [4].

Fenoprofen. This drug has caused pruritus, urticaria, vesicobullous eruption, thrombocytopenic purpura and TEN [5].

Ibuprofen. Pruritus is the only common cutaneous reaction. When used in rheumatoid arthritis, rashes are rare, but patients with systemic LE are liable to develop a generalized rash with fever and abdominal symptoms [6]. Angio-oedema/urticaria [7], fixed eruptions, vesicobullous rashes, erythema multiforme, vasculitis and alopecia [8] occur. Psoriasis has been reported to be exacerbated [9]. This drug is available over the counter in the UK.

Ketoprofen. Topical application has caused photo-allergic contact dermatitis [10] and systemic ketoprofen has caused pseudoporphyria.

Naproxen. The incidence of side-effects is low given the widespread and long-term use of naproxen. Rashes occur in about 5% of patients; pruritus is the commonest symptom. Naproxen is associated with a photosensitivity dermatitis [11] and pseudoporphyria [12–16]; most naproxen photo-urticarial reactions are evoked by the UVA band. Urticaria/angio-oedema, anaphylaxis [17], purpura and thrombocytopenia [18], hyperhidrosis, acneiform problems in women [19], vasculitis [20,21], vesicobullous and fixed drug eruptions [22], erythema multiforme, a pustular reaction [23] and lichen planus-like reaction [24] have all been reported, as has recurrent allergic sialadenitis [25].

Tiaprofenic acid. This drug may cause photosensitivity [26].

REFERENCES

1 Merot Y, Harms M, Saurat JH. Photosensibilisation au carprofén (imadyl), un nouvel anti-inflammatoire non stéroidien. *Dermatologica* 1983; **166**: 301–7.
2 Peacock A, Ledingham J. Fenbufen-induced erythema multiforme. *Br Med J* 1981; **283**: 582.
3 Muthiah MM. Severe hypersensitivity reaction to fenbufen. *Br Med J* 1988; **297**: 1614.
4 Burton GH. Rash and pulmonary eosinophilia associated with fenbufen. *Br Med J* 1990; **300**: 82–3.
5 Stotts JS, Fang ML, Dannaker CJ, Steinman HK. Fenoprofen-induced toxic epidermal necrolysis. *J Am Acad Dermatol* 1988; **18**: 755–7.
6 Shoenfeld Y, Livni E, Shaklai M, Pinkhas J. Sensitization to ibuprofen in SLE. *JAMA* 1980; **244**: 547–8.
7 Shelley ED, Shelley WB. Ibuprofen urticaria. *J Am Acad Dermatol* 1987; **17**: 1057–8.
8 Meyer HC. Alopecia associated with ibuprofen. *JAMA* 1979; **242**: 142.
9 Ben-Chetrit E, Rubinow A. Exacerbation of psoriasis by ibuprofen. *Cutis* 1986; **38**: 45.
10 Alomar A. Ketoprofen photodermatitis. *Contact Dermatitis* 1985; **12**: 112–13.
11 Shelley WB, Elpern DJ, Shelley ED. Naproxen photosensitization demonstrated by challenge. *Cutis* 1986; **38**: 169–70.
12 Farr PM, Diffey BL. Pseudoporphyria due to naproxen. *Lancet* 1985; **i**: 1166–7.
13 Judd LE, Henderson DW, Hill DC. Naproxen-induced pseudoporphyria: a clinical and ultrastructural study. *Arch Dermatol* 1986; **122**: 451–4.
14 Mayou S, Black MM. Pseudoporphyria due to naproxen. *Br J Dermatol* 1986; **114**: 519–20.
15 Burns DA. Naproxen pseudoporphyria in a patient with vitiligo. *Clin Exp Dermatol* 1987; **12**: 296–7.
16 Levy ML, Barron KS, Eichenfield A, Honig PJ. Naproxen-induced pseudoporphyria: a distinctive photodermatitis. *J Pediatr* 1990; **117**: 660–4.
17 Cistero A, Urias S, Guindo J et al. Coronary artery spasm and acute myocardial infarction in naproxen-associated anaphylactic reaction. *Allergy* 1992; **47**: 576–8.
18 Hunt PJ, Gibbons SS. Naproxen induced thrombocytopenia: a case report. *NZ Med J* 1995; **108**: 483–4.
19 Hamman CO. Severe primary dysmenorrhea treated with naproxen. A prospective, double-blind crossover investigation. *Prostaglandins* 1980; **19**: 651–7.
20 Grennan DM, Jolly J, Holloway LJ, Palmer DG. Vasculitis in a patient receiving naproxen. *NZ Med J* 1979; **89**: 48–9.
21 Singhal PC, Faulkner M, Venkatesham J, Molho L. Hypersensitivity angiitis associated with naproxen. *Ann Allergy* 1989; **63**: 107–9.
22 Habbema L, Bruynzeel DP. Fixed drug eruption due to naproxen. *Dermatologica* 1987; **174**: 184–5.
23 Grattan CEH. Generalized pustular drug rash due to naproxen. *Dermatologica* 1989; **179**: 57–8.
24 Heymann WR, Lerman JS, Luftschein S. Naproxen-induced lichen planus. *J Am Acad Dermatol* 1984; **10**: 299–301.
25 Knulst AC, Stengs CJ, Baart de la Faille H et al. Salivary gland swelling following naproxen therapy. *Br J Dermatol* 1995; **133**: 647–9.
26 Neumann RA, Knobler RM, Lindemayr H. Tiaprofenic acid-induced photosensitivity. *Contact Dermatitis* 1989; **20**: 270–3.

Phenylacetic acids

Diclofenac. A variety of cutaneous adverse effects [1,2], including pruritus, urticaria, various exanthemata, papulo-vesicular eruptions [3], delayed allergy [4], vasculitis [5], a bullous eruption associated with linear basement-membrane deposition of IgA [6] and fatal erythema multiforme [1] have been recorded.

REFERENCES

1 Ciucci AG. A review of spontaneously reported adverse drug reactions with diclofenac sodium (voltarol). *Rheum Rehabil* 1979; **Suppl. 2**: 116–21.
2 O'Brien WM. Adverse reactions to nonsteroidal antiinflammatory drugs. Diclofenac compared with other nonsteroidal antiinflammatory drugs. *Am J Med* 1986; **80**: 70–80.
3 Seigneuric C, Nougué J, Plantavid M. Érythème polymorphe avec atteinte muqueuse: responsabilité du diclofénac? *Ann Dermatol Vénéréol* 1982; **109**: 287.
4 Schiavino D, Papa G, Nucera E et al. Delayed allergy to diclofenac. *Contact Dermatitis* 1992; **26**: 357–8.
5 Bonafé J-L, Mazières B, Bouteiller G. Trisymptôme de Gougerot induit par les anti-inflammatoires. Rôle du diclofénac? *Ann Dermatol Vénéréol* 1982; **109**: 283–4.
6 Gabrielson TØ, Staerfelt F, Thune PO. Drug induced bullous dermatosis with linear IgA deposits along the basement membrane. *Acta Derm Venereol (Stockh)* 1981; **61**: 439–41.

Oxicams

Piroxicam. This drug may cause adverse cutaneous reactions in 2–3% of patients [1,2]. More than two-thirds of affected patients have photosensitivity; lesions may be vesicobullous or eczematous, and occur within 3 days of starting therapy in 50% of cases [3–10]. Photosensitivity may result from phototoxic metabolites [7]. Photocontact dermatitis developed in three patients after the application of a gel containing 0.5% piroxicam. Patch tests were positive to thiomersal and thiosalicylic acid and photopatch tests with piroxicam were positive. Patch tests in patients with systemic photosensitivity to piroxicam were also positive for thiomersal and thiosalicylic acid. Contact allergic sensitivity to the latter is a marker for patients with a high risk of developing photosensitivity reactions to piroxicam [10].

Other eruptions include urticaria, maculopapular [11] or lichenoid rashes, alopecia, erythema multiforme [12] and vasculitis [13]. Piroxicam was well tolerated in patients with an urticarial reaction to a single NSAID, but provoked urticaria in 27% of patients with allergy to at least two different NSAIDs, indicating that mechanisms other than interference with prostaglandin synthesis and release of inflammatory mediators participate in allergic reactions to NSAIDs [14]. Classical fixed drug eruption [15,16] and a non-pigmenting fixed drug reaction [17], with cross-sensitivity among piroxicam, tenoxicam, and droxicam in one case [18], have also been reported. Contact sensitivity to piroxicam is recorded [19]. Piroxicam was thought to have triggered subacute LE in a patient with Sjögren's syndrome and seronegative arthritis [20]. Isolated case reports of fatal pemphigus vulgaris [21] and fatal TEN [22] have appeared. The drug has caused peripheral neuropathy and erythroderma [23]. Blood dyscrasias have been reported.

REFERENCES

1 Pitts N. Efficacy and safety of piroxicam. *Am J Med* 1982; **72** (Suppl. 2A): 77–87.
2 Gerber D. Adverse reactions of piroxicam. *Drug Intell Clin Pharmacol* 1987; **21**: 707–10.
3 Stern RS. Phototoxic reactions to piroxicam and other nonsteroidal antiinflammatory agents. *N Engl J Med* 1983; **309**: 186–7.
4 Diffey BL, Daymond TJ, Fairgreaves H. Phototoxic reactions to piroxicam, naproxen and tiaprofenic acid. *Br J Rheumatol* 1983; **22**: 239–42.
5 Serrano G, Bonillo J, Aliaga A *et al*. Piroxicam-induced photosensitivity. *J Am Acad Dermatol* 1984; **11**: 113–20.
6 McKerrow KJ, Greig DE. Piroxicam-induced photosensitive dermatitis. *J Am Acad Dermatol* 1986; **15**: 1237–41.
7 Kochevar IE, Morison WL, Lamm JL *et al*. Possible mechanism of piroxicam-induced photosensitivity. *Arch Dermatol* 1986; **122**: 1283–7.
8 Kaidbey KH, Mitchell FN. Photosensitizing potential of certain nonsteroidal anti-inflammatory agents. *Arch Dermatol* 1989; **125**: 783–6.
9 Kochevar IE. Photoxicity of nonsteroidal inflammatory drugs. Coincidence or specific mechanism? *Arch Dermatol* 1989; **125**: 824–6.
10 Serrano G, Bonillo J, Aliaga AET *et al*. Piroxicam-induced photosensitivity and contact sensitivity to thiosalicylic acid. *J Am Acad Dermatol* 1990; **23**: 479–83.
11 Faure M, Goujon C, Perrot H *et al*. Accidents cutanés provoqués par le piroxicam. A propos de trois observations. *Ann Dermatol Vénéréol* 1982; **109**: 255–8.
12 Bertail M-A, Cavelier B, Civatte J. Réaction au piroxicam (Feldène®). A type d'ectoderme érosive pluri-orificielle. *Ann Dermatol Vénéréol* 1982; **109**: 261–2.
13 Goebel KN, Mueller-Brodman W. Reversible overt nephropathy with Henoch-Schönlein purpura due to piroxicam. *Br Med J* 1982; **284**: 311–12.
14 Carmona MJ, Blanca M, Garcia A *et al*. Intolerance to piroxicam in patients with adverse reactions to nonsteroidal antiinflammatory drugs. *J Allergy Clin Immunol* 1992; **90**: 873–9.
15 Stubb S, Reitamo S. Fixed drug eruption caused by piroxicam. *J Am Acad Dermatol* 1990; **22**: 1111–12.
16 de la Hoz B, Soria C, Fraj J *et al*. Fixed drug eruption due to piroxicam. *Int J Dermatol* 1990; **29**: 672–3.
17 Valsecchi R, Cainelli T. Nonpigmenting fixed drug reaction to piroxicam. *J Am Acad Dermatol* 1989; **21**: 1300.
18 Ordoqui E, De Barrio M, Rodriguez VM *et al*. Cross-sensitivity among oxicams in piroxicam-caused fixed drug eruption: two case reports. *Allergy* 1995; **50**: 741–4.
19 Valsecchi R, Pansera B, di Landro A, Cainelli T. Contact sensitivity to piroxicam. *Contact Dermatitis* 1993; **29**: 167.
20 Roura M, Lopez-Gil F, Umbert P. Systemic lupus erythematosus exacerbated by piroxicam. *Dermatologica* 1991; **182**: 56–8.
21 Martin RL, McSweeny GW, Schneider J. Fatal pemphigus vulgaris in a patient taking piroxicam. *N Engl J Med* 1983; **309**: 795–6.
22 Roujeau JC, Revuz I, Touraine R *et al*. Syndrome de Lyell au cours d'un traitement par un nouvel antiinflammatoire. *Nouv Presse Med* 1981; **10**: 3407–8.
23 Sangla I, Blin O, Jouglard J *et al*. Neuropathic axonale et toxidermie iatrogene par le piroxicam. Manifestations d'hypersensibilite? *Rev Neurol* 1993; **149**: 217–18.

Anthranilic acids

Meclofenate sodium. Rashes occur in up to 9% of patients. More than two-thirds of reactions have been exanthematous, with prominent pruritus; vasculitic, purpuric or petechial reactions are also noted, as well as occasional urticaria, fixed drug eruption, erythema multiforme [1], exfoliative erythroderma and a vesicobullous reaction. It has been reported to exacerbate psoriasis [2]. Selective adverse reactions to glafenine and meclofenamate occurred in a patient tolerating aspirin and other cyclo-oxygenase inhibitors [3].

Mefenamic acid. Urticaria, a morbilliform eruption, fixed drug eruption [4,5] and generalized exfoliative dermatitis are documented. Acute renal failure, severe thrombocytopenia and jaundice developed after a small dose of mefenamic acid in one patient with drug-dependent antibodies reacting against platelets [6].

REFERENCES

1 Harrington T, Davis D. Erythema multiforme induced by meclofenamate sodium. *J Rheumatol* 1983; **10**: 169–70.
2 Meyerhoff JO. Exacerbation of psoriasis with meclofenamate. *N Engl J Med* 1983; **309**: 496.
3 Fernandez-Rivas M, de la Hoz B, Cuevas M *et al*. Hypersensitivity reactions to anthranilic acid derivatives. *Ann Allergy* 1993; **71**: 515–18.
4 Wilson DL, Otter A. Fixed drug eruption associated with mefenamic acid. *Br Med J* 1986; **293**: 1243.
5 Watson A, Watt G. Fixed drug eruption to mefenamic acid. *Australas J Dermatol* 1986; **27**: 6–7.
6 Schwartz D, Gremmel F, Kurz R *et al*. Case report: acute renal failure, thrombocytopenia and nonhemolytic icterus probably caused by mefenamic acid (Parkemed)-dependent antibodies. *Beitrage Infusionsther* 1992; **30**: 413–15.

Heterocyclic acetic acids

Indomethacin. Allergic reactions are very uncommon, but pruritus, urticaria, purpura and morbilliform eruptions are documented. Stomatitis [1] and thrombocytopenia occur rarely, as well as a generalized exfoliative dermatitis and TEN necrolysis [2]. Vasculitis has been documented [3]. There have been rare reports of exacerbation of psoriasis [4,5]; however, indomethacin in a standard dose of 75 mg/day had no significant harmful effect on psoriasis in a series of patients treated with the Ingram regimen of coal-tar bath, suberythemal UV B phototherapy and dithranol in Lassar's paste [6]. Exacerbation of dermatitis herpetiformis has been recorded [7].

REFERENCES

1 Guggenheimer J, Ismail YH. Oral ulcerations associated with indomethacin therapy: report of three cases. *J Am Dent Assoc* 1975; **90**: 632–4.
2 O'Sullivan M, Hanly JG, Molloy M. A case of toxic epidermal necrolysis secondary to indomethacin. *Br J Rheumatol* 1983; **22**: 47–9.
3 Marsh FP, Almeyda JR, Levy IS. Non-thrombocytopenic purpura and acute glomerulonephritis after indomethacin therapy. *Ann Rheum Dis* 1971; **30**: 501–5.
4 Katayama H, Kawada A. Exacerbation of psoriasis induced by indomethacin. *J Dermatol (Tokyo)* 1981; **8**: 323–7.
5 Powles AV, Griffiths CEM, Seifert MH, Fry L. Exacerbation of psoriasis by indomethacin. *Br J Dermatol* 1987; **117**: 799–800.
6 Sheehan-Dare RA, Goodfield MJD, Rowell NR. The effect of oral indomethacin on psoriasis treated with the Ingram regime. *Br J Dermatol* 1991; **125**: 253–5.
7 Griffiths CEM, Leonard JN, Fry L. Dermatitis herpetiformis exacerbated by indomethacin. *Br J Dermatol* 1985; **112**: 443–5.

Sulindac. Rashes occur in up to 9% of patients. The drug has caused anaphylaxis [1] and anaphylactoid reactions [2], photosensitivity [3], facial and oral erythema, a pernio-like reaction [4] and fixed drug eruption [5].

Stevens–Johnson syndrome [6–8], TEN [6,9], serum sickness and exfoliative erythroderma are documented. Blood dyscrasias, toxic hepatitis, pancreatitis, and aseptic meningitis in patients with systemic LE are recorded.

Tolmetin. Anaphylactoid reactions are well recognized [10]. TEN has been recorded.

REFERENCES

1 Smith F, Lindberg P. Life-threatening hypersensitivity to sulindac. *JAMA* 1980; **244**: 269–70.
2 Hyson CP, Kazakoff MA. A severe multisystem reaction to sulindac. *Arch Intern Med* 1991; **151**: 387–8.
3 Jeanmougin M, Manciet J-R, Duterque M *et al*. Photosensibilisation au sulindac. *Ann Dermatol Vénéréol* 1987; **114**: 1400–1.
4 Reinertsen J. Unusual pernio-like reaction to sulindac. *Arthritis Rheum* 1981; **24**: 1215.
5 Aram HA. Fixed drug eruption due to sulindac. *Int J Dermatol* 1984; **23**: 421.
6 Levitt L, Pearson RW. Sulindac-induced Stevens–Johnson toxic epidermal necrolysis syndrome. *JAMA* 1980; **243**: 1262–3.
7 Husain Z, Runge LA, Jabbs JM, Hyla JA. Sulindac-induced Stevens–Johnson syndrome: report of 3 cases. *J Rheumatol* 1981; **8**: 176–9.
8 Maguire FW. Stevens–Johnson syndrome due to sulindac: a case report and review of the literature. *Del Med J* 1981; **53**: 193–7.
9 Chevrant Breton J, Pibouin M, Allain H *et al*. Toxic epidermal necrolysis induced by sulindac. *Thérapie* 1985; **40**: 67–9.
10 Rossi A, Knapp D. Tolmetin-induced anaphylactoid reactions. *N Engl J Med* 1982; **307**: 499–500.

Pyrazolones

Amidopyrine (aminophenazone). This is the most dangerous of all analgesics and has caused hundreds of deaths due to blood dyscrasias. It has been withdrawn from western Europe and North America but is still available in certain parts of the world. TEN, exfoliative dermatitis and erythema multiforme are all well known.

Azapropazone. Photosensitivity is recognized [1]. A multi-focal bullous fixed drug eruption resembling erythema multiforme, has been reported [2]. A bullous eruption on the face and extremities, with histological features suggestive of pemphigoid but negative immunofluorescence was reported [3]. The drug is contraindicated in patients receiving warfarin, as the latter medication is potentiated [4].

REFERENCES

1 Olsson S, Biriell C, Boman G. Photosensitivity during treatment with azapropazone. *Br Med J* 1985; **291**: 939.
2 Sowden JM, Smith AG. Multifocal fixed drug eruption mimicking erythema multiforme. *Clin Exp Dermatol* 1990; **15**: 387–8.
3 Barker DJ, Cotterill JA. Skin eruptions due to azapropazone. *Lancet* 1977; **i**: 90.
4 Win N, Mitchell DC. Azapropazone and warfarin. *Br Med J* 1991; **302**: 969–70.

Phenylbutazone and oxyphenbutazone. Reactions have been frequent and often fatal [1,2]. Therefore, in the UK oxyphenbutazone has been withdrawn and phenyl-butazone is restricted to hospital usage for ankylosing spondylitis. Pruritus, morbilliform eruptions, urticaria, and buccal ulceration are the commonest; erythema multiforme, fixed eruptions (especially with oxyphenbutazone), generalized exfoliative dermatitis and TEN [3] are all well-documented hazards. Drug exanthemata or erythro-derma may occur in up to 4% of treated patients with phenylbutazone. Occasional reports of exacerbation of psoriasis have occurred [4]. Rarer reactions have included generalized lymphadenopathy, a Sjögren-like syndrome, non-thrombocytopenic purpura, allergic vasculitis [5] and polyarteritis nodosa. Provocation of temporal arteritis has been reported. A haemorrhagic bullous eruption of the hands was observed in three patients [6]. Cutaneous necrosis has been seen after intramuscular injection. Phenylbutazone causes fluid retention, gastrointestinal bleeding and bone-marrow depression [2]; the hazards of the latter are greatly increased if the dose exceeds 200 mg/day.

REFERENCES

1 Van Joost T, Asghar SS, Cormane RH. Skin reactions caused by phenyl-butazone. Immunologic studies. *Arch Dermatol* 1974; **110**: 929–33.
2 Inman WHW. Study of fatal bone marrow depression with special reference to phenylbutazone and oxyphenbutazone. *Br Med J* 1977; **i**: 1500–5.
3 Montgomery PR. Toxic epidermal necrolysis due to phenylbutazone. *Br J Dermatol* 1970; **83**: 220.
4 Reshad H, Hargreaves GK, Vickers CFH. Generalized pustular psoriasis precipitated by phenylbutazone and oxyphenbutazone. *Br J Dermatol* 1983; **109**: 111–13.
5 Von Paschoud J-M. Vasculitis allergica cutis durch phenylbutazon. *Dermatologica* 1966; **133**: 76–86.
6 Millard LG. A haemorrhagic bullous eruption of the hands caused by phenylbutazone: a report of 3 cases. *Acta Derm Venereol (Stockh)* 1977; **57**: 83–6.

Miscellaneous anti-inflammatory agents

Benzydamin

Photo-allergy has been described to both topical and systemic administration of this drug [1].

REFERENCE

1 Frosch PJ, Weickel R. Photokontakallergie durch Benzydamin (Tantum). *Hautarzt* 1989; **40**: 771–3.

Allopurinol

Dermatological complications occur in up to 10% of cases [1–7]. Acute sensitivity reactions are well known, including scarlatiniform erythema, morbilliform rashes, urticaria or generalized exfoliative dermatitis, which may be associated with fever, eosinophilia, hepatic abnormalities and a nephropathy. Vasculitis (perhaps triggered by oxypurinol, the principal metabolite of allopurinol, which has a long half-life and accumulates in renal failure [5]), erythema multiforme [7], Stevens–Johnson syndrome and TEN [5,8,9] have been reported. Cell-mediated immunity directed towards allopurinol and more importantly to its oxypurinol metabolite is thought to be involved in the pathogenesis of allopurinol-induced hypersensitivity [10]. Hypersensitivity reactions occur on average within 2–6 weeks of starting the drug, although the interval may be much longer. Eruptions are commoner in the setting of impaired renal function [11] and with concomitant thiazide therapy [12], and may first appear up to 3 weeks after the drug has been discontinued [13]. The mortality is about 20% [5]. Other allopurinol-induced cutaneous changes include alopecia [14] and ichthyosis [14]. Allopurinol potentiates the risk of a reaction to ampicillin [15], and increases blood cyclosporin levels [16]. Desensitization may be successful in cases with minor rashes induced by allopurinol [17–19].

REFERENCES

1 Lupton GP. The allopurinol hypersensitivity syndrome. *J Am Acad Dermatol* 1979; **1**: 365–74.
2 McInnes GT, Lawson DH, Jick H. Acute adverse reactions attributed to allopurinol in hospitalised patients. *Ann Rheum Dis* 1981; **40**: 245–9.
3 Singer JZ, Wallace SL. The allopurinol hypersensitivity syndrome. Unnecessary morbidity and mortality. *Arthritis Rheum* 1986; **29**: 82–7.
4 Foucault V, Pibouin M, Lehry D *et al*. Accidents médicamenteux sévères et allopurinol. *Ann Dermatol Vénéréol* 1988; **115**: 1169–72.
5 Arellano F, Sacristan JA. Allopurinol hypersensitivity syndrome: a review. *Ann Pharmacotherapy* 1993; **27**: 337–43.
6 Elasy T, Kaminsky D, Tracy M, Mehler PS. Allopurinol hypersensitivity syndrome revisited. *West J Med* 1995; **162**: 360–1.
7 Kumar A, Edward N, White MI *et al*. Allopurinol, erythema multiforme, and renal insufficiency. *Br Med J* 1996; **312**: 173–4.
8 Bennett TO, Sugar J, Sahgal S. Ocular manifestations of toxic epidermal necrolysis associated with allopurinol use. *Arch Ophthalmol* 1977; **95**: 1362–4.
9 Dan M, Jedwab M, Peled M *et al*. Allopurinol-induced toxic epidermal necrolysis. *Int J Dermatol* 1984; **23**: 142–4.
10 Braden GL, Warzynski MJ, Golightly M, Ballow M. Cell-mediated immunity in allopurinol-induced hypersensitivity. *Clin Immunol Immunopathol* 1994; **70**: 145–51.
11 Handke KR, Noone RM, Stone WJ. Severe allopurinol toxicity. Description and guidelines for prevention in patients with renal insufficiency. *Am J Med* 1984; **76**: 47–56.
12 Handke KR. Evaluation of a thiazide allopurinol drug interaction. *Am J Med Sci* 1986; **292**: 213–16.
13 Bigby M, Jick S, Jick H, Arndt K. Drug-induced cutaneous reactions. A report from the Boston Collaborative Drug Surveillance Program on 15 438 consecutive inpatients, 1975 to 1982. *JAMA* 1986; **256**: 3358–63.
14 Auerbach R, Orentreich N. Alopecia and ichthyosis secondary to allopurinol. *Arch Dermatol* 1968; **98**: 104.
15 Jick H, Slone D, Shapiro S *et al*. Excess of ampicillin rashes associated with allopurinol or hyperuricemia. A report from the Boston Collaborative Drug Surveillance Program, Boston University Medical Center. *N Engl J Med* 1972; **286**: 505–7.
16 Gorrie M, Beaman M, Nicholls A, Backwell A. Allopurinol interaction with cyclosporin. *Br Med J* 1994; **308**: 113.
17 Fam AG, Lewtas J, Stein J, Paton TW. Desensitization to allopurinol in patients with gout and cutaneous reactions. *Am J Med* 1992; **93**: 299–302.
18 Kelso JM, Keating RM. Successful desensitization for treatment of a fixed drug eruption to allopurinol. *J Allergy Clin Immunol* 1996; **97**: 1171–2.
19 Walz-LeBlanc BA, Reynolds WJ, MacFadden DK. Allopurinol sensitivity in a patient with chronic tophaceous gout: success of intravenous desensitization after failure of oral desensitization. *Arthritis Rheum* 1991; **34**: 1329–31.

Drugs acting on the central nervous system

The adverse effects of psychotropic medication have been reviewed [1,2]; the prevalence of skin reactions to psychotropic medications is about 5% [2].

REFERENCES

1 Gupta MA, Gupta AK, Haberman HF. Psychotropic drugs in dermatology. A review and guidelines for use. *J Am Acad Dermatol* 1986; **14**: 633–45.
2 Srebrnik A, Hes JP, Brenner S. Adverse cutaneous reactions to psychotropic drugs. *Acta Derm Venereol (Stockh)* 1991; Suppl. **158**: 1–12.

Antidepressants

Tricyclics and related compounds

Antidepressants are associated with a range of idiosyncratic reactions affecting the liver, skin, haematological and central nervous systems; reactions mediated by chemically reactive metabolites formed by the cytochrome P-450 enzyme system either directly or indirectly via an immune mechanism. Individual susceptibility is determined by genetic and environmental factors, which result in inadequate detoxication of the chemically reactive metabolite [1]. Sedative, cardiovascular, anticholinergic and gastrointestinal side-effects are well known [2,3]. Agranulocytosis may occur occasionally. Cutaneous reactions are rare [2], but include maculopapular rashes, photosensitivity (protriptyline and imipramine), urticaria, pruritus, hyperhidrosis, vasculitis or acne (maprotiline), and TEN (amoxapine).

Amineptine. Severe acne [4] and rosacea [5] have been reported.

Amitriptyline. A bullous reaction in a patient with overdosage of amitriptyline and chlorazepate dipotassium has been reported [6]. Alopecia is documented.

Clomipramine. A photo-allergic eruption has been documented [7].

Imipramine. This drug has caused urticarial or exanthematic eruptions occasionally [8] and agranulocytosis has occurred. Oedema of the feet is seen in older people. Glossitis and stomatitis are rare, as are transient erythema of the face, photosensitivity and exfoliative dermatitis. Slate-grey pigmentation of exposed skin may develop; golden-yellow granules, which ultrastructurally are electron dense inclusion bodies in phagocytes, fibroblasts and dendrocytes, are seen in the papillary dermis [9]. Cutaneous vasculitis is well documented. Atypical cutaneous lymphoid hyperplasia has been documented [10].

Maprotiline. Acne [11] and vasculitis [12] are recorded.

Mianserin. Erythema multiforme has recently been reported [13], as has a severe allergic reaction [14].

Trazodone. This drug has caused leukonychia [15], erythema multiforme [16] and vasculitis [17], and has been implicated in causing a psoriasiform eruption. Skin swelling is recorded [18].

REFERENCES

1 Pirmohamed M, Kitteringham NR, Park BK. Idiosyncratic reactions to antidepressants: a review of the possible mechanisms and predisposing factors. *Pharmacol Ther* 1992; **53**: 105–25.
2 Gupta MA, Gupta AK, Haberman HF. Psychotropic drugs in dermatology. A review and guidelines for use. *J Am Acad Dermatol* 1986; **14**: 633–45.
3 Gupta MA, Gupta AK, Ellis CN. Antidepressant drugs in dermatology. An update. *Arch Dermatol* 1987; **123**: 647–52.
4 Thioly-Bensoussan D, Edelson Y, Cardinne A, Grupper C. Acné monstrueuse iatrogène provoquée par le Survector®: première observation mondiale à propos de deux cas. *Nouv Dermatol* 1987; **6**: 535–7.
5 Jeanmougin M, Civatte J, Cavelier-Balloy B. Toxiderme rosaceiforme a l'amineptine (Survector). *Ann Dermatol Vénéréol* 1988; **115**: 1185–6.
6 Herschtal D, Robinson MJ. Blisters of the skin in coma induced by amitriptyline and chlorazepate dipotassium. Report of a case with underlying sweat gland necrosis. *Arch Dermatol* 1979; **115**: 499.
7 Ljunggren B, Bojs G. A case of photosensitivity and contact allergy to systemic tricyclic drugs, with unusual features. *Contact Dermatitis* 1991; **24**: 259–65.
8 Almeyda J. Drug reactions XIII. Cutaneous reactions to imipramine and chlordiazepoxide. *Br J Dermatol* 1971; **84**: 298–9.
9 Hashimoto K, Joselow SA, Tye MJ. Imipramine hyperpigmentation: a slate-gray discoloration caused by long-term imipramine administration. *J Am Acad Dermatol* 1991; **25**: 357–61.
10 Crowson AN, Magro CM. Antidepressant therapy. A possible cause of atypical cutaneous lymphoid hyperplasia. *Arch Dermatol* 1995; **131**: 925–9.
11 Ponte CD. Maprotiline-induced acne. *Am J Psychiatry* 1982; **139**: 141.
12 Oakley AM, Hodge L. Cutaneous vasculitis from maprotiline. *Aust NZ J Med* 1985; **15**: 256–7.
13 Quraishy E. Erythema multiforme during treatment with mianserin. *Br J Dermatol* 1981; **104**: 481.
14 Bazin N, Beaufils B, Feline A. A severe allergic reaction to mianserin. *Am J Psychiatry* 1991; **148**: 1088–9.
15 Longstreth GF, Hershman J. Trazodone-induced hepatotoxicity and leukonychia. *J Am Acad Dermatol* 1985; **13**: 149–50.
16 Ford HE, Jenike MA. Erythema multiforme associated with trazodone therapy. *J Clin Psychiatry* 1985; **46**: 294–5.
17 Mann SC, Walker MM, Messenger GG et al. Leukocytoclastic vasculitis secondary to trazodone treatment. *J Am Acad Dermatol* 1984; **10**: 669–70.
18 Fisher S, Bryant SG, Kent TA. Postmarketing surveillance by patient self-monitoring: trazodone versus fluoxetine. *J Clin Psychopharmacol* 1993; **13**: 235–42.

Monoamine-oxidase inhibitors

Iproniazid. Vasculitis and peripheral neuritis are documented.

Phenelzine. Hypersensitivity skin reactions are rare.

Selective serotonin reuptake inhibitors

Fluoxetine

This drug has caused urticaria [1], urticarial vasculitis [2]

and hypersensitivity [3]; familial cases are documented [4]. Atypical cutaneous lymphoid hyperplasia [5], including pseudomycosis fungoides [5–7], is recorded.

Miscellaneous other SSRIs

The 5-hydroxytryptamine(3)-receptor antagonists, granisetron, ondansetron and tropisetron, are antiemetic medications used during chemotherapy. Effects include headache and gastrointestinal symptoms, and rarely hypersensitivity reactions [8]. There were no crossover reactions to citalopram or paroxetine among patients hypersensitive to zimeldine [9].

REFERENCES

1 Leznoff A, Binkley KE, Joffee RT et al. Adverse cutaneous reactions associated with fluoxetine strategy for reintroduction of this drug in selected patients. *J Clin Psychopharmacol* 1992; **12**: 355–7.
2 Roger D, Rolle F, Mausset J et al. Urticarial vasculitis induced by fluoxetine. *Dermatology* 1995; **191**: 164.
3 Beer K, Albertini J, Medenica M, Busbey S. Fluoxetine-induced hypersensitivity. *Arch Dermatol* 1994; **130**: 803–4.
4 Olfson M, Wilner MT. A family case history of fluoxetine-induced skin reactions. *J Nerv Ment Dis* 1991; **179**: 504–5.
5 Crowson AN, Magro CM. Antidepressant therapy. A possible cause of atypical cutaneous lymphoid hyperplasia. *Arch Dermatol* 1995; **131**: 925–9.
6 Gordon KB, Guitart J, Kuzel T et al. Pseudo-mycosis fungoides in a patient taking clonazepam and fluoxetine. *J Am Acad Dermatol* 1996; **34**: 304–6.
7 Vermeer MH, Willemze R. Is mycosis fungoides exacerbated by fluoxetine? *J Am Acad Dermatol* 1996; **35**: 635–6.
8 Kataja V, de Bruijn KM. Hypersensitivity reactions associated with 5-hydroxytryptamine(3)-receptor antagonists: a class effect? *Lancet* 1996; **347**: 584–5.
9 Bengtsson BO, Lundmark J, Walinder J. No crossover reactions to citalopram or paroxetine among patients hypersensitive to zimeldine. *Br J Psychiatry* 1991; **158**: 853–5.

Lithium

Skin reactions [1–5] are relatively uncommon. Pustular and psoriasiform lesions induced by this drug have received particular attention. The pustular propensities of lithium have been attributed to lysosomal enzyme release and increased neutrophil chemotaxis [2]. Tetracycline should be avoided in treating these pustular eruptions as it may precipitate serious lithium toxicity. The acneiform 'erysipelas' eruption consists of monomorphic pustules on an erythematous base, tends to affect mainly the arms and legs, is not associated with comedones or cystic lesions, and may be very persistent. Various patterns of folliculitis may occur. Lithium can aggravate pre-existing psoriasis, making it more difficult to control [6–9], and may precipitate a palmoplantar pustular reaction [10] or even generalized pustular psoriasis [11]. Psychiatrists should avoid the use of lithium in psoriatics if possible. Darier's disease may also be exacerbated or initiated [12,13].

Additional reactions described include morbilliform rashes, erythema multiforme [14], a dermatitis herpetiformis-like rash [15], linear IgA bullous dermatosis

[16] and a generalized exfoliative eruption [17]. An LE-like syndrome [18] with increased prevalence of antinuclear antibodies [19], toenail dystrophy [20] and hair loss [21,22] have been reported. Keratoderma has been documented [23], as has hidradenitis suppurativa [24]. None of these effects is related to excessive blood levels of lithium or other evidence of toxicity.

REFERENCES

1 Callaway CL, Hendrie HC, Luby ED. Cutaneous conditions observed in patients during treatment with lithium. *Am J Psychiatry* 1968; **124**: 1124–5.
2 Heng MCY. Cutaneous manifestations of lithium toxicity. *Br J Dermatol* 1982; **106**: 107–9.
3 Deandrea D, Walker N, Mehlmauer M, White K. Dermatological reactions to lithium: a review. *J Clin Psychopharmacol* 1982; **2**: 199–204.
4 Sarantidis D, Waters B. A review and controlled study of cutaneous conditions associated with lithium carbonate. *Br J Psychiatry* 1983; **143**: 42–50.
5 Albrecht G. Unerwünschte Wirkungen von Lithium an der Haut. *Hautarzt* 1985; **36**: 77–82.
6 Lazarus GS, Gilgor RS. Psoriasis, polymorphonuclear leukocytes, and lithium carbonate. An important clue. *Arch Dermatol* 1979; **115**: 1183–4.
7 Skoven I, Thormann J. Lithium compound treatment and psoriasis. *Arch Dermatol* 1979; **115**: 1185–7.
8 Abel EA, Dicicco LM, Orenberg EK *et al.* Drugs in exacerbation of psoriasis. *J Am Acad Dermatol* 1986; **15**: 1007–22.
9 Sasaki T, Saito S, Aihara M *et al.* Exacerbation of psoriasis during lithium treatment. *J Dermatol (Tokyo)* 1989; **16**: 59–63.
10 White SW. Palmoplantar pustular psoriasis provoked by lithium therapy. *J Am Acad Dermatol* 1982; **7**: 660–2.
11 Lowe NJ, Ridgway HB. Generalized pustular psoriasis precipitated by lithium. *Arch Dermatol* 1978; **114**: 1788–9.
12 Milton GP, Peck GL, Fu J-J *et al.* Exacerbation of Darier's disease by lithium carbonate. *J Am Acad Dermatol* 1990; **23**: 926–8.
13 Rubin MB. Lithium-induced Darier's disease. *J Am Acad Dermatol* 1996; **32**: 674–5.
14 Balldin J, Berggren U, Heijer A, Mobacken H. Erythema multiforme caused by lithium. *J Am Acad Dermatol* 1991; **24**: 1015–16.
15 Meinhold JM, West DP, Gurwich E *et al.* Cutaneous reaction to lithium carbonate: a case report. *J Clin Psychiatry* 1980; **41**: 395–6.
16 McWhirter JD, Hashimoto K, Fayne S *et al.* Linear IgA bullous dermatosis related to lithium carbonate. *Arch Dermatol* 1987; **123**: 1120–2.
17 Kuhnley EJ, Granoff AL. Exfoliative dermatitis during lithium treatment. *Am J Psychiatry* 1979; **136**: 1340–1.
18 Shukla VR, Borison RL. Lithium and lupus-like syndrome. *JAMA* 1982; **248**: 921–2.
19 Presley AP, Kahn A, Williamson N. Antinuclear antibodies in patients on lithium carbonate. *Br Med J* 1976; **ii**: 280–1.
20 Hooper JF. Lithium carbonate and toenails. *Am J Psychiatry* 1981; **138**: 1519.
21 Dawber R, Mortimer P. Hair loss during lithium treatment. *Br J Dermatol* 1982; **107**: 124–5.
22 Orwin A. Hair loss following lithium therapy. *Br J Dermatol* 1983; **108**: 503–4.
23 Labelle A, Lapierre YD. Keratodermia: side effects of lithium. *J Clin Psychopharmacol* 1991; **11**: 149–50.
24 Gupta AK, Knowles SR, Gupta MA *et al.* Lithium therapy associated with hidradenitis suppurativa: case report and a review of the dermatologic side effects of lithium. *J Am Acad Dermatol* 1995; **32**: 382–6.

Hypnotics, sedatives and anxiolytics

Barbiturates

A toxic bullous eruption may appear at pressure points in comatose patients after overdosage [1–4]. In one series, 8% of patients admitted with drug-induced coma had such bullae [3] (Fig. 77.5). The bullae are few, large and may lead to ulceration [2]. Necrotic lesions are seen in 4% of patients recovering from, and in 40% of fatalities related to, a barbiturate-induced coma [4]. Allergic reactions are very uncommon and may be scarlatiniform or morbilliform. Exfoliative dermatitis has proved fatal [5], as has erythema multiforme. Urticaria and serum sickness are very rare as is purpuric capillaritis. Fixed eruptions are well known [6] and particularly occur on the glans penis. TEN, LE-like syndrome, purpura and photosensitivity are recorded [7]. Phenobarbital is one cause of the anticonvulsant hypersensitivity syndrome (see below) [8,9]. In one case, a syndrome resembling Langerhans' cell histiocytosis was produced [10]. Hypopigmentation may follow a severe reaction [11]. Exfoliative dermatitis is recorded [12].

REFERENCES

1 Beveridge GW, Lawson AAH. Occurrence of bullous lesions in acute barbiturate intoxication. *Br Med J* 1965; **i** 835–7.
2 Gröschel D, Gerstein AR, Rosenbaum JM. Skin lesions as a diagnostic aid in barbiturate poisoning. *N Engl J Med* 1970; **283**: 409–10.
3 Pinkus NB. Skin eruptions in drug-induced coma. *Med J Aust* 1971; **2**: 886–8.
4 Almeyda J, Levantine A. Drug reactions XVII. Cutaneous reactions to barbiturates, chloralhydrate and its derivatives. *Br J Dermatol* 1972; **86**: 313–16.
5 Sneddon IB, Leishman AWD. Severe and fatal phenobarbitone eruptions. *Br Med J* 1952; **i**: 1276–8.
6 Korkij W, Soltani K. Fixed drug eruption. A brief review. *Arch Dermatol* 1984; **120**: 520–4.
7 Gupta MA, Gupta AK, Haberman HF. Psychotropic drugs in dermatology. A review and guidelines for use. *J Am Acad Dermatol* 1986; **14**: 633–45.
8 Vittorio CC, Muglia JJ. Anticonvulsant hypersensitivity syndrome. *Arch Intern Med* 1995; **155**: 2285–90.
9 De Vriese AS, Philippe J, Van Renterghem DM *et al.* Carbamazepine hypersensitivity syndrome: report of 4 cases and review of the literature. *Medicine* 1995; **74**: 144–51.
10 Nagata T, Kawamura N, Motoyama T *et al.* A case of hypersensitivity syndrome resembling Langerhans cell histiocytosis during phenobarbital prophylaxis for convulsion. *Jpn J Clin Oncol* 1992; **22**: 421–7.
11 Mion N, Fusade T, Mathelier-Fusade P *et al.* Depigmentation cutaneo-phanerienne consecutive a une toxidermie au phenobarbital. *Ann Dermatol Vénéréol* 1992; **119**: 927–9.
12 Sawaishi Y, Komatsu K, Takeda O *et al.* A case of tubulo-interstitial nephritis with exfoliative dermatitis and hepatitis due to phenobarbital hypersensitivity. *Eur J Pediatr* 1992; **151**: 69–72.

Benzodiazepines

Allergic reactions are very rare [1].

Alprazolam. Photosensitivity has been recorded with this newer benzodiazepine [2].

Chlordiazepoxide. Morbilliform erythema, urticaria [3], fixed eruption [4], photo-allergic eczema [5] and exacerbation of porphyria have been recorded. Erythema multiforme and chronic pigmented purpuric eruption occur rarely [6].

Clobazam. A generalized erythematous pruritic eruption

[7] and TEN confined to light-exposed areas [8] have been reported.

Diazepam and nitrazepam. Bullae similar to those seen after barbiturates may occur in comatose patients after overdosage [9,10]. Thrombophlebitis may follow intravenous injection of diazepam [11]. Hyperpigmentation in previously dermabraded scars has been attributed to diazepam [12]. An eruption comprising oedema, moon face and generalized erythema, with erosions of cheeks, axillae and the genitocrural area was attributed to nitrazepam; a provocation test was positive [13].

Lormetazepam. A fixed drug eruption has been reported [14].

Temazepam. An extensive fixed drug reaction has been reported [15]. Extravasation following attempted femoral vein injection of a suspension of the contents of capsules in tap water, by an addict, resulted in extensive necrosis of genital and pubic skin [16].

REFERENCES

1 Edwards JG. Adverse effects of antianxiety drugs. *Drugs* 1981; **22**: 495–514.
2 Kanwar AJ, Gupta R, Das Mehta S, Kaur S. Photosensitivity to alprazolam. *Dermatologica* 1990; **181**: 75.
3 Almeyda J. Drug reactions XIII. Cutaneous reactions to imipramine and chlordiazepoxide. *Br J Dermatol* 1971; **84**: 298–9.
4 Blair HM, III. Fixed drug eruption from chlordiazepoxide: report of a case. *Arch Dermatol* 1974; **109**: 914.
5 Luton EF, Finchum RN. Photosensitivity reaction to chlordiazepoxide. *Arch Dermatol* 1965; **91**: 362–3.
6 Nishioka K, Katayama I, Masuzawa M *et al.* Drug-induced chronic pigmented purpura. *J Dermatol (Tokyo)* 1989; **16**: 220–2.
7 Machet L, Vaillant L, Dardaine V, Lorette G. Patch testing with clobazam: relapse of generalised drug eruption. *Contact Dermatitis* 1992; **26**: 347–8.
8 Redondo P, Vicente J, España A *et al.* Photo-induced toxic epidermal necrolysis caused by clobazam. *Br J Dermatol* 1996; **135**: 999–1002.
9 Ridley CM. Bullous lesions in nitrazepam-overdosage. *Br Med J* 1971; **iii**: 28.
10 Varma AJ, Fisher BK, Sarin MK. Diazepam-induced coma with bullae and eccrine sweat gland necrosis. *Arch Intern Med* 1977; **137**: 1207–10.
11 Langdon DE, Harlan JR, Bailey RL. Thrombophlebitis with diazepam used intravenously. *JAMA* 1973; **223**: 184–5.
12 Fereira JA. The role of diazepam in skin hyperpigmentation. *Aesthetic Plast Surg* 1980; **4**: 343–8.
13 Shoji A, Kitajima J, Hamada T. Drug eruption caused by nitrazepam in a patient with severe pustular psoriasis successfully treated with methotrexate and etretinate. *J Dermatol (Tokyo)* 1987; **14**: 274–8.
14 Jafferany M, Haroon TS. Fixed drug eruption with lormetazepam (Noctamid). *Dermatologica* 1988; **177**: 386.
15 Archer CB, English JSC. Extensive fixed drug eruption induced by temazepam. *Clin Exp Dermatol* 1988; **13**: 336–8.
16 Meshikhes AN, Duthie JS. Untitled report. *Br Med J* 1991; **303**: 478.

Miscellaneous drugs

Carbromal

This drug, now rarely used, commonly produced a characteristic capillaritis with punctate purpura and haemosiderin giving a golden-brown discoloration of the skin, especially on the legs [1].

Chloral hydrate

Hypersensitivity reactions are very rare. Chloral is now virtually given only in tablet form as dichloralphenazone, in which the phenazone may cause a fixed eruption [2].

Ethchlorvynol

Overdose has caused bullous lesions [3].

Glutethimide

Dermographism with subsequent erythema, and vesicles that lasted several days, were reported in one comatose patient [4], and bullae in another patient [5] following overdosage. Fixed eruptions are recorded [6].

Meprobamate

Anorexia, drowsiness, dizziness, flushing and gastrointestinal symptoms may occur, especially with high doses. Fixed eruptions may occur [7]. The most characteristic cutaneous reaction, preceded by itching, malaise and fever, is an erythema, starting in the limb flexures which rapidly gives way to a fierce non-thrombocytopenic purpura [8]. A widespread toxic erythema was associated with an anaphylactoid reaction, in a patient in whom patch testing proved useful in diagnosis [9].

REFERENCES

1 Peterson WC, Jr, Manick KP. Purpuric eruptions associated with use of carbromal and meprobamate. *Arch Dermatol* 1967; **95**: 40–2.
2 McCulloch H, Zeligman I. Fixed drug eruption and epididymitis due to antipyrine. *Arch Dermatol Syphilol* 1951; **64**: 198–9.
3 Brodin MD, Redmon WJ. Bullous eruptions due to Ethchlorvynol. *J Cutan Pathol* 1980; **7**: 326–9.
4 Leavell UW, Jr, Coyer JR, Taylor RJ. Dermographism and erythematous lines in glutethimide overdose. *Arch Dermatol* 1972; **106**: 724–5.
5 Burdon JGW, Cade JF. 'Barbiturate burns' caused by glutethimide. *Med J Aust* 1979; **1**: 101–2.
6 Fisher M, Lerman JS. Fixed eruption due to glutethimide. *Arch Dermatol* 1971; **104**: 87–9.
7 Gore HC, Jr. Fixed drug eruption cross reaction of meprobamate and carisoprodol. *Arch Dermatol* 1965; **91**: 627.
8 Levan NE. Meprobamate reaction. *Arch Dermatol* 1957; **75**: 437–8.
9 Felix RH, Comaish JS. The value of patch and other skin tests in drug eruptions. *Lancet* 1974; **i**: 1017–19.

Antipsychotics

The most important clinical side-effects include those on the central nervous and cardiovascular systems and the ocular effects [1,2]. Drugs with high potency, such as haloperidol and pimozide, tend to have fewer cardiovascular and anticholinergic effects and are less sedating, but have more neurological effects. Long-term use of antipsychotic agents results in tardive dyskinesia.

Phenothiazines

The side-effects of this group of drugs have been reviewed [1–4].

Chlorpromazine. This drug is still widely used, but many related compounds are now available. Pigmentation of the skin in light-exposed areas after chronic usage may be a problem, especially in women and black people [5–11]. Rarely, a purplish or slate-grey pigmentation develops [6]. There may be brown discoloration of cornea and lens [5], and bulbar conjunctiva [7]. Chlorpromazine has an affinity for melanin *in vitro* [8]. Electron microscopy shows many melanosome complexes within lysosomes of dermal macrophages, and electron dense 'chlorpromazine bodies' in macrophages, endothelial cells and Schwann cells [9,10]; energy-dispersive X-ray microanalysis has revealed the abundant presence of sulphur in these granules, found in the chlorpromazine molecule [10]. Similar pigmentary deposits are found in internal organs [11] and in blood neutrophils and monocytes.

Chlorpromazine has caused lichenoid eruptions [12], exfoliative dermatitis, erythema multiforme, an LE-like illness [13] with positive antinuclear factor [14] and the lupus anticoagulant [15], and Henoch–Schönlein vasculitis [16]. Phototoxicity is well known [17–19] and phenothiazine-derived antihistamines may cause photosensitivity in atopics and subsequent development of actinic reticuloid [19]. Photocontact urticaria has been documented [20]. A pustular reaction is recorded [21]. Cholestatic jaundice is an important hazard.

Fluspirilene. Subcutaneous nodules may develop at injection sites after long-term high doses of this depot preparation [22].

Thiothixene. A sensitivity reaction has been recorded [23].

Trifluoperazine. A fixed eruption has been recorded [24].

Loxapine. Dermatitis, pruritus and seborrhoea have been recorded, and photosensitivity eruptions may occur occasionally [25].

Levomepromazin. An erythema annulare centrifugum-like pseudolymphomatous eruption has been reported [26].

REFERENCES

1 Simpson GM, Pi EH, Sramek JJ, Jr. Adverse effects of antipsychotic agents. *Drugs* 1981; **21**: 138–51.

2 Gupta MA, Gupta AK, Haberman HF. Psychotropic drugs in dermatology. A review and guidelines for use. *J Am Acad Dermatol* 1986; **14**: 633–45.
3 Hägermark Ö, Wennersten G, Almeyda J. Drug reactions XIV. Cutaneous side effects of phenothiazines. *Br J Dermatol* 1971; **84**: 605–7.
4 Bond WS, Yee GC. Ocular and cutaneous effects of chronic phenothiazine therapy. *Am J Hosp Pharm* 1980; **37**: 74–8.
5 Greiner AC, Berry K. Skin pigmentation and corneal and lens opacities with prolonged chlorpromazine therapy. *Can Med Assoc J* 1964; **90**: 663–5.
6 Hays GB, Lyle CB, Jr, Wheeler CE, Jr. Slate-grey color in patients receiving chlorpromazine. *Arch Dermatol* 1964; **90**: 471–6.
7 Satanove A. Pigmentation due to phenothiazines in high and prolonged dosage. *JAMA* 1965; **191**: 263–8.
8 Blois MS, Jr. On chlorpromazine binding *in vivo. J Invest Dermatol* 1965; **45**: 475–81.
9 Hashimoto K, Wiener W, Albert J, Nelson RG. An electron microscopic study of chlorpromazine pigmentation. *J Invest Dermatol* 1966; **47**: 296–306.
10 Benning TL, McCormack KM, Ingram P *et al.* Microprobe analysis of chlorpromazine pigmentation. *Arch Dermatol* 1988; **124**: 1541–4.
11 Greiner AC, Nicolson GA. Pigment deposition in viscera associated with prolonged chlorpromazine therapy. *Can Med Assoc J* 1964; **90**: 627–35.
12 Matsuo I, Ozawa A, Niizuma K, Ohkido M. Lichenoid dermatitis due to chlorpromazine phototoxicity. *Dermatologica* 1979; **159**: 46–9.
13 Pavlidakey GP, Hashimoto K, Heller GL, Daneshvar S. Chlorpromazine-induced lupuslike disease: case report and review of the literature. *J Am Acad Dermatol* 1985; **13**: 109–15.
14 Zarrabi MH, Zucker S, Miller F *et al.* Immunologic and coagulation disorders in chlorpromazine-treated patients. *Ann Intern Med* 1979; **91**: 194–9.
15 Canoso RT, Sise HS. Chlorpromazine-induced lupus anticoagulant and associated immunologic abnormalities. *Am J Hematol* 1982; **13**: 121–9.
16 Aram H. Henoch–Schönlein purpura induced by chlorpromazine. *J Am Acad Dermatol* 1987; **17**: 139–40.
17 Johnson BE. Cellular mechanisms of chlorpromazine photosensitivity. *Proc R Soc Med* 1974; **67**: 871–3.
18 Ljunggren B. Phenothiazine phototoxicity: toxic chlorpromazine photoproducts. *J Invest Dermatol* 1977; **69**: 383–6.
19 Amblard P, Beani J-C, Reymond J-L. Photo-allergie rémanente aux phénothiazines chez l'atopique. *Ann Dermatol Vénéréol* 1982; **109**: 225–8.
20 Lovell CR, Cronin E, Rhodes EL. Photocontact urticaria from chlorpromazine. *Contact Dermatitis* 1986; **14**: 290–1.
21 Burrows NP, Ratnavel RC, Norris PG. Pustular eruptions after chlorpromazine. *Br Med J* 1994; **309**: 97.
22 UK Committee of Safety of Medicines. *Curr Probl* 1981; **7**.
23 Matsuoka LY. Thiothixene drug sensitivity. *J Am Acad Dermatol* 1982; **7**: 405–6.
24 Kanwar AJ, Singh M, El-Sheriff AK, Belhaj MS. Fixed eruption due to trifluoperazine hydrochloride. *Br J Dermatol* 1987; **117**: 798–9.
25 Anon. Cloxapine and loxapine for schizophrenia. *Drug Ther Bull* 1991; **29**: 41–2.
26 Blazejak T, Hölzle E. Phenothiazin-induziertes Pseudolymphom. *Hautarzt* 1990; **41**: 161–3.

Miscellaneous antipsychotic agents

Clozapine. An acute severe adverse reaction resembling systemic LE is recorded [1].

Haloperidol. This drug causes reactions at injection sites [2,3].

REFERENCES

1 Reinke M, Wiesert KN. High incidence of haloperidol decanoate injection site reactions (Letter). *J Clin Psychiatry* 1992; **53**: 415–16.
2 Maharaj K, Guttmacher LB, Moeller R. Haloperidol decanoate: injection site reactions. *J Clin Psychiatry* 1995; **56**: 172–3.

3 Wickert WA, Campbell NR, Martin L. Acute severe adverse clozapine reaction resembling systemic lupus erythematosus. *Postgrad Med J* 1994; **70**: 940–1.

Drugs for alcoholism

Cyanamide

This inhibitor of alcohol dehydrogenase, used in the treatment of alcoholism, has been implicated in the development of a lichen planus-like eruption with oesophageal involvement [1].

Disulfiram

This drug causes vasomotor flushing, morbilliform rash and urticaria, as well as eczema in patients sensitized to rubber; it cross-reacts with rubber [2–4]. A toxic pustular eruption is recorded [5].

REFERENCES

1 Torrelo A, Soria C, Rocamora A *et al.* Lichen planus-like eruption with esophageal involvement as a result of cyanamide. *J Am Acad Dermatol* 1990; **23**: 1168–9.
2 Webb PK, Gibbs SC, Mathias CT *et al.* Disulfiram hypersensitivity and rubber contact dermatitis. *JAMA* 1979; **241**: 2061.
3 Fischer AA. Dermatologic aspects of disulfiram use. *Cutis* 1982; **30**; 461–524.
4 Minet A, Frankart M, Eggers S *et al.* Réactions allergiques aux implants de disulfirame. *Ann Dermatol Vénéréol* 1989; **116**: 543–5.
5 Larbre B, Larbre JP, Nicolas JF *et al.* Toxicodermie pustuleuse aus disulfirame. A propos d'un cas. *Ann Dermatol Vénéréol* 1990; **117**: 721–2.

Anticonvulsants

Allergic rashes to antiepileptic drugs are usually mild; the rare occurrence of a severe reaction indicates that the drug should be ceased, and this can be done abruptly with minimal risk of status epilepticus [1]. There may be cross-reactivity in terms of clinical reactions to the aromatic anticonvulsants (phenytoin, phenobarbital, carbamazepine, primidone and clonazepam), which may all cause the so-called *anticonvulsant hypersensitivity syndrome*, with fever, mucocutaneous eruptions, lymphadenopathy and hepatitis, 1 week to 3 months into therapy; there may be multiorgan involvement with renal and pulmonary lesions [2–9]. The reaction may develop into TEN. Arene oxide metabolites may be involved in the pathogenesis of these eruptions [2]. Sodium valproate may be substituted safely. The anticonvulsant hypersensitivity syndrome reportedly occurs at a rate of between one in 1000 and one in 10 000 exposures; siblings of patients may be at an increased risk of developing this syndrome [8]. Generalized pustulation may be a manifestation of the anticonvulsant hypersensitivity syndrome [10]. A severe form of hypersensitivity vasculitis, with extensive visceral involvement and poor prognosis, is seen very rarely with phenytoin and in isolated cases with carbamazepine and trimethadione [11].

Drug-induced systemic LE is much more frequent, and has been described with most anticonvulsants in clinical use (phenytoin, carbamazepine, ethosuximide, trimethadione, primidone and valproate) [11]. Of the newer anticonvulsant drugs, vigabatrin is usually well tolerated, but lamotrigine is associated with rashes [12,13].

REFERENCES

1 Pelekanos J, Camfield P, Camfield C, Gordon K. Allergic rash due to antiepileptic drugs: clinical features and management. *Epilepsia* 1991; **32**: 554–9.
2 Shear N, Spielberg S. Anticonvulsant hypersensitivity syndrome. *In vitro* assessment of risk. *J Clin Invest* 1989; **82**: 1826–32.
3 Chang DK, Shear NH. Cutaneous reactions to anticonvulsants. *Semin Neurol* 1992; **12**: 329–37.
4 Handfield-Jones SE, Jenkins RE, Whittaker SJ *et al.* The anticonvulsant hypersensitivity syndrome. *Br J Dermatol* 1993; **129**: 175–7.
5 Gall H, Merk H, Scherb W, Sterry W. Anticonvulsiva-Hyper-sensitivitats-Syndrom auf Carbamazepin. *Hautarzt* 1994; **45**: 494–8.
6 Richens A, Davidson DL, Cartlidge NE, Easter DJ. A multicentre comparative trial of sodium valproate and carbamazepine in adult onset epilepsy. Adult EPITEG Collaborative Group. *J Neurol Neurosurg Psychiatry* 1994; **57**: 682–7.
7 Alldredge BK, Knutsen AP, Ferriero D. Antiepileptic drug hypersensitivity syndrome: *in vitro* and clinical observations. *Pediatr Neurol* 1994; **10**: 169–71.
8 Vittorio CC, Muglia JJ. Anticonvulsant hypersensitivity syndrome. *Arch Intern Med* 1995; **155**: 2285–90.
9 Licata AL, Louis ED. Anticonvulsant hypersensitivity syndrome. *Comprehen Ther* 1996; **22**: 152–5.
10 Kleier RS, Breneman DL, Boiko S. Generalized pustulation as a manifestation of the anticonvulsant hypersensitivity syndrome. *Arch Dermatol* 1991; **127**: 1361–4.
11 Drory VE, Korczyn AD. Hypersensitivity vasculitis and systemic lupus erythematosus induced by anticonvulsants. *Clin Neuropharmacol* 1993; **16**: 19–29.
12 Schmidt D, Kramer G. The new anticonvulsant drugs. Implications for avoidance of adverse effects. *Drug Saf* 1994; **11**: 422–31.
13 Brodie MJ. Lamotrigine versus other antiepileptic drugs: a star rating system is born. *Epilepsia* 1994; **35**: (Suppl. 5): S41–6.

Carbamazepine

Eruptions occur in between 3% [1–4] and 12% [5–7] of patients and include: diffuse erythema; miliary exanthema; maculopapular or speckled, morbilliform, reddish rash; urticaria; purpuric petechiae; or a mucocutaneous syndrome; from the eighth to the 60th day. The anticonvulsant hypersensitivity syndrome [8–10], erythroderma and exfoliative dermatitis, and TEN [2,3,11] are well recognized. Eczema and photosensitivity [12], an LE-like syndrome, dermatomyositis and erythema multiforme [13], as well as a pustular [14,15] and a lichenoid reaction [2,16], are very rare. Lesions with clinical and histological features suggestive of mycosis fungoides have been reported [17,18]. Patch testing has been advocated for the diagnosis of carbamazepine eruptions [8,9,19,20], but has resulted in reinduction of exfoliative dermatitis [21]. A psoriasiform eruption has been reported [22], as has thrombocytopenia and leukopenia complicated by Henoch–Schönlein purpura [23]. Cross-reactivity may occur with oxcarbazepine [24,25]. Other adverse effects include nausea, vomiting, ataxia, vertigo and drowsiness. Abnormal liver function [26] and bone-marrow suppression with occasional deaths due to aplastic anaemia have been recorded [2]. Development of a rash may act as an early warning of marrow toxicity. Carbamazepine therapy during pregnancy carries a 1% risk of development of spina bifida in the offspring [27].

Oral steroid therapy enabled 16 of 20 patients successfully to continue on carbamazepine after development of a rash shortly after introduction of the drug [28]. Desensitization has been achieved by induction of tolerance in patients in whom there was no suitable alternative therapy [29,30].

REFERENCES

1 Harman PRM. Carbamazepine (Tegretol) drug eruptions. *Br J Dermatol* 1967; **79**; 500–1.
2 Roberts DL, Marks R. Skin reactions to carbamazepine. *Arch Dermatol* 1981; **117**: 273–5.
3 Breathnach SM, McGibbon DH, Ive FA *et al*. Carbamazepine ('Tegretol') and toxic epidermal necrolysis: report of three cases with histopathological observations. *Clin Exp Dermatol* 1982; **7**; 585–91.
4 Chadwick D, Shan M, Foy P *et al*. Serum anticonvulsant concentrations and the risk of drug-induced skin eruptions. *J Neurol Neurosurg Psychiatry* 1984; **47**: 642–4.
5 Richens A, Davidson DL, Cartlidge NE, Easter DJ. A multicentre comparative trial of sodium valproate and carbamazepine in adult onset epilepsy. Adult EPITEG Collaborative Group. *J Neurol Neurosurg Psychiatry* 1994; **57**: 682–7.
6 Kramlinger KG, Phillips KA, Post RM. Rash complicating carbamazepine treatment. *J Clin Psychopharmacol* 1994; **14**: 408–13.
7 Konishi T, Naganuma Y, Hongo K *et al*. Carbamazepine-induced skin rash in children with epilepsy. *Eur J Pediatr* 1993; **152**: 605–8.
8 Scerri L, Shall L, Zaki I. Carbamazepine-induced anticonvulsant hypersensitivity syndrome—pathogenic and diagnostic considerations. *Clin Exp Dermatol* 1993; **18**: 540–2.
9 De Vriese AS, Philippe J, Van Renterghem DM *et al*. Carbamazepine hypersensitivity syndrome: report of 4 cases and review of the literature. *Medicine* 1995; **74**: 144–51.
10 Okuyama R, Ichinohasama R, Tagami H. Carbamazepine induced erythroderma with systemic lymphadenopathy. *J Dermatol* 1996; **23**: 489–94.
11 Reed MD, Bertino JA, Blumer JL. Carbamazepine-associated exfoliative dermatitis. *Clin Pharmacol* 1982; **1**: 78–9.
12 Terui T, Tagami H. Eczematous drug eruption from carbamazepine: coexistence of contact and photocontact sensitivity. *Contact Dermatitis* 1989; **20**: 260–4.
13 Simpson JR. 'Collagen disease' due to carbamazepine (Tegretol). *Br Med J* 1966; **ii**: 1434.
14 Staughton RCD, Harper JI, Rowland Payne CME *et al*. Toxic pustuloderma: a new entity? *J R Soc Med* 1984; **77**: 6–8.
15 Commens CA, Fischer GO. Toxic pustuloderma following carbamazepine therapy. *Arch Dermatol* 1988; **124**: 178–9.
16 Atkin SL, McKenzie TMM, Stevenson CJ. Carbamazepine-induced lichenoid eruption. *Clin Exp Dermatol* 1990; **15**: 382–3.
17 Welykyj S, Gradini R, Nakao J, Massa M. Carbamazepine-induced eruption histologically mimicking mycosis fungoides. *J Cutan Pathol* 1990; **17**: 111–16.
18 Rijlaarsdam U, Scheffer E, Meijer CJLM *et al*. Mycosis fungoides-like lesions associated with phenytoin and carbamazepine therapy. *J Am Acad Dermatol* 1991; **24**: 216–20.
19 Houwerzijl J, De Gast GC, Nater JP *et al*. Lymphocyte-stimulation tests and patch tests in carbamazepine hypersensitivity. *Clin Exp Immunol* 1977; **29**: 272–7.
20 Silva R, Machado A, Brandao M, Gonçalo S. Patch test diagnosis in carbamazepine erythroderma. *Contact Dermatitis* 1986; **15**: 254–5.
21 Vaillant L, Camenen I, Lorette G. Patch testing with carbamazepine: reinduction of an exfoliative dermatitis. *Arch Dermatol* 1989; **125**: 299.
22 Brenner S, Wolf R, Landau M, Politi Y. Psoriasiform eruption induced by anticonvulsants. *Israel J Med Sci* 1994; **30**: 283–6.
23 Kaneko K, Igarashi J, Suzuki Y *et al*. Carbamazepine-induced thrombocytopenia and leucopenia complicated by Henoch–Schönlein purpura symptoms. *Eur J Pediatr* 1993; **152**: 769–70.
24 Beran RG. Cross-reactive skin eruption with both carbamazepine and oxcarbazepine. *Epilepsia* 1993; **34**: 163–5.
25 Dam M. Practical aspects of oxcarbazepine treatment. *Epilepsia* 1994; **35** (Suppl. 3): S23–5.
26 Ramsey ID. Carbamazepine-induced jaundice. *Br Med J* 1967; **4**: 155.
27 Rosa FW. Spina bifida in infants of women treated with carbamazepine during pregnancy. *N Engl J Med* 1991; **324**: 674–7.
28 Murphy JM, Mashman J, Miller JD, Bell JB. Suppression of carbamazepine-induced rash with prednisone. *Neurology* 1991; **41**: 144–5.
29 Eames P. Adverse reaction to carbamazepine managed by desensitization. *Lancet* 1989; **i**: 509–10.
30 Boyle N, Lawlor BA. Desensitization to carbamazepine-induced skin rash. *Am J Psychiatry* 1996; **153**: 1234.

Diphenylhydantoin (phenytoin, dilantin)

Cutaneous manifestations related to phenytoin have been reviewed [1–7]. The various diverse presentations share certain histopathological findings: adhesion of the infiltrated cells to the basal layer of the epidermis, cell infiltration into the epidermis, vacuolation of the basal cells, and dyskeratotic cells in the epidermis and epidermal necrosis, with CD8+ T cells predominant in the epidermis [5].

About 5% of children develop a mild transient maculopapular rash within 3 weeks of starting treatment. This is more likely to occur if high loading doses are given initially [3,4]. In other series, between 8.5% [8] and 19% [9] of patients receiving phenytoin developed exanthematic rashes [10]. A phenytoin-induced hypersensitivity state, with generalized lymphadenopathy, hepatosplenomegaly, fever, arthralgia and eosinophilia occurs in about 1% of patients, and may be accompanied by hepatitis, nephritis and haematological abnormalities [7,11–13]. Skin involvement may lead to a suspicion of lymphoma, the phenytoin-induced pseudolymphoma syndrome [14–19]. Cutaneous lesions may be restricted to a few erythematous plaques [18], or cutaneous nodules [15], or consist of a generalized erythematous maculopapular rash [14], generalized exfoliative dermatitis [16,20] or TEN [21,22]. Generalized pustulation has been recorded as a manifestation of the anticonvulsant hypersensitivity syndrome [23]. Universal depigmentation has resulted from TEN [24]. Cutaneous histopathology in the pseudolymphoma syndrome is often indistinguishable from that of mycosis fungoides, with infiltrating cells having cerebriform nuclei and Pautrier microabscesses [17,19]. The rash resolves after cessation of the drug; systemic corticosteroids may aid resolution [25]. However, there is a threefold risk of true lymphoma on long-term therapy [26–28], and T-cell lymphoma has been reported in an adult [29].

Long-term treatment causes fibroblast proliferation, and may result in dose-dependent gingival hyperplasia [30,31] or coarsening of the features [32]; hypertrophic retro-auricular folds were reported in an isolated case [33].

Hypertrichosis may be seen. Other reactions have included fixed eruptions [34], including a widespread fixed drug eruption mimicking TEN [35], erythema multiforme [1,3], TEN with cholestasis [36], cutaneous vasculitis [37], an LE-like syndrome [38] and eosinophilic fasciitis [39]. Localized reactions to intravenous phenytoin have included delayed bluish discoloration, erythema and oedema, sometimes with bullae, distal to the site of injection [40]; immediate burning pain and swelling, and a delayed erythematous eruption with superficial sloughing, partial epidermal necrosis, and frequent multinucleate keratinocytes on histology have also been reported [41].

Treatment during pregnancy may lead to a characteristic 'fetal syndrome', with general underdevelopment and hypoplasia of phalanges and nails [42]; neonatal acne may be associated [43]. However, recent controlled observations suggest that acne is neither caused nor worsened by hydantoins [44], despite reports to the contrary [45].

REFERENCES

1 Silverman AK, Fairley J, Wong RC. Cutaneous and immunologic reactions to phenytoin. *J Am Acad Dermatol* 1988; **18**: 721–41.
2 Levantine A, Almeyda J. Drug reactions XX. Cutaneous reactions to anticonvulsants. *Br J Dermatol* 1972; **87**: 646–9.
3 Pollack MA, Burk PG, Nathanson G. Mucocutaneous eruptions due to anti epileptic drug therapy in children. *Ann Neurol* 1979; **5**: 262–7.
4 Wilson JT, Höjer B, Tomson G et al. High incidence of a concentration-dependent skin reaction in children treated with phenytoin. *Br Med J* 1978; **i**: 1583–6.
5 Tone T, Nishioka K, Kameyama K et al. Common histopathological processes of phenytoin drug eruption. *J Dermatol* 1992; **19**: 27–34.
6 Potter T, DiGregorio F, Stiff M, Hashimoto K. Dilantin hypersensitivity syndrome imitating staphylococcal toxic shock. *Arch Dermatol* 1994; **130**: 856–8.
7 Conger LA, Jr, Grabski WJ. Dilantin hypersensitivity reaction. *Cutis* 1996; **57**: 223–6.
8 Leppik IE, Lapora A, Loewenson R. Seasonal incidence of phenytoin allergy unrelated to plasma levels. *Arch Neurol* 1985; **42**: 120–2.
9 Rapp RP, Norton JA, Young B, Tibbs PA. Cutaneous reactions in head-injured patients receiving phenytoin for seizure prophylaxis. *Neurosurgery* 1983; **13**: 272–5.
10 Robinson HM, Stone JH. Exanthem due to diphenylhydantoin therapy. *Arch Dermatol* 1970; **101**: 462–5.
11 Stanley J, Fallon-Pellici V. Phenytoin hypersensitivity reaction. *Arch Dermatol* 1978; **114**: 1350–3.
12 Brown M, Schubert T. Phenytoin hypersensitivity hepatitis and mononucleosis syndrome. *J Clin Gastroenterol* 1986; **8**: 469–77.
13 Shear N, Spielberg S. Anticonvulsant hypersensitivity syndrome. *In vitro* assessment of risk. *J Clin Invest* 1989; **82**: 1826–32.
14 Charlesworth EN. Phenytoin-induced pseudolymphoma syndrome. An immunologic study. *Arch Dermatol* 1977; **113**; 477–80.
15 Adams JD. Localized cutaneous pseudolymphoma associated with phenytoin therapy: a case report. *Australas J Dermatol* 1981; **22**: 28–9.
16 Rosenthal CJ, Noguera CA, Coppola A, Kapelner SN. Pseudolymphoma with mycosis fungoides manifestations, hyperresponsiveness to diphenylhydantoin, and lymphocyte disregulation. *Cancer* 1982; **49**: 2305–14.
17 Kardaun SH, Scheffer E, Vermeer BJ. Drug-induced pseudolymphomatous skin reactions. *Br J Dermatol* 1988; **118**: 545–52.
18 Wolf R, Kahane E, Sandbank M. Mycosis fungoides-like lesions associated with phenytoin therapy. *Arch Dermatol* 1985; **121**: 1181–2.
19 Rijlaarsdam U, Scheffer E, Meijer CJLM et al. Mycosis fungoides-like lesions associated with phenytoin and carbamazepine therapy. *J Am Acad Dermatol* 1991; **24**: 216–20.
20 Danno K, Kume M, Ohta M et al. Erythroderma with generalized lymphadenopathy induced by phenytoin. *J Dermatol (Tokyo)* 1989; **16**: 392–6.
21 Sherertz EF, Jegasothy BV, Lazarus GS. Phenytoin hypersensitivity reaction presenting with toxic epidermal necrolysis and severe hepatitis: report of a patient treated with corticosteroid 'pulse therapy'. *J Am Acad Dermatol* 1985; **12**: 178–81.
22 Schmidt D, Kluge W. Fatal toxic epidermal necrolysis following reexposure to phenytoin. A case report. *Epilepsia* 1983; **24**: 440–3.
23 Kleier RS, Breneman DL, Boiko S. Generalized pustulation as a manifestation of the anticonvulsant hypersensitivity syndrome. *Arch Dermatol* 1991; **127**: 1361–4.
24 Smith DA, Burgdorf WHC. Universal cutaneous depigmentation following phenytoin-induced toxic epidermal necrolysis. *J Am Acad Dermatol* 1984; **10**: 106–9.
25 Chopra S, Levell NJ, Cowley G, Gilkes JJ. Systemic corticosteroids in the phenytoin hypersensitivity syndrome. *Br J Dermatol* 1996; **134**; 1109–12.
26 Tashima CK, De Los Santos R. Lymphoma and anticonvulsant therapy. *JAMA* 1974; **228**: 287–8.
27 Bichel J. Hydantoin derivatives and malignancies of the haemopoietic system. *Acta Med Scand* 1975; **198**: 327–8.
28 Li FP, Willard DR, Goodman R et al. Malignant lymphoma after diphenylhydantoin (Dilantin) therapy. *Cancer* 1975; **36**: 1359–62.
29 Isobe T, Horimatsu T, Fujita T et al. Adult T cell lymphoma following diphenylhydantoin therapy. *Acta Haematol Jpn* 1980; **43**: 711–14.
30 Angelopoulos AP, Goaz PW. Incidence of diphenylhydantoin gingival hyperplasia. *Oral Surg* 1972; **34**: 898–906.
31 Hassell TM, Page RC, Narayanan AS, Cooper CG. Diphenylhydantoin (dilantin) gingival hyperplasia: drug induced abnormality of connective tissue. *Proc Natl Acad Sci USA* 1976; **73**: 2909–12.
32 Lefebvre EB, Haining RG, Labbé RF. Coarse facies, calvarial thickening and hyperphosphatasia associated with long-term anticonvulsant therapy. *N Engl J Med* 1972; **286**: 1301–2.
33 Trunnell TN, Waisman M. Hypertrophic retroauricular folds attributable to diphenylhydantoin. *Cutis* 1982; **30**: 207–9.
34 Sweet RD. Fixed skin eruption due to phenytoin sodium. *Lancet* 1950; **i**: 68.
35 Baird BJ, De Villez RL. Widespread bullous fixed drug eruption mimicking toxic epidermal necrolysis. *Int J Dermatol* 1988; **27**: 170–4.
36 Spechler SJ, Sperber H, Doos WG, Koff RS. Cholestasis and toxic epidermal necrolysis associated with phenytoin sodium ingestion: the role of bile duct injury. *Ann Intern Med* 1981; **95**: 455–6.
37 Yermakov VM, Hitti IF, Sutton AL. Necrotizing vasculitis associated with diphenylhydantoin: two fatal cases. *Hum Pathol* 1983; **14**: 182–4.
38 Gleichman H. Systemic lupus erythematosus triggered by diphenyl-hydantoin. *Arthritis Rheum* 1982; **25**: 1387–8.
39 Buchanan RR, Gordon DA, Muckle TJ et al. The eosinophilic fasciitis syndrome after phenytoin (Dilantin) therapy. *J Rheumatol* 1980; **7**: 733–6.
40 Kilarski DJ, Buchanan C, Von Behren L. Soft tissue damage associated with intravenous phenytoin. *N Engl J Med* 1984; **311**: 1186–7.
41 Hunt SJ. Cutaneous necrosis and multinucleate epidermal cells associated with intravenous phenytoin. *Am J Dermatopathol* 1995; **17**: 399–402.
42 Nagy R. Fetal hydantoin syndrome. *Arch Dermatol* 1981; **117**: 593–5.
43 Stankler L, Campbell AGM. Neonatal acne vulgaris: a possible feature of the fetal hydantoin syndrome. *Br J Dermatol* 1980; **103**: 453–5.
44 Greenwood R, Fenwick PBC, Cunliffe WJ. Acne and anticonvulsants. *Br Med J* 1983; **287**: 1669–70.
45 Jenkins RB, Ratner AC. Diphenylhydantoin and acne. *N Engl J Med* 1972; **287**: 148.

Lamotrigine

Dosage-related allergic skin rashes occur in about 5% of patients [1], leading to a withdrawal rate of 2% of patient exposures [2]; the rash rarely is severe enough to require hospitalization. However, in one study, six of eight patients with a prior lamotrigine-related rash had no recurrence on rechallenge, and two other patients had only mild rashes [3]. TEN is recorded [4]. Serious skin reactions including

Stevens–Johnson syndrome and TEN occur in about one in 100 adults and between one in 100 and one in 300 children [5].

REFERENCES

1 Richens A. Safety of lamotrigine. *Epilepsia* 1994; **35** (Suppl. 5): S37–40.
2 Messenheimer JA. Lamotrigine *Epilepsia* 1995; **36** (Suppl. 2): S87–94.
3 Tavernor SJ, Wong IC, Newton R, Brown SW. Rechallenge with lamotrigine after initial rash. *Seizure* 1995; **4**: 67–71.
4 Sterker M, Berrouschot J, Schneider D. Fatal course of toxic epidermal necrolysis under treatment with lamotrigine. *Int J Clin Pharmacol Ther* 1995; **33**: 595–7.
5 Anonymous. Lamotrigine (Lamictal): increased risk of serious skin reactions in children. *Curr Probl Pharmacovig* 1997; **23**: 8.

Sodium valproate

Occasional transient rashes and stomatitis are documented. Temporary hair loss may be followed by increasing curliness of the regrowing hair [1]. Alteration in hair colour has been noted [2]. One case of generalized morphoea [3], and two of cutaneous leukocytoclastic vasculitis recurring on challenge [4] have been reported. An extrapyramidal syndrome may be induced [5], and the drug may be teratogenic [6].

REFERENCES

1 Jeavons PM, Clark JE, Harding GFA. Valproate and curly hair. *Lancet* 1977; **i**: 359.
2 Herranz JL, Arteaga R, Armijo JA. Change in hair colour induced by valproic acid. *Dev Med Child Neurol* 1981; **23**: 386–7.
3 Goihman-Yahr M, Leal H, Essenfeld-Yahr E. Generalized morphea: a side effect of valproate sodium? *Arch Dermatol* 1980; **116**: 621.
4 Kamper AM, Valentijn RM, Stricker BHC, Purcell PM. Cutaneous vasculitis induced by sodium valproate. *Lancet* 1991; **337**: 497–8.
5 Lautin A, Stanley M, Angrist B, Gershon S. Extrapyramidal syndrome with sodium valproate. *Br Med J* 1979; **ii**: 1035–6.
6 Gomez MR. Possible teratogenicity of valproic acid. *J Paediatr* 1981; **98**: 508–9.

Trimethadione

Serious hypersensitivity reactions may occur, including erythema multiforme, urticaria and generalized exfoliative dermatitis.

Vigabatrin

An allergic vasculitis developed in one patient 6 months after commencement of this drug [1].

REFERENCE

1 Dieterle L, Becker EW, Berg PA *et al.* Allergische Vaskulitis durch Vigabatrin. *Nervenarzt* 1994; **65**: 122–4.

Opioid analgesics and amphetamine

Cutaneous side-effects common to drug abuse, most frequently cocaine, heroin and pentazocine, following parenteral injection include [1,2]: infections, abscesses, septic phlebitis, subcutaneous and deep dermal cellulitis, necrosis, tetanus, widespread urticaria; cutaneous manifestations of primary and secondary syphilis, HIV infection and endocarditis. Starch and talc granulomas, lymphangitis and lymphadenitis in draining lymph nodes, pigmentary abnormalities including hyperpigmentation over the injected veins, accidental 'soot' tattoos where needles were sterilized over an open flame, scarring, ulceration, necrotizing angiitis and leukocytoclastic vasculitis may supervene. *Skin popping* refers to injection of drugs beneath the skin without concern for vascular access; this may result in ulcers being delayed for a number of years [3].

REFERENCES

1 Rosen VJ. Cutaneous manifestations of drug abuse by parenteral injections. *Am J Dermatopathol* 1985; **7**: 79–83.
2 Smith DJ, Busito MJ, Velanovich V *et al.* Drug injection injuries of the upper extremity. *Ann Plastic Surg* 1989; **22**: 19–24.
3 Pardes JB, Falanga V, Kerdel FA. Delayed cutaneous ulcerations arising at sites of prior parenteral drug abuse. *J Am Acad Dermatol* 1993; **29**: 1052–4.

Buprenorphine

An addict accidentally injected a suspension of crushed tablets into the superficial pudendal artery instead of the femoral vein, and developed pain, oedema and mottling of the penis [1].

REFERENCE

1 Naylor AR, Gordon M, Jenkins AMcL. Untitled report. *Br Med J* 1991; **303**: 478.

Codeine

This drug has been associated with pruritus, urticaria (usually due to non-immunological release of histamine) [1,2], macular and maculopapular eruptions, scarlatiniform rashes [1,3], angio-oedema, fixed eruption, a bullous eruption, erythema multiforme and erythema nodosum.

REFERENCES

1 Hunskaar S, Dragsund S. Scarlatiniform rash and urticaria due to codeine. *Ann Allergy* 1985; **54**: 240–1.
2 De Groot AC, Conemans J. Allergic urticarial rash from oral codeine. *Contact Dermatitis* 1986; **14**: 209–14.
3 Voohost R, Sparreboom S. Four cases of recurrent pseudo-scarlet fever caused by phenanthrene alkaloids with a 6-hydroxy group (codeine and morphine). *Ann Allergy* 1980; **44**: 116–20.

Heroin

Use of the dorsal vein of the penis for administration of the drug has produced ulceration [1]. Systemic infections, such as candidiasis, may supervene [2]. Leukocytoclastic vasculitis and necrotizing angiitis have been reported in drug abusers [3–5]. Pigmentation of the tongue may occur as a form of fixed drug eruption in heroin addicts [6]. A possible association with development of pemphigus erythematosus has been suggested [7].

REFERENCES

1 White WB, Barrett S. Penile ulcer in heroin abuse: a case report. *Cutis* 1982; **29**: 62–3.
2 Bielsa I, Miro JM, Herrero C *et al*. Systemic candidiasis in heroin abusers. *Int J Dermatol* 1987; **26**: 314–19.
3 Citron BP, Halpern M, McCarron M *et al*. Necrotizing angiitis associated with drug abuse. *N Engl J Med* 1970; **283**: 1003–11.
4 Lignelli GJ, Bucheit WA. Angiitis in drug abusers. *N Engl J Med* 1971; **284**: 112–13.
5 Gendelman H, Linzer M, Barland P *et al*. Leukocytoclastic vasculitis in an intravenous heroin abuser. *NY State J Med* 1983; **83**: 984–6.
6 Westerhof W, Wolters EC, Brookbakker JTW *et al*. Pigmented lesions of the tongue in heroin addicts—fixed drug eruption. *Br J Dermatol* 1983; **109**: 605–10.
7 Fellner MJ, Winiger J. Pemphigus erythematosus and heroin addiction. *Int J Dermatol* 1978; **17**: 308–11.

Morphine

Morphine is a potent histamine releaser and may cause pruritus and urticaria [1]. Profuse sweating is a common effect. Morphine provokes facial flushing blocked by naloxone [2]. Local skin irritation during subcutaneous morphine infusion is recorded [3].

REFERENCES

1 McLelland J. The mechanism of morphine-induced urticaria. *Arch Dermatol* 1986; **122**: 138–9.
2 Cohen RA, Coffman JD. Naloxone reversal of morphine-induced peripheral vasodilatation. *Clin Pharmacol Ther* 1980; **28**: 541–4.
3 Shvartzman P, Bonneh D. Local skin irritation in the course of subcutaneous morphine infusion: a challenge. *J Pall Care* 1994; **10**: 44–5.

Pentazocine

Woody induration of the skin and subcutaneous tissues at injection sites, perhaps with central ulceration and peripheral pigmentation, and a granulomatous histology, is well recognized [1–7]. Pigmentation, ulceration and a chronic panniculitis have supervened after many years of use. Phlebitis, cellulitis, fibrous myopathy [8] and limb contractures can complicate these changes. Generalized eruptions are rare [9]. There is an isolated report of TEN [10].

REFERENCES

1 Parks DL, Perry HO, Muller SA. Cutaneous complications of pentazocine injections. *Arch Dermatol* 1971; **104**: 231–5.
2 Schlicher JE, Zuehlke RL, Lynch PJ. Local changes at the site of pentazocine injection. *Arch Dermatol* 1971; **104**: 90–1.
3 Swanson DW, Weddige RL, Morse RM. Hospitalised pentazocine abusers. *Mayo Clin Proc* 1973; **48**: 85–93.
4 Schiff BL, Kern AB. Unusual cutaneous manifestations of pentazocine addiction. *JAMA* 1977; **238**: 1542–3.
5 Padilla RS, Becker LE, Hoffman H, Long G. Cutaneous and venous complications of pentazocine abuse. *Arch Dermatol* 1979; **115**: 975–7.
6 Palestine RF, Millns JL, Spigel GT *et al*. Skin manifestations of pentazocine abuse. *J Am Acad Dermatol* 1980; **2**: 47–55.
7 Mann RJ, Gostelow BE, Meacock DJ, Kennedy CTC. Pentazocine ulcers. *J R Soc Med* 1982; **75**: 903–5.
8 Johnson KR, Hsueh WA, Glusman SM, Arnett FC. Fibrous myopathy: A rheumatic complication of drug abuse. *Arthritis Rheum* 1976; **19**: 923–6.
9 Pedragosa R, Vidal J, Fuentes R, Huguet P. Tricotropism by pentazocine. *Arch Dermatol* 1987; **123**: 297–8.
10 Hunter JAA, Davison AM. Toxic epidermal necrolysis associated with pentazocine therapy and severe reversible renal failure. *Br J Dermatol* 1973; **88**: 287–90.

Methylamphetamine

A link with necrotizing angiitis has been recorded when this drug is used alone or with heroin or D-lysergic acid diethylamide [1].

REFERENCE

1 Citron BP, Halpern M, McCarron M *et al*. Necrotizing angiitis associated with drug abuse. *N Engl J Med* 1970; **283**: 1003–11.

Anti-Parkinsonian drugs

Amantadine

Reversible livedo reticularis has occurred in a high percentage of patients receiving amantadine, a tricyclic amine used in the treatment of Parkinson's disease [1,2].

Bromocryptine

Transient livedo reticularis [3], erythromelalgia [4], acrocyanosis with Raynaud's phenomenon [5,6], morphea [7] and swelling of the legs with a sclerodermatous histology [8] have been reported rarely, as has alopecia [9] and psychosis.

Carbidopa

Scleroderma-like reactions have occurred when this drug has been given in conjunction with tryptophan [10,11].

Levodopa

There have been several isolated reports of the occurrence of malignant melanoma [12–14], in certain instances involving multiple primaries, but the association may be by chance alone.

REFERENCES

1 Shealy CN, Weeth JB, Mercier D. Livedo reticularis in patients with parkinsonism receiving amantadine. *JAMA* 1970; **212**: 1522–3.
2 Vollum DI, Parkes JD, Doyle D. Livedo reticularis during amantadine treatment. *Br Med J* 1971; **ii**: 627–8.
3 Calne DB, Plotkin C, Neophytides A *et al.* Long-term treatment of Parkinsonism with bromocriptine. *Lancet* 1978; **i**: 735–7.
4 Eisler T, Hall RP, Kalavar KAR, Calne DB. Erythromelalgia-like eruption in Parkinsonian patients treated with bromocriptine. *Neurology* 1981; **37**: 1368–70.
5 Duvoisin RC. Digital vasospasm with bromocryptine. *Lancet* 1976; **ii**: 204.
6 Pearce I, Pearce JMS. Bromocriptine in Parkinsonism. *Br Med J* 1978; **i**: 1402–4.
7 Leshin B, Piette WW, Caplin RM. Morphea after bromocriptine therapy. *Int J Dermatol* 1989; **28**: 177–9.
8 Dupont E, Olivarius B, Strong MJ. Bromocriptine-induced collagenosis-like symptomatology in Parkinson's disease. *Lancet* 1982; **i**: 850–1.
9 Blum I, Leiba S. Increased hair loss as a side effect of bromocriptine treatment. *N Engl J Med* 1980; **303**: 1418.
10 Sternberg EM, Van Woert MH, Young SN *et al.* Development of a scleroderma-like illness during therapy with L-5-Hydroxytryptophan and Carbidopa. *N Engl J Med* 1980; **303**: 782–7.
11 Chamson A, Périer C, Frey J. Syndrome sclérodermiforme et poïkilodermique observé au cours d'un traitement par carbidopa et 5-hydroxytryptophane. Culture de fibroblastes avec analyse biochimique du métabolisme du collagene. *Ann Derm Vénéréol* 1986; **113**: 71.
12 Sober AJ, Wick MM. Levodopa therapy and malignant melanoma. *JAMA* 1978; **240**: 554–5.
13 Bernstein JE, Medenica M, Soltani K *et al.* Levodopa administration and multiple primary cutaneous melanomas. *Arch Dermatol* 1980; **116**: 1041–4.
14 Rosin MA, Braun M, III. Malignant melanoma and levodopa. *Cutis* 1984; **33**: 572–4.

Antivertigo drugs and cerebrovascular dilators

Cinnarazine

This drug [1], and its derivative flunarizine [2], have been implicated in the precipitation of lichenoid eruptions. In the case of cinnarazine, clinical and immunofluorescence features of lichen planus were combined with the presence of a circulating antibasement-membrane zone IgG antibody [2]. Other side-effects include drowsiness, depression, and parkinsonism.

REFERENCES

1 Miyagawa W, Ohi H, Muramatsu T *et al.* Lichen planus pemphigoides-like lesions induced by cinnarizine. *Br J Dermatol* 1985; **112**: 607–13.
2 Suys E, De Coninck A, De Pauw I, Roseeuw D. Lichen planus induced by flunarizine. *Dermatologica* 1990; **181**: 71–2.

Miscellaneous nervous system drugs

Appetite suppressants and stimulants

Centrally acting appetite suppressants may induce urticarial vasculitis [1]. Megestrol, a synthetic orally active progesterone derivative used to stimulate appetite and weight gain in cachetic patients, caused a generalized morbilliform rash in a man; skin testing with progesterone acetate was positive [2].

Pyritinol

This drug, given for cerebral concussion, caused an unusual erythema multiforme-like eruption and severe headache after 10 days' treatment [3].

REFERENCES

1 Papadavid E, Yu RC, Tay A, Chu AC. Urticarial vasculitis induced by centrally acting appetite suppressants. *Br J Dermatol* 1996; **134**: 990–1.
2 Fisher DA. Drug-induced progesterone dermatitis. *J Am Acad Dermatol* 1996; **34**: 863–4.
3 Nachbar F, Korting HC, Vogl T. Erythema multiforme-like eruption in association with severe headache following pyritinol. *Dermatology* 1993; **187**: 42–6.

Drugs acting on the cardiovascular system

Adverse cutaneous reactions from cardiovascular drug therapy, and from antiarrhythmic drugs, have been reviewed [1,2].

REFERENCES

1 Reiner DM, Frishman WH, Luftschein S, Grossman M. Adverse cutaneous reactions from cardiovascular drug therapy. *NY State J Med* 1992; **92**: 137–47.
2 Sun DK, Reiner D, Frishman W *et al.* Adverse dermatologic reactions from antiarrhythmic drug therapy. *J Clin Pharmacol* 1994; **34**: 953–66.

Cardiac antiarrhythmic drugs

Amiodarone

This iodinated antiarrhythmic drug causes photosensitivity in around 40% of patients [1–13]. Symptoms develop within 2 h of sun exposure as a burning sensation followed by erythema; the action spectrum is UVA extending to a degree into visible light wavebands above 400 nm [4]. Light sensitivity may persist for up to 4 months after the drug is stopped [1,2]. Blue or grey pigmentation of the face and other sun-exposed areas, resembling that in argyria, is a much less common late effect, occurring in 2–5% of cases; non-sun-exposed areas may also be involved [3,6–12]. It is induced by a phototoxic reaction involving both UVB and UVA [3,6], and is related to both duration and dosage of the drug [11]. However, although cutaneous side-effects are more likely with increasing duration of treatment and cumulative dosage, neither the serum amiodarone level nor the serum metabolite level have any predictive power [13]. Amiodarone-pigmented skin contains the drug and its metabolites in higher concentrations than non-pigmented skin [3]. Iodine-rich amiodarone and its metabolites have been detected bound to lipofuscin within secondary lysosomes in perivascular dermal macrophages [7–10]. Electron dense granules and myelin-like bodies are also found in peripheral blood leukocytes [12]. The cutaneous pigmentation slowly fades after discontinuation of therapy, but may persist for months to years [8].

Iododerma has occurred with long-term therapy. Vasculitis [14] and linear IgA disease [15] have been recorded. A fatal case of TEN has been reported [16]. The most severe adverse side-effect seen with amiodarone is pulmonary fibrosis, which occurs in 5–10% of exposed patients, and which has a 10% mortality rate. Other problems have been cardiac dysrhythmias, thyroid dysfunction, peripheral neuropathy and reversible corneal deposits [17].

REFERENCES

1 Marcus FI, Fontaine GH, Frank R, Grosgogeat Y. Clinical pharmacology and therapeutic applications of the antiarrhythmic agent amiodarone. *Am Heart J* 1981; **101**: 480–93.
2 Chalmers RJ, Muston HL, Srinivas V, Bennett DH. High incidence of amiodarone-induced photosensitivity in North-west England. *Br Med J* 1982; **285**: 341.
3 Zachary CB, Slater DN, Holt DW *et al.* The pathogenesis of amiodarone-induced pigmentation and photosensitivity. *Br J Dermatol* 1984; **110**: 451–6.
4 Ferguson J, Addo HA, Jones S *et al.* A study of cutaneous photosensitivity induced by amiodarone. *Br J Dermatol* 1985; **113**: 537–49.
5 Roupe G, Larkö O, Olsson SB *et al.* Amiodarone photoreactions. *Acta Derm Venereol (Stockh)* 1987; **67**: 76–9.
6 Waitzer S, Butany J, From L *et al.* Cutaneous ultrastructural changes and photosensitivity associated with amiodarone therapy. *J Am Acad Dermatol* 1987; **16**: 779–87.
7 McGovern B, Garan H, Kelly E, Ruskin JN. Adverse reactions during treatment with amiodarone hydrochloride. *Br Med J* 1983; **287**: 175–9.
8 Miller RAW, McDonald ATJ. Dermal lipofuscinois associated with amiodarone therapy. Report of a case. *Arch Dermatol* 1984; **120**: 646–9.
9 Holt DW, Adams PC, Campbell RWF *et al.* Amiodarone and its desethyl-metabolite: tissue distribution and ultrastructural changes in amiodarone treated patients. *Br J Clin Pharmacol* 1984; **17**: 195–6.
10 Török L, Szekeres L, Lakatos A, Szücs M. Amiodaronebedingte Hyperpigmentierung. *Hautarzt* 1986; **37**: 507–10.
11 Heger JJ, Prystowsky EN, Zipes DP. Relationships between amiodarone dosage, drug concentrations, and adverse side effects. *Am Heart J* 1983; **106**: 931–5.
12 Rappersberger K, Konrad K, Wieser E *et al.* Morphological changes in peripheral blood cells and skin in amiodarone-treated patients. *Br J Dermatol* 1986; **114**: 189–96.
13 Shukla R, Jowett NI, Thompson DR, Pohl JE. Side effects with amiodarone therapy. *Postgrad Med J* 1994; **70**: 492–8.
14 Staubli M, Zimmerman A, Bircher J. Amiodarone-induced vasculitis and polyserositis. *Postgrad Med J* 1985; **61**: 245–7.
15 Primka EJ, III, Liranzo MO, Bergfeld W *et al.* Amiodarone-induced linear IgA disease. *J Am Acad Dermatol* 1996; **31**: 809–11.
16 Bencini PL, Crosti C, Sala F *et al.* Toxic epidermal necrolysis and amiodarone. *Arch Dermatol* 1985; **121**: 838.
17 Morgan DJR. Adverse reactions profile: 3. Amiodarone. *Drug Ther Bull* 1991; **31**: 104–11.

Digoxin

Allergic reactions are very rare [1], but exanthematic erythema, urticaria, bullous eruptions and thrombocytopenic purpura are documented. In one patient, a psoriasiform rash occurred, confirmed by later re-exposure [2].

REFERENCES

1 Martin SJ, Shah D. Cutaneous hypersensitivity reaction to digoxin. *JAMA* 1994; **271**: 1905.
2 David M, Livni E, Stern E *et al.* Psoriasiform eruption induced by digoxin: confirmed by re-exposure. *J Am Acad Dermatol* 1981; **5**: 702–3.

Procainamide

This drug is well known to precipitate an LE-like syndrome [1–6], perhaps in part as a result of binding of the hydroxylamine metabolite of procainamide to complement component C4, with resultant impaired complement-mediated clearance of immune complexes [5,6]. A lichenoid eruption followed the occurrence of drug-induced LE in one case [7]. Urticarial vasculitis has been reported [8].

REFERENCES

1 Dubois EL. Procainamide induction of a systemic lupus erythematosus-like syndrome. Presentation of six cases, review of the literature, and analysis and follow-up of reported cases. *Medicine* 1969; **48**: 217–18.
2 Blomgren SE, Condemi JJ, Vaughan JH. Procainamide-induced lupus erythematosus. Clinical and laboratory observations. *Am J Med* 1972; **52**: 338–48.
3 Whittle TS, Jr, Ainsworth SK. Procainamide-induced systemic lupus erythematosus. Renal involvement with deposition of immune complexes. *Arch Pathol Lab Med* 1976; **100**: 469–74.
4 Tan EM, Rubin RL. Autoallergic reactions induced by procainamide. *J Allergy Clin Immunol* 1984; **74**: 631–4.
5 Sim E, Stanley L, Gill EW, Jones A. Metabolites of procainamide and practolol inhibit complement components C3 and C4. *Biochem J* 1988; **251**: 323–6.
6 Sim E. Drug-induced immune complex disease. *Complement Inflamm* 1989; **6**: 119–26.
7 Sherertz EF. Lichen planus following procainamide-induced lupus erythematosus. *Cutis* 1988; **42**: 51–3.
8 Knox JP, Welykyj SE, Gradini R, Massa MC. Procainamide-induced urticarial vasculitis. *Cutis* 1988; **42**: 469–72.

Quinidine

An eczematous photosensitivity is well described [1–5]; fever is common. Thrombocytopenic purpura may be induced, resulting from antibodies to drug–platelet conjugates [6,7]. Urticarial, scarlatiniform and morbilliform eruptions occur; the latter may proceed to generalized exfoliative dermatitis if the drug is continued. Fixed, and lichenoid eruptions [8–14], often light-induced, are recorded, as well as an acneiform rash [15]. Livedo reticularis has been documented; the mechanism is unknown, although recent sunlight exposure was a feature common to all cases [16–18]. Drug-induced LE [19–21] and Henoch–Schönlein vasculitis [22,23] have been seen. Psoriasis may be exacerbated [24,25]. Localized blue–grey pigmentation of the shins, hard palate, nails, nose, ears and forearms has been recorded [26].

REFERENCES

1 Berger TG, Sesody SJ. Quinidine-induced lichenoid photodermatitis. *Cutis* 1982; **29**: 595–8.
2 Marx JL, Eisenstat BA, Gladstein AH. Quinidine photosensitivity. *Arch Dermatol* 1983; **119**: 39–43.
3 Armstrong RB, Leach EE, Whitman G *et al*. Quinidine photosensitivity. *Arch Dermatol* 1985; **121**: 525–8.
4 Jeanmougin M, Sigal M, Djian B *et al*. Photo-allergie à la quinidine. *Ann Dermatol Vénéréol* 1986; **113**: 985–7.
5 Schürer NY, Lehmann P, Plewig G. Chinidininduzierte Photoallergie. Eine klinische und experimentelle Studie. *Hautarzt* 1991; **42**: 158–61.
6 Christie DJ, Weber RW, Mullen PC *et al*. Structural features of the quinidine and quinine molecules necessary for binding of drug-induced antibodies to human platelets. *J Lab Clin Med* 1984; **104**: 730–40.
7 Gary M, Ilfeld D, Kelton JG. Correlation of a quinidine-induced platelet-specific antibody with development of thrombocytopenia. *Am J Med* 1985; **79**: 253–5.
8 Anderson TE. Lichen planus following quinidine therapy. *Br J Dermatol* 1967; **79**: 500.
9 Pegum JS. Lichenoid quinidine eruption. *Br J Dermatol* 1968; **80**: 343.
10 Maltz BL, Becker LE. Quinidine-induced lichen planus. *Int J Dermatol* 1980; **19**: 96–7.
11 Bonnetblanc J-M, Bernard P, Catanzano G, Souyri N. Eruptions lichénoides photinduites aux quinidiniques. *Ann Dermatol Vénéréol* 1987; **114**: 957–61.
12 Wolf R, Dorfman B, Krakowski A. Quinidine induced lichenoid and eczematous photodermatitis. *Dermatologica* 1987; **174**: 285–9.
13 De Larrard G, Jeanmougin M, Moulonguet I *et al*. Toxidermie lichénoide alopéciante à la quinidine. *Ann Dermatol Vénéréol* 1988; **115**: 1172–4.
14 Jeanmougin M, Elkara-Marrak H, Pons A *et al*. Éruption lichénoïde photo-induite a l'hydroxyquinidine. *Ann Dermatol Vénéréol* 1987; **114**: 1397–9.
15 Burckhart CG. Quinidine-induced acne. *Arch Dermatol* 1987; **117**: 603–4.
16 Marion DF, Terrien CM. Photosensitive livedo reticularis. *Arch Dermatol* 1973; **108**: 100–1.
17 De Groot WP, Wuite J. Livedo racemosa-like photosensitivity reaction during quinidine durettes medication. *Dermatologica* 1974; **148**: 371–6.
18 Bruce S, Wolf JE, Jr. Quinidine-induced photosensitive livedo reticularis-like eruption. *J Am Acad Dermatol* 1985; **12**: 332–6.
19 Lavie CJ, Biundo J, Quinet RJ, Waxman J. Systemic lupus erythematosus (SLE) induced by quinidine. *Arch Intern Med* 1985; **145**: 446–8.
20 McCormack GD, Barth WF. Quinidine induced lupus syndrome. *Semin Arthritis Rheum* 1985; **15**: 73–9.
21 Cohen MG, Kevat S, Prowse MV *et al*. Two distinct quinidine-induced rheumatic syndromes. *Ann Intern Med* 1988; **108**: 369–71.
22 Aviram A. Henoch–Schönlein syndrome associated with quinidine. *JAMA* 1980; **243**: 432–4.
23 Zax RH, Hodge SJ, Callen JP. Cutaneous leukocytoclastic vasculitis. Serial histopathologic evaluation demonstrates the dynamic nature of the infiltrate. *Arch Dermatol* 1990; **126**: 69–72.
24 Baker H. The influence of chloroquine and related drugs on psoriasis and keratoderma blenorrhagicum. *Br J Dermatol* 1966; **78**: 161–6.
25 Brenner S, Cabili S, Wolf R. Widespread erythematous scaly plaques in an adult. Psoriasiform eruption induced by quinidine. *Arch Dermatol* 1993; **129**: 1331–2, 1334–5.
26 Mahler R, Sissons W, Watters K. Pigmentation induced by quinidine therapy. *Arch Dermatol* 1986; **122**: 1062–4.

Beta-adrenoceptor-blocking agents

This group of drugs shares in common certain potential side-effects [1,2]. Peripheral ischaemia may be aggravated, and cold extremities and Raynaud's phenomenon [3] may present as new symptoms. Peripheral gangrene and peripheral skin necrosis [4,5] have been reported. An LE-like syndrome [6], and eczematous or lichenoid [1,2] eruptions may be induced rarely. Psoriasis vulgaris is occasionally aggravated or precipitated by a number of β-blockers including atenolol, oxprenolol and propranolol [7–13]. Cross-sensitivity is not usual [14], but cross-reactivity between atenolol, oxprenolol and propranolol has been reported [15]. Peyronie's disease (induratio penis plastica) has been attributed to labetalol, metoprolol and propranolol [16,17]. Beta-blockers may enhance anaphylactic reactions caused by other allergens, and may make resuscitation more difficult [18–20]. Alopecia has been attributed to topical ophthalmic β-blockers, especially timolol [21]. Vitiligo may be exacerbated [22].

REFERENCES

1 Felix RH, Ive FA, Dahl MGC. Skin reactions to beta-blockers. *Br Med J* 1975; **i**: 626.
2 Hödl S. Nebenwirkungen der Betarezeptorenblocker an der Haut. Übersicht und eigene Beobachtungen. *Hautarzt* 1985; **36**: 549–57.
3 Marshall AJ, Roberts CJC, Barritt DW. Raynaud's phenomenon as a side effect of beta-blockers in hypertension. *Br Med J* 1976; **i**: 1498–9.
4 Gokal R, Dornan TL, Ledingham JGG. Peripheral skin necrosis complicating beta-blockade. *Br Med J* 1979; **i**: 721–2.
5 Hoffbrand BI. Peripheral skin necrosis complicating beta-blockade. *Br Med J* 1979; **i**: 1082.
6 Hughes GRV. Hypotensive agents, beta-blockers, and drug-induced lupus. *Br Med J* 1982; **284**: 1358–9.
7 Arntzen N, Kavli G, Volden G. Psoriasis provoked by β-blocking agents. *Acta Dermatol Venereol (Stockh)* 1984; **64**: 346–8.
8 Abel EA, Dicicco LM, Orenberg EK *et al*. Drugs in exacerbation of psoriasis. *J Am Acad Dermatol* 1986; **15**: 1007–22.
9 Heng MCY, Heng MK. Beta-adrenoceptor antagonist-induced psoriasiform eruption. Clinical and pathogenetic aspects. *Int J Dermatol* 1988; **27**: 619–27.
10 Gold MH, Holy AK, Roenigk HH, Jr. Beta-blocking drugs and psoriasis. A review of cutaneous side effects and retrospective analysis of their effects on psoriasis. *J Am Acad Dermatol* 1988; **19**: 837–41.
11 Halevy S, Livni E. Psoriasis and psoriasiform eruptions associated with propranolol: the role of an immunologic mechanism. *Arch Dermatol Res* 1990; **283**: 472–3.
12 Steinkraus V, Steinfath M, Mensing H. Beta-adrenergic blocking drugs and psoriasis. *J Am Acad Dermatol* 1992; **27**: 266–7.
13 Halevy S, Livni E. Beta-adrenergic blocking drugs and psoriasis: the role of an immunologic mechanism. *J Am Acad Dermatol* 1993; **29**: 504–5.
14 Furhoff A-K, Norlander M, Peterson C. Cross-sensitivity between practolol and other beta-blockers? *Br Med J* 1976; **i**: 831.
15 Van Joost T, Smitt JHS. Skin reactions to propranolol and cross sensitivity to β-adrenoreceptor blocking agents. *Arch Dermatol* 1981; **117**: 600–1.
16 Yudkin JS. Peyronie's disease in association with metoprolol. *Lancet* 1977; **ii**: 1355.
17 Jones HA, Castleden WM. Peyronie's disease. *Med J Aust* 1981; **ii**: 514–15.
18 Hannaway PJ, Hopper GDK. Severe anaphylaxis and drug-induced beta-blockade. *N Engl J Med* 1983; **308**: 1536.
19 Toogood JH. Risk of anaphylaxis in patients receiving beta-blocker drugs. *J Allergy Clin Immunol* 1988; **81**: 1–5.
20 Hepner MJ, Ownby DR, Anderson JA *et al*. Risk of systemic reactions in patients taking beta-blocker drugs receiving allergen immunotherapy injections. *J Allergy Clin Immunol* 1990; **86**: 407–11.
21 Fraunfelder FT, Meyer SM, Menacker SJ. Alopecia possibly secondary to topical ophthalmic β-blockers. *JAMA* 1990; **263**: 1493–4.
22 Schallreuter KU. Beta-adrenergic blocking drugs may exacerbate vitiligo. *Br J Dermatol* 1995; **132**: 168–9.

Acebutolol

Rashes with mixed lichenoid and LE-like features have been reported [1]. The LE syndrome may have pleuro-pulmonary features [2].

Atenolol

Conjunctivitis and a periocular dermatitis [3], as well as a psoriasiform rash [4], pseudolymphomatous reaction [5] and vasculitis [6] are recorded.

Cetamolol

A psoriasiform eruption has been documented [7].

Labetalol

Mixed eruptions with psoriasiform and pityriasis rubra pilaris-like changes [8], a bullous lichenoid eruption [9] and a systemic LE-like syndrome [10] are documented.

Metoprolol

Various psoriasiform or eczematous rashes may follow long-term therapy [11,12]. Conjunctivitis and periocular dermatitis have occurred [3]. Peyronie's disease appears to be a rare but confirmed side-effect and may be reversible. Telogen effluvium has been noted [13].

Oxprenolol

This drug, like practolol, has caused an oculocutaneous syndrome [14]. An eruption combining well-defined, eroded or scaly, red rings with a lichenoid histology [15,16] is recognized. Acute psoriasis with arthropathy has been described [17]. Peripheral skin necrosis associated with Raynaud's phenomenon, an LE syndrome, various patterns of dermatitis [3] and generalized pigmentation [18] are all documented.

Practolol

This drug has been withdrawn, but is discussed in view of its important side-effect profile. It caused an oculo-cutaneous syndrome comprising dry eyes and scarring, fibrosis and metaplasia of the conjunctiva; a psoriasiform, lichenoid or mixed eruption with a characteristic histology; pleural and pericardial reactions; fibrinous peritonitis and serous otitis media [19,20]. Subsequent treatment with another β-blocker did not elicit cross-sensitivity reactivation of the syndrome [21]. Ocular cicatricial pemphigoid was seen [22], and exacerbation of psoriasis was recorded [23].

Pindolol

Psoriasiform [24] and lichenoid rashes with pemphigus-like antibodies demonstrated by immunofluorescence have been seen, as well as a systemic LE syndrome [25].

Propranolol

This is probably the most widely used β-blocker, and many adverse cutaneous reactions have been reported [26–29]. Rashes may be lichenoid [30], psoriasiform [29] or generalized and exfoliative. Other miscellaneous reported reactions have been alopecia [31], erythema multiforme [32] and a cheilostomatitis with ulceration of the lips. Peyronie's disease has developed. Generalized pustular psoriasis [33] and pemphigus [34] have occurred.

REFERENCES

1 Taylor AEM, Hindson C, Wacks H. A drug eruption due to acebutolol with combined lichenoid and lupus erythematosus features. *Clin Exp Dermatol* 1982; **7**: 219–21.
2 Record NB. Acebutolol-induced pleuropulmonary lupus syndrome. *Ann Intern Med* 1981; **95**: 326–7.
3 Van Joost T, Middelkamp Hup H, Ros FE. Dermatitis as a side-effect of long-term topical treatment with certain beta-blocking agents. *Br J Dermatol* 1979; **101**: 171–6.
4 Gawkrodger DJ, Beveridge GW. Psoriasiform reaction to atenolol. *Clin Exp Dermatol* 1984; **9**: 92–4.
5 Henderson CA, Shamy HK. Atenolol-induced pseudolymphoma. *Clin Exp Dermatol* 1990; **15**: 119–20.
6 Wolf R, Ophir J, Elman M, Krakowski A. Atenolol-induced cutaneous vasculitis. *Cutis* 1989; **43**: 231–3.
7 White WB, Schulman P, McCabe EJ. Psoriasiform cutaneous eruptions induced by cetamolol hydrochloride. *Arch Dermatol* 1986; **122**: 857–8.
8 Finlay AY, Waddington E, Savage RL *et al.* Cutaneous reactions to labetalol. *Br Med J* 1978; **i**: 987.
9 Gange RW, Wilson Jones E. Bullous lichen planus caused by labetalol. *Br Med J* 1978; **i**: 816–17.
10 Brown RC, Cooke M, Losowsky MS. SLE syndrome, probably induced by labetalol. *Postgrad Med J* 1981; **57**: 189–90.
11 Neumann HAM, van Joost T, Westerhof W. Dermatitis as a side-effect of long-term metoprolol. *Lancet* 1979; **ii**: 745.
12 Neumann HAM, van Joost T. Adverse reactions of the skin to metoprolol and other beta-adrenergic-blocking agents. *Dermatologica* 1981; **162**: 330–5.
13 Graeber CW, Lapkin RA. Metoprolol and alopecia. *Cutis* 1981; **28**: 633–4.
14 Holt PJA, Waddington E. Oculocutaneous reaction to oxprenolol. *Br Med J* 1975; **ii**: 539–40.
15 Levene GM, Gange RW. Eruption during treatment with oxprenolol. *Br Med J* 1978; **i**: 784.
16 Gange RW, Levene GM. A distinctive eruption in patients receiving oxprenolol. *Clin Exp Dermatol* 1979; **4**: 87–97.
17 MacFarlane DG, Settas L. Acute psoriatic arthropathy precipitated by oxprenolol. *Ann Rheum Dis* 1984; **43**: 102–4.
18 Harrower ADB, Strong JA. Hyperpigmentation associated with oxprenolol administration. *Br Med J* 1977; **ii**: 296.
19 Felix RH, Ive FA, Dahl MGC. Cutaneous and ocular reactions to practolol. *Br Med J* 1974; **iv**: 321–4.
20 Wright P. Untoward effects associated with practolol administration: oculomucocutaneous syndrome. *Br Med J* 1975; **i**: 595–8.
21 Furhoff A-K, Norlander M, Peterson C. Cross-sensitivity between practolol and other beta-blockers? *Br Med J* 1976; **i**: 831.
22 Van Joost T, Crone RA, Overdijk AD. Ocular cicatricial pemphigoid associated with practolol therapy. *Br J Dermatol* 1976; **94**: 447–50.
23 Søndergaard J, Wadskov S, Ærenlund-Jensen H, Mikkelsen HI. Aggravation of psoriasis and occurrence of psoriasiform cutaneous eruptions induced by practolol (Eraldin®). *Acta Dermatol Venereol (Stockh)* 1976; **56**: 239–43.
24 Bonerandi J-J, Follana J, Privat Y. Apparition d'un psoriasis au cours d'un traitement par bêta-bloquants (Pindolol). *Ann Dermatol Syphiligr* 1976; **103**: 604–6.
25 Bensaid J, Aldigier J-C, Gualde N. Systemic lupus erythematosus syndrome induced by pindolol. *Br Med J* 1979; **i**: 1603–4.
26 Ærenlund-Jensen H, Mikkelsen HI, Wadskov S, Søndergaard J. Cutaneous reactions to propranolol (Inderal®). *Acta Med Scand* 1976; **199**: 363–7.

27 Cochran REI, Thomson J, McQueen A, Beevers DG. Skin reactions associated with propranolol. *Arch Dermatol* 1976; **112**: 1173–4.
28 Scribner MD. Propranolol therapy. *Arch Dermatol* 1977; **113**: 1303.
29 Faure M, Hermier C, Perrot H. Accidents cutanés provoqués par le propranolol. *Ann Dermatol Vénéréol* 1979; **106**: 161–5.
30 Hawk JLM. Lichenoid drug eruption induced by propranolol. *Clin Exp Dermatol* 1980; **5**: 93–6.
31 Hilder RJ. Propranolol and alopecia. *Cutis* 1979; **24**: 63–4.
32 Pimstone B, Joffe B, Pimstone N *et al.* Clinical response to long-term propranolol therapy in hyperthyroidism. *S Afr Med J* 1969; **43**: 1203–5.
33 Hu C-H, Miller AC, Peppercorn R, Farber EM. Generalized pustular psoriasis provoked by propranolol. *Arch Dermatol* 1985; **121**: 1326–7.
34 Godard W, Lambert D, Gavanou J, Chapuis J-L. Pemphigus induit après traitement par l'association propranolol-méprobamate. *Ann Dermatol Vénéréol* 1980; **107**: 1213–16.

Antihypertensive drugs and vasodilators

The dermatological side-effects of antihypertensive agents have been reviewed [1].

REFERENCE

1 Thestrup-Pedersen K. Adverse reactions in the skin from antihypertensive drugs. *Dan Med Bull* 1987; **34**: 3–5.

Angiotensin-converting enzyme (ACE) inhibitors

In addition to dematological problems, these drugs may be nephrotoxic, cause cough and electrolyte disturbances, and are teratogenic [1,2]. Angio-oedema has been reported with captopril, enalapril maleate and lisinopril [3–10]. The cumulative incidence of angio-oedema, almost always on the head and neck, has been estimated at between 0.1 and 0.7% of cases treated; it usually occurs in the first week of treatment [4,8], but onset more than 6 weeks after starting treatment occurs in 20% of patients [5]. In addition, increased frequency, intensity and duration of bouts of angio-oedema has been recorded during long-term use of ACE inhibitors [6–8]. There may be cross-reactivity between drugs; angio-oedema has developed after substituting lisinopril for captopril [9]. Fatal angio-oedema occurred in a patient on captopril for 2 years [10]. Anaphylactoid reactions have been reported during haemodialysis with AN69 membranes in patients receiving ACE inhibitors; the role of bacterial contamination of dialysate is controversial [11–13]. Anaphylactoid reactions have also occurred with LDL-apheresis with dextran sulphate [14]. ACE inhibitors have been implicated in both the exacerbation and induction of psoriasis [15–18]. ACE inhibitors most commonly produce a dose-related pruritic maculopapular eruption on the upper trunk and arms, especially with captopril (2.4–7%) and less with enalapril (1.5%), which is often transitory and rarely requires discontinuation. Urticaria, a pemphigoid-like reaction, a pityriasis rosea-like reaction, a lichenoid eruption, erythroderma, alopecia and Stevens–Johnson syndrome have been reported [19]. Captopril and enalapril may produce eruptions with histological similarities to mycosis fungoides [20].

REFERENCES

1 Ferner RE. Adverse effects of angiotensin-converting-enzyme inhibitors. *Adverse Drug React Bull* 1990; **141**: 528–31.
2 Parish RC, Miller LJ. Adverse effects of angiotensin converting enzyme inhibitors: an update. *Drug Saf* 1992; **7**: 14–31.
3 Orfan N, Patterson R, Dykewicz MS. Severe angioedema related to ACE inhibitors in patients with a history of idiopathic angioedema. *JAMA* 1990; **264**: 1287–9.
4 Slater EE, Merill DD, Guess HA *et al.* Clinical profile of angioedema associated with angiotensin converting-enzyme inhibition. *JAMA* 1988; **260**: 967–70.
5 Hedner T, Samuelsson O, Lindholm L *et al.* Angio-oedema in relation to treatment with angiotensin converting enzyme inhibitors. *Br Med J* 1992; **304**: 941–6.
6 Chin HL. Severe angioedema after long-term use of an angiotensin-converting enzyme inhibitor. *Ann Intern Med* 1990; **112**: 312.
7 Kozel MMA, Mekkes JR, Bos JD. Increased frequency and severity of angio-oedema related to long-term therapy with angiotensin-converting enzyme inhibitor in two patients. *Clin Exp Dermatol* 1995; **20**: 60–1.
8 Sabroe RA, Kobza Black A. Angiotensin-converting enzyme (ACE) inhibitors and angio-oedema. *Br J Dermatol* 1997; **136**: 153–8.
9 McElligott S, Perlroth M, Raish L. Angioedema after substituting lisinopril for captopril. *Ann Intern Med* 1992; **116**: 426–7.
10 Jason DR. Fatal angioedema associated with captopril. *J Forensic Sci* 1992; **37**: 1418–21.
11 Verresen L, Waer M, Vanrenterghem Y, Michielsen P. Angiotensin-converting-enzyme inhibitors and anaphylactoid reactions to high-flex membrane dialysis. *Lancet* 1990; **336**: 1360–2.
12 Tielemans C, Madhoun P, Lenears M *et al.* Anaphylactoid reactions during hemodialysis on AN69 membranes in patients receiving ACE inhibitors. *Kidney Int* 1990; **38**: 982–4.
13 Verresen L, Waer M, Vanrenterghem Y, Michielsen P. Anaphylactoid reactions, haemodialysis, and ACE inhibitors. *Lancet* 1991; **337**: 1294.
14 Keller C, Grutzmacher P, Bahr F *et al.* LDL-apheresis with dextran sulphate and anaphylactoid reactions to ACE inhibitors. *Lancet* 1993; **341**: 60–1.
15 Wolf R, Tamir A, Brenner S. Psoriasis related to angiotensin-converting enzyme inhibitors. *Dermatologica* 1990; **181**: 51–3.
16 Coulter DM, Pillans PI. Angiotensin-converting enzyme inhibitors and psoriasis. *NZ Med J* 1993; **106**: 392–3.
17 Tamir A, Wolf R, Brenner S. Exacerbation and induction of psoriasis by angiotensin-converting enzyme inhibitors. *J Am Acad Dermatol* 1994; **30**: 1045.
18 Ikai K. Exacerbation and induction of psoriasis by angiotensin-converting enzyme inhibitors. *J Am Acad Dermatol* 1996; **32**: 819.
19 Vollenweider Roten S, Mainetti C, Donath R, Saurat J-H. Enalapril-induced lichen planus-like eruption. *J Am Acad Dermatol* 1995; **32**: 293–5.
20 Furness PN, Goodfield MJ, MacLennan KA *et al.* Severe cutaneous reactions to captopril and enalapril: histological study and comparison with early mycosis fungoides. *J Clin Pathol* 1986; **39**: 902–7.

Captopril. Dermatological complications occur in between 4% [1] and 12% [2] of patients treated with captopril, and less commonly with other ACE inhibitors; side-effects are more likely with renal impairment. Loss of sense of taste, or a metallic taste (augesia), ulceration of the tongue and aphthous stomatitis [3] are reported. Early changes within the first months [4–6] include pruritus, urticaria [7] and angio-oedema, which occurs in about one in 1000 patients and may occasionally be fatal [8], pityriasis rosea-like [9] and morbilliform rashes. These are dose dependent and have a good prognosis. Late changes [4–6] consist of pemphigus-like [10–12] and lichenoid [13–17] eruptions. Systemic LE-like eruptions have been recorded [18,19]. Antinuclear antibodies may develop [20,21]. Oral changes may be due to a leukocytoclastic vasculitis [22], and a serum sickness-like syndrome has been induced [23]. Psoriasis has been reported to be exacerbated or triggered [24,25].

Severe reactions [26,27] have included exfoliative dermatitis [28–30], and marrow depression with neutropenia or agranulocytosis [31]. Lymphadenopathy may be induced [32]. Alopecia [33] and an acquired IgA deficiency [34] have been reported. The merits of skin testing in the prediction of captopril reactions have been discussed [35]. It has been postulated that some toxic effects are related to the presence of a sulphydryl group, as enalapril (another ACE inhibitor lacking this group) has been safely substituted in certain cases of captopril hypersensitivity [36].

Cilazapril. Cilazapril had more neurological (mainly headache) but fewer skin reactions than the other ACE inhibitors, lisinopril, enalapril and captopril [37].

Enalapril. Enalapril produces rashes in approximately 1.4%, requiring discontinuation in approximately 0.4%, of patients [38]. Toxic pustuloderma is recorded [38]. A single report of pemphigus foliaceus has appeared; part of the structure of this drug is identical to that of captopril, although it does not contain a sulphydryl group [39]. Bullous eruptions [40] and lichenoid eruptions [41] occur.

Lisinopril. Vasculitis has been recorded [42], as has pallor, flushing and oedema [43].

REFERENCES

1 Williams GH. Converting-enzyme inhibitors in the treatment of hypertension. *N Engl J Med* 1988; **319**: 1517–25.
2 Wilkin JK, Hammond JJ, Kirkendall WM. The captopril-induced eruption. A possible mechanism: cutaneous kinin potentiation. *Arch Dermatol* 1980; **116**: 902–5.
3 Seedat YK. Aphthous ulcers of mouth from captopril. *Lancet* 1979; **ii**: 1297–8.
4 Clement M. Captopril-induced eruptions. *Arch Dermatol* 1981; **117**: 525–6.
5 Luderer JR, Lookingbill DP, Schneck DW *et al.* Captopril-induced skin eruptions. *J Clin Pharmacol* 1982; **22**: 151–9.
6 Daniel F, Foix C, Barbet M *et al.* Captopril-induced eruptions: occurrence over a three-year period. *Ann Dermatol Vénéréol* 1983; **110**: 441–6.
7 Wood SM, Mann RD, Rawlins MD. Angio-oedema and urticaria associated with angiotensin converting enzyme inhibitors. *Br Med J* 1987; **294**: 91–2.
8 Slater EE, Merrill DD, Guess HA *et al.* Clinical profile of angioedema associated with angiotensin converting-enzyme inhibition. *JAMA* 1988; **260**: 967–70.
9 Wilkin JK, Kirkendall WM. Pityriasis rosea-like rash from captopril. *Arch Dermatol* 1982; **118**: 186–7.
10 Parfrey PS, Clement M, Vandenburg MJ, Wright P. Captopril-induced pemphigus. *Br Med J* 1980; **281**: 194.
11 Katz RA, Hood AF, Anhalt GJ. Pemphigus-like eruption from captopril. *Arch Dermatol* 1987; **123**: 20–1.
12 Korman NJ, Eyre RW, Stanley JR. Drug-induced pemphigus: autoantibodies directed against the pemphigus antigen complexes are present in penicillamine and captopril-induced pemphigus. *J Invest Dermatol* 1991; **96**: 273–6.
13 Reinhardt LA, Wilkin JK, Kirkendall WM. Lichenoid eruption produced by captopril. *Cutis* 1983; **31**: 98–9.
14 Bravard P, Barbet M, Eich D *et al.* Éruption lichénoïde au captopril. *Ann Dermatol Vénéréol* 1983; **110**: 433–8.
15 Flageul B, Foldes C, Wallach D *et al.* Captopril-induced lichen planus pemphigoides with pemphigus-like features. A case report. *Dermatologica* 1986; **173**: 248–55.
16 Bretin N, Dreno B, Bureau B, Litoux P. Immunohistological study of captopril-induced late cutaneous reactions. *Dermatologica* 1988; **177**: 11–15.
17 Rotstein E, Rotstein H. Drug eruptions with lichenoid histology produced by captopril. *Australas J Dermatol* 1989; **30**: 9–14.
18 Patri P, Nigro A, Rebora A. Lupus erythematosus-like eruption from captopril. *Acta Derm Venereol (Stockh)* 1985; **65**: 447–8.
19 Sieber C, Grimm E, Follath F. Captopril and systemic lupus erythematosus syndrome. *Br Med J* 1990; **301**: 669.
20 Reidenberg MM, Case DB, Drayer DE *et al.* Development of antinuclear antibodies in patients treated with high doses of captopril. *Arthritis Rheum* 1984; **27**: 579–81.
21 Kallenberg CGM. Autoantibodies during captopril treatment. *Arthritis Rheum* 1985; **28**: 597–8.
22 Viraben R, Adoue D, Dupre A, Touron P. Erosions and ulcers of the mouth. *Arch Dermatol* 1982; **118**: 959.
23 Hoorntje SJ, Weening JJ, Kallenberg GGM *et al.* Serum-sickness-like syndrome with membranous glomerulopathy in a patient on captopril. *Lancet* 1979; **ii**: 1297.
24 Hauschild TT, Bauer R, Kreysel HW. Erstmanifestation einer eruptiv-exanthematischen Psoriasis vulgaris unter Captoprilmedikation. *Hautarzt* 1986; **37**: 274–7.
25 Wolf R, Dorfman B, Krakowski A. Psoriasiform eruption induced by captopril and chlorthalidone. *Cutis* 1987; **40**: 162–4.
26 Goodfield MJ, Millard LG. Severe cutaneous reactions to captopril. *Br Med J* 1985; **290**: 1111.
27 Furness PN, Goodfield MJ, MacLennan KA *et al.* Severe cutaneous reactions to captopril and enalapril; histological study and comparison with early mycosis fungoides. *J Clin Pathol* 1986; **39**: 902–7.
28 Solinger AM. Exfoliative dermatitis from captopril. *Cutis* 1982; **29**: 473–4.
29 O'Neill PG, Rajan N, Charlat ML, Bolli R. Captopril-related exfoliative dermatitis. *Texas Med* 1989; **85**: 40–1.
30 Daniel F, Foix C, Barbet M *et al.* Toxidermies au captopril: incidences au cours d'un traitement de 1321 mois/patients. *Ann Dermatol Vénéréol* 1983; **110**: 441–6.
31 Edwards CRW, Drury P, Penketh A, Damluji SA. Successful reintroduction of captopril following neutropenia. *Lancet* 1981; **i**: 723.
32 Åberg H, Mörlin C, Frithz G. Captopril-associated lymphadenopathy. *Br Med J* 1981; **283**: 1297–8.
33 Motel PJ. Captopril and alopecia: a case report and review of known cutaneous reactions in captopril use. *J Am Acad Dermatol* 1990; **23**: 124–5.
34 Hammarström L, Smith CIE, Berg U. Captopril-induced IgA deficiency. *Lancet* 1991; **337**: 436.
35 Smit AJ, van der Laan S, De Monchy J *et al.* Cutaneous reactions to captopril. Predictive values of skin tests. *Clin Allergy* 1984; **14**: 413–19.
36 Gavras I, Gavras H. Captopril and enalapril. *Ann Intern Med* 1983; **98**: 556–7.
37 Coulter DM. Short term safety assessment of cilazapril. *NZ Med J* 1993; **106**: 497–9.
38 Ferguson JE, Chalmers RJ. Enalapril-induced toxic pustuloderma. *Clin Exp Dermatol* 1996; **21**: 54–5.
39 Shelto RM. Pemphigus foliaceus associated with enalapril. *J Am Acad Dermatol* 1991; **24**: 503–4.
40 Mullins PD, Choudhury SL. Enalapril and bullous eruptions. *Br Med J* 1994; **309**: 1411.
41 Vollenweider Roten S, Mainetti C, Donath R, Saurat J-H. Enalapril-induced lichen planus-like eruption. *J Am Acad Dermatol* 1995; **32**: 293–5.
42 Barlow RJ, Schulz EJ. Lisinopril-induced vasculitis. *Clin Exp Dermatol* 1988; **13**: 117–20.
43 Fallowfield JM, Blenkinsopp J, Raza A *et al.* Post-marketing surveillance of lisinopril in general practice in the UK. *Br J Clin Pract* 1993; **47**: 296–304.

Calcium channel blockers

Cutaneous reactions are rare and have been reported in 6/million prescriptions of nifedipine, 17/million prescriptions of verapamil, and 6/million prescriptions of diltiazem [1,2]. In one study, reactions to the dihydropiridine drugs (including nicardipine, nifedipine, nisoldipine), verapamil and diltiazem occurred after an average of 95 days (range 7 days to 10 years) [3]. Pruritus, maculopapular rashes, and urticaria/angio-oedema have been described with all these drugs, as have Stevens–Johnson syndrome and erythema multiforme; TEN has occurred with diltiazem. There is a suggestion that the more severe reactions are commoner with diltiazem. Peripheral oedema as a side-effect is common to the dihydropyridine calcium antagonists, including nifedipine, nicardipine, isradipine and amlodipine; it occurs in 7–30% of patients depending on the specific drug, but is usually mild [4]. Psoriasiform eruptions are described [3].

REFERENCES

1 Stern R, Khalsa JH. Cutaneous adverse reactions associated with calcium channel blockers. *Arch Intern Med* 1989; **149**: 829–32.
2 Sadick NS, Katz AS, Schreiber TL. Angioedema from calcium channel blockers. *J Am Acad Dermatol* 1989; **21**: 132–3.
3 Kitamura K, Kanasashi M, Suga C et al. Cutaneous reactions induced by calcium channel blockers: high frequency of psoriasiform eruptions. *J Dermatol* 1993; **20**: 279–86.
4 Maclean D, MacConnachie AM. Selected side-effects: 1. Peripheral oedema with dihydropyridine calcium antagonists. *Prescribers' J* 1991; **31**: 4–6.

Diltiazem. Cutaneous reactions to diltiazem have been reviewed [1,2]. They include macular exanthem, toxic erythema with fever and on occasion facial angio-oedema [3–5], generalized cutaneous reactions [6], erythema multiforme [7], subcorneal pustular dermatosis, a photo-sensitive erythroderma [8], vasculitis [9] and vasculitic leg ulcers [10], a generalized pustular dermatitis [11], psoriasiform eruptions [2], exfoliative dermatitis in a patient with psoriasis [12], a subacute cutaneous LE-like syndrome [13], recurrent nail dystrophy, hyperplastic gingivitis [14], and proptosis and periorbital oedema [15] are recorded. Generalized lymphadenopathy has occurred [16]. Patch tests may be positive in diltiazem reactions [4,5]. Dermatological cross-sensitivity between diltiazem and amlodipine is reported [17].

REFERENCES

1 Wittal RA, Fischer GO, Georgouras KE, Baird PJ. Skin reactions to diltiazem. *Australas J Dermatol* 1992; **33**: 11–18.
2 Kitamura K, Kanasashi M, Suga C et al. Cutaneous reactions induced by calcium channel blocker: high frequency of psoriasiform eruptions. *J Dermatol* 1993; **20**: 279–86.
3 Wakeel RA, Gavin MP, Keefe M. Severe toxic erythema caused by Diltiazem. *Br Med J* 1988; **296**: 1071.
4 Hammentgen R, Lutz G, Köhler U, Nitsch J. Makulopapulöses Exanthem bei Diltiazem-Therapie. *Dtsch Med Wschr* 1988; **113**: 1283–5.
5 Romano A, Pietrantonio F, Garcovich A et al. Delayed hypersensitivity to diltiazem in two patients. *Ann Allergy* 1992; **69**: 31–2.
6 Sousa-Basto A, Azenha A, Duarte ML, Pardal-Oliveira F. Generalized cutaneous reaction to diltiazem. *Contact Dermatitis* 1993; **29**: 44–5.
7 Berbis P, Alfonso MJ, Levy JL, Privat Y. Diltiazem associated erythema multiforme. *Dermatologica* 1990; **179**: 90.

8 Hashimoto M, Tanaka S, Horio T. Photosensibility due to diltiazem hydrochloride. *Acta Dermatol* 1979; **74**: 181–4.
9 Sheehan-Dare RA, Goodfield MJ. Severe cutaneous vasculitis induced by diltiazem. *Br J Dermatol* 1988; **119**: 134.
10 Carmichael AJ, Paul CJ. Vasculitic leg ulcers associated with diltiazem. *Br Med J* 1988; **297**: 562.
11 Lambert DG, Dalac S, Beer F et al. Acute generalized exanthematous pustular dermatitis induced by diltiazem. *Br J Dermatol* 1988; **118**: 308–9.
12 Larvijsen APM, Van Dijke C, Vermeer B-J. Diltiazem-associated exfoliative dermatitis in a patient with psoriasis. *Acta Derm Venereol (Stockh)* 1986; **66**: 536–8.
13 Crowson AN, Magro CM. Diltiazem and subacute cutaneous lupus erythematosus-like lesions. *N Engl J Med* 1995; **333**: 1429.
14 Giustiniani S, Robustelli della Cuna F, Marieni M. Hyperplastic gingivitis during diltiazem therapy. *Int J Cardiol* 1987; **15**: 247–9.
15 Friedland S, Kaplan S, Lahav M, Shapiro A. Proptosis and periorbital edema due to diltiazem treatment. *Arch Ophthalmol* 1993; **111**: 1027–8.
16 Scolnick B, Brinberg D. Diltiazem and generalized lymphadenopathy. *Ann Intern Med* 1985; **102**: 558.
17 Baker BA, Cacchione JG. Dermatologic cross-sensitivity between diltiazem and amlodipine. *Ann Pharmacother* 1994; **28**: 118–19.

Nicardipine. Erythromelalgia is recorded [1].

Nifedipine. Headache, tachycardia and flushing are common side-effects. Gingival hyperplasia is well recognized [2]. Burning sensations, erythema, painful oedema and erythromelalgia have been described [3–6]. There have been isolated reports of a truncal morbilliform rash [7], fixed drug reaction [8], a generalized bullous eruption, vasculitis [9], purpura, photosensitivity [10] in one case confirmed by rechallenge [11], gynaecomastia [12], erysipelas-like lesions on the shins with erythematous plaques on the trunk [13] and exfoliative dermatitis [14,15].

Verapamil. Erythema multiforme has been reported [16], as have gingival hyperplasia, gynaecomastia [17], alopecia, maculopapular eruptions, ecchymosis, vasculitis, urticaria and hyperkeratosis [17].

REFERENCES

1 Levesque H, Moore N, Wolfe LM, Courtoid H. Erythromelalgia induced by nicardipine (inverse Raynaud's phenomenon?). *Br Med J* 1989; **298**: 1252–3.
2 Benini PL, Crosti C, Sala F et al. Gingival hyperplasia by nifedipine. Report of a case. *Acta Derm Venereol (Stockh)* 1985; **65**: 362–5.
3 Bridgman JF. Erythematous edema of the legs due to nifedipine. *Br Med J* 1978; **i**: 578.
4 Fisher JR, Padnick MB, Olstein S. Nifedipine and erythromelalgia. *Ann Intern Med* 1983; **98**: 671–2.
5 Brodmerkel GJ, Jr. Nifedipine and erythromelalgia. *Ann Intern Med* 1983; **99**: 415.
6 Alcalay J, David M, Sandbank M. Cutaneous reactions to nifedipine. *Dermatologica* 1987; **175**: 191–3.
7 Parish LC, Witkowski JA. Truncal morbilliform eruption due to nifedipine. *Cutis* 1992; **49**: 113–14.
8 Alcalay J, David M. Generalized fixed drug eruptions associated with nifedipine. *Br Med J* 1986; **292**: 450.
9 Brenner S, Brau S. Vasculitis following nifedipine. *Harefuah* 1985; **108**: 139–40.
10 Thomas SE, Wood ML. Photosensitivity reactions associated with nifedipine. *Br Med J* 1986; **292**: 992.

11 Zenarola P, Gatti S, Lomuto M. Photodermatitis due to nifedipine: report of 2 cases. *Dermatologica* 1991; **182**: 196–8.
12 Clyne CAC. Unilateral gynaecomastia and nifedipine. *Br Med J* 1986; **292**: 380.
13 Leibovici V, Zlotogorski A, Heyman A *et al*. Polymorphous drug eruption due to nifedipine. *Cutis* 1988; **41**: 367.
14 Reynolds NJ, Jones SK, Crossley J, Harman RRM. Exfoliative dermatitis due to nifedipine. *Br J Dermatol* 1989; **121**: 401–4.
15 Mohammed KN. Nifedipine-induced exfoliative dermatitis and pedal edema. *Ann Pharmacother* 1994; **28**: 967.
16 Kürkçüoglu N, Alaybeyi F. Erythema multiforme after verapamil treatment. *J Am Acad Dermatol* 1991; **24**: 511–12.
17 Rodriguez LaG, Jick H. Risk of gynaecomastia associated with cimetidine, omeprazole, and other antiulcer drugs. *Br Med J* 1994; **308**: 503–6.

Centrally acting antihypertensive drugs

Clonidine. Hypersensitivity rashes occur in up to 5% of patients. A pityriasis rosea-like and LE-like syndrome, exacerbation of psoriasis [1] and an isolated instance of anogenital cicatricial pemphigoid [2] have been documented. Transdermally administered clonidine has caused allergic contact dermatitis.

REFERENCES

1 Wilkin JK. Exacerbation of psoriasis during clonidine therapy. *Arch Dermatol* 1981; **117**: 4.
2 Van Joost T, Faber WR, Manuel HR. Drug-induced anogenital cicatricial pemphigoid. *Br J Dermatol* 1980; **102**: 715–18.

Methyldopa. An eczematous eruption of discoid or seborrhoeic pattern is characteristic, is more likely to occur in previously eczematous subjects and persists until the drug is stopped [1]. Eczema of the palms and soles has also been described and may become widespread. The reaction is probably allergic as it may be dose related. Purpuric, erythematous and lichenoid rashes occur, sometimes in association with fever and other allergic symptoms [2,3]. Lichenoid eruptions may be ulcerated [4,5] and persistent ulceration of the tongue has been described. Fixed eruptions are very rare. An LE-like syndrome is documented [6,7] and an autoimmune haemolytic anaemia is well known [5]. Psoriasis may be precipitated. An extensive erythematous skin eruption, fever, lymphadenopathy and eosinophilia due to methyldopa, recurrent on re-exposure has been recorded [8].

REFERENCES

1 Church R. Eczema provoked by methyldopa. *Br J Dermatol* 1974; **91**: 373–8.
2 Stevenson CJ. Lichenoid eruptions due to methyldopa. *Br J Dermatol* 1971; **85**: 600.
3 Burry JN, Kirk J. Lichenoid drug reaction from methyldopa. *Br J Dermatol* 1974; **91**: 475–6.
4 Burry JN. Ulcerative lichenoid eruption from methyldopa. *Arch Dermatol* 1976; **112**: 880.
5 Furhoff A-K. Adverse reactions with methyldopa–a decade's reports. *Acta Med Scand* 1978; **203**: 425–8.
6 Harrington TM, Davis DE. Systemic lupus-like syndrome induced by methyldopa therapy. *Chest* 1981; **79**: 696–7.
7 Dupont A, Six R. Lupus-like syndrome induced by methyldopa. *Br Med J* 1982; **285**: 693–4.
8 Wolf R, Tamir A, Werbin N, Brenner S. Methyldopa hypersensitivity syndrome. *Ann Allergy* 1993; **71**: 166–8.

Adrenergic neurone-blocking agents

Guanethidine. Hypersensitivity eruptions are very rare but polyarteritis nodosa has been attributed to this drug [1].

REFERENCES

1 Dewar HA, Peaston MJT. Three cases resembling polyarteritis nodosa arising during treatment with guanethidine. *Br Med J* 1964; **ii**: 609–11.

Vasodilator antihypertensive drugs

Diazoxide. Transient flushing is common. During long-term treatment up to half the patients develop hirsutism without other signs of virilization [1]. A clinical picture resembling hypertrichosis lanuginosa may develop [2,3]. Oedema occurs in at least 10% of patients; photosensitivity is very uncommon but well recognized. Lichenoid [3,4] and other rashes occur rarely.

REFERENCES

1 Burton JL, Schutt WH, Caldwell JW. Hypertrichosis due to diazoxide. *Br J Dermatol* 1975; **93**: 707–11.
2 Koblenzer PJ, Baker J. Hypertrichosis lanuginosa associated with diazoxide therapy in prepubertal children: a clinicopathologic study. *Ann NY Acad Sci* 1968; **150**: 373–82.
3 Menter MA. Hypertrichosis lanuginosa and a lichenoid eruption due to diazoxide therapy. *Proc R Soc Med* 1973; **66**: 326–7.
4 Okun R, Russell RP, Wilson WR. Use of diazoxide with trichlormethiazide for hypertension. *Arch Intern Med* 1963; **112**: 882–6.

Hydralazine. The LE-like syndrome due to this drug is well known [1–7]. Hydralazine binds to complement component C4 and inhibits its function; this may impair clearance of immune complexes, and predispose to development of an LE syndrome [6,7].

Orogenital ulceration may be part of the picture [8] and the syndrome has presented as a leg ulcer [9]. Cutaneous vasculitis may be severe and necrotizing [10,11]. An association between a hydralazine-induced LE syndrome and the development of Sweet's syndrome has been noted rarely [12]. Fixed drug eruption has been reported [13]. Characteristic lung changes are attributed to the drug [14].

REFERENCES

1 Alarcon-Segovia D, Wakin KG, Worthington JW *et al*. Clinical and experimental studies on the hydralazine syndrome and its relationship to systemic lupus erythematosus. *Medicine* 1967; **46**: 1–33.
2 Batchelor JR, Welsh KI, Mansilla Tinoco R *et al*. Hydralazine-induced systemic

lupus erythematosus: influence of HLA-DR and sex upon susceptibility. *Lancet* 1980; **i**: 1107–9.

3 Dubroff LM, Reid R, Jr, Papalian M. Molecular models for hydralazine-related systemic lupus erythematosus. *Arthritis Rheum* 1981; **24**: 1082–5.
4 Perry HM, Jr. Possible mechanisms of the hydralazine-related lupus-like syndrome. *Arthritis Rheum* 1981; **24**: 1093–1105.
5 Mansilla Tinoco R, Harland SJ, Ryan P *et al*. Hydralazine, antinuclear antibodies, and the lupus syndrome. *Br Med J* 1982; **284**: 936–9.
6 Sim E, Law S-KA. Hydralazine binds covalently to complement component C4. Different reactivity of C4A and C4B gene products. *FEBS Lett* 1985; **184**: 323–7.
7 Sim E. Drug-induced immune complex disease. *Complement Inflamm* 1989; **6**: 119–26.
8 Neville E, Graham PY, Brewis RA. Orogenital ulcers, SLE and hydralazine. *Postgrad Med J* 1981; **57**: 378–9.
9 Kissin MW, Williamson RCN. Hydrallazine-induced SLE-like syndrome presenting as a leg ulcer. *Br Med J* 1979; **ii**: 1330.
10 Bernstein RM, Egerton-Vernon J, Webster J. Hydrallazine-induced cutaneous vasculitis. *Br Med J* 1980; **280**: 156–7.
11 Peacock A, Weatherall D. Hydralazine-induced necrotising vasculitis. *Br Med J* 1981; **282**: 1121–2.
12 Servitje O, Ribera M, Juanola X, Rodriguez-Moreno J. Acute neutrophilic dermatosis associated with hydralazine-induced lupus. *Arch Dermatol* 1988; **123**: 1435–6.
13 Sehgal VN, Gangwani OP. Hydralazine-induced fixed drug eruption. *Int J Dermatol* 1986; **25**: 394.
14 Bass BH. Hydralazine lung. *Thorax* 1981; **36**: 695–6.

Minoxidil. This arterial vasodilator causes hypertrichosis, especially of the arms and face, which may be unacceptable to women [1,2]; the hair disappears slowly after the drug is withdrawn. Fluid retention may require diuretic therapy to control it. Thrombocytopenia [3], bullous eruptions [4] and erythema multiforme or Stevens–Johnson syndrome [5] have been described.

REFERENCES

1 Burton JL, Marshall A. Hypertrichosis due to minoxidil. *Br J Dermatol* 1979; **101**: 593–5.
2 Ryckmanns F. Hypertrichose durch Minoxidil. *Hautarzt* 1980; **31**: 205–6.
3 Peitzmann SJ, Martin C. Thrombocytopenia and minoxidil. *Ann Intern Med* 1980; **92**: 874.
4 Rosenthal T, Teicher A, Swartz J, Boichis H. Minoxidil-induced bullous eruption. *Arch Intern Med* 1978; **138**: 1856–7.
5 DiSantis DJ, Flanagan J. Minoxidil-induced Stevens–Johnson syndrome. *Arch Intern Med* 1981; **141**: 1515.

Nitrate vasodilators

Glyceryl and penta-erythritol tetranitrate. Reactions to nitrate vasodilators are rare, but erythroderma with cross-reactivity to glyceryl trinitrate has been caused by this drug [1].

REFERENCE

1 Ryan FP. Erythroderma due to peritrate and glyceryl trinitrate. *Br J Dermatol* 1972; **87**: 498–500.

Diuretics

Carbonic anhydrase inhibitor

Acetazolamide. This drug has caused hirsutism in a child [1]. Hypersensitivity reactions are rare.

REFERENCE

1 Weiss IS. Hirsutism after chronic administration of acetazolamide. *Am J Ophthalmol* 1974; **78**: 327–8.

Loop diuretics

Bumetanide. Occasional hypersensitivity rashes occur. Pseudoporphyria has been reported wih this sulphonamide-derived drug [1].

Ethacrynic acid. A Henoch-Schönlein type of vasculitis has been documented.

Frusemide (furosemide). Reactions are rare: only two patients of 3830 receiving this medication in a recent study developed cutaneous complications [2]. Phototoxic blistering has followed very high dosage (2.0 g/day) in chronic renal failure [3] but erythema multiforme [4,5], bullous pemphigoid [6,7], other bullous haemorrhagic eruptions [8] and an acquired blistering disorder with skin fragility [9] have apparently been precipitated by conventional dosage. The skin changes may mimic those of porphyria. Several cases of generalized exfoliative dermatitis have been documented. Anaphylaxis [10], a necrotizing vasculitis [11] and an eruption resembling Sweet's syndrome [12] have been reported. Cross-reactivity between frusemide, hydrochlorothiazide and sulphonamides is recorded, but the use of one of these drugs in a patient known to have allergy to another involves only low risk [13].

REFERENCES

1 Leitao EA, Person JR. Bumetanide-induced pseudoporphyria. *J Am Acad Dermatol* 1990; **23**: 129–30.
2 Bigby M, Jick S, Jick H, Arndt K. Drug-induced cutaneous reactions. A report from the Boston Collaborative Drug Surveillance Program on 15438 consecutive inpatients, 1975 to 1982. *JAMA* 1986; **256**: 3358–63.
3 Burry JN, Lawrence JR. Phototoxic blisters from high frusemide dosage. *Br J Dermatol* 1976; **94**: 493–9.
4 Gibson TP, Blue P. Erythema multiforme and furosemide therapy. *JAMA* 1970; **212**: 1709.
5 Zugerman C, La Voo EJ. Erythema multiforme caused by oral furosemide. *Arch Dermatol* 1980; **116**: 518–19.
6 Fellner MI, Katz JM. Occurrence of bullous pemphigoid after furosemide therapy. *Arch Dermatol* 1976; **112**: 75–7.
7 Castel T, Gratacos R, Castro J *et al*. Bullous pemphigoid induced by frusemide. *Clin Exp Dermatol* 1981; **6**: 635–8.
8 Ebringer A, Adam WR, Parkin JD. Bullous haemorrhagic eruption associated with frusemide. *Med J Aust* 1969; 1: 768–71.

9 Kennedy AC, Lyell A. Acquired epidermolysis bullosa due to high dose frusemide. *Br Med J* 1976; **i**: 1509–10.
10 Hansbrough JR, Wedner HJ, Chaplin DD. Anaphylaxis to intravenous furosemide. *J Allergy Clin Immunol* 1987; **80**: 538–41.
11 Hendricks WM, Ader RS. Furosemide-induced cutaneous necrotizing vasculitis. *Arch Dermatol* 1977; **113**: 375.
12 Cobb MW. Furosemide-induced eruption simulating Sweet's syndrome. *J Am Acad Dermatol* 1989; **21**: 339–43.
13 Sullivan TJ. Cross-reactions among furosemide, hydrochlorothiazide, and sulfonamides. *JAMA* 1991; **265**: 120–1.

Potassium-sparing diuretics

Spironolactone. This drug, which is also used for the treatment of acne vulgaris and hirsutism [1], may cause gynaecomastia [2–4], gastrointestinal upset, hyperkalaemia and rarely agranulocytosis [1]. Spironolactone has an antiandrogen effect [4] and may result in loss of libido and impotence or menstrual irregularities. A maculopapular eruption [5], LE-like syndrome [6], annular LE [7], erythema annulare centrifugum [8] and a lichenoid eruption [9] have been seen.

REFERENCES

1 Shaw JC. Spironolactone in dermatologic therapy. *J Am Acad Dermatol* 1991; **24**: 236–43.
2 Clarke E. Spironolactone therapy and gynecomastia. *JAMA* 1965; **193**: 157–8.
3 Loriaux DL, Meuard R, Taylor A *et al.* Spironolactone and endocrine dysfunction. *Ann Intern Med* 1976; **85**: 630–6.
4 Rose LI, Underwood RH, Newmark SR *et al.* Pathophysiology of spironolactone-induced gynecomastia. *Ann Intern Med* 1977; **87**: 398–403.
5 Gupta AK, Knowles SR, Shear NH. Spironolactone-associated cutaneous effects: a case report and a review of the literature. *Dermatology* 1994; **189**: 402–5.
6 Uddin MS, Lynfield YL, Grosberg SJ, Stiefler R. Cutaneous reaction to spironolactone resembling lupus erythematosus. *Cutis* 1979; **24**: 198–200.
7 Leroy D, Dompmartin A, Le Jean S *et al.* Toxidermie a l'aldactone® à type d'érythème annulaire centrifuge lupique. *Ann Dermatol Vénéréol* 1987; **114**: 1237–40.
8 Carsuzaa F, Pierre C, Dubegny M. Erytheme annulaire centrifuge à l'aldactone. *Ann Dermatol Vénéréol* 1987; **114**: 375–6.
9 Downham TF, III. Spironolactone-induced lichen planus. *JAMA* 1978; **240**: 1138.

Thiazides and related diuretics

Photosensitivity is uncommon, occurring in one in 1000 to one in 100 000 prescriptions [1–7]. Hydrochlorothiazide causes considerably more reactions than bendroflumethiazide. The mechanism is unknown, and both phototoxic [1,4,7] and photo-allergic [2,3] mechanisms have been proposed. The commonest reaction is lichenoid, but petechial and erythematous eruptions may occur in exposed skin. Xerostomia has been reported, as has a vasculitis [8]. An eruption resembling subacute cutaneous LE has been described in patients taking a combination of hydrochlorothiazide and triamterene [9,10] and with hydrochlorothiazide alone [11]. Other side-effects include hypokalaemia, short-term elevation of low-density lipoprotein cholesterol, impotence, a diabetogenic effect and exacerbation of gout [12].

Chlorthalidone. Pseudoporphyria has been documented with this thiazide-related diuretic [13]. Psoriasis has been triggered in a patient also receiving captopril [14].

REFERENCES

1 Diffey BL, Langtry J. Phototoxic potential of thiazide diuretics in normal subjects. *Arch Dermatol* 1989; **125**: 1355–8.
2 Harber LC, Lashinsky AM, Baer RL. Photosensitivity to chlorothiazide and hydrochlorothiazide. *N Engl J Med* 1959; **261**: 1378–81.
3 Torinuki W. Photosensitivity due to hydrochlorothiazide. *J Dermatol (Tokyo)* 1980; **7**: 293–6.
4 Rosén K, Swanbeck G. Phototoxic reactions from some common drugs provoked by a high-intensity UVA lamp. *Acta Derm Venereol (Stockh)* 1982; **62**: 246–8.
5 Hawk JLM. Photosensitizing agents used in the United Kingdom. *Clin Exp Dermatol* 1984; **9**: 300–2.
6 Robinson HN, Morison WL, Hood AF. Thiazide diuretic therapy and chronic photosensitivity. *Arch Dermatol* 1985; **121**: 522–4.
7 Addo HA, Ferguson J, Frain-Bell W. Thiazide-induced photosensitivity: a study of 33 subjects. *Br J Dermatol* 1987; **116**: 749–60.
8 Björnberg A, Gisslén H. Thiazides: a cause of necrotising vasculitis? *Lancet* 1965; **ii**: 982–3.
9 Berbis P, Vernay-Vaisse C, Privat Y. Lupus cutané subaigu observé au cours d'un traitement par diurétiques thiazidiques. *Ann Dermatol Vénéréol* 1986; **113**: 1245–8.
10 Darken M, McBurney EI. Subacute cutaneous lupus erythematosus-like drug eruption due to combination diuretic hydrochlorothiazide and triamterene. *J Am Acad Dermatol* 1988; **18**: 38–42.
11 Reed BR, Huff JC, Jones SK *et al.* Subacute cutaneous lupus erythematosus associated with hydrochlorothiazide therapy. *Ann Intern Med* 1985; **103**: 49–51.
12 Orme M. Thiazides in the 1990s. The risk: benefit ratio still favours the drug. *Br Med J* 1990; **300**: 1168–9.
13 Baker EJ, Reed KD, Dixon SL. Chlorthalidone-induced pseudoporphyria: clinical and microscopic findings of a case. *J Am Acad Dermatol* 1989; **21**: 1026–9.
14 Wolf R, Dorfman B, Krakowski A. Psoriasiform eruption induced by captopril and chlorthalidone. *Cutis* 1987; **40**: 162–4.

Miscellaneous cardiovascular drugs

Dobutamine

Two patients with local dermal hypersensitivity at the site of dobutamine hydrochloride injection, consisting of erythema, pruritus and phlebitis with or without bullae, have been described [1]. Dermal cellulitis has also been reported [2].

Dopamine

This positive inotropic agent has caused local skin necrosis, due to extravasation at the site of an intravenous cannula [3], and acral gangrene secondary to distal vasoconstriction [4]. Localized piloerection and vasoconstriction proximal to the site of infusion have been documented [5]. Allergic reactions may occur [6].

REFERENCES

1 Wu CC, Chen WJ, Cheng J. Local dermal hypersensitivity from dobutamine hydrochloride (Dobutrex solution) injection. *Chest* 1991; **99**: 1547–8.

2 Cernek PK. Dermal cellulitis—a hypersensitivity reaction from dobutamine hydrochloride. *Ann Pharmacother* 1994; **28**: 964.
3 Green SI, Smith JW. Dopamine gangrene. *N Engl J Med* 1976; **294**: 114.
4 Boltax RS, Dineen JP, Scarpa FJ. Gangrene resulting from infiltrated dopamine solution. *N Engl J Med* 1977; **296**: 823.
5 Ross M. Dopamine-induced localized cutaneous vasoconstriction and piloerection. *Arch Dermatol* 1991; **127**: 586–7.
6 Merola B, Sarnacchiaro F, Colao A *et al*. Allergy to ergot-derived dopamine agonists. *Lancet* 1992; **339**; 620.

Vasopressin

This drug, when used intravenously for control of bleeding oesophageal varices or as a local vasoconstrictor agent, has caused cutaneous necrosis at sites of extravasation, and occasionally at distant sites, with a bullous eruption [1]. Mottling, cyanosis, ecchymoses, bullae, ulcers and gangrene are often preceded by coolness and paraesthesiae [2].

REFERENCES

1 Korenberg RJ, Landau-Price D, Penneys NS. Vasopressin-induced bullous disease and cutaneous necrosis. *J Am Acad Dermatol* 1986; **15**: 393–8.
2 Maceyko RF, Vidimos AT, Steck WD. Vasopressin-associated cutaneous infarcts, alopecia, and neuropathy. *J Am Acad Dermatol* 1994; **31**: 111–13.

Rutosides (Paroven)

This mixture of oxerutins, used for relief of symptoms of oedema related to chronic venous insufficiency and for reduction of lymphoedema, has been associated with transient urticaria [1].

REFERENCE

1 Anonymous. Paroven: not much effect in trials. *Drug Ther Bull* 1992; **30**: 7–8.

Drugs acting on the respiratory system

Beta-agonist drugs

Albuterol

Patchy erythema of the hands developed in a pregnant patient following infusion [1].

Salbutamol

LE-like acral erythema developed after infusion in three pregnant patients with premature labour [2].

Salmeterol

An urticarial reaction which recurred on challenge was attributed to this drug administered from a metered dose inhaler [3].

REFERENCES

1 Morin Leport LRM, Loisel JC, Feuilly C. Hand erythema due to infusion of sympathomimetics. *Br J Dermatol* 1990; **122**: 116–17.
2 Reygagne P, Lacour JP, Ortonne J-P. Palmar and plantar erythema due to infusion of sympathomimetics in pregnant women. *Br J Dermatol* 1991; **124**: 210.
3 Hatton MQF, Allen MB, Mellor EJ, Cooke NJ. Salmeterol rash. *Lancet* 1991; **337**: 1169–70.

Antimuscarinic bronchodilators

Aminophylline

This drug is a mixture of theophylline and ethylenediamine. Urticaria, generalized erythema and exfoliative dermatitis have followed systemic administration, probably as a result of reactions to the ethylenediamine component, rather than of theophylline itself [1]. Cross-reactions may occur with ethylenediamine in antihistamines and topical preparations [1,2]. Patch tests may or may not be positive [3].

REFERENCES

1 Gibb W, Thompson PJ. Allergy to aminophylline. *Br Med J* 1983; **287**: 501.
2 Elias JA, Levinson AI. Hypersensitivity reactions to ethylenediamine in aminophylline. *Am Rev Respir Dis* 1981; **123**: 550–2.
3 Kradjan WA, Lakshminarayan S. Allergy to aminophylline: lack of predictability by skin testing. *Am J Hosp Pharm* 1981; **38**: 1031–3.

Miscellaneous respiratory system drugs

Sodium cromoglycate

Hypersensitivity reactions are rare, but urticaria, angiooedema and anaphylactic shock are recorded [1].

REFERENCE

1 Scheffer AL, Rocklin RE, Goetzl EJ. Immunologic components of hypersensitivity reactions to cromolyn sodium. *N Engl J Med* 1975; **293**: 1220–4.

Pseudoephedrine

This drug is present in nasal decongestants and has caused a fixed drug eruption [1–3], recurrent pseudoscarlatina [4,5], allergic reactions [6], systemic contact dermatitis [7] and a reaction simulating recurrent toxic shock syndrome [8].

REFERENCES

1 Shelley WB, Shelley ED. Nonpigmenting fixed drug reaction pattern: examples caused by sensitivity to pseudoephedrine hydrochloride and tetrahydrozoline. *J Am Acad Dermatol* 1987; **17**: 403–7.

2 Hauken M. Fixed drug eruption and pseudoephedrine. *Ann Intern Med* 1994; **120**: 442.

3 Quan MB, Chow WC. Nonpigmenting fixed drug eruption after pseudoephedrine. *Int J Dermatol* 1996; **35**: 367–70.

4 Taylor BJ, Duffill MB. Recurrent pseudo-scarlatina and allergy to pseudoephedrine hydrochloride. *Br J Dermatol* 1988; **118**: 827–9.

5 Rochina A, Burches E, Morales C *et al.* Adverse reaction to pseudoephedrine. *J Invest Allergol Clin Immunol* 1995; **5**: 235–6.

6 Heydon J, Pillans P. Allergic reaction to pseudoephedrine. *NZ Med J* 1995; **108**: 112–13.

7 Tomb RR, Lepoittevin JP, Espinassouze F *et al.* Systemic contact dermatitis from pseudoephedrine. *Contact Dermatitis* 1991; **24**: 86–8.

8 Cavanah DK, Ballas ZK. Pseudoephedrine reaction presenting as recurrent toxic shock syndrome. *Ann Intern Med* 1993; **119**: 302–3.

Metals and metal antagonists

Metals

Arsenic

Bullous eruptions, photosensitivity, exfoliative dermatitis and alopecia may be acute manifestations of arsenic toxicity. Occupational exposure may occur, especially in agriculture. Fowler's solution (containing 1% potassium arsenite) and sodium arsenate were used in the past for psoriasis; as little as 0.19 g has been carcinogenic and the interval between exposure and tumour induction may be as long as 47 years [1]. Subjects with an abnormally high retention of ingested arsenic may be at particular risk [2]. The cutaneous manifestations of arsenic exposure, including pigmentation, palmoplantar punctate keratoses and intraepidermal (Bowen's disease), basal cell or squamous carcinomas of the skin, are well known [1–9]. Keratoses and tumours may be present without pigmentation. In one series of patients, there was a dose-related development of palmar and plantar keratoses in 40%, and carcinomas of the skin in 8%, of patients who received arsenic in the form of Fowler's solution for 6–26 years; the minimum latent period before development of keratoses was 2.5 years, and the average was 6 years [3]. Bowen's disease occurred within 10 years, and invasive carcinomas within 20 years, in another series [7]. Arsenic contamination of well water in Taiwan resulted in numerous affected individuals with arsenical keratoses and cutaneous carcinomas [5]. Carcinomas may arise in the arsenical keratoses [5]. Cutaneous electron microscopic changes are said to be characteristic [8]. The diagnostic significance of the skin arsenic content is disputed. A 42-year-old man who took arsenic for 35 years for psoriasis developed melanoderma, keratoses, muscular dystrophies, hyperlipidaemia, testicular atrophy, gynaecomastia, skin tumours and an obliterating angiitis of leg vessels, which led to amputation [4]. The role of arsenic in causing internal malignancy is the subject of controversy [7,10,11].

REFERENCES

1 Evans S. Arsenic and cancer. *Br J Dermatol* 1977; **97** (Suppl. 15): 13–14.

2 Bettley FR, O'Shea JA. The absorption of arsenic and its relation to carcinoma. *Br J Dermatol* 1975; **92**: 563–8.

3 Fierz U. Katamnestische Untersuchungen über die Nebenwirkungen der Therapie mit anorganischem Arsen bei Hautkrankheiten. *Dermatologica* 1965; **131**: 41–58.

4 Meyhofer W, Knoth W. Über die Auswirkung einer langjährigen antipsoriatischen Arsentherapie auf mehrere Organe unter besonderer Berücksichtigung androligscher Befunde. *Hautarzt* 117: 309–13.

5 Yeh S. Skin cancer in chronic arsenicism. *Hum Pathol* 1973; **4**: 469–85.

6 Weiss J, Jänner M. Multiple Basaliome und Menigiom nach mehrjähriger Arsentherapie. *Hautarzt* 1980; **31**: 654–6.

7 Miki Y, Kawatsu T, Matsuda K *et al.* Cutaneous and pulmonary cancers associated with Bowen's disease. *J Am Acad Dermatol* 1982; **6**: 26–31.

8 Ohyama K, Sonoda K, Kuwahara H. Electron microscopic observations of arsenical keratoses and Bowen's disease associated with chronic arsenicism. *Dermatologica* 1982; **64**: 161–6.

9 Ratnam KV, Espy MJ, Muller SA *et al.* Clinicopathologic study of arsenic-induced skin lesions: no definite association with human papillomavirus. *J Am Acad Dermatol* 1992; **27**: 120–2.

10 Reymann F, Møller R, Nielsen A. Relationship between arsenic intake and internal malignant neoplasms. *Arch Dermatol* 1978; **114**: 378–81.

11 Callen JP, Headington J. Bowen's and non-Bowen's squamous intraepidermal neoplasia of the skin. Relationship to internal malignancy. *Arch Dermatol* 1980; **116**: 422–6.

Gold

The use of gold in rheumatoid arthritis is associated with a 23–30% incidence of reactions [1–3]; most of these are minor, but about 15% may be severe or even fatal [4]. Possession of the HLA-DR3 and -B8 phenotypes reportedly predisposes to thrombocytopenia, leukopenia and nephrotoxicity, -DR4 is linked to leukopenia, and HLA-B7 is associated with cutaneous adverse reactions [2]. In another study, HLA-DR5 was significantly associated with mucocutaneous lesions, while -B8 and -DR3 antigens were associated with proteinuria in rheumatoid arthritis patients after gold therapy; -DR7 was negatively associated with reactions and may confer protection, while -B27 was associated with chrysiasis due to gold therapy [5]. A further study showed that gold dermatitis in patients with rheumatoid arthritis was associated with HLA-B35 and disease duration [6].

Rashes and mouth ulcers are common [1,2,7–12], representing about 50% of all complications with parenteral gold and 35% with oral gold. Localized or generalized pruritus is an important warning sign of potential toxicity. Gold reactions may simulate exanthematic eruptions [13], erythema annulare centrifugum [14], seborrheic dermatitis or lichen planus [15,16]; a mixture of these patterns, sometimes with discoid eczematoid lesions, is characteristic. Lichen planus is often of the hypertrophic variety especially on the scalp, and severe and irreversible alopecia may follow [17]. There may be striking and persistent postinflammatory hyperpigmention. Permanent nail dystrophy has followed onycholysis [18].

In one study, eczematous or lichenoid rashes persisted up to 11 months after cessation of therapy [19]. Histology was characterized by a sparse dermal perivascular infiltrate, predominantly of CD4+ HLA-DR+ helper T lymphocytes, an increase in the number of dermal Langerhans' cells and epidermal macrophage-like cells, and Langerhans' cell apposition to mononuclear cells. A patient with a lichenoid and seborrhoeic dermatitis-like rash on gold sodium thiomalate therapy had a positive intradermal test to gold thiomalate; patch tests were positive to thiomalate (the thiol carrier of gold thiomalate), but negative to gold itself [20]. Interestingly, the same patient subsequently developed a seborrhoeic dermatitis-like eruption, but not a lichenoid eruption, while on auranofin; this time, patch tests were positive to both auranofin and to gold. A previous contact dermatitis from gold jewellery may be reactivated [21].

Other reactions documented include erythema nodosum [22], severe hypersensitivity reactions [23], vasculitis [24], polyarteritis, a systemic LE like syndrome, generalized exfoliative dermatitis and TEN. Psoriasis was reported to be exacerbated in a patient with arthritis treated with gold [25].

Prolonged administration may cause a distinct grey, blue or purple pigmentation of exposed skin (chrysiasis), which is a dose-dependent reaction, occurring above a threshold of 20 mg/kg gold; gold granules are seen within dermal endothelial cells and macrophages [26–30]. Even in the absence of pigmentation, gold can be detected histochemically in the skin up to 20 years after therapy. Localized argyria with chrysiasis has been caused by implanted acupuncture needles [31]. An unusual late cutaneous reaction involved appearance of widespread keloid-like angiofibromatoid lesions [32].

A benign vasodilatory 'nitritoid' reaction, consisting of flushing, light headedness and transient hypotension, may occur immediately after the first injection of gold [2]. Non-vasomotor effects, including arthralgia, myalgia and constitutional symptoms within the first 24 h, are recognized. Mucous membrane symptoms include loss of taste, metallic taste, stomatitis, glossitis and diarrhoea. Punctate stomatitis may occur with or without skin lesions. Gold is also deposited in the cornea and may cause a keratitis with ulceration. A polyneuropathy is recorded. In general, auronofin is less toxic than intramuscular gold [2]. Eosinophilia is common and may sometimes herald another complication; serum IgE may be raised [33]. Other immunological reactions are rare, although pulmonary fibrosis is recorded [34]. Blood dyscrasias, especially thrombocytopenic purpura, and occasionally fatal neutropenia or aplastic anaemia occur in a small proportion of cases and usually present within the first 6 months of therapy. Jaundice occurs in about 3% of cases, and may result from idiosyncratic intrahepatic cholestasis [35]. Proteinuria and renal damage are well known.

REFERENCES

1 Thomas I. Gold therapy and its indications in dermatology. A review. *J Am Acad Dermatol* 1987; **16**: 845–54.
2 Pullar T. Adverse reactions profile: 1. Gold. *Prescribers' J* 1991; **31**: 22–6.
3 Lemmel EM. Comparison of pyritinol and auranofin in the treatment of rheumatoid arthritis. The European Multicentre Study Group. *Br J Rheumatol* 1993; **32**: 375–82.
4 Girdwood RH. Death after taking medicaments. *Br Med J* 1974; **i**: 501–4.
5 Rodriguez-Perez M, Gonzalez-Dominguez J, Mataran L *et al*. Association of HLA-DR5 with mucocutaneous lesions in patients with rheumatoid arthritis receiving gold sodium thiomalate. *J Rheumatol* 1994; **21**: 41–3.
6 van Gestel A, Koopman R, Wijnands M *et al*. Mucocutaneous reactions to gold: a prospective study of 74 patients with rheumatoid arthritis. *J Rheumatol* 1994; **21**: 1814–19.
7 Almeyda J, Baker H. Drug reactions XII. Cutaneous reactions to anti-rheumatic drugs. *Br J Dermatol* 1970; **83**: 707–11.
8 Penneys NS, Ackerman AB, Gottlieb NL. Gold dermatitis: a clinical and histopathological study. *Arch Dermatol* 1974; **109**: 372–6.
9 Penneys NS. Gold therapy: dermatologic uses and toxicities. *J Am Acad Dermatol* 1979; **1**: 315–20.
10 Webster CG, Burnett JW. Gold dermatitis. *Cutis* 1994; **54**: 25–8.
11 Lizeaux-Parmeix V, Bedane C, Lavignac C *et al*. Reactions cutanées aux sels d'or. *Ann Dermatol Vénéréol* 1994; **121**: 793–7.
12 Laeijendecker R, van Joost T. Oral manifestations of gold allergy. *J Am Acad Dermatol* 1994; **30**: 205–9.
13 Möller H, Björkner B, Bruze M. Clinical reactions to systemic provocation with gold sodium thiomalate in patients with contact allergy to gold. *Br J Dermatol* 1996; **135**: 423–7.
14 Tsuji T, Nishimura M, Kimura S. Erythema annulare centrifugum associated with gold sodium thiomalate therapy. *J Am Acad Dermatol* 1992; **27**: 284–7.
15 Lasarowa AZ, Tsankov NK, Stoimenov AP. Lichenoide Eruptionen nach Goldtherapie. Bericht uber zwei Falle. *Hautarzt* 1992; **43**: 514–16.
16 Russell MA, King LE, Jr, Boyd AS. Lichen planus after consumption of a gold-containing liquor. *N Engl J Med* 1996; **334**: 603.
17 Burrows NP, Grant JW, Crisp AJ, Roberts SO. Scarring alopecia following gold therapy. *Acta Derm Venereol (Stockh)* 1994; **74**: 486.
18 Voigt K, Holzegel K. Bleibende nagelveränderungen nach Goldtherapie. *Hautarzt* 1977; **28**: 421–3.
19 Ranki A, Niemi K-M, Kanerva L. Clinical, immunohistochemical, and electron-microscopic findings in gold dermatitis. *Am J Dermatopathol* 1989; **11**: 22–8.
20 Ikezawa Z, Kitamura K, Nakajima H. Gold sodium thiomalate (GTM) induces hypersensitivity to thiomalate, the thiol carrier of GTM. *J Dermatol (Tokyo)* 1990; **17**: 550–4.
21 Rennie T. Local gold toxicity. *Br Med J* 1976; **ii**: 1294.
22 Stone RL, Claflin A, Penneys NS. Erythema nodosum following gold sodium thiomalate therapy. *Arch Dermatol* 1973; **107**: 603–4.
23 Walzer RA, Feinstein R, Shapiro L, Einbinder J. Severe hypersensitivity reaction to gold. Positive lymphocyte transformation test. *Arch Dermatol* 1972; **106**: 231–4.
24 Roenigk HR, Handel D. Gold vasculitis. *Arch Dermatol* 1974; **109**: 253–5.
25 Smith DL, Wernick R. Exacerbation of psoriasis by chrysotherapy. *Arch Dermatol* 1991; **127**: 268–70.
26 Beckett VL, Doyle JA, Hadley GA *et al*. Chrysiasis resulting from gold therapy in rheumatoid arthritis: Identification of gold by X-ray microanalysis. *Mayo Clin Proc* 1982; **57**: 773–5.
27 Pelachyk IM, Bergfeld WF, McMahon JT. Chrysiasis following gold therapy for rheumatoid arthritis. *J Cutan Pathol* 1984; **11**: 491–4.
28 Smith RW, Leppard B, Barnett NL *et al*. Chrysiasis revisited: a clinical and pathological study. *Br J Dermatol* 1995; **133**: 671–8.
29 Fleming CJ, Salisbury ELC, Kirwan P *et al*. Chrysiasis after low-dose gold and UV light exposure. *J Am Acad Dermatol* 1996; **34**: 349–51.
30 Keen CE, Brady K, Kirkham N, Levison DA. Gold in the dermis following chrysotherapy: histopathology and microanalysis. *Histopathology* 1993; **23**: 355–60.
31 Suzuki H, Baba S, Uchigasaki S, Murase M. Localized argyria with chrysiasis caused by implanted acupuncture needles. Distribution and chemical forms of silver and gold in cutaneous tissue by electron microscopy and X-ray microanalysis. *J Am Acad Dermatol* 1993; **29**: 833–7.

32 Herbst WM, Hornstein OP, Grießmeyer G. Ungewöhnliche kutane Angiofibromatose nach Goldtherapie einer primär chronischen Polyarthritis. *Hautarzt* 1989; **40**: 568–72.
33 Davis P, Ezeoke A, Munro J et al. Immunological studies on the mechanism of gold hypersensitivity reactions. *Br Med J* 1973; **iii**: 676–8.
34 Morley TF, Komansky HJ, Adelizzi RA et al. Pulmonary gold toxicity. *Eur J Respir Dis* 1984; **65**: 627–32.
35 Favreau M, Tannebaum H, Lough J. Hepatic toxicity associated with gold therapy. *Ann Intern Med* 1977; **87**: 717–19.

Iron

Iron-induced brownish discoloration has been noted at the site of local injection (local siderosis) [1].

REFERENCE

1 Bork K. Lokalisierte kutane Siderose nach intramuskulären Eiseninjekition. *Hautarzt* 1984; **35**: 598–9.

Mercury

Mercury-containing teething powders have long been banned, but occasional occupational or environmental exposure can occur. Mercury amalgam in dental fillings has caused buccal pigmentation. Stomatitis may occur as a toxic reaction. Allergic reactions may be scarlatiniform or morbilliform, and can progress to generalized exfoliative dermatitis. Pink disease or acrodynia, a distinctive pattern of reaction to chronic exposure to mercury in young infants and children, is now very rare [1]. Painful extremities, pinkish acral discoloration, peeling of the palms and soles, gingivitis and various systemic complications may occur. Acrodynia developed in a child following inhalation of mercury-containing vapours from phenyl-mercuric acetate contained in latex paint [2]. A mercury-containing drug given for 3 weeks to a patient with long-standing pustular psoriasis of the palms was associated with development of generalized pustular psoriasis [3]. See also page 3506; exogenous ochronosis from topical mercury-containing preparations.

REFERENCES

1 Dinehart SM, Dillard R, Raimer SS et al. Cutaneous manifestations of acrodynia (pink disease). *Arch Dermatol* 1988; **124**: 107–9.
2 From the MMWR. Mercury exposure from interior latex paint—Michigan. *Arch Dermatol* 1990; **126**: 577.
3 Wehner-Caroli J, Scherwitz C, Schweinsberg F, Fierlbeck G. Exazerbation einer Psoriasis pustulosa bei Quecksilber-Intoxikation. *Hautarzt* 1994; **45**: 708–10.

Silver

Ingestion of, or topical application of, silver preparations to the oral mucosa or upper respiratory tract can produce slate-blue discoloration, especially of exposed skin, including oral and conjunctival mucosae [1–8]. Topical application may also cause systemic argyria, in which visceral organs are also discoloured [9]. Localized argyria can result from earring backs becoming embedded [10]. In some patients, the nailbeds of the fingers but not the toes may show bluish discoloration [11]. Silver granules are found free within the dermis; the melanin may be increased in the epidermis or within melanophages [12,13].

REFERENCES

1 Pariser RJ. Generalized argyria. Clinicopathologic features and histochemical studies. *Arch Dermatol* 1978; **114**:373–7.
2 Reynold J-L, Stoebner P, Amblard P. Argyrie cutanée. Étude en microscopie electronique et en microanalyse X de 4 cas. *Ann Dermatol Vénéréol* 1980; **107**: 251–5.
3 Johansson EA, Kanerva L, Niemi K-M et al. Generalized argyria with low ceruloplasmin and copper levels in the serum. A case report with clinical and microscopical findings and a trial of penicillamine treatment. *Clin Exp Dermatol* 1982; 7: 169–76.
4 Pezzarossa E, Alinovi A, Ferrari C. Generalized argyria. *J Cutan Pathol* 1983; **10**: 361–3.
5 Gherardi R, Brochard P, Chamak B et al. Human generalized argyria. *Arch Pathol Lab Med* 1984; **108**: 181–2.
6 Jurecka W. Generalisierte Argyrose. *Hautarzt* 1986; **37**: 628–31.
7 Mittag H, Knecht J, Arnold R et al. Zur Frage der Argyrie. Ein klinische, analytisch-chemische und mikromorphologische Untersuchung. *Hautarzt* 1987; **38**: 670–7.
8 Tanner LS, Gross DJ. Generalized argyria. *Cutis* 1990; **45**: 237–9.
9 Marshall IP, Schneider RP. Systemic argyria secondary to topical silver nitrate. *Arch Dermatol* 1977; **113**: 1077–9.
10 van den Nieuwenhijsen IJ, Calame JJ, Bruynzeel DP. Localized argyria caused by silver earrings. *Dermatologica* 1988; **177**: 189–91.
11 Plewig G, Lincke H, Wolff HH. Silver-blue nails. *Acta Derm Venereol (Stockh)* 1977; **57**: 413–19.
12 Hönigsmann H, Konrad K, Wolff K. Argyrose (Histologie und Ultrastruktur). *Hautarzt* 1973; **24**: 24–30.
13 Shelley WB, Shelley ED, Burmeister V. Argyria: The intradermal 'photograph', a manifestation of passive photosensitivity. *J Am Acad Dermatol* 1987; **16**: 211–17.

Metal antagonists

Desferrioxamine

Itching, erythema and urticaria are occasionally seen [1]. An indurated erythema with oedema lasting 2 weeks has been reported following infusion of desferrioxamine [2].

REFERENCES

1 Bousquet J, Navarra M, Robert G et al. Rapid desensitisation for desferrioxamine anaphylactoid reactions. *Lancet* 1983; **ii**: 859–60.
2 Venencie P-Y, Rain B, Blanc A, Tertian G. Toxidermie a la déféroxamine (Desféral). *Ann Derm Vénéréol* 1988; **115**: 1174.

Penicillamine

There is a fourfold increase in toxicity with this drug in patients with rheumatoid arthritis with a genetically determined poor capacity to sulphoxidate the structurally related mucolytic agent, carbocysteine [1,2]. In addition, penicillamine toxicity is independently associated with HLA phenotype [1–3]. HLA-DR3 and -B8 are associated with renal toxicity, -DR3, -B7 and -DR2 with haematological toxicity, and -A1 and -DR4 with thrombocytopenia. Cutaneous adverse reactions are linked to HLA-DRW6. Anti-Ro(SSA)-positive patients with rheumatoid arthritis more often expressed rashes and acute febrile reactions [4].

The cutaneous side-effects of this chelating agent are of three distinct types, namely acute hypersensitivity reactions occurring early during treatment, late reactions including disturbances of autoimmune mechanisms leading to pemphigus foliaceus or erythematosus and cicatricial pemphigoid, and lathyrogenic effects on connective tissue [5–10]. Hypersensitivity reactions are common and consist of urticarial or morbilliform rashes appearing within the first few weeks; the eruption clears on drug withdrawal and does not always recur on re-exposure. It is possible to densitize patients to penicillamine [11].

Autoimmune syndromes caused by penicillamine are well documented. The development of pemphigus during the treatment of both Wilson's disease and rheumatoid arthritis with penicillamine was first noted in the French literature [12,13]. Since then, there have been numerous case reports [14–26]; about 7% of patients receiving

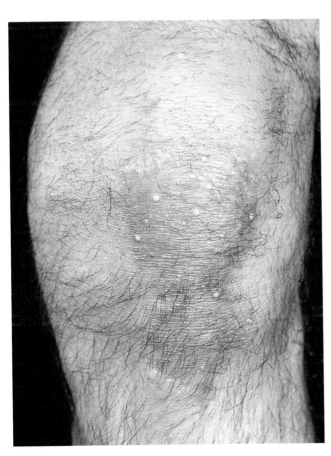

Fig. 77.6 Penicillamine dermopathy with milia. (Courtesy of St John's Institute of Dermatology, London, UK.)

penicillamine for more than 6 months develop drug-induced pemphigus [14]. The reader is referred to the section on drug-induced pemphigus above. Direct immunofluorescence findings mimic the idiopathic disorder, with epidermal intracellular deposition of immunoreactants [17]. Most patients develop pemphigus foliaceus, although there have been isolated reports of pemphigus vulgaris [15] and of pemphigus erythematosus with both epidermal intracellular and subepidermal deposition of IgG [16,18]. In some patients clinical appearances may resemble dermatitis herpetiformis [22,23]. Oral lesions may be indistinguishable from those seen in the idiopathic disease, causing cheilosis, glossitis and stomatitis [24]. Painful erosive vulvovaginitis may lead to scarring. Penicillamine-induced pemphigus usually subsides rapidly after cessation of the drug; occasionally it may be more persistent [14] and fatalities have occurred [25,26]. A curious bullous dermatosis without the features of pemphigus has been described recently [27]. Other autoimmune manifestations include a bullous pemphigoid-like reaction [28], cicatricial pemphigoid [29,30], both discoid and systemic LE [31–34], dermatomyositis [35–38], and both morphea and systemic sclerosis [39,40]. Pre-existing lichen planus [41] may be exacerbated, and lichenoid eruptions develop *de novo* [42,43]. Alopecia, facial dryness and scaling, nail changes and hypertrichosis are recorded. The yellow-nail syndrome has been reported frequently in association with penicillamine [44].

Prolonged high dose therapy for more than a year, as for Wilson's disease, has effects on collagen and elastin, resulting from inhibition of the condensation of soluble tropocollagen to insoluble collagen. There is anisodiametricity of connective tissue fibres, resulting in the 'lumpy-bumpy elastic fibre' [45–47]. The skin becomes wrinkled and thin, aged looking and abnormally fragile; asymptomatic violaceous, friable, haemorrhagic macules, papules and plaques develop on pressure sites, and minor trauma causes ecchymoses [48]. There may be light-blue anetoderma-like lesions [49], and small, white papules at venepuncture sites. Lymphangiectasis may develop [48]. Blisters may occur, with a picture resembling epidermolysis bullosa with scarring and milia formation (Fig. 77.6) [50]. Cutis laxa and elastosis perforans serpiginosa [51–56], which may be verruciform [51–54], are described. Lesions resembling pseudoxanthoma elasticum have been documented rarely [57–60].

Penicillamine may induce impaired taste sensation in up to 25% of patients, but other gastrointestinal effects are usually minor. Important non-dermatological complications [5,61] include marrow suppression; various renal problems, such as reversible proteinuria, in up to 30% of patients on therapy for more than 6 months; established nephrotic syndrome; and Goodpasture's syndrome. Thrombocytopenia occurs in up to 3% of patients, and may be either of gradual or precipitous onset. Immunological abnormalities include acquired IgA deficiency [62] and development of myasthenia gravis [63]. The bones may be involved in the connective tissue disorder. A chronic broncho-alveolitis is recognized [64]. Breast enlargement and breast gigantism [65] are documented.

REFERENCES

1 Emery P, Panayi GS, Huston G *et al.* D penicillamine-induced toxicity in rheumatoid arthritis: the role of sulphoxidation status and HLA-DR3. *J Rheumatol* 1984; **11**: 626–32.

2 Dasgupta B. Adverse reactions profile: 2. Penicillamine. *Prescribers' J* 1991; **31**: 72–7.

3 Wooley PH, Griffin J, Panayi GS *et al.* HLA-DR antigens and toxic reaction to sodium aurothiomalate and D-penicillamine in patients with rheumatoid arthritis. *N Engl J Med* 1980; **303**: 300–2.

4 Vlachoyiannopoulos PG, Zerva LV, Skopouli FN *et al.* D-penicillamine toxicity in Greek patients with rheumatoid arthritis: anti-Ro(SSA) antibodies and cryoglobulinemia are predictive factors. *J Rheumatol* 1991; **18**: 44–9.

5 Dasgupta B. Adverse reactions profile: 2. Penicillamine. *Prescribers' J* 1991; **31**: 72–7.

6 Katz R. Penicillamine-induced skin lesions. Occurrence in a patient with hepatolenticular degeneration (Wilson's disease). *Arch Dermatol* 1967; **95**: 196–8.

7 Greer KE, Askew FC, Richardson DR. Skin lesions induced by penicillamine. *Arch Dermatol* 1976; **112**: 1267–9.

8 Sternlieb I, Fisher M, Scheinberg IH. Penicillamine-induced skin lesions. *J Rheumatol* 1981; **8** (Suppl. 7): 149–54.

9 Levy RS, Fisher M, Alter JN. Penicillamine: Review and cutaneous manifestations. *J Am Acad Dermatol* 1983; **8**: 548–58.

10 Bialy-Golan A, Brenner S. Penicillamine-induced bullous dermatoses. *J Am Acad Dermatol* 1996; **35**: 732–42.

11 Chan CY, Baker AL. Penicillamine hypersensitivity: successful desensitization of a patient with severe hepatic Wilson's disease. *Am J Gastroenterol* 1994; **89**: 442–3.

12 Degos R, Touraine R, Belaïch S *et al.* Pemphigus chez un malade traité par pénicillamine pour maladie de Wilson. *Bull Soc Fr Dermatol Syphiligr* 1969; **76**: 751–3.

13 Benveniste M, Crouzet J, Homberg JC *et al.* Pemphigus induits par la D-pénicillamine dans la polyarthrite rhumatoïde. *Nouv Presse Med* 1975; **4**: 3125–8.

14 Marsden RA, Ryan TJ, Vanhegan RI *et al.* Pemphigus foliaceus induced by penicillamine. *Br Med J* 1976; **ii**: 1423–4.

15 From E, Frederiksen P. Pemphigus vulgaris following D-penicillamine. *Dermatologica* 1976; **152**: 358–62.

16 Thorvaldsen J. Two cases of penicillamine-induced pemphigus erythematosus. *Dermatologica* 1979; **159**: 167–70.

17 Santa Cruz DJ, Prioleau PG, Marcus MD, Uitto J. Pemphigus-like lesions induced by D-penicillamine. Analysis of clinical, histopathological, and immunofluorescence features in 34 cases. *Am J Dermatopathol* 1981; **3**: 85–92.

18 Yung CW, Hambrick GW, Jr. D-penicillamine-induced pemphigus syndrome. *J Am Acad Dermatol* 1982; **6**: 317–24.

19 Bahmer FA, Bambauer R, Stenger D. Penicillamine-induced pemphigus foliaceus-like dermatosis. A case with unusual features, successfully treated by plasmapheresis. *Arch Dermatol* 1985; **121**: 665–8.

20 Kind P, Goerz G, Gleichmann E, Plewig G. Penicillamininduzierter Pemphigus. *Hautarzt* 1987; **38**: 548–52.

21 Civatte J. Durch Medikamente induzierte Pemphigus-Erkrankungen. *Dermatol Mschr* 1989; **175**: 1–7.

22 Marsden RA, Dawber RPR, Millard PR, Mowat AG. Herpetiform pemphigus induced by penicillamine. *Br J Dermatol* 1977; **97**: 451–2.

23 Weltfriend S, Ingber A, David M, Sandbank M. Pemphigus herpetiformis nach D-Penicillamin bei einem Patienten mit HLA B8. *Hautarzt* 1988; **39**: 587–8.

24 Eisenberg E, Ballow M, Wolfe SH *et al.* Pemphigus-like mucosal lesions: a side effect of penicillamine therapy. *Oral Surg* 1981; **51**: 409–14.

25 Sparrow GP. Penicillamine pemphigus and the nephrotic syndrome occurring simultaneously. *Br J Dermatol* 1978; **98**: 103–5.

26 Matkaluk RM, Bailin PL. Penicillamine-induced pemphigus foliaceus. A fatal outcome. *Arch Dermatol* 1981; **117**: 156–7.

27 Fulton RA, Thomson J. Penicillamine-induced bullous dermatosis. *Br J Dermatol* 1982; **107** (Suppl. 22): 95–6.

28 Brown MD, Dubin HV. Penicillamine-induced bullous pemphigoid-like eruption. *Arch Dermatol* 1987; **123**: 1119–20.

29 Pegum JS, Pembroke AC. Benign mucous membrane pemphigoid associated with penicillamine treatment. *Br Med J* 1977; **i**: 1473.

30 Shuttleworth D, Graham-Brown RAC, Hutchinson PE, Jolliffe DS. Cicatricial pemphigoid in D-penicillamine treated patients with rheumatoid arthritis—a report of three cases. *Clin Exp Dermatol* 1985; **10**: 392–7.

31 Burns DA, Sarkany I. Penicillamine induced discoid lupus erythematosus. *Clin Exp Dermatol* 1979; **4**: 389–92.

32 Walshe JM. Penicillamine and the SLE syndrome. *J Rheumatol* 1981; **8** (Suppl. 7): 155–60.

33 Chalmers A, Thompson D, Stein HE *et al.* Systemic lupus erythematosus during penicillamine therapy for rheumatoid arthritis. *Ann Intern Med* 1982; **97**: 659–63.

34 Tsankov NK, Lazarov AZ, Vasileva S, Obreshkova EV. Lupus erythematosus-like eruption due to D-penicillamine in progressive systemic sclerosis. *Int J Dermatol* 1990; **29**: 571–4.

35 Simpson NB, Golding JR. Dermatomyositis induced by penicillamine. *Acta Derm Venereol (Stockh)* 1979; **59**: 543–4.

36 Wojnarowska F. Dermatomyositis induced by penicillamine. *J R Soc Med* 1980; **73**: 884–6.

37 Carroll GC, Will RK, Peter JB *et al.* Penicillamine induced polymyositis and dermatomyositis. *J Rheumatol* 1987; **14**: 995–1001.

38 Wilson CL, Bradlow A, Wojnarowska F. Cutaneous problems with drug therapy in rheumatoid arthritis. *Int J Dermatol* 1991; **30**: 148–9.

39 Bernstein RM, Hall MA, Gostelow BE. Morphea-like reaction to D-penicillamine therapy. *Ann Rheum Dis* 1981; **40**: 42–4.

40 Miyagawa S, Yoshioka A, Hatoko M *et al.* Systemic sclerosis-like lesions during long-term penicillamine therapy for Wilson's disease. *Br J Dermatol* 1987; **116**: 95–100.

41 Powell FC, Rogers RS, III, Dickson ER. Lichen planus, primary biliary cirrhosis and penicillamine. *Br J Dermatol* 1982; **107**: 616.

42 Seehafer JR, Rogers RS, III, Fleming R, Dickson ER. Lichen planus-like lesions caused by penicillamine in primary biliary cirrhosis. *Arch Dermatol* 1981; **117**: 140–2.

43 Van Hecke E, Kint A, Temmerman L. A lichenoid eruption induced by penicillamine. *Arch Dermatol* 1981; **117**: 676–7.

44 Ilchyshyn A, Vickers CFH. Yellow nail syndrome associated with penicillamine therapy. *Acta Derm Venereol (Stockh)* 1983; **63**: 554–5.

45 Bardach H, Gebhart W, Niebauer G. 'Lumpy-bumpy' elastic fibers in the skin and lungs of a patient with a penicillamine-induced elastosis perforans serpiginosa. *J Cutan Pathol* 1979; **6**: 243–52.

46 Gebhart W, Bardach H. The 'lumpy-bumpy' elastic fiber: A marker for long-term administration of penicillamine. *Am J Dermatopathol* 1981; **3**: 33–9.

47 Hashimoto K, McEvoy B, Belcher R. Ultrastructure of penicillamine-induced skin lesions. *J Am Acad Dermatol* 1981; **4**: 300–15.

48 Goldstein JB, McNutt S, Hambrick GW. Penicillamine dermatopathy with lymphangiectases. A clinical, immunohistologic, and ultrastructural study. *Arch Dermatol* 1989; **125**: 92–7.

49 Davis W. Wilson's disease and penicillamine-induced anetoderma. *Arch Dermatol* 1977; **113**: 976.

50 Beer WE, Cooke KB. Epidermolysis bullosa induced by penicillamine. *Br J Dermatol* 1967; **79**: 123–5.

51 Guilane J, Benhamou JP, Molas G. Élastome perforant verruciforme chez un malade traité par pénicillamine pour maladie de Wilson. *Bull Soc Fr Derm Syph* 1972; **79**: 450–3.

52 Reymond JL, Stoebner P, Zambelli P *et al.* Penicillamine induced elastosis perforans serpiginosa: an ultrastructural study of two cases. *J Cutan Pathol* 1982; **9**: 352–7.

53 Sfar Z, Lakhua M, Kamoun MR *et al.* Deux cas d'élastomes verruciforme après administration prolongée de D-pénicillamine. *Ann Dermatol Vénéréol* 1982; **109**: 813–14.

54 Price RG, Prentice RSA. Penicillamine-induced elastosis perforans serpiginosa. Tip of the iceberg? *Am J Dermatopathol* 1986; **8**: 314–20.

55 Sahn EE, Maize JC, Garen PD *et al.* D-Penicillamine-induced elastosis perforans serpiginosa in a child with juvenile rheumatoid arthritis. Report of a case and review of the literature. *J Am Acad Dermatol* 1989; **20**: 979–88.

56 Wilhelm K, Wolff HH. Penicillamin-induzierte Elastosis perforans serpiginosa. *Hautarzt* 1994; **45**: 45–7.
57 Meyrick-Thomas RH, Light N, Stephens AD *et al.* Pseudoxanthoma elasticum-like skin changes induced by penicillamine. *J R Soc Med* 1984; **77**: 794–8.
58 Meyrick-Thomas RH, Kirby JDT. Elastosis perforans serpiginosa and pseudoxanthoma elasticum-like skin change due to D-penicillamine. *Clin Exp Dermatol* 1985; **10**: 386–91.
59 Light N, Meyrick Thomas RH, Stephens A *et al.* Collagen and elastin changes in D-penicillamine-induced pseudoxanthoma elasticum. *Br J Dermatol* 1986; **114**: 381–8.
60 Burge S, Ryan T. Penicillamine-induced pseudo-pseudoxanthoma elasticum in a patient with rheumatoid arthritis. *Clin Exp Dermatol* 1988; **13**: 255–8.
61 Levy RS, Fisher M, Alter JN. Penicillamine: review and cutaneous manifestations *J Am Acad Dermatol* 1983; **8**: 548–58.
62 Hjalmarson O, Hanson L-Å. IgA deficiency during D-penicillamine treatment. *Br Med J* 1977; **i**: 549.
63 Garlepp MJ, Dawkins RL, Christiansen FT. HLA antigens and acetylcholine receptor antibodies in penicillamine induced myasthenia gravis. *Br Med J* 1983; **286**: 338–40.
64 Murphy KC, Atkins CJ, Offer RC *et al.* Obliterative bronchiolitis in two rheumatoid arthritis patients treated with penicillamine. *Arthritis Rheum* 1981; **24**: 557–60.
65 Passas C, Weinstein A. Breast gigantism with penicillamine therapy. *Arthritis Rheum* 1978; **21**: 167–8.

Tiopronin (N-(2-mercaptopropionyl) glycine)

This drug, used in Japan for the treatment of liver disease, mercury intoxication, cataracts and allergic dermatoses, dissociates disulphide bonds, like penicillamine. Morbilliform, urticarial and lichenoid eruptions, bullous in one case, have occurred [1].

REFERENCE

1 Hsiao L, Yoshinaga A, Ono T. Drug-induced bullous lichen planus in a patient with diabetes mellitus and liver disease. *J Am Acad Dermatol* 1986; **15**: 103–5.

Anticoagulants, fibrinolytic agents and antiplatelet drugs

Oral anticoagulants

Adverse reactions to oral anticoagulant drugs have been reviewed [1–3].

REFERENCES

1 Baker H, Levene GM. Drug reactions V. Cutaneous reactions to anticoagulants. *Br J Dermatol* 1969; **81**: 236–8.
2 Hirsh J. Oral anticoagulant drugs. *N Engl J Med* 1991; **324**: 1865–75.
3 Gallerani M, Manfredini R, Moratelli S. Non-haemorrhagic adverse reactions of oral anticoagulant therapy. *Int J Cardiol* 1995; **49**: 1–7.

Coumarins

There may be cross-sensitivity across the group of acenocoumarol, phenprocoumon and warfarin [1].

Phenprocoumon. A patient on long-term anticoagulation developed repeated episodes of skin and subcutaneous fat necrosis related to episodes of overanticoagulation with acquired functional deficiency of protein C, thought to be due to hepatic dysfunction resulting from congestive cardiac failure [2].

Warfarin. Haemorrhage is the commonest adverse reaction. Maculopapular rashes occur [1], and may be seen after a single dose of warfarin [3]. Rarely, an oral loading dose may lead to one or more areas of painful erythema and ecchymosis, which rapidly progress to central blistering and massive cutaneous and subcutaneous necrosis (Fig. 77.7) [4–12]; if extensive, the condition may be fatal [3]. The lesions usually start between the second and 14th day of treatment (usually third to fifth day), tend to be symmetrical, and occur over fatty areas, for example the breasts, buttocks, thighs, calves and abdomen. Most patients have been women, but lesions of the penis may occur [6]. Warfarin necrosis has been associated with the heterozygous state for deficiency of protein C, a vitamin K-dependent serine protease [8–10]. Activated protein C is a potent anticoagulant that selectively inactivates cofactors Va and VIIIa and inhibits platelet coagulant activity by inactivation of platelet factor Va. Continued coumarin therapy does not aggravate the condition, but resumption of therapy with loading doses may lead to new lesions [7]. The condition is preventable by vitamin K_1 injections. Other side-effects are rare, and include urticaria [13], dermatitis, gastrointestinal upset, purple erythema of the dependent parts (the purple-toe syndrome) [14–16], acral purpura [17] and alopecia [18].

Oral anticoagulants and quinidine act synergistically to depress vitamin K-sensitive hepatic clotting synthesis [19]. Their combined use can precipitate serious hypoprothrombinaemic haemorrhage. Azapropazone displaces warfarin from protein-binding sites and also alters renal

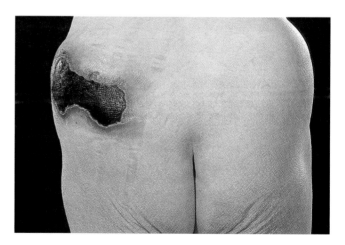

Fig. 77.7 Warfarin necrosis. (Courtesy of A. Ive, Dryburn Hospital, Durham, UK.)

clearance of R and S isomers of warfarin; this may lead to effective warfarin overdosage [20]. Itraconazole may potentiate the action of warfarin [21].

REFERENCES

1 Kruis-de Vries MH, Stricker BHC, Coenraads PJ, Nater JP. Maculopapular rash due to coumarin derivatives. *Dermatologica* 1989; **178**: 109–11.
2 Teepe RGC, Broekmans AW, Vermeer BJ et al. Recurrent coumarin-induced skin necrosis in a patient with an acquired functional protein C deficiency. *Arch Dermatol* 1986; **122**: 1408–12.
3 Antony SJ, Krick SK, Mehta PM. Unusual cutaneous adverse reaction to warfarin therapy. *South Med J* 1993; **86**: 1413–14.
4 Lacy JP, Goodin RR. Warfarin-induced necrosis of skin. *Ann Intern Med* 1975; **82**: 381–2.
5 Schleicher SM, Fricker MP. Coumarin necrosis. *Arch Dermatol* 1980; **116**: 444–5.
6 Weinberg AC, Lieskovsky G, McGehee WG, Skinner DG. Warfarin necrosis of the skin and subcutaneous tissue of the male external genitalia. *J Urol* 1983; **130**: 352–4.
7 Slutzki S, Bogokowsky H, Gilboa Y, Halpern Z. Coumadin-induced skin necrosis. *Int J Dermatol* 1984; **23**: 117–19.
8 Kazmier FJ. Thromboembolism, coumarin necrosis, and protein C. *Mayo Clin Proc* 1985; **60**: 673–4.
9 Gladson CL, Groncy P, Griffin JH. Coumarin necrosis, neonatal purpura fulminans, and protein C deficiency. *Arch Dermatol* 1988; **123**: 1701a–6a.
10 Auletta MJ, Headington JT. Purpura fulminans. A cutaneous manifestation of severe protein C deficiency. *Arch Dermatol* 1988; **124**: 1387–91.
11 Sharafuddin MJ, Sanaknaki BA, Kibbi AG. Erythematous, hemorrhagic, and necrotic plaques in an elderly man. Coumarin-induced skin necrosis. *Arch Dermatol* 1992; **128**: 105, 108.
12 Comp PC. Coumarin-induced skin necrosis. Incidence, mechanisms, management and avoidance. *Drug Saf* 1993; **8**: 128–35.
13 Sheps ES, Gifford RW. Urticaria after administration of warfarin sodium. *Am J Cardiol* 1959; **3**: 118–20.
14 Feder W, Auerbach R. 'Purple toes': an uncommon sequela of oral coumarin drug therapy. *Ann Intern Med* 1961; **55**: 911–17.
15 Akle CA, Joiner CL. Purple toe syndrome. *J R Soc Med* 1981; **74**: 219.
16 Lebsack CS, Weibert RT. Purple toes syndrome. *Postgrad Med* 1982; **71**: 81–4.
17 Stone MS, Rosen T. Acral purpura: an unusual sign of coumarin necrosis. *J Am Acad Dermatol* 1986; **14**: 797–802.
18 Umlas J, Harken DE. Warfarin-induced alopecia. *Cutis* 1988; **42**: 63–4.
19 Koch-Weser J. Quinidine-induced hypoprothrombinemic hemorrhage in patients on chronic warfarin therapy. *Ann Intern Med* 1968; **68**: 511–17.
20 Win N, Mitchell DC. Azapropazone and warfarin. *Br Med J* 1991; **302**: 969–70.
21 Yeh J, Soo SC, Summerton C, Richardson C. Potentiation of action of warfarin by itraconazole. *Br Med J* 1990; **301**: 669.

Indandiones

Hypersensitivity reactions occur in up to 0.3% of patients within 3 months of onset of treatment of phenindione. Scarlatiniform, eczematous, erythema multiforme-like or generalized exfoliative eruptions are seen [1,2]. Alopecia and a stomatitis may accompany the rash. Brownish-yellow or orange discoloration of the palmar or finger skin on handling the tablets develops after contact with soap alkali [3]. Cutaneous necrosis occurs rarely.

REFERENCES

1 Hollman A, Wong HO. Phenindione sensitivity. *Br Med J* 1964; **ii**: 730–2.
2 Copeman PWM. Phenindione toxicity. *Br Med J* 1965; **ii**: 305.
3 Silverton NH. Skin pigmentation by phenindione. *Br Med J* 1966; **i**: 675.

Heparin: parenteral anticoagulant

The most frequent side-effect is haemorrhage [1,2]. Other common side-effects include osteoporosis and (temporary) telogen effluvium 6–16 weeks after administration. Hypoaldosteronism may occur. Hypersensitivity reactions including urticaria and anaphylactic shock are well documented but very uncommon [3]. Rapid desensitization was achieved in a patient with heparin urticarial hypersensitivity requiring cardiac surgery [4]. Hypereosinophilia is recorded [5]. Vasospastic reactions, including pain, cyanosis and severe itching or burning plantar sensations, are described.

Erythematous infiltrated plaques developing 3–21 days after commencement of heparin therapy [6–14] may closely mimic contact dermatitis both clinically and histologically, and patch tests may be positive [8,9]. A subcutaneous provocation test may be a useful diagnostic measure. Low-molecular-weight heparin analogues may be satisfactorily substituted in some patients with this reaction [6,15], but are not always tolerated [7,16,17]; a panel of different low-molecular-weight heparin preparations should be checked by subcutaneous provocation tests before reinstitution of heparin therapy. Chlorocresol may be responsible for some reactions attributed to heparin [7,18], including anaphylactoid reactions.

Skin necrosis occurring 6–8 days after onset of subcutaneous heparin is rare, but may occur at injection sites and occasionally at distal sites elsewhere [19–27]. Diabetic women on high-dose antibiotics are predisposed to this complication. A scleroderma-like evolution has been recorded [22]. Clinically, the skin necrosis resembles that of coumarin necrosis [25]. It may occur with use of low-molecular-weight heparin [23,26].

Heparin may cause an allergic thrombocytopenia [28–35]. Thrombocytopenia is usually asymptomatic, but may be associated with arterial or venous thrombosis in about 0.4% of cases [29,33,34]; thromboembolism may occasionally be lethal [30]. Thrombocytopenia usually begins 3–15 days after initiation of therapy, may occur within hours in previously exposed patients and is thought to be caused by an IgG–heparin immune complex involving both the Fab and Fc portions of the IgG molecule [29]. Heparin-induced antiendothelial cell antibodies, which recognize heparin-like glycans on the cell surface of platelets and endothelial cells, may lead to platelet aggregation and endothelial cell expression of procoagulant tissue factor, with resultant thrombocytopenia and thrombosis [21]. Thrombocytopenia may occur with both unfractionated and with low-molecular-weight heparin [20]. Clinical cross-reactivity between heparin and the polysulphated chondroitin-like substance, Arteparon, used for treatment of degenerative joint disease, has been described [32].

REFERENCES

1 Tuneu A, Moreno A, de Moragas JM. Cutaneous reactions secondary to heparin injections. *J Am Acad Dermatol* 1985; **12**: 1072–7.
2 Hirsh J. Heparin. *N Engl J Med* 1991; **324**: 1565–74.
3 Curry N, Bandana EJ, Pirofsky B. Heparin sensitivity: report of a case. *Arch Intern Med* 1973; **132**: 744–5.
4 Patriarca G, Rossi M, Schiavino D *et al*. Rush desensitization in heparin hypersensitivity: a case report. *Allergy* 1994; **49**: 292–4.
5 Bircher AJ, Itin PH, Buchner SA. Skin lesions, hypereosinophilia, and subcutaneous heparin. *Lancet* 1994; **343**: 861.
6 Zimmermann R, Harenberg J, Weber E *et al*. Behandlung bei heparin-induzierter kutaner Reaktion mit einem niedermolekularen Heparin-Analog. *Dtsch Med Wschr* 1984; **109**: 1326–8.
7 Klein GF, Kofler H, Wol H, Fritsch PO. Eczema-like, erythematous, infiltrated plaques: a common side-effect of subcutaneous heparin therapy. *J Am Acad Dermatol* 1989; **21**: 703–7.
8 Guillet G, Delaire P, Plantin P, Guillet MH. Eczema as a complication of heparin therapy. *J Am Acad Dermatol* 1989; **21**: 1130.
9 Bircher AJ, Flückiger R, Buchner SA. Eczematous infiltrated plaques to subcutaneous heparin: a type IV allergic reaction. *Br J Dermatol* 1990; **123**: 507–14.
10 O'Donnell BF, Tan CY. Delayed hypersensitivity reaction to heparin. *Br J Dermatol* 1993; **129**: 634–6.
11 Sivakumaran M, Ghosh K, Munks R *et al*. Delayed cutaneous reaction to unfractionated heparin, low molecular weight heparin and danaparoid. *Br J Haematol* 1994; **86**: 893–4.
12 Mathelier-Fusade P, Deschamps A, Abuaf N, Leynadier F. Reactions cutanées a l'héparine: aspects immunologiques et cliniques. *Presse Med* 1995; **24**: 323–5.
13 Koch P, Hindi S, Landwehr D. Delayed allergic skin reactions due to subcutaneous heparin-calcium, enoxaparin-sodium, pentosan polysulfate and acute skin lesions from systemic sodium-heparin. *Contact Dermatitis* 1996; **34**: 156–8.
14 Gallais V, Bredoux H, Rancourt MF *et al*. Toxidermie a l'heparine. *Presse Med* 1996; **25**: 1040.
15 Koch P, Bahmer FA, Schafer H. Tolerance of intravenous low-molecular-weight heparin after eczematous reaction to subcutaneous heparin. *Contact Dermatitis* 1991; **25**: 205–6.
16 Bosch A, Las Heras G, Martin E, Oller G. Skin reaction with low molecular weight heparins. *Br J Haematol* 1993; **85**: 637.
17 Phillips JK, Majumdar G, Hunt BJ, Savidge GF. Heparin-induced skin reaction due to two different preparations of low molecular weight heparin (LMWH). *Br J Haematol* 1993; **84**: 349–50.
18 Ainley EJ, Mackie IG, MacArthur D. Adverse reaction to chlorocresol-preserved heparin. *Lancet* 1977; **i**: 705.
19 Shelley WB, Säyen JJ. Heparin necrosis: an anticoagulant-induced cutaneous infarct. *J Am Acad Dermatol* 1982; **7**: 674–7.
20 Levine LE, Bernstein JE, Soltani K *et al*. Heparin-induced skin necrosis unrelated to injection sites; a sign of potentially lethal complications. *Arch Dermatol* 1983; **119**: 400–3.
21 Mathieu A, Avril MF, Schlumberger M *et al*. Un cas de nécrose cutanée induite par l'héparine. *Ann Dermatol Vénéréol* 1984; **111**: 733–4.
22 Barthelemy H, Hermier C, Perrot H. Nécrose cutanée avec évolution scléridermiforme après l'injection souscutanée d'heparinate de calcium. *Ann Dermatol Vénéréol* 1985; **112**: 245–7.
23 Cordoliani F, Saiag P, Guillaume J-C *et al*. Nécrose cutanés étendues induites par la fraxiparine. *Ann Dermatol Vénéréol* 1987; **114**: 1366–8.
24 Rongioletti F, Pisani S, Ciaccio M, Rebora A. Skin necrosis due to intravenous heparin. *Dermatologica* 1989; **178**: 47–50.
25 Gold JA, Watters AK, O'Brien E. Coumadin versus heparin necrosis. *J Am Acad Dermatol* 1987; **16**: 148–50.
26 Ojeda E, Perez MC, Mataix R *et al*. Skin necrosis with a low molecular weight heparin. *Br J Haematol* 1992; **82**: 620.
27 Yates P, Jones S. Heparin skin necrosis—an important indicator of potentially fatal heparin hypersensitivity. *Clin Exp Dermatol* 1993; **18**: 138–41.
28 Cine DB, Tomaski A, Tannenbaum S. Immune endothelial cell injury in heparin-associated thrombocytopenia. *N Engl J Med* 1987; **316**: 581–9.
29 Warkentin TE, Kelton JG. Heparin-induced thrombocytopenia. *Annu Rev Med* 1989; **40**: 31–44.
30 Jaffray B, Welch GH, Cooke TG. Fatal venous thrombosis after heparin therapy. *Lancet* 1991; **337**: 561.
31 Eichinger S, Kyrle PA, Brenner B *et al*. Thrombocytopenia associated with low-molecular-weight heparin. *Lancet* 1991; **337**: 1425–6.
32 Greinacher A, Michels I, Schafer M *et al*. Heparin-associated thrombocytopenia in a patient treated with polysulphated chondroitin sulphate: evidence for immunological crossreactivity between heparin and polysulphated glycosaminoglycan. *Br J Haematol* 1992; **81**: 252–4.
33 Gross AS, Thompson FL, Arzubiaga MC *et al*. Heparin-associated thrombocytopenia and thrombosis (HATT) presenting with livedo reticularis. *Int J Dermatol* 1993; **32**: 276–9.
34 O'Bryan-Tear G. Heparin induced thrombosis. Datasheet warns of risk. *Br Med J* 1993; **307**: 561.
35 Ouellette D, Menkis AH. Heparin-induced thrombocytopenia. *Ann Thorac Surg* 1993; **55**: 809.

Protamine: heparin antagonist

This low-molecular-weight protein, derived from salmon sperm and/or testes, is used for neutralization of heparin anticoagulation after cardiac surgery. Adverse reactions have been reviewed [1]. Idiosyncratic responses or those related to complement generation of anaphylatoxins are recorded [2]. IgE-dependent anaphylaxis [3], as well as delayed reactions causing skin nodules [4–6], which may be granulomatous [6], may occur in diabetics treated with protamine-containing insulin.

REFERENCES

1 Cormack JG, Levy JH. Adverse reactions to protamine. *Coron Artery Dis* 1993; **4**: 420–5.
2 Sussman GL, Dolovich J. Prevention of anaphylaxis. *Semin Dermatol* 1989; **8**: 158–65.
3 Kim R. Anaphylaxis to protamine masquerading as an insulin allergy. *Del Med J* 1993; **65**: 17–23.
4 Sarche MB, Paolillo M, Chacon RS *et al*. Protamine as a cause of generalized allergic reactions to NPH insulin. *Lancet* 1982; **i**: 1243.
5 Kollner A, Senff H, Engelmann L *et al*. Protaminallergie vom Spattyp und Insulinallergie vom Soforttyp. *Dtsch Med Wochenschr* 1991; **116**: 1234–8.
6 Hulshof MM, Faber WR, Kniestedt WF *et al*. Granulomatous hypersensitivity to protamine as a complication of insulin therapy. *Br J Dermatol* 1992; **127**: 286–8.

Fibrinolytic drugs

Haemorrhage is the most common untoward effect from use of thrombolysins [1]. Allergic complications are rare, particularly with alteplase or urokinase. These agents should be used electively in all patients previously exposed to streptokinase or anistreplase [2].

Alteplase (tissue plasminogen activator)

Painful purpura occurring within hours of administration has been recorded [3].

Aminocaproic acid

A maculopapular eruption occurring 12–72h after administration of ε-aminocaproic acid, with positive patch tests to the drug, has been described [4]. A transient, non-inflammatory, subepidermal, bullous eruption on the legs, with fibrin thrombi in papillary dermal vessels, has also been recorded [5].

Anistreplase

Anistreplase anisoylated plasminogen streptokinase activator complex given for an acute myocardial infarction was associated with leukocytoclastic vasculities [6]. Maculopapular rashes and urticaria are described; patients with maculopapular rashes had significantly higher rises in serum IgM, IgG, IgA and IgE antistreptokinase level [7].

REFERENCES

1 Chesebro JH, Knatterud G, Roberts R *et al.* Thrombolysis in myocardial infarction (TIMI) trial, phase I: a comparison between intravenous tissue plasminogen activator and intravenous streptokinase. *Circulation* 1987; **76**: 142–54.
2 de Bono DP. Complications of thrombolysis and their clinical management. *Zeitschr Kardiol* 1993; **82** (Suppl. 2): 147–51.
3 DeTrana C, Hurwitz RM. Painful purpura: an adverse effect to a thrombolysin. *Arch Dermatol* 1990; **126**: 690–1.
4 Gonzalez Gutierrez ML, Esteban Lopez MI, Ruiz Ruiz MD. Positivity of patch tests in cutaneous reaction to aminocaproic acid: two case reports. *Allergy* 1995; **50**: 745–6.
5 Brooke CP, Spiers EM, Omura EF. Noninflammatory bullae associated with epsilon-aminocaproic acid infusion. *J Am Acad Dermatol* 1992; **27**: 880–2.
6 Burrows N, Russell Jones R. Vasculitis occurring after intravenous anistreplase. *J Am Acad Dermatol* 1992; **26**: 508.
7 Dykewicz MS, McMorrow NK, Davison R *et al.* Drug eruptions and isotypic antibody responses to streptokinase after infusions of anisoylated plasminogen-streptokinase complex (APSAC, anistreplase). *J Allergy Clin Immunol* 1995; **95**: 1020–8.

Streptokinase

Allergic reactions have been reported in up to 6% of patients [1–3], ranging from minor skin rashes to angio-oedema or anaphylaxis (which may be fatal [4–6]), bleeding, strokes, and a syndrome resembling adult respiratory distress syndrome [3]. Patients who develop reactions to streptokinase cannot be predicted on the basis of antistreptokinase IgG antibody titres at presentation; minor reactions to streptokinase would not appear to be antibody mediated [7]. However, streptokinase-related thrombolytic agents should be avoided in reinfarction thrombolysis therapy in patients with raised antistreptokinase antibody titres, as hypersensitivity reactions including serum sickness may occur [8–10]. This drug has been reported in association with a hypersensitivity vasculitis [11,12], serum sickness with leukocytoclastic vasculitis [13,14] and a lymphocytic angiitis [15]. Skin necrosis is recorded [16].

Urokinase

Haemorrhagic bullae occurred as a complication of urokinase therapy for haemodialysis catheter thrombosis [17].

REFERENCES

1 Dykewicz MS, McGratt KG, Davison R *et al.* Identification of patients at risk for anaphylaxis due to streptokinase. *Arch Intern Med* 1986; **146**: 305–7.
2 ISIS-2 (Second International Study of Infarct Survival). Collaborative Group. Randomized trial of intravenous streptokinase, oral aspirin, both, or neither among 17187 cases of suspected acute myocardial infarction: ISIS-2. *Lancet* 1988; **2**: 349–60.
3 Siebert WJ, Ayres RW, Bulling MT *et al.* Streptokinase morbidity—more common than previously recognised. *Aust NZ J Med* 1992; **22**: 129–33.
4 Allpress SM, Cluroe AD, Vuletic JC, Kolemeyer TD. Death after streptokinase. *NZ Med J* 1993; **106**: 295.
5 Hohage H, Schulte B, Pfeiff B, Pullmann H. Anaphylaktische Reaktion unter Streptokinase-Therapie. *Wien Klin Wochenschr* 1993; **105**: 176–8.
6 Cooper JP, Quarry DP, Beale DJ, Chappell AG. Life-threatening, localized angio-oedema associated with streptokinase. *Postgrad Med J* 1994; **70**: 592–3.
7 Lynch M, Pentecost BL, Littler WA, Stockley RA. Why do patients develop reactions to streptokinase? *Clin Exp Immunol* 1993; **94**: 279–85.
8 Lee HS, Yule S, McKenzie A *et al.* Hypersensitivity reactions to streptokinase in patients with high pretreatment antistreptokinase antibody and neutralisation titres. *Eur Heart J* 1993; **14**: 1640–3.
9 Cross DB. Should streptokinase be readministered? Insights from recent studies of antistreptokinase antibodies. *Med J Aust* 1994; **161**: 100–1.
10 Jennings K. Antibodies to streptokinase. *Br Med J* 1996; **312**: 393–4.
11 Ong ACM, Handler CE, Walker JM. Hypersensitivity vasculitis complicating intravenous streptokinase therapy in acute myocardial infarction. *Int J Cardiol* 1988; **21**: 71–3.
12 Thompson RF, Stratton MA, Heffron WA. Hypersensitivity vasculitis associated with streptokinase. *Clin Pharmacol* 1985; **4**: 383–8.
13 Patel IA, Prussick R, Buchanan WW, Sauder DN. Serum sickness-like illness and leukocytoclastic vasculitis after intravenous streptokinase. *J Am Acad Dermatol* 1991; **24**: 652–3.
14 Totto WG, Romano T, Benian GM *et al.* Serum sickness following streptokinase therapy. *Am J Rheumatol* 1982; **138**: 143–4.
15 Sorber WA, Herbst V. Lymphocytic angiitis following streptokinase therapy. *Cutis* 1988; **42**: 57–8.
16 Penswick J, Wright AL. Skin necrosis induced by streptokinase. *Br Med J* 1994; **309**: 378.
17 Ejaz AA, Aijaz M, Nawab ZM *et al.* Hemorrhagic bullae as a complication of urokinase therapy for hemodialysis catheter thrombosis. *Am J Nephrol* 1995; **15**: 178–9.

Antiplatelet drugs

Ticlopidine

This antiplatelet drug, indicated for coronary artery disease, cerebrovascular disease, peripheral vascular disease and diabetic retinopathy, is a thienopyridine derivative [1,2]; it is not licensed in the UK. Gastrointestinal symptoms, thrombocytopenia with minor bleeding including bruising, neutropenia, rashes in 10–15% of patients, and hepatic dysfunction in 4% of cases, have been reported. Thrombotic thrombocytopenic purpura has also been documented [3].

REFERENCES

1 McTavish D, Faulds D, Goa KL. Ticlopidine. An updated review of its pharmacology and therapeutic use in platelet-dependent disorders. *Drugs* 1990; **40**: 238–59.
2 Editorial. Ticlopidine. *Lancet* 1991; **337**: 459–60.
3 Page Y, Tardy B, Zeni F *et al*. Thrombotic thrombocytopenic purpura related to ticlopidine. *Lancet* 1991; **337**: 774–6.

Vitamins including retinoids

Vitamin A

Generalized peeling may be a delayed manifestation of acute intoxication [1]. Chronic intoxication produces the following epithelial problems: pruritus; erythema; hyperkeratosis; dryness of mouth, nose and eyes; epistaxis; fissuring; dryness and scaling of the lips; peeling of the palms and soles; and alopecia. A yellow-orange skin discoloration, photosensitivity and nail changes have also been observed [2–5]. Headache, pseudotumour cerebri, anaemia, hepatomegaly and skeletal pain may be present. Cortical hyperostoses and periosteal reaction of tubular bone [6], and more rarely premature epiphyseal closure and change in the contour of long bones [7], are seen.

REFERENCES

1 Nater P, Doeglas HMG. Halibut liver poisoning in 11 fishermen. *Acta Derm Venereol (Stockh)* 1970; **50**: 109–13.
2 Oliver TK. Chronic vitamin A intoxication. Report of a case in an older child and a review of the literature. *Am J Dis Child* 1959; **95**: 57–67.
3 Muenter MD, Perry HO, Ludwig J. Chronic vitamin A intoxication in adults. Hepatic, neurologic and dermatologic complications. *Am J Med* 1971; **50**: 129–36.
4 Teo ST, Newth J, Pascoe BJ. Chronic vitamin A intoxication. *Med J Aust* 1973; **2**: 324–6.
5 Bobb R, Kieraldo JH. Cirrhosis due to hypervitaminosis A. *West J Med* 1978; **128**: 244–6.
6 Frame B, Jackson CE, Reynolds WA, Umphrey JE. Hypercalcemia and skeletal effects in chronic hypervitaminosis A. *Ann Intern* 1974; **80**: 44–8.
7 Ruby LK, Mital MA. Skeletal deformities following chronic hypervitaminosis A. *J Bone Joint Surg* 1974; **56**: 1283–7.

Retinoids

The cutaneous and systemic side-effects of these synthetic vitamin A-related compounds resemble those of hypervitaminosis A, and have been extensively reviewed [1–12].

REFERENCES

1 Orfanos CE, Braun-Falco O, Farber EM *et al.*, eds. *Retinoids. Advances in Basic Research and Therapy*. Berlin: Springer-Verlag, 1981.
2 Foged E, Jacobsen F. Side-effects due to Ro 10-3959 (Tigason). *Dermatologica* 1982; **164**: 395–403.
3 Windhorst DB, Nigra T. General clinical toxicology of oral retinoids. *J Am Acad Dermatol* 1982; **4**: 675–82.
4 Cunliffe WJ, Miller AJ, eds. *Retinoid Therapy: A Review of Clinical and Laboratory Research*. Lancaster: MTP Press Ltd, 1984.
5 Saurat JH, ed. *Retinoids: New Trends in Research and Therapy*. Basel: Karger, 1985

6 Yob EH, Pochi PE. Side effects and long-term toxicity of synthetic retinoids. *Arch Dermatol* 1987; **123**: 1375–8.
7 Bigby M, Stern RS. Adverse reactions to isotretinoin. A report from the Adverse Drug Reaction Reporting System. *J Am Acad Dermatol* 1988; **18**: 543–52.
8 Saurat J-H. Side effects of systemic retinoids and their clinical management. *J Am Acad Dermatol* 1992; **27**: S23–8.
9 Vahlquist A. Long-term safety of retinoid therapy. *J Am Acad Dermatol* 1992; **27**: S29–33.
10 Gollnick HPM. Oral retinoids—efficacy and toxicity in psoriasis. *Br J Dermatol* 1996; **135** (Suppl. 49): 6–17.
11 Mørk N-J, Kolbenstvedt A, Austad J. Skeletal side-effects of 5 years' acitretin treatment. *Br J Dermatol* 1996; **134**: 1156–7.
12 Hermann G, Jungblut RM, Goerz G. Skeletal changes after long-term therapy with synthetic retinoids. *Br J Dermatol* 1997; **136**: 469–70.

Acitretin

The side-effects of this principal metabolite of etretinate are similar to those of the parent compound [1–5], comprising cheilitis, conjunctivitis, peeling of the palms and soles, xerosis, myalgia and alopecia; elevated serum triglyceride, cholesterol and liver transaminase levels are seen. Alopecia is particularly frequent [4], and scaling of the palms and soles appears more prominent than with etretinate [5]. There is a higher occurrence of vulvovaginal candidiasis during acitretin exposure [6]. Multiple milia have occurred [7]. Skeletal effects may be significant, but are not an absolute contraindication to therapy [8]. Persistent levels of etretinate have been detected in plasma following changing therapy to acitretin [9]. Detectable etretinate is present in 45% and 83% of plasma and subcutaneous tissue, respectively, in current acitretin users and in 18% and 86% of those who have stopped acitretin [9]. Inability to detect plasma etretinate is therefore a poor predictor of the absence of etretinate in fat. Acitretin and/or etretinate were detectable in fat and in some cases plasma from women who had ceased acitretin therapy for up to 29 months [9]. It has been proposed that acitretin and etretinate should be monitored in subcutaneous tissue when plasma measurements are negative, and that the recommended contraception period of 2 years after cessation of acitretin therapy should be reconsidered to avoid the risk of teratogenicity [10].

REFERENCES

1 Geiger J-M, Czarnetzki BM. Acitretin (Ro 10-1670, Etretin): overall evaluation of clinical studies. *Dermatologica* 1988; **176**: 182–90.
2 Gupta AK, Goldfarb MT, Ellis CN, Voorhees JJ. Side-effect profile of acitretin therapy in psoriasis. *J Am Acad Dermatol* 1989; **21**: 1088–93.
3 Ruzicka T, Sommerburg C, Braun-Falco O *et al*. Efficiency of acitretin in combination with UV-B in the treatment of severe psoriasis. *Arch Dermatol* 1990; **126**: 482–6.
4 Murray HE, Anhalt AW, Lessard R *et al*. A 12-month treatment of severe psoriasis with acitretin: results of a Canadian open multicenter study. *J Am Acad Dermatol* 1991; **24**: 598–602.
5 Blanchet-Bardon C, Nazzaro V, Rognin C *et al*. Acitretin in the treatment of severe disorders of keratinization. Results of an open study. *J Am Acad Dermatol* 1991; **24**: 982–6.
6 Sturkenboom MC, Middelbeek A, de Jong van den Berg LT *et al*. Vulvo-vaginal candidiasis associated with acitretin. *J Clin Epidemiol* 1995; **48**: 991–7.

7 Chang A, Kuligowski ME, van de Kerkhof PC. Multiple milia during treatment with acitretin for mycosis fungoides. *Acta Derm Venereol (Stockh)* 1993; **73**: 235.
8 Mørk N-J, Kolbenstvedt A, Austad J. Skeletal side-effects of 5 years' acitretin treatment. *Br J Dermatol* 1996; **134**: 1156–7.
9 Lambert WE, De Leenheer AP, De Bersaques JP, Kint A. Persistent etretinate levels in plasma after changing the therapy to acitretin. *Arch Dermatol* Res 1990; **282**: 343–4.
10 Sturkenboom MC, de Jong Van Den Berg LT, van Voorst Vader PC *et al.* Inability to detect plasma etretinate and acitretin is a poor predictor of the absence of these teratogens in tissue after stopping acitretin treatment. *Br J Clin Pharmacol* 1994; **38**: 229–35.

Etretinate

This drug has been largely superseded by acitretin. The dermatological side-effects are dose dependent, and resemble those associated with isotretinoin therapy [1–3]. With dosage over 0.5 mg/kg, cheilitis with dryness, scaling and fissuring of the lips is almost universal. There may be pruritus; a dry mouth; dry nose; epistaxis; meatitis; desquamation including the face, hands and feet; and reduced tolerance of sunlight [4] and therapeutic products such as tar or dithranol. Pseudoporphyria has been reported in a renal transplant recipient treated with etretinate to suppress cutaneous neoplasia [5]. A 'retinoid dermatitis' resembling asteatotic eczema may develop in up to 50% of patients [6]. Increased stickiness of the palms and soles, possibly due to increased quantities of carcinoembryonic antigen and other glycoproteins in eccrine sweat [7,8], has been reported. Mucosal erosions, conjunctivitis, paronychia, alopecia [9] and curling, kinking or darkening of hair [10] are all well documented. Intertriginous erosions have also been described [11]. Oedema [12], excess granulation tissue [13] and multiple pyogenic granulomas [14] develop rarely. Erythroderma has been reported [15].

Prolonged therapy may lead to skin fragility [16,17]; blistering, erosions and scarring have been reported in one patient [18]. Softening of the nails is seen [19], and chronic paronychia, onycholysis, onychomadesis, nail shedding, onychoschizia and fragility may occur [20,21]. Parakeratotic digitate keratoses appearing after treatment of disseminated superficial actinic porokeratosis may arise as a result of etretinate-resistant regions in the ring of the cornoid lamella [22]. There has been a single case of generalization of palmoplantar pustulosis following cessation of etretinate therapy [23].

Systemic side-effects of etretinate include benign intracranial hypertension [24]. Minor disturbances of tests of liver function are not uncommon, and may not always be reversible; liver changes range from non-specific reactive hepatitis, to acute hepatitis, chronic active hepatitis, and severe fibrosis or cirrhosis [25–28]. Fatal liver necrosis occurred in a patient with ichthyosiform erythroderma [29], but other factors may have been relevant. Several studies involving liver biopsies have, however, indicated good tolerance of etretinate without significant hepatotoxic side-effects [30–32]; in one study, patients were followed for 3 years [32]. Etretinate, like isotretinoin, can cause increase in triglycerides and cholesterol [33–36] but to a lesser extent [36]. There have been isolated reports of possible etretinate-related thrombocytopenia [37]. Retinal toxicity has been postulated [38], although a recent report has not confirmed this [39]. Erectile dysfunction has been documented occasionally [40].

Skeletal abnormalities, such as periosteal thickening, vertebral hyperostosis, disk degeneration, osteoporosis and calcification of spinal ligaments, occur in a significant number of adults receiving long-term therapy for disorders of keratinization, but the severity of the changes is minor [41,42]. Radiological evidence of thinning of long bones may be seen in children [43], and premature epiphyseal closure has been recorded [44].

Etretinate is, like isotretinoin, grossly teratogenic, and because of its deposition in body fat stores it is excreted only very slowly, especially in the obese [45]. Detectable serum levels have been found in some patients more than 2 years following discontinuation of therapy. It is therefore recommended that female patients of child-bearing years should be advised to prevent pregnancy not only during the course of treatment, but also for at least 2 years after stopping therapy; if pregnancy is contemplated after this period of time, estimation of circulating levels of retinoid metabolites should be obtained.

REFERENCES

1 Foged E, Jacobsen F. Side-effects due to Ro 10-3959 (Tigason). *Dermatologica* 1982; **164**: 395–403.
2 Ellis CN, Voorhees JJ. Etretinate therapy. *J Am Acad Dermatol* 1987; **16**: 267–91.
3 Halioua B, Saurat J-H. Risk: benefit ratio in the treatment of psoriasis with systemic retinoids. *Br J Dermatol* 1990; **122** (Suppl. 36): 135–50.
4 Collins MRL, James WD, Rodman OG. Etretinate photosensitivity. *J Am Acad Dermatol* 1986; **14**: 274.
5 McDonagh AJG, Harrington CI. Pseudoporphyria complicating etretinate therapy. *Clin Exp Dermatol* 1989; **14**: 437–8.
6 Taieb A, Maleville J. Retinoid dermatitis mimicking 'eczéma craquelé'. *Acta Derm Venereol (Stockh)* 1985; **65**: 570.
7 Pennys NS, Hernandez D. A sticky problem with etretinate. *N Engl J Med* 1991; **325**: 521.
8 Higgins EM, Pembroke AC. Sticky palms—an unusual side-effect of etretinate therapy. *Clin Exp Dermatol* 1993; **18**: 389–90.
9 Berth-Jones J, Shuttleworth D, Hutchinson PE. A study of etretinate alopecia. *Br J Dermatol* 1990; **122**: 751–5.
10 Vesper JL, Fenske A. Hair darkening and new growth associated with etretinate therapy. *J Am Acad Dermatol* 1996; **34**: 860.
11 Shelley ED, Shelley WB. Inframammary, intertriginous, and decubital erosion due to etretinate. *Cutis* 1991; **47**: 111–13.
12 Allan S, Christmas T. Severe edema associated with etretinate. *J Am Acad Dermatol* 1988; **19**: 140.
13 Hodak E, David M, Feuerman EJ. Excess granulation tissue during etretinate therapy. *J Am Acad Dermatol* 1984; **11**: 1166–7.
14 Williamson DM, Creenwood R. Multiple pyogenic granulomata occurring during etretinate therapy. *Br J Dermatol* 1983; **109**: 615–17.
15 Levin J, Almeyda J. Erythroderma due to etretinate. *Br J Dermatol* 1985; **112**: 373.
16 Williams ML, Elias PM. Nature of skin fragility in patients receiving retinoids for systemic effect. *Arch Dermatol* 1981; **117**: 611–19.
17 Neild VS, Moss RF, Marsden RA *et al.* Retinoid-induced skin fragility in a patient with hepatic disease. *Clin Exp Dermatol* 1985; **10**: 459–65.

18 Ramsay B, Bloxham C, Eldred A *et al*. Blistering, erosions and scarring in a patient on etretinate. *Br J Dermatol* 1989; **121**: 397–400.

19 Lindskov R. Soft nails after treatment with aromatic retinoids. *Arch Dermatol* 1982; **118**: 535–6.

20 Baran R. Action thérapeutique et complications du rétinoïde aromatique sur l'appareil unguéal. *Ann Dermatol Vénéréol* 1982; **109**: 367–71.

21 Baran R. Etretinate and the nails (study of 130 cases): possible mechanisms of some side-effects. *Clin Exp Dermatol* 1986; **11**: 148–52.

22 Carmichael AJ, Tan CY. Digitate keratoses—a complication of etretinate used in the treatment of disseminated superficial actinic porokeratosis. *Clin Exp Dermatol* 1990; **15**: 370–1.

23 Miyagawa S, Muramatsu T, Shirai T. Generalization of palmoplantar pustulosis after withdrawal of etretinate. *J Am Acad Dermatol* 1991; **24**: 305–6.

24 Viraben R, Mathieu C. Benign intracranial hypertension during etretinate therapy for mycosis fungoides. *J Am Acad Dermatol* 1985; **13**: 515–17.

25 Schmidt H, Foged E. Some hepatotoxic side effects observed in patients treated with aromatic retinoid (Ro 10-9359). In: Orfanos CE, Braun-Falco O, Farber EM *et al*., eds. *Retinoids. Advances in Basic Research and Therapy*. Berlin: Springer-Verlag, 1981: 359–62.

26 Van Voorst Vader P, Houthoff H, Eggink H, Gips C. Etretinate (Tigason) hepatitis in two patients. *Dermatologica* 1984; **168**: 41–6.

27 Kano Y, Fukuda M, Shiohara T, Nagashima M. Cholestatic hepatitis occurring shortly after etretinate therapy. *J Am Acad Dermatol* 1994; **31**: 133–4.

28 Sanchez MR, Ross B, Rotterdam H *et al*. Retinoid hepatitis. *J Am Acad Dermatol* 1993; **28**: 853–8.

29 Thune P, Mørk NJ. A case of centrolobular necrosis of the liver due to aromatic retinoid—Tigason (Ro-10-9359). *Dermatologica* 1980; **160**: 405–8.

30 Foged E, Bjerring P, Kragballe K *et al*. Histologic changes in the liver during etretinate treatment. *J Am Acad Dermatol* 1984; **11**: 580–3.

31 Zachariae H, Foged E, Bjerring P *et al*. Liver biopsy during etretinate (Tigason®) treatment. In: Saurat JH, ed. *Retinoids: New Trends in Research and Therapy*. Basel: Karger, 1985: 494–7.

32 Roenigk HH, Jr. Retinoids: effect on the liver. In: Saurat JH, ed. *Retinoids: New Trends in Research and Therapy*. Basel: Karger, 1985: 476–88.

33 Ellis CN, Swanson NA, Grekin RC *et al*. Etretinate therapy causes increases in lipid levels in patients with psoriasis. *Arch Dermatol* 1982; **118**: 559–62.

34 Michaëlsson G, Bergquist A, Vahlquist A, Vessby B. The influence of Tigason (R 10-9359) on the serum lipoproteins in man. *Br J Dermatol* 1981; **105**: 201–5.

35 Vahlquist C, Michaëlsson G, Vahlquist A, Vessby B. A sequential comparison of etretinate (Tigason) and isotretinoin (Roaccutane) with special regard to their effects on serum lipoproteins. *Br J Dermatol* 1985; **112**: 69–76.

36 Marsden J. Hyperlipidaemia due to isotretinoin and etretinate: possible mechanisms and consequences. *Br J Dermatol* 1986; **114**: 401–7.

37 Naldi L, Rozzoni M, Finazzi G *et al*. Etretinate therapy and thrombocytopenia. *Br J Dermatol* 1991; **124**: 395.

38 Weber U, Melink B, Goerz G, Michaelis L. Abnormal retinal function associated with long-term etretinate? *Lancet* 1988; **i**: 235–6.

39 Pitts JF, MacKie RM, Dutton GN *et al*. Etretinate and visual function: a 1-year follow-up study. *Br J Dermatol* 1991; **125**: 53–5.

40 Reynolds OD. Erectile dysfunction in etretinate treatment. *Arch Dermatol* 1991; **127**: 425–6.

41 DiGiovanna JJ, Gerber LH, Helfgott RK *et al*. Extraspinal tendon and ligament calcification associated with long-term therapy with etretinate. *N Engl J Med* 1986; **315**: 1177–82.

42 Halkier-Sørensen L, Andresen J. A retrospective study of bone changes in adults treated with etretinate. *J Am Acad Dermatol* 1989; **20**: 83–7.

43 Halkier-Sørensen L, Laurberg G, Andresen J. Bone changes in children on long-term treatment with etretinate. *J Am Acad Dermatol* 1987; **16**: 999–1006.

44 Prendiville J, Bingham EA, Burrows D. Premature epiphyseal closure—a complication of etretinate therapy in children. *J Am Acad Dermatol* 1986; **15**: 1259–62.

45 DiGiovanna JJ, Zech LA, Ruddel ME *et al*. Etretinate: persistent serum levels after long-term therapy. *Arch Dermatol* 1989; **125**: 246–51.

Isotretinoin (13-cis-retinoic acid)

Dermatological complications have been reviewed [1,2]; erythema and scaling of the face, generalized xerosis, skin fragility, pruritus, epistaxis, dry nose and dry mouth may be seen in up to 80% of cystic acne patients. A dose-related cheilitis occurs in over 90%, while conjunctivitis occurs in about 40% of patients. Transient exacerbation of acne may occur, especially in the early stages of therapy. Exuberant granulation tissue, or pyogenic granuloma at the site of healing acne lesions, has been reported frequently [3–7].

Rashes, including erythema, and thinning of the hair (in rare cases persistent) occur in fewer than 10% of patients. Both isotretinoin and etretinate may cause curliness or kinking of hair [8]. The following have occurred in approximately 5% of cases: peeling of the palms and soles, skin infections and possible increased susceptibility to sunburn. Phototesting confirmed photosensitivity in some patients in one [9] but not another [10] study. A photo-aggravated allergic reaction has been documented in which the patient had positive patch tests to isotretinoin [11]. Reversible melasma is recorded [12], as is facial cellulitis [13]. Scarring, which may be keloidal, may occur following dermabrasion or laser therapy within a year of isotretinoin therapy; such procedures are best postponed during this period [14–16].

Systemic side-effects of isotretinoin include headache, which is not uncommon, and anorexia, nausea and vomiting are much more common than with etretinate, as are lethargy and fatigue [17]. Isotretinoin therapy has been associated with benign intracranial hypertension [18]; in some cases, there was concomitant use of tetracyclines, so this combination should be avoided. A variety of central nervous system reactions have been reported, but may bear no relationship to therapy. Depression with recurrence following rechallenge has been recorded [19]. Patients treated for disorders of keratinization have developed corneal opacities, which improved when the drug was withdrawn [20]. Blepharoconjunctivitis, dry eyes with decreased tolerance of contact lenses and blurred vision due to myopia may occur [5]. Decreased night vision has been documented rarely, as have cataracts and other visual disturbances [21–25]; decreased night vision after isotretinoin therapy may be more permanent than generally suspected [25], and many asymptomatic patients have abnormal electroretinograms [22]. Loss of sense of taste is recorded [26].

Transient chest pain is uncommon. Non-specific urogenital findings and non-specific gastrointestinal symptoms have occurred in approximately 5% of cases. Isotretinoin therapy has been associated with onset of inflammatory bowel disease [27] and with impairment of pulmonary function in patients with systemic sclerosis [28,29].

Approximately 16% of patients develop musculoskeletal symptoms, including arthralgia, of mild to moderate degree; cases of acute knee aseptic arthritis have been documented [30]. High-dose prolonged therapy in a child for epidermolytic hyperkeratosis was associated with premature closure of epiphyses [31]. A high prevalence of skeletal hyperostosis has been noted in patients on prolonged (1 year or more), relatively high-dose (2 mg/kg/day) isotretinoin therapy for disorders of keratinization [32–36]. The syndrome of *diffuse idiopathic interstitial hyperostosis* (DISH) includes ossification of ligaments and accretion of bone onto vertebral bodies, especially of the cervical spine. Mild osteoporosis has also been seen. X-ray changes have been minimal in prospective studies of patients with cystic acne treated with a single course of isotretinoin at recommended doses [37–39]. Nasal bone osteophytosis has been described with short-term therapy for acne [40].

Mild to moderate elevation of liver enzymes occurs in about 15% of cases; in some patients these return to normal despite continued administration of the drug. A single report of fatty liver developing in a patient, with low to normal levels of α_1-antitrypsin, on low-dose isotretinoin has been reported [41]. Elevated sedimentation rates occur in about 40% of patients. Between 10 and 20% of patients show decreased red-blood-cell parameters and white-blood-cell counts, elevated platelet counts and pyuria. There has been a single report of thrombocytopenia [42].

Isotretinoin induces reversible changes in serum lipids in a significant number of treated subjects [43–48]. A dose-related increase in triglycerides occurs in about 25% of individuals according to the Roche data sheet. Five of 135 cystic acne patients, and 32 of 298 patients treated for all diagnoses, showed triglyceride levels above 500 mg%. In another study, 17% of patients taking isotretinoin for 20 weeks exhibited hypertriglyceridaemia, but in 15% this was of only mild to moderate degree [46]. About 15% showed a mild to moderate decrease in serum high-density lipoprotein levels, and 7% experienced minimal elevations of serum cholesterol during therapy; some patients had increases in low-density lipoprotein cholesterol [46]. Lipid abnormalities peaked within 4 weeks in men, but not until 12 weeks in women. If sustained over a long period, these alterations in lipoproteins might be risk factors for coronary artery disease. Patients with an increased tendency to develop hypertriglyceridaemia include those with diabetes mellitus, obesity, increased alcohol intake or a familial history. Some patients have been able to reverse triglyceride elevation by reduction in weight, restriction of dietary fat and alcohol, and reduction in dose while continuing the drug. An obese male patient with Darier's disease developed elevated triglycerides and subsequent eruptive xanthomas [49].

Major human fetal abnormalities related to isotretinoin therapy during pregnancy have been documented [50–53]. The most frequently reported abnormalities involve the central nervous system (microcephaly or hydrocephalus and cerebellar malformation) and cardiovascular system (anomalies of the great vessels). Microtia or absence of external ears, microphthalmia, facial dysmorphia and

thymus gland abnormalities have also been reported. There is an increased risk of spontaneous abortion. Women of child-bearing potential should sign a consent form and be instructed that they should not be pregnant when Roaccutane therapy is started (preferably on the second or third day of the next normal menstrual period), and should use effective contraception during, and for 1 month after stopping, therapy. Roaccutane has a much shorter half-life than etretinate, so that pregnancy is permissible 1 month after stopping therapy. Analysis of data voluntarily reported to Hoffmann–La Roche Inc in the USA enabled prospective study of 88 patients who had completed or discontinued isotretinoin therapy prior to becoming pregnant: 90% of all pregnancies occurred within 2 months after cessation of therapy, and 64% within 1 month [54]. There were no significant increases in the rates of spontaneous abortion or of congenital malformations among the live births. There appears to be no adverse effect of isotretinoin on male reproductive function [55,56].

REFERENCES

1 Yob EH, Pochi PE. Side effects and long-term toxicity of synthetic retinoids. *Arch Dermatol* 1987; **123**: 1375–8.
2 Bigby M, Stern RS. Adverse reactions to isotretinoin. A report from the Adverse Drug Reaction Reporting System. *J Am Acad Dermatol* 1988; **18**: 543–52.
3 Campbell JP, Grekin RC, Ellis CN *et al.* Retinoid therapy is associated with excess granulation tissue responses. *J Am Acad Dermatol* 1983; **9**: 708–13.
4 Exner JH, Dahod S, Pochi PE. Pyogenic granuloma-like acne lesions during isotretinoin therapy. *Arch Dermatol* 1983; **119**: 808–11.
5 Valentic JP, Barr RJ, Weinstein GD. Inflammatory neovascular nodules associated with oral isotretinoin treatment of severe acne. *Arch Dermatol* 1983; **119**: 871–2.
6 Stary A. Acne conglobata: Ungewöhnlicher Verlauf unter 13-*cis*-Retinsäuretherapie. *Hautarzt* 1986; **37**: 28–30.
7 Blanc D, Zultak M, Wendling P, Lonchampt F. Eruptive pyogenic granulomas and acne fulminans in two siblings treated with isotretinoin. A possible common pathogenesis. *Dermatologica* 1988; **177**: 16–18.
8 Bunker CB, Maurice PDL, Dowd PM. Isotretinoin and curly hair. *Clin Exp Dermatol* 1990; **15**: 143–5.
9 Ferguson J, Johnson BE. Photosensitivity due to retinoids: clinical and laboratory studies. *Br J Dermatol* 1986; **115**: 275–83.
10 Wong RC, Gilber M, Woo TY *et al.* Photosensitivity and isotretinoin therapy. *J Am Acad Dermatol* 1986; **15**: 1095–6.
11 Auffret N, Bruley C, Brunetiere RA *et al.* Photoaggravated allergic reaction to isotretinoin. *J Am Acad Dermatol* 1990; **23**: 321–2.
12 Burke H, Carmichael AJ. Reversible melasma associated with isotretinoin. *Br J Dermatol* 1996; **135**: 862.
13 Boffa MJ, Dave VK. Facial cellulitis during oral isotretinoin treatment for acne. *J Am Acad Dermatol* 1994; **31**: 800–2.
14 Rubenstein R, Roenigk HH, Jr, Stegman SJ *et al.* Atypical keloids after dermabrasion of patients taking isotretinoin. *J Am Acad Dermatol* 1986; **15**: 280–5.
15 Zachariae H. Delayed wound healing and keloid formation following argon laser treatment or dermabrasion during isotretinoin treatment. *Br J Dermatol* 1988; **118**: 703–6.
16 Katz BE, MacFarlane DF. Atypical facial scarring after isotretinoin therapy in a patient with previous dermabrasion. *J Am Acad Dermatol* 1994; **30**: 852–3.
17 Windhorst DB, Nigra T. General clinical toxicology of oral retinoids. *J Am Acad Dermatol* 1982; **4**: 675–82.
18 Anon. Adverse effects with isotretinoin. *J Am Acad Dermatol* 1984; **10**: 519–20.
19 Scheiman PL, Peck GL, Rubinow DR *et al.* Acute depression from isotretinoin. *J Am Acad Dermatol* 1990; **23**: 1112–14.

20 Cunningham WJ. Use of isotretinoin in the ichthyoses. In: Cunliffe WJ, Miller AJ, eds. *Retinoid Therapy. A Review of Clinical and Laboratory Research.* Lancaster: MTP Press, 1984: 321–5.

21 Fraunfelder FT, La Braico JM, Meyer SM. Adverse ocular reactions possibly associated with isotretinoin. *Am J Ophthalmol* 1985; **100**: 534–7.

22 Brown RD, Grattan CEH. Visual toxicity of synthetic retinoids. *Br J Ophthalmol* 1989; **73**: 286–8.

23 Gold JA, Shupack JL, Nemec MA. Ocular side effects of the retinoids. *Int J Dermatol* 1989; **28**: 218–25.

24 Denman ST, Welebar RG, Hanifin JM *et al.* Abnormal night vision and altered dark adaptometry in patients treated with isotretinoin for acne. *J Am Acad Dermatol* 1986; **14**: 692–3.

25 Maclean H, Wright M, Choie D, Tidman MJ. Abnormal night vision with isotretinoin therapy for acne. *Clin Exp Dermatol* 1995; **20**: 86.

26 Halpern SM, Todd PM, Kirby JD. Loss of taste associated with isotretinoin. *Br J Dermatol* 1996; **134**: 378.

27 Gold MH, Roenigk HH. The retinoids and inflammatory bowel disease. *Arch Dermatol* 1988; **124**: 325–6.

28 Bunker CB, Sheron N, Maurice PDL *et al.* Isotretinoin and eosinophilic pleural effusion. *Lancet* 1989; **i**: 435–6.

29 Bunker CB, Maurice PDL, Little S *et al.* Isotretinoin and lung function in systemic sclerosis. *Clin Exp Dermatol* 1991; **16**: 11–13.

30 Matsuoka LY, Wortsman J, Pepper JJ. Acute arthritis during isotretinoin treatment for acne. *Arch Intern Med* 1984; **144**: 1870–1.

31 Milstone LM, McGuire J, Ablow RC. Premature epiphyseal closure in a child receiving oral 13-*cis*-retinoic acid. *J Am Acad Dermatol* 1982; **7**: 663–6.

32 Pittsley R, Yoder K. Retinoid hyperostosis. Skeletal toxicity associated with long-term administration of 13 *cis*-retinoic acid for refractory ichthyosis. *N Engl J Med* 1983; **308**: 1012–14.

33 Ellis CN, Madison KC, Pennes DR *et al.* Isotretinoin is associated with early skeletal radiographic changes. *J Am Acad Dermatol* 1984; **10**: 1024–9.

34 Gerber L, Helfgott R, Gross E *et al.* Vertebral abnormalities associated with synthetic retinoid use. *J Am Acad Dermatol* 1984; **10**: 817–23.

35 Pennes D, Ellis C, Madison K *et al.* Early skeletal hyperostosis secondary to 13-*cis*-retinoic acid. *Am J Roentgenol* 1984; **142**: 979–83.

36 McGuire J, Milstone L, Lawson J. Isotretinoin administration alters juvenile and adult bone. In: Saurat JH, ed. *Retinoids: New Trends in Research and Therapy.* Basel: Karger, 1985: 419–39.

37 Ellis CN, Pennes DR, Madison KC *et al.* Skeletal radiographic changes during retinoid therapy. In: Saurat JH, ed. *Retinoids: New Trends in Research and Therapy,* Basel: Karger, 1985: 440–4.

38 Kilcoyne RF, Cope R, Cunningham W *et al.* Minimal spinal hyperostosis with low-dose isotretinoin therapy. *Invest Radiol* 1986; **21**: 41–4.

39 Carey BM, Parkin GJS, Cunliffe WJ, Pritlove J. Skeletal toxicity with isotretinoin therapy: a clinico-radiological evaluation. *Br J Dermatol* 1988; **119**: 609–14.

40 Novick NL, Lawson W, Schwartz IS. Bilateral nasal bone osteophytosis associated with short-term oral isotretinoin therapy for cystic acne vulgaris. *Am J Med* 1984; **77**: 736–9.

41 Taylor AEM, Mitchison H. Fatty liver following isotretinoin. *Br J Dermatol* 1991; **124**: 505–6.

42 Johnson TM, Rainin R. Isotretinoin-induced thrombocytopenia. *J Am Acad Dermatol* 1987; **17**: 838–9.

43 Nigra TP, Katz RA, Jorgensen H. Elevation of serum triglyceride levels from oral 13-*cis*-retinoic acid. In: Orfanos CE, Braun-Falco O, Farber EM *et al.*, eds. *Retinoids. Advances in Basic Research and Therapy.* Berlin: Springer-Verlag, 1981: 363–9.

44 Lyons F, Laker MF, Marsden JR *et al.* Effect of oral 13-*cis*-retinoic acid on serum lipids. *Br J Dermatol* 1982; **107**: 591–5.

45 Zech LA, Gross EG, Peck GL, Brewer HB. Changes in plasma cholesterol and triglyceride levels after treatment with oral isotretinoin. A prospective study. *Arch Dermatol* 1983; **119**: 987–93.

46 Bershad S, Rubinstein A, Paterniti JR, Jr *et al.* Changes in plasma lipids and lipoproteins during isotretinoin therapy for acne. *N Engl J Med* 1985; **313**: 981–5.

47 Gollnick H, Schwartzkopff W, Pröschle W *et al.* Retinoids and blood lipids: an update and review. In: Saurat JH, ed. *Retinoids: New Trends in Research and Therapy,* Basel: Karger, 1985, 445–60.

48 Marsden J. Hyperlipidaemia due to isotretinoin and etretinate: possible mechanisms and consequences. *Br J Dermatol* 1986; **114**: 401–7.

49 Dicken CH, Connolly SM. Eruptive xanthomas associated with isotretinoin (13-*cis*-retinoic acid). *Arch Dermatol* 1980; **16**: 951–2.

50 Hill RM. Isotretinoin teratogenicity. *Lancet* 1984; **i**: 1465.

51 Stern RS, Rosa F, Baum C. Isotretinoin and pregnancy. *J Am Acad Dermatol* 1984; **10**: 851–4.

52 Chen DT. Human pregnancy experience with the retinoids. In: Saurat JH, ed. *Retinoids: New Trends in Research and Therapy.* Basel: Karger, 1985: 398–406.

53 Rosa FW, Wilk AL, Kelsey FO. Teratogen update: vitamin A cogeners, the outcome of pregnancies in patients who had taken isotretinoin. *Teratology* 1986; **33**: 355–64.

54 Dai WS, Hsu M-A, Itri L. Safety of pregnancy after discontinuation of isotretinoin. *Arch Dermatol* 1989; **125**: 362–5.

55 Schill W-B, Wagner A, Nikolowski J, Plewig G. Aromatic retinoid and 13-*cis*-retinoic acid: spermatological investigations. In: Orfanos CE, Braun-Falco O, Farber EM *et al.*, eds. *Retinoids. Advances in Basic Research and Therapy.* Berlin: Springer-Verlag, 1981: 389–95.

56 Töröck L, Kása M. Spermatological and endocrinological examinations connected with isotretinoin treatment. In: Saurat JH, ed. *Retinoids: New Trends in Research and Therapy.* Basel: Karger, 1985: 407–10.

Tretinoin

Oral tretinoin administered as differentiation therapy of acute promyelocytic leukaemia was associated with mild skin rashes, the nature of which was unspecified [1]. An acute neutrophilic dermatosis with a myeloblastic infiltrate occurred in a leukemia patient receiving all-*trans*-retinoic acid therapy [2].

REFERENCES

1 Warrell RP, Frankel SR, Miller WH *et al.* Differentiation therapy of acute promyelocytic leukemia with tretinin (all-trans-retinoic acid). *N Engl J Med* 1991; **324**: 1385–93.

2 Piette WW, Trapp JF, O'Donnell MJ *et al.* Acute neutrophilic dermatosis with myeloblastic infiltrate in a leukemia patient receiving all-*trans*-retinoic acid therapy. *J Am Acad Dermatol* 1994; **30**: 293–7.

Vitamin B

Vitamin B_1

Anaphylaxis following intravenous administration has occurred [1].

Vitamin B_6 (pyridoxine)

Vasculitis is recorded [2], as is a pseudoporphyria syndrome with megadosage [3].

Nicotinic acid

Flushing is common; other transient rashes, urticaria, pruritus, scaling, hyperpigmentation and an acanthosis nigricans-like eruption [4,5] are all documented. Persistent rashes and hair loss have rarely occurred.

REFERENCES

1 Kolz R, Lonsdorf G, Burg G. Unverträglichkeitsreaktionen nach parenteraler Gabe von Vitamin B₁. *Hautarzt* 1980; **31**: 657–9.

2 Ruzicka T, Ring J, Braun-Falco O. Vasculitis allergica durch Vitamin B₆. *Hautarzt* 1984; **35**: 197–9.

3 Baer R, Stilman MA. Cutaneous skin changes probably due to pyridoxine abuse. *J Am Acad Dermatol* 1984; **10**: 527–8.
4 Tromovitch TA, Jacobs PH, Kern S. Acanthosis nigricans-like lesions from nicotinic acid. *Arch Dermatol* 1964; **89**: 222–3.
5 Elgart ML. Acanthosis nigricans and nicotinic acid. *J Am Acad Dermatol* 1981; **5**: 709–10.

Vitamin C (ascorbic acid)

Patients with cutaneous and respiratory allergy have been described.

Vitamin E (α-tocopherol)

White hair developed at injection sites in infants given intramuscular vitamin E for epidermolysis bullosa, probably due to quinones formed during vitamin E degradation [1].

REFERENCE

1 Sehgal VN. Vitamin E—a melanotoxic agent. A preliminary report. *Dermatologica* 1972; **145**: 56–9.

Vitamin K

Skin reactions with vitamin K have been reviewed [1–9]. Eruption may occur after a single intramuscular injection of 10 mg of vitamin K_1. The pruritic erythematous macular lesions or plaques, localized to the site of injection, appear 4–16 days later, and may last for up to 6 months [1–9]. Patch and intradermal skin tests may be positive, suggesting an immunological basis. Most, but not all [3,6,8], cases have occurred in patients with liver disease. In addition, a proportion of these reactions progress to produce scleroderma-like changes [9–14]. An annular erythema has been documented [15].

REFERENCES

1 Barnes HM, Sarkany I. Adverse skin reactions from vitamin K_1. *Br J Dermatol* 1976; **95**: 653–6.
2 Bullen AW, Miller JP, Cunliffe WJ, Losowsky MS. Skin reactions caused by vitamin K in patients with liver disease. *Br J Dermatol* 1978; **98**: 561–5.
3 Sanders MN, Winkelmann RK. Cutaneous reactions to vitamin K. *J Am Acad Dermatol* 1988; **19**: 699–704.
4 Mosser C, Janin-Mercier A, Souteyrand P. Les réactions cutanées apres administration parentérale de vitamine K. *Ann Dermatol Vénéréol* 1987; **114**: 243–51.
5 Finkelstein H, Champion MC, Adam JE. Cutaneous hypersensitivity to vitamin K_1 injection. *J Am Acad Dermatol* 1987; **16**: 540–5.
6 Joyce JP, Hood AF, Weiss MM. Persistent cutaneous reaction to intramuscular vitamin K injection. *Arch Dermatol* 1988; **124**: 27–8.
7 Tuppal R, Tremaine R. Cutaneous eruption from vitamin K_1 injection. *J Am Acad Dermatol* 1992; **27**: 105–6.
8 Lee MM, Gellis S, Dover JS. Eczematous plaques in a patient with liver failure. Fat-soluble vitamin K hypersensitivity. *Arch Dermatol* 1992; **128**: 257, 260.
9 Lemlich G, Green M, Phelps R *et al.* Cutaneous reactions to vitamin K_1 injections. *J Am Acad Dermatol* 1993; **28**: 345–7.
10 Texier L, Gendre PH, Gauthier O *et al.* Hypodermites sclérodermiformes lombo-fessières induites par des injections médicamenteuses intramusculaires associées a la vitamine K_1. *Ann Dermatol Syphiligr* 1972; **99**: 363–71.
11 Janin-Mercier A, Mosser C, Souteyrand P, Bourges M. Subcutaneous sclerosis with fasciitis and eosinophilia after phytonadione injections. *Arch Dermatol* 1985; **121**: 1421–3.
12 Brunskill NJ, Berth-Jones J, Graham-Brown RAC. Pseudosclerodermatous reaction to phytomenadione injection (Texier's syndrome). *Clin Exp Dermatol* 1988; **13**: 276–8.
13 Pujol RM, Puig L, Moreno A *et al.* Pseudoscleroderma secondary to phytonadione (vitamin K1) injections. *Cutis* 1989; **43**: 365–8.
14 Guidetti MS, Vincenzi C, Papi M, Tosti A. Sclerodermatous skin reaction after vitamin K1 injections. *Contact Dermatitis* 1994; **31**: 45–6.
15 Kay MH, Duvic M. Reactive annular erythema after intramuscular vitamin K. *Cutis* 1986; **37**: 445–8.

Hormones and related compounds

ACTH and systemic corticosteroids

The side-effects of these agents have been reviewed [1–13]. Well-known side-effects include acne, cutaneous thinning and atrophy, telangiectasia, striae distensae, purpura and ecchymoses, hypertrichosis, impaired wound healing, pigmentary changes, Cushingoid (moon) facies, truncal adiposity [14] and buffalo hump of the upper back. Other systemic side-effects include fluid and electrolyte abnormalities, weight gain, oedema, hypertension, cardiac failure, peptic ulcer disease, pancreatitis, diabetes, muscular weakness, myopathy, tendon rupture, glaucoma, posterior subcapsular cataracts, mental changes including psychosis, osteoporosis, vertebral collapse, necrosis of the femoral head, growth suppression in children, opportunistic infection, masking of infection or reactivation of a dormant infection (e.g. tuberculosis), polycythaemia and suppression of the hypothalamic–pituitary axis. Pulse steroid therapy with systemic methylprednisolone has resulted in sudden death due to anaphylaxis, arrhythmia, or ischaemic heart disease, but not particularly in dermatological patients [15].

Adrenocorticotrophic hormone

Allergic reactions to ACTH are recorded but are uncommon. Urticaria and dizziness, nausea and weakness are the most frequent, but severe anaphylactic shock has occurred. Synthetic ACTH is usually tolerated by patients sensitive to animal ACTH [16]. Depot preparations (tetracosactrin adsorbed on a zinc phosphate complex) have produced reactions [17,18] and may induce melanoderma [18].

REFERENCES

1 Lucky AW. Principles of the use of glucocorticosteroids in the growing child. *Pediatr Dermatol* 1984; **1**: 226–35.
2 Fritz KA, Weston WL. Systemic glucocorticosteroid therapy of skin disease in children. *Pediatr Dermatol* 1984; **1**: 236–45.
3 Davis GF. Adverse effects of corticosteroids: II. Systemic. *Clin Dermatol* 1986; **4**: 161–9.
4 Gallant C, Kenny P. Oral glucocorticoids and their complications. A review. *J Am Acad Dermatol* 1986; **14**: 161–77.
5 Seale PS, Compton MR. Side-effects of corticosteroid agents. *Med J Aust* 1986; **144**: 139–42.

6 Chosidow O, Étienne SD, Herson S, Puech AJ. Pharmacologie des corticoides. Notions classiques et nouvelles. *Ann Dermatol Vénéréol* 1989; **116**: 147–66.
7 Fine R. Glucocorticoids (1989). *Int J Dermatol* 1990; **29**: 377–9.
8 Kyle V, Hazleman BL. Treatment of polymyalgia rheumatica and giant cell arteritis: II. Relation between steroid dose and steroid associated side effects. *Ann Rheum Dis* 1989; **48**: 662–6.
9 Truhan AP, Ahmed AR. Corticosteroids: a review with emphasis on complications of prolonged systemic therapy. *Ann Allergy* 1989; **62**: 375–90.
10 Weiss MM. Corticosteroids in rheumatoid arthritis. *Semin Arthritis Rheum* 1989; **19**: 9–21.
11 Rasanen L, Hasan T. Allergy to systemic and intralesional corticosteroids. *Br J Dermatol* 1993; **128**: 407–11.
12 Dooms-Goossens A. Sensitisation to corticosteroids. Consequences for anti-inflammatory therapy. *Drug Saf* 1995; **13**: 123–9.
13 Imam AP, Halpern GM. Uses, adverse effects of abuse of corticosteroids. Part II. *Allergol Immunopathol* 1995; **23**: 2–15.
14 Horber HH, Xurcher RM, Herren H *et al.* Altered body fat distribution in patients with glucocorticoid treatment and in patients on long-term dialysis. *Am J Clin Nutr* 1986; **43**: 758–69.
15 White KP, Driscoll MS, Rothe MJ, Grant-Kels JM. Severe adverse cadiovascular effects of pulse steroid therapy: is continuous cardiac monitoring necessary? *J Am Acad Dermatol* 1994; **30**: 768–73.
16 Patriarca G. Allergy to tetracosactrin-depot. *Lancet* 1971; **i**: 138.
17 Clee MD, Ferguson J, Browning MCK *et al.* Glucocorticoid hypersensitivity in an asthmatic patient: presentation and treatment. *Thorax* 1985; **40**: 477–8.
18 Khan SA. Melanoderma caused by depot tetracosactrin. *Trans St John's Hosp Dermatol Soc* 1970; **56**: 168–71.

Systemic corticosteroids

Cutaneous side-effects of systemic corticosteroids include allergic and immediate reactions [1,2]. In one study, seven of 25 patients with cutaneous delayed-type hypersensitivity to hydrocortisone had an immediate reaction following intradermal injection of hydrocortisone sodium succinate, and had significantly increased levels of IgG antibodies to hydrocortisone. These patients are at risk of developing type III and possibly type I reactions following systemic hydrocortisone [3].

Protein binding of hydrocortisone or a degradation product may be important in the development of corticosteroid allergy [4]. Urticarial reactions have followed the intra-arterial injection of prednisone, prednisolone or hydrocortisone [5], but are rare. Anaphylactoid reactions have been reported to topical and parenteral hydrocortisone, but may represent pseudoallergic reactions rather than IgE-mediated immediate hypersensitivity [6,7].

Generalized skin reactions, including urticaria and maculopapular eruptions, developed in patients after therapy respectively with oral triamcinolone acetonide [8], prednisone [9], or dexamethasone and betamethasone [10]; the patients were subsequently shown to be patch-test positive to these corticosteroids. In another study, five patients reacted with diffuse erythema principally on the trunk or on the face, within a few hours to 24 h, and fading in 1–3 days, with systemic or intralesional hydrocortisone, methylprednisolone, prednisolone or betamethasone [2]. One patient reacted to prednisolone and methylprednisolone, and two patients were positive to pivalone, on patch testing. Patients sensitive to hydrocortisone or methylprednisolone reacted to these corticosteroids in

intradermal tests. A combination of intradermal and patch tests is recommended when allergy to systemic or intralesional corticosteroids is suspected [2].

Other cases of generalized delayed systemic corticosteroid reactions, including eczematous or exanthematous eruptions and erythroderma, with or without bullae or purpura, often with positive patch or intradermal testing, have been recorded [11–15]. Systemic administration of hydrocortisone, and provocation of endogenous cortisol secretion by means of injection of the ACTH analogue tetracosactide, provoked dose-dependent allergic skin reactions at sites of previous allergic reactions to topical steroids in two patients with proven topical corticosteroid sensitivity (i.e. systemic allergic contact type dermatitis); in one case, this was at a positive patch-test site to hydrocortisone-17-butyrate [16]. Thus, it has been postulated that high stress levels, which cause increased secretion of endogenous adrenal cortical hormones, could be implicated in exacerbations of eczema in corticosteroid-sensitive patients, and a persistent autoimmune skin reaction to cortisol might occur following topical sensitization to topical hydrocortisone [16]. The fact that systemic provocation testing with hydrocortisone results in a reaction confined to the skin, in steroid-sensitive patients, may be partly explained by the observation *in vitro* that only enriched Langerhans' cells, and not peripheral blood mononuclear antigen-presenting cells, are capable of presenting corticosteroid to T cells of corticosteroid-sensitive subjects [17].

Perioral dermatitis has been recorded in renal transplant recipients on corticosteroids and immunosuppressive therapy [18]. Panniculitis following short-term high dose steroid therapy in children manifests as subcutaneous nodules on the cheeks, arms and trunk [19]. Reversible panniculitis occurred in a child treated with steroids for hepatic encephalopathy [20]. Juxta-articular adiposis dolorosa developed in a patient treated with high doses of prednisone for the L-tryptophan-induced eosinophilia myalgia syndrome [21]. Acanthosis nigricans may occur with corticosteroid therapy [22]. Immunosuppression with corticosteroids has been associated with the development of Kaposi's sarcoma during the treatment of temporal arteritis [23].

Inhaled corticosteroids have been associated with purpura and dermal thinning [24] as well as acne [25], allergic reactions [26] and an eczematous dermatitis [27]. Intralesional corticosteroid injection may also lead to allergic reactions [28], including a disseminated morbilliform and persistent urticarial dermatitis following intra-articular triamcinolone acetonide [29], erythroderma following intradermal budesonide [30] and erythema multiforme after intradural injection of prednisolone acetate [31]. Facial flushing and/or generalized erythema has followed epidural steroid injection [32]. Anaphylactic shock has been recorded after intra-articular injections of corticosteroids, containing carboxymethylcellulose, benzylic acid, polysorbate 80 and merthiolate; skin tests to carboxymethylcellulose were positive [33].

REFERENCES

1 Preuss L. Allergic reactions to systemic glucocorticoids: a review. *Ann Allergy* 1985; **55**: 772–5.
2 Rasanen L, Hasan T. Allergy to systemic and intralesional corticosteroids. *Br J Dermatol* 1993; **128**: 407–11.
3 Wilkinson SM, Mattey DL, Beck MH. IgG antibodies and early intradermal reactions to hydrocortisone in patients with cutaneous delayed-type hypersensitivity to hydrocortisone. *Br J Dermatol* 1994; **131**: 495–8.
4 Wilkinson SM, English JS, Mattey DL. *In vitro* evidence of delayed-type hypersensitivity to hydrocortisone. *Contact Dermatitis* 1993; **29**: 241–5.
5 Ashford RF, Bailey A. Angioneurotic oedema and urticaria following hydrocortisone—a further case. *Postgrad Med J* 1980; **56**: 437.
6 King RA. A severe anaphylactoid reaction to hydrocortisone. *Lancet* 1960; **ii**: 1093–4.
7 Peller JS, Bardana EL, Jr. Anaphylactoid reaction to corticosteroid: Case report and review of the literature. *Ann Allergy* 1985; **54**: 302–5.
8 Brambilla L, Boneschi V, Chiappino G *et al.* Allergic reactions to topical desoxymethasone and oral triamcinolone. *Contact Dermatitis* 1989; **21**: 272–3
9 De Corres LF, Bernaola G, Urrutia I *et al.* Allergic dermatitis from systemic treatment with corticosteroids. *Contact Dermatitis* 1990; **22**: 104–5.
10 Maucher O, Faber M, Knipper H *et al.* Kortikoidallergie. *Hautarzt* 1987; **38**: 577–82.
11 Whitmore SE. Delayed systemic allergic reactions to corticosteroids. *Contact Dermatitis* 1995; **32**: 193–8.
12 Torres V, Tavares-Bello R, Melo H, Soares AP. Systemic contact dermatitis from hydrocortisone. *Contact Dermatitis* 1993; **29**: 106.
13 Vidal C, Tome S, Fernandex-Redondo V, Tato F. Systemic allergic reaction to corticosteroids. *Contact Dermatitis* 1994; **31**: 273–4.
14 Whitmore SE. Dexamethasone injection-induced generalised dermatitis. *Br J Dermatol* 1994; **131**: 296–7.
15 Fernandez de Corres L, Urrutia I, Audicana M *et al.* Erythroderma after intravenous injection of methylprednisolone. *Contact Dermatitis* 1991; **25**: 68–70.
16 Lauerma AI, Reitamo S, Maibach HI. Systemic hydrocortisone/cortisol induces allergic skin reactions in presensitized subjects. *J Am Acad Dermatol* 1991; **24**: 182–5.
17 Lauerma AI, Räsänen L, Reunala T, Reitamo S. Langerhans cells but not monocytes are capable of antigen presentation *in vitro* in corticosteroid contact hypersensitivity. *Br J Dermatol* 1991; **123**: 699–705.
18 Adams SJ, Davison AM, Cunliffe WJ, Giles GR. Perioral dermatitis in renal transplant recipients maintained on corticosteroids and immunosuppressive therapy. *Br J Dermatol* 1982; **106**: 589–92.
19 Roenigk HH, Haserick JR, Arundell FD. Poststeroid panniculitis. *Arch Dermatol* 1964; **90**: 387–91.
20 Saxena AK, Nigam PK. Panniculitis following steroid therapy. *Cutis* 1988; **42**: 341–2.
21 Greenbaum SS, Varga J. Corticosteroid-induced juxta-articular adiposis dolorosa. *Arch Dermatol* 1991; **127**: 231–3.
22 Brown J, Winkelmann RK. Acanthosis nigricans: a study of 90 cases. *Medicine* 1968; **47**: 33–51.
23 Leung F, Fam AG, Osoba D. Kaposi's sarcoma complicating corticosteroid therapy for temporal arteritis. *Am J Med* 1981; **71**: 320–2.
24 Capewell S, Reynolds S, Shuttleworth D *et al.* Purpura and dermal thinning associated with high-dose inhaled corticosteroids. *Br Med J* 1990; **300**: 1548–51.
25 Monk B, Cunliffe WJ, Layton AM, Rhodes DJ. Acne induced by inhaled corticosteroids. *Clin Exp Dermatol* 1993; **18**: 148–50.
26 Lauerma AH, Kiistala R, Makinen-Kiljunen S *et al.* Allergic skin reaction after inhalation of budesonide. *Clin Exp Allergy* 1993; **23**: 232–3.
27 Holmes P, Cowen P. Spongiotic (eczematous-type) dermatitis after inhaled budesonide. *Aust NZ J Med* 1992; **22**: 511.
28 Saff DM, Taylor JS, Vidimos AT. Allergic reaction to intralesional triamcinolone acetonide: a case report. *Arch Dermatol* 1995; **131**: 742–3.
29 Ijsselmuiden OE, Knegt-Junk KJ, van Wijk RG, van Joost T. Cutaneous adverse reactions after intra-articular injection of triamcinolone acetonide. *Acta Derm Venereol (Stockh)* 1995; **75**: 57–8.
30 Wilkinson SM, Smith AG, English JS. Erythroderma following the intradermal injection of the corticosteroid budesonide. *Contact Dermatitis* 1992; **27**: 121–2.
31 Lavabre C, Chevalier X, Larget-Piet B. Erythema multiforme after intradural injection of prednisolone acetate. *Br J Rheumatol* 1992; **31**: 717–18.
32 DeSio JM, Kahn CH, Warfield CA. Facial flushing and/or generalized erythema after epidural steroid injection *Anesth Analg* 1995; **80**: 617–19.
33 Beaudouin E, Kanny G, Gueant JL, Moneret-Vautrin DA. Anaphylaxie à la carboxymethylcellulose: à propos de deux cas de chocs à des corticoides injectables. *Allerg Immunol* 1992; **24**: 333–5.

Topical corticosteroids

The dermatological complications of topical corticosteroids have been reviewed [1–4]. Many of the adverse reactions are related to the potency of the preparation; thus, in general, fluorinated steroids are associated with more significant side-effects. Topical steroids cause decreased epidermal kinetic activity [5], decreased dermal collagen and ground-substance synthesis, and thinning of the dermis and epidermis [6–8]. Initial vasoconstriction of the superficial small vessels is followed by rebound vasodilatation, which becomes permanent in later stages. There are resultant striae, easy bruising, purpura, hypertrichosis and telangiectasia; stellate pseudoscars or ulcerated areas may be seen. Reversible hypopigmentation may develop. Local injection of a potent steroid may result in atrophy with telangiectasia, and localized lipoatrophy may occur. Perilymphatic atrophy is recorded following intradermal steroid injection. Long-term daily use of a potent steroid, especially under plastic occlusion as for fingertip eczema, may result in acroatrophy of terminal phalanges of the fingers [9,10].

Topical steroids may exacerbate acne, or lead to acne rosacea, with papules, pustules and telangiectasia, or perioral dermatitis, characterized by erythema, papules and pustules at the perioral area [11–13]. They decrease the number and antigen-presenting capacity of epidermal Langerhans' cells [14], and mask or potentiate skin infections, including fungal (tinea incognito) and bacterial infections and verruca vulgaris. Their withdrawal may provoke conversion of plaque to pustular type psoriasis [15]. Topical steroid therapy around the eye has been associated with development of glaucoma.

Topical corticosteroids may induce allergic contact dermatitis [16–28]. The prevalence of positive patch tests to corticosteroids in contact dermatitis clinics ranges from 2 up to 5% [21,22]. The allergen may be the steroid itself, or a preservative or stabilizer such as ethylene diamine. There may be cross-reactivity between different steroids [24,26,27]. Cross-reactivity is more likely between steroids with similar substitutions at C6 and C9 positions. Intradermal tests may be a more sensitive means of detecting corticosteroid hypersensitivity than patch testing [28].

Systemic side-effects of topical corticosteroids occur

particularly from the use of large amounts of high potency topical corticosteroids, especially under plastic occlusion [29,30]. Oedema from sodium retention occurs more frequently with halogenated corticosteroids [30]. Hypothalamic–pituitary axis suppression may occur [31,32]; a single application of 25g of 0.05% clobetasol propionate ointment suppressed plasma cortisol for 96h [33]. Cushing's syndrome [34,35] may result, and growth retardation in children is a hazard [36]. Glycosuria and hyperglycaemia may rarely occur [37].

REFERENCES

1 Miller JA, Munro DD. Topical corticosteroids: clinical pharmacology and therapeutic use. *Drugs* 1980; **19**: 119–34.
2 Behrendt H, Korting HC. Klinische Prüfung von erwünschten und unerwünschten Wirkungen topisch applizierbarer Glukokortikosteroide am Menschen. *Hautarzt* 1990: **41**: 2–8.
3 Coskey RJ. Adverse effects of corticosteroids: I. Topical and intralesional. *Clin Dermatol* 1986; **4**: 155–60.
4 Kligman AM. Adverse effects of topical corticosteroids. In: Christophers E, Schöpf E, Kligman AM, Stoughton RB, eds. *Topical Corticosteroid Therapy: A Novel Approach to Safer Drugs*. New York: Raven Press, 1988: 181–7.
5 Marshall RC, Du Vivier RA. The effects on epidermal DNA synthesis of the butyrate esters of clobetasone and clobetasol, and the propionate ester of clobetasol. *Br J Dermatol* 1978; **98**: 355–9.
6 Smith JG, Wehr RF, Chalker DK. Corticosteroid-induced cutaneous atrophy and telangiectasia. *Arch Dermatol* 1976; **112**: 1115–17.
7 Winter GD, Burton JL. Experimentally induced steroid atrophy in the domestic pig and man. *Br J Dermatol* 1976; **94**: 107–9.
8 Lehmann P, Zheng P, Lacker RM, Kligman AM. Corticosteroid atrophy in human skin: a study by light, scanning and transmission electron microscopy. *J Invest Dermatol* 1983; **81**: 169–76.
9 Requena L, Zamora E, Martin L. Acroatrophy secondary to long-standing applications of topical steroids. *Arch Dermatol* 1990; **126**: 1013–14.
10 Wolf R, Tur E, Brenner S. Corticosteroid-induced 'disappearing digit'. *J Am Acad Dermatol* 1990 **23**: 755–6.
11 Sneddon I. Perioral dermatitis. *Br J Dermatol* 1972; **87**: 430–2.
12 Cotterill JA. Perioral dermatitis. *Br J Dermatol* 1979; **101**: 259–62.
13 Edwards EK, Jr, Edwards ED, Sr. Perioral dermatitis secondary to the use of a corticosteroid ointment as moustache wax. *Int J Dermatol* 1987; **26**: 649.
14 Ashworth J, Booker J, Breathnach SM. Effect of topical corticosteroid therapy on Langerhans cell function in human skin. *Br J Dermatol* 1988; **118**: 457–69.
15 Boxley JD, Dawber RPR, Summerly R. Generalised pustular psoriasis on withdrawal of clobetasol propionate ointment. *Br Med J* 1975; **2**: 225–6.
16 Ashworth J, White IR, Rycroft RJG, Cronin E. Contact sensitivity to topical corticosteroids. *Br J Dermatol* 1990; **123** (Suppl. 37): 24.
17 Elsner P. Contact allergy to topical glucocorticoids. *Curr Probl Dermatol* 1993; **21**: 170–9.
18 Hohler T, Worz K, Himmler V. Adverse drug reactions to various topical glucocorticosteroids: quantitative aspects. *Curr Probl Dermatol* 1993; **21**: 180–5.
19 Belsito DV. Allergic contact dermatitis to topical glucocorticosteroids. *Cutis* 1993; **52**: 291–4.
20 Dooms-Goossens A. Kontaktallergie auf topische Glukokortikoide. *Hautarzt* 1994; **45**: 196.
21 Wilkinson SM. Hypersensitivity to topical corticosteroids. *Clin Exp Dermatol* 1994; **19**: 1–11.
22 Bircher AJ, Thurlimann W, Hunziker T *et al.* Contact hypersensitivity to corticosteroids in routine patch test patients. A multi-centre study of the Swiss Contact Dermatitis Research Group. *Dermatology* 1995; **191**: 109–14.
23 Almond-Roesler B, Blume-Peytavi U, Orfanos CE. Kontaktallergien auf Kortikosteroide. Pravalenz, Kreuzsensibilisierung und Nachweismoglichkeiten. *Hautarzt* 1995; **46**: 228–33.
24 Lepoittevin JP, Drieghe J, Dooms-Goossens A. Studies in patients with corticosteroid contact allergy. Understanding cross-reactivity among different steroids. *Arch Dermatol* 1995; **131**: 31–7.
25 Rietschel RL. Patch testing for corticosteroid allergy in the United States. *Arch Dermatol* 1995; **131**: 91–2.
26 Wilkinson SM, Hollis S, Beck MH. Cross-reaction patterns in patients with allergic contact dermatitis from hydrocortisone. *Br J Dermatol* 1995; **132**: 766–71.
27 Wilkinson M, Hollis S, Beck M. Reactions to other corticosteroids in patients with positive patch test reactions to budesonide. *J Am Acad Dermatol* 1995; **33**: 963–8.
28 Wilkinson SM, Heagerty AHM, English JSC. A prospective study into the value of patch and intradermal tests in identifying topical corticosteroid allergy. *Br J Dermatol* 1992; **127**: 22–5.
29 Vickers CFH, Fritsch WC. A hazard of plastic film therapy. *Arch Dermatol* 1963; **87**: 633–5.
30 Fitzpatrick TB, Griswold MC, Hicks JH. Sodium retention and edema from percutaneous absorption of fluorcortisone acetate. *JAMA* 1955; **158**: 1149–52.
31 Carruthers JA, August PJ, Staughton RCD. Observations on the systemic effect of topical clobetasol propionate (Dermovate). *Br Med J* 1975; **4**: 203–4.
32 Weston WL, Fennessey PV, Morelli J *et al.* Comparison of hypothalamus–pituitary–adrenal axis suppression from superpotent topical steroids by standard endocrine function testing and gas chromatographic mass spectrometry. *J Invest Dermatol* 1988; **90**: 532–5.
33 Hehir M, du Vivier A, Eilon L *et al.* Investigation of the pharmacokinetics of clobetasol propionate and clobetasone butyrate after a single application of ointment. *Clin Exp Dermatol* 1983; **8**: 143–51.
34 May P, Stein ES, Ryler RJ *et al.* Cushing syndrome from percutaneous absorption of triamcinolone cream. *Arch Intern Med* 1976; **136**: 612–13.
35 Himathongkam T, Dasanabhairochana P, Pitchayayothin N, Sriphrapradang A. Florid Cushing's syndrome and hirsutism induced by desoximetasone. *JAMA* 1978; **239**: 430–1.
36 Bode HH. Dwarfism following long-term topical corticosteroid therapy. *JAMA* 1980; **244**: 813–14.
37 Gomez EC, Frost P. Induction of glycosuria and hyperglycemia by topical corticosteroid therapy. *Arch Dermatol* 1976; **112**: 1559–62.

Sex hormones

Gonadotrophins

These drugs may cause allergic reactions [1]. Menotrophin (Pergonal) has been associated with localized keratosis follicularis (Darier's disease) [2]. Intracutaneous administration of two human menopausal gonadotrophin preparations (Organon and Pergonal) caused local induration and erythema [3].

REFERENCES

1 Dore PC, Rice C, Killick S. Human gonadotrophin preparations may cause allergic reaction. *Br Med J* 1994; **308**: 1509.
2 Telang GH. Atillasoy E, Stierstorfer M. Localized keratosis follicularis associated with menotropin treatment and pregnancy. *J Am Acad Dermatol* 1994; **30**: 271–2.
3 Odink J, Zuiderwijk PB, Schoen ED, Gan RA. A prospective, double-blind, split-subject study on local skin reactions after administration of human menopausal gonadotrophin preparations to healthy female volunteers. *Hum Reprod* 1995; **10**: 1045–7.

Gonadorelin analogues

Leuprorelin. This drug, given for precocious puberty, has caused anaphylaxis [1], rashes [2] and local reactions [3].

REFERENCES

1 Taylor JD. Anaphylactic reaction to LHRH analogue, leuprorelin. *Med J Aust* 1994; **161**: 455.
2 Carel JC, Lahlou N, Guazzarotti L *et al*. Treatment of central precocious puberty with depot leuprorelin. French Leuprorelin Trial Group. *Eur J Endocrinol* 1995; **132**: 699–704.
3 Manasco PK, Pescovitz OH, Blizzard RM. Local reactions to depot leuprolide therapy for central precocious puberty. *J Pediatr* 1993; **123**: 334–5.

Oestrogens and related compounds

Oestrogens. Spider naevi and melanocytic naevi may develop under oestrogen therapy, as may chloasma. Severe premenstrual exacerbation of papulovesicular eruptions, urticaria, eczema or generalized pruritus occurred in seven women; several had a positive delayed tuberculin-type skin test to oestrogen [1]. Patients with generalized chronic urticaria had an urticarial reaction to intradermal oestrogens. Elimination of oral oestrogen therapy or anti-oestrogen therapy with tamoxifen proved effective [1]. Stilboestrol therapy of pregnant women has been associated with female and male genital tract abnormalities in the offspring. Stilboestrol is a transplacental carcinogen and has caused adenocarcinoma of the vagina 20 years later in young women whose mothers took the drug in the first 18 weeks of pregnancy [2–4]. Acanthosis nigricans has resulted from diethylstilboestrol [5]. Hyperkeratosis of the nipples developed in a man treated for adenocarcinoma of the prostate with stilboestrol [6]. Porphyria cutanea tarda may also be precipitated [7,8].

REFERENCES

1 Shelley WB, Shelley ED, Talanin NY, Santoso-Pham J. Estrogen dermatitis. *J Am Acad Dermatol* 1995; **32**: 25–31.
2 Monaghan JM, Sirisena LAW. Stilboestrol and vaginal clear-cell adenocarcinoma syndrome. *Br Med J* 1978; **i**: 1588–90.
3 Wingfield M. The daughters of stilboestrol. Grown up now but still at risk. *Br Med J* 1991; **302**: 1414–15.
4 Anonymous. Diethylstilboestrol—effects of exposure *in utero*. *Drug Ther Bull* 1991; **29**: 49–50.
5 Banuchi SR, Cohen L, Lorincz AL, Morgan J. Acanthosis nigricans following diethylstilbestrol therapy. *Arch Dermatol* 1974; **109**: 544–6.
6 Mold DE, Jegasothy BV. Estrogen-induced hyperkeratosis of the nipple. *Cutis* 1980; **26**: 95–6.
7 Becker FT. Porphyria cutanea tarda induced by estrogens. *Arch Dermatol* 1965; **92**: 252–6.
8 Roenigk HH, Gottlob ME. Estrogen-induced porphyria cutanea tarda. *Arch Dermatol* 1970; **102**: 260–6.

Oral contraceptives. Cutaneous complications of oral contraceptives have been reviewed [1–4]. These drugs combine an oestrogen with a progestogen. Candidiasis is common; the sexual partner may suffer penile irritation after coitus without physical signs or frank candidal balanoposthitis. Genital warts may increase. Facial hyperpigmentation (chloasma) is well recognized [5,6], as are hirsutism and acne. Gingival epithelial melanosis has been recorded [7]. Alopecia related to contraceptive therapy may be of either androgenic or postpartum telogen pattern following withdrawal of the drug. Erythema nodosum is a well-recognized but rare complication [8,9].

The relapse of herpes gestationis is well documented [10]. Rare lichenoid, eczematous and fixed eruptions have been described, as has a lymphocytic cutaneous vasculitis, and an eruption resembling Sweet's syndrome [11]. Oral contraceptives have been implicated in both the provocation [12] and induction of remission of pityriasis lichenoides. A systemic LE-like reaction has also been reported [13]. An oral contraceptive-induced LE-like eruption, with erythematous lesions on the palms and feet in association with a weakly positive antinuclear factor and C1q deposition at the dermo-epidermal junction on direct immunofluorescence, developed in a patient. It resolved on cessation of medication [14].

The jaundice rarely induced by these drugs resembles cholestatic jaundice of pregnancy. The hepatotoxic effects may result in provocation of variegate porphyria, porphyria cutanea tarda [15,16] and hereditary coproporphyria [17]; onycholysis may occur [16]. Photosensitivity unrelated to porphyrin disturbances has also been reported [17]. Benign hepatomas may also be a hazard [18].

Other hormonal contraceptives. Keloid formation has followed levonorgestrel implantion [19]. Vaginal erythematous areas were associated with use of a levonorgestrel-releasing contraceptive ring in 48 of 139 subjects [20].

REFERENCES

1 Baker H. Drug reactions VIII. Adverse cutaneous reaction to oral contraceptives. *Br J Dermatol* 1969; **81**: 946–9.
2 Jelinek JE. Cutaneous complications of oral contraceptives. *Arch Dermatol* 1970; **101**: 181–6.
3 Coskey RJ. Eruptions due to oral contraceptives. *Arch Dermatol* 1977; **113**: 333–4.
4 Girard M. Évaluation des risques cutanés de la pilule. *Ann Dermatol Vénéréol* 1990; **117**: 436–40.
5 Resnik S. Melasma induced by oral contraceptive drugs. *JAMA* 1967; **199**: 601.
6 Smith AG, Shuster S, Thody AJ *et al*. Chloasma, oral contraceptives, and plasma immunoreactive beta melanocyte-stimulating hormone. *J Invest Dermatol* 1977; **68**: 169–70.
7 Hertz RS, Beckstead PC, Brown WJ. Epithelial melanosis of the gingiva possibly resulting from the use of oral contraceptives. *J Am Dent Assoc* 1980; **100**: 713–14.
8 Posternal F, Orusco MMM, Laugier P. Eythème noueux et contraceptifs oraux. *Bull Dermatol* 1974; **81**: 642–5.
9 Bombardieri S, Di Munno O, Di Punzio C, Pasero G. Erythema nodosum associated with pregnancy and oral contraceptives. *Br Med J* 1977; **i**: 1509–10.
10 Morgan JK. Herpes gestationis influenced by an oral contraceptive. *Br J Dermatol* 1968; **80**: 456–8.
11 Tefany FJ, Georgouras K. A neutrophilic reaction of Sweet's syndrome type associated with the oral contraceptive. *Australas J Dermatol* 1991; **32**: 55–9.
12 Hollander A, Grotts IA. Mucha–Habermann disease following estrogen-progesterone therapy. *Arch Dermatol* 1973; **107**: 465.
13 Garrovich M, Agudelo C, Pisko E. Oral contraceptives and systemic lupus erythematosus. *Arthritis Rheum* 1980; **23**: 1396–8.
14 Furukawa F, Tachibana T, Imamura S, Tamura T. Oral contraceptive-induced lupus erythematosus in a Japanese woman. *J Dermatol (Tokyo)* 1991; **18**: 56–8.

15 Degos R, Touraine R, Kalis B *et al.* Porphyrie cutanée tardive après prise prolongé de contraceptifs oraux. *Ann Dermatol Syphiligr* 1969; **96**: 5–14.

16 Byrne JPH, Boss JM, Dawber RPR. Contraceptive pill-induced porphyria cutanea tarda presenting with onycholysis of the finger nails. *Postgrad Med J* 1976; **52**: 535–8.

17 Roberts DT, Brodie MJ, Moore MR *et al.* Hereditary coproporphyria presenting with photosensitivity induced by the contraceptive pill. *Br J Dermatol* 1977; **96**: 549–54.

17 Erickson LR, Peterka ES. Sunlight sensitivity from oral contraceptives. *JAMA* 1968; **203**: 980–1.

18 Baum JK, Holtz F, Bookstein JJ, Klein EW. Possible association between benign hepatomas and oral contraceptives. *Lancet* 1973; **ii**: 926–8.

19 Nuovo J, Sweha A. Keloid formation from levonorgestrel implant (Norplant System) insertion. *J Am Board Family Pract* 1994; **7**: 152–4.

20 Bounds W, Szarewski A, Lowe D, Guillebaud J. Preliminary report of unexpected local reactions to a progestogen-releasing contraceptive vaginal ring. *Eur J Obst Gynecol Repr Biol* 1993; **48**: 123–5.

Anti-oestrogen drugs

Clomiphene. Hot flushes [1] and recurrent petechiae and palpable purpura of the legs with neutrophilic infiltration in a woman treated for infertility with multiple courses of clomiphene [2] have been reported.

REFERENCES

1 Derman SG, Adashi EY. Adverse effects of fertility drugs. *Drug Saf* 1994; **11**: 408–21.

2 Coots NV, McCoy CE, Gehlbach DL, Becker LE. A neutrophilic drug reaction to Clomid. *Cutis* 1996; **57**: 91–3.

Tamoxifen. This oestrogen receptor antagonist used in the therapy of breast cancer in women has caused hirsutism, hair loss, dry skin and a variety of rashes.

Progesterone and progestogens

Autoimmune progesterone dermatitis. A number of eruptions, including urticaria, eczema, pompholyx, and erythema multiforme, have been reported to recur cyclically in the second, luteal phase of the menstrual cycle, with pre-menstrual peaking in severity. Oral and perineal lesions may occur [1–7]. It has been proposed that they result from sensitization to endogenous progesterone. There is frequently, but not always, a history of prior exposure to synthetic progesterones [1,3]. Confirmation is with a positive intradermal test with progesterone preferably in an aqueous or aqueous alcohol solution, and/or existence of a circulating antibody to progesterone, and by sup-pression of symptoms with agents that inhibit ovulation and result in decreased serum progesterone [7]. Two patients with recurrent premenstrual erythema multiforme and autoreactivity to 17α-hydroxyprogesterone have been described [5,6]; in one case, the eruption spread in pregnancy, cleared after abortion and was associated with a high-affinity binding factor to 17α-hydroxyprogesterone in the serum [6]. In one patient, a premenstrual urticarial reaction was exacerbated by oestrogen, rather than progesterone [8].

Megestrol. A generalized morbilliform rash developed in a cachectic man treated with this synthetic orally active progesterone derivative to stimulate appetite and weight gain; skin testing with progesterone acetate was positive [9].

REFERENCES

1 Hart R. Autoimmune progesterone dermatitis. *Arch Dermatol* 1977; **113**: 426–30.

2 Wojnarowska F, Greaves MW, Peachey RDG *et al.* Progesterone-induced erythema multiforme. *J R Soc Med* 1985; **78**: 407–8.

3 Stephens CJM, Black MM. Perimenstrual eruptions: autoimmune progesterone dermatitis. *Semin Dermatol* 1989; **8**: 26–9.

4 Yee KC, Cunliffe WJ. Progesterone-induced urticaria: response to buserelin. *Br J Dermatol* 1994; **130**: 121–3.

5 Cheesman KL, Gaynor LV, Chatterton RT, Jr *et al.* Identification of a 17α-hydroxyprogesterone-binding immunoglobulin in the serum of a woman with periodic rashes. *J Clin Endocrinol Metabol* 1982; **55**: 597–9.

6 Pinta JS, Sobrinho L, da Silva MB *et al.* Erythema multiforme associated with autoreactivity to 17α-hydroxyprogesterone. *Dermatologica* 1990; **180**: 146–50.

7 Herzberg AJ, Strohmeyer CR, Cirillo-Hyland VA. Autoimmune progesterone dermatitis. *J Am Acad Dermatol* 1995; **32**: 333–8.

8 Mayou SC, Charles-Holmes R, Kenney A *et al.* A premenstrual urticarial eruption treated with bilateral oophorectomy and hysterectomy. *Clin Exp Dermatol* 1988; **13**: 114–16.

9 Fisher DA. Drug-induced progesterone dermatitis. *J Am Acad Dermatol* 1996; **34**: 863–4.

Androgens

Anabolic steroids. Exacerbation of acne vulgaris with de-velopment of acne conglobata has been reported [1]. Both the size of sebaceous glands and the rate of sebum secretion are increased [2,3]. A lichenoid eruption was reported in a patient with aplastic anaemia treated with nandrolone furylpropionate (Cemelon) [4].

Danazol. This 17-ethinyltestosterone derivative, which is an inhibitor of pituitary gonadotropin, is a very weak androgen. Twenty-nine per cent of 530 recipients of danazol reported at least one adverse event within 45 days after receiving the drug, but there were no known long-term sequelae [5]. Acne, hirsutism, seborrhoea, rash and generalized alopecia are documented [6–8]. Exacerbation of LE-like eruptions has been reported in patients receiving this drug for non-C1-esterase inhibitor-dependent angio-oedema [9] or for hereditary angio-oedema [10].

Gestrinone. This derivative of 19-nortestosterone, like danazol, may cause weight gain, hirsutism, acne, voice change or irregular menstrual bleeding [11].

Testosterone. Severe acne or acne fulminans has followed therapy with testosterone, with [2,12] or without [13] anabolic steroids.

Yohimbine. Yohimbine is an indole alkaloid obtained from the yohimbe tree in West Africa which is used in the treatment of male impotence. A case of generalized erythrodermic skin eruption, progressive renal failure and LE-like syndrome is recorded [14].

REFERENCES

1 Merkle T, Landthaler M, Braun-Falco O. Acne-conglobata-artige Exazerbation einer Acne vulgaris nach Einnahme von Anabolika und Vitamin-B-Komplex-haltigen Präparaten. *Hautarzt* 1990; **41**: 280–2.
2 Király CL, Collan Y, Alén M. Effect of testosterone and anabolic steroids on the size of sebaceous glands in power athletes. *Am J Dermatopathol* 1987; **9**: 515–19.
3 Király CL, Alén M, Rahkila P, Horsmanheimo M. Effect of androgenic and anabolic steroids on the sebaceous gland in power athletes. *Acta Derm Venereol (Stockh)* 1987; **67**: 36–40.
4 Aihara M, Kitamura K, Ikezawa Z. Lichenoid drug eruption due to nandrolone furylpropionate (Cemelon). *J Dermatol (Tokyo)* 1989; **16**: 330–4.
5 Jick SS, Myers MW. A study of danazol's safety. *Pharmacotherapy* 1995; **15**: 40–1.
6 Spooner JB. Classification of side-effects to danazol therapy. *J Int Med Res* 1977; **5** (Suppl. 3): 15–17.
7 Greenberg RD. Acne vulgaris associated with antigonadotrophic (Danazol) therapy. *Cutis* 1979; **24**: 431–2.
8 Duff P, Mayer AR. Generalized alopecia: an unusual complication of danazol therapy. *Am J Obstet Gynecol* 1981; **141**: 349–50.
9 Fretwell MD, Altman LC. Exacerbation of a lupus-erythematosus-like syndrome during treatment of non-C1-esterase-inhibitor dependent angioedema with danazol. *J Allergy Clin Immunol* 1982; **69**: 306–10.
10 Sassolas B, Guillet G. Lupus, hereditary angioneurotic oedema and the risks of danazol treatment. *Br J Dermatol* 1991; **125**: 190–1.
11 Anonymous. Gestrinone (Dimetriose)—another option in endometriosis. *Drug Ther Bull* 1991; **29**: 45.
12 Heydenreich G. Testosterone and anabolic steroids and acne fulminans. *Arch Dermatol* 1989; **125**: 571–2.
13 Traupe H, von Mühlendahl KE, Brämswig J, Happle R. Acne of the fulminans type following testosterone therapy in three excessively tall boys. *Arch Dermatol* 1988; **124**: 414–17.
14 Sandler B, Aronson P. Yohimbine-induced cutaneous drug eruption, progressive renal failure, and lupus-like syndrome. *Urology* 1993; **41**: 343–5.

Insulin

Adverse reactions to insulin [1–5] used to be relatively common, with bovine insulin having the most potential for production of allergic reactions, followed by porcine and human insulin. Insulin allergy and other local cutaneous reactions are rarely seen with highly purified and biosynthetic preparations [3,4], but local symptoms still occur in approximately 5% of patients [3]. Lipoatrophy, which was reported in 10–55% of patients treated with non-purified bovine/porcine insulin preparations, has almost disappeared since the advent of exclusive human insulin treatment. Allergic symptoms to human insulin are found in less than 1% of *de novo*-treated patients, but still occur when human insulin is used in the insulin-allergic patient [3]. Anaphylaxis may occur with recombinant human insulin [6]. Local allergic reactions are often of immediate hypersensitivity type; they are more common in the first few months, and usually subside with continued therapy. Generalized pruritus and urticaria occur rarely. Typically, more severe anaphylactoid reactions follow reintroduction of insulin in patients who previously have received long-term therapy. Delayed reactions may also occur, and take the form of pruritic erythema and induration, sometimes with papulation, within 24 h of injection [7]. Biphasic responses may be seen in the same individual, with initial immediate urticaria and a delayed reaction after 4–6 h. Allergy may develop to the insulin itself (i.e. bovine or porcine protein), or to preservatives such as parabens and zinc [8,9], or to protamine (surfen) present in depot preparations [10–12]. Sterile furunculoid lesions at injection sites, which heal with scars and which have a granulomatous histology, may result. Lipoatrophy at injection sites, or more rarely distally, occurred especially with longer-acting preparations; affected patients had lesional immunoglobulin deposits and circulating anti-insulin antibodies [13]. Exceptionally, hypertrophic lipodystrophy [14], or hyperkeratotic verrucous plaques at the site of repeated injections [15], may develop.

REFERENCES

1 Grammer L. Insulin allergy. *Clin Rev Allergy* 1986; **4**: 189–200.
2 De Shazo RD, Mather P, Grant W *et al.* Evaluation of patients with local reactions to insulin with skin tests and *in vitro* techniques. *Diabetes Care* 1987; **10**: 330–6.
3 Schernthaner G. Immunogenicity and allergenic potential of animal and human insulins. *Diabetes Care* 1993; **16** (Suppl. 3): 155–65.
4 Patrick AW, Williams G. Adverse effects of exogenous insulin. Clinical features, management and prevention. *Drug Saf* 1993; **8**: 427–44.
5 Barbaud A, Got I, Trechot P *et al.* Allergies cutanées et insulinothérapie. Aspects recents, conduite a tenir. *Ann Dermatol Vénéréol* 1996; **123**: 214–18.
6 Fineberg SE, Galloway JA, Fineberg NS *et al.* Immunogenicity of recombinant human insulin. *Diabetologica* 1983; **25**: 465–9.
7 White WN, DeMartino SA, Yoshida T. Severe delayed inflammatory reactions from injected insulin. *Am J Med* 1983; **74**: 909–13.
8 Feinglos MN, Jegasothy BV. 'Insulin' allergy due to zinc. *Lancet* 1979; **i**: 122–4.
9 Jordaan HF, Sandler M. Zinc-induced granuloma—a unique complication of insulin therapy. *Clin Exp Dermatol* 1989; **14**: 227–9.
10 Anaphylaxis to protamine masquerading as an insulin allergy. *Del Med J* 1993; **65**: 17–23.
11 Kollner A, Senff H, Engelmann L *et al.* Protaminallergie vom Spattyp und Insulinallergie vom Soforttyp. *Dtsch Med Wochenschr* 1991; **116**: 1234–8.
12 Hulshof MM, Faber WR, Kniestedt WF *et al.* Granulomatous hypersensitivity to protamine as a complication of insulin therapy. *Br J Dermatol* 1992; **127**: 286–8.
13 Reeves WG, Allen BR, Tattersal RB. Insulin-induced lipoatrophy: evidence for an immune pathogenesis. *Br Med J* 1980; **280**: 1500–3.
14 Johnson DA, Parlette HL. Insulin-induced hypertrophic lipodystrophy. *Cutis* 1983; **32**: 273–4.
15 Fleming MG, Simon SI. Cutaneous insulin reaction resembling acanthosis nigricans. *Arch Dermatol* 1986; **122**: 1054–6.

Thyroxine

Chronic urticaria and angio-oedema was reported in a patient, associated with exogenous thyrotoxicosis, related to thyroid replacement therapy [1].

REFERENCE

1 Pandya AG, Beaudoing DL. Chronic urticaria associated with exogenous thyroid use. *Arch Dermatol* 1990; **126**: 1238–9.

Antithyroid drugs

Thiouracils

Hypersensitivity reactions include drug fever, pruritus, urticaria, angio-oedema, exanthemata, acneiform rashes, depigmentation of hair and LE-like syndromes. Propylthiouracil has caused allergic vasculitis [1,2], and methylthiouracil has resulted in erythema multiforme. Thiouracils may cause excessive hair loss. These drugs may cause marrow failure [3].

REFERENCES

1 Vasily DB, Tyler WB. Propylthiouracil-induced cutaneous vasculitis. *JAMA* 1980; **243**: 458–60.
2 Gammeltoft M, Kristensen JK. Propylthiouracil-induced cutaneous vasculitis. *Acta Derm Venereol (Stockh)* 1982; **62**: 171–3.
3 The International Agranulocytosis and Aplastic Anemia Study. Risk of agranulocytosis and aplastic anemia in relation to use of antithyroid drugs. *Br Med J* 1988; **287**: 262–5.

Chemotherapeutic (cytotoxic) agents

General side-effects

There have been a number of excellent reviews of the dermatological complications of these compounds [1–8], including histopathological reactions [9,10]. Bone-marrow depression, with aplastic anaemia, agranulocytosis or thrombocytopenia, and gastrointestinal intolerance may occur with any of these drugs. Mucocutaneous surfaces are especially vulnerable to the toxic effects of this group of drugs on rapidly dividing cells. Common side-effects therefore include alopecia (see above) and stomatitis [11]. Cytotoxic drugs may cause alopecia by either anagen or telogen effluvium. Severe alopecia of anagen type within 2 weeks of administration of the drug is frequently seen with cyclophosphamide, doxorubicin and the nitrosureas; it is usually reversible with cessation of therapy. Other chemotherapeutic agents implicated in the production of alopecia include amsacrine, bleomycin, cyclophosphamide, cytarabine, dactinomycin, daunorubicin, etoposide, fluorouracil and methotrexate. Stomatitis occurs most frequently with acridinyl anisidide, dactinomycin, daunorubicin, doxorubicin, fluorouracil and methotrexate; it may respond to reduced dosage. Similarly, a number of drugs may cause pigmentation of the buccal mucosa [12] or of the nails [13–15]. Onycholysis may be induced [16].

Hypersensitivity or allergic reactions such as urticaria and angio-oedema [17,18] occur with all cancer chemotherapeutic agents except altretamine, the nitrosoureas and dactinomycin. With L-asparaginase and mitomycin (administered intravesically) they occur in about 10% of patients, and they are relatively frequent with cisplatin; they are very rare with methotrexate. Type I reactions are commonest, but all four types of reactions are represented. Many of these agents have distinctive cutaneous side-effects, ranging from localized or diffuse hyperpigmentation to less usual ones, including radiation enhancement and recall phenomena, photosensitivity and hypersensitivity reactions, and phlebitis or chemical cellulitis. Photosensitivity reactions occur with dacarbazine, fluorouracil, mitomycin and vinblastine. Radiation recall effects involve reactivation of an inflammatory response in areas irradiated months or years previously. Clinically, these range from erythema to vesiculation, with erosions and subsequent hyperpigmentation.

They have most often been reported in association with dactinomycin and doxorubicin therapy [19]; but also with edatrexate [20]; melphalan, etoposide, vinblastine, bleomycin, fluorouracil, hydroxyurea and methotrexate may also cause radiation enhancement. UV recall is recorded with mitomycin and the combination of etoposide and cyclophosphamide [21]. Rare complications such as diffuse sclerosis of the hands and feet, Raynaud's phenomenon [22], sterile folliculitis and flushing reactions may also occur. Multiple drug regimens may pose special problems in trying to elucidate the cause of a specific reaction, such as white-banded nails [23] or multiple Beau's lines [24]. A pityriasis lichenoides-like eruption occurred during therapy for myelogenous leukemia with vincristine and mercaptopurine, antibiotics and aciclovir [25]. Fingertip necrosis occurred during chemotherapy with bleomycin, vincristine and methotrexate for HIV-related Kaposi's sarcoma [26].

Most cytotoxic drugs are teratogenic, and are contraindicated during pregnancy, especially during the first trimester. Alkylating drugs usually cause sterility in males, and may shorten reproductive life in women.

REFERENCES

1 Weiss RB. Hypersensitivity reactions to cancer chemotherapy. *Semin Oncol* 1982; **9**: 5–13.
2 Bronner AK, Hood AF. Cutaneous complications of chemotherapeutic agents. *J Am Acad Dermatol* 1983; **9**: 645–63.
3 McDonald CJ. Cytotoxic agents for use in dermatology. I. *J Am Acad Dermatol* 1985; **12**: 753–5.
4 McDonald CJ. Use of cytotoxic drugs in dermatologic diseases. II. *J Am Acad Dermatol* 1985; **12**: 965–75.
5 Hood AF. Cutaneous side effects of cancer chemotherapy. *Med Clin North Am* 1986; **70**: 187–209.
6 Delaunay M. Effets cutanés indésirables de la chimiothérapie antitumorale. *Ann Dermatol Vénéréol* 1989; **116**: 347–61.
7 Kerker BJ, Hood AF. Chemotherapy-induced cutaneous reactions. *Semin Dermatol* 1989; **8**: 173–81.
8 Rapini RP. Cytotoxic drugs in the treatment of skin disease. *Int J Dermatol* 1991; **30**: 313–22.
9 Fitzpatrick JE, Hood AF. Histopathologic reactions to chemotherapeutic agents. *Adv Dermatol* 1988; **3**: 161–84.
10 Fitzpatrick JE. The cutaneous histopathology of chemotherapeutic reactions. *J Cutan Pathol* 1993; **20**: 1–14.
11 Bottomley WK, Perlin E, Ross GR. Antineoplastic agents and their oral manifestations. *Oral Surg* 1977; **44**: 527–34.
12 Krutchik AN, Buzdar AU. Pigmentation of the tongue and mucous

membranes associated with cancer chemotherapy. *South Med J* 1979; **72**: 1615–16.

13 Sulis E, Floris C. Nail pigmentation following cancer chemotherapy: a new genetic entity? *Eur J Cancer* 1980; **16**: 1517–19.

14 Daniel CR, III, Scher RK. Nail changes secondary to systemic drugs or ingestants. *J Am Acad Dermatol* 1984; **10**: 250–8.

15 Daniel CR, III, Scher PK. Nail changes secondary to systemic drugs or ingestants. In: Scher RK, Daniel CR, III, eds. *Nails: Therapy, Diagnosis, Surgery.* Philadelphia: WB Saunders, 1990; 192–201.

16 Makris A, Mortimer P, Powles TJ. Chemotherapy-induced onycholysis. *Eur J Cancer* 1996; **32A**: 374–5.

17 Weiss RB. Hypersensitivity reactions. *Semin Oncol* 1992; **19**: 458–77.

18 O'Brien ME, Souberbielle BE. Allergic reactions to cytotoxic drugs—an update. *Ann Oncol* 1992; **3**: 605–10.

19 Solberg LA, Jr, Wick MR, Bruckman JE. Doxorubicin-enhanced skin reaction after whole-body electron beam irradiation for leukemia cutis. *Mayo Clin Proc* 1980; **55**: 711–15.

20 Perez EA, Campbell DL, Ryu JK. Radiation recall dermatitis induced by edatrexate in a patient with breast cancer. *Cancer Invest* 1995; **13**: 604–7.

21 Williams BJ, Roth DJ, Callen JP. Ultraviolet recall associated with etoposide and cyclophosphamide therapy. *Clin Exp Dermatol* 1993; **18**: 452–3.

22 Vogelzang NJ, Bosl GJ, Johnson D *et al.* Raynaud's phenomenon: a common toxicity after combination chemotherapy for testicular cancer. *Ann Intern Med* 1981; **95**: 288–92.

23 James WD, Odom RB. Chemotherapy-induced transverse white lines in the fingernails. *Arch Dermatol* 1983; **119**: 334–5.

24 Singh M, Kaur S. Chemotherapy-induced multiple Beau's lines. *Int J Dermatol* 1986; **25**: 590–1.

25 Isoda M. Pityriasis lichenoides-like eruption occurring during therapy for myelogenous leukemia. *J Dermatol (Tokyo)* 1989; **16**: 73–5.

26 Pechère M, Zulian GB, Vogel J-J *et al.* Fingertip necrosis during chemotherapy with bleomycin, vincristine and methotrexate for HIV-related Kaposi's sarcoma. *Br J Dermatol* 1996; **134**: 378–9.

Extravasation

Extravasation, leading to skin necrosis with ulceration, occurs with several agents [1–5]. Phlebitis and chemical cellulitis have been recorded with most antimitotic agents. Residual drug should be aspirated, and the limb elevated; plastic surgical advice should be sought as soon as possible. High dermal concentrations of doxorubicin have been documented as late as 28 days after accidental extravasation [6]. Histological examination of doxorubicin-related extravasation lesions demonstrated exaggerated interface-type dermatitis with thrombosis of venous tributaries [7].

REFERENCES

1 Ignoffo RJ, Friedman MA. Therapy of local toxicities caused by extravasation of cancer chemotherapeutic drugs. *Cancer Treat Rev* 1980; **7**: 17–27.

2 Vansvloten Harwood K, Aisner J. Treatment of chemotherapeutic extravasation: current status. *Cancer Treat Rep* 1984; **86**: 939–45.

3 Banerjee A, Brotherston TM, Lamberty BGH *et al.* Cancer chemotherapy agent-induced perivenous extravasation injury. *J Postgrad Med* 1987; **63**: 5–9.

4 Rudolph R, Larson DL. Etiology and treatment of chemotherapeutic agent extravasation injuries: a review. *J Clin Oncol* 1987; **5**: 1116–26.

5 Dufresne RG, Jr. Skin necrosis from intravenously infused materials. *Cutis* 1989; **39**: 197–8.

6 Sonneveld P, Wassenaar HA, Nooter K. Long persistence of doxorubicin in human skin after extravasation. *Cancer Treat Rep* 1984; **68**: 895–6.

7 Bhawan J, Petry J, Rybak ME. Histologic changes induced in skin by extravasation of doxorubicin (adriamycin). *J Cutan Pathol* 1989; **16**: 158–63.

Acral erythema

Several cytotoxic drugs (especially cytosine arabinoside, fluorouracil and doxorubicin, and rarely cyclophosphamide, hydroxyurea, mercaptopurine, methotrexate and mitotane) can cause dose-dependent acral erythema, either alone or in combination [1–12]. Bulla formation, desquamation, and subsequent re-epithelialization may occur. Reactions may occur sooner (from 24 h to 3 weeks) and more severely with bolus or short-term chemotherapy than with low-dose continuous infusion, and are usually reproducible on challenge. Intravenous cyclosporine, given in bone-marrow transplant patients, reportedly worsens the pain of the acral erythema [12]. The condition should be distinguished from graft-versus-host disease in patients who receive chemotherapy followed by bone marrow transplantation, and from chemotherapy-induced Raynaud's phenomenon. This may not be easy, as histological changes may suggest graft-versus-host disease [13].

REFERENCES

1 Doyle LA, Berg C, Bottino G, Chabner E. Erythema and desquamation after high-dose methotrexate. *Ann Intern Med* 1983; **98**: 611–12.

2 Feldman LD, Jaffer A. Fluorouracil-associated palmar-plantar erythrodysesthesia syndrome. *JAMA* 1985; **254**: 3479.

3 Crider MK, Jansen J, Norins AL, McHale MS. Chemotherapy-induced acral erythema in patients receiving bone marrow transplantation. *Arch Dermatol* 1986; **122**: 1023–7.

4 Cox GJ, Robertson DB. Toxic erythema of palms and soles associated with high-dose mercaptopurine chemotherapy. *Arch Dermatol* 1986; **122**: 1413–14.

5 Guillaume J-C, Carp E, Rougier P *et al.* Effets secondaires cutanéo-muqueux des perfusions continues de 5-fluorouracile: 12 observations. *Ann Dermatol Vénéréol* 1988; **115**: 1167–9.

6 Horwitz LJ, Dreizen S. Acral erythemas induced by chemotherapy and graft-versus-host disease in adults with hematogenous malignancies. *Cutis* 1990; **46**: 397–404.

7 Baack BR, Burgdorf WHC. Chemotherapy-induced acral erythema. *J Am Acad Dermatol* 1991; **24**: 457–61.

8 Reynaert H, De Coninck A, Neven AM *et al.* Chemotherapy-induced acral erythema and acute graft-versus-host disease after allogeneic bone marrow transplantation. *Bone Marrow Transplant* 1992; **10**: 185–7.

9 Cohen PR. Acral erythema: a clinical review. *Cutis* 1993; **51**: 175–9.

10 Pirisi M, Soardo G. Images in clinical medicine. Chemotherapy-induced acral erythema. *N Engl J Med* 1994; **330**: 1279.

11 Komamura H, Higashiyama M, Hashimoto K *et al.* Three cases of chemotherapy-induced acral erythema. *J Dermatol* 1995; **22**: 116–21.

12 Kampmann KK, Graves T, Rogers SD. Acral erythema secondary to high-dose cytosine arabinoside with pain worsened by cyclosporin infusions. *Cancer* 1989; **63**: 2482–5.

13 Beard JS, Smith KJ, Skelton HG. Combination chemotherapy with 5-fluorouracil, folinic acid, and α-interferon producing histologic features of graft-versus-host disease. *J Am Acad Dermatol* 1993; **29**: 325–30.

Neutrophilic eccrine hidradenitis

Neutrophilic eccrine hidradenitis may represent a reaction pattern to a variety of chemotherapeutic agents [1–8], but particularly cytarabine and bleomycin. Clinically, erythematous papules or plaques or nodules are most frequent, although hyperpigmented plaques, pustules, purpura and urticaria have been described. Lesions resolve spontaneously over several days. The histology is characterized by infiltration of eccrine coils with neutrophils and necrosis of the secretory epithelium. The condition has also been described in a patient receiving haemodialysis without chemotherapy [9] and in a patient without a malignancy who was taking acetominophen [10].

REFERENCES

1 Fitzpatrick JE, Bennion SD, Reed OM *et al.* Neutrophilic eccrine hidradenitis associated with induction chemotherapy. *J Cutan Pathol* 1987; **14**: 272–8.
2 Scallan PJ, Kettler AH, Levy ML *et al.* Neutrophilic eccrine hidradenitis. *Cancer* 1988; **62**: 2532–6.
3 Fernández Cogolludo E, Ambrojo Antunez P, Aguilar Martínez A *et al.* Neutrophil eccrine hidradenitis—a report of two additional cases. *Clin Exp Dermatol* 1989; **14**: 341–6.
4 Burg G, Bieber T, Langecker P. Lokalisierte neutrophile ekkrien Hidradenitis unter Mitoxantron: eine typische Zytostatikanebenwirkung. *Hautarzt* 1988; **39**: 233–6.
5 Allegue F, Soria C, Rocamora A *et al.* Neutrophilic eccrine hidradenitis in two neutropenic patients. *J Am Acad Dermatol* 1990; **23**: 1110–13.
6 Margolis DJ, Gross PR. Neutrophilic eccrine hidradenitis: a case report and review of the literature. *Cutis* 1991; **48**: 198–2000.
7 Thorisdottir K, Tomecki KJ, Bergfeld WF *et al.* Neutrophilic eccrine hidradenitis. *J Am Acad Dermatol* 1993; **28**: 775–7.
8 Kanzki H, Takashi O, Makino E *et al.* Neutrophilic eccrine hidradenitis: report of two cases. *J Dermatol* 1995; **22**: 137–42.
9 Moreno A, Barnadas MA, Ravella A, Moragas JM. Infectious eccrine hidradenitis in a patient undergoing hemodialysis. *Arch Dermatol* 1985; **121**: 1106–7.
10 Kuttner BJ, Kurban RS. Neutrophilic eccrine hidradenitis in the absence of an underlying malignancy. *Cutis* 1988; **41**: 403–5.

Syringosquamous metaplasia

A related but distinct entity termed syringosquamous metaplasia, which may be confused with well-differentiated squamous cell carcinoma histologically, has been described in patients receiving chemotherapy for leukaemia and other cancers [1–3]. Clinically, this may appear as an erythematous, blanching, papular crusted eruption.

REFERENCES

1 Bhawan J, Malhotra R. Syringosquamous metaplasia. A distinctive eruption in patients receiving chemotherapy. *Am J Dermatopathol* 1990; **12**: 1–6.
2 Hurt MA, Halvorson RD, Petr FC, Jr *et al.* Eccrine squamous syringometaplasia. A cutaneous sweat gland reaction in the histologic spectrum of 'chemotherapy-associated eccrine hidradenitis' and 'neutrophilic eccrine hidradenitis'. *Arch Dermatol* 1990; **126**: 73–7.
3 Valks R, Buezo GF, Dauden E *et al.* Eccrine squamous syringometaplasia in intertriginous areas. *Br J Dermatol* 1996; **134**: 984–6.

Side-effects related to immunosuppression

The cutaneous manifestations of immunosuppression have been reviewed [1–4]. Immunosuppressive therapy, such as azathioprine and prednisone for renal transplant patients, may encourage skin infections of various types, for example warts, herpes simplex and herpes zoster [5],

pityriasis versicolor and fungal infections [6]. Development of disseminated superficial actinic porokeratosis [7–9], porokeratosis of Mibelli [10–13] and increased numbers of benign [14,15] or eruptive, dysplastic [16] melanocytic naevi may be promoted.

REFERENCES

1 Cohen EB, Komorowski RA, Clowry LJ. Cutaneous complications in renal transplant recipients. *Am J Clin Pathol* 1987; **88**: 32–7.
2 Abel EA. Cutaneous manifestations of immunosuppression in organ transplant recipients. *J Am Acad Dermatol* 1989; **21**: 167–79.
3 Boitard C, Nach J-F. Long-term complications of conventional immunosuppressive treatment. *Adv Nephrol* 1989; **18**: 335–54.
4 Paller AS, Mallory SB. Acquired forms of immunosuppression. *J Am Acad Dermatol* 1991; **24**: 482–8.
5 Spencer ES, Anderson HK. Viral infections in renal allograft recipients treated with long-term immunosuppression. *Br Med J* 1979; **2**: 829–30.
6 Shelley WB. Induction of tinea cruris by topical nitrogen mustard and systemic chemotherapy. *Acta Derm Venereol (Stockh)* 1981; **61**: 164–5.
7 Bencini PL, Crosti C, Sala F. Porokeratosis: immunosuppression and exposure to sunlight. *Br J Dermatol* 1987; **116**: 113–16.
8 Neumann RA, Knobler RM, Metze D, Jurecka W. Disseminated superficial porokeratosis and immunosuppression. *Br J Dermatol* 1988; **119**: 375–80.
9 Lederman JS, Sober AJ, Lederman GS. Immunosuppression: a cause of porokeratosis? *J Am Acad Dermatol* 1985; **13**: 75–9.
10 Grattan CEH, Christopher AP. Porokeratosis and immunosuppression. *J R Soc Med* 1987; **80**: 597–8.
11 Tatnall FM, Sarkany I. Porokeratosis of Mibelli in an immunosuppressed patient. *J R Soc Med* 1987; **80**: 180–1.
12 Wilkinson SM, Cartwright PH, English JSC. Porokeratosis of Mibelli and immunosuppression. *Clin Exp Dermatol* 1991; **16**: 61–2.
13 Herranz P, Pizarro A, De Lucas R *et al.* High incidence of porokeratosis in renal transplant recipients. *Br J Dermatol* 1997; **136**: 176–9.
14 McGregor JM, Barker JNWN, MacDonald DM. The development of excess numbers of melanocytic naevi in an immunosuppressed identical twin. *Clin Exp Dermatol* 1991; **16**: 131–2.
15 Hughes BR, Cunliffe WJ, Bailey CC. Excess benign melanocytic naevi after chemotherapy for malignancy in childhood. *Br Med J* 1989; **299**: 88–91.
16 Barker JNWN, MacDonald DM. Eruptive dysplastic naevi following renal transplantation. *Clin Exp Dermatol* 1988; **13**: 123–5.

Internal malignancy

The frequency of internal cancers common in the general population is not increased in transplant patients. However, that of a variety of otherwise uncommon malignancies is increased [1–3], including non-Hodgkin's type lymphoma (mostly B-cell, with 14% of T-cell, and less than 1% of null-cell, origin), which accounts for 21% of cancers in transplant recipients; Kaposi's sarcoma; other sarcomas; carcinoma of the vulva and perineum; carcinoma of the kidney; and hepatobiliary tumours. Non-Hodgkin's lymphoma appears commoner and develops earlier where potent immunosuppressive agents such as cyclosporin and/or the monoclonal antibody OKT3 have been used; however, although cancer develops in 6% of all transplant recipients, only 1% of patients die from this complication [3]. Leukaemia may develop following chemotherapy [4], and bladder cancer has been associated with cyclophosphamide therapy [5].

Skin cancers

Actinic keratoses, squamous cell and basal cell cancer of the lip and skin [6–12], and malignant melanoma [13] have been reported to be more common, especially in immunosuppressed renal transplant patients. The majority of these patients have received azathioprine and corticosteroids. Interestingly, the immunosuppressed recipients of renal transplant recipients have been reported to be at a high risk for skin cancer unless they express the HLA class I allele, A11 [14]. Furthermore, patients with longstanding renal grafts mismatched for HLA-B have a significantly higher incidence of squamous cell cancers than other mismatches, and patients who are homozygous for HLA-DR are at an increased risk for actinic keratoses and skin cancer [15]. These findings imply that major histocompatibility complex gene products participate in the pathogenesis of skin cancer in immunosuppressed patients, probably via influences on T-cell recognition of neoantigens [16]. There was no difference from control levels in the number of CD1+HLA-DR+ antigen-presenting Langerhans cells in the epidermis of immunosuppressed renal transplant recipients treated with either azathioprine/prednisone or cyclosporin/prednisone [17].

REFERENCES

1 Penn I. Depressed immunity and the development of cancer. *Clin Exp Immunol* 1981; **146**: 459–74.
2 Penn I. Tumors of the immunocompromised patient. *Annu Rev Med* 1988; **39**: 63–73.
3 Penn I. Cancers complicating organ transplantation. *N Engl J Med* 1990; **323**: 1767–9.
4 Williams CJ. Leukaemia and cancer chemotherapy. The risk is acceptably small but may be reducible further. *Br Med J* 1990; **301**: 73–4.
5 Elliot RW, Essenhigh DM, Morley AR. Cyclophosphamide treatment of systemic lupus erythematosus: risk of bladder cancer exceeds benefit. *Blood* 1970; **35**: 543–8.
6 Walder BK, Robertson MR, Jeremy D. Skin cancer and immunosuppression. *Lancet* 1971; **ii**: 1282–3.
7 Lowney ED. Antimitotic drugs and aggressive squamous cell tumors. *Arch Dermatol* 1972; **105**: 924.
8 Kinlen LJ, Sheil AGR, Peto J, Doll R. Collaborative United Kingdom—Australasian study of cancer in patients treated with immunosuppressive drugs. *Br Med J* 1979; **ii**: 1461–6.
9 Boyle J, Briggs JD, MacKie RM et al. Cancer, warts and sunshine in renal transplant patients. *Lancet* 1984; **i**: 702–5.
10 McLelland J, Rees A, Williams G et al. The incidence of immunosuppression-related skin disease in long-term transplant patients. *Transplantation* 1988; **46**: 871–4.
11 Gupta AK, Cardella CJ, Haberman HF. Cutaneous malignant neoplasms in patients with renal transplants. *Arch Dermatol* 1986; **122**: 1288–93.
12 Hintner H, Fritsch P. Skin neoplasia in the immunodeficient host. *Curr Probl Dermatol* 1989; **18**: 210–17.
13 Greene MH, Young TI. Malignant melanoma in renal transplant recipients. *Lancet* 1981; **i**: 1196–9.
14 Bouwes Bavinck JN, Koottee AMM, van der Woude FJ et al. HLA-A11-associated resistance to skin cancer in renal-transplant recipients. *N Engl J Med* 1990; **323**: 1350.
15 Bouwes Bavinck JM, Vermeer BJ, vans der Woude FJ et al. Relation between skin cancer and HLA antigens in renal-transplant recipients. *N Engl J Med* 1991; **325**: 843–8.
16 Streilein JW. Immunogenetic factors in skin cancer. *N Engl J Med* 1991; **325**: 884–7.
17 Scheibner KG, Murray A, Sheil R et al. T6+ and HLA-DR+ cell numbers in epidermis of immunosuppressed renal transplant recipients. *J Cutan Pathol* 1987; **14**: 202–6.

Alkylating agents

These drugs act by interfering with cell replication by damaging DNA. Gametogenesis is often severely affected, and their use is associated with a marked increase in non-lymphocytic leukaemia, especially when used in conjunction with radiotherapy.

Alkyl sulphonates

Busulphan. Reactions are rare, but have included urticaria, bullous erythema multiforme [1], Addisonian-like pigmentation [2,3] due to increased epidermal and dermal melanin, and drug-induced porphyria cutanea tarda [4]. Vasculitis has been reported. Keratinocyte nuclear abnormalities with abundant pale cytoplasm have been described [5]. Progressive pulmonary fibrosis may occur.

REFERENCES

1 Dosik H, Hurewitz DJ, Rosner F, Schwartz JM. Bullous eruptions and elevated leukocyte alkaline phosphatase in the course of busulphan-treated chronic granulocytic leukaemia. *Blood* 1970; **35**: 543–8.
2 Harrold BP. Syndrome resembling Addison's disease following prolonged treatment with busulphan. *Br Med J* 1966; **1**: 463–4.
3 Burns WA, McFarland W, Matthews MJ. Toxic manifestations of busulfan therapy. *Med Ann DC* 1971; **40**: 567–9.
4 Kyle RA, Dameshek W. Porphyria cutanea tarda associated with chronic granulocytic leukemia treated with busulfan. *Blood* 1964; **23**: 776–85.
5 Hymes SR, Simonton SC, Farmer ER et al. Cutaneous busulfan effect in patients receiving bone marrow transplanation. *J Cutan Pathol* 1985; **12**: 125–9.

Nitrogen mustard derivatives

Chlorambucil. Morbilliform rashes occur; urticarial plaques and periorbital oedema have been described rarely [1–4]. A delayed allergic reaction on the third cycle of chemotherapy, with generalized erythroderma with exfoliation and oedema of the face and arms, as well as immune haemolytic anemia and TEN, have been described [5]. Alopecia is uncommon. Sterility with azoospermia and amenorrhea is documented.

REFERENCES

1 Knisely RE, Settipane GA, Albala MM. Unusual reaction to chlorambucil in a patient with chronic lymphocytic leukemia. *Arch Dermatol* 1971 **104**: 77–9.
2 Millard LG, Rajah SM. Cutaneous reaction to chlorambucil. *Arch Dermatol* 1977; **113**: 1298.
3 Peterman A, Braunstein B. Cutaneous reaction to chlorambucil therapy. *Arch Dermatol* 1986; **122**: 1358–60.
4 Zervas J, Karkantaris C, Kapiri E et al. Allergic reaction to chlorambucil in chronic lymphocytic leukaemia: case report. *Leuk Res* 1992; **16**: 329–30.
5 Torricelli R, Kurer SB, Kroner T, Wuthrich B. Allergie vom Spattyp auf Chlorambucil (Leukeran). Fallbeschreibung und Literaturubersicht. *Schweiz Med Wochenschr* 1995; **125**: 1870–3.

Cyclophosphamide and mesna. Alopecia is common and occurs in 5–30% of cases [1]. Pigmentation, which may be widespread or localized to the palms, soles or nails, is well documented and usually reversible [2,3]. Nail dystrophy may be seen. Allergic exanthemata are rare, but anaphylactic and urticarial reactions are less so [4–7]. Type I hypersensitivity with a markedly delayed onset (from 8 to 16 h up to 10 days, associated with immediate skin-test results to cyclophosphamide metabolites but not the parent drug, have been documented [7]. There may be cross-sensitivity to other alkylating agents, especially mechlorethamine and chlorambucil [8]. Sterility may supervene.

Haemorrhagic cystitis, the result of toxicity of the metabolite acrolein, is a complication in up to 40% of cases if cyclophosphamide is used alone. Introduction of the thiol compound, mesna (2-mercaptoethane sulphonate), has virtually eliminated this complication. There have been recent reports of urticaria, angio-oedema, allergic maculo-papular pruritic rashes, generalized fixed drug eruption, and occasional more severe reactions with flushing, widespread erythema, and ulceration or blistering of mucous membranes related to mesna; patch tests may be positive [9–13].

REFERENCES

1 Ahmed AR, Hombal SM. Cyclophosphamide (Cytoxan). *J Am Acad Dermatol* 1984; **11**: 1115–26.
2 Harrison BM, Wood CBS. Cyclophosphamide and pigmentation. *Br Med J* 1972; **1**: 352.
3 Shah PC, Rao KRP, Patel AR. Cyclophosphamide induced nail pigmentation. *Br J Dermatol* 1978; **98**: 675–80.
4 Murti L, Horsman LR. Acute hypersensitivity reaction to cyclophosphamide. *J Pediatr* 1979; **94**: 844–5.
5 Lakin JD, Cahill RA. Generalized urticaria to cyclophosphamide: Type I hypersensitivity to an immunsuppressive agent. *J Allergy Clin Immunol* 1976; **58**: 160–71.
6 Knysak DJ, McLean JA, Solomon WR *et al.* Immediate hypersensitivity reaction to cyclophosphamide. *Arthritis Rheum* 1994; **37**: 1101–4.
7 Popescu NA, Sheehan MG, Kouides PA *et al.* Allergic reactions to cyclophosphamide: delayed clinical expression associated with positive immediate skin tests to drug metabolites in five patients. *J Allergy Clin Immunol* 1996; **97**: 26–33.
8 Kritharides L, Lawrie K, Varigos GA. Cyclophosphamide hypersensitivity and cross-reactivity with chlorambucil. *Cancer Treat Rep* 1987; **71**: 1323–4.
9 Pratt CB, Sandlund JT, Meyer WH, Cain AM. Mesna-induced urticaria. *Drug Intell Clin Pharm* 1988; **22**: 914.
10 Seidel A, Andrassy K, Ritz E *et al.* Allergic reactions to mesna. *Lancet* 1991; **338**: 381.
11 Gross WL, Mohr J, Christophers E. Allergic reactions to mesna. *Lancet* 1991; **338**: 381.
12 D'Cruz D, Haga H-J, Hughes GRV. Allergic reactions to mesna. *Lancet* 1991; **338**: 705–6.
13 Zonzits E, Aberer W, Tappeiner G. Drug eruptions from mesna. After cyclophosphamide treatment of patients with systemic lupus erythematosus and dermatomyositis. *Arch Dermatol* 1992; **128**: 80–2.

Lomustine. Flushing has been reported.

Mechlorethamine. Angio-oedema and pruritus have been recorded [1], but in view of the large number of patients receiving this drug as part of the MOPP (mechlorethamine, oncovin, procarbazine, prednisone) regimen for lymphoma, it must be exceedingly rare. Topical mechlorethamine [2] used to treat psoriasis or mycosis fungoides may cause hyperpigmentation of involved and uninvolved skin [3], contact sensitization [4,5] and rarely immediate-type hypersensitivity with urticaria or anaphylactoid reactions [6].

REFERENCES

1 Wilson KS, Alexander S. Hypersensitivity to mechlorethamine. *Ann Intern Med* 1981; **94**: 823.
2 Price NM, Deneau DG, Hoppe RT. The treatment of mycosis fungoides with ointment-based mechlorethamine. *Arch Dermatol* 1982; **118**: 234–7.
3 Flaxman BA, Sosis AC, Van Scott EJ. Changes in melanosome distribution in Caucasoid skin following topical application of nitrogen mustard. *J Invest Dermatol* 1973; **60**: 321–6.
4 Van Scott EJ, Winters PL. Responses of mycosis fungoides to intensive external treatment with nitrogen mustard. *Arch Dermatol* 1970; **102**: 507–14.
5 Ramsay DL, Halperin PS, Zeleniuch-Jacquotte A. Topical mechlorethamine therapy for early stage mycosis fungoides. *J Am Acad Dermatol* 1988; **19**: 684–91.
6 Daughters D, Zackheim H, Maibach H. Urticaria and anaphylactoid reactions after topical application of mechlorethamine. *Arch Dermatol* 1973; **107**: 429–30.

Melphalan. Trivial morbilliform rashes are relatively common [1]. Severe anaphylactic reactions may occur after intravenous use, especially in patients with IgA κ myeloma [2]. Urticaria or angio-oedema after oral use is very rare [3]. Vasculitis has been documented, and melanonychia striata has been recorded [4]. Radiation recall is uncommon [5]. Sterility with azoospermia and amenorrhea are recorded.

REFERENCES

1 Costa GG, Engle RL, Jr, Schilling A *et al.* Melphalan and prednisone: an effective combination for the treatment of multiple myeloma. *Am J Med* 1973; **54**: 589–99.
2 Cornwell GG, Pajak TF, McIntyre OR. Hypersensitivity reactions to i.v. melphalan during the treatment of multiple myeloma: cancer and leukemia group B experience. *Cancer Treat Rep* 1979; **63**: 399–403.
3 Lawrence BV, Harvey HA, Lipton A. Anaphylaxis due to oral melphalan. *Cancer Treat Rep* 1980; **64**: 731–2
4 Malacarne P, Zavagli G. Melphalan-induced melanonychia striata. *Arch Dermatol Res* 1977; **258**: 81–3.
5 Kellie SJ, Plowman PN, Malpas JS. Radiation recall and radio-sensitization with alkylating agents. *Lancet* 1987; **i**: 1149–50.

Ethylenemine derivatives

Thio-TEPA (triethylenethiophosphoramide)

Intravesical installation caused pruritus, urticaria or angio-oedema in five of 164 patients with bladder carcinoma [1]. Intravenous administration resulted in patterned hyperpigmentation confined to skin occluded by adhesive bandages or electrocardiograph pads, probably due to secretion of the drug in sweat [2]. By contrast, topical thiotepa has produced periorbital leukoderma [3].

REFERENCES

1 Veenema RJ, Dean AL, Uson AC *et al*. Thiotepa bladder installations: therapy and prophylaxis for superfical bladder tumors. *J Urol* 1969; **101**: 711–15.
2 Horn TD, Beveridge RA, Egorine MJ *et al*. Observations and proposed mechanism of N,N',N''-triethylenethiophosphoramide (thiotepa)-induced hyperpigmentation. *Arch Dermatol* 1989; **125**: 524–7.
3 Harben DJ, Cooper PH, Rodman OG. Thiotepa-induced leukoderma. *Arch Dermatol* 1979; **115**: 973–4.

Nitrosureas

Carmustine

Topical carmustine (BCNU) used for the treatment of cutaneous T-cell lymphoma may result in erythema, skin tenderness, telangiectasia. Contact sensitization may develop [1]. Mild bone-marrow suppression has been recorded.

REFERENCE

1 Zackheim HS, Epstein EH, Jr, Crain WR. Topical carmustine (BCNU) for cutaneous T cell lymphoma: a 15-year experience in 143 patients. *J Am Acad Dermatol* 1990; **22**: 802–10.

Dacarbazine (DTIC)

Photosensitivity [1,2] and a fixed eruption-like rash [3] have been reported. A patient with malignant melanoma treated with DTIC developed sudden hepatic vein thrombosis (Budd–Chiari syndrome) following intravenous administration [4]. Increasing blood eosinophilia appears to be a sign of the imminent development of this DTIC complication. Chemical cellulitis occurs following extravasation.

REFERENCES

1 Bolling R, Meyer-Hamme S, Schauder S. Lichtsensibilisierung unter DTIC-Therapie beim metastasierenden malignen Melanom. *Hautarzt* 1980; **31**: 602–5.
2 Yung CW, Winston EM, Lorincz AL. Dacarbazine-induced photosensitivity reaction. *J Am Acad Dermatol* 1981; **4**: 451–3.
3 Koehn GG, Balizet LR. Unusual local cutaneous reaction to dacarbazine. *Arch Dermatol* 1982; **118**: 1018–19.
4 Swensson-Beck H, Trettel WH. Budd–Chiari-Syndrom bei DTIC-Therapie. *Hautarzt* 1981; **33**: 30–1.

Procarbazine

Type I reactions are rare; recurrent angio-oedema, urticaria and arthralgia with decreased serum complement have been reported [1,2]. Hypersensitivity to procarbazine in patients treated with mechlorethamine, vincristine and procarbazine (MOP) for high-grade glioma manifested as a maculopapular rash, fever, reversible abnormal liver function and interstitial pneumonitis [3].

REFERENCES

1 Glovsky MM, Braunwald J, Opelz G, Alenty A. Hypersensitivity to procarbazine associated with angio-edema, urticaria and low serum complement activity. *J Allergy Clin Immunol* 1976; **57**: 134–40.
2 Andersen E, Videbaeck A. Procarbazine-induced skin reactions in Hodgkin's disease and other malignant lymphomas. *Scand J Haematol* 1980; **24**: 149–51.
3 Coyle T, Bushunow P, Winfield J *et al*. Hypersensitivity reactions to procarbazine with mechlorethamine, vincristine, and procarbazine chemotherapy in the treatment of glioma. *Cancer* 1992; **69**: 2532–40.

Cytotoxic antibiotics

Bleomycin

Alopecia, glossitis and buccal ulceration occur, and drug fever is common, usually 1–4 h after injection. Distinctive, localized, erythematous, tender, macules, nodules or infiltrated plaques on the hands, elbows, knees and buttocks have been documented [1–3]. Their causation is uncertain, since the rash may resolve despite continued therapy [4]. Raynaud's phenomenon with or without ischaemic ulcerations, and systemic sclerosis-like changes in men, have been described [5–7]. Capillary microscopy has been advocated for the investigation of bleomycin acral vascular toxicity [8]. Intradermal bleomycin into normal human skin induced a localized time- and dose-dependent inflammatory reaction and persistent postinflammatory hyperpigmentation; histology showed neutrophilic eccrine hidradenitis, with keratinocyte necrosis, HLA-DR and ICAM-1 expression, and endothelial cell ICAM-1 up-regulation and E-selectin induction [9]. Intralesional bleomycin therapy for warts induced keratinocyte apoptosis and complete epidermal necrosis with diffuse neutrophil accumulation and microabscess formation at the granular layer [10]. Clinically, intralesional therapy may cause persistent Raynaud's phenomenon [11,12] and loss of nails [13].

Cutaneous erythema or hyperpigmentation, which may be diffuse [14], patchy or linear, and prominent over pressure areas, especially the elbows or in striae distensae [15], is seen in approximately 30% of patients [16]. 'Flagellate' streaked erythema or pigmentation [17–21] on the trunk and proximal extremities is common (Fig. 77.8); it recurs in previously involved sites, and develops in new sites, within 24 h of rechallenge [21]. It has been proposed that trauma from scratching induces localized vasodilatation, with increased concentration of cutaneous bleomycin; hyperpigmentation has been documented in a patient treated with bleomycin where a heating pad had been applied [22]. There may be darkening of the nail

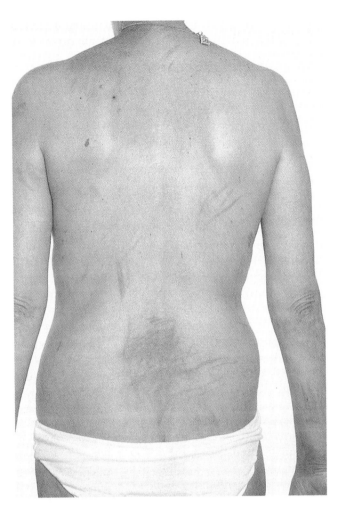

Fig. 77.8 Flagellate pigmentation caused by bleomycin. (Courtesy of Dr A. Ilchyshyn, Coventry and Warwickshire Hospital, Coventry, UK.)

cuticle and palmar creases. The principal problem of systemic therapy is progressive pulmonary fibrosis.

REFERENCES

1 Lincke-Plewig H. Bleomycin-Exanthem. *Hautarzt* 1980; **31**: 616–18.
2 Cohen IS, Mosher MB, O'Keefe EJ. Cutaneous toxicity of bleomycin therapy. *Arch Dermatol* 1973; **107**: 553–5.
3 Haerslev T, Avnstorp C, Joergensen M. Sudden onset of adverse effects du to low-dosage bleomycin indicates an idiosyncratic reaction. *Cutis* 1993; **52**: 45–6.
4 Bennett JP, Burns CP. Absence of progression of recurrent bleomycin skin toxicity without postponement or attenuation of therapy. *Am J Med* 1988; **85**: 585–6.
5 Finch WR, Rodnan GP, Buckingham RB *et al*. Bleomycin-induced scleroderma. *J Rheumatol* 1980; **7**: 651–9.
6 Bork K, Korting GW. Symptomatische Sklerodermie durch Bleomyzin. *Hautarzt* 1983; **34**: 10–12.
7 Snauwaert J, Degreef H. Bleomycin-induced Raynaud's phenomenon and acral sclerosis. *Dermatologica* 1984; **169**: 172–4.
8 Bellmunt J, Navarro M, Morales S *et al*. Capillary microscopy is a potentially useful method for detecting bleomycin vascular toxicity. *Cancer* 1990; **65**: 303–9.
9 Templeton SF, Solomon AR, Swerlick RA. Intradermal bleomycin injections into normal human skin. A histopathologic and immunopathologic study. *Arch Dermatol* 1994; **130**: 577–83.
10 James MP, Collier PM, Aherne W *et al*. Histologic, pharmacologic, and immunocytochemical effects of injection of bleomycin into viral warts. *J Am Acad Dermatol* 1993; **28**: 933–7.
11 Epstein E, O'Keefe EJ, Hayes M, Bovenmyer DA. Persisting Raynaud's phenomenon following intralesional bleomycin treatment of finger warts. *J Am Acad Dermatol* 1985; **13**: 468–71.
12 Epstein E. Intralesional bleomycin and Raynaud's phenomenon. *J Am Acad Dermatol* 1991; **24**: 785–6.
13 Gonzalez FU, Gil MCC, Martinez AA *et al*. Cutaneous toxicity of intralesional bleomycin in the treatment of periungual warts. *Arch Dermatol* 1986; **122**: 974–5.
14 Wright AL, Bleehen SS, Champion AE. Reticulate pigmentation due to bleomycin: light- and electron-microscopic studies. *Dermatologica* 1990; **181**: 255–7.
15 Tsuji T, Sawabe M. Hyperpigmentation in striae distensae after bleomycin treatment *J Am Acad Dermatol* 1993; **28**: 503–5.
16 Ohnuma T, Selawry OS, Holland JF *et al*. Clinical study with bleomycin: tolerance to twice weekly dosage. *Cancer* 1972; **30**: 914–22.
17 Cortina P, Garrido JA, Tomas JF *et al*. 'Flagellate' erythema from bleomycin, with histopathological findings suggestive of inflammatory oncotaxis. *Dermatologica* 1990; **180**: 106–9.
18 Fernandez-Obregon AC, Hogan KP, Bibro MK. Flagellate pigmentation from intrapleural bleomycin. A light and electron microscopic study. *J Am Acad Dermatol* 1985; **13**: 464–8.
19 Polla BS, Saurat JG, Merot Y, Slosman D. Flagellate pigmentation from bleomycin. *J Am Acad Dermatol* 1986; **14**: 690.
20 Rademaker M, Meyrick Thomas RH, Lowe DG, Munro DD. Linear streaking due to bleomycin. *Clin Exp Dermatol* 1987; **12**: 457–9.
21 Mowad CM, Nguyen TV, Elenitsas R, Leyden JJ. Bleomycin-induced flagellate dermatitis: a clinical and histopathological review. *Br J Dermatol* 1994; **131**: 700–2.
22 Kukla LJ, McGuire WP. Heat-induced recall of bleomycin skin changes. *Cancer* 1982; **50**: 2283–4.

Dactinomycin (actinomycin D)

A papulopustular acneiform sterile folliculitis, spreading from the face to the trunk and buttocks, and which may mimic septic cutaneous emboli, is common [1]. Dactinomycin-related lesions with the histology of an interface dermatitis with syringometaplasia developed in the axillae, groins and central line exit site of two children [2].

REFERENCES

1 Epstein EH, Lutzner MA. Folliculitis induced by actinomycin D. *N Engl J Med* 1969; **281**: 1094–6.
2 Kanwar VS, Gajjar A, Ribeiro RC *et al*. Unusual cutaneous toxicity following treatment with dactinomycin: a report of two cases. *Med Pediatr Oncol* 1995; **24**: 329–33.

Daunorubicin

Angio-oedema with generalized urticaria [1], and hyperpigmentation of the oral mucosa, skin and nails [2,3] have been described.

REFERENCES

1 Freeman AI. Clinical note. Allergic reaction to daunomycin (NSC-82151). *Cancer Chemother Rep* 1970; **54**: 475–6.
2 Kelly TM, Fishman LM, Lessner HE. Hyperpigmentation with Daunorubicin therapy. *Arch Dermatol* 1984; **120**: 262–3.
3 Anderson LL, Thomas ED, Berger TG *et al*. Cutaneous pigmentation after daunorubicin chemotherapy. *J Am Acad Dermatol* 1992; **26**: 255–6.

Doxorubicin (Adriamycin)

Short-lived localized erythema or urticaria with pruritus along the vein proximal to the injection site may occur in up to 3% of patients [1]. Angio-oedema, generalized urticaria with or without anaphylaxis and chronic urticaria have been reported rarely [2]. Cutaneous and nail pigmentation are well recognized [3,4]. Erythema and desquamation of palmar and plantar skin, with or without onycholysis, occurs frequently in patients receiving doxorubicin [5–7]. Liposomal doxorubicin was associated with a dose-limiting hand–foot syndrome and stomatitis [8,9]. Allergic cross-reaction occurs with daunorubicin. Toxic epidermal injury after intra-arterial injection [10], phlebitis and chemical cellulitis with extensive tissue necrosis and ulceration following extravasation [11] are well documented.

REFERENCES

1 Vogelzang NJ. 'Adriamycin flare': a skin reaction resembling extravasation. *Cancer Treat Rep* 1979; **63**: 2067–9.
2 Hatfield AK, Harder L, Abderhalden RT. Chronic urticarial reactions caused by doxorubicin-containing regimens. *Cancer Chemother Rep* 1981; **65**: 353–4.
3 Giacobetti R, Estely NB, Morgan ER. Nail hyperpigmentation secondary to therapy with doxorubicin. *Am J Dis Child* 1981; **135**: 317–18.
4 Curran CF. Doxorubicin-associated hyperpigmentation. *NZ Med J* 1990; **103**: 517.
5 Vogelzang NJ, Ratain MJ. Cancer chemotherapy and skin changes. *Ann Intern Med* 1985; **103**: 303–4.
6 Jones AP, Crawford SM. Anthracycline-induced toxicity affecting palmar and plantar skin. *Br J Cancer* 1989; **59**: 814.
7 Curran CF. Onycholysis in doxorubicin-treated patients. *Arch Dermatol* 1990; **126**: 1244.
8 Uziely B, Jeffers S, Isacson R *et al*. Liposomal doxorubicin: antitumor activity and unique toxicities during two complementary phase I studies. *J Clin Oncol* 1995; **13**: 1777–85.
9 Gordon KB, Tajuddin A, Guitart J *et al*. Hand–foot syndrome associated with liposome-encapsulated doxorubicin therapy. *Cancer* 1995; **75**: 2169–73.
10 Von Eyben FE, Bruze M, Eksborg S *et al*. Toxic epidermal injury following intraarterial adriamycin treatment. *Cancer* 1981; **48**: 1535–8.
11 Reilly JJ, Neifeld JP, Rosenberg SA. Clinical course and management of accidental Adriamycin extravasation. *Cancer* 1977; **40**: 2053–6.

Mitomycin

Urticaria and dermatitis [1–3], particularly on the face, palms and soles, or genitals and sometimes more generalized, have been reported after intravesical therapy. Sunlight-induced recall of ulceration following extravasation has been recorded [4].

REFERENCES

1 Colver GB, Inglis JA, McVittie E *et al*. Dermatitis due to intravesical mitomycin C: a delayed-type hypersensitivity reaction? *Br J Dermatol* 1990; **122**: 217–24.
2 De Groot AC, Conemans JMH. Systemic allergic contact dermatitis from intravesical instillation of the antitumor antibiotic mitomycin C. *Contact Dermatitis* 1991; **24**: 201–9.
3 Arregui MA, Aguirre A, Gil N *et al*. Dermatitis due to mitomycin C bladder instillations: study of 2 cases. *Contact Dermatitis* 1991; **24**: 368–70.
4 Fuller B, Lind M, Bonomi P. Mitomycin C extravasation exacerbated by sunlight. *Ann Intern Med* 1981; **94**: 542.

Antimetabolites

Aminoglutethimide

This inhibitor of adrenal steroid synthesis has been reported to induce systemic LE [1].

REFERENCE

1 McCraken M, Benson EA, Hickling P. Systemic lupus erythematosus induced by aminoglutethimide. *Br Med J* 1980; **281**: 1254.

Azathioprine

Dermatological aspects of this derivative of the antimetabolite mercaptopurine have been reviewed [1–3]. Bone-marrow suppression is the main problem; blood counts should be performed weekly for the first month, then monthly thereafter. Homozygotes for the low-activity allele for thiopurine methyltransferase are at risk for myelosuppression [4,5]. It has therefore been suggested that thiopurine methyltransferase levels should be measured before commencing patients on azathioprine [6]. Gastrointestinal upset is common and may necessitate discontinuation of therapy. Hypersensitivity reactions [7–9], including fever [10], maculopapular rashes, urticaria, vasculitis, erythema multiforme or erythema nodosum, cholestatic jaundice, hepatitis, liver necrosis, interstitial pneumonitis, polyneuropathy, pancreatitis, and shock [11] with hypotension, nephritis and oliguria are well recognized.

An acneiform exanthem has been described, confirmed on challenge [12]. Multiple large resistant warts are common on the hands of renal transplant recipients maintained on long-term azathioprine and prednisolone therapy; herpes simplex and herpes zoster infection may occur [13], and Norwegian scabies may be promoted [14]. Disseminated superficial actinic porokeratosis [15] and porokeratosis of Mibelli [16] have been documented. Keratoacanthomas and squamous cell carcinomas may develop [17]. Long-term therapy may predispose to the development of malignancy, especially of non-Hodgkin's lymphoma [18]. Azathioprine crosses the placenta, but there is little evidence that azathioprine is teratogenic in humans, and detailed analysis of successful pregnancies notified to the European Dialysis and Transplant Association did not suggest an excessive congenital abnormality rate [19]. However, depressed fetal haemopoiesis and resultant neonatal thrombocytopenia and leukopenia have been documented [20]. Pregnancy may be best avoided in patients receiving this drug [21]. Allopurinol may potentiate the effect of azathioprine by inhibiting its metabolism; the dose of azathioprine should therefore be reduced to one-quarter of the regular dose.

REFERENCES

1 Speerstra F, Boerbooms AM, van de Putte LB *et al*. Side effects of azathioprine treatment in rheumatoid arthritis: analysis of ten years of experience. *Ann Rheum Dis* 1982; **41**: 37–9.

2 Gendler E. Azathioprine for use in dermatology. *J Dermatol Surg Oncol* 1984; **10**: 462–4.

3 Younger IR, Harris DWS, Colver GB. Azathioprine in dermatology. *J Am Acad Dermatol* 1991; **25**: 281–6.

4 Snow JL, Gibson LE. The role of genetic variation in thiopurine methltransferase activity and the efficacy and/or side effects of azathioprine therapy in dermatologic patients. *Arch Dermatol* 1995; **131**: 193–7.

5 Snow JL, Gibson LE. A pharmacogenetic basis for the safe and effective use of azathioprine and other thiopurine drugs in dermatologic patients. *J Am Acad Dermatol* 1995; **32**: 114–16.

6 Jackson AP, Hall AG, McLelland J. Thiopurine methyltransferase levels should be measured before commencing patients on azathioprine. *Br J Dermatol* 1997; **136**: 133–4.

7 Stetter M, Schmidl M, Krapf R. Azathioprine hypersensitivity mimicking Goodpasture's syndrome. *Am J Kidney Dis* 1994; **23**: 874–7.

8 Knowles SR, Gupta AK, Shear NH, Sauder D. Azathioprine hypersensitivity-like reactions—a case report and a review of the literature. *Clin Exp Dermatol* 1995; **20**: 353–6.

9 Parnham AP, Dittmer I, Mathieson PW *et al*. Acute allergic reactions associated with azathioprine. *Lancet* 1996; **348**: 542–3.

10 Smak Gregoor PJ, van Saase JL, Weimar W, Kramer P. Fever and rigors as sole symptoms of azathioprine hypersensitivity. *Netherlands J Med* 1995; **47**: 288–90.

11 Jones JJ, Ashworth J. Azathioprine-induced shock in dermatology patients. *J Am Acad Dermatol* 1993; **29**: 795–6.

12 Schmoeckel C, von Liebe V. Akneiformes Exanthem durch Azathioprin. *Hautarzt* 1983; **34**: 413–15.

13 Spencer ES, Anderson HK. Viral infections in renal allograft recipients treated with long-term immunosuppression. *Br Med J* 1979; **2**: 829–30.

14 Paterson WD, Allen BR, Beveridge GW. Norwegian scabies during immunosuppressive therapy. *Br Med J* 1983; **4**: 211–12.

15 Neumann RA, Knobler RM, Metze D *et al*. Disseminated superficial porokeratosis and immunosuppression. *Br J Dermatol* 1988; **119**: 375–80.

16 Tatnell FM, Sarkany I. Porokeratosis of Mibelli in an immunosuppressed patient. *J R Soc Med* 1987; **80**: 180–1.

17 McLelland J, Rees A, Williams G *et al*. The incidence of immunosuppression-related skin disease in long-term transplant patients. *Transplantation* 1988; **46**: 871–4.

18 Phillips LT, Salisbury J, Leigh I, Baker H. Non-Hodgkin's lymphoma associated with long-term azathioprine therapy. *Clin Exp Dermatol* 1987; **12**: 444–5.

19 The Registration Committee of the European Dialysis and transplant Association. Successful pregnancies in women treated by dialysis and kidney transplantation. *Br J Obstet Gynaecol* 1980; **87**: 839–45.

20 Davison JM, Dellagrammatikas H, Parkin JM. Maternal azathioprine therapy and depressed haemopoiesis in the babies of rental allograft patients. *Br J Obstet Gynaecol* 1985; **92**: 233–9.

21 Gebhart DOE. Azathioprine teratogenicity: review of the literature and case report. *Obstet Gynecol* 1983; **61**: 270.

Cytosine arabinoside

This drug interferes with pyrimidine synthesis. A self-limited palmoplantar erythema, occasionally with bullae, may occur [1–4]. Neutrophilic eccrine hidradenitis has been reported [5]. A syndrome with fever, malaise, arthralgia, conjunctivitis and diffuse erythematous maculopapular rash is documented [6].

REFERENCES

1 Walker IR, Wilson WEB, Sauder DN *et al*. Cytarabine-induced palmar-plantar erythema. *Arch Dermatol* 1985; **121**: 1240–1.

2 Shall L, Lucas GS, Whittaker JA, Holt PJA. Painful red hands: a side-effect of leukaemia therapy. *Br J Dermatol* 1988; **119**: 249–53.

3 Brown J, Burck K, Black D, Collins C. Treatment of cytarabine acral erythema with corticosteroids. *J Am Acad Dermatol* 1991; **24**: 1023–5.

4 Richards C, Wujcik D. Cutaneous toxicity associated with high-dose cytosine arabinoside. *Oncol Nurs Forum* 1992; **19**: 1191–5.

5 Flynn TC, Harrist TJ, Murphy GF *et al*. Neutrophilic eccrine hidradenitis: a distinctive type of neutrophilic dermatosis associated with cytarabine therapy and acute leukemia. *J Am Acad Dermatol* 1984; **11**: 584–90.

6 Shah SS, Rybak ME, Griffin TW. The cytarabine syndrome in an adult. *Cancer Treat Rep* 1983; **67**: 405–6.

Fluorouracil

Anaphylaxis is rare; alopecia and recall phenomena [1] may be seen. Erythema followed by hyperpigmentation of sun-exposed areas occurs in up to 5% of patients [2]. Photosensitivity is recorded; pellagra may be caused by direct inhibition of the transformation of tryptophan into nicotinamide. Rarely, hyperpigmented streaks, 'serpentine supravenous hyperpigmentation', develop over arm veins used for injection [2–4]. Continuous infusion may be followed by the development of erythema, oedema and desquamation of the hands [5–7]. Pyridoxine may decrease the intensity and pain of fluorouracil-induced acral erythema [7]. Oral administration resulted in painful erythema multiforme-like erosions and blisters on the soles and arms in one case [8]. Systemic fluorouracil may result in marked inflammation of metastatic skin lesions [9] and of solar keratoses [10]. Topical application may lead to hyperpigmentation with or without a preceding irritant or allergic contact dermatitis [11].

REFERENCES

1 Prussick R, Thibault A, Turner ML. Recall of cutaneous toxicity from fluorouracil. *Arch Dermatol* 1993; **129**: 644–5.

2 Hrushesky WJ. Unusual pigmentary changes associated with 5-fluorouracil therapy. *Cutis* 1980; **26**: 181–2.

3 Hrushesky WJ. Serpentine supravenous 5-fluorouracil (NSC-19893) hyperpigmentation. *Cancer Treat Rep* 1976; **60**: 639.

4 Vukelja SJ, Bonner MW, McCollough M *et al*. Unusual serpentine hyperpigmentation associated with 5-fluorouracil. Case report and review of cutaneous manifestations associated with systemic 5-fluorouracil. *J Am Acad Dermatol* 1991; **25**; 905–8.

5 Feldman LD, Jaffer A. Fluorouracil-associated palmar-plantar erythrodysesthesia syndrome. *JAMA* 1985; **254**: 3479.

6 Guillaume J-C, Carp E, Rougier P *et al*. Effects secondaires cutanéo-muqueux des perfusions continues de 5-fluorouracile: 12 observations. *Ann Dermatol Vénéréol* 1988; **115**: 1167–9.

7 Vukelja SJ, Lombardo RA, James WD *et al*. Pyridoxine for the palmar-plantar erythrodysesthesia syndrome. *Ann Intern Med* 1989; **111**: 688–9.

8 Ueki H, Namba M. Arzneimittelexanthem durch ein neues 5-Fluorourazilderivat. *Hautarzt* 1980; **31**: 207–8.

9 Schlang HA. Inflammation of malignant skin involvement with fluorouracil. *JAMA* 1977; **238**: 1722.

10 Bataille V, Cunningham D, Mansi J, Mortimer P. Inflammation of solar keratoses following systemic 5-fluorouracil. *Br J Dermatol* 1996; **135**: 478–80.

11 Goette DK, Odom RB. Allergic contact dermatitis to topical fluorouracil. *Arch Dermatol* 1977; **113**: 1058–61.

Methotrexate

Dermatological aspects of methotrexate have been reviewed [1–3]. This drug is a folic-acid analogue and antagonist, which inactivates dihydrofolate reductase. There is marked individual variation in absorption from the gastrointestinal tract, and hence in expression of toxic effects. Alopecia occurs in 6% of patients receiving low-dose therapy for psoriasis, and in 8% of patients on high-dose regimens for malignancy, and is usually the result of telogen effluvium. Intermittent high dosage has resulted in horizontal pigmented banding of hair (the 'flag sign' of chemotherapy) [4]. Urticaria develops in about 4% of patients on low-dose oral or parenteral therapy for psoriasis [5]. Photosensitivity occurs in up to 5% of cases. Methotrexate use has been associated with severe reactivation of sunburn [6,7]; in one case, there was sparing of chronically sun-exposed skin [7]. Chronic viral wart and molluscum infections may result from immunosuppression. Cutaneous toxicity with epidermal necrosis may occasionally occur [8,9]. A macular erythema occurring in 15% of patients, and biopsy-proven capillaritis, have been reported with high-dose therapy [3]. Anaphylactic reactions [10], and pain, burning, erythema and desquamation of the palms and soles [11–13], are seen with high-dose intravenous methotrexate, but are extremely rare. Vasculitis has been very rarely documented with both intermediate dosage therapy for leukaemia [14] and high-dose therapy [15]. TEN is recorded [16].

Because folic acid is an essential cofactor for DNA synthesis and cell division, bone-marrow suppression may occur even on low-dose therapy [17–20]. Severe bone-marrow suppression [21] with the dosage used in the therapy of psoriasis is fortunately not common. Stomatitis may be a warning sign of overdosage. The risk of myelosuppression is much greater in the presence of renal impairment. Gastrointestinal upset is common. Abnormalities of taste sensation occur rarely [22].

The main hazard is hepatotoxicity with long-term use [23]. The risk of developing severe hepatotoxicity is related to the daily dose, the dose frequency and the cumulative dose [24]. Alcohol consumption, underlying liver disease and obesity, especially in the presence of diabetes, are aggravating factors. Recommendations include obtaining baseline haematological, renal and hepatic function tests and a liver biopsy before or within 4 months of starting therapy, and repeating after every 1.5 g [25]. Liver-function tests may be unreliable indicators of fibrosis of cirrhosis. These guidelines appear prudent but have never been rigorously tested, and are variously applied in clinical practice [25,26]. There seems to be a discrepancy between the degree of hepatotoxicity in rheumatoid arthritis and psoriasis, and many rheumatologists do not routinely carry out liver biopsy [26]. The requirement for liver biopsies in psoriasis patients on long-term low-dose once-weekly oral methotrexate has been questioned [27]. Radionucleotide liver scans are thought to be of little value in the detection of methotrexate-induced liver disease, but liver ultrasound may be of some assistance [28]. Abnormal liver biopsy may improve after cessation of therapy [29]. Acute renal failure may follow high-dose methotrexate therapy, but renal damage is rare in patients treated for psoriasis. Pulmonary complications, such as pneumonitis or fibrosis, are rare [30,31]. There do not appear to be adverse effects on humoral or cellular immunity from low weekly doses as given for rheumatoid arthritis or psoriasis [32].

Methotrexate is a known teratogen, and may cause oligospermia [33,34]. It is recommended that patients avoid pregnancy or impregnation during and for 12 weeks after cessation of methotrexate therapy [35].

Care must be taken with regard to potential drug interactions with methotrexate [36,37]. Drugs that also interfere with folate metabolism, such as trimethoprim–sulphamethoxazole [38–40], may cause pancytopenia; both trimethoprim and sulphamethoxazole bind to dihydrofolate reductase. Drugs that displace methotrexate from plasma protein-binding sites, such as salicylates, sulphonamides and diphenylhydantoin, as well as drugs that impair the renal clearance of methotrexate, such as NSAIDs and sulphonamides, may also cause pancytopenia.

REFERENCES

1 Plantin P, Saraux A, Guillet G. Méthotrexate en dermatologie: aspects actuels. *Ann Dermatol Vénéréol* 1989; **116**: 109–15.
2 Zachariae H. Methotrexate side-effects. *Br J Dermatol* 1990; **122** (Suppl. 36): 127–33.
3 Olsen EA. The pharmacology of methotrexate. *J Am Acad Dermatol* 1991; **25**: 306–18.
4 Wheeland RG, Burgdorf WH, Humphrey GB. The flag sign of chemotherapy. *Cancer* 1983; **51**: 1356–8.
5 Weinstein GD, Frost P. Methotrexate for psoriasis. A new therapeutic schedule. *Arch Dermatol* 1971; **103**: 33–8.
6 Mallory SB, Berry DH. Severe reactivation of sunburn following methotrexate use. *Pediatrics* 1986; **78**: 514–15.
7 Westwick TJ, Sherertz EF, McCarley D, Flowers FP. Delayed reactivation of sunburn by methotrexate: sparing of chronically sun-exposed skin. *Cutis* 1987; **39**: 49–51.
8 Harrison PV. Methotrexate-induced epidermal necrosis. *Br J Dermatol* 1987; **116**: 867–9.
9 Kaplan DL, Olsen EA. Erosion of psoriatic plaques after chronic methotrexate administration. *Int J Dermatol* 1988; **27**: 59–62.
10 Klimo P, Ibrahim E. Anaphylactic reaction to methotrexate used in high doses as an adjuvant treatment of osteogenic sarcoma. *Cancer Treat Rep* 1981; **65**: 725.
11 Doyle LA, Berg C, Bottino G *et al.* Erythema and desquamation after high-dose methotrexate. *Ann Intern Med* 1983; **98**: 611–12.
12 Martins da Cunha AC, Rappersberger K, Gadner H. Toxic skin reaction restricted to palms and soles after high-dose methotrexate. *Pediatr Hematol Oncol* 1991; **8**: 277–80.
13 Aractingi S, Briant E, Marolleau J *et al.* Décollements cutanés induits par le méthotrexate. *Presse Med* 1992; **21**: 1668–70.
14 Fondevila CG, Milone GA, Pavlovsky S. Cutaneous vasculitis after intermediate dose of methotrexate (IDMTX). *Br J Haematol* 1989; **72**: 591–2.
15 Navarro M, Pedragosa R, Lafuerza A *et al.* Leukocytoclastic vasculitis after high-dose methotrexate. *Ann Intern Med* 1986; **105**: 471–2.

16 Collins P, Rogers S. The efficacy of methotrexate in psoriasis—a review of 40 cases. *Clin Exp Dermatol* 1992; **17**: 257–60.

17 MacKinnon SK, Starkebaum G, Wilkens RF. Pancytopenia associated with low-dose pulse methotrexate in the treatment of rheumatoid arthritis. *Semin Arthitis Rheum* 1985; **15**: 119–26.

18 Shupack JL, Webster GF. Pancytopenia following low-dose oral methotrexate therapy for psoriasis. *JAMA* 1988; **259**: 3594–6.

19 Abel EA, Farber EM. Pancytopenia following low-dose methotrexate therapy. *JAMA* 1988; **259**: 3612.

20 Copur S, Dahut W, Chu E, Allegra CJ. Bone marrow aplasia and severe skin rash after a single low dose of methotrexate. *Anti-Cancer Drugs* 1995; **6**: 154–7.

21 Takami M, Kuniyoshi Y, Oomukai T *et al*. Severe complications after high-dose methotrexate treatment. *Acta Oncol* 1995; **34**: 611–12.

22 Duhra P, Foulds IS. Methotrexate-induced impairment of taste acuity. *Clin Exp Dermatol* 1988; **13**: 126–7.

23 Zachariae H, Kragballe K, Søgaard H. Methotrexate induced liver cirrhosis: studies including serial liver biopsies during continued treatment. *Br J Dermatol* 1980; **102**: 407–12.

24 Lewis JH, Schiff E. ACG Committee on FDA-Related Matters. Methotrexate-induced chronic liver injury: guidelines for detection and prevention. *Am J Gastroenterol* 1988; **88**: 1337–45.

25 Roenigk HH, Jr, Auerbach R, Maibach HI, Weinstein GD. Methotrexate in psoriasis: revised guidelines. *J Am Acad Dermatol* 1988; **19**: 145–56.

26 Petrazzuoli M, Rothe MJ, Grin-Jorgensen C *et al*. Monitoring patients taking methotrexate for hepatotoxicity. Does the standard of care match published guidelines? *J Am Acad Dermatol* 1994; **31**: 969–77.

27 Boffa MJ, Chalmers RJG, Haboubi NY *et al*. Sequential liver biopsies during long-term methotrexate treatment for psoriasis: a reappraisal. *Br J Dermatol* 1995; **133**: 774–8.

28 Coulson IH, McKenzie J, Neild VS *et al*. A comparison of liver ultrasound with liver biopsy histology in psoriatics receiving long-term methotrexate therapy. *Br J Dermatol* 1987; **116**: 491–5.

29 Newman M, Auerbach R, Feiner H *et al*. The role of liver biopsies in psoriatic patients receiving long-term methotrexate treatment. Improvement in liver abnormalities after cessation of therapy. *Arch Dermatol* 1989; **125**: 1218–24.

30 Phillips TJ, Jones DH, Baker H. Pulmonary complications following methotrexate therapy. *J Am Acad Dermatol* 1987; **16**: 373–5.

31 Carson CW, Cannon GW, Egger MJ *et al*. Pulmonary disease during the treatment of rheumatoid arthritis with low dose pulse methotrexate. *Semin Arthitis Rheum* 1987; **16**: 186–95.

32 Andersen PA, West SG, O'Dell JR *et al*. Weekly pulse methotrexate in rheumatoid arthritis: clinical and immunologic effects in a randomized, double-blind study. *Ann Intern Med* 1985; **103**: 489–96.

33 Sussman A, Leonard JM. Psoriasis, methotrexate, and oligospermia. *Arch Dermatol* 1980; **116**: 215–17.

34 Shamberger RC, Rosenberg SA, Seipp CA *et al*. Effects of high-dose methotrexate and vincristine on ovarian and testicular functions in patients undergoing postoperative adjuvant treatment of osteosarcoma. *Cancer Treat Rep* 1981; **65**: 739–46.

35 Morris LF, Harrod MJ, Menter MA, Silverman AK. Methotrexate and reproduction in men: case report and recommendations. *J Am Acad Dermatol* 1993; **29**: 913–16.

36 Evans WE, Christensen ML. Drug interactions with methotrexate. *J Rheumatol* 1985; **12** (Suppl. 12): 15–20.

37 Liddle BJ, Marsden JR. Drug interactions with methotrexate. *Br J Dermatol* 1989; **120**: 582–3.

38 Thomas DR, Dover JS, Camp RDR. Pancytopenia induced by the interaction between methotrexate and trimethoprim-sulfamethoxazole. *J Am Acad Dermatol* 1987; **17**: 1055–6.

39 Ferrazzini G, Klein J, Sulh H *et al*. Interaction between trimethoprim-sulfamethoxazole and methotrexate in children with leukemia. *J Pediatr* 1990; **117**: 823–6.

40 Groenendal H, Rampen FHJ. Methotrexate and trimethoprim–sulphamethoxazole—a potentially hazardous combination. *Clin Exp Dermatol* 1990; **15**: 358–60.

Vinca alkaloids and etoposide

These drugs cause metaphase arrest by interfering with microtubule assembly.

Etoposide (VP-16)

This semisynthetic podophyllotoxin derivative causes bone-marrow suppression, alopecia, and gastrointestinal symptoms. It has caused Stevens–Johnson syndrome and radiation recall. Four cases of a diffuse erythematous maculopapular rash occurring 5–9 days after initiation of therapy, with spontaneous resolution within 3 weeks, have been reported [1]. On histology, scattered, markedly enlarged individual keratinocytes with a 'starburst' nuclear chromatin pattern were seen. Hypersensitivity reactions are generally held to be rare [2–4], but 51% of patients with newly diagnosed Hodgkin's disease had one or more acute hypersensitivity reactions to etoposide administration, including flushing, respiratory problems, changes in blood pressure and abdominal pain [5].

Vincristine

Peripheral neuropathy is well recognized with long-term therapy [6].

Vinblastine

Photosensitivity is common [7]. Acute alopecia and radiation recall are documented. Erythema multiforme-like reactions are described following intravenous injection [8].

REFERENCES

1 Yokel BK, Friedman KJ, Farmer ER, Hood AF. Cutaneous pathology following etoposide therapy. *J Cutan Pathol* 1987; **14**: 326–30.

2 Kasperek C, Black CD. Two cases of suspected immunologic-based hypersensitivity reactions to etoposide therapy. *Ann Pharmacother* 1992; **26**: 1227–30.

3 de Souza P, Friedlander M, Wilde C *et al*. Hypersensitivity reactions to etoposide. A report of three cases and review of the literature. *Am J Clin Oncol* 1994; **17**: 387–9.

4 Hoetelmans RM, Schornagel JH, ten Bokkel Huinink WW, Beijnen JH. Hypersensitivity reactions to etoposide. *Ann Pharmacother* 1996; **30**: 367–71.

5 Hudson MM, Weinstein HJ, Donaldson SS *et al*. Acute hypersensitivity reactions to etoposide in a VEPA regimen for Hodgkin's disease. *J Clin Oncol* 1993; **11**: 1080–4.

6 Watkins SM, Griffin JP. High incidence of vincristine-induced neuropathy in lymphomas. *Br Med J* 1978; **i**: 610–12.

7 Breza TS, Halprin KM, Taylor JR. Photosensitivity reaction to vinblastine. *Arch Dermatol* 1975; **111**: 1168–70.

8 Arias D, Requena L, Hasson A *et al*. Localized epidermal necrolysis (erythema multiforme-like reactions) following intravenous injection of vinblastine. *J Cutan Pathol* 1991; **18**: 344–6.

Enzymes

L-Asparaginase

Dose-dependent IgE-mediated hypersensitivity reactions, including urticaria and anaphylaxis, are frequent, especially when the drug is used alone [1]. Allergic reactions to intramuscular L-asparaginase include local painful erythema, and urticaria or a general exanthem; continuous infusion is better tolerated [2].

REFERENCES

1 Ertel IJ, Nesbit ME, Hammond D *et al.* Effective dose of L-asparaginase for induction of remission in previously treated children with acute lymphocytic leukemia: a report from Children's Cancer Study Group. *Cancer Res* 1979; **39**: 3893–6.
2 Rodriguez T, Baumgarten E, Fengler R *et al.* Langzeitinfusion von L-Asparaginase—eine Alternative zur intramuskularen Injektion? *Klin Ped* 1995; **207**: 207–10.

Miscellaneous chemotherapeutic agents

Acridinyl anisidide (AMSA)

Skin reactions are rare, but widespread erythema has been reported [1].

REFERENCE

1 Rosenfelt FP, Rosenbloom BE, Weinstein IM. Allergic reaction following administration of AMSA. *Cancer Treat Rep* 1982; **66**: 549–5.

Bromodeoxyuridine

A distinctive eruption comprising linear supravenous papules and erythroderma has been described with bromodeoxyuridine given in combination with radiotherapy for central nervous system tumours [1]. Ipsilateral facial dermatitis with epilation of eyebrows and eyelashes, ocular irritation, bilateral nail dystrophy, oral ulceration, exanthem or erythema multiforme have also been described [2].

REFERENCES

1 Fine J-D, Breathnach SM. Distinctive eruption characterized by linear supravenous papules and erythroderma following broxuridine (Bromodeoxyuridine) therapy and radiotherapy. *Arch Dermatol* 1986; **122**: 199–200.
2 McCuaig CM, Ellis CN, Greenberg HS *et al.* Mucocutaneous complications of intra-arterial 5-bromodeoxyuridine and radiation. *J Am Acad Dermatol* 1989; **21**: 1235–40.

Carboplatin

Hypersensitivity reactions occur in 1–30% of patients [1–5]; acute allergic reactions include urticaria, bronchospasm, hypotension, facial erythema and facial swelling. Desensitization can be successful [5]. A pruritic maculopapular rash occurred in 10 of 40 patients treated with carboplatin, etoposide and ifosfamide plus mesna followed by autologous stem-cell reinfusion; the rash was distributed at the extremities or was confluent on the trunk and face, with facial oedema and painful swelling of hands and feet, and resolved spontaneously in all patients with hyperpigmentation [6].

REFERENCES

1 Hendrick AM, Simmons D, Cantwell BM. Allergic reactions to carboplatin. *Ann Oncol* 1992; **3**: 239–40.
2 Tonkin KS, Rubin P, Levin L. Carboplatin hypersensitivity: case reports and review of the literature. *Eur J Cancer* 1993; **29A**: 1356–7.
3 Weidmann B, Mulleneisen N, Bojko P, Niederle N. Hypersensitivity reactions to carboplatin. Report of two patients, review of the literature, and discussion of diagnostic procedures and management. *Cancer* 1994; **73**: 2218–22.
4 Chang SM, Fryberger S, Crouse V *et al.* Carboplatin hypersensitivity in children. A report of five patients with brain tumors. *Cancer* 1995; **75**: 1171–5.
5 Broome CB, Schiff RI, Friedman HS. Successful desensitization to carboplatin in patients with systemic hypersensitivity reactions. *Med Pediatr Oncol* 1996; **26**: 105–10.
6 Beyer J, Grabbe J, Lenz K *et al.* Cutaneous toxicity of high-dose carboplatin, etoposide and ifosfamide followed by autologous stem cell reinfusion. *Bone Marrow Transplant* 1992; **10**: 491–4.

Cisplatin

Severe hypersensitivity reactions, including flushing, erythema, maculopapular eruptions, urticaria and anaphylaxis occur in about 5% of cases when this drug is used as a single agent, and in up to 20% when given with other chemotherapeutic agents [1,2]. Cross-reactivity with carboplatin may occur [2]. Atopic subjects are especially at risk. Local reactions follow extravasation [3]. Severe allergic exfoliative dermatitis with ischaemia and necrosis of the hands developed in a patient who had received multiple doses of cisplatin [4].

REFERENCES

1 Vogl SE, Zaravinos T, Kaplan BH. Toxicity of cis-diaminedichloro-platinum II given in a two-hour outpatient regimen of diuresis and hydration. *Cancer* 1980; **45**: 11–15.
2 Shlebak AA, Clark PI, Green JA. Hypersensitivity and cross-reactivity to cisplatin and analogues. *Cancer Chemother Pharmacol* 1995; **35**: 349–51.
3 Fields S, Koeller J, Topper RL *et al.* Local soft tissue toxicity following cisplatin extravasation. *J Natl Cancer Inst* 1990; **82**: 1649–50.
4 Lee TC, Hook CC, Long HJ. Severe exfoliative dermatitis associated with hand ischemia during cisplatin therapy. *Mayo Clin Proc* 1994; **69**: 80–2.

Colchicine

Alopecia is recorded [1].

REFERENCE

1 Haarms M. Haarausfall und Haarveränderungen nach Kolchizintherapie. *Hautarzt* 1980; **31**: 161–3.

Flutamide

A photosensitive dermatitis has been reported with this non-steroid antiandrogen used in the treatment of prostatic carcinoma [1].

REFERENCE

1 Fujimoto M, Kikuchi K, Imakado S, Furue M. Photosensitive dermatitis induced by flutamide. *Br J Dermatol* 1996; **135**: 496–7.

Hydroxyurea

Dermatological aspects of this drug have been reviewed [1–4]. A modest fall in haemoglobin and development of macrocytosis is almost constant. Stomatitis occurs especially with high dose therapy and has been accompanied by soreness, violet erythema, and oedema of the palms and soles with subsequent intense universal hyperpigmentation [5], but alopecia is rare. Morbilliform erythema occurs, and hyperpigmentation, generalized or localized to pressure areas, is recorded in up to 5% of cases [2]. Nail changes such as multiple, pigmented nail bands [6] or onycholysis with nail dystrophy occur. Fixed drug eruption has been reported [3]. Dermatomyositis-like acral erythema, scaling, and atrophy especially on the dorsum of the hands with lesser involvement of the feet [1,4,7–9], and palmar and plantar keratoderma have been rarely described with long-term therapy for chronic myeloid leukaemia. Photosensitivity is documented, and LE [10] and vasculitis have been reported. Accelerated development of skin malignancies occurs, and eruptive squamous and basal cell cancers on light-exposed areas may be seen [11]. An ulcerative lichen planus-like dermatitis has been recorded [12]. Radiation recall occurs [13]. Leg ulcers that improved following cessation of therapy have been described in patients treated for chronic myeloid leukaemia [14]. Impaired renal function has been reported in some, but not all, studies [3].

REFERENCES

1 Kennedy BJ, Smith LR, Goltz RW. Skin changes secondary to hydroxyurea therapy. *Arch Dermatol* 1975; **111**: 183–7.
2 Layton AM, Sheehan-Dare RA, Goodfield MJD, Cotterill JA. Hydroxyurea in the management of therapy resistant psoriasis. *Br J Dermatol* 1989; **121**: 647–53.
3 Boyd AS, Neldner KH. Hydroxyurea therapy. *J Am Acad Dermatol* 1991; **25**: 518–24.
4 Kelly RI, Bull RH, Marsden A. Cutaneous manifestations of long-term hydroxyurea therapy. *Australas J Dermatol* 1994; **35**: 61–4.
5 Brincker H, Christensen BE. Acute mucocutaneous toxicity following high-dose hydroxyurea. *Cancer Chemother Pharmacol* 1993; **32**: 496–7.
6 Vomvouras S, Pakula AS, Shaw JM. Multiple pigmented nail bands during hydroxyurea therapy: an uncommon finding. *J Am Acad Dermatol* 1991; **24**: 1016–17.
7 Richard M, Truchetet F, Friedel J *et al*. Skin lesions simulating chronic dermatomyositis during long-term hydroxyurea therapy. *J Am Acad Dermatol* 1989; **21**: 797–9.
8 Senet P, Aractingi S, Porneuf M *et al*. Hydroxyurea-induced dermatomyositis-like eruption. *Br J Dermatol* 1995; **133**: 455–9.
9 Bahadoran P, Castanet J, Lacour JP *et al*. Pseudo-dermatomyositis induced by long-term hydroxyurea therapy: report of two cases. *Br J Dermatol* 1996; **134**: 1161–3.
10 Layton AM, Cotterill JA, Tomlinson IW. Hydroxyurea-induced lupus erythematosus. *Br J Dermatol* 1994; **130**: 687–8.
11 Papi M, Didona B, DePita O *et al*. Multiple skin tumors on light-exposed areas during long-term treatment with hydroxyurea. *J Am Acad Dermatol* 1993; **28**: 485–6.
12 Renfro L, Kamino H, Raphael B *et al*. Ulcerative lichen planus-like dermatitis associated with hydroxyurea. *J Am Acad Dermatol* 1991; **24**: 143–5.
13 Sears ME. Erythema in areas of previous irradiation in patients treated with hydroxyurea (NSC-32065). *Cancer Chemother Rep* 1964; **40**: 31–2.
14 Montefusco E, Alimena G, Gastaldi R *et al*. Unusual dermatologic toxicity of long-term therapy with hydroxyurea in chronic myelogenous leukemia. *Tumori* 1986; **72**: 317–21.

OKT3

Orthoclone OKT3, a murine monoclonal antibody directed against the CD3 subset of T lymphocytes, has been used as an immunosuppressive agent in renal transplant recipients, and has been anecdotally associated with anaphylaxis [1].

REFERENCE

1 Werier J, Cheung AHS, Matas AJ. Anaphylactic hypersensitivity reaction after repeat OKT3 treatment. *Lancet* 1991; **337**: 1351.

Taxanes

Docetaxel. Docetaxel, a semisynthetic analogue of paclitaxel from the needles of the European yew, *Taxus baccata*, used in the treatment of advanced and/or metastatic cancer, caused neutropenia, skin reactions (81%) and nail changes (41%), neurosensory toxicity (59%), fluid retention with oedema and hypersensitivity reactions (16–55%) [1–3]. The commonest skin reaction is characterized by discrete erythematous to violaceous patches or oedematous plaques similar to acral erythema [4].

REFERENCES

1 ten Bokkel Huinink WW, Prove AM, Piccard M *et al*. A phase II trial with docetaxel (Taxotene) in second line treatment with chemotherapy for advanced breast cancer. A study of the EORTC Early Clinical Trials Group. *Ann Oncol* 1994; **5**: 527–32.
2 Pazdur R, Lassere Y, Soh LT *et al*. Phase II trial of docetaxel (Taxotere) in metastatic colorectal carcinoma. *Ann Oncol* 1994; **5**: 468–70.
3 Mertens WC, Eisenhauer EA, Jolivet J *et al*. Docetaxel in advanced renal carcinoma. A phase II trial of the National Cancer Institute of Canada Clinical Trials Group. *Ann Oncol* 1994; **5**: 185–7.
4 Zimmerman GC, Keeling JH, Burris HA *et al*. Acute cutaneous reactions to docetaxel, a new chemotherapeutic agent. *Arch Dermatol* 1995; **131**: 202–6.

Paclitaxel. Paclitaxel is a diterpenoid taxane derivative found in the bark and needles of the western yew, *Taxus brevifolia*, which interrupts mitosis by promoting and stabilizing microtubule formation, and shows substantial activity against advanced, refractory cancer. Neutropenia is the major dose-limiting toxic effect; other adverse effects include severe hypersensitivity reactions including anaphylaxis, cardiac toxicity, neurotoxicity, arthralgia or myalgia, mucositis, nausea and vomiting, and alopecia [1–6]. Desensitization is possible [7]. Bullous fixed drug eruption is recorded [8].

Local necrosis has followed accidental subcutaneous extravasation of paclitaxel [9], and administration via a central vein has produced a recall reaction at a site of prior extravasation [10].

REFERENCES

1 Onetto N, Canetta R, Winograd B *et al.* Overview of Taxol safety. *Monogr Natl Cancer Inst* 1993; **15**: 131–9.
2 Schiller JH, Storer B, Tutsch K *et al.* A phase I trial of 3-hour infusions of paclitaxel (Taxol) with or without granulocyte colony-stimulating factor. *Semin Oncol* 1994; **21** (Suppl. 8): 9–14.
3 Gelmon K. The taxoids: paclitaxel and docetaxel. *Lancet* 1994; **344**: 1267–72.
4 van Herpen CM, van Hoesel QG, Punt CJ. Paclitaxel-induced severe hypersensitivity reaction occurring as a late toxicity. *Ann Oncol* 1995; **6**: 852.
5 Berghmans T, Klastersky J. Paclitaxel-induced cutaneous toxicity. *Support Care Cancer* 1995; **3**: 203–4.
6 Payne JY, Holmes F, Cohen P *et al.* Paclitaxel: severe mucocutaneous toxicity in a patient with hyperbilirubinemia. *South Med J* 1996; **89**: 542–5.
7 Essayan DM, Kagey-Sobotka A, Colarusso PJ *et al.* Successful parenteral desensitization to paclitaxel. *J Allergy Clin Immunol* 1996; **97**: 42–6.
8 Young PC, Montemarano AD, Lee N *et al.* Hypersensitivity to paclitaxel manifested as a bullous fixed drug eruption. *J Am Acad Dermatol* 1996; **34**: 313–14.
9 Raymond E, Cartier S, Canuel C *et al.* Extravasation de paclitaxel (Taxol). *Rev Med Int* 1995; **16**: 141–2.
10 Meehan JL, Sporn JR. Case report of Taxol administration via central vein producing a recall reaction at a site of prior Taxol extravasation. *J Natl Cancer Inst* 1994; **86**: 1250–1.

Suramin

Suramin sodium, a polysulphonated naphthylurea used in the treatment of onchocerciasis and trypanosomiasis and for metastatic prostatic and other cancers, has caused generalized, erythematous, maculopapular eruptions within the first 24h of therapy, which were self-limited despite continued drug infusion; keratoacanthoma; and disseminated superficial actinic porokeratosis [1–3]. Distinctive findings include scaling erythematous papules (suramin keratoses) and a predilection for previously sun-exposed areas (UV recall). Severe cutaneous reactions occur in 10% of cases [3]. Histopathological findings have included hyperkeratosis, parakeratosis, spongiosis, acanthosis, exocytosis, apoptosis, a perivascular lympho-histiocytic infiltrate, upper dermal oedema and increased dermal mucin [3]. Erythema multiforme [4] and TEN [5,6] are recorded.

REFERENCES

1 O'Donnell BP, Dawson NA, Weiss RB *et al.* Suramin-induced skin reactions. *Arch Dermatol* 1992; **128**: 75–9.
2 Wichterich K, Tebbe B, Handke A *et al.* Kutane Arzneimittelreaktion durch Suramin bei 4 Patienten mit metastasierendem Prostata-Karzinom. *Hautarzt* 1994; **45**: 84–7.
3 Lowitt MH, Eisenberger M, Sina B, Kao GF. Cutaneous eruptions from suramin. A clinical and histopathologic study of 60 patients. *Arch Dermatol* 1995; **131**: 1147–53.
4 Katz SK, Medenica MM, Kobayashi K *et al.* Erythema multiforme induced by suramin. *J Am Acad Dermatol* 1995; **32**: 292–3.
5 May E, Allolio B. Fatal toxic epidermal necrolysis during suramin therapy. *Eur J Cancer* 1991; **28A**: 1294.
6 Falkson G, Rapoport BL. Lethal toxic epidermal necrolysis during suramin therapy. *Eur J Cancer* 1992; **27**: 1338.

Triazinate

Acanthosis nigricans-like hyperpigmentation has been recorded [1].

REFERENCE

1 Greenspan AH, Shupack JL, Foo S-H. Acanthosis nigricans-like hyper-pigmentation secondary to triazinate therapy. *Arch Dermatol* 1985; **121**: 232–5.

Topical nitrogen mustard

Urticaria, anaphylactoid reactions, and a local bullous reaction have been recorded [1,2]. Contact dermatitis is well recognized.

REFERENCES

1 Daughters D, Zackheim H, Maibach H. Urticaria and anaphylactoid reactions after topical application of mechlorethamine. *Arch Dermatol* 1973; **107**: 429–30.
2 Goday JJ, Aguirre A, Raton JA *et al.* Local bullous reaction to topical mechlorethamine (mustine). *Contact Dermatitis* 1990; **22**: 306–7.

Drugs affecting the immune response

Cyclosporin A

Cyclosporin A is a ligand for the immunophilin, cyclophilin A, and is thought to block early events in T-cell gene activation, by interfering with the intracellular translocation of a substance known as nuclear factor of activated T cells [1,2]. It selectively inhibits antigen-induced activation of, and IL-2 production by, CD4+-helper T lymphocytes, thereby blocking T-cell proliferation [3,4]. It inhibits transcription of genes encoding for IL-2 and IFN-γ [5], and blocks expression of IL-2 receptors. Cyclosporin also inhibits Langerhans' cell antigen-presenting function [6–8], and suppresses ICAM-1 expression by papillary endothelium in inflamed skin, thus reducing T-cell recruitment [9]. Much of the information on side-effects is derived from patients who have undergone organ transplants, and in diseases such as rheumatoid arthritis [10]. However, this drug is now being increasingly used by dermatologists [11–18], especially in the management of difficult psoriasis [13–16], but also in refractory atopic eczema [17] and a number of other conditions [16].

Hypertrichosis develops in a high proportion of patients; it affects especially the face and eyebrows, the upper back along the spinal column and the lateral upper arms [18–23]. The hypertrichosis is reversible, and children and adolescents seem to be at a greater risk of developing this complication [23]. Other cutaneous complications include gingival hyperplasia [21,24], angio-oedema [25] and hyperplastic pseudofolliculitis barbae [26]. Anaphylaxis may occur in response to intravenous cyclosporin [11], probably due to the solvent. A mild capillary leak syndrome has resulted in purpuric lesions in the flexures and at pressure points [27].

There have been isolated reports of the development of benign lymphocytic infiltrates in patients with psoriasis or alopecia areata [28,29], of pseudolymphoma after therapy of actinic reticuloid [30], and of an aggressive T-cell lymphoma after cyclosporin therapy for Sézary syndrome [31]. Squamous cell skin cancer may develop [32–34] and could potentially be predisposed to by previous PUVA [6]. A recent study showed no difference in the incidence of cutaneous malignancy between renal allograft recipients treated either with cyclosporin or azathioprine [34]. Kaposi's sarcoma may occur; a renal transplant patient treated with cyclosporin and methylprednisolone developed a Kaposi's sarcoma, which completely regressed on reducing the dosage of both drugs [35]. There have been isolated reports of development of malignant melanoma in cyclosporin-treated patients, but the incidence of this complication does not seem to be increased above the risk in the general population [36,37].

Headache and rarely seizures [38], gastrointestinal and musculoskeletal symptoms are well recognized. There is an increased risk of nephrotoxicity [39,40], which appears to be caused by arteriolar vasoconstriction due to local thromboxane A_2 release [41], and consequent hypertension [42]. Impaired renal function may develop after short- as well as long-term treatment for psoriasis [43]. Both renal dysfunction and hypertension are reversible, and lymphoma development is unlikely, in patients on short-term low-dose (less than 5 mg/kg) therapy. Adverse effects on renal function and systolic blood pressure appear greater in psoriasis patients receiving higher doses [15]. Rarely, a serious capillary leak syndrome, which may be fatal, occurs, with marked fluid retention and periorbital oedema; there may be associated gastrointestinal bleeding, pneumonitis, uraemia and urinary sodium loss followed by hypertension and convulsions [21]. Hepatotoxicity is a complication [44], and hypercholesterolemia is recorded [45]. Cyclosporin may be associated with myopathy without rhabdomyolysis, or with rhabdomyolysis; the latter occurs in the setting of concomitant lovastatin or colchicine therapy [46]. Lymphoma and other cancers have developed on high dosage as for organ grafting [19,47]. Transplant patients treated with cyclosporin have not been shown to have a higher incidence of neoplasms than those receiving other immunosuppressive agents.

A successful pregnancy occurred in a patient receiving cyclosporin for psoriasis [48]. There is no evidence of a teratogenic effect in humans, based on the experience of 107 transplant recipients [49].

Interactions with cyclosporine and other drugs have been reviewed [50]. Cyclosporin blood levels may be increased by concomitant therapy with erythromycin or ketoconazole, as a result of inhibition of the hepatic microsomal cytochrome P-450 enzyme system [51], as well as by danazol and norethindrone, oral contraceptives and calcium-channel antagonists. Decreased blood levels may be caused by drugs that induce hepatic enzymes, including phenytoin, phenobarbital, and tuberculostatic therapy with rifampicin and isoniazid. Aminoglycoside antibiotics, melphalan, amphotericin B and trimethoprim alone or in combination with sulphamethoxazole, interact with cyclosporin by altering renal function. Patients should avoid grapefruit juice taken within 1 h of oral cyclosporin, as it contains a psoralen that inhibits the CYP3A subfamily of cytochrome P-450 and reduces metabolism of cyclosporin [52].

REFERENCES

1 Gallagher RB, Cambier JC. Signal transmission pathways and lymphocyte function. *Immunol Today* 1990; **11**: 187–9.

2 Anon. Unmasking immunosuppression. *Lancet* 1991; **338**: 789.

3 Ryffel B. Pharmacology of cyclosporine. 6. Cellular activation: regulation of intracellular events by cyclosporine. *Pharmacol Rev* 1989; **41**: 407–22.

4 Borel JF. Pharmacology of cyclosporin (Sandimmune). 4. Pharmacological properties *in vivo*. *Pharmacol Rev* 1989; **41**: 259–371.

5 Granelli-Piperno A. Lymphokine gene expression *in vivo* is inhibited by cyclosporin A. *J Exp Med* 1990; **171**: 533–44.

6 Furue M, Katz SI. The effects of cyclosporin on epidermal cells. I. Cyclosporin inhibits accessory cell functions of epidermal Langerhans cells *in vitro*. *J Immunol* 1988; **140**: 4139–43.

7 Demidem A, Taylor JR, Grammer SF, Streilein JW. Comparison of effects of transforming growth factor-beta and cyclosporin A on antigen-presenting cells of blood and epidermis. *J Invest Dermatol* 1991; **96**: 401–7.

8 Dupuy P, Bagot M, Michel L *et al*. Cyclosporin A inhibits the antigen-presenting functions of freshly isolated human Langerhans cells *in vitro*. *J Invest Dermatol* 1991; **96**: 408–13.

9 Petzelbauer P, Stingl G, Wolff K, Volc-Platzer B. Cyclosporin A suppresses ICAM-1 expression by papillary endothelium in healing psoriatic plaques. *J Invest Dermatol* 1991; **96**: 362–9.

10 Dougados M, Awada H, Amor B. Cyclosporin in rheumatoid arthritis: a double blind placebo controlled study in 52 patients. *Ann Rheum Dis* 1988; **47**: 127–33.

11 Gupta AK, Brown MD, Ellis CN *et al*. Cyclosporine in dermatology. *J Am Acad Dermatol* 1989; **21**: 1245–56.

12 Fradin MS, Ellis CN, Voorhees JJ. Management of patients and side effects during cyclosporine therapy for cutaneous disorders. *J Am Acad Dermatol* 1990; **23**: 1265–74.

13 De Rie MA, Meinardi MMHM, Bos JD. Analysis of side-effects of medium- and low-dose cyclosporin maintenance therapy in psoriasis. *Br J Dermatol* 1990; **123**: 347–53.

14 Mihatsch MJ, Wolff K, eds. Risk/benefit ratio of cyclosporin A (Sandimmun®) in psoriasis. *Br J Dermatol* 1990; **122** (Suppl. 36): 1–115.

15 Ellis CN, Fradin MS, Messana JM *et al*. Cyclosporine for plaque-type psoriasis. Results of a multidose, double-blind trial. *N Engl J Med* 1991; **324**: 277–84.

16 Ellis CN, ed. Cyclosporine in dermatology. Proceedings of a symposium. *J Am Acad Dermatol* 1991; **23**: 1231–4.

17 Sowden JM, Berth-Jones J, Ross JS *et al*. Double-blind, controlled, crossover study of cyclosporin in adults with severe refractory atopic dermatitis. *Lancet* 1991; **338**: 137–40.

18 Fradin MS, Ellis CN, Voorhees JJ. Management of patients and side effects during cyclosporine therapy for cutaneous disorders. *J Am Acad Dermatol* 1990; **23**: 1265–75.

19 European Multicentre Trial. Cyclosporin A as sole immunosuppressive agent in recipients of kidney allografts from cadaver donors. Preliminary results. *Lancet* 1982; **ii**: 57–60.

20 Mortimer PS, Thompson JF, Dawber RP *et al.* Hypertrichosies and multiple cutaneous squamous cell carcinomas in association with cyclosporin A therapy. *J R Soc Med* 1983; **76**: 786–7.

21 Harper JI, Kendra JR, Desai S *et al.* Dermatological aspects of the use of Cyclosporin A for prophylaxis of graft-versus-host disease. *Br J Dermatol* 1984; **110**: 469–74.

22 Bencini PL, Montagnino G, Sala F *et al.* Cutaneous lesions in 67 cyclosporin-treated renal transplant recipients. *Dermatologica* 1986; **172**: 24–30.

23 Wysocki GP, Daley TD. Hypertrichosis in patients receiving cyclosporine therapy. *Clin Exp Dermatol* 1987; **12**: 191–6.

24 Bennett JA, Christian JM. Cyclosporin-induced gingival hyperplasia: case report and literature review. *J Am Dent Assoc* 1985; **3**: 272–3.

25 Isenberg DA, Snaith ML, Al-Khader AA *et al.* Cyclosporin relieves arthralgia, causes angioedema. *N Engl J Med* 1980; **303**: 754.

26 Lear J, Bourke JF, Burns DA. Hyperplastic pseudofolliculitis barbae associated with cyclosporin. *Br J Dermatol* 1997; **136**: 132–3.

27 Ramon D, Bettloch E, Jimenez A *et al.* Remission of Sézary's syndrome with cyclosporin A. Mild capillary leak syndrome as an unusual side effect. *Acta Derm Venereol (Stockh)* 1986; **66**: 80–2.

28 Brown MD, Ellis CN, Billings J *et al.* Rapid occurrence of nodular cutaneous T-lymphocyte infiltrates with cyclosporine therapy. *Arch Dermatol* 1988; **124**: 1097–100.

29 Gupta AK, Cooper KD, Ellis CN *et al.* Lymphocytic infiltrates of the skin in association with cyclosporine therapy. *J Am Acad Dermatol* 1990; **23**: 1137–41.

30 Thestrup-Pedersen K, Zachariae C, Kaltoft K *et al.* Development of cutaneous pseudolymphoma following ciclosporin therapy of actinic reticuloid. *Dermatologica* 1988; **177**: 376–81.

31 Catterall MD, Addis BJ, Smith JL, Coode PE. Sézary syndrome: transformation to a high grade T-cell lymphoma after treatment with Cyclosporin A. *Clin Exp Dermatol* 1983; **8**: 159–69.

32 Thompson JF, Allen R, Morris PJ, Wood R. Skin cancer in renal transplant patients treated with cyclosporin. *Lancet* 1985; **i**: 158–9.

33 Stern RS. Risk assessment of PUVA and cyclosporine. Lessons from the past: challenges for the future. *Arch Dermatol* 1989; **125**: 545–7.

34 Bunney MH, Benton EC, Barr BB *et al.* The prevalence of skin disorders in renal allograft recipients receiving cyclosporin A compared with those receiving azathioprine. *Nephrol Dial Transplant* 1990; **5**: 379–82.

35 Pilgrim M. Spontane Manifestation und Regression eines Kaposi-Sarkoms unter Cyclosporin A. *Hautarzt* 1988; **39**: 368–70.

36 Mérot Y, Miescher PA, Balsiger F *et al.* Cutaneous malignant melanomas occurring under cyclosporin A therapy: a report of two cases. *Br J Dermatol* 1990; **123**: 237–9.

37 Arellano F, Krupp PF. Cutaneous malignant melanoma occurring after cyclosporin A therapy. *Br J Dermatol* 1991; **124**: 611.

38 Humphreys TR, Leyden JJ. Acute reversible central nervous system toxicity associated with low-dose oral cyclosporin therapy. *J Am Acad Dermatol* 1993; **29**: 490–2.

39 Myers BD, Ross J, Newton L *et al.* Cyclosporine-associated chronic nephropathy. *N Engl J Med* 1984; **311**: 699–705.

40 Myers BD, Sibley R, Newton L *et al.* The long-term course of cyclosporine-associated chronic nephropathy. *Kidney Int* 1988; **33**: 590–600.

41 Coffman TM, Carr DR, Yarger WE, Klotman PE. Evidence that renal prostaglandin and thromboxane production is stimulated in chronic cyclosporine nephrotoxicity. *Transplantation* 1987; **43**: 282–5.

42 Porter GAM, Bennett WM, Sheps SG. Cyclosporine-associated hypertension. *Arch Intern Med* 1990; **150**: 280–3.

43 Powles AV, Carmichael D, Julme B *et al.* Renal function after long-term low-dose cyclosporin for psoriasis. *Br J Dermatol* 1990; **122**: 665–9.

44 Lorber MI, Van Buren CT, Flechner SM *et al.* Hepatobiliary and pancreatic complications of cyclosporine therapy in 466 renal transplant recipients. *Transplantation* 1987; **43**: 35–40.

45 Ballantyne CM, Podet EJ, Patsch WP *et al.* Effects of cyclosporine therapy on plasma lipoprotein levels. *JAMA* 1989; **262**: 53–6.

46 Arellano F, Krupp P. Muscular disorders associated with cyclosporin. *Lancet* 1991; **337**: 915.

47 Penn I, First MR. Development and incidence of cancer following cyclosporin therapy. *Transplant Proc* 1986; **18** (Suppl. 1): 210–13.

48 Wright S, Glover M, Baker H. Psoriasis, cyclosporine, and pregnancy. *Arch Dermatol* 1991; **127**: 426.

49 Cockburn I, Krupp P, Monka C. Present experience of Sandimmune in pregnancy. *Transplant Proc* 1989; **21**: 3730–2.

50 Yee GC, McGuire TR. Pharmacokinetic drug interactions with cyclosporin (Part I). *Clin Pharmacokinet* 1990; **19**: 319–32.

51 Abel EA. Isotretinoin treatment of severe cystic acne in a heart transplant patient receiving cyclosporine: consideration of drug interactions. *J Am Acad Dermatol* 1991; **24**: 511.

52 Anonymous. Drug interactions with grapefruit. *Curr Probl Pharmacovig* 1997; **23**: 2.

PUVA therapy

See Chapter 35.

Immunotherapy

Sera

Animal immune sera can produce any type of early or late hypersensitivity reactions, from urticaria, asthma or fatal anaphylaxis to serum sickness. Clinical manifestations of serum sickness include fever, arthritis, nephritis, neuritis, myocarditis, uveitis, oedema and an urticarial or papular rash. A characteristic serpiginous, erythematous and purpuric eruption developed on the hands and feet, at the borders of palmar and plantar skin, in patients treated with equine antithymocyte globulin [1,2]. Low serum C4 and C3 levels, elevated plasma C3a anaphylatoxin levels, and circulating immune complexes were found. Immunoreactants, including IgM, C3, IgE, and IgA, were deposited in the walls of dermal blood vessels on direct immunofluorescence [1,2]. Patients with autoimmune disease may have a particular liability to react to anti-lymphocyte globulin.

REFERENCES

1 Lawley TJ, Bielory L, Gascon P *et al.* A prospective clinical and immunologic analysis of patients with serum sickness. *N Engl J Med* 1984; **311**: 1407–13.

2 Bielory L, Yancey KB, Young NS *et al.* Cutaneous manifestations of serum sickness in patients receiving antithymocyte globulin. *J Am Acad Dermatol* 1985; **13**: 411–17.

Vaccines

Overall the incidence of significant side-effects is very low. There were 2832 reports of adverse events associated with immunizing agents received by the Childhood Immunization Division of the Laboratory Centre for Disease Control, from more than 12 million doses of vaccines, in Canada during 1990 [1]. Only 39 of 43 618 Alaskan natives who received 101 360 doses of hepatitis B plasma-derived vaccine developed side-effects, including myalgia/arthralgia lasting longer than 3 days, skin rashes (eight patients) and dizziness [2]. Influenza vaccination in the elderly is, however, reported to cause no more systemic side-effects than placebo [3]. Another study, by contrast, found local reactions in 17.5% of patients, including swelling, itching and pain [4]. Measles and measles–mumps–rubella vaccine, hepatitis B vaccine, and diphtheria and tetanus toxoids have been statistically associated with anaphylaxis [5], and measles–mumps–rubella vaccine with thrombocytopenia and purpura [5,6]. Local reactions include erythema, swelling and tenderness, which may result from an Arthus reaction [7–9]. Keloid scarring may develop. Local inflammatory reactions, fever, lymphadenopathy, urticaria and lichenoid rashes have been observed following vaccination in patients sensitive to the preservative merthiolate; patch testing and intradermal testing may be positive [10,11]. Inflammatory nodular reactions may occur as a result of aluminium sensitization, as with hepatitis B, diphtheria and tetanus vaccination [12,13]; patch testing to aluminium may be positive [12]. Itching, eczema and circumscribed hypertrichosis developed over nodules following immunization with vaccines absorbed on aluminium hydroxide in three children [13]. Transient subcutaneous nodule formation at the injection site, and increased regional adenopathy, have been rarely noted in patients with HIV infection treated with gp160 vaccination [14].

Urticaria, angio-oedema or anaphylaxis may occur in patients vaccinated with live measles vaccine, who are allergic to egg protein. However, in a series of children with egg allergy and a positive skin-prick test with egg white, 0.98% developed a mild reaction not requiring therapy following immunization with a full dose of vaccine [15]. Three per cent of 98 patients with a history of previous human diploid cell rabies vaccine inoculations developed generalized urticaria or wheezing within 1 day, and a further 3% developed urticaria 6–14 days, after booster vaccination [16]. Urticaria and systemic symptoms including malaise and fever, or Stevens–Johnson syndrome may follow tetanus toxoid vaccination [17,18]. Vaccination may result in development of an autoimmune state; dermatomyositis has been provoked. Fatalities have rarely occurred following vaccination as a result of anaphylaxis [19,20]. Vaccination against Japanese encephalitis caused serious adverse reactions, including urticaria, angio-oedema, hypotension and collapse [21]. An association with vaccination for influenza and with tetanus toxoid and induction of bullous pemphigoid has been noted rarely [22–24].

REFERENCES

1 Duclos P, Pless R, Koch J, Hardy M. Adverse events temporally associated with immunizing agents. *Can Fam Psysician* 1993; **39**: 1907–13.
2 McMahon BJ, Helminiak C, Wainwright RB *et al*. Frequency of adverse reactions to hepatitis B vaccine in 43,618 persons. *Am J Med* 1992; **92**: 254–6.
3 Margolis KL, Nichol KL, Poland GA, Pluhar RE. Frequency of adverse reactions to influenza vaccine in the elderly. A randomized, placebo-controlled trial. *JAMA* 1990; **264**: 1139–41.
4 Govaert TME, Dinant GJ, Aretz K *et al*. Adverse reactions to influenza vaccine in elderly people: randomised double blind placebo controlled trial. *Br Med J* 1993; **307**: 988–90.
5 Stratton KR, Howe CJ, Johnson RB, Jr. Adverse events associated with childhood vaccines other than pertussis and rubella. Summary of a report from the Institute of Medicine. *JAMA* 1994; **271**: 1602–5.
6 Farrington P, Pugh S, Colville A *et al*. A new method for active surveillance of adverse events from diphtheria/tetanus/pertussis and measles/mumps/rubella vaccines. *Lancet* 1995; **345**: 567–9.
7 Jacobs RL, Lowe RS, Lanier BQ. Adverse reactions to tetanus toxoid. *JAMA* 1982; **247**: 40–2.
8 Sutter RW. Adverse reactions to tetanus toxoid. *JAMA* 1994; **271**: 1629.
9 Marrinan LM, Andrews G, Alsop-Shields L, Dugdale AE. Side effects of rubella immunisation in teenage girls. *Med J Aust* 1990; **153**: 631–2.
10 Noel I, Galloway A, Ive FA. Hypersensitivity to thiomersal in hepatitis B vaccine. *Lancet* 1991; **338**: 705.
11 Rueff F. Nebenwirkungen durch Thiomersal und Huhnereiweiss bei Impfungen. *Hautarzt* 1994; **45**: 879–81.
12 Cosnes A, Flechet M-L, Revuz J. Inflammatory nodular reactions after hepatitis B vaccination due to aluminium sensitization. *Contact Dermatitis* 1990; **23**: 65–7.
13 Pembroke AC, Marten RH. Unusual cutaneous reactions following diphtheria and tetanus immunization. *Clin Exp Dermatol* 1979; **4**: 345–8.
14 Redfield RR, Birx DL, Ketter N *et al*. A phase I evaluation of the safety and immunogenicity of vaccination with recombinant gp160 in patients with early human immunodeficiency virus infection. *N Engl J Med* 1991; **324**: 1677–84.
15 Aickin R, Hill D, Kemp A. Measles immunisation in children with allergy to egg. *Br Med J* 1994; **309**: 223–5.
16 Fishbein DB, Yenne KM, Dreesen DW *et al*. Risk factors for systemic hypersensitivity reactions after booster vaccinations with human diploid cell rabies vaccine: a nationwide prospective study. *Vaccine* 1993; **11**: 1390–4.
17 Kuhlwein A, Bleyl A. Tetanusantitoxintiter und Reaktionen nach Tetanusimpfungen. *Hautarzt* 1985; **36**: 462–4.
18 Weisse ME, Bass JW. Tetanus toxoid allergy. *JAMA* 1990; **264**: 2448.
19 Boston Collaborative Drug Surveillance Program. Drug-induced anaphylaxis. A cooperative study. *JAMA* 1973; **224**: 613–15.
20 Lockey RF, Benedict LM, Turkeltaub PC, Bukantz SC. Fatalities from immunotherapy (IT) and skin testing (ST). *J Allergy Clin Immunol* 1987; **79**: 660–77.
21 Ruff TA, Eisen D, Fuller A, Kass R. Adverse reactions to Japanese encephalitis vaccine. *Lancet* 1991; **338**: 881–2.
22 Bodokh I, Lacour JP, Bourdet JF *et al*. Réactivation de pemphigoïde bulleuse apres vaccination antigrippale. *Thérapie* 1994; **49**: 154.
23 Venning VA, Wojnarowska F. Induced bullous pemphigoid. *Br J Dermatol* 1995; **132**: 831–2.
24 Fournier B, Descamps V, Bouscarat F *et al*. Bullous pemphigoid induced by vaccination. *Br J Dermatol* 1996; **135**: 153–4.

Hyposensitization immunotherapy

Hyposensitization immunotherapy is a standard therapy for recalcitrant hayfever and bee or wasp stings in many countries in the world, including the US, Scandinavia, and the continent of Europe [1]. However, in the UK, allergen-injection immunotherapy for IgE-mediated diseases has been largely discontinued, following the recommendations of the Committee on Safety of Medicines in 1986 [2], because of concern about deaths related to bronchospasm and anaphylaxis. The Committee recommended that immunotherapy be given only where full facilities for cardiopulmonary resuscitation are available, and that patients be kept under medical observation for at least 2 h. The necessity for the latter recommendation has been questioned recently, since serious reactions occur within minutes [1]. The British Society for Allergy and

Clinical Immunology Working Party concluded that specific allergen immunotherapy for summer hayfever uncontrolled by conventional medication and for wasp and bee venom hypersensitivity has an acceptable risk/benefit ratio, provided that treatment is given by experienced practitioners in a clinic where full resuscitative facilities are immediately available; a symptom-free observation period of 60 min after injection is sufficient [3,4]. Patients with asthma should be excluded however, in view of an increased frequency of reactions [4,5]. Fatalities from allergen immunotherapy are extremely rare [6]. Beta-blocker drugs did not increase the frequency of systemic reactions in patients receiving allergen immunotherapy in one series, but patients developed more severe systemic reactions that were more refractory to therapy [7].

Local urticarial reactions are by contrast common [1]. Desensitization injections for hayfever have resulted in occasional tender nodules lasting for several months or years [8,9]; these are thought to develop as a result of allergy to aluminium, as it is present in the lesions and patch tests may be positive [9]. Inflammatory nodules at injection sites, first developing several years later, have also been described [10]. Injections of mixtures of grass pollens, cereal pollens and dust-mite allergens have resulted in multiple cutaneous B-cell pseudolymphomas [11]. Vasculitis [12–14] and serum sickness [15] have been described following hyposensitization therapy as for pollen and house-dust-mite allergy. Cold urticaria developed during the course of hyposensitization to wasp venom [16].

REFERENCES

1 Varney VA, Gaga M, Frew AJ *et al.* Usefulness of immunotherapy in patients with severe summer hay fever uncontrolled by antiallergic drugs. *Br Med J* 1991; **302**: 265–9.
2 Anonymous. CSM update. Desensitising Vaccines. *Br Med J* 1986; **293**: 948.
3 Anonymous. Position paper on allergen immunotherapy. Report of a BSACI working party. January–October 1992. *Clin Exp Allergy* 1993; **23** (Suppl. 3): 1–44.
4 British Society for Allergy and Clinical Immunology Working Party. Injection immunotherapy. *Br Med J* 1993; **307**: 919–23.
5 Bousquet J, Michel FB. Safety considerations in assessing the role of immunotherapy in allergic disorders. *Drug Saf* 1994; **10**: 5–17.
6 Lockey RF, Benedict LM, Turkeltaub PC, Bukantz SC. Fatalities from immunotherapy and skin testing. *J Allergy Clin Immunol* 1987; **79**: 660–77.
7 Hepner MJ, Ownby DR, Anderson JA *et al.* Risk of systemic reactions in patients taking beta-blocker drugs receiving allergen immunotherapy injections. *J Allergy Clin Immunol* 1990; **86**: 407–11.
8 Osterballe O. Side effects during immunotherapy with purified grass pollen extracts. *Allergy* 1982; **37**: 553–62.
9 Frost L, Johansen S, Pedersen S *et al.* Persistent subcutaneous nodules in children hypo-sensitised with aluminium-containing allergen extracts. *Allergy* 1985; **40**: 368–72.
10 Jones SK, Lovell CR, Peachey RDG. Delayed onset of inflammatory nodules following hay fever desensitization injections. *Clin Exp Dermatol* 1988; **13**: 376–8.
11 Goerdt S, Spieker T, Wölffer L-U *et al.* Multiple cutaneous B-cell pseudolymphomas after allergen injections. *J Am Acad Dermatol* 1996; **35**: 1072–4.
12 Phanuphak P, Kohler PF. Onset of polyarteritis nodosa during allergic hyposensitisation treatment. *Am J Med* 1980; **68**: 479–85.
13 Merk H, Kober ML. Vasculitis nach spezifischer Hyposensibilisierung. *Z Hautkr* 1982; **57**: 1682–5.
14 Berbis P, Carena MC, Auffranc JC, Privat Y. Vascularite nécrosante cutanéo-systémique survenue en cours de désensibilisation. *Ann Dermatol Vénéréol* 1986; **113**: 805–9.
15 Umetsu DT, Hahn JS, Perez-Atayde AR, Geha RS. Serum sickness triggered by anaphylaxis: a complication of immunotherapy. *J Allergy Clin Immunol* 1985; **76**: 713–16.
16 Anfosso-Capra F, Philip-Joet F, Reynaud-Gaubert M, Arnaud A. Occurrence of cold urticaria during venom desensitization. *Dermatologica* 1990; **181**: 276–7.

BCG vaccination

Vaccination with BCG causes a benign, self-limiting lesion consisting of a small papule, pustule or ulcer, which heals to leave a small scar within weeks. Axillary lymphadenitis and abscesses occurred after vaccination of rural Haitian children [1], and disseminated BCG infection in children born to HIV-1-infected women [2]. Occasionally, local abscess formation may follow vaccination of strongly tuberculin positive individuals, administration of too much vaccine; or injecting it too deeply [3–5]. BCG abscesses may also rarely arise following needlestick injury in health-care professionals [6]. In Austria, where the Ministry of Health's recommendation is for all neonates to be vaccinated, the normal complication rate is between 0.3 and 0.6%, with suppurative lymphadenitis, generalized lymphadenopathy and osteitis [7]. This rate temporarily increased substantially, with 5% of 659 children vaccinated at the University Hospital, Innsbruck, requiring surgical excision of suppurating lymph nodes, following a change to use of a more virulent strain [7]. Anaphylactoid reactions to BCG vaccine, probably as a result of immune complex reactions mediated by antibodies to dextran in the vaccine, have been reported [8]. A papulonecrotic type of vasculitis has been documented [9]. Dermatomyositis may occasionally be a complication [10].

BCG immunotherapy for malignant melanoma has been associated with [11]: local ulceration [11,12], local recurrent erysipelas, keloid formation, influenza-like symptoms, lymphadenopathy, urticaria and angio-oedema, granulomatous hepatitis, arthritis [13] and reactivation of pulmonary tuberculosis. Widespread miliary granulomas were present in a patient with fatal disseminated infection following intralesional immunotherapy of cutaneous malignant melanoma [14].

REFERENCES

1 Bonnlander H, Rossignol AM. Complications of BCG vaccinations in rural Haiti. *Am J Public Health* 1993; **83**: 583–5.
2 O'Brien KL, Andrae JR, Marie AL *et al.* Bacillus Calmette-Guérin complications in children born to HIV-1-infected women with a review of literature. *Pediatrics* 1995; **95**: 414–17.
3 Lotte A, Wasz-Hockert O, Poisson N *et al.* BCG complications. *Adv Tuberculosis Res* 1984; **21**: 107–93, 194–245.
4 de Souza GRM, Sant'anna CC, Lapa e Silva JR *et al.* Intradermal BCG complications—analysis of 51 cases. *Tubercle* 1983; **64**: 23–7.

5 Puliyel JM, Hughes A, Chiswick ML, Mughal MZ. Adverse local reactions from accidental BCG overdose in infants. *Br Med J* 1996; **313**: 528–9.

6 Warren JP, Nairn DS, Robertson MH. Cold abscess after accidental BCG inoculation. *Lancet* 1984; **ii**: 289.

7 Hengster P, Fille M, Menardi G. Suppurative lymphadenitis in newborn babies after change of BCG vaccine. *Lancet* 1991; **337**: 1168–9.

8 Rudin C, Amacher A, Berglund A. Anaphylactoid reactions to BCG vaccination. *Lancet* 1991; **337**: 377.

9 Lübbe D. Vasculitis allergica vom papulonekrotischen Typ nach BCG-Impfung. *Dermatol Mschr* 1982; **168**: 186–92.

10 Kass E, Staume S, Mellbye OJ *et al.* Dermatomyositis associated with BCG vaccination. *Scand J Rheumatol* 1979; **8**: 187–91.

11 Schult C. Nebenwirkungen der BCG-Immuntherapie bei 511 Patienten mit malignen Melanom. *Hautarzt* 1984; **35**: 78–83.

12 Korting HC, Strasser S, Konz B. Multiple BCG-Ulzera nach subkutaner Impfstoffapplikation im Rahmen der Immunochemotherapie des malignen Melanoms. *Hautarzt* 1988; **39**: 170–3.

13 Torisu M, Miyahara T, Shinohara A *et al.* A new side effect of BCG immunotherapy: BCG-induced arthritis in man. *Cancer Immunol Immunother* 1978; **5**: 77–83.

14 de la Monte SM, Hutchins GM. Fatal disseminated bacillus Calmette-Guérin infection and arrested growth of cutaneous malignant melanoma following intralesional immunotherapy. *Am J Dermatopathol* 1986; **8**: 331–5.

Cytokines

Cytokines are being increasingly used in the management of neoplastic and haematological disorders and AIDS, and in addition are starting to be used for the therapy of specific dermatological disorders; side-effects have been reviewed [1]. Reactions range from minor injection site reactions, pruritus and flushing to life-threatening autoimmune disorders, severe erythroderma or bullous skin reactions [2].

REFERENCES

1 Luger TA, Schwarz T. Therapeutic use of cytokines in dermatology. *J Am Acad Dermatol* 1991; **24**: 915–26.

2 Asnis LA, Gaspari AA. Cutaneous reactions to recombinant cytokine therapy. *J Am Acad Dermatol* 1995; **33**: 393–410.

Colony-stimulating factors

Recombinant haematopoietic colony-stimulating factors used in the treatment of haematological disorders are usually well tolerated, but may induce itching and erythema at the site of subcutaneous injection, thrombophlebitis with intravenous infusion, facial flushing and a transient maculopapular eruption, fever, chills, myalgias, arthralgia and bone pain, transient leukopenia, decreased appetite, nausea, and mild elevation of transaminase levels [1]. Two types of recombinant human granulocyte colony-stimulating factor (G-CSF) are in use for neutropenia; one is a glycosylated natural product from mammalian cells, and the other a non-glycosylated form from *Escherichia coli*. A drug eruption may occur with either type without detectable antibodies; intradermal tests may be useful and there may not be cross-reactivity [2]. Both local reactions at the site of injection and diffuse maculopapular eruptions may be seen [2–5]. Local pustular reactions [6] or subcorneal pustular dermatosis [7] are documented. Intravenous recombinant granulocyte–macrophage colony-stimulating factor (GM-CSF) therapy for leukaemia resulted in a widespread confluent maculopapular eruption in three patients, associated with a dermal lymphocyte, macrophage and granulocyte infiltration, exocytosis, and keratinocyte ICAM-1 expression [8]. Nine of 23 patients with advanced malignancy treated with GM-CSF had a cutaneous eruption characterized by local erythema and pruritus at the injection site, recall erythema at previous injection sites or a generalized maculopapular rash [9]. Other studies have reported widespread rashes [10,11], in one series manifested as annular erythematous papules and plaques on the extremities, becoming generalized and clearing with fine desquamation [11]. Recurrent exacerbation of acne [12], widespread folliculitis [13] and a Sweet's syndrome-like rash [14–16] have been recorded. A capillary-leak syndrome with pleural and pericardial effusions, ascites and large-vessel thrombosis has been noted only with high-dose GM-CSF therapy [17]. Necrotizing vasculitis developed at GM-CSF injection sites in one patient with white-cell aplasia, but not in over 150 other neutropenic patients who received the drug [18]. However, vasculitis was reported in a large series [19]. Psoriasis [20], and arthritis in Felty's syndrome with rheumatoid arthritis [21], have been reported to deteriorate.

REFERENCES

1 Wakefield PE, James WD, Samlaska CP, Meltzer MS. Colony-stimulating factors. *J Am Acad Dermatol* 1990; **23**: 903–12.

2 Sasaki O, Yokoyama A, Uemura S *et al.* Drug eruption caused by recombinant human G-CSF. *Int Med* 1994; **33**: 641–3.

3 Schiro JA, Kupper TS. Cutaneous eruptions during GM-CSF infusion. Clues for cytokine biology. *Arch Dermatol* 1991; **127**: 110–12.

4 Samlaska CP, Noyes DK. Localized cutaneous reactions to granulocyte colony-stimulating factor. *Arch Dermatol* 1993; **129**: 645–6.

5 Scott GA. Report of three cases of cutaneous reactions to granulocyte macrophage-colony-stimulating factor and a review of the literature. *Am J Dermatopathol* 1995; **17**: 107–14.

6 Passweg J, Buser U, Tichelli A *et al.* Pustular eruption at the site of subcutaneous injection of recombinant human granulocyte-macrophage colony-stimulating factor. *Ann Hematol* 1991; **63**: 326–7.

7 Lautenschlager S, Itin PH, Hirsbrunner P, Büchner SA. Subcorneal pustular dermatosis at the injection site of recombinant human granulocyte-macrophage colony-stimulating fator in a patient with IgA myeloma. *J Am Acad Dermatol* 1994; **30**: 783–9.

8 Horn TD, Burke PJ, Karp JE, Hood AF. Intravenous administration of recombinant human granulocyte–macrophage colony-stimulating factor causes a cutaneous eruption. *Arch Dermatol* 1991; **127**: 49–52.

9 Lieschke GJ, Maher D, Cebon J *et al.* Effects of bacterially synthesized recombinant human granulocyte–macrophage colony-stimulating factor in patients with advanced malignancy. *Ann Intern Med* 1989; **110**: 357–64.

10 Yamashita N, Natsuaki M, Morita H *et al.* Cutaneous eruptions induced by granulocyte colony-stimulating factor in two cases of acute myelogenous leukemia. *J Dermatol* 1993; **20**: 473–7.

11 Glass LF, Fotopoulos T, Messina JL. A generalized cutaneous reaction induced by granulocyte colony-stimulating factor. *J Am Acad Dermatol* 1996; **34**: 455–9.

12 Lee PK, Dover JS. Recurrent exacerbation of acne by granulocyte colony-stimulating factor administration. *J Am Acad Dermatol* 1996; **34**: 855–6.

13 Ostlere LS, Harris D, Prentice HG, Rustin MH. Widespread folliculitis

induced by human granulocyte-colony-stimulating factor therapy. *Br J Dermatol* 1992; **127**: 193–4.

14 Karp DL. The Sweet syndrome or G-CSF reaction? *Ann Intern Med* 1992; **117**: 875–6.

15 Richard MA, Grob JJ, Laurans R *et al.* Sweet's syndrome induced by granulocyte colony-stimulating factor in a woman with congenital neutropenia. *J Am Acad Dermatol* 1996; **35**: 629–31.

16 Prevost-Blank PL, Shwayder AT. Sweet's syndrome secondary to granulocyte colony-stimulating factor. *J Am Acad Dermatol* 1996; **35**: 995–7.

17 Antman KS, Griffin JD, Elias A *et al.* Effect of recombinant human granulocyte–macrophage colony-stimulating factor on chemotherapy-induced myelosuppression. *N Engl J Med* 1988; **319**: 593–8.

18 Farmer KL, Kurzrock R, Duvic M. Necrotizing vasculitis at granulocyte–macrophage-colony-stimulating factor injection sites. *Arch Dermatol* 1990; **126**: 1243–4.

19 Jain KK. Cutaneous vasculitis associated with granulocyte colony-stimulating factor. *J Am Acad Dermatol* 1994; **31**: 213–15.

20 Kelly RI, Marsden RA. Granulocyte–macrophage colony-stimulating factor and psoriasis. *J Am Acad Dermatol* 1994; **30**: 144.

21 McMullin MF, Finch MB. Felty's syndrome treated with rhG-CSF associated with flare of arthritis and skin rash. *Clin Rheumatol* 1995; **14**: 204–8.

Interferon (IFN)

Cutaneous reactions to recombinant IFN given to patients with cancer or AIDS are frequent (5–10%) but usually of moderate degree. Most patients experience influenza-like symptoms following systemic therapy; reversible leukopenia and thrombocytopenia is recorded with higher dosage. Local reactions consist of erythema or induration at injection sites or urticaria [1–3]. One of 63 patients treated with IFN-γ for prophylaxis of infection in chronic granulomatous disease had a severe cutaneous reaction (unspecified), and rashes or injection-site erythema or tenderness occurred in 17% and 14% of cases, respectively [1]. Side-effects of intralesional injection of a sustained release formulation of IFN-α2b for the treatment of basal cell carcinomas in 33 patients included, in addition to various influenza-like systemic complaints, a rash in 6%, as well as local inflammation in 85% and local pruritus in 22% of cases [4]. Patch testing to IFN was positive in one case [3]. Transient, localized or disseminated oedematous, erythematous and/or papular changes, vesicles or petechiae were seen in six patients during intravenous IFN-α for chronic active hepatitis C, 5–14 days after starting therapy [5]. Eruptions disappeared in 10–14 days despite continuation of IFN-α; histology revealed upper dermal perivascular CD4+ lymphoid infiltration and oedema, with endothelial cell but not keratinocyte ICAM-I and E-selectin expression, suggesting a non-allergic mechanism. Skin ulceration or necrosis may be a serious problem with both IFN-α and -β [6–9]. Raynaud's phenomenon and digital necrosis induced by IFN-α is recorded [10]. Lichen planus had been documented during recombinant IFN-α therapy [11]. Reactivation of oral herpes simplex, and enhanced radiation toxicity have been recorded [12]. IFN-α2a for the treatment of cutaneous T-cell lymphoma has induced temporary alopecia [13]. By contrast, IFN-α therapy has caused increased growth of eyelashes [14]. No adverse cutaneous side-effects resulted from intralesional injection of IFN-γ in 10 patients treated for keloid scarring [15].

IFN-α used in the teatment of disseminated carcinoma [16,17] or intralesionally for viral warts [18], and IFN-β for multiple sclerosis [7], has been reported to exacerbate or trigger onset of psoriasis; psoriatic arthritis has also been triggered by IFN-α [19] and IFN-γ [20], and Reiter's syndrome by IFN-α [21]. Psoriasis appeared at the site of subcutaneous injection of recombinant IFN-γ in patients with psoriatic arthritis [22], and at the site of intralesional injection in a patient receiving recombinant IFN-β for a basal cell carcinoma [23]. Exacerbation of underlying autoimmune disease is documented with IFN-α [24]. Neutralizing antibodies to recombinant IFN-α may be produced [25]. Systemic LE has been recorded following IFN therapy of myelogenous leukaemia [26], and pemphigus vulgaris after IFN-β and IL-2 therapy for lymphoma [27].

REFERENCES

1 The International Chronic Granulomatous Disease Cooperative Study Group. A controlled trial of interferon gamma to prevent infection in chronic granulomatous disease. *N Engl J Med* 1991; **324**: 509–16.

2 Kerker BJ, Hood AF. Chemotherapy-induced cutaneous reactions. *Semin Dermatol* 1989; **8**: 173–81.

3 Detmar U, Agathos M, Nerl C. Allergy of delayed type to recombinant interferon α 2c. *Contact Dermatitis* 1989; **20**: 149–50.

4 Edwards L, Tucker SB, Perednia D *et al.* The effect of an intralesional sustained-release formulation of interferon alfa-2b on basal cell carcinomas. *Arch Dermatol* 1990; **126**: 1029–32.

5 Toyofuku K, Imayama S, Yasumoto S *et al.* Clinical and immunohistochemical studies of skin eruptions: relationship to administration of interferon-alpha. *J Dermatol* 1994; **21**: 732–7.

6 Cnudde F, Gharakhanian S, Luboinski J *et al.* Cutaneous local necrosis following interferon injections. *Int J Dermatol* 1991; **30**: 147.

7 Webster GF, Knobler RL, Lublin FD *et al.* Cutaneous ulcerations and pustular psoriasis flare caused by recombinant interferon beta injections in patients with multiple sclerosis. *J Am Acad Dermatol* 1996; **34**: 365–7.

8 Sheremata WA, Taylor JR, Elgart GW. Severe necrotizing cutaneous lesions complicating treatment with interferon beta-1b. *N Engl J Med* 1995; **332**: 1584.

9 Levesque H, Cailleux N, Moore N *et al.* Autoimmune phenomena associated with cutaneous aseptic necrosis during interferon-alpha treatment for chronic myelogenous leukaemia. *Br J Rheumatol* 1995; **34**: 582–3.

10 Bachmeyer C, Farge D, Gluckman E *et al.* Raynaud's phenomenon and digital necrosis induced by interferon-alpha. *Br J Dermatol* 1996; **135**: 481–3.

11 Papini M, Bruni PL. Cutaneous reactions to recombinant cytokine therapy. *J Am Acad Dermatol* 1996; **35**: 1021.

12 Kerker BJ, Hood AF. Chemotherapy-induced cutaneous reactions. *Semin Dermatol* 1989; **8**: 173–81.

13 Olsen EA, Rosen ST, Vollmer RT *et al.* Interferon alfa-2a in the treatment of cutaneous T cell lymphoma. *J Am Acad Dermatol* 1989; **20**: 395–407.

14 Foon KA, Dougher G. Increased growth of eyelashes in a patient given leukocyte A Interferon. *N Engl J Med* 1984; **311**: 1259.

15 Granstein RD, Rook A, Flotte RJ *et al.* A controlled trial of intralesional recombinant interferon-γ in the treatment of keloidal scarring. *Arch Dermatol* 1990; **126**: 1295–302.

16 Quesada JR, Gutterman JU. Psoriasis and alpha-interferon. *Lancet* 1986; **i**: 1466–8.

17 Hartmann F, von Wussow P, Deicher H. Psoriasis—exacerbation bei therapie mit alpha-Interferon. *Dtsch Med Wochenschr* 1989; **114**: 96–8.

18 Shiohara T, Kobayashi M, Abe K, Nagashima M. Psoriasis occurring predominantly on warts. Possible involvement of interferon alpha. *Arch Dermatol* 1988; **124**: 1816–21.

19 Jucgla A, Marcoval J, Curco N, Servitje O. Psoriasis with articular involvement induced by interferon alfa. *Arch Dermatol* 1991; **127**: 910–11.

20 O'Connell PG, Gerber LH, Digiovanna JJ, Peck GL. Arthritis in patients with

psoriasis treated with gamma-interferon. *J Rheumatol* 1992; **19**: 80–2.

21 Cleveland MG, Mallory SB. Incomplete Reiter's syndrome induced by systemic interferon alpha treatment. *J Am Acad Dermatol* 1993; **29**: 788–9.

22 Fierlbeck G, Rassner G, Müller C. Psoriasis induced at the injection site of recombinant interferon gamma. *Arch Dermatol* 1990; **126**: 351–5.

23 Kowalzick L, Weyer U. Psoriasis induced at the injection site of recombinant interferons. *Arch Dermatol* 1990; **126**: 1515–16.

24 Conlon KC, Urba WJ, Smith JW, II, *et al.* Exacerbation of symptoms of autoimmune disease in patients receiving alpha-interferon therapy. *Cancer* 1990; **65**: 2237–42.

25 Steis RG, Smith JW, Urba WJ. Resistance to recombinant interferon alfa-2a in hairy-cell leukemia associated with neutralizing anti-interferon antibodies. *N Engl J Med* 1988; **318**: 1409–13.

26 Ramseur WL, Richards F, Duggan DB. A case of fatal pemphigus vulgaris in association with beta interferon and interleukin-2 therapy. *Cancer* 1989; **63**: 2005–7.

27 Shilling PJ, Kurzrock P, Kantarijian H *et al.* Development of systemic lupus erythematosus after interferon therapy for chronic myelogenous leukemia. *Cancer* 1991; **68**: 1536–7.

Interleukins (IL)

Interleukin 1. Mucositis and an erythematous eruption with erosions in intertriginous areas and under occlusive tape have been documented [1].

Interleukin 2. Immunotherapy with IL-2 either alone or in conjunction with lymphokine-activated killer cells, is used in the treatment of metastatic cancer; mild influenza-like symptoms are common. Cutaneous complications [2–8] include mucositis, macular erythema (principally restricted to the head, neck and upper chest), burning and pruritus, which resolves with mild desquamation, erythroderma and petechiae. Transient urticaria, necrotic lesions and blisters may be seen [8]. Type I hypersensitivity reactions, ranging from pruritus, erythema and oedema to hypotension, within hours of chemotherapy in patients previously treated with high-dose IL-2 have occurred [9]. A generalized capillary leak syndrome, with non-pitting oedema and diffuse pulmonary infiltrate on chest X-ray is recorded [6]. Exacerbation of psoriasis (including erythroderma) has been described [2–6]. IL-2 treatment predisposes to acute hypersensitivity reactions to iodine-containing contrast media [6]. Glossitis, telogen effluvium, punctate superficial ulcers and erosions in scars may be seen. Erythema nodosum has been documented [10]. Local inflammatory painful nodules with a central multiloculated vesicle have occurred at the site of subcutaneous injections of IL-2 and IFN-α [11]. Linear IgA bullous dermatosis has been associated with IL-2 therapy [12]. TEN is a rare complication [13]. It is of interest that lymphocytes activated by IL-2 can non-specifically destroy keratinocytes *in vitro* [14].

Other side-effects include hypothyroidism (antithyroid antibodies are present in 50% of patients), neurological and psychiatric disturbances, musculoskeletal disorders, impaired renal function, cardiovascular injuries, cholestasis, pancreatitis, anaemia, thrombocytopenia, lymphocytopenia and eosinophilia [6].

Interleukin 3. Erythema and purpura at the site of injection, and urticaria [15] may be induced.

Interleukin 4. Transient acantholytic dermatosis is recorded [16].

Interleukin 6. Coalescent, erythematous, scaling macules and papules occurred [17].

REFERENCES

1 Prussick R, Horn TD, Wilson WH, Turner MC. A characteristic eruption associated with ifosfamide, carboplatin, and etoposide chemotherapy after pretreatment with recombinant interleukin-1α. *J Am Acad Dermatol* 1996; **35**: 705–9.

2 Rosenberg SA, Lotze MT, Muul LM *et al.* Clinical experience with the treatment of 157 patients with advanced cancer using lymphokine-activated killer cells and interleukin-2 or high dose interleukin 2 alone. *N Engl J Med* 1987; **316**: 889–97.

3 Gaspari A, Lotze MT, Rosenberg SA *et al.* Dermatologic changes associated with interleukin-2 administration. *JAMA* 1987; **258**: 1624–9.

4 Rosenberg SA. Immunotherapy of cancer using interleukin 2: current status and future prospects. *Immunol Today* 1988; **9**: 58–62.

5 Lee RE, Gaspari AA, Lotze MT *et al.* Interleukin 2 and psoriasis. *Arch Dermatol* 1988; **124**: 1811–15.

6 Vial T, Descotes J. Clinical toxicity of interleukin-2. *Drug Saf* 1992; **7**: 417–33.

7 Larbre B, Nicolas JF, Sarret Y *et al.* Immunotherapie par interleukine 2 et manifestations cutanées. *Ann Dermatol Vénéréol* 1993; **120**: 528–33.

8 Wolkenstein P, Chosidow O, Wechster J *et al.* Cutaneous side effects associated with interleukin 2 administration for metastatic melanoma. *J Am Acad Dermatol* 1993; **28**: 66–70.

9 Heywood GR, Rosenberg SA, Weber JS. Hypersensitivity reactions to chemotherapy agents in patients receiving chemoimmunotherapy with high-dose interleukin 2. *J Natl Cancer Inst* 1995; **87**: 915–22.

10 Weinstein A, Bujak D, Mittelman A *et al.* Erythema nodosum in a patient with renal cell carcinoma treated with interleukin 2 and lymphokine-activated killer cells. *JAMA* 1987; **258**: 3120–1.

11 Klapholz L, Ackerstein A, Goldenhersh MA *et al.* Local cutaneous reaction induced by subcutaneous interleukin-2 and interferon alpha-2a immunotherapy following ABMT. *Bone Marrow Transplant* 1993; **11**: 443–6.

12 Tranvan A, Pezen DS, Medenica M *et al.* Interleukin-2 associated linear IgA bullous dermatosis. *J Am Acad Dermatol* 1996; **35**: 865–7.

13 Wiener JS, Tucker JA, Jr, Walther PJ. Interleukin-2-induced dermatotoxicity resembling toxic epidermal necrolysis. *South Med J* 1992; **82**: 656–9.

14 Kalish RS. Non-specifically activated human peripheral blood mononuclear cells are cytotoxic for human keratinocytes *in vitro. J Immunol* 1989; **142**: 74–80.

15 Bridges AG, Helm TN, Bergfeld WF *et al.* Interleukin-3-induced urticaria-like eruption. *J Am Acad Dermatol* 1996; **34**: 1076–8.

16 Mahler SJ, De Villez RL, Pulitzer DR. Transient acantholytic dermatosis induced by recombinant human interleukin 4. *J Am Acad Dermatol* 1993; **29**: 206–9.

17 Fleming TE, Mirando WS, Soohoo LF *et al.* An inflammatory eruption associated with recombinant human IL-6. *Br J Dermatol* 1994; **130**: 534–6.

Stem-cell factor

Human recombinant stem-cell factor, a cytokine that acts on haematopoietic progenitor cells and that is used for human anaemic disorders, and for speeding haematological recovery after chemotherapy, causes reversible hyperpigmentation at sites of injection; there are increases in melanocyte numbers, dendrite extension and melanin [1].

REFERENCE

1 Grichnik JM, Crawford J, Jimenez F *et al*. Human recombinant stem-cell factor induces melanocytic hyperplasia in susceptible patients. *J Am Acad Dermatol* 1995; **33**: 577–83.

Tumour necrosis factor (TNF)

Subcutaneous or intramuscular administration of TNF for advanced malignancy is limited by local pain, erythema and swelling or frank ulceration, while intravenous infusion may cause hypotension [1].

REFERENCE

1 Wakefield PE, James WD, Samlaska CP, Meltzer MS. Tumor necrosis factor. *J Am Acad Dermatol* 1991; **24**: 675–85.

Erythropoietin

This drug has caused a generalized eczematous reaction [1].

REFERENCE

1 Hardwick N, King CM. Generalized eczematous reaction to erythropoietin. *Contact Dermatitis* 1993; **28**: 123.

Miscellaneous drugs affecting the immune response

Diphencyprone

Diphencyprone [1] used for alopecia areata has resulted in urticaria [2] and erythema multiforme [3], and it has been linked to development of vitiligo [4–6]. Severe contact dermatitis reactions may be induced.

REFERENCES

1 Shah M, Lewis FM, Messenger AG. Hazards in the use of diphencyprone. *Br J Dermatol* 1996; **134**; 1153.
2 van der Steen PHM, van Baar HMJ, Perret CM, Happle R. Treatment of alopecia areata with diphenylcyclopropenone. *J Am Acad Dermatol* 1991; **24**: 253–7.
3 Perret CM, Steijlen PM, Zaun H, Happle R. Erythema multiforme-like eruptions: a rare side effect of topical immunotherapy with diphenyl-cyclopropenone. *Dermatologica* 1990; **180**: 5–7.
4 Hatzis J, Gourgiotou K, Tosca A *et al*. Vitiligo as a reaction to topical treatment with diphencyprone. *Dermatologica* 1988; **177**: 146–8.
5 Duhra P, Foulds IS. Persistent vitiligo induced by diphencyprone. *Br J Dermatol* 1990; **123**: 415–16.
6 Henderson CA, Ilchyshyn A. Vitiligo complicating diphencyprone sensitization therapy for alopecia universalis. *Br J Dermatol* 1995; **133**: 496–7.

Roquinimex

Autologous graft-versus-host reactions occurred in three of eight patients treated with the cytokine inducer carboxamide–quinoline immunotherapeutic agent roquinimex (Linomide), used for post-transplantation immunotherapy in autologous bone-marrow transplantation for acute and chronic myelogenous leukaemia [1]. Localized or widespread violaceous papules histologically compatible with a grade II graft-versus-host reaction were associated with eccrine sweat-gland necrosis.

REFERENCE

1 Gaspari AA, Cheng SF, DiPersio JF, Rowe JM. Roquinimex-induced graft-versus-host reaction after autologous bone marrow transplantation. *J Am Acad Dermatol* 1995; **33**: 711–17.

Antihistamines

H_1 antihistamines

All traditional H_1 antagonists cause side-effects [1–4], especially sedation, most marked with the amino-alkyl ether and phenothiazine groups. Dizziness, poor coordination, blurred vision and diplopia, as well as nervousness, insomnia and tremor may occur. In addition, atropine-like anticholinergic effects including dryness of mucous membranes, urinary retention, palpitations, agitation, increased intraocular pressure and gastro-intestinal upset are seen. Phenothiazine-derived drugs may cause photosensitivity or cholestatic jaundice. The effects of nervous system depressants, such as alcohol, hypnotics, sedatives, analgesics and anxiolytics, may be potentiated. Decreased efficacy of drugs metabolized by the liver microsomal enzyme system, including oral anticoagulants, phenytoin and griseofulvin, may occur as a result of liver-enzyme induction by antihistamines. The newer anti-histamine drugs (e.g. terfenadine, astemizole, loratadine, cetirizine) are much less likely to cause sedation [1–4].

Terfenadine and astemizole rarely cause QT interval prolongation and *torsades de pointes*. Arrhythmias occur when metabolism of terfenadine is impaired, as with inhibition of the metabolizing enzyme P-450 isoform CYP3A4 by ketoconazole, itraconazole and related imidazole antifungals, erythromycin, clarithromycin and related macrolide antibiotics, or grapefruit juice, or by liver disease [5–7]. Patients on terfenadine or astemizole should be instructed accordingly. The UK Committee on Safety of Medicines has issued guidance, and has withdrawn terfenadine from over-the-counter sale, as has the US Food and Drug Administration. However, no increased risk of life-threatening ventricular arrhythmic events or cardiac arrest with terfenadine compared with over-the-counter antihistamines, ibuprofen or clemastine was found in one study [8].

True hypersensitivity reactions are rare. Fixed eruptions have been caused by thonzylamine and cyclizine [9]. Skin eruptions have been documented with terfenadine [10,11], including possible exacerbation of psoriasis [12]; alopecia has been reported rarely [13]. A pityriasis-lichenoides-et-varioliformis-acuta-like drug exanthem was reportedly caused by astemizole, with a positive challenge test [14]. Antihistamines are associated with atypical lymphoid hyperplasia, presenting as solitary or multiple nodules and plaques, or multiple papules, in some patients [15].

REFERENCES

1 Woodward JK. Pharmacology and toxicology of nonclassical antihistamines. *Cutis* 1988; **42**: 5–9.
2 Lichtenstein LM, Simons FER, eds. Advancements in antiallergic therapy: beyond conventional antihistamines. *J Allergy Clin Immunol* 1990; **86** (Suppl.): 995–1046.
3 Kennard CD, Ellis CN. Pharmacologic therapy for urticaria. *J Am Acad Dermatol* 1991; **25**: 176–89.
4 Soter NA. Treatment of urticaria and angioedema: low-sedating H1-type antihistamines. *J Am Acad Dermatol* 1991; **24**: 1084–7.
5 Thomas SHL. Drugs, QT interval abnormalities and ventricular arrhythmias. *Adverse Drug Reactions Acute Toxicol Rev* 1994; **13**: 77–102.
6 Woosley RL. Cardiac actions of antihistamines. *Annu Rev Pharmacol Toxicol* 1996; **36**: 233–52.
7 Thomas SHL. Drugs and the QT interval. *Adverse Drug Reaction Bull* 1997; **182**: 691–4.
8 Pratt CM, Hertz RP, Ellis BE *et al.* Risk of developing life-threatening ventricular arrhythmia associated with terfenadine in comparison with over-the-counter antihistamines, ibuprofen and clemastine. *Am J Cardiol* 1994; **73**: 346–52.
9 Griffiths WAD, Peachey RDG. Fixed drug eruption due to cyclizine. *Br J Dermatol* 1970; **82**: 616–17.
10 Stricker BHCH, Van Dijke CHP, Isaacs AJ, Lindquist M. Skin reactions to terfenadine. *Br Med J* 1986; **293**: 536.
11 McClintock AD, Ching DW, Hutchinson C. Skin reactions and terfenadine. *NZ Med J* 1995; **108**: 208.
12 Harrison PV, Stones RN. Severe exacerbation of psoriasis due to terfenadine. *Clin Exp Dermatol* 1988; **13**: 275.
13 Jones S, Morley W. Terfenadine causing hair loss (unreviewed report). *Br Med J* 1985; **291**: 940.
14 Stosiek N, Peters KP, von den Driesch P. Pityriasis-lichenoides-et-varioliformis-acuta-ähnliches Arzneiexanthem durch Astemizol. *Hautarzt* 1993; **44**: 235–7.
15 Magro CM, Crowson AN. Drugs with antihistaminic properties as a cause of atypical cutaneous lymphoid hyperplasia. *J Am Acad Dermatol* 1995; **32**: 419–28.

H$_2$ antihistamines

Severe adverse reactions are rare with cimetidine, ranitidine, nizatidine and famotidine [1]. Gastrointestinal upset, headache, drowsiness, fatigue or muscular pain occur in fewer than 3% of patients. Confusion, dizziness, somnolence, gynaecomastia or galactorrhea with increased prolactin levels (cimetidine and ranitidine only), impotence and loss of libido (with cimetidine), bone-marrow depression, hepatitis, abnormal renal function or nephritis, arthralgia, myalgia, cardiac abnormalities, and minor or severe skin reactions occur in fewer than 1% of patients.

Cimetidine. Mucocutaneous reactions are rare in relation to the enormous worldwide use of this drug. Reported reactions include a seborrhoeic dermatitis-like rash [2] and asteatotic dermatitis [3], erythema annulare centrifugum [4], erythrosis [5], giant urticaria [6], transitory alopecia [7], erythema multiforme [8] and exfoliative dermatitis [9]. Other effects have included thrombocytopenia [10] and a leukocytoclastic vasculitis [11]. Exacerbation of cutaneous LE [12] and systemic LE with granulocytopenia [13] are documented. Cimetidine binds to, and therefore blocks the binding of dihydrotestosterone to, androgen receptors, and gynaecomastia and hypogonadism are now well known side-effects [14]. The drug augments cell-mediated immunity *in vitro*, by blockade of H$_2$ receptors on T lymphocytes [15].

REFERENCES

1 Feldman M, Burton ME. Histamine$_2$-receptor antagonists. Standard therapy for acid-peptic diseases (First of two parts). *N Engl J Med* 1990; **323**: 1672–80.
2 Kanwar A, Majid A, Garg MP, Singh G. Seborrheic dermatitis-like eruption caused by cimetidine. *Arch Dermatol* 1981; **117**: 65–6.
3 Greist MC, Epinette WW. Cimetidine-induced xerosis and asteatotic dermatitis. *Arch Dermatol* 1982; **118**: 253–4.
4 Merrett AC, Marks R, Dudley FJ. Cimetidine-induced erythema annulare centrifugum: no cross-sensitivity with ranitidine. *Br Med J* 1981; **283**: 698.
5 Angelini G, Bovo P, Vaona B, Cavallini G. Cimetidine and erythrosis-like lesions. *Br Med J* 1979; **i**: 1147–8.
6 Hadfield WA, Jr. Cimetidine and giant urticaria. *Ann Intern Med* 1979; **91**: 128–9.
7 Vircburger MI, Prelevic GM, Brkic S *et al.* Transitory alopecia and hypergonadotrophic hypogonadism during cimetidine treatment. *Lancet* 1981; **i**: 1160–1.
8 Ahmed AH, McLarly DG, Sharma SK, Masawe AEJ. Stevens–Johnson syndrome during treatment with cimetidine. *Lancet* 1979; **ii**: 433.
9 Yantis PL, Bridges ME, Pittman FE. Cimetidine-induced exfoliative dermatitis. *Dig Dis Sci* 1980; **25**: 73–4.
10 Rate R, Bonnell M, Chervenak C, Pavinich G. Cimetidine and hematologic effects. *Ann Intern Med* 1979; **91**: 795.
11 Dernbach WK, Taylor G. Leukocytoclastic vasculitis from cimetidine. *JAMA* 1981; **246**: 331.
12 Davidson BL, Gilliam JN, Lipsky PE. Cimetidine-associated exacerbation of cutaneous lupus erythematosus. *Arch Intern Med* 1982; **142**: 166–7.
13 Littlejohn GO, Urowitz MB. Cimetidine, lupus erythematosus, and granulocytopenia. *Ann Intern Med* 1979; **91**: 317–18.
14 Jensen RT, Collen MJ, Pandol SJ *et al.* Cimetidine-induced impotence and breast changes in patients with gastric hypersecretory states. *N Engl J Med* 1983; **308**: 883–7.
15 Mavligit GM. Immunologic effects of cimetidine: potential uses. *Pharmacotherapy* 1987; **7** (Suppl. 2): S120–4.

Famotidine. This drug has been associated with the development of symptomatic dermographism [1], pruritic exanthem [2–4], contact eczema [4], leukocytoclastic vasculitis [5] and TEN.

REFERENCES

1 McCarley Warner D, Ramos-Caro FA, Flowers FP. Famotidine (Pepcid)-induced symptomatic dermatographism. *J Am Acad Dermatol* 1994; **31**: 677–8.
2 Reynolds JC. Famotidine in the management of duodenal ulcer: an analysis of multicenter findings worldwide. *Clin Ther* 1988; **10**: 436–49.
3 Dragosics B, Weiss W, Okulski G. Zur Therapie peptischer Ulzera mit Famotidin. Erfahrungsbericht einer offenen klinischen Studie. *Wien Med Wochenschr* 1992; **142**: 408–13.
4 Monteseirin J, Conde J. Contact eczema from famotidine. *Contact Dermatitis* 1990; **22**: 290.

5 Andreo JA, Vivancos F, Lopez VM *et al*. Vasculitis leucocitoclastica y famotidina. *Med Clin Barc* 1990; **95**: 234–5.

Ranitidine. Urticaria [1] and anaphylaxis [2] are recorded, as are allergic dermatitis and allergic contact dermatitis [3,4]. Immune-complex-mediated rashes [5], lichenoid eruptions [6] and photosensitivity with UVA sensitivity on monochromator light testing [7] have been documented, as has cholestatic hepatitis [8]. This drug has a less marked effect on androgen receptors than cimetidine, but gynaecomastia has occurred [9].

REFERENCES

1 Picardo M, Santucci B. Urticaria from ranitidine. *Contact Dermatitis* 1983; **9**: 327.
2 Lazaro M, Compaired JA, De La Hoz B *et al*. Anaphylactic reaction to ranitidine. *Allergy* 1993; **48**: 385–7.
3 Juste S, Blanco J, Garces M, Rodriguez G. Allergic dermatitis due to oral ranitidine. *Contact Dermatitis* 1992; **27**: 339–40.
4 Alomar A, Puig L, Vilaltella I. Allergic contact dermatitis due to ranitidine. *Contact Dermatitis* 1987; **17**: 54–5.
5 Haboub N. Rash mediated by immune complexes associated with ranitidine treatment. *Br Med J* 1988; **296**: 897.
6 Horiuchi Y, Katagiri T. Lichenoid eruptions due to the H2-receptor antagonists roxatidine and ranitidine. *J Dermatol* 1996; **23**: 510–12.
7 Todd P, Norris P, Hawk JLM, du Vivier AWP. Ranitidine-induced photosensitivity. *Clin Exp Dermatol* 1995; **20**: 146–8.
8 Devuyst O, Lefebvre C, Geubel A, Coche E. Acute cholestatic hepatitis with rash and hypereosinophilia associated with ranitidine treatment. *Acta Clin Belg* 1993; **48**: 109–14.
9 Tosti S, Cagnoli M. Painful gynaecomastia with ranitidine. *Lancet* 1982; **ii**: 160.

Injections, infusions and procedures

Radiographic contrast media and radiopharmaceuticals

Radiographic contrast media

Reactions to radiographic contrast media were previously reported to occur in about 4–8% of cases; severe reactions occurred in one in 1000 administrations, and occasionally fatal anaphylactoid reactions (one in 3000 for intravenous cholangiograms and between one in 10000 and one in 100000 for intravenous urography) developed [1–3]. Although IgE-mediated mechanisms may be involved [4], the vast majority of contrast reactions are not due to iodine allergy, but rather to non-immunological release of mast-cell mediators or to direct complement activation [5,6]. The risk of severe reactions is increased in atopics, asthmatics, those taking β-blockers, and with higher doses; up to 40% of patients with a previous reaction may develop a recurrence [7,8].

Newer lower osmolality radiocontrast media are associated with fewer reactions [8–14], for example administration of iohexol in 50660 patients undergoing excretory urography resulted in a frequency of adverse reactions of any type of 2.1% [9]. There was a 7.0% incidence of mild adverse reactions to low osmolar iodine contrast medium in 4550 radiological procedures including computed tomography (CT), intravenous urography, arteriography, venography and myelography in one series [12]. There were only two cases of severe anaphylactoid reactions during 783 consecutive cases undergoing voiding cystourethrography or retrograde pyelography [14]. The incidence of contrast media complications in the catheterization laboratory is 0.23% with one death per 55000 [15].

Lower osmolality radiocontrast media (e.g. iohexol or iopamidol) should be the contrast media of choice for patients with a prior immediate generalized reaction to conventional contrast media, and in addition patients should receive H_1 antihistamines and corticosteroid prophylaxis therapy [8,13,15]. However, although the relative risk for all adverse drug reactions was three to six times higher for ionic versus non-ionic contrast media in one study [16], in another study, mortality was not lower with newer, low osmolar media than with the older, high osmolar media [17]. In this latter large study, the overall mortality was 13 per million intravenous injections of radiocontrast media, rising to 35 per million in those over 65 years [17]. A further study in the USA found that 19% of 1004 patients in a clinical trial comparing the safety of low-versus high-osmolality radiologic contrast media in patients who underwent either cardiac angiography or contrast-enhanced body CT had at least one adverse reaction [18]. The mean cost per patient of treating adverse reactions was $459 (range, $0–39057).

In addition to immediate reactions, wide-spread erythema and oedema at 6h, reaching a maximum at 9–12h, followed intravenous injection of a CT contrast medium (iotrolan) [19]. Isolated cases of bullous lichen planus [20] and vasculitis [21] have been recorded. There has been a single case report of fatal TEN following the second exposure to diatrizoate solution for excretory pyelography [22].

REFERENCES

1 Lieberman P, Siegle RL, Treadwell G. Radiocontrast reactions. *Clin Rev Allergy* 1986; **4**: 229–45.
2 Grammer LC, Patterson R. Adverse reactions to radiographic contrast material. *Clin Dermatol* 1986; **4**: 149–54.
3 Katayama H, Tanaka T. Clinical survey of adverse reactions to contrast media. *Invest Radiol* 1988; **23** (Suppl.): S88–9.
4 Kanny G, Maria Y, Mentre B, Moneret-Vautrin DA. Case report: recurrent anaphylactic shock to radiographic contrast media. Evidence supporting an exceptional IgE-mediated reaction. *Allerg Immunol* 1993; **25**: 425–30.
5 Arroyave CM, Bhatt KN, Crown NR. Activation of the alternative pathway of the complement system by radiocontrast media. *J Immunol* 1976; **117**: 1866–9.
6 Rice MC, Lieberman P, Siegle RL, Mason J. *In vitro* histamine release induced by radiocontrast media and various chemical analogs in reactor and control subjects. *J Allergol Clin Immunol* 1983; **72**: 180–6.
7 Enright T, Chua-Lim A, Duda E, Lim DT. The role of a documented allergic profile as a risk factor for radiographic contrast media reaction. *Ann Allergy* 1989; **62**: 302–5.
8 Porri F, Vervloet D. Les reactions aux produits de contraste iodes. *Allerg Immunol* 1994; **26**: 374–6.
9 Schrott KM, Behrends B, Clauss W *et al*. Iohexol in excretory urography: results of the drug monitoring programs. *Fortschr Med* 1986; **104**: 153–6.

10 Greenberger PA, Patterson R. The prevention of immediate generalized reactions to contrast media in high-risk patients. *J Allergy Clin Immunol* 1991; **87**: 867–71.

11 Gertz EW, Wisneski JA, Miller R *et al*. Adverse reactions of low osmolality contrast media during cardiac angiography: a prospective randomized multicenter study. *J Am Coll Cardiol* 1992; **19**: 899–906.

12 Kuwatsuru R, Katayama H, Tomita T *et al*. Adverse reactions to low osmolar iodine contrast media (second report). [Japanese] *Nippon Acta Radiologica* 1992; **52**: 1233–46.

13 Porri F, Pradal M, Fontaine JL *et al*. Reactions aux produits de contraste iodes. *Presse Med* 1993; **22**: 543–9.

14 Weese DL, Greenberg HM, Zimmern PE. Contrast media reactions during voiding cystourethrography or retrograde pyelography. *Urology* 1993; **41**: 81–4.

15 Goss JE, Chambers CE, Heupler FA, Jr. Systemic anaphylactoid reactions to iodinated contrast media during cardiac catheterization procedures: guidelines for prevention, diagnosis, and treatment. Laboratory Performance Standards Committee of the Society for Cardiac Angiography and Interventions. *Cath Cardiovasc Diag* 1995; **34**: 99–105.

16 Andrew E, Haider T. Incidence of roentgen contrast medium reactions after intravenous injection in pre-registration trials and post-marketing surveillances. *Acta Radiol* 1993; **34**: 210–13.

17 Cashman JD, McCredie J, Henry DA. Intravenous contrast media: use and associated mortality. *Med J Aust* 1991; **155**: 618–23.

18 Powe NR, Moore RD, Steinberg EP. Adverse reactions to contrast media: factors that determine the cost of treatment. *Am J Roentgenol* 1993; **161**: 1089–95.

19 Kanzaki T, Sakagami H. Late phase allergic reaction to a CT contrast medium (iotrolan). *J Dermatol* 1991; **18**: 528–31.

20 Grunwald MH, Halevy S, Livni E, Feuerman EJ. Bullous lichen planus after intravenous pyelography. *J Am Acad Dermatol* 1985; **13**: 512–13.

21 Kerdel FA, Fraker DL, Haynes HA. Necrotizing vasculitis from radiographic contrast media. *J Am Acad Dermatol* 1984; **10**: 25–9.

22 Kaftori JK, Abraham Z, Gilhar A. Toxic epidermal necrolysis after excretory pyelography. Immunologic-mediated contrast medium reaction? *Int J Dermatol* 1988; **27**: 346–7.

Radiopharmaceuticals

The reported incidence of reactions to agents used in nuclear medicine is low; these usually take the form of immediate urticaria or angio-oedema [1–3]. Urticarial or anaphylactic reactions to technetium (^{99m}Tc) sulphur colloid and ^{99m}Tc human albumin microspheres together accounted for 50% of reported reactions [2]. The bone-scanning agent ^{99m}Tc methylene diphosphonate produces a delayed-onset erythematous pruritic eruption within 4–24 h [4].

REFERENCES

1 Rhodes BA, Cordova MA. Adverse reactions to radio-pharmaceuticals: Incidence in 1978, and associated symptoms. *J Nucl Med* 1980; **2**: 1107.

2 Cordova MA, Hladik WB, III, Rhodes BA. Validation and characterization of adverse reactions to radiopharmaceuticals. *Noninv Med Imag* 1984; **1**: 17–24.

3 Keeling D, Sampson CB. Adverse reactions to radiopharmaceuticals: incidence, reporting, symptoms, treatment. *Nuklearmedizin* 1986; **23** (Suppl.): 478–82.

4 Collins MRL, James WD, Rodman OG. Adverse cutaneous reaction to technetium Tc 99m methylene diphosphonate. *Arch Dermatol* 1988; **124**: 180–1.

Halides

Bromides

Bromides have a long half-life and are excreted slowly by the kidney; bromism may develop in patients with impaired renal function, and eruptions may not develop until as much as 2 months after the drug has been discontinued. Acneiform and vegetating lesions occur more often, and bullae less frequently, than with iodism [1,2]. Vegetating bromoderma presents as single or multiple papillomatous nodules or plaques, studded with small pustules, on the face or limbs. Bromoderma tuberosum has been caused by anticonvulsive treatment with potassium bromide [3]. Bromism is also characterized by weakness, restlessness, headache, ataxia and personality changes [2].

Iodides

Serious and even fatal reactions of anaphylactic type have been caused by radiographic contrast media containing organic iodine [4]. Iodism, nasal congestion and conjunctivitis, often accompanied by an exanthematic eruption, may be associated with a wide variety of systemic symptoms [5,6]. Prolonged administration of small doses of iodide, as in many cough mixtures, may provoke eruptions with or without mucosal or systemic symptoms. Lesions may first develop some days after the drug is discontinued. The following may occur: urticaria, an acneiform rash, papulopustular lesions, nodules, anthracoid or carbuncular lesions, or clear or haemorrhagic bullae on the face, forearms, neck and flexures, or buccal mucosa [6]. If the iodine is continued, the bullae may be replaced by vegetating masses, which simulate pemphigus vegetans or a granulomatous infection [7]. Iododerma has developed after administration of oral [8] and intravenous [9,10] radiographic contrast media, and during thyroid protection treatment [11]. Iododerma seems more frequent in patients with renal failure, and may be accompanied by leuko-cytoclastic vasculitis [2]. The eruption recurs within days of re-administration in a sensitized individual [12]. Cell-mediated [5] and 'hyperinflammatory' [13] mechanisms have been postulated. Vegetating iododerma may be an idiosyncratic response which is commoner in patients with polyarteritis nodosa or paraproteinemia [14]. Fixed eruptions occur rarely [15]. Generalized pustular psoriasis has been reportedly provoked by potassium iodide [16].

Histology of bromoderma and iododerma

In bromoderma, verrucous pseudoepitheliomatous hyperplasia is associated with abscesses containing neutrophils and eosinophils in the epidermis, and a dense dermal infiltrate initially consisting mainly of neutrophils and eosinophils, and later containing many lymphocytes, plasma cells and histiocytes. The abundant dilated blood vessels may show endothelial proliferation. In iododermas, ulceration is more marked, but there is usually less epithelial hyperplasia. Both conditions must be differentiated from blastomycosis and coccidiomycosis, and from pemphigus vegetans [17].

REFERENCES

1 Blasik LG, Spencer SK. Fluoroderma. *Arch Dermatol* 1979; **115**: 1334–5.
2 Carney MWP. Five cases of bromism. *Lancet* 1971; **ii**: 523–4.
3 Pfeifle J, Grieben U, Bork K. Bromoderma tuberosum durch antikonvulsive Behandlung mit Kaliumbromid. *Hautarzt* 1992; **43**: 792–4.
4 Vaillant L, Pengloan J, Blanchier D *et al.* Iododerma and acute respiratory distress with leucocytoclastic vasculitis following the intravenous injection of contrast medium. *Clin Exp Dermatol* 1990; **15**: 232–3.
5 Kincaid MC, Green WR, Hoover RE, Farmer ER. Iododerma of the conjunctiva and skin. *Ophthalmology* 1981; **88**: 1216–20.
6 O'Brien TJ. Iodic eruptions. *Australas J Dermatol* 1987; **28**: 119–22.
7 Rosenberg FR, Einbinder J, Walzer RA, Nelson CT. Vegetating iododerma. An immunologic mechanism. *Arch Dermatol* 1972; **105**: 900–5.
8 Boudoulas O, Siegle RJ, Grinwood RE. Iododerma occurring after orally administered iopanoic acid. *Arch Dermatol* 1987; **123**: 387–8.
9 Heydenreich G, Larsen PO. Iododerma after high dose urography in an oliguric patient. *Br J Dermatol* 1977; **97**: 567–9.
10 Lauret P, Godin M, Bravard P. Vegetating iodides after an intravenous pyelogram. *Dermatologica* 1985; **71**: 463–8.
11 Wilkin JK, Strobel D. Iododerma during thyroid protection treatment. *Cutis* 1985; **36**: 335–7.
12 Jones LE, Pariser H, Murray PF. Recurrent iododerma. *Arch Dermatol* 1958; **28**: 353–8.
13 Stone OJ. Proliferative iododerma: a possible mechanism. *Int J Dermatol* 1985; **24**: 565–6.
14 Soria C, Allegue F, España A *et al.* Vegetating iododerma with underlying systemic diseases: report of three cases. *J Am Acad Dermatol* 1990; **22**: 418–22.
15 Baker H. Fixed drug eruption due to iodide and antipyrine. *Br J Dermatol* 1962; **74**: 310–16.
16 Shelley WB. Generalized pustular psoriasis induced by potassium iodide. *JAMA* 1967; **201**: 1009–14.
17 Elder D, Elenitsas R, Jaworsky C, Johnson B, Jr, eds. *Lever's Histopathology of the Skin*, 8th edn. Philadelphia: JB Lippincott, 1997.

Agents used in general anaesthesia

Neuromuscular blocking agents, skeletal muscle relaxants and general anaesthetics

The incidence of life-threatening anaphylactic or anaphylactoid reactions during anaesthesia has been variously reported to occur in one in 1000 to one in 20 000, and minor reactions probably occur in more than 1% of cases; neuromuscular blocking agents are the triggering agents in about 50% of these reactions [1–9]. The mortality rate in anaphylactic reactions to drugs used in general anaesthesia is between 4 and 6% [8]. Reactions appear most likely with suxamethonium and gallamine, then δ-tubocurarine and alcuronium, and least likely with pancuronium and vecuronium [3,6,9]. Mucocutaneous manifestations including erythema, urticaria, and angio-oedema, are reported in up to 80% of reactions, but may only be recognized after the acute phase has passed. Reactions are more frequent in women and in atopic patients. Proposed mechanisms for anaphylactic reactions include type I (IgE antibody-mediated) hypersensitivity [9–12], with antibodies persisting for up to 29 years [11], and direct histamine release. Only one reaction in three is likely to be IgE-mediated (type 1) anaphylaxis, but non-immune reactions are no less hazardous than type 1 reactions [9]. Cross-reactivity is widespread with most of the drugs but is least with pancuronium. It has been suggested that pancuronium should be used where muscle relaxation during anaesthesia is essential but sensitivity to another relaxant exists [3], although others have questioned the safety of this procedure [7]. IgE-dependent sensitivity to thiopental may result in anaphylactic reactions [5].

REFERENCES

1 Fisher MMcD. Intradermal testing in the diagnosis of acute anaphylaxis during anaesthesia—results of five years experience. *Anaesth Intensive Care* 1979; **7**: 58–61.
2 Fisher M McD. The diagnosis of acute anaphylactoid reactions to neuromuscular blocking agents: a commonly undiagnosed condition. *Anaesth Intensive Care* 1981; **9**: 235–41.
3 Galletly DC, Treuren BC. Anaphylactoid reactions during anaesthesia. Seven years' experience of intradermal testing. *Anaesthesia* 1985; **40**: 329–33.
4 Leynadier F, Sansarricq M, Didier JM, Dry J. Prick tests in the diagnosis of anaphylaxis to general anaesthetics. *Br J Anaesth* 1987; **59**: 683–9.
5 Cheema AL, Sussman GL, Jancelewicz Z *et al.* Update: Pentothal-induced anaphylaxis. *J Allergy Clin Immunol* 1988; **81**: 220.
6 Fisher MM, Baldo BA. The incidence and clinical features of anaphylactic reactions during anesthesia in Australia. *Ann Franc D'Anesthes Reanimation* 1993; **12**: 97–104.
7 Moneret-Vautrin DA, Laxenaire MC. Anaphylaxis to muscle relaxants: predictive tests. *Anaesthesia* 1990; **45**: 246–7.
8 Moscicki RA, Sockin SM, Corsello BF *et al.* Anaphylaxis during induction of general anesthesia: subsequent evaluation and management. *J Allergy Clin Immunol* 1990; **86**: 325–32.
9 Watkins J. Adverse reaction to neuromuscular blockers: frequency, investigation, and epidemiology. *Acta Anaesthesiol Scand (Suppl.)* 1994; **102**: 6–10.
10 Baldo BA, Fisher MM. Mechanisms in IgE-dependent anaphylaxis to anesthetic drugs. *Ann Franc D'Anesthes Reanimation* 1993; **12**: 131–40.
11 Fisher MM, Baldo BA. Persistence of allergy to anaesthetic drugs. *Anaesth Intensive Care* 1992; **20**: 143–6.
12 Assem ES. Anaphylactoid reactions to neuromuscular blockers: major role of IgE antibodies and possible contribution of IgE-independent mechanisms. *Monogr Allergy* 1992; **30**: 24–53.

Local anaesthetic agents

Local anaesthetics may cause both immediate anaphylactic reactions and contact dermatitis [1–10]. True allergic reactions caused by local anaesthetics are extremely rare [9,11]; more often, the allergic response is caused by a metabolite, preservative or unrelated substance. Acute anaphylactic reactions are uncommon, but are probably less likely to occur when amide linkage agents are used [4,5]. Necrosis of the fingertip has followed local injection for nail extraction [12].

Amethocaine. Amethocaine in the form of a self-adhesive patch caused slight or moderate erythema at the site of application in 26% of patients, and slight oedema in 5% [13].

EMLA cream (proprietary name). A eutectic mixture of prilocaine and lignocaine (lidocaine) in a cream base (EMLA cream) has been associated with methaemoglobinaemia [14–16]; two metabolites of prilocaine, namely 4-hydroxy-2-methylaniline and 2-methylaniline (*o*-toluidine), have been incriminated. A 3-month-old infant became cyanosed after application of 5 g, but this may have been contributed to by concomitant sulphonamide therapy [14]. Small but significant increases in met-haemoglobin levels have been reported in children 1–6 years old following routine administration of 5 g before surgery, and may persist for at least 24 h [15], so that it is recommended that the minimum effective dose be used in children requiring daily application. Blanching following application of EMLA is common [17]. Contact dermatitis can arise to both lignocaine and prilocaine [18–20]. Severe lignocaine intoxication with progressive neurological and psychiatric abnormalities and cardiorespiratory arrest occurred following topical application to painful ulcerated areas in a patient with cutaneous T-cell lymphoma [21].

Bupivacaine. A delayed hypersensitivity rash may occur after injection of arthroscopy portals with bupivacine [22].

REFERENCES

1 Schatz M. Skin testing and incremental challenge in the evaluation of adverse reactions to local anesthetics. *J Allergy Clin Immunol* 1984; **74**: 606–16.
2 Fisher MMcD, Graham R. Adverse responses to local anaesthetics. *Anaesth Intensive Care* 1984; **12**: 325–7.
3 Ruzicka T, Gerstmeier M, Przybilla B, Ring J. Allergy to local anesthetics: comparison of patch test with prick and intradermal test results. *J Am Acad Dermatol* 1987; **16**: 1202–8.
4 Christie JL. Fatal consequences of local anesthesia: report of five cases and a review of the literature. *J Forensic Sci* 1975; **21**: 671–9.
5 Kennedy KS, Cave RH. Anaphylactic reaction to lidocaine. *Arch Otolaryngol Head Neck Surg* 1986; **112**: 671–3.
6 Glinert RJ, Zachary CB. Local anesthetic allergy. Its recognition and avoidance. *J Dermatol Surg Oncol* 1991; **17**: 491–6.
7 Grognard C. Complications des anesthesiques locaux. *Ann Dermatol Vénéréol* 1993; **120**: 172–4.
8 Skidmore RA, Patterson JD, Tomsick RS. Local anesthetics. *Dermatol Surg* 1996; **22**: 511–22.
9 Gall H, Kaufmann R, Kalveram CM. Adverse reactions to local anesthetics: analysis of 197 cases. *J Allergy Clin Immunol* 1996; **97**: 933–7.
10 Kajimoto Y, Rosenberg ME, Kytta J *et al.* Anaphylactoid skin reactions after intravenous regional anaesthesia using 0.5% prilocaine with or without preservative—a double-blind study. *Acta Anaesthesiol Scand* 1995; **39**: 782–4.
11 Jackson D, Chen AH, Bennett CR. Identifying true lidocaine allergy. *J Am Dent Assoc* 1994; **125**: 1362–6.
12 Roser-Maaß E. Nekrosen an Fingerendgliedern nach Lokalanästhesie bei Nagelextraktion. *Hautarzt* 1981; **32**: 39–41.
13 Doyle E, Freeman J, Im NT, Morton NS. An evaluation of a new self-adhesive patch preparation of amethocaine for topical anaesthesia prior to venous cannulation in children. *Anaesthesia* 1993; **48**: 1050–2.
14 Jakobson B, Nilsson A. Methaemoglobinaemia associated with a prilocaine–lidocaine cream and trimethoprim–sulphamethoxazole. A case report. *Acta Anaesthesiol Scand* 1985; **29**: 453–5.
15 Frayling IM, Addison GM, Chattergee K, Meakin G. Methaemoglobinaemia in children treated with prilocaine–lignocaine cream. *Br Med J* 1990; **301**: 153–4.
16 Nilsson A, Engberg G, Henneberg S *et al.* Inverse relationship between age-dependent erythrocyte activity of methaemoglobin reductase and prilocaine-induced methaemoglobinaemia during infancy. *Br J Anaesth* 1990; **64**: 72–6.
17 Villada G, Zetlaoui J, Revuz J. Local blanching after epicutaneous application of EMLA cream. *Dermatologica* 1990; **181**: 38–40.
18 Duggan M, Burns D, Henry M, Mitchell T. Reaction to topical lignocaine in a patient with contact dermatitis. *Contact Dermatitis* 1993; **28**: 190–1.
19 van den Hove J, Decroix J, Tennstedt D, Lachapelle JM. Allergic contact

dermatitis from prilocaine, one of the local anaesthetics in EMLA cream. *Contact Dermatitis* 1994; **30**: 239.
20 Thakur BK, Murali MR. EMLA cream-induced allergic contact dermatitis: a role for prilocaine as an immunogen. *J Allergy Clin Immunol* 1995; **95**: 776–8.
21 Lie RL, Vermeer BJ, Edelbroek PM. Severe lidocaine intoxication by cutaneous absorption. *J Am Acad Dermatol* 1990; **23**: 1026–8.
22 Magsamen BF. Delayed hypersensitivity rash to the knee after injection of arthroscopy portals with bupivacine (Marcaine). *Arthroscopy* 1995; **11**: 512–13.

Infusions and injections

Intravenous infusion

Pain, oedema, induration and thrombophlebitis are well-recognized complications [1,4,5,9]. Localized bullous eruptions following infusion of commonly used non-vesicant fluids, such as saline, have been described [2]. Extravasation was reported to occur in 11% of 16 380 administrations to children monitored over a 6-month period [3]. Skin necrosis following intravenous infusion of chemotherapeutic agents occurs in up to 6% of patients [1,2,3,5–8].

REFERENCES

1 Barton A. Adverse reactions to intravenous catheters and other devices. *Lancet* 1993; **342**: 683.
2 Robijns BJL, de Wit WM, Bosma NJ, van Vloten WA. Localized bullous eruptions caused by extravasation of commonly used intravenous infusion fluids. *Dermatologica* 1991; **182**: 39–42.
3 Brown AS, Hoelzer DJ, Piercy SA. Skin necrosis from extravasation of intravenous fluids in children. *Plast Reconstr Surg* 1979; **64**: 145–50.
4 Dufresne RG. Skin necrosis from intravenously infused materials. *Cutis* 1987; **39**: 197–8.
5 MacCara E. Extravasation: A hazard of intravenous therapy. *Drug Intell Clin Pharm* 1987; **17**: 713–17.
6 Ignoffo RJ, Friedman MA. Therapy of local toxicities caused by extravasation of cancer chemotherapeutic drugs. *Cancer Treat Rev* 1980; **7**: 17–27.
7 Harwood KV, Aisner J. Treatment of chemotherapeutic extravasation: current status. *Cancer Treat Rep* 1984; **68**: 939–45.
8 Banerjee A, Brotherston TM, Lamberty BGH *et al.* Cancer chemotherapy agent-induced perivenous extravasation injury. *J Postgrad Med* 1987; **63**: 5–9.
9 Rudolph R, Larson DL. Etiology and treatment of chemotherapeutic agent extravasation injuries. A review. *J Clin Oncol* 1987; **5**: 1116–26.

Blood transfusion

Urticaria occurs in about 1% of transfusions [1], and may be the result of allergy to soluble proteins in donor plasma. Post-transfusion purpura may rarely occur as a result of profound thrombocytopenia about 1 week after transfusion, and is associated with antiplatelet alloantibodies. Other potential side-effects include transmission of infectious diseases, including syphilis, hepatitis B, and HIV-related syndromes (AIDS).

Graft-versus-host disease may develop following transfusion of unirradiated blood in immunosuppressed patients [2–8], including those with malignancies [2], and infants with severe congenital immunodeficiency [3]. Isolated reports of fatal transfusion-associated graft-versus-host disease in presumed immunocompetent hosts receiving fresh unirradiated blood have been reported [9–11]. This paradoxical situation may be in part explained by situations in which recipients heterozygous for a given major histocompatibility complex haplotype receive a transfusion from a donor homozygous for this haplotype, since the recipient would not react to the donor haplotype, but the donor lymphocytes would react to the non-identical recipient haplotype [8]. Thus, some recipients of non-irradiated blood from their offspring may be at risk of developing graft-versus-host disease. An acute fatal illness, characterized by fever, diffuse erythematous rash, and progressive leukopenia, has been described in Japanese patients 10 days after surgical operation, under the name postoperative erythroderma [12]. Histologically, scattered single-cell epidermal cell eosinophilic necrosis, satellite-cell necrosis, basal cell liquefaction degeneration and a scanty dermal infiltrate may be seen; the reaction is compatible with an acute graft-versus-host reaction following blood transfusion [12].

REFERENCES

1 Shulman IA. Adverse reactions to blood transfusion. *Texas Med* 1990; **85**: 35–42.
2 Decoste SD, Boudreaux C, Dover JS. Transfusion-associated graft-vs-host disease in patients with malignancies. Report of two cases and review of the literature. *Arch Dermatol* 1990; **126**: 1324–9.
3 Hathaway WE, Githens JH, Blackburn WR *et al.* Aplastic anemia, histiocytosis and erythrodermia in immunologically deficient children. *N Engl J Med* 1965; **273**: 953–8.
4 Brubaker DB. Human posttransfusion graft-versus-host disease. *Vox Sang* 1983; **45**: 401–20.
5 Leitman SF, Holland PV. Irradiation of blood products: indications and guidelines. *Transfusion* 1985; **25**: 292–300.
6 Anderson KC, Weinstein HJ. Transfusion-associated graft-versus-host disease. *N Engl J Med* 1990; **323**: 315–21.
7 Ray TL. Blood transfusions and graft-vs-host disease. *Arch Dermatol* 1990; **126**: 1347–50.
8 Ferrara JLM, Deeg HJ. Graft-versus-host disease. *N Engl J Med* 1991; **324**: 667–74.
9 Arsura EL, Bertelle A, Minkowitz S *et al.* Transfusion-associated graft-vs-host disease in a presumed immunocompetent patient. *Arch Intern Med* 1988; **148**: 1941–4.
10 Capond SM, DePond WD, Tyan DB *et al.* Transfusion-associated graft-versus-host disease in an immunocompetent patient. *Ann Intern Med* 1991; **114**: 1025–6.
11 Juji T, Takahashi K, Shibata Y *et al.* Post-transfusion graft-versus-host disease in immunocompetent patients after cardiac surgery in Japan. *N Engl J Med* 1989; **321**: 56.
12 Hidano A, Yamashita N, Mizuguchi M, Toyoda H. Clinical, histological, and immunohistological studies of postoperative erythroderma. *J Dermatol* 1989; **16**: 20–30.

Hydroxyethyl starch

Hydroxyethyl starch (hetastarch) is used as a plasma expander for hypovolaemia, to prime cardiopulmonary bypass machines, as a sedimenting agent to increase the yield of granulocytes during leukopheresis, and to improve microcirculation as in the treatment of sudden deafness. It has been implicated in the development of lichen planus [1], and severe generalized pruritus in up to 32% of recipients, beginning 2 weeks after exposure and taking up to 2 years to settle [2–5].

REFERENCES

1 Bode U, Deisseroth AB. Donor toxicity in granulocyte collections: association of lichen planus with the use of hydroxyethyl starch leukapheresis. *Transfusion* 1981; **21**: 83–5.
2 Parker NE, Porter JB, Williams HJM, Leftley N. Pruritus after administration of hetastarch. *Br Med J* 1982; **284**: 385–6.
3 Gall H, Kaufmann R, von Ehr M *et al.* Persistierender Pruritus nach Hydroxyathylstarke-Infusionen. Retrospektive Langzeitstudie an 266 Fallen. *Hautarzt* 1993; **44**: 713–16.
4 Cox NH, Popple AW. Persistent erythema and pruritus, with a confluent histiocytic skin infiltrate, following the use of a hydroxyethylstarch plasma expander. *Br J Dermatol* 1996; **134**: 353–7.
5 Speight EL, MacSween RM, Stevens A. Persistent itching due to etherified starch plasma expander. *Br Med J* 1997; **314**: 1466–7.

Renal dialysis

Dermatological complications of renal dialysis have been reviewed [1,2]. These include marked premature ageing, hyperpigmentation, xeroderma, decreased sebaceous and sweat-gland secretion, Raynaud's syndrome, generalized pruritus and carpal tunnel syndrome due to amyloid β deposition [1]. Extravasation, phlebitis and bacterial infection of the cannula, with resulting septicaemia, may occur; related to the site of insertion of the cannula into the arteriovenous fistula. A bullous dermatosis of haemodialysis has been described [2,3]. This resembles porphyria clinically and histologically, and porphyrins may be elevated [3], although cases with pseudoporphyria in which there are no abnormalities of porphyrin metabolism have also been documented [2]. Two-thirds of patients with dialysis-associated anaphylaxis have IgE antibodies to ethylene oxide/human serum albumin [4]. Allergic contact dermatitis due to rubber chemicals in the haemodialysis equipment may be seen around the arteriovenous shunt [5]. Porokeratosis localized to the access region for haemodialysis has also been reported [6].

REFERENCES

1 Altmeyer P, Kachel H-G, Jünger M *et al.* Hautveränderungen bei Langzeitdialysepatienten. *Hautarzt* 1982; **33**: 303–9.
2 Gupta AK, Gupta MA, Cardella CJ, Haberman HF. Cutaneous complications of chronic renal failure and dialysis. *Int J Dermatol* 1986; **25**: 498–504.
3 Poh-Fitzpatrick MB, Bellet N, DeLeo VA *et al.* Porphyria cutanea tarda in two patients treated with hemodialysis for chronic renal failure. *N Engl J Med* 1978; **299**: 292–4.
4 Grammer LC, Roberts M, Wiggins CA *et al.* A comparison of cutaneous testing and ELISA testing for assessing reactivity to ethylene oxide-human serum albumin in hemodialysis patients with anaphylactic reactions. *J Allergy Clin Immunol* 1991; **87**: 674–6.
5 Kruis-De Vries MH, Coenraads PJ, Nater JP. Allergic contact dermatitis due to rubber chemicals in haemodialysis equipment. *Contact Dermatitis* 1987; **17**: 303–5.
6 Nakazawa A, Matsuo I, Ohkido M. Porokeratosis localized to the access region for hemodialysis. *J Am Acad Dermatol* 1991; **25**: 338–40.

Necrosis from intramuscular injections

Severe painful local necrosis at the site of an injected medicament (embolia cutis medicamentosa, also known as the *Nicolau syndrome*) may follow intramuscular therapeutic injections and was originally described with bismuth. It occurs particularly with preparations containing corticosteroids, local anaesthetics, antirheumatic drugs and antihistamines; more rarely, chlorpromazine, penicillin, phenobarbitone and sulphonamides have been implicated [1,2]. Clinically, stellate erythema and infiltration are followed by central deep necrosis which heals with scarring.

REFERENCES

1 Bork K. *Cutaneous Side Effects of Drugs*. Philadelphia: WB Saunders, 1988.
2 Faucher L, Marcoux D. What syndrome is this? Nicolau syndrome. *Pediatr Dermatol* 1995; **12**: 187–90.

Polidocanol

The sclerosing solution polidocanol is said to cause allergic reactions in up to 0.06% of cases, but systemic allergic reactions may be more common than previously recognized [1].

REFERENCE

1 Feied CF, Jackson JJ, Bren TS *et al.* Allergic reactions to polidocanol for vein sclerosis. Two case reports. *J Dermatol Surg Oncol* 1994; **20**: 466–8.

Drugs affecting metabolism or gastrointestinal function

Hypoglycaemic drugs

Dermatological aspects of the oral hypoglycaemic drugs have been reviewed [1–4].

Biguanides

Rashes are much less frequent with metformin and phenformin than with sulphonylureas. Transient erythemas, pruritus and urticaria have been noted.

Sulphonylureas

Chlorpropamide and tolbutamide are most often prescribed, and both can give rise to toxic or allergic reactions. Angio-oedema with glibornuride, urticaria with glibenclamide and a bullous dermatitis with carbutamide have been described [5]; there was no cross-reactivity between first- and second-generation sulphonylureas.

Chlorpropamide. Eruptions occur in 2–3% of patients on chlorpropamide [2]. These include maculopapular rashes, photosensitivity [6], erythema annulare, Stevens–Johnson syndrome [7], erythema nodosum [1], lichenoid eruptions [8,9], purpura and exfoliative dermatitis [10]. Porphyria has been provoked [11]. A disulfiram-like effect, with flushing of the face, headache and palpitations after taking alcohol, occurs in up to 30% of patients [12,13]. The fact that the flush is blocked by naloxone suggests that opioids may be involved in the response.

Glibenclamide. Bullae and cholestasis have occurred together [14].

REFERENCES

1 Beurey J, Jeandidier P, Bermont A. Les complications dermatologiques des traitements antidiabétiques. *Ann Dermatol Syphiligr* 1966; **93**: 13–42.
2 Almeyda J, Baker H. Drug reactions. X. Adverse cutaneous reactions to hypoglycaemic agents. *Br J Dermatol* 1970; **82**: 634–6.
3 Harris EL. Adverse reactions to oral antidiabetic agents. *Br Med J* 1971; **3**: 29–30.
4 Perez MI, Kohn SR. Cutaneous manifestations of diabetes mellitus. *J Am Acad Dermatol* 1994; **30**: 519–31.
5 Chichmanian RM, Papasseudi G, Hieronimus S *et al.* Allergies aux sulfonylurees hypoglycemiantes. Les reactions croisées existent-elles? *Thérapie* 1991; **46**: 163–7.
6 Hitselberger JF, Fosnaugh RP. Photosensitivity due to chlorpropamide. *JAMA* 1962; **180**: 62–3.
7 Yaffee HS. Stevens–Johnson syndrome caused by chlorpropamide: report of a case. *Arch Dermatol* 1960; **82**: 636–7.
8 Dinsdale RCW, Ormerod TP, Walker AE. Lichenoid eruption due to chlorpropamide. *Br Med J* 1968; **i**: 100.
9 Barnett JH, Barnett SM. Lichenoid drug reactions to chlorpropamide and tolazamide. *Cutis* 1984; **34**: 542–4.
10 Rothfeld EL, Goldman J, Goldberg HH, Einhorn S. Severe chlorpropamide toxicity. *JAMA* 1960; **172**: 54–6.
11 Zarowitz H, Newhouse S. Coproporphyrinuria with a cutaneous reaction induced by chlorpropamide. *NY State J Med* 1965; **65**: 2385–7.
12 Stakosch CR, Jefferys DB, Keen H. Blockade of chlorpropamide alcohol flush by aspirin. *Lancet* 1980; **i**: 394–6.
13 Medback S, Wass JAH, Clement-Jones V *et al.* Chlorpropamide alcohol flush and circulating met-enkephalin: a positive link. *Br Med J* 1981; **283**: 937–9.
14 Wongpaitoon V, Mills PR, Russell RI, Patrick RS. Intra-hepatic cholestasis and cutaneous bullae associated with glibenclamide therapy. *Postgrad Med J* 1981; **57**: 244–6.

Lipid-lowering drugs

Acipimox

This nicotinic acid analogue causes less prostaglandin-mediated flushing and itching than nicotinic acid [1].

Clofibrate

Erythema multiforme and a variety of other erythematous rashes have been described [2].

Gemfibrozil

This lipid-lowering drug, which mainly lowers triglycerides, has been associated with exacerbation of psoriasis [3,4].

HMG-CoA reductase inhibitors

The lipid-lowering drugs lovastatin, simvastatin and pravastatin can cause eczema [4,5]; these drugs inhibit an early step of cholesterol biosynthesis, i.e. 3-hydroxy-3-methylglutaryl coenzyme A (HMG-CoA) reductase activity. Simvastatin has caused a lichenoid eruption with skin and mucosal involvement [6,7].

Triparanol and diazacholesterol

These drugs inhibit a late step in cholesterol biosynthesis, δ-24-sterol reductase, and can induce ichthyosis or palmoplantar hyperkeratosis [4].

REFERENCES

1 Anonymous. Acipimox—a nicotinic acid analogue for hyperlipidaemia. *Drug Ther Bull* 1991; **29**: 57–9.
2 Murata Y, Tani M, Amano M. Erythema multiforme due to clofibrate. *J Am Acad Dermatol* 1988; **18**: 381–2.
3 Fisher DA, Elias PM, LeBoit PL. Exacerbation of psoriasis by the hypolipidemic agent, gemfibrozil. *Arch Dermatol* 1988; **124**: 854–5.
4 Proksch E. Lipidsenker-induzierte Nebenwirkungen an der Haut. *Hautarzt* 1995; **46**: 76–80.
5 Krasovec M, Elsner P, Burg G. Generalized eczematous skin rash possibly due to HMG-CoA reductase inhibitors. *Dermatology* 1993; **186**: 248–52.
6 Feldmann R, Mainetti C, Saurat JH. Skin lesions due to treatment with simvastatin (Zocor). *Dermatology* 1993; **186**: 272.
7 Roger D, Rolle F, Labrousse F *et al*. Simvastatin-induced lichenoid drug eruption. *Clin Exp Dermatol* 1994; **19**: 88–9.

Drugs for gastrointestinal ulceration

Omeprazole

This proton pump inhibitor, a substituted benzimidazole, has gained widespread use in the treatment of gastric and duodenal ulceration and reflux oesophagitis. Adverse events with the drug are rare and involve mainly the gastrointestinal and central nervous systems with diarrhoea, headache and dizziness, and confusion in the elderly, moderate elevation of aminotransferases and possible leukopenia [1–3]. The prevalence of cutaneous reactions to omeprazole is approximately 0.5–1.5% [1–4]. A variety of eruptions are recorded, including angio-oedema and urticaria [4,5], anaphylaxis [6], maculopapular rashes, lichen planus [7], pityriasiform eruption [8], exfoliative dermatitis [9], bullous eruption [10], erythema multiforme and photosensitivity. Gynaecomastia is recorded [11].

Tripotassium dicitratobismuthate (De-Nol)

The Netherlands Centre for Monitoring of Adverse Reactions to Drugs has received several reports of skin reactions, on average 2 days after starting treatment, including maculopapular exanthema, angio-oedema and erythema [12].

REFERENCES

1 McTavish D, Buckley MM, Heel RC. Omeprazole: an update review of its pharmacology and therapeutic use in acid related disorders. *Drugs* 1991; **42**: 138–70.
2 Castot A, Bidault I, Dahan R, Efthymiou ML. Bilan des effets inattendus et toxiques de l'omeprazole (Mopral) rapportés aux centres regionaux de pharmacovigilance, au cours des 22 premiers mois de commercialisation. *Thérapie* 1993; **48**: 469–74.
3 Yeomans ND. Omeprazole: short- and long-term safety. *Adv Drug React Toxicol Rev* 1994; **13**: 145–56.
4 Bowlby HA, Dickens GR. Angioedema and urticaria associated with omeprazole confirmed by drug rechallenge. *Pharmacotherapy* 1994; **14**: 119–22.
5 Haeney MR. Angio-oedema and urticaria associated with omeprazole. *Br Med J* 1992; **305**: 870.
6 Ottervanger JP, Phaff RA, Vermeulen EG, Stricker BH. Anaphylaxis to omeprazole. *J Allergy Clin Immunol* 1996; **97**: 1413–14.
7 Sharma BK, Walt RP, Pounder RE *et al*. Optimal dose of oral omeprazole for maximal 24 hour decrease of intragastric acidity. *Gut* 1984; **25**: 957–64.
8 Buckley C. Pityriasis rosea-like eruption in a patient receiving omeprazole. *Br J Dermatol* 1996; **135**: 660–1.
9 Epelde Gonzalo FD, Boada Montagut L, Thomas Vecina S. Exfoliative dermatitis related to omeprazole. *Ann Pharmacother* 1995; **29**: 82–3.
10 Stenier C, Fiasse R, Bourlond J *et al*. Bullous skin reaction induced by omeprazole. *Br J Dermatol* 1995; **133**: 343–4.
11 Lindquist M, Edwards IR. Endocrine effects of omeprazole. *Br Med J* 1992; **305**: 451–2.
12 Ottervanger JP, Stricker BH. Huidafwijkingen door bismutoxide (De-Nol). *Ned Tijdschr Geneesk* 1994; **138**: 152–3.

Laxatives

Side-effects of laxatives have been reviewed [1].

Danthron

A highly characteristic irritant erythema of the buttocks and thighs has been observed in patients who are partially incontinent. The erythema results from skin soiling by faecal matter containing a dithranol (anthralin)-like breakdown product [2].

Phenolphthalein

Fixed eruptions are well known [3–5]. Bullous erythema multiforme and an LE-like reaction are documented.

REFERENCES

1 Ruoff H-J. Unerwünschte Wirkungen und Wechselwirkungen von Abführmitteln. *Med Klin* 1980; **75**: 214–18.
2 Barth JH, Reshad H, Darley CR, Gibson JRA. A cutaneous complication of Dorbanex therapy. *Clin Exp Dermatol* 1984; **9**: 95–6.
3 Shelley WB, Schlappner OL, Heiss HB. Demonstration of intercellular immunofluorescence and epidermal hysteresis in bullous fixed drug eruption due to phenolphthalein. *Br J Dermatol* 1972; **6**: 118–25.
4 Wyatt E, Greaves M, Sondergaard J. Fixed drug eruption (phenolphthalein). Evidence for a blood-borne mediator. *Arch Dermatol* 1972; **106**: 671–3.
5 Zanolli MD, McAlvany J, Krowchuk DP. Phenolphthalein-induced fixed drug eruption: a cutaneous complication of laxative use in a child. *Pediatrics* 1993; **91**: 1199–201.

Miscellaneous drugs

Food and drug additives

Dermatological complications of food and drug additives have been reviewed [1–14]. These substances have been implicated in the causation of urticaria [4–7], anaphylaxis, purpura and vasculitis [8–12]. However, one study suggested that common food additives are seldom if ever of significance in urticaria [11]. In another study, only 0.63% of food additive provocation tests resulted in exacerbation in 1110 patients with urticaria; tests were not again positive on reprovocation [13]. The prevalance of adverse reactions to food additives is estimated to be 0.03–0.23% [15]. The necessity for double-blind, placebo-controlled testing to substantiate alleged food additive allergy has been emphasized [16]. Information about excipients ('inert ingredients'), such as sweeteners, flavourings, dyes, and preservatives for chewable and liquid preparations of 102 over-the-counter and prescription products of antidiarrhoea, cough and cold, antihistamine/decongestant, analgesic/antipyretic and liquid theophylline medications, has been presented [17]. An average preparation contained two sweeteners; especially saccharin and sucrose, followed by sorbitol, glucose, fructose and others. The type of flavouring was not specified in 36 of the 102 preparations; cherry was the most common flavouring, followed by vanilla and lemon. Twenty-one different dyes and colouring agents were used; red dye No. 40 was the most common, followed by yellow No. 6. Sodium benzoate and methylparabens were the commonest of eight preservatives used. Mandatory labelling of excipients in all pharmaceutical preparations is the only way that physicians and patients can be fully informed [17]. It is important to appreciate that peanut oil, to which patients may be strongly allergic, is found in certain medications [18]. Caffeine in coffee and cola beverages caused urticaria in a 10-year-old child, confirmed by prick test and oral challenge test with caffeine [19].

REFERENCES

1 Levantine AJ, Almeyda J. Cutaneous reactions to food and drug additives. *Br J Dermatol* 1977; **91**: 359–62.
2 Simon RA. Adverse reactions to drug additives. *J Allergy Clin Immunol* 1984; **74**: 623–30.
3 Ruzicka T. Diagnostik von Nahrungsmittelallergien. *Hautarzt* 1987; **38**: 10–15.
4 Juhlin LG, Michäelsson G, Zetterström O. Urticaria and asthma induced by food-and-drug additives in patients with aspirin hypersensitivity. *J Allergy* 1972; **50**: 92–8.
5 Doeglas HMG. Reactions to aspirin and food additives in patients with chronic urticaria, including the physical urticarias. *Br J Dermatol* 1975; **93**: 135–44.
6 Supramaniam G, Warner JO. Artificial food additive intolerance in patients with angio-oedema and urticaria. *Lancet* 1986; **ii**: 907–9.
7 Juhlin L. Additives and chronic urticaria. *Ann Allergy* 1987; **59**: 119–23.
8 Michäelsson G, Petterson L, Juhlin L. Purpura caused by food and drug additives. *Arch Dermatol* 1974; **109**: 49–52.
9 Kubba R, Champion RI. Anaphylactoid purpura caused by tartrazine and benzoates. *Br J Dermatol* 1975; **93** (Suppl. 2): 61–2.
10 Eisenmann A, Ring J, von der Helm D *et al*. Vasculitis allergica durch Nahrungsmittelallergie. *Hautarzt* 1988; **39**: 319–21.
11 Veien NK, Krogdahl A. Cutaneous vasculitis induced by food additives. *Acta Derm Venereol (Stockh)* 1991; **71**: 73–4.
12 Lowry MD, Hudson CF, Callen FP. Leukocytoclastic vasculitis caused by drug additives. *J Am Acad Dermatol* 1994; **30**: 854–5.
13 Hernandez Garcia J, Garcia Selles J, Negro Alvarez JM *et al*. Incidencias de reacciones adversas con aditivos. Nuestra experiencia de 10 anos. *Allergol Immunopathol* 1994; **22**: 233–42.
14 Barbaud A. Place of excipients in drug-related allergy. *Clin Rev Allergy Immunol* 1995; **13**: 253–63.
15 Wuthrich B. Adverse reactions to food additives. *Ann Allergy* 1993; **71**: 379–84.
16 Goodman DL, McDonnell JT, Nelson HS *et al*. Chronic urticaria exacerbated by the antioxidant food preservatives, butylated hydroxyanisole (BHA) and butylated hydroxytoluene (BHT). *J Allergy Clin Immunol* 1990; **86**: 570–5.
17 Kumar A, Rawlings RD, Beaman DC. The mystery ingredients: sweeteners, flavorings, dyes, and preservatives in analgesic/antipyretic, antihistamine/decongestant, cough and cold, antidiarrheal, and liquid theophylline preparations. *Pediatrics* 1993; **91**: 927–33.
18 Weeks R. Peanut oil in medications. *Lancet* 1996; **348**: 759–60.
19 Caballero T, Garcia-Ara C, Pascual C *et al*. Urticaria induced by caffeine. *J Invest Allergol Clin Immunol* 1993; **3**: 160–2.

Colouring agents

Colourings in food and in medications, including some antihistamines, such as tartrazine, sunset yellow and other azo dyes, have been reported to cause adverse reactions [1,2] including urticaria [3,4] or vasculitis [5,6].

REFERENCES

1 Vandelle C, Belegaud D, Bidault I, Castol A. Allergie aux colorants des medicaments. Confrontation des cas publiés et de l'experience du Centre Regional de Pharmacovigilance. *Thérapie* 1993; **48**: 484–5.
2 Gracey-Whitman L, Ell S. Artificial colourings and adverse reactions. *Br Med J* 1995; **311**: 1204.
3 Neuman I, Elian R, Nahum H *et al*. The danger of 'yellow dyes' (tartrazine) to allergic subjects. *J Allergy* 1972; **50**: 92–8.
4 Miller K. Sensitivity to tartrazine. *Br Med J* 1982; **285**: 1597–8.
5 Lowry MD, Hudson CF, Callen FP. Leukocytoclastic vasculitis caused by drug additives. *J Am Acad Dermatol* 1994; **30**: 854–5.
6 Wuthrich B. Adverse reactions to food additives. *Ann Allergy* 1993; **71**: 379–84.

Flavouring agents

Aspartame. Aspartame, a synthetic dipeptide composed of aspartic acid and the methyl ester of phenylalanine used under the trade name of NutraSweet (G.D. Searle & Co., Skokie, Illinois, USA) as a low-calorie artifical sweetener, has been associated with relatively few adverse side-effects despite its widespread usage [1]. Cutaneous side-effects reported include urticaria, angio-oedema and other nondescript 'rashes' [2], granulomatous septal panniculitis [3] and lobular panniculitis [4]. However, in a recent study of patients with a history of aspartame sensitivity, it was not possible to identify any subject with a clearly reproducible adverse reaction [5]. Similarly, a multicentre, placebo-controlled challenge study showed that aspartame and its conversion products are no more likely than placebo to cause urticaria and/or angio-oedema reactions in subjects with a history consistent with hypersensitivity to aspartame [6].

Cyclamates. Cyclamates, used as sweeteners in soft drinks, have caused photosensitivity [7].

Quinine. Quinine in tonic water and other bitter drinks may cause fixed eruptions [8].

REFERENCES

1 US Food and Drug Administration. Food additives permitted for direct addition to food for human consumption: aspartame. *Federal Register* 1983; **48**: 31376–82.
2 Kulczycki A, Jr. Aspartame-induced urticaria. *Ann Intern Med* 1986; **104**: 207–8.
3 Novick NL. Aspartame-induced granulomatous panniculitis. *Ann Intern Med* 1985; **102**: 206–7.
4 McCauliffe DP, Poitras K. Aspartame-induced lobular panniculitis. *J Am Acad Dermatol* 1991; **24**: 298–300.
5 Garriga MM, Berkebile C, Metcalfe DD. A combined single-blind, double-blind, placebo-controlled study to determine the reproducibility of hypersensitivity reactions to aspartame. *J Allergy Clin Immunol* 1991; **87**: 821–7.
6 Geha R, Buckley CE, Greenberger P *et al*. Aspartame is no more likely than placebo to cause urticaria/angioedema: results of a multicenter, randomized, double-blind, placebo-controlled, crossover study. *J Allergy Clin Immunol* 1993; **92**: 513–20.
7 Lambert SI. A new photosensitizer. The artificial sweetener cyclamate. *JAMA* 1967; **201**: 747–50.
8 Commens C. Fixed drug eruption. *Aust J Dermatol* 1983; **24**: 1–8.

Preservatives

The antioxidant food preservatives, butylated hydroxyanisole (BHA) and butylated hydroxytoluene (BHT), have been reported to exacerbate chronic urticaria [1]. Sodium benzoate has been associated with urticaria, angio-oedema, asthma and rarely anaphylaxis [2]. Parabens used as a preservative may also cause urticaria [3].

Sulphiting agents are commonly used in parenteral emergency drugs, including adrenaline (epinephrine), dexamethasone, dobutamine, dopamine, noradrenaline (norepinephrine), phenylephrine, procainamide and physostigmine [4]. Published anaphylactic or asthmatic reactions have been associated with sulphited local anaesthetics, gentamicin, metoclopramide, doxycycline and vitamin B complex. The reactions have a rapid onset, and do not always coincide with a positive oral challenge, but patients with a history of positive oral challenge to 5–10 mg of sulphite may be   at increased risk of developing a reaction to parenteral sulphites. Sulphites added as antioxidant preservatives may provoke urticaria, asthma, anaphylaxis and shock [4–10] as well as urticarial vasculitis [11]. Intolerance due to metabisulphite as an antioxidant in a dental anaesthetic has led to angio-oedema; patch tests were positive [12]. Basophil activation induced by sulphites may be IgE dependent [13]. It has been claimed that there is a high specificity of patch testing in the diagnosis of patients with sulphite sensitivity [14].

REFERENCES

1 Goodman DL, McDonnell JT, Nelson HS *et al*. Chronic urticaria exacerbated by the antioxidant food preservatives, butylated hydroxyanisole (BHA) and butylated hydroxytoluene (BHT). *J Allergy Clin Immunol* 1990; **86**: 570–5.
2 Michils A, Vandermoten G, Duchateau J, Yernault J-C. Anaphylaxis with sodium benzoate. *Lancet* 1991; **337**: 1424–5.
3 Nagel JE, Fuscaldo JT, Fireman P. Paraben allergy. *JAMA* 1977; **237**: 1594–5.
4 Smolinske SC. Review of parenteral sulfite reactions. *J Toxicol Clin Toxicol* 1992; **30**: 597–606.
5 Habenicht HA, Preuss L, Lovell RG. Sensitivity to ingested metabisulfites: cause of bronchospasm and urticaria. *Immunol Allergy Pract* 1983; **5**: 243–5.
6 Settipane GA. Adverse reactions to sulfites in drugs and foods. *J Am Acad Dermatol* 1984; **10**: 1077–80.
7 Belchi-Hernandez J, Florido-Lopez JF, Estrada-Rodriguez JL *et al*. Sulfite-induced urticaria. *Ann Allergy* 1993; **71**: 230–2.
8 Twarog FJ, Leung DYM. Anaphylaxis to a component of isoetharine (sodium bisulfite). *JAMA* 1982; **248**: 2030–1.
9 Przybilla B, Ring J. Sulfit-Überempfindlichkeit. *Hautarzt* 1987; **38**: 445–8.
10 Hassoun S, Bonneau JC, Drouet M, Sabbah A. Enquete sur pathologies induites par les sulfites en allergologie. *Allerg Immunol* 1994; **26**: 184, 187–8.
11 Wuthrich B. Adverse reactions to food additives. *Ann Allergy* 1993; **71**: 379–84.
12 Dooms-Goosens A, Gidi de Alan A, Degreef H, Kochuyt A. Local anaesthetic intolerance due to metabisulfite. *Contact Dermatitis* 1989; **20**: 124–6.
13 Sainte-Laudy J, Vallon C, Guerin JC. Mise en evidence des IgE specifiques du groupe des sulfites chez les intolerants à ces conservateurs. *Allerg Immunol* 1994; **26**: 132–4, 137–8.
14 Gay G, Sabbah A, Drouet M. Valeur diagnostique de l'epidermotest aux sulfites. *Allerg Immunol* 1994; **26**: 139–40.

Miscellaneous food additives

Agricultural or veterinary chemicals may leave residues in animal and plants used as human food, for example penicillin in milk or meat, with resultant urticaria [1,2]. The exposure of a rural Turkish population to flour contaminated with hexachlorobenzene induced an outbreak of cutaneous porphyria [3]. Contaminated rapeseed cooking oil containing acetanilide resulted in the Spanish 'toxic oil syndrome'; the central feature of the illness was a toxic pneumonitis, but fixed rashes and scleroderma-like changes in survivors were seen [4–6]. Outbreaks of atypical erythema multiforme and other exanthemata in Holland were attributed to an additive in margarine [7,8]. The high arsenic content of a rural water supply in Taiwan caused arsenism [9]. Chemicals added to tobacco, for example menthol in cigarettes, have caused urticaria [10]. *N*-nitroso compounds, which are known to be carcinogenic in animals, occur in food products and certain alcoholic drinks, but there is no direct proof as yet of a causal role in human disease [11].

REFERENCES

1 Boonk WJ, Van Ketel WG. The role of penicillin in the pathogenesis of chronic urticaria. *Br J Dermatol* 1982; **106**: 183–90.
2 Kanny G, Puygrenier J, Beaudoin E, Moneret-Vautrin DA. Choc anaphylactique alimentaire: implication des residus de penicilline. *Allerg Immunol* 1994; **26**: 181–3.
3 Peters HA, Gocmen A, Cripps DJ *et al*. Epidemiology of hexachlorobenzene-induced porphyria in Turkey. *Arch Neurol* 1982; **39**: 744–9.

4 Martinez-Tello FJ, Navas-Palacios JJ, Ricoy JR *et al.* Pathology of a new toxic syndrome caused by ingestion of adulterated oil in Spain. *Virchows Arch A Pathol Anat Histopathol* 1982; **397**: 261–85.

5 Leading Article. Toxic oil syndrome. *Lancet* 1983; **i**: 1257–8.

6 Rush PJ, Bell MJ, Fam AG. Toxic oil syndrome (Spanish oil disease) and chemically induced scleroderma-like conditions. *J Rheumatol* 1984; **11**: 262–4.

7 Sternberg TH, Bierman SM. Unique syndromes involving the skin induced by drugs, food additives, and environmental contaminants. *Arch Dermatol* 1963; **88**: 779–88.

8 Mali JW, Malten KE. The epidemic of polymorphic toxic erythema in the Netherlands in 1960. The so-called margarine disease. *Acta Derm Venereol (Stockh)* 1966; **46**: 123–35.

9 Yeh S. Skin cancer in chronic arsenicism. *Hum Pathol* 1973; **4**: 469–85.

10 McGowan EM. Menthol urticaria. *Arch Dermatol* 1966; **94**: 62–3.

11 Tannenbaum SR. N-nitroso compounds: a perspective on human exposure. *Lancet* 1983; **i**: 628–30.

Herbal remedies, homeopathy and naturopathy

Chinese herbal medicine

Adverse effects of Chinese herbal medicines, including life-threatening 'dazao'-induced angio-oedema and liquorice-induced hypokalaemic periodic paralysis, accounted for 0.2% of medical admissions to a hospital in Hong Kong over an 8 month period [1]. Herbal poisoning in Hong Kong, Taipei and Kuala Lumpur has occurred as a result of addition of adulterants (*Podophyllum emodi*) or erroneous substitutes (*Datura metel*) [2]. A fatality due to total liver necrosis associated with ingestion of Chinese herbal medicines is believed to have occurred because the patient prepared a decoction from a herbal mixture containing *Eurysolen gracilis* Prain (*Labiatae*), a herb not used in Chinese medicine [3]. A multisystem illness developed in a patient after ingestion of Chinese herbal medicines containing the potentially toxic compounds benzaldehyde, cinnamoyl alcohol and ephedrine [4]. Some Chinese patent medicines contain mercurial ingredients, cinnabar (red mercuric sulphide) and calomel (mercurous chloride) [5]. Alopecia and sensory polyneuropathy from thallium in a Chinese herbal medication has been reported [6]. Chinese herbal medicine may contain camouflaged prescription anti-inflammatory drugs, corticosteroids and lead [7], and some practitioners of Chinese medicine supply 'herbal creams', which actually contain potent topical steroid ointments [8,9]. There are major concerns about hepatotoxicity [10–14] and nephrotoxicity [15–21] of Chinese herbal medicine. In one case, hepatotoxicity was associated with ingestion of the Chinese herbal product jin bu huan anodyne tablets (*Lycopodium serratum*) [12]. A rapidly progressive fibrosing interstitial nephritis developed in young women who followed the same slimming regimen containing two Chinese herbs (*Stephania tetrandra* and *Magnolia officinalis*) [15–17]. The known carcinogen, aristolochic acid, has been suspected in some cases of nephropathy [17,18]. Urothelial malignancy has supervened [20]. An acquired Fanconi syndrome was induced by a mixture of Chinese crude drugs [21].

The need for correct identification of herbs in herbal poisoning [22], and for monitoring of the safety of herbal medicines [23], has been emphasized. Greater awareness of their toxicity is required [24,25]. Special licensing of herbal remedies exists in Germany, France and Australia and has been advocated in the UK [26].

Analgesic and anti-inflammatory Chinese medicinal materials, especially those containing fragrance, may cause contact sensitization, and can cause systemic contact dermatitis [27,28]. Erythema multiforme [28], exanthema [29], and erythroderma [30] are described. Fever with oedematous erythema was caused by a decoction of the crude drug Boi of Kampo (Sino-Japanese traditional) medicine for the alleviation of arthralgia; oral ingestion tests incriminated the constituent sinomenine [31].

A 'tea' prepared from a decoction of herbs has been reported to be of benefit in eczema [32,33]. The decoction contains paenol (2'-hydroxy-4'-methoxyacetophenone), which is known to have platelet antiaggregatory, analgesic and antipyretic properties [34]. Hepatotoxicity was described in a 9-year-old girl who consumed a Chinese herbal tea for 6 months [35] and was reported in a further patient [36]. Reversible abnormal liver-function tests have been reported in two children receiving Chinese herbal therapy (Zemaphyte) [37]. Toxicology screening in a group of adults on Zemaphyte for 1 year revealed no abnormalities in haematological or biochemical parameters; transient nausea and abdominal distension, with a mild laxative effect, was noted in about one-third of patients [38].

REFERENCES

1 Chan TY, Chan AY, Critchley JA. Hospital admissions due to adverse reactions to Chinese herbal medicines. *J Trop Med Hyg* 1992; **95**: 296–8.

2 But PP. Herbal poisoning caused by adulterants or erroneous substitutes. *J Trop Med Hyg* 1994; **947**: 371–4.

3 Perharic-Walton L, Murray V. Toxicity of Chinese herbal remedies. *Lancet* 1992; **340**: 674.

4 Gorey JD, Wahlqvist ML, Boyce NW. Adverse reaction to a Chinese herbal remedy. *Med J Aust* 1992; **157**: 484–6.

5 Kang-Yum E, Oransky SH. Chinese patent medicine as a potential source of mercury poisoning. *Vet Hum Toxicol* 1992; **34**: 235–8.

6 Schaumburg HH, Berger A. Alopecia and sensory polyneuropathy from thallium in a Chinese herbal medication. *JAMA* 1992; **268**: 3430–1.

7 Goldman JA, Myerson G. Chinese herbal medicine: camouflaged prescription anti-inflammatory drugs, corticosteroids, and lead. *Arthritis Rheum* 1991; **34**: 1207.

8 Allen BR, Parkinson R. Chinese herbs for eczema. *Lancet* 1990; **336**: 177.

9 O'Driscoll J, Burden AD, Kingston TP. Potent topical steroid obtained from a Chinese herbalist. *Br J Dermatol* 1992; **127**: 543–4.

10 Mostefa-Kara N, Pauwels A, Pinus E *et al.* Fatal hepatitis after herbal tea. *Lancet* 1992; **340**: 674.

11 Graham-Brown R. Toxicity of chinese herbal remedies. *Lancet* 1992; **340**: 673.

12 Woolf GM, Petrovic LM, Rojter SE *et al.* Acute hepatitis associated with the Chinese herbal product jin bu huan. *Ann Int Med* 1994; **121**: 729–35.

13 Pillans PI. Toxicity of herbal products. *NZ Med J* 1995; **108**: 469–71.

14 Larrey D, Pageaux GP. Hepatotoxicity of herbal remedies and mushrooms. *Semin Liver Dis* 1995; **15**: 183–8.

15 Vanherweghem JL, Depierreux M, Tielemans C *et al.* Rapidly progressive

interstitial renal fibrosis in young women: association with slimming regimen including Chinese herbs. *Lancet* 1993; **341**; 387–91.

16 Depierreux M, Van Damme B, Vanden Houte K, Vanherweghem JL. Pathologic aspects of a newly described nephropathy related to the prolonged use of Chinese herbs. *Am J Kidney Dis* 1994; **24**: 172–80.

17 Cosyns JP, Jadoul M, Squifflet JP *et al*. Chinese herbs nephropathy: a clue to Balkan endemic nephropathy? *Kidney Int* 1994; **45**: 1680–8.

18 Vanhaelen M, Vanhaelen-Fastre R, But P, Vanherweghem JL. Identification of aristolochic acid in Chinese herbs. *Lancet* 1994; **343**: 174.

19 Diamond JR, Pallone TL. Acute interstitial nephritis following use of tung shueh pills. *Am J Kidney Dis* 1994; **24**: 219–21.

20 Cosyns JP, Jadoul M, Squifflet JP *et al*. Urothelial malignancy in nephropathy due to Chinese herbs. *Lancet* 1994; **344**: 188.

21 Izumotani T, Ishimura E, Tsumura K *et al*. An adult case of Fanconi syndrome due to a mixture of Chinese crude drugs. *Nephron* 1993; **65**: 137–40.

22 But PP. Need for correct identification of herbs in herbal poisoning. *Lancet* 1993; **341**: 637.

23 Mills SY. Monitoring the safety of herbal remedies. European pilot studies are under way. *Br Med J* 1995; **311**: 1570.

24 Atherton DJ. Towards the safer use of traditional remedies. Greater awareness of toxicity is needed. *Br Med J* 1994; **308**: 673–4.

25 Harper J. Traditional Chinese medicine for eczema. Seemingly effective, but caution must prevail. *Br Med J* 1994; **308**: 489–90.

26 De Smet PAGM. Should herbal medicine-like products be licensed as medicines. Special licensing seems the best way forward. *Br Med J* 1995; **310**: 1023–4.

27 Li LF. A clinical and patch test study of contact dermatitis from traditional Chinese medicinal materials. *Contact Dermatitis* 1995; **33**: 392–5.

28 Mateo MP, Velasco M, Miquel FJ, de la Cuadra J. Erythema-multiforme-like eruption following allergic contact dermatitis from sesquiterpene lactones in herbal medicine. *Contact Dermatitis* 1995; **33**: 449–50.

29 Li LF, Zhao J, Li SY. Exanthematous drug eruption due to Chinese herbal medicines sanjieling capsule and huoxuexiaoyan pill. *Contact Dermatitis* 1994; **30**: 252–3.

30 Catlin DH, Sekera M, Adelman DC. Erythroderma associated with ingestion of an herbal product. *West J Med* 1993; **159**: 491–3.

31 Okuda T, Umezawa Y, Ichikawa M *et al*. A case of drug eruption caused by the crude drug Boi (Sinomenium stem (*Sinomeni caulis et Rhizoma*). *J Dermatol* 1995; **22**: 795–800.

32 Atherton D, Sheehan M, Rustin MHA *et al*. Chinese herbs for eczema. *Lancet* 1990; **336**: 1254.

33 Sheehan MP, Atherton DJ, Luo HD. Controlled trial of traditional Chinese medicinal plants in widespread non-exudative atopic eczema. *Br J Dermatol* 1991; **125** (Suppl. 38): 17 (Abstract).

34 Galloway JH, Marsh ID, Bittiner SB *et al*. Chinese herbs for eczema, the active compound? *Lancet* 1991; **337**: 566.

35 Davies EG, Pollock I, Steel HM. Chinese herbs for eczema. *Lancet* 1990; **336**: 177.

36 Carlsson C. Herbs and hepatitis. *Lancet* 1990; **336**: 1068.

37 Sheehan MP, Atherton DJ. One year follow-up of children with atopic eczema treated with traditional Chinese medicinal plants. *Br J Dermatol* 1992; **127** (Suppl. 40): 13.

38 Sheehan MP, Stevens H, Ostlere LS *et al*. Follow-up of adult patients with atopic eczema treated with Chinese herbal therapy for 1 year. *Clin Exp Dermatol* 1995; **20**: 136–40.

Kava dermopathy

The kava plant, a member of the black-pepper family, is used ceremonially by many traditional societies of the Southern Pacific in the form of an intoxicant beverage prepared from roots to induce relaxation, sociability and promote sleep. Herbal drugs containing kava are sold for insomnia, nervousness and depression. A reversible ichthyosiform kava dermopathy may result from excessive use of kava [1,2]. Systemic contact-type dermatitis has occurred after oral administration of kava extract [2].

REFERENCES

1 Norton SA, Ruze P. Kava dermopathy. *J Am Acad Dermatol* 1994; **31**: 89–97.

2 Suss R, Lehmann P. Hamatogenes Kontaktekzem durch pflanzliche Medikamente am Beispiel des Kavawurzel-extraktes. *Hautarzt* 1996; **47**: 459–61.

Homeopathic drugs

Cases of erythroderma, confluent urticaria and anaphylaxis have been reported following homeopathic medication [1]. Treatment of a diaper dermatitis and mild respiratory and enteral infections with homeopathic mercurial medicine—Mercurius 6a (cinnabar dilute $1 \times 10(6)$)—was followed by dissemination of the dermatitis, irritability and albuminuria [2].

REFERENCES

1 Aberer W, Strohal R. Homeopathic preparations—severe adverse effects, unproven benefits. *Dermatologica* 1991; **182**: 253.

2 Montoya-Cabrera MA, Rubio-Rodriguez S, Velazquez-Gonzalez E, Avila Montoya S. Intoxicacion mercurial causada por un medicamento homeopatico. *Gaceta Med Mex* 1991; **127**: 267–70.

Naturopathy

Bizarre and unpredictable cutaneous reactions may follow topical application or ingestion of naturally occurring substances. A curious gyrate erythematous eruption was seen in a patient following local application of onion rings as a home remedy for arthralgia [1]. Substantial amounts of psoralen may be absorbed from vegetables; a patient who consumed a large quantity of celery root (*Apium graveolens*) 1h before a visit to a suntan parlour developed a severe generalized phototoxic reaction [2]. Phototoxicity has been reported from herbal remedies for vitiligo containing powdered seeds of *Psoralea corylifolia*, which contains psoralen, isopsoralen and psoralidin [3]. Contact sensitization has been caused by alternative topical medicaments containing plant extracts [4–7], including tea-tree oil [5,6], which has caused systemic contact dermatitis [5], and allergic airborne contact dermatitis from benzaldehyde, eucalyptus oil, laurel oil, pomerance flower oil, lavender oil, rosewood oil and jasmine oil used for aromatherapy [7].

REFERENCES

1 Breathnach SM, Hintner H. *Adverse Drug Reactions and the Skin*. Oxford: Blackwell Scientific Publications, 1992

2 Ljunggren B. Severe phototoxic burn following celery ingestion. *Arch Dermatol* 1990; **126**: 1334–6.

3 Maurice PDL, Cream JJ. The dangers of herbalism. *Br Med J* 1989; **299**: 1204.

4 Bruynzeel DP, van Ketel WG, Young E *et al*. Contact sensitization by alternative topical medicaments containing plant extracts. The Dutch Contact Dermatoses Group. *Contact Dermatitis* 1992; **27**: 278–9.

5 de Groot AC, Weyland JW. Systemic contact dermatitis from tea tree oil. *Contact Dermatitis* 1992; **27**: 279–80.

6 Knight TE, Hausen BM. Melaleuca oil (tea tree oil) dermatitis. *J Am Acad Dermatol* 1994; **30**: 423–7.
7 Schaller M, Korting HC. Allergic airborne contact dermatitis from essential oils used in aromatherapy. *Clin Exp Dermatol* 1995; **20**: 143–5.

Miscellaneous

Canthaxanthin, a synthetic non-provitamin A carotenoid deposited in epidermis and subcutaneous fat, caused fatal aplastic anaemia when ingested to promote tanning [1].

REFERENCE

1 Bluhm R, Branch R, Johnston P, Stein R. Aplastic anemia associated with canthaxanthin ingested for 'tanning' purposes. *JAMA* 1990; **264**: 1141–2.

Industrial and other exposure to chemicals

The reader is referred above for discussion of sclero-dermatous reactions to environmental agents. A form of fluoride toxicity occurred due to industrial poisoning in the Italian town of Chizzolo, resulting in pinkish brown, round or oval macules seen in hundreds of the local population [1]. Similar small outbreaks have occurred in North America [2]. Exfoliative dermatitis has been recorded with trichloroethylene [3]. Occupational exposure to trichloroethylene has also caused Stevens–Johnson syndrome [4].

Patients exposed to dioxin after an industrial accident at Seveso, Italy, developed early irritative lesions, comprising erythema and oedema of exposed areas, vesicobullous and necrotic lesions of the palms and fingertips, and papulonodular lesions; later lesions were those of chloracne [5]. Contamination of rice-bran cooking oil with polychlorinated biphenyls in Taiwan resulted in chloracne, and congenital abnormalities in offspring [6].

Pruritus, urticaria, and discoid and diffuse eczema may occur following the use of brominated disinfectant compounds such as 1-bromo-3-chlor 5, 5-dimethyl hydantoin (Di-halo, Aquabrome) in public swimming pools [7]. Accidental occupational exposure to high concentrations of methyl bromide during a fumigation procedure resulted in erythema with multiple vesicles and large bullae, with predeliction for moist flexures and pressure areas [8]. Idiopathic thrombocytopenic purpura has been associated with industrial exposure to wood preservatives [9], turpentine [10], and to insecticides such as chlordane and heptachlor [11].

REFERENCES

1 Waldbott GC, Cecilioni VA. 'Chizzolo' maculae. *Cutis* 1970; **6**: 331–4.
2 Tabuenca JM. Toxic-allergic syndrome caused by ingestion of rapeseed oil denatured with aniline. *Lancet* 1981; **ii**: 567–8.
3 Nakayama H, Kobayashi M, Takahashi M *et al.* Generalized eruption with severe liver dysfunction associated with occupational exposure to trichloroethylene. *Contact Dermatitis* 1988; **19**: 48–51.
4 Phoon WH, Chan MOY, Rahan VS *et al.* Stevens–Johnson syndrome associated with occupational exposure to trichloroethylene. *Contact Dermatitis* 1984; **10**: 270–6.
5 Caputo R, Monti M, Ermacora E *et al.* Cutaneous manifestations of tetrachlorodibenzo-*p*-dioxin in children and adolescents. *J Am Acad Dermatol* 1988; **19**: 812–19.
6 Gladen BC, Taylor JS, Wu Y-C *et al.* Dermatological findings in children exposed transplacentally to heat-degraded polychlorinated biphenyls in Taiwan. *Br J Dermatol* 1990; **122**: 799–808.
7 Rycroft RJG, Penny PT. Dermatoses associated with brominated swimming pools. *Br Med J* 1983; **28**: 462.
8 Hezemans-Boer M, Toonstra J, Meulenbelt J *et al.* Skin lesions due to exposure to methyl bromide. *Arch Dermatol* 1988; **124**: 917–21.
9 Hay A, Singer CRJ. Wood preservatives, solvents, and thrombocytopenic purpura. *Lancet* 1991; **338**: 766.
10 Wahlberg P, Nyman D. Turpentine and thrombocytopenic purpura. *Lancet* 1969; **ii**: 215–16.
11 Epstein SS, Ozonoff D. Leukemias and blood dyscrasias following exposure to chloradone and heptachlor. *Carcinogen Mutagen Teratogen* 1987; **7**: 527–40.

Local and systemic effects of topical applications

Many topical therapeutic agents may cause serious or even dangerous systemic side-effects if absorbed in sufficient quantity; such absorption may be facilitated through diseased skin, and with use of newer vehicles or occlusive polythene dressings. The risk of serious systemic effects is greatest in infancy and in the old and frail. The quantity absorbed in relation to body weight is greatest in infancy, when the surface area is relatively greater; moreover, neonatal skin is more permeable. Most dangerous or fatal reactions have occurred either because the physician was unaware of the potential hazard or because the patient has continued self-treatment without medical supervision.

Topical therapy

Anthralin (dithranol)

Topical anthralin used in the therapy of stable plaque psoriasis is well-known to cause erythema, irritation and a sensation of burning in normal skin; it stains the skin and clothing [1]. Application of 10% triethanolamine following short contact dithranol treatment has been reported to inhibit the anthralin-induced inflammation without preventing the therapeutic effect [2]. Allergic contact dermatitis to anthralin is very rare. The natural and synthetic anthranols have toxic effects on liver, intestines and the central nervous system, but systemic toxicity in humans under therapeutic conditions has not been established [3].

REFERENCES

1 Paramsothy Y, Lawrence CM. Time course and intensity of anthralin inflammation on involved and uninvolved psoriatic skin. *Br J Dermatol* 1987; **116**: 517–19.
2 Ramsay B, Lawrence CM, Bruce JM, Shuster S. The effect of triethanolamine application on anthralin-induced inflammation and therapeutic effect in psoriasis. *J Am Acad Dermatol* 1990: **23**: 73–6.

3 Ippen H. Basic questions on toxicology and pharmacology of anthralin. *Br J Dermatol* 1981; **105** (Suppl. 20): 72–6.

Boric acid

Poisoning has usually occurred in infants treated for napkin eruptions. Almost all cases have been caused by the use of boric ointments or lotions. However, use of borated talc proved fatal in one infant [1]. Wet boric dressings caused the death of an adult woman [2].

REFERENCES

1 Brooke C, Boggs T. Boric-acid poisoning: report of a case and review of the literature. *Am J Dis Child* 1951; **82**: 465–72.
2 Jordan JW, Crissey JT. Boric acid poisoning: report of fatal adult case from cutaneous use. A critical evaluation of this drug in dermatologic practice. *Arch Dermatol* 1957; **75**: 720–8.

Calcipotriol

This vitamin D$_3$ analogue has been reported to cause transient local irritation, and facial or perioral dermatitis [1]. Contact allergy is recorded [2]. Topical application of calcipotriol for 5 weeks to a mean of 16% of the body surface of psoriatics did not result in detectable systemic alteration of calcium metabolism [3]. The manufacturer's data sheet (Leo Laboratories) states that increased serum calcium may occur with application in daily doses of 50–100 g of the 50 µg/g ointment. Severe symptomatic hypercalcaemia developed after application of about 200 g of the ointment over 1 week to exfoliative psoriasis covering 40% of the body surface [4]. It is recommended that treatment be confined to stable mild to moderate psoriasis, and that the recommended dose of 100 g/week should not be exceeded.

REFERENCES

1 Kragballe K, Gjertsen BT, De Hoop D *et al*. Double-blind, right/left comparison of calcipotriol and betamethasone valerate in treatment of psoriasis vulgaris. *Lancet* 1991; **337**: 193–6.
2 de Groot AC. Contact allergy to calcipotriol. *Contact Dermatitis* 1994; **30**: 242–3.
3 Saurat J-H, Gumowski Sunek D, Rizzoli R. Topical calcipotriol and hypercalcaemia. *Lancet* 1991; **337**: 1287.
4 Dwyer C, Chapman RS. Calcipotriol and hypercalcaemia. *Lancet* 1991; **338**: 764–5.

Coal tar

Coal tar vapour inhalation precipitated severe symptomatic bronchoconstriction in an atopic asthmatic subject following application of coal-tar bandages for treatment of eczema, confirmed by challenge [1].

REFERENCE

1 Ibbotson SH, Stenton SC, Simpson NB. Acute severe bronchoconstriction precipitated by coal tar bandages. *Clin Exp Dermatol* 1995; **20**: 58–9.

Chlorhexidine gluconate (Hibitane)

Urticaria, dyspnoea and anaphylactic shock have occurred following topical application as a disinfectant [1], as have contact urticaria, photosensitive dermatitis [2] and deafness.

REFERENCES

1 Okano M, Nomura M, Hata S *et al*. Anaphylactic symptoms due to chlorhexidine gluconate. *Arch Dermatol* 1989; **125**: 50–2.
2 Wahlberg JE, Wennersten G. Hypersensitivity and photosensitivity to chlorhexidine. *Dermatologica* 1971; **143**: 376–9.

Dequalinium chloride

Necrotic lesions have occurred following its use in the treatment of balanitis [1].

REFERENCE

1 Coles RB, Simpson WT, Wilkinson DS. Dequalinium: a possible complication of its use in balanitis. *Lancet* 1964; **ii**: 531.

Dimethyl sulphoxide

Topical application can cause erythema, pruritus and urticaria, but systemic reactions are very rare; a generalized contact-dermatitis-like reaction followed intravesical instillation in a sensitized individual [1].

REFERENCE

1 Nishimura M, Takano Y, Toshitani Y. Systemic contact dermatitis medicamentosa occurring after intravesical dimethyl sulfoxide treatment for interstitial cystitis. *Arch Dermatol* 1988; **124**: 182–3.

Doxepin

Doxepin cream causes allergic contact dermatitis and systemic contact dermatitis [1,2].

REFERENCES

1 Taylor JS, Praditsuwan P, Handel D, Kuffner G. Allergic contact dermatitis from doxepin cream. One-year patch test clinic experience. *Arch Dermatol* 1996; **132**: 515–18.
2 Shelley W, Shelley ED, Talanin NY. Self-potentiating allergic contact dermatitis caused by doxepin hydrochloride cream. *J Am Acad Dermatol* 1996; **34**: 143–4.

Formaldehyde

Industrial exposure is recognized to be a health hazard, and a threshold limit value of 2 ppm is allowed in the UK and the USA [1]. Irritant or allergic dermatitis is common in exposed workers [2]. Systemic symptoms including breathlessness, headache and drowsiness have been attributed to prolonged exposure to very low levels in the home [3].

REFERENCES

1 Leading Article. The health hazards of formaldehyde. *Lancet* 1981; **i**: 926–7.
2 Glass WI. An outbreak of formaldehyde dermatitis. *NZ Med J* 1961; **60**: 423.
3 Harris JC, Rumack BH, Aldrich FD. Toxicology of urea formaldehyde and polyurethane foam insulation. *JAMA* 1981; **245**: 243–6.

Gamma-benzene hexachloride (lindane)

Lindane therapy for scabies has potential toxicity, which includes neurotoxicity with convulsions, especially in children [1–7]. Most reports have occurred with over-exposure or misuse, but side–effects have followed single applications, particularly when the epidermal barrier has been compromised. Whether this constitutes a significant problem in normal individuals is doubtful [6]. Nevertheless, it has been suggested that permethrin may be a safer and less toxic alternative [7].

REFERENCES

1 Lee B, Groth P. Scabies: transcutaneous poisoning during treatment. *Arch Dermatol* 1979; **115**: 124–5.
2 Pramanik AK, Hansen RC. Transcutaneous gamma benzene hexachloride absorption and toxicity in infants and children. *Arch Dermatol* 1979; **115**: 124–5.
3 Matsuoka LY. Convulsions following application of gamma benzene hexachloride. *J Am Acad Dermatol* 1981; **5**: 98–9.
4 Rasmussen JE. The problem of lindane. *J Am Acad Dermatol* 1981; **5**: 507–16.
5 Davies JE, Dehdia HV, Morgade C *et al*. Lindane poisonings. *Arch Dermatol* 1983; **119**: 142–4.
6 Rasmussen J. Lindane: A prudent approach. *Arch Dermatol* 1987; **123**: 1008–10.
7 Friedman SJ. Lindane neurotoxic reaction in nonbullous ichthyosiform erythroderma. *Arch Dermatol* 1987; **123**: 1056–8.
8 Schultz MW, Gomez M, Hansen RC *et al*. Comparative study of 5% permethrin cream and 1% lindane lotion for the treatment of scabies. *Arch Dermatol* 1990; **126**: 167–70.

Hexachlorophane

This substance has potential neurotoxicity. Exposure of babies to a talc containing 6.3% of hexachlorophane due to a manufacturing error resulted in deaths with ulceration, skin lesions and a characteristic demyelinating encephalopathy [1]. A 3% emulsion has produced milder neurological changes but a 0.33% concentration in talc is apparently safe. Encephalopathy has occurred in burns patients [2].

REFERENCES

1 Martin-Bouyer G, Lebreton R, Toga M *et al*. Outbreak of accidental hexachlorophene poisoning in France. *Lancet* 1982; **i**: 91–5.
2 Larson DL. Studies show hexachlorophene causes burn syndrome. *J Am Hosp Assoc* 1968; **42**: 63–4.

Hydroquinone

Depigmenting creams containing 6–8% of hydroquinone, used especially by black South African women, have caused rebound hyperpigmentation and coarsening of the skin, with ochronotic changes in the dermis, colloid degeneration and colloid milium [1–6]. Collagen degeneration may be seen histologically [2]. Similar changes have been seen in black women in the USA [3] and in a Mexican American woman [4]. Interestingly, ochronosis does not develop in areas of vitiligo [7]. The nails may be pigmented [8].

REFERENCES

1 Findlay GH, Morrison JGL, Simson IW. Exogenous ochronosis and pigmented colloid milium from hydroquinone bleaching creams. *Br J Dermatol* 1975; **93**: 613–22.
2 Phillips JI, Isaacson C, Carman H. Ochronosis in Black South Africans who used skin lighteners. *Am J Dermatopathol* 1986; **8**: 14–21.
3 Lawrence N, Bligard CA, Reed R, Perret WJ. Exogenous ochronosis in the United States. *J Am Acad Dermatol* 1988; **18**: 1207–11.
4 Howard KL, Furner BB. Exogenous ochronosis in a Mexican-American woman. *Cutis* 1990; **45**: 180–2.
5 Camarasa JG, Serra-Baldrich E. Exogenous ochronosis with allergic contact dermatitis from hydroquinone. *Contact Dermatitis* 1994; **31**: 57–8.
6 Snider RL, Thiers BH. Exogenous ochronosis. *J Am Acad Dermatol* 1993; **28**: 662–4.
7 Hull PR, Procter PR. The melanocyte: An essential link in hydroquinone-induced ochronosis. *J Am Acad Dermatol* 1990; **22**: 529–31.
8 Garcia RL, White JW, Willis WF. Hydroquinone nail pigmentation. *Arch Dermatol* 1978; **114**: 1402–3.

Iodine

Povidone–iodine scrub for acne (Betadine) induced hyperthyroidism [1].

REFERENCE

1 Smit E, Whiting DA, Feld S. Iodine-induced hyperthyroidism caused by acne treatment. *J Am Acad Dermatol* 1994; **31**: 115–17.

Lead lotions

The continued use of wet dressings of lead subacetate in the treatment of exfoliative dermatitis caused lead poisoning with punctate basophilia and an elevated urinary lead level [1].

REFERENCE

1 Kennedy CC, Lynas HA. Lead poisoning by cutaneous absorption from lead dressings. *Lancet* 1949; **i**: 650–2.

Mercury

Poisoning is now fortunately rare, but was seen from continued application of large amounts of a topical application, as for psoriasis [1,2]. Idiosyncratic poisoning after much smaller doses is also recognized [3]. Intoxication has followed the use of a mercury dusting powder [4] and poisoning of a suckling infant has followed the use of perchloride of mercury lotion for cracked nipples [5]. Fever, a generalized morbilliform rash and oedema of the extremities have been the usual clinical features. Exfoliative dermatitis and encephalopathy have developed; permanent damage to the renal tubules is manifest as persistent albuminuria or frank nephrotic syndrome [6]. Rarely, gross symptoms, such as loose teeth [7], swollen, bleeding gums and weight loss may be observed.

Application of a mercury-containing cream to the face over many years can produce slate-grey pigmentation, especially on the eyelids, nasolabial folds and neck folds (exogenous ochronosis) [8–10]; mercury granules lie free in the dermis or within macrophages [11]. Mercury is a moderate sensitizer and leads to contact sensitivity.

REFERENCES

1 Inman PM, Gordon B, Trinder P. Mercury absorption and psoriasis. *Br Med J* 1956; **ii**: 1202–6.
2 Young E. Ammoniated mercury poisoning. *Br J Dermatol* 1960; **72**: 449–55.
3 Williams BH, Beach WC. Idiosyncrasy to ammoniated mercury: treatment with 2,3-dimercapto-propanol (BAL). *JAMA* 1950; **142**; 1286–8.
4 MacGregor ME, Rayner PHW. Pink disease and primary renal tubular acidosis: a common cause. *Lancet* 1964; **ii**: 1083–5.
5 Hunt GM. Mercury poisoning in infancy. *Br Med J* 1966; **i**: 1482.
6 Silverberg DS, McCall JT, Hunt JC. Nephrotic syndrome with use of ammoniated mercury. *Arch Intern Med* 1967; **20**: 581–6.
7 Bourgeois M, Dooms-Goossens A, Knockaert D *et al*. Mercury intoxication after topical application of a metallic mercury ointment. *Dermatologica* 1986; **172**: 48–51.
8 Lamar LM, Bliss BO. Localized pigmentation of the skin due to topical mercury. *Arch Dermatol* 1966; **93**: 450–3.
9 Prigent F, Cohen J, Civatte J. Pigmentation des paupieres probablement secondaire l'application prolongée d'une pomade ophtalmologique contenant du mercure. *Ann Dermatol Vénéréol* 1986; **113**: 357–8.
10 Aberer W. Topical mercury should be banned—dangerous, outmoded but still popular. *J Am Acad Dermatol* 1991; **24**: 150–1.
11 Burge KM, Winkelmann RK. Mercury pigmentation. An electron microscopic study. *Arch Dermatol* 1970; **102**: 51–61.

Methyl salicylate (oil of wintergreen)

Topical application of methyl salicylate and menthol as a rubifacient, with use of a heating pad, resulted in local skin necrosis and interstitial nephritis [1].

REFERENCE

1 Heng MCY. Local necrosis and interstitial nephritis due to topical methyl salicylate and menthol. *Cutis* 1987; **39**: 442–4.

Mexiletine

Mexiletine hydrochloride induced contact uriticaria in a patient receiving iontophoresis [1]. A generalized drug eruption followed topical provocation on previously involved skin [2].

REFERENCES

1 Yamazaki S, Katayama I, Kurumaji Y *et al*. Contact urticaria induced by mexiletine hydrochloride in a patient receiving iontophoresis. *Br J Dermatol* 1994; **130**: 538–40.
2 Kikuchi K, Tsunoda T, Tagami H. Generalized drug eruption due to mexiletine hydrochloride: topical provocation on previously involved skin. *Contact Dermatitis* 1991; **25**: 70–2.

Minoxidil

Topical minoxidil, as used for androgenetic alopecia, is associated with cutaneous problems in up to 10% of patients, with allergic contact dermatitis occurring in 4% of individuals [1]. Diffuse hypertrichosis occurred during treatment with 5% topical minoxidil in female patients [2]. Acute, non-allergic eruptions of the scalp resulted from combined use of minoxidil and retinoic acid [3].

REFERENCES

1 Wilson C, Walkden V, Powell S *et al*. Contact dermatitis in reaction to 2% topical minoxidil solution. *J Am Acad Dermatol* 1991; **24**: 661–2.
2 Peluso AM, Misciali C, Vincenzi C, Tosti A. Diffuse hypertrichosis during treatment with 5% topical minoxidil. *Br J Dermatol* 1997; **136**: 118–20.
3 Fisher AA. Unusual acute, nonallergic eruptions of the scalp from combined use of minoxidil and retinoic acid. *Cutis* 1993; **51**: 17–8.

Non-steroidal anti-inflammatory drugs

Allergic and photo-allergic contact dermatitis and photo-toxicity have resulted from topical NSAIDs [1–3]. An erythema-multiforme-like reaction followed acute contact dermatitis from two different bufexamac-containing topical preparations [4].

REFERENCES

1 Ophaswongse S, Maibach H. Topical nonsteroidal antiinflammatory drugs: allergic and photoallergic contact dermatitis and phototoxicity. *Contact Dermatitis* 1993; **29**: 57–64.
2 Oh VM. Ketoprofen gel and delayed hypersensitivity dermatitis. *Br Med J* 1994; **309**: 512.
3 Valsecchi R, Pansera B, Leghissa P, Reseghetti A. Allergic contact dermatitis of the eyelids and conjunctivitis from diclofenac. *Contact Dermatitis* 1996; **34**: 150–1.
4 Koch P, Bahmer FA. Erythema-multiforme-like, urticarial papular and plaque eruptions from bufexamac: report of 4 cases. *Contact Dermatitis* 1994; **31**: 97–101.

Phenol

Severe systemic reactions, such as abdominal pain, dizziness, haemoglobinuria, cyanosis and sometimes fatal coma have followed the application of phenol to extensive wounds. Accidental application of pure phenol to a small area of skin in an infant has proved fatal. The prolonged use of phenol as a dressing for a large ulcer may give rise to exogenous ochronosis, with darkening of the cornea and of the skin of face and hands.

Podophyllin

Excessive application may lead to severe local irritation or ulceration [1]. There have been occasional reports of confusional states, coma, peripheral neuropathy, vomiting and even death following painting of this resin on large areas of genital warts, especially in pregnancy [2,3]. However, careful review of the reports suggests that in the majority the effects could not be attributed with certainty to podophyllin [2]. Animal experiments suggest teratogenicity; although teratogenicity is controversial in humans, it is best avoided in pregnancy.

REFERENCES

1 Higgins SP, Stedman YF, Chandiok P. Severe genital ulceration in two females following self-treatment with podophyllin solutions. *Genitourin Med* 1994; **70**: 146–7.
2 Bargman H. Is podophyllin a safe drug to use and can it be used in pregnancy? *Arch Dermatol* 1988; **124**: 1718–20.
3 Sundharam JA, Bargman H. Is podophyllin safe for use in pregnancy? *Arch Dermatol* 1989; **125**: 1000–1.

Resorcinol

Acute resorcinol poisoning is very rare, but an ointment containing 12.5% resorcinol applied to the napkin area produced dusky cyanosis, a maculopapular eruption, haemolytic anaemia and haemoglobinuria in an infant [1]. The continued application to large leg ulcers of ointments containing resorcinol has caused myxoedema and widespread blue–grey pigmentation mimicking ochronosis [2]. Application for warts caused generalized urticaria with angio-oedema, pompholyx of palms and soles, or papulovesicular eczema with pompholyx [3].

REFERENCES

1 Cunningham AA. Resorcin poisoning. *Arch Dis Child* 1956; **31**: 173–6.
2 Thomas AE, Gisburn MA. Exogenous ochronosis and myxoedema from resorcinol. *Br J Dermatol* 1961; **73**: 378–81.
3 Barbaud A, Modiano P, Cocciale M *et al.* The topical application of resorcinol can provoke a systemic allergic reaction. *Br J Dermatol* 1996; **135**: 1014–15.

Salicylic acid and salicylates

The frequent application of salicylic acid ointments to extensive lesions will produce symptoms of salicylism even in adults [1–6]. Most cases of poisoning have occurred in children with psoriasis or ichthyosis [1,2]; fatal cases have been recorded [4]. Drowsiness and delusions are followed by acidosis, coma and death from respiratory failure.

REFERENCES

1 Young CJ. Salicylate intoxication from cutaneous absorption of salicylate acid: review of the literature and report of a case. *South Med J* 1952; **45**: 1075–7.
2 Cawley EP, Peterson NT, Wheeler CE. Salicylic acid poisoning in dermatological therapy. *JAMA* 1953; **151**: 372–4.
3 Von Weiss JF, Lever WF. Percutaneous salicylic acid intoxication in psoriasis. *Arch Dermatol* 1964; **90**: 614–19.
4 Lindsey LP. Two cases of fatal salicylate poisoning after topical application of an anti-fungal solution. *Med J Aust* 1969; **1**: 353–4.
5 Davies MG, Vella Briffa D, Greaves MW. Systemic toxicity from topically applied salicylic acid. *Br Med J* 1979; **i**: 661.
6 Anderson JAR, Ead RD. Percutaneous salicylate poisoning. *Clin Exp Dermatol* 1979; **4**: 349–51.
7 Pec J, Strmenova M, Palencarova E *et al.* Salicylate intoxication after use of topical salicylic acid ointment by a patient with psoriasis. *Cutis* 1992; **50**: 307–9.

Silver sulphadiazine

Topical application has caused hyperpigmentation [1], contact sensitivity [2] and dermatitis [3].

REFERENCES

1 Dupuis LL, Shear NH, Zucker RM. Hyperpigmentation due to topical application of silver sulfadiazine cream. *J Am Acad Dermatol* 1985; **12**: 1112–14.
2 Fraser-Moodie A. Sensitivity to silver in a patient treated with silver sulphadiazine (Flamazine). *Burns* 1992; **18**: 74–5.
3 McKenna SR, Latenser BA, Jones LM *et al.* Serious silver sulphadiazine and mafenide acetate dermatitis. *Burns* 1995; **21**: 310–12.

Tretinoin

Topical tretinoin, used for the management of photo-aged skin, may cause erythema, peeling, burning and itching of the skin within days [1,2]. Pink discoloration without other signs may also develop, as may inflammation in solar keratoses.

REFERENCES

1 Weiss JS, Ellis CN, Headington JT *et al.* Topical tretinoin improves photoaged skin: a double-blind, vehicle-controlled study. *JAMA* 1988; **259**: 527–32.
2 Weinstein GD, Nigra TP, Pochi PE *et al.* Topical tretinoin for treatment of photodamaged skin. *Arch Dermatol* 1991; **127**: 659–65.

Vitamin E

Vitamin E in deodorants has caused contact dermatitis [1].

REFERENCE

1 Minkin W, Cohen HJ, Frank SB. Contact dermatitis from deodorants. *Arch Dermatol* 1973; **107**: 774–5.

Warfarin

An epidemic of haemorrhagic disease with fatalities occurred due to warfarin-contaminated talcs [1]. Poisoning has also been attributed to preparation of rodent baits [2].

REFERENCES

1 Martin-Bouyer G, Linh PD, Tuan LC *et al*. Epidemic of haemorrhagic disease in Vietnamese infants caused by warfarin-contaminated talcs. *Lancet* 1983; **i**: 230–2.
2 Fristedt B, Sterner N. Warfarin intoxication from percutaneous absorption. *Arch Environ Health* 1965; **11**: 205–8.

Transdermal drug-delivery systems

Transdermal delivery systems are available for clonidine, oestradiol, nitroglycerin, scopolamine and nicotine, and systems for other drugs are being developed. Erythema, irritancy, and contact sensitization are not uncommon; the occlusive element may lead to miliaria rubra [1–12]. Systemic reactions may occur. Allergic skin reactions occur in up to 50% of patients with clonidine, but with nitroglycerin, scopolamine, oestradiol and testosterone they are much less frequent [2]. Reactivation of an area of contact dermatitis may develop via oral medication rarely [2]. Transdermal compared with oral metoprolol had comparable efficacy, and systemic side-effects were comparable; 69% of patients had local side-effects at the patch site (erythema, papular exanthema, pruritus, localized urticarial exanthema) [4]. Allergic contact dermatitis is recorded with nicotine [8–11], nitroglycerin and oestradiol [12]. Use of transdermal oestrogen patches resulted in systemic sensitization to ethanol [13]. Transdermal fentanyl patches have been associated with a diffuse rash [14].

REFERENCES

1 Hogan DJ, Maibach HI. Adverse dermatologic reactions to transdermal drug delivery systems. *J Am Acad Dermatol* 1990; **22**: 811–14.
2 Holdiness MR. A review of contact dermatitis associated wih transdermal therapeutic systems. *Contact Dermatitis* 1989; **20**: 3–9.
3 Berti JJ, Lipsky JJ. Transcutaneous drug delivery: a practical review. *Mayo Clin Proc* 1995; **70**: 581–6.
4 Jeck T, Edmonds D, Mengden T *et al*. Betablocking drugs in essential hypertension: transdermal bupranolol compared with oral metoprolol. *Int J Clin Pharmacol Res* 1992; **12**: 139–48.
5 Kolloch RE, Mehlburger L, Schumacher H, Gobel BO. Efficacy and safety of two different galenic formulations of a transdermal clonidine system in the treatment of hypertension. *Clin Autonomic Res* 1993; **3**: 373–8.
6 Anonymous. One year efficacy and tolerability of clonidine administered by the transdermal route in patients with mild to moderate essential hypertension—a multicentre open label study. The Antihypertensive Patch Italian Study (APIS) Investigators. *Clin Autonomic Res* 1993; **3**: 379–83.
7 Breidthardt J, Schumacher H, Mehlburger L. Long-term (5 year) experience with transdermal clonidine in the treatment of mild to moderate hypertension. *Clin Autonomic Res* 1993; **3**: 385–90.
8 Bircher AJ, Howard H, Rufli T. Adverse skin reactions to nicotine in a transdermal therapeutic system. *Contact Dermatitis* 1991; **25**: 230–6.
9 Farm G. Contact allergy to nicotine from a nicotine patch. *Contact Dermatitis* 1993; **29**: 214–15.
10 Dwyer CM, Forsyth A. Allergic contact dermatitis from methacrylates in a nicotine transdermal patch. *Contact Dermatitis* 1994; **30**: 309–10.
11 Sudan BJ. Nicotine skin patch treatment and adverse reactions: skin irritation, skin sensitization, and nicotine as a hapten. *J Clin Psychopharmacol* 1995; **15**: 145–6.
12 Torres V, Lopes JC, Leite L. Allergic contact dermatitis from nitroglycerin and estradiol transdermal therapeutic systems. *Contact Dermatitis* 1992; **26**: 53–4.
13 Grebe SK, Adams JD, Feek CM. Systemic sensitization to ethanol by transdermal estrogen patches. *Arch Dermatol* 1993; **129**: 379–80.
14 Stoukides CA, Stegman M. Diffuse rash associated with transdermal fentanyl. *Clin Pharm* 1992; **11**: 222.

The management of drug reactions

Diagnosis

Drug reactions, apart from fixed drug eruption, have non-specific clinical features, and it is often impossible to identify the offending chemical with certainty, especially when a patient with a suspected reaction is receiving many drugs simultaneously. Drug reactions may be mistaken for naturally occurring conditions, and may therefore be overlooked. By the same token, it may on occasion be very difficult to state that a given eruption is drug induced. Experience with the type of reaction most commonly caused by particular drugs may enable the range of suspects to be narrowed, but familiar drugs may occasionally produce unfamiliar reactions, and new drugs may mimic the reactions of the familiar. The assessment of a potential adverse drug reaction always necessitates taking a careful history, and may involve a trial of drug elimination, skin tests, *in vitro* tests, and challenge by re-exposure.

A drug reaction may first become evident after the offending medication has been stopped, and depot injections may have delayed effects. Interpretation of elimination tests should be tempered by the knowledge that drug reactions may take weeks to settle. *In vivo* and *in vitro* tests are only applicable to truly allergic reactions. Skin tests, including prick and intradermal testing, and patch testing, are for the most part unreliable, even when apparently appropriate antigens are used; they may be hazardous [1]. *In vitro* tests are not widely available and are currently essentially research tools.

All too frequently, therefore, the diagnosis is no more than an assessment of probability. The fact that major disagreements occurred between clinical pharmacologists asked to assess the likelihood of adverse drug reaction in two series [2,3] confirms that identification of a responsible drug is often a subjective judgement. An algorithm that provides detailed criteria for ranking the probability of whether a given drug is responsible for a reaction, based on: (i) previous experience; (ii) the alternative aetiological candidates; (iii) timing of events; (iv) drug level; and (v) the results of drug withdrawal and rechallenge, has been reported [4,5]. A number of other algorithms have been developed to assist in the diagnosis of which, if any, drug is the cause of a given eruption [6–9]. The difficulties inherent in the diagnosis of drug reactions have recently been reviewed [10,11].

REFERENCES

1 Bruynzeel D, van Ketel W. Skin tests in the diagnosis of maculopapular drug eruptions. *Semin Dermatol* 1987; **6**: 119–24.
2 Karch FE, Smith CL, Kerzner B *et al.* Adverse drug reactions—a matter of opinion. *Clin Pharmacol Ther* 1976; **19**: 489–92.
3 Koch-Weser J, Sellers EM, Zacest R. The ambiguity of adverse drug reactions. *Eur J Clin Pharmacol* 1977; **11**: 75–8.
4 Kramer MS, Leventhal JM, Hutchinson TA, Feinstein AR. An algorithm for the operational assessment of adverse drug reactions. I. Background, description, and instructions for use. *JAMA* 1979; **242**: 623–32.
5 Leventhal JM, Hutchinson TA, Kramer MS, Feinstein AR. An algorithm for the operational assessment of adverse drug reactions. III. Results of tests among clinicians. *JAMA* 1979; **242**: 1991–4.
6 Naranjo CA, Busto U, Sellers EM *et al.* A method for estimating the probability of adverse drug reactions. *Clin Pharmacol Ther* 1981; **27**: 239–45.
7 Louick C, Lacouture P, Mitchell A *et al.* A study of adverse reaction algorithms in a drug surveillance program. *Clin Pharmacol Ther* 1985; **38**: 183–7.
8 Pere J, Begaud B, Harramburu F, Albin H. Computerized comparison of six adverse drug reaction assessment procedures. *Clin Pharmacol Ther* 1986; **40**: 451–61.
9 Ghajar BM, Lanctôt KL, Shear NH, Naranjo CA. Bayesian differential diagnosis of a cutaneous reaction associated with the administration of sulfonamides. *Semin Dermatol* 1989; **8**: 213–18.
10 Ring J. Diagnostik von Arzneimittel-bedingten Unverträglichkeitsreaktionen. *Hautarzt* 1987; **38**: S16–S22.
11 Shear NH. Diagnosing cutaneous adverse reactions to drugs. *Arch Dermatol* 1990; **126**: 94–7.

Drug history

Patients should be specifically questioned about laxatives, oral contraceptives, vaccines, homeopathic medicines, etc. as these may not be volunteered as medications. They should be asked when they last took a tablet for any reason. The history should include information on when each drug was first taken relative to the onset of the reaction, whether the same or a related drug has been administered previously, and whether there is a prior history of drug sensitivity or contact dermatitis. Allergic drug reactions do not usually develop for at least 4 days, and more commonly 7–10 days, after initial drug administration in a previously unsensitized individual. However, this time relationship cannot be relied on to differentiate between allergic and non-allergic reactions, since a previous sensitizing exposure may not have produced a clinically evident reaction.

Drug elimination

Resolution of a reaction on withdrawal of a drug is supportive incriminatory evidence but not diagnostic. Failure of a rash to subside on drug withdrawal does not necessarily exonerate it, since traces of the drug may persist for long periods, and some reactions, once initiated, continue for many days without re-exposure to the drug. The unwitting substitution of a drug that is chemically closely related may perpetuate a reaction, as when an antihistamine of phenothiazine structure is prescribed to

alleviate the symptoms of a reaction caused by another phenothiazine. Elimination diets have been advocated for diagnosis of food additive intolerance leading to urticaria [1,2].

REFERENCES

1 Rudzki E, Czubalski K, Grzywa Z. Detection of urticaria with food additives intolerance by means of diet. *Dermatologica* 1980; **161**: 57–62.
2 Metcalfe DD, Sampson HA, eds. Workshop on experimental methodology for clinical studies of adverse reactions to foods and food additives. *J Allergy Clin Immunol* 1990; **86** (Suppl.): 421–42.

Skin testing

Skin testing, including prick testing and intradermal testing, may be useful in the identification of patients who present with immediate hypersensitivity reactions and are sensitive to one of a number of drugs, including penicillin and other β-lactam antibiotics, agents used in general anaesthesia, tetanus toxoid, streptokinase, chymopapain, heterologous sera or insulin, and may thus aid in the prevention of anaphylaxis [1]. The results of skin test reactions, including intradermal testing and patch testing, were evaluated in 242 patients with delayed type (non-immediate) drug eruptions [2]. Intradermal testing was positive in 89.7% of patients, and patch tests were positive in 31.5% of cases; overall, 62% of patients had either a positive intradermal or patch test. Intradermal testing was more frequently positive in maculopapular rashes, erythema multiforme and erythrodermic rashes than in eczematous reactions, whereas positive patch tests were comparatively frequent in erythroderma, eczematous reactions and anticonvulsant-induced reactions. It was concluded that a combination of patch testing and intradermal testing is useful in the demonstration of causative agents in delayed type drug eruptions [2]. Unfortunately, the usefulness of this approach is limited, because the significant antigenic determinants are unknown for most drugs [1]. Moreover, intradermal testing is not always safe. False-negative skin testing may occur because of poor absorption through the skin, because a metabolite rather than the substance administered in the test is the sensitizing antigen, or because testing is performed either too soon after a reaction, in a refractory period, or too late, so that the patient no longer demonstrates skin test reactivity.

REFERENCES

1 Sussman GL, Dolovich J. Prevention of anaphylaxis. *Semin Dermatol* 1989; **8**: 158–65.
2 Osawa J, Naito S, Aihara M *et al.* Evaluation of skin test reactions in patients with non-immediate type drug eruptions. *J Dermatol (Tokyo)* 1990; **17**: 235–9.

Patch testing

Patch testing in drug eruptions may be helpful in identifying the drug responsible, especially in systemic contact-type dermatitis medicamentosa, in photosensitivity (photo-patch testing) or fixed drug reactions [1–6]. Positive patch tests have been found overall in about 15% of patients with drug eruptions [3,4] and 25% of patients with penicillin allergy [3,4,7]. Patch testing in a previously involved site, but not in normal skin, may yield a positive response in a proportion of cases of fixed drug eruption, especially with phenazone (pyrazolone) derivatives (e.g. phenylbutazone), but also a sulphonamide, doxycycline, trimethoprim, chlormezanone, a barbiturate and carbamazepine [8]. In a series of 30 patients [9], positive reactions were always seen with phenazone salicylate (16 patients) and carbamazepine (three patients), and in one case from chlormezanone. Both positive and negative reactions were seen with trimethoprim (three and two, respectively), doxycycline (two and one) and sulfadiazine (one and one). The vehicle used as a diluent for the drug may be important in determining whether or not a reaction is seen [8]. However, most reports in the literature do not suggest that patch testing is helpful in fixed drug eruption [10]. Topical provocation of a fixed drug eruption due to sulphamethoxazole was reported [11].

Patch testing has supported a diagnosis of allergy, in the absence of topical sensitization, to diazepam, meprobamate and practolol [1], carbamazepine [12–14] (but only in patients with exfoliative dermatitis and maculo-papular exanthema and not with fixed drug eruption), erythema multiforme or urticaria [13], tartrazine dyes [15], chloramphenicol [16], diclofenac maculopapular eruption [17], and in TEN induced by ampicillin [18]. Antibiotics (especially penicillin, ampicillin and other β-lactam antibiotics [19,20], aminoglycosides), NSAIDs (pyrazolone derivatives and occasionally aspirin), anticonvulsants (carbamazepine, hydantoin derivatives), neuroleptics (phenothiazines, barbiturates, meprobamate, benzodiazepines), β-blockers, gold salts, carbimazole, amantidine, corticosteroids, mitomycin C, heparin and amide anaesthetics have all been associated with positive patch tests in allergic subjects [2]. However, care must be exercised, because anaphylactoid responses may occur even in response to the small amounts of drug absorbed from a patch test. Moreover, patch testing has produced exfoliative dermatitis in a patient sensitized to carbamazepine [21] and relapse of a generalized drug eruption in the case of clobazam [22]. A patch test with a solution of the drug will sometimes induce a generalized petechial reaction in patients with purpura caused by drug sensitivity, for example in carbromal or Sedormid purpura.

REFERENCES

1 Felix RE, Comaish JS. The value of patch and other skin tests in drug eruptions. *Lancet* 1984; i: 1017–19.
2 Van Ketel WG. Immunological investigations in patients with drug-induced skin eruptions. *Arch Dermatol* 1984; **110**: 112–13.
3 Bruynzeel DP, van Ketel WG. Skin tests in the diagnosis of maculo-papular drug eruptions. *Semin Dermatol* 1987; **6**: 119–24.
4 Bruynzeel DP, van Ketel WG. Patch testing in drug eruptions. *Semin Dermatol* 1989; **8**: 196–203.
5 Le Sellin J. Interet des tests epicutanes dans l'allergie medicamenteuse. *Allergol Immunol* 1994; **26**: 315–17.
6 Calkin JM, Maibach HI. Delayed hypersensitivity drug reactions diagnosed by patch testing. *Contact Dermatitis* 1993; **29**: 223–33.
7 Bruynzeel DP, von Blomberg-van der Flier M, Scheper RJ *et al.* Allergy for penicillin and the relevance of epicutaneous tests. *Dermatologica* 1985; **171**: 429–34.
8 Alanko K, Stubb S, Reitamo S. Topical provocation of fixed drug eruption. *Br J Dermatol* 1987; **116**: 561–7.
9 Alanko K. Topical provocation of fixed drug eruption. A study of 30 patients. *Contact Dermatitis* 1994; **31**: 25–7.
10 Sehgal VN, Gangwani OP. Fixed drug eruption. Current concepts. *Int J Dermatol* 1987; **26**: 67–74.
11 Oleaga JM, Aguirre A, Gonzalez M, Diaz-Perez JL. Topical provocation of fixed drug eruption due to sulphamethoxazole. *Contact Dermatitis* 1993; **29**: 155.
12 Houwerzijl J, de Gast GC, Nater JP. Patch test in drug eruptions. *Contact Dermatitis* 1982; **8**: 155–8.
13 Alanko K. Patch testing in cutaneous reactions caused by carbamazepine. *Contact Dermatitis* 1993; **29**: 254–7.
14 Jones M, Fernandez-Herrera J, Dorado JM *et al.* Epicutaneous test in carbamazepine cutaneous reactions. *Dermatology* 1994; **188**: 18–20.
15 Roeleveld CG, Van Ketel WG. Positive patch tests to the azo dye tartrazine. *Contact Dermatitis* 1976; **2**: 180.
16 Rudzki E, Grzywa Z, Maciejowska E. Drug reaction with positive patch tests to chloramphenicol. *Contact Dermatitis* 1976; **2**: 181.
17 Romano A, Pietrantonio F, Di Fonso M *et al.* Positivity of patch tests in cutaneous reaction to diclofenac. Two case reports. *Allergy* 1994; **49**: 57–9.
18 Tagami H, Tatsuda K, Iwatski K, Yamada M. Delayed hypersensitivity in ampicillin-induced toxic epidermal necrolysis. *Arch Dermatol* 1983; **119**: 910–14.
19 Galindo Bonilla PA, Garcia Rodriguez R, Feo Brito F *et al.* Patch testing for allergy to beta-lactam antibiotics. *Contact Dermatitis* 1994; **31**: 319–20.
20 Romano A, Di Fonso M, Pietrantonio F *et al.* Repeated patch testing in delayed hypersensitivity to beta-lactam antibiotics. *Contact Dermatitis* 1993; **28**: 190.
21 Vaillant L, Camenen I, Lorette G. Patch testing with carbamazepine: reinduction of an exfoliative dermatitis. *Arch Dermatol* 1989; **125**: 299.
22 Machet L, Vaillant L, Dardaine V, Lorette G. Patch testing with clobazam: relapse of generalized drug eruption. *Contact Dermatitis* 1992; **26**: 347–8.

Penicillin

It is clearly important to exclude from treatment with penicillin those patients truly at risk of developing hypotensive episodes or fatal anaphylaxis. The role of skin testing in this situation has been reviewed [1–12]. Skin tests should be carried out using major determinant (benzylpenicilloyl polylysine, PPL) and minor determinant mixture (benzyl penicillin, benzyl penicilloate and benzyl penilloate) antigens [13]. Procedures have been published, and the reader is referred to the original articles for details as to methodology [13,14]. Epicutaneous testing should precede intradermal testing, and positive (histamine or opiate) and negative (diluent) controls should be included. False-negative results may be found after a systemic allergic reaction, as a result of a refractory period or temporary desensitization, so that skin testing should be postponed for at least 4–6 weeks [13].

There is a high incidence of wrongly diagnosed penicillin allergy on the basis of history, and a considerable proportion of patients who have had proven allergic reactions to penicillins eventually stop producing the IgE antibody responsible. In a large study, only 1% of 566 patients with a history of penicillin allergy, and negative skin tests to major determinant (octa-benzylpenicilloyl-ocytalysine) and minor determinant mixture and its components (potassium benzylpenicillin, benzylpenicilloate, and benzylpenicilloyl-*N*-propylamine), had possibly IgE-mediated reactions [4]. In another study [7], 7% of 776 individuals with a previous history of penicillin allergy and 2% of 4287 subjects negative by history, had positive skin tests to major determinant (PPL) and/or to a minor-determinant mixture. Positive skin tests were seen in 17% and 12% of patients with a history of anaphylaxis or urticaria, respectively, but in only 4% with a history of an exanthem. Mild adverse reactions to skin tests occurred in 1% of patients positive by history and 9% of those with positive skin tests. In patients with negative skin tests who received benzylpenicillin or ampicillin, mild acute allergic reactions occurred in 0.5% of subjects negative by history, and 3% of subjects positive by history. Thus, routine penicillin skin testing can facilitate the safe use of penicillin in 90% of individuals with a previous history of allergy [7]. Positive skin tests, an average of 5 years later, to major and minor determinants of benzylpenicillin and/or minor determinant mixtures of ampicillin, amoxicillin or cloxacillin, were found in 19% of 112 patients with a history of urticaria and angio-oedema or exanthem to penicillins and other semisynthetic penicillins (most frequently ampicillin and amoxicillin) [8]. Skin test reactivity was limited in about half to the semisynthetic penicillin reagents derived from ampicillin, amoxicillin or cloxacillin. The existence of isolated skin-test positivity to reagents specific for ampicillin or amoxycillin, with good tolerance of major and minor penicillin determinants, has been confirmed in other reports [9,15,16], emphasizing the necessity for using reagents specific for the side chains of these aminopenicillin drugs to exclude possible immediate hypersensitivity in patients who reacted to these antibiotics clinically [8–11,15,16]. Thus 7% of 288 patients with a history of penicillin allergy reacted only to skin testing with amoxycillin and not to benzyl or phenoxymethyl-penicillin diagnostic reagents determinants [15]; these would have been missed if the latter agents had been used alone.

Patients treated with penicillin after a negative skin test to benzyl penicilloyl polylysine and to minor determinant mixture develop IgE-mediated reactions only very rarely, and these are almost always mild and self-limited [1,4,7]. Thus, when adequately performed, negative skin tests indicate that the risk of a life-threatening reaction is almost negligible, and that any β-lactam antibiotic may be safely given. By contrast, the risk of an acute allergic reaction, including respiratory obstruction or hypotension, with a positive history and positive skin test is 50–70%; the risk in a patient with a negative history but a positive skin test is about 10% [1,13,17].

Intradermal testing is in general safe with few reactions, and does not appear to result in sensitization [13]. There is, however, a risk, albeit very small, of fatality from skin testing [18]. A more major problem with skin testing is that use of the major determinant, penicilloyl polylysine, alone misses about 10–25% of all positive subjects, and that even addition of benzyl penicillin G as the sole minor determinant antigen misses 5–10% of positive subjects [19,20]. This is significant because patients with reactivity to minor antigenic determinants are thought to be at a higher risk for anaphylaxis [13,21]. Moreover, minor determinant antigen mixture is not available commercially; mixtures of minor determinants are unstable [22]. In addition, as detailed above, reagents to detect sensitivity to aminopenicillins may be necessary. Comprehensive skin testing is therefore only practicable in specialized centres. Skin tests can give both false-positive and false-negative reactions [17,18]. Thus, it has been argued that a positive or negative result in an individual patient cannot be used to entirely reliably predict outcome [23].

Further difficulties are that skin tests have no predictive value in non IgE-mediated reactions such as serum sickness, haemolytic anaemia, drug fever, interstitial nephritis, contact dermatitis, maculopapular exanthemata or exfoliative dermatitis. Accelerated or late IgE-mediated reactions may occur despite a negative pretreatment skin test [1,13]. Positive intradermal skin test reactions occurred in only 87% of patients with a history of delayed type rashes induced by penicillins and cephalosporins and who had positive oral provocation tests [24]. Oral challenge was positive in 18 of 33 patients with positive delayed skin testing and patch testing to ampicillin or amoxicillin, but also in 16 of 27 patients with negative allergy tests [25]. Skin testing is contraindicated where there is a history of exfoliative dermatitis, Stevens–Johnson syndrome or TEN.

There is clearly individual variation in the approach to the diagnosis and management of β-lactam allergy [12], based on a survey of 3500 physician members and fellows of the American Academy of Allergy and Immunology, and of allergy training programme directors in the USA. Benzylpenicilloyl-polylysine and fresh penicillin G are used for skin testing by more than 86% of both respondent groups, whereas minor determinant mixtures are used by only 40%. Epicutaneous followed by intradermal injection was the skin-test technique used by 86% of these allergists.

REFERENCES

1 Weiss ME, Adkinson NF. Immediate hypersensitivity reactions to penicillin

and related antibiotics. *Clin Allergy* 1988; **18**: 515–40.

2 Torricelli R, Wuthrich B. Diagnostisches Vorgehen bei Verdacht auf Soforttypallergie auf Penicilline. *Hautarzt* 1996; **47**: 392–3.

3 Shepherd G, Mendelson L. The role of skin testing for penicillin allergy. *Arch Intern Med* 1992; **152**: 2505.

4 Sogn DD, Evans R III, Shepherd GM *et al*. Results of the National Institute of Allergy and Infectious Diseases Collaborative Clinical Trial to test the predictive value of skin testing with major and minor penicillin derivatives in hospitalized adults. *Arch Intern Med* 1992; **152**: 1025–32.

5 Lin RY. A perspective on penicillin allergy. *Arch Intern Med* 1992; **152**: 930–7.

6 Weiss ME. Evaluation and treatment of patients with prior reactions to beta-lactam antibiotics. *Curr Clin Topics Infect Dis* 1993; **3**: 131–45.

7 Gadde J, Spence M, Wheeler B, Adkinson NF, Jr. Clinical experience with penicillin skin testing in a large inner-city STD clinic. *JAMA* 1993; **270**: 2456–63.

8 Silviu-Dan F, McPhillips S, Warrington RJ. The frequency of skin test reactions to side-chain penicillin determinants. *J Allergy Clin Immunol* 1993; **91**: 694–701.

9 Audicana M, Bernaola G, Urrutia I *et al*. Allergic reactions to betalactams: studies in a group of patients allergic to penicillin and evaluation of cross-reactivity with cephalosporin. *Allergy* 1994; **49**: 108–13.

10 Blanca M. The contribution of the side chain of penicillins in the induction of allergic reactions. *J Allergy Clin Immunol* 1994; **94**: 562–3.

11 Warrington RJ. The contribution of the side chain of penicillins in the induction of allergic reactions. *J Allergy Clin Immunol* 1995; **95**: 640.

12 Wickern GM, Nish WA, Bitner AS, Freeman TM. Allergy to beta-lactams: a survey of current practices. *J Allergy Clin Immunol* 1994; **94**: 725–31.

13 Weber EA, Knight A. Testing for allergy to antibiotics. *Semin Dermatol* 1989; **8**: 204–12.

14 Adkinson NF, Jr. Tests for immunoglobulin drug reactions. In: Rose NF, Friedman H, eds. *Manual of Clinical Immunology*. Washington DC: American Society for Microbiology, 1986: 692–7.

15 Blanca M, Vega JM, Garcia J *et al*. Allergy to penicillin with good tolerance to other penicillins; study of the incidence in subjects allergic to beta-lactams. *Clin Exp Allergy* 1990; **20**: 475–81.

16 Vega JM, Blanca M, Garcia JJ *et al*. Immediate allergic reactions to amoxicillin. *Allergy* 1994; **49**: 317–22.

17 Green GR, Rosenblum AH, Sweet LC. Evaluation of penicillin hypersensitivity: value of clinical history and skin testing with penicilloyl-polylysine and penicillin G: a cooperative prospective study of the penicillin study group of the American Academy of Allergy. *J Allergy Clin Immunol* 1977; **60**: 339–45.

18 Dogliotti M. An instance of fatal reaction to the penicillin scratch test. *Dermatologica* 1968; **136**: 489–96.

19 Gorevic PD, Levine BB. Desensitization of anaphylactic hypersensitivity specific for the penicilloate minor determinant of penicillin and carbenicillin. *J Allergy Clin Immunol* 1981; **68**: 267–72.

20 Sogn DD. Penicillin allergy. *J Allergy Clin Immunol* 1984; **74**: 589–93.

21 Adkinson NF, Jr. Risk factors for drug allergy. *J Allergy Clin Immunol* 1984; **74**: 567–72.

22 Saxon A, Bell GN, Rohr AS, Adelman DC. Immediate hypersensitivity reactions to beta-lactam antibiotics. *Ann Intern Med* 1987; **107**: 204–15.

23 Ewan P. Allergy to penicillin. *Br Med J* 1991; **302**: 1462.

24 Aihara M, Ikezawa Z. Evaluation of the skin test reactions in patients with delayed type rash induced by penicillins and cephalosporins. *J Dermatol (Tokyo)* 1987; **14**: 440–8.

25 Romano A, Di Fonso M, Papa G *et al*. Evaluation of adverse cutaneous reactions to aminopenicillins with emphasis on those manifested by maculopapular rashes. *Allergy* 1995; **50**: 113–18.

Agents used in general anaesthesia

Intradermal [1–3] or prick [4–5] testing may be helpful in identifying the causative drug [6], and is essential in confirming lack of sensitivity to pancuronium before use in cases of documented sensitivity to other relaxants [3]. In one series [7] of patients with a history of anaphylaxis during induction of general anaesthesia, skin testing was performed by the prick and intracutaneous methods with dilutions of thiobarbiturates, muscle relaxants or β-lactam antibiotics. No patient experienced a recurrence of anaphylaxis during subsequent general anaesthesia when agents producing positive skin tests were avoided, provided a premedication regimen of prednisone and diphenhydramine was given [7].

REFERENCES

1 Fisher MMcD. Intradermal testing in the diagnosis of acute anaphylaxis during anaesthesia—results of five years experience. *Anaesth Intensive Care* 1979; **7**: 58–61.

2 Fisher MMcD. The diagnosis of acute anaphylactoid reactions to neuromuscular blocking agents: a commonly undiagnosed condition. *Anaesth Intensive Care* 1981; **9**: 235–41.

3 Galletly DC, Treuren BC. Anaphylactoid reactions during anaesthesia. Seven years' experience of intradermal testing. *Anaesthesia* 1985; **40**: 329–33.

4 Leynadier F, Sansarricq M, Didier JM, Dry J. Prick tests in the diagnosis of anaphylaxis to general anaesthetics. *Br J Anaesth* 1987; **59**: 683–9.

5 Moneret-Vautrin DA, Laxenaire MC. Anaphylaxis to muscle relaxants: predictive tests. *Anaesthesia* 1990; **45**: 246–7.

6 Moneret-Vautrin DA, Laxenaire MC. Skin tests in diagnosis of allergy to muscle relaxants and other anesthetic drugs. *Monogr Allergy* 1992; **30**: 145–55.

7 Moscicki RA, Sockin SM, Corsello BF *et al*. Anaphylaxis during induction of general anesthesia: Subsequent evaluation and management. *J Allergy Clin Immunol* 1990; **86**: 325–32.

Local anaesthetics

Avoidance of local anaesthetics on the basis of a vague or equivocal history of a prior adverse reaction may result in substantial increased pain and risk. True allergic reactions probably constitute no more than 1% of all adverse reactions to these drugs, some but not the majority of which are due to preservatives, especially parabens. Skin testing and/or incremental challenge beginning with diluted drug is a safe and effective method for identifying a drug that a patient with a history of adverse drug reaction can tolerate [1–7]. Patients with positive patch tests to local anaesthetics and a negative history of anaphylactoid reactions rarely have positive intradermal skin tests. The risk of anaphylactic reactions with amide local anaesthetics (except butanilicaine) is therefore low in such patients [3]. Conversely, patients with anaphylactic reactions to local anaesthetics are usually patch-test negative [3]. Skin testing may produce systemic adverse reactions, especially with undiluted drug. False-positive reactions occur, but false-negative reactions have not been reported, and most skin-tested patients who tolerate a local anaesthetic are skin-test negative to the drug. The choice of a drug for use in skin testing and incremental challenge may be facilitated by current concepts of non-cross-reacting groups of local anaesthetics. Thus, benzoic acid esters, both those with and without *p*-aminobenzoyl groups, do not cross-react with amide local anaesthetic agents.

REFERENCES

1 Schatz M. Skin testing and incremental challenge in the evaluation of

adverse reactions of local anesthetics. *J Allergy Clin Immunol* 1984; **74**: 606–16.

2 Fisher MMcD, Graham R. Adverse responses to local anaesthetics. *Anaesth Intensive Care* 1984; **12**: 325–7.
3 Ruzicka T, Gerstmeier M, Przybilla B, Ring J. Allergy to local anesthetics: comparison of patch test with prick and intradermal test results. *J Am Acad Dermatol* 1987; **16**: 1202–8.
4 Glinert RJ, Zachary CB. Local anesthetic allergy. Its recognition and avoidance. *J Dermatol Surg Oncol* 1991; **17**: 491–6.
5 Hodgson TA, Shirlaw PJ, Challacombe SJ. Skin testing after anaphylactoid reactions to dental local anesthetics. A comparison with controls. *Oral Surg Oral Med Oral Pathol* 1993; **75**: 706–11.
6 Wasserfallen JB, Frei PC. Long-term evaluation of usefulness of skin and incremental challenge tests in patients with history of adverse reaction to local anesthetics. *Allergy* 1995; **50**: 162–5.
7 Gall H, Kaufmann R, Kalveram CM. Adverse reactions to local anesthetics: analysis of 197 cases. *J Allergy Clin Immunol* 1996; **97**: 933–7.

Analgesics and NSAIDs

Prick tests were positive only in 13% of 117 patients with a history suggestive of anaphylactoid reactions to a variety of mild analgesics including NSAIDs [1].

REFERENCE

1 Przybilla B, Ring J, Harle R, Galosi A. Hauttestung mit Schmerz-mittelinhaltsstoffen bei Patienten mit anaphylaktoiden Unverträgli-chkeitsreaktionen auf 'leichte' Analgetika. *Hautarzt* 1985; **36**: 682–7.

Heparin

Provocation testing may be a useful diagnostic measure [1,2]. Low-molecular-weight heparin analogues may be satisfactorily substituted in some patients with this reaction [1], but are not always tolerated [2]; a panel of different low-molecular-weight heparin preparations should be checked by subcutaneous provocation tests before re-institution of heparin therapy.

REFERENCES

1 Zimmermann R, Harenberg J, Weber E *et al.* Behandlung bei heparin-induzierter kutaner Reaktion mit einem niedermolekularen Heparin-Analog. *Dtsch Med Wschr* 1984; **109**: 1326–8.
2 Klein GF, Kofler H, Wol H, Fritsch PO. Eczema-like, erythematous, infiltrated plaques: a common side effect of subcutaneous heparin therapy. *J Am Acad Dermatol* 1989; **21**: 703–7.

Skin testing in urticaria

Skin tests have been advocated as useful in the investigation of chronic urticaria [1,2]. Patch testing with a series of penicillins was positive in 6.9% of patients in one study [1], and there were positive intracutaneous tests to cilligen and/or penicillin G in 21.5% of patients. Avoidance of dietary dairy produce, which potentially might have contained penicillin, alleviated the urticaria in 50% of the penicillin-allergic patients. The reported prevalence of positive intracutaneous tests to penicillin was much higher in this study than in other reported series in the literature.

REFERENCES

1 Boonk WJ, van Ketel WG. Skin testing in chronic urticaria. *Dermatologica* 1981; **163**: 151–9.
2 Antony SJ, Fisher RH. Association of penicillin allergy with idiopathic anaphylaxis. *J Fam Practitioner* 1993; **37**: 499–502.

In vitro tests

Tests for IgE antibody

The detection of drug-specific circulating antibodies does not prove an allergy. It is important to record when a blood test is taken in relation to the evolution of a drug reaction, as the antibody response to a drug has a finite duration. For example, antipenicillin IgE antibodies begin to disappear within 10–30 days. Radioallergosorbent (RAST) tests for drug-specific IgE class antibody are available for penicillin, insulin and ACTH. The RAST test detects specific IgE antibody to the penicilloyl determinant, and is positive in 60–90% of patients with a positive skin test to penicilloyl polylysine [1,2]; however, there is no *in vitro* test for minor determinant antigens, and therefore in practice this test is of very limited use [2,3]. Investigation of cross-reactivity of antibodies to penicillin in 123 patients with a history of penicillin allergy, using enzyme-linked immunosorbent assay (ELISA) tests, detected IgE antibodies specific to amoxycillin, ampicillin or flucloxacillin, respectively, in three patients [4]. These antibodies did not cross-react with other penicillin antigens, and would have been missed had testing involved only use of benzylpenicillin. Thus, allergy to semisynthetic penicillins can occur without allergy to benzyl penicillin, negative tests specific for benzylpenicillin or phenoxymethylpenicillin cannot be generalized to other penicillins, and exclusive reliance on benzylpenicilloyl RAST tests to detect allergy to semisynthetic penicillins could lead to serious adverse consequences [5]. IgE antibodies specific for 1-phenyl-2,3-dimethyl-3-pyrazoline-5-one were found in 17 of 19 serum samples from individuals sensitive to pyrazoline drugs with 4-aminoantipyrine discs by RAST testing [6].

REFERENCES

1 Wide L, Juhlin L. Detection of penicillin allergy of the immediate type by radioimmunoassay of reagins (IgE) to penicilloyl conjugates. *Clin Allergy* 1971; **1**: 171–7.
2 Weiss ME, Adkinson NF. Immediate hypersensitivity reactions to penicillin and related antibiotics. *Clin Allergy* 1988; **18**: 515–40.
3 Ewan P. Allergy to penicillin. *Br Med J* 1991; **302**: 1462.
4 Christie G, Coleman J, Newby S *et al.* A survey of the prevalence of penicillin specific IgG, IgM and IgE antibodies detected by ELISA and defined by hapten inhibition in patients with suspected penicillin allergy and in healthy volunteers. *Br J Clin Pharmacol* 1988; **25**: 381–6.
5 Walley T, Coleman J. Allergy to penicillin. *Br Med J* 1991; **302**: 1462–3.
6 Zhu D, Becker WM, Schulz KH *et al.* Detection of IgE antibodies specific for 1-phenyl-2,3-dimethyl-3-pyrazoline-5-one by RAST: a serological diagnostic method for sensitivity to pyrazoline drugs. *Asian Pacific J Allergy Immunol* 1992; **10**: 95–101.

Miscellaneous in vitro tests

The histamine-release test [1], the basophil degranulation test [2–4], the passive haemagglutination test [5], and the lymphocyte transformation test [6–11] are of strictly limited use. A positive basophil degranulation assay, which involves binding of drug to specific IgE on the basophil surface, has been reported with penicillin, erythromycin, sulphonamides and aspirin, but false-negative results are common [3,4]. A number of drugs have been reported to induce lymphocyte proliferation, as determined by incorporation of ^{3}H-thymidine, in patients with drug eruptions, including penicillin, carbamazepine, phenytoin, frusemide (furosemide), sulphamethoxazole and hydrochlorothiazide [7,9–11]. However, in general only low levels of stimulation are observed, perhaps because the antigen responsible for the reaction is a drug metabolite rather than the parent compound, and the significance of the test is difficult to interpret. While the leukocyte and macrophage migration inhibition tests [12,13] and the lymphocyte toxicity assay [14–17] are the subject of investigation, they are essentially research tools. A patient with a fixed drug eruption to multiple drugs (codeine, tetracycline, ampicillin, dimenhydrinate, penicillin V and co-trimoxazole), confirmed by challenge testing, showed positive macrophage migration inhibition (MIF) test results to all these, but was negative on both challenge and MIF testing to erythromycin; it was concluded that MIF testing correlated well with the results of challenge testing and could be useful in identifying causative agents [18]. In another study, platelet-activating factor (PAF) release from white blood cells after antigenic challenge as tested by platelet aggregation correlated with skin tests (75% agreement), lymphocyte transformation (68% agreement) and a positive penicillin IgE-RAST (66% agreement) [19].

REFERENCES

1 Perelmutter L, Eisen AH. Studies on histamine release from leukocytes of penicillin-sensitive individuals. *Int Arch Allergy* 1970; **38**: 104–12.
2 Shelley WB. Indirect basophil degranulation test for allergy to penicillin and other drugs. *JAMA* 1963; **184**: 171–8.
3 Sastre Dominguez J, Sastre Castillo A. Human basophil degranulation test in drug allergy. *Allergol Immunopathol* 1986; **14**: 221–8.
4 Harrabi S, Loiseau P, Dehenry J. A technic for human basophil degranulation. *Allerg Immunol* 1987; **19**: 287–9.
5 Thiel JA, Mitchell S, Parker CW. The specificity of hemagglutination reactions in human and experimental penicillin hypersensitivity. *J Allergy* 1964; **35**: 399–424.
6 Rocklin RE, David JR. Detection *in vitro* of cellular hypersensitivity to drugs. *J Allergy Clin Immunol* 1971; **48**: 276–82.
7 Gimenez-Camarasa JM, Garcia-Calderon P, de Moragas JM. Lymphocyte transformation test in fixed drug eruption. *N Engl J Med* 1975; **292**: 819–21.
8 Dobozy A, Hunyadi J, Kenderessy AS, Simon N. Lymphocyte transformation test in detection of drug hypersensitivity. *Clin Exp Dermatol* 1981; **6**: 367–72.
9 Sarkany I. Role of lymphocyte transformation in drug allergy. *Int J Dermatol* 1981; **8**: 544–5.
10 Roujeau JC, Albengres E, Moritz S *et al.* Lymphocyte transformation test in drug-induced toxic epidermal necrolysis. *Int Arch Allergy Appl Immunol* 1985; **78**: 22–4.
11 Zakrzewska JM, Ivanyi L. *In vitro* lymphocyte proliferation by carbamazepine, carbamazepine-10, 11-epoxide, and oxcarbazepine in the diagnosis of drug-induced hypersensitivity. *J Allergy Clin Immunol* 1988; **82**: 1826–32.
12 David JR, al-Askari S, Lawrence HS, Thomae L. Delayed hypersensitivity *in vitro*. I. The specificity of inhibition of cell migration by antigens. *J Immunol* 1964; **93**: 264–73.
13 Halevy S, Grunwald MH, Sandbank M *et al.* Macrophage migration inhibition factor (MIF) in drug eruption. *Arch Dermatol* 1990; **126**: 48–51.
14 Shear N, Spielberg S, Grant D *et al.* Differences in metabolism of sulfonamides predisposing to idiosyncratic toxicity. *Ann Intern Med* 1986; **105**: 179–84.
15 Shear N, Spielberg S. Anticonvulsant hypersensitivity syndrome. *In vitro* assessment of risk. *J Clin Invest* 1989; **82**: 1826–32.
16 Rieder MJ, Uetrecht J, Shear NH *et al.* Diagnosis of sulfonamide hypersensitivity reactions by *in-vitro* 'rechallenge' with hydroxylamine metabolites. *Ann Intern Med* 1989; **110**: 286–9.
17 Shear NH. Diagnosing cutaneous adverse reactions to drugs. *Arch Dermatol* 1990; **126**: 94–7.
18 Kivity S. Fixed drug eruption to multiple drugs: clinical and laboratory investigation. *Int J Dermatol* 1991; **30**: 149–51.
19 Dunoyer-Geindre S, Ludi F *et al.* PAF acether release on antigenic challenge. A method for the investigation of drug allergic reactions. *Allergy* 1992; **47**: 50–4.

Challenge tests

A drug suspected of causing a drug eruption may be reliably incriminated by the reaction in response to a test dose administered after recovery. However, fatal reactions have occurred to test doses, as for example to penicillin and quinine, and provocation tests should only be performed in exceptional circumstances [1–6]. A history of Stevens–Johnson syndrome or of TEN constitutes an absolute contraindication to drug challenge, and test dosing in reactions of anaphylactic type, blood dyscrasia or systemic LE-like reaction is seldom advisable. Challenge tests are open to misinterpretation [6], because a very small challenge dose may fail to elicit a reaction that a therapeutic dose would provoke, because of false positives, and because false negatives may occur as a result of a refractory period following a reaction [7].

Test dosing in patients with drug reactions such as fixed drug eruption, which are not potentially fatal, may be helpful [5]. Topical challenge in the form of patch testing in a previously involved site may yield a positive response in a high proportion of such cases [8]. Oral provocation tests using tartrazine, and other food additives such as sodium benzoate, have been advocated for the investigation of chronic urticaria or food intolerance [9–12]. Protocols for the analysis of adverse reactions to foods and food additives have been published [13].

REFERENCES

1 Kauppinen K. Cutaneous reactions to drugs. With special reference to severe mucocutaneous bullous eruptions and sulphonamides. *Acta Derm Venereol (Stockh)* 1972; **52** (Suppl. 68): 1–89.
2 Kauppinen K. Rational performance of drug challenge in cutaneous hypersensitivity. *Semin Dermatol* 1983; **2**: 117–230.
3 Kauppinen K, Stubb S. Drug eruptions. Causative agents and clinical types. *Acta Derm Venereol (Stockh)* 1984; **64**: 320–4.
4 Girard M. Conclusiveness of rechallenge in the interpretation of adverse

drug reactions. *Br J Clin Pharmacol* 1987; **23**: 73–9.

5 Kauppinen K, Alanko K. Oral provocation: uses. *Semin Dermatol* 1989; **8**: 187–91.

6 Girard M. Oral provocation: limitations. *Semin Dermatol* 1989; **8**: 192–5.

7 Stevenson DD, Simon RA, Mathison DA. Aspirin-sensitive asthma: tolerance to aspirin after positive oral aspirin challenges. *J Allergy Clin Immunol* 1980; **66**: 82–8.

8 Alanko K, Stubb S, Reitamo S. Topical provocation of fixed drug eruption. *Br J Dermatol* 1987; **116**: 561–7.

9 Warin RP, Smith RJ. Challenge test battery in chronic urticaria. *Br J Dermatol* 1976; **94**: 401–6.

10 Supramaniam G, Warner JO. Artificial food additive intolerance in patients with angio-oedema and urticaria. *Lancet* 1986; **ii**: 907–9.

11 Wilson N, Scott A. A double blind assessment of additive intolerance in children using a 12 day challenge period at home. *Clin Exp Allergy* 1989; **19**: 267–72.

12 Michils A, Vandermoten G, Duchateau J, Yemault J-C. Anaphylaxis with sodium benzoate. *Lancet* 1991; **337**: 1424–5.

13 Metcalfe DD, Sampson HA, eds. Workshop on experimental methodology for clinical studies of adverse reactions to foods and food additives. *J Allergy Clin Immunol* 1990; **86** (Suppl.): 421–42.

Treatment

Clearly, prevention is better than cure [1,2]. Drugs implicated in a previous reaction should be avoided; the patient should be asked about allergies, and hypersensitivity records in the notes and on prescription charts should be checked. In the case of suspected penicillin allergy, an alternative antibiotic, preferably with a non-β-lactam structure, such as erythromycin, should be substituted; use of griseofulvin should be avoided, as it has a 5–10% cross-reactivity based on non-structural mechanisms [2]. However, lack of a positive history does not eliminate the possibility of an allergic reaction, as in the case of penicillin hypersensitivity [3]. Where it is essential to readminister one of a group of drugs to a patient with a previous history of an adverse reaction to a related medication, as with radiographic contrast media and agents used in general anaesthesia, then if possible preliminary skin testing should be carried out, to enable identification of safe alternative therapy. In addition, the procedure should be covered by premedication with oral corticosteroids and antihistamines, with or without adrenalin, in order to obtund the onset of an anaphylactic reaction. In the situation where there is no acceptable alternative for an essential drug, then rapid desensitization therapy should be considered.

The approach to treatment of an established presumed drug eruption obviously depends on the severity of the reaction. For many minor conditions, withdrawal of the suspected drug, and symptomatic therapy with emollients, mild to moderately potent topical corticosteroids, and systemic antihistamines where indicated, is all that is necessary. When a patient is receiving multiple drugs, it is wise to withdraw all but the essential medications, and to consider substituting alternative non-cross-reacting drugs for the remainder. Because of the wide variety of patterns of drug reaction, it is only possible to summarize the therapy of individual reactions here. The reader is referred to the discussion of the more serious conditions in this textbook and elsewhere [1–7].

REFERENCES

1 Sheffer AL, Pennoyer MD. Management of adverse drug reactions. *J Allergy Clin Immunol* 1984; **74**: 580–8.

2 Fellner MJ, Ledesma GN. Current comments on cutaneous allergy. Management of antibiotic allergies. *Int J Dermatol* 1991; **30**: 184–5.

3 Weber EA, Knight A. Testing for allergy to antibiotics. *Semin Dermatol* 1989; **8**: 204–12.

4 Braun-Falco O, Plewig G, Wolff HH, Winkelmann RK. *Dermatology*. Berlin: Springer-Verlag, 1991.

5 Breathnach SM, Hintner H. *Adverse Drug Reactions and the Skin*. Oxford: Blackwell Scientific Publications, 1992.

6 Breathnach SM. Management of drug eruptions: Part II. Diagnosis and treatment. *Australas J Dermatol* 1995; **36**: 187–91.

7 Drake LA, Dinehart SM, Farmer ER *et al.* Guidelines of care for cutaneous adverse drug reactions. American Academy of Dermatology. *J Am Acad Dermatol* 1996; **35**: 458–61.

Anaphylaxis

The management of severe acute urticaria and anaphylaxis is detailed in Table 77.23.

Table 77.23 Management of anaphlyaxis.

Stop drug administration
Give i.m. 0.5–1 ml 1 : 1000 adrenaline immediately
Check airway and give oxygen
Antihistamines
   Chlorpheniramine maleate 10–20 mg i.v.
   or hydroxyzine 25–50 mg i.m. and four times daily orally
   or H₁ and H₂ antagonists
   or cimetidine 300 mg i.v. 6 hourly
Corticosteroids
   Hydrocortisone 250 mg i.v. and 100 mg 6 hourly
   Prednisolone 40 mg/day for 3 days
Give i.v. 0.9% NaCl or 5% glucose
Monitor BP and pulse
For bronchospasm:
   aminophylline 250 mg i.v. over 5 mins and
   250 mg in 500 ml 0.9% NaCl over 6 hours
   or nebulized terbutaline, salbutamol or metaproterenol

Exfoliative dermatitis / erythroderma

The complications of this potentially serious drug-induced condition include: hypothermia, fluid and electrolyte loss, infection, high-output cardiac failure, stress ulceration and gastrointestinal haemorrhage, malabsorption and venous thrombosis. The management [1,2] includes maintenance of body temperature and fluid and electrolyte balance, treatment of cardiac failure by use of digitalization and diuretics (avoiding vasodilator drugs), and administration of intravenous albumin for hypoalbuminaemia. If the patient does not respond rapidly to potent topical corticosteroids, prednisolone 40–60 mg/day should be given. This approach also applies to the anticonvulsant hypersensitivity syndrome; oral corticosteroid therapy has been helpful [3,4].

REFERENCES

1 Marks J. Erythroderma and its management. *Clin Exp Dermatol* 1982; **7**: 415–22.
2 Roujeau JC, Revuz J. Intensive care in dermatology. In: Champion RH, Pye RJ, eds. *Recent Advances in Dermatology*, Vol. 8. Edinburgh: Churchill Livingstone, 1990: 85–99.
3 Murphy JM, Mashman J, Miller JD, Bell JB. Suppression of carbamazepine-induced rash with prednisone. *Neurology* 1991; **41**: 144–5.
4 Chopra S, Levell NJ, Cowley G, Gilkes JJ. Systemic corticosteroids in the phenytoin hypersensitivity syndrome. *Br J Dermatol* 1996; **134**: 1109–12.

Toxic epidermal necrolysis

The management of TEN is summarized in Table 77.24, and is perhaps best carried out on an intensive care or burns unit. The mortality is of the order of 20–30% despite intensive therapy, and may be related to septicaemia, pneumonia or pneumonitis, hypovolaemia, gastrointestinal haemorrhage, pulmonary emboli and disseminated intra-vascular coagulation. Lymphopenia or neutropenia are poor prognostic signs. There is a significant incidence of disabling long-term complications, especially in relation to ocular and other mucous membranes, in survivors. It is therefore particularly important to be aware of these and to take preventative measures.

There is no consensus on the merits of therapy with moderately high-dose corticosteroids for TEN. Some authorities maintain that high-dose steroid therapy promotes or masks the signs of infection, delays healing, precipitates gastrointestinal bleeding, prolongs hospital-

Table 77.24 Management of toxic epidermal necrolysis.

Intensive therapy: ITU or burns unit
Air-fluidized bed
Maintain fluid and electrolyte balance (replace up to 5 l/day)
Maintain body temperature
Maintain nutrition; oral hygiene
Frequent ophthalmological assessment
  Antiseptic/antibiotic eye drops 2 hourly
  Disrupt synechiae frequently
Limitation of infection
  Neutropenia: reverse barrier nursing
  Frequent cultures of erosions, and blood cultures
  Culture tips of Foley catheters and intravenous lines
  Prophylactic broad-spectrum systemic antibiotics (controversial)
Topical cleansing/antibacterial agents
  0.5% silver nitrate solution on gauze
  or 10% chlorhexidine gluconate washes
  or saline washes
  or polymixin/bacitracin or 2% mupirocin
  Avoid silver sulphadiazine
Wound care
  Remove necrotic epidermis
  Paraffin gauze or hydrogel dressings
  Biological dressings (xenografts, allografts, skin substitutes)

ization and increases mortality [1,2]. However, others favour steroid therapy on the basis that it may reduce inflammation and keratinocyte necrosis. It was generally agreed at the First International Congress on Cutaneous Drug Reactions in Créteil, France in 1994 that if steroids, or any other immunosuppressive agent, are to be given, then they should be administered as early as possible in the evolution of the disease. There have been anecdotal reports on the use of plasmapheresis [3], cyclosporin A [4] and cyclophosphamide [5] in TEN. Because of the rarity of the condition, controlled trials assessing these different treatment approaches are very difficult to carry out.

REFERENCES

1 Halebian PH, Corder VJ, Madden MR *et al*. Improved burn center survival of patients with toxic epidermal necrolysis managed without corticosteroids. *Ann Surg* 1986; **204**: 503–12.
2 Rzany B, Schmitt H, Schöpf E. Toxic epidermal necrolysis in patients receiving glucocorticosteroids. *Acta Derm Venereol (Stockh)* 1991; **71**: 171–2.
3 Kamanabroo D, Schmitz-Landgraf W, Czartnetski BM. Plasmapheresis in severe drug-induced toxic epidermal necrolysis. *Arch Dermatol* 1985; **121**: 1548–9.
4 Renfro L, Grant-Kels JM, Daman L.A. Drug-induced toxic epidermal necrolysis treated with cyclosporin. *Int J Dermatol* 1989; **28**: 441–4.
5 Heng MC, Allen SG. Efficacy of cyclophosphamide in toxic epidermal necrolysis: clinical and pathophysiologic aspects. *J Am Acad Dermatol* 1991; **25**: 778–86.

Desensitization

It is possible to induce a state of antigen-specific mast-cell unresponsiveness, in patients with type I IgE-mediated reactions, if a drug is essential for a patient's well-being and no alternative is available. Desensitization markedly diminishes the risk of anaphylactic reactions, but not of non-IgE-mediated reactions; it should only be carried out in an intensive care unit setting. Mechanisms proposed to explain the development of tolerance following desensitization procedures include mediator depletion, tachyphylaxis, production of blocking antibodies, or change in the level of specific IgE antibodies.

Desensitization is most frequently carried out for patients with penicillin allergy, with increasing doses of penicillin being administered over 3–5 h [1–3]. The drug is usually given orally; increasing doses are given, starting with a very weak concentration (e.g. 1/1 000 000 of the therapeutic dose) and working up to a full dose. There have been no severe allergic reactions recorded in patients who completed oral desensitization to penicillin; about 35% experience minor cutaneous reactions including pruritus or urticaria. While the protection is usually short lived, tolerance can be maintained by long-term administration of low doses of oral penicillin. Patients with vancomycin sensitivity who require the drug have been successfully desensitized [4].

Patients with HIV infection with previous cutaneous reactions to sulphonamides have also been desensitized [5–7]. A 10-day oral desensitization regimen has been described for trimethoprim–sulphamethoxazole in 28 HIV-infected patients [6]; 82% were successfully desensitized, and four of the 28 patients had relatively severe rashes (three maculopapular, one erythroderma) during the desensitization phase. Four patients subsequently had rashes 12–33 weeks after desensitization [6].

REFERENCES

1 Wendel GD, Stark BJ, Jamison RB *et al.* Penicillin allergy and desensitization in serious infections during pregnancy. *N Engl J Med* 1985; **312**: 1229–32.
2 Stark BJ, Earl HS, Gross GN *et al.* Acute and chronic desensitization of pencillin-allergic patients using oral penicillin. *J Allergy Clin Immunol* 1987; **79**: 523–32.
3 Weiss ME, Adkinson NF. Immediate hypersensitivity reactions to penicillin and related antibiotics. *Clin Allergy* 1988; **18**: 515–40.
4 Wong JT, Ripple RE, MacLean JA *et al.* Vancomycin hypersensitivity: synergism with narcotics and 'desensitization' by a rapid continuous intravenous protocol. *J Allergy Clin Immunol* 1994; **94**: 189–94.
5 Torgovnick J. Desensitization to sulfonamides in patients with HIV infection. *Am J Med* 1990; **88**: 548–9.
6 Absar N, Daneshvar H, Beall G. Desensitization to trimethoprim/sulfamethoxazole in HIV-infected patients. *J Allergy Clin Immunol* 1994; **93**: 1001–5.
7 Belchi-Hernandez J, Espinosa-Parra FJ. Management of adverse reactions to prophylactic trimethoprim–sulfamethoxazole in patients with human immunodeficiency virus infection. *Ann Allergy Asthma Immunol* 1996; **76**: 355–8.

Chapter 78
Topical Therapy

W.A.D.GRIFFITHS & J.D.WILKINSON

General considerations [1–4]

Much dermatological topical therapy has developed empirically with favourite mixtures and remedies, the so-called magisterial formulations occupying a prominent place. Although the formulations listed in the official monographs had been tried and tested over many years, a properly controlled evaluation led to major deletions in more recent editions of these pharmacopoeias [2,5–8]. Stricter control over the inclusion of toxic ingredients and the conditions of manufacture have both contributed to a reduction in the range of such formulations in current use. Economical factors have contributed to the difficulties in finding pharmacists capable and willing to provide 'ad hoc' prescriptions. Mindful of the differing conditions in the developed and the emerging countries we have, where possible in this chapter, retained notes on many of the traditional basic ingredients of dermatological formulations.

In earlier times, there were only a few 'active' ingredients, and most traditional dermatological treatments relied on physical rather than chemical properties for their effect. Such active ingredients as did exist were mixed together, according to the physician's prescription, in a suitable carrier substance, vehicle or base. The influence exerted by the vehicle was often underestimated, *both* its physical effect *and* its effect on drug penetration and performance [4,9–11]. Even specific remedies were used in a somewhat random and haphazard way and might, at times, be incorporated into totally inappropriate vehicles. The importance of the vehicle is now well-recognized [12,13], not only for its

physical properties but also as a delivery system for the many new active topical drugs that have been developed over the last 50 years. These new drugs are far more active than their predecessors and include both specific therapeutic agents and drugs with more general effects. The vehicles are frequently tailor-made and chosen as carefully as the drug for which they are intended. Many of these new drugs are unstable unless used in the prescribed concentration and vehicle, and attempts at modifying or altering these complex drug–vehicle systems will often adversely affect penetration, absorption and performance. With topical corticosteroids, different concentrations of active drug may still apparently have the same biological effect [14].

When dilutions are required, reference may be made to the *External Diluent Directory* [15]. There are many topical preparations, however, where dilution is neither practical nor possible after manufacture and packaging. Where a patient finds the lowest strength still too potent, the physician will then have to advise the use of smaller quantities applied at less frequent intervals.

Although extemporaneous formulations are now less frequently recommended, and several traditional treatments have been discarded because of toxicity, sensitivity or lack of demonstrable effect, new remedies have not entirely replaced older ones [1,4,10,16] which are often still very effective, and whose side-effects are at least well recognized. The complexity of modern formulations, coupled with stricter safety and efficacy requirements, increased legislative controls and a reluctance among some pharmacists to prepare extemporaneous formulations will make it increasingly difficult, however, for the physician to obtain traditional or 'personalized' prescriptions. One notable disadvantage of proprietary preparations is the limited description of their constituents on packaging. Every topical preparation should, *as a minimum*, declare the concentration of any active ingredient and list (qualitatively) all other ingredients and excipients. Full ingredient labelling of all topical pharmaceutical preparations and toiletries is already mandatory in several countries. International efforts to extend this requirement to other countries have included negotiations with the European Commission.

REFERENCES

1 Arndt KA. *Manual of Dermatologic Therapeutics*, 3rd edn. Boston: Little, Brown & Co, 1983.
2 *British Pharmacopoeia*. London: HMSO, 1993.
3 Collen SI. Effective topical dermatologic therapy. *Dermatol Clin* 1989; **7**: 37–42.
4 Polano MK. *Topical Skin Therapeutics*. Edinburgh: Churchill Livingstone, 1984.
5 *British National Formulary*, No. 32. London: British Medical Association and The Pharmaceutical Society of Great Britain, 1996.
6 Pharmaceutical Society of Great Britain. *Pharmaceutical Codex*, 12th edn. London: Pharmaceutical Press, 1994.
7 Reynolds JEF, ed. *Martindale: the Extra Pharmacopoeia*, 31st edn. London: Pharmaceutical Press, 1996.
8 *United States Pharmacopoeia National Formulary*, 22nd edn. Rockville, Maryland: United States Pharmacopoeial Convention Inc., 1990.
9 Barry BW. *Dermatologic Formulations: Percutaneous Absorption. Drugs and The Pharmaceutical Sciences*, Vol. 18. New York: Marcel Dekker, 1983.
10 Flynn GL. In: Banker GS, Rhodes CT, eds. *Modern Pharmaceutics in Drugs and The Pharmaceutical Sciences*, Vol. 7. New York: Marcel Dekker, 1979.
11 Mauvais-Jarvis P, Vickers CFH, Wepierre J, eds. *Percutaneous Absorption of Steroids*. London: Academic Press, 1980.
12 Munro DD. The relationship between percutaneous absorption and stratum corneum retention. *Br J Dermatol* 1969; **81** (Suppl. 4): 92–7.
13 Sarkany I, Hadgraft JW. In: Hibbott HW, ed. *Handbook of Cosmetic Science*. Oxford: Pergamon Press, 1969: 98.
14 Stoughton RB, Wullich K. Same glucocorticoid in brand-name products. *Arch Dermatol* 1989; **125**: 1509–11.
15 *External Diluent Directory*. London: The National Pharmaceutical Association, 1989 and Supplement 1995.
16 Litt JZ. Alternative topical therapy. *Dermatol Clin* 1989; **7**: 37–42.

Therapeutic implications of percutaneous absorption [1]

The nature of the skin barrier has been fully discussed in Chapter 4. In general, drugs penetrate at rates determined largely by their lipid–water coefficients [1–3], water-soluble ions and polar molecules (except for the very smallest) being excluded. In diseased skin, where the stratum corneum is improperly formed, drug absorption may be much increased but, as clinical improvement occurs and a normal stratum corneum emerges, absorption may slow down and the concentration of active drug may need to be increased or steps may need to be taken to facilitate drug penetration.

Treatment by topical application means that there is intimate contact between the drug and the target tissue, and the risks of *systemic side-effects* are minimized. It is often difficult, however, for the clinician to regulate the amount

of drug applied, and patient compliance may at times be a problem.

Complex physical laws govern the absorption of substances through the skin [1,2,4] (Chapter 4), but a major stimulus to research into the penetration of active agents was the recognition that the absorption of corticosteroids produces vasoconstriction, and this can be used as a 'marker' of penetration [3,5]. Permeability of the skin can also be increased by the use of 'accelerants', for example the addition of tetrafurfuryl alcohol or propylene glycol to a weak corticosteroid produces a vasoconstrictive effect equivalent to that of a stronger corticosteroid. Among many such agents, dimethyl sulphoxide (DMSO) is outstanding in this ability [6,7]. In practice, the degree of penetration depends on the nature of the vehicle used, the behaviour of the active agent in this vehicle and the method of application employed, for example occlusion and hydration enhance penetration.

The basic principles of prescribing and formulating topical applications are unfortunately often neglected in the medical curriculum. However, a doctor today must not only ensure that treatment is in the right form and contains the most appropriate active ingredient, but must also be able to instruct the patient how to use the treatment and advise as to any likely side-effects [8].

REFERENCES

1 Barry BW. *Dermatological Formulations: Percutaneous Absorption. Drugs and the Pharmaceutical Sciences*, Vol. 18. New York: Marcel Dekker, 1983.
2 Flynn GL. In: Banker GS, Rhodes CT, eds. *Modern Pharmaceuticals in Drugs and The Pharmaceutical Sciences*, Vol. 17. New York: Marcel Dekker, 1979: 263.
3 Mauvais-Jarvis P *et al.*, eds. *Percutaneous Absorption of Steroids*. New York: Academic Press, 1980.
4 Blank JH, Scheuplein RJ. In: Hibbott HW, ed. *Handbook of Cosmetic Science*. Oxford: Pergamon, 1989: 47.
5 McKenzie AW, Stoughton RB. Method for comparing percutaneous absorption of steroids. *Arch Dermatol* 1962; **86**: 608–10.
6 Leake CD, Rosenbaum EE, Jacob SW. Summary of the New York Academy of Science symposium on 'Biological Actions of Dimethyl Sulfoxide'. *Ann NY Acad Sci* 1967; **141**: 670–1.
7 Martin D, Hauthal HG. *Dimethyl Sulfoxide*. New York: Von Nostrand Reinhold, 1976.
8 Poland MK. *Topical Skin Therapeutics*. Edinburgh: Churchill Livingstone, 1984.

The vehicle

SYN. BASE

In dermatology, a drug is very rarely, if ever, applied to the skin in the form of a pure chemical substance, but is normally incorporated into a vehicle. The term 'vehicle' is now preferred to the older term 'base' for the sum of the excipients in which an active agent is offered to the skin. An 'ideal' vehicle should be easy to apply and remove, non-toxic, non-irritant, non-allergenic, chemically stable, homogeneous, bacteriostatic, cosmetically acceptable [1,2] and pharmacologically inert [3,4]. In addition, one has to consider the properties of the vehicle in relation to the active agent. For effective drug delivery, a vehicle should ensure chemical stability of the active drug, its efficient release from the formulation, its easy partition into the outer layer of the skin and the efficient permeation of the drug through the epidermis.

Many attempts have been made to produce a comprehensive classification of external formulations but the simplest system consists of an initial division into liquid, semisolid and powder (Table 78.1) [5]. The liquid preparations may be divided into monophasic solutions, emulsions and suspensions. Solutions can be usefully separated into aqueous, alcoholic, alcoholic–aqueous and oily. The emulsions are classified into oil in water (O/W) and water in oil (W/O). The semisolid preparations divide into water-free and water-containing systems. Highly concentrated non-aqueous systems are called ointments and water-containing semisolid preparations are classified as either hydrogels, creams or emulsions. Semisolid suspensions are called pastes. Ointments can be classified as non-polar (generally tenside-free systems), polar (containing tensides with a hydrophilic–lipophilic balance (HLB) of less than 10) and strongly polar systems (with tensides with an HLB value of over 10). In the aqueous system, monophasic and multiphasic systems are differentiated, and aqueous gels are placed with the monophasics. The multiphasic systems are termed creams. They are similar to emulsions and so, here again, classification into O/W or W/O is possible, depending upon whether they can be washed off with water or not. Ambiphilic creams are intermediate, combining some features of both. All commonly used external preparations fit into one of the categories listed in Table 78.1, and are shown, diagrammatically, in Fig. 78.1.

Table 78.1 Classification system for external preparations.

Liquid
Monophasic = solutions
    Pure aqueous
        Low viscosity—lotions
        High viscosity, pseudoplastic—gels
    Alcoholic, alcoholic–aqueous—paints
    Oily—oils
Emulsions
    Oil in water (O/W)
    Water in oil (W/O)
Suspensions

Semisolid
Water-free ointments
    Non-polar
    Polar (tensides up to HLB 10)
    Strongly polar (HLB of greater than 10)
Containing water
    Monophasic (hydrogels)
    Multiphasic (emulsions, creams)
        Washable (O/W)—aqueous creams
        Non-washable (W/O)—oily creams
        Intermediate type—ambiphilic
Highly concentrated suspensions—pastes

Powders

HLB, hydrophilic–lipophilic balance.

Basic materials [3,6–9]

These are discussed fully in specialized texts, such as

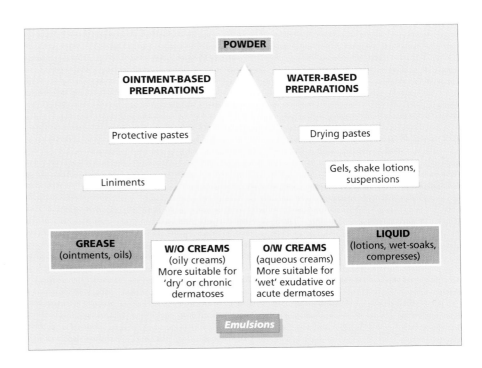

Fig. 78.1 A practical guide to the choice and performance of dermatological vehicles. (From Polano [4].)

that of Polano [4], and will be mentioned only briefly here.

Powders

Inorganic powders are an important component of many dermatological treatments and include zinc oxide, titanium dioxide, talc, bentonite and calamine. Organic powders include various starches and zinc stearate. *Zinc oxide* is widely used as a component of many dusting powders, shake lotions and pastes. It has covering and protective properties, gives consistency to creams and pastes, and is said to have cooling and slightly astringent properties. *Titanium dioxide* is chemically very inert and for this reason it can be used instead of zinc oxide in pastes containing salicylic acid. It is also superior to zinc oxide in its UV-reflecting properties. *Talc* is inert magnesium polysilicate, with a very low specific gravity. It contributes 'slip' and has a cooling effect. *Calamine* may be either zinc carbonate or zinc oxide, coloured with a little ferric oxide, and has bland, soothing and antipruritic properties. *Starch* is more absorbent than inorganic powders, but tends to deteriorate and is prone to microbiological decomposition. Some powders, for example *bentonite* (colloidal hydrated aluminium silicate), *aluminium magnesium silicate, tragacanth, methylcellulose* and *carbomer* are used in gels or as stabilizers in shake lotions.

Greases

These can be divided into true fats and oils, waxes, mineral greases and macrogols. *True fats and oils* are the triglycerides of saturated and non-saturated fatty acids with a small amount of free fatty acid. There are many varieties, for example arachis oil, olive oil, lanolin, cetyl and stearyl alcohol, Wool Fat BP, Anhydrous Lanolin USP. Purified wool fat [10,11] is a mixture of higher fatty acids esterified with monohydric alcohols, including cholesterol esters and related alcohols. It may be mixed with other fats or greases to improve their flow properties and enable them to emulsify water. Although still widely used, patients may become sensitized to the wool alcohol fraction, and therefore the use of a purified, less sensitizing, lanolin extract has been proposed [12]: Hydrous Wool Fat BP, Lanolin USP, is wool fat with 25–30% water. It is used both as an emollient and as a protective. Eucerin (Wool Alcohols BP) is the wool alcohol fraction of wool fat, and contains cholesterol and isocholesterol. It is mixed with liquid, soft and hard paraffin to form Ointment of Wool Alcohols BP, which, on the addition of water, produces Hydrous Ointment BP, a vehicle for many W/O creams. Theobroma Oil BP, Cocoa Butter USP, consists chiefly of the triglycerides of palmitic, stearic and oleic acids. It is a solid fat which melts at between 30 and 35°C. Other true fats include Cetyl Esters Wax NF, Stearyl Alcohol NF and Cetostearyl Alcohol BP. They are mainly used as stabilizing agents in creams.

Waxes include Beeswax BP, to stiffen ointments for lip salves, and Emulsifying Wax BP, Lanette Wax 5X, which is a mixture of one part sodium lauryl sulphate and nine parts cetostearyl alcohol. It is an important emulsifying agent in anionic O/W creams.

Mineral greases may be fluid, soft or solid [13].

Fluid greases include Liquid Paraffin BP, Mineral Oil USP or low molecular weight *macrogols* such as polyethylene glycol 300. They can be used to soften ointments and pastes or to clean debris and crust from the skin.

Soft greases include Yellow and White Soft Paraffin BP, Petrolatum USP, Vaseline, Plastibase—a suspension of mineral oil in polyethylene—and mixed liquid and solid macrogols (having molecular weights of 300 and 4000 respectively). Cetomacrogol 1000 BP is a condensation of cetostearyl alcohol with ethylene oxide. It is useful as a non-ionic emulsifying agent.

Liquids

In common use are Purified Water BP, USP, Glycerol BP, Glycerine USP (a thick hygroscopic liquid used in some lotions and gels), Ethanol USP (which is 95–96% ethyl alcohol) and other solvents such as Ether BP, USP and Chloroform BP, USP. Industrial Methylated Spirits BP, Rubbing Alcohol USP or Isopropyl Alcohol BP can be substituted. Calcium Hydroxide Solution BP, USP, or limewater, is a 0.15% aqueous solution of calcium hydroxide. It is considered to have anti-inflammatory and soothing properties, and is used in cooling pastes and other soothing preparations. Sorbitol Solution BP, USP, is a 70% solution of Sorbitol BP, a polyalcohol in water. It is often used as a humectant in O/W creams. Propylene Glycol BP, USP, is a useful solvent and good penetrant, especially for corticosteroid creams and ointments [14–16]. It may also act as a keratolytic and preservative in water-containing creams. At high concentration, it is hygroscopic and may be irritant [17,18]. It may also, albeit rarely, sensitize [19] as do may other excipients [20–22].

REFERENCES

1 Cussler EL. In: Brewer MM, ed. *Cosmetic Science*, 3rd edn. London: Academic Press, 1978: 117.
2 Weinstein S. New methods for the *in vivo* assessment of skin smoothness and skin softness. *J Soc Cosmet Chem* 1978; **29**: 99–115.
3 *British National Formulary*, No. 32. London: British Medical Association and The Pharmaceutical Society of Great Britain, 1996.
4 Polano MK. *Topical Skin Therapeutics*. Edinburgh: Churchill Livingstone, 1984.
5 Brandau R, Lippold BH. *Dermal and Transdermal Absorption*. Stuttgart: Widden-schaftliche Verlagsgesellschaft, 1982: 16.
6 Arndt KA. *Manual of Dermatologic Therapeutics*, 3rd edn. Boston: Little, Brown & Co., 1983.
7 British Pharmacopoeic Commission. *British Pharmacopoeia* 1993.
8 Reynolds JEF, ed. *Martindale: The Extra Pharmacopoeia*, 31st edn. London: Pharmaceutical Press, 1996.
9 *United States Pharmacopoeia National Formulary*. Rockville, Maryland: United States Pharmacopoeial Convention Inc., 1990.

10 Conrad LI, Maso MF, Deragon SA. Surface modifying effects of lanolin derivatives. *J Soc Cosmet Chem* 1966; **17**: 157–69.

11 Guillot JP, Ginuffret JY, Martin MC. Etude toxicologique chez l'animal de differents échantillons de lanoline anhydre, de lanoline modifiée et de dérivés de lanoline. *Int J Cosmet* 1980; **2**: 1–38.

12 Clarke EW, Cronin E, Wilkinson DS. Lanolin with reduced sensitizing potential—a preliminary note. *Contact Dermatitis* 1977; **3**: 69–74.

13 Seville RH. Simplified dithranol treatment of psoriasis. *Br J Dermatol* 1975; **93**: 205–8.

14 Ostrenga JJ, Haleblian J, Poulsen B *et al*. Vehicle design for a new topical steroid. Fluocinonide. *J Invest Dermatol* 1971; **56**: 392–9.

15 Ponec N. Penetration of corticosteroids through the skin in relation to the vehicle. *Dermatologica* 1976; **152** (Suppl.): 37–46.

16 Reinstein J, Ostrenga J, Haleblian J *et al*. Design of optimal topical system for fluocinonide. *Acta Derm Venereol (Stockh)* 1972; **52** (Suppl 67):13–18.

17 Angelini G, Meninghini CL. Contact allergy from propylene glycol. *Contact Dermatitis* 1981; **7**: 197–8.

18 Hjorth N. Contact dermatitis. *Br J Dermatol* 1980; **103** (Suppl. 18): 19–20.

19 Hannuksela M, Kousa M, Pirila V. Allergy to ingredients of vehicles. *Contact Dermatitis* 1976; **2**: 105–10.

20 Cronin E. *Contact Dermatitis*. Edinburgh: Churchill Livingstone, 1980.

21 Fisher AA. *Contact Dermatitis*. Philadelphia: Lea & Febiger, 1986.

22 Nater JP, De Groot AC. *Unwanted Effects of Cosmetics and Drugs used in Dermatology*. Amsterdam: Elsevier, 1985.

Principles of formulation [1–9]

Only the most general principles of pharmaceutical formulation will be dealt with here. For more detailed information readers are referred to the work of Polano [9] or other standard reference books [1–4,8,10,11].

All topical preparations can be considered as being monophasic (e.g. lotions, powder or grease), biphasic (e.g. creams and protective or drying pastes) or triphasic (e.g. cream pastes or cooling pastes) (Fig. 78.1).

Monophasic vehicles

Powders, now mainly used as toiletries or for prophylaxis, absorb moisture, reduce friction, have good covering properties and can be used to increase surface area. They are best applied to normal skins and therefore have limited dermatological use. *Greases* are emollient, protective and hydrating. They are the principal component of ointments and lip salves; their occlusiveness tends to enhance penetration of active ingredients. Some ointments have added emulsifiers to improve drug incorporation and to help them emulsify sweat and sebum. Simple Ointment BP, for example, contains wool fat and cetostearyl alcohol. White Ointment USP contains 5% beeswax and is therefore useful for those who are lanolin sensitive. Oils can be used as emollients or as a means for removing grease or fatty pastes from the skin or, with added surfactant, as bath emollients. *Liquids* evaporate and tend therefore to be cooling, soothing and drying. Alcoholic or hydroalcoholic solutions are, in addition, astringent and antiseptic. These basic elements can be combined to form biphasic or triphasic preparations.

Biphasic vehicles

The combination of powder with water gives either a drying paste or a shake lotion, according to the proportion of each component. Grease or oil and powder will form either a liniment or a protective (fatty) paste. Water and grease, however, will mix to form stable or semistable emulsions only in the presence of a surfactant or emulsifier. These then form O/W or W/O creams according to the type of emulsifier used and the relative proportions of the two components. In general, the characteristics of a biphasic vehicle are those of its continuous phase modified by its disperse phase.

Triphasic vehicles

These are represented by cream pastes or cooling pastes, and are often simply referred to as creams in the UK, for example Zinc Cream BP. They combine some of the advantages of all their ingredients, and can be used in even the most acute dermatoses.

Choice of vehicle

It is a basic dermatological precept that the more acute the dermatosis the blander the treatment. The application of a cooling paste and the use of frequent wet compresses, with or without topical steroids, remains an indispensable part of the management of acute or exudative dermatoses. The principle of 'wet on wet' and the use of occlusive ointments for dry or chronic dermatoses is also axiomatic. As the condition improves, a 'wet' dermatosis may subsequently be treated with either a drying paste or an O/W cream, and a 'dry' dermatosis may have a hydrous ointment or W/O cream applied. The additional powder in liniments or protective pastes allows the skin to 'breathe' and makes them less occlusive than plain ointments.

Cold creams and *cooling pastes* rely for their effect on their inherent instability, the water tending to separate out and evaporate. Cream pastes and ordinary W/O (oily) creams are more stable and hence less cooling.

Aqueous or *water-based preparations* (Fig. 78.1), for example lotions, O/W creams, gels and drying pastes tend to be cooling, soothing and drying due to their evaporative water loss.

Lotions, wet soaks, wet compresses and O/W creams can be used to clean or redissolve dried exudate and crust and may, at times, be antiseptic and mildly astringent (e.g. Potassium Permanganate Solution BNF diluted 1 in 10 with water or Aluminium Subacetate Solution USP). Aqueous-based preparations need to be used frequently if they are to retain their physical effects. They are particularly helpful in the initial management of acute dermatoses and intertrigo.

Shake lotions, such as Calamine Lotion BP, are able to cover large areas of the body with a thin coating of powder, and, because of the increased evaporative surface, are even more soothing and cooling than ordinary lotions. The well-established anti-inflammatory and soothing effects of calamine are therefore simply a reflection of its physical characteristics. However, because of its drying properties, it would not be a rational treatment for those with xerotic pruritus.

Gels are semisolid preparations gelled with high-molecular-weight polymers, such as carboxypolymethylene (Carbomer BP) or methylcellulose, and can be regarded as semiplastic aqueous lotions. They are non-greasy, water miscible, easy to apply and wash off, and are especially suitable for treating hairy parts of the body.

Ointments have oil or grease as their continuous phase (Fig. 78.1). They are semisolid, anhydrous substances, and are occlusive, emollient and protective. They restrict transepidermal water loss, and are therefore hydrating and moisturizing. Ointments can be divided into two main groups: fatty, for example White Soft Paraffin BP (Petrolatum, Vaseline), and water soluble, for example Macrogol (polyethylene glycol) Ointment BP. The latter have the advantage of being less greasy, with good solvent properties, and are easily washed off. Both types of ointment are emollient and lubricant, but the fatty bases are obviously more occlusive, and as a result have greater protective and hydrating properties.

Creams are semisolid emulsion systems containing both oil and water. O/W (aqueous or vanishing) creams, for example Aqueous Cream BP, are water miscible, cooling and soothing, and are well absorbed into the skin. They are not occlusive but, because of the dispersed lipid phase, they also have a mild moisturizing and emollient effect. W/O creams, for example Oily Cream BP, are immiscible with water and, therefore, more difficult to wash off. They are emollient, lubricant, moisturizing and mildly occlusive (but less so than ointments). Both systems require the addition of either a natural or a synthetic surfactant or emulsifier. O/W creams always contain a preservative to prevent secondary bacterial and fungal colonization. Many W/O creams contain lanolin.

Pastes are semisolid stiff preparations containing a high proportion of finely powdered material. The characteristic features of a paste are substantivity, 'inertness' and 'blandness'. There are drying pastes, cream pastes and protective pastes. They can also be used as a delivery system for drugs, and because of their substantivity the drug effect can be limited to a well-defined area. Protective (fatty) pastes are greasy and therefore messy and water insoluble. They are difficult to apply and remove, but their very stiffness permits accurate localization. They are occlusive, protective and hydrating. Drying (non-greasy) pastes are water miscible and more easily removed. They are drying and soothing, and are often used in conjunction with dressings as paste bandages or as vehicles for active medicaments. Pastes can be 'softened' by the addition of 10% arachis oil or 'hardened' by the addition of hard paraffin [12]. Cream pastes, for example Zinc Cream BP, combine some of the features

of powders, liquids and fats, and can be used on acute conditions.

Dusting powders usually contain a mixture of two or more substances in fine powder form, free from grittiness. They are usually applied only to normal, intact skin as a preventative or protective measure. They are used to reduce friction (talc) or excessive moisture (starch), and tend therefore to be used in areas prone to moisture and friction, for example intertriginous areas, feet, etc. They have a slightly drying and lubricating effect, but are nowadays regarded as a somewhat inefficient means of delivery of active drugs.

Paints are liquid preparations, either aqueous, hydroalcoholic or alcoholic (tinctures), which are usually applied with a brush to the skin or mucous membranes. They evaporate, and are therefore cooling as well as astringent and antiseptic. Alcoholic paints often sting.

Collodions, for example Flexible Collodion BP, are liquid preparations consisting of pyroxylin (cellulose nitrate) in organic solvent. They evaporate to leave a flexible film which can hold medicaments in contact with the skin. They may also be used as protectives to seal minor cuts and abrasions. They are easy to apply and water repellent, but also often inflammable, irritant to the eyes and mucous membranes, and only really suitable for small areas.

REFERENCES

1 Arndt KA. *Manual of Dermatologic Therapeutics*, 3rd edn. Boston: Little, Brown & Co., 1983.
2 Barry BW. *Dermatological Formulations: Percutaneous Absorption. Drugs and The Pharmaceutical Sciences*, Vol. 18. New York: Marcel Dekker, 1983.
3 *British National Formulary*, No 32. London: British Medical Association and The Pharmaceutical Society of Great Britain, 1996.
4 British Pharmacopoeia Commission. *British Pharmacopoeia*. London: HMSO, 1993.
5 Fuhrer C. In: Praudau R, Lippold BH, eds. *Dermal and Transdermal Absorption*. Stuttgart: Wissenschaftliche Veragsgesellschaft, 1982.
6 Katz M. In: Ariens EJ, ed. *Drug Design*. New York: Academic Press, 1973: 117.
7 Nurnberg E. Welche galenische Grundlagen werden heute die Hautbehandlung Eingesetz? *Hautarzt* 1978; **29**: 61–7.
8 Pharmaceutical Society of Great Britain. *Pharmaceutical Codex*, 12th edn. London: Pharmaceutical Press, 1994.
9 Polano MK. *Topical Skin Therapeutics*. Edinburgh: Churchill Livingstone, 1984.
10 Reynolds JEF, ed. *Martindale: The Extra Pharmacopoeia*, 31st edn. London: Pharmaceutical Press, 1996.
11 *United States Pharmacopoeia National Formulary*. Rockville, Maryland: United States Pharmacopoeial Convention Inc, 1980.
12 Seville RH. Simplified dithranol treatment for psoriasis. *Br J Dermatol* 1975; **93**: 205–8.

Emulsions [1–9]

An emulsion is a two-phase system consisting of two immiscible components, one (the dispersed or inner phase) being suspended in the other (the continuous or outer phase) as small droplets 0.2–0.50 μm in size. One phase is aqueous, the other oily. Stable emulsions remain in this form; unstable emulsions, with a large droplet size, tend to separate as cream does from milk. Emulsions can be diluted with the outer (continuous) phase only. When the diameter of the droplets of the dispersed phase is very small, microemulsions ('transparent systems') are formed with different properties [2,9].

Emulsification of immiscible phases is produced by the addition of an emulsifying agent, which is a large molecule with both strongly polar (i.e. water soluble) and non-polar (i.e. oil soluble) groups allowing it to bridge the gap between polar and non-polar substances.

W/O systems result from the dispersion of an aqueous phase in an oily phase, as in Oily Cream BP. O/W systems are formed when oil is the disperse phase and water the continuous phase, as in Aqueous Cream BP. The former constitute, in general, oily creams or 'cold creams', the latter aqueous or 'vanishing creams'. It is sometimes possible to produce both types of emulsion in the same system [2]: these are called ambiphilic creams. A simple method of determining the nature of an emulsion is to interpose on a filter paper a drop of the emulsion between one of oil and one of water. In 15 min the continuous phase will mix with, or be dispersed by, one or other of the neighbouring drops. Alternatively, it may be tested by adding a larger quantity of water. If the emulsion separates, it is of W/O type; if not, it is of O/W type, the continuous phase being (within limits) able to expand and still retain its contained disperse phase.

General theory [2,5,9–11]

This is a highly specialized and complicated branch of pharmaceutics. The brief outline given here relates to those emulsions likely to be encountered in dermatological rather than cosmetic practice, but it is in the latter field that the art of emulsification has become specially developed.

All molecular substances possess electrical charges. When the molecules are symmetrical these are balanced and the molecule is electrically neutral (non-polar), for example benzene. Non-polar substances are insoluble in water but soluble in other non-polar solvents. They are referred to as being hydrophobic, because they cannot be mixed with water. Polar substances, for example acetic acid and alcohols, in contrast, have asymmetrical formulae with unbalanced electrical charges, and are soluble in water (hydrophilic) but insoluble in organic solvents and oils. Some substances, however, have dual characteristics, being hydrophobic at one end and hydrophilic at the other. As they dissolve partly in water and partly in oil they act as emulsifying agents by binding the two phases together. Depending on the attractive force of the two portions of the molecule, one or other phase will predominate. If the hydrophilic attraction is dominant, an O/W emulsion results; if hydrophobic forces are dominant, then a W/O emulsion is formed. These forces also determine their relative solubility in oil or water. On balance, sodium stearate (soap) is hydrophilic and thus mixes with water and forms an O/W emulsion, whereas calcium stearate, which contains two long-chain fatty acids, is hydrophobic, mixing with fats and oils to form W/O emulsions.

In general, the ease of emulsification and thus the stability of the emulsion depends on the interfacial tension existing between the two phases involved in the emulsion, those with a low interfacial tension emulsifying easily and those with a high interfacial tension requiring considerable mechanical energy to enlarge the surface area between the dissimilar molecules; small droplets having considerably less surface tension are therefore less likely to conglomerate or precipitate out of suspension. The ionic situation at the interface and the electrical properties of repulsion and attraction are of fundamental importance in the theory of emulsification [2]. Concentration, temperature and the addition of electrolytes have a critical effect on this balance and the stability of the emulsion. These considerations are of special practical importance when emulsions are used as bases for ionic and electrically active preparations in topical dermatological therapy.

Properties

The term 'emulsion' is sometimes used loosely. The aqueous phase may vary from water to a solid gel; and the oily phase from a liquid to solid. The emulsifier may be regarded as a third, interfacial phase. Added ingredients may considerably modify the properties. Emulsions are easily disturbed by an excess of the dispersed phase. Thus, Oily Cream BP may separate in the presence of excess water. Even perfume and preservatives may act as surface-active agents and destabilize the emulsion. The degree of homogenization and particle dispersion are obviously important. In dermatological practice, stability and compatibility with additives are paramount. 'Creaming', flocculation and coalescence may occur. Phase inversion may occur from the addition of bivalent- or trivalent-phase electrolytes. Less attention has been paid to the rheological properties of dermatological as opposed to cosmetic preparations, but an even flow of the emulsion on the skin is obviously desirable in both cases [10].

Choice of emulsion

Emulsions follow the characteristics of the external phase, O/W emulsions being readily diluted with water, W/O emulsions with oil. O/W emulsions are generally more acceptable on the skin than W/O emulsions. Aqueous Cream BP is the standard example of such an O/W emulsion. Emulsification greatly increases the surface area of the dispersed phase and thus may alter its chemical or pharmaceutical properties. W/O emulsions provide a greasy residue with some 'cooling' effect. O/W emulsons aid penetration of lipophilic substances [11], and, apart from their cosmetic acceptability and cooling and soothing properties, also leave a thin film of lipid on the surface as an emollient.

Emulsifying agents [1,4,8,12,13,15]

The activity of an emulsifying agent depends upon its ability to alter the interfacial angle of physically dissimilar substances (the contact or wetting angle). This in turn depends upon the strength of the relative cohesive forces involved. In dermatology, three-part systems also occur, i.e. water–oil–solid (skin or hair), but these are modified by the natural surface emulsion of amino and fatty acids derived from sweat and sebum. An extreme example of emulsifying action is seen in cleansers, shampoos and detergents.

HLB value [14]

The relative affinity of an emulsifier for water (hydrophilic) and for oil (lipophilic) has a value in denoting its emulsification tendency. Emulsifiers with an HLB value of 3–6 tend to give W/O systems and those with higher values O/W systems (Table 78.2). The HLB value only indicates this one character of the emulsifier and has no other relevance.

Amphipathic agents [11]

These are substances with molecules or ions, part of which have an affinity, and part a repulsion for, the medium in which they are dissolved. They form the great bulk of emulsifying agents and consist of five groups, based on the character of the polar attachment to the hydrophobic portion of the molecule. These are:

1 anionic;
2 cationic;
3 non-ionic (these do not dissociate in water);
4 ampholytic, the activity depending on the pH of the solution;
5 miscellaneous.

Table 78.2 Some common emulsifiers [2,9].

Producing W/O systems (HLB 3–6)
Polyvalent metallic soaps
(Oil-soluble quaternary ammonium cationics)
Propylene glycol fatty acid esters and monostearate
Sorbitan monopalmitate and mono-oleate
Glyceryl monostearate

Producing O/W systems (HLB 7–17)
Alkyl sulphates and sulphonates
Synthetic phosphoric acid esters
Cationic emulsifiers
Sorbitan monolaurate
Most polyoxyethylene compounds
Triethanolamine oleate

W/O, water in oil; O/W, oil in water; HLB, hydrophilic–lipophilic balance.

Anionic emulsifiers

These include the soaps and the sulphated compounds. The hydrophilic portion of the molecule provides the anion.

In soaps, O/W emulsions are formed from the monovalent alkaline salts of long-chain fatty acids, and have the general formula RCOOM (alkali soaps), as in, for example, sodium stearate. Metallic soaps have the general formula $(RCOO)_N M$, where M is a polyvalent metal and N is valency. The most common metals are calcium or magnesium, and these form W/O emulsions. Calamine Liniment BPC is such a 'soap'; calcium oleate being formed by the action of limewater on the oleic acid. Organic soaps, for example triethanolamine stearate, are formed by the substitution of hydrogen ions in fatty acids by organic basic groups. They produce stable O/W emulsions, little affected by acids or calcium ions. If the amines are volatile, the emulsion dries out and cannot be re-emulsified by water. They thus produce water-resistant coatings.

In sulphates and sulphonated emulsifiers, a sulphate compound results from esterification of a fatty alcohol with sulphuric acid followed by neutralization with an alkali, for example sodium lauryl sulphate, triethanolamine lauryl sulphate. A slightly different process produces sulphonated derivatives, for example sodium secondary dodecyl sulphonate (Teepol). Both types of preparation are widely used as emulsifiers for O/W systems, and have the advantage of being tolerant to calcium, thus avoiding the creation of a scum with hard water. For emulsification, a stabilizer has to be added and this is normally a fatty alcohol, for example cetostearyl alcohol as in Emulsifying Wax BP, a self-emulsifying anionic wax for emulsions containing 10% sodium lauryl sulphate and 90% cetostearyl alcohol. Sulphonated compounds are less used for emulsions but, being effective wetting agents, find an important place in detergents.

Cationic emulsifiers

Here, the cation provides the surface activity (reverse soaps) and the compounds used are quaternary ammonium salts. They are less efficient than anionic emulsifiers, and are chiefly used where antiseptic properties of the formulation are required as they inhibit the growth of many microorganisms.

Non-ionic emulsifiers

These are esters or ethers with balanced hydrophilic and hydrophobic groups, and, as they do not dissociate, they show considerable stability to acids and alkalis. They are derived from alcohols, such as cetyl alcohol, glycerol, mannitol, sorbitol and include cetomacrogol, Spans and Tweens. Their physical behaviour and chemistry vary with individual members of the groups. Cetomacrogol 1000 BP is an ether of cetyl alcohol and polyethylene oxide. It is a component of Cetomacrogol Emulsifying Wax BP, which contains 10% Cetomacrogol 1000 and 90% cetostearyl alcohol; polyoxethylene sorbitol mono-oleate (polysorbate 80 or Span 80) is an ester of sorbitol containing polyethylene oxide (about 20 groups) and oleic acid. Both these preparations are widely used for O/W emulsions.

Ampholytic emulsifiers

Their behaviour depends on the pH of the emulsion. They are anionic above pH 9, cationic below pH 5 and non-ionic at pH 7. They tolerate electrolytes, and are compatible with phenols and quaternary ammonium agents.

Other emulsifiers

These include the older animal and vegetable emulsifiers, such as gum acacia, tragacanth, starches, dextrins and lecithin. The wool fats and alcohols are of special importance as W/O emulsifiers.

REFERENCES

1 Becher P. *Emulsions: Theory and Practice.* New York: Reinhold, 1957.
2 Clark R In: Hibbot HW, ed. *Handbook of Cosmetic Science.* Oxford: Pergamon Press, 1963: 175–204.
3 Flynn GL. Topical drug absorption and topical pharmaceutical systems. In: Banker GS, Rhodes CT, eds. *Modern Pharmaceutics: Drugs and The Pharmaceutical Sciences,* Vol. 7. New York: Marcel Dekker, 1979: 263–327.
4 Hollis GL. *Directory of Surface Active Chemicals: Surfactants UK,* 2nd edn. Darlington, UK: TergoData, 1980.
5 Jellinek JS. *Formulation and Function of Cosmetics.* New York: Wiley, 1970: 32–74, 133–8.
6 Katz M. In: Ariens EJ, ed. *Drug Design (Medicinal Chemistry),* Vol. 4. New York: Academic Press, 1973: 93.
7 Sumner GG. *Clayton's The Theory of Emulsions and their Technical Treatment.* London: Churchill Livingstone, 1954.
8 White RF. *Pharmaceutical Emulsions and Emulsifying Agents,* 4th edn. London: Chemist & Druggist, 1964.
9 Wilkinson JB, ed. *Harry's Cosmeticology,* 6th edn. London: Hill, 1979.
10 Barry BW. *Dermatological Formulations: Percutaneous Absorption. Drugs and The Pharmaceutical Sciences,* Vol. 18. New York: Marcel Dekker, 1983.
11 Polano MK. *Topical Skin Therapeutics.* Edinburgh: Churchill Livingstone, 1984.
12 Bickerman JJ. *Surface Chemistry.* New York: Academic Press, 1958.
13 Moilliet JL, Collie B, Black W. *Surface Activity,* 2nd edn. London: Spon, 1969.
14 Griffin WC. Calculation of HLB values of non-ionic surfactant. *J Soc Cosmet Chem* 1954; **5**: 249–56.
15 Scott BA. The physical chemistry of surface active agents. In: Hibbot HW, ed. *Handbook of Cosmetic Science.* Oxford: Pergamon Press, 1963: 145–74.

Preservatives [1–5]

Minerals, oils, greases and W/O creams with oil as the continuous phase do not usually require preservatives. Lotions, O/W creams and gels, however, because they have water as their continuous phase, are easily contaminated with both moulds and bacteria, and animal and vegetable oils, unless protected from biological decomposition, may deteriorate or become rancid [6]. The ideal preservative should be non-toxic, non-irritant, non-sensitizing, odourless, colourless and effective even at very low concentrations and under conditions of normal usage [7]. In addition, it must be compatible with both the vehicle and the active ingredients [8]. Although topical preparations do not need to be sterile, they should be free from pathogens and contain only acceptable numbers of non-pathogenic microbes.

The parahydroxybenzoic acid esters are effective and widely used preservatives [9]. They can be used singly [10] or in combination. Considering their widespread use, their sensitizing potential appears to be low [4]. Because, individually, they are only sparingly water soluble and as their effects are additive, mixtures are usually preferred. This also increases their spectrum of activity and lowers the risk of sensitization. As little as 0.4% parabens may be enough to preserve an O/W cream [9]. Their activity is reduced in the presence of oils and non-ionic emulsifiers.

Chlorocresol is a preservative used especially in the UK. It is more effective in acid than in alkaline solution. It has a low sensitizing potential. It was for many years the preservative in Aqueous Cream BP, but has now been replaced by phenoxyethanol. It is the preservative in a widely prescribed range of topical corticosteroids.

Sorbic acid (2.4 hexadienoic acid) is also a good preservative, which maintains its activity in the presence of non-ionic detergents. It also has a low sensitization index. It can only be used, however, in preparations with a pH of less than 6.5.

Propylene glycol can inhibit the growth of moulds and fungi, and can therefore be used as a preservative.

Organic mercurials are used as preservatives in many ophthalmic preparations and in some vaccines and skin test solutions [11] but may rarely also be incorporated in some topical preparations [12]. Ethylenediaminetetraacetate is a widely used preservative in ear, nose and eye drops. Gallates and other antioxidants such as butylhydroxyanisole (BHA) and butylhydroxytoluene (BHT) are used to prevent rancidity in oily and fatty preparations.

Other preservatives, including those mainly used in cosmetic products, are discussed in Chapters 19 and 20.

Lanolin [13–15]

Lanolin will absorb about 30% of water. It is therefore a useful W/O emulsifier and is widely used in many therapeutic and cosmetic preparations [14]. Its composition varies qualitatively and quantitatively with humidity, temperature and method of collection. It is composed of alcohol and acid esters and a very variable proportion of free fatty alcohols and acids. Small quantities of anionic detergent may also be present [16]; the amount in 20 samples of wool grease varied from 0.55 to 2.4% [17]. These may increase the detectable incidence of hypersensitivity significantly [18].

The proportion of free fatty alcohols found in over 30 different samples of lanolin varied from 6.1 to 12.6% [18]. Lanolin derivatives result from acetylation, ethoxylation, solvent fractionation, saponification and acidolysis. They are highly effective wetting agents for finely ground solids in liquid vehicles, powerful emulsifiers, solubilizers of colloidal dispersal systems and spreading agents.

Nomenclature [19]. The nomenclature of the various types of lanolin is confusing and is discussed on page 3522. Wool fat and wool alcohols both contain small quantities of BHA or BHT as antioxidants.

Amerchols are a proprietary range of surface-active emulsifying agents based on wool fat and containing free sterol and higher alcohols.

Lanesta is the name given to a range of isopropyl esters of wool fat alcohols.

Solulan comprises a range of polyoxyethylene derivatives of wool fat or wool alcohols, some wholly or partly acetylated.

Lanolin-free bases

Among bases free of lanolin may be mentioned Emulsifying Wax and Ointment BP, Lanette Wax, Macrogol Ointment BP, and the paraffins. Lanolin has been replaced in many proprietary ointments in recent years, by cetyl, stearyl and cetostearyl alcohol.

Sensitization [20,21]

Although the incidence of sensitization to preservatives in medicaments is low when compared with their widespread usage [2], allergy to preservatives and other ingredients of topical medicaments may be due to a wide range of ingredients and is not restricted to fragrance, biocides and lanolin [2,11,22]. Sensitivity to an ingredient of the vehicle may be 'occult', and is easily overlooked [23].

Nearly all components of the base may be sensitizers. These include ethylenediamine [3], propylene glycol [24], emulsifiers [25], sorbic acid [26,27], cetyl, stearyl and cetostearyl alcohols and fragrance [28].

Most cases of sensitivity to vehicle components are a result of medical rather than cosmetic usage [2]. Patients with chronic stasis eczema or leg ulcers appear to be particularly susceptible [13,29].

Unfortunately, because there is as yet no product labelling in Europe [30], and topical medicaments only list 'active ingredients', it is still often very difficult to advise a patient with a sensitivity.

REFERENCES

1 Bloomfield SF. A review. The use of disinfectants in the home. *J Appl Bacteriol* 1978; **45**: 1–38.

2 Cronin E. *Contact Dermatitis*. Edinburgh: Churchill Livingstone, 1980.
3 Fisher AA. Instructions for the ethylene diamine-sensitive patient. *Cutis* 1974; **13**: 27–8.
4 Hjorth N. Contact dermatitis. *Br J Dermatol* 1980; **103** (Suppl. 18): 19–20.
5 Katz M. In: Ariens EJ, ed. *Drug Design (Medicinal Chemistry)*, Vol. 4. New York: Academic Press, 1973: 93.
6 Polano MK. *Topical Skin Therapeutics*. Edinburgh: Churchill Livingstone, 1984.
7 Noble WC, Savin JA. Steroid cream contaminated with *Pseudomonas aeruginosa*. *Lancet* 1966; **i**: 347–9.
8 Crowshaw B. Preservatives for cosmetics and toiletries. *J Soc Cosmet Chem* 1977; **28**: 3–16.
9 Evans S. Epidermal sensitivity to 'lanolin' and 'parabens': occurrence in pharmaceutical and cosmetic products. *Br J Dermatol* 1970; **82**: 625.
10 O'Neill JJ, Peelor PL, Peterson AF. Selection of parabens as preservatives. *J Soc Cosmet Chem* 1979; **30**: 25–38.
11 Fisher AA. *Contact Dermatitis*, 3rd edn. Philadelphia: Lea & Febiger, 1986.
12 Wilkinson DS. Thiomersal. *Contact Dermatitis* 1978; **5**: 58–9.
13 Breit R, Bandmann HJ. Contact Dermatitis XXII—Dermatitis from lanolin. *Br J Dermatol* 1973; **88**: 414–15.
14 Cronin E. Lanolin dermatitis. *Br J Dermatol* 1966; **78**: 167–74.
15 Scholossman MC, McCarthy JP. Lanolin derivatives, chemistry: relationship to allergic contact dermatitis. *Contact Dermatitis* 1979; **6**: 65–72.
16 Clarke EW. The water absorption properties of lanolin. *J Soc Cosmet Chem* 1971; **22**: 421–37.
17 Anderson CA, Ganly RG, Wood GF. The determination of nonylphenol ethylene oxide detergents in wool grease. *J Pharm Pharmacol* 1966; **18**: 809–14.
18 Clarke EW, Cronin E, Wilkinson DS. Lanolin with reduced sensitizing potential—a preliminary note. *Contact Dermatitis* 1977; **3**: 69–76.
19 Reynolds JEF, ed. *Martindale: The Extra Pharmacopoeia*, 31st edn. London: Pharmaceutical Press, 1996.
20 Fregert S, Hjorth N, Magnusson B. Epidemiology of contact dermatitis. *Trans St Johns Hosp Derm Soc* 1969; **55**: 17–35.
21 North American Contact Dermatitis Group. Epidemiology of contact dermatitis in North America: 1972. *Arch Dermatol* 1973; **108**: 537–40.
22 Nater JP, De Groot AC. *Unwanted Effect of Cosmetics and Drugs Used in Dermatology*. Amsterdam: Elsevier, 1985.
23 Fisher AA, Pascher F, Kanof NB. Allergic contact dermatitis due to ingredients of vehicles. *Arch Dermatol* 1971; **104**: 286–90.
24 Hannuksela M, Pirilä V, Salo OP. Skin reactions to propylene glycol. *Contact Dermatitis* 1975; **1**: 112–16.
25 Hannuksela M, Kousa M, Pirilä V. Contact sensitivity to emulsifiers. *Contact Dermatitis* 1976; **2**: 201–4.
26 Brown R. Another case of sorbic acid sensitivity. *Contact Dermatitis* 1979; **5**: 268.
27 Saihan EM, Harman RRM. Contact sensitivity to sorbic acid in 'Unguentum Merck'. *Br J Dermatol* 1978; **99**: 583–4.
28 Larsen WG. Perfume dermatitis. A study of 20 patients. *Arch Dermatol* 1977; **113**: 623–5.
29 Wilkinson JD, Hambly EM, Wilkinson DS. Comparison of patch test results in two adjacent areas of England. II—Medicaments. *Acta Derm Venereol (Stockh)* 1980; **60**: 245–9.
30 De Groot AC. Labelling cosmetics with their ingredients. *Br Med J* 1990; **300**: 1636–8.

Incorporation of active ingredients [1,2]

The effect of any topical application is the sum of the non-specific effects of the vehicle and the specific effects of the active ingredients. The response to any topically applied drug is dependent on three factors [3,4].

1 *Availability for absorption*: the drug must be readily released from the vehicle. Concentration and partition coefficients are important.

2 *Penetration*: penetration and permeation of the drug through the skin.

3 *Interaction and degradation*: the effect of the active drug on its target receptors and the rate at which it is degraded or removed from the skin.

An active drug and its vehicle must be compatible. An unsuitable combination may either inactivate the active drug or prevent its efficient release from the vehicle. If the active drug is to be added to a vehicle then the final formulation should be adjusted so as not to upset the liquid/solid balance of the preparation. If a liquid-active agent is added, the liquid component of the vehicle should be proportionately reduced; if a solid agent, the solid should be adjusted accordingly. In this way, the consistency of the final product will remain unaltered [1].

Some active agents are rapidly degraded if mixed in an inappropriate base. Thus, a proportion of the salicylic acid in Lassar's paste may be rapidly converted to inactive zinc salicylate. This has little specific effect on its own but is able to 'protect' dithranol from being oxidized by the zinc oxide [1].

Suitable vehicles for dilution of ionic agents

A dilution of a topical formulation containing ingredients which are ionic or cationic must be made in a non-ionic vehicle to avoid upsetting the activity or stability of the preparation. Among such substances are triphenylmethane dyes, polyvalent metals, many antibiotics and corticosteroids.

Suitable emulsifying agents and bases which can be used for this purpose are detailed in the pharmacopoeias [2,5]. W/O emulsions may be prepared with sorbitan monostearate and O/W emulsions with sorbitan esters and polyoxyethylene derivatives. Cetomacrogols are commonly used in the UK [5].

Some commonly used agents and preservatives [6,7] are incompatible with non-ionic bases, for example phenols, resorcinol and salicylic acid.

When dilution or mixing of ionic agents is desirable, the advice of a pharmacist should be sought.

REFERENCES

1 Polano MK. *Topical Skin Therapeutics*. Edinburgh: Churchill Livingstone, 1984.
2 Reynolds JEF, ed. *Martindale: The Extra Pharmacopoeia*, 31st edn. London: Pharmaceutical Press, 1996.
3 Barry BW. *Dermatological Formulations: Percutaneous Absorption. Drugs and The Pharmaceutical Sciences*, Vol. 18. New York: Marcel Dekker, 1983.
4 Katz M. In: Ariens EJ, ed. *Drug Design (Medicinal in Chemistry)*, Vol. 4. New York: Academic Press, 1973: 93.
5 *British National Formulary*, No. 32 London: British Medical Association and The Pharmaceutical Society of Great Britain, 1996.
6 Browne MRW. Turbidimetric method for the rapid evaluation of antimicrobial agents. Inactivation of preservatives by non-ionic agents. *J Soc Cosmet Chem* 1966; **17**: 185–9.
7 Patel NK, Foss NE. Interaction of some pharmaceuticals with macro-molecules: I. Effect of temperature on the binding of parabens and phenols by Polysorbate 80 and Polyethylene glycol 4000. *J Pharm Sci* 1964; **53**: 94–7.

Modifying factors [1–8]

The absorption of drugs can be influenced in various ways, for example by chemical modification, to obtain a more favourable lipid–water partition coefficient, by modification of the size of the molecule, by micronization (to increase the rate of dissolution), by suitable choice of the point of application and the form in which the drug is applied, and by the use of absorption promoters. Propylene glycol [9,10], azone [11], urea [12], salicylic acid [13] and DMSO and related drugs [13–16] have all been shown to be promoters of drug penetration. The mechanism by which these drugs work remains unclear, although some may act as marginal irritants [17] and hence facilitate penetration through the stratum corneum. Liposomes may also prove to be useful as a drug delivery system [18].

Dimethylsulphoxide [19–24]

DMSO is a highly polar, stable substance with exceptional solvent properties. It releases histamine *in vivo* and may induce weals when applied topically. It reacts with water, liberating heat.

DMSO acts as a penetrant, enhancing the penetration of drug substance through the skin [24–26], and it can induce the formation of a steroid reservoir [15]. The stratum corneum retains significant amounts of DMSO and, as most drugs are more soluble in DMSO than water, the high concentration of drug attained within the stratum corneum tends to further promote percutaneous absorption [22]. This quality has been shown to be of particular value in increasing the effectiveness of idoxuridine in herpes simplex [27] and zoster [28]. It may similarly enhance the action of other drugs. In the past, toxicological considerations have precluded its more widespread use.

Dimethylformamide and dimethylacetamide act similarly but are less effective [14,25,29]. These and many other penetration enhancers are fully discussed by Barry [1].

Physiological factors affecting the delivery of active drug [1,30–32]

Epidermal hydration and occlusion significantly increase drug penetration [33–35], and other factors such as age [29,36], skin condition [37,38], temperature [39], skin type [40,41] and site of application are also important [32,42,43] and have a significant effect on absorption rates. These and other factors are discussed in more detail in Chapter 4.

Transdermal drug delivery [44]

This new technique has not yet found much use in dermatology, but has important applications in cardiology with nitroglycerine and isosorbide available in patch form, and in other areas of medicine with clonidine, oestradiol and scopolamine. The advantages of the system include the avoidance of hepatic 'first-pass' metabolism, the maintenance of steady-state plasma levels of drug, and convenience.

REFERENCES

1 Barry BW. *Dermatological Formulations: Percutaneous Absorption. Drugs and The Pharmaceutical Sciences*, Vol. 18. New York: Marcel Dekker, 1983.

2 Flynn GL. Topical drug absorption and topical pharmaceutical systems. In: Banker GS, Rhodes CT, eds. *Modern Pharmaceuticals*. New York: Marcel Dekker, 1979: 263–327.

3 Higuchi T. In: Rocher B, ed. *Design of Biopharmaceutical Properties through Pro-Drugs and Analogy*. Washington, DC: American Pharmaceutical Association, 1977.

4 Katz M. In: Ariens EJ, ed. *Drug Design (Medicinal Chemistry)*, Vol. 14. New York: Academic Press, 1973: 93.

5 Polano MK. *Topical Skin Therapeutics*. Edinburgh: Churchill Livingstone, 1984.

6 Polano MK, Ponec M. Bioavailability and effects of various vehicles on percutaneous absorption. In: Mauvais-Jarvis P, Vickers CFH, Wepierre J, eds. *Percutaneous Absorption of Steroids*. New York: Academic Press, 1980: 67–79.

7 Scheuplein RJ. Percutaneous absorption: theoretical aspects. In: Mauvais-Jarvis P, Vickers CFH, Wepierre J, eds. *Percutaneous Absorption of Steroids*. New York: Academic Press, 1980: 1–17.

8 Wester RC, Maibach HI. In: Drill VA, Lasar P, eds. *Cutaneous Toxicity*. New York: Academic Press, 1977: 63.

9 Ostrenga J, Haleblan J, Poulsen B *et al*. Vehicle for a new topical steroid, floucinonide. *J Invest Dermatol* 1971; **56**: 392–9.

10 Polano MK, Ponec M. Dependence of corticosteroid penetration on the vehicle. *Arch Dermatol* 1976; **112**: 675–80.

11 Spruance SL, McKeough M, Sugibayashi K *et al*. Effect of azone and pro-pylene glycol on penetration of trifluorothymidine through skin and efficacy of different topical formulations against cutaneous herpes simplex virus infections in guinea pigs. *Antimicrob Agents Chemother* 1984; **26**: 819–23.

12 Feldman RJ, Maibach HI. Percutaneous penetration of hydrocortisone with urea. *Arch Dermatol* 1974; **109**: 58–9.

13 Munro DD, Stoughton RB. Dimethylacetamide (DMAC) and dimethylform-amide (DMF) effect on cutaneous absorption. *Arch Dermatol* 1965; **92**: 585–6.

14 Feldman RJ, Maibach HI. Percutaneous penetration of C^{14} hydrocortisone in man. *Arch Dermatol* 1966; **94**: 649–51.

15 Stoughton RB. Dimethylsulfoxide (DMSO) induction of a steroid reservoir in human skin. *Arch Dermatol* 1965; **91**: 657–60.

16 Stoughton RB. Hexachlorophane deposition in human stratum corneum. Enhancement by dimethylacetamide, dimethylsulfoxide and methylethylether. *Arch Dermatol* 1966; **94**: 646–8.

17 Chaudrasekarau SK, Shaw EJE. Factors influencing the percutaneous absorption of drugs. *Curr Probl Dermatol* 1978; **7**: 142.

18 Schaefer H, Korting M, Korting HC *et al*. Liposome preparations: a step forward in topical drug therapy for skin disease? A review. *J Am Acad Dermatol* 1989; **21**: 1271–5.

19 Beger I, Lorenz D. Purification of analysis of dimethylsulphoxide. In: Martin D, Hauthal HG, eds. *Dimethyl Sulphoxide*. New York: Van Nostrand Reinhold, 1976: 41–8.

20 Jacob SW, Herschler R, eds. Biological actions of dimethyl sulphoxide. *Ann NY Acad Sci* 1975; **23**: 243.

21 Jacob SW, Bischel M, Herschler RJ. Dimethyl sulfoxide (DMSO): a new concept in pharmacotherapy. *Curr Ther Res* 1964; **6**: 134–5.

22 Katz M, Poulsen BJ. Absorption of drugs through the skin. In: Brodie BB, Gillette J, eds. *Handbook of Experimental Pharmacology*, Vol. 28. New York: Springer, 1971: 103–74.

23 Kligman AM. Dimethylsulfoxide—Part 2. *JAMA* 1965; **193**: 923–8.

24 Landahu G, Schloss Hauer HJ, eds. *Dimethylsulphoxide—DMSO Symposium*. Berlin: Saladruck, 1965.

25 Baker H. The effects of dimethylsulfoxide, dimethylformamide and dimethylacetamide on the cutaneous barrier to water in human skin. *J Invest Dermatol* 1968; **50**: 283–8.

26 Stoughton RB, Fritsch WC. Influence of dimethylsulfoxide (DMSO) on human percutaneous absorption. *Arch Dermatol* 1964; **90**: 512–17.

27 MacCallum FO, Juel-Jensen BE. Herpes simplex virus skin infection in man treated with idoxuridine in dimethylsulphoxide. Results of a double-blind controlled trial. *Br Med J* 1966; **ii**: 805–7.

28 Juel-Jensen BE, MacCallum FO, MacKenzie AMR. Treatment of zoster with idoxuridine in dimethylsulphoxide. Results of two double-blind controlled trials. *Br Med J* 1970; **iv**: 776–80.

29 Rasmussen JE. In: Dobson RL, ed. *The Year Book of Dermatology 1979*. Chicago: Year Book Medical Publishers, 1979: 15.

30 Idson B. Hydration and percutaneous absorption. *Curr Probl Dermatol* 1978; **7**: 132–41.

31 McKenzie AW, Stoughton RB. Method for comparing percutaneous absorption of steroids. *Arch Dermatol* 1962; **86**: 608–10.

32 Scheuplein RJ, Black IH. Permeability of the skin. *Physiol Rev* 1971; **5**: 702–47.

33 Fritsch WC, Stoughton RB. The effect of temperature and humidity on the penetration of C acetyl salicylic acid in excised human skin. *J Invest Dermatol* 1963; **41**: 307–11.

34 Scheuplein RJ. In: Jarrett A, ed. *Physiology and Pathology of the Skin*, Vol. 5. New York: Academic Press, 1978: 1669–92.

35 Sulzberger MB, Witten VH. Thin pliable plastic films in topical dermatologic therapy. *Arch Dermatol* 1961; **84**: 1027–8.

36 Kligman AM. Cutaneous toxicology: an overview from the underside. *Curr Probl Dermatol* 1978; **7**: 1–25.

37 Schaefer H. *Percutaneous Absorption of Steroids*. Paris: International Symposium, 1979.

38 Solomon AE, Lowe NJ. Percutaneous absorption in experimental epidermal disease. *Br J Dermatol* 1979; **100**: 717–22.

39 Shaw JE, Taskovitch L, Chandrasekaran SK. Properties of skin in relation to drug absorption *in vitro* and *in vivo*. In: Drill VA, Lasar P, eds. *Current Concepts in Cutaneous Toxicity*. New York: Academic Press, 1980: 127–33.

40 Frosch PJ, Kligman AM. Rapid blister formation in human skin with ammonium hydroxide. *Br J Dermatol* 1977; **96**: 461–73.

41 Weigand DA, Haygood C, Gaylor JR *et al*. Radical variations in the cutaneous barrier. In: Drill VA, Lasar P, eds. *Current Concepts in Cutaneous Toxicity*. New York: Academic Press, 1980: 221–35.

42 Feldman RJ, Maibach HI. Regional percutaneous penetration of C^{14} cortisol in man. *J Invest Dermatol* 1967; **48**: 181–3.

43 Maibach HI, Feldman RJ, Milby TH *et al*. Regional variation in percutaneous penetration in man. *Arch Environ Health* 1971; **23**: 208–11.

44 Kydonieus AF, Berner B. *Transdermal Delivery of Drugs*. Boca Raton, Florida: CRC Press, 1987.

Dosage [1,2]

In dermatology, an active ingredient is usually prescribed as a percentage of the total prescription, whereas the quantities used are governed by the total surface areas to be covered and the likely duration of treatment. The total dose, however, still has to be considered, especially with regard to possible toxicity, for example phenol, salicylic acid, podophyllin, and the local and systemic effects of topically applied steroids.

Important variables include concentration, the total amount applied, the frequency of application and the total area treated. Other factors, such as drug penetration, site, hydration and occlusion, have already been discussed. It should be noted, however, that dose–response curves are frequently non-linear, and penetration and clinical effect depend less on the total amount of drug applied and more on the actual amount of active drug in contact with the skin [3,4]. Penetration of steroid creams and ointments is not enhanced by simply increasing the amount applied above an optimum thickness [5], and change in concentration is not always reflected by a parallel change in efficacy. For instance, 2.5% hydrocortisone preparations are no more effective than those containing 1%, and extemporaneously diluted steroids cannot be presumed to produce a pro rata decrease in effect. Some dilutions may show very little reduction in efficacy because of their dose–response curve and depot effect [6], whereas others may have far less effect than anticipated, especially if they are incorporated into an inappropriate base.

Table 78.3 A guide to suitable quantities of a topically applied drug for 1 week's treatment.

	To use sparingly	To use liberally	Lotions
Whole body	100 g	250–500 g	500 ml
Localized disease	15–30 g	50–100 g	25–100 ml

Frequency of application

Very little is known about optimal frequency of application. Bland applications obviously have to be applied frequently enough to maintain their physical effect, but most active preparations are usually applied just once or twice a day. With topical steroids, because of their depot effect, it may be possible to reduce this to alternate days or less.

Steroid creams and ointments should be applied sparingly. Dilute or less potent steroids can be used when larger areas of the body need to be covered. Non-steroid creams, liniments and pastes, however, are used thickly to allow for their different physical modes of action.

Quantitative aspects of topical prescribing [7–9]

This is often overlooked. The amount prescribed should last the patient until the next visit or should be adequate for the intended duration of treatment. Polano [2] recommends 10 g cream or ointment per application per day as the minimum amount feasible for whole-body application. Schlagel and Sanborn [10] found 12 g/day the minimum amount necessary, and 'liberal' applications of emollients may entail using more than 100 g/day. A 'thick' layer of cream or ointment is usually 0.05–0.1 mm in thickness and a 'thin' layer 0.005–0.01 mm [1,2]. The *British National Formulary* [11] makes some suggestions as to appropriate quantities of topical applications to be prescribed for both regional or whole-body use. The quantities that the authors find to be adequate in general for 1 week's treatment are given in Table 78.3.

REFERENCES

1 Arndt KA. *Manual of Dermatologic Therapeutics*, 3rd edn. Little Brown & Co., 1983: 11.
2 Polano MK. *Topical Skin Therapeutics*. Edinburgh: Churchill Livingstone, 1984.
3 Wester RC, Maibach HI. Relationship of topical delivery and percutaneous absorption in rhesus monkeys and man. *J Invest Dermatol* 1976; **67**: 518–20.
4 Wester RCA, Nolonan PK, Maibach HI. Frequency of application on percutaneous absorption of hydrocortisone. *Arch Dermatol* 1977; **113**: 620–2.
5 Ponec M. *Chemical and biochemical aspects of topical psoriasis treatment*. Thesis, Leiden, 1977: 49.
6 Gibson JR, Kirsch J, Saihan EM *et al*. The dilution of proprietary corticosteroid ointments: an attempt to evaluate relative clinical potencies. *Br J Dermatol* 1982; **106**: 445–88.
7 Friedrickson T, Lassus A, Bleeker J. Treatment of psoriasis and atopic dermatitis with halcinonide cream applied once to three times daily. *Br J Dermatol* 1980; **102**: 575–7.
8 Hradil E, Lindstrom C, Moller H. Intermittent treatment of psoriasis with clobetasone propionate. *Acta Derm Venereol (Stockh)* 1979; **58**: 375–7.
9 Van der Harst CA, De Jonghe H, Pot F *et al*. Comparison of two application schedules for clobetasol propionate. *Acta Derm Venereol (Stockh)* 1982; **62**: 270–3.
10 Schlagel CA, Sanborn EC. The weights of topical preparations required for total and partial inunction. *J Invest Dermatol* 1964; **42**: 253–6.
11 *British National Formulary*, No. 32. London: British Medical Association and The Pharmaceutical Society of Great Britain, 1996.

Topical agents

Simple remedies [1,2]

Advances in the science of formulation of topical agents have resulted in a number of very sophisticated applications that are available to cover almost every need in topical prescribing, but these may be expensive or not in worldwide supply. It may therefore be useful to remember the benefits that may still be obtained from the judicious use of simple, inexpensive agents that are readily available. They are not as elegant and may not be quite as effective in all cases, but they have a considerable overall value, especially in remote areas.

The almost forgotten pumice stone [3], used alone when the skin is wet or after applying a simple salicylic acid–propylene glycol gel [4], is very valuable for hyperkeratotic conditions and, of course, for removing the protective coating of verrucae. One of our patients with considerable hyperkeratosis of the heels preferred a 'corn rasp' to all keratolytics. A simple aid for applying creams to inaccessible areas has been designed [5].

Various combinations of powder, glycerine, water and alcohol will produce shake lotions or 'cooling pastes'. Zinc paste with 1% phenol is an effective antipruritic and protective agent for pruritus ani. Potassium permanganate crystals can be diluted to form antiseptic soaks or wet dressings (see Formulary, Chapter 82). The triphenylmethane dyes and Castellani's paint, used correctly, may not be aesthetic but they are effective, particularly for mixed bacterial or fungal infections. Simple non-steroidal creams, pastes and lotions are still useful for inflammatory dermatoses [6].

Leg ulcers are often as satisfactorily treated with saline, 3–6% hydrogen peroxide solution, 5% acetic acid solution, or with Eusol or Eusol and paraffin as by the many, more expensive, applications and dressings now available. 'Samaritan mixture' (Chapter 82) combines acetic acid with oil: the authors have used it as a home dressing for leg ulcers, particularly if infected by *Pseudomonas pyocyaneus*. 'Black wash' (0.5% aqueous silver nitrate) is also used for leg ulcers and for burns (although its hypotonicity makes it unsuitable for large burned areas).

Zinc cream, zinc and castor oil or a zinc paste are very effective in napkin (diaper) dermatitis, provided the occlusive effect of plastic covering is removed.

Sodium chloride 0.9% with a preservative has been said to be a non-painful local anaesthetic [7] (but of short duration).

REFERENCES

1 Arndt KA. *Manual of Dermatologic Therapeutics*, 2nd edn. Boston: Little, Brown & Co., 1978.
2 Polano MK. *Topical Skin Therapeutics*. Edinburgh: Churchill Livingstone, 1984.
3 Baden HP. The pumice stone in dermatologic therapy. *J Am Acad Dermatol* 1980; **2**: 29–30
4 Baden HP, Alper JC. A keratolytic gel containing salicylic acid in propylene glycol. *J Invest Dermatol* 1973; **61**: 330–3.
5 Goolamali SK. A simple aid for the application of skin preparations. *Br J Dermatol* 1979; **101**: 723–4.
6 Perret WJ. Nonsteroidal topical treatment of inflammatory dermatoses. *Cutis* 1980; **26**: 172–3, 176.
7 Wiener SG. Injectable sodium chloride as a local anesthetic for skin surgery. *Cutis* 1979; **23**: 342–3.

Traditional agents [1,2]

The substances discussed below are not intended to provide a complete dermatological formulary but merely a brief guide to those traditional agents and their derivatives that are in common topical use. Drugs with specific or particular activities or indications are discussed in separate sections later.

Details of preparations can be found in the Formulary (Chapter 82).

Aluminium

As a thin foil, it has been used as a protective dressing. It is used in Baltimore paste as an inert protective application, and as aluminium acetotartrate (subacetate) for wet dressings, or as non-sensitizing eardrops in moist and exudative otitis externa. Twenty per cent solutions of the chloride and chlorhydrate in alcohol are now commercially available as axillary antiperspirants [3]. Bentonite, widely used as a gelling agent in shake lotions and emulsions, is colloidal hydrated aluminium silicate. Aluminium oxide in a graded particulate form is used as an abrasive cleanser in some cases of acne.

Benzoic acid

This is an antiseptic, preservative and antifungal agent. Benzoic acid compound ointment BNF (Whitfield's ointment) contains 6% benzoic acid and 3% salicylic acid in emulsifying ointment. It is also used as a tincture. Benzoic acid is a permitted food preservative.

Benzyl benzoate, as a 25% emulsion, is a standard treatment for scabies.

Ethyl-*p*-aminobenzoate (benzocaine) is best avoided because of its sensitization risk. The parahydroxybenzoates are widely used as preservatives in topical applications.

Calcium

This is used as calcium hydroxide (limewater) in the production of several local preparations, such as zinc cream and oily calamine lotion. With oleic acid it forms a soap.

Camphor

This is sometimes added to lotions for its antipruritic and cooling effects. It is widely used in proprietary chilblain preparations.

Ichthammol

Originally a shale oil treated with sulphuric acid and ammonia, ichthammol (ammonium ichthysulphonate) is a viscous black substance containing no less than 10% organically combined sulphur. It is soluble in water and glycerin, but becomes viscous and hard on standing. Its physical properties lead to difficulties in formulation. It is still used as an anti-inflammatory and vasoconstrictive agent for eczema, seborrhoeic dermatitis and rosacea, although without indisputable evidence of its effectiveness. It is also used with glycerin in external otitis.

Iodine (p. 3541)

This can be used as an antiseptic.

Magnesium

The oxide is used in dusting powders and, as the hydrous polysilicate (talc), in shake lotions and pastes. It adds 'slip' to the former and adhesive qualities to the latter. Magnesium sulphate in 25% solution or as a paste is used in inflammatory lesions for its osmotic effect.

Menthol [4]

This has been added to calamine and other lotions and creams to relieve pruritus. The sensation of cold it induces is thought to suppress itch by competitive stimulation of the nerve receptors.

Mercury

Although mercury has been used in the past for the treatment of psoriasis and eczema, toxic effects from absorption are frequent. It is a parasiticide, and has some antibacterial action. Organic mercurial compounds, such as phenylmercuric acetate, are used as preservatives. Sensitization to all these preparations is not uncommon.

Phenol

This is a potent but toxic bactericide. In a strength of 0.5–1%, it is often added to calamine or other lotions for its antipruritic effect. It exerts an analgesic effect on the pain receptors. It is used as phenol hydrate for its caustic action (Chapter 80). It is absorbed through the skin, especially in infancy [5], and excreted in the urine. It has caused severe toxic effects and death when used to excess.

Resorcinol (*m*-dihydroxybenzene)

As the advantages of this are less apparent than its dangers, there is little justification for its continued use.

Selenium disulphide

This is used for the treatment of *seborrhoea* of the scalp and the control of pityriasis versicolor. Although absorption was found to occur on prolonged contact with normal skin [2] no significant absorption occurred after shampooing diseased scalps [6]. It is also used as an intermittent '10 minute body shampoo' [7], for the suppression of pityriasis versicolor [8], and in treating confluent and reticulate papillomatosis [9]. Used in this way, the risk of toxicity is low [10].

Silver

The nitrate is used in solid form as a caustic/haemostatic. Solutions of 0.5–2% inhibit the growth of *Pseudomonas aeruginosa*. It is used for burns [11,12] and leg ulcers. Argyria may follow its prolonged administration.

Silver sulphadiazine

First introduced over 20 years ago [13,14], this compound has become established as a safe and convenient dressing for burns [14]. Even when applied over wide areas, systemic absorption is minimal and the risk of renal damage is thought to be slight [15]. It is applied as a 1% cream. It appears to have a low potential for sensitization and is useful in the management of leg ulcers where it provides good prophylaxis against *Staphylococcus aureus* and some Gram-negative organisms. Some patients may become sensitive to the cetyl alcohol contained in the base of one proprietary formulation. When sulphonamide-resistant Gram-negative bacilli were present, a silver nitrate/chlorhexidine cream was found to be of value [16].

Sulphur

This is still widely used for acne, seborrhoeic conditions and rosacea, despite some doubt about its activity [17], and even allegations of comedogenicity [18], although these have lacked subsequent confirmation [19]. Sodium thiosulphate 20% in a 1% cetrimide solution is a useful treatment for extensive pityriasis versicolor infections.

A 2% sulphur and 2% salicylic acid shampoo has been shown to be of benefit in the treatment of dandruff [20], and topical sulphur-containing preparations have also been shown to be effective in rosacea [21].

Tars

See below.

Titanium

Used as a dioxide it is a chemically inert and useful substitute for zinc oxide when salicylic acid is also required [22]. It has been recommended as the active ingredient of some photoprotective creams.

Urea BP [23–25]
SYN. CARBAMIDE

This accelerates the digestion of fibrin at about 15% and is proteolytic at 40% strength, solubilizing and denaturing protein. This property, together with its antibacterial activity, has encouraged its use in infected and crusted necrotic sloughs [26], but its most popular current use is as 10% O/W cream for ichthyosis [27] and dry skin conditions requiring emollients. Combinations with hydrocortisone may be useful for the dry, itching skin of atopics or those with asteatotic eczema. It has also been used as a 40% aqueous solution for the treatment of black, hairy tongue [28], and for acne conglobata [29]. Pretreatment with urea enhanced the subsequent effect of 5-fluorouracil in treating solar keratoses [25]. This was due to epidermal thinning, which may equally enhance the absorption of many other topically applied substances. It may also be used in lymph-ostatic hyperkeratosis and papillomatosis, in psoriasis, and in the treatment of mycoses [30].

Zinc

Zinc oxide is present in a large number of dermatological and cosmetic formulations. Zinc peroxide 50% in water, freshly prepared, constitutes Meleney's paste.

The calamine now in use consists of zinc carbonate coloured with ferrous oxide, although many naturally pink zinc ores have been used in the past 350 years.

Zinc pyrithione (zinc omadine) is a fungicide and bactericide. It is incorporated in shampoos [31] as an antidandruff agent. Some, but by no means all, of its success may be due to the prevention of aggregation of horn cells into visible flakes [32]. Zinc undecylenate is also used.

Topically applied zinc has also been reported to be of benefit in recurrent herpes simplex [33] and topical zinc oxide improved healing rates in patients with leg ulcers [34].

Oral zinc sulphate is discussed in Chapter 59.

REFERENCES

1 Polano MK. *Skin Therapeutics, Prescription and Preparation*. Amsterdam: Elsevier, 1952.

2 Suskind RR. Percutaneous toxicity. In: Sternberg TH, Newcomer VD, eds. *The Evaluation of Therapeutic Agents and Cosmetics.* New York: McGraw-Hill, 1964: 171–85.

3 Scholes KT, Crow KD, Ellis JP. Axillary hyperhidrosis treated with alcoholic solution of aluminium chloride hexahydrate. *Br Med J* 1978; **ii**: 84–5.

4 Symposium on Menthol. *Proceedings of an International Symposium.* Paris: Georg Theime, 1967.

5 Rogers SCF, Burrows D, Neill D. Percutaneous absorption of phenol and methylalcohol in magenta paint (BPC). *Br J Dermatol* 1978; **98**: 559–60.

6 Slinger WN, Hubbard DM. Treatment of seborrhoeic dermatitis with a shampoo containing selenium disulfide. *Arch Dermatol* 1951; **64**: 41–8.

7 Sanchez JL, Torres VM. Double blind study of selenium sulphide in tinea versicolor. *J Am Acad Dermatol* 1984; **11**: 235–8.

8 Hersle K. Selenium sulphide treatment of tinea versicolor. *Acta Derm Venereol (Stockh)* 1971; **51**: 476–8.

9 Kirby JD, Borrie PF. Confluent and reticulate papillomatosis (two cases). *Proc R Soc Med* 1975; **68**: 532–4.

10 Henschler D, Kirschner W. Zur resorption und Toxizität von Selensulfid. *Arch Toxikol* 1969; **24**: 341–4.

11 Cason JS, Jackson DM, Lowbury EJL. Antiseptic and aseptic prophylaxis for burns—use of silver nitrate and of isolators. *Br Med J* 1966; **ii**: 1288–94.

12 Richards RME, Mahlangu GN. Therapy for burn wound infection. *J Clin Hosp Pharm* 1981; **6**: 233–43.

13 Fox CL. Pharmacodynamics of sulfadiazine and related topical antimicrobial agents. In: Frost P, Gomez EC, Zaias N, eds. *Recent Advances in Dermato Pharmacology.* New York: Spectrum, 1978: 441–56.

14 Fox CL. Silver sulfadiazide—a new topical therapy for *Pseudomonas* in burns. *Arch Surg* 1978; **96**: 184–8.

15 Delaveau P, Friedrich-Nove P. Absorption cutanée et l'elimination urinaire d'une combinaison sulfadiazine-argent utilisée dans le traitement de brûlures. *Therapie* 1977; **32**: 563–72.

16 Lowbury EJL, Babb JR, Bridges K. Topical chemoprophylaxis with silver sulfadiazine and silver nitrate chlorhexidine creams: emergence of sulphon-amide-resistant Gram-negative bacilli. *Br Med J* 1976; **i**: 493–6.

17 Pullman H, Koenan H, Steigleder GK. On the effect of topically applied sulphur. *Arch Dermatol Res* 1977; **257**: 237–8.

18 Mills RA, Jr, Kligman AM. Is sulphur helpful or harmful in acne vulgaris? *Br J Dermatol* 1972; **86**: 620–7.

19 Strauss JS, Goldman PH, Nacht S *et al.* Re-examination of the comedogenicity of sulphur. *Arch Dermatol* 1978; **114**: 1340–2.

20 Leyden JJ, McGinley KJ, Mills OH *et al.* Effects of sulphur and salicylic acid in a shampoo in the treatment of dandruff; a doubleblind study using corneocyte counts and clinical grading. *Cutis* 1987; **39**: 557–61.

21 Blom I, Hornmark AM. Topical treatment with sulphur 10% for rosacea. *Acta Derm Venereol (Stockh)* 1984; **64**: 358–9.

22 De Vries HR. Substitution of zinc oxide by titanium dioxide in salicylic acid pastes. *Br J Dermatol* 1961; **73**: 371–5.

23 Ashton H, Frenk E, Stevenson CJ. Therapeutics: III. Urea as a topical agent. *Br J Dermatol* 1971; **85**: 194–6.

24 Rohde BT. Urea and urea combinations in psoriasis. *Hautarzt* 1981; (Suppl. 9): 74–5.

25 Thomas E. Urea in dermatologic therapy. *Cutis* 1972; **12**: 782–3.

26 Kligman AM. Dermatologic uses of urea. *Acta Derm Venereol (Stockh)* 1957; **37**: 155–9.

27 Swanbeck G. A new treatment of ichthyosis and other hyperkeratotic conditions. *Acta Derm Venereol (Stockh)* 1968; **48**: 123–7.

28 Pegum J. Urea in the treatment of black hairy tongue (Letter). *Br J Dermatol* 1971; **84**: 602.

29 Williamson DM, Cunliffe WJ, Gatecliff M *et al.* Acute ulcerative acne con-globata (acne fulminans) with erythema nodosum. *Clin Exp Dermatol* 1977; **2**: 351–4.

30 Nolting S. Urea treatment of mycoses. *Hautarzt* 1989; **40** (Suppl. 9): 76–7.

31 Brauer EW, Opdyke DL, Burnett CM. The anti-seborrhoeic qualities of zinc pyrithione (zinc pyridine-2-thiol-iroxide) in cream vehicle. *J Invest Dermatol* 1966; **47**: 174–5.

32 Leyden JJ, McGinley KJ, Kligman AM. Shorter methods of evaluating antidandruff agents. *J Soc Cosmet Chem* 1975; **26**: 573–80.

33 Eby GA, Halcomb WW. Use of topical zinc to prevent recurrent herpes simplex infections: review of literature and suggested protocols. *Med Hypotheses* 1985; **17**: 157–65.

34 Stromberg HE, Agren MS. Topical zinc oxide treatment improves arterial and venous leg ulcers. *Br J Dermatol* 1984; **111**: 461–8.

Dyes

The acridine dyes proflavine and acriflavine should be avoided because of their sensitizing potential. The tri-phenylmethane (rosaniline) dyes are now rarely used because of fears over their safety. They have been shown to interact with cellular DNA [1] and thus to be mutagenic and, by inference, possibly carcinogenic. They had excellent anticandidal properties and were effective against Gram-negative organisms. They were cheap, and rarely sensitized [2]. Methylrosaniline chloride (crystal, gentian violet) and *p*-diethylamine triphenylmethanol (brilliant green) were normally used as 0.5–1% aqueous or alcoholic solutions or in pastes, gels or cetomacrogol creams. They were also used as indelible skin markers prior to surgery [3] or for marking patch-test sites for later reference.

Necrotic lesions induced by triphenylmethane dyes on stripped skin or scarification were investigated by Mobacken and coworkers [4–6], who found a reduced synthesis of protein and collagen, and of DNA, with delay in fibroplasia and collagen formation. This may account for some reports of ulcer formation in infants' mouths being treated for thrush [7,8].

REFERENCES

1 Rosenkranz HS, Carr HS. Possible hazard in the use of Gentian violet. *Br Med J* 1971; **iii**: 702–3.

2 Bielicky T, Novak M. Contact group sensitization to triphenylmethane dyes. *Arch Dermatol* 1969; **100**: 540–3.

3 Asscher AW, Chant ADB, Marshall R. Improved skin marking (Letter). *Lancet* 1968; **ii**: 638

4 Bjornberg A, Mobacken H. Necrotic skin reactions caused by 1 per cent gentian violet and brilliant green. *Acta Derm Venereol (Stockh)* 1972; **52**: 55–60.

5 Mobacken H, Ahonen J, Zederfeldt D. The effect of cationic triphenylmethane dye (crystal violet) on rabbit granulation tissue oxygen consumption and RNA and protein synthesis in tissue slices. *Acta Derm Venereol (Stockh)* 1972; **54**: 343–7.

6 Norby K, Mobacken H. Effect of tryphenylmethane dyes (brilliant green, crystal violet, methyl violet) on proliferation in human normal fibroblast-like and established epithelial-like cell lines. *Acta Derm Venereol (Stockh)* 1972; **52**: 476–83.

7 Horsfield P, Logan FA, Newey JA. Oral irritation with gentian violet. *Br Med J* 1976; **ii**: 528.

8 John RW. Necrosis of oral mucosa after local application of crystal violet. *Br Med J* 1968; **i**: 157–8.

Benzoyl peroxide

Benzoyl peroxide is a powerful oxidizing agent, used also as a catalyst for resins and a bleaching agent for flour. Topical applications have been shown to be absorbed in considerable amounts [1]. However, the drug has been reported as non-toxic to humans [2], although unconfirmed reference has been made to its tumour-promoting activity in mice [3]. Its effectiveness as a peeling agent and comedo-lytic is the main basis for its successful use in the treatment of acne [4,5]. It has been shown to be germicidal [6], and the reduction in facial microbial flora is equal to that attained by systemic tetracycline [7].

Autoradiographic studies have shown that it also has a direct sebostatic effect on the sebaceous gland [8]. It is available in lotion, cream or gel form, alone, with sulphur, and with hydrocortisone. When combined with miconazole or erythromycin it is said to be more effective than benzoyl peroxide alone [9,10]. Although a potential irritant, it is well tolerated by most patients if applied with care in the early stages of treatment. Improved formulation may lessen the irritancy [11]. A study comparing 2.5%, 5% and 10% benzoyl peroxide gels found the 2.5% to be as effective but significantly less irritating [12]. Sensitization may occur [13], and bleaching of clothes, hair [14], and, to a lesser extent, the skin [15] may follow its use.

A 20% lotion has been used to promote rapid re-epithelialization of wounds [16]. It has also been found helpful in the desloughing of leg ulcers and pressure sores [17].

Superoxide dismutase

Free superoxide dismutase (SOD) creams and low-molecular-weight antioxidants have been used in the treatment of burns and skin ulcers [18].

REFERENCES

1 Nacht S, Yeung D, Beasley JN. Benzoyl peroxide: percutaneous penetration and metabolic disposition. *J Am Acad Dermatol* 1981; **4**: 31–7.
2 Holzman J, Morsches B, Benes P. The absorption of benzoyl peroxide from leg ulcers. *Arzneimittelforsch* 1979; **29**: 1180–3.
3 Slaga TH, Klein-Szanto AJP, Triplett LL. Skin tumour promoting activity of benzoyl peroxide, a widely used free-radical generating compound. *Science* 1981; **213**: 1023–5.
4 Lyons RE. Comparative effectiveness of benzoyl peroxide and tretinoin in acne vulgaris. *Int J Dermatol* 1978; **17**: 246–51.
5 Vasarinsh P. Benzoyl peroxide—sulfur lotions. *Arch Dermatol* 1968; **98**: 183–7.
6 Leyden JJ, Stewart R, Kligman AM. Updated *in vivo* methods for evaluating topical antimicrobial agents on human skin. *J Invest Dermatol* 1979; **72**: 165–70.
7 Fulton JE, Farzad-Bakhshandeh A, Bradley S. Studies on the mechanism of action of topical benzoyl peroxide and vitamin A acid in acne vulgaris. *J Cutan Pathol* 1977; **1**: 191–200.
8 Fanta D, Jurecka W. Autoradiographic investigation on benzoyl-peroxide treated skin. *Acta Derm Venereol (Stockh)* 1978; **58**: 361–3.
9 Mesquita-Guimaraes J, Ramos S, Taveres MR *et al.* A double-blind clinical trial with a lotion containing 5% benzoyl peroxide and 2% miconazole in patients with acne vulgaris. *Clin Exp Dermatol* 1989; **14**: 357–60.
10 Reinel B, Beierdorffer H. A new drug combination for the treatment of acne. Miconazole 2% + benzoyl peroxide 5% versus benzoyl peroxide 5%—a double-blind study. *Z Hautkr* 1985; **60**: 648–56.
11 Lovenzetti OJ, Werner T, McDonald DT. Some comparisons of benzoyl peroxide formulations. *J Soc Cosmet Chem* 1977; **28**: 533–49.
12 Mills OH, Jr, Kligman AM, Pochi P *et al.* Comparison of 2.5%, 5% and 10% benzoyl peroxide on inflammatory acne vulgaris. *Int J Dermatol* 1986; **25**: 644–7.
13 Poole RL, Griffith JL, MacMillan FSK. Experimental contact sensitization with benzoyl peroxide. *Arch Dermatol* 1970; **102**: 635–9.
14 Bleiberg J, Brodkin RH, Abbey A. Bleaching of hair after use of benzoyl peroxide acne lotions. *Arch Dermatol* 1973; **108**: 583.
15 Buskell LL. Bleaching by benzoyl peroxide. *Arch Dermatol* 1974; **110**: 461.
16 Alvarez OM, Hetz PM, Eaglestein WH. Benzoyl peroxide and epidermal wound healing. *Arch Dermatol* 1983; **119**: 222–5.
17 Pace WE. Treatment of cutaneous ulcers with benzoyl peroxide. *Can Med Assoc J* 1976; **115**: 1101–3.
18 Niwa Y. Lipid peroxides and superoxide dismutase (SOD) induction in skin inflammatory diseases and treatment with SOD preparations. *Dermatologica* 1989; **179** (Suppl. 1): 101–6.

Tars

A tar is a product of the destructive distillation of organic substances. Four groups of substances are sources of therapeutic tars: wood, coal, bitumen and crude petroleum.

Wood tars

Oils of cade, beech, birch and pine are widely used, particularly in Scandinavian countries. Wood tars lack certain basic chemical structures characteristic of coal tars, such as pyridine, quinoline and quinaline rings [1]. They may sensitize but do not photosensitize.

These tars are normally applied in 1–10% strength in ointments or pastes, or as a paint in 95% alcohol.

Bituminous tars

These were originally obtained from the distillation of shale deposits containing fossilized fish, hence 'ichthyol', ammonium ichthosulphonate. The sulphur content of ichthyol (about 10%) is present as compounds of thiopen, which is itself inert. Bituminous tars are less effective than coal tars and may have a different mode of action. They are not photosensitizers.

Petroleum tars

These are of no therapeutic importance.

Coal tar [2–4]

Coal tar is a black, viscous fluid with a characteristic smell. Attempts to remove the colour, odour, photosensitizing property and carcinogenicity have not been entirely successful [5], and variations in this natural product have made the assessment of active ingredients particularly difficult [3,4]. Of some 10000 different constituents believed to make up coal tar, only 400 have been identified. These constitute 55% of the whole.

All coal tars are products of different distillates of heated coal. The content of the tar depends on the type used and the temperature of the distillation. 'Low-temperature' tar was found to contain a greater number of components but to be less effective in producing orthokeratosis in mouse-tail skin than 'high-temperature' tar [3,4]. It was also more irritating. However, a comparison of high- and low-temperature tars showed no eventual difference in effect in the treatment of psoriasis itself, although crude (high-temperature) coal tar gave quicker results [6]. This suggests that the reversal of parakeratosis is only one factor in the control of psoriasis. The authors of this study point out that dithranol was not very effective in the mouse-tail test [7].

The hydrocarbons, which constitute about half the composition of tar, include benzol, naphthalene and anthracene. The high-boiling-point tar acids (phenolics) include isomers of substituted polyhydroxyphenols, and it seems likely that it is such phenols which may be responsible for the therapeutic effect of tar [3,4,8]. However, the exact mechanism by which tar exerts its effect remains unknown. These high-temperature fractions may have a direct effect on the granular layer by release of lysosomes followed by mitotic stimulation. Low-temperature extracts appear to cause epidermal thickening without restitution of the granular layer [3,4], and may be the reason for the indifferent action of some synthetic and proprietary tar preparations [3,4,9].

Until a more suitable preparation is available, many dermatologists will continue to believe that crude tar remains therapeutically superior [9,10].

The combination of tar with UV light (the Goeckerman regimen) has long been known to be helpful in psoriasis.

In recent years, attempts have been made to identify the critical wavelengths of radiation involved [11,12]. Generally, UVB radiation has been found to be more effective than UVA [13,14]. Refined tars are less phototoxic than the crude product, but phototoxicity is directly related to therapeutic efficacy. UVA [15] did not appear to be a useful adjunct to tar and UVB, in the treatment of psoriasis in one study.

Laboratory studies have shown that tar plus UV light reduces epidermal DNA synthesis [12,16]. This may be related to the formation of cross-links between opposite strands on the DNA double helix [17].

A cytostatic effect of crude coal tar has also been postulated [18] following the finding that prolonged application to normal skin produces epidermal thinning associated with retention hyperkeratosis. More studies are still required, particularly to identify the more active fractions of tar distillates.

Carcinogenicity

The well-established carcinogenicity of pitch and heavy tar fractions has aroused renewed interest in the current climate of therapeutic conservatism, concerns about the oncogenic potential of polycyclic hydrocarbons [20], and consumer protection [19,21], fuelled perhaps by reports which show urine from psoriatics using crude coal tar to be mutagenic to certain bacterial strains [5]. Reports of malignant tumours in humans in relation to tar therapy are rare. Rook *et al.* reported five cases [22] and Greither *et al.* 13 [23]. Most had genital or groin involvement, but these are nowadays unlikely sites for tar application. Several large, long-term follow-up studies have shown, reassuringly, no increased incidence of skin tumours [14,24–27].

Uses

The chief use of coal-tar preparations is their keratoplastic and antipruritic activity in atopic dermatitis and chronic eczema, and in psoriasis, where tar is the basis of the Goeckerman regimen (Chapter 35). Wood tars are widely used for much the same purpose in some countries, but their effect is not enhanced by UV light. Oil of Cade is particularly used in scalp preparations (Chapter 82) or when tar preparations are needed on the face.

REFERENCES

1 Obermeyer ME, Becker SA. A study of crude coal tar and allied substances. *Arch Dermatol Syphilol* 1935; **31**: 796–810.
2 Muller SA, Kierland RR. Crude coal tar in dermatologic therapy. *Mayo Clin Proc* 1964; **39**: 275–80.
3 Wrench R, Britten AZ. Evaluation of coal tar fractions for use in psoriasiform diseases using the mouse tail test (i). High and low temperature tars and their constituents. *Br J Dermatol* 1975; **92**: 569–74.
4 Wrench R, Britten AZ. Evaluation of coal tar fractions for use in psoriasiform diseases using the mouse tail test (ii). Tar oil, acids. *Br J Dermatol* 1975; **92**: 575–9.
5 Wheeler LA, Soperstein MD, Lowe NJ *et al.* Mutagenicity of urine from psoriatic patients undergoing treatment with coal tar and ultraviolet light. *J Invest Dermatol* 1981; **77**: 181–5.
6 Chapman RS, Finn OR. An assessment of high and low temperature tars in psoriasis. *Br J Dermatol* 1976; **94**: 71–4.
7 Wrench R, Britten AZ. Evaluation of dithranol and a 'synthetic tar' as antipsoriatic treatments using the mouse tail test. *Br J Dermatol* 1975; **93**: 75–8.
8 Hellier FF, Whitefield M. The treatment of psoriasis with triacetoxyanthracene. *Br J Dermatol* 1967; **79**: 491–6.
9 Young E. An external treatment of psoriasis. A controlled investigation of the effects of coal tar. *Br J Dermatol* 1970; **82**: 510–15.
10 Champion RH. Treatment of psoriasis. *Br Med J* 1966; **ii**: 993–5.
11 Fischer T. Comparative treatment of psoriasis with UV-light, trioxsalen plus UV-light and coal tar plus UV-light. *Acta Derm Venereol (Stockh)* 1971; **57**: 345–50.
12 Stoughton RB, Dequoy P, Walters JF. Crude coal tar plus near ultraviolet light suppresses DNA synthesis in epidermis. *Arch Dermatol* 1978; **114**: 43–5.
13 Parrish JA, Morison WL, Gonzalez E. Therapy of psoriasis by tar sensitization. *J Invest Dermatol* 1978; **70**: 111–12.
14 Petrozzi JK, Barton JO, Kaidbey KK. Updating of the Goeckerman regime for psoriasis. *Br J Dermatol* 1978; **98**: 437–44.
15 Diette KM, Momtaz K, Stern RS *et al.* Role of ultraviolet A in phototherapy for psoriasis. *J Am Acad Dermatol* 1984; **11**: 441–7.
16 Walter JF, Stoughton RB, Dequoy PR. Suppression of epidermal proliferation by ultraviolet light, coal tar and anthralin. *Br J Dermatol* 1978; **99**: 89–96.
17 Pathak MA, Biswas RK. Skin photosensitization and DNA cross linking ability of photochemotherapeutic agents. *J Invest Dermatol* 1977; **68**: 236.
18 Lavker RM, Grove GL, Kligman AM. The atrophogenic effect of crude coal tar on human epidermis. *Br J Dermatol* 1981; **105**: 77–82.
19 Zackheim HS. Should therapeutic coal tar preparations be available over-the-counter? *Arch Dermatol* 1978; **14**: 125–6.
20 Gilman AG, Rall TW, Nies AS *et al.* (eds). *Goodman and Gilman's The Pharmacological Basis of Therapeutics*, 8th edn. New York: Pergamon, 1990.
21 Stern RS, Laird N. Carcinogenic risk of treatments for severe psoriasis. *Cancer* 1994; **73**: 2760–3.
22 Rook AJ, Gresham GA, Davis RA. Epithelioma possibly induced by therapeutic application of tar. *Br J Cancer* 1967; **10**: 17–23.
23 Greither A, Gisbertz C, Ippen H. Teerbehandlung und Krebs. *Zeitschr Haut Geschlkr* 1967; **42**: 631–5.
24 Jones SK, Mackie RM, Holt DJ *et al.* Further evidence of the safety of tar in the management of psoriasis. *Br J Dermatol* 1985; **113**: 97–101.
25 Pittelkow MR, Perry HO, Muller SA *et al.* Psoriasis treated with coal tar — 25-year follow-up study. *Arch Dermatol* 1981; **117**: 465–8.

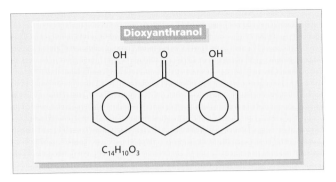

Fig. 78.2 Dioxyanthranol.

26 Maughan WZ, Muller SA, Perry HO *et al.* Incidence of skin cancers in patients with atopic dermatitis treated with coal tar. *J Am Acad Dermatol* 1980; **3**: 612–15.
27 Schmid MH, Korting HC. Coal tar, pine tar and sulphonated shale oil preparations: comparative activity, efficacy and safety. *Dermatology* 1996; **193**: 1–5.

Dithranol [1]

SYN. ANTHRALIN

Dithranol and dioxyanthranol (Fig. 78.2) differ only in the position of the hydroxy group, and are comparable in effect.

Dithranol is similar in its irritating and staining properties to chrysarobin but is stronger in effect. It is used in ointments, pastes, creams, or as a paint in acetone and benzene.

The mechanism of the action of dithranol is still uncertain. It inhibits glycolytic enzymes *in vitro* [2]. It has been suggested that enzyme inactivation may result from lipoid peroxidation leading to cross-linkage of enzyme proteins [3]. Arachidonic acid levels are also reduced [4]. Mitotic inhibition [5] appears to be preceded by a paradoxical acanthogenic effect [6,7]. Mitochondrial DNA production is reduced in the animal model [8,9] and this antimitotic effect has been shown to be equipotent with methotrexate [10]. *In vitro* studies with human skin showed decreased oxygen consumption and inhibition of the pentose phosphate shunt [11]. The level of cyclic guanosine monophosphate is known to be increased in psoriasis. Dithranol has been shown to restore cyclic nucleosides in skin to normal levels [12].

There is no evidence that the use of dithranol or anthralin in paste vehicles causes systemic toxicity. Nor is dithranol a carcinogen in humans, although it induced respiratory-deficient mutants in yeasts [13]. Whatever its mode of activity, it is well-recognized that dithranol must be kept in its reduced state until delivered to the skin, where oxidation is allowed to occur and therapeutic effect attained. Dithranol, especially when incorporated in zinc oxide, is slowly oxidized by alkaline impurities to an inactive pink anthrone [14]. The effect of salicylic acid in preventing this has been known for a long time [15–17]. Salicylic acid neutralizes hydroxyl ions in an alkaline medium, and perhaps reacts with free zinc ions to form an inactive zinc–dithranol complex. It was also found [11] that zinc ions and salicylic acid, as well as dithranol itself, inhibit glucose-6-phosphate dehydrogenase, thus justifying the time-honoured combination of these three agents.

An improved formulation of dithranol in zinc and salicylic acid paste (Chapter 82) is claimed to have a longer shelf-life and may be easier for patients to apply [18].

The use of a water-soluble antioxidant, ascorbic acid, has allowed the production of a series of stable dithranol cream preparations [14]. These are not as therapeutically potent as equivalent strengths of pastes or ointments but show much greater patient acceptability for home usage [19]. The combination of tar with dithranol is said to reduce dithranol irritancy without inhibiting therapeutic effect [20].

Recent advocacy of short-duration applications of strong dithranol pastes or creams on an outpatient basis should reduce the patient's resistance to the home use of these preparations [21–23].

Dithranol has also been used to stimulate an inflammatory response and regrowth of hair in patients with alopecia areata [24], and for the treatment of warts [25].

REFERENCES

1 Shroot B, Schaefer J, Juhlin L. Editorial: anthralin—the challenge. *Br J Dermatol* 1981; **105** (Suppl. 20): 3–5.
2 Rassner G. Enzymaktivitätshemmung *in vitro* durch Dithranol (Cignolin). *Arch Dermatol Res* 1972; **243**: 47–51.
3 Diezel W, Mefferth H, Sonnichsen N. Untersuchungen zum Wirkungsmechanisms von Dithranol: Erhöhte Lipidperoxidation und Enzymhemmung. *Dermatologica* 1975; **150**: 154–62.
4 Barr RM, Wong E, Cunningham FM *et al.* Effect of dithranol treatment on arachidonic acid and its lipoxygenase products in psoriasis. *Arch Dermatol Res* 1989; **280**: 474–6.
5 Fisher LB, Maibach HI. The effect of anthralin and its derivatives on epidermal cell kinetics. *J Invest Dermatol* 1975; **64**: 338–41.
6 Braun-Falco O, Burg G, Schoefinius HH. Uber die Wirkung von Dithranol (Cignolin) bei Psoriasis vulgaris. Cyto- und histochemische Untersuchungen. *Arch Dermatol Res* 1971; **241**: 217–36.
7 Cox AJ, Watson W. Histological variations in lesions of psoriasis. *Arch Dermatol* 1972; **106**: 503–6.
8 Lowe NJ, Breeding J. Anthralin; different concentration effects on epidermal cell DNA synthesis rates in mice and clinical responses in human psoriasis. *Arch Dermatol* 1981; **117**: 698–700.
9 Walter JF, Stoughton RB, Dequoy P. Suppression of epidermal proliferation by ultraviolet light, coal tar and anthralin. *Br J Dermatol* 1978; **99**: 89–96.
10 Klem EB. Effects of antipsoriasis drugs and metabolic inhibitors on the growth of epidermal cells in culture. *J Invest Dermatol* 1977; **70**: 27–32.
11 Raab WP. Dithranol (anthralin) versus triacetoxyanthracene. *Br J Dermatol* 1976; **95**: 193–6.
12 Saihan EM, Albano J, Burton JL. The effect of steroid and dithranol therapy on cyclic nucleotides in psoriasis epidermis. *Br J Dermatol* 1980; **102**: 565–9.
13 Zetterberg G, Swanbeck G. Studies on dithranol and dithranol-like compounds. *Acta Derm Venereol (Stockh)* 1971; **51**: 45–9.
14 Whitefield M. Pharmaceutical formulations of anthralin. *Br J Dermatol* 1981; **105** (Suppl 20): 28–32.
15 Luckacs S, Braun-Falco O. Uber das Verhalten von Dithranol (Cignolin) in Pasten und Lösungen und seine Beeingflussbarkeit durch Salicylsäure. *Hautarzt* 1973; **24**: 304–9.
16 Ponec-Waelsh M, Hulsebotsch HJ. Further studies on the interaction between anthralin, salicylic acid and zinc oxide in pastes. *Arch Dermatol Res* 1974; **249**: 141–52.
17 Raab WP, Gmeiner B. The inhibition of glucose-6-phosphate dehydrogenase activity by dithranol (anthralin), zinc ions and/or salicylic acid. *Arch Dermatol Res* 1974; **251**: 87–94.

18 Seville RH. Dithranol paste for psoriasis. *Br J Dermatol* 1966; **78**: 269–72.

19 Wilson PD, Ive FA. Dithrocream in psoriasis. *Br J Dermatol* 1980; **103**: 105–6.

20 Schulz HJ, Schander S, Mahrle G *et al*. Combined tar-anthralin versus anthralin treatment lowers irritancy with unchanged antipsoriatic efficacy. *J Am Acad Dermatol* 1987; **17**: 19–24.

21 Runne V, Kunze J. Short duration ('minutes') therapy with dithranol for psoriasis: a new out-patient regimen. *Br J Dermatol* 1982; **106**: 135–9.

22 Runne V, Kunze J. Minute therapy of psoriasis with dithranol and its modifications. A critical evaluation based on 315 patients. *Hautarzt* 1985; **36**: 40–6.

23 Ryatt KS, Statham BN, Rowell NR. Short-contact modification of the Ingram regime. *Br J Dermatol* 1984; **111**: 455–9.

24 Fiedler-Weiss VC, Buys CM. Evaluation of anthralin in the treatment of alopecia areata. *Arch Dermatol* 1987; **123**: 1491–3.

25 Flindt-Hansen H, Tikjob G, Brandrup F. Wart treatment with anthralin. *Acta Derm Venereol (Stockh)* 1984; **64**: 177–9.

Keratolytics

The majority of the agents used as keratolytics have moisturizing effects on the skin when used in low concentration, and keratolytic activity in higher concentration. Several, such as lactic acid and urea, which occur in human metabolism, are known as *natural moisturizing factors*, and are popular ingredients in cosmetic formulations. Keratolytics are used in a number of protocols for cosmetic skin peeling, and for the prevention and reduction of photo-ageing. The cosmeceutical use of these agents is beyond the scope of this book, but guidance is readily available from other sources [1,2]. Notes on individual compounds follow.

REFERENCES

1 Roenigk RK, Brodland DG. Facial chemical peel. In: Baran R, Maibach HI, eds. *Cosmetic Dermatology*. London: Martin Dunitz, 1994; 439–49.

2 Moy LS, Peace S, Moy RL. Comparison of the effect of various chemical peeling agents in a mini-pig model. *Dermatol Surg* 1996; **22**: 429–32.

Alpha-hydroxy acids [1–3]

A series of weak mono- or dicarboxylic acids. They are used as moisturizers, preservatives in creams and peeling agents. They are being used increasingly to 'freshen' the complexion and reverse the histological changes of photo-ageing. The most important are lactic, malic and glycollic (α-hydroxy-acetic) acids. Some preparations contain salts of the acids such as ammonium lactate 5–15%.

REFERENCES

1 Rubin MG. The clinical use of alpha hydroxy acids. *Australas J Dermatol* 1994; **35**: 29–33.

2 Van Scott EJ, Yu RJ. Alpha hydroxy acids: procedures for use in clinical practice. *Cutis* 1989; **43**: 222–8.

3 Ditre CM, Griffin TD, Murphy GF *et al*. Effects of alpha-hydroxy acids on photoaged skin: a pilot clinical, histologic, and ultrastructural study. *J Am Acad Dermatol* 1996; **34**: 187–95.

Glycerol
SYN. GLYCERIN [1,2]

This is a trihydric alcohol, which is miscible with water and alcohol. It is usually presented as a clear, viscous liquid with a sweet taste. It is strongly hygroscopic, making it useful in cosmetic emollient preparations. It is also used for its antiviral and preservative effects in cadaver skin.

REFERENCES

1 Rawlings A, Harding C, Watkinson A *et al*. The effect of glycerol and humidity on desmosome degradation in stratum corneum. *Arch Dermatol Res* 1995; **287**: 457–64.

2 Harry RG. Humectants. In: Wilkinson JB, Moore RJ, eds. *Harry's Cosmeticology*, 7th edn. Singapore: Longman, 1982: 641–52.

Propylene glycol [1,2]

This is the second in the series of dihydric alcohols including ethylene glycol, α/β-propylene glycol, α/γ-propylene glycol, β/γ-butylene glycol. Propylene glycol is a sweet, viscous fluid, readily soluble in water. It is used as a keratolytic either alone or in combination with other keratolytics and emollients in a concentration of 10–20%. In higher concentrations, irritation is marked [3]. In addition to its use as a keratolytic, it is also employed as a preservative and a penetration enhancer.

REFERENCES

1 Kinnunen T, Koskela M. Antibacterial and antifungal properties of propylene glycol, hexylene glycol and 1,3-butylene glycol *in vitro*. *Acta Derm Venereol (Stockh)* 1991; **71**: 148–50.

2 Hilton J, Woollen BH, Scott RC *et al*. Vehicle effects on *in vitro* percutaneous absorption through rat and human skin. *Pharmacol Res* 1994; **11**: 1396–400.

3 Funk JO, Maibach HI. Propylene glycol dermatitis: re-evaluation of an old problem. *Contact Dermatitis* 1994; **31**: 236–41.

Salicylic acid
SYN. O-HYDROXYBENZOIC ACID

This is the best known of the keratolytic agents in dermatological therapy. It is used on its own or in combination with other agents in a wide range of formulae. Its use has been advocated in a 60% propylene glycol gel as a keratolytic [1]. Together with benzoic acid, it constitutes Whitfield's ointment or lotion, an effective fungicide. In zinc paste, it prevents the oxidation of dithranol to danthron.

The application of salicylic acid to extensive areas, particularly in children, may involve a risk of toxicity from absorption [2,3].

At the concentration normally used, salicylic acid may exert a direct solubilizing effect on the stratum corneum, with dissolution of the intercellular cement [4,5]. Its main effect appears to be a reduction of intercellular stickiness, perhaps by an action on the cement substances [6]. This results in enhanced shedding of corneocytes, and has no recordable effect on mitotic activity [7]. Salicylic acid 2% applied for 6h reduced intrastratum-corneum adhesive forces. No effect was seen at 3h, nor with 10% urea at 3h and 6h [8].

The addition of 10% salicylic acid has been shown to increase the rate of passage of steroids across a membrane [9]. Clinically, this effect has been confirmed with some potent steroids [10], but not with flucortolone [11] or hydrocortisone [12]. A direct anti-inflammatory effect has also been claimed [13], but has yet to be confirmed. Salicyclic acid 16–40% has also been traditionally used in wart paint or in wart/corn plasters. Cure rates in such delivery systems approach 70% [14].

REFERENCES

1 Baden HP. Treatment of hyperkeratotic dermatitis of the palms. Sequential treatment with a keratolytic gel and corticosteroid ointment. *Arch Dermatol* 1974; **110**: 737–8.
2 Pascher F. Systemic reactions to topically applied drugs. *Int J Dermatol* 1978; **17**: 768–75.
3 Pec J, Strmenova M, Palencarova E *et al.* Salicylate intoxication after use of topical salicylic acid ointment by a patient with psoriasis. *Cutis* 1992; **50**: 307–9.
4 Davies MG, Marks R. Studies on the effect of salicylic acid on normal skin. *Br J Dermatol* 1976; **95**: 187–92.
5 Marks R, Davies M, Cattell A. An explanation for the keratolytic effect of salicylic acid. *J Invest Dermatol* 1975; **64**: 283 (Abstract).
6 Huber C, Christophers E. Keratolytics: effect of salicylic acid. *Arch Dermatol Res* 1977; **257**: 293–7.
7 Roberts DL, Marshall R, Marks R. Detection of the action of salicylic acid on the normal stratum corneum. *Br J Dermatol* 1980; **103**: 191–6.
8 Loden M, Bostrom P, Kneczke M. Distribution and keratolytic effect of salicylic acid and urea in human skin. *Skin Pharmacol* 1995; **8**: 173–8.
9 Polano MK, Ponec M. Dependence of corticosteroid penetration on the vehicle. *Arch Dermatol* 1976; **112**: 675–80.
10 Weinert V, Blazek V. Der Einfluss der Salicylsaure auf den Abblassungseffekt von Corticosteroid Dermatica, dargestellt am Beispiel des Flumestason-pivalat. *Arch Dermatol Res* 1981; **271**: 19–27.
11 Tauber U, Weiss C, Matthes H. Does salicylic acid increase the percutaneous absorption of diflucortolone-21-valerate? *Skin Pharmacol* 1993; **6**: 276–81.
12 Weirich EG, Longauer JK, Kirkwood AM. Dermatopharmacology of salicylic acid. II. Epidermal anti-hyperplastic effect of salicylic acid in animals. *Dermatologica* 1975; **151**: 321–32.
13 Weirich EG, Longauer JK, Kirkwood AM. Dermatopharmacology of salicylic acid. III. Topical contra-inflammatory effect of salicylic acid and other drugs in animal experiments. *Dermatologica* 1976; **152**: 87–99.
14 Bart BJ, Biglow J, Vance JC *et al.* Salicylic acid in Karayagum patch as a treatment for verruca vulgaris. *J Am Acad Dermatol* 1989; **20**: 74–6.

Urea [1]

This crystalline, slightly salty compound is freely soluble in water and alcohol. It has marked hydrating properties and is used in dry skin conditions. It is used best in a cream base in a concentration of 5–10%, above which crystallization tends to impart a gritty feel. Formulation in a greasy base may cause a burning sensation [1]. Both 3 and 10% urea creams have been reported to be effective in improving skin hydration and reduction of scaling, and 10% produced improvement of disordered transepidermal water loss in patients with dry skins [2]. One study did not find a significant keratolytic effect with 10% urea [3]. Its benefit in dry skin may well be due to its dipolar character and hydrating properties [4]. It has proved useful in non-surgical avulsion of the nail [5,6]. A 20% urea and 10% salicylic acid preparation in emulsifying ointment or zinc oxide paste is applied to the nail, occluded, and changed at weekly intervals until the nail plate softens sufficiently for it to be removed with forceps or a curette.

REFERENCES

1 Swanbeck G. Harnstoff als monotherpeutikum bei trockener Haut. *Hautarzt* 1989; **40** (Suppl. 9): 42–3.
2 Serup J. A double-blind comparison of two creams containing urea as the active ingredient. Assessment of efficacy and side-effects by non-invasive techniques and a clinical scoring scheme. *Acta Derm Venereol Suppl (Stockh)* 1992; **177**: 34–43.
3 Loden M, Bostrom P, Kneczke M. Distribution and keratolytic effect of salicylic acid and urea in human skin. *Skin Pharmacol* 1995; **8**: 173–8.
4 Swanbeck G. Urea in the treatment of dry skin. *Acta Derm Venereol Suppl (Stockh)* 1992; **177**: 7–8.
5 South DA, Farber EM. Urea ointment in the non-surgical avulsion of nail dystrophies—a reappraisal. *Cutis* 1980; **25**: 609–12.
6 Farber EM, South DA. Urea ointment in the non-surgical avulsion of nail dystrophies. *Cutis* 1978; **22**: 689–92.

Germicides and antibacterial agents [1–4]

Disinfectants and antiseptics are generally used to destroy or inhibit the growth of pathogenic organisms in the nonsporing or vegetative state. An antiseptic (or germicide) kills or prevents the growth of microorganisms, usually in relation to living tissue. A disinfectant destroys pathogens in the environment. Germicides are more closely defined as bactericides, fungicides, etc. Bacteriostatic agents inhibit the growth of bacteria; bactericidal agents kill them. Most bactericidal substances are bacteriostatic in low concentrations but some bacteriostatics are never bactericidal.

Their efficiency *in vivo* may not correspond with that obtained *in vitro* because of tissue toxicity and inhibition by serum, tissue proteins and pus. Chlorine, metals and certain dyes are highly effective in low concentrations, but their action is depressed in the presence of proteins. The use of otherwise efficient agents may also be limited by toxicity, sensitization [5], staining or odour. Disinfectants should be rapidly effective, non-corrosive, able to penetrate well, compatible with soaps and not inhibited by serum or faeces. Antiseptics may be allowed a less rapid action, except in preoperative preparation of the skin; a sustained action is important. Bactericidal agents with a broad spectrum of activity are preferred.

Antiseptic agents of value on the normal skin may be inhibited or even detrimental when applied to broken skin or under particular conditions of moisture or occlusion [5,6].

Principles of selection and use

It is better to use two or three antiseptic agents well than to change them frequently. They should be used for the purpose for which they were designed, in the recommended strength and vehicle, and for no longer than is necessary to achieve their purpose. The emergence of microorganisms against which they have no activity may be as deleterious as the original bacteria they were used to suppress. Sensitization reactions may follow prolonged use; their frequency varies with different groups. The inclusion of antiseptics in cosmetics is common practice and, despite careful testing, sensitization does occur [7,8].

Classification

The following groups contain substances of dermatological importance:

1 phenols, halogenated phenols, alkyl-substituted phenols and resorcinols;
2 alcohols;
3 aldehydes;
4 acids;
5 halogens and halogenated compounds;
6 oxidizing agents;
7 heavy metals and their salts;
8 surface-active agents;
9 dyes;
10 hydroxyquinolines;
11 miscellaneous agents.

Phenols and chlorinated phenols

These have a bactericidal action in appropriate concentrations, but they rapidly lose their effect either on dilution or in the presence of organic matter. Although phenol itself is the prototype of this group, several of its compounds are more effective and less toxic.

Phenol (carbolic acid). Liquefied phenol consists of an 80% w/w solution of phenol in water. It is also used as a skin caustic. It is soluble in oils and fats, and may be removed rapidly from the skin with glycerin, vegetable oils or 50% alcohol. The addition of salt increases its action by reducing its solubility in water; alcohol has the opposite effect. It is readily absorbed through the skin [9,10], and has been found in the urine of infants treated with Castellani's paint (carbofuchsin solution) [11]. It is clinically bacteriostatic in a strength of 1%, and fungicidal at 1.3%. In a strength of 1–2% it has a reputation as an antipruritic.

Cresol. This is a mixture of *o*-, *m*- and *p*-cresol, alkyl derivatives of phenol with similar but more powerful bactericidal activity than phenol. Saponated cresol solutions such as lysol have been used as disinfectants (50% in saponified linseed oil). The use of cresols as germicides is declining because of the development of less irritant phenolics.

Thymol, also an anthelmintic, is traditionally used as an oral antiseptic. Although it is a more potent antiseptic than phenol, its low water solubility and irritancy tend to limit its use.

Choroxylenol. This is marketed in the UK as Dettol and is one of the commonest British household antiseptics. It is bactericidal against most Gram-positive organisms, but less active against staphylococci and Gram-negative bacteria. A 5% solution dissolved in soap forms Chloroxylenol Solution BP. This can be applied undiluted to the skin. *Pseudomonas pyocyanea has* been isolated from the corks of bottles containing chloroxylenol. Enhancement of its activity against *Pseudomonas* can be achieved by the addition of 0.1% acetic acid [12].

Hexachlorophane. This is a chlorinated bisphenol which is currently used as a skin and hand disinfectant. Although it has a slow bacteriostatic action against Gram-positive organisms, it has the advantage of accumulating in the stratum corneum after repeated usage [13,14]. Previously widely used in medicinals and toiletries, it has fallen into disfavour following reports of toxicity from absorption when used in exceptional conditions. In 1968, vacuolar degeneration of the white matter of the brain was found in two children with burns and two with ichthyosis who died in hospital after routine bathing with hexachlorophane. In another report, four out of eighteen children with normal skin died following accidental intoxication with talc containing 6% hexachlorophane. In these cases, the clinical picture was of intracranial hypertension and spinal cord damage [15]. It is known that hexachlorophane may be absorbed from the skin and can cross the placenta. The possibility of teratogenicity has been raised, and its use in pregnancy is discouraged [16]. Although it should not be used on badly burned or excoriated skin, there is no evidence that moderate and sensible use of this agent is harmful to adults. However, premature and low-birth-weight infants may be suceptible to toxic effects. Hexachlorophane has been used for the treatment of staphylococcal sepsis in the newborn where other measures are not effective: in the UK the concentration used for this purpose is 0.33%. It is available as a 3% cream, which may also be used as a preoperative scrub for health-care workers, and as a 0.33% dusting powder, which is used in neonates to prevent sepsis of the cord stump. Prolonged use, especially in obsessional washers, should be discouraged, and there seems little justification for its regular use as a face and body cleanser in patients with acne. Primary sensitization is rare [9].

Triclosan is a chlorinated bisphenol, which is found in many proprietary skin cleansers in concentrations up to 2%. It is effective against Gram-positive and most Gram-negative organisms except *Pseudomonas* species. A hand wash containing 0.3% triclosan was found to be less effective in eradication of hand surface bacteria than non-medicated soap [17].

Alcohols

The bactericidal activity of the aliphatic alcohols increases with their molecular weight. Seventy per cent ethyl alcohol is effective, and isopropyl alcohol slightly more so.

A 10-sec application of 70% isopropyl alcohol was found to be as effective as a 60-sec application of povidone–iodine in reducing aerobic bacteria on the skin for 5 min. After 60 min, the reduction was found to be better maintained by povidone–iodine [18]. In relation to the safety of health-care workers, it has been noted that ethanol and isopropanol tend to alter the structure of latex and vinyl gloves, and permeate through the gloves [19].

Aldehydes

In contrast with alcohols, the simpler compounds are more active.

Formaldehyde solution (formalin). Formalin contains about 40% formaldehyde gas. It has a high degree of chemical reactivity with proteins, and has the property of converting toxins to toxoids, enabling the antigenic reactions to be retained. Although employed chiefly as a disinfectant, it has also been used in fungus infection, hyperhidrosis, and in the treatment of veruccae. As a treatment, it is usually employed in a 3–10% concentration. Sensitization is not uncommon.

Hexamethylenetetramine. This liberates formaldehyde, and is sometimes used in dusting powders for the feet.

Acids

Benzoic acid is one of the more commonly used preservatives in foodstuffs, cosmetics and drug preparations. It has fungicidal properties.

Acetic acid (in 1–5% concentration) has a bactericidal effect on *Pseudomonas aeruginosa*, and has been used in the management of burns and soft-tissue wounds [20].

Azelaic acid. Among its many properties is broad-spectrum antibacterial activity (see below).

Halogens and halogenated compounds

Iodine and chlorine are powerful germicidal agents.

Iodine. The mode of action is unknown. Effective concentrations also kill spores. Its action is rapid, most bacteria being killed within 1 min of exposure to a 1:20 000 concentration. A 1% aqueous solution of iodine has been shown to be viricidal when used as a hand wash [21].

Weak Iodine Solution BP contains 2.5%, with 2.5% potassium iodide, in an alcoholic solution.

Iodoform. This releases iodine, and has a mild antibacterial action. It is incorporated in bismuth–iodoform paste.

Iodophors. These are complexes of iodine and a solubilizer or carrier that liberate iodine in solution.

Povidone–iodine (Betadine). This is an iodophore, i.e. a complex of iodine and a carrier polymer, which slowly liberates inorganic iodine onto the skin or mucous membranes. The activity of the iodine is preserved without the irritative effects of the free tincture. It was found to be effective in reducing postoperative sepsis [22], and has replaced hexachlorophane in the UK in many areas of use. It is well tolerated and easily removed with water. Despite some favourable reports, it is probably of less value in preventing sepsis in burns [23]. Severe metabolic acidosis has been reported in two patients with extensive burns [24]. The authors have found it an acceptable treatment for leg ulcers, and it has been recommended as a skin cleanser in acne [25]. It can also be used as a shampoo in cases of seborrhoeic dermatitis. It is preferable to hexachlorophane for use on areas of inflamed and broken skin, for example in the perianal and perigenital regions. It is available in several forms.

Povidine–iodine has a low rate of sensitization. In eight patients with allergic contact sensitivity five were negative to potassium iodide [26].

Cadexomer iodine. Cadexomers differ from iodophores in that no chemical bond exists between the carrier and the active agent. A three-dimensional lattice of cross-linked glucose chains entraps the iodine molecule and releases it only in the presence of moisture. This compound has been found useful in absorbing moist exudates from the surfaces of chronic venous ulcers and in reducing bacterial contamination [27].

Chlorine. Chlorine is easily bound by organic matter, and its clinical use is limited to hypochlorite solutions.

Eusol (Edinburgh University solution), a solution of calcium hypochlorite and boric acid, is still used alone or with liquid paraffin, although it has lost favour because of evidence of delayed wound healing caused by direct toxicity to re-epithelializing tissues [5]. However, the case against it is much stronger in opinion and reviews than in convincing clinical data.

Chloramines. These are chloramide derivatives of toluene. They are also used for water sterilization.

Chlorhexidine. This became the natural successor to hexachlorophane. It has been particularly studied by Lowbury *et al.* [28,29], who found it more effective in reducing skin flora, especially in a detergent or alcoholic vehicle. In powder form, it has been shown to be as effective as hexachlorophane in preventing colonization of the skin of neonates with coagulase-positive staphylococci [30]. As a skin-preparation solution, it proved the equal of povidone–iodine in the prevention of postoperative infections [31].

Sensitization appears to be infrequent. It is inactivated by soap and by the tannin of corks.

Chlorhexidine has been found to support growth of *Pseudomonas cepacia* when in a diluted form [32]. Both its acetate and gluconate preparations are used in disinfection of the skin and oral cavity, and inanimate objects. It is available in concentrations ranging from 0.0015% to 7.5% (concentrate), and has been used in combination with cetrimide.

Hydroxyquinolines. See page 3543.

Oxidizing agents

Only two need to be considered.

Hydrogen peroxide. Hydrogen peroxide 5–7% in water (Hydrogen Peroxide Solution BP) gives up to 20 times its volume of oxygen (20 vol). At this strength it bleaches hair and kills most organisms. The effervescence caused helps remove slough and tissue debris. It is also available as a 1.5% cream for use in the treatment of leg ulcers. Hydrogen peroxide solution is also used in the treatment of anaerobic infection, especially Vincent's infection.

As a cream, hydrogen peroxide has been shown to be equivalent in efficacy to topical fusidic acid in the treatment of impetigo [33].

Potassium permanganate. This is used as a mildly antiseptic application in the form of cold compresses at a dilution of 1:5000, and in a bath at a dilution of 1:10 000. It stains keratin (and also bath porcelain, from which it may be removed with dilute sulphuric acid or hydrogen peroxide).

Heavy metals

These have poor bactericidal properties and are relatively toxic. Although they are strong protein precipitants, their activity may be due to sulphydryl enzyme inhibition.

Mercury is no longer used. Sensitization reactions were common, and toxic reactions, such as nephrotic syndrome, acrodynia [34] and aplastic anaemia [35], have been recorded.

Silver. See above.

Surface-active agents (cationic surfactants)

These are quaternary ammonium or pyridinium compounds with bactericidal activity against many Gram-positive and some Gram-negative organisms.

Benzalkonium chloride is a freely soluble quaternary ammonium antiseptic. It has been used as a sterilizing and preoperative solution or tincture, and is also used as lozenges, a proprietary cream, an antiseptic in some shampoos, bath oils and feminine hygiene sprays, and a preservative in cleaning solutions for hard contact lenses.

Cetrimide. Cetrimide is a quaternary ammonium antiseptic, which, as well as having detergent properties, has bactericidal activity against Gram-positive and some Gram-negative bacteria. It is commonly combined in solution with chlorhexidine. Cetrimide Cream BP contains 0.5% cetrimide and is used for minor cuts and abrasions. Like benzalkonium, it is also used as a preservative in eyedrops and contact-lens disinfectants. Cases of irritant contact dermatitis attributed to cetrimide have occurred after application of 3% cetrimide with 0.3% chlorhexidine to the genital and the flexural areas [36].

Dequalinium chloride was a widely and successfully used cream and lotion [8], but necrotic reactions in naturally occluded body areas were found to occur [37]. Other members of the group, such as cetylpyridinium chloride, have not been widely used in the UK. A lozenge containing dequalinium is available as a mouth and throat antiseptic.

Dyes

Gentian (crystal) violet is a triphenylmethane dye, which has antiseptic properties against some Gram-positive bacteria and yeasts. Employed for many years as a topical treatment for bacterial and fungal skin infections, its use was drastically curtailed after experimental studies demonstrated that it interacted with DNA of living cells [38] and was linked to malignancies in mice [39]. No reports of human malignancy attributed to the use of gentian violet on the skin have been found in the recent literature. It is now licensed for topical application to unbroken skin only, and is not recommended for application to mucous membranes or open wounds.

Brilliant green, also a triphenylmethane dye with actions similar to gentian violet, has suffered similar restrictions in usage, as have other members of the group, such as malachite green. An *in-vitro* study found it to be less effective than gentian violet in its antimicrobial activity, requiring a higher critical concentration [40].

Magenta, or basic fuchsin, is a major component of Castellani's paint. It is known to have activity against Gram-positive bacteria and fungi, but is no longer used because of potential carcinogenicity. Colourless Castellani's paint, the same formula without the magenta (boric acid, resorcinol, phenol), is still used to reduce secondary bacterial contamination in onycholysis and in chronic paronychia.

Miscellaneous

Polynoxylin. Polyoxymethylene is a condensation product

of formaldehyde and urea, and is used (10%) in paste, cream, powder or gel form or as oral lozenges and eardrops.

Cyclic salicylanilides. The halogen and trifluoromethyl-substituted salicylanilides have received much attention. The halogenated salicylanilides, notably tetrachlorosalicyl-anilide (TCS), were found to produce photodermatitis when incorporated in a soap [41]. Trichlorocarbanilide, a related non-fluorescing compound, is without this risk [42].

REFERENCES

1 Karamer A. Aktuelle gesichtspunkte der Antiseptik in der Dermatologie und Venerologie. *Hautarzt* 1994; **45**: 207–21.
2 Sinclair RD, Ryan TJ. A great war for antiseptics. *Australas J Dermatol* 1993; **34**: 115–18.
3 Ford-Jones EL. Topical antiseptics. *Clin Dermatol* 1989; **7**: 142–55.
4 Anon. Topical antibiotics and antiseptics for the skin. *Drug Ther Bull* 1987; **25**: 97–9.
5 Tatnall FM, Leigh IM, Gibson JR. Comparative study of antiseptic toxicity on basal keratinocytes, transformed human keratinocytes and fibroblasts. *Skin Pharmacol* 1990; **3**: 157–63.
6 Tilseley DA, Wilkinson DS. Necrosis and dequalinium. II. Vulval and extra-genital ulceration. *Trans St John's Hosp Derm Soc* 1965; **51**: 49–54.
7 De Groot AC. Labelling cosmetics with their ingredients. *Br Med J* 1990; **300**: 1636–8.
8 Nater JP, De Groot AC. *Unwanted Effects of Cosmetics and Drugs used in Dermatology.* Amsterdam: Elsevier, 1985.
9 Lewin JF, Cleary WT. An accidental death caused by the absorption of phenol through the skin. A case report. *Forensic Sci Int* 1982; **19**: 177–9.
10 Pascher F. Systemic reactions to topically applied drugs. *Int J Dermatol* 1978; **17**: 768–75.
11 Rogers SCF, Burrows D, Niell D. Percutaneous absorption of phenol and methyl alcohol in Magenta Paint BPC. *Br J Dermatol* 1978; **98**: 559–60.
12 Russell AD, Furr JR. The antibacterial activity of a new chloroxylenol prep-aration containing ethylene diamine tetracetic acid. *J Appl Bacteriol* 1977; **43**: 253–60.
13 Black JG, Sprott WE, Howes D *et al.* Percutaneous absorption of hexachloro-phane. *Toxicology* 1974; **2**: 127–39.
14 Manowitz M, Johnston VD. Depositions of hexachlorophene on the skin. *J Soc Cosmet Chem* 1967; **18**: 527–36.
15 Goutieres F, Aicardi J. Accidental percutaneous hexachlorophane intoxication in children. *Br Med J* 1997; **ii**: 663–5.
16 Halling H. Suspected link between exposure to hexachlorophane and malformed infants. *Ann N Y Acad Sci* 1979; **320**: 426–35.
17 Namura S, Nishijima S, McGinlery KJ *et al.* A study of the efficacy of anti-microbial detergents for hand washing: using the full-hand touch plates method. *J Dermatol* 1993; **20**: 88–93.
18 Dzubow LM, Halper AC, Leyden JJ *et al.* Comparison of preoperative skin preparations for the face. *J Am Acad Dermatol* 1988; **19**: 737–41.
19 Mellstrom GA, Lindberg M, Boman A. Permeation and destructive effects of disinfectants on protective gloves. *Contact Dermatitis* 1992; **26**: 163–70.
20 Sloss JM, Cumberland N, Milner SM. Acetic acid used for the elimination of *Pseudomonas aeruginosa* from burn and soft tissue wounds. *J R Army Med Corps* 1993; **139**: 49–51.
21 Hendlev JO, Mika LA, Cwaltney JM. Evaluation of virucidal compounds for inactivation of Rhinoviruses on hands. *Antimicrob Agents Chemother* 1978; **14**: 690–4.
22 Berry AR, Watt B, Goldacre MJ *et al.* A comparison of the use of povidone iodine and chlorhexidine in the prophylaxis of post-operative wound infection. *J Hosp Infect* 1982; **3**: 55–63.
23 Calland RB, Saunders JH, Mosley JC *et al.* Prevention of wound infections in operations by pre-operative antibiotics or povidone iodine—a controlled trial. *Lancet* 1977; **ii**: 1043–5.
24 Pietsch J, Meakins JL. Complications of povidone-iodine absorption in topically treated burns patients. *Lancet* 1976; **i**: 280–2.
25 Millikan LE. A double-blind study of Betadine skin cleanser in acne vulgaris. *Cutis* 1976; **17**: 394–6.

26 Van Ketel WG, Van den Berg WH. Sensitization to povidone-iodine. *Dermatol Clin* 1990; **8**: 107–9.
27 Skog E, Arnesjö B, Troëng T *et al.* A randomized trial comparing cadexomer iodine and standard treatment in the out-patient management of chronic venous ulcers. *Br J Dermatol* 1983; **109**: 77–83.
28 Lowbury EJL, Lilly HA. Use of 4% chlorhexidine detergent solution (Hibiscrub) and other methods of skin disinfection. *Br Med J* 1973; **iv**: 510–15.
29 Lowbury EJL, Lilly HA, Ayliffe CAJ. Preoperative disinfection of surgeons' hands: use of alcoholic solutions and effects of gloves on skin flora. *Br Med J* 1974; **iv**: 369–72.
30 Alder VG, Burman VG, Simpson RA *et al.* Comparison of hexachlorophane and chlorhexidine powders in prevention of neonatal infection. *Arch Dis Child* 1980; **55**: 277–80.
31 Black JG, Sprott WE, Howes D *et al.* Percutaneous absorption of hexachloro-phane. *Toxicology* 1974; **2**: 127–39.
32 Gosden PE, Norman P. Pseudobacteraemia associated with contaminated skin cleansing agent. *Lancet* 1986; **1**: 209.
33 Christensen OB, Anehus S. Hydrogen peroxide cream: an alternative to topical antibiotics in the treatment of impetigo contagiosa. *Acta Derm Venereol (Stockh)* 1994; **74**: 460–2.
34 Pascher F. Systemic reactions to topically applied drugs. *Int J Dermatol* 1978; **17**: 768–75.
35 Slee PHTJ, den Ottlander JJ, de Wolff FA. A case of Merbromin® intoxication possibly resulting in aplastic anemia. *Acta Med Scand* 1979; **205**: 463–6.
36 Lee JY, Wang BJ. Contact dermatitis caused by cetrimide in antiseptics. *Contact Dermatitis* 1995; **33**: 168–71.
37 Manowitz M, Johnston VD. Depositions of hexachlorophene on the skin. *J Soc Cosmet Chem* 1967; **18**: 527–36.
38 Rosenkranz HS, Carr HS. Possible hazard in use of gentian violet. *Br Med J* 1971; **3**: 702–3.
39 Food Advisory Committee. Final report on the review of the Colouring Matter in Food Regulations 1973:Fd AC\REP\4. London, HM Stationery Office, 1987.
40 Bakker P, Van Doorne H, Booskens V *et al.* Activity of gentian violet and brilliant green against some microorganisms associated with skin infections. *Int J Dermatol* 1992; **31**: 210–13.
41 Wilkinson DS. Hexachlorophene bath hazard. *Contact Dermatitis* 1978; **4**: 172.
42 Crow KD, Wilkinson DS, Osmundsen PE. A review of photo-reactions to halogenated salicylanilides. *Br J Dermatol* 1969; **81**: 180–5.

Hydroxyquinolines [1,2]

These have a wide range of antibacterial activity. Some are also used as intestinal antiseptics. They are very poorly absorbed. On the skin, the more powerful compounds have the disadvantage of staining; sensitization reactions may also occur. Overall, however, they are safe, and an acceptable alternative to antibiotics, especially when used in com-bination with topical steroids [3]. The nomenclature is confusing.

REFERENCES

1 De Groot AC. Labelling cosmetics with their ingredients. *Br Med J* 1990; **300**: 1636–8.
2 Nater JP, De Groot AC. *Unwanted Effects of Cosmetics and Drugs used in Dermatology.* Amsterdam: Elsevier, 1985.
3 Maibach HI. Iodochlorhydroxyquinolin–hydrocortisone treatment of fungal infections. A double-blind trial. *Arch Dermatol* 1978; **114**: 1773–5.

Topical antibiotics

The scope, choice and indications for antibiotics in skin dis-ease are fully discussed in Chapter 76. Topical antibiotics are most frequently used for the prevention of postoperative wound infections [1], leg ulcers [2], superficial wound infections [3,4], impetigo and acne [5,6]. Further details may be found under the relevant headings.

Whenever possible, the sensitivity of the infecting organism should be determined before treatment. Where this is not possible, the choice will depend on the nature of the infection and the prevailing patterns of drug resistance. Staphylococcal resistance to tetracyclines is well known. The value of many antibiotics is limited by their tendency to sensitize when used topically, for example chloramphenicol and neomycin.

Penicillin and streptomycin

These are potent skin sensitizers. Incautious handling by medical staff was once a frequent cause of a disabling dermatitis until a 'no touch' technique was enforced.

Tetracyclines [7]

These are used alone in the topical treatment of acne [8], but are also present in several proprietary topical corticosteroid preparations. Bacterial resistance is common, and they tend to stain skin and clothing. They were nevertheless effective in 90% of 85 patients with acne, and were considered cosmetically acceptable by 90% of the patients [9]. No adverse reactions were seen in a group of 300 patients treated over 13 weeks [10].

Neomycin and framycetin
SYN. SOFRAMYCIN

Many preparations containing one or other of these are marketed in the UK, and are widely used, although sensitization reactions are common, especially around leg ulcers, under occlusion and in patients with chronic otitis externa, pruritus ani/vulvae, and in those with recurrent eye problems. Neomycin was among the commonest sensitizers reported by Wilkinson *et al.* [11]. Simultaneous contact allergy to neomycin, bacitracin, and polymyxin has been reported [12].

Sodium fusidate

Derived from *Fusidium coccineum*, this is active against staphylococcal infections and effective in erythrasma [13].

Sensitization occurs only very rarely [14,15], but bacterial resistance is more common. It is used alone for superficial staphylococcal infections, and in combination with topical steroids in the treatment of infected eczema.

Gentamicin sulphate

The particular dermatological value of gentamicin sulphate lies in its broad spectrum of activity, including against *Pseudomonas aeruginosa*. Contact allergy is fairly frequent in patients with chronic otitis externa [16] and, compared with other agents, it remains a common sensitizer [17]. Cross-sensitivity within the aminoglycosides occurs [18].

Metronidazole [19]

Metronidazole 0.75–1% has been shown to be a safe and effective treatment for rosacea [20,21]. Topical metronidazole appears to be as effective as low-dose oral oxytetracycline [22], although tetracycline had a more rapid effect and was more likely to produce complete resolution of papules and pustules. Moderate improvement with minimal side-effects was seen in six patients [23]. Topical metronidazole has also been used with some success in patients with decubitus and other ulcers, eliminating malodour in 36h [24]. In a double-blind, placebo-controlled trial, topical metronidazole was ineffective in reducing the inflammatory lesions of acne [25].

Bacitracin

This is too toxic for systemic use. Its antibacterial action is principally against Gram-positive organisms, so it is usually used topically in combination with other antibiotics, such as neomycin or polymyxin B. Allergic reactions of an anaphylactoid nature have been recorded [26]. In leg-ulcer patients it was reported to be the most potent sensitizer of all the topical antibiotics tested [27].

Polymyxin B

This has no activity against Gram-positive organisms, but is effective against most Gram-negative organisms. Ototoxicity has followed its use in otitis externa associated with drum perforation [28].

Mupirocin [29]

This topical antibiotic is derived from *Pseudomonas fluorescens*. It is chemically unrelated to other antibiotics, and its mode of action in arresting bacterial protein synthesis is novel [30]. Cross-resistance with other antibiotics is therefore not seen. It is active against a wide range of Gram-positive organisms and some Gram-negative organisms [31]. Its usefulness both in cutaneous bacterial infections [32,33] and in the elimination of nasal carriage of staphylococci has been demonstrated [34]. It would appear to be as clinically active against staphylococci as sodium fusidate but with fewer problems of emergent resistant bacterial strains [35].

REFERENCES

1 Gette MT, Marks JG, Jr, Malonwy ME. Frequency of postoperative allergic contact dermatitis to topical antibiotics. *Arch Dermatol* 1992; **128**: 365–7.

2 Wilson CL, Cameron J, Powell SM *et al.* High incidence of contact dermatitis in leg-ulcer patients—implications for management. *Clin Exp Dermatol* 1991; **16**: 250–3.

3 White DG, Collins PO, Rowsell RB. Topical antibiotics in the treatment of superficial infections in general practice—a comparison of mupirocin with sodium fusidate. *J Infect* 1989; **18**: 221–9.

4 Dire DJ, Coppola M, Swyer DA *et al.* Prospective evaluation of topical antibiotics for preventing infections in uncomplicated soft-tissue wounds repaired in the ED. *Acad Emerg Med* 1995; **2**: 4–10.

5 Sykes NL, Jr, Webster GF. Acne. A review of optimum treatment. *Drugs* 1994; **48**: 59–70.

6 Yee KC, Cunliffe WJ. Itching in acne—an unusual complication of therapy. *Dermatology* 1994; **189**: 117–19.

7 Verbov JL. Tetracyclines in dermatology. *Trans St John's Hosp Derm Soc* 1969; **55**: 78–84.

8 Norris JF, Hughes BR, Basey AJ *et al.* A comparison of the effectiveness of topical tetracycline, benzoyl-peroxide gel and oral oxytetracycline in the treatment of acne. *Clin Exp Dermatol* 1991; **16**: 31–3.

9 Burton J. A placebo-controlled study to evaluate the efficacy of topical tetracycline and oral tetracycline in the treatment of mild to moderate acne. *J Int Med Res* 1990; **18**: 94–103.

10 Frank SB. Topical treatment of acne with a tetracycline preparation: results of a multi-group study. *Cutis* 1976; **17**: 539–45.

11 Wilkinson JD, Hambly EM, Wilkinson DS. Comparison of patch test results in two adjacent areas of England. II. Medicaments. *Acta Derm Venereol (Stockh)* 1980; **60**: 245–9.

12 Grandinetti PJ, Fowler JF, Jr. Simultaneous contact allergy to neomycin, bacitracin, and polymyxin. *J Am Acad Dermatol* 1990; **23**: 646–7.

13 MacMillan AL, Sarkany I. Specific topical therapy for erythrasma. *Br J Dermatol* 1970; **82**: 507–9.

14 Baptista A, Barros MA. Contact dermatitis from sodium fusidate. *Contact Dermatitis* 1990; **23**: 186–7.

15 Romaguera C, Grimalt F. Contact dermatitis to sodium fusidate. *Contact Dermatitis* 1985; **12**: 176–7.

16 Holmes RC, Johns AN, Wilkinson JD *et al.* Medicament contact dermatitis in patients with chronic inflammatory ear disease. *J R Soc Med* 1982; **75**: 27–30.

17 Gollhausen R, Enders F, Przybilla B *et al.* Trends in allergic contact sensitization. *Contact Dermatitis* 1988; **18**: 147–54.

18 Forstrom L, Pirila V, Pirila L. Cross-sensitivity within the neomycin group of antibiotics. *Acta Derm Venereol Suppl (Stockh)* 1979; **59**: 67–9.

19 Schmadel CK, McEvoy GK. Topical metronidazole: a new therapy for rosacea. *Clin Pharm* 1990; **9**: 94–101.

20 Aronson IK, Rumsfield JA, West EP *et al.* Evaluation of topical metronidazole gel in acne rosacea. *Drug Intell Clin Pharmacol* 1987; **21**: 346–51.

21 Erikson G, Nor CE. Impact of metronidazole on skin and colon microflora in patients with rosacea. *Infection* 1987; **15**: 8–10.

22 Veien NK, Christiansen JE, Hjorth N *et al.* Topical metronidazole in the treatment of rosacea. *Cutis* 1986; **38**: 209–10.

23 Signore RJ. A pilot study of 5 per cent permethrin cream versus 0.75 per cent metronidazole gel in acne rosacea. *Cutis* 1995; **56**: 177–9.

24 Witkowski JA, Parish LC. Topical metronidazole gel. The bacteriology of decubitus ulcers. *Int J Dermatol* 1991; **30**: 660–1.

25 Tong D, Peters W, Barnetson RS. Evaluation of 0.75% metronidazole gel in acne—a double-blind study. *Clin Exp Dermatol* 1994; **19**: 221–3.

26 Vale MA, Connolly A, Epstein A. Metal/bacitracin induced anaphylaxis. (Letter.) *Arch Dermatol* 1978; **114**: 800.

27 Zaki I, Shall L, Dalziel KL. Bacitracin: a significant sensitizer in leg ulcer patients? *Contact Dermatitis* 1994; **31**: 92–4.

28 Erikson G, Nor CE. Impact of metronidazole on skin and colon microflora in patients with rosacea. *Infection* 1987; **15**: 8–10.

29 Chain EB, Mellows C. Pseudomonic acid—Part 1. The structure of pseudomonic CID A: a novel antibiotic produced by *Pseudomonas fluorescens. J Chem Soc Perkin Trans* 1977; **1**: 294–309.

30 Hughes J, Mellowes C. Interaction of pseudomonic acid A with *Escherichia coli* B isoleucyl t-RNA synthetase. *Biochem J* 1980; **191**: 209–10.

31 White AR, Beale AS, Boon RJ *et al.* Antibacterial activity of mupirocin, an antibiotic produced by *Pseudomonas fluorescens. R Soc Med Int Congr **Symp** Ser* 1984; **80**: 43–55.

32 Lever R, Hadley K, Downey D, MacKie R. Staphylococcal colonisation in atopic dermatitis and the effect of topical mupirocin therapy. *Br J Dermatol* 1988; **119**: 189–98.

33 Mertz PM, Marshall DA, Eaglstein WH *et al.* Topical mupirocin treatment of impetigo is equal to oral erythromycin therapy. *Arch Dermatol* 1989; **125**: 1069–73.

34 Dacre JE, Emmerson AM, Jenner EA. Nasal carriage of gentamicin and methicillin resistant *Staphylococcus aureus* treated with topical pseudomonic acid (Letter). *Lancet* 1983; **ii**: 1036.

35 Lewis-Jones CA, Hart CA, Vickers CFH. The evaluation of mupirocin in the treatment of acute skin infections in childhood. *R Soc Med Int Congr Symp Ser* 1984; **80**: 103–8.

Topical antibiotics in acne [1,2]

The benefits of oral antibiotic therapy on acne must be weighed against the risks and possible adverse effects of long-term administration [3]. Even though the tetracyclines in particular appear to be very safe drugs [4], it was logical to investigate the topical use of these agents.

In general, topical antibiotics work about as well as benzoyl peroxide or tretinoin in acne, but in view of the risk of bacterial resistance, a degree of caution should be exercised in their use [5]. Attention has centred on three topical antibiotics.

Tetracycline hydrochloride

See page 3544.

Erythromycin

Only the lipid-soluble forms, for example the base, propionate or stearate, are effective. Several authors have considered the problem of erythromycin-resistant propionibacteria [6,7]. It is equivalent in effect to topical clindamycin, is safe and well tolerated [8,9]. A topical 2% erythromycin gel has been shown to be as effective as 1% clindamycin phosphate in patients with mild to moderate acne [10], and 1.5% erythromycin and 1% clindamycin phosphate solutions were found to be equally effective [9].

Clindamycin

This is an effective preparation in acne [11]. It is as effective as oral minocycline 50 mg twice a day [12], and oral tetracyline [13]. It was somewhat less effective than topical nicotinamide 45 gel in a trial involving 76 patients [14]. A 1% solution of this drug was found to be more effective than topical tetracyline or erythromycin [15]. It was found to be as effective as 5% benzoyl peroxide gel in patients with papular or pustular acne [16]; fewer side-effects were seen with topical clindamycin.

REFERENCES

1 Sykes NL, Jr, Webster GF. Acne. A review of optimum treatment. *Drugs* 1994; **48**: 59–70.

2 Anon. Topical antibiotics for acne. *Drug Ther Bull* 1992; **30**: 33–5.

3 Akers WA, Maibach HI. Relative safety of long-term administration of tetracycline in acne vulgaris. *Cutis* 1976; **17**: 531–4.

4 Ad Hoc Committee on the Use of Antibiotics in Dermatology. Systemic

antibiotics for treatment of acne vulgaris: efficacy and safety. *Arch Dermatol* 1975; **111**: 1630–6.

5 Eady EA, Holland KT, Cunliffe WJ. Should topical antibiotics be used for the treatment of acne vulgaris? *Br J Dermatol* 1982; **107**: 235–46.

6 Bojar RA, Eady EA, Jones CE *et al*. Inhibition of erythromycin-resistant propionibacteria on the skin of acne patients by topical erythromycin with and without zinc. *Br J Dermatol* 1994; **130**: 329–36.

7 Harkaway KS, McGinley KJ, Foglia AN *et al*. Antibiotic resistance patterns in coagulase-negative staphylococci after treatment with topical erythromycin, benzoyl peroxide, and combination therapy. *Br J Dermatol* 1992; **126**: 586–90.

8 Schachner L, Pestana A, Kittles C. A clinical trial comparing the safety and efficacy of a topical erythromycin-zinc formulation with a topical clindamycin formulation. *J Am Acad Dermatol* 1990; **22**: 489–95.

9 Shalita AR, Smith EB, Bauer E. Topical erythromycin v clindamycin therapy for acne. A multicenter, double-blind comparison. *Arch Dermatol* 1984; **120**: 351–5.

10 Leyden JJ, Shalita AR, Saajian CD *et al*. Erythromycin 2% gel in comparison with clindamycin phosphate 1% solution in acne vulgaris. *J Am Acad Dermatol* 1987; **16**: 822–7.

11 Kuhlman DS, Callen JP. A comparison of clindamycin phosphate 1 percent topical lotion and placebo in the treatment of acne vulgaris. *Cutis* 1986; **38**: 203–6.

12 Sheehan-Dare RA, Papworth-Smith J, Cunliffe WJ. A double-blind comparison of topical clindamycin and oral minocycline in the treatment of acne vulgaris. *Acta Derm Venereol (Stockh)* 1990; **70**: 543–7.

13 Katsambas A, Towaky AA, Stratigos J. Topical clindamycin phosphate compared with oral tetracycline in the treatment of acne vulgaris. *Br J Dermatol* 1987; **116**: 387–91.

14 Shalita AR, Smith JG, Parish LC *et al*. Topical nicotinamide compared with clindamycin gel in the treatment of inflammatory acne vulgaris. *Int J Dermatol* 1995; **34**: 434–7.

15 Resh W, Stoughton RB. Topically applied antibiotics for acne vulgaris. *Arch Dermatol* 1976; **112**: 182–4.

16 Schmidt JB, Neuman R, Fanta D *et al*. 1% clindamycin phosphate solution versus 5% benzoyl peroxide gel in papular pustular acne. *Z Hautkr* 1988; **63**: 374–6.

Antifungal agents

These are discussed in detail in Chapters 31 and 76. This section is confined to notes on the newer antifungal agents [1,2]. These topical agents are suitable for treating tinea pedis, and tinea corporis of limited extent. For more extensive infections, and for treating hair and nails, systemic therapy is preferred [3].

There are three classes of compound to be considered.

Imidazoles

These act by inhibiting synthesis of ergosterol, which is necessary for the formation of fungal cell membranes. They are fungistatic. Clotrimazole and miconazole are the best known. Newer related compounds are now available for which individual improvements are claimed, but there is little effective difference. They include *bif-, fenti-, tio-, ter-, iso-, sul-, e-, keto-, oxy*-conazole, and doubtless others will appear.

Allylamines

These also act by inhibiting the formation of ergosterol but block synthesis at an earlier stage in the pathway than imidazoles, namely between squalene and squalene epoxide.

They are fungicidal. The two representatives of this class commonly available are naftifine (USA) and terbinafine (Europe). They are rapidly effective in superficial dermatophyte infections. Naftifine also possesses some anti-inflammatory activity.

Morpholines

Amorolfine, the only representative, acts by inhibiting two separate stages in the ergosterol pathway, and is fungicidal. In addition to treatment of superficial fungal infections this drug shows promise in treating the difficult problem of distal toe-nail infection. A formulation in a lacquer for once- or twice-weekly application is available [4].

For an in depth review and consideration of comparative trials see Gupta *et al*. [2].

REFERENCES

1 Stiller MJ, Shupack JL, Rosenthal SA. Treatment of dermatophytosis. II. Newer topical antifungal drugs. *Int J Dermatol* 1993; **32**: 638–41.

2 Gupta AK, Sauder DN, Shear NH. Antifungal agents: an overview. Part II. *J Am Acad Dermatol* 1994; **30**: 911–33.

3 Hay RJ. Current treatment of dermatophytoses. *Acta Derm Venereol Suppl (Stockh)* 1986; **121**: 117–23.

4 Reinel D, Clarke C. Comparative efficacy and safety of amorolfine nail lacquer 5% in onychomycosis, once-weekly versus twice-weekly. *Clin Exp Dermatol* 1992; **17** (Suppl. 1): 44–9.

Antiviral agents

Unfortunately, little progress has been made in this important field in recent years. Topical antiviral therapy offers a number of advantages over systemic therapy. These include convenience, higher target tissue drug levels and greater efficacy, specific targeting of the drug to the site of infection, reduced cost, and reduced exposure of the remainder of the body to drug side-effects [1]. Topical aciclovir is well established in the treatment of primary and recurrent herpes simplex infections [2]. Some protective effect may be obtained by regular application [3].

Podophyllin

Traditionally, 0.5–25% is used to treat genital warts; 0.5% podophyllin in ethanol may be used on a daily basis (3 days a week) to treat penile warts [4]. Podophyllin 10–25% in tincture of benzoin compound may be applied once or twice a week to genital or perianal warts (washed off after 6–12 h). One of the main active components of podophyllin—podophyllotoxin—has now been isolated and can be used at a 0.5% concentration in ethanol as a once-daily application. It will clear 60–70% of genital warts within 3–5 days [5].

Idoxuridine

For the treatment of herpes simplex and herpes zoster

infections, 5–15% is used topically. Both idoxuridine and topical aciclovir must be applied frequently early in an attack to have optimal effect [6].

5-Fluorouracil cream 5%

Although most commonly used as an antineoplastic agent to treat solar keratosis, Bowen's disease or superficial multifocal basal cell carcinoma, topical fluorouracil cream (applied once or twice a week) has also been shown to be effective in curing many resistant vulval or vaginal condylomas [7]. A proprietary combination of 5-fluorouracil and salicylic acid, applied on a daily basis, resulted in complete healing of genital warts in an average of 12 days [8]. The same combination has been used with success prior to curettage of warts under local anaesthetic [9].

Monochloracetic acid

This can either be used alone or in combination with 60% salicylic acid as a treatment for simple or mosaic plantar warts, and for simple plantar warts a cure rate of over 60% at 6 weeks has been obtained [10]. Care must be taken in using this agent, as a chemical cellulitis may sometimes develop if acid enters any cracks or splits.

REFERENCES

1 Spruance SL, Freeman DJ. Topical treatment of cutaneous herpes simplex virus infections. *Antiviral Res* 1990; **14**: 305–21.
2 Kinghorn CR. Topical acyclovir in the treatment of recurrent herpes simplex virus infections. *Scand J Infect Dis Suppl* 1985; **47**: 58–62.
3 Gibson JR, Klaber MR, Harvey SG *et al*. Prophylaxis against herpes labialis with acyclovir cream—a placebo-controlled study. *Dermatologica* 1986; **172**: 104–7.
4 Maiti H, Hayl KR. Treatment of condyloma accuminata with podophyllin resin. *Practitioner* 1985; **229**: 37–9.
5 Von Krogh G. Topical self-treatment of penile warts with a 0.5% podophyllotoxin in ethanol for 4–5 days. *Sex Transm Dis* 1987; **14**: 135–40.
6 Spruance SL, Stewart JC, Freeman DJ. Early application of topical 15% idoxuridine in dimethylsulfoxide shortens the course of herpes simplex labialis: a multicenter placebo-controlled trial. *J Infect Dis* 1990; **161**: 191–7.
7 Krebs HB. The use of topical 5-fluorouracil in the treatment of genital condylomata. *Obstet Gynecol Clin N Am* 1987; **14**: 559–68.
8 Djawari D. Fluorouracil treatment on condyloma accuminata. *Z Hautkr* 1986; **61**: 463–9.
9 Seuff H, Reine ID, Matthies C *et al*. Topical fluorouracil solution in the treatment of warts—clinical experience and percutaneous absorption. *Br J Dermatol* 1988; **118**: 409–14.
10 Steele K, Shirodaria P, O'Hare M *et al*. Monochloracetic acid in 60% salicylic acid as a treatment for simple plantar warts: effectiveness and mode of action. *Br J Dermatol* 1988; **118**: 537–44.

Topical steroids

The revolution brought about in dermatological therapy by the introduction of topical steroids, which started with compound F or hydrocortisone in 1952 [1], is well known. Cortisone itself has been shown to be effective in some dermatoses when given systemically. It was found to be inactive when applied topically. During the 1950s further

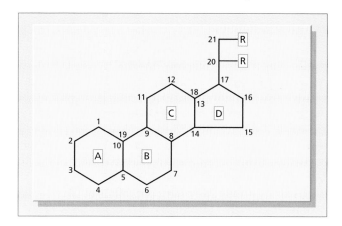

Fig. 78.3 The configuration of the basic corticosteroid structure.

derivatives were produced with enhanced topical activity. The basic structure of the steroid moiety is shown in Fig. 78.3. Modification of both the ring structure and the side chains produced dramatic changes in the effectiveness of the steroid. Thus, fluorination of the 9 position, the introduction of an unsaturated bond between the first two carbon atoms and the nature of the side chains, particularly in the 21 position, enhanced activity [2].

During the 1960s the full therapeutic possibilities of topical steroids were explored, and those dermatoses most responsive to them were identified. In the following decade, the adverse effects of treatment were encountered with increasing frequency. The greater the efficacy of the topical steroid in treating the inflammatory dermatoses the greater appeared to be the side-effects. The first need demonstrated was a suitable method for ranking topical steroids in order of potency [3]. This may be assessed by therapeutic trial, but the method is slow and expensive and is not suitable for predicting the effect of newer products. The introduction of the vasoconstrictor assay [4] and its subsequent modifications [5] have proved of great value. The assay depends upon the property of glucocorticosteroids to produce transient vasoconstriction. The degree of pallor produced following application of a steroid in varying dilution for a standard length of time increases with the concentration of the steroid.

Despite the fact that this assay depends upon only one of the numerous biological effects of corticosteroids, it has repeatedly been demonstrated to correlate well with clinical effectiveness. This and other aspects of steroid assessment have been discussed in detail by Barry [5]. Another method of assessing steroid potency employs the Duhring chamber [6].

The second need was for a product that was therapeutically effective but without adverse effects [7]. Despite numerous claims to the contrary, such a product has not appeared, although several have a reduced capacity to cause adrenal suppression [8].

Percutaneous absorption

The application of a corticosteroid is followed by absorption through the skin (percutaneous absorption), during which time it must exert all its beneficial effects. In theory, the absorbed steroid distributed in the circulation may affect the skin 'on a second pass' by perfusion outwards from the cutaneous capillaries. This is rarely of clinical importance but must be considered in side-to-side comparisons in therapeutic trials. The percutaneous absorption of topical steroids is a multistage process. Barry [5] has indicated 17 different stages between the application of the steroid and its effect on the skin cell. A considerable body of data has accumulated on the various stages of absorption. The essential features are that the corticosteroid is normally crystalline and must be suspended in a suitable vehicle (see below).

The steroid diffuses into the stratum corneum or its constituents. Interaction with any other skin treatment which has been applied may also be important. It appears that the whole stratum corneum contributes to the barrier through which the steroid must penetrate, representing the probable rate-limiting step. Vickers [9] introduced the concept of a reservoir for corticosteroids within the stratum corneum, which permits the absorption of steroid up to a certain level but not more. The rate of penetration into the stratum corneum is greater the more hydrophilic the steroid, i.e. water solubility favours rapid penetration. Within the viable epidermis, the converse holds true. Penetration into the living keratinocytes is fastest with lipophilic steroids. Hydrocortisone has low solubility in lipids and fluocinolone acetonide relatively high lipid solubility. In experimental assays, it generally holds true that the higher lipid-soluble steroids are clinically the more potent. The dichotomy between the rapid rate of penetration into the stratum corneum with low lipid solubility and the slow rate of intracellular penetration with low lipid solubility explains why there are such wide differences in clinical effectiveness between individual steroids. Receptor binding by the cytoplasm is also greater with increasing lipid solubility. Studies to determine the strength of binding indicate that clinical potency is also related to high receptor binding. Furthermore, binding appears to be specific for glucocorticoids without cross-binding of other steroids such as β-oestradiol or nandrolone. Receptor binding affinity is sensitive to structural alterations in the steroid. Thus, the introduction of a double bond in the A ring, esterification in the 17α position, and fluorination at position 9α increase binding affinity, whereas esterification in the 21 position reduces binding affinity (Fig. 78.3). The steroid–receptor complexes are translocated to the nucleus where they modulate messenger RNA (mRNA) production.

Exposure to UV radiation enhances percutaneous steroid absorption [10]. The mechanism of anti-inflammatory activity of glucocorticoids is still incompletely understood.

REFERENCES

1 Sulzberger MB, Witten VH. The effect of topically applied compound F in selected dermatoses. *J Invest Dermatol* 1952; **19**: 101–2.
2 Elks J. Steroid structure and steroid activity. *Br J Dermatol* 1976; **94** (Suppl. 12): 3–13.
3 *Monthly Index of Medical Specialities.* London: Haymarket Publishing Services, 1996.
4 McKenzie AW, Stoughton RB. Method for comparing percutaneous absorption of steroids. *Arch Dermatol* 1962; **86**: 608–10.
5 Barry BW. *Dermatological Formulations: Percutaneous Absorption. Drugs and Pharmaceutical Sciences*, Vol. 18. New York: Marcel Dekker, 1983.
6 Frosch PJ, Behrenbeck EM, Frosch K *et al.* The Duhring chamber assay for corticosteroid atrophy. *Br J Dermatol* 1981; **104**: 57–65.
7 Dipetrillo T, Cutroneo KR. Anti-inflammatory adrenal steroids that neither inhibit skin collagen nor cause dermal atrophy. *Arch Dermatol* 1984; **120**: 878–83.
8 Thalen A, Brattsand R, Andersson PH. Development of glucocorticosteroids with enhanced ratio between topical and systemic effects. *Acta Derm Venereol (Stockh)* 1989; **69** (Suppl. 151): 11–19.
9 Vickers CFH. Existence of reservoir in the stratum corneum. *Arch Dermatol* 1963; **88**: 20–3.
10 Lamaud E, Schalla W. Influence of UV irradiation on penetration of hydrocortisone. *In vivo* study in hairless rat skin. *Br J Dermatol* 1984; **111** (Suppl. 27): 152–7.

Mechanism of action

Corticosteroids have anti-inflammatory, immunosuppressive, and anti-mitogenic activity due to their ability to exert multiple effects on the various functions of leukocytes, epidermal and dermal cells. The exact mechanism of these effects is still under investigation. The currently accepted general model of steroid action incorporates three major steps: receptor binding, synthesis of specific mRNA (transcription), and the synthesis of protein [1]. Hydrophobic glucocorticosteroid molecules diffuse across the plasma membrane of the cell and reversibly bind to a specific receptor protein that is present in the cell cytoplasm [2]. This hormone binding to the receptor causes increased DNA-binding affinity due to allosteric changes in the structure of the receptor, leading to accumulation of the steroid–receptor complex in the cell nucleus [1]. Gene transcription can be modulated by the hormone complex binding to certain sequences on nuclear DNA termed hormone response elements (HREs), which result in production of new proteins by RNA molecules using the new DNA complex as a template [3,4]. Some of the new proteins produced include: lipocortin, interleukin-1 and lymphokines (e.g. interleukin-2). Lipocortin, a family of glycoproteins, plays an important role in regulating the activity of phospholipase A_2 which subsequently effects the production and release of arachidonic acid, which is the precursor for leukotrienes and phospholipids [5]. Corticosteroids have the ability to block the production of all arachidonate derivatives (eicosanoids) by restricting the availability of arachidonic acid through inducing the production of lipocortin [6,7]. Although the gene-modification model of protein transcription and translation is currently favoured because of findings from experimental systems, it still cannot explain all the properties of glucocorticosteroids. It may, however, lay the groundwork for future studies.

REFERENCES

1 Kragballe K. Topical corticosteroids: mechanisms of action. *Acta Derm Venereol (Stockh)* 1989; **69**: 7–10.
2 Carson-Jurica MA, Schrader WT, O'Malley BW. Steroid receptor family: structure and functions. *Endocr Rev* 1990; **11**: 201–20.
3 Evans RM. The steroid and thyroid hormone receptor superfamily. *Science* 1988; **240**: 889–95.
4 Williams GR, Franklyn JA. Physiology of the steroid–thyroid hormone nuclear receptor superfamily. *Clin Endocrinol Metab* 1994; **8**: 241–66.
5 Kragballe K, Voorhees JJ. Arachidonic acid and leukotrienes in dermatology. *J Invest Dermatol* 1983; **81**: 293–6.
6 Blackwell GJ, Canuccio R, Di Rosa M *et al.* Macrocortin: a polypeptide causing the anti-phospholipase effect of glucocorticoids. *Nature* 1980; **287**: 147–9.
7 Hammarstrom S, Hamberg M, Duell EA *et al.* Glucocorticoid in inflammatory proliferative skin disease reduces arachidonic and hydroxyeicosatetraenoic acids. *Science* 1977; **197**: 994–5.

Vehicle

The choice of vehicle is of the greatest importance in the formulation of topical steroids [1]. The foregoing discussion should make it apparent that solubilities and partition coefficients profoundly alter bioavailability. It also follows that disturbance of the physicochemical composition of the vehicle will alter bioavailability [2]. This is of particular importance to the *ex tempore* dilution of a proprietary manufactured product. The practice of diluting or of adding other medicaments should be discouraged [3]. If dilution is considered necessary, the manufacturer's own recommended diluent should be used. A further problem arises regarding alteration of the formulation of a manufacturer's product. Taking the example of betamethasone-17-valerate, the addition of tar, salicylic acid or extemporaneous dilution hastens isomerization to the 21-valerate, which is considerably less potent as a corticosteroid [4]. The importance of this finding to other steroids has recently been re-examined and discussed [5]. The stability of the steroid in relation to the additives used is a subject of much research. Some, for example propylene glycol, may, according to the manufacturer, enhance penetration without impairing steroid stability. Steroid-impregnated tape may also be used with success in some more localized skin conditions [6].

Alteration of the vehicle of the potent steroid clobetasol propionate significantly reduced percutaneous absorption and the potential for producing systemic toxicity, without reducing the vasoconstrictor assay parameters [7].

Clinical dermatologists, and perhaps more frequently patients, are impressed that a topical steroid is more active at the beginning of treatment than later. To achieve the same effect, the patient may need to apply the steroid after ever-shortening intervals. This process is called tachyphylaxis [8]. Evidence has been presented that intermittent application may avoid tachyphylaxis [9,10], but a recent study showed that dermal thinning also occurred with intermittent use

and, even when the no-treatment interval was extended, any protective effect was also subject to tachyphylaxis [11].

REFERENCES

1 Polano MK, Ponec M. Dependence of corticosteroid penetration on the vehicle. *Arch Dermatol* 1976; **112**: 675–80.
2 Woodford R, Barry BW. Optimization of bioavailability of topical steroids: thermodynamic control. *J Invest Dermatol* 1982; **79**: 388–91.
3 Gibson JR, Kirsch J, Darley CR. An assessment of the relationship between vasoconstrictor assay findings, clinical efficiency and thinning effects of a variety of undiluted and diluted corticosteroid preparations. *Br J Dermatol* 1984; **111** (Suppl. 27): 204–12.
4 Ryatt KS, Feather JW, Mehta A *et al.* The stability and blanching efficacy of betamethasone-17-valerate in emulsifying ointment. *Br J Dermatol* 1982; **107**: 71–6.
5 Gibson JR, Kirsch J, Darley CR. An attempt to evaluate the relative clinical potencies of various diluted and undiluted proprietary corticosteroid preparations. *Clin Exp Dermatol* 1983; **8**: 489–93.
6 Cattaneo M, Betti R, Lodi A. Evaluation of efficacy and tolerability of K-SA floucinolone acetonide tape. *Ind J Clin Pharmacol Res* 1987; **7**: 279–82.
7 Harding SM, Sohail S, Busse MJ. Percutaneous absorption of clobetasol propionate from novel ointment and cream foundations. *Clin Exp Dermatol* 1985; **10**: 13–21.
8 Du Vivier A. Tachyphylaxis to topically applied steroids. *Arch Dermatol* 1976; **112**: 1245–8.
9 Clement M, Phillips SH, Du Vivier A. Is steroid tachyphylaxis preventable? *Clin Exp Dermatol* 1985; **10**: 22–9.
10 Marghescu S. Externe Kortikoidtherapie: Kontinuierliche versus diskontinuierliche Anwendung. *Hautarzt* 1983; **34**: 114–17.
11 Lubach D, Bensmann A, Bornemann U. Steroid-induced dermal atrophy. Investigations on discontinuous application. *Dermatologica* 1989; **179**: 67–72.

Unwanted effects of topical steroids

The unwanted effects of topical steroids are directly related to their potencies. To date, it has not proved possible to dissociate side-effects from potency, except perhaps with regard to systemic adrenocortical suppression. Side-effects can therefore only be avoided either by relying on weaker steroids or by acquiring a clear appreciation of how, when and where to use the more potent preparations (see also below under Precautions).

The side-effects can be considered at several levels.

Epidermal effects

These include the following.
1 Epidermal thinning is associated with a decrease in epidermal kinetic activity [1], a decrease in mean keratinocyte layer thickness, and a general flattening of the dermo-epidermal convolutions. This effect can be partially prevented by the concomitant use of topical tretinoin [2].
2 Melanocyte inhibition, a vitiligo-like condition, has been described. This complication is more likely to occur with steroids under occlusion or with intracutaneous steroid injections [3,4].

Dermal effects [5,6]

Collagen synthesis is reduced and there is a reduction in

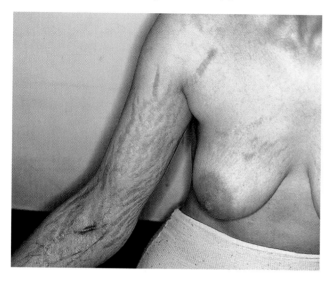

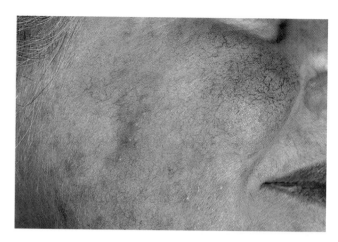

Fig. 78.6 Steroid-induced telangiectasia and atrophy. (Courtesy of Wycombe General Hospital, UK.)

Fig. 78.4 Atrophy and striae induced by topical steroids. (Courtesy of St John's Institute of Dermatology, London, UK.)

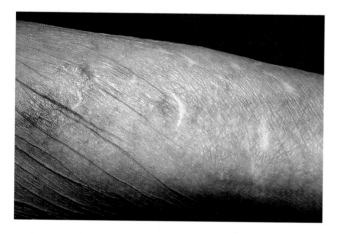

Fig. 78.5 Atrophy and scars induced by topical steroids. (Courtesy of St John's Institute of Dermatology, London, UK.)

ground substance. This results in the formation of striae, and poor support of dermal vasculature leads to easy rupture on trauma or shearing (Fig. 78.4). The resulting intradermal bleeding spreads relatively unimpeded to produce a blot haemorrhage. This resolves with the formation of a stellate scar (Fig. 78.5). The appearance is that of prematurely aged skin.

Vascular effects

These may include the following.
1 Fixed vasodilatation. Corticosteroids at first produce vasoconstriction of the superficial small vessels, followed by a phase of rebound vasodilatation, which in later stages is fixed (Fig. 78.6) [7].

2 Rebound phenomenon. As vasoconstriction wears off, the small vessels overdilate, allowing oedema, enhanced inflammation and sometimes pustulation.

Systemic absorption

Inhibition of the pituitary–adrenal axis by excessive application of moderately potent topical steroids or by relatively modest use of stronger steroids is well documented [8]. Temporary reversible suppression was seen after using 49 g of superpotent steroids per week for 2 weeks [9] in eight out of 40 patients, and similar results were seen in two further studies [10,11]. Significant suppression was reported in three patients using less than 50 g/week [12]. Recommended weekly dosage is less than 50 g of superpotent steroids and 100 g of potent steroids. In addition, prolonged usage at this level is best avoided. Even hydrocortisone applied topically may suppress the adrenocortical response in some children [13]. Cushingoid features may be seen in infants inappropriately treated [14]. Severe medical problems are fortunately rare despite alarmingly abnormal biochemical parameters. Stunting of growth in a child treated with long-term fluorinated steroids has been observed, but the weaker steroids are considered safe in children [15,16].

Posterior subcapsular cataracts and glaucoma [17–19] are other hazards. Allergic contact dermatitis to the steroid molecule may also occur, and may easily be overlooked [20,21].

A number of iatrogenic clinical syndromes have been defined as largely due to the use of topical steroids.
1 Perioral dermatitis (Fig. 78.7).
2 Tinea incognito [22]. Topical steroids reduce the inflammation and itching of tinea without clearing the fungus (Fig. 78.8). The clinical signs of fungal infection are confusingly obscured.
3 Impetigo incognito. Topical corticosteroids may impair the host's immunological response against the infection and obscure other clinical signs of inflammation.

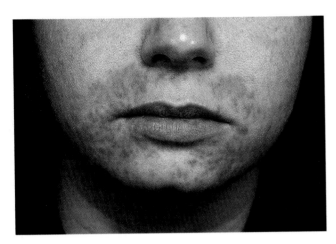

Fig. 78.7 Perioral dermatitis induced by topical steroids. (Courtesy of St John's Institute of Dermatology, London, UK.)

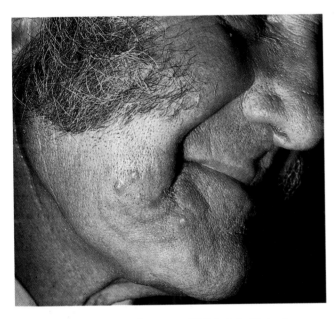

Fig. 78.8 Tinea incognito. (Courtesy of St John's Institute of Dermatology, London, UK.)

4 Infantile gluteal granuloma [23] (Chapter 14). This curious condition is found only in infants who wear napkins (diapers)—an alteration of host response to *Candida* under the influence of steroids has been suggested.

5 Pustular psoriasis. In the UK, topical steroids are used much less than elsewhere for treating chronic plaque psoriasis, because the rebound phenomenon following cessation of treatment or reduction of the amount of topical steroid applied may, in a few patients, be followed by the onset of an acute pustular stage [24–26].

Clinical experience in Europe, where tar and/or dithranol have been used by many dermatologists in preference to topical steroids, suggests that the plaques of psoriasis in a patient treated with topical steroids appear very unstable and less well-defined at the margins, and become more likely to spread as sheets. It is also the authors' experience that patients are less easy to treat subsequently with dithranol than those who have not been treated with topical steroids.

Comedones have been induced by the application of fluorinated steroids to the perianal skin [27]. The symptoms of anogenital pruritus may change to marked soreness under the influence of topical steroids. All cutaneous infections may be exacerbated by the injudicious application of topical steroids [28]. The combination of a steroid with an antibiotic is discussed below.

Precautions

Care should be exercised in prescribing topical steroids, and especially in repeating prescriptions. Plain hydrocortisone 1% is safe to use in most circumstances. The more potent steroids are more hazardous. Facial skin is especially susceptible to steroid damage. The more potent steroids should be reserved for treating severe facial dermatoses such as chronic discoid lupus erythematosus.

Dermatologists have perhaps been too successful in making general practitioners and the public aware of the hazards of topical corticosteroids. Patients are frequently encountered whose dermatosis requires strong steroids but who are denied effective treatment by the inappropriate prescription of hydrocortisone or simple emollients. Public awareness of their potential to produce unwanted side-effects, fostered by reports in the lay press, has led to a reluctance by some to use topical steroids. Such a view is based upon misconceptions stemming from past abuses. The aim should be to encourage the understanding of when and where to use topical steroids safely.

The corticosteroids are assessed for potency on the basis of the vasoconstrictor assay [29], and in clinical trials and atrophogenicity assays [30]. A combination of these and other methods is used to produce a grouping of steroids of roughly equivalent potency. Such groupings are clinically very helpful but can be regarded as only a rough guide [31]. Individual response, the circumstances of use, and occasional reports in the literature of adverse reactions, make the assessment of the relative strengths of topical steroids uncertain.

The classification recommended in the *British National Formulary* contains only four categories of potency, whereas the American classification includes seven groups. The more comprehensive classification provided in the *Monthly Index of Medical Specialities (MIMS)* is widely adopted in the UK. Further discussion is provided by Polano and August [32]. The classification suggested (Table 78.4) is based on the *MIMS* list. More objective assay studies indicate that some degree of reclassification may ultimately be necessary. Children and babies have delicate, easily damaged skin,

Mildly potent	*Potent*
Aclometasone dipropionate 0.05%	Beclomethasone dipropionate 0.025%
Fluocinolone acetonide 0.0025%	Betamethasone dipropionate 0.05%
Hydrocortisone base or acetate 0.1%–2.5%	Betamethasone valerate 0.025%
Hydrocortisone 0.5% with sodium chloride and urea	Betamethasone valerate 0.1%
Methylprednisolone 0.25%	Budesonide 0.025%
	Desoxymethasone 0.25%
Moderately potent	Diflucortolone valerate 0.1%
Clobetasone butyrate 0.05%	Fluclorolone acetonide 0.025%
Desoxymethasone 0.05%	Fluocinolone acetonide 0.025%
Fluocinolone acetonide 0.00625%	Fluocinonide 0.05%
Fluocortonone hexanoate 0.1%	Hydrocortisone 17-butyrate 0.1%
Fluocortolone pivalate 0.1%	Triamcinolone acetonide 0.1%
Fluocortolone 0.25%	
Fluocortolone hexanoate 0.25%	*Very potent*
Flurandrenolone 0.0125%	Clobetasol propionate 0.05%
Flurandrenolone 0.05%	Diflucortolone valerate 0.03%
Hydrocortisone 1% with urea	Halcinonide 0.1%

Table 78.4 A suggested classification of topical steroids according to their potencies.

and because they have a high surface area to body volume may easily show pituitary–adrenal suppression as a result of systemic absorption.

Combinations of steroid–antimicrobial agents [33]

These combinations have not in the past been readily accepted by dermatologists because the broad spectrum of therapeutic activity encourages laxity in diagnosis. Some of the older antimicrobial agents were also notorious topical sensitizers. The flexural areas of the body, for which combination treatments are often advocated, provide conditions in which the likelihood of the occurrence of adverse effects is increased. The case for use of these combinations is much stronger in the treatment of eczemas with evidence of secondary infection, although many dermatologists still prefer to give an antibiotic systemically.

Additives, preservatives, fragrances, stabilizers and antioxidants are components of many topical preparations, and adverse reactions to any of these should be considered in a patient whose dermatosis exacerbates during therapy. True allergy to the steroid itself may also occur [21].

Occlusion and topical corticosteroids

The incorporation of a corticosteroid such as flurandrenolone into the adhesive of a plastic tape with high occlusiveness enhances the potency of the topical steroid by encouraging hydration of the stratum corneum. A similar effect is obtained using polythene gloves, plastic film, or by occlusion with bio-occlusive dressings [30].

Whole-body occlusion was formerly widely used, but adverse effects were so common it fell into disrepute.

Intralesional steroids

A few recalcitrant dermatoses (e.g. nodular prurigo, lichen simplex) may respond to injection of steroid into the lesions. Triamcinolone is often used, but dermal atrophy and leukoderma may occur. Blindness has been reported following intralesional injection of the eyebrow skin [19].

The individual conditions for which topical steroids are used are numerous, and are considered in the relevant sections of this text.

REFERENCES

1 Marshall RC, Du Vivier A. The effects on epidermal DNA synthesis of the butyrate esters of clobetasone and clobetasol and the propionate ester of clobetasol. *Br J Dermatol* 1978; **98**: 355–9.
2 Lesnik RH, Mezick JA, Capetola R *et al*. Topical all-*trans*-retinoic acid prevents corticosteroid-induced skin atrophy without abrogating the anti-inflammatory effect. *J Am Acad Dermatol* 1989; **21**: 186–90.
3 Arnold J, Anthonioz P, Marchand JP. Depigmenting action of corticosteroids. *Dermatologica* 1975; **151**: 274–80.
4 McCormack PG, Ledesma CN, Vaillant JC. Linear hypopigmentation after intra-articular corticosteroid injection. *Arch Dermatol* 1984; **120**: 708–9.
5 Lehman P, Zheng P, Lavker RM. Corticosteroid atrophy in human skin. A study by light, scanning and transmission electron microscopy. *J Invest Dermatol* 1983; **81**: 169–76.
6 Tan CY, Marks R, Payne P. Comparison of xeroradiographic and ultrasound detection of corticosteroid induced dermal thinning. *J Invest Dermatol* 1981; **76**: 126–8.
7 Smith JG, Wehr RF, Chalker DK. Corticosteroid induced cutaneous atrophy and telangiectasia. *Arch Dermatol* 1976; **112**: 1115–17.
8 Cornell RC, Stoughton RB. Six month controlled study of effect of desoximetasone and betamethasone-17-valerate on the pituitary–adrenal axis. *Br J Dermatol* 1981; **105**: 91–5.
9 Katz HI, Hien NT, Prawer SE *et al*. Superpotent topical steroid treatment of psoriasis vulgaris—clinical efficacy and adrenal function. *J Am Acad Dermatol* 1987; **16**: 804–11.
10 Walsh P, Aeling JL, Huff L *et al*. Hypothalamus-pituitary-adrenal axis suppression by superpotent topical steroids. *J Am Acad Dermatol* 1993; **29**: 501–3.
11 Weston WL, Fennessey PV, Morelli J *et al*. Comparison of hypothalamus-pituitary-adrenal axis suppression from superpotent topical steroids by standard

12 Ohman EM, Rogers S, Meenan FO *et al.* Adrenal suppression following low-dose topical clobetasol propionate. *J R Soc Med* 1987; **80**: 422–4.
13 Turpeinen M. Adrenocortical response to adrenocorticotrophic hormone in relation to duration of topical therapy and percutaneous absorption of hydrocortisone in children with dermatitis. *Eur J Paediatr* 1989; **148**: 729–31.
14 Borzykowski M, Grant DB, Wells RS. Cushing's syndrome induced by topical steroids used for the treatment of non-bullous ichthyosiform erythroderma. *Clin Exp Dermatol* 1976; **1**: 337–42.
15 Krafchik BR. The use of topical steroids in children. *Semin Dermatol* 1995; **14**: 70–4.
16 Massarano AA, Hollis S, Devlin J *et al.* Growth in atopic eczema. *Arch Dis Child* 1993; **68**: 677–9.
17 Cubey RB. Glaucoma following the application of corticosteroid to the skin of the eyelids. *Br J Dermatol* 1976; **95**: 207–8.
18 Nielsen NW, Sorensen PN. Glaucoma induced by application of corticosteroids to the periorbital region. *Arch Dermatol* 1978; **114**: 953–4.
19 Zugerman C, Saunders D, Levit F. Glaucoma from topically applied steroids (Letter). *Arch Dermatol* 1976; **112**: 1326.
20 Coh CL. Cross sensitivity to multiple topical corticosteroids. *Contact Dermatitis* 1989; **20**: 65–7.
21 Wilkinson SM, English JS. Hydrocortisone sensitivity: clinical features of fifty-nine cases. *J Am Acad Dermatol* 1992; **27**: 683–7.
22 Ive FA, Marks R. Tinea incognito. *Br Med J* 1968; **iii**: 149–52.
23 Bonifazi E, Garofalo L, Lospalluti M. Granuloma gluteale infantum with atrophic scars: clinical and histological observations in eleven cases. *Clin Exp Dermatol* 1981; **6**: 23–9.
24 Arbiser JL, Grossman K, Kaye E *et al.* Use of short-course class 1 topical glucocorticoid under occlusion for the rapid control of erythrodermic psoriasis. *Arch Dermatol* 1994; **130**: 704–6.
25 Menter A. Occlusion of potent topical steroids. *Arch Dermatol* 1995; **131**: 226–7.
26 Yen A. Occlusion of potent topical steroids. *Arch Dermatol* 1995; **131**: 227.
27 Oliet EJ, Estes SA. Perianal comedones associated with chronic topical fluorinated steroid use (Letter). *J Am Acad Dermatol* 1982; **7**: 407.
28 Marples RR, Rebora A, Kligman AM. Topical steroid–antibiotic combinations. *Arch Dermatol* 1973; **108**: 237–40.
29 McKenzie AW, Stoughton RB. Method for comparing percutaneous absorption of steroids. *Arch Dermatol* 1962; **86**: 608–10.
30 David M, Lowe NJ. Psoriasis therapy: comparative studies with a hydrocolloid dressing, plastic film occlusion and triamcinolone cream. *J Am Acad Dermatol* 1989; **21**: 511–14.
31 Gibson JR, Kirsch J, Darley CR. An attempt to evaluate the relative clinical potencies of various diluted and undiluted proprietary corticosteroid preparations. *Clin Exp Dermatol* 1983; **8**: 489–93.
32 Polano MK, August PJ. Corticosteroids for topical use. In: Polano MK, ed. *Topical Skin Therapeutics*. Edinburgh: Churchill Livingstone, 1984: 112–18.
33 Leyden JJ, Kligman AM. The case for steroid–antibiotic combinations. *Br J Dermatol* 1977; **96**: 179–87.

Topical cytotoxic drugs and immunotherapy

A number of cytotoxic agents have been used topically for the eradication of superficial malignant conditions of the skin. These are discussed in Chapters 36 and 80. The use of these agents in proliferative but benign conditions is considered here.

Azelaic acid

This dicarboxylic acid, derived from *Pityrosporum* yeasts, is used as a depigmenting agent in melasma, postinflammatory hyperpigmentation and lentigo maligna. Azelaic acid 20% is superior to hydroquinone 2% and as effective as hydroquinone 4%. The addition of tretinoin enhances its depigmenting effect [1,2]. It is also useful in mild to moderate acne [3]. It may also prove to have a role as an antimycotic [4,5], and as a topical antimicrobial agent [6].

REFERENCES

1 Breathnach AS. Melanin hyperpigmentation of skin: melasma, topical treatment with azelaic acid, and other therapies. *Cutis* 1996; **57** (Suppl. 1): 36–45.
2 Grimes PE. Melasma. Etiologic and therapeutic considerations. *Arch Dermatol* 1995; **131**: 1453–7.
3 Graupe K, Cunliffe WJ, Gollnick HP *et al.* Efficacy and safety of topical azelaic acid (20% cream): an overview of results from European clinical trials and experimental reports. *Cutis* 1996; **57** (Suppl. 1): 20–35.
4 Brasch J, Friege B. Dicarboxylic acids affect the growth of dermatophytes *in vitro. Acta Derm Venereol (Stockh)* 1994; **74**: 347–50.
5 Brasch J, Christophers E. Azelaic acid has antimycotic properties *in vitro. Dermatology* 1993; **186**: 55–8.
6 Maple PA, Hamilton-Miller JM, Brumfitt W. Comparison of the *in-vitro* activities of the topical antimicrobials azelaic acid, nitrofurazone, silver sulphadiazine and mupirocin against methicillin-resistant *Staphylococcus aureus. J Antimicrob Chemother* 1992; **29**: 661–8.

Bleomycin

A number of reports have appeared on the successful treatment of recalcitrant viral warts with intralesional injections of 0.1% bleomycin [1–3]. Two large, double-blind, placebo-controlled trials gave similar results [2,3]. Seventy-five to ninety-five per cent of warts on the hands and 60% of plantar warts cleared following one to three injections. Local pain is significant, but tolerated by patients who had previously received many unsuccessful treatments.

A 1% solution in dimethyl sulphoxide administered for 5 min over 14 consecutive days reduced the size of lesions and histological appearance of dysplasia in 22 patients with oral leukoplakia [4].

Bleomycin has antitumour, antibacterial and antiviral activity. It binds to DNA, causing strand scission and elimination of pyrimidine and purine bases. The mechanism of action in warts is not yet known. The small volumes used do not cause systemic toxicity. Treatment of a periungual wart resulted in a permanent nail dystrophy [5]. The compound must be handled with care.

REFERENCES

1 Cordero AA, Guglielmi HA, Woscoff A. The common wart: intra-lesional treatment with bleomycin sulfate. *Cutis* 1980; **26**: 319–20.
2 Bunney HH, Nolan MW, Buxton PK *et al.* The treatment of resistant warts with intralesional bleomycin: a controlled clinical trial. *Br J Dermatol* 1984; **110**: 197–207.
3 Shumer SM, O'Keefe EJ. Bleomycin in the treatment of recalcitrant warts. *J Am Acad Dermatol* 1983; **9**: 91–6.
4 Epstein JB, Wong FL, Millner A *et al.* Topical bleomycin treatment of oral leukoplakia: a randomized double-blind clinical trial. *Head Neck* 1994; **16**: 539–44.
5 Miller RAW. Nail dystrophy following intralesional injections of bleomycin for periungual wart. *Arch Dermatol* 1984; **120**: 963–4.

Cyclosporin

Early hopes that the systemically highly effective drug cyclosporin might also be effective topically have in general not been fulfilled. In psoriasis, penetration of the drug is known to occur in sufficient amounts, but it remains ineffective by this route. Penetration-enhancing vehicles failed to influence activity [1–3]. It is not effective in oral lichen planus [4], contact dermatitis [5,6], atopic dermatitis [6], alopecia areata and male-pattern alopecia [7,8]. There are a few reports of benefit in cicatricial pemphigoid [9] and Hailey–Hailey disease [10].

REFERENCES

1 Duncan JI, Wakeel RA, Winfield AJ et al. Immunomodulation of psoriasis with a topical cyclosporin A formulation. *Acta Derm Venereol (Stockh)* 1993; **73**: 84–7.
2 Delfino M, Brunetti B, Fabbrocini G. Topical cyclosporine is ineffective in the treatment of psoriasis. *Int J Dermatol* 1992; **31**: 895.
3 Schulze HJ, Mahrle G, Steigleder GK. Topical cyclosporin A in psoriasis. *Br J Dermatol* 1990; **122**: 113–14.
4 Sieg P, Von Domarus H, Von Zitzewitz V et al. Topical cyclosporin in oral lichen planus: a controlled, randomized, prospective trial. *Br J Dermatol* 1995; **132**: 790–4.
5 Surber C, Itin P, Buchner S et al. Effect of a new topical cyclosporin formulation on human allergic contact dermatitis. *Contact Dermatitis* 1992; **26**: 116–19.
6 De Rie MA, Meinardi MM, Bos JD. Lack of efficacy of topical cyclosporin A in atopic dermatitis and allergic contact dermatitis. *Acta Derm Venereol (Stockh)* 1991; **71**: 452–4.
7 Gilhar A, Pillar T, Etzioni A. Topical cyclosporin A in alopecia areata. *Acta Derm Venereol (Stockh)* 1989; **69**: 252–3.
8 Gilhar A, Pillar T, Etzione A. Topical cyclosporine in male pattern alopecia. *J Am Acad Dermatol* 1990; **22**: 251–3.
9 Azana JM, de Misa RF, Bioxeda JP et al. Topical cyclosporine for cicatricial pemphigoid. *J Am Acad Dermatol* 1993; **28**: 134.
10 Jitsukawa K, Ring J, Weyer U et al. Topical cyclosporine in chronic benign familial pemphigus (Hailey–Hailey disease). *J Am Acad Dermatol* 1992; **27**: 625–6.

Dinitrochlorobenzene, squaric acid and diphencyprone

The potent topical sensitizer dinitrochlorobenzene (DNCB) 0.1% in acetone has been used to treat alopecia areata [1] and viral warts [2–4] by inducing an inflammatory response containing a high proportion of immunocompetent lymphocytes. Doubts over the mutagenicity potential of DNCB led to the use of other agents, such as squaric acid dibutylester [5], *Primula* [6] and diphenylcyclopropenone [7,8]. The reaction in alopecia areata was compared with that induced by a simple irritant, croton oil, which did not induce regrowth of hair [9]. Phenolics, cantharides, camphor and other irritants have been used for many years, mostly without controlled trials [10].

Diphencyprone completely cleared warts in 20 of 44 patients, and a further 17 showed improvement [11]. Squaric acid dibutyl ester cleared warts in 12 of 20 patients [12]. In alopecia areata, diphencyprone produced total hair regrowth in 54 of 139 patients, and a further six showed a partial but cosmetically acceptable regrowth, with a follow-up of 19 months [13]. Squaric acid dibutyl ester was used in 33 children with alopecia totalis or universalis, and complete hair regrowth occurred in 10, of whom seven subsequently had severe relapses [14].

REFERENCES

1 Happle R, Cebulla K, Echternach-Happle K. Dinitrochlorobenzene therapy for alopecia areata. *Arch Dermatol* 1978; **114**: 1629–31.
2 Buckner D, Price NM. Immunotherapy of verrucae vulgares with dinitrochlorobenzene. *Br J Dermatol* 1978; **98**: 451–5.
3 Sanders BB, Smith KW. Dinitrochlorobenzene immunotherapy of human warts. *Cutis* 1981; **27**: 389–92.
4 Weiss VC, West DP. Topical minoxidil therapy and hair regrowth. *Arch Dermatol* 1985; **121**: 191–2.
5 Happle R, Kalveran KJ, Buchner V. Contact allergy as a therapeutic tool for alopecia areata: application of squaric acid dibutylester. *Dermatologica* 1980; **161**: 289–97.
6 Rhodes EL, Dolman W, Kennedy C et al. Alopecia areata regrowth induced by *Primula obconica*. *Br J Dermatol* 1981; **104**: 339–40.
7 Happle R, Hausen BM, Wiesner-Menzel L. Diphencyprone in the treatment of alopecia areata. *Acta Derm Venereol (Stockh)* 1993; **63**: 49–52.
8 Wilkerson MC, Henkin J, Wilkin JK. Diphenylcyclopropenone: examination for potential contaminants, mechanism of sensitization and photochemical stability. *J Am Acad Dermatol* 1984; **11**: 802–7.
9 Swanson NA, Mitchell AJ, Leahy MS et al. Topical treatment of alopecia areata. *Arch Dermatol* 1981; **117**: 384–7.
10 Mitchell AJ, Krull EA. Alopecia areata: pathogenesis and treatment. *J Am Acad Dermatol* 1984; **11**: 763–75.
11 Orrechia G, Douville H, Santagostino L et al. Treatment of multiple relapsing warts with diphencyprone. *Dermatologica* 1988; **177**: 225–31.
12 Iijima A, Otsuka F. Contact immunotherapy with squaric acid dibutylester for warts. *Dermatology* 1993; **187**: 115–18 (erratum 1993; **197**: 314).
13 Van der Steen PH, Boezeman JB, Happle R. Topical immunotherapy for alopecia areata: re-evaluation of 139 cases after an additional follow-up period of 19 months. *Dermatology* 1992; **184**: 198–201.
14 Tosti A, Guidetti MS, Bardazzi F et al. Long-term results of topical immunotherapy in children with alopecia totalis or alopecia universalis. *J Am Acad Dermatol* 1996; **35**: 199–201.

5-Fluorouracil [1,2]

In the form of a 5% cream, this is a very effective treatment for multiple solar keratoses. Lesions on the scalp and face respond more readily than lesions on the limbs. The cream is applied twice a day for 2 weeks. A brisk inflammatory response should occur within the keratoses, otherwise clearing is incomplete. Severe ulcerative reactions occur in a few patients. Combination with a fluorinated steroid has been shown to limit the intensity of the inflammatory response without reducing the efficacy of the 5-fluorouracil [3]. Some patients require longer periods of treatment, and others are cleared only by occlusion of the agent with polyethylene film. The complications of treatment have been reviewed [4].

5-Fluorouracil works well in Bowen's disease, extramammary Paget's disease [5] and superficial genital neoplasia and preneoplasia. It proved successful in reducing the number of lesions appearing in the basal cell naevus syndrome [6]. It has a limited role in the treatment of viral warts [7]. It has been used with variable results in naevoid keratotic conditions including Darier's disease [8], and in superficial actinic porokeratosis.

REFERENCES

1 Goette DK. Topical chemotherapy with 5-fluorouracil. A review. *J Am Acad Dermatol* 1981; **4**: 633–49.
2 Jansen GT. Commentary: use of topical fluorouracil. *Arch Dermatol* 1983; **119**: 784–5.
3 Breza T, Taylor R, Eaglestein WH. Non-inflammatory destruction of actinic keratoses by fluorouracil. *Arch Dermatol* 1977; **112**: 1256–8.
4 Kurtis B, Rosen T. Squamous cell carcinoma arising in a basal cell epithelioma treated with 5-fluorouracil. *J Dermatol Surg Oncol* 1979; **5**: 394–6.
5 Bewley AP, Bracka A, Staughton RC *et al.* Extramammary Paget's disease of the scrotum: treatment with topical 5-fluorouracil and plastic surgery. *Br J Dermatol* 1994; **131**: 445–6.
6 Strange PR, Lang PG, Jr. Long-term management of basal cell nevus syndrome with topical tretinoin and 5-fluorouracil. *J Am Acad Dermatol* 1992; **27**: 842–5.
7 Senff H, Reinel D, Matthies C *et al.* Topical 5-fluorouracil solution in the treatment of warts—clinical experience and percutaneous absorption. *Br J Dermatol* 1988; **118**: 409–14.
8 Knulst AC, De La Faille HB, Van Vloten WA. Topical 5-fluorouracil in the treatment of Darier's disease. *Br J Dermatol* 1995; **133**: 463–6.

Methotrexate. Poor penetration of topical methotrexate limits its usefulness in psoriasis. Improved results have been reported when methotrexate is used with a penetration enhancer [1,2].

REFERENCES

1 Weinstein CD, McCulloch JL, Olsen E. Topical methotrexate therapy for psoriasis. *Arch Dermatol* 1989; **125**: 227–30.
2 Ball MA, McCullough JL, Weinstein GD. Percutaneous absorption of methotrexate: effect on epidermal DNA synthesis in hairless mice. *J Invest Dermatol* 1982; **79**: 7–10.

Podophyllin [1]

This is an extract of the dried rhizome and the roots of *Podophyllum peltatum* (North America) or of *Podophyllum emodi* (India), commonly known as the mandrake or Mayapple. The chief constituents of the resin are lignans, which are C_{18} compounds. The most important ones are podophyllotoxin and β-peltatin. Podophyllin resin 10–40%, depending on the source, is available in various vehicles such as compound benzoin tincture, alcohol or flexible collodion, and is effective in clearing anogenital warts. Three batches of 20% podophyllin were analysed by high-performance liquid chromatography (HPLC) and were found to contain quercetin 2.5–3.8% and kaempherol 6.0–6.4% of dry substance. In comparison, podophyllotoxin consists of 12.7–13.8% of podophyllin dry substance. As these two constituents represent 10% of the dry weight of podophyllin 20% the authors suggest that extraction and purification may lead to a more effective preparation [2].

It should not be used on the buccal mucosa or tongue, or in pregnancy [3]. Adverse reactions include polyneuropathy, coma, urticaria, leukopenia and thrombocytopenia. Severe ulcerative local reactions are not uncommon, and a test dose of 5–10% washed off after 1h is an advisable precaution. A newer, low-concentration podophyllotoxin is available for the patient's own use [4]. In one study, 82% of warts were cleared in 6 weeks [5]. The cytotoxic effect may cause confusion in the histological interpretation of biopsy material from treated warts.

REFERENCES

1 Trease GE, Evans WC. Podophyllum and podophyllum resins. In: *Pharmacognosy*, 12th edn. London: Bailliére Tindall, 1983: 643–7.
2 Petersen CS, Weismann K. Quercetin and kaempherol: an argument against the use of podophyllin? *Genitourin Med* 1995; **71**: 92–3.
3 Fisher AA. Severe systemic and local reactions to topical *Podophyllum* resin. *Cutis* 1981; **28**: 233–6 and 242 *passim*.
4 Von Krogh C. Topical self-treatment of penile warts with a 0.5% podophyllin in ethanol for 4–5 days. *Sex Transm Dis* 1987; **14**: 135–40.
5 Bentner KR, Conant MA, Friedman-Kien AE *et al.* Patient applied podophyllin for the treatment of genital warts. *Lancet* 1989; **i**: 831–4.

Tacrolimus

Tacrolimus is a macrolide antibiotic produced by *Streptomyces tsukubaensis* which has potent T-cell-specific immuno-suppressant activity [1]. At the cellular level, its effects are similar to cyclosporin A, but it penetrates skin better than cyclosporin A, perhaps because of its lower molecular weight [2]. Tacrolimus strongly inhibits interleukin 2 (IL-2) production, without a prominent effect on IL-2 responsiveness [3], and inhibits IL-5 induction *in vitro* [4]. It is effective in psoriasis when given systemically [5]. These properties make it a very promising topical agent in dermatology. Preliminary trials of its topical use have been reported in psoriasis [6], skin grafting [7], allergic contact dermatitis [3,8], atopy [4,9], and stimulation of anagen hair growth in mice [1,10,11].

REFERENCES

1 Yamamoto S, Jiang H, Kato R. Stimulation of hair growth by topical application of FK506, a potent immunosuppressive agent. *J Invest Dermatol* 1994; **102**: 160–4.
2 Lauerma AI, Maibach HI. Topical FK506—clinical potential or laboratory curiosity? *Dermatology* 1994; **188**: 173–6.
3 Furue M, Osada A, Chang CH *et al.* Immunosuppressive effects of azelastine hydrochloride on contact hypersensitivity and T-cell proliferative response: a comparative study with FK506. *J Invest Dermatol* 1994; **103**: 49–53.
4 Mori A, Suo M, Nishizaki Y *et al.* Regulation of interleukin-5 production by peripheral blood mononuclear cells from atopic patients with FK506, cyclosporin A and glucocorticoid. *Int Arch Allergy Immunol* 1994; **104** (Suppl.1): 32–5.
5 Jegasothy BV, Ackerman CD, Todo S *et al.* Tacrolimus (FK506)—a new therapeutic agent for severe recalcitrant psoriasis. *Arch Dermato* 1992; **128**: 781–5.
6 Rappersberger K, Meingassner JG, Fialla R *et al.* Clearing of psoriasis by a novel immunosuppressive macrolide. *J Invest Dermatol* 1996; **106**: 701–10.
7 Yuzawa K, Taniguchi H, Seino K *et al.* Topical immunosuppression in skin grafting with FK506 ointment. *Transplant Proc* 1996; **28**: 137–9.
8 Funk JO, Maibach HI. Horizons in pharmacologic intervention in allergic contact dermatitis. *J Am Acad Dermatol* 1994; **31**: 999–1014.
9 Nakagawa H, Etoh T, Ishibashi Y *et al.* Tacrolimus ointment for atopic dermatitis. *Lancet* 1994; **344**: 883.
10 Iwabuchi T, Maruyama T, Sei Y *et al.* Effects of immunosuppressive peptidyl-prolyl *cis-trans* isomerase (PPIase) inhibitors, cyclosporin A, FK506, ascomycin and rapamycin, on hair growth initiation in mouse: immunosuppression is not required for new hair growth. *J Dermatol Sci* 1995; **9**: 64–9.
11 Jiang H, Yamamoto S, Kato R. Induction of anagen in telogen mouse skin by topical application of FK506, a potent immunosuppressant. *J Invest Dermatol* 1995; **104**: 523–5.

Miscellaneous agents

Minoxidil

Topical 2% minoxidil has been used over the last decade for androgenetic alopecia in females and male-pattern alopecia in males. It has been used to a lesser extent in alopecia areata. To summarize the data, the effect is positive but not impressive. In a double-blind multicentre trial in the USA, 256 females with androgenetic alopecia were treated for 32 weeks. They obtained a mean increase in non-vellus hairs of $23/cm^2$ compared with $11/cm^2$ in the placebo group. Objective assessment reported 13% with moderate and 50% with minimum regrowth, whereas the patients' assessment was more optimistic, with 60% in the active group reporting regrowth and 40% in the placebo group [1]. In a similar European trial involving 294 patients, there was an increase in non-vellus hair of $33/cm^2$ in the active group and $19/cm^2$ in the placebo group [2]. Objective assessment in an Australian trial showed that only 12% had moderate regrowth in a 48-week period [3]. More accurate assessment is claimed by weighing the hair growing from a given area over a period of time [4]. In a follow-up study over 5 years, hair regrowth tended to peak at 1 year, with a slow decline in regrowth over subsequent years. However, at $4\frac{1}{2}$ –5 years, maintenance of non-vellus hairs beyond that seen at baseline was still evident [5].

REFERENCES

1 DeVillez RL, Jacobs JP, Szpunar CA *et al*. Androgenetic alopecia in the female. Treatment with 2% minoxidil solution. *Arch Dermatol* 1994; **130**: 303–7.
2 Jacobs JP, Szpunar CA, Warner ML. Use of topical minoxidil therapy for androgenetic alopecia in women. *Int J Dermatol* 1993; **32**: 758–62.
3 Connors TJ, Cooke DE, De Launey WE *et al*. Australasian trial of topical minoxidil and placebo in early male pattern baldness. *Australas J Dermatol* 1990; **31**: 17–25.
4 Price VH, Menefee E. Quantitative estimation of hair growth. I. Androgenetic alopecia in women: effect of minoxidil. *J Invest Dermatol* 1990; **95**: 683–7.
5 Olsen EA, Weiner MS, Amara IA *et al*. Five-year follow-up of men with androgenetic alopecia treated with topical minoxidil. *J Am Acad Dermatol* 1990; **22**: 643–6.

Nicotinamide [1]

The marked anti-inflammatory properties of topical nicotinamide, the amide derivative of vitamin B_3 (niacin), have been used to treat acne vulgaris. A 4% alcoholic gel is available. It is not yet certain by what mechanism the preparation exerts its anti-inflammatory effect. In a multicentre trial, it gave a global reduction in acne of 82% compared with 68% for 1% clindamycin gel over an 8-week period. An advantage of nicotinamide is that the problem of antibiotic resistance does not arise.

REFERENCE

1 Shalita AR, Smith JG, Parish LC *et al*. Topical nicotinamide compared with clindamycin gel in the treatment of inflammatory acne vulgaris. *Int J Dermatol* 1995; **34**: 434–7.

Vitamin A acid

SYN. TRETINOIN; ALL-*TRANS*-RETINOIC ACID

Vitamin A has been used topically for over 20 years but originally in the form of the alcohol or ester.

Mode of action. Topical application of all-*trans*-retinoic acid is followed by partial isomerization to 9-*cis*- and 13-*cis*-retinoic acid [1]. Different isomers vary in activity, but have similar effects on the epidermis [2]. The main action is restoration of normal keratinization in conditions in which this is disturbed. It enhances DNA synthesis in the germinative epithelium and increases the mitotic rate. It also has a regulating effect on epidermal cell differentiation, leading to a thickening of the granular layer and a normalization of parakeratosis.

Binding proteins for retinoids are widely distributed throughout the body in many cell types. Cellular retinoic acid binding protein II (CRABP-II) predominates in skin, and is found in keratinocytes and fibroblasts. Following transport to the nucleus, retinoid binds to retinoic acid receptors (RAR) and retinoid X receptor (RXR). Receptor interaction with DNA response elements stimulates promoter regions to induce transcriptional and translational activity. The resultant protein synthesis can in turn mediate structural and functional activity of cells, and modulate transcription of other genes [3].

Electron microscopy studies have shown replacement of disorganized dermal collagen fibres, an increase in viable epidermal thickness, and a return to a more uniform size and electron density of the basal and spinous keratinocytes. These changes occurred in both photodamaged and intrinsically aged non-photodamaged skin. At least 6 months of treatment was required [4,5]. The predominance of one or other of these effects depends on the concentration used. Much of the difficulty encountered in assessing the preparation in practice stems from this, and from the erythema and irritancy that higher concentrations may produce.

Uses. Vitamin A acid has been used for a number of skin disorders characterized by follicular plugging, parakeratosis and hyperkeratosis, and as a treatment intended partially to reverse the changes associated with sun-induced skin ageing [6].

Acne. The pre-eminent use of topical vitamin A acid is in the treatment of acne. Numerous reports attest to its value [7,8]. It is normally applied at a concentration of 0.025–0.5% in a lotion, cream or gel (although stronger preparations have been tolerated in dark-skinned races). After an initial exacerbation [9], it causes softening and expulsion of comedones in 3–4 weeks, and will prevent these reforming if its use is continued. Neither erythema nor peeling are necessary for this to be achieved [10]. It is also effective in steroid-induced acne and other acneiform eruptions. Topical isotretinoin 0.05% gel has also been shown to be effective in acne [11]. Adapalene is a synthetic retinoid with similar therapeutic efficacy to isotretinoin, which produces less irritation than all-*trans*-retinoic acid [12].

Psoriasis. Despite theoretical indications of potential value, local applications of vitamin A acid have not been particularly impressive in their effect on psoriasis [13]. Tazarotene is the first of a new generation of topical receptor-selective acetylenic retinoids which has been shown to modulate the three main pathological characteristics of psoriasis: keratinocyte hyperproliferation, abnormal keratinocyte differentiation and infiltration of inflammatory cells into the skin [14].

Skin cancer/solar ageing. Tretinoin has both a therapeutic and prophylactic effect on chemically induced skin tumours, and may be both a promoter and inhibitor of UVB carcinogenesis. Clinically, it appears to have a mainly antineoplastic effect, and may be used to treat small solar keratoses [15]. It also has a 'normalizing' effect on the histological appearance of dysplastic naevi [16]. Topical all-*trans*-retinoic acid and 13-*cis*-retinoic acid improve the features of photoageing [17–19]. Accompanying these clinical changes is histological evidence of epidermal hyperproliferation, stratum corneum compaction, deposition of glycosaminoglycans in all layers of the epidermis and reduced levels of epidermal melanin [20].

Other conditions. A number of other conditions have been treated with varying success. It is of value in the treatment of senile comedones. Comedo and warty naevi also show some response, as may plane warts and reactive perforating collagenosis.

Darier's disease was an obvious candidate for vitamin A therapy in topical form. Some cases do respond, especially if mild or localized. Keratosis pilaris responds better to topical vitamin A than to other measures. Of the ichthyoses, the lamellar variety appears to be helped most, although ichthyosis vulgaris was also responsive in a four-centre trial [21], as was erythrokeratoderma variabilis [22].

Vitamin A acid has been used with success in lichen planus, but we have not found it of practical value except in oral lesions [23], where it is surprisingly well tolerated. Similar observations have been made on its usefulness in geographic tongue, a disorder which has always been a therapeutic challenge [24].

Fox–Fordyce disease (apocrine miliaria) has been effectively treated with a 0.1% solution [25]. Hydrocortisone cream (1%) has been recommended to control the associated axillary discomfort [26]. Hypertrophic scars and keloids have been reported to respond to a daily application of a 0.05% solution [27,28].

The ability of topical all-*trans*-retinoic acid to decrease epidermal melanin without melanocyte loss has resulted in its application as a depigmenting agent [29]. Melasma has been bleached successfully with a combination of vitamin A acid 0.1%, hydroquinone 5% and dexamethasone 0.1% in a fatty acid propylene glycol base, applied daily to affected areas [30], but treatment should be limited to 6 months to avoid hydroquinone-induced pseudo-ochronosis. Similar good results have been obtained using 2% hydroquinone plus 0.1% tretinoin in equal parts propylene glycol/ethyl alcohol [29].

Sensitization. Despite very widespread use, the risk of sensitization seems to be very small, although it may be masked by irritant reactions [31,32].

REFERENCES

1 MacKenzie RM, Hellwege DM, McGregor ML *et al.* Separation and identification of geometric isomers of retinoic acid and methyl retinoate. *J Chromatogr* 1978; **155**: 379–87.
2 Spearman RIC, Jarrett A. Biological comparison of isomers and chemical forms of vitamin A (retinol). *Br J Dermatol* 1974; **90**: 553–60.
3 Craven NM, Griffiths CEM. Topical retinoids and cutaneous biology. *Clin Exp Dermatol* 1996; **21**: 1–10.
4 Yamamoto O, Bhawan J, Solars G *et al.* Ultrastructural effects of topical tretinoin on dermo-epidermal junction and papillary dermis in photodamaged skin. A controlled study. *Exp Dermatol* 1995; **4**: 146–54.
5 Kligman AM, Dogadkina D, Lavker RM. Effects of topical tretinoin on non-sun-exposed protected skin of the elderly. *J Am Acad Dermatol* 1993; **29**: 25–33.
6 Weiss JS, Ellis CN, Headington JT *et al.* Topical tretinoin improves photoaged skin. A double-blind vehicle-controlled study. *JAMA* 1988; **259**: 527–32.
7 Shalita A, Weiss JS, Chalker DK *et al.* A comparison of the efficacy and safety of adapalene gel 0.1% and tretinoin gel 0.025% in the treatment of acne vulgaris: a multicenter trial. *J Am Acad Dermatol* 1996; **34**: 482–5.
8 Elbaum DJ. Comparison of the stability of topical isotretinoin and topical tretinoin and their efficacy in acne. *J Am Acad Dermatol* 1988; **19**: 486–91.
9 Kligman AM. Effect of all-*trans*-retinoic acid on the dermis of hairless mice. *J Am Acad Dermatol* 1986; **15**: 779–85.
10 Gunther S. Vitamin-A acid in acne vulgaris: association between effect and improvement. *Dermatol Wochenschr* 1974; **160**: 215–18.
11 Chalker DK, Leisher JL, Graham Smith J, Jr *et al.* Efficacy of topical isotretinoin 0.05% gel in acne vulgaris: results of a multicenter double-blind investigation. *J Am Acad Dermatol* 1987; **17**: 251–4.
12 Griffiths CEM, Elder JT, Bernard BA *et al.* Comparison of CD271 (adapalene) and all-*trans* retinoic acid in human skin: dissociation of epidermal effects and CRABP II m-RNA expression. *J Invest Dermatol* 1993; **101**: 325–8.
13 Gunther S. The therapeutic value of retinoic acid in chronic discoid, acute guttate and erythrodermic psoriasis: clinical observations on twenty-five patients. *Br J Dermatol* 1973; **89**: 515–17.
14 Esgleyes-Ribot T, Chandaratna RA, Lew-Kaya DA *et al.* Response of psoriasis to a new topical retinoic acid AGN 190168. *J Am Acad Dermatol* 1994; **30**: 581–90.
15 Epstein JH. All-*trans*-retinoic acid and cutaneous cancers. *J Am Acad Dermatol* 1986; **15**: 772–8.
16 Meyskens FL, Jr, Edwards L, Levine MS. Role of topical tretinoin in melanoma and dysplastic naevi. *J Am Acad Dermatol* 1986; **15**: 822–5.
17 Kligman AM, Grove GL, Hirose RL *et al.* Topical tretinoin for photodamaged skin. *J Am Acad Dermatol* 1986; **15**: 836–59.
18 Kligman AM, Leyden JJ. Treatment of photoaged skin with topical tretinoin. *Skin Pharmacol* 1993; **6** (Suppl. 1): 78–82.

19 Green LJ, McCormick A, Weinstein GD. Photoaging and the skin. The effects of tretinoin. *Dermatol Clin* 1993; **11**: 97–105.

20 Bhawan J, Gonzales-Serva A, Nehal K *et al.* Effects of tretinoin on photo-damaged skin. A histologic study. *Arch Dermatol* 1991; **127**: 666–72.

21 Muller SA, Belcher RW, Esterley NB. Keratinizing dermatoses. *Arch Dermatol* 1977; **113**: 1052–4.

22 Van der Wateren AR, Cormane RH. Oral retinoic acid as therapy for erythro-keratoderma variabilis. *Br J Dermatol* 1977; **97**: 83–5.

23 Gunther S. Vitamin-A acid in treatment of oral lichen planus. *Arch Dermatol* 1973; **107**: 277.

24 Helfman RJ. The treatment of geographic tongue with topical retinoic acid. *Cutis* 1979; **24**: 179.

25 Tkach JR. Tretinoin treatment of Fox–Fordyce disease (Letter). *Arch Dermatol* 1979; **15**: 1285.

26 Giacobetti R, Caro WA, Roenigk JR. Fox–Fordyce disease—control with tretinoin cream. *Arch Dermatol* 1979; **115**: 1365–6.

27 Janssen De Limpens AMP. The local treatment of hypertrophic scars and keloids with topical retinoic acid. *Br J Dermatol* 1980; **103**: 319–23.

28 Panagerie-Castaings H. Retinoic acid in the treatment of keloids. *J Dermatol Surg Oncol* 1988; **14**: 1275–6.

29 Pathak MA, Fitzpatrick TB, Kraus EW. Usefulness of retinoic acid in the treatment of melasma. *J Am Acad Dermatol* 1986; **15**: 894–9.

30 Kligman AM, Willis I. A new formula for depigmenting the human skin. *Arch Dermatol* 1975; **111**: 40–8.

31 Tomb R, Dolfus A, Couppie P. Eczema par allergie de contact à la tretinoine. *Ann Dermatol Vénéréol* 1992; **119**: 761–4.

32 Lindgren S, Groth O, Molin L. Allergic contact response to vitamin A acid. *Contact Dermatitis* 1976; **2**: 212–17.

Depigmenting agents [1,2]

There is a need for a safe, non-toxic, depigmenting agent for patients with melasma and postinflammatory hyper-pigmentation. Mercury, once widely used, persists as a 'folklore' remedy in 'skin-bleach' creams, but legislation is eliminating its use in most countries. The daily uptake from absorption following topical application has been calculated as 20 times that taken in food [3]. A case of membranous nephropathy has been reported [4].

Current treatment mainly consists of hydroquinone alone in a 2–4% concentration, or in combination with 0.025% retinoic acid [5]. The addition of a weak topical steroid reduces the irritant effect [6]. Hydroquinone is unstable and rapidly darkens, making it difficult to use. The addition of buthionine sulfoximine to hydroquinone has an enhancing effect on the depigmentation [7]. Irritation is not infrequent, and exogenous ochronosis, characterized by darkening of the treated area [8], and pigmented colloid milium [9], have been reported. The use of monobenzyl ether of hydroquinone is now largely restricted to depigmenting the remaining pigmented areas in patients with extensive vitiligo. The depigmentation produced was believed to be permanent, but cases of repigmentation have been recorded [10]. Controversy exists as to whether azelaic acid has a depigmenting effect on the skin [11–13]. Newer agents under investigation are promising. These include N-acetyl-4-S-cysteaminylphenol (N-Ac-4-S-CAP), which produces reversible depigmentation in the Yucatan pig model [14,15]. In one report of its use in melasma, 8% of patients showed complete depigmentation, 66% marked improvement, and 25% moderate improvement [16].

REFERENCES

1 Benmaman O, Sanchez JL. Treatment and camouflaging of pigmentary disorders. *Clin Dermatol* 1988; **6**: 50–61.

2 Engasser PC, Maibach HI. Cosmetic dermatology: bleaching creams. *J Am Acad Dermatol* 1981; **5**: 143–7.

3 Marzulli FN, Brown DWC. Potential systemic hazards of topically applied mercurials. *J Soc Cosmet Chem* 1972; **23**: 875–86.

4 Kibukamusoke JW, Davies DR, Hutt MSR. Membranous nephropathy due to skin-lightening cream. *Br Med J* 1974; **ii**: 646–7.

5 Pathak MA, Fitzpatrick TB, Kraus EW. Usefulness of retinoic acid in the treatment of melasma. *J Am Acad Dermatol* 1986; **15**: 894–9.

6 Kligman AM, Willis I. A new formula for depigmenting human skin. *Arch Dermatol* 1975; **111**: 40–8.

7 Bolognia JL, Sodi SA, Osber MP *et al.* Enhancement of the depigmenting effect of hydroquinone by cystamine and buthionine sulfoximine. *Br J Dermatol* 1995; **133**: 349–57.

8 Hardwick N, van Celder LW, van der Merwe CA *et al.* Exogenous ochronosis: an epidemiological study. *Br J Dermatol* 1989; **120**: 229–38.

9 Findlay CH, Morrison JCL, Simson IW. Exogenous ochronosis and pigmented colloid milium from hydroquinone bleaching creams. *Br J Dermatol* 1975; **93**: 613–22.

10 Oakley AM. Rapid repigmentation after depigmentation therapy: vitiligo treated with monobenzyl ether of hydroquinone. *Australas J Dermatol* 1996; **37**: 96–8.

11 Duteil L, Ortonne JP. Colorimetric assessment of the effects of azelaic acid on light-induced skin pigmentation. *Photodermatol Photoimmunol Photomed* 1992; **9**: 67–71.

12 Nazzaro-Porro M, Zina G, Breathnach AS. The depigmenting effect of azelaic acid (Letter). *Arch Dermatol* 1990; **126**: 1649–50.

13 Wilderson MG. The depigmenting effect of azelaic acid. *Arch Dermatol* 1990; **126**: 1650–1.

14 Jimbow M, Marusyk H, Jimbow K. The *in vivo* melanocytotoxicity and depigmenting potency of N-2,4-acetoxyphenyl thioethyl acetamide in the skin and hair. *Br J Dermatol* 1995; **133**: 526–36.

15 Alena F, Dixon W, Thomas P *et al.* Glutathione plays a key role in the depigmenting and melanocytotoxic action of N-acetyl-4-S-cysteaminylphenol in black and yellow hair follicles. *J Invest Dermatol* 1995; **104**: 792–7.

16 Jimbow K. N-acetyl-4-S-cysteaminylphenol as a new type of depigmenting agent for the melanoderma of patients with melasma. *Arch Dermatol* 1991; **127**: 1528–34.

Antiperspirants [1]

Aluminium salts have long been used for topical control of hyperhidrosis. Weaker preparations are rarely helpful for the more severely affected patient. A series of papers [2–5] demonstrated the effectiveness of 20% aluminium chloride hexahydrate in absolute alcohol applied under occlusion at night, provided the skin is thoroughly dried before application. The mechanism of action is probably by inducing blockage of the sweat ducts [2,6]. Irritation can be a problem, but usually responds to a weak to medium-strength topical steroid and reduced frequency of application. Anhydrous aluminium chloride 6.25% has also been used in the treatment of acne [7].

Aldehydes have a similar mode of action. Aqueous glutaraldehyde solution (10%) can be applied on a swab to the soles of the feet [8,9]. The keratin stains orange–brown. Formaldehyde Solution BP (1–3%), used as a twice-daily soak, helps mild cases. Both are frequent sensitizers, and may be unsuitable for prolonged use.

Zinc, starch and talc dusting powder dries moist skin by adsorption and absorption. The formulation also provides some measure of lubrication of the surfaces. Too much starch in the formulation risks the formation of cement-like particles with an effect opposite to that intended. Most over-the-counter antiperspirant preparations contain aluminium chlorhydroxide. Some also contain antiseptic agents, such as triclosan, zinc phenol-sulphonate or quaternary ammonium preparations. Fragrances are usually included. These preparations should not be applied to recently shaved skin.

Anticholinergic agents are best applied topically to minimize systemic side-effects. Poldine methylsulphate [10] and glycopyrronium bromide [11] can be very effective for up to 1 month. The latter has fewer central effects than atropine, but some difficulty in swallowing and in visual accommodation is usual for 24–48h following treatment. They are administered by iontophoresis. Iontophoresis of tap water is also effective, by an unknown mechanism [12, 13] that does not appear to be due to ductal occlusion. Glycopyrrolate cream 2% or lotion has been used with success in patients suffering from severe gustatory sweating following parotidectomy [14].

Surgical treatments are considered in Chapter 43.

REFERENCES

1 Walder D, Penneys NS. Antiperspirants and deodorizers. *Clin Dermatol* 1988; **6**: 29–36.
2 Holzle E, Kligman AM. Mechanism of antiperspirant action of aluminium salts. *Br J Dermatol* 1979; **30**: 279–95.
3 Papa CM, Kligman AM. Mechanisms of eccrine anidrosis: II. The antiperspirant effects of aluminium salts. *J Invest Dermatol* 1967; **49**: 139–45.
4 Shelley WB, Hurley KJ. The allergic origin of zirconium deodorant granulomas. *Br J Dermatol* 1958; **70**: 75–101.
5 Shelley WB, Hurley HJ, Jr. Studies on topical antiperspirant control of axillary hyperhidrosis. *Acta Derm Venereol (Stockh)* 1975; **55**: 241–60.
6 Holzle E, Kligman AM. The pathogenesis of miliaria rubra. Role of the resident microflora. *Br J Dermatol* 1978; **99**: 117–37.
7 Hjorth N, Storm D, Dela K. Topical anhydrous aluminium chloride formulation in the treatment of acne vulgaris: a double-blind study. *Cutis* 1985; **35**: 499–500.
8 Juhlin L. Topical glutaraldehyde for plantar hyperhidrosis. *Arch Dermatol* 1968; **97**: 327–30.
9 Sato K, Dobson RL. Mechanism of the antiperspirant effect of topical glutaraldehyde. *Arch Dermatol* 1969; **100**: 564–9.
10 Hill BHR. Poldine iontophoresis in the treatment of palmar and plantar hyperhidrosis. *Aust J Dermatol* 1976; **17**: 92–3.
11 Abell E, Morgan K. The treatment of idiopathic hyperhidrosis by glycopyrrhonium bromide and tapwater iontophoresis. *Br J Dermatol* 1974; **911**: 87–91.
12 Grice K, Sattar H, Baker H. Treatment of idiopathic hyperhidrosis with iontophoresis of tap water and poldine methosulphate. *Br J Dermatol* 1972; **86**: 72–8.
13 Shrivastava SN, Singh G. Tap water iontophoresis in palmoplantar hyperhidrosis. *Br J Dermatol* 1977; **96**: 189–95.
14 May JS, McGuirt WF. Frey's syndrome: treatment with topical glycopyrrolate. *Head Neck* 1989; **11**: 85–9.

Epilatories and depilatories [1,2]

Epilation refers to complete removal of the hair from the follicle, depilation to removal of the hair at the skin level [3]. Epilation can be brought about only by plucking or wax epilatories. These are based on resin and beeswax.

X-rays in a dose sufficient to cause permanent epilation should always be condemned. Electrolysis and short-wave diathermy destruction of individual hairs can, in skilled hands [4], be very effective, but may otherwise cause pitting. Focal postinflammatory pigmentation is troublesome in black and Latin skins. As vellus hair-follicle density on the face is approximately $400/cm^2$ and about 100 hairs are usually treated at one sitting, treatment may have to be prolonged. Some patients find local pain unbearable. Local anaesthesia may be necessary.

Depilatory creams depend upon breaking the disulphide bonds in hair. Three main classes are currently used. The oldest are various sulphides, which have a powerful effect but may irritate, and in the presence of water generate hydrogen sulphide which has an unpleasant odour. Strontium or barium sulphide 20% (for instance in a talc, methylcellulose, glycerine and water base) are widely used. They are effective on the terminal hair in the axillae.

Thioglycollates are being used more frequently, but they are slower to work than sulphides. Concentrations of 2.5–4% produce an effect in 5–15 minutes.

Substituted mercaptans (thioalcohols) are most widely used. They work slowly, but are suitable for use on the face.

Bleaching with 10–20 vol. hydrogen peroxide and sufficient ammonia to turn litmus blue is a simple and safe alternative to these measures.

REFERENCES

1 Harry RG. Depilatories. In: Wilkinson JB, Moore RJ, eds. *Harry's Cosmeticology*, 7th edn. Singapore: Longman, 1982: 142–55.
2 Klein AE, Rish DC. Depilatory and shaving products. *Clin Dermatol* 1978; **6**: 68–70.
3 Spoor HJ. Depilation and epilation. *Cutis* 1978; **21**: 283–7.
4 Callant A. *Principles and Techniques for the Electrologist.* Cheltenham: Stanley Thorne, 1983.

Insect repellents and parasiticides [1–5]

These are also discussed in Chapter 33.

Repellents

Despite considerable research in recent years, the ideal repellent has not yet been discovered. It must combine seemingly opposed qualities—persistence on the skin, sustained volatility and lack of toxicity [2]. A high ambient temperature, washing and sweating, clothing friction and exercise all limit effectiveness [2,6], but the most important factor remains the variability of individual 'attractiveness' to mosquitoes. Many factors have been studied that increase the attractiveness of an individual to the bites of insects, and they vary with the insect species. They include ambient level of carbon dioxide, probably exhaled rather than from the skin, sweat, particularly that produced below the waist, age and gender [7]. An Australian study revealed that patients with eczema believed that they were much more prone to be bitten by insects than individuals without eczema (30% versus 8%) [8]. The interested reader is recommended to consult the recent comprehensive review by Combemale *et al.* [1], from which the following notes and recommendations are largely drawn.

The ideal of a systemic insect repellent has not been realized. Ultrasound devices worn by the subject are ineffective. There are two categories of topical repellents. Natural products, mostly essential oils, such as oil of citronella or spike lavender, have been used for centuries and have a weak protective effect. They are prone to produce contact dermatitis and photocontact dermatitis [9].

The insecticide pyrethrin is weakly repellent.

Synthetic insect repellents comprise amides, imides, alcohols and phenols. The most potent is diethyl toluamide (DEET). These products are thought to be non-teratogenic, non-carcinogenic and non-mutagenic, but data are very limited, especially for 35/35, the most recent addition.

Dimethyl phthalate (DMP). Mean duration of protection is 90 min, and the recommended concentration is 40%.

2-ethyl hexanediol. Mean duration of protection is 1.8 h, and optimal concentration is 30–50%. Weak concentrations may actually attract insects. Irritancy and a burning sensation may occur.

Diethyl toluamide. Mean duration of protection is 4.2 h, which can be increased to 4–6 weeks by impregnating clothing. Optimal concentration is 35–50%. In addition to the toluamide, succinamate and benzamide derivatives are sometimes used. The addition of polymers to reduce volatility may prolong the efficacy. Toxic encephalopathy has been reported in young children, with two deaths.

N-butyl-N-acetyl-3-ethylaminopropionate (35/35) is being used increasingly, but data relating to it are limited. Mean duration of protection is 6 h, and the optimal concentration is 20%.

Indalone and MGK repellents are used in a few products.

DEET protects poorly against *Anopheles*, whereas ethyl hexanediol, which is very active against this species, protects poorly against *Aedes*. A combination of DEET and ethyl hexanediol provides the broadest protection. The following recommendations have been made [1].

In non-tropical countries

Adults
DEET, not less than 15%
Combination of DMP and ethylhexanediol
35/35 with the above reservations on toxicology

Children
Avoid DEET and rely on:
DMP-ethylhexanediol
35/35 in reserve

Pregnant women
As safety data regarding synthetic repellents are limited, citronella or other natural oils are recommended.

In the tropics

The risk of transmissible diseases necessitates greater protection.

Adults
DEET (35–50%) plus ethylhexanediol

Children
DEET (<15%) plus ethylhexanediol

Pregnant women
The choice is uncertain in the present state of knowledge.

In conditions of extreme exposure (safaris, tropical forests, etc.)

The above advice, plus impregnation of clothing, mosquito nets and tents with pyrethrin monthly.

New formulations in different bases, such as lotions, creams and gels, have no influence on the effectiveness of the repellent.

Butopyronoxyl is effective for repelling ticks [5].

Ectoparasiticides

These fall into two groups: parasiticides, used in the treatment of the affected patient, and insecticides used mainly for environmental control. The distinction, however, is arbitrary.

Parasiticides

Most hospitals and local authorities in the UK now have policies for the treatment of head lice, usually rotating the agents to avoid the development of resistance. Synthetic pyrethroids, malathion or carbaryl may be used to treat head lice. A review of published trials suggested that permethrin was the most effective [10,11], but permethrin resistance has been reported [12]. Topical ivermectin was successful after a single application [13]. For scabies, benzyl benzoate is effective and inexpensive. It may cause stinging in the flexures. Permethrin 5% is an alternative [11]. Both topical and oral ivermectin can be used [13,14]. Crotamiton has weak scabicidal activity and is an antipruritic. It is sometimes used as a follow-up treatment to other therapies.

Insecticides

Advice on safe and effective insecticides is restricted by toxicological and environmental considerations, as these agents are commonly used in the form of powders or aerosols, and may be widely disseminated.

Nicotine, pyrethrum and derris are used in pest control and general insect suppression. Pyrethrum extract contains about 25% w/w of pyrethrins. Its action can be enhanced by piperonyl butoxide, and this combination is available in over-the-counter preparations in the USA [15].

Many of the repellents already mentioned are used as insecticides. A number of newer organophosphorus compounds have attracted increasing interest. They can be used to spray the environment as well as parasitized animals, and include dichlorvos and iodofenphos.

REFERENCES

1 Combemale P, Deruaz D, Villanova D *et al.* Les insectifuges ou les repellents. *Ann Dermatol Vénéréol* 1992; **119**: 411–34.
2 Feldman RJ, Maibach HI. Absorption of some organic compounds through the skin in man. *J Invest Dermatol* 1970; **54**: 399–404.
3 Maibach HI, Khan AA, Aker W. Use of insect repellents for maximum efficacy. *Arch Dermatol* 1974; **109**: 32–5.
4 Reynolds JEF, ed. *Martindale: The Extra Pharmacopoeia*, 31st edn. London: Pharmaceutical Press, 1996.
5 World Health Organization. *Insecticide Resistance and Vector Control: 17th report of the WHO Expert Committee on Insecticides.* WHO Technical Report Series no 443. Geneva: WHO, 1970.
6 Khan AA, Maibach HI, Skidmore DL. A study of insect repellents. 2. Effect of temperature on protection time. *J Econ Entomol* 1973; **66**: 437–8.
7 Keystone JS. Of bites and body odour. *Lancet* 1996; **347**: 1423.
8 Harford-Cross M. Tendency to being bitten by insects among patients with eczema and with other dermatoses. *Br J Gen Pract* 1993; **43**: 339–40.
9 Cronin E. Cosmetics—oil of citronella. In: *Contact Dermatis.* Edinburgh: Churchill Livingstone, 1980: 159–62.
10 Vander-Stichele RH, Dezeure EM, Bogaert MG. Systematic review of clinical efficacy of topical treatments for head lice. *Br Med J* 1995; **311**: 604–8.
11 Brown S, Becher J, Brady W. Treatment of ectoparasitic infections: review of the English-language literature, 1982–1992. *Clin Infect Dis* 1995; **20** (Suppl. 1): 104–9.
12 Rupes V, Moravec J, Chmela J *et al.* A resistance of head lice (Pediculus capitis) to permethrin in Czech republic. *Cent Eur J Public Health* 1995; **3**: 30–2.
13 Youssef MY, Sadaka HA, Eissa MM *et al.* Topical application of ivermectin for human ectoparasites. *Am J Trop Med Hyg* 1995; **53**: 652–3.
14 Glaziou P, Cartel JL, Alzieu P *et al.* Comparison of ivermectin and benzyl benzoate for treatment of scabies. *Trop Med Parasitol* 1993; **44**: 331–2.
15 Lynfield YK, O'Donoghue MN. Pediculosis therapy. *J Am Acad Dermatol* 1982; **6**: 949–50.

Sunscreens

The steady increase in the incidence of malignant melanomas, the increased incidence of non-melanoma skin cancer and preneoplastic disorders, and the heightened awareness of the premature ageing effects of UV irradiation have contributed to the demand for more effective protection from the sun. This can be achieved by:

1 totally blocking the UV irradiation reaching the skin by physical means such as thick clothing or creams containing powders acting as a mechanical barrier;

2 screening out or absorbing the rays by application of a medicament containing a photo-absorbing chemical. Whichever is used, the degree of protection is only partial, and there is no such thing as a truly total sun block or 100% efficient sunscreening agent. The applications currently in use have been refined to improve cosmetic acceptability, effectiveness, and water resistance or durability. Nevertheless, adverse reactions can occur, which may be irritant, allergic, phototoxic or photo-allergic. Reactions may occur to the base, the active absorber, or to one of a number of additives such as fragrances or stabilizers. It follows from the second law of thermodynamics that in any system scattering or chemically absorbing irradiant energy, the net loss of energy is converted into energy of other forms, principally heat. For a discussion of the basic aspects of photobiology see Chapter 25. Sunscreens have been widely promoted by health groups and manufacturers alike for the prevention of sun-induced skin cancers. Appropriate-strength sunscreens have been found to be effective in the reduction of the incidence of actinic keratoses [1] and in the prevention of UVB-induced immunosuppression [2], which is considered to play a role in cutaneous carcinogenesis. The prevention of melanoma by the use of sunscreens is a controversial topic, and there have been two recent case–control studies that linked sunscreen usage to a higher incidence of melanoma [3,4]. This may be related in part to the likelihood that the subjects studied had previously used sunscreens that provided protection against UVB radiation alone, and exposed themselves to higher doses of solar radiation than those who did not use sunscreen. A valid point suggested by McGregor and Young [5] is the risk of loss of photoprotective efficacy if sunscreens are used as a means to prolong the time spent in the sun. Marketing of sunscreens has much to do with usage habits of consumers, who should be made aware of other modes of photoprotection, including the avoidance of unnecessary sun exposure.

Physical blockers absorb and scatter all UV rays, infrared rays and visible light. Inert compounds are ground to a wide variety of particle sizes and suspended in a range of bases. They are now frequently combined with a chemical sunscreen. Titanium oxide, zinc oxide and red petrolatum are frequently used ingredients. Their main disadvantage is lack of cosmetic acceptability.

Chemical sunscreens are arbitrarily divided into UVA blockers active in the range 320–360 nm, and UVB blockers active in the range 290–320 nm. Some compounds are effective in both ranges, and many modern formulations aim to cover most of the range and are termed 'broad-spectrum' blockers. The efficiency of each agent is related to the spectrum of wavelengths absorbed and the resistance to washing off during swimming or sweating [6–9]. The main classes of UV absorbers have been grouped as follows [10].

1 Cinnamates—UVB.
2 PABA—UVB.
3 Salicylates—UVB.

4 Benzophenones—UVA.

5 Camphor—UVA.

6 Dibenzoylmethane—UVA.

7 Anthralin—UVA.

8 Miscellaneous, mainly UVB.

A wide range of derivatives of these compounds is employed, and lists of those compounds which have been approved for use in the USA or Europe are included in the monographs referenced [10–12].

The concept of sun protection factors (SPF) was introduced to guide users in selecting a more 'efficient' sunscreen [13–15]. Unfortunately, different systems of assay are used in different countries, making direct comparisons very misleading. However, all depend on deriving a ratio of the time or the amount of energy to reach a given end-point, such as minimal erythema, when using the screen to that required without using the screen.

$$ SPF = \frac{\text{Dose UV radiation to produce minimal erythema with sunscreen}}{\text{Dose UV radiation to produce minimal erythema without sunscreen}} $$

Some degree of commercial licence is evident in claims about products with very high protection factors. As a guide, SPFs of up to 10 can be regarded as mild, 10–15 as medium, and over 15 as strong protectors. International agreement about light sources, end-points and conditions of testing is needed. Assessment of resistance to water has been attempted by several methods [8,16].

REFERENCES

1 Naylor MF, Boyd A, Smith DW *et al.* High sun protection factor sunscreens in the suppression of actinic neoplasia. *Arch Dermatol* 1995; **131**: 170–5.

2 Whitmore SE, Morison WL. Prevention of UVB-induced immunosuppression in humans by a high Sun Protection Factor sunscreen. *Arch Dermatol* 1995; **131**: 1128–33.

3 Westerdahl J, Olsson H, Masback A *et al.* Is the use of sunscreens a risk factor for malignant melanoma? *Melanoma Res* 1995; **5**: 59–65.

4 Autier P, Dore JF, Schifflers E *et al.* Melanoma and use of sunscreens: an EORTC case-control study in Germany, Belgium and France. *Int J Cancer* 1995; **61**: 749–55.

5 McGregor JM, Young AR. Sunscreens, suntans, and skin cancer. *Br Med J* 1996; **312**: 1621–2.

6 Catalano PM, Fulghum DD. A water resistant sunscreen. *Clin Exp Dermatol* 1977; **2**: 127–30.

7 Hawk J, Challoner AVJ, Chaddock L. The efficacy of sunscreening agents: protection factors and transmission spectra. *Clin Exp Dermatol* 1982; **7**: 21–31.

8 Kraft ER, Hoch SG, Quisno RA *et al.* The importance of the vehicle. *J Soc Cosmet Chem* 1982; **23**: 383–91.

9 MacLeod TM, Frain-Bell W. A study of chemical light-screening agents. *Br J Dermatol* 1975; **92**: 417–25.

10 Shaath NA. The chemistry of sunscreens. In: Lowe NJ, Shaath NA, eds. *Sunscreens: Development, Evaluation and Regulatory Aspects.* New York: Marcel Dekker, 1990: 211–33.

11 Kaidbey KH, Kligman AM. An appraisal of the efficacy and substantivity of the new high-protection sunscreens. *J Am Acad Dermatol* 1981; **4**: 566–70.

12 Klein K. Formulating suncreen products. In: Lowe NJ, Shaath NA, eds. *Sunscreens: Development, Evaluation and Regulatory Aspects.* New York: Marcel Dekker, 1990: 235–66.

13 Bickers DR. Photoprotection of human skin. *J Am Acad Dermatol* 1982; **7**: 402–4.

14 Farr PM, Diffey BL. How reliable are sunscreen protection factors? *Br J Dermatol* 1985; **112**: 113–18.

15 Roelandts R, van Hee J, Bonamie A *et al.* A survey of ultraviolet absorbers in commercially available sun products. *Int J Dermatol* 1983; **22**: 247–55.

16 Thompson C, Maibach H, Epstein J. Allergic contact dermatitis from sunscreen preparations complicating photodermatitis. *Arch Dermatol* 1977; **113**: 1252–3.

Cleansing agents

Skin cleansers [1–3]

Normal human skin has its own natural cleaning action resulting from the continuous outward flow of epidermal cells in epidermopoeisis. Natural sebum has both emollient and mild antibacterial properties. In modern society, cleaning the skin is both socially desirable and in many occupations necessary. The term 'cleansing' is often used in preference to 'cleaning', with the covert implication of a more cosmetic or gentle procedure. The objectives of skin cleansing differ according to the circumstances. They include the following.

1 Removal of extraneous dirt and contaminants.

2 Removal of endogenous sebum.

3 Removal of endogenous sweat.

4 Removal of bacteria and other microorganisms.

5 Removal of stratum corneum cells (exfoliation).

The recommendation of a particular cleansing routine should take into account which of these objectives is of special importance to the user or patient. Cleansers have differing and definite roles in the following circumstances:

1 Normal social skin cleansing.

2 Cleansing in an industrial setting [4].

3 Presurgical skin cleansing.

4 Prephlebotomy skin cleansing.

5 Acne cleansing routines.

6 Skin cleansing in patients with eczema, psoriasis and other dermatoses.

Soaps

Soaps are manufactured from fatty acids and alkalis, and are, to a greater or lesser degree, irritant [1,5]. 'Gentle' soaps have been manufactured to reduce the irritant qualities, and methods devised to assess them objectively [6–8].

Emollients

For routine cleansing in patients with dry skin or inflammatory dermatoses, aqueous cream or emulsifying ointment are widely used, and have the advantages of ready availability and low cost. It should be noted that aqueous cream may sting when applied to inflamed or fissured skin (e.g. children with atopic eczema). A wide range of commercial cleansers with emollient properties are available that contain lipids such as liquid paraffin or soya oil. Many contain antiseptics, fragrances and other additives to which an individual patient may be sensitive.

Synthetic detergents (syndets)

These are available in bars and lotions. Irritation may be marked with sodium lauryl sulphate, but improved formulations give better results in objective tests [8]. Combinations with higher alcohols reduce the irritant properties. A claimed advantage of syndets with a neutral pH is the absence of alteration of the skin microflora [9].

Oils

In most hyperkeratotic conditions, cleansing can be combined with a mild emollient and keratolytic effect using synthetic or naturally occurring oils such as liquid paraffin, arachis oil, coconut oil and almond oil. Sensitization may occur with natural or essential oils.

Medicated cleansers

Chlorhexidine is widely used in acne preparations, and has been shown to be of benefit [10]. It was superior to povidone–iodine and a lotion soap in reducing skin staphylococci in a presurgical shower routine [11]. A review of surgical cleansing commended alcohol, iodophores and chlorhexidine, rather than the older metallic compounds, halogen compounds and tincture of iodine [12].

Swabs

For phlebotomy, various alcohols, such as methyl-ethylisopropyl alcohol, are used. Contact sensitivity to the latter may occur [13]. The use of isopropanol as a cleanser during phlebotomy for blood alcohol levels in drink–driving offences does not interfere with the accuracy of the results when correct phlebotomy technique is used [14].

Abrasive cleansers

Cleansers containing finely ground minerals or synthetic beads combined with emollients, detergents and antiseptics are a useful adjunct to the management of milder grades of acne.

REFERENCES

1 Bettley FR, Donoghue E. The irritant effect of soap upon the normal skin. *Br J Dermatol* 1960; **72**: 67–76.
2 Wortzman MS. Evaluation of mild skin cleansers. *Dermatol Clin* 1991; **9**: 35–44.
3 White IR. Skin tolerance to cleansing agents. *Wien Med Wochenschr* 1990; **108** (Suppl.): 13–16.
4 Ortonne JP. Skin cleansing: an important problem in occupational dermatology. *Wien Med Wochenschr* 1990; **108**: 19–21.
5 Frosch PJ. Irritancy of soaps and detergent bars. In: Frosch P, Horowitz SN, eds. *Principles of Cosmetics for the Dermatologist*. St Louis: CV Mosby, 1982.
6 Symposium on skin cleansing. *Trans St John's Hosp Derm Soc* 1965; **51**: 133–257.
7 Frosch PJ, Kligman AM. The soap chamber test, a new method for assessing the irritancy of soaps. *J Am Acad Dermatol* 1979; **1**: 35–41.
8 Kresken J, Eckert J, Wassilew SW. Zur Problematik von Hautvertraglichkeitsprufungen. Untersuchung von Hautreinigungsmitteln in Modiikationen des Duhring-Kammer-Tests. *Derm Beruf Umwelt* 1989; **37**: 63–6.
9 Shmid MH, Korting HC. The concept of the acid mantle of the skin: its relevance for the choice of skin cleansers. *Dermatology* 1995; **191**: 276–80.
10 Stoughton RB, Leyden JJ. Efficacy of 4 per cent chlorhexidine gluconate skin cleanser in the treatment of acne vulgaris. *Cutis* 1987; **39**: 551–3.
11 Kaiser AB, Kernodle DS, Barg NL *et al.* Influence of preoperative showers on staphylococci skin colonization: a comparative trial of antiseptic skin cleansers. *Ann Thorac Surg* 1988; **45**: 35–8.
12 Laufman H. Current use of skin and wound cleansers and antiseptics. *Am J Surg* 1989; **157**: 359–65.
13 Cronin E. *Contact Dermatitis*. Edinburgh: Churchill Livingstone, 1980.
14 Ryder KW, Glick MR. The effect of skin cleansing agents on ethanol results measured with the Du Pont automatic clinical analyzer. *J Forensic Sci* 1986; **31**: 574–9.

Chapter 79
Radiotherapy and Reactions to Ionizing Radiation

MARGARET F.SPITTLE

Introduction

The clinical effects of ionizing radiation on the skin have been known since the discovery of X-rays in 1895 [1]. At first, the physical aspects of dosimetry were little understood, a fact that did not hamper the enthusiasm with which both benign and malignant disease were irradiated. Both the dosage and indications for irradiation were initially empirical, and the dermatologist may still see the late effects on the skin and subcutaneous tissues of overdosage due to inexperience. This was especially obvious when irradiation was used for cosmetic purposes by paramedical personnel. Indications for treating benign disease by irradiation have declined since the elaboration of topical steroids. If the effect of irradiation is understood, this treatment still has a specific place in the dermatologist's armamentarium for patients otherwise refractory to treatment [2,3].

Orthovoltage irradiation necessarily treats the surface of the skin to the maximum incident dose. As these effects can be monitored and scored, systems have been used to compare differing voltage and fractionation regimens. In view of its superficial nature, orthovoltage irradiation is employed when the skin is to be treated. Since the introduction of supervoltage irradiation, which gives a maximum dose below the surface of the skin, the acute skin reaction is rarely seen in the treatment of deep-seated malignant disease. However, if the skin is particularly at risk from recurrence as, for example, in the primary treatment of breast cancer, it can be fully treated. The effect of high-dose irradiation given to tissue tolerance may then be seen. Radiation is most frequently used in the management of cancer, and where skin malignancies are concerned is an important pillar of the multidisciplinary oncology approach. Indeed, it is in the best interest of patients suffering from skin tumours to be seen in a clinic where the expertise of specialists in radiotherapy and oncology, plastic surgery and micrographic surgery as well as dermatology are present.

In this chapter, the discussion of the indications for radiation treatment and types of radiation available will be restricted to the management of benign dermatological disease.

REFERENCES

1 Goldschmidt H, Sherwin WK. Reactions to ionizing radiation. *J Am Acad Dermatol* 1980; **3**: 551–79.
2 Rowell NR. A follow-up study of superficial radiotherapy for benign dermatoses: recommendations for the use of X-rays in dermatology. *Br J Dermatol* 1973; **88**: 583–90.
3 Rowell NR. In: Rook AJ, ed. Ionizing radiation in benign dermatoses. In: *Recent Advances in Dermatology*, Vol. 4. Edinburgh: Churchill Livingstone, 1977: 329–50.

Protection and safety

Dermatological radiotherapy apparatus is now rarely found outside the large radiotherapy centres where radiation protection and maintenance is the responsibility of a team of dedicated physicists. The regulations in the Code of Practice are strict. [1]. The occasional use of ionizing radiation by the non-specialist practitioner can be hazardous, especially with low-voltage X-ray apparatus that may incorporate several variables of voltage, filtration and treatment distance in its range. Radiation accidents should not be allowed to happen, and are less likely to occur when techniques are used frequently by expert radiographers and with regular quality assurance. An error is particularly sad when radiation is being used to treat benign disease.

Benign disease should only be treated by radiation when it has proved to be resistant to standard dermatological care. It is therefore important for the radiotherapist to confirm with a dermatologist that this is the case. To limit radiation to the treatment of malignant disease only would be facile, and would deny it to a patient with serious disabling palmar eczema while supporting the treatment of a small basal cell epithelioma that is not adversely affecting the quality of life. Much older literature describes the late radiation effects and possible carcinogenesis attributed to radiation given when protection standards and dosimetry were little understood. To make a statement on radiation therapy of benign disease the Food and Drug Administration (FDA) set up a multidisciplinary committee in 1978. Although not formalized in the UK, the recommendations of that committee endorsed by the FDA are as described by Goldschmidt [1,2].

1 The potential risk of treatment with any form of radiation of a benign, non-life-threatening disease must be recognized. Ionizing radiation therapy may be considered if other safer methods have not succeeded in alleviating the condition, and if the consequences of no further treatment are unacceptable. This should not lead to an overreaction to the presumed risk of radiation where known risks of radiation may be traded off against the unknown risk of some other therapeutic modality.

2 The committee strongly endorsed the concept that it must remain the prerogative of the physician to have available for use any form of therapy—radiation, drugs, or others—in which the benefits accruing to the patient from its use are considered to outweigh the risks inherent in its use.

3 Infants and children should be treated with ionizing radiation only in very exceptional cases.

4 Direct irradiation of the skin areas overlying organs that are particularly prone to late effects, for example thyroid, eyes, gonads, bone marrow and breast, should be avoided.

5 Medical practitioners using ionizing radiation should be adequately trained in both the practical and the theoretical aspects of radiation therapy and protection.

6 Meticulous radiation protection techniques should be used in all instances.

7 The less penetrating X-ray qualities, for example Grenz rays, offer a wider margin of safety. Wherever possible, the depth of the penetration of the X-ray beam should be chosen in accordance with the depth of the pathological process.

8 Laboratory and epidemiological studies should be initiated and/or continued to fill the gaps in our knowledge of the effects of ionizing radiation at the doses used in the past and currently.

Types of ionizing radiation

X-rays are part of the electromagnetic spectrum. They have a shorter wavelength and are more energetic and penetrating than UV radiation.

Orthovoltage radiation includes beams softer than 1 million electron volts (meV).

Superficial X-rays, up to 100 kV, are used in the management of benign skin disease. The higher voltages are used for hypertrophic disease needing treatment to a greater depth, for example keloids.

Grenz rays, German for borderline, describes the most poorly penetrating ionizing rays, which are 6–15 kV, and

are at the borderline with non-ionizing radiation. As 90% of this radiation is absorbed in the upper 1 mm of the skin, it is important to treat only diseases of very superficial pathology with this beam. Dose-dependent pigmentation of the skin may occur, but alopecia will not, as the energy of the beam does not reach the depth of the hair follicle. Doses of 100–300 Gy have rarely been associated with malignancy [3], but there is a wide margin of safety with Grenz rays. However, the minimum voltage consistent with the depth of pathology should be chosen.

Half-value depth (HVD) is the depth in tissue at which the X-ray beam intensity is reduced to one-half of the incident dose. As guidance, the HVD chosen in X-ray therapy should coincide with the greatest depth of the pathological process [2].

Half-value thickness (HVT) is defined as that thickness of an appropriate filter material (usually aluminium) that reduces the beam intensity to half.

Gamma rays are produced by the decay of radioactive substances—either naturally occurring material such as radium, or artificial isotopes such as radioactive cobalt and iridium. Radioactive isotopes may be used for interstitial therapy, utilizing the rapid decrease in dose with distance from the source to achieve a restricted high-dose area in tissues. Radium or caesium needles and iridium wire are used for interstitial irradiation [4].

Alpha rays are particles, being the nuclei of helium. They have a high linear energy transfer and are poorly penetrating. Thorium X is an α-emitter, and was used in the treatment of capillary haemangiomas. The results of treatment were unconvincing and, as the isotope is difficult to handle, it is now not used clinically [5].

Beta rays are electrons and can be derived from radioactive isotopes, such as ^{90}strontium or be produced by a linear accelerator. The energy of electrons is almost totally absorbed at a depth proportional to the given voltage. It is possible to irradiate the whole skin area with an electron beam. The minimal depth dose characteristics that may be achieved avoid the irradiation of subcutaneous structures, which would occur if X-ray therapy that is absorbed exponentially was used. This technique is used in the treatment of mycosis fungoides [6]. Multiple radiation fields are combined to give a homogenous dose to the whole skin down to a depth of approximately 1 cm.

Electron-beam therapy is used to irradiate skin cancers in sites where the malignant lesion to be treated is large or overlying cartilage or bone. The mode of absorption of high-energy X-rays produced from a linear accelerator or of γ-rays is relatively independent of the atomic number of the tissue irradiated. Low-voltage X-rays are absorbed disproportionately in high-atomic-number materials. If this fact is not understood, necrosis may occur in cartilage or bone underlying large superficial lesions. Therefore, superficial X-ray therapy should be avoided when treating lesions overlying the nose, ear, hand and tibia to a radical dose.

Modern high-voltage electron therapy is indicated in these sites [7].

Fast neutron beams have a higher relative biological efficiency than X-rays or γ-rays, but seem to have little dermatological potential. Large tumour volumes may have potentially necrotic and anoxic cells in the centre. Well oxygenated cells are approximately three times more radio-sensitive than poorly oxygenated cells when irradiated with X-rays, which may contribute to the radioresistance of some tumours. However, neutron damage is less dependent on this 'oxygen effect', and neutrons are therefore more effective in destroying anoxic cells.

REFERENCES

1 Goldschmidt H. FDA recommendations on radiation of benign diseases. *Arch Dermatol* 1978; **114**(8): 1149.
2 Goldschmidt H, Sherwin WK. Reactions to ionizing radiation. *J Am Acad Dermatol* 1980; **3**: 551–79.
3 Mortensen AC, Kjeldsen H. Carcinomas following Grenz ray treatment of benign dermatoses. *Acta Derm Venereol (Stockh)* 1987; **67**: 523–5.
4 Nicolas J, Daly NJ, De Lafontan B. Results and treatment of 165 lid carcinomas by iridium wire implant. *Int J Rad Oncol Biol Phys* 1984; **10**: 455–9.
5 Fleischmajer R, Witten VH. Thorium X applied to human skin: clinical and autoradiographic findings following introduction by iontophoresis. *J Invest Dermatol* 1955; **25**: 223–32.
6 Fuks A, Bagshaw MA. Total-skin electron treatment of mycosis fungoides. *Radiology* 1971; **100**: 145–50.
7 Spittle MF. Mycosis Fungoides. Electron beam therapy in England. *Cancer Treat Rep* 1979; **63**: 639–41.

Dose

The SI unit of absorbed dose is 1 J/kg and is called the Gray. Note that 100 rad = 1 J/kg = 1 Gy; 1 rad = 1 cGy (centiGray). The dose prescription is only complete if it defines the total dose, the number of fractions of radiation and the time in days over which the radiation is to be given. The voltage and penetration characteristics of the beam chosen should be accurately prescribed. Unless this is correctly detailed, the biological effectiveness of the radiation cannot be assessed. The time–dose relationship must be understood.

In trying to reduce to a minimum any deleterious effects of radiation, the dose given in one course of irradiation should be as low as is consistent with the required effect. Two hundred centiGray given weekly for 4 weeks, or 100–500 cGy given every 3 weeks for 9 weeks, are accepted regimens. Although no rigid rule can be applied in this, as in other branches of medicine, it seems reasonable neither to repeat the dose to the same area more than once in a year, since a successful treatment would surely have avoided need for repetition within this time, nor to repeat the course to the same area more than twice in a lifetime. These recommendations are made in an attempt to prevent adverse radiation effects. However, when using radiation it is important to treat with a dose and penetration appropriate to the disease process. The patient's informed consent to treat must be obtained. Accurate records of treatment details must be made. It is important that the patient understands that radiation is being given, and should disclose any previous treatment with ionizing rays to this or other sites. Special consideration should be given before using irradiation in children since this may prevent normal growth of irradiated tissue.

Radiosensitivity

All radiation is destructive. Abnormal cells repair radiation damage less well than normal cells. This inability to repair is reflected in death at mitosis. Anaplastic cells and those with a high mitotic index are more radioresponsive than differentiated cells. Radioresponsiveness and radiocurability are dissimilar and are functions of differences in cell population kinetics. Radiotherapy is usually given as a fractionated course, as the intervals between doses allow for the recovery of normal cells. The effect of a dose of radiation is reduced by increasing the number of fractions in which it is given or by lengthening the total overall treatment time. The effect of irradiation can be modified by anoxia, infection, oedema, trauma and any inborn genetic susceptibility. The face tolerates irradiation well and radical dosages may be accompanied by good cosmetic results [1].

When irradiating benign conditions, the minimum dose and the lowest voltage appropriate to achieve the desired effect should be chosen. The threat of radiation carcinogenesis must clearly be seen in the context of the clinical indication for treatment. There is a threshold for somatic radiation changes which need not be breached in the treatment of benign conditions. The late radiation sequelae of treatment given many years ago are inexcusable with modern standards of dosimetry and equipment, and should not be seen in the treatment of benign diseases [2].

REFERENCES

1 Fitzpatrick PJ, Thompson GA, Easterbrook WM *et al.* Basal and squamous cell carcinoma of the eyelids and their treatment by radiotherapy. *Int J Rad Oncol Biol Phys* 1984; **10**: 449–54.
2 Traenkle HL. X-ray induced skin cancer in man. *Natl Cancer Inst Monogr* 1963; **10**: 423–32.

Indications for radiotherapy

Lymphocytoma cutis

Lymphocytes are acutely sensitive to radiation, undergoing interphase death. Three treatments of 300 cGy in 1 week at 50 kV is sufficient dose to cause complete regression of these lesions.

Keratoacanthoma

This is a self-limiting disease and the lesions should regress with observation. Occasionally a lesion persists, recurs or is cosmetically disfiguring and the subsequent scarring following spontaneous regression would be unacceptable. Radiation may then be used. The diagnosis is largely clinical, and the histological appearance is notoriously similar to a squamous cell carcinoma. For this reason some authors [1–3] prefer to give doses of radiation that would cure a squamous cell carcinoma in spite of the possibility of the late radiation sequelae and a poorer cosmetic result that will occur.

Keloids

Intractable keloids resistant to intralesional steroids or other conventional treatment may respond to radiation. Excision of the keloid with early irradiation of the scar and stitch marks is more successful, but in some sites, for example tip of shoulder, upper middle chest, where surgery is inadvisable, good response of pain, itch and redness can be achieved with some regression of the keloid itself. Relatively high doses are necessary; these will cause temporary pigmentation, which will remain for many months in pigmented skin. Doornbos *et al.* [4] noted that 17 of 18 unexcised keloids that were less than a year old regressed with 1500 cGy given in three treatments over 6 days at 120 kV. Older keloids respond less well to irradiation. The most satisfactory management of keloids is postexcision irradiation where a dose–response relationship can be seen. Total doses less than 900 cGy, irrespective of fractionation and postsurgical interval, did not prevent recurrence. Three doses of 400 cGy were given by Kovalic [5] with a 73% success rate. Using the commonly employed dose of 900 cGy, Lo *et al.* [6] described an 85% success rate and Borok [7] a 96% response rate. No late sequelae or carcinogenesis was described by any of the previously quoted authors with follow up in excess of 30 years.

Darier's disease and familial benign chronic pemphigus (Hailey–Hailey disease)

These diseases respond well to fractionated courses of Grenz rays. However, since prolonged remission is often the most that can be expected in these conditions, it is important to establish the dose of radiation previously given before considering further treatment. Although very high total doses of Grenz rays have been given without complications, carcinogenesis is described [8]. In cases where the disease process is more thickened, 30 kV or 50 kV may be used.

Palmoplantar psoriasis and eczema

In intractable, persistent disease, irradiation may be tried, and while a good temporary response is seen in up to 80% of patients and lasting response in some, many patients will have relapsed before 6 months. This often calls into question the advisability of repeating the treatment. In general, feet respond to a higher voltage than hands, and eczema responds more readily with improvement especially in cracking and fissuring than does pustular psoriasis. Psoriatic lesions should be treated at 30–50 kV and eczema at 10–30 kV; a dose of 100–200 cGy weekly for 4 weeks is appropriate. Patches of lichenified eczema or psoriasis may also respond to radiotherapy at the higher voltage range. The voltage appropriate to the depth of pathology should be chosen [9]. Irradiation is indicated when treatments such as systemic steroids or cytotoxic therapy might be avoided.

Acrodermatitis of Hallopeau

This resistant condition involving the nailbed responds well to irradiation and to little else. Five doses of 300 cGy over 1 or 2 weeks at 50–150 kV produces an excellent response with slow normalization of nail growth and resolution of pustules. This dose is higher than often employed for benign disease and should not be repeated to the same phalanx.

Acne and rosacea

Such important advances in the medical management of these diseases have been made that the indications for radiation are rare. As the disease process is deep, Grenz rays have no part to play in the management of acne [10]. 100 cGy weekly for 4 weeks at 30–50 kV can be employed for intractable cases, but extensive shielding of the thyroid [11] and parotid glands [12] is necessary. The administration of high doses over long periods given 30–50 years ago to patients with recurrent acne caused many of the disastrous radiation sequelae so often described in the world literature.

This is a memorial not only to the ignorance of both medical and lay practitioners, but to the fact that worthwhile short-term gains were seen from the irradiation of many forms of benign dermatological disease. Late radiation changes should never be seen with the doses of radiation employed for the management of acne.

Herpes simplex

Although it is difficult to indicate the mechanism, Knight [13] has described a reduction in frequency and severity of recurrence and in some cases cure of herpes simplex attacks by Grenz rays. Two hundred centiGray weekly for 4 weeks is given to the area of usual expression of the vesicles.

Cavernous haemangiomas

In general, these improve during childhoosd and are rarely irradiated. The occasional lesion in a life-threatening site, growing faster than the infant (e.g. vocal cord or mouth), may need urgent consideration by a radiotherapist [14].

Epilation

Irradiation can cause epilation and, depending on dose, this can be permanent or temporary. This fact has been employed in the management of sycosis barbae and pilonidal sinuses to prevent ingrowing hair. Doses in excess of 600 cGy in one treatment are necessary.

The treatment of *Microsporum audouini* infections with radiation had a vogue prior to the elaboration of griseo-fulvin. When carried out as prescribed in the traditional Kienboch–Adamson technique, good temporary epilation with regrowth of hair and loss of the organism was achieved. A temporary change of hair colour and texture frequently occurred following irradiation. Many children were irradiated and a few show the sequelae of a much higher dose than the 700 cGy prescribed in areas of field overlap. Whilst in the great majority of cases this was a successful treatment, in a few patients adverse long-term results including a greater incidence of malignancy, both in the scalp and in underlying tissues, developed [15]. The alternative past treatment of this condition with systemic hormones or ineffective topical remedies, resulting in years wasted in absence from school, highlights the scourge of this historic epidemic.

REFERENCES

1 Caccialanza M, Sopelana N. Radiation therapy of keratoacanthomas: results in 55 patients. *Int J Rad Oncol Biol Phys* 1988; **16**: 475–7.
2 Donahue B, Cooper JS, Rush S. Treatment of aggressive keratoacanthomas by radiotherapy. *J Am Acad Dermatol* 1990; **23**: 489–93.
3 Koster W, Nasemann T, Reimlinger S *et al.* Rontgendifferentialtherapie des Keratoakanthoms—ein kasuistischer Beitrag. *Z Hautkr* 1985; **60**: 215–18.
4 Doornbos JF, Stoffel SJ, Hass AC *et al.* The role of kelovoltage irradiation in the treatment of keloids. *Int J Rad Oncol Biol Phys* 1990; **18**: 833–9.
5 Kovalic JJ, Perez C. Radiation therapy following keloidectomy: a 20-year experience. *Int J Rad Oncol Biol Phys* 1989; **17**: 77–80.
6 Lo TCM, Seckel BR, Salzman FA *et al.* Single-dose electron beam irradiation in treatment and prevention of keloids and hypertrophic scars. *J Radiother Oncol* 1990; **19**: 267–72.
7 Borok TL, Bray M, Sinclair I *et al.* Role of ionizing irradiation for 393 keloids. *Int J Rad Oncol Biol Phys* 1988; **15**: 865–70.
8 Mortensen AC, Kjeldsen H. Carcinomas following Grenz ray treatment of benign dermatoses. *Acta Derm Venereol (Stockh)* 1987; **67**: 523–5.
9 Fairris GM, Jones DH, Mack DP *et al.* Conventional superficial X-ray versus Grenz ray therapy in the treatment of constitutional eczema of the hands. *Br J Dermatol* 1985; **112**: 339–41.
10 Jelliffe AM, Soutter C, Meara RH. An investigation into the treatment of acne vulgaris with Grenz rays. *Br J Dermatol* 1969; **81**: 617–20.
11 Favus MJ, Schneider AB, Stachura ME *et al.* Thyroid cancer occurring as a late consequence of head and neck irradiation. *N Engl J Med* 1976; **294**: 1019–25.
12 Preston-Martin S. Prior X-ray therapy for acne related to tumors of the parotid gland. *Arch Dermatol* 1989; **125**: 921–4.
13 Knight AG. Grenz ray treatment of recurrent herpes simplex. *Br J Dermatol* 1972; **86**: 172–4.
14 Furst CJ, Silfversward C, Holm LE. Mortality in a cohort of radiation treated childhood skin hemangiomas. *Acta Oncol* 1989; **28**: 789–94.
15 Ridley CM. Basal-cell carcinoma following X-ray epilation of the scalp. *Br J Dermatol* 1962; **74**: 222.

Acute radiodermatitis

Acute radiation reaction [1]

The minimal single dose that produces an observed erythema is called the 'erythema dose' and before the existence of other measurements much importance was placed on the dose needed to achieve this end. However, there is a great personal variation, and field size, quality of radiation, area of skin irradiated, sex, race and age of the patient are some of the many factors affecting this parameter. The erythema dose was superseded by the roentgen and then the rad. The international unit of radiation dose is now the Gray—the centiGray is often used clinically.

The clinical course of the acute radiation reaction depends on the size of the dose and fractionation used. Large single fractions of irradiation are rarely given in clinical practice. An initial erythema and oedema may be seen within 24 h of irradiating the skin, and then a secondary and progressive erythema is manifest on the third to the sixth day. If the dose has been sufficiently high, vesicles and bullae may be formed, which subsequently dry and desquamate. The desquamated skin is usually dark. The perifollicular cells appear more resistant to radiation, and re-epithelialization is initiated in the perifollicular areas, which coalesce to cover the denuded surface. Postinflammatory pigmentation may occur at the periphery of the field and within the field in dark skins, when this pigmentation may last for many months. If the epithelium is irradiated to a high dose, it will appear atrophic and smooth, unable to form pigment and with no hair, sweat or sebaceous glands. This thin epithelium reacts poorly to trauma and has less tolerance to further radiation. Hyper-keratosis, telangiectasia, dyspigmentation and atrophy may eventually occur, and malignant lesions supervene.

Treatment. Little treatment has been found which affects the natural history of the acute radiation reaction. However, trauma, heat, cold, friction and infection may cause ulceration, as such skin cannot readily repair damage. Mild steroid creams may give some symptomatic relief. Vigorous and repeated washing should be avoided in the acute stage.

Histopathology

In acute radiodermatitis, there is oedema and sparseness of connective tissue beneath the epidermis. There may be flattening and loss of epidermal rete ridges with separation of the elastic tissue from the basal layer. Capillary endothelium may be hypertrophic and congested capillaries a feature. Haemorrhage and thrombosis are often observed.

Special stains may show subtle changes in the DNA–RNA structure of epithelial cells as early as the third day [1,2]. During the healing phase, the patchiness of the pathology is a striking feature. Atrophy may be bordered by epidermal hyperplasia, pigmentation is very irregular, and blood vessels are of variable size and shape; deeper vessels may be fibrosed. The fundamental pathology of chronic radiodermatitis is fibrosis of the vessels, with occlusion and varying degrees of homogenization of the connective tissue. Residual vessels may be enormously dilated. Bizarre, large, stellate fibroblasts may be seen in the dermal connective tissue in some cases. Fibrosis of the deep dermis and subcutaneous tissue may occasionally occur after supervoltage radiotherapy [3].

The changes in the epidermis vary from simple atrophy to acanthosis and extreme dyskeratosis. There is usually loss of adnexae such as hair follicles.

Chronic radiodermatitis

The skin is atrophic and shows telangiectasia due to dilatation of a reduced or poorly supported skin vasculature. Dyspigmentation occurs; pigmentation usually is reduced or absent, but there may be small islands of increased pigment production and retention. Decreased sebaceous activity is invariable. The skin is usually atrophic, but increased fibrosis occasionally causes stiffening and tethering. Radionecrotic ulceration may occur, especially in areas of moisture and trauma, and is found in the most poorly vascularized central area of the irradiation scar. Areas of ulceration often show irregular new vessel growth, and histological examination may reveal pseudoepitheliomatous hypertrophy at the edge of an area of extreme atrophy or necrosis. Where there is underlying bone sequestration, radical surgery is necessary to obtain healing.

Chronic radiation change may be confused with a recurrence of a malignant lesion, but the severe pain associated with radiation necrosis is seldom seen with the malignant disease. The effects of normal ageing and sun exposure may combine with the effects of ionizing radiation, and produce accelerated changes of atrophy, necrosis or malignant change. This may also be seen when psoralens and UVA (PUVA) is used on irradiated skin.

Late radiation changes leading to necrosis should never be seen when modern techniques of fractionation to a radical dose for skin malignancies are used. Orthovoltage irradiation of skin overlying subcutaneous bone or cartilage, as in the lower leg, nose and ear, may occasionally result in radionecrosis, as there is a disproportionate absorption of radiation in these high-density tissues, and as cartilage has a particularly poor blood supply. Thus, supervoltage irradiation should be used in these sites. Radionecrosis typically occurs approximately 1 year following complete healing of the skin after radiotherapy, and is often precipitated by trauma or infection. Excision and grafting provide the only satisfactory treatment of extensive radionecrosis. Small areas may slowly heal with conservative management.

REFERENCES

1 Kurban AK, Farah FS. Effects of X-irradiation of the skin. *Acta Derm Venereol (Stockh)* 1969; **49**: 64–71.
2 Black MM, Wilson Jones E. Dermal cylindroma following X-ray epilation of the scalp. *Br J Dermatol* 1971; **85**: 70–2.
3 James WD, Odom RB. Late subcutaneous fibrosis following megavoltage radiotherapy. *J Am Acad Dermatol* 1980; **3**: 616–18.

Radiation-induced tumours

The type of tumour induced by radiation depends on both the cellular structure and the anatomical location of the damaged tissues. Basal cell epitheliomas occur following radiation to the face, scalp and trunk, whereas on the hands squamous cell tumours may occur. These are much more rarely seen since the development of more sophisticated radiotherapy machinery and a greater knowledge of radiobiology. It has not been possible to demonstrate any precise quantitative relationship between the development of cutaneous epitheliomas and the amount of radiation received on the skin surface, nor is it known what total dose or fractionation regimen would be most carcinogenic. It has long been known that carcinomas occur more profusely in areas subjected to many small doses administered at intervals over a long period. Multiple basal cell epitheliomas in the lumbar region following radiotherapy to the lumbar spine for ankylosing spondylitis have been reported [1]. Some may show the histological appearances of the pre-malignant fibroepithelioma of Pinkus. Radiation-induced basal cell epitheliomas of the scalp may be seen 20–50 years following X-ray treatment of the scalp for ringworm infection. Late radiation changes are not always visible, so that pre-existing clinical irradiation damage is not necessary for radiation-induced tumours to occur on the scalp of these patients, where hair growth may be relatively normal.

The doses of radiation used to treat benign dermatological conditions should never produce late radiation damage of even mild type [2]. In general, radiation-induced cancers have occurred after inappropriate doses, often of many thousands of centiGray, given over a long period, frequently by lay therapists for conditions such as hirsutism or greasy skin and large pores [3], which are not treated as such today. Shielding of structures especially sensitive to irradiation, for example the adolescent thyroid [4], was not routinely carried out. Although a greater knowledge of the limitations and effectiveness of radiation should prevent the occurrence of late radiation damage including carcinogenicity, the long latent period often demonstrated in those cases warns against early complacency [5,6].

Treatment. Most radiation induced tumours should be excised. However, where there is no radiation damage evident on the skin, a subsequent radical dose of radiotherapy can be tolerated.

Atypical fibroxanthoma

SYN. PSEUDOSARCOMA OF THE SKIN

This tumour, seen particularly in fair-skinned males who have suffered actinic damage, may also follow radiation damage [7–9]. It usually occurs on the face, occasionally on the trunk or limbs. The clinical course is benign, despite the highly anaplastic histological appearance. Twenty-one tumours initially labelled as spindle-cell squamous carcinomas were found by Hudson and Winkelmann [7] to be atypical fibroxanthoma.

Fibrosarcoma

Sarcoma appears to arise in irradiated skin much less frequently than carcinoma, and many of the tumours are low grade, showing no tendency to produce distant metastases [10]. Some authors have given the term pseudosarcoma to these cases [11]. At least some of the reported sarcomas are in reality spindle-cell carcinomas [12]; this may be shown by the attachment of the tumour to the epidermis or by the presence of horny pearls. Radiation fibromatosis [13] is a diffuse proliferation in which bizarre and sometimes monstrous fibroblasts appear in the dermal connective tissue; the appearance can easily be mistaken for fibrosarcoma. Only exceptionally does fibromatosis undergo a malignant change. It does appear that irradiation of an already chronically inflamed skin is more likely to be followed by a fibrosarcoma than the irradiation of normal skin.

The fibrosarcomas, like the carcinomas following radiation, appear usually after repeated exposures to low-voltage rays and rarely from supervoltage radiation. The latent period in one series [14] averaged 26 years.

REFERENCES

1 Meara RH. Superficial basal-cell epitheliomata following radiotherapy. *Br J Dermatol* 1964; **76**: 294–96.
2 Lukacs S, Goldschmidt H. Radiotherapy of benign dermatoses: indications, practice and results. *J Dermatol Surg Oncol* 1978; **4**: 620–5.
3 Martin H, Strong E, Spiro RH. Radiation induced skin cancer of the head and neck. *Cancer* 1970; **25**: 61–71.
4 Goldschmidt H. Dermatologic radiotherapy and thyroid cancer. *Arch Dermatol* 1977; **113**: 362–4.
5 Fuks A, Bagshaw MA. Total-skin electron treatment of mycosis fungoides. *Radiology* 1971; **100**: 145–50.
6 Martin H, Strong E, Spiro RH. Radiation induced skin cancer of the head and neck. *Cancer* 1970; **25**: 61–71.
7 Hudson AW, Winkelmann RK. Atypical fibroxanthoma of the skin: a reappraisal of 19 cases in which the original diagnosis was spindle-cell squamous carcinoma. *Cancer* 1972; **29**: 413–22.
8 Kemmett D, Gawkrodger DJ, McLaren KM *et al.* Two atypical fibroxanthomas arising separately in X-irradiated skin. *Clin Exp Dermatol* 1988; **13**: 382–4.
9 Kempson RL, McGavran MH. Atypical fibroxanthomas of the skin. *Cancer* 1964; **17**: 1463–71.
10 Stout AP. Fibrosarcoma: the malignant tumor of fibroblasts. *Cancer* 1948; **1**: 30–63.
11 Michalowski R. Cheilite glandulaire suppurée en surface ou Maladie de Baelz. *Acta Derm Venereol (Stockh)* 1946; **31** (Suppl. 27): 31–8.
12 Traenkle HL. X-ray induced skin cancer in man. *Natl Cancer Inst Monogr* 1963; **10**: 423–32.
13 Stout AP. Juvenile fibromatosis. *Cancer* 1954; **7**: 953–78.
14 Russell B. Fibrosarcomata of the skin and subcutaneous tissues. *Trans St John's Hosp Dermatol Soc* 1959; **42**: 15–18.

Chapter 80
Physical and Laser Therapies

R.P.R.DAWBER, N.P.J.WALKER & C.M.LAWRENCE

Cryosurgery
Curettage
Electrosurgery
Infrared coagulation
Caustics and chemical peeling
Topical cytotoxic therapy
Intralesional therapy

Lasers
Sclerotherapy

Miscellaneous physical procedures
Keloid therapy

Minor surgical procedures
Haemostasis
Tattoo removal by salabrasion
Soft-tissue augmentation and facial line correction

Introduction

The extent to which the dermatologist now bestrides both medicine and surgery is well shown in the approach to treatment of benign and malignant lesions of the skin. Some will devote much time and thought to surgical procedures, and to them dermatological surgery becomes almost a specialty in its own right. Others with different interests or outlooks will restrict themselves to those minor procedures at which they have become adept, preferring to refer more complicated problems to colleagues who have an interest in dermatological surgery, or those in other specialties.

In all developed countries, dermatological surgery training is now mandatory—which is important because up to 50% of a dermatologist's workload may involve surgical procedures. This chapter describes the main physical procedures, other than excisional ones, which constitute the variety of modalities used in dermatological surgery, as opposed to the 'pure' excisional and reconstructive skills of plastic surgery. The dermatological surgeon needs diagnostic acumen and the ability to judge which of the many possible modes of treatment is appropriate for a particular lesion—in a particular site in a patient whose general health has been assessed and whose skin type and degree of atrophy and elasticity have been qualitatively assessed. Cryosurgery, curettage, electrosurgery and laser surgery will at times be more appropriate, even for malignant lesions, than formal excision. A simple technique done well will often give a better result than a more advanced technique performed badly!

Ideally, dermatological surgery and plastic surgery skills should be complementary, not in competition. In many centres around the world, there are now combined clinics and theatre lists. This type of collaboration should lead to more balanced judgements, and needs to be encouraged and expanded.

Cryosurgery [1–4]

The earliest freezing agent used in the 'modern' treatment of skin diseases was the salt–ice mixture (–20°C) advocated by Arnott in 1851. By 1913, the clinical effectiveness of liquid air and solid carbon dioxide (carbon dioxide snow) was well known. Increasing knowledge in the field of cryobiology, together with the development of sophisticated cryoprobes and liquid gas jets, has led to a great increase in the use of cryosurgery during the last 25 years [2].

Liquid nitrogen is now most commonly used throughout the world; its boiling point is –196°C. Nitrous oxide gas is also used as a refrigerant in closed probe systems (applying the Joule–Thompson effect), giving a working temperature of –70°C.

Histopathology. Histological changes are evident within 30 min of freezing. Cells show pyknotic nuclei, oedema and coarsely granular and often vacuolated cytoplasm. At the edge of the frozen area, the cells have eosinophilic cytoplasm and small basophilic nuclei. By 1 h, dermal vascular damage and oedema appear. Later changes are those seen in any acutely ischaemic area. The cellular infiltrate is mainly of polymorphonuclear leukocytes, with some lymphocytes and plasma cells most obvious at the edge of the frozen area. Resolution begins within 3 days, and healing usually occurs without scarring or contraction [5]. Hair follicles are easily damaged with relatively brief freeze times [6].

Clinical methods [1,2,7]. Carbon dioxide snow is little used now, but if no other refrigerant is available satisfactory results can be obtained, mainly for benign lesions. It is made by releasing gas from a cylinder into a chamois leather bag, and the solid 'snow' is then transferred to a plastic funnel tube in which it is compressed. Alternatively, small cylinders of gas may be discharged through a narrow opening into a collecting tube. Such apparatus is useful for superficial lesions; deeper destruction can only be achieved by applying greater pressure with special applicators.

Liquid nitrogen is universally available owing to its widespread use in industry, hospital and research establishments. It is very cheap. The liquid is unstable at room temperature, but 1 litre stored in an unsealed (Dewar) flask will last a full day and treat 50–60 patients. Cotton-wool swabs or copper discs are dipped into the liquid and applied to the skin for 5–30 sec. Liquid nitrogen sprays and probes are now commercially available for use when greater tissue destruction is required, and have become standard equipment in clinical practice.

Nitrous oxide cryoprobes are also available. The gas is easily obtained because of its use in anaesthesia. This refrigerant is less appropriate than liquid nitrogen for treating malignancy.

Clinical uses [1–3,7]. A wide spectrum of skin lesions have been treated with freezing. Table 80.1 shows a list of many of the conditions in which cure has been reported. The simplicity and speed of cryosurgery treatment makes it particularly attractive for dermatological practice. It must be stressed that, for most lesions in Table 80.1 other modes of treatment may be equally effective, but are often less convenient and typically give inferior cosmetic results.

Lesions that are superficial, benign or flat can be treated by the liquid nitrogen cotton-wool swab method. To obtain cure of preneoplastic and neoplastic conditions, the lower temperature and more consistently destructive properties of liquid nitrogen spray or probe equipment are desirable. Cryosurgical treatment of basal cell epitheliomas gives cure rates that compare favourably with other modes of therapy [1,2,8,9]. High cure rates depend on adequate technique and correct choice of lesion and site—the inner canthus of the eye, nasolabial and retro-auricular folds and the hair-bearing scalp are less favoured sites. The temperature reached and the number of freeze–thaw cycles are also critical. Repeat freeze–thaw cycles give more reliable cell death, whichever method is adopted [2,9].

Side-effects [1]. Pain is minimal compared with surgery and is usually transient, due to the anaesthetizing effect of freezing. Pronounced oedema is not uncommon in the lax tissue around the eyes, lips, tongue and labia. Haemorrhagic blisters may occur. It is important to note that blister formation is not necessary for the cure of lesions

Table 80.1 Skin conditions responsive to cryosurgery [2,7,8].

Naevi	Pigmented
	Epidermal
Lentigo	Benign and malignant
Vascular lesions	Telangiectasia
	Spider naevus
	Pyogenic granuloma
	Pseudopyogenic granuloma
	Kaposi's sarcoma
	Haemangioma
	Lymphangioma
Keratotic and preneoplastic [1]	Viral warts
	Molluscum contagiosum
	Seborrhoeic keratosis
	Solar keratosis [11]
	Cutaneous horn
	Keratoacanthoma
	Bowen's disease
Carcinoma [2,8,9]	Basal cell epithelioma
	Squamous cell epithelioma
	Lentigo maligna
Cysts	Epidermal
	Synovial
	Acne
	Mucous cyst
Leukoplakia	
Axillary hyperhidrosis	
Scarring	Keloid [10]
	Acne (carbon dioxide snow, acetone 'slush')
Sebaceous hyperplasia	
Rhinophyma	

such as viral warts. Sun-damaged and senile atrophic skin, and areas previously treated with topical steroids or X-irradiation, are more likely to blister or become necrotic after freezing. Skin necrosis is a desirable part of the treatment of neoplastic and many preneoplastic lesions, and several weeks may elapse before healing is complete. Hypopigmentation is common after low-temperature liquid nitrogen cryosurgery (probe or jet), particularly in dark-skinned patients [5]. Temporary postinflammatory hyperpigmentation is to be expected following less severe freezing. Paraesthesiae and, rarely, anaesthesia occur, and may be troublesome because of the local effect of freezing on nerve endings. Care must be taken to avoid damage to major nerves, as distal anaesthesia and motor paralysis may occur; however, these rare effects are temporary [5]. Similarly, deep freezing over the lacrimal ducts may, very rarely, lead to permanent ductal obstruction. Adventitious glands are sensitive to freezing, and temporary hair loss and hypohidrosis are common; both can occasionally be permanent. In the treatment of axillary hyperhidrosis, the depilation may be regarded by the patient as a 'bonus'.

REFERENCES

1 Dawber RPR, Colver G, Jackson A. *Cutaneous Cryosurgery*, 2nd edn. London: M. Dunitz, 1997.
2 Kuflik EG. Cryosurgery updated. *J Am Acad Dermatol* 1994; **31**: 925–44.
3 Graham GF, Detlefs RL, Garrett AB *et al*. Guidelines of care for cryosurgery. *J Am Acad Dermatol* 1994; **31**: 648–53.
4 Dawber RPR. Cryosurgery. In: Lask GP, Moy RL, eds. *Principles and Techniques of Cutaneous Surgery*. New York: McGraw-Hill: 153–64.
5 Dawber RPR. Cold kills! *Clin Exp Dermatol* 1988; **13**: 137–50.
6 Burge SM, Dawber RPR. Hair follicle destruction and regeneration in guinea pig skin and cutaneous freeze injury. *Cryobiology* 1990; **27**: 153–63.
7 Sinclair RD, Tzermias C, Dawber RPR. Cosmetic cryosurgery. In: Baran R, Maibach HI, eds. *Cosmetic Dermatology*. London: M. Dunitz, 541–50.
8 Sinclair RD, Dawber RPR. Cryosurgery of malignant and pre-malignant diseases of the skin: a simple approach. *Australas J Dermatol* 1995; **36**: 133–42.
9 Mallon E, Dawber RPR. Cryosurgery treatment for basal cell carcinoma. *Dermatol Surg* 1997 (in press).
10 Zouboulis CC, Blume U, Buttner P. Outcome of cryosurgical treatment in patients with keloids and hypertrophic scars. *Arch Dermatol* 1993; **129**: 1146–51.
11 Schwartz RA. Therapeutic perspectives in actinic and other keratoses. *Int J Dermatol* 1996; **35**: 533–8.

Curettage

Benign lesions

Curettage of *viral warts*, like all therapies, is not totally effective. The treatment is painful and there is a risk of scarring and recurrence. Solitary warts on the face of adults can usually be removed effectively using curettage. Otherwise, curettage of viral warts should only be performed when other methods have failed. Plantar warts may be removed by curettage but the local anaesthetic injections are painful unless nerve-block anaesthesia is successful [1]. Recurrences can be a problem, as patients are unlikely to tolerate repeat treatment. Curettage is probably justifiable in painful, solitary, plantar warts, which have not responded to other therapies, although the patient should be warned of the risk of permanent, potentially painful, scar formation. Periungual warts are difficult to curette off and curettage should only be employed as a last resort; the nail may have to be avulsed to allow adequate access for curettage. Multiple finger warts should not be treated by curettage unless all else has failed. Genital or perianal warts that have not responded to cryotherapy or podophyllin can be curetted off.

Multiple *seborrhoeic warts* are best treated by cryotherapy. Solitary warts or those that have not responded to cryotherapy can be curetted off if necessary.

Other lesions such as *pyogenic granulomas* and *actinic keratoses* (Fig. 80.1) are commonly treated using curettage.

Curettage is only possible if the material being scraped off is more frail than the surrounding skin, or where there is a natural cleavage plane between the lesion and the surrounding normal tissue. The resulting shallow wound heals by a combination of wound shrinkage and re-epithelialization from the follicular and edge epithelium.

Tense and fix the numbed skin using the finger and thumb. Scrape off the lesion with the edge of a sharp spoon or ring curette until a smooth surface remains. On mobile areas, first fulgurize or incise the wart margin to obtain a plane of cleavage. Stop bleeding using either cautery, electrodesiccation or a chemical haemostatic agent. Do not use alcohol-based skin-cleansing solutions when using cautery or electrodesiccation because of the risk of fire.

Non-melanoma skin cancers

Basal cell carcinoma

Curettage of basal cell carcinomas (BCCs) depends on the tumour being less robust and hence easier to scrape off than the surrounding normal tissue. Thus, if strands of fibrous tissue separate clumps of tumour, as occurs in morphoeic, recurrent or locally invasive BCCs, curettage will fail. Similarly, if the adjacent skin tears easily, cannot be tensed or hair roots impede curettage, the results will be poor and curettage should be avoided. When small [2–5] (less than 20 mm diameter), non-recurrent tumours [6–8] on suitable sites (Table 80.2) are curetted by experts [9,10], the 5-year cure rate is 95% or better (Table 80.3). Higher recurrence rates occur after curettage of recurrent [6], morphoeic [3] or large tumours [2,3], or treatment by inexperienced operators [9] (Table 80.4). Cautery and electrodesiccation can be used interchangeably and are an important component of successful treatment; higher recurrence rates are reported if curettage alone is used [11]. Paradoxically, despite these high cure rates, careful histological examination of skin excised immediately after curettage and electrodesiccation of appropriately selected BCCs shows that residual tumour is present in almost 30% of cases [12,13]. Thus, cure must also depend on other factors, such as residual tumour cell mass, inflammatory reaction and healing responses.

Squamous cell carcinoma

Experience suggests that well-differentiated, primary, slow-growing tumours arising on sun-exposed sites can be removed by curettage, although there is little published data relating to outcome after curettage of different clinical tumour types (Table 80.5). Because of the higher risk of recurrence or metastasis with scar cancers and squamous cell carcinomas (SCCs) on the ears and lips [14], curettage and cautery is not recommended at these sites.

The technique is the same in both BCC and SCC. Tense the anaesthetized skin around the lesion and scrape off the bulk of the tumour using a small, sharp curette [15]; the curette should not be so sharp that there is a risk of

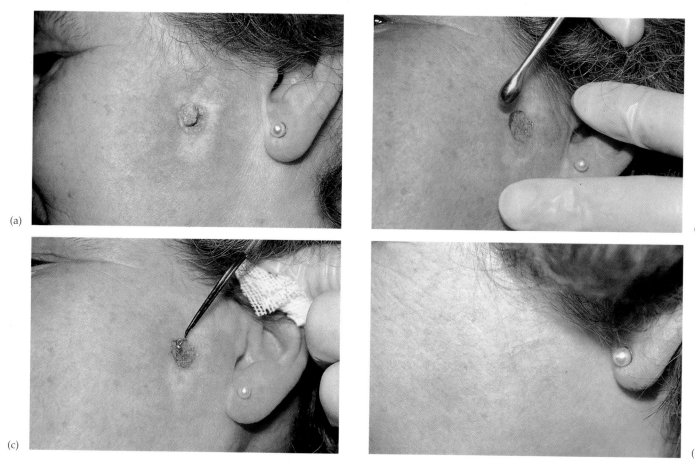

(a)

(b)

(c)

(d)

Fig. 80.1 Curettage and cautery of an actinic keratosis. After local anaesthetic injection, this hyperkeratotic actinic keratosis (a) was curetted off (b) and the wound cauterized (c). At 4 months the wound had healed leaving a barely visible scar (d).

Table 80.2 Sites to avoid curettage and cautery of basal cell carcinomas.

Sites with a high recurrence rate after all treatment modalities	Sites where curettage is technically difficult	Sites associated with poor cosmesis after curettage
Nose	Lips	Vermilion border
Nasolabial fold	Eyelid	Ala rim
Around the eye	Hair-bearing scalp	Nose tip
Around the ear		Chin
Scalp		

it slicing through the underlying dermis (Fig. 80.2). The fragmented specimen should be mounted on a small piece of filter paper where it is allowed to congeal slightly before being dropped into formalin. In this way the pathologist receives a single sample rather than multiple small floating fragments. Cauterize, using a hot wire with a beaded tip, or electrodesiccate the wound surface. Repeat the curettage using a smaller curette to search for residual pockets of tumour. At this stage the curette will be scraping against the normal dermis and less material will be removed. If

the curette penetrates the dermis and enters fat, curettage should be abandoned and the area excised down to and including fat, as it is impossible to distinguish between the softer tumour tissue and the underlying fat. Perforation of the dermis is particularly likely to occur if an incisional biopsy has been taken prior to treatment. Repeat the cautery or electrodesiccation. Consider the need for a third cycle of curettage and cautery if a large amount of material is removed at the second stage. The histological specimen only confirms the diagnosis; it provides no indication about

Table 80.3 Cure rates following curettage and cautery/electrodesiccation of primary basal cell carcinoma.

Author Year of publication	Number of tumours	Duration of follow-up (years)	Number of recurrences (%)	Tumour size
Simpson [7] 1966	495	2–5	35 (7)	ns
Williamson and Jackson [10] 1962	287	3	22 (7.6)	ns
Knox et al. [5] 1967	282	5	4 (1.4)	<20 mm
Sweet [3] 1963	268	≥3	19 (7.1)	<20 mm
Spiller and Spiller [4] 1984	208	5	3 (1.4)	<20 mm
Tromovitch [8] 1965	75	≥5	(4)	ns

ns, not stated.

Table 80.4 Types of basal cell carcinoma (BCC) not to treat by curettage.

Large tumours, i.e. ≥2 cm diameter
Tumours at sites where curettage produces a poor cosmetic result, is technically difficult, or is associated with a high risk of recurrence
Morphoeic, infiltrating or basisquamous BCCs
Recurrent tumours
Ill-defined tumours
Tumours penetrating muscle, fat, bone, etc.
Tumours where an incisional biopsy has been performed

Table 80.5 Cure rates following curettage and cautery of primary squamous cell carcinoma (SCC).

Author Year of publication	Number of tumours	Duration of follow-up (years)	Number of recurrences (% cure rate)	Metastasis?	Tumour size (number greater and smaller than 2 cm)
Knox et al. [5] 1967	213	5	1 (99)	No record	185 < 2 cm 28 > 2 cm
Knox et al. [5] 1967	545	>1 year	3 (99)	1	495 < 2 cm 50 > 2 cm
Tromovitch [8] 1965	29	5	(96.6)	Nil	No record
Freeman et al. [16] 1964	407	1–5	(96–100)	Nil	355 < 2 cm 52 > 2 cm

the adequacy of treatment. Ideally, the patient should be followed up yearly for 5 years. If the tumour recurs, consider the need for Mohs surgery, as cure rates are poor after curettage of recurrent tumours [6].

Intraepidermal carcinoma (Bowen's disease)

Intraepidermal carcinoma, especially on the lower leg, can be treated by curettage. Although all wounds at this site heal slowly, particularly if there is coexisting oedema or poor peripheral circulation, curettage is probably superior to radiotherapy, 5-fluorouracil or cryotherapy, as the extent of treatment is more predictably determined by the operator.

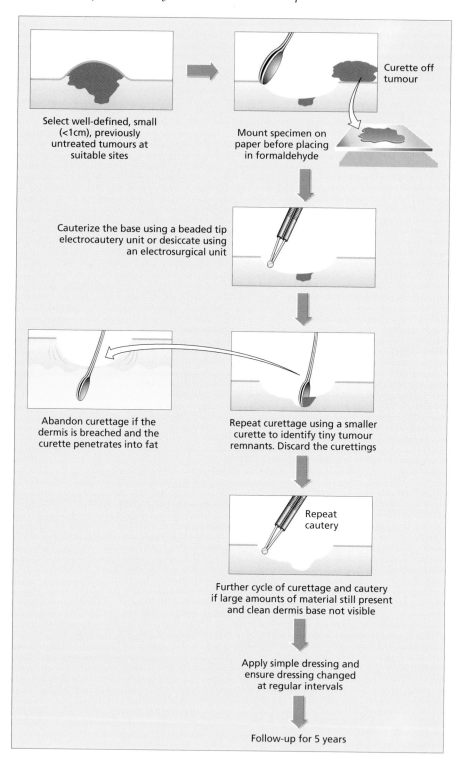

Select well-defined, small (<1cm), previously untreated tumours at suitable sites

Mount specimen on paper before placing in formaldehyde

Curette off tumour

Cauterize the base using a beaded tip electrocautery unit or desiccate using an electrosurgical unit

Abandon curettage if the dermis is breached and the curette penetrates into fat

Repeat curettage using a smaller curette to identify tiny tumour remnants. Discard the curettings

Repeat cautery

Further cycle of curettage and cautery if large amounts of material still present and clean dermis base not visible

Apply simple dressing and ensure dressing changed at regular intervals

Follow-up for 5 years

Fig. 80.2 Schematic diagram of the stages of curettage and cautery of a basal cell carcinoma. (From Lawrence [17].)

REFERENCES

1 Eriksson E. *Illustrated Handbook in Local Anaesthesia*, 2nd edn. Philadelphia: WB Saunders, 1980: 112–14.
2 Dubin N, Kopf AW. Multivariate risk score for recurrence of cutaneous basal cell carcinomas. *Arch Dermatol* 1983; **119**: 373–7.
3 Sweet RD. The treatment of basal cell carcinoma by curettage. *Br J Dermatol* 1963; **75**: 137–48.

4 Spiller WF, Spiller RF. Treatment of basal cell carcinoma by curettage and electrodesiccation. *J Am Acad Dermatol* 1984; **11**: 808–14.
5 Knox JM, Freeman RG, Duncan WC, Heaton CL. Treatment of skin cancer. *South Med J* 1967; **60**: 241–6.
6 Menn H, Robins P, Knopf AW, Bart RS. The recurrent basal cell epithelioma: a study of 100 cases of recurrent retreated basal cell epithelioma. *Arch Dermatol* 1971; **103**: 628–31.
7 Simpson JR. The management of rodent ulcers by curettage and cauterisation. *Br J Dermatol* 1966; **78**: 147–8.

8 Tromovitch TA. Skin cancer. Treatment by curettage and desiccation. *Calif Med* 1965; **103**: 107–8.
9 Kopf AW, Bart RS, Schrager D *et al.* Curettage-electrodesiccation treatment of basal cell carcinoma. *Arch Dermatol* 1977; **113**: 439–43.
10 Williamson GS, Jackson R. Treatment of basal cell carcinoma by electrodesiccation and curettage. *Can Med Assoc J* 1962; **86**: 855–62.
11 Reymann F. Treatment of basal cell carcinoma of the skin with curettage. II. A follow-up study. *Arch Dermatol* 1973; **108**: 528–31.
12 Salasche SJ. Curettage and electrodesiccation in the treatment of mid-facial basal cell epithelioma. *J Am Acad Dermatol* 1983; **8**: 496–503.
13 Edens BL, Bartlow GA, Haghigi P *et al.* Effectiveness of curettage and electrodesiccation in the removal of basal cell carcinoma. *J Am Acad Dermatol* 1983; **9**: 383–8.
14 Rowe DE, Carroll RJ, Day CL. Prognostic factors for local recurrence, metastasis, and survival rates in squamous cell carcinoma of the skin, ear and lip. *J Am Acad Dermatol* 1992; **26**: 976–90.
15 Bennett RG. *Fundamentals of Cutaneous Surgery.* St Louis: Mosby, 1988: 536–43.
16 Freeman RG, Knox JM, Heaton CL. The treatment of skin cancer. A statistical study of 1,341 skin tumours comparing results obtained with irradiation, surgery and curettage followed by electrodesiccation. *Cancer* 1964; **17**: 535–8.
17 Lawrence CM. *An Introduction to Dermatological Surgery.* London: Blackwell Healthcare Communications, 1996: 160 pp.

Electrosurgery

Electrosurgery includes electrodesiccation, electrofulguration, cutting diathermy (syn. electrosection, electroresection) and electrolysis [1,2]. Coagulation or tissue destruction is produced by the heat created as the electrical current passes through the tissue. Although not strictly an electrosurgical technique, electrocautery is usually also included because of its development from the age-old method of using heat in the form of hot oils, cautery irons, etc., to control bleeding.

Electrocautery

SYN. CAUTERY; HEAT CAUTERY; HOT-WIRE CAUTERY

The cautery machine power output should be controllable so that the tip temperature can be adjusted rather than being dependent on the battery power. A variety of tips are available. The *beaded tip* is best for haemostasis after curettage and shave biopsy; this should be just hot enough to char a cotton swab, but not red hot as the platinum tip may melt. If the beaded tip drags on the tissue as it is drawn across the wound, the tip temperature is too low. After use, any remaining debris should be burnt off by briefly allowing the tip to become red hot. The needle-like end of the *cold point cautery tip* is heated, by conduction, via a wire coil, and is used to treat spider naevi. The *flat blade* can be used for pedunculated lesions or shave excisions, but has to be glowing red hot to cut through tissue, producing a heating artefact on the excised material. Furthermore, the red-hot blade has to be quickly passed through the skin to avoid excessive heat damage at the wound site, so the direction and depth of the cut cannot be adjusted easily and the blade may accidentally cut or burn deeper into the tissue than required.

Electrosurgery

SYN. SURGICAL DIATHERMY; COLD ELECTROCAUTERY

Waveform. Electrosurgical equipment converts domestic alternating current into high-frequency alternating current. When this passes through a high-resistance medium, such as the skin and fat, heat is produced resulting in tissue coagulation, desiccation or cutting, depending on the electrical waveform. A highly damped waveform (i.e. intermittent pulses), results in electrodesiccation/fulguration, a continuous waveform produces a cutting effect and coagulation is produced by a slightly damped waveform [3]. There is overlap between these effects.

Unipolar/monoterminal/bipolar diathermy. Apart from the waveform produced, electrosurgery equipment also varies in the way it discharges and collects the current. Unipolar (monopolar) current is delivered via an active electrode, usually a needle or ball tip, resulting in a high concentration of current at the electrode tip. The current disperses through the patient's body and is collected via a dispersive (syn. indifferent, passive, return, ground) electrode with a large surface area. The current density falls with increasing distance from the active electrode and there is minimal risk of tissue damage as the current is collected over the large area of the dispersive electrode. If, due to faulty application or equipment, there is only a small area of skin/electrode contact, a burn may occur at the dispersive electrode. Also, if the current is channelled at narrow points along its path, for example the penis, an area of high-current density leading to tissue damage can occur. Bipolar electrodes avoid these hazards by producing and collecting the current via a pair of forceps so that current only travels in the tissue held between the tips of the forceps, not through the whole patient. Monoterminal electrosurgical equipment (e.g. Birtcher Hyfrecator) produces a high-voltage, low-amperage current, and is designed to be used without a dispersive electrode. There is, however, a risk of a small but painful discharge occurring between the patient and the operator or some other grounded or earthed point, for example the edge of a metal table, if the patient is lying on an electrically insulated couch [4]. This can be prevented by maintaining a large area of skin contact between the operator and patient during use, or using a dispersive electrode.

Electrodesiccation/electrofulguration. This is produced using a monoterminal or unipolar electrode. Electrodesiccation occurs when the needle remains in contact with the skin and no spark occurs. Because the current concentration is greater at the point of contact, the tissue damage is slightly deeper compared with electrofulguration. During the latter, the needle tip is not in contact with the skin and a spark jumps between the skin and the needle, but its energy is spread over a greater area. The resulting heat causes superficial damage to the tissues and is an effective way of stopping bleeding from capillaries. Various needle tips have been developed for specific circumstances [5]. Because of the risk of virus transmission, a different clean needle must be used for each patient [6].

Pacemakers and electrosurgery

Using an electrosurgical unit may stop a pacemaker working temporarily, so that the patient's heart may stop beating briefly if there is no underlying cardiac rhythm. Alternatively, the pacemaker may deviate from a demand to a fixed-rate mode as this is not affected by the electrosurgical current [7]. The effect lasts only as long as the unit is being operated. When diathermy finishes, the pacemaker reverts to normal function. There are also anecdotal reports of the pacemaker failing shortly after electrosurgery [8]. Diathermy used directly over a pacemaker may rarely cause its permanent reprogramming, but permanent inhibition is very rare. All pacemakers, particularly older versions, are vulnerable. All types of electrosurgical equipment, apart from electrocautery, can cause the problem. Bipolar diathermy is least hazardous, and where possible should be used in preference to mono-terminal or monopolar diathemy. With both monopolar and bipolar diathermy, only short bursts (less than 5 sec) should be used, the patient's heart rate should be monitored and resuscitation equipment should be available. Diathermy should not be performed within 15 cm of the heart, the pacemaker or its leads. If monopolar diathermy has to be used, the path from the active electrode (diathermy tip) to the dispersive electrode must also be at least 15 cm from the heart, the pacemaker and its leads.

Spider naevi

Spider naevi can be destroyed using either cold point cautery or electrodesiccation. With both modalities check correct positioning before treatment by pressing the tip downwards to ensure that the spider naevus blanches. The cold point cautery tip should be just hot enough to scorch a cotton swab. Insert the hot tip into the central feeding blood vessel and hold in place for approximately 1–2 seconds. The treatment can be repeated 4–6 weeks later if necessary. Low-dose electrodesiccation is similarly effective. Blanching may not be complete initially, but treatment should not be repeated more than once at each visit because of the risk of scarring. Assess the result after 6 weeks and repeat the treatment if required. Treatment can usually be tolerated without local anaesthetic, but if this is required use plain lignocaine.

Telangiectatic vessels

Facial, particularly nasal, telangiectases, can be destroyed by electrodesiccation. Local anaesthetic is not required. The needle tip is traced along the vessel, which should blanch. There is a risk of linear scarring, which may not be noticeable on the sebaceous skin of the nose but is visible on a smooth skin surface [9].

Xanthelasma

Eyelid xanthelasma can be excised or destroyed in a variety of ways. Electrodesiccation and curettage of the fatty deposits is relatively simple to perform, and there is minimal risk of damage to other structures. After local anaesthetic injection, the skin over the xanthelasma is electrodesiccated and fulgurized. When the surface is breached, some of the underlying fatty deposits can be scraped off using a sharp curette. The area is then electrodesiccated again and left to heal by second intention. Cosmetic results are good and the technique has the advantage over trichloroacetic acid in being predictably effective after one treatment.

Small seborrhoeic and plane warts

Eyelid viral or seborrhoeic warts can be treated by electrodesiccation with little risk of conjunctival damage if the eyelid margin is everted or pulled away from the conjunctiva. Alternatively, an eye shield or eyelid (chalazion) clamp can be used; the latter immobilizes the lid, creates a bloodless field and protects the conjunctiva [10]. After local anaesthetic injection and gentle electro-desiccation warts are easy to curette off.

Surgical paring and electrofulguration of rhinophyma

Cutting diathermy or electrosection of tissue is particularly useful for treatment of rhinophyma, where bleeding can be a problem [11]. Alternatively, shave excision of redundant tissue, with subsequent sculpturing using electrodesiccation and fulguration, is effective. Re-epithelialization takes place, with minimal scarring, from the abundant pilosebaceous follicles which remain in the dermis (Fig. 80.3). Carbon dioxide laser resection is also effective.

Electrolysis

Hair is not an electrical conductor and thus electronic tweezers do not produce permanent hair removal; this can only be achieved if the electrical current reaches the germinal bulb via a needle inserted to the correct depth [12]. Galvanic electrolysis involves the use of low-voltage, low-amperage direct current passed down a

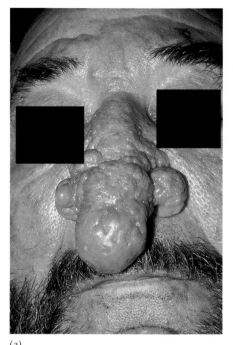

(a)

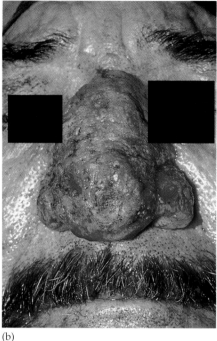

(b)

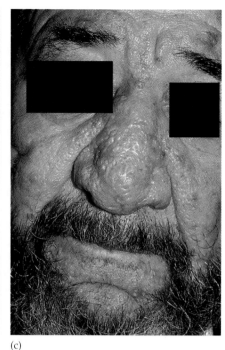

(c)

Fig. 80.3 Shave excision and electrosurgery of a rhinophyma. This disfiguring rhinophyma (a) was reduced in size and the nose shape recreated by shave excision and electrodesiccation of the bleeding surface under local anaesthetic (b), resulting in an acceptable cosmetic result at 4 months (c).

needle inserted into the follicle. The resulting current induces the formation of hydroxides, which cause dissolution of the follicular epithelium and hence detachment of the hair shaft. This technique is effective but time consuming. High-frequency electrodesiccation is a faster alternative, which destroys the follicle by heating. Insulated needles deliver the electrical current more precisely to the base of the follicle, but the wider needle is difficult to insert and the insulation may break. Side-effects of electrolysis include self-limiting redness and wealing, postinflammatory pigmentation, and scarring caused by too high a current.

REFERENCES

1 Jackson R. Basic principles of electrosurgery. A review. *Can J Surg* 1970; **13**: 354–61.
2 Elliott JA. Electrosurgery. Its use in dermatology with a review of its development and technologic aspects. *Arch Dermatol* 1966; **94**: 340–9.
3 Boughton RS, Spencer SK. Electrosurgical fundamentals. *J Am Acad Dermatol* 1987; **16**: 862–7.
4 Sebben JE. Patient 'grounding'. *J Dermatol Surg Oncol* 1988; **14**: 926–31.
5 Sebben JE. Modifications of electrosurgery electrodes. *J Dermatol Surg Oncol* 1992; **18**: 908–12.
6 Sheretz EF, Davis GL, Rice RW *et al.* Transfer of hepatitis B virus by contaminated reusable needle electrodes after electrodesiccation in simulated use. *J Am Acad Dermatol* 1986; **15**: 1242–6.

7 Sebben JE. Electrosurgery and cardiac pacemakers. *J Am Acad Dermatol* 1983; **9**: 457–63.
8 Wajszczuk WJ, Mowry FM, Dugan NL. Deactivation of a dermal pacemaker by transurethral electrocautery. *N Engl J Med* 1969; **280**: 34–5.
9 Fewkes JL, Cheney ML, Pollack SV. *Atlas of Cutaneous Surgery.* Philadelphia: JB Lippincott, 1992.
10 Bennett RG. *Fundamentals of Cutaneous Surgery.* St Louis: CV Mosby, 1988: 257, 429.
11 Greenbaum SS, Krull EA, Watnick K. Comparison of CO₂ laser and electrosurgery in the treatment of rhinophyma. *J Am Acad Dermatol* 1988; **18**: 363–8.
12 Richards RN, Meharg GE. Electrolysis: observations from 13 years and 140 000 hours of experience. *J Am Acad Dermatol* 1995; **33**: 662–6.

Infrared coagulation [1–3]

The infrared coagulator produces ordinary light (non-coherent) with a spectrum of 400–2700 nm. Power is generated from a tungsten halogen bulb and is transmitted along a quartz glass light guide—at its end this has a sapphire cap, which is placed in contact with the skin. The heat imparted causes thermal injury to a depth dependent on the duration of exposure, which can be set on an automatic timer and varied from 0 to 1.5 sec, for example a 1-sec exposure will remove tissue to a depth of approximately 0.75 mm.

The major characteristics are:

1 non-laser radiation of maximum output 960 nm (near infrared);
2 tungsten halogen bulb power source—15 V, 150 W;
3 pulsed energy;
4 solid quartz glass light guide;
5 diameter of treated area 2–10 mm, the larger diameters enabling more rapid treatment;
6 sapphire cap to light guide—sapphire is transparent to

near infrared but rapidly conducts away heat generated in the upper dermis;

7 minimum optical hazard—the appearance of bright visible radiation causes aversion of the eyes if it is pointing in their direction, thus preventing infrared damage;

8 it is portable, and relatively cheap.

It has been used mainly for tattoos [1], a variety of superficial vascular lesions [2], warts and myxoid cysts of the digit. Tattoos [1] can be treated with remarkably little morbidity. The area to be treated is mapped into overlapping circles similar in diameter to the sapphire tip, and each circle is treated with a pulsed exposure of approximately 1.25 sec. An ice cube applied to the skin for 5 sec before and after treatment is used to minimize conducted heat damage to surrounding skin. The immediate appearance of the coagulated tissue is white and slightly contracted; the eschar that develops over several days drops off in 2–3 weeks. Serous exudate, pain and swelling during the healing phase are generally insignificant.

Telangiectases, port-wine stains and angioma serpiginosum have been treated using short exposure times, for example 0.75–0.875 sec (also with ice). It is evidently less specific and probably less effective, with a greater risk of scarring, than an appropriate laser.

REFERENCES

1 Colver GB, Cherry GW, Dawber RPR, Ryan TJ. Tattoo removal using infrared coagulation. *Br J Dermatol* 1985; **112**: 481–5.
2 Colver GB, Cherry GW, Dawber RPR, Ryan TJ. Infra-red coagulation for removing tattoos and vascular naevi. *Br J Dermatol* 1984; **111** (Suppl. 26): 27.
3 Burge S, Colver GB, Rayment R. *Simple Skin Surgery*, 2nd edn. Oxford: Blackwell Science, 1996: 69–70.

Caustics and chemical peeling

Caustics

In experienced hands, caustics provide a simple and readily available means of destroying many superficial skin lesions. The operator should be well acquainted with the action and degree of penetration of individual caustics, and the toxic effects that may result from absorption, especially if they are to be used on large areas, and particularly when applied to the face [1,2]. In treating individual lesions, caustics are usually applied by means of a cotton-bud applicator or a wool-tipped orange stick, pointed if necessary.

Aluminium chloride hexahydrate

A 20% solution (Drichlor; Anhydrol Forte) usually applied on a cotton-bud is a very useful styptic for superficial wounds such as those following shave excision. Ferric subsulphate (Monsel's solution) is widely used, but may leave a pigmented scar.

Silver nitrate [3]

This is used in the form of a pencil or as a strong solution to suppress exuberant granulation. It is haemostatic and may be used to arrest bleeding after curettage. Repeated use tends to lead to unsightly staining of the skin.

Phenol (liquefied phenol)

This is a valuable superficial caustic, which should, however, be used cautiously. It should not be diluted as this increases its absorption and potency [4,5] and thus also its nephrotoxicity. Ochronosis may occur from prolonged absorption. It is not a haemostatic, and bleeding limits its effectiveness. When used as a treatment for ingrown toenails it is important that the phenol is applied to a 'dry' nailbed and that sufficient time is allowed for it to take effect [6].

Potential toxicity and cardiac arrhythmias remain a major concern, especially with more extensive use, and it should not be used during pregnancy. Phenol is used in a soap/croton oil/water mix for chemical face peels (see below). A glycol-spirit solution can be used for neutralization if required.

Trichloroacetic acid

This is an effective haemostatic caustic, which has many uses. The 30–50% concentration can be used as a styptic, and is frequently employed in conjunction with superficial curettage in the treatment of solar keratoses, seborrhoeic warts, etc. The supersaturated solution can also be used on its own to treat many benign and dysplastic skin lesions. Trichloroacetic acid 50% is similar to phenol in its destructive effect on the epidermis.

Trichloroacetic acid may be a useful treatment for xanthelasmata and solar lentigos. It must be applied with great care, however, especially around the eyes. Its action is rapid, and a white 'frosting' occurs within a few seconds of application. The caustic action can be partially neutralized by applying alcohol, water or sodium bicarbonate-soaked gauze, but this is unlikely to have any effect once the acid has penetrated the skin.

Excess sebum should first be removed using detergent, ether or acetone. Trichloroacetic acid should then be applied with an 'almost dry' cotton applicator. The concentration to be used will vary according to site, the condition to be treated and whether the trichloroacetic acid is being used as a styptic or a superficial skin caustic.

Weaker solutions of trichloroacetic acid are sometimes used for treating wider areas of skin (see below). Because of deliquescence, trichloroacetic acid should be kept in a closed, coloured and corrosion-resistant bottle.

Dichloroacetic acid

This is also a powerful caustic and skin styptic.

Monochloroacetic acid

This should not be considered as a superficial caustic. It penetrates rapidly and may remove the whole epidermis by blister formation. It may be used for mosaic warts, and can also be used for resistant periungual warts.

Alpha-hydroxyacids

These acids, for example glycolic acid, can be used to produce superficial or freshening peels and, at high concentration, medium-depth chemical peels.

Zinc chloride

This is a very powerful caustic [7].

Chemical peeling [1,2,8–10]

This procedure can be used to improve the appearance of ageing, wrinkled or sun-damaged skin. It is less effective in dealing with acne scars but is a valid dermatological manoeuvre for these and other superficial lesions on the face.

Chemical face peeling is used in conjunction with, or as an alternative to, dermabrasion. Patients with a dry skin and a fair complexion are the best subjects. A variety of preparations in differing concentration can be used alone or in combination depending on the desired outcome [11]. Trichloroacetic acid is probably the most commonly used agent. Weak preparations (10–15%) may be used for light 'freshening' peels and higher concentrations for medium-depth or deep peels. Alpha-hydroxy acids (mild), Jessner's solution (mild) and phenol (deep) may also be used. The neck should only be included with caution as the skin in this area is more prone to scarring and hyperpigmentation. Weaker preparations are generally used on eyelids, and care must be taken not to cause hypertrophic scars, which may occur around the mouth or mandible. Prolonged erythema and increased sensitivity to sunlight, and pigmentary changes (both hyperpigmentation and hypopigmentation), may follow the procedure.

REFERENCES

1 Brody HJ. *Chemical Peeling*. St Louis: Mosby Year Book, 1992.
2 Rubin MG. *Manual of Chemical Peels, Superficial and Medium Depth*. Philadelphia: JB Lippincott, 1995.
3 Jarson PO. Topical hemostatic agents for dermatologic surgery. *J Dermatol Surg Oncol* 1988; **14**: 623–32.
4 Conning DM, Hayes MJ. The dermal toxicity of phenol. *Br J Ind Med* 1970; **27**: 155–9.
5 Truppmann ES, Ellenberg JD. Major ECG changes during chemical facial peeling. *Plast Reconstr Surg* 1979; **63**: 44–8.
6 Frumkin A. Phenol cauterisation of nail matrix remnants. *J Dermatol Surg Oncol* 1987; **13**: 1324–5.
7 Falanga V, Friondon M. Zinc chloride paste for the debridement of chronic leg ulcers. *J Dermatol Surg Oncol* 1990; **16**: 658–62.
8 Lask GP, Parish LC, eds. *Aesthetic Dermatology*. New York: McGraw-Hill, 1991: 128–38.
9 McCollough G, Langsdon PR. *Dermabrasion and Chemical Peel*. New York: Thieme, 1988.
10 Stegman SJ, Tromovitch TA. *Cosmetic Dermatologic Surgery*, 2nd edn. Chicago: Year Book Medical Publishers, 1990.
11 Coleman WP, Futrell JM. The glycolic acid-trichloroacetic acid peel. *J Dermatol Surg Oncol* 1994; **20**: 76–80.

Topical cytotoxic therapy [1–4]

Unfortunately, apart from 5-fluorouracil, efforts to develop clinically useful topical agents to deal effectively with superficial skin malignancy have been disappointing. Their use in the therapy of non-malignant conditions, for example condylomas, is discussed in Chapter 26.

5-Fluorouracil [2,3]

This has a long-established record, that has stood the test of time. Not only does it effectively destroy keratoses but it also appears able to deal with less obvious areas of actinic damage, giving a 'field effect' around treated lesions. Concentrations of 1–5% applied twice a day for 1–4 weeks can be used to treat areas of skin that have a large number of keratoses. A pronounced inflammatory reaction develops, which can be reduced by using topical steroids. Treatment may be repeated at a later date if any lesions persist after the inflammatory phase has regressed.

The reaction can be largely avoided if 5-fluorouracil is applied weekly over a prolonged period [5]. The results are excellent, although the response is less impressive on the hands and forearms than on the face and scalp. It has been suggested that the addition of keratolytics or topical vitamin A acid may be of value in this situation; 5-fluorouracil may also be combined with cryotherapy [6].

Allergic contact and photosensitivity reactions have been associated with 5-fluorouracil [7]. Onycholysis has followed its application around nails [1,3]

It is also of value in superficial malignancies of the skin such as Bowen's disease [8] and erythroplasia of the penis [9]. It should only be used for the most superficial type of skin malignancy [2–4]; even when applied with occlusion, recurrences are frequent, but reasonable results have been obtained. There is a risk, even when treating superficial basal cell carcinomas, that deep tumour 'nests' will remain and lead to late and initially occult recurrence.

Colchicine [1,2]

Derivatives of the parent substance are less toxic; *N*-desacetylmethyl colchicine (Colcemid omacine) has been used in strengths of 0.25–1.00% or more. It inhibits mitosis in metaphase. It is applied, once or twice a day, for 4 weeks, covered by an adhesive dressing, and has been used for BCCs, Bowen's disease, leukoplakia and solar keratoses. Keratoacanthomas may also respond [2]. It has been used as an accessory treatment after curettage and cauterization of BCCs in situations where recurrences might be expected. Its use leads to more scarring than would otherwise occur, but it may be a useful adjunct to therapy. Thiocolsiran is similar.

Nitrogen mustard (mechlorethamine) [2]

This has been used topically in patients suffering from mycosis fungoides, Langerhans' cell histiocytosis and multicentric reticulohistiocytosis, [2,5–7,10,11]. It has also been reported as useful in the treatment of acropustulosis [12].

REFERENCES

1 Bennett RG. *Fundamentals of Cutaneous Surgery*. St Louis: Mosby, 1988: 627–701.
2 Du Vivier A. Topical cytostatic drugs in the treatment of skin cancer. *Clin Exp Dermatol* 1982; **7**: 89–92.
3 Goette DK. Topical chemotherapy with 5-fluorouracil: a review. *J Am Acad Dermatol* 1981; **4**: 633–49.
4 Goldes JA, Kao GF. Premalignant lesions. In: Roenigk RK, Roenigk HH, eds. *Dermatologic Surgery*, 2nd edn. New York: Marcel Dekker, 1996: 439–63.
5 Pearlman DL. Weekly pulse dosing: effective and comfortable topical 5-fluorouracil treatment of multiple facial actinic keratoses. *J Am Acad Dermatol* 1991; **25**: 665–7.
6 Abadir DR. Combination of topical 5-fluorouracil with cryotherapy for treatment of actinic keratoses. *J Dermatol Surg Oncol* 1982; **9**: 403–6.
7 Sams WM. Unwanted responses with topical 5-fluorouracil. *Arch Dermatol* 1968; **97**: 14–22.
8 Sturm HM. Bowen's disease and 5-fluorouracil. *J Am Acad Dermatol* 1979; **1**: 513–22.
9 Lewis RJ, Bendl BJ. Erythroplasia of Queyrat: treatment with topical 5-fluorouracil. *Can Med Assoc J* 1971; **104**: 148–9.
10 Du Vivier A, Vollum DI. Photochemotherapy and topical nitrogen mustard in the treatment of mycosis fungoides. *Br J Dermatol* 1980; **102**: 319–22.
11 Nethercott JR, Murray AH, Medwidsky W. Histiocytosis X in two adults: treatment with topical mechlorethamine. *Arch Dermatol* 1983; **119**: 157–61.
12 Notowicz A, Stolz E, Heuvel NVD. Treatment of Hallopeau's acrodermatitis with topical mechlorethamine. *Arch Dermatol* 1978; **114**: 129.

Intralesional therapy

Intralesional triamcinolone

Several preparations for intralesional use are available [1]. An aqueous suspension of triamcinolone acetonide 10 mg/ml is commonly used, and can be diluted with saline or lignocaine. Triamcinolone hexacetonide 5 mg/ml is also available. There is no difference with regard to efficacy between the hexacetonide and acetonide salts [2].

Triamcinolone 5–10 mg/ml is sufficient for all conditions except keloids, for which a higher concentration may be required. Intralesional hydrocortisone acetate (25 mg/ml) can also be used. The amount injected ranges from 0.1 to 0.5 ml of 10 mg/ml solution, depending on the size and nature of the lesion. The injection should be given using a 27–30-gauge needle deep in the dermis when possible, to minimize the risk of collagen atrophy. The manufacturers recommend that no more than 30 mg of triamcinolone should be given in one session, and a maximum of 5 mg at any one site. (Steroid equivalence: 5 mg prednisolone = 4 mg triamcinolone = 20 mg hydrocortisone.) Plasma cortisol levels are suppressed for a few days by 20 mg of intralesional triamcinolone acetonide given into various sites; higher doses suppress cortisol levels for longer [3]. Systemic symptoms have been reported in children after a single injection of 240 mg triamcinolone diacetate and after five fortnightly 25-mg triamcinolone diacetate injections [4]. Local side-effects include collagen atrophy [5], hypopigmentation [6], skin necrosis [6], perilymphatic linear depigmented and atrophic streaks [7,8], and telangiectasia [9].

Needleless injection of steroids

Intralesional triamcinolone is also given using a needleless injector (Dermojet or Portojet). The injection is slightly less painful but is principally employed because injections can be given quickly [10]. The risk of intraocular injection must be considered if this technique is used around the eye [11]. Dose-for-dose needleless injection of steroid appears to be less effective than needle injection, probably because some of the steroid solution is lost as it spills onto the skin with the former.

Uses

Resolution of inflammatory acne cysts may be speeded by injection of triamcinolone. It is usually best to express a portion of the cyst contents before injection of sufficient triamcinolone 5–10 mg/ml to fill the cyst.

Virtually any steroid-responsive dermatosis will respond well to intralesional triamcinolone. Use of such therapy is time consuming, temporary and potentially associated with localized collagen atrophy, and should only be used with caution. Responsive dermatoses include psoriasis, lichen planus, lichen simplex, lupus erythematosus [12], chondrodermatitis [13], orofacial granulomatosis [14], granuloma annulare and alopecia areata. The last mentioned is particularly disappointing, as, although small tufts of hair may grow at the injection sites, the effect is temporary and the treatment does not affect disease outcome [15]. Necrobiosis lipoidica improves but may ulcerate. Nail psoriasis may respond to intralesional steroid injection into the matrix and nailbed [16].

REFERENCES

1 Callen JP. Intralesional corticosteroids. *J Am Acad Dermatol* 1981; **4**: 149–51.
2 Porter D, Burton JL. A comparison of intralesional triamcinolone hexacetonide and triamcinolone acetonide in alopecia areata. *Br J Dermatol* 1971: **85**: 272–3.
3 Potter RA. Intralesional triamcinolone and adrenal suppression in acne vulgaris. *J Invest Dermatol* 1971; **57**: 364–70.
4 Curtis JA, Cormode E, Laski B *et al.* Endocrine complications of topical and intralesional corticosteroid therapy. *Arch Dis Child* 1982; **57**: 204–7.
5 Krusche T, Worret WI. Mechanical properties of keloids *in vivo* during treatment with intralesional triamcinolone acetonide. *Arch Dermatol Res* 1995; **287**: 289–93.
6 Jarratt MT, Spark RF, Arndt KA. The effects of intradermal steroids on the pituitary-adrenal axis and the skin. *J Invest Dermatol* 1974; **62**: 463–6.
7 Kikuchi I, Horikawa S. Perilymphatic atrophy of the skin: a side effect of topical corticosteroid injection therapy. *Arch Dermatol* 1974; **109**: 558–9.
8 Gupta AK, Rasmussen JE. Peri-lesional linear atrophic streaks associated with intralesional corticosteroid injections in a psoriatic plaque. *Pediatr Dermatol* 1987; **4**: 259–60.
9 Schetman D, Hambrick GW, Wilson CE. Cutaneous changes following local injection of triamcinolone. *Arch Dermatol* 1963; **88**: 820–8.
10 Abell E, Munro DD. Intralesional treatment of alopecia areata with triamcinolone acetonide by jet injector. *Br J Dermatol* 1973; **88**: 55–9.
11 Perry HT, Cohn BT, Nauheim JS. Accidental intra-ocular injection with Dermojet syringe. *Arch Dermatol* 1977; **113**: 1131.
12 Callen JP. Chronic cutaneous lupus erythematosus. Clinical, laboratory, therapeutic and prognostic examination of 62 patients. *Arch Dermatol* 1982; **118**: 412–16.
13 Lawrence CM. The treatment of chondrodermatitis nodularis with cartilage removal alone. *Arch Dermatol* 1991; **127**: 530–5.
14 Sakuntabhai A, MacLeod RI, Lawrence CM. Intralesional steroid injection after nerve block anaesthesia in the treatment of orofacial granulomatosis. *Arch Dermatol* 1993; **129**: 477–80.
15 Anonymous. Alopecia areata. *Br Med J* 1979; **1**: 505–6.
16 de Berker D, Lawrence CM. A simplified protocol of steroid injection for psoriatic nail dystrophy. *Br J Dermatol* 1995; **133** (Suppl. 45): 15.

Intralesional therapies for skin malignancies

Intralesional *methotrexate* is reported to be a painless and effective method of treating keratoacanthoma, with faster than spontaneous resolution [1,2]. Topical 5-fluorouracil has long been used to treat superficial BCC and actinic keratoses. Recent reports suggest that repeated intralesional *5-fluorouracil* injections for 3 weeks destroys almost 90% of small, nodular BCCs, although the injections are extremely painful [3]. Intralesional *interferon-α2b* has been used to treat T-cell lymphomas of skin [4], condylomata acuminata, Bowenoid papulosis [5], melanoma [6], BCC [7,8] and SCC [9]. Up to 80% of small, solid or superficial BCCs injected using high-dose therapy appear to resolve, although adverse effects occur in 80% of patients at this dose. In contrast, only a minority of aggressive pattern invasive BCCs respond [10]. Intralesional *cisplatin* has been used to treat SCC in animals [11], and given by iontophoresis has been used for SCC and BCC in humans [12]. Intralesional *vincristine* and *bleomycin* have been used with some success in Kaposi's sarcoma [13,14].

REFERENCES

1 Melton JL, Nelson BR, Stough DB *et al.* Treatment of keratoacanthomas with intralesional methotrexate. *J Am Acad Dermatol* 1991; **25**: 1017–23.
2 Hurst LN, Gan BS. Intralesional methotrexate in keratoacanthoma of the nose. *Br J Plast Surg* 1995; **48**: 243–6.
3 Orenberg EK, Miller BH, Greenway T *et al.* The effect of intralesional 5-fluorouracil therapeutic implant (MPI 5003) for treatment of basal cell carcinoma. *J Am Acad Dermatol* 1992; **27**: 723–8.
4 Bunn PA, Jr, Ihde DC, Foon KA. The role of recombinant interferon alpha-2a in the therapy of cutaneous T-cell lymphoma. *Cancer* 1986; **57**: 1689–95.
5 Gross G, Roussaki A, Schöpf E *et al.* Successful treatment of condylomata acuminata and Bowenoid papulosis with subcutaneous injections of low-dose recombinant interferon alpha. *Arch Dermatol* 1986; **122**: 749–50.
6 Ishihara K, Hayasaka K, Yamazaki N. Current status of melanoma treatment with interferon, cytokines and other biologic response modifiers in Japan. *J Invest Dermatol* 1989; **92**: 326s–8s.
7 Edwards I, Tucker SB, Perednia D *et al.* The effect of an intralesional sustained-release formulation of interferon alpha-2b on basal cell carcinomas. *Arch Dermatol* 1990; **126**: 1029–32.
8 Cornell RC, Greenway HT, Tucker SB *et al.* Intralesional interferon therapy for basal cell carcinoma. *J Am Acad Dermatol* 1990; **23**: 694–700.
9 Wickramasinghe L, Hindson TC, Wacks H. Treatment of neoplastic skin lesions with intralesional interferon. *J Am Acad Dermatol* 1989; **20**: 71–4.
10 Stenquist B, Wennberg AM, Gisslén H, Larkö O. Treatment of aggressive basal cell carcinoma with intralesional interferon: evaluation of efficacy by Mohs surgery. *J Am Acad Dermatol* 1992; **27**: 65–9.
11 Kitchell BK, Orenberg EK, Brown DM *et al.* Intralesional sustained release chemotherapy with therapeutic implants for treatment of canine sun-induced squamous cell carcinoma. *Eur J Cancer* 1995; **31A**: 2093–8.
12 Chang BK, Guthrie TH, Hayakawa K, Gangarosa LP. A pilot study of iontophoretic cisplatin chemotherapy of basal and squamous cell carcinoma. *Arch Dermatol* 1993; **129**: 425–7.
13 Brambilla L, Boneschi V, Beretta G, Finzi AF. Intralesional chemotherapy for Kaposi's sarcoma. *Dermatologica* 1984; **169**: 150–5.
14 Poignonec S, Lachiver LD. Intralesional bleomycin for acquired immunodeficiency syndrome-associated cutaneous Kaposi's sarcoma. *Arch Dermatol* 1995; **131**: 228–30.

Other intralesional therapies

OK-432 is a lyophilized mixture of low virulence Su strain of *Streptococcus pyogenes*. This damages endothelial linings, and given intralesionally has been used to destroy lymphangiomas [1] with few significant side-effects and good response in half of the patients treated. Intralesional *bleomycin* is a treatment of last resort for unresponsive warts [2,3]. The injections are extremely painful and followed by inflammation lasting for up to 72h [4]. Pricking the bleomycin solution into the wart may be as successful, and is better tolerated [5].

REFERENCES

1 Ogita S, Tsuto T, Nakamura K *et al.* OK-432 therapy in 64 patients with lymphangioma. *J Pediatr Surg* 1994; **29**: 784–5.
2 Bunney MH, Nolan MW, Buxton PK *et al.* The treatment of resistant warts with intralesional bleomycin: a controlled clinical trial. *Br J Dermatol* 1984; **111**: 197–207.
3 Amer M, Diab N, Ramadan A *et al.* Therapeutic evaluation for intralesional injection of bleomycin sulphate in 143 resistant warts. *J Am Acad Dermatol* 1988; **18**: 1313–16.
4 Templeton SF, Solomon AR, Swerlick RA. Intradermal bleomycin injections into normal human skin. *Arch Dermatol* 1994; **130**: 577–83.
5 Munn SE, Higgins E, Marshall M, Clement M. A new method of intralesional bleomycin therapy in the treatment of recalcitrant warts. *Br J Dermatol* 1996; **135**: 969–71.

Lasers [1,2]

Lasers of various types are used extensively for the treatment of many cutaneous lesions. They are characterized by the active medium, which can be gas, solid or liquid. The therapeutic applications depend on wavelength and energy, the choice depending on the desired effect and absorption characteristics of the target tissue.

General principles. Laser is an acronym for *l*ight *a*mplification by the *s*timulated *e*mission of *r*adiation. Stimulated emission occurs when a photon causes an excited atom to return to a lower energy state and release a second photon in phase and of the same wavelength as the stimulating photon. The resultant output is characterized by certain properties which make laser radiation potentially useful:

1 monochromaticity;
2 coherence—spatial and temporal;
3 collimation.

The very high degree of coherence and the lack of divergence of the beam enable extremely high and precise power densities to be achieved. Laser light can produce different tissue effects (Table 80.6) depending on wavelength, power density (W/cm^2), length of exposure and tissue absorption. In dermatology, thermal effects are most important.

Selective photothermolysis [3]. This is the term used to describe the process by which light can be used to produce precise thermal injury. The process depends on the wavelength of light, the colour of the target and its size, which determines the thermal relaxation time. The thermal relaxation time is a measure of the time it takes a heated object to cool, and increases with target size (Table 80.7). Most clinical lasers are now configured to ensure spatial confinement of the thermal effect to the target tissue. The risk of injury to surrounding normal tissue and unwanted side-effects are therefore reduced.

Table 80.6 Biological effects of lasers.

Biostimulation
Thermal
Ionization
Photodynamic
Acoustic

Table 80.7 Examples of thermal relaxation times.

Target	Size	Thermal relaxation time
Melanosome	0.5–1 μm	0.25–1 μsec
Dermal capillary	0.1 mm	10 msec
Whole skin	–	0.8 msec

Safety. Lasers are powerful energy sources, which can scar and maim if used incorrectly. They should be used only in properly controlled sites by trained personnel who are taking all the necessary precautions to protect themselves and their patients from accidental exposure. A thorough practical understanding of laser–tissue interactions is most important.

Low-power lasers. Lasers operating at energies that do not produce any thermal effect are reported as being able to produce photobioactivation, and have been advocated for the treatment of leg ulcers and other chronic wounds. There is a paucity of well-controlled studies, and evidence for their usefulness is slight [4,5].

REFERENCES

1 Alster TS, Lewis AB. Dermatologic laser surgery. *Dermatol Surg* 1996; **22**: 797–805.
2 Spicer MS, Goldberg DJ. Lasers in dermatology. *J Am Acad Dermatol* 1996; **34**: 1–25.
3 Anderson RR, Parish JA. Selective photothermolysis: precise microsurgery by selective absorption of pulsed radiation. *Science* 1983; **220**: 524–7.
4 Colver GB, Priestley GC. Failure of a helium-neon laser to affect components of wound healing *in vitro*. *Br J Dermatol* 1989; **121**: 179–86.
5 Oshiro T, Calderhead RG. *Low-level Laser Therapy*. Chichester: John Wiley & Sons, 1988.

Vascular lesions [1,2]

Vascular lesions have generally been treated with lasers which target the haemoglobin absorption spectrum. However, there are theoretical reasons for looking at longer wavelengths whose absorption may be reduced but which have a greater tissue penetration. There are two main types of laser currently employed in treating vascular lesions: those which appear to work by sealing the vessels thermally and those which appear physically to disrupt the vessels—a process which is seen clinically as purpura. There is as yet no ideal system. Lesions should always be treated cautiously, in the knowledge that further treatment can be given if necessary.

Efforts to develop a laser which would provide selective thermolysis led to the production of flashlamp-pumped pulsed dye lasers with a pulse duration of 450 μsec. Most systems are tuned to an output of 585 nm, which is currently thought to provide the best combination of vascular specificity and tissue penetration. As technology has advanced, the treatment spot size has increased from 5 to 10 mm. This has reduced treatment times and possibly enhanced penetration. The major indication has been in the treatment of capillary malformations. They require several treatments at intervals of 8 weeks or more to produce the maximum improvement [1]. Only 10% of such lesions resolve completely, although a majority are significantly improved in terms of texture, colour and papular degenerative changes. A few may not respond and others may show progressive ectasia and require retreatment [3]. The risk of scarring is small. Superficial capillary haemangiomas which warrant treatment usually respond [4], and pulsed dye lasers can be used to treat a whole range of cutaneous vascular anomalies [5].

There are a number of laser systems which have been developed to deliver light of low-peak powers. The argon laser (488–514 nm) was the first to be used in treating vascular lesions. Argon lasers are relatively low powered continuous wave machines, but although many lesions were improved, there was a significant risk of scarring [2]. The development of robotized devices to scan narrow-diameter beams of high intensity in a controlled way within the putative thermal relaxation time, so that there is reduced thermal damage, has allowed these lasers to be used safely [6]. Most lasers of this type (Table 80.8) also provide an output from a narrow, single beam, which allows telangiectases and small vascular lesions to be treated without purpura, thereby reducing post-treatment morbidity.

There are now so many lasers, and even devices which are filtered flashlamps [7,8], available for treating vascular lesions that it is at times difficult, even for an experienced practitioner, to say definitively which laser is best for which clinical indication. When presented with a clinical problem, an assessment should be made of whether treatment is appropriate or necessary, and the options considered. It is usual for small areas to be treated initially to determine whether a satisfactory outcome is likely.

REFERENCES

1 Geronemus RG. Pulsed dye laser treatment of vascular lesions in children. *J Dermatol Surg Oncol* 1993; **19**: 303–10.
2 McBurney EI. Clinical usefulness of the argon laser for the 1990s. *J Dermatol Surg Oncol* 1993; **19**: 352–62.
3 Alster TS, Wilson F. Treatment of port-wine stains with the flashlamp-pumped pulsed dye laser: extended clinical experience in children and adults. *Ann Plast Surg* 1994; **32**: 478–84.
4 Barlow RJ, Walker NPJ, Markey AC. Treatment of proliferative haemangiomas with the 585 nm pulsed dye laser. *Br J Dermatol* 1996; **134**: 700–4.
5 Garden JM, Bakus AD. Clinical efficacy of the pulsed dye laser in the treatment of vascular lesions. *J Dermatol Surg Oncol* 1993; **19**: 321–6.
6 McDaniel DH. Clinical usefulness of Hexascan. Treatment of cutaneous vascular and melanocytic disorders. *J Dermatol Surg Oncol* 1993; **19**: 312–19.
7 Strempel H, Klein G. Laser therapy without laser: a controlled trial comparing the flashlamp-pumped pulsed dye laser with the photoderm high-energy gas discharge lamp. *Lasers Med Sci* 1996; **11**: 185–7.
8 Jernbeck J, Malm M. Calcitonin gene-related peptide increases the blood flow of port-wine stains and improves continuous-wave dye laser treatment. *Plast Reconstr Surg* 1993; **91**: 245–51.

Pigmented lesions [1,2]

Melanin can be selectively targeted with ultrashort high-energy pulsed lasers, although, as with vascular lesions, low-power continuous wave (CW) lasers of appropriate wavelength can also be used successfully to treat melanin-containing lesions [3]. There are various laser systems (Table 80.8) that have been reported to be effective, particularly for benign epidermal pigmentation. Dermal lesions respond less predictably, and the long-term efficacy has yet to be determined [4]. Some results can be very dramatic, but unfortunately it is not yet possible to produce significant long-term improvement in the majority of congenital melanocytic naevi.

Tattoos [5–7]

Implanted dermal pigment may be treated with lasers—either the carbon dioxide laser, [8] or by employing the principles of selective photothermolysis to fragment the pigment and allow its removal by phagocytosis, as an alternative to dermabrasion, salabrasion, or excision with or without grafting. Carbon dioxide laser vaporization essentially produces a burn which heals by secondary intention. The healing may result in a satisfactory scar, or excessive dermal injury may lead to a hypertrophic or keloidal scar. It remains to be seen whether the newer carbon dioxide laser delivery systems, which cause less thermal damage, will enable tattoos to be treated with a better cosmetic outcome. The three Q-switched laser systems, which can be used to treat pigmented lesions,

Table 80.8 Characteristics of laser systems in clinical use.

Laser	Wavelength (nm)	Target tissue/effect	Output
Argon	488–514	Melanin, haemoglobin	Continuous
Ruby	694	Melanin, dark pigment	Q-switched
Alexandrite	755	Melanin, dark pigment	Q-switched
Nd:YAG	1064	Melanin, dark pigment	Q-switched
Frequency-doubled ND:YAG	532	Melanin, yellow/red pigment	Q-switched
Carbon dioxide	10600	Tissue ablation and incision	Continuous/pulsed
Flashlamp-pumped pulsed dye	585	Haemoglobin	Pulsed
Copper vapour/ bromide	510	Melanin	Quasi-continuous
	578	Haemoglobin	Quasi-continuous

Table 80.9 Response of tattoo pigments to laser treatment.

Pigment	Q-switched ruby 694 nm	Q-switched alexandrite 755 nm	Q-switched Nd:YAG 1064 nm	Frequency-doubled Nd:YAG 532 nm	Flashlamp-pumped pulsed dye 585 nm
Black	+++	+++	+++	–	–
Green	++	+++	+	–	–
Red	–	–	–	+++	+++

+++, excellent response; ++, good response; +, fair response; –, no response.

can also be employed to treat tattoos (Table 80.9). The manufacturers are continually exploring ways of targeting the various colours which may be present. The final outcome of treatment depends on the type of tattoo, the colour and depth of the pigment, and the number of treatments. It is not possible to guarantee complete removal. Small, tentatively applied amateur tattoos almost always respond completely, but large, multicoloured professional ones may persist, at least in part, after multiple treatments. Persistent hypopigmentation may follow treatment, and scarring is possible if high fluences are used.

REFERENCES

1 Alster TS, Lewis AB. Dermatologic laser surgery. *Dermatol Surg* 1996; **22**: 797–805.
2 Spicer MS, Goldberg DJ. Lasers in dermatology. *J Am Acad Dermatol* 1996; **34**: 1–25.
3 McDaniel DH. Clinical usefulness of Hexascan. Treatment of cutaneous vascular and melanocytic disorders. *J Dermatol Surg Oncol* 1993; **19**: 312–19.
4 Alster TS, Williams CM. Treatment of nevus of Ota by the Q-switched alexandrite laser. *Dermatol Surg* 1995; **21**: 592–6.
5 Ashinoff R, Geronemus RG. Rapid response of traumatic and medical tattoos to treatment with the Q-switched ruby laser. *Plast Reconstr Surg* 1993; **91**: 841–5.
6 Kilmer SL, Lee MS, Grevelink JM *et al.* The Q-switched Nd:YAG laser (1064 nm) effectively treats tattoos: a controlled, dose-response study. *Arch Dermatol* 1993; **129**: 971–8.
7 Fitzpatrick RE, Goldman MP. Tattoo removal using the alexandrite laser. *Arch Dermatol* 1994; **130**: 1508–14.
8 Wheeland RG, Walker NPJ. Lasers—twenty-five years later. *Int J Dermatol* 1986; **25**: 209–16.

Cutaneous ablation [1,2]

Light in the mid and far infrared region of the spectrum is rapidly absorbed by water and therefore by body tissue. There is no selectivity of effect. When the light strikes the body tissue, the cells are vaporized almost instantaneously. Although vaporization is limited to those cells immediately in the path of the beam, there is a narrow band of thermal damage around the treatment site whose width depends on the laser type, the power density and the exposure times. The carbon dioxide laser was the first laser to be used extensively in this way. Although initially the outcome could be compromised by unwanted thermal damage and scarring, this risk has been markedly reduced by the

development of a variety of scanning devices. The carbon dioxide laser is the archetypal surgical laser. Using a high-power density, via a focusing handpiece, the depth of an incision is controlled by the speed with which the beam is moved over the surface, enabling excisions to be performed as easily as with a scalpel. Lower densities are now achieved by using a scanner, and this allows a variety of skin lesions to be treated (Table 80.10).

Resurfacing

The development of scanning systems has allowed the carbon dioxide laser to be used to treat extensive areas of skin damaged by photo-ageing or scarred by acne, with good results [3,4]. This procedure is associated with prolonged morbidity, and lasers with even higher tissue absorption (i.e. erbium YAG 2940 nm), and therefore even less dermal damage, may offer advantages [5].

Table 80.10 Some therapeutic applications of carbon dioxide laser radiation.

Keloids
Seborrhoeic keratoses
Epidermal naevi
Tumours
Warts, condylomas
Cheilitis
Tattoos

REFERENCES

1 Alster TS, Lewis AB. Dermatologic laser surgery. *Dermatol Surg* 1996; **22**: 797–805.
2 Spicer MS, Goldberg DJ. Lasers in dermatology. *J Am Acad Dermatol* 1996; **34**: 1–25.
3 Alster TS, West TB. Resurfacing of atrophic facial acne scars with a high-energy, pulsed carbon dioxide laser. *Dermatol Surg* 1996; **22**: 151–5.
4 Dover JS, Hruza GJ. Laser skin resurfacing. *Semin Cutan Med Surg* 1996; **15**: 177–88.
5 Kaufmann R, Hibst R. Pulsed 2.94 μm erbium—YAG laser skin ablation—experimental results and first clinical application. *Clin Exp Dermatol* 1990; **15**: 389–93.

The future

Lasers and allied technology are developing rapidly. New clinical indications are continually being proposed, only some of which have been confirmed by well-controlled trials and the passage of time. Currently, other than cutaneous resurfacing, there is considerable interest in exploiting selective laser/tissue effects for hair removal [1] and for the treatment of a variety of essentially aesthetic conditions [2].

Photodynamic therapy using topical photosensitizers and lasers or other light sources to treat superficial tumours is at last showing promise [3,4].

REFERENCES

1 Grossman MC, Dierickx C, Farinelli W *et al.* Damage to hair follicles by normal-mode ruby laser pulses. *J Am Acad Dermatol* 1996; **35**: 889–94.
2 Alster TS, Apfelberg DB, eds. *Cosmetic Laser Surgery.* New York: John Wiley & Sons, 1996.
3 Meijnders PJN, Star WM, De Bruijn RS *et al.* Clinical results of photodynamic therapy for superficial skin malignancies or actinic keratosis using topical 5-aminolaevulinic acid. *Lasers Med Sci* 1996; **11**: 123–32.
4 Stables GI, Stringer MR, Robinson DJ *et al.* Large patches of Bowen's disease treated by topical aminolaevulinic acid photodynamic therapy. *Br J Dermatol* 1997; **136**: 957–60.

Sclerotherapy (see also Chapter 50)

The injection of sclerosant chemicals is a useful means of obliterating dilated superficial veins, particularly on the legs. The superficial vessels should only be treated after any proximal points of reflux have been dealt with. Patients who seek treatment therefore require a thorough assessment of their venous system, and the history and physical examination may be supplemented with non-invasive venous assessment using ultrasonography.

There are a variety of solutions which can be used, and some are available in different concentrations. The solutions may be divided into detergents (i.e. sodium morrhuate, sodium tetradecyl sulphate, polidocanol), osmotic solutions (i.e. hypertonic saline) and chemical irritants (i.e. chromated glycerin). They each have their advantages and disadvantages.

Side-effects [3] include telangiectatic matting, post-inflammatory hyperpigmentation, ulceration, thrombophlebitis and, rarely, systemic reactions (urticaria, anaphylaxis).

REFERENCES

1 Goldman MP. Sclerotherapy. In: Roenigk RK, Roenigk HH, eds. *Dermatologic Surgery.* New York: Marcel Dekker, 1996: 1169–82.
2 Guex JJ. Indications for the sclerosing agent polidocanol (aetoxisclerol). *J Dermatol Surg Oncol* 1993; **19**: 959–61.
3 Goldman MP, Saddick NS, Weiss RA. Cutaneous necrosis, telangiectatic matting and hyperpigmentation following sclerotherapy. Etiology, prevention and treatment. *Dermatol Surg* 1995; **21**: 19–29.

Miscellaneous physical procedures

Keloid therapy

Keloids spread beyond the original wound and remain elevated, whereas hypertrophic scars are localized to the injured area and flatten spontaneously with time [1]. Both are commoner in young individuals, Afro-Caribbeans and at particular sites, including principally the central chest, back and posterior neck, followed by the ears, deltoid areas, anterior chest, beard area and the rest of the neck [2,3]. Patients with one keloid, except those on the earlobe [4], are believed to be at risk of further keloids. A huge variety of treatments have been promoted, including excision, superficial X-ray therapy (although this may provoke malignant tumours [5]), cryotherapy [6,7], pressure [8,9], ultrasound, laser excision [10], and medical therapies including intralesional steroids, interferon-α2b [11] and verapamil [12]. Most reports have claimed partial benefit, few have admitted failure. Despite systemic or local side-effects [13], intralesional steroid, in the form of triamcinolone 10–40 mg/ml, injected into the scar every 2–3 weeks, is probably the most effective therapy, particularly for presternal and small keloids. High pressure is required to inject steroids into hard keloids, and this often results in the needle and syringe separating, spraying steroid solution everywhere. Therefore, a Luer-lock glass syringe with finger holes is preferred to a plastic syringe [14].

Pedunculated or easily excised keloids, for example on the earlobe, are best treated by intramarginal excision and pre- and postoperative steroid injection [15]. On the earlobe, part of the skin covering the keloid can be salvaged to cover the defect created by removal of the latter [16]. Most authorities recommend a combination of surgery and triamcinolone injections. Some suggest that triamcinolone should be given before, during and after surgery [4], others use steroids during and after surgery [17], whereas others only use steroids postoperatively, to avoid the risk of wound dehiscence [18]. All agree that triamcinolone 40 mg/ml is usually required. On balance, it seems best to give steroids both intra- and postoperatively—approximately four times at 2–3-week intervals, starting 2–3 weeks after suture removal (which should be delayed for 10–14 days because of the risk of steroid-induced wound dehiscence). Cryotherapy is also combined with triamcinolone in order to make the injection easier [19]. Freeze the keloid for 10–15 sec using liquid nitrogen. Fifteen minutes later the tissue oedema created allows the injection to be given more easily. With repeated injections it becomes possible to inject more triamcinolone into the keloid, which can be felt to expand slightly as the steroid is injected. Remember that cryotherapy may produce hypopigmentation of pigmented skin. Triamcinolone injections may also produce temporary hypopigmentation

[4]. Alternative therapies include the application of potent topical steroids, for example clobetasol propionate cream or flurandrenolone tape. The latter carries less risk of steroid atrophy of the adjacent skin because only the keloid is covered. Intralesional interferon-α2b appears to reduce keloid size and inhibit collagen production [11]. Intralesional verapamil is said to reduce keloid size [12] by inhibiting proline incorporation into collagen [20]. Silicone gel sheeting is probably the only practical therapy for larger lesions, particularly new keloids [21]. No pressure is required. Adhesive tape is used to hold the sheeting in place, and the latter is cleaned regularly and applied daily for 12–20 h. Folliculitis may occur on hair-bearing skin [22].

REFERENCES

1 Berman B, Bieley HC. Keloids. *J Am Acad Dermatol* 1995; **33**: 117–23.
2 Nemeth AJ. Keloids and hypertrophic scars. *J Dermatol Surg Oncol* 1993; **19**: 738–46.
3 Datubo-Brown DD. Keloids: a review of the literature. *Br J Plast Surg* 1990; **43**: 70–7.
4 Kelly AP. Keloid surgery. In: Robinson, Arndt, LeBoit, Wintroub, eds. *Atlas of Cutaneous Surgery*. Philadelphia: WB Saunders, 1996.
5 Hoffman S. Radiotherapy for keloids? *Ann Plast Surg* 1982; **9**: 265.
6 Rusciani L, Rossi G, Bono R. Use of cryotherapy in the treatment of keloids. *J Dermatol Surg Oncol* 1993; **19**: 529–34.
7 Shepherd JP, Dawber RP. The response of keloid scars to cryosurgery. 1982; **70**: 677–9.
8 Nicolai JPA, Bos MY, Bronkhorst FB *et al.* A protocol for the treatment of hypertrophic scars and keloids. *Aesthetic Plast Surg* 1987; **11**: 29–32.
9 Mercer DM, Studd DM. 'Oyster splints' a new compression device for the treatment of keloid scars. *Br J Plast Surg* 1983; **36**: 75–6.
10 Kantor GR, Wheeland RG, Bailin PL *et al.* Treatment of earlobe keloid with carbon dioxide laser excision: a report of 16 cases. *J Dermatol Surg Oncol* 1985; **11**: 1063–5.
11 Granstein RD, Rook A, Flotte TJ *et al.* A controlled trial of intralesional recombinant interferon gamma in the treatment of keloidal scarring, clinical and histological findings. *Arch Dermatol* 1990; **126**: 1295–302.
12 Lawrence WT. Treatment of earlobe keloids with surgery plus adjuvant intralesional verapamil and pressure earring. *Ann Plast Surg* 1996; **37**: 167–9.
13 Krusche T, Worret WI. Mechanical properties of keloids *in vivo* during treatment with intralesional triamcinolone acetonide. *Arch Dermatol Res* 1995; **287**: 289–93.
14 Lawrence CM. *An Introduction to Dermatological Surgery*. Oxford: Blackwell Science, 1996.
15 Sharma BC. Keloids: a prospective study of 57 cases. *Med J Zambia* 1980; **14**: 66–9.
16 Salasche SJ, Grabski WJ. Keloids of the earlobes: a surgical technique. *J Dermatol Surg Oncol* 1983; **9**: 552–6.
17 Fewkes JL, Cheney L, Pollack SV. *Illustrated Atlas of Cutaneous Surgery*. Philadelphia: JB Lippincott, 1992: 22.5.
18 Bennett RG. *Fundamentals of Cutaneous Surgery*. St Louis: Mosby, 1988: 716–17.
19 Ceilley RI, Babin RW. The combined use of cryosurgery and intralesional injections of suspensions of fluorinated adrenocorticosteroids for reducing keloids and hypertrophic scars. *J Dermatol Surg Oncol* 1979; **5**: 54–6.
20 Lee RC, Ping J. Calcium antagonists retard extracellular matrix production in connective tissue equivalent. *J Surg Res* 1990; **49**: 463–6.
21 Hirshowitz B, Ullmann Y, Har-Shai Y *et al.* Silicone occlusive sheeting (SOS) in the management of hypertrophic and keloid scarring including possible mode of action by static electricity. *Eur J Plast Surg* 1993; **16**: 5–9.
22 Mercers NSG. Silicone gel in the treatment of keloid scars. *Br J Plast Surg* 1993; **42**: 83–7.

Minor surgical procedures

Using an orange stick small quantities of caustic agents can be precisely applied. When 90% liquid phenol is used to treat molluscum contagiosum or small cysts, the orange stick tip may need to be sharpened so that it just fits the cavity being treated. Do not wrap cotton-wool around the tip, as the greater volume of caustic liquid may drip onto the skin with disastrous consequences. If a small quantity of phenol is poured into a container before use, ensure that a metal, not plastic, receptacle is used, as phenol may melt plastic. Ensure that the phenol-containing receptacle is easily distinguished from others, and dispose of the remaining solution carefully.

Mollusca can be squeezed to express the cellular debris from the centre of the lesion before phenol application. The tip of the orange stick is dipped into the phenol, any excess wiped off, and the stick is then placed in the centre of the lesion and gently twisted. The solution does not need to be neutralized. After initial whitening the molluscum becomes inflamed and then resolves 7–10 days later. Treatment is painful and not usually tolerated by small children.

Xanthelasma can be treated using the blunt end of an orange stick, wet but not dripping with trichloroacetic acid, dabbed onto the affected area. *Multiple small facial epidermoid* or *acne cysts* can be treated in a similar way. The cyst is incised, the contents expressed and phenol carefully applied to the cyst lining using an orange stick. No dressing is required, but a local anaesthetic is necessary.

Milia are tiny, keratin-filled, epithelial-lined cysts with no connection to the overlying skin. They can be removed via a small skin incision made with a sterile #21 or #19 venesection needle. No anaesthetic is required. Prick the needle tip into the skin and, by pulling the cutting edge upwards, incise the skin overlying the milium. Hook or squeeze out the cyst through the skin incision.

Comedones may be emptied by gentle pressure using a comedone expressor—a small metal instrument with a cup-shaped end, which has a central hole. Comedone expression does not alter the natural history of acne but will improve the patient's self-confidence early in treatment. Steaming, warm, moist compresses, and topical tretinoin application soften comedones prior to removal.

Haemostasis

Bleeding from open wounds can be stopped readily using an absorbable haemostatic dressing such as Surgicel (glucosic copolymer), Kaltostat (calcium alginate), Oxycel (oxidized cellulose) or Gelfoam (porous gelatin matrix), although the mechanism of action of these agents is poorly understood. These materials may behave like a foreign body whilst dissolving in the wound and increase the risk of infection, so large pieces should be removed before wound closure.

Chemical haemostatic agents [1] are effective on oozing skin wounds, for example after curettage and shave excision, but are ineffective in the presence of arterial bleeding, and should not be used in sutured wounds as they cause cell death, which predisposes to infection. Application should be followed by pressure on the wound for 2–3 min to allow haemostasis to occur without the chemical being washed away. Ferric subsulphate (Monsel's) solution carries the risk of iron tattooing [2]. Silver nitrate sticks are effective but caustic, and may leave scars. Aluminium chloride, either 35% in isopropyl alcohol or 20% in ethyl alcohol, is effective; occasionally, it causes histiocytic reactions in treated skin [3].

REFERENCES

1 Larson PO. Topical haemostatic agents for dermatologic surgery. *J Dermatol Surg Oncol* 1988; **14**: 623–32.
2 Olmstead PM, Lund HZ, Leonard DD. Monsel's solution: a histologic nuisance. *J Am Acad Dermatol* 1980; **3**: 492–8.
3 Barr RJ, Alpern KS, Jay S. Histiocytic reaction associated with topical aluminium chloride (Drysol reaction). *J Dermatol Surg Oncol* 1993; **19**: 1017–21.

Tattoo removal by salabrasion

Tattoos can be excised, removed by laser therapy (see above), or the skin containing the tattoo can be destroyed using caustic applications [1], cryotherapy, dermabrasion and salabrasion [2]. The abrasive effect of the salt crystals is enhanced by the caustic action of salt application as is evident by slower wound healing and greater pigment removal than in equivalent wounds produced by derma-brasion. Salabrasion involves local anaesthetic injection and repeated rubbing of the skin using common table salt to produce an erosion over the tattoo. This is exhausting for the operator, and mechanical alternatives have been described [3]. Little tattoo pigment is removed during the rubbing phase. Thereafter, a dressing is placed over the wound and the top layer of damaged dermis containing the tattoo is shed into this as the wound heals. Pigment removal and scarring are greater if salt is left on the wound after salabrasion [4]. As with all destructive therapies, the cosmetic results are unpredictable and an ugly scar may remain.

REFERENCES

1 Piggot TA, Norris RW. The treatment of tattoos with trichloracetic acid: experience with 670 patients. *Br J Plast Surg* 1988; **41**: 112–17.
2 Crittenden FM, Jr. Salabrasion removal of tattoos. In: Epstein E, Epstein E, Jr, eds. *Skin Surgery*, 5th edn. Springfield: Thomas, 1982.
3 Shelley WB, Shelley ED. Focal salabrasion for removal of linear tattoos. *J Dermatol Surg Oncol* 1984; **10**: 216–18.
4 Koerber WA, Price NM. Salabrasion of tattoos. *Arch Dermatol* 1978; **114**: 884–8.

Soft-tissue augmentation and facial line correction

As fat is an autograft, *autologous fat implantation (microlipoinjection)* is potentially a useful method of soft-tissue augmentation, but it can only be placed sub-cutaneously. Fat injected into dermis does not survive [1]. The fat is harvested using a syringe via a wide-bore needle. Any contaminating blood is washed off and the fat reinjected using a 16–18-gauge needle. Intravascular injection, and infection, must be avoided. Microlipo-injection is used to increase lip size, obliterate age-related guttering on the hands, or in breast enlargement, but cannot be used for small or superficial scars. Grafted fat persists for 1–2 years, although this varies with site and the cosmetic defect treated [2,3].

Bovine collagen (Zyderm I 35 mg/ml collagen and Zyderm II 65 mg/ml) has been used to correct superficial facial scars and wrinkles. The effect is temporary; after 6 months, top-up treatment is required. Glutaraldehyde cross-linked collagen (Zyplast) was introduced with the aim of prolonging the effect, but appears to be little different [4]. Approximately 3% of patients react to the test injection [5]. Late allergic reactions are rare but may occur years after collagen injections [6,7]. Soft and distensible postsurgery, chicken pox and acne scars respond well [8], unlike rigid fibrotic or ice-pick scars.

Injectable medical grade *silicon* (polymerized dimethyl-siloxane) has been used for age-related wrinkles and facial scarring. Injection (with 1-ml quantities/session) is believed to carry little risk, although the reports of connective tissue disease in breast-augmentation patients [10] may limit further use of this material.

Gelatin matrix implant (Fibrel) is a mixture of gelatin powder and ε-aminocaproic acid reconstituted with saline and the patient's plasma. The matrix is placed in the dermis and is thought to promote new collagen formation, which ultimately replaces the implant. Its elevating effect on depressed scars lasts 1–2 years [11], and it can be used in depressed acne scars [12]. Lip-contour irregularities and deep nasolabial fold creases can be improved permanently by inserting *polytetrafluoroethylene (Gore-Tex)* strips [13] under the defect. Frown lines over the brow are the result of prolonged contraction of the facial muscle corrugator supercilii. The muscle action can be paralysed by injecting *botulinum toxin (Botox)* into the muscle, and the frown line disappears for approximately 6 months.

REFERENCES

1 Coleman WP, Lawrence N, Sherman RN *et al.* Autologous collagen? Lipocytic dermal augmentation: a histopathological study. *J Dermatol Surg Oncol* 1993; **19**: 1032–40.
2 Pinski KS, Roenigk HH. Autologous fat transplantation, long term follow-up. *J Dermatol Surg Oncol* 1992; **18**: 179–84.
3 Bircoll M, Novack BH. Autologous fat transplantation employing liposuction

techniques. *Ann Plast Surg* 1987; **18**: 327–9.

4 Matti BA, Nicolle FV. Clinical use of Zyplast in correction of age and disease related contour deficiencies of the face. *Aesthetic Plast Surg* 1990; **14**: 227–34.

5 Elson ML. Clinical assessment of Zyplast implant: a year of experience for soft tissue contour correction. *J Am Acad Dermatol* 1988; **18**: 707–13.

6 Hanke CW, Highley HR, Jolivette DM *et al*. Abscess formation and local necrosis after treatment with Zyderm or Zyplast collagen implant. *J Am Acad Dermatol* 1991; **25**: 319–26.

7 Moscona RR, Bergman R, Friedman-Birnbaum R. An unusual late reaction to Zyderm I injections: a challenge for treatment. *Plast Reconstr Surg* 1993; **92**: 331–4.

8 Varnavides CK, Forster RA, Cunliffe WJ. The role of bovine collagen in the treatment of acne scars. *Br J Dermatol* 1987; **116**: 199–206.

9 Clark DP, Hanke CW, Swanson NA. Dermal implants: safety of products injected for soft tissue augmentation. *J Dermatol Surg Oncol* 1989; **21**: 992–8.

10 Silver RM, Sahn EE, Allen JA *et al*. Demonstration of silicon in sites of connective-tissue disease in patients with silicone-gel breast implants. *Arch Dermatol* 1993; **129**: 63–8.

11 Multicentre Study. Treatment of depressed cutaneous scars with gelatin matrix implant: a multicenter study. *J Am Acad Dermatol* 1987; **16**: 1155–62.

12 Millikan L, Banks K, Purkait B, Chungi V. A 5-year safety and efficacy evaluation with Fibrel in the correction of cutaneous scars following one or two treatments. *J Dermatol Surg Oncol* 1991; **17**: 223–9.

13 Cisneros JL, Singla R. Intradermal augmentation with expanded poly-tetrafluoroethylene (Gore-Tex) for facial lines and wrinkles. *J Dermatol Surg Oncol* 1993; **19**: 539–42.

Chapter 81
Dermatological Surgery

N.P.J.WALKER, C.M.LAWRENCE & R.P.R.DAWBER

Introduction

The acquisition of basic dermatological surgery skills is an important component of dermatological training. In this chapter we aim to cover the techniques used for simple excisional surgery and also provide an introduction to more advanced techniques with which dermatologists should be familiar, even if they do not employ such techniques, so that they may discuss them with their patients. The interested reader will already be aware of the relevant literature, including those journals devoted wholly to this subject, such as *Dermatologic Surgery*. Bennett's textbook [1] is of particular value, as are other texts such as *Simple Skin Surgery* [2], *Dermatologic Surgery* [3] and *Surgical Dermatology* [4], which could reasonably be regarded as defining the range of dermatological surgery as practised at present in the UK. Other books deal more specifically with cosmetic dermatological surgery [5,6], or general aspects of plastic surgery [7–9]. There is much to be said for dermatologists carrying out as many of the surgical and physical procedures as possible, providing they acknowledge their own limitations.

REFERENCES

1 Bennett RG. *Fundamentals of Cutaneous Surgery*. St Louis: Mosby, 1988.
2 Burge S, Colver GB, Rayment R. *Simple Skin Surgery*, 2nd edn. Oxford: Blackwell Science, 1996.
3 Roenigk RK, Roenigk HH, eds. *Dermatologic Surgery*, 2nd edn. New York: Marcel Dekker, 1996.
4 Eedy DJ, Breathnach SM, Walker NPJ. *Surgical Dermatology*. Oxford: Blackwell Science, 1996.
5 Parish LC, Lask GP. *Aesthetic Dermatology*. New York: McGraw-Hill, 1991.
6 Stegman SJ, Tromovitch TA. *Cosmetic Dermatologic Surgery*, 2nd edn. Chicago: Year Book Medical Publishers, 1990.
7 Grabbe WC, Smith JW. *Plastic Surgery*, 3rd edn. Boston: Little, Brown & Co, 1979.
8 McGregor IA. *Fundamental Techniques of Plastic Surgery and their Surgical Applications*. New York: Churchill Livingstone, 1975.
9 Sisson GA, Tardy MJ. *Plastic and Reconstructive Surgery of the Face and Neck*. New York: Grune & Stratton, 1977.

Critical anatomical areas

It is essential to have a working knowledge of the important clinical anatomy of each operation site. The following is only a brief introduction to some of the critical anatomical details with which the operator must be familiar. Excisions down to superficial fat will rarely result in exposure of or potential damage to functionally important structures, except in a very thin subject. Incisions to deep fat or fascia and the removal of large cysts or lipomas may result in exposure of important arteries, veins, lymphatics, sensory or motor nerves and other structures. On the head and neck, division of larger arteries and veins will not cause vascular complications because of the extensive collateral circulation. However, it is important to be aware of the position of large arteries and veins in order to be prepared to deal with bleeding from such vessels. Division of sensory nerves may produce annoying sensory loss, but this will have little functional impact. Knowledge of the anatomy of the supraorbital, infraorbital and mental sensory nerves is important, as these are commonly used in peripheral nerve blocks. Division of motor nerves is potentially disabling and thus it is essential to know the anatomy of the vulnerable cranial and peripheral nerves; such nerves share few cross-connections with adjacent nerves and run a superficial course.

Skin tension lines and the orientation of scars

Incisions should be designed to follow the wrinkles or

relaxed skin tension lines (syn. stress lines, favourable skin tension lines, maximal skin tension lines) as the scars will be stronger and less likely to stretch [1]. Relaxed skin tension lines run perpendicular to the direction of contraction of the underlying muscles and parallel to the dermal collagen bundles [2]; cutting across these transversely weakens the skin much more than a cut running parallel to the collagen bundles [3]. In the absence of wrinkles, relaxed skin tension lines can be identified by getting the patient to smile and close their eyes tightly, or by manipulating the skin. Langer's lines [4] (syn. resting stress lines) were mapped on cadaver skin, and are different from relaxed skin tension lines on large parts of the body [3]; they should not be used for identifying the elective direction of excision.

Head and neck

Cosmetic units

Cosmetic results of surgery are better if all the incisions remain within a cosmetic unit [5]. These are areas of skin which share similar characteristics, for example the nose, cheek, periorbital skin. The junction lines separating these areas are also important because scars placed in junction lines are usually unobtrusive whereas scars which cross a junction line, i.e. bridge two cosmetic units, are very obvious. It is thus important to try to design a repair so that the scars follow relaxed skin tension lines and remain within the same cosmetic unit, or run in the junction lines if close to a boundary between two adjacent cosmetic units.

Blood vessels and lymphatic supply of face

Larger vessels, particularly the temporal artery, can be avoided by hydrodissection (see p. 3625). The facial artery (Fig. 81.1) at the nasolabial fold, and its continuation into the angular artery at the medial canthus, are frequently divided when excising tumours at these sites. The external jugular vein runs under the platysma muscle but on top of the sternocleidomastoid muscle, and may be easily damaged during superficial incisions on the neck at this site (Fig. 81.2a). In a proportion of individuals, emissary veins, connecting the intracranial and extracranial venous circulation, run across the subgaleal space towards the back of the scalp (parietal emissary vein) and just above the forehead (frontal emissary vein) [6], and may be damaged when undermining the subgaleal space at these sites. Lymphatic drainage sites should be examined for metastases during follow-up of patients treated for squamous cell carcinoma or melanoma [7]. Division of skin lymphatics during incisions along the eyelid may result in temporary but unavoidable lower eyelid lymphoedema.

Sensory nerves of face

Nerve blocks. Sensation to the face is supplied by the Vth or trigeminal cranial nerve. The three branches readily blocked in skin surgical procedures on the head and neck include the supraorbital, infraorbital and mental nerves (Fig. 81.3). These emerge from the skull via palpable foramina, which all lie in the same plane, just medial to a vertical line running through the pupil [8]. Blocking the great auricular, transverse cervical and lesser occipital

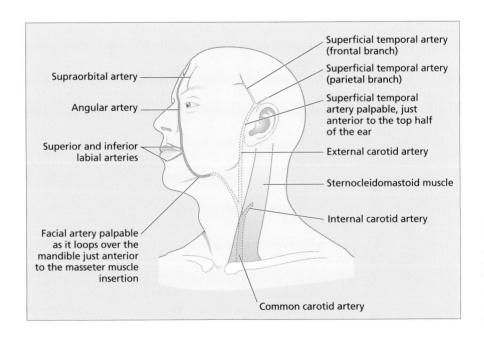

Fig. 81.1 Arteries of the head and neck encountered in skin surgery. The labial artery lies on the inside (mucosal) surface of the lip approximately 5 mm from the visible vermilion border. (- - -) Arteries rarely encountered; (—) arteries frequently identified during superficial skin surgery on the face.

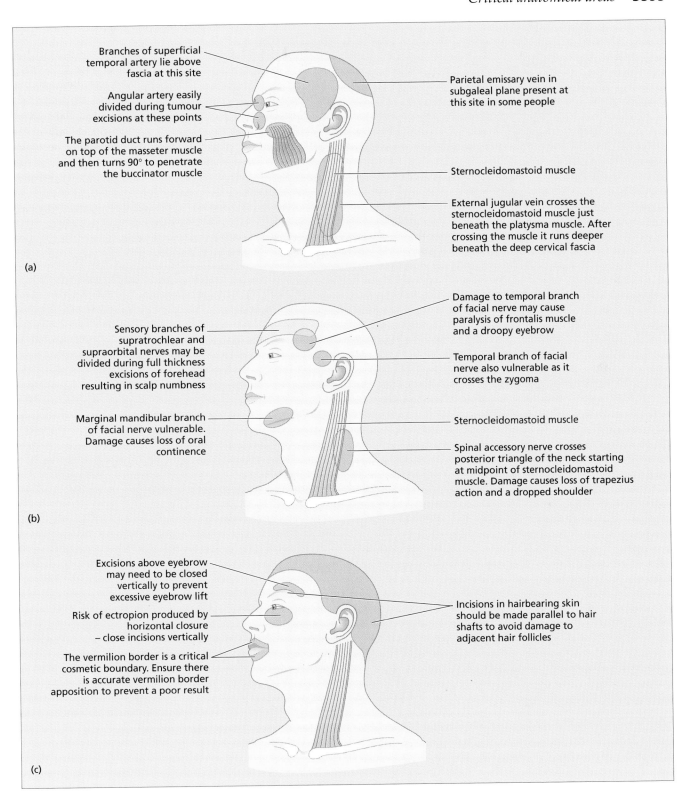

Fig. 81.2 Potential surgical hazard sites during skin surgery on the head. Potential blood vessel and duct (a), nerve (b) and cosmetic hazards (c) on the head and neck. (From Lawrence [9].)

nerves as they emerge from the posterior border of the middle third of the sternocleidomastoid muscle [10] produces anaesthesia of a large portion of the scalp, neck and ear. The focal point of the injection is indicated by Erb's point; this is identified by finding the midpoint on a line between

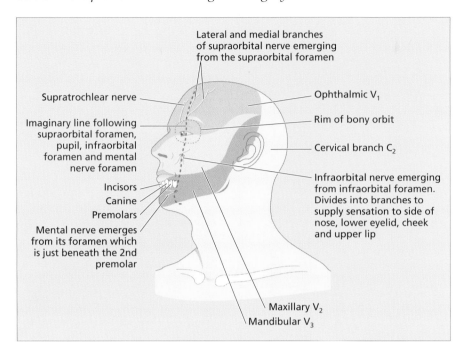

Fig. 81.3 Sensory nerves on the face used in nerve-block anaesthesia. Sensation on the face is served by the three main divisions of the trigeminal nerve—the ophthalmic, maxillary and mandibular divisions. Three important branches of these nerves—the supraorbital, infraorbital and mental nerves—emerge in the same plane along a vertical line running through the pupil.

the angle of the jaw and the mastoid process, taking a vertical line downwards, and where this line crosses the posterior border of the sternocleidomastoid muscle is Erb's point. Here the spinal accessory nerve also emerges from behind the sternocleidomastoid muscle. This motor nerve is rarely affected by the anaesthesia, as it lies deeper, on the floor of the posterior triangle, whereas the three named sensory branches of the cervical plexus curl round to lie on top of the sternocleidomastoid muscle [11].

Division of small sensory nerves is of little consequence, with the possible exception of scalp numbness following incisions on the forehead. Improvement in sensory loss can be expected for up to 1 year.

Motor nerves

Two branches of the facial nerve, the marginal mandibular branch and the temporal branch, are vulnerable during skin surgery (Fig. 81.4). The temporal branch of the facial nerve supplies the frontalis and orbicularis muscles. Damage to the nerve to the frontalis muscle makes it impossible to raise the eyebrow and the forehead furrows disappear. This can easily occur during excision of large

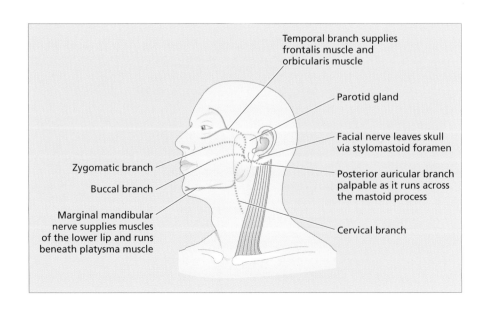

Fig. 81.4 Motor branches of the facial nerve vulnerable in skin surgery. (---) Nerves rarely encountered; (—) nerves at risk during superficial skin surgery on the face.

tumours on the temple, and particularly as the nerve crosses the zygomatic arch where there is little tissue between the skin and periosteum (see Fig. 81.2b). The marginal mandibular branch innervates muscles that move the lower lip. Damage can be devastating because it results in weakness of the lips, with dribbling when eating and drinking. The nerve is superficial and vulnerable as it emerges from under the parotid gland at the angle of the jaw, at the point where the facial artery can be palpated as it crosses the mandible. More anteriorly, the nerve runs beneath the platysma muscle, which is reassuring if this thin muscle sheet can be identified [12]. Variations in nerve position with age and neck position must also be considered. The remaining branches of the facial nerve are less vulnerable because they share several cross-connections and lie deeper. The other important motor cranial nerve is the accessory (XIth) nerve, which supplies the trapezius and sternocleidomastoid muscles. This may be damaged during dissection in the posterior triangle of the neck, causing weakness of the trapezius muscle and producing a dropped shoulder.

Undermining levels

When undermining to increase skin mobility, different levels are appropriate at different sites (Table 81.1).

Specific facial sites

If an incision runs across the vermilion of the *lip*, the vermilion border must be carefully marked before anaesthetic injection to avoid a poor cosmetic result (see Fig. 81.2c). In older patients with poor lid elasticity, operations around the *lower eyelid* may result in ectropion if any downwards tension is applied to the lower eyelid. In a patient with poor lid elasticity, the procedure should be designed to increase rather than reduce eyelid tension; this usually means closing the wound vertically rather than horizontally. If an incision goes across the *hair line*, ensure that the scalp margin is reconstructed so that a smooth contour remains. Because hairs grow obliquely through the skin, any incision

Table 81.1 Undermining levels.

Site	Undermining level
Face	Mid-fat
Nose	Just above the periosteum and perichondrium
Forehead	Beneath the deep frontalis fascia (i.e. equivalent to the subgaleal plane)
Scalp	Subgaleal plane
Trunk and limb—small excisions	Deep fat
Trunk and limb—large excisions	Just above the deep fascia

through *hair-bearing skin* should be made parallel to the hair shafts, rather than vertically through the scalp, so that as few follicles as possible are damaged.

Limbs

The only truly vulnerable motor nerve on the limbs is on the lateral aspect of the knee, where the common peroneal nerve (lateral popliteal) can be damaged as it winds round the neck of the fibula. Here the nerve can be palpated against the bone. Injury to the nerve at this site will produce a foot drop due to paralysis of foot dorsiflexors and elevators.

REFERENCES

1 Salasche SJ, Bernstein G, Senkarik M. *Surgical Anatomy of the Skin.* Norwalk: Appleton & Lange, 1988.
2 Borges AF, Alexander JE. Relaxed skin tension lines, z-plasty on scars and fusiform excision of lesions. *Br J Plast Surg* 1962; **15**: 242–54.
3 Kraissl CJ. The selection of appropriate lines for elective surgical incision. *Plast Reconstr Surg* 1951; **8**: 1–28.
4 Langer K. On the anatomy and physiology of the skin. I. The cleavability of the cutis. Translated and republished in *Br J Plast Surg* 1978; **31**: 3–8, with covering editorial 1–2.
5 Summers BK, Siegle RJ. Facial cutaneous reconstructive surgery: general aesthetic principles. *J Am Acad Dermatol* 1993; **29**: 669–81.
6 Sobotta J. Head, neck upper limbs and skin. In: Staubesand J, ed. *Atlas of Human Anatomy.* Munich: Urban & Schwarzenberg, 1989.
7 Romanes GJ. *Cunningham's Manual of Practical Anatomy,* 15th edn, Vol. 3. *Head and Neck and Brain.* Oxford: Oxford University Press, 1986.
8 Scott DB. *Techniques of Regional Anaesthesia.* Norwalk: Appleton & Lange/Mediglobe, 1989.
9 Lawrence CM. *An Introduction to Dermatological Surgery.* Oxford: Blackwell Science, 1996.
10 Lumley JSP. *Surface Anatomy, the Anatomical Basis of Clinical Examination.* Edinburgh: Churchill Livingstone, 1990.
11 Williams PL, Bannister LH, Berry M *et al.*, eds. *Gray's Anatomy,* 38th edn. New York: Churchill Livingstone, 1995.
12 Summers BK, Siegle RJ. Facial cutaneous reconstructive surgery: facial flaps. *J Am Acad Dermatol* 1993; **29**: 917–41.

Equipment and sterilization [1–5]

Skin is visible, 'mobile', easily removed, and generally heals well with minimal scarring after injury. In the past, this often led to simple skin surgery being undertaken by ill-trained medical practitioners, with inadequate facilities, often using 'improvised' operating equipment. Hippocrates wrote [3] 'all instruments ought to be well-suited for the purpose in hand as regards their size, weight and delicacy', and this is a fundamental tenet of surgery.

Surgical excision involves certain basic steps which are common to all cutaneous surgery: incision and excision, undermining, haemostasis, tissue movement for closure, suturing and suture removal. The correct facilities and equipment must be available for each of these. Certain basic instruments are appropriate for most cutaneous surgery, and these are given particular attention here.

The basic equipment, with optional items which should be available if required, is shown in Table 81.2 [1]. Skin

Table 81.2 Essential and optional equipment. From Burge *et al.* [1].

Essential	Optional	Essential	Optional
THE ROOM		*Skin hook:*	
An examination couch with adjustable backrest	Theatre table	Can easily be constructed by pushing a sterile needle onto a sterile moistened cotton wool bud on an orange stick. Bend the needle into a curve	
A stool for the surgeon			
Good lighting: anglepoise lights	Overhead theatre lights		
		Scissors:	
EQUIPMENT—PREOPERATIVE PREPARATION		Curved pointed iris scissors	
Autoclave for steam sterilization or electric oven for dry heat sterilization		Blunt straight scissors	
		Needle holders	
Skin preparation:		Small artery clamps	
Chlorhexidine solution		Various sizes of absorbable and non-absorbable sutures attached to needles	Skin punch for biopsies, 3 mm and 4 mm
Chlorhexidine detergent (Hibiscrub)			Sharp ring curettes in various sizes
Surgical gloves			
Sterile paper towels:	Re-usable drapes	HAEMOSTASIS	
A window can be cut in the centre and the towel placed over the lesion		Gauze swabs	Hyfrecator
		30–50% aluminium chloride in alcohol or Monsel's solution (67.5% basic ferric sulphate)	Electrocautery
Skin markers:	Sterile pen and Indian ink		Diathermy
Gentian violet and pointed orange stick			Bipolar electrocoagulation
Skin marker pen			Cryosurgery gun
Indelible felt-tip pen			Supply of liquid nitrogen
			Silver nitrate sticks
ANAESTHETIC		DRESSINGS	
Disposable syringes 2 ml, 5 ml fine needles	Dental syringe and fine needles	Steri-strips	Opsite
	Dental syringe vials	Compound Benzoin tincture BP (Friar's balsam) for sticking plaster to skin	
Lignocaine:		Elastoplast	
1% and 2% plain and with adrenaline 1:100 000 or 1:200 000		Micropore	
		Gauze	
		Jelonet	
INSTRUMENTS		HISTOPATHOLOGY	
Scalpel blades:		Specimen pots	EM fixative 4% glutaraldehyde
No. 15 for excision			
No. 22 for shave biopsy		*Fixative:*	Fixative or liquid nitrogen to store specimens for immunohistology
Scalpel handle		10% buffered formalin	
Forceps:			
Fine-toothed (e.g. Adson–Brown)			
Non-toothed			

EM, electron microscopy.

surgeons involved in the complex removal of tumours, performance of flaps and grafts, etc., should have facilities at their disposal equivalent to those in any plastic surgery or general operating theatre.

Most wound infections are associated with necrotic tissue, haematoma formation and the presence of foreign bodies. However, the skin has a good blood supply, and postoperative infection is rare—skin infection following surgery is thus often due to poor surgical technique rather than primarily due to poor sterility and sterilization. The tradition of protracted 'scrubbing up' is not mandatory, or even necessarily desirable—two washes in running water using 4% chlorhexidine or 10% povidine–iodine solution are satisfactory. Surgical gloves should always be worn, mainly for the surgeon's own protection against hepatitis B infection.

Dried pus or blood on instruments may be associated with potentially dangerous organisms, and instruments should always be washed before sterilizing in an autoclave or an electric oven. Ultrasonic cleaners are now widely available. It is important to note that water boiling at atmospheric pressure does not adequately sterilize, as bacteria are not consistently killed by moist heat at 100°C [4,5]. Instruments must never be left lying in 'antiseptic sterilizing liquids', because these easily become contaminated; they should be kept in sterile packs.

Human immunodeficiency virus (HIV) and hepatitis B are easily inactivated by even the mildest form of sterilization.

Inadequate sterilization of instruments which are not prepacked or adequately cleaned is the main danger, apart from the obvious risk of contact with infected blood if the surgeon receives a penetrating wound from any of the instruments used.

REFERENCES

1 Burge S, Colver GB, Rayment R. *Simple Skin Surgery*, 2nd edn. Oxford: Blackwell Science, 1996: 5–9.
2 Grande DJ, Neuberg M. Instrumentation for the dermatologic surgeon. *J Dermatol Surg Oncol* 1989; **15**: 288–97.
3 Diwan R. Instruments for dermatologic surgery. In: Lask GP, Moy RL, eds. *Principles and Techniques of Cutaneous Surgery*. New York: McGraw-Hill, 1996: 85–100.
4 Sebben JE. Survey of sterile technique in dermatological surgeons. *J Am Acad Dermatol* 1988; **18**: 1107–14.
5 Sebben JE, Fazio MJ. Sterilisation of equipment for dermatologic surgery. In: Lask GP, Moy RL, eds. *Principles and Techniques of Cutaneous Surgery*. New York: McGraw-Hill, 1996: 47–56.

Safety aspects

Safety factors relating to the procedures described in this chapter are detailed for each particular treatment modality. This section outlines some of the necessary general safety measures directed at minimizing infection risk to the patient, surgeon and assistants; the availability of appropriate equipment for the operation, and potential complications from the operative procedures; correct patient preparation and fitness for the procedure; and protection of the surgeon against the hazards of surgical practice [1].

'Aseptic technique' is an impossible aim. The objective should be to reduce bacterial colonization to a minimum at the operation site, and to prevent contamination from adjacent sites. Antisepsis and sterilization are discussed elsewhere (see above). There are two components to the precautions employed in the control of blood-borne infections, especially HIV and hepatitis—prevention of transmission from patient to patient, and protection of the surgical team. Most hospitals now insist that medical and nursing staff have adequate immunity against hepatitis B, and each unit has its own infection control staff and protocols. The methods of the US Centers for Disease Control and Prevention are useful, in general [2]. The basic tenet is that all patients should be managed during an operative procedure as if they have HIV, hepatitis B or other blood-borne pathogens—universal precautions are mandatory for every patient.

All members of a surgical team should be at liberty to draw the attention of other members of the team to any deficiencies in standards.

Needle-stick injuries and other sharp instrument cuts are particularly important. It should be a rule that no uncapped needle is left on the instrument tray and that no needle is recapped by the two-handed method. All sharp disposable instruments must be removed from the tray after the operation by the surgeon, who should put these directly into the 'sharps disposal' boxes now provided almost universally. Clothing should be specific for the operating room, i.e. 'street clothes' should not be worn. Apart from potentially introducing a variety of organisms to the operating room, they may become contaminated.

Operating rooms should have rigid 'conduct protocols' for each procedure (most of these are a combination of common sense and aseptic technique), even superficial skin surgery. Once the patient is in the operating room, those not directly concerned with the procedure should be excluded.

It is mandatory that all patients should have a full medical history taken (e.g. electrosurgery may be inappropriate in those with cardiac pacemakers [3]). A full drug history is imperative (e.g. aspirin and anticoagulants promote bleeding; interaction between non-selective β-blockers and the adrenaline in local anaesthetics may rarely cause malignant hypertension). Most people know if they have a propensity to faint, and an epileptic individual may be aware of various precipitants of attacks. As there is always a risk of patient collapse in operating rooms, adequate space for an emergency resuscitation team to work is necessary, and appropriate equipment and an oxygen supply should be readily available [4]. All theatre personnel should be trained in first aid and basic resuscitation techniques, and every doctor and nurse should be able to carry out an electrocardiogram and perform defibrillation [5].

REFERENCES

1 Jackson M, Lynch P. An attempt to make an issue less murky: a comparison of four systems for infection prevention. *Infect Control Hosp Epidemiol* 1991; **12**: 48–9.
2 Maloney ME. Infection control. In: Lask GP, Moy RL, eds. *Principles and Techniques of Cutaneous Surgery*. New York: McGraw-Hill, 1996: 57–62.
3 Sebben JE. The hazards of electrosurgery. *J Am Acad Dermatol* 1987; **16**: 869–71.
4 Nagi C, Greenway HT. Emergency airway assessment and management: guide for office practice. *J Assoc Milit Dermatol* 1985; **9**: 66–8.
5 Cummins RO, Thesis W. Encouraging early defibrillation: the AHA and automatic defibrillators. *Ann Emerg Med* 1990; **19**: 1245–7.

Complications [1]

The outcome of any surgical procedure may be affected by complications (Table 81.3). Sometimes, these may be the unforeseen end result of a cascade of events, but much more

Complications	Predisposing factors	Prevention
Infection	Infected lesions Poor sterility Steroids Adjacent infectious source Occlusive dressings Poor blood supply Fat, haematoma and foreign material Sutures Poor technique Excessive devitalized tissue from careless handling or electrocoagulation	Careful preoperative and operative techniques Sutureless closure Antibiotic sprays Prophylactic antibiotics for infected or potentially infected wounds
Delay in closure	Poor blood supply Excess movement Infection Tension Steroids Debilitated patient Poor nutritional status	Layered closure Gentle tissue handling Minimize devitalization of tissues Care in decision to operate Warmth Careful postoperative dressings
'Gaping scar'	Inadequate apposition Dermal instability Excess movement Infection Tension	Careful apposition Subcutaneous or subcuticular sutures Adequate postoperative support, e.g. antitension dressings
Painful scars	Feet and fingers especially	Avoid pressure sites if possible Dressings to reduce subsequent pressure and/or movement Careful apposition
Hypertrophic scars	Site Tension Reaction to embedded material Trauma Individual susceptibility	Avoid 'cape' area if possible Good surgical technique including undermining of edges where necessary
Keloids	Previous history Black skin Upper half of body Tension	Avoid surgery where possible Antitension measures for 3 weeks Watch and prepare to treat
'Railroad tracks'	Skin sutures under too much tension	Good suture technique Use of 'non-reactive' suture material
Stitch marks 'abscess'	Sutures left in too long	Early suture removal
Wound edge inversion	Poor technique	Good surgical technique Occlusive or semi-occlusive dressings
Bleeding and/or haematoma formation	Bleeding tendency Aspirin NSAIDs Alcohol	Preoperative screening Good haemostasis Use of adrenaline in local anaesthetic

Table 81.3 Complications in wound healing.

commonly complications can be anticipated, and therefore often prevented by thorough operative assessment, careful planning and meticulous technique. Good surgical practice requires a thorough and precise routine, and the development of complications often stems from deviation from this routine.

The common complications are bleeding, infection and wound dehiscence.

Aspirin and alcohol both potentiate bleeding, and they should be avoided in the pre- and perioperative period. It is routine practice to combine a local anaesthetic with adrenaline to produce vasoconstriction. This helps during the procedure, but as the effect of the adrenaline wanes, bleeding may start. Intraoperatively, bleeding is controlled by a combination of electrosurgery, pressure and ligation. During the procedure, traction and pressure may control bleeding until haemostasis is obtained, and sometimes suction is useful. For most procedures these measures suffice, but in some circumstances a drain may be left in the wound, particularly if there is a potential cavity. Layered dressings and immobilizing the wound may be helpful postoperatively. If a haematoma develops despite these measures, it will be heralded by the development of pain and swelling, and patients should be told to seek medical advice if such a change occurs. A decision must then be made whether to open the wound, evacuate the haematoma and obtain haemostasis, or to manage conservatively. An important consideration is whether the presence of a haematoma will act as a nidus for infection, and if there is undue wound tension, healing will be compromised.

The second most common complication is infection. A clean wound in healthy tissue will normally resist infection. In certain situations there may be a potential for infection, for example warm, moist site, ulcerated lesion, prolonged procedure, and prophylactic antibiotics should be considered in these circumstances. Postoperative infection usually becomes apparent 4–8 days after the procedure as erythema, pain, swelling and heat around the site. The early prescription of antibiotics may be all that is required, but a decision may have to be made to incise, drain and pack a wound if there is obviously a collection of pus.

Other significant problems are fortunately rare and usually relate to the appearance of the scar. Often of greatest concern is alteration in nerve function. Both sensory and motor nerves may be damaged during cutaneous surgery, but fortunately this is usually neuropraxia and resolves over several months. There are sites where nerve damage is more common (pp. 3594–3597), and care should be taken when operating in these sites.

REFERENCE

1 Stasko T. Complications of cutaneous procedures. In: Roenigk RK, Roenigk HH, eds. *Dermatologic Surgery*, 2nd edn. New York: Marcel Dekker, 1996: 149–75.

Local anaesthetics [1–4]

Principles and types

The prime considerations are effectiveness, rapid action and relative freedom from toxicity and sensitization. These qualities are found in lignocaine hydrochloride (lidocaine), an amide-type local anaesthetic, which is the agent of choice for most dermatologists. Procaine (ester of *p*-aminobenzoic acid) is recommended [2,5] chiefly by anaesthetists because of its lower toxicity, but the amounts used by dermatologists in standard procedures are usually small, and its cross-reactivity with other drugs of the *p*-aminobenzoic acid ester type is a strong disincentive to its use. Of three other preparations of the same general amino group as lignocaine [3], mepivacaine and bupivacaine are similar but have a more sustained action (up to 480 min with adrenaline), whereas prilocaine has a rather briefer effect (60–400 min) [1]. Most local anaesthetics also contain parabens preservative.

Adrenaline (epinephrine) 1:80 000 to 1:200 000 is added to prolong anaesthesia and to reduce immediate bleeding. By reducing absorption, it also reduces the risk of systemic toxicity. However, it should not, in general, be used for operations on fingers and toes or in other sites where the blood supply is likely to be impaired. If a larger amount of local anaesthetic is to be used, the concentration of both local anaesthetic and adrenaline should be reduced, and adrenaline should be avoided entirely in patients with hypertension or cardiac disease, and in those receiving psychotropic drugs, especially phenothiazines or monoamine oxidase inhibitors.

Toxic reactions [1]

Toxic reactions with small quantities of local anaesthetics are rare. They are more likely to occur if the injection is inadvertently given intravenously. Amide-type anaesthetics should be used with care in those with hepatic disease, and ester-type anaesthetics, such as procaine, with caution in those with renal impairment or with a history of allergy to benzocaine, sulphonamides, paraphenylenediamine or other *para*-type chemicals. Amide-type anaesthetics such as lignocaine are generally preferred nowadays because of the very low incidence of allergic reactions to this type of anaesthetic. For patients genuinely sensitive to this group, local anaesthesia may be obtained using injection of antihistamine or normal saline [3].

Overdosage usually presents as a sensation of numbness or tingling. Systemic reactions include vasodilatation, cardiac or respiratory depression, or central nervous system manifestations such as dizziness, drowsiness, tinnitus, slurred speech, muscle twitching and tonic seizures. These side-effects are, to some extent, reversible with diazepam (Valium).

The use of adrenaline may be associated with mild tachycardia and an excited state, and it should not be used during pregnancy, in combination with inhalation anaesthesia, or in patients suffering from glaucoma. Interaction with non-selective β-blockers (e.g. propranolol) may rarely cause malignant hypertension, but this does not occur with cardioselective β-blockers (e.g. atenolol, metoprolol) [1].

Allergic or anaphylactic reactions are sometimes unexpected and always disconcerting. They require immediate counter-measures, and resuscitation equipment and appropriate drugs should always be available. Patients should always be asked if they have had any untoward reactions to local anaesthetics, for example in dental procedures. These may have been nothing more than fainting, but in cases of doubt a test dose can be given or an alternative method of anaesthesia chosen.

Vasovagal attacks associated with the use of anaesthesia are common and should not be confused with the more serious toxic or allergic reactions.

Local complications include bruising, and a temporary sensation of stinging or burning, which is quite common. More persistent sensory anaesthesia or temporary motor nerve palsies may occur. Very rarely, there may be tissue necrosis.

Methods

Local anaesthesia may be achieved *topically* using either amethocaine cream (Ametop) or a eutectic lignocaine–prilocaine cream (EMLA) [5], or by *local infiltration*. Both EMLA and Ametop are applied under occlusion, the former for 2 h and the latter for 1 h. Other methods of anaesthesia include *field block* or *regional anaesthesia* [2,6], which produce temporary interruption of sensory nerve conductivity in a given area. Field block involves infiltration of local anaesthetic at several points around the lesion to be excised, and nerve block involves infiltration close to the nerve supplying the operative field. The choice of which type of local anaesthetic to use depends not only on the method of anaesthesia and the site and expected duration of operation but also on the patient's general condition and the physician's own preference and experience.

The maximum recommended dosage for lignocaine with adrenaline (epinephrine) is 7 mg/kg or approximately 50 ml of a 1% lignocaine solution. In practice, most dermatologists use substantially less. Children should receive smaller amounts of more dilute preparations. Before injecting any local anaesthetic, it is a wise precaution to aspirate first. This should be mandatory when attempting nerve blocks, especially in the head and neck region. Commonly used nerve blocks in dermatology include supraorbital, supratrochlear, infraorbital and mental blocks [3,6]. There are also simple combination blocks for the nose and ear [1]. Adrenaline should never be used when performing 'ring blocks', such as digital nerve blocks, or when anaesthetizing circumferentially around a structure such as the ear.

Other anaesthetic agents include the following.

1 Ethylchloride, dichlorotetrafluorethane (Freon), solid carbon dioxide snow and liquid nitrogen spray give short-lived periods of anaesthesia with refrigeration. They are suitable for the incision of small cysts, abscesses or superficial skin lesions, and for the curettage of multiple small warts or milia.

2 The anaesthetic effect of *antihistamines* can be used when hypersensitivity to other agents is present. Diphenhydramine hydrochloride as a 1% solution is suitable.

3 The injection into the skin of sufficient *normal saline* to cause a weal may be used to produce an anaesthetic effect [1].

4 Benzodiazepines such as intravenous *diazepam* (2.5–10 mg) are useful to allay anxiety, particularly in children, but are not specifically anaesthetic at 'sedative' doses. However, small procedures such as the removal of a molluscum contagiosum can often be carried out with less distress following its administration. Topical local anaesthesia may be adequate for minor lesions in children [5].

5 *Hypnosis* and acupuncture may be useful when performed by an experienced practitioner and in a suitable subject. Apparently painless minor surgery can be carried out on difficult sites, particularly in those sensitive to local anaesthetics.

6 *General anaesthesia* will not be discussed here. An anaesthetist's advice will normally be sought. Patients requiring a general anaesthetic, especially children, are best admitted to hospital either as a day case or overnight. Written consent should always be obtained.

Some reassurance about the relative painlessness of the planned procedure should always be given, particularly to those who are fearful of injections. Pain is said to be less when neutralized lignocaine is used [3].

Young children should not have their trust abused, however, by being told that 'it will not hurt'. Some children are notably braver when their parents are not present. Time, patience and gentleness are the guiding principles for successful anaesthesia. Preliminary sedation is often helpful. In older children who have not been taught a reasonable amount of self-control and stoicism, firmness may have to be allied to kindness and tricks of distraction.

REFERENCES

1 Skidmore RA, Patterson JD, Tomsick RS. Local anaesthetics. *Dermatol Surg* 1996; **22**: 511–22.
2 Auletta MJ. Local anaesthesia for dermatologic surgery. *Semin Dermatol* 1994; **13**: 35–42.
3 Matarasso SL, Glogau RS. Local anaesthesia. In: Lask GP, Moy RL, eds. *Principles and Techniques of Cutaneous Surgery*. New York: McGraw-Hill, 1996: 63–75.
4 Auletta MJ, Grekin RC. *Local Anesthesia for Dermatologic Surgery*. New York: Churchill-Livingstone, 1991.
5 Buckley MM, Benfield P. Eutectic lidocaine/prilocaine cream: a review of the topical anaesthetic/analgesic efficacy of EMLA. *Drugs* 1993; **46**: 126–51.
6 Adriani J. *Regional Anaesthesia—Techniques in Clinical Practice*. Springfield: Thomas, 1970.

Biopsy techniques

Incisional and excisional elliptical biopsy

Elliptical excision biopsy is used for tumour or suspect mole removal. Incisional biopsy is used to take diagnostic biopsies of rashes and tumours before treatment is started. The technique has the advantage that the entire thickness of skin down to fat is excised. An appropriate margin can be selected if required and the incision line placed in the optimum direction [1].

For lesions on the face orientate the ellipse so that the scar runs parallel to or within an existing skin crease or wrinkle line, with the patient seated rather than lying

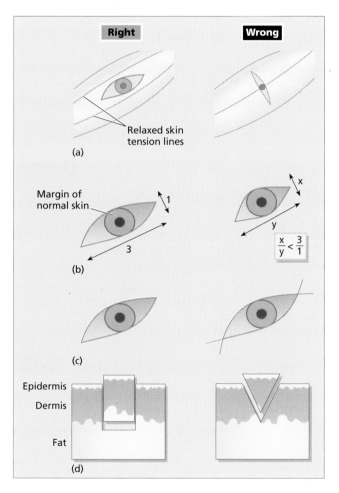

(a) Relaxed skin tension lines

(b) Margin of normal skin   1   3   x   y $\frac{x}{y} < \frac{3}{1}$

(c)

(d) Epidermis   Dermis   Fat

Fig. 81.5 Principles of elliptical excision. The ellipse is designed to follow skin-crease lines (a), and should be approximately three times as long as it is wide (b). Ensure that an appropriate margin of normal skin is also excised (b). At the ends of the ellipse, hold the blade vertically so that the incision lines do not cross over (c). The blade should be held at 90° to the skin when cutting the ellipse so that the wound has vertical sides down to fat. Do not bevel the blade towards the specimen as this makes the wound more difficult to close and may cut into the dermal component of the lesion (d). (From Lawrence [3].)

flat so that the effect of gravity on the skin crease lines is apparent. Wrinkle or smile lines can be exaggerated by asking the patient to grimace or smile, or by manipulating the skin [2]. In an excisional biopsy, measure the margin to be excised and mark the optimal line of closure before injecting the anaesthetic. When drawing on the skin, use a skin marker or Bonney's blue ink (a mixture of crystal violet and brilliant green), as other inks may tattoo the skin.

The ellipse length should be approximately three times as long as the width, to produce an ellipse angle of approximately 30°, so that buckling does not occur when the wound is sutured (Fig. 81.5). A larger angle may suffice at some sites or in older people [4]. Make the incisions as a single continuous sweep rather than a series of small nicks and hold the blade at 90° to the skin, not angled inwards, so that the ellipse sides are vertical [5]. Ensure that the incision lines meet neatly without crossing over at the tip by starting and finishing each sweep with the blade held vertically. Incise down to fat. When the ellipse sides and tips are completely separate from the surrounding skin the ellipse should be sitting on a bed of fat. The fat under the ellipse should be cut through using scissors, while the ellipse is gently pulled away from the skin using a skin hook [6]. Undermine the edge at the appropriate level if there is any tension. Close the wound using both subcutaneous and surface sutures if necessary, using the correct suture technique. If required, the junction between involved and uninvolved skin can be marked using typists' correction fluid, which persists during histological processing.

Punch biopsy

Punch biopsy produces a core of skin down to fat. It is quick and easy to perform, and leaves only a small wound. The disadvantages include the potential for sampling error and the difficulty in stopping bleeding if a small arteriole is punctured at the base of the wound. Punch biopsies can also be used to excise naevi on the back. At this site, wounds can be allowed to heal by second intention, with better cosmetic results than primary closure produces [7]. Subcutaneous tissue lesions can be sampled using a punch biopsy by pinching up a fold of skin to include the subcutaneous tissue before the biopsy is taken [8].

Disposable and reusable 2–8 mm diameter punches are available; 3 and 4 mm are most frequently used. When the skin is numb, drill the blade down to fat with gentle downward pressure [5]. To minimize the scar size, stretch the skin at right angles to the wrinkle lines while taking the biopsy so that, when the tension is relaxed, an oval rather than a round wound is produced, with its long axis parallel to the wrinkle lines [6]. The skin core may pop up when the surrounding skin is pressed down, or it can be hooked out using a needle. Cut through the fat at the base with scissors and remove carefully to avoid crushing the specimen. The wound can be sutured or allowed to granulate; the latter produces an acceptable small round or oval scar. If the wound is to be allowed to heal by second intention, stopping bleeding using a collagen matrix dressing results in a better cosmetic result than using Monsel's solution [9], particularly if the collagen matrix is coated with elastin [10].

Shave

Shave excision is a simple, rapid and effective method of removing benign papular naevi. It can also be used to obtain a tissue diagnosis in protuberant nodular skin tumours. Shave biopsy of dermatoses affecting the epidermis or high dermis results in adequate tissue for diagnosis, and the subsequent re-epithelialization from follicular epithelium produces a good cosmetic result.

Naevi

Inject the local anaesthetic directly into the naevus, as this stiffens the tissue and makes it easier to slice off. Holding a no. 15 blade horizontally, shave off the naevus flush with the skin. Stop bleeding using cautery, electrodesiccation

or a chemical haemostatic agent. Cautery or electrodesiccation is preferred, as they can be used to destroy remaining wound edge tissue fragments. The wound will take 2–3 weeks to heal. In approximately 45% of head and neck and 30% of trunk naevi, no visible scar remains (Fig. 81.6). In the remainder, the scar is smaller than the original naevus on head, neck and limb sites and a little larger than the naevus on trunk sites. Pigmentation at the scar edge or centre remains in approximately 25% of initially pigmented naevi after shave excision; non-pigmented naevi rarely, if ever, leave a pigmented scar [11]. Persistent pigmentation is even more common when aluminium chloride haemostasis is used rather than cautery [12]. Retained pigment does not need to be excised. If a further specimen is sent, the pathologist must be given the full history in order to interpret the changes correctly. Hairs remain in 25% of initially hairy naevi; these can be destroyed by electrolysis if necessary.

Skin tumours

Shave biopsy of a solid tumour is faster and easier than an incisional biopsy, which needs to be sutured. A fragment can be shaved off to confirm the diagnosis prior to

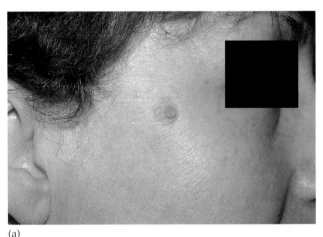

(a)

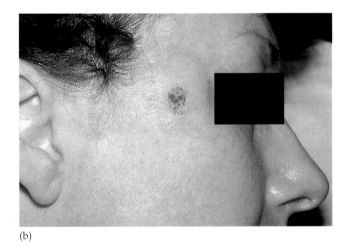

(b)

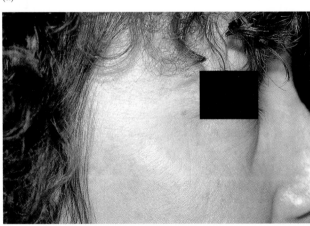

(c)

Fig. 81.6 Shave biopsy of benign papular naevi. This patient had a benign, tan-coloured naevus on the face (a) removed by shave excision followed by cautery (b), resulting in a good cosmetic result 6 months later (c).

definitive treatment. This type of biopsy will not help to distinguish a keratoacanthoma from a squamous cell carcinoma, and is unsuitable if histological examination of the deep margin or edge of a tumour is required to confirm the diagnosis. A large exophytic tumour can sometimes be shave biopsied painlessly without the need for local anaesthesia. Bleeding can be stopped using silver-nitrate stick coagulation, as the cosmetic outcome will be determined by the subsequent treatment. The fragile specimen should be mounted on paper before being placed in formalin.

REFERENCES

1 Borges AF, Alexander JE. Relaxed skin tension lines, z-plasty in scars and fusiform excisions of lesions. *Br J Plast Surg* 1962; **15**: 242–54.
2 Summers BK, Siegle RJ. Facial cutaneous reconstructive surgery: general aesthetic principles. *J Am Acad Dermatol* 1993; **29**: 669–81.
3 Lawrence CM. *An Introduction to Dermatological Surgery.* Oxford: Blackwell Science, 1996: 80.
4 Hudson-Peacock MJ, Lawrence CM. Comparison of wound closure by means of dog ear repair and elliptical excision. *J Am Acad Dermatol* 1995; **32**: 627–30.
5 Zachary CB. *Basic Cutaneous Surgery: A Primer in Technique.* New York: Churchill Livingstone, 1991.
6 Fewkes JL, Cheney ML, Pollack SV. *Illustrated Atlas of Cutaneous Surgery.* Philadelphia: JB Lippincott, 1992.
7 Barnett R, Stranc M. A method of producing improved scars following excision of small lesions of the back. *Ann Plast Surg* 1979; **5**: 391–4, 435.
8 Crollick JS, Klein LE. Punch biopsy diagnostic technique. *J Dermatol Surg Oncol* 1987; **13**: 839.
9 Armstrong RB, Nichols J, Pachance J. Punch biopsy wounds treated with Monsel's solution or a collagen matrix. *Arch Dermatol* 1986; **122**: 546–9.
10 de Vries HJC, Zeegelaar JE, Middelkoop E *et al.* Reduced wound contraction and scar formation in punch biopsy wounds. Native collagen dermal substitutes. A clinical study. *Br J Dermatol* 1995; **132**: 690–7.
11 Hudson-Peacock MJ, Bishop J, Lawrence CM. Shave excision of benign papular naevocytic naevi. *Br J Plast Surg* 1995; **48**: 318–22.
12 Hudson-Peacock MJ, Lawrence CM. Cosmetic outcome following shave excision of benign papular naevi using either electrocautery or aluminium chloride for haemostasis. *Br J Dermatol* 1995; **133** (Suppl. 45): 47.

Simple excision, suture technique and wound closure

Excision [1–3]

The aim of an excision should be to remove completely the lesion in question and to leave as inconspicuous a scar as possible. The nature of the lesion and the probable effects of alternative treatment help to determine the amount of scarring that is acceptable. An ugly scar may be justified if the patient has a malignant melanoma but not if he/she has a benign naevus. Most lesions fall well within these extremes, and the choice of excision or other forms of treatment is a matter of judgement, experience and, to some extent, convenience.

Surgeon preparation

The surgeon should be confident the proposed procedure and any possible complications are within his or her competence, and should not be reserved about referring for a second opinion. The surgeon should be immunized against hepatitis B, and should be cognizant of and observe safe practices with regard to handling sharps and probably infectious material. Gloves should always be worn and eye protection considered, if appropriate [4].

Patient preparation

Patients should be aware of the limitations of surgery and the fact that complications may and do occur, and that these cannot always be predicted or avoided. The patient's informed consent [5] should be obtained in writing. Parental consent should be obtained in the case of minors. Prior to surgery, the patient should have had the procedure fully explained to him/her, and the probable benefits and potential risks of the operation should be discussed. Most patients attending for surgery are anxious and will require reassurance. A preoperative sedative may be useful for particularly anxious patients.

Re-examination and palpation of the lesion will reveal its extent, probable depth and proximity to large blood vessels, nerves or other important structures. Langer's lines of skin tension [6] were previously used as a guide to incision, but the best cosmetic results are usually obtained by following the wrinkle lines [1,7], which run perpendicular to the major underlying muscles. The two often coincide, as on the neck. When they do not, as on the limbs, the choice depends on other factors. Small excisions on the lower leg, for instance, can be more securely apposed and kept free of tension if they are longitudinal. Testing for skin laxity with the fingers usually clarifies the best direction in which to make an excision. The size and type of excision made will also depend upon many factors, including the site and nature of the lesion to be excised and the nature of the planned skin closure.

The skin surface should be cleaned prior to operation with either a detergent–antibacterial combination, preferably one containing chlorhexidine [8] or an iodophor (povidone–iodine) scrub, or with a surface antiseptic skin preparation such as 0.5% chlorhexidine in 70% isopropyl alcohol or an iodine paint. The purpose of the skin preparation is to remove pathogens and to reduce the resident flora so that the risk of surgical infection is slight [9].

General technique [2,3]

The planned lines of excision should be marked, and local anaesthesia obtained. If a vasoconstrictor has been used, allow sufficient time for the skin to blanch before incising.

A small, round-ended blade (Gillette no. 15) is best used for the excision, which should be performed with two elliptical incisions perpendicular through the skin. The length of the wound should be at least three times its breadth, so that the angles at the tips of the excision should never exceed 30°. The lesion is held firmly but gently with fine-toothed forceps or a skin hook, and separated from its base. Ideally, for histological purposes, it should contain some subcutaneous fat.

The specimen is placed immediately in a formol–saline specimen bottle or, for immunofluorescence or frozen section studies, on aluminium foil and suspended in liquid nitrogen. To prevent curling of small biopsy or excision samples, these may be placed on small squares of filter paper and floated into the formalin solution.

Venous bleeding is staunched initially by pressure. Any persistent bleeding points must be sealed using electrosurgery before closure. Arterial bleeding may require clamping and ligation of vessels. Chemical styptics should not be used if the wound is to be sutured.

If the skin is lax, nothing further is required. However, undercutting of the skin may be necessary to reduce wound tension. In regions such as the thigh and leg, excess fat may have to be removed to facilitate wound closure. In these areas, and whenever a wound is likely to be infected or avascular, an antibiotic powder spray may be used once bleeding has been stopped.

Subcutaneous absorbable sutures are used for large excisions or at sites of probable tension. The final procedure is to appose the wound edges exactly and neatly.

Good cosmetic results depend on careful suturing, and the operator should be conversant with the various suturing techniques [2,3].

REFERENCES

1 Baer RL, Kopf AW. Dermatologic office surgery. In: *Year Book of Dermatology 1963–64*. Chicago: Year Book Medical Publishers, 1964: 7–47.
2 Epstein E, Epstein E, Jr, eds. *Skin Surgery*, 5th edn. Springfield: Thomas, 1982.
3 Stegman SJ. *Basics of Dermatologic Surgery*. Chicago: Year Book Medical Publishers, 1982.
4 Smith JG, Chalker DK. A glove upon that hand. *South Med J* 1982; **75**: 129–31.
5 Redden EM, Baker DC. Coping with the complexities of informed consent in dermatologic surgery. *J Dermatol Surg Oncol* 1984; **10**: 111–16.
6 Ridge MD, Wright V. The directional effects of skin. A bioengineering study of skin with particular reference to Langer's lines. *J Invest Dermatol* 1966; **46**: 341–6.
7 Kraissl CJ. The selection of appropriate lines for elective surgical excision. *Plast Reconstr Surg* 1951; **8**: 1–28.
8 Kaul AF, Jewitt JF. Agents and techniques for disinfection of the skin. *Surg Gynecol Obstet* 1981; **152**: 677–85.
9 Selwyn S, Ellis H. Skin bacteria and skin disinfection reconsidered. *Br Med J* 1972; **i**: 136–40.

Sutures [1–4]

Skin sutures are of two main types: *absorbable* and *non-absorbable*. Both types of suture should ideally have very low tissue reactivity, high tensile strength and good knot security, and should provide easy handling.

Absorbable sutures are represented by plain and chromic catgut, Vicryl (polyglactin-910), Dexon (polyglycolic acid), PDS (polydioxane sulphate) and Maxon (polyglyconate). Plain catgut loses its strength in 4–5 days and is rarely used nowadays. *Chromic catgut*, to all intents and purposes, has been replaced by the newer *synthetic absorbable sutures* (Vicryl, Dexon, PDS, Maxon), which cause very little tissue reaction and which dissolve completely in 90–120 days. Absorbable sutures are usually used as 'deep' suture materials, for example subcutaneous or subcuticular.

Non-absorbable sutures include silk, nylon and polypropylene (Prolene). Again, the newer synthetic sutures have better tensile strength and cause less tissue reactivity, and are generally to be preferred. Braided nylon and Dacron (also braided) have better knot-tying properties but there is possibly, as with silk, an increased risk of infection due to the braided nature of the suture material. For wounds that are likely to remain under constant tension, such as those on the back or shoulders, one can use non-absorbable suture material such as nylon to close the deep subcutaneous layer, or leave a subcuticular prolene suture in for several weeks. However, most dermatologists prefer absorbable sutures.

In general, skin suture needles are of the reverse cutting type. Suture size usually varies from 3/0 to 6/0, depending on site and function.

Suture technique [2,3,5]

Several suture techniques are necessary if one is to become proficient in dermatological surgery. A *simple interrupted suture* is usually the preferred method of final skin closure, although some surgeons favour a *running subcuticular stitch* with a broad piece of porous or semiporous tape applied to the skin surface to give extra support and stability to the wound. The tape can be replaced after the subcuticular suture has been removed, and will continue to keep the skin edges approximated until it peels off. Interrupted non-absorbable nylon sutures, however, are normally preferred. Skin sutures should not be applied under any tension. They are normally 4/0 to 6/0, and are placed close to the skin edge for fine approximation. If the wound tends to invert, then the deeper component of the suture can be placed more laterally to help evert the edges. Interrupted skin sutures are all that are required for most superficial biopsies or excisions.

If there is tension across the wound, or a significant tendency to inversion, then it may be advisable to insert one or two *vertical mattress* sutures first. A modification of this suture, the *half-buried mattress*, is also useful as a corner stitch when anchoring the apices of flaps. The *horizontal mattress* suture (with bolsters) [6] can also be used to approximate long wounds or wounds under tension.

However, there is a risk of tissue necrosis or scarring if the suture is pulled too tight or left in too long.

There are various forms of *buried suture* which are used to close off 'dead space' in a deep wound. Normally, one would use interrupted *deep subcutaneous* or buried dermal sutures [7], but a variant of the horizontal mattress known as a '*purse-string*' suture can also be used with similar effect. Running sutures, both cutaneous and subcutaneous, can be used to save time, but are less secure than interrupted sutures. The running subcuticular suture—in reality a running superficial horizontal mattress—is difficult to do well, but is an elegant suture for shallow wounds or when there are already deep subcutaneous sutures in place.

Tape closures may be used in conjunction with interrupted sutures or on their own if there is good approximation and adequate subcutaneous or subcuticular support. They are not suitable for wounds under tension. Another use of tape closures is as an additional skin support both while skin sutures are in place and for the 2–3 weeks following their removal. Cyanoacrylates may also be useful, especially in children [8].

Stainless steel staples are a rapid and effective way to close longer skin incisions. They are strong, and incite very little tissue reaction, but are perhaps not fine or flexible enough to cope with the contours and irregularities of surgical excisions on the face [9].

REFERENCES

1 Aston SJ. The choice of suture material for skin closure. *J Dermatol Surg Oncol* 1976; **2**: 57–61.
2 Dingman RO, Watanabe MJ, Izenberg PH. General principles of skin surgery. In: Epstein E, Epstein E, Jr, eds. *Skin Surgery*, 5th edn. Springfield: Thomas, 1982: 74–107.
3 Stegman SJ. Suturing techniques for dermatologic surgery. *J Dermatol Surg Oncol* 1978; **4**: 63–8.
4 Swanson NA, Tromovitch TA. Suture materials, 1980s: properties, uses, and abuses. *Int J Dermatol* 1982; **21**: 373–8.
5 Stegman SJ, Tromovitch TA, Glogau RG. *Basics of Dermatologic Surgery.* Chicago: Year Book Medical Publishers, 1982.
6 Simmonds WL. Surgical gems: uses of bolsters in dermatologic surgery. *J Dermatol Surg Oncol* 1977; **3**: 281–2.
7 Albom MJ. Surgical gems: dermo-subdermal sutures for long, deep surgical wounds. *J Dermatol Surg Oncol* 1977; **3**: 504–5.
8 Ellis DAF, Shaikh A. The ideal tissue adhesive in facial plastic and reconstructive surgery. *J Otolaryngol* 1990; **19**: 68–72.
9 Stegmaier OC. Use of skin stapler in dermatologic surgery. *J Am Acad Dermatol* 1982; **6**: 305–9.

Particular forms of excision

Variations in detail and technique apply to particular lesions and areas of the body. A few examples only are given.

Pilar or epidermoid cysts [1]

Small cysts are often deeper than they appear and may be difficult to locate after infiltration with local anaesthetic. Larger, tense cysts of the scalp often extend deeply and their removal may be accompanied by arterial bleeding, which must be located and dealt with. Most cysts are best removed by traditional elliptical incision and blunt dissection with scissors or a haemostat, while pulling gently on the ellipse and the attached cyst. If the cyst ruptures, the remaining contents should be expressed and the whole of the cyst wall removed.

Lesions on the shoulder and upper back

Dermatologists are frequently consulted about lesions in these areas. Although excision is simple, the greatest care should be taken to appose the wound with the least tension, and to apply firm antitension dressings. Subcutaneous or subcuticular sutures may be required, and movement and tension across the scar should be restricted as far as possible. When the lesion is large, or when there is any reason to anticipate an unsightly scar, the patient should be warned of this and excision performed only if absolutely necessary. In some circumstances it may be appropriate to excise the lesion with a narrow margin of normal skin and allow healing by secondary intention [2].

Benign moles

These are best left alone. The patient or parent should be told that the results of intervention may well be worse than the original blemish.

Basal cell and squamous cell carcinomas [3]

Small basal cell carcinomas are often best excised. The choice of treatment, however, depends on the patient's age, and on the site, size and type of lesion. An adequate margin should always be obtained, and prior skin marking following careful examination in good lighting is advisable [4].

In patients with chronic actinic damage, some keratoses justify biopsy excision, especially if they are beginning to 'heap up' or if there is a suspicion of malignant change. All specimens should be sent for histological examination. Squamous cell carcinomas usually require wide excision, although in some cases a preliminary biopsy may be necessary. If this or local excision reveals an anaplastic or undifferentiated carcinoma, further excision has to be considered and regional lymph nodes kept under close observation.

Cure rates for basal cell carcinoma treated by surgical excision vary from 90 to 98% [5–7]. Some sites, such as the lips, ear, scalp and periocular and nasolabial areas, have a higher rate of recurrence, and management of lesions in these sites, particularly those with infiltrative growth patterns, requires particular care [3,8].

Chondrodermatitis nodularis helicis (see also p. 3627)

A thick elliptical incision is made around the lesion, the skin is eased back gently, and the nodule and underlying cartilage are removed by a shave excision. The surrounding skin is then gently undermined and reapposed with fine skin sutures and tape closures.

Mucous membranes

Excision of lesions in the mouth and on the tongue, lips and genitalia is difficult only in that access may be restricted and bleeding profuse. If a semicircular suture needle is inserted first, the excision (or biopsy) may be conveniently carried out onto this as a base, and the edges of the wound brought quickly together. Electrodiathermy on cut or cut-coagulation mode is also of use when performing surgery in the mouth. The application of pressure on surrounding tissues by an assistant, the use of adrenaline in the local anaesthetic, and tongue or tissue clamps are all helpful.

Excision of axillary vault [9,10] (see also p. 3627)

This very satisfactory form of treatment for severe axillary sweating is simple to carry out under local anaesthesia. A transverse elliptical excision is made in the dome of the axilla to remove a 4.5 cm × 1.5 cm area of skin. It should be deep enough to remove the sweat glands, which lie up to 0.6 cm below the surface. Apposition without tension can usually be achieved without much undercutting. A light pressure dressing is applied for 24–48 h, and the wound is then left undressed and cleansed daily with a bactericidal antiseptic.

More extensive surgical removal [11,12] may give better long-term results. Radical excision of all the sweat glands, with Z-plasty repair, proved successful in all but seven of 123 cases [13].

Keratoacanthoma

If it cannot be excised *in toto*, a biopsy for confirmation of the diagnosis must include the centre, edge and a portion of normal adjacent skin.

Excision of pigmented lesions (Chapter 38)

The management of pigmented lesions demands diagnostic acumen, skill and decisiveness. Blue naevi, pigmented basal cell carcinomas, seborrhoeic warts and histiocytomas are usually easily recognizable, although diagnostic difficulties occasionally occur. If there is any doubt about the diagnosis the lesion should be excised locally, if its size permits this, and an urgent histopathological opinion requested. Frozen section examination is usually not suf-

ficiently definitive in the doubtful, and thus most important, cases. When the lesion is too large to excise without primary closure, the dermatologist may have to decide whether or not to biopsy. Available evidence suggests that this does not adversely influence the prognosis. The subject is discussed fully by Epstein *et al.* [14]. It is better to err on the side of safety and to treat the lesion as malignant until proved otherwise.

The majority of darkly pigmented skin lesions are benign [14], but when a lesion is obviously a malignant melanoma, it is the duty of the dermatologist to act rapidly and arrange for its urgent excision.

Hypertrophic scars

These will often resolve with time. Intralesional steroid injections are helpful. They may be treated (and could often be prevented) by Z-plasty techniques [15], by sustained pressure, or using silicone gel sheet dressings [16].

REFERENCES

1 Roxburgh RA. Excision of sebaceous cysts and lipomas. *Br J Hosp Med* 1969; **2**: 866–7.
2 Barnett R, Stranc M. A method of producing improved scars following excision of small lesions of the back. *Ann Plast Surg* 1979; **3**: 391–4.
3 Randle HW. Basal cell carcinoma: identification and treatment of the high-risk patient. *Dermatol Surg* 1996; **22**: 255–61.
4 Breuninger H, Dietz K. Prediction of subclinical tumour infiltration in basal cell carcinoma. *J Dermatol Surg Oncol* 1991; **17**: 574–8.
5 Chernosky ME. Squamous cell and basal cell carcinomas: preliminary study of 3817 primary skin cancers. *South Med J* 1978; **71**: 802–3.
6 Marchac D, Papadopoulos O, Duport G. Curative and aesthetic results of surgical treatment of 138 basal-cell carcinomas. *J Dermatol Surg Oncol* 1982; **8**: 379–87.
7 Porte A, Molle B, Zumer L *et al*. Résultat du traitement de 250 épithéliomas cutanés. *Ann Chirurg Plast* 1979; **24**: 253–6 (Abstract).
8 Bart RS, Schrager D, Kopf AW *et al*. Scalpel excision of basal cell carcinomas. *Arch Dermatol* 1978; **114**: 739–42.
9 Hurley HJ, Shelley WB. A simple surgical approach to the management of axillary hyperhidrosis. *JAMA* 1963; **186**: 109–12.
10 Hurley HJ, Shelley WB. Axillary hyperhidrosis. Clinical features and local surgical management. *Br J Dermatol* 1966; **78**: 127–40.
11 Skoog T, Thyresson N. Hyperhidrosis of the axillae. A method of surgical treatment. *Acta Chirurg Scand* 1962; **124**: 531–8.
12 Skoog T, Thyresson N. The surgical treatment of axillary hyperhidrosis. *Br J Dermatol* 1966; **78**: 551.
13 Bretteville-Jensen G, Mossing N, Albrechtsen R. Surgical treatment of axillary hyperhidrosis in 123 patients. *Acta Derm Venereol (Stockh)* 1975; **55**: 73–7.
14 Epstein E, Bragg K, Linden G. Biopsy and prognosis of malignant melanoma. *JAMA* 1969; **208**: 1369–71.
15 Longacre JJ. *Scar Tissue. Its Use and Abuse*. Springfield: Thomas, 1972.
16 Sproat JE, Dalcin A, Weitauer N *et al*. Hypertrophic sternal scars: silicone gel sheet versus Kenalog injection treatment. *Plast Reconstr Surg* 1992; **90**: 988–92.

Wound closure [1–3]

A fundamental requirement of those involved in dermatological surgery is the ability to repair the surgical wound that they create. In addition, their surgery should leave the least conspicuous scar possible. Although 'open wounds' left to heal by secondary intention do so surprisingly well, especially when small and superficial, dermatological surgeons should have a range of closure techniques at their disposal in order to be able to cope with all but the most unexpected situations. Careful planning and meticulous technique are of the utmost importance.

The *side-to-side* closure is the most frequently used and often the most cosmetically satisfying technique for the majority of surgical repairs. The basic method of closing a simple wedge biopsy or ellipse is, of course, well known to all doctors. Undermining of the free skin edges will assist in bringing them together without undue tension. This is normally best done at the level of the superficial fat, but deeper planes may be required on the scalp (where it is best to undermine the galea) and elsewhere.

Closure may require additional buried (absorbable) sutures if the wound is deep, or if there is excessive movement or tension across the wound.

When histological confirmation of clearance is required, it is often advisable to 'colour code' or otherwise mark the surgical specimen on removal. This helps to plan re-excision if this later proves necessary.

Suture removal depends on the site and the amount of tension across the wound. With additional supporting surface tapes and buried sutures where appropriate, 4–5 days is usually sufficient for skin sutures on the face, 5–7 days for the scalp and neck and 10–14 days elsewhere.

The M-plasty [4]

This is particularly useful if one end of an elliptical excision will cross an important anatomical or cosmetic line. In this situation, an M-plasty will help to reduce the overall length of excision required by bringing the apex of the excision back within the original area to be excised. Obviously, for malignant lesions, there should still be an adequate margin of clearance at the inverted apex.

'Dog-ear' repairs [5]

'Dog-ears' occur when the length to width ratio of an excision is insufficient to prevent the skin at the poles from buckling when the opposing skin edges are brought together. It occurs more commonly when there is insufficient laxity or movement in the surrounding tissues. Excisions where the angle at the apex exceeds 30° are also liable to produce 'dog-ears'. 'Pseudo-dog-ears' occur if too much fat is left at the poles of an excision.

There are several ways in which this problem can be surmounted [3].
1 The excision can be extended and the redundant overlapping skin excised.
2 One side of the pucker can be cut back flush with the skin and the excess skin from the other side identified by drawing it across the wound; this can then be cut off.
3 The excess skin of the 'dog-ear' can be removed by converting it into a T-plasty or an M-plasty. This is a useful technique when the length of the wound cannot be extended [6].

Wound edges of unequal lengths

This problem can frequently be overcome simply by using a halving technique whereby a suture is placed across the centre of the wound and subsequent sutures continue to divide the resultant defects into ever smaller compartments. Because of local skin elasticity, the shorter side tends to stretch to match the longer. For more disproportionate edges, a wedge may have to be removed from the longer side in order to make the sides of the resultant ellipse more equal, or the wound can be sutured in the normal way and a 'dog-ear' repair performed to remove the excess skin from one side.

Z-plasty

This is a technique which is used to treat contractures and to break up or alter the direction of linear scars to improve the cosmetic appearance. The angle size used governs the increased lengthening of the scar that will result. Conventionally, an angle of 60° is used, which theoretically produces a 75% increase in scar length (Figs 81.7 & 81.8).

Fig. 81.7 Technique of Z-plasty. (From Eedy *et al.* [7].)

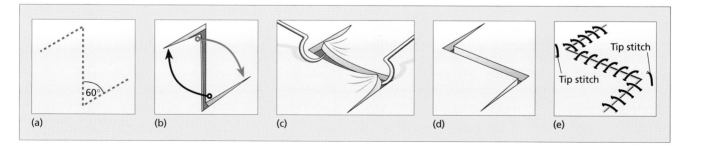

(a) (b) (c) (d) (e)

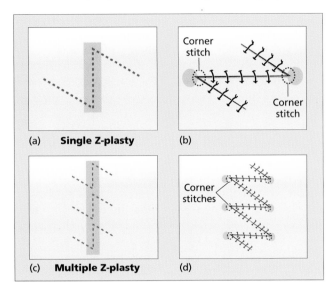

(a) **Single Z-plasty**

(b) Corner stitch / Corner stitch

(c) **Multiple Z-plasty**

(d) Corner stitches

Fig. 81.8 Technique of Z-plasty. (a,b) Single Z-plasty. (c,d) Multiple Z-plasty. Note breaking up of zone of lateral tension (shaded areas) with multiple Z-plasty. (From Eedy *et al.* [7].)

REFERENCES

1 Chernosky ME. Scalpel and scissor surgery as seen by the dermatologist. In: Epstein E, Epstein E, Jr, eds. *Skin Surgery*, 5th edn. Springfield: Thomas, 1982: 189–229.

2 Stegman SJ. Planning closure of a surgical wound. *J Dermatol Surg Oncol* 1978; **4**: 390–3.

3 Stegman SJ. *Basics of Dermatologic Surgery*. Chicago: Year Book Medical Publishers, 1982.

4 Webster RC, Davidson TM, Smith RC *et al.* M-plasty techniques. *J Dermatol Surg Oncol* 1976; **2**: 393–6.

5 Gormley DE. The dog-ear: causes, prevention and correction. *J Dermatol Surg Oncol* 1977; **3**: 194–8.

6 Salasche SJ, Roberts LC. Dog-ear correction by M-plasty. *J Dermatol Surg Oncol* 1984; **10**: 478–82.

7 Eedy DJ, Breathnach SM, Walker NPJ. *Surgical Dermatology*. Oxford: Blackwell Science, 1996.

Dressings

Wound dressings are not essential [1], although optimizing wound care by using an appropriate dressing probably produces a predictably better result. An ideal dressing should meet the following criteria.

1 Soaks up excess exudate from the wound surface, thereby reducing the risk of bacterial penetration.

2 Maintains a moist wound–dressing interface to encourage migration of epidermal cells over the granulating tissue. Covered split-thickness wounds heal faster than dry wounds [2]. A scab is a poor barrier against loss of moisture from the dermal surface because it allows the surface to dry out, thus forcing the epidermis to grow under the dry wound surface. As the epidermal cells migrate, they secrete a proteolytic enzyme which dissolves the base of the scab; migration ceases when cell–cell contact occurs [3].

3 Does not contain organisms or fibres which may con-

taminate the wound. Cellulose-derived dressings may shed fibre fragments into the wound [4], causing a foreign-body reaction and leading to increased risk of infection.

4 Is impermeable to bacteria.

5 Causes minimal injury to healing tissue when removed.

It is often claimed that a dressing that permits increased oxygen permeability aids wound healing. Such dressings do aid healing in split-thickness wounds [5]. However, in full-thickness wounds the same synthetic wound dressings create hypoxic conditions at the healing surface [6]. Paradoxically, tissue hypoxia in full-thickness wounds appears to stimulate rather than retard granulation tissue formation [7].

Basic dressing [8]

This includes contact, absorbent and outer layers [9]. The layer in contact with the wound is non-adherent, either because it contains a greasy ointment (e.g. tulle dressing) or because it is made from a specially designed low-adherence material [10] (e.g. polyethylene). The absorbent layer (e.g. cotton-wool, gauze) soaks up the excess wound exudate and cushions the wound. The outer layer (e.g. tubular bandage, elasticated tape) holds the other two layers in place and applies slight pressure. The basic dressing is left in place until suture removal, but needs to be changed if it gets wet or becomes saturated with exudate [11], as this greatly increases bacterial penetration. Many proprietary dressings combine two or all three components (e.g. Melolin contains a polyethylene non-adherent layer attached to an absorbent cellulose component). The hydrogels (e.g. Vigilon), hydrocolloid (e.g. Granuflex), xerogel (e.g. dextranomer starch polymer), alginate (e.g. Kaltostat) and synthetic foam dressings are designed to provide all three components, and these can also be used on pressure sores [12,13], leg ulcers [14] and full-thickness surgical wounds [15].

Pressure dressings

These are placed over the basic dressing. Most commonly, and on suitable sites, a piece of compressible padded dressing (e.g. cotton-wool, sponge, eye pad) is pressed down onto the wound with an elasticated or *crepe bandage* for 48 h. Where bandage application is difficult, a *multi-tape dressing* can be used. Dental rolls are placed over and pressed down onto the dressing by using adhesive tape strips, and additional adhesive (e.g. collodion or tinct benz co.) is used to increase the tape adhesion. A *tie-over pressure dressing* is commonly applied over skin grafts, but can be used on any wound. Several paired sutures are placed around the wound and tied together to hold down a three-layered contact, absorbent and compression dressing, so that the graft is held down onto the recipient site to prevent a haematoma forming beneath it.

Suggested dressing for wound types

Small full- or partial thickness wounds (shave and curettage sites) require a simple, low-adherent dressing or paraffin tulle held in place with a conforming adhesive tape. Unsutured punch biopsy sites do not appear to benefit from occlusive dressings [16], but heal better with a collagen matrix dressing than they do after simply applying Monsel's solution to stop bleeding [17]. *Sutured wounds* (side-to-side closures and flaps) require a greasy antiseptic ointment application and an absorbent-backed, low-adherent dressing held in place with a conforming adhesive tape. A pressure dressing may also be required. After suture removal, apply adhesive tape strips for 5 days. On a *full-thickness graft* apply a simple contact dressing (e.g. greasy antiseptic ointment and paraffin tulle) and then a tie-over pressure dressing which includes a sponge or cotton-wool compressible pad. On *full-thickness wounds* a variety of wound management methods are used. If acceptable to the patient, the wound can be left without a dressing and simply cleaned two to three times a day and smeared with sterile white soft paraffin or a greasy antiseptic ointment. Alternatively, the wound can be cleaned less frequently if a combination contact/absorbent dressing is applied. These wounds need to be re-dressed less frequently as they heal. During the initial exudative stage, i.e. the first 4 days, the dressing will need to be changed at least once a day. Thereafter, the dressing should be changed if the wound surface starts to dry out or the dressing becomes saturated, wet or otherwise dirty. The wound should be cleaned with a simple antiseptic (e.g. aqueous chlorhexidine, 10 vol. hydrogen peroxide) before being re-dressed using a greasy antiseptic ointment application, and simple contact dressing (e.g. polyethylene/cellulose dressing (Melolin)) held in place with adhesive tape. Alternatively, a semipermeable adhesive polyurethane [18] or gel or colloid dressing can be used and changed as necessary. *Split-skin graft donor sites* heal faster with a dressing that maintains a moist wound–dressing interface, for example calcium alginate [19] and semipermeable adhesive polyurethane film [20]. A pressure bandage applied over the wound is also required, but bleeding will still occur, and the blood-stained exudate can either be allowed to drain through puncture wounds made in the lower portion of the film, or can be removed by changing the dressing more frequently, although this may introduce infection and is painful.

Other factors believed to enhance wound healing include topical tretinoin on full-thickness wounds [21], amniotic membrane used as a biological dressing for micro-skin grafts [22], topical zinc [23], and application of epidermal growth factor [24]. Wound healing is delayed by topical steroid application [25], tobacco smoking [26], and possibly age [27] via a decrease in skin blood flow with increasing arteriosclerosis [28]. Topical bovine collagen [29] has no effect on facial wound healing.

REFERENCES

1 Mengert WF, Hermes RL. Simplified gynecologic care. *Am J Obstet Gynecol* 1949; **58**: 1109–16.
2 Hinman CD, Maibach H. Effect of air exposure and occlusion on experimental human skin wounds. *Nature* 1963; **200**: 377–8.
3 Harris DR. Healing of the surgical wound. 1. Basic considerations. *J Am Acad Dermatol* 1979; **1**: 197–207.
4 Wood RAB. Disintegration of cellulose dressings in open granulating wounds. *Br Med J* 1976; **1**: 1444–5.
5 Silver IA. Oxygen tension and epithelialisation. In: Maibach HI, Rovee DT, eds. *Epidermal Wound Healing*. Chicago: Year Book Publishers, 1972.
6 Varghese MC, Balin AK, Carer M, Caldwell D. Local environment of chronic wounds under synthetic dressings. *Arch Dermatol* 1986; **122**: 52–7.
7 Knighton DR, Silver IA, Hunt TK. Regulation of wound healing angiogenesis—effect of oxygen gradients and inspired oxygen concentration. *Surgery* 1981; **90**: 262–70.
8 Bennett RG. *Fundamentals of Cutaneous Surgery*. St Louis: Mosby, 1988: 310–51.
9 Telfer NR, Moy RL. Wound care after office procedures. *J Dermatol Surg Oncol* 1993; **19**: 722–31.
10 Local applications to wounds—II. Dressings for wounds and ulcers. *Drug Ther Bull* 1991; **29**: 97–100.
11 Colebrook L, Hood AM. Infection through soaked dressings. *Lancet* 1948; **ii**: 682–3.
12 Engdahl E. Clinical evaluation of Debrisan on pressure sores. *Curr Ther Res* 1980; **28**: 377–80.
13 Gorse GJ, Messner RL. Improved pressure sore healing with hydrocolloid dressings. *Arch Dermatol* 1987; **123**: 766–71.
14 Handfield-Jones SE, Grattan CEH, Simpson RA, Kennedy CTC. Comparison of a hydrocolloid dressing and paraffin gauze in the treatment of venous ulcers. *Br J Dermatol* 1988; **118**: 425–7.
15 Eaglstein WH. Occlusive dressings. *J Dermatol Surg Oncol* 1993; **19**: 716–20.
16 Knudsen EA, Snitker G. Wound healing under plastic coated pads. *Acta Derm Venereol (Stockh)* 1969; **49**: 438–41.
17 Armstrong RB, Nichols J, Pachance J. Punch biopsy wounds treated with Monsel's solution or a collagen matrix. *Arch Dermatol* 1986; **122**: 546–9.
18 Hien NT, Prawer SE, Katz HI. Facilitated wound healing using transparent film dressing following Mohs micrographic surgery. *Arch Dermatol* 1988; **124**: 903–6.
19 Attwood AI. Calcium alginate dressing accelerates split skin graft donor site healing. *Br J Plast Surg* 1989; **42**: 373–9.
20 James JH, Watson ACH. The use of Op-site, a vapour permeable dressing on skin graft donor sites. *Br J Plast Surg* 1975; **28**: 107–10.
21 Popp C, Kligman AM, Stoudemayer TJ. Pre-treatment of photo-aged forearm skin with topical tretinoin accelerates healing of full thickness wounds. *Br J Dermatol* 1995; **132**: 46–53.
22 Subrahmanyam M. Amniotic membrane as a cover for micro-skin grafts. *Br J Plast Surg* 1995; **48**: 477–8.
23 Agren MS. Studies on zinc in wound healing. *Acta Derm Venereol Suppl (Stockh)* 1990; **154**: 1–36.
24 Brown GL, Nanney LB, Griffen J et al. Enhancement of wound healing by topical treatment with epidermal growth factor. *N Engl J Med* 1989; **321**: 76–9.
25 Eaglstein WH, Mertz PM. New method for assessing epidermal wound healing: the effects of triamcinolone acetonide and polyethylene film occlusion. *J Invest Dermatol* 1978; **71**: 382–4.
26 Silverstein P. Smoking and wound healing. *Am J Med* 1992; **93** (1A): 22S–24S.
27 Ashcroft GS, Horan MA, Ferguson MW. The effect of ageing on cutaneous wound healing in mammals. *J Anat* 1995; **187**: 1–26.
28 Tsuchida Y. The effect of ageing and arteriosclerosis on human skin blood flow. *J Dermatol Sci* 1995; **5**: 175–81.
29 Becker GD, Adams LA, Hackett J. Collagen assisted healing of facial wounds after Mohs surgery. *Laryngoscope* 1994; **104**: 1267–70.

Secondary intention healing

Full-thickness wounds remaining after malignant [1,2] or benign [3] tumour excision can be left to heal by second intention. The cosmetic result depends on wound site and patient age. The nasolabial fold, medical canthus, scalp and

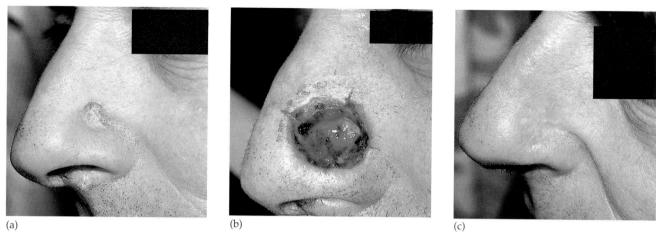

(a) (b) (c)

Fig. 81.9 This man had a basal cell carcinoma on the side of the nose (a); this was excised (b) and the wound was allowed to heal by second intention. The cosmetic result 4 months later was good (c).

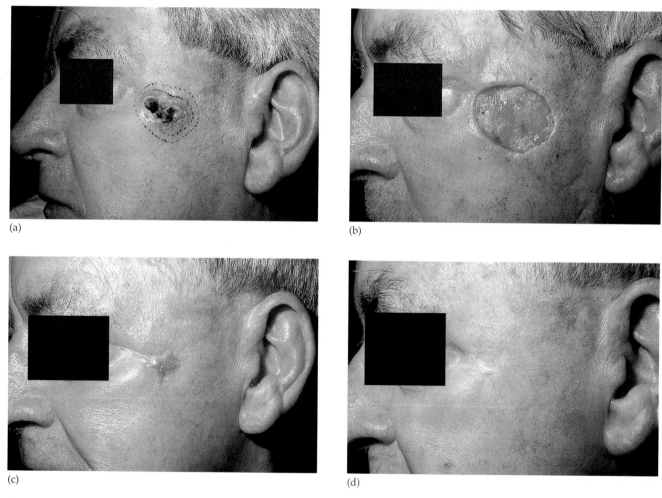

(a) (b)

(c) (d)

Fig. 81.10 This man had a basal cell carcinoma on the temple (a) excised (b). Three months later the wound had healed but the scar was thick and red (c). 15 months later this scar had become considerably less conspicuous (d).

pre- and post-auricular skin produce particularly good results, although the technique can be used in many sites, including the fingers [4]. Almost half of the reduction in wound size occurs because of scar contraction [5] and subsequent stretching of surrounding tissues [6]. Therefore, if the wound is next to a mucocutaneous junction, such as the lip, ala nasa or eyelid, scar contraction may distort this free margin, producing an ugly and potentially poorly functioning wound. Most other head and neck sites heal well, although in general the cosmetic results are best on concave rather than convex skin surfaces [7]. The older the patient the better the result, probably because wound contraction is aided by the availability of loose adjacent skin and because hypertrophic scarring is less common in older patients. The method can be used if there is doubt about the adequacy of excision, or closure of the defect requires a larger or more complex procedure, which the patient does not desire. In some situations, such as excision of naevi on the back [3], or the treatment of acne keloidalis nuchae [8] and hidradenitis [9], secondary intention healing is the preferred method as it results in a superior cosmetic result.

When a tumour is being excised, the specimen is orientated with a marking suture before complete removal, so that if further excision is required the correct margin can be identified. When bleeding is controlled, a contact dressing is applied, and this is covered by a pressure dressing for 24–48h. Thereafter, the dressing can be changed at 2–4-day intervals, depending on the amount of exudate. At each dressing change, the wound is cleaned to remove crust or debris and a greasy antiseptic ointment (e.g. Polyfax, Flamazine or Betadine ointment) and non-adherent dressing are applied. On average, a 25-mm-diameter head and neck wound takes approximately 35 days to heal [10]. If histology shows that the tumour has been incompletely excised the involved margin can be re-excised 1–2 weeks after the first excision. Because vertical sections are taken and the entire excision margin is not examined, the technique does not provide the same complete excision margin control as the horizontal sections of Mohs surgery [1]. These wounds are surprisingly pain-free. Bacterial contamination may occur, but tissue infection is rare; when present the wound edge is tender, red and swollen. A yellow exudate is common in the first few days. Before granulation tissue appears, a yellowish fibrin clot covers the wound. Bone and cartilage can be left exposed, but must be carefully dressed to reduce the risk of desiccation and ultimately necrosis [11]. Alternatively, the exposed bone can be fenestrated or abraded, to encourage the formation of granulation tissue and hence enhance re-epithelialization [12]. When the wound first heals, the scar often contains large looped vessels, which slowly disappear as the scar thickens. A slightly elevated, red, hypertrophic scar is then present, and the cosmetic result is not optimum until approximately 1 year (Figs 81.9 & 81.10).

REFERENCES

1 Mohs FE. *Chemosurgery. Microscopically Controlled Surgery for Skin Cancer.* Springfield: Thomas, 1978.
2 Goldwyn RM, Rueckert F. The value of healing by secondary intention for sizeable defects of the face. *Arch Surg* 1977; **112**: 285–92.
3 Barnett R, Stranc M. A method of producing improved scars following excision of small lesions of the back. *Ann Plast Surg* 1979; **3**: 391–4, 435.
4 de Berker DAR, Dahl MGC, Malcolm AJ, Lawrence CM. Micrographic surgery for subungual squamous cell carcinoma. *Br J Plast Surg* 1996; **49**: 414–19.
5 Catty RHC. Healing and contraction of experimental full thickness wounds in the human. *Br J Surg* 1965; **52**: 542–8.
6 Lawrence CM, Comaish JS, Dahl MGC. Excision of skin malignancies without wound closure. *Br J Dermatol* 1986; **115**: 563–71.
7 Zitelli JA. Wound healing by secondary intention. *J Am Acad Dermatol* 1983; **9**: 407–15.
8 Glenn MJ, Bennett RG, Kelly AP. Acne keloidalis nuchae: treatment with excision and secondary intention healing. *J Am Acad Dermatol* 1995; **33**: 243–6.
9 Silverberg B, Smoot CE, Landa SJF, Parsons RW. Hidradenitis suppurativa: patients' satisfaction with wound healing by second intention. *Plast Reconstr Surg* 1987; **79**: 555–9.
10 Lawrence CM, Matthews JNS, Cox NH. The effect of ketanserin on healing of fresh surgical wounds. *Br J Dermatol* 1995; **132**: 580–6.
11 Snow SN, Stiff MA, Bullen R et al. Second intention healing of exposed facial-scalp bone after Mohs surgery for skin cancer: a review of 91 cases. *J Am Acad Dermatol* 1994; **31**: 450–4.
12 Latenser J, Snow SNP, Mohs FE et al. Power drills to fenestrate exposed bone to stimulate wound healing. *J Dermatol Surg Oncol* 1991; **17**: 265–70.

Skin grafts

Skin of varying thickness can be used for skin grafting. A split-skin graft is not limited in size because the donor site regenerates. Full-thickness and composite skin grafts potentially produce better cosmetic results than split-skin grafts, but are limited in size by the amount of skin that can be excised at the donor site without creating problems. In comparison with flaps, grafts are technically easier to perform, but generally produce inferior cosmetic results.

Full-thickness grafts

A full-thickness graft is used, in preference to a split-skin graft, when the cosmetic result and strength of the repair are important. Any site with matching and spare skin is a potential donor site [1]. Common donor sites include the skin behind and in front of the ear, nasolabial fold [2], upper eyelid, inner aspect of the upper arm, lower abdomen and supraclavicular fossa. The donor and graft sites should match for skin thickness, adnexal structures, surface markings, weathering and texture. After carefully assessing the amount and shape of skin required, the donor skin is excised down to fat [3]. The fat is then trimmed off the under surface of the graft to prevent it hindering new blood-vessel penetration. Edge sutures are used to prevent shearing forces dislodging the graft, and a pressure dressing, usually held in place using tie-over sutures, is employed to prevent a haematoma lifting the graft off the recipient site (Fig. 81.11). There is no theoretical limitation to the size of a full-thickness graft; this depends on how much donor

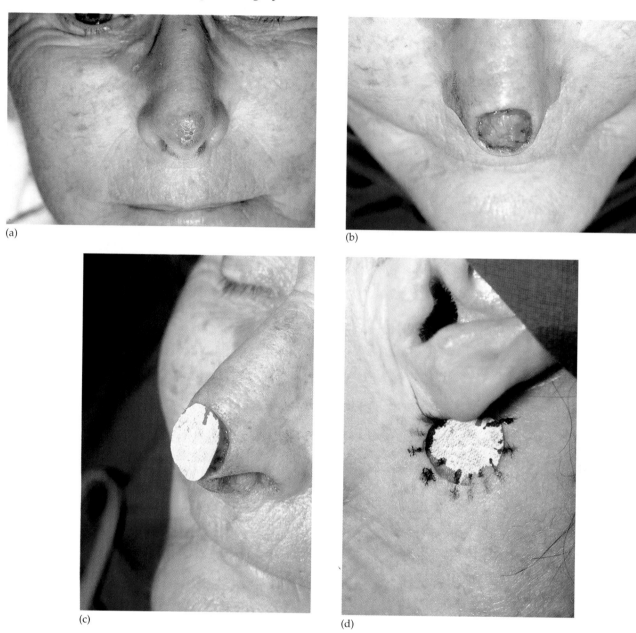

(a)

(b)

(c)

(d)

Fig. 81.11 Full-thickness graft on the nose. This basal cell carcinoma on the tip of the nose (a) was excised (b). The defect size and shape was recorded using a sterile paper template (c), the template was placed on the donor skin site (d) and the appropriate-sized piece of skin excised. The fat was trimmed off the undersurface of the donor skin, and this was sutured into place on the wound (e). A tie-over dressing was applied (f). Seven days later the dressing was removed and the graft was pink and had clearly taken (g). The subsequent cosmetic result at 3 months was excellent (h).

skin can be harvested. In most instances, the donor site is chosen because there are redundant folds of skin present and the skin edges can be sutured easily after donor skin excision. At other sites, for example behind the ear, the defect can be allowed to heal by second intention. Grafts take best on dermis and granulation tissue, will just survive on fat, perichondrium and periosteum, but will perish on exposed bone or cartilage. Grafts fail because of infection or poor blood supply. The latter occurs because of faulty technique, for example incorrect haemostasis, suturing or wound care, or because the recipient site has an inadequate blood supply, for example on the lower leg, or at sites previously treated by radiotherapy. All grafts contract, and this may lead to ectropion of the lower eyelid. Hence, at this and other critical sites grafts should be 10–25% larger than the defect to compensate for this. Depressed graft scars can be elevated by injection of autograft fat under the graft [4].

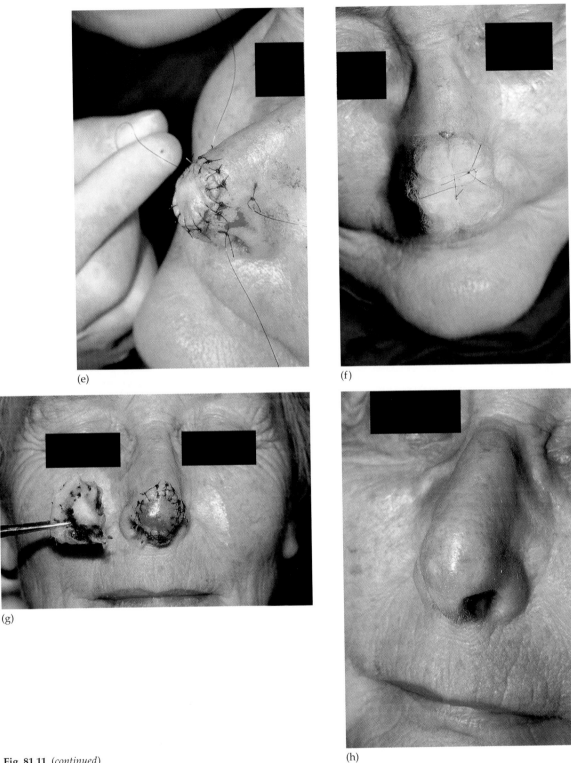

(e)

(f)

(g)

(h)

Fig. 81.11 (*continued*)

Composite grafts

Composite grafts are defined as those comprising two or more germ layers. In dermatology, these are grafts containing skin and cartilage components. When used to repair full-thickness ala rim defects using skin taken from the helix rim, graft survival is unpredictable [5]. In contrast, composite grafts containing skin and perichondrium, or perichondrial cutaneous grafts, are claimed to be better than full-thickness grafts for nose, ear and periocular defects, as they contract less, induce new cartilage formation, and maintain their thickness and epidermal appendages [6].

Split-skin graft

Except in extreme circumstances (e.g. extensive burns) split-skin graft size is not limited by the amount of donor skin that can be harvested because the donor skin site will re-epithelialize by regeneration from retained follicular remnants. Split-skin grafts can therefore be used to cover very large wounds. Because the skin is thin and relatively transparent split grafts are also sometimes used to cover tumour excision sites where the adequacy of excision is dubious, because recurrence is more easily identified through the thinner graft than it would be after full-thickness or flap closure. The disadvantages of split-skin grafts compared with full-thickness grafts are the relatively poor cosmetic result and greater graft shrinkage [1]. When a split graft is taken, skin is sliced off through the dermis, leaving behind parts of the adenexal and follicular structures from which epidermis migrates to cover the donor site. Grafts can be taken using a hand-held knife or a mechanical dermatome (Fig. 81.12a). The latter is easier to use and produces a predictably good graft. *Meshing*, or cutting multiple parallel slits in the graft, allows it to expand rather like a fishnet stocking when stretched (Fig. 81.12b). The gaps are covered by epithelium migrating from the adjacent strips of the graft (Fig. 81.12c). A meshed graft will therefore cover a wider area, allow exudate to drain through the gaps (e.g. on the leg), and will conform to an uneven contour (e.g. ear). The common donor sites include the upper arm, upper thigh and abdominal wall. These sites are best anaesthetized using EMLA cream [7] rather than injected anaesthetic. The donor sites heal faster with a dressing that maintains a moist wound–dressing interface, for example calcium alginate [8] and semi-permeable adhesive polyurethane film (Opsite) [9].

Pinch grafts

Pinch grafts are occasionally useful for wounds of the lower leg, although the donor site heals leaving unsightly scars. The technique is simple [10] but without careful aseptic technique success rates are low [11]. The skin is elevated on a needle tip, the apex sliced off, and when multiple skin shaves have been harvested the grafts are placed at regular intervals on the clean granulating ulcer. As with

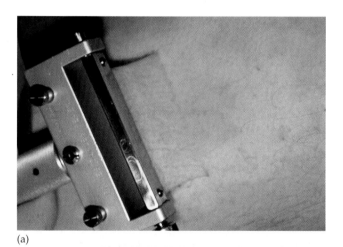

(a)

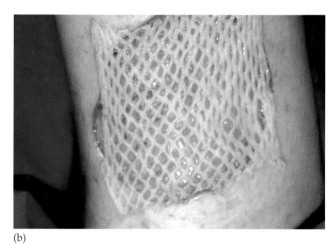

(b)

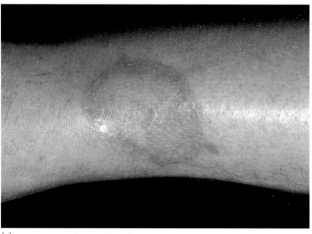

(c)

Fig. 81.12 Meshed split-skin graft. A split-skin graft was harvested from the thigh skin using a power dermatome (a). The skin was meshed on a mesher, and the meshed graft applied to the defect (b). This was the appearance of the graft 11 months later (c).

all leg-ulcer skin grafting, if the causative factors are not eradicated before grafting, the ulcer will recur even if the graft is initially successful.

Grafting techniques used for repigmentation of inactive vitiligo

Epidermal grafts containing viable melanocytes can be harvested using suction blisters [12], or very thin split-skin grafts [13]. Before grafting, the epidermis is removed from the hypopigmented skin by freezing to create a blister [12], or by dermabrasion [13]. Alternatively, *mini-grafts*, or tiny (1.2-mm-diameter) full-thickness punch grafts of normally pigmented skin are grafted, at 2-mm intervals, into similar-sized punch wounds sited in the depigmented skin [14]. Because melanocytes migrate approximately 2mm away from the graft site, there is no need to graft the whole area, and because the punch grafts are so small there is minimal cobblestone effect at the recipient site. In both techniques, a hidden donor site, such as the upper inner thigh or lower back, is used.

Acne scar punch grafts

Ice-pick acne scars can be excised using a punch biopsy blade and the wound filled with a slightly bigger punch biopsy-shaped piece of donor skin taken from a matching but unobtrusive site (e.g. behind the ear). Dermabrasion is usually subsequently required to reduce the cobblestone effect [15].

REFERENCES

1 Skouge JW. *Skin Grafting. Practical Manuals in Dermatologic Surgery.* New York: Churchill Livingstone, 1991.
2 Booth SA, Zalla MJ, Roenigk RK, Phillips PK. The naso-labial fold donor site for full thickness skin grafts of nasal tip defects. *J Dermatol Surg Oncol* 1993; **19**: 553–9.
3 Roenigk RK, Zalla MJ. Full-thickness grafts. In: Robinson JK, Arndt KA, LeBoit PE, Wintroub BU, eds. *Atlas of Cutaneous Surgery.* Philadelphia: WB Saunders, 1996.
4 Hambley RM, Carruthers JA. Microlipoinjection for the elevation of depressed full-thickness grafts on the nose. *J Dermatol Surg Oncol* 1992; **18**: 963–8.
5 Lipman SH, Roth RJ. Composite grafts from earlobes for reconstruction of defects in noses. *J Dermatol Surg Oncol* 1982; **8**: 135–7.
6 Rohrer TE, Dzubow LM. Conchal bowl skin grafting in nasal tip reconstruction: clinical and histologic evaluation. *J Am Acad Dermatol* 1995; **33**: 476–81.
7 Goodacre TEE, Sanders R, Watts DA, Stoker M. Split skin grafting using topical local anaesthesia (EMLA): a comparison with infiltrative anaesthesia. *Br J Plast Surg* 1988; **41**: 533–8.
8 Attwood AI. Calcium alginate dressing accelerates split skin graft donor site healing. *Br J Plast Surg* 1989; **42**: 373–9.
9 James JH, Watson ACH. The use of Opsite, a vapour permeable dressing on skin graft donor sites. *Br J Plast Surg* 1975; **28**: 107–10.
10 Ceilley RI, Rinek MA, Zuehlke RL. Pinch grafting for chronic ulcers on the lower extremities. *J Dermatol Surg Oncol* 1977; **3**: 303–9.
11 Kirsner RS, Falanga V. Techniques of split skin grafting for lower extremity ulcerations. *J Dermatol Surg Oncol* 1993; **19**: 779–83.
12 Falabella R. Surgical techniques for repigmentation. In: Robinson JK, Arndt KA, LeBoit PE, Wintroub BU, eds. *Atlas of Cutaneous Surgery.* Philadelphia: WB Saunders, 1996.
13 Kahn AM, Cohen MJ. Vitiligo: treatment by dermabrasion and epithelial sheet grafting. *J Am Acad Dermatol* 1995; **33**: 646–8.
14 Boersma BR, Westerhof W, Bos JD. Repigmentation in vitiligo vulgaris by autologous minigrafting: results in 19 patients. *J Am Acad Dermatol* 1995; **33**: 990–5.
15 Johnson WC. Treatment of pitted scars: punch transplant technique. *J Dermatol Surg Oncol* 1986; **12**: 260–5.

Flaps (Figs 81.13–81.16)

A flap is a section of full-thickness skin in which one portion, the pedicle, remains attached to the skin while the distal portion is undermined and moved to cover the defect [1]. The blood supply of any flap is therefore at least initially provided via its pedicle, and the broader the pedicle the better the blood supply. The length to width ratio of a flap should rarely exceed 3:1. Good haemostasis also allows new blood-vessel formation to occur, and the more closely a flap resembles a graft (i.e. thin, defatted skin) the greater is the contribution to its blood supply from the recipient site rather than the flap pedicle. The disadvantage, however, is that the thinner the flap the greater the contraction, and this is particularly important when using thin skin around the eye. Different techniques can be used for many repairs [2], although some techniques [3] are inherently suited to the nose [4,5], chin [6], eyelid [7,8], ear [9,10], forehead [11], scalp [12], cheeks [13] and lip [14,15].

Flaps can be confusingly categorized by the direction of movement, the name of the surgeon who first described the flap, the blood supply or the type of tissue moved. The most useful method relates to how the skin was moved to cover the defect—hence the description of advancement, rotation or transposition flaps (Table 81.4). Classification according to blood supply shows that dermatologists almost exclusively use random pattern flaps, i.e. the blood supply is inherent in the skin being moved. This may come from the dermal blood supply (reticular—the type most widely used by dermatologists), or the perforating vessels from the subdermal plexus (segmental, e.g. island pedicle flaps). In contrast, axial pattern flaps are designed to obtain their blood supply from one named artery. With the exception of the midline forehead flap [4], which is based on the supratrochlear artery, axial flaps are rarely used in dermatological surgery. Island pedicle flaps do not have a skin pedicle but get their blood supply from the tissue on the underside of the flap. This may be subcutaneous tissue, muscle or a named vessel.

As skin is moved to close the primary or original defect, a secondary defect is created which in turn also has to be covered. The essence of flap repair is to design the flap so that this secondary defect is created at a site where there is sufficient spare or loose skin to permit closure. On the face, loose skin is usually present in the

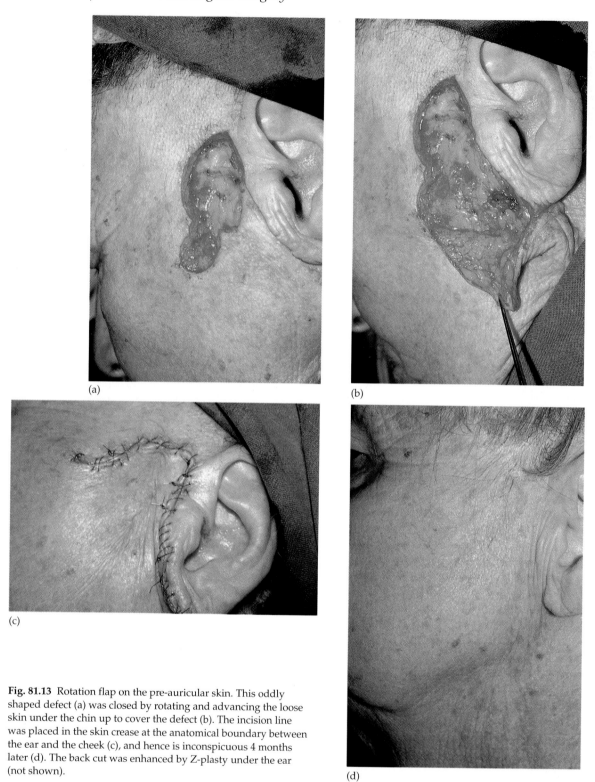

Fig. 81.13 Rotation flap on the pre-auricular skin. This oddly shaped defect (a) was closed by rotating and advancing the loose skin under the chin up to cover the defect (b). The incision line was placed in the skin crease at the anatomical boundary between the ear and the cheek (c), and hence is inconspicuous 4 months later (d). The back cut was enhanced by Z-plasty under the ear (not shown).

middle of the forehead, the glabellar region and bridge of the nose, the nasolabial fold, the front of the ear, and the cheek. Hence, these areas of laxity will be exploited for most flaps.

Advancement flaps are used where skin must move in one direction from an area of laxity to cover the defect. Although simple to conceptualize they have limited use. The secondary defect is closed last and the flaps have

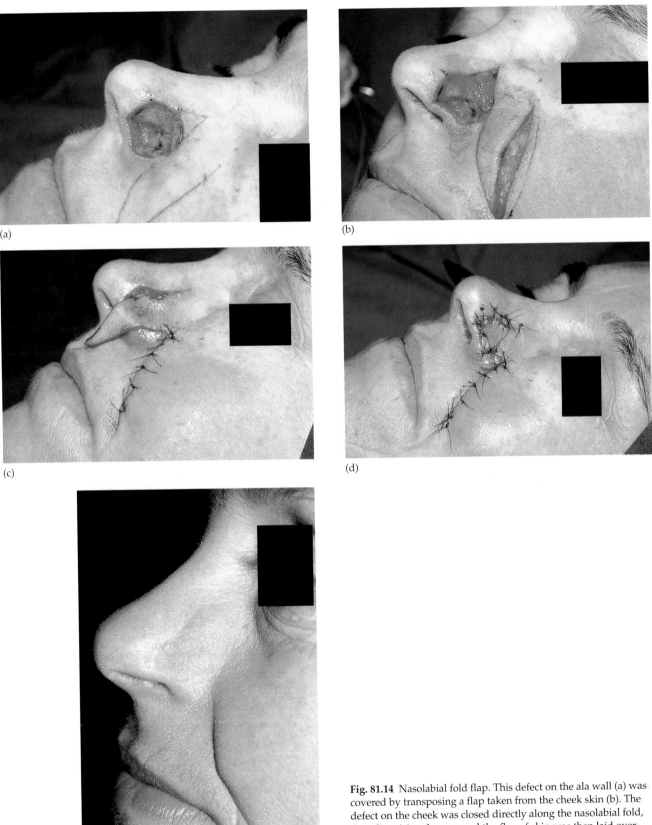

(a)

(b)

(c)

(d)

(e)

Fig. 81.14 Nasolabial fold flap. This defect on the ala wall (a) was covered by transposing a flap taken from the cheek skin (b). The defect on the cheek was closed directly along the nasolabial fold, thus disguising the scar, and the flap of skin was then laid over the defect (c). The flap was trimmed to shape and sutured into place (d). The result 12 months later was good (e).

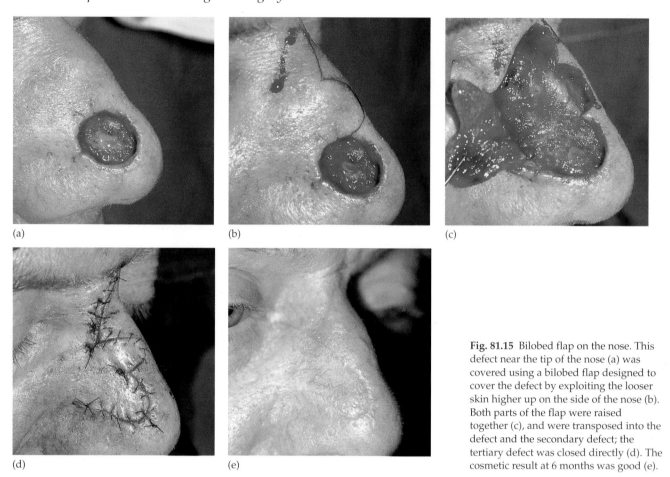

(a)

(b)

(c)

(d)

(e)

Fig. 81.15 Bilobed flap on the nose. This defect near the tip of the nose (a) was covered using a bilobed flap designed to cover the defect by exploiting the looser skin higher up on the side of the nose (b). Both parts of the flap were raised together (c), and were transposed into the defect and the secondary defect; the tertiary defect was closed directly (d). The cosmetic result at 6 months was good (e).

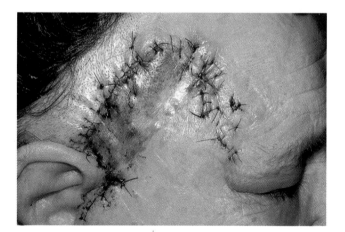

Fig. 81.16 Complications—flap necrosis in a cigarette smoker. Despite warnings, this patient continued to smoke before and after surgery. Possibly because of this, the rotation flap on her temple necrosed at 7 days.

limited mobility. In many instances, defect coverage is only achieved by stretching the flap rather than transferring the tension to an area of lax skin. *Rotation flaps* usually require both advancement and rotation about a pivotal point on a broad pedicle (Fig. 81.13). Mobility is frequently limited,

and long incisions and extensive undermining may be required to mobilize sufficient tissue; the secondary defect is closed last. *Transposition flaps* provide the greatest mobility, and are different because the secondary defect is closed first (Fig. 81.14). As a result, the flap is pushed rather than dragged into the defect, so that if a transposition flap is designed properly virtually all the tension can be placed on the secondary defect rather than the flap, thus reducing the risk of ischaemic necrosis. These advantages make transposition flaps the most widely used (Fig. 81.15). A wide variety of flaps based on these three simple designs have been described, each with careful refinements for different sites (Table 81.4).

Complications. Ischaemic necrosis of the flap usually occurs because of excessive tension resulting from poor design or mobility. Secondary infection is also more common if the flap has a poor blood supply [16]. On the head and neck blood supply is excellent at all sites, but on the trunk, and especially on the lower limb, attempts at flap repair frequently result in failure because of relatively poor blood supply. Cigarette smokers are more likely to suffer from flap or graft necrosis than non-smokers (Fig. 81.16), although this can be reversed if smokers significantly

Table 81.4 Flap types and uses.

Flap type	Random pattern flaps (synonym/s)	Uses	Comments
Advancement	Crescentic advancement flap [21]	Cheek/nose, cheek/upper lip closures	In effect side-to-side closure with special attention to cosmetic boundaries. A useful technique
	Single advancement (U-plasty)	Cheek, temple, forehead [6], upper lip [15]	If designed with a broad base can be very effective on the cheek
	Double advancement (H-plasty)	Forehead defects, eyebrow repairs	Little mobility, multiple scars, numb scalp. Conceptually easy but difficult to get right
	Bipedical advancement [22]	Forehead, nasal side wall, chin	In effect side-to-side closure with parallel or V–Y relaxing incisions
	O–T-plasty (A–T-plasty, V–T-plasty, Dieffenbach's winged V-plasty [23])	Lower eyelid, upper lip [24], forehead [6]	A bilateral advancement flap useful around the eye, lip, nose [3] and hair margin
	Midline forehead island flap [25]	Medial canthus	A variety of island pedicle flap with a random pattern blood supply. Flap is tunnelled under the skin into the defect
	Island pedicle flap [26] (kite flap of Dufourmentel)	Upper lip [14] Trunk and limb	Two pedicles can be used on the trunk and limb; one is used on repairs of the upper lip. The blood supply comes from the subcutaneous tissue attached to the underside of the skin. A similar design is used in an axial flap employed for defects on the nose tip and ala. The pedicle is based on the branch of the angular artery that supplies the nasalis muscle [27]
	Single advancement (unilateral Burow's wedge flap) [3]	Upper lip, temple, cheek, forehead	A useful flap which is both advanced and rotated into position and the redundant skin removed using a Burow's triangle
Rotation	Single rotation with back-cut (hatchet flap)	Cheek, temple, medial canthus	A useful technique [28] (Fig. 81.13)
	Sliding glabella rotation flap (V–Y advancement)	Medial canthus, dorsal nose [29]	Exploits the redundant skin in the glabella area. Skin movement includes both advancement and rotation as do many rotation or advancement flaps
	Double rotation (O–Z-plasty)	Forehead, scalp, chin [6]	Large area of undermining required. Only works on lax scalp
	Multiple rotation flaps (pinwheel design)	Scalp	Variant of O–Z-plasty
Transposition	Nasolabial flap [30]	Ala rim or side wall of the nose	Good results with careful attention to detail. Pincushioning can be a problem (Fig. 81.14)
	Basic transposition/ rhombic flap	Cheek, nose, chin, medial canthus, upper lip	Rarely if ever used as the true geometric rhomboid. Basic transposition flaps are very useful and generally exploit the natural elasticity of the skin so that the flap shape adapts to fit the defect [31]. A Z-plasty adaptation [32] may enhance flap mobility [33]. The glabellar transposition flap (banner flap) [34] is a named variant
	Median forehead pedicle flap	Nose tip or lower third of nose	Axial flap. Two stage procedure; the flap knuckle or pedicle has to be separated later
	30° angle transposition flap [4] (Webster flap)	Dorsum of the nose	Not difficult. Bilateral and single flaps can be used
	Bilobed [35]	Nose side wall	A double transposition flap. Not as difficult to do as might appear (Fig. 81.15)

reduce cigarette consumption 2 days before and 7 days after surgery [17]. If the flap scar is obtrusive, particularly on the nose, it can be revised by dermabrasion, which is best performed 6 weeks after surgery [18]. Manual dermabrasion [19] or scalpel sculpturing [20] may be less hazardous to the operator and equally effective.

REFERENCES

1 Tromovitch TA, Stegman SJ, Glogau RG. *Flaps and Grafts in Dermatologic Surgery*. Chicago: Year Book Publishers, 1989.
2 Field LM. Combining flaps. Medial canthal/lateral nasal root reconstruction utilising glabellar 'fan' and cheek rotation flaps—an O–Z variation. *J Dermatol Surg Oncol* 1994; **20**: 205–8.
3 Summers BK, Siegle RJ. Facial cutaneous reconstructive surgery: facial flaps. *J Am Acad Dermatol* 1993; **29**: 917–41.
4 Salasche SJ, Grabski WJ. *Flaps for the Central Face*. New York: Churchill Livingstone, 1990.
5 Zitelli JA, Fazio MJ. Reconstruction of the nose with local flaps. *J Dermatol Surg Oncol* 1991; **17**: 184–9.
6 Wheeland RG. Reconstruction of the lower lip and chin using local and random pattern flaps. *J Dermatol Surg Oncol* 1991; **17**: 605–15.
7 Moy RL, Ashjian AA. Periorbital reconstruction. *J Dermatol Surg Oncol* 1991; **17**: 153–9.
8 Ross JJ, Pham R. Closure of eyelid defects. *J Dermatol Surg Oncol* 1992; **18**: 1061–4.
9 Cavanaugh EB. Management of lesions of the helical rim using a chondro-cutaneous advancement flap. *J Dermatol Surg Oncol* 1982; **8**: 691–6.
10 Mellette JR. Ear reconstruction with local flaps. *J Dermatol Surg Oncol* 1991; **17**: 176–82.
11 Siegel RJ. Forehead reconstruction. *J Dermatol Surg Oncol* 1991; **17**: 200–4.
12 Field LM. Scalp flaps. *J Dermatol Surg Oncol* 1991; **17**: 190–9.
13 Bennett RG. Local skin flaps on the cheeks. *J Dermatol Surg Oncol* 1991; **17**: 161–5.
14 Zitelli JA, Brodland DG. A regional approach to reconstruction of the upper lip. *J Dermatol Surg Oncol* 1991; **17**: 143–8.
15 Spinowitz AL, Stegman SJ. Partial-thickness wedge and advancement flap for upper lip repair. *J Dermatol Surg Oncol* 1991; **17**: 581–6.
16 Salasche SJ, Grabski WJ. Complications of flaps. *J Dermatol Surg Oncol* 1991; **17**: 132–40.
17 Goldminz D, Bennett RG. Cigarette smoking and flap and full thickness graft necrosis. *Arch Dermatol* 1991; **127**: 1012–15.
18 Yarborough JM. Ablation of facial scars by programmed dermabrasion. *J Dermatol Surg Oncol* 1988; **14**: 292–4.
19 Zisser M, Kaplan B, Moy RL. Surgical pearl: manual dermabrasion. *J Am Acad Dermatol* 1995; **33**: 105–6.
20 Snow SNP, Stiff MA, Lambert DR. Scalpel sculpturing techniques for graft revision and dermatologic surgery. *J Dermatol Surg Oncol* 1994; **20**: 120–6.
21 Mellette JR, Harrington AC. Applications of the crescentic advancement flap. *J Dermatol Surg Oncol* 1991; **17**: 447–54.
22 Flint ID, Siegle RJ. The bipedical flap revisited. *J Dermatol Surg Oncol* 1994; **20**: 394–400.
23 Field LM. The forehead V to T plasty (Dieffenbach's winged V-plasty). *J Dermatol Surg Oncol* 1986; **12**: 560–2.
24 Spinowitz AL, Stegman SJ. Partial thickness wedge and advancement flap for upper lip repair. *J Dermatol Surg Oncol* 1991; **17**: 581–6.
25 Field LM. Midline forehead island flap. *J Dermatol Surg Oncol* 1987; **13**: 243–6.
26 Skouge JW. Upper lip repair: the subcutaneous island pedicle flap. *J Dermatol Surg Oncol* 1980; **16**: 63–8.
27 Constantine VS. Nasalis myocutaneous sliding flap. *J Dermatol Surg Oncol* 1991; **17**: 439–44.
28 Tromovitch TA, Stegman SJ, Glogau RG. *Flaps and Grafts in Dermatologic Surgery*. Chicago: Year Book Publishers, 1989.
29 Marchac D, Toth B. The axial frontonasal flap revisited. *Plast Reconstr Surg* 1985; **76**: 686–94.
30 Zitelli JA. The nasolabial flap as a single stage procedure. *Arch Dermatol* 1990; **126**: 1445–8.
31 Holt PJA, Motley RJ. A modified rhombic transposition flap and its

application in dermatology. *J Dermatol Surg Oncol* 1991; **17**: 287–92.
32 Zachary CB. *Basic Cutaneous Surgery: A Primer in Technique*. New York: Churchill Livingstone, 1991: 87.
33 Johnson SC, Bennett RG. Double Z-plasty to enhance rhombic flap mobility. *J Dermatol Surg Oncol* 1994; **20**: 128–32.
34 Field LM. The glabellar transposition 'banner' flap. *J Dermatol Surg Oncol* 1988; **14**: 376–8.
35 Zitelli JA. The bilobed flap for nasal reconstruction. *Arch Dermatol* 1989; **125**: 957–9.

Micrographic (Mohs') surgery [1–4]

The concept of controlling the excision margins of infiltrative skin tumours by microscopic examination of horizontal sections cut from the periphery of an excision specimen that had previously been fixed *in vivo* was developed by Mohs in the 1940s [5]. This fixed-tissue technique, which produced excellent cure rates even in some of the most difficult of tumours, has now largely been replaced by the fresh-tissue technique [6]. There are other techniques and adaptations, which aim to achieve 100% histological margin control, that may be more appropriate for tumours with difficult morphology or because of local circumstances [7,8].

The principle of the technique is that the maximum confidence as regards tumour clearance is combined with the minimum loss of surrounding normal tissue. This is particularly important for tumours with an infiltrative growth pattern, especially in critical anatomical sites, and for recurrent lesions. Essentially, the technique involves excision of the lesion and microscopic examination of sections cut from marked, anatomically orientated, segments of tissue, so that the entire periphery of the excision specimen is examined [9] (Fig. 81.17). Immunofluorescence or immunoperoxidose staining with cytokeratin antibodies may help in the histological interpretation of infiltrative lesions [10].

One of the major disadvantages of Mohs' original technique, other than the prolonged nature of the procedure (possibly continuing over several days) and the pain and discomfort of the *in vivo* fixative, was the presence of a postoperative eschar, which precluded immediate reconstruction and necessitated healing by secondary intention. With the fresh-tissue technique all but the most extensive lesions can be excised in one session, usually under local anaesthesia, and the area can be repaired immediately. If paraffin sections are used, repair is best delayed until the microscopic sections have been examined. This is not to deny the value of secondary-intention healing in appropriate situations [11].

The results of micrographic surgery are impressive, with a 98–99% 5-year cure rate for basal cell carcinomas and a 94.4% 5-year cure rate for squamous cell carcinomas [12]. It should be considered the treatment of choice for the management of certain lesions. Tumours with infiltrative growth patterns or morphoeic histology may extend 7–10 mm beyond the clinically defined margins [13], and if

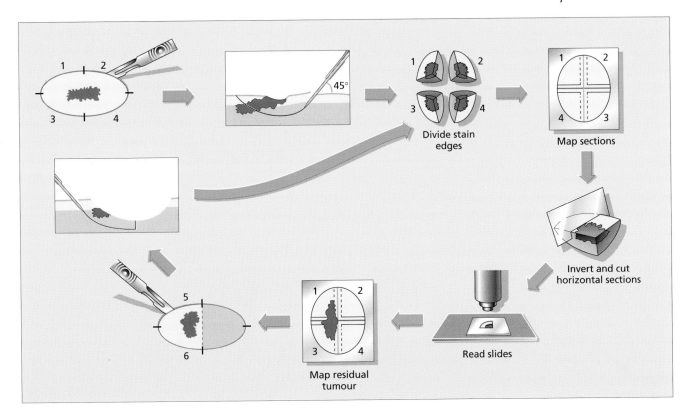

Fig. 81.17 The stages of Mohs' micrographic surgery.

such a tumour overlies a putative anatomical fusion plane, for example ala base, the use of horizontal frozen sections may be crucial in ensuring complete resection. Although the main indication is for basal cell carcinoma, the technique has been used for a wide variety of cutaneous malignancies [14].

REFERENCES

1 Bennett RG. Mohs' surgery. In: Bailin PL, Ratz JL, Wheeland RG, eds. *Advanced Dermatologic Surgery*. Philadelphia: WB Saunders, 1987: 409–28.
2 Drake LA, Dinehart SM, Goltz RW *et al.* Guidelines of care for Mohs' micrographic surgery. *J Am Acad Dermatol* 1995; **33**: 271–8.
3 Lawrence CM. Mohs' surgery of basal cell carcinoma—a critical review. *Br J Plast Surg* 1993; **46**: 599–606.
4 Swanson NA. Mohs' surgery. *Arch Dermatol* 1983; **119**: 761–73.
5 Mohs FE. Chemosurgery: a microscopically controlled method of cancer excision. *Arch Surg* 1941; **42**: 279–95.
6 Tromovitch TA, Stegman SJ. Microscopic-controlled excision of cutaneous tumours. Chemosurgery, fresh tissue technique. *Cancer* 1978; **41**: 653–8.
7 Breuninger H, Schaumburg-Lever G. Control of excisional margins by conventional histo-patholological techniques in the treatment of skin tumours. An alternative to Mohs' technique. *J Pathol* 1988; **154**: 167–71.
8 Picoto A, Camacho F, Walker NPJ *et al.* Mohs' micrographic surgery: European experience. In: Roenigk RK, Roenigk HH, eds. *Surgical Dermatology*. London: Dunitz, 1993: 125–9.
9 Walker NPJ, Bailin PL. Dermatological surgery. In: Champion RH, ed. *Recent Advances in Dermatology*, Vol. 7. Edinburgh: Churchill Livingstone, 1986: 211–31.
10 Ramnarain N, Walker NPJ, Markey AC. Basal cell carcinoma: rapid techniques using cytokeratin markers to assist treatment by micrographic (Mohs') surgery. *Br J Biomed Sci* 1995; **52**: 184–7.
11 Zitelli JA. Wound healing by secondary intention. *J Am Acad Dermatol* 1983; **9**: 407–15.
12 Mohs FE. Chemosurgery: microscopically controlled surgery for skin cancer—past, present and future. *J Dermatol Surg Oncol* 1978; **4**: 41–54.
13 Lang PG, Maize JC. Histologic evolution of recurrent basal cell carcinoma and treatment implications. *J Am Acad Dermatol* 1986; **14**: 186–96.
14 Randle HW, Roenigk RK. Indications for Mohs' micrographic surgery. In: Roenigk RK, Roenigk HH, eds. *Dermatologic Surgery*, 2nd edn. New York: Marcel Dekker, 1996: 703–29.

Nail surgery

See Chapter 65.

Hair transplantation [1,2]

The punch autograft was for many years the major procedure in this field, but many other surgical techniques have been developed that may sometimes be used alone or as adjuncts to punch grafting. In addition to a range of techniques, including strip and fusiform grafting, scalp reduction of balding areas with or without tissue expansion, and a variety of scalp flaps, mini- and micrografts have recently become very popular because of the more natural appearance that can be achieved. The major condition for which these techniques are used remains androgenic alopecia in its various forms. Areas of focal scarring can also be treated.

Careful preoperative assessment of the mental and physical status of the patient is crucial. It is imperative to exclude those subjects with known functional psychoses, those who are dysmorphophobic or cannot comprehend the nature of the treatment and its effects, and those with physical illness which might compromise healing or satisfactory hair regrowth, for example bleeding disorders, steroid therapy and previous hypertrophic or keloid scars. Every patient accepted for transplantation or other surgical corrective treatment must have received clear instructions on the details of the operation and its potential side-effects, and have a realistic expectation of outcome.

The details of the techniques will not be considered here. In treating androgenic alopecia, the exact techniques used will depend on the pattern of loss. Grafts are inserted from the frontal margin, working towards the crown. Improvements in technique now allow from 60 to 150 punch graft transfers or many hundred mini- and micrografts to be carried out per session, with relatively few failures. Some patients are happy with frontal density correction and less dense grafting on other more posterior vertex areas. Several sessions may be required to achieve a satisfactory result.

In general, most patients detect early hair growth in the eighth to 12th week after treatment, good growth usually being established at about the sixth month after graft insertion.

Complications are rare, and include arterial bleeding, arteriovenous and venous aneurysms, foreign-body reactions, infection, poor graft survival and hypertrophic scarring.

Other procedures

It is now commonplace for skilled scalp surgeons to use punch grafting with other grafting, reduction and flap procedures. For details of these methods, the reader is referred to more detailed texts [2].

In the UK, many dermatologists remain nihilistic with regard to surgical correction of alopecia, but with careful patient selection and adequate surgical skill good results can be obtained.

REFERENCES

1 Norwood OT, Shiell RC. *Hair Transplant Surgery*, 2nd edn. Springfield: Thomas, 1984.
2 Unger WP. *Hair Transplantation*, 3rd edn. New York: Marcel Dekker, 1997.

Dermabrasion (surgical skin planing) [1–4]

The abrasive (planing) technique for the removal of superficial lesions, rhinophyma, pitted or depressed scars, tattoos and foreign bodies was first clearly described by Kromayer [1]. Its main value lies in treating lesions on the face where regeneration of the epidermis proceeds rapidly, generally without scarring, because of the abundance of pilosebaceous structures from which repair occurs as long as destruction does not extend to the subcutis.

Considerable advances in the technique have taken place in the last 25 years, due especially to the high-speed rotary drill and the use of more efficient refrigeration [2]. Care must be taken to follow details of the technique rigidly to avoid damage to the patient or operator. Briefly, the technique (allowing for many individual modifications) is as follows [2,4].

1 The patient is sedated, with, for example, 10–20 mg i.v. diazepam.
2 The area is prechilled with cold packs.
3 The skin is cleansed with spirit or some suitable substitute after washing with soap and water.
4 The ears and nostrils are plugged with ointment-impregnated gauze, and the hair and ears are carefully protected by clipped towels.
5 The eyes are carefully protected, for example by ointment and lead shields, by thick gauze held by an assistant, or by the plastic cups used by sunbathers to protect the eyes.
6 The area to be treated is frozen by a continuous stream of Freon (dichlorotetrafluoroethane), and the skin is abraded to the required depth. The degree of freezing and of abrasion necessary must be learnt by experience. The abrading wheels ('brushes') may be of stainless steel wires or diamond fraizes.

Bleeding occurs for 15–30 min after treatment. Paraffin gauze, dry dressings or non-adherent dressings are applied and removed in 1–24 h. The crusts separate in 7–10 days. Healing is usually completed within 3 weeks, particularly if the wound is left open and dry. The pain and crusting can be minimized and the rate of healing improved by the application of a biosynthetic dressing such as Opsite, Biobrane or Vigilon. Preoperative topical retinoic acid may reduce the risk of postoperative milia formation and promote healing.

Infection following dermabrasion is rare, although herpes simplex can be devastating and aciclovir prophylaxis should be given to those at risk. Mild irritation or discomfort from sunlight or cosmetics may occur for a few weeks. Persistent erythema, hyperpigmentation, hypertrophic scars and dermatitis are occasional complications.

Dermabrasion can be considered as a very useful part of cosmetic dermatological practice. Its value in the minimizing of pitted acne scars of the face is undoubted (although the small 'ice-pick' scars respond less satisfactorily than coarse irregular scars). Other conditions for which it has been recommended include traumatic and surgical scars, tattoos, telangiectasia, melasma, epidermal naevi, angiofibromas in epiloia, actinic keratoses, syringomas, wrinkles, cysts and multiple milia [2]. It has been combined with topical steroids in hypertrophic lichen planus, lichen simplex and localized lichenified psoriasis.

REFERENCES

1 Kromayer E. *The Cosmetic Treatment of Skin Complaints*. Oxford: Oxford University Press, 1930.
2 Mandy SH. Dermabrasion. In: Lask GP, Moy RL, eds. *Principles and Techniques of Cutaneous Surgery*. New York: McGraw-Hill, 1996: 495–504.
3 Yarborough JM. Dermabrasion by wire brush. *J Dermatol Surg Oncol* 1987; **13**: 610–12.
4 Roenigk HH. Dermabrasion for rejuvenation and scar revision. In: Baran R, Maibach HI, eds. *Cosmetic Dermatology*. London: Dunitz, 1994: 451–66.

Botulinum toxin [1–3]

This potent neurotoxin has been used since 1979 for the treatment of strabismus and blepharospasm. It has been shown to be useful in the treatment of frown lines, disorders of the muscles of facial expression and hyperhidrosis [4]. The preparation of the toxin and its administration require great care, and some authors advocate electromyographic guidance [5]. The effect of a single treatment may last up to 6 months, and with repeated injections the effect may become permanent.

REFERENCES

1 Carruthers JDA, Carruthers JA. Treatment of glabellar frown lines with *C. botulinum*-A exotoxin. *J Dermatol Surg Oncol* 1992; **18**: 17–21.
2 Garcia A, Fulton E. Cosmetic denervation of the muscles of facial expression with botulinum toxin. *Dermatol Surg* 1996; **22**: 39–43.
3 Klein AW. Cosmetic therapy with botulinum toxin. *Dermatol Surg* 1996; **22**: 757–9.
4 Naumann M, Flachenecker P, Bröcker E *et al*. Botulinum toxin for palmar hyperhidrosis. *Lancet* 1997; **349**: 252.
5 Lowe NJ, Maxwell A, Harper H. Botulinum-A exotoxin for glabellar folds: a double-blind, placebo controlled study with an electromyographic injection technique. *J Am Acad Dermatol* 1996; **35**: 569–72.

Miscellaneous surgical procedures

Techniques

Hydrodissection

The skin can be lifted away from underlying critical arteries and veins by hydrodissection. Approximately 20 ml of saline is injected into loose tissue below the lesion, thereby lifting the area to be excised off any underlying vital structures. The injection must be given after local anaesthesia, just before excision. The technique works best where there is a boundary that will delay the spread of the saline, for example on the temple and the ear [1].

Snip excision

Small tags can be snipped off with a pair of sharp scissors without the need for local anaesthetic [2]. The tag should be pulled away from the skin and snipped off at its base; bleeding usually stops spontaneously. Haemostasis may be a problem with larger polyps with a well-developed blood supply; hence, an anaesthetic will be required. The wounds can be left to heal by second intention, with excellent cosmetic results [3].

Relaxing incisions

Relaxing incisions are one of several techniques used to increase skin mobility. Multiple, small, full-thickness incisions are made parallel to the skin edge at the site of greatest wound tension [4]. These allow the skin to stretch like a meshed graft, resulting in small elliptical defects, which heal by second intention. The technique is particularly useful for excisions on the lower leg, where it produces surprisingly good cosmetic results with less morbidity than split- or full-thickness grafts. The technique can be used with other ways of improving skin mobility [5]. Other types of relaxing incision include the V–Y-plasty [6], which should not be confused with the V–Y island pedicle advancement flap (Table 81.4).

Wedge excision—lip, lid and ear

On the eyelid, lip and ear, a tumour can be excised and the defect readily closed by removing a full-thickness wedge with an appropriate margin of uninvolved skin. The different tissues at the edges of the defect are then sutured, and thus the technique varies with the site. The inherent tissue elasticity of the eyelid and lip allows considerable defects to be repaired by direct closure without distorting the free margins of these structures. On the lip, defects smaller than one-third of the lip length can be closed directly following a wedge excision [7], if necessary using a W-plasty correction on the lower lip to avoid excessive distortion [8]. On the eyelid, defects of up to 50% can be closed directly, provided the correct technique is used [9]. However, a wedge excision on the ear reduces its size considerably, and buckling of the ear may occur unless the technique is modified to avoid this [10]. In most instances this type of defect is not a problem, as spectacles can still be supported by the ear and differences in ear size are not cosmetically unacceptable.

Lipoma removal

Simple skin incision and lipoma excision ensures complete removal but produces an unnecessarily large scar. A subfrontalis lipoma (Fig. 81.18) can be particularly difficult to remove because of its site beneath the frontalis muscle of the forehead [11]. Lipomas in this situation are usually confused with epidermoid cysts preoperatively.

Scar size can be minimized by breaking up the lipoma into smaller fragments using blunt-ended forceps or a needle-holder inserted via a 4–6-mm punch biopsy wound made over the centre of the lipoma. The fragmented

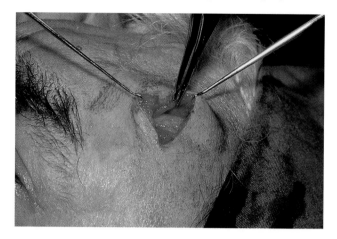

Fig. 81.18 Subfrontalis lipoma. This lipoma lies beneath the frontalis muscle. The muscle has been split vertically and is held back with forceps to reveal the lipoma.

contents can then be squeezed out through the small wound. The fat can also be removed using liposuction [12]. A further development of this technique involves emulsification of the lipoma using an ultrasonic suction scalpel and removal of the debris under endoscopic control [13].

Tissue expansion

Tissue expansion may be helpful if there is insufficient local skin laxity to allow immediate closure and a graft would produce a relatively poor cosmetic result. The skin needed to fill the defect can be stretched to the required size by steadily expanding saline-filled plastic bags placed under the skin adjacent to the proposed defect. For 8–12 weeks after insertion the bags are filled at intervals to produce a mound that stretches the overlying skin. When the defect is excised, the adjacent distended skin is then available to cover the resulting defect [14]. Because the skin used is almost identical to the piece excised, the cosmetic result is potentially excellent. Expansion does not simply stretch existing skin but actually appears to induce basal layer mitotic activity, an increase in dermal collagen, and development of an enhanced blood supply from the fibrous capsule around the implant. Atrophy of adjacent fat and muscle also occurs. Immediate tissue expansion or stretching the skin at the time of operation using skin hooks, Foley catheters [15] or sutures [16] increases available skin in the short term but appears to result in greater shrinkage and hence scar stretching.

Circumcision

This is a simple surgical procedure [17], and may be indicated in the management of lichen sclerosus et atrophicus.

REFERENCES

1 Salasche SJ, Giancola JM, Trookman NS. Surgical pearl: hydroexpansion with local anaesthetic. *J Am Acad Dermatol* 1995; **33**: 510–12.
2 Lawrence CM. *An Introduction to Dermatological Surgery.* Oxford: Blackwell Science, 1996: 66–8.
3 Fewkes JL, Cheney ML, Pollack SV. *Illustrated Atlas of Cutaneous Surgery.* Philadelphia: JB Lippincott, 1992.
4 Motley RJ, Holt PJA. The use of meshed advancement flaps in the treatment of lesions of the lower leg. *J Dermatol Surg Oncol* 1990; **16**: 346–8.
5 Kolbusz RV, Bielinski KB. The combined use of immediate intraoperative tissue expansion and meshing technique. *Arch Dermatol* 1993; **129**: 152–3.
6 Comaish JS. Dermatological surgery. In: Verbov JL, ed. *Dermatological Surgery.* Lancaster: MTP Press, 1986: 18.
7 Wheeland RG. Reconstruction of the lower lip and chin using local and random pattern flaps. *J Dermatol Surg Oncol* 1991; **17**: 605–15.
8 Jemec BIE. A short review of some methods of excisions from and reconstructions of lower lips. *J Dermatol Surg Oncol* 1981; **7**: 576–9.
9 Ross JJ, Pham R. Closure of eyelid defects. *J Dermatol Surg Oncol* 1992; **18**: 1061–4.
10 Tebbetts JB. Auricular reconstruction: selected single stage techniques. *J Dermatol Surg Oncol* 1982; **8**: 557–66.
11 Salasche SJ, McCollough ML, Angeloni VL, Grabski WJ. Frontalis associated lipoma of the forehead. *J Am Acad Dermatol* 1989; **20**: 462–8.
12 Kaneko T, Tokushige H, Kimura N *et al.* The treatment of multiple angiolipomas by liposuction surgery. *J Dermatol Surg Oncol* 1994; **20**: 690–2.
13 Sawaizumi M, Maruyama Y, Onishi K *et al.* Endoscopic extraction of lipomas using an ultrasonic suction scalpel. *Ann Plast Surg* 1996; **36**: 124–8.
14 Baker SR, Swanson NA. Reconstruction of midfacial defects following surgical management of skin cancer. *J Dermatol Surg Oncol* 1994; **20**: 133–40.
15 Auletta MJ, Matarasso SL, Glogau RG, Tromovitch TA. Comparison of skin hooks and Foley catheters for immediate tissue expansion. *J Dermatol Surg Oncol* 1993; **19**: 1084–8.
16 Liang MD, Briggs P, Heckler FR, Futrell JW. Pre-suturing—a new technique for closing large skin defects: clinical and experimental studies. *Plast Reconstr Surg* 1988; **81**: 694–702.
17 Harahap ML, Siregar AS. Circumcision: a review and a new technique. *J Dermatol Surg Oncol* 1986; **14**: 383–6.

Specific diseases

Epidermoid cysts

Epidermoid cysts (sometimes incorrectly called sebaceous cysts) are lined by a keratinizing epithelium, which produces the cheesy, keratinous contents. Epidermoid cysts require excision if they are disfiguring or repeatedly infected. The inflamed tissue around an infected epidermoid cyst is friable, making it difficult to excise without fragmenting the cyst wall. An infected cyst should therefore be drained, and the patient treated with an appropriate antibiotic. When the inflammation settles the cyst can be excised. Cysts inflamed as a result of a foreign-body giant-cell reaction to released keratin are best treated by triamcinolone injection followed by subsequent removal. Freely mobile cysts can be easily shelled out through the smooth tissue plane that separates the very thin cyst wall from the surrounding tissue, although at this plane the cyst wall is easily punctured and must be handled gently. In all cases the entire cyst wall and punctum should be removed, the latter at the centre of a small skin ellipse, which can also be used to manipulate the cyst during removal. If the cyst punctures during extraction, every effort should be made to remove residual wall fragments to prevent recurrence. To avoid long scars, very large cysts can be decompressed via a 4-mm punch biopsy before excision [1]. The wound is either left to heal for 4–6 weeks before definitive removal of the shrunken cyst or an attempt can be made to pull the cyst inside out through the circular wound using artery forceps [2]. Immobile cysts are surrounded by extensive scar tissue and usually have to be excised with the surrounding fibrotic tissue and overlying skin.

Hidradenitis

If medical treatment of hidradenitis suppurativa has failed, involved areas can be excised and the defects covered with skin grafts or flaps. However, cure rates of less than 20% are reported [3] and secondary infection is a frequent problem [4]. Alternatives such as excision followed by healing by second intention are well tolerated by the patient and produce good results [5]. An even simpler procedure involves deroofing the fistula leaving the floor of the track to re-epithelialize the wounded area. Excised tissue or suspect areas should be sent for histology because of the recognized complication of malignant change [6].

Vermilionectomy

This is sometimes called a mucosal advancement [7,8]. The vermilion, usually of the lower lip, is excised, principally because of actinic damage, and replaced by lip mucosa pulled forward and sutured at the vermilion/skin border.

Split ear lobe

Split ear lobes are either congenital or a result of having earrings torn out. Simply de-epithelializing the sides of the cleft and suturing the exposed edges usually results in a notch appearing at the lobe edge. A full thickness or single-sided Z-plasty correction of the cut edges, depending on lobe thickness [9], is advocated as the best way to ensure good cosmesis, although many other methods are described [10].

Partial or incomplete clefts can be repaired by excising and suturing the enlarged hole. If, however, there is only a narrow band of skin separating the hole from the lower pole of the lobe, it is probably best to create a complete defect by cutting the small bridge of skin and closing the defect accordingly. Earrings can be worn again only in patients with thick lobes. Some repairs incorporate reconstruction of a new earring hole at the same time as repair of the defect [11].

Chondrodermatitis nodularis

Intralesional and topical steroids help in approximately 25% of cases. Surgical excision of the affected cartilage

without removal of skin (Fig. 81.19) will result in cure in over 90% of helix lesions and 70% of those on the antihelix [12]. Recurrences will occur if rough or protuberant edges of cartilage are left at operation, but can be treated using the same technique [13]. Other methods, including cryotherapy, curettage and laser ablation, have been used, but with mixed and unpredictable results.

Myxoid cysts

Myxoid cysts around the nail unit can be treated using a variety of procedures. The principle of treatment is that the connection between the cyst and the adjacent joint must be disrupted to prevent the cyst refilling. This is presumably what happens after successful cryotherapy [14], intralesional steroid therapy or curettage, although the cure rate of these procedures is relatively poor. The definitive surgical procedure involves identification of the connection between the joint and the cyst by injection of dye into the joint, followed by exploration of the region between the joint capsule and the cyst to identify and tie off the dye-containing connection (Fig. 81.20) [15]. There is probably no need to excise any skin but the direction of the skin incision is important [16].

Axillary vault excision and other remedies for hyperhidrosis

Axilla. After the failure of medical treatments [17], axillary hyperhidrosis is best treated by excision of the sweat-gland-bearing axillary skin [18] (p. 3608). If malodour is also a problem the apocrine glands, which lie in the subcutaneous fat, have to be removed. If hyperhidrosis is the principal problem, the eccrine glands need to be removed, and these lie more superficially in the dermis and superficial fat. The operation is not difficult, but the resulting scars invariably stretch, and infections are common [19,20]. Various methods have been devised to overcome these problems, and in general a single or several transverse incisions parallel to the normal skin creases are used [17]. Access is easier if a longitudinal incision is used but the scar from this invariably stretches. It is not necessary to remove all the hair-bearing skin. Sweat glands in the adjacent skin can be removed by trimming off the subcutaneous fat on its underside with scissors, so that it becomes a full-thickness skin flap. Wound complications are less frequent because the defect is narrower. Methods which attempt removal of the sweat glands using subcutaneous curettage [21] or liposuction [22], leaving the skin intact, are also described. The earlier methods were not particularly successful, but liposuction removal is claimed to be very effective, although only small numbers of patients have been treated.

Palmar hyperhidrosis in adults and children is now best treated surgically by endoscopic transthoracic sympathectomy

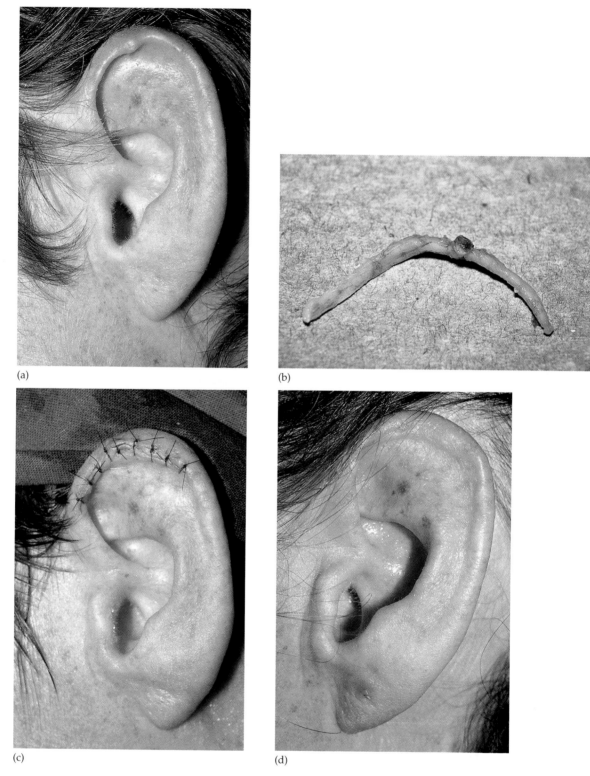

(a)

(b)

(c)

(d)

Fig. 81.19 Excision of chondrodermatitis nodularis helicis. This helix nodule (a) was treated by cartilage excision. An incision was made along the helix rim and the skin reflected to expose the cartilage. A sliver of cartilage was taken to include the 3-mm punch biopsy of the skin nodule (b). Care was taken to ensure that the cartilage edges were smooth and gently shelving up to the uninvolved cartilage. The skin edges were then sutured (c). The result at 6 months (d) was good.

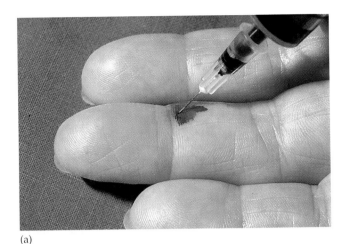

(a)

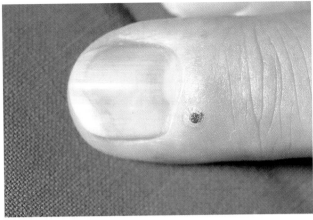

(b)

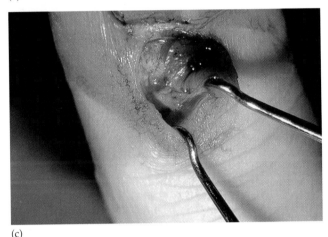

(c)

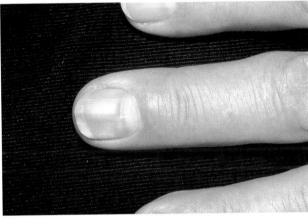

(d)

Fig. 81.20 Myxoid cyst excision. After methylene blue injection into the distal interphalangeal joint (a), dye penetrates to the myxoid cyst on the proximal nail fold (b). When the skin around the cyst is elevated the connection between the cyst and the joint can be identified (c) and ligated. Two months later the cosmetic result was good and the nail gutter had started to resolve proximally (d).

[23]. This involves division of the sympathetic trunk on the second rib. Success rates of 98% are reported. Side-effects include compensatory and gustatory sweating [24], and there is a risk of developing Horner's syndrome and pneumothorax, although the incidence of both is very low in experienced hands. In approximately 10% of cases [25], some recurrence of sweating occurs 1–2 years after surgery. The technique can also be useful in Raynaud's disease [26]. A similar approach can be used to reduce axillary sweating, when the 2nd to the 6th thoracic ganglia have to be destroyed. Access below the third thoracic ganglion is difficult, and this is believed to account for the poorer cure rate for axillary sweating [27]. Plantar hyperhidrosis may respond to open or chemical lumbar sympathectomy [17].

REFERENCES

1 O'Keeffe PJ. Trephining sebaceous cysts. *Br J Plast Surg* 1972; **25**: 411–15.
2 Patton HS. An alternative method for removing sebaceous cysts. *Surg Gynecol*

Obstet 1963; **117**: 645–6.
3 Jemec GBE. Effect of localised surgical excisions in hidradenitis suppurativa. *J Am Acad Dermatol* 1988; **18**: 1103–7.
4 Banerjee AK. Surgical treatment of hidradenitis suppurativa. *Br J Surg* 1992; **79**: 863–6.
5 Silverberg B, Smoot CE, Landa SJF, Parsons RW. Hidradenitis suppurativa: patients' satisfaction with wound healing by second intention. *Plast Reconstr Surg* 1987; **79**: 555–9.
6 Brown SCW, Kazzazi N, Lord PH. Surgical treatment of perineal hidradenitis suppurativa with special reference to recognition of the perianal form. *Br J Surg* 1986; **73**: 978–80.
7 Wheeland RG. Reconstruction of the lower lip and chin using local and random pattern flaps. *J Dermatol Surg Oncol* 1991; **17**: 605–15.
8 Field LM. An improved design for vermilionectomy with a mucous membrane advancement flap. *J Dermatol Surg Oncol* 1991; **17**: 833–4.
9 Reiter D, Alford EL. Torn earlobe: a new approach to management with a review of 68 cases. *Ann Otol Rhinol Laryngol* 1994; **103**: 879–84.
10 Blanco-Dávila F, Vásconez HC. The cleft earlobe: a review of methods of treatment. *Ann Plast Surg* 1994; **33**: 677–80.
11 Fayman MS. Split earlobe repair. *Br J Plast Surg* 1994; **47**: 293.
12 Lawrence CM. The treatment of chondrodermatitis nodularis with cartilage removal alone. *Arch Dermatol* 1991; **127**: 530–5.
13 Lawrence CM. Surgical treatment of chondrodermatitis nodularis. In: Robinson JK, Arndt KA, LeBoit PE, Wintroub BU, eds. *Atlas of Cutaneous Surgery*. Philadelphia: WB Saunders, 1996: 201–6.
14 Dawber RPR, Sonnex T, Leonard J, Ralfs I. Myxoid cysts of the finger: treatment by liquid nitrogen spray cryosurgery. *Clin Exp Dermatol* 1983; **8**: 153–7.
15 Miller PK, Roenigk RK, Amadio PC. Focal mucinosis (myxoid cysts). *J Dermatol Surg Oncol* 1991; **118**: 716–19.
16 Field LM. Electrodesiccation at the DIP for myxoid cyst and skin flaps in proximity to the interphalangeal joints. *J Dermatol Surg Oncol* 1993; **19**: 388–9.

17 Moran KT, Brady MP. Surgical management of primary hyperhidrosis. *Br J Surg* 1991; **78**: 279–83.

18 Wen-Horng Wu, Sheih Ma, Jin-Teh Lin *et al*. Surgical treatment of axillary osmidrosis: analysis of 343 cases. *Plast Reconstr Surg* 1994; **94**: 288–94.

19 Hurley HJ, Shelley WB. A simple surgical approach to the management of axillary hyperhidrosis. *JAMA* 1963; **186**: 109–12.

20 Bretteville-Jensen G, Mossing N, Albrechtsen R. Surgical treatment of axillary hyperhidrosis in 123 patients. *Acta Derm Venereol (Stockh)* 1975; **55**: 73–7.

21 Jemec B. Abrasio axillae in hyperhidrosis. *Scand J Plast Reconstr Surg* 1975; **9**: 44–6.

22 Shenaq SM, Spira MS. Treatment of bilateral axillary hyperhidrosis by suction assisted lipolysis technique. *Ann Plast Surg* 1987; **19**: 548–51.

23 Drott C, Göthberg G, Claes G. Endoscopic transthoracic sympathectomy: an efficient and safe method for the treatment of hyperhidrosis. *J Am Acad Dermatol* 1995; **33**: 78–81.

24 Quraishy MS, Giddings AEB. Treating hyperhidrosis. *Br Med J* 1993; **306**: 1221–2.

25 Byrne J, Walsh TN, Hederman WP. Endoscopic transthoracic electrocautery of the sympathetic chain for palmar and axillary hyperhidrosis. *Br J Surg* 1990; **77**: 1046–9.

26 Nicholson ML, Hopkinson BR, Dennis MJS. Endoscopic transthoracic sympathectomy: successful in hyperhidrosis but can the indications be extended? *Ann R Coll Surg Engl* 1994; **76**: 311–14.

27 Gordon A, Colin J. Treating hyperhidrosis. *Br Med J* 1993; **306**: 1752.

Cosmetic procedures

Scar revision including acne scar correction

Pitted or 'ice-pick' acne scars can be treated by dermabrasion [1], very deep pitted scars do well with punch grafting [2] and the wide, depressed scars respond to soft-tissue augmentation techniques including collagen [3] and Fibrel injections [4]. The flat, purple–pink scars are best left to improve with time. Scar revision after surgery includes dermabrasion, which is best done 6 weeks postoperatively [5], and the treatment of keloids or hypertrophic scars [6].

Liposuction (lipectomy)

This involves selective removal of subcutaneous fat using a small cannula and suction equipment to produce a slimmer body shape [7]. The technique can be used at almost any body site, and can produce impressive results with an experienced physician. Tumescent anaesthesia [8] evolved from the need to do liposuction under local anaesthesia; as a consequence it has become apparent that higher maximal lignocaine doses are possible using dilute anaesthetic solutions [9]. Liposuction has also been used to treat lipomas [10] and insulin-induced fat hypertrophy [11], in flap undermining, lymphoedema [12], breast reduction, lipodystrophy [13] and axillary hyperhidrosis [14], and to remove haematomas or extravasated corrosive drugs [15].

Blepharoplasty

This involves the removal of redundant skin and orbital fat from the upper [16] and lower [17] eyelids in order to correct unsightly bags or skin folds. Selection of the correct procedure to take account of individual variations in eyelid anatomy, identification of pre-existing eye disease, meticulous technique, and the ability to adapt or include other procedures depending on the co-existing abnormalities present make this an operation for the expert [18]. Complications include blindness [19], excessive sclera show or ectropion, and failure to correct the original defect.

REFERENCES

1 Alt TA. Technical aids for dermabrasion. *J Dermatol Surg Oncol* 1987; **13**: 638–48.

2 Solotoff SA. Treatment of pitted acne scarring—post-auricular punch grafts followed by dermabrasion. *J Dermatol Surg Oncol* 1986; **12**: 1079–84.

3 Varnavides CK, Forster RA, Cunliffe WJ. The role of bovine collagen in the treatment of acne scars. *Br J Dermatol* 1987; **116**: 199–206.

4 Millikan H, Banks K, Purkait B, Chungi V. A 5-year safety and efficacy evaluation with Fibrel in the correction of cutaneous scars following one or two treatments. *J Dermatol Surg Oncol* 1991; **17**: 223–9.

5 Yarborough JM. Ablation of facial scars by programmed dermabrasion. *J Dermatol Surg Oncol* 1988; **14**: 292–4.

6 Harahap M. Revision of a depressed scar. *J Dermatol Surg Oncol* 1984; **10**: 206–9.

7 Fournier PF. Why the syringe and not the suction machine. *J Dermatol Surg Oncol* 1988; **14**: 1062–71.

8 Coleman WP, Klein JA. Use of the tumescent technique for scalp surgery, dermabrasion and soft tissue reconstruction. *J Dermatol Surg Oncol* 1992; **18**: 130–5.

9 Samdal F, Amland PF, Bugge JF. Plasma lidocaine levels during suction-assisted lipectomy using large doses of dilute lidocaine with adrenaline. *Plast Reconstr Surg* 1994; **93**: 1217–23.

10 Kaneko T, Tokushige H, Kimura N *et al*. The treatment of multiple angiolipomas by liposuction surgery. *J Dermatol Surg Oncol* 1994; **20**: 690–2.

11 Hardy KJ, Gill GV, Bryson JR. Severe insulin-induced lipohypertrophy successfully treated by liposuction. *Diabetes Care* 1993; **16**: 929–30.

12 McO'Brien B, Khazanchi RK, Kumar PAV *et al*. Liposuction in the treatment of lymphoedema: a preliminary report. *Br J Plast Surg* 1989; **42**: 530–3.

13 Ketterings C. Lipodystrophy and its treatment. *Ann Plast Surg* 1988; **21**: 536–43.

14 Coleman WP. Non-cosmetic applications of liposuction. *J Dermatol Surg Oncol* 1988; **14**: 1085–90.

15 Martin PH, Carver N, Petros AJ. Use of liposuction and saline washout for the treatment of extensive subcutaneous extravasation of corrosive drugs. *Br J Anaesth* 1994; **72**: 702–4.

16 Perman KI. Upper eyelid blepharoplasty. *J Dermatol Surg Oncol* 1992; **18**: 1096–9.

17 Neuhaus RW. Lower eyelid blepharoplasty. *J Dermatol Surg Oncol* 1992; **18**: 1100–9.

18 Flowers RS. Blepharoplasty and periorbital aesthetic surgery. *Clin Plast Surg* 1993; **20**: 209–30.

19 Mahaffey PJ, Wallace AF. Blindness following cosmetic blepharoplasty—a review. *Br J Plast Surg* 1986; **39**: 213–21.

Chapter 82
Formulary of Topical Applications

J. D. WILKINSON

Vehicles and bland
   preparations
Wet dressings and baths
Lotions
Paints, varnishes and
   tinctures

Emollients
Creams
Gels
Ointments
Pastes
Scalp preparations

Cleansing agents and
   shampoos
Protective and screening
   applications
Aural preparations
Oral preparations
Miscellaneous formulae

The standard reference book for prescribing in the UK is the *British National Formulary* (BNF). It is published twice a year in pocket-book form and contains not only a complete list of official preparations but also those proprietary preparations on the British market at the time of publication. The BNF therefore contains virtually all the topical formulations which the dermatologist needs, and there seems little point in duplicating them here. Although the detailed formulation of some agents in everyday use, zinc, sulphur, salicylic acid, etc., may vary slightly from country to country, dermatologists will also have their own National Formu-laries or lists to refer to.

There are a small number of particular formulae, however, which have been evolved by individual dermatologists or used with success over long periods in particular hospitals; some of these fill a void; others involve variations in the vehicle or active agents. As these are all of potential and continuing value, especially in countries where proprietary preparations may not always be available or affordable, they form the basis of this Formulary. Also included, however, is a small selection of the most commonly used official BNF preparations (marked *), as they are frequently referred to in other chapters.

The whole field of topical dermatological formulation has been covered in detail by Polano in *Topical Skin Therapeutics* [1]—a comprehensive guide to the subject. The principles of topical therapy are discussed in Chapter 78. Other British sources of information are mentioned in the references. Other readers—notably in other European countries and the USA—will have their own handbooks, which will repair the deficiencies of this small selection, for which the author takes full responsibility.

The author is particularly indebted to the editors of the BNF for permission to include some of their material, and to all those contributors who have given the formulations used in their own hospitals.

The preparations are grouped conventionally according to their physical type or use. The following abbreviations are used:

APF   *Australian Pharmaceutical Formulary and Handbook,* 1988
BP   *British Pharmacopoeia,* 1993
BPC   *British Pharmaceutical Codex,* Supplement
BRI   *Bristol Royal Infirmary,* UK
GOS   Hospital for Sick Children, Gt Ormond Street, London, UK
LGI   Leeds General Infirmary, UK
PC   *Pharmaceutical Codex,* incorporating the BPC
PN   *Pharmacopoeia Nordica*
Pr.   Proprietary preparation
RVI   Royal Victoria Infirmary, Newcastle upon Tyne, UK
SGH   St George's Hospital, London, UK
SRI   Sheffield Royal Infirmary, UK
STH   St Thomas' Hospital, London, UK
USP   *United States Pharmacopoeia*
WGH   Wycombe General Hospital, UK

Vehicles and bland preparations

Vehicles (or bases) are powders, oils, greases or liquids, which alone or in biphasic or triphasic mixtures form relatively stable agents which have two functions: they act as vehicles for the incorporation of active ingredients, and they often have soothing and emollient qualities of their own. Because of their widespread use, a number of official (*) formulae are included in this section.

Aqueous Cream BP* 1993

An oil-in-water emulsion of 30% emulsifying ointment

with phenoxyethanol 1% as a preservative and purified water to 100%. It can be used as a soap substitute skin cleanser, as a vehicle, and as an emollient.

Cetomacrogol Cream BP* 1988 (Formula A)

Cetomacrogol emulsifying ointment	30 g
Chlorocresol	0.1 g
Freshly boiled and cooled purified water	to 100 g

A diluent, for example for corticosteroid creams.

Cetomacrogol Cream BP* 1988 (Formula B)

Cetomacrogol emulsifying ointment	30 g
Methyl hydroxybenzoate	0.15 g
Propyl hydroxybenzoate	0.08 g
Benzyl alcohol	1.5 g
Freshly boiled and cooled purified water	to 100 g

As above. Note the difference in preservative.

Emulsifying Ointment BP* 1993

Emulsifying wax	30 g
Liquid paraffin	20 g
White soft paraffin	50 g

Can be used as a soap substitute skin cleanser or as an emollient. May be diluted with water but, without preservative, has a short shelf-life.

Emulsifying Wax BP* 1993

Cetostearyl alcohol	90 g
Sodium lauryl sulphate	10 g
Water	4 ml

Hydrophilic Ointment USP

White soft paraffin	250 g
Stearyl alcohol	250 g
Propylene glycol	120 g
Sodium lauryl sulphate	10 g
Methyl paraben	0.25 g
Propyl paraben	0.15 g
Water	to 1000 g

Hydrous Wool Fat Ointment BPC* 1973

Hydrous wool fat and yellow soft paraffin, equal parts.

Orabase, Orahesive (Pr.)

A gel or adhesive powder of carboxymethylcellulose, pectin and gelatin as a protective or vehicle for use on the oral mucosa.

Stomahesive (Pr.) [2]

Pectin, gelatin, carboxymethylcellulose and polyisobutylene on a polythene backing. For stoma care.

Topical antibiotic vehicle (BRI)

Propylene glycol	4
Water for irrigation	8
Isopropyl alcohol	to 40 parts

Add contents of capsules to make a 1% (or as desired) solution.

Topical antibiotic vehicle (WGH)

Industrial Methylated Spirit BP (95%)	66
Propylene glycol	4.5
Distilled water	to 90

Add contents of capsules to make a 1–1.5% solution. Shelf-life 4 weeks.

Wet dressings and baths

Aluminium acetate is widely used for wet dressings in the USA and elsewhere. In the UK, potassium permanganate is favoured, despite its staining.

Aluminium acetate lotion* (Burow's solution APF) 1988

Aluminium acetate solution	5 ml
Purified water, freshly boiled and cooled	to 100 ml

It contains about 0.65% of the salts. It must be freshly prepared and is used undiluted.

Burow's Solution BP 1993

Aluminium sulphate	225 g
Acetic acid (33%)	250 ml
Tartaric acid	45 g
Calcium carbonate	100 g
Purified water	750 ml

Solution as used in Burow's paste (p. 3635)

Chlorinated Lime and Boric Acid Solution BP 1993 (Eusol)

Chlorinated lime	1.25 g
Boric acid	1.25 g
Water	to 100 ml

Contains not less than 0.25% available chlorine. It is applied as wet dressings, especially for the initial cleaning of wounds and ulcers. Use within 1 week.

Eusol and liquid paraffin (LGI)

Eusol and liquid paraffin, equal parts, with 1% bees-wax (this can be omitted if the mixture is shaken before use (WGH)). For infected leg ulcers. Use within 2 weeks.

Formaldehyde lotion*

Formaldehyde Solution BP, 3% in water. It must be freshly prepared. Glutaraldehyde 10% solution, buffered with sodium bicarbonate 10%, is also used for hyperhidrosis of hands and feet, but stains brown temporarily.

Potassium permanganate solution*

A 0.1% solution in distilled water is usually dispensed. This must be diluted to 1:7 to 1:10 with water before use for wet dressings. If crystals are used, these must first be dissolved in water and diluted until this becomes a pale-pink colour.

Dilute Sodium Hypochlorite Solution BP 1993

Contains about 1% available chlorine. Use only diluted solutions containing no more than 0.5% available chlorine on skin or in wounds.

Lotions

Calamine liniment (LGI)

Calamine	8g
Lanolin	7g
Limewater	50 ml
Arachis oil	to 100 ml

Less drying than calamine lotion (see also Calamine lotion, oily, PC*).

Calamine lotion (STH)

Calamine	15g
Zinc oxide	5g
Glycerol	5 ml
Water	to 100 ml

To which may be added, usually in the strengths indicated, liquefied phenol 1%, precipitated sulphur 2%, etc.

Copper and Zinc Sulphate Lotion BPC (Dalibour Water)

Copper sulphate 1% and zinc sulphate 1.5% in camphor water 2.5%; water to 100%. An astringent application.

Zinc Liniment PN 1963

Zinc oxide	12.5
Talc	12.5
Alcohol (70%)	12.5
Glycerol	12.5
Water	to 100

An official example of a shake lotion.

Paints, varnishes and tinctures

Brilliant Green and Crystal Violet Paint BP* 1980†

0.5% of each in equal parts of alcohol (90%) and water. To be used undiluted. Either dye may be used alone or in an aqueous or alcoholic base.

Wart applications

Cantharidin wart paint

Cantharidin 0.7% in equal parts of acetone and collodion. Apply with a small brush and allow to dry. For periungual warts.

Podophyllin Compound Paint BP 1993†

Podophyllin resin 15% in compound benzoin tincture. Various modifications of strength (10–25%) and base (industrial methylated spirit) abound in various formulae. If a spirit base is used, the surrounding skin should be protected with yellow soft paraffin. Contraindicated in pregnancy.

Wart paint (BRI)

Formaldehyde solution	25 ml
Acetone	60 ml
Salicylic acid	60 g
Flexible collodion	to 500 ml

Wart paint [3]

Lactic acid	16
Salicylic acid	16
Flexible collodion	to 100

Wart paste (BRI)

Trichloroacetic acid	5 g
(or liquefied trichloroacetic acid	3.1 ml)
Salicylic acid	12 g
Glycerol	5 ml

† NB: Certain toxicological considerations apply to the use of crystal violet, podophyllin and products containing salicylic acid.

Several proprietary formulae are marketed, notably paints similar to wart paint [4] above. Glutaraldehyde, 10% aqueous, and more preparations based on salicylic acid are also available. Other therapeutic agents are discussed in Chapter 78.

Emollients

These are designed to soften or to give the impression of softening or smoothing the surface of the skin. A wide variety of different preparations are now available as proprietary products or cosmetic 'moisturizers'. Some of the formulae listed under Vehicles are also used for this purpose by patients. A small selection of other emollients are listed here.

Bath emollient (WGH)

Liquid paraffin	55
Anhydrous lanolin	5.5
Cetomacrogol Emulsifying Wax BP	1
Nipagin M	0.1
Distilled water	to 100

Add two tablespoonfuls (30 ml) to bath and mix well.

Glycerol–water lotion (WGH)

Tragacanth powder	0.5 g
Absolute alcohol (99%)	1.0 ml
Glycerol	25 ml
Water	to 100 ml

The only application tolerated by a patient with an excessively sensitive unstable psoriasis.

Creams

Acetic acid ('Samaritan') cream (WGH)

Acetic acid	30
Nipagen M	0.03
Arachis oil	20
Emulsifying Wax BP	15
Distilled water	35

A dressing for leg ulcers.

Crystal violet cream (WGH)†

Crystal Violet (or Brilliant Green) BP	0.1–1.0
Cetomacrogol cream (Formula A)	to 100

For acute infected eczemas of hands and feet.

Lanette wax cream [1]

Lanette wax SX	10
Arachis oil	10

† NB: Certain toxicological considerations apply to the use of crystal violet, podophyllin and products containing salicylic acid.

Methyl paraben	0.5
Water	to 100

A simple oil-in-water cream. Emulsifying Wax BP can be substituted for lanette wax.

Zinc cream (STH)

Zinc oxide	10
Wool fat	2.5
Arachis oil	37.5
Emulsifying wax	2.5
Water	to 100

To which ichthammol 2% may be added ('Ichthammol cream').

Molloy's mix (WGH)

Liquor picis carbonis 3% v/w
Salicylic acid 3% w/v in Aqueous Cream BP
A useful, general purpose, relatively clean tar preparation for psoriasis.

Gels

Glycerin of Starch BPC 1958 (starch glycerin)

Wheat starch 8.5% heated with water and glycerol until it gelatinizes. (The formula varies in different countries.)

Salicylic acid gel (SGH, BRI)

Salicylic acid	60 g
Propylene glycol	200 ml
Industrial Methylated Spirit BP (95%)	250 ml
Glycerin	50 ml
Tragacanth	50 g
Water for irrigation	410 ml

Ointments

These more or less greasy applications are used for non-exudative lesions, or for those in which a protective or keratolytic effect is required. They may also form vehicles for delivery of active agents to the skin. Modern emulsifying agents have blurred the distinction between creams and ointments, but as the latter usually have no water content they seldom require the addition of preservatives.

Greasy ointments may be divided into true fats, waxes, mineral greases and macrogols. They are well represented in National Formularies.

Aluminium Subacetate Ointment PN 1963

Aluminium subacetate	1.6
Water	18.4

Wool fat	40
Yellow soft paraffin	40

Benzoic Acid Compound Ointment BP 1993 (Whitfield's Ointment)

Benzoic acid 6% and salicylic acid 3% in Emulsifying Ointment BP. Still an effective and cheap antifungal preparation. Use half-strength in the flexures.

Coal tar ointment (STH)

Solution of coal tar	12
Lanolin	10
Yellow soft paraffin	to 100

Coal Tar and Salicylic Acid Ointment BP* 1993

Coal tar and salicylic acid, 2% of each, in a complex paraffin–coconut oil emulsified base. A useful but little used preparation.

50:50 mix (GOS)

White soft paraffin	50
Liquid paraffin	50

A useful emollient for dry atopic eczema.

Paraffin Ointment BP 1993

Hard paraffin	3 g
White beeswax	2 g
Cetostearyl alcohol	5 g
White soft paraffin	90 g

A protective for fissured skin or lips.

Pastes

These are either greasy pastes, for example powder in a greasy vehicle, or drying or cooling pastes, for example powder in a liquid base. The latter are not used in the UK as much as elsewhere, and their useful properties are somewhat neglected.

Burow's paste (1, 2, 3 Paste) [1]

Burow's Solution BP 1993	1
Lanolin	2
Zinc paste	3

There are many variations on this theme.

Coal tar solution paste (LGI)

Coal tar solution	25
Zinc oxide	5
Yellow soft paraffin	to 100

For chronic eczema. To clean, use arachis oil or aqueous cream.

Coal Tar Paste BP 1993*

Strong solution of coal tar	7.5 g
Compound Zinc Paste BP 1993	92.5 g
(Zinc oxide	25 g
Starch	25 g
White soft paraffin	50 g)

Magnesium Sulphate Paste BP 1993 (Morison's paste)

Magnesium sulphate 45% and phenol 0.5% in anhydrous glycerol. Keep in an airtight container. Stir before use.

Titanium Dioxide Paste PC* 1979

Titanium dioxide 20%, zinc oxide 25%, kaolin 10%, with red precipitated ferric oxide, glycerin, chlorocresol and water. A greaseless paste, UV repellent. Salicylic acid remains active in this vehicle.

Vioform and Zinc Paste (STH)

Vioform 1% in zinc paste BPC.

Zinc and Salicylic Acid Paste BP 1993 ('Lassar's paste')

Salicylic acid	2 g
Zinc oxide	24 g
Starch	24 g
White soft paraffin	50 g

See [1] with regard to inactivation of salicylic acid in this formula. But it is a necessary ingredient when this is used as a paste base for dithranol.

Zinc Paste PN 1963

Zinc oxide 40%, yellow soft paraffin 60%.

Paste vehicles for dithranol (anthralin)

Modifications on the original Lassar's paste are designed to give greater adhesion or flexibility in different climatic conditions, chiefly by varying the amount of hard and soft paraffin.

Dithranol paste, standard [4,5]

Dithranol	0.1–1.0 g
Salicylic acid	2 g
Zinc oxide	25 g
Starch	25 g

White soft paraffin of melting point 46°C
(for UK)   to 100 g
5–15% hard paraffin (melting point 49°C) can be substituted with advantage, for example 7.5% at WGH.

Lassar's paste for dithranol (RVI; STH)

Salicylic acid	2 g
Zinc oxide	24 g
Starch	24 g
Hard paraffin	10 g
Yellow soft paraffin	40 g

An example of the stiffer paste.

Starch-dithranol paste [1]

Starch	40 g
Soft paraffin	to 100 g

Avoids the interaction of zinc oxide and dithranol.

Scalp preparations

The relative paucity of official preparations for the scalp contrasts with the variety of unofficial formulations used by different skin departments in the UK, and underlines the difficulty in obtaining an effective and acceptable vehicle, particularly for women with long hair. Those containing cade oil, tar or salicylic acid are used in any crusted or scaly scalp condition; those containing dithranol are specifically for psoriasis. They are normally applied overnight before shampooing the following morning.

Tar pomade (LGI)

Coal tar solution	6 g
Salicylic acid	2 g
Tween 20	1 g
Emulsifying ointment	to 100 g

Coconut oil compound ointment (STH)

Coal tar solution	12
Precipitated sulphur	4
Salicylic acid	2
Coconut oil	60
Yellow soft paraffin	9
Emulsifying Wax BP	13

Compound coconut oil ointment

Coconut Oil BP	30%
Strong Coal Tar Solution BPC	6.25%
Precipitated Sulphur BP	2%
Salicylic acid	4%
Emulsifying ointment	to 100%

Cradle cap ointment (STH)

Salicylic acid	2
Precipitated sulphur	2
Coal tar solution	2
Emulsifying ointment	to 100

As implied, but also for mildly crusted lesions in adults.

Dithranol pomade (BRI)

Dithranol	0.3
Salicylic acid	0.3
Yellow soft paraffin	4.3
Emulsifying Ointment PC	to 100

Incorporate dithranol and then salicylic acid into the paraffin by trituration. Add to warmed emulsifying ointment. (Proprietary pomades are also marketed.)

Dithranol pomade 1%

Emulsifying wax	25 g
Dithranol	0.5–1 g
Embanox 6	0.5 g
Ascorbic acid	0.1 g
Liquid paraffin	to 100 g

New pomade (BRI)

Salicylic acid	2
Coal tar solution	6
Polysorbate (Tween) 20	1
Emulsifying Ointment PC	91

Cade oil ointment (WGH)

Cade oil	6
Precipitated sulphur	3
Salicylic acid	2
Emulsifying Ointment PC	89

Salicylated scalp oil

1–2% salicylic acid in arachis or castor oil, or in a proprietary baby oil. Useful for mild scaling conditions.

Cleansing agents and shampoos

Cleansing agents

Emulsifying Ointment BPC or Aqueous Cream BPC are commonly prescribed in the UK. Arachis or other vegetable oils are useful for cleaning off pastes. Several antiseptic and antibacterial solutions, creams, lotions and concentrates are available commercially and are widely used.

Some simple agents, still widely used, are noted below. See also the section on wet dressings and soaks.

Hydrogen Peroxide BPC*

Solutions of 3% (10 vol), 6% (20 vol) and 27% (about 90 vol) are available. Bleaches fabric. Solutions above 6% should be diluted before being applied to the skin.

Soap Spirit BPC* (soft soap)

Soft soap 65% wt/vol in Industrial Methylated Spirit BP.

Zinc peroxide paste [6]

Sterilized zinc peroxide 50% powder in *sterile* distilled water freshly prepared for each treatment. Prepared packs can be made available for immediate ward mixing.

Shampoos

The enormous variety of cosmetic and proprietary medicated shampoos will serve almost every purpose, but there are rare occasions when a non-perfumed scalp cleanser may be required.

Cade oil shampoo [7]

Cade oil	10
Triethanolamine	10
Spirit soap	to 100

Leave on for 2 h before washing off.

Detergent shampoo

Lanette wax SX	1
Sodium lauryl sulphate	6.5
Water	to 100

Not particularly elegant, but simple to prepare in bulk and free from perfume.

Protective and screening applications

Bland protective agents may be used around infected wounds and ulcers, natural exudates or artificial openings discharging intestinal fluid. They may also be used around patches of psoriasis which are being treated with dithranol.

Screening against UV light is now well provided by cosmetic and proprietary preparations. A general purpose UV screen is included, however.

All-purpose light barrier (Dundee light screen) [8]

Titanium dioxide	20
Zinc oxide	6
Kaolin	2
Red ferric oxide	1
Mexenone	4
Cream base	to 100

Modify colour with brown ferric oxide to match skin.

Aluminium Compound Paste BP 1993 (Baltimore paste)

Aluminium powder 20%, zinc oxide 40% and liquid paraffin 40%. A bland protective paste.

Aluminium protective paste [9]

Aluminium hydroxide	4
Tragacanth powder	2.5
Glycerin	25
Water	to 100

For ileostomies and colostomies.

Compound zinc paste and aqueous cream (BRI)

Compound Zinc Paste BP	
Aqueous Cream BP	equal parts

A water-repellent application for napkin erythemas, etc. Several other proprietary preparations based on dimethicone, etc., are also available.

Drying paste (WGH) [1]

Zinc oxide (or titanium), talc, equal parts	30–50
Glycerol, distilled water, equal parts	to 100

There are many variations and additions.

Titanium Dioxide Paste BPC* 1973

Titanium dioxide	20 g
Chlorocresol	0.1 g
Red ferric oxide	2 g
Glycerol	15 g
Light kaolin	10 g
Zinc oxide	25 g
Water	to 100 g

An example of a glycerol–water–powder drying paste. It can be diluted with Emulsifying Ointment BPC, equal parts (LGI).

Pâté à l'eau (LGI)

Zinc oxide, purified talc, glycerol and calcium hydroxide solution, equal parts. A simple soothing watery paste without lanolin or preservatives.

Aural preparations

Wax may be softened before syringing by inserting a few

drops of warm oil for a night or two or by the use of proprietary wax softeners and solvents.

The external auditory meatus should be cleaned gently and cleared of debris before drops or paints are applied. If a swab is used, this must be tipped with a *loose*, free wisp of wool beyond the swab to avoid injuring the ear drum.

Acetic acid paint [10]

2.5% acetic acid in isopropyl alcohol.

Aluminium Acetate Ear Drops* BP 1993

Solution of aluminium acetate (about 13%).

Brilliant Green and Crystal Violet Paint BP 1980

See page 3633.

Phenol Eardrops BPC* 1973

Phenol glycerol	40 ml
Glycerol	to 100 ml

Sodium Bicarbonate Eardrops BP 1993

Sodium bicarbonate	5 g
Glycerol	30 ml
Purified water	to 100 ml

For removal of wax.

Oral preparations

There are many official and proprietary mouthwashes and mildly anaesthetic preparations available. The following have been used for persistent or very painful lesions of the mouth and tongue.

Analgesic mouthwash (WGH)

Aspirin powder	15 g
Amethocaine HCl powder	0.5 g
Compound powder of tragacanth	10 g
Mucilage of tragacanth	50 ml
Chloroform water	to 200 ml

Hold in the mouth as long as possible and swallow if necessary, if throat ulcers are present.

Betamethasone mouthwash (LGI)

Dissolve one Betnesol 500 mg tablet in 20 ml of water, and use immediately as mouthwash. Hold in the mouth for 10 min, then spit out. Use three times a day.

Modified Knox formula mouthwash

Triamcinolone acetonide injection 10 mg/ml	50 mg
Erythromycin syrup 250 mg/5 ml	to 100 ml

For children use erythromycin 125 mg/5 ml. Use twice a day as a mouthwash.

Miscellaneous formulae

Axillary antiperspirant lotion [11]

Aluminium chloride hexahydrate	25% (or less)
Industrial Methylated Spirit BP	to 100%

Allow to dissolve at room temperature for 3 weeks, shaking daily. Proprietary 'roll-ons' available.

Depigmenting lotion (SRI)

Hydroquinone	5 g
All-*trans*-retinoic acid	0.1 g
Hydrocortisone	1 g
Sodium metabisulphite	0.1 g
Butylated hydroxytoluene	0.05 g
Base—50/50 polyethylene glycol 400 : methylated spirit 99%	to 100 ml

Depigmentation cream [12]

Vitamin A (retinoic acid)	5
Hydroquinone	0.1
Dexamethasone (or equivalent)	0.1
Hydrophilic Ointment USP	to 100

(or ethanol, propylene glycol, equal parts)

Bland face powder [1]

Zinc oxide	18–24
Zinc stearate	4–6
Prepared chalk	6
Purified talc	to 100

Colour with ochre, carmine or iron oxide if desired. The oilier the skin, the less the stearate.

Nail avulsion ointment [13,14]

Urea	40 g
Salicylic acid	20 g
Distilled water	30 ml
Aquaphor	110 g

Aquaphor contains 10% lanolin, 20% petrolatum, 30% mineral oil and 40% water. See references for mode of use.

Powder for Balanitis [1]

Tannic acid	equal parts to 25
Zinc oxide	
Talc	to 100

Zinc Oil [1]

Zinc oxide	50–60
Olive (or arachis) oil	to 100

The properties of this seemingly simple formula are complex. It should be nearly liquid. Fluids or solids may be added but the balance should be retained.

Postoperative styptic [15]

Ferric chloride 10% in water. Monsel's solution is also widely used.

BIBLIOGRAPHY

British National Formulary, No 32 (1996). London: British Medical Association and The Pharmaceutical Society of Great Britain. Issued twice a year. References marked* in text.

British Pharmacopoeia, 1993, London.

Pharmaceutical Codex incorporating the British Pharmaceutical Codex. London: Pharmaceutical Press.

REFERENCES

1 Polano MK. *Topical Skin Therapeutics*. Edinburgh: Churchill Livingstone, 1984.
2 Gross E, Irving M. Protection of the skin around intestinal fistulas. *Br J Surg* 1977; **64**: 258–63.
3 Bunney MH, Nolan MW, Williams DA. An assessment of methods of treating viral warts by comparative treatment trials based on a standard design. *Br J Dermatol* 1976; **94**: 667–79.
4 Comaish JG. Ingram method of treating psoriasis. *Arch Dermatol* 1965; **92**: 56–8.
5 Seville RH. Dithranol paste for psoriasis. *Br J Dermatol* 1966; **78**: 269–72.
6 Meleney FL, Johnson BA. Prophylactic and active treatment of surgical infections with zinc peroxide. *Surg Gynecol Obstet* 1937; **64**: 387–92.
7 Readett M. Seborrheic dermatitis. *Practitioner* 1966; **196**: 627–33.
8 MacLeod TM, Frain-Bell W. A study of chemical light screening agents. *Br J Dermatol* 1975; **92**: 417–25.
9 Belisario JC. Circumileostomy skin difficulties (Letter). *Arch Dermatol* 1965; **91**: 93.
10 Jones EM. *External Otitis*. Springfield: Thomas, 1965.
11 Shelley WB, Hurley HJ. Studies on topical antiperspirant control of axillary hyperhidrosis. *Acta Derm Venereol (Stockh)* 1975; **55**: 241–60.
12 Kligman AM, Willis I. A new formula for depigmenting human skin. *Arch Dermatol* 1975; **111**: 40–8.
13 Buselmher TJ. Combination urea and salicyclic acid ointment nail avulsion in nondystrophic nails: a follow-up observation. *Cutis* 1980; **25**: 397, 405.
14 Farber EM, South DA. Urea ointment in the nonsurgical avulsion of nail dystrophies. *Cutis* 1978; **22**: 689–92.
15 Goldberg HC. Monsel's solution (Letter). *J Am Acad Dermatol* 1981; **5**: 613.

Chapter 83
Glossary of Dermatological Terms

D.S.WILKINSON

Introduction

The compilation of any glossary of terms used in dermatology involves a number of decisions: how much to include and what to omit; how far to pursue derivations without seeming to be pedantic; how seriously to regard acronyms; and how far to pursue the life histories of authors of eponymous diseases. Some dermatologists, such as Tilbury Fox, have provided a *Glossarial Index*; others, such as Radcliffe-Crocker, have given the derivation of each term used; Prosser White used footnotes in the manner of Gibbon. Changing times and the exigencies of publishing have rendered these methods obsolete. So great has been the expansion of scientific knowledge and the terms needed to describe new concepts and new entities that medical dictionaries have taken their place. These are necessarily voluminous; the *International Dictionary of Medicine and Biology* fills 3200 pages. Dermatology is relatively young as a speciality—Robert Willan's seminal work *On Cutaneous Diseases (Part I)* was only published in 1808—but since then it has accumulated more than its fair share of Graeco-Latin terms and eponymous diseases.

Words are the means by which we communicate thoughts. Imprecision in their use or a lack of knowledge of their origin detracts from their value. A debased currency buys bad goods. Being a visible—and a highly emotive—organ, the skin and its diseases have acquired a rich vocabulary of descriptive terms, many with vernacular roots (in our case, Anglo-Saxon). Those for whom English is not a mother tongue may find them difficult to interpret. But, above all, it is the Graeco-Roman influence on Western medicine, the heritage of Hippocrates and Galen, that has dominated medical terminology and which is still providing us with new terms through the richness and subtlety of the Greek language and the pertinence of the Latin. Now that these languages have ceased to be part of the cultural background of many European countries, it has become necessary to define the meaning of many words that would once have been readily understood by all doctors.

There have been few recent attempts at providing glossaries for dermatological terms. Winkelmann's admirable and concise *Glossary of Basic Dermatology Lesions* covers exactly what the title suggests. At the other end of the scale, the very entertaining and comprehensive dermatological dictionary of Leider and Rosenblum fills 495 pages with erudite knowledge but gives no details of the authors of the eponymous diseases it lists. In attempting to fulfil the brief presented to him, the author has tried to steer a middle course.

Eponymous diseases have proliferated, especially in the genetic field. It is often of interest to the reader to know the provenance of some of the diseases so described but where several names are conjoined it has not always been possible to establish this with the accuracy the author would have wished.

Acronyms form an increasingly common private language for those engaged in any branch of science and technology. Though the art of dermatology is still best spelled out in words, it is understandable that its technology should be expressed in acronyms. It would, however, be out of place to attempt to include all of these coined short-cuts of communication in this glossary. Like all forms of jargon, their use is subject to changing fashion and any selection is bound to be incomplete. It is hoped that all those in most frequent use have been included.

There will inevitably be a number of omissions relating to new syndromes. Several of these have been omitted for reasons of space and prudence. It is easy to create a syndrome and to call it a disease, but its acceptance as such depends on the judgement of time.

Changes in current edition

There has been no change in the principles or format, though it has been considerably enlarged. It continues to be based, necessarily, on the contents and index of the preceding edition, with the addition of such new material as has been provided. Most of the new entries are concerned with 20th-century authors and their syndromes. Again, only names with such eponymous links are included, thus omitting, with regret, many prominent dermatologists of this and previous centuries.

Some errors in attribution or dates have been corrected but, despite every effort to establish these accurately, a few remain uncertain or unfilled. The number of acronyms continues to increase. For reasons of space, those which relate to immunological terms and inflammatory mediators have been excluded; they will be familiar enough to those working in these fields and are adequately explained in the relevant chapters.

There has been some debate recently both on the misuse of the term 'syndrome' and on the language of eponyms, particularly the use of the possessive genitive. The matter is still open and the author has taken a pragmatic and empirical line based on common usage at the present time. Though still commonly used in many parts of the world, eponyms are becoming displaced in the Anglo-Saxon countries and the situation may have become very different in another five years.

Notes on the text

Definitions

The definitions are for the most part based on those used in the textbook. The author takes responsibility for any errors that may have resulted from the need to keep them as short as possible. When a particular definition requires elaboration, a reference is given to the appropriate source. In some cases a term is of sufficient interest also to merit a numbered reference, but these have been kept to a minimum for reasons of space.

Other definitions have been taken from the *Glossary of Dermatology Lesions* and are appropriately indicated.

Derivations

The genitive case of Greek and Latin derivations is usually given after the nominative as a better indication of the root from which the medical term stems.

Occasional reference is made to the early classical medical writers when these authors have employed a particular term in a specific medical sense that may not be reflected in the general classical literature.

Where a word has an African or Caribbean origin, it has sometimes been necessary to give a local dialect or patois; in those deriving from the Arabic, the transliteration must be approximate.

Eponyms

It has at times been difficult to establish accurately the specialty in which authors of eponymous diseases practised. In much of the 19th century, before dermatology became established in its own right, these authors would have been physicians, surgeons or pathologists. Others described dermatological syndromes early in their careers and then changed course. In recent decades, the difficulties have stemmed from the proliferation of special interests within dermatology (and paediatrics) and it is sometimes impossible to determine whether an author is, for instance, a paediatric dermatologist, a paediatrician, a geneticist or a dermatologist with an interest in genetics.

Etymology

Information on the derivation of a word is given in brackets and in italics after the meaning. Where the word or its combining form is more closely related to the stem, the genitive case is given after the nominative.

Transliteration of Greek characters follows traditional lines. Most letters remain the same; the exceptions are as follows:

‘ (rough breathing) = h
γγ = ng
γξ = nx
γχ = nk
ζ = Z
η = ē
θ = th
κ = k,c
ξ = x
ou = u
ρ = rh when initial letter
ρρ = rrh in compounds
υ = y
φ = ph
χ = ch (hard pronunciation)
ψ = ps
ω = ō

Abbreviations

AD = Anno Domini
BC = before Christ
Fr = French
Gk = Greek
L = Latin
LL = Late Latin (3rd–6th cent.)
Med L = Medieval Latin (7th–15th cent.)
ME = Middle English (*c.* 1150–1500)
New L = New Latin (16th cent.–)
OE = Old English (5th cent.–*c.* 1150)
OF = Old French
OHG = Old High German

a-priv. = *a*-privative
adj. = adjective
b. = born
c. = circa
Cels = Celsus
cent. = century
cf. = compare (L *confer*)
colloq. = colloquial
comb. form = combining form

dim. = diminutive
e.g. = for example (L *exempli gratia*)
et al. = and others (L *et alia*)
etc. = et cetera
fl. = flourished, active in
Gal = Galen
Hipp = Hippocrates
irreg. = irregular
lit. = literally
N = North, Northern
obs. = obsolete
OED = *Oxford English Dictionary*
orig. = originally
part. = participle
pl. = plural
pref. = prefix
pres. = present
q.v. = refer to (L *quod vide*)
S = South, Southern
sing. = singular
sp. = species
suff. = suffix
US = United States
USA = United States of America

The glossary

a-, an- pref. privative in sense of lack of or removal of term; opposite to (L *privatio*, from *privare* to deprive), e.g. *a*sepsis but not *an*aphylaxis.

Aarskog DJ Norwegian paediatrician *fl.* 20th cent.

Aarskog's syndrome faciodigitogenital syndrome; orofaciodigital dysostosis.

Abriskosov (Abriskossoff) AI Russian pathologist 1875–1955.

Abriskosov's tumour granular cell myoblastoma.

abscedens ('et suffodiens') as of perifolliculitis capitis. Decayed material separating from sound tissue; abscess-forming (L pres. part. *abscedere* depart, fall away).

abscess a localized collection of pus in a cavity formed by disintegration or necrosis of tissues [1]. (L *abscessus* abscess [Cels], from past part. of *abscedere* to go away, form an abscess.)

acantho- comb. form indicating spine or thorn (Gk *akantha* thorn).

acantholysis separation of epidermal keratinocytes by loss of their intercellular connections causing the cells to become round and hyaline [1] (Gk *akantha* thorn, *lysis* loosening).

acanthosis increase in prickle-cell layer of skin (Gk *akantha* thorn, prickle).

Acarus genus of small MITE in family Arachnidae (New L from Gk *akari* a kind of mite, from *akarēs* tiny).

ACE Angiotensin Converting Enzyme.

Achard EC French physician 1860–1944. Coined the term 'paratyphoid fever'.

Achard-Thiers syndrome diabetes mellitus and hirsutism in postmenopausal women. An ill-defined entity.

Achenbach W German physician *fl.* 20th cent.

Achenbach's syndrome paroxysmal haematoma of the finger.

acne term properly used for a chronic inflammatory disease of the pilosebaceous follicles, showing a keratinous plug; variously qualified, but commonly referring to acne vulgaris. Derivation obscure. *Aknas* first used by Aëtius *c.* 542 AD, but origin of term unknown. '*Acmas*' (Cassius, 3rd cent. AD) refers to spots appearing at *akmē* puberty, prime. Or perhaps from Gk *achnē* something coming from the surface, chaff or from *a-knēsis* a coined term for not itching. See [2] for full account.

acnitis little-used term for acne agminata or pustular form of lupus miliaris disseminatus faciei. A slowly resolving facial eruption of unknown aetiology (ACNE, *itis*).

acro- comb. form meaning tip, extremity or top (Gk *akros* outermost, extreme).

acrochordon skin tag (Gk *akro(s)* tip, *chordē* string, cord).

acrodynia pink disease (Gk *akro(s)* at extremities, *odynē* pain, *ia*).

acrogeria a syndrome of premature ageing predominantly affecting the extremities of the skin (Gk *akro(s)* tip, *gero(n)* old).

acrokeratosis hyperkeratosis affecting the extremities (Gk *akro(s)* tip, *keras, keratos* horn, *osis*).

acrokeratoelastoidosis horny papules on borders of hands and feet showing dermal elastic tissue changes (Gk *akro(s)* outermost, *keras, keratos* horn, *elast* Epic Aorist *elassa*, from *elaunein* to drive on, *oid*).

acromegaly hypertrophy of skin, subcutaneous tissue and bone affecting the extremities caused by increased secretion of growth hormone in adults (Gk *akro(s)* tip, *megalo-* great).

acropathy a disease or injury of the extremities (Gk *akro(s)* tip, *pathos* suffering, hence disease).

actinic pertaining to rays or beams of light (Gk *aktis, aktinos* ray).

actino- comb. form relating to effect of light (Gk *aktis, aktinos* ray).

actinomycosis a chronic suppurative infection of man and animals due to a species of *Actinomyces*. Ray-fungus disease (Gk *aktis, aktinos* ray, *mykēs* fungus).

acuminate sharp, pointed (L *acuminatus* pointed, sharpened).

acupuncture originally Oriental, a method of treating disease, relieving pain or inducing anaesthesia by the insertion of needles at specified body points (L *acus* needle, L *punctum* a prick, puncture, from past part. *pungere* to prick).

Adams PH US paediatrician *fl.* 20th cent.

Adams-Oliver syndrome congenital scalp defects with distal limb anomalies.

ADCC Antibody-Dependent Cell-mediated Cytotoxicity.

Addison T British physician and 'demonstrator of cutaneous diseases' 1793–1860. Described 'true keloid' and xanthelasmata. See KELOID.

Addison's disease, syndrome adrenocortical insufficiency syndrome.

Addison's keloid obs. thought now to have been morphoea.

aden(o)- comb. form meaning gland (Gk *adēn, adenos* gland).

ADI Autosomal Dominant Ichthyosis.

Adie WJ British neurologist 1886–1935. HOLMES-ADIE SYNDROME.

adiposis obesity, fat deposition (L *adeps* fat, *osis*).

adrenarche onset of increased adrenocortical secretion ushering in puberty (L *ad-ren*, compound word from *renes* kidney; Gk *archē* beginning).

AEC Ankyloblepharon, Ectodermal defects, Cleft lip and palate.

aestivalis, -e pertaining to summer (L *aestivalis* summer).

Aëtius Amidenus (Medicus) Greek physician b. Mesopotamia early 6th cent. AD. Court physician at Byzantium. Wrote a 16-volume medical work. First to use terms '*ekzemata*' and '*aknae*'.

agminata clustered lesions (adj. from L *agmen, agminis* group).

AIDS *A*cquired *I*mmuno*D*eficiency *S*yndrome.

ainhum spontaneous separation of digit by constricting fibrous band. Dactylolysis spontanea (Portuguese, from Yoruba Nigerian *eyon, in-yoon* to saw).

AIP *A*cute *I*ntermittent *P*orphyria.

Aird RB US neurologist *fl.* 20th cent. FLYNN-AIRD SYNDROME.

AKE *A*cro*K*erato*E*lastoidosis.

-al, -ale, -alis Gk, suff. meaning relating to, process of (L-*alis*).

ALA δ-*A*mino*L*aevulinic *A*cid.

albinism congenital hypopigmentation of skin, hair and eyes (Portuguese *albino*, from L *albus* white).

Albright F US endocrinologist 1900–69. One of the founders of modern endocrinology.

Albright's syndrome pigmentation of the skin with monostotic or polyostotic fibrous dysplasia.

Aldous HE US surgeon *fl.* 20th cent. WOOLF-DOLOWITZ-ALDOUS SYNDROME.

Aldrich RA US paediatrician *fl.* 20th cent. WISKOTT-ALDRICH SYNDROME.

Alezzandrini AA Argentinian ophthalmologist *fl.* 20th cent.

Alezzandrini's syndrome unilateral retinitis, ipsilateral poliosis and vitiligo; occasional deafness

-algia suff. state of pain (Gk *algos* pain).

algodystrophy reflex sympathetic syndrome (Gk *algo*(s) pain, *dys, trophē* nurture; faulty nourishment, maldevelopment).

Alibert JL, Baron founder of French dermatology 1768–1837. 'Family tree' of dermatoses. Described mycosis fungoides.

Alibert's cheloid see CHELOID.

alkaptonuria an inborn error of tyrosine metabolism leading to deposition of oxidized homogentisic acid in fibrous and cartilaginous tissue and characterized by dark urine (*al*, from Arabic *alqaliy* soda ash; Gk *kaptein* to suck up greedily, consume, *ouron* urine).

allelo- pref. reciprocal, mutual (Gk *allelōn* genitive pl. from reduplication of *allos* of one another).

allergy originally 'altered immunological reactivity to antigens' (von Pirquet (q.v.) 1906); now **1** immune response in a primed or sensitized individual (synonym immunity) or **2** exaggerated immune response which, when harmful, causes allergic disorders [3] (Gk *allos* other, *ergon* work).

alloknesis intense itching caused by mechanical stimulation of the skin (Gk *allos* other, different, *knēsis* scratching, rubbing).

allotrichia a term used to describe a specific type of change in the character of the hair (Gk *allo*(s) other, *thrix, trichos* hair).

alopecia loss of hair from normally hairy regions of the body; hair-fall. In common usage, loss of hair from the scalp for any of several causes (Gk *alōpekia* a disease like the mange of foxes; bald patches, from *alōpēx, alōpekis* fox).

Alström CH Swedish psychiatrist 1907–94.

Alström's syndrome congenital amaurosis and retinal degeneration, infantile obesity, deafness, insulin-dependent diabetes mellitus, renal dysfunction and other defects.

ambi- pref. both (L *ambo* both).

ameloblastoma a benign but locally invasive tumour of the odontogenic epithelium (OF *amel* enamel, *blastoma*, Gk *blastos* germ, seed, *oma*).

amelogenesis dental enamel formation (Anglo-French *amel*, from Fr *émail* enamel, Gk *genesis* origin, generation).

amiantacea (pityriasis) name given to a condition in which soft, asbestos-like scales adhere to scalp hairs (Gk *amiantos* undefiled; *amiantos lithos* asbestos stone).

amniocentesis puncturing the amniotic sac as prenatal diagnostic procedure (Gk *amnion* inner membrane round the fetus, *kentēsis*, from *kentein* to prick, puncture).

amphi- pref. about, on both sides (Gk *amphis* on both sides).

amphoteric partaking of both characters of properties, equally balanced (Gk *amphoteros* comparative of *ampho* both).

amyloid a complex proteinaceous substance with a distinctive fibrillar ultrastructure and characteristic physiochemical properties (Gk *amylon* starch and *oid* starch-like).

ana- pref. up, back, again (Gk *ana* up, upwards, throughout).

anamnesis clinical history obtained from the patient (Gk *ana* back, *mnēsis* calling to mind).

anaphylaxis allergic reaction in which antigen releases mediators from antibody-sensitized mast cells or basophils (Gk *ana* back, *phylaxis* guard, protection, from *phylassein* to keep watch; hence reversed protection).

ANCA *A*nti*N*eutrophil *C*ytoplasmic *A*ntibody.

Anderson W British surgeon and dermatologist 1842–1900.

Anderson–Fabry disease angiokeratoma corporis diffusum.

Åndrä A German faciomaxillary surgeon *fl.* 20th cent. SANDMANN–ANDRÄ SYNDROME.

anetoderma macular atrophy of the skin; slack skin (Gk *anetos* slack, as of a bow, *derma* skin).

ANG *A*cute *N*ectrotizing *G*ingivitis.

angio- comb. form meaning blood vessels (Gk *angeion* vessel, blood vessel [Gal]).

angiodyskinesia term coined for condition of disordered blood vessel function (Gk *angeion* blood vessel, *dyskinēsia* difficulty in moving [Hipp], from *dys* difficult, *kinēsis* motion).

angiokeratoma a vascular lesion combining ectasia of dermal blood vessels with hyperkeratosis (Gk *angeion* blood vessel, *keras, keratos,* horn, *oma*).

angiolupoid a rare form of sarcoidosis consisting of a soft, reddish hemispherical nodule with a marked vascular component.

anhidrosis lack of sweating (Gk *a*-priv., *hidrōs* sweat).

aniline (phenylamine) an organic base first obtained from indigo in 1826 and from coal residue in 1834, so named by Fritzsche in 1841 (Sanskrit *nili* indigo, Arabic *an-nil* the indigo plant).

ankyloblepharon fusion of eyelid margins (Gk *ankylos* crooked, bent, *blepharon* eyelid).

ankyrin a cytoskeletal protein on the inner surface of the plasma membrane, serving as an anchorage (Gk *ankyra* anchor).

anorexia lack of desire for food (Gk *an*-priv., *orexis* yearning, desiring, *ia*).

ANOTHER syndrome *A*lopecia, *N*ail dystrophy, *O*phthalmic complications, *T*hyroid dysfunction, *H*ypohidrosis, *E*phelides and *E*nteropathy and *R*espiratory tract infections.

ante- pref. before in time, order or position (L *ante* before).

anthrax acute infective zoonosis of herbivorous animals, sometimes transmitted to man (L *anthrax*, from Gk *anthrax* charcoal, hence carbuncle, a dark red stone, or boil, malignant pustule [Hipp]).

anthropophilic preferring humans as host, thriving on or benefiting from human environment (Gk *anthrōpos* man, *philos* loving, dear to, cf. philanthropic, loving mankind).

anti- pref. against, opposite to, counteracting (Gk *anti* against).

APECED *A*utoimmune *P*oly*E*ndocrinopathy-*C*andidiasis-*E*ctodermal *D*ystrophy syndrome.

Apert E French paediatrician 1868–1940.

Apert–Crouzon syndrome acrocephalosyndactyly Type II.

Apert's syndrome acrocephalosyndactyly Type I.

aphthae painful ulcers of the mucosae, often multiple and recurrent (Gk *aphtha* an eruption in the mouth [Hipp]).

aplasia failure or lack of growth or development (Gk *a*-priv., *plasis* a forming, shaping).

apo- pref. to indicate separate, derived from, formed from (Gk *apo* away, from).

apocrine relating to a gland or secretion containing separated cellular material (Gk *apo* from, *crinein* to separate).

APOD *Acute Papular OnchoDermatitis.*

apoptosis a type of cell degeneration and death in which keratinocytes become homogeneous and eosinophilic (Gk *apo* away from, *ptōsis* a falling).

APUD *Amine Precursor Uptake Decarboxylase.* Designation for group of cells in different organs secreting polypeptide hormones.

aquagenic caused by contact with water (L *aqua* water, Gk *genos*, *genikos* producing, creating).

arachnidism reaction to bites of venomous members of Arachnida, especially spiders (Gk *arachnēs* spider).

arachnodactyly increased length of fingers and toes, from resemblance to spider's legs (Gk *arachnēs* spider, *dactylos* finger).

arborizing branching ramification, as of a tree's branching, especially of superficial blood vessels; arborizing telangiectasia (L *arbor* tree).

argyria ashen-grey discoloration of the skin and conjunctivae, resulting from chronic exposure to silver or its salts (Gk *argyros* silver).

-aria suff. forming generic and group names (New L from L *-arias*).

Arthus NM French physiologist 1862–1945.

Arthus phenomenon, reaction the formation of tissue-damaging complexes by injection of antigen into sensitized animals or man combining with antibody at the site. The mechanism of immune complex diseases.

Ascher KW Czech-born US ophthalmologist 1887–1971.

Ascher's syndrome blepharochalasis with progressive hypertrophy of upper lip.

-asma suff., as English *ism*.

-ato suff. indicating state of, pertaining to.

atopy state of excessive formation of IgE antibody following exposure to common environmental allergens (Pepys 1975) (Gk *a*-priv., *topos* place, out of place, strange) [3].

ATP *Autoimmune (idiopathic) Thrombocytopenic Purpura.*

atrichia absence of hair (Gk *a*-priv., *thrix*, *trichos* hair). Atrichial also describes cutaneous glands unrelated to hair follicles.

atrophoderma of Pasini and Pierini see PASINI AND PIERINI

atrophy a wasting, shrinkage, diminution or lack of tissue (Gk *atrophia*, from *a*-priv., *trophē* nourishment, nurture).

Audouin JG French entomologist and parasitologist 1794–1841. *Microsporon audouinii.*

Auspitz H Austrian dermatologist 1835–86.

Auspitz sign evocation of a glistening red membrane and punctate haemorrhages on removal of successive psoriatic scales.

Bacillus Calmette–Guérin CALMETTE–GUÉRIN BACILLUS.

Bäfverstedt BE Swedish dermatologist 1905–90.

Bäfverstedt's ichthyosis a form of ichthyosis hystrix.

Bäfverstedt's syndrome benign lymphocytoma cutis.

Baker WM British surgeon 1839–96.

Baker's cyst ('Morrant Baker's cyst') a synovial-lined cyst in popliteal fossa; popliteal bursitis.

balanitis inflammation of glans penis (or glans clitoris). Loosely but incorrectly used for balanoposthitis (Gk *balano*(s) acorn, glans penis [Gal]).

balanoposthitis inflammation of glans penis and prepuce (Gk *balano*(s) glans penis, *posthē* prepuce).

balm an aromatic substance with soothing or healing powers (corruption of BALSAM).

balm of Gilead (Mecca balsam) an ancient substance with mystical attributions for healing. Commonly, from *Commiphora opobalsamum*, a tree near the Red Sea, later grown on Mount Gilead. In the USA applied to buds of *Populus candicans* and related sp., but exact nature disputed. Also applied to an ulcer dressing of honey and butter or of sugar, polyethylene glycol and hydrogen peroxide—'sugar paste'. (ME *baume*, from L *balsumum* resin of balsam tree, Gilead, a luxuriant area in Judea between the river Jordan and the desert plateau.)

balsam properly, a resin or oleoresin containing benzoic or cinnamic acid or both but commonly applied to a variety of fragrant resins found in various tropical and subtropical trees (Gk *balsamon*, prob. from Hebrew *borsmin* 'chief of oils' or *bāsām* spice).

balsam of Peru mixture of volatile oil and resin obtained from *Myroxylon pereirae*, originally from El Salvador and so-named when this country belonged to the Peruvian Viceroy.

balsam of Tolu obtained from *Myroxylon balsamum*, originally from Santiago de Tolu in Columbia.

Bannayan GA US pathologist *fl.* 20th cent.

Bannayan–Zonana syndrome macrocephaly, multiple lipomas and haemangiomas.

Baraitser M British paediatrician *fl.* 20th cent.

Baraitser's syndrome 1 premature ageing with short stature and pigmented naevi; 2 almost total alopecia of all sites with mental and physical retardation.

Barcoo rot parochial name for pyodermatous ulceration. Desert or Veld sore. Named after a river in Queensland, Australia.

Barlow, Sir Thomas, Bart British physician 1845–1945.

Barlow's disease infantile scurvy.

Barmah forest virus a togavirus infection, so named from a forest in Queensland, Australia.

Barr ML Canadian histologist b. 1908.

Barr body X-chromatin; sex chromatin.

Barr YM British virologist *fl.* 20th cent. EPSTEIN–BARR VIRUS.

Barraquer Roviralta, L Spanish neurologist *fl.* early 20th cent.

Barraquer-Simons disease partial lipoatrophy, partial lipodystrophy.

Barrière H French dermatologist 1921–89. BUREAU–BARRIÈRE SYNDROME.

Bart BJ US dermatologist *fl.* 20th cent.

Bart's syndrome localized absence of skin, blistering and nail abnormalities, resembling epidermolysis bullosa.

Bart RS US dermatologist *fl.* 20th cent.

Bart–Pumphrey syndrome knuckle pads, leuconychia and deafness.

Bartholin C secundus Danish anatomist 1655–1738. One of a distinguished Copenhagen family of physicians, physicists and philosophers.

Bartholin's duct major sublingual duct arising in anterior pair of sublingual glands.

Bartholin's gland greater vestibular gland.

Barton AL Peruvian physician 1871–1950.

Barton's syndrome Bartonellosis.

Bartonella genus of small Gram-negative bacilli that parasitize red blood cells.

Bartonellosis (synonyms Carrion's disease, Oroya fever, verruga peruana) infection with *Bartonella baccilliformis* transmitted by the sand fly, occurring in Peru, Colombia and Ecuador.

Basan M German dermatologist *fl*. 20th cent.

Basan's syndrome a form of ectodemal dysplasia with dryness of skin, mouth and vulva, hypohidrosis, dental caries, sparse hair and nail ridging.

basidiobolomycosis disease caused by a genus of fungus causing subcutaneous phycomycosis (New L *basidium*, dim. of Gk *basis* a base and *idium*, diminishing suff. *bolo-*, from Gk *bōlus* a clod of earth, lump, *mykēs* fungus). Refers to club-like distal surface bearing basidiospores.

Bateman T one of the pioneers of British dermatology 1778–1821. Pupil of Willan (q.v.) and compiler of his works.

Bateman's purpura senile purpura.

Bazex A French dermatologist 1911–88.

Bazex syndrome 1 follicular atrophoderma and basal-cell carcinomata; **2** paraneoplastic acrokeratosis; **3** benign circinate pityriasiform erythema of childhood.

Bazin APE French dermatologist 1807–78. One of the great figures of 19th-century dermatology. Pioneered cutaneous parasitology.

Bazin's disease (tuberculous) erythema induratum affecting legs of young women.

BBS sarcoidosis (Besnier–Boeck–Schaumann disease).

BCG CALMETTE–GUÉRIN BACILLUS.

Beals RK US orthopaedic surgeon *fl*. 20th cent.

Beals–Hecht syndrome contractural arachnodactyly.

Beau JHS French physician 1806–65.

Beau's lines transverse depressions on the nails following acute illnesses or debilitating medical events.

Becker SW US dermatologist 1894–1964.

Becker's naevus (synonym naevus spilus tardus) pigmented epidermal hairy naevus.

Becker's syndrome familial, discrete or confluent brown macules on neck, forearms or elsewhere.

Beckwith JB US paediatric pathologist *fl*. 20th cent.

Beckwith–Wiedemann syndrome (synonym EMG syndrome) exophthalmos, macroglossia and gigantism.

Bednář B Czechoslovakian pathologist *fl*. 20th cent.

Bednář tumour a form of dermatofibrosarcoma protuberans containing melanin.

Behçet H (Bēhchet) Turkish dermatologist 1889–1948.

Behçet's syndrome triple complex syndrome of recurrent ulceration of mouth and genitalia, and iritis. Pyoderma may occur and central nervous system and other organs may be involved.

bejel form of endemic nonvenereal syphilis similar to yaws and due to *Treponema pallidum* (Arabic *bajlak* syphilis).

Bence-Jones H British physician 1814–73.

Bence-Jones protein a low-molecular-weight protein found in urine of patients with myeloma.

Berardinelli W Argentinian physician 1903–56.

Berardinelli syndrome see LAWRENCE–SEIP SYNDROME.

beriberi a nutritional deficiency disease due to lack of thiamin and other B vitamins (Singhalese *beri* weak, *beriberi* extreme weakness).

Berlin C Israeli dermatologist *fl*. 20th cent.

Berlin syndrome stunted growth, mental retardation, 'leopard skin' and other anomalies.

berlock obs. term for berloque (German *berlocke*).

berloque dermatitis, a streaky form of pigmented contact photo-dermatitis, usually seen in the neck but occasionally elsewhere, due to psoralens, as in bergamot oil in perfume (Fr *berloque* or *breloque* a pendant, something hanging from a chain; origin uncertain).

Besnier E French dermatologist 1831–1909. A leading dermatologist of late 19th cent. Successor to Bazin (q.v.). First description of sarcoidosis (lupus pernio) 1889.

Besnier–Boeck Schaumann disease sarcoidosis.

Besnier's prurigo flexural form of atopic dermatitis.

BIDS Brittle hair, Impaired intelligence, Decreased fertility, Short stature.

BIE Bullous Ichthyosiform Erythroderma.

Bier AKG German physician 1861–1949.

Bier's spots red or white spots occurring on the cyanotic congestion caused by occlusion of a tourniquet, or occasionally in those with a perniotic circulation. A physiological phenomenon.

Biett LT Swiss-born French dermatologist 1784–1840. 'The father of lupus erythematosus.'

Biett's collar (collarette) ring of scales around papules of secondary syphilis.

Bilharz TM German parasitologist 1825–62.

Bilharzia (sis) schistosomiasis.

Birbeck MSC British research biologist *fl*. 20th cent.

Birbeck granules rod-shaped trilaminate cytoplasmic organelles, a specific feature of LANGERHANS' CELLS.

Birt AR Canadian dermatologist 1906–95.

Birt–Hogg–Dubé syndrome fibrofolliculomas, trichodiscomas and acrochordons.

Bixler D US oral surgeon and geneticist *fl*. 20th cent.

Bixler syndrome hyperteleorism, meatal atresia and facial clefting.

Björnstad RT Norwegian dermatologist *fl*. 20th cent.

Björnstad syndrome pili torti with sensorineural deafness.

B-K mole syndrome dysplastic naevus syndrome. (Named after initials of first two patients in whom the condition was recorded.)

blackthorn the prickly shrub or small tree *Prunus spinosa* (L sloe).

Blanc E French ophthalmologist 1901–52. BONNET–DECHAUME–BLANC SYNDROME.

Blandford fly *Simulium posticatum*, widely distributed in Europe, found near rivers in Oxfordshire and Dorset in the UK. Named after Blandford Forum, Dorset.

Blaschko A German venereologist, leprologist and scientist 1858–1922.

Blaschko's lines a system of skin markers represented by the pattern of systemized naevi. Unrelated to any known anatomical system, they have been interpreted as the result of tissue mosaicism [4].

blasto- comb. form meaning bud, germ; relating to early growth (Gk *blastos* sprout, germ). Hence blastomycosis, blastospore, etc.

Blau EB US paediatrician *fl*. 20th cent.

Blau's syndrome familial granulomatous arthritis, uveitis and skin granulomas.

blenorrhagia urethral flow or conjunctival mucoid discharge (Gk *blenna* [Hipp] mucous matter, *errhagēn* passive aorist of *rhēgnymi* to burst forth).

blepharitis inflammation of the eyelid (Gk *blephar(on)* eyelid, *itis*).

blepharochalasis drooping or sagging of upper eyelids (Gk *blephar(on)* eyelid, *chalasis* slackening, loosening).

Blizzard RM US paediatrician *fl.* 20th cent. JOHANSON–BLIZZARD SYNDROME.

Bloch B Swiss dermatologist 1878–1933.

Bloch–Sulzberger, Bloch–Siemens syndrome incontinentia pigmenti.

Bloom D Polish-born US dermatologist 1892–1985.

Bloom's syndrome congenital telangiectatic erythema and stunted growth.

blueberry-muffin baby (BMB) neonatal foci of dermal erythropoiesis seen in congenital rubella or other congenital infections. From resemblance of the purple-red colour to the American blueberry, *Vaccinium corymbosum* or *angustifolium*.

Blum P French dermatologist 1878–1933. GOUGEROT–BLUM SYNDROME.

Bockenheimer P German surgeon 1875–1933.

Bockenheimer's syndrome diffuse phlebectasia.

Bockhart M German dermatologist 1831–97.

Bockhart's impetigo superficial staphylococcal follicular pustules.

Boeck CPM Norwegian dermatologist 1845–1917. Outstanding diagnostician and teacher. Studied tuberculosis and designated sarcoidosis.

Boeck's sarcoid sarcoidosis.

boil colloq. term for furuncle (ME *bile*, OE *byl*).

Bonnet P French ophthalmologist 1884–1959.

Bonnet–Dechaume–Blanc syndrome unilateral retinocephalic arteriovenous malformation similar to WYBURN–MASON SYNDROME.

Böök JA (Booek) Swedish geneticist *fl.* 20th cent.

Böök's syndrome hyperhidrosis, premature canities and premolar aplasia.

Borrel A French bacteriologist 1867–1936.

Borrelia genus of spirochaete named after Borrel. A cause of endemic relapsing fever and the cause of LYME DISEASE.

Borst M German pathologist 1869–1946.

Borst-Jadassohn phenomenon localised intraepidermal foci of abnormal, immature or foreign cells in a whorled pattern. No longer regarded as an entity or of especial diagnostic significance.

Boston exanthem due to infection with echovirus 16. Named after town in Massachusetts, USA (Gk *exanthema* pustule, eruption).

botryomycosis a chronic granulomatous reaction resembling actinomycosis affecting horses, cattle, camels and, rarely man and due to infection with *Staphylococci, Pseudomonas* or other organisms. *Botryomycome* is a French term for *pyogenic granuloma* (Gk *botrys* a cluster or bunch of grapes, *mykēs* fungus).

Bourneville DM French neurologist 1840–1909.

Bourneville–Pringle syndrome tuberous sclerosis; epiloia.

Bowen JT US dermatologist 1857–1940.

Bowen's disease precancerous dermatosis; a form of carcinoma *in situ*.

Branham HH US surgeon 1862–1936.

Branham's sign slowing of the heart rate on compression of arteriovenous fistula.

branny desquamation of small scales of skin (OF *bran, bren* husk of grain, perhaps Celtic).

Brauer A German dermatologist 1883–1945. BUSCHKE–FISCHER–BRAUER SYNDROME.

Brauer's syndrome familial focal facial dermal dysplasia.

Brearley LJ US oral surgeon *fl.* 20th cent. WITKOP–BREARLEY–GENTRY SYNDROME.

Brégeat P French ophthalmologist 1909–89.

Brégeat's syndrome oculo-orbital-thalamo-encephalic angiomatosis.

Briquet P French psychiatrist 1796–1881. Wrote important monograph on hysteria.

Briquet's syndrome a chronic factitious disorder of young persons resembling MÜNCHHAUSEN'S SYNDROME but of an hysterical not consciously deceptive nature; also, syndrome of hysterical dyspnoea, often with dysphonia.

Brill NE US physician 1860–1925.

Brill–Symmers disease nodular lymphosarcoma.

Brill–Zinsser disease sporadic typhus; recrudescence of symptoms of endemic typhus, often after several years.

Brocq LAJ French dermatologist 1856–1928. An astute observer who made immense contributions to dermatological literature. DUHRING–BROCQ DISEASE, pseudopelade, lupoid sycosis, etc.

Brocq's erythrose peribuccale pigmentaire pigmented peribuccal erythema predominantly affecting middle-aged women (Gk *erythros* red).

Brodie, Sir Benjamin C British surgeon 1783–1862.

Brodie-Trendelenburg test a clinical manoeuvre to detect venous incompetence in the leg.

bromhidrosis foul-smelling sweat, usually of axillary apocrine origin (Gk *brōmos* stench, especially of beasts at rut; *hidrōs* sweat, *osis*).

Brooke HAG British dermatologist 1854–1919. Pioneered dermatology in Midlands; 'Brooke of Manchester'. Noted for his wit. Described keratosis follicularis contagiosa.

Brooke's tumour trichoepithelioma, epithelioma adenoides cysticum.

Brown Kelly A British laryngologist 1865–1941. PATERSON–BROWN KELLY SYNDROME.

Bruch KBWL German anatomist 1819–84.

Bruch's membrane (layer) basal lamina complex of choroid, the thin innermost layer of the choroid proper.

Brushfield T British ophthalmologist 1858–1937.

Brushfield's spots white or yellowish spots in concentric rings on anterior iris, seen commonly in fair-eyed patients with DOWN SYNDROME.

Bruton OC US paediatrician b. 1908.

Bruton's disease infantile sex-linked hypogammaglobulinaemia.

buba madre mamanpian, mother yaws. The primary stage of yaws (Spanish *buba* pustule, *madre* mother).

bubo obs. term for a swollen inflamed lymphatic gland, especially in neck, axilla or groin (Late L *bubo* swelling, from Gk *boubōn* groin). Swellings especially in groins as in the plague (first described in England 1398).

Buckley RH US paediatrician and allergist *fl.* 20th cent.

Buckley's syndrome hyperimmunoglobulin E syndrome, 'Job's dermatitis'.

Bucky GP German-born US radiologist 1880–1963.

Bucky rays Grenz rays; soft X-rays.

Buehler EV US immunologist and toxicologist *fl.* 20th cent.

Buehler test a test procedure for delayed contact hypersensitivity in the guinea pig.

Buerger L Austrian-born US urological surgeon 1879–1943.

Buerger's disease thromboangiitis obliterans.

bulla colloq. term for bleb, blister. An elevated lesion of the skin containing fluid and over 0.5 cm diameter (arbitrary) (L *bulla* a bubble) [1].

bulimia insatiable appetite for food. Usually applied to eating disorder ('binge eating') leading to abdominal pain and vomiting (Gk *bulimia* ravenous hunger, from *bous* ox, *limos* hunger, *ia*).

bulleetus round or oval bodies sometimes inserted under the skin of the penis in the Far East (Phillipino ball-bearing).

Bunnell WW US physician 1902–66. PAUL–BUNNELL TEST.

Bureau Y French dermatologist 1900–93.

Bureau–Barrière syndrome ulcerating and mutilating trophic lesions of the lower limbs and feet ('acropathie ulcero-mutilante').

Burkitt DP British physician active in Uganda 1911–93.

Burkitt's tumour African lymphoma. A malignant lymphoma affecting extranodal sites and caused by the EPSTEIN–BARR VIRUS.

Burnet, Sir Frank Macfarlane Australian virologist and immunologist 1899–1985. Nobel prize-winner. Discoverer of *Coxiella burnetii*.

Burow KA German surgeon 1809–74.

Burow's solution aluminium acetate, frequently used as wet dressings.

Burow's paste (1, 2, 3 Paste) a mixture of Burow's solution, lanolin and zinc paste.

burrow a cuniculus, passage or tunnel in the skin that houses a metazoal parasite, particularly the acarus of scabies [1] (origin obscure; perhaps variant of *borough*, from OE *burg* fortress, from *beorgan* to shelter, protect).

bursa a closed sac lined by synovial membrane and containing fluid (Late L *bursa*, from Gk *byrsa*, skin stripped off, a hide).

Buruli ulcer mycobacterium ulcerans infection, named after an area of the Nile valley in Uganda.

Buschke A Polish-born German dermatologist 1868–1943.

Buschke–Fischer–Brauer syndrome punctate (disseminate) keratoderma.

Buschke–Loewenstein tumour giant condyloma acuminatum.

Buschke–Ollendorf syndrome disseminate lenticular dermatofibrosis, connective tissue naevus of skin and osteopoikilosis.

Buschke's syndrome scleroedema adultorum, originally described by Piffard in 1876.

Busse OEFU German pathologist 1867–1922.

Busse–Buschke disease (synonyms torulosis, European blastomycosis, BUSCHKE'S SYNDROME) cryptococcosis.

Buzzi F German dermatologist *fl.* late 19th cent. SCHWENINGER–BUZZI ANETODERMA.

B virus *Herpesvirus simiae*, an herpetic eruption transmitted by Macaca monkeys.

Bwamba fever a bunyaviral infection named after Bwamba, an area in Western Uganda.

Bywaters EGL British physician and rheumatologist *fl.* 20th cent.

Bywaters' lesion infarctive vasculitic lesion of pulp of fingers or nail folds characteristic of rheumatoid arthritis but also seen in other forms of small-vessel vasculitis.

Cacchione A Italian physician *fl.* 20th cent. DE SANCTIS–CACCHIONE SYNDROME.

cacoguesia unpleasant taste in the mouth (Gk *kako(s)* bad, *geusis* taste).

Calabar swellings shifting oedematous swellings seen in loiasis. Named after town in Nigeria.

calciphylaxis induction of systemic or localized deposits of calcium following challenge of hypersensitive host (L *calx, calcis* lime, Gk *phylaxis*, a guarding, watching).

callus hyperplasia of the stratum corneum (keratoderma) due to physical pressure (L *callus* [Cels] hardened skin) [1].

Calmette LCA French bacteriologist 1863–1933. Pupil of Pasteur.

Calmette–Guérin bacillus (synonyms BCG vaccine, Calmette vaccine) an avirulent strain of *Mycobacterium bovis* with diminished pathogenicity.

cAMP cyclic Adenosine MonoPhosphate.

Campbell de Morgan see DE MORGAN.

camptodactyly fixed flexion deformity of the fingers (Gk *kamptos* bent, *dactylos* finger).

Canada WJ US radiologist *fl.* 20th cent. CRONKHITE–CANADA SYNDROME.

cancrum oris, nasi gangrenous lesion of the mouth or nose, canker (New L from L *cancer* crab, eroding ulcer).

canker obs. term for spreading ulcer, especially of the mouth, see CANCRUM ORIS. Also in veterinary use (ME *canker, cancre*, from OF *cancre* crab, from L *cancer* crab).

canities greying or whitening of hair (L *canities* grey hair).

Cannon AB US dermatologist 1888–1950.

Cannon's disease white sponge naevus.

canthariasis invasion of body by beetles or their larvae (Gk *kantharos* beetle).

Cantú JM Mexican haematologist and geneticist *fl.* 20th cent.

Cantú's syndrome brown macules of face, forearms and feet with hyperkeratosis of palms and soles.

caput Medusae coiled, tortuous enlarged veins of abdominal wall seen in portal obstruction, fancifully resembling the snakes on the head of Medusa (L *caput* head, Medusa, a mythical Gorgon with hissing serpents as hair).

carate (caraate) pinta infection with *Treponema carateum* (Quechuan for brown spot, synonymous with Spanish *pinta*).

carbuncle a necrotizing infection of the skin and subcutaneous tissue composed of a group of furuncles (boils) (L *carbunculus* dim. of *carbo* coal, charcoal) [1].

Carney JA Irish-born US pathologist *fl.* 20th cent.

Carney syndrome pigmented multinodular adrenocortical dysplasia. Atrial myxomas, spotty pigmentation and endocrine overactivity. Probably same as LAMB and NAME.

Caroli J French gastroenterologist 1902–79.

Caroli's disease congenital cystic dilatation of the intrahepatic bile ducts.

Caroli's triad (in French usage) urticaria, arthralgia and headaches as prodrome of hepatitis B infection.

Carrión DA Peruvian medical student 1859–85. Inoculated himself with blood of patient with verruga peruana and later died of Oroya fever.

Carrión's disease see BARTONELLOSIS.

Carteaud A French dermatologist *fl.* 20th cent. GOUGEROT–CARTEAUD SYNDROME.

Casal C Spanish physician 1679–1759.

Casal's necklace, collar area of erythema and pigmentation around neck seen in pellagra.

Castellani, Sir Aldo Italian physician 1877–1971. Active in field of tropical dermatology and mycology. Discovered *Treponema pertenue* and described dermatitis papulosa nigra.

Castellani's paint basic fuchsin, carbolic and boric acids, acetone and resorcinol. Carbolfuchsin paint. Once widely used for epidermophytosis, now less so, or in modified form.

Castleman B US pathologist 1906–82.

Castleman's disease (giant lymph node hyperplasia, angiofollicular lymph node hyperplasia, etc.). A lympoproliferative disease of unknown pathogenesis.

cata-, kata- pref. down, against (Gk *kata, kath* down).

causalgia intense burning pain, often with smooth, shiny skin, profuse sweating and hypersensitivity, following incomplete lesion of a peripheral nerve (Gk *kausis* a burning, *algos* pain).

CBCL Cutaneous *B*-Cell Lymphoma.

CBG Corticosteroid-Binding Globulin.

Ceboidea superfamily of suborder Anthropoidea of order Primates (Gk *kēbos* long-tailed monkey).

Celsus Aulus (Aurelius) Cornelius *fl.* early 1st cent. AD. Roman aristocrat and encyclopaedist who included eight books on medicine in his 'Artes'. 'A Hippocratic eclectic'.

Celsus' four cardinal signs of inflammation *calor, tumor, rubor, dolor*: heat, swelling, redness, pain.

CEP Congenital *E*rythropoietic *P*orphyria.

cephalic index the breadth of the head as a percentage of the length; a measurement used by anthropologists (Gk *kephalē* head).

cerulae (maculae) dark-blue azure macules (L *caeruleus* sky-colour blue).

ceruloderma dermal melanocytosis, often showing a slate-grey, blue or steel-like colour (L *caeruleus* azure, or blue, from *caelum* sky, possibly via *caeluleus*).

cerumen the waxy secretion of the ceruminous (modified sweat) glands of the external auditory meatus (New L from *cera*, Gk *kēros* wax).

chaeta stiff bristle formed of keratin-like substance (Gk *chaetē* long flowing hair).

Chagas CRJ Brazilian parasitologist and community physician 1879–1934.

Chagas' disease, (South) American trypanosomiasis infection by *Trypanosoma cruzi*, spread by cone-nosed reduviid bugs.

chagoma a primary inoculation lesion of American trypanosomiasis (see CHAGAS' DISEASE).

chalazion granulomatous cyst of Meibomian glands of eyelid (Gk *chalazion* dim. of *chalaza* hailstone).

Chanarin I British haematologist *fl.* 20th cent. DORFMAN–CHANARIN SYNDROME.

chancre usually, syphilitic ulcer developing at site of infection with *Treponema pallidum*; also, rarely, for lesion at inoculation site of sporotrichosis, tularaemia or tuberculosis.

CHANDS *C*urly *H*air, *A*nkyloblepharon, *N*ail *D*ysplasia *S*yndrome.

chap to fissure or become fissured or cracked; a dryness or fissuring of the skin due to cold and wind (ME *chappen* but origin uncertain).

Charcot JM renowned French neurologist 1825–93.

Charcot's joints painless distortion of the hips, knees or ankles in tabes dorsalis.

Chase W Merrill US microbiologist and immunologist *fl.* 20th cent. SULZBERGER–CHASE PHENOMENON.

Chaudhry AP US faciomaxillary surgeon *fl.* 20th cent. GORLIN–CHAUDHRY–MOSS SYNDROME.

Chédiak M Cuban physician *fl.* 20th cent.

Chédiak–Higashi syndrome autosomal recessive disorder of lysosomes and melanosomes showing as hypopigmentation, hepatosplenomegaly and susceptibility to infections.

cheilitis inflammation of the lips (Gk *cheilos* lip, edge, *itis*).

cheiro- comb. form meaning hand (Gk *cheir, cheiros* hand).

cheiropompholyx blistering eruption of the hands. Name given by Hutchinson (q.v.) to TILBURY FOX'S DYSIDROSIS (Gk *cheir* hand, *pompholyx* bubble). See POMPHOLYX.

chelation binding of a metal ion by more than one group on the same molecule, the chelating agent (Gk *chēlē* claw, pincer, talon, forked probe; thus, to bring together two notches).

cheloid a more correctly derived spelling for Alibert's KELOID (prob. from Gk *chēlē* claw, talon, forked probe, as Alibert noted resemblance to claws of crayfish or crabs).

Chester porphyria variety of acute porphyria. After city in N England from which a large kindred were reported.

chigger six-legged larva of trombicular (harvest) MITE (African related to Wolof *chiga* of Sudan).

chigoe (synonym jigger) flea of sp. *Tunga penetrans* (Fr *chique*, Spanish *chigo*, both of Carib origin; a tropical sand flea).

chikungunya fever a togaviral infection originally found in Tanzania (Swahili form for 'that which binds up', from the position of patients with joint symptoms).

chilblain lesion chiefly affecting fingers, toes and ears caused by a vascular response to low temperature and humidity (ME *chile* coldness, from OE *ciele* cold, and OE *blegen* inflammatory sore, pustule).

CHILD syndrome *C*ongenital *H*emidysplasia with *I*chthyosiform erythroderma and *L*imb *D*efects.

chilopoda a class of arthropods comprising the centipedes (Gk *cheilos* lip, rim *pous, podos* foot).

chimaera an organism composed of cells of more than one genotype (L *chimaera*, from Gk *chimaera* a she-goat). Mythologically, Chimaera, fire-breathing creature with head of lion, body of goat and tail of serpent.

Chizzole maculae form of industrial fluoride toxicity. From small town in N Italy near fluoride smelting plant.

Chlamydia genus of tiny intracellular parasites classified as bacteria; the cause of psittacosis—lymphogranuloma venereum—trachoma group of infection (Gk *chlamys, chlamydos* a horseman's short mantle or cloak).

chloasma (melasma) patchy pigmentation, particularly of face (Gk *chloazein* to be or to become green).

chondro- comb. form meaning cartilage (Gk *chondros* grain, small round mass, groat; = L *alica*, hence cartilage [Hipp], from gelatinous appearance like washed groats).

choristia state of having small aggregates of normal tissue in an abnormal location; ectopic formation (Gk *chōrista*, pl. of *chōristos* separable, *-ia* state).

Chotzen F German neuropsychiatrist born 1871. SAETHRE–CHOTZEN SYNDROME.

Christ J German physician and dentist 1871–1947.

Christ–Siemens–Touraine syndrome hypohidrotic ectodermal dysplasia, X-linked.

Christian HA US physician 1876–1951. WEBER–CHRISTIAN DISEASE, HAND–SCHÜLLER–CHRISTIAN SYNDROME.

chrysiasis deposition of gold within tissue (Gk *chry(sos)* gold, *iasis*).

Churg J US pathologist *fl.* 20th cent.

Churg–Strauss granulomatosis allergic granulomatosis, allergic granulomatous angiitis.

chyle a milky or turbid lymphatic fluid taken up by lacteals from the intestine during digestion (Gk *chylos* juice, animal juice [Hipp] or produced by ingestion of food [Gal]).

CIN Cervical *I*ntra-epithelial *N*eoplasia.

CINCA syndrome *C*hronic *I*nfantile *N*eurological *C*utaneous *A*rticular syndrome.

cinnabar mercuric sulphide, vermilion (Gk *kinnabair*, from Persian).

circumscriptum a well-defined, enclosed (L *circumscriptum*, past part. of *circumscribere* to draw a line around, confine).

cirrhosis a chronic disease of the liver, of varied aetiology (Gk *kirrhos* tawny, *osis*).

Civatte A French dermatologist 1877–1956.

Civatte's bodies eosinophilic dead keratinocytes extruded into superficial dermis; colloid bodies.

Civatte's poikiloderma stippled and reticulate pigmentation with telangiectasia and atrophy of skin of sides of face and neck in women (Gk *poikilos* dappled).

Clarke, Sir Cyril A British physician *fl.* 20th cent. HOWEL EVANS–CLARKE SYNDROME.

Clarkson B US physician *fl.* 20th cent.

Clarkson's syndrome capillary leak syndrome.

clavus corn (L *clavus* nail).

clegs large blood-sucking flies of *Haematopota* sp., gadflies, horse-flies (ME from Old Norse *kleggi* horsefly).

Clouston HR Canadian paediatrician 1889–1950.

Clouston's syndrome a form of hidrotic ectodermal dysplasia.

Clutton HH British surgeon 1850–1909.

Clutton's joints painless joint effusion in congenital syphilis.

Coats G British ophthalmologist 1876–1915.

Coats' disease retinal telangiectasia, often with cutaneous telangiectasia.

Cobb S US neuropathologist 1887–1968.

Cobb's syndrome cutaneomeningospinal angiomatosis.

Coccidia a subclass of protozoan class Sporozoa, responsible for important diseases of domesticated animals and fowls (New L *coccidium*, dim. of *coccum* or *coccus* scarlet berry, from Gk *kokkos* berry).

coccidioides a genus of fungus of which one species causes coccidioidomycosis (New L *coccidi(um)*, Gk *oid* berry-like).

coccus, cocci spherical bacillus grouped in pairs, chains or clusters (L *coccum*, from Gk *kokkos* a berry, granular seed, as of a pomegranate).

coccyx the coccygeal bone (Gk *kokkyx* a cuckoo (onomatopoeic), from supposed resemblance of shape to a cuckoo's beak) (Gk *kokkygia*, L *os coccygis*).

cockade a lesion having concentric rings of different colour; en cocarde (Fr *cocarde*, from OF *coquarde* a vain person, from *coq* a cock; hence cockade (cockscomb) rosette worn in hat as part of livery or badge of office. See KOKARDEN NAEVUS).

Cockayne EA British paediatrician and geneticist 1880–1956. Pioneer in field of genodermatoses. Noted entomologist.

Cockayne's syndrome short stature, large extremities, mental deficiency, photosensitivity and other defects.

Cockayne–Touraine syndrome form of hyperplastic epidermolysis bullosa simplex; see WEBER–COCKAYNE SYNDROME.

cockroach insect of the primitive order of Dictyoptera, common in warm human habitats (Spanish *cucharacha*, origin uncertain).

coeliac relating to the abdominal cavity (Late L *coeliacus*, from Gk *koiliakos* suffering in the bowel [Gal], from *koilia* the hollow of the belly).

Coffin GS US paediatrician *fl.* 20th cent.

Coffin–Lowry syndrome a form of ectodermal dysplasia, possibly due to lysosomal storage disease.

Coffin–Siris syndrome a syndrome combining abnormalities of hair, teeth, nails and skeleton.

Cohen MM, Jr US orthodontist *fl.* 20th cent.

Cohen's syndrome hypostomia, obesity, mental retardation and facial, oral, dental and limb abnormalities.

Cole HN US dermatologist 1884–1966. COLE–ENGMAN-ZINSSER SYNDROME *diskeratosis congenita*.

collagen the main connective tissue protein, forming fibres of great tensile strength (Gk *kolla* glue, *gen* origin).

Collins, E Treacher see TREACHER COLLINS.

colophony rosin, obtained from trees of genus *Pinus*. After Colophon, on west coast of Asia Minor, famous for production of this substance.

comedo a greasy plug in a sebaceous follicle (L *comedo* glutton, from *comedere* to devour). Term formerly used for a worm that devours the body, hence for the worm-like thread on expression of the plug [Hebra].

Comèl M Italian dermatologist and angiologist 1902–95.

Comèl–Netherton syndrome ichthyosis linearis circumflexa and trichorrexis invaginata; NETHERTON'S SYNDROME.

concha any structure resembling the form of a shell but especially the auricle: hollow of the ear (L *concha*, from Gk *konchē* shell, mussel).

condyloma a wart-like growth due to hypertrophy of prickle-cell layer, commonly used for genital and perianal lesions of viral (acuminatum) or syphilitic (latum) origin (Gk *kondylōma*, from *kondylos* knuckle).

conglobata clumped in a mass, clustered (L *conglobatus* past part. of *conglobare* to gather into a rounded form).

Conradi E German physician b. 1882.

Conradi's syndrome, Conradi–Hünermann syndrome chondro-dysplasia congenita punctata.

Cornelia C de Lange see DE LANGE.

Costa OG Brazilian dermatologist *fl.* 20th cent. ACROKERATOELASTOIDOSIS.

Cowden family name of first-recorded patient with Cowden's syndrome.

Cowden's syndrome multiple tricholemmas, often associated with breast and pancreatic carcinomas. Multiple hamartoma syndrome.

Coxsackie virus enterovirus, Groups A and B. Named after a town in New York State, USA.

CPLS syndrome *C*left *P*alate-*L*ateral *S*ynechia syndrome

CPOD *C*hronic *P*apular *O*ncho*D*ermatitis.

Crandall BF US paediatrician *fl.* 20th cent.

Crandall's syndrome pili torti, deafness and hypogonadism.

craquelé cracked, resembling 'crazy-paving' (Fr *craquelé* crackly, cracked as of special type of china and porcelain or of soil affected by dryness).

Creveld S van see VAN CREVELD.

cribriform sieve-like, perforated by small openings (L *cribrum* sieve, *forma* shape).

crinkle wrinkle, corrugation (Low German *krinkel* curve, dim. of *krink* circle).

Crocker H Radcliffe see RADCLIFFE CROCKER.

Crohn BB US gastroenterologist 1884–1983.

Crohn's disease (synonym regional ileitis) a chronic inflammatory bowel disease characterized by transmural inflammation, linear ulceration and granuloma formation.

Cri du chat syndrome chromosome 5, short arm deletion syndrome. Named after the cat-like mewing cry in infancy (Fr).

Cronkhite LW, Jr US physician *fl.* 20th cent.

Cronkhite–Canada syndrome pigmentation of hands, gastro-intestinal polyposis, patchy alopecia and nail changes.

Cross HE US ophthalmologist *fl.* 20th cent.

Cross' syndrome oculocerebral syndrome with hypopigmentation.

Crosti A Italian dermatologist 1896–1988. GIANOTTI–CROSTI SYNDROME.

Crosti's lymphoma a T-cell lymphoma affecting backs of elderly males.

Crouzon O French neurologist 1874–1938. Craniofacial dysostosis. APERT–CROUZON SYNDROME.

Crow RS British physician *fl.* 20th cent.

Crow–Fukase syndrome (synonyms TAKATSUKI SYNDROME, Shimpo's syndrome, PEP, POEMS) peripheral neuropathy with dysproteinaemia, skin changes and endocrinopathy.

Crowe FW US physician 1919–87.

Crowe's sign axillary freckling, an important aid in the diagnosis of neurofibromatosis.

CRST (CREST) syndrome Calcinosis, Raynaud's phenomenon, (*E*sophageal involvement), *S*clerodactyly, *T*elangiectasia.

cryo- comb. form meaning cold (Gk *kryos* cold).

crypto- comb. form meaning hidden, disguised (Gk *kryptos* hidden).

CTCL Cutaneous *T*-Cell *L*ymphoma.

Cullen TS US gynaecologist 1868–1953.

Cullen's sign bluish staining around umbilicus usually denoting acute pancreatitis or ruptured ectopic pregnancy.

cuniculatus in the form of a tube or tunnel (LL from *cuniculum* underground passage such as made by a rabbit).

cuniculus a burrow, such as that formed by the *Acarus scabiei* (L *cuniculus* rabbit, or its burrow).

Curry CJR US geneticist *fl.* 20th cent.

Curry–Hall syndrome small conical deciduous teeth, short limbs, polydactyly and nail dysplasia.

Cushing HW US neurosurgeon 1869–1939. Friend of Osler (q.v.) and outstanding clinician whose name is attached to several syndromes and signs.

Cushing's syndrome adrenocortical hypertrophy. The term 'Cushingoid' is applied to the appearance caused by high-dose corticosteroid therapy.

cutis laxa laxity or fold-like formation of skin (L *cutis* skin, *laxa* loose). See DERMATOCHALASIS.

cylindroma tumour having cylinder-like vacuoles of stroma surrounded by epithelial cells (Gk *kylindros* cylinder, *oma*). Outmoded term for adenoid cystic carcinoma and eccrine dermal cylindroma.

cyst any closed cavity or sac (normal or abnormal) with an epithelial, endothelial or membranous lining and containing fluid or semisolid material (Gk *kystis* bladder [1]).

cytophagic the ability of one cell to ingest another (Gk *kytos* hollow vessel, body; also comb. form meaning cell, *phagein* to eat, feed on).

Dabska M Polish oncologist *fl.* 20th cent.

Dabska's tumour endovascular papillary angioendothelioma.

da Costa S Mendes see MENDES DA COSTA.

dacro-, dacryo- relating to the lacrimal apparatus (Gk *dacryon* tear).

dactylitis inflammation or infection of a finger (Gk *dactylos* finger, *itis*).

Dalibour J French surgeon late 17th cent.–1735.

Dalibour water a solution of copper and zinc sulphates originally used for war wounds. Resurrected by SABOURAUD. Often wrongly referred to as d'Alibour.

dandruff popular term for pityriasis capitis: 'scurfy scalp' (*dander* origin unknown, *hurf* dialectical from Scandinavian akin to Old Norse *hrufa* scale, crust).

Danlos HA French dermatologist 1844–1912. EHLERS-DANLOS SYNDROME.

Darier F-J French dermatologist 1856–1938. Last surviving member of the 'Big Five'—Besnier (q.v.), Brocq (q.v.), Darier, Sabouraud (q.v.) and Fournier (q.v.). Outstanding clinician and teacher. His name has been attached to pseudoxanthoma elasticum, erythema annulare centifugum and benign familial PEMPHIGUS. Now commonly reserved for:

Darier's disease keratosis follicularis.

Darier's sign evocation of local erythema, wealing and itching on rubbing lesions of urticaria pigmentosa.

Darier-Roussy sarcoid a misleading term, now obs., for a nonspecific subcutaneous lesion showing an epithelial-cell tuberculoid histology.

Darling ST US pathologist 1872–1925.

Darling's disease histoplasmosis.

dartre obs. Fr term for TETTER.

Day RL US paediatrician 1905–89. RILEY–DAY SYNDROME.

de Barsey AM Belgian paediatrician *fl.* 20th cent.

de Barsey's syndrome elastic tissue hypoplasia with dwarfism and oligophrenia.

decalvans causing loss of hair, e.g. folliculitis decalvans of Quinquaud (q.v.) (Fr *décalvant*, from *dé* intensive; L *calv(us)* bald, *decalvare* to make bald).

Dechaume JA French neurologist 1896–1968. BONNET–DECHAUME-BLANC SYNDROME.

Dechaume MR French dermatologist 1897–1991. DEGOS–DECHAUME SYNDROME.

decubitus the position of a person lying down, qualified by the part of the body lying on a surface (L past part. of *decumbere* to lie down, lying down).

decubitus ulcer bedsore; pressure sore due to prolonged recumbency without movement.

Degos R French dermatologist 1904–88. Outstanding clinician, teacher and writer.

Degos' acanthoma clear-cell acanthoma.

Degos' syndrome 1 malignant atrophic papulosis; **2** erythro-keratoderma en cocardes.

Degos–Dechaume syndrome depapillating glossitis, fissured cheilitis, xerostoma, koilonychia and hypochlorhydria.

Degos–Touraine syndrome incontinentia pigmenti and poikilo-derma of light-exposed areas.

de Lange Cornelia C eminent Dutch paediatrician 1871–1950.

de Lange's syndrome, Cornelia de Lange's syndrome, Amsterdam dwarf a short stature syndrome with mental retardation, a grim mask-like facies and a high incidence of chromosomal abnormalities.

Delhi boil one of many local names for lesion of cutaneous leishmaniasis. After Delhi in India.

Delleman JW Dutch ophthalmologist and geneticist *fl.* 20th cent.

Delleman–Oorthuys syndrome oculo-cerebrocutaneous syndrome: multiple asymmetric cutaneous, cerebral and ophthalmic abnormalities.

d'emblée appearing suddenly, without prodromes (Fr *d'emblée* at the very outset).

de Meijere JCH Dutch zoologist 1866–1947. MEIJERE'S HAIR TRIO.

de Morgan, Campbell British physician 1811–76.

de Morgan spots, Campbell de Morgan spots cherry angiomata.

dengue a togavirus transmitted by mosquitoes (Swahili *ka dinga pepo*); a sudden febrile seizure, later identified with Spanish *dengue* affectation, from the delicate gait imposed by the pain of movement.

Dennie CC US dermatologist 1883–1971.

Dennie–Morgan folds see MORGAN'S FOLDS.

Denny–Brown DE New Zealand-born US neurologist 1901–81.

Denny–Brown syndrome paraneoplastic sensory neuropathy.

Dercum FX US neurologist 1856–1931.

Dercum's disease neurolipomatosis (adiposis) dolorosa.

-derma, derm-, dermat- comb. forms denoting skin or affection of this (a complex origin via Gk *derma*, from Proto-Indo-European *der* to flay, peel).

dermabrasion surgical technique of removal of superficial lesions of the skin by abrasive methods such as with high-speed rotary drills.

dermatitis cinerensis ashy dermatosis (L *derma* skin, *itis, cinis, cineris* ashes).

dermatitis repens term used by Radcliffe Crocker for acral pustulosis, probably synonymous with or closely related to acrodermatitis continua of Hallopeau.

dermatochalasis cutis laxa; loose skin (Gk *derma, dermatos* skin, *chalasis* loosening).

dermatoglyphics the highly characteristic epidermal ridge patterns of the volar skin of palms, soles, fingers and toes; the study of such (Gk *derma, dermatos* skin, *glyphein* to engrave, etch).

-dermia a more accurate but increasingly less-used comb. term for a pathological state of the skin (*derma* skin, *ia* state). Feminine in declension in contrast to *derma-* (neuter).

dermis term now used to denote the connective tissue layer of the skin, as opposed to the *epidermis* (new L from Gk *dermis*, comb. form of *derm-*).

de Sanctis C Italian psychiatrist 1862–1935.

de Sanctis–Cacchione syndrome xeroderma pigmentosum with microcephaly, dwarfism, mental deficiency and ataxia.

desmoplastic a term first introduced for the development of a thick, sclerosing, collagenous stroma around trichoepitheliomas; now applied to other naevoid and malignant lesions (Gk *desmos* bond, yoke, *plastos* formed).

Devergie MGA French dermatologist 1798–1879.

Devergie's disease pityriasis rubra pilaris. Puits de Devergie are the minute depressions on the eroded skin surface seen in exudative forms of eczema.

dhobi (dhobie, dhoby) Indian washerman (Hindi *dhōbi*, from *dhōb* washing); 'dhobie itch' colloq. term used by servicemen for tinea cruris.

di- twice, double (Gk *dis* double).

dia- (di-) through, between, across; completely (Gk *dia* through).

Diamond LK US paediatrician *fl.* 20th cent. GARDNER–DIAMOND SYNDROME.

diapedesis passage of cells through intact blood-vessel walls (Gk *diapēdēsis*, from *dia* through, *pēdan* to leap, *ēsis* a leaping through or across).

diascopy examination of skin with exclusion of blood by firm pressure of glass, etc.; vitropression (Gk *dia, skopein* observe).

DIC Disseminated Intravascular Coagulation.

dicuchwa endemic syphilis. Colloq. term in Botswana (Setswana *dicuchwa* syphilitic sore**).

Dieulafoy G French physician 1839–1911.

Dieulafoy's malformation, disease submucosal gastric bleeding due to erosion over a calibre-persistent artery running parallel to the surface.

DiGeorge AM US paediatrician *fl.* 20th cent.

DiGeorge syndrome thymic-parathyroid aplasia. Third and fourth pharyngeal arch syndrome.

dimple a small hollow or dent in any plump part of the human body surface (ME *dympull*, origin uncertain but cognizant with OHG *dumphilo* and German *tumpel* pool).

diphtheria an acute infection caused by *Corynebacterium diphtheriae* (Gk *diphthera*, from *dephein* to tan hides; a 'leathering', after the dense membrane produced).

DISH Diffuse Idiopathic Skeletal Hyperostosis.

distichiasis presence of a double row of eyelashes (Gk *distich(os)* of two rows, *iasis*).

diutinum prolonged, protracted, of long duration (L *diutinum*).

Divry P Belgian neuropsychiatrist 1889–1967.

Divry–van Bogaert syndrome diffuse corticomeningeal angiomatosis and progressive demyelination.

Dohi K Japanese dermatologist 1866–1931. Founder of modern Japanese dermatology.

Dohi's acropigmentation symmetrical dyschromatosis of the extremities.

Dolowitz DA US otolaryngologist *fl.* 20th cent. WOOLF–DOLOWITZ–ALDOUS SYNDROME.

Donohue WL Canadian pathologist 1906–85.

Donohue's syndrome leprechaunism.

Donovan C, Lt Col Irish-born British physician 1863–1951. Served in Indian Medical Service. LEISHMAN–DONOVAN BODIES.

DOOR syndrome Deafness, Onychodystrophy, Osteodystrophy, Retardation.

Doppler CJ Austrian physicist and mathematician 1803–53.

Doppler effect the change in the perceived wavelength or pitch when a rapidly moving source of light or sound approaches or recedes from the receiver.

Dorfman ML Israeli dermatologist *fl.* 20th cent.

Dorfman–Chanarin syndrome an autosomal recessive multisystem lipid storage disorder, with ichthyosiform erythroderma and characteristic red-staining lipid vacuoles in white blood cells.

Dorfman RF US pathologist *fl.* 20th cent. ROSAI–DORFMAN DISEASE.

Dowling GB British dermatologist 1892–1976. Outstanding figure mid-20th cent. British dermatology. An acute clinician and outstanding diagnostician. Exerted a major influence on British dermatology 1945–75.

Dowling–Degos syndrome reticulate pigmented anomaly of the flexures.

Dowling–Meara syndrome herpetiform simple epidermolysis bullosa.

Down JLH British physician 1828–96. Established the model form of care for mentally ill patients.

Down (Down's) syndrome mongolism (obs.) trisomy 21.

Drescher E Polish paediatric surgeon 1887–1961. MURRAY–PURETIC´–DRESCHER SYNDROME.

DSAP Disseminated Superficial Actinic Porokeratosis.

Dubé WJ Canadian pathologist *fl.* 20th cent. BIRT–HOGG––DUBÉ SYNDROME.

Dubowitz V British paediatrician *fl.* 20th cent.

Dubowitz syndrome familial low birthweight, dwarfism with unusual facies, mental retardation, high-pitched voice and eczema.

Dubreuilh MW French dermatologist 1857–1935.

Dubreuilh, precancerous melanosis of HUTCHINSON'S MELANOTIC FRECKLE (LENTIGO MALIGNA).

Ducrey A Italian dermatologist 1860–1940.

Ducrey's bacillus *Haemophilus ducreyi*, the cause of chancroid.

Duhring L US dermatologist 1845–1913. A founder of the American Dermatological Association. Described prurigo hiemalis.

Duhring–Brocq disease dermatitis herpetiformis.

Duncan's disease X-linked lymphoproliferative disease. So-named from the family in whom it was first recognized.

Dupuytren G, Baron French surgeon and anatomist 1777–1835.

Dupuytren's contracture fibrous thickening of palmar fascia causing a characteristic flexural deformity of the fingers.

dys- pref. indicating difficult, abnormal, impaired (Gk *dys* difficult, wrong).

dysaesthesia state of altered sensory perception (Gk *dys* abnormal, *aisthēsia* feeling).

dysautonomia dysfunction of the autonomic nervous system, autonomic independence (Gk *dys*, *auto(s)* self, *nemein* to control, possess).

dyschromatosis abnormal pigmentation (Gk *dys* incorrect, *chrōma* colour).

dysidrosis (better, **dyshidrosis**) lit. difficult sweating. Name given by Tilbury Fox (q.v.) in 1873 for an acute vesicular eruption of palms and/or fingers resembling 'small boiled sago grains' and thought by him to be due to poral occlusion and sweat retention (Gk *dys*, *hidrōs* sweat).

dyskeratotic abnormal or premature keratinization of epidermal cells (Gk *dys*, *keras*, *keratos* horn, *osis*).

dysmorphophobia correctly, morbid fear of developing physical deformity, but in current use to describe state of disturbance of perception of body image (Gk *dysmorphos* misshapen, from *dys*, *morphē* shape, form, *phobos* fear).

dystrophy faulty nourishment, maldevelopment, abnormal form of growth (Gk *dys* abnormal, *trophē* nurture, rearing).

Ebola virus a rhabdovirus named after a river in Zaire.

Ebstein WE German physician and pathologist 1836–1912. PEL–EBSTEIN FEVER.

EB virus EPSTEIN–BARR VIRUS.

ec-, ex- pref. meaning from, out of, without (Gk *ek-*, *ex-*).

ecchymosis (synonym bruise) a macular red or purple or coloured haemorrhage in skin or mucous membrane more than 2 mm in diameter [1] (Gk *ekchymōsis* [Hipp], from *ekchymosthai* to extravasate blood, from *ek* out, *chymos* juice).

ECHO virus Enteric Cytopathic Human Orphan.

ECP Erythropoietic CoproPorphyria.

ectasia dilatation of a duct or vessel; dermatologically, usually of blood or lymphatic vessel (Gk *ek* out, *tasis* a stretching, from *teinein* to stretch).

ecthyma a deep, crusted pyogenic infection, usually on legs (Gk *ekthyma* breaking out, pustule [Hipp]).

ecto- comb. form meaning outside external to (from Gk *ektos* outside, without).

ectopic displaced, out of usual site or range (Gk *ek* out, *topos* place).

eczema an inflammatory skin reaction characterized histologically by spongiosis and clinically by a variety of features, notably vesiculation (Gk *ek* out, *zeein* to boil, seethe).

Edwards JH British geneticist *fl.* 20th cent.

Edwards' syndrome trisomy 18 (lobster-claw deformity).

EEC Ectodactyly, Ectodermal dysplasia, Cleft lip and palate.

EGF Epidermal Growth Factor.

Ehlers EL Danish dermatologist 1863–1937.

Ehlers–Danlos syndrome a group of heritable disorders of connective tissue, characterized by hyperextensibility, fragility, easy bruising and poor skin healing, to varying degrees in different types.

Ekbom K-A Swedish neurologist 1907–77.

Ekbom's disease delusions of parasitosis.

elastorrhexis breaking up of elastic fibres (New L *elasticus*, from Gk *elastikos* set in motion, from *elasa* Epic Gk aorist of *elaunein* to drive on, *rhexis*, from *rhēgnymi* to break).

ELISA Enzyme-Linked ImmunoSorbent Assay.

Ellis RWB British paediatrician 1902–66.

Ellis–van Creveld syndrome chondroectodermal dysplasia with polydactyly, congenital heart disease, etc.

Ellison EH US surgeon 1918–70. ZOLLINGER–ELLISON SYNDROME.

ELND Elective Lymph Node Dissection. Used particularly with reference to treatment of malignant melanoma.

EMG 1 ElectroMyoGram; **2** Exophthalmos, Macroglossia and Gigantism, BECKWITH–WIEDEMANN SYNDROME.

EMLA Eutectic Mixture of Local Anaesthetics.

empiricism properly used as a system that is based or relying on observation, testing and experience rather than on theory; paradoxically, also sometimes used in derogatory sense of an unscientific procedure, 'guilty of quackery' (*OED*) (L *empiricus*, from Gk *empeirikos*, whence the Emperikoi, a sect of physicians who believed that practice was all-important) [5].

encephalins a group of opioid neuropeptides (Gk *en* in, *cephalē* head, brain).

endorphins a group of opioid neuropeptides (Gk *en* inner, *orphin* contracted from *morphine*, from Gk god Morpheus).

Engman MF US dermatologist 1869–1953. COLE–ENGMAN-ZINSSER SYNDROME.

ENL Erythema Nodosum Leprosum.

ephelis commonly, a freckle (Gk, origin uncertain; *eph-* (*epi-* on, *hēlios* sun seems more likely than *hēlos* a stud, nail or wart).

epi- pref. upon, above, over; next, near (Gk *epi*, *eph*).

epidermotropism movement towards the epidermis (Gk *epi*, *derma* skin, *tropos* direction, way, *ia*).

epiloia a telescopic word from *Epi*lepsy, *Lo*w *I*ntelligence and *A*denoma sebaceum, embracing the cardinal features of tuberous sclerosis.

epithelium the cellular covering of the skin and mucous membranes (New L from Gk *epi* on, *thēlē* teat, nipple, L *ium*, noun suff.). From the nipple-like surface of the papillary dermis.

epitrichial (layer) the embryonic periderm. A term used for the outer layers of the fetal epidermis (Gk *epi* on, *thrix*, *trichos* hair).

EPP Erythropoietic ProtoPorphyria.

Epstein A Czechoslovakian paediatrician 1849–1918.

Epstein's pearls gingival cysts of the newborn; dental lamina cysts. Self-resolving keratin-filled cysts on mid-palatinal raphe.

Epstein, Sir Anthony M British virologist *fl.* 20th cent.

Epstein–Barr virus a herpes virus causing infectious mononucleosis.

epulis a term used inconsistently for any localized swelling of the gingiva, inflammatory or tumorous in nature (Gk *epi*, *oulon* the gum).

equina GLANDERS (L *equinus* of horses).

erucism ill-effects of contact with the larvae (caterpillars) of Lepidoptera (L *eruca* caterpillar).

erysipelas an acute infection of the skin by the haemolytic streptococcus, St Anthony's fire (Gk *erysipelas* [Hipp], of uncertain origin; possibly from *erysi* reddening and *pella* skin, though both forms abnormal; or akin to *erysibē* the red blight of corn).

erysipeloid ('fish handler's disease') an infection due to *Erysipelothrix insidiosa*. From resemblance to ERYSIPELAS.

erythema redness of the skin produced by vascular congestion or perfusion [1] (Gk *erythēma* redness, flush upon the skin [Hipp]).

erythermalgia a synonym for ERYTHROMELALGIA or a particular form of this (Gk *eryth(ros)* red, *thermē* heat, *algos* pain) [6].

erythralgia ERYTHROMELALGIA (Gk *erythros* red, *algos* pain).

erythrasma infection by *Corynebacterium minutissimum* (Gk *erythros* red, *-asma* process, state).

erythro- comb. form meaning red (Gk *erythros* red).

erythromelalgia painful erythema of extremities, triggered by exercise or heat (Gk *erythros* red, *melos* limb, *algos* pain).

erythroplasia painless localized erythema of mucous membranes, e.g. ERYTHROPLASIA OF QUEYRAT (Gk *erythro(s)* red, *plasis* a forming, moulding).

espundia form of mucocutaneous (American) leishmaniasis affecting nasal and oral mucous membranes (Spanish, from L *spongia* sponge).

esthiomène obs. term for a destructive lesion of vulva or clitoris occurring in lymphogranuloma venereum (Gk *esthiomai*, passive part. of *esthiein* to eat).

ex- pref. out of, from, away. See EC-.

exo- pref. out of, outside, external to (Gk *exō* -out, out of, without).

exorphens term given to food peptides having an opiate-like activity (Gk *ex-* out, outer, *orphin*, contracted from *morphine*, from Gk god Morpheus).

exostosis benign bony protuberance growing from bone in response to inflammation or trauma (Gk *ex*, *osteon* bone, *osis*).

Fabry J German dermatologist 1860–1930. ANDERSON–FABRY DISEASE.

Fabry's disease see ANDERSON–FABRY DISEASE.

FACE Facial Afrocaribbean Childhood Eruption.

factitial artificial or contrived (L *factitius* made by art, from *facere* make).

FAH Focal Acral Hyperkeratosis.

Fairbank, Sir Thomas HR British orthopaedic surgeon 1876–1961.

Fairbank's syndrome multiple epiphyseal dysplasia with keratosis pilaris.

FAMMM Familial Atypical Mole-Malignant Melanoma syndrome. B-K mole syndrome; dysplastic naevus syndrome.

Fanconi G Swiss paediatrician 1892–1979. Name attached to more than 15 syndromes. One of the founders of modern paediatric medicine. WISSLER–FANCONI SYNDROME, etc.

Fanconi's anaemia a hereditary pancytopenia with growth retardation and skeletal and other anomalies.

'Fanconi–like syndrome' immunological deficiency, pancytopenia and cutaneous malignancies, resembling FANCONI'S ANAEMIA.

Farber S US paediatric pathologist 1903–73.

Farber's disease disseminated lipogranulomatosis.

farcy form of GLANDERS involving skin and lymphatics (Fr *farcir*, from L *farciminum* a disease of horses, from *farcire* to stuff, fill up, from Gk *phrassein* to block up).

Favre MJ French physician and dermatologist 1876–1954. NICHOLAS–FAVRE DISEASE.

Favre's dermite ochre acroangiodermatitis; gravitational purpura.

Favre–Racouchot syndrome nodular elastosis of the skin. Irregularly thickened skin with comedones and follicular cysts; a chronic solar degenerative elastosis.

favus a fungal infection of the scalp, usually caused by *Trichophyton schoenleinii*. It forms a characteristic cup-shaped crust (scutula) which, on removal, exposes an oozing red surface (L *favus* honeycomb, from its appearance).

felon little-used term for acute purulent infection of finger pad or nail fold; whitlow (OF *felon*, but source uncertain; perhaps akin to L *fel* gall, poison).

Felty AR US physician 1895–1964.

Felty's syndrome rheumatoid arthritis, splenomegaly and leucopenia.

Fendt H German dermatologist b. 1872. SPIEGLER–FENDT SARCOID.

Ferguson Smith J British dermatologist 1888–1978.

Ferguson Smith's self-healing epithelioma an inherited condition of multiple self-healing tumours resembling squamous-cell carcinomas, usually in light-exposed skin.

Fernandez JMM Argentinian dermatologist and leprologist 1902–65.

Fernandez reaction delayed-type hypersensitivity reaction to Dharmendra antigen in LEPROSY.

fetoscopy the technique of inserting a fibreoptic endoscope into the pregnant uterus to visualize the contents and for blood or tissue sampling.

Feuerstein RC, Capt. US Air Force physician *fl.* 20th cent.

Feuerstein–Mims–Schimmelpenning syndrome epidermal naevi with defects of central nervous system, eye or skeleton (akin to naevus phakomatosis of Jadassohn (q.v.)).

fibroma a benign tumour of fibroblasts forming collagen (L *fibra* fibre, *oma*).

Fick AE German physiologist and mathematician 1829–1901.

Fick's first law of diffusion the flux (or rate of flow) of a fluid is the product of the average concentration of molecules and their average velocity. Relevant to the permeability of the skin barrier to a penetrant.

Fiessinger MN French bacteriologist 1881–1946.

Fiessinger–Leroy syndrome see REITER'S SYNDROME.

Fiessinger–Rendu syndrome see STEVENS–JOHNSON SYNDROME.

Finsen NR Danish physicist 1860–1904, b. in Faroes. Pioneer of heliotherapy for lupus vulgaris.

Finsen light light produced by a Finsen lamp, a carbon-arc lamp producing concentrated ultraviolet radiation.

Fisch L Czech-born British otorhinolaryngologist *fl*. 20th cent.

Fisch's syndrome white forelock, heterochromia iridium and perceptive deafness.

Fischer E German dermatologist early 20th cent. BUSCHKE–FISCHER–BRAUER SYNDROME.

Fleck F German dermatologist 1909–95.

Fleck syndrome hypohidrosis with diabetes insipidus.

Flegel H German dermatologist *fl*. 20th cent.

Flegel's disease hyperkeratosis lenticularis perstans.

Fleischer B German ophthalmologist 1874–1965. KAYSER–FLEISCHER RINGS.

Flynn P US neurologist *fl*. 20th cent.

Flynn–Aird syndrome a neuroectodermal syndrome with skin atrophy, ulceration, atrophy and dental caries.

fogo selvagem Brazilian, S American or wildfire PEMPHIGUS, an endemic bullous disease of S America (Portuguese, wild fire).

Fölling IA Norwegian physician 1888–1973.

Fölling's disease phenylketonuria.

Fong EE US radiologist *fl*. 20th cent. Described iliac horns, a feature of NAIL–PATELLA SYNDROME.

Fong's syndrome nail-patella syndrome (hereditary osteo-onychodysplasia).

Fordyce JA US dermatologist 1858–1925. FOX–FORDYCE DISEASE.

Fordyce angiomata scrotal angiomata.

Fordyce spots ectopic sebaceous glands of inner surface and vermilion of lip and oral mucosa, appearing as creamy-coloured symptomless lesions; an anatomical variant of the normal.

-form having the form or shape of (L *forma* shape; akin to Gk *morphē*).

Forscheimer F US paediatrician 1853–1913.

Forscheimer's sign a maculopapular eruption on the palate in prodromal or early stages of rubella.

Fort Bragg fever (synonym pretibial fever) a febrile systemic illness showing an ill-defined pretibial erythematous rash; due to a leptospiral infection. Named after town in N Carolina USA where an epidemic of 'pretibial fever' occurred among soldiers in 1942–43.

Fournier JA French dermatologist 1832–1914. Dominated French dermatology at end of 19th cent. Instigated dermatovenereology at St Louis Hospital, Paris.

Fournier's gangrene fulminating gangrene of the external genitalia.

Fournier's sign bowing of the tibia seen in osteitis deformans, syphilis and yaws.

Fournier's teeth malformation of teeth in congenital syphilis.

Fowler T British physician 1736–1801.

Fowler's solution liquor arsenicalis; potassium arsenite solution.

Fox GH US dermatologist 1846–1937. A founder of the American Dermatological Association and a prolific writer.

Fox–Fordyce disease (synonyms lichen axillaris, apocrine miliaria) intensely pruritic papular eruption involving aprocrine ducts in axillae, breasts or genital area.

framboesia yaws (New L from Fr *framboise* raspberry, after supposed resemblance).

framboesiform resembling the florid lesions of yaws.

Franceschetti A Swiss ophthalmologist 1896–1968.

Franceschetti–Jadassohn syndrome (synonym Naegeli syndrome) reticular pigmentation, hypotrichosis and palmoplantar keratoderma.

Franceschetti–Klein syndrome see TREACHER COLLINS–FRANCESCHETTI SYNDROME.

François J Belgian ophthalmologist 1907–84.

François syndrome dermochondrocorneal dystrophy. HALLERMANN–STREIFF SYNDROME.

Frank ST US physician *fl*. 20th cent.

Frank's sign acquired oblique earlobe groove which, when of full extent, is said to indicate increased risk of diabetes or coronary disease.

Franklin EC US physician 1929–82.

Franklin's disease heavy-chain disease.

Fraser FC Canadian paediatrician and geneticist *fl*. 20th cent. MELNICK–FRASER SYNDROME.

Fraser GR British geneticist *fl*. 20th cent.

Fraser's syndrome cryptophthalmia-syndactyly.

freckle (synonym ephelis) light-brown macules developing in sun-exposed skin, especially in fair-skinned persons (ME *freckel*, from Scandinavian). See HUTCHINSON'S MELANOTIC FRECKLE.

Frei WS German dermatologist 1885–1943.

Frei's disease lymphogranuloma venereum.

Frei's test a diagnostic intradermal test of limited value for lymphogranuloma venereum.

Freire-Maia N Brazilian geneticist *fl*. 20th cent.

Freire-Maia type of ectodermal dysplasia. Equivalent to HOHD SYNDROME.

Freund JT Hungarian-born US immunologist 1891–1960.

Freund's (complete) adjuvant an emulsion of killed mycobacteria in paraffin oil and detergent used in animals to enhance immunological responses to antigenic determinants.

Frey L Polish neurologist 1889–1943.

Frey's syndrome auriculotemporal syndrome.

Frias L US paediatrician and geneticist *fl*. 20th cent. OPITZ–FRIAS SYNDROME.

Friderichsen C Danish paediatrician 1886–1982. WATERHOUSE–FRIDERICHSEN SYNDROME.

Fried K Israeli geneticist *fl*. 20th cent.

Fried's syndrome fine hair, tooth and nail defects.

fucosidosis an inherited lysosomal storage disorder caused by a deficiency of α-fucosidase. Fucose, 6-deoxygalactose, an aldose, is found in some seaweeds (Gk *phykos* seaweed, *id, osis*).

Fukase M Japanese physician 1914–88. CROW–FUKASE SYNDROME.

furuncle a localized pyogenic infection originating in a hair follicle (L *furunculus* a petty thief) [1].

Futcher PH US physician *fl*. 20th cent.

Futcher's lines (synonym Voigt's lines) sharply demarcated lines of pigmentation on anterolateral junction of upper arms or posteromedial aspect of lower legs. Common in those with darkly pigmented skin.

Galen, Claudius Greek physician active in Rome *c*. 130–200 AD. Outstanding medical figure of his time. His influence ensured the survival of medicine throughout the dark ages but his authority was such that its subsequent development was hindered for several centuries.

galenicals term given to **1** use of herbs or vegetable remedies, as opposed to minerals or chemicals; **2** use of crude drugs and preparations made from them and the formulae derived from them; 'simples'.

GALT system *G*astrointestinal *A*ssociated *L*ymphoid *T*issue system.

ganglion an aggregation of neurone cell bodies in the peripheral nervous system or a cystic mass related to joints or tendons (Gk *ganglion* a tumour under the skin).

gangosa deforming rhinopharyngitis; a mutilating destruction of the centre of the face seen in yaws and American leishmaniasis (Spanish, from *gangoso* speech with a nasal twang, onomatopoeic).

gangrene commonly used to describe necrotizing and sloughing lesions but more properly referring to death of tissue resulting from ischaemia (L *gangraena*, from Gk *gangraina* an eating sore [Cels]).

GAPO *G*rowth retardation, *A*lopecia, *P*seudo-anodontia and *O*ptic atrophy.

Garbe W Canadian dermatologist *fl.* 20th cent. SULZBERGER–GARBE SYNDROME.

Gardner EJ US zoologist and geneticist 1909–87.

Gardner's syndrome epidermoid cysts, fibromas and osteomas with polyposis of the colon.

Gardner FH US haematologist *fl.* 20th cent.

Gardner–Diamond syndrome painful bruising syndrome; auto-erythrocyte sensitization syndrome.

gargoylism outmoded term for **1** mucopolysaccharidosis 1H; **2** any of the severe mucopolysaccharide or mucolipid storage diseases that produce a coarse facies and dysostosis multiplex (OF *gargouille* throat, L *gurgulio* gullet; later a grotesque projection from gutters of buildings to carry rainwater. 'The bare vgly gargyle faces' 1532 [*OED*]).

Gaucher PCE French physician 1854–1918.

Gaucher's cells histiocytes with a small nucleus, voluminous pale cytoplasm and containing characteristic elongated tubular structures.

Gaucher's disease a group of inborn errors of glycosphingolipid metabolism.

Gedde-Dahl T, Jr Norwegian geneticist *fl.* 20th cent. Epidermolysis bullosa simplex (type Ogna).

-gen comb. form meaning producing or produced by (Gk *genos*, *genikos* race, descendant; thus, producing).

Gentry WC, Jr US dermatologist *fl.* 20th cent. WITKOP–BREARLEY–GENTRY SYNDROME.

Ghon A Czechoslovakian pathologist 1866–1936.

Ghon's focus primary tuberculous complex of the lung.

Gianotti F Italian paediatric dermatologist 1920–84.

Gianotti–Crosti syndrome infantile papular acrodermatitis.

Gibert CM French dermatologist 1797–1866. Established the infectious nature of syphilis.

Gibert's disease pityriasis rosea.

Giedion A Swiss radiologist *fl.* 20th cent. LANGER–GIEDION SYNDROME, SCHINZEL–GIEDION SYNDROME.

Gilchrist TC US dermatologist 1862–1927.

Gilchrist's syndrome N American blastomycosis.

Gilford H British physician 1861–1941. HUTCHINSON–GILFORD SYNDROME.

glabrous smooth; commonly used to designate smooth hairless skin; properly, skin without any hair follicles (L *glaber*, *glabris* smooth, bald).

glanders a contagious disease of horses, mules and donkeys caused by *Pseudomonas mallei*. When nodules and abscesses form, known as FARCY. May have been the cause of havoc among Greek horses and men in the Trojan War [7] (OF *glanders*, from L *glandulae* little glands dim. of *glans* acorn; thus, glands, swellings).

glaucoma increased intraocular pressure (Gk *glaukoma*, from *glauk(os)* grey-blue, green, *oma*), from the bluish tint of the cornea.

glomus a ball-shaped neurovascular body containing richly innervated arterioles (L *glomus*, a ball of thread, skein, similar to L *globus*).

glomus tumour (synonym globangioma) an encapsulated and often painful tumour of the glomus usually affecting the extremities.

gnathophyma inflamed rosaceous nodule of the jaw, usually on the tip of the chin (Gk *gnathos* jaw, *phyma* tumour).

Gnathostoma a genus of spiruroid nematodes parasitic in the stomach wall of some predatory mammals and, occasionally, humans (Gk *gnathos* jaw, *stoma* mouth. Hence, gnathostomiasis, infection with *Gnathostoma*).

Goeckerman WH US dermatologist 1884–1954.

Goeckerman regime (for psoriasis) combined tar and UVB light.

Goldenhar M Swiss physician *fl.* 20th cent.

Goldenhar's syndrome oculoauriculovertebral dysplasia.

Golé L French dermatologist 1832–1905. TOURAINE–SOLENTE–GOLÉ SYNDROME.

Golgi C Italian histologist and anatomist 1844–1926.

Golgi apparatus a cytoplasmic organelle situated near the nucleus, which accepts, modifies and distributes the products of the vesicles of the endoplasmic reticulum.

Golgi-Mazzoni corpuscle a laminate sensory nerve ending found in the fingers.

Goltz RW US dermatologist *fl.* 20th cent. GORLIN–GOLTZ SYNDROME.

Goltz's syndrome focal dermal hypoplasia.

Golubatz fly *Simulium columbaschense*, a notorious blackfly formerly common in the Balkans, named after Golubatz, a town on the Danube.

Good RA US physician *fl.* 20th cent.

Good's syndrome an immune deficiency state occurring with thymoma.

Goodman RM Israeli geneticist 1932–87.

Goodman syndrome a form of acrocephalopolysyndactyly Type IV.

Gorham LW US physician 1885–1968.

Gorham's syndrome angiomatous naevi with osteolysis; disappearing bone disease.

Gorlin RJ US oral pathologist and surgeon *fl.* 20th cent.

Gorlin's syndrome, Gorlin-Goltz syndrome naevoid basal-cell-carcinoma syndrome.

Gorlin–Chaudhry–Moss syndrome craniofacial dysostosis with patent ductus arteriosus, hypertrichosis, microphthalmia, hypodontia, etc.

Gottron HA German dermatologist 1890–1974.

Gottron's sign erythematous papules over metacarpal and proximal interphalangeal joints in dermatomyositis.

Gottron's syndrome 1 familial acrogeria; **2** scleromyxoedema; **3** symmetrical progressive erythrokeratoderma.

Gougerot H French dermatologist 1881–1955. One of the leading figures in 20th-century dermatology and a renowned teacher.

Gougerot–Carteaud syndrome confluent and reticulate papillomatosis.

Gougerot–Blum syndrome (purpura) pigmented purpuric lichenoid dermatitis.

Gougerot–Houwer–Sjögren syndrome see SJÖGREN'S SYNDROME.

Gougerot–Ruiter syndrome ('trisymptome', 'pentasymptome', etc.) leucocytoclastic angiitis.

goundou (synonyms anákhré, gorondou, dog-nose) nasal osteoblastic periostitis occurring in yaws (Fr, from W African native name).

Gowers, Sir William R British neurologist 1845–1915. A leading medical figure of late 19th cent.

Gowers' panatrophy localized areas of loss of subcutaneous tissue without accompanying sclerotic changes.

Graham-Little, Sir Ernest G British dermatologist 1867–1950.

Graham-Little syndrome see PICCARDI–LASSUEUR–GRAHAM-LITTLE SYNDROME.

granuloma a chronic inflammatory lesion showing accumulations of macrophages which have undergone epithelioid transformation, with or without lymphocytes and multinuclear giant cells; more loosely, a nodular chronic inflammatory lesion arising in response to a variety of stimuli (L *granulum* a little grain, dim. of *granum* grain).

granulosa granular, as of granular layer of epidermis (derived term from LL *granulum* a small grain).

Graves RJ Irish physician 1796–1853. A founder of the Irish School of Medicine and reformer of clinical teaching. At his request his epitaph read 'He Fed Fevers'.

Graves' disease hyperthyroidism due to diffuse toxic goitre.

Great Rift Valley see RIFT VALLEY FEVER.

Greither A German dermatologist 1914–86.

Greither's syndrome progressive palmoplantar keratoderma.

Greither–type ectodermal dysplasia (Greither–Tritsch syndrome) transgredient palmo-plantar keratoderma with hypohidrosis, alopecia, eye, tooth and nail deformities.

Grey Turner G British surgeon 1877–1951.

Grey Turner's sign bruise-like discoloration of skin of left flank in acute pancreatitis.

Grenz(e) rays (Bucky rays) borderline (X-) rays (German *Grenze* borderline).

Grenz(e) zone a zone of normal dermis overlying deeper pathological changes.

Griscelli C French immunologist *fl.* 20th cent.

Griscelli's syndrome immunodeficiency and partial albinism.

Grönblad Ester E Swedish ophthalmologist 1898–1970.

Grönblad–Strandberg syndrome pseudoxanthoma elasticum.

Grossman AJ US plastic surgeon *fl.* 20th cent.

Grover RW US dermatologist *fl.* 20th cent.

Grover's disease originally, transient acantholytic dermatosis; subsequently, also includes persistent forms.

Grzybowski M Polish dermatologist 1895–1949.

Grzybowski's disease generalized eruptive keratoacanthoma.

Guérin C French bacteriologist 1872–1961. CALMETTE–GUÉRIN BACILLUS.

Gulienetti R Italian plastic surgeon *fl.* 20th cent. ROSELLI–GULIENETTI SYNDROME.

gumma characteristic though inconstant lesion of tertiary syphilis, of a rubbery consistency and with a fibrous capsule, it consists of necrotic tissue and epithelioid, multinucleated and plasma cells. Also (rarely) used for tuberculous gumma (New L from L *gummi* gum, equivalent to Gk *kommi* gum, gummy substance).

Günther H German physician 1884–1956.

Günther's disease congenital erythropoietic porphyria.

Guthrie R US paediatrician *fl.* 20th cent.

Guthrie's test a screening test for detecting phenylketonuria.

Gutmann C German pathologist 1876–1930. MICHAELIS–GUTMANN BODIES.

GVHD *Graft-Versus-Host Disease*.

gynaecomastia enlargement of breasts **(**Gk *gynē*, *gynaikos* woman, *mast(os)*, from earlier *mazos* breast).

Haber H Czech-born British dermatologist and histopathologist 1901–62.

Haber's syndrome familial rosacea-like eruption and keratotic plaques.

Habermann R German dermatologist 1884–1941. MUCHA-HABERMANN DISEASE.

Hailey HE US dermatologist b. 1909.

Hailey WH US dermatologist 1898–1967.

Hailey–Hailey disease benign familial PEMPHIGUS.

HAIR–AN syndrome *HyperAndrogenism, Insulin Resistance, Acanthosis Nigricans.* Type A syndrome of insulin resistance. Affected women have marked virilism.

halitosis oral malodour (L *halitus* breath)**.**

Hall BD US paediatrician *fl.* 20th cent. CURRY–HALL SYNDROME.

Hallermann W German forensic physician 1901–75.

Hallermann–Streiff syndrome mandibulo-oculofacial dyscephaly with other defects. FRANÇOIS SYNDROME.

Hallopeau FH French dermatologist and pathologist 1842–1919. One of the great figures of late-19th-century dermatology. Acrodermatitis continua, pyodermite végétante, etc.

Hallopeau–Siemens syndrome recessive form of generalized dystrophic epidermolysis bullosa.

hamartoma a benign tumour or tumour-like lesion composed of tissue normal for the body but inappropriate for the site; or abnormally mixed or overgrown. Broadly, naevoid anomaly (New L from Gk *hamartia* failure, fault, *hamartanein* miss the mark, do wrong, *oma*). In theology hamartiology is the doctrine of sin.

Hand A US paediatrician 1868–1949. Found yellow deposits in skull of patient with polyuria.

Hand–Schüller–Christian syndrome multifocal eosinophilic granuloma, form of LANGERHANS' CELL HISTIOCYTOSIS.

Hanhart E Swiss physician and geneticist 1891–1973. Studied isolated communities in the Alps. RICHNER–HANHART SYNDROME.

Hansemann DP von German pathologist 1858–1920.

Hansemann cells large histiocytes with fine eosinophil granules seen in malakoplakia.

Hansen GHA Norwegian bacteriologist and leprologist 1841–1912. Discovered the *Mycobacterium leprae* bacillus in 1873.

Hansen's disease LEPROSY.

Hantaan, Hanta virus a bunyavirus causing haemorrhagic fever, named after a river near Songnaeri in S Korea.

Harada E Japanese ophthalmologist 1892–1947.

Harada's syndrome see VOGT–KOYANAGI SYNDROME.

harara Middle-East term for urticaria multiformis endemica conveyed by the *Phlebotomus* fly (Arabic *harara* fever, frenzy and applied to any hot, red and itchy or urticarial condition).

Hartnup name of an English hospital patient in whom the disease was first recognized.

Hartnup disease a rare metabolic disorder comprising pellagra, cerebellar ataxia and indicanuria.

Hashimoto K US dermatologist *fl*. 20th cent.

Hashimoto–Pritzker syndrome a spontaneously regressing variant of Langerhans cell histiocytosis.

Haverhill fever infection with *Streptobacillus moniliformis* in absence of rat bite. Named after a town in Massachusetts, USA where the first epidemic of Haverhill fever was recorded in 1926.

Haxthausen H Danish dermatologist 1892–1959.

Haxthausen's disease cold panniculitis of the newborn.

Haxthausen's syndrome keratoderma climactericum.

Hay RJ British dermatologist and mycologist *fl*. 20th cent.

Hay–Wells syndrome (synonym AEC syndrome) ankyloblepharon, ectodermal defects, cleft lip and palate defects.

HCP *H*ereditary *C*opro*P*orphyria.

Heaf FRG British physician 1894–1973.

Heaf test an intradermal multiple-puncture test for tuberculosis.

Heberden W British physician 1710–1801. One of the outstanding clinicians of his era, 'the last of the learned physicians'.

Heberden's nodes bony swellings of the distal interphalangeal joints of the hands, indicative of osteoarthritis.

Heberden's purpura see HENOCH–SCHÖNLEIN PURPURA.

Hebra F, Ritter von Austrian dermatologist 1816–80. An outstanding figure among 19th-century dermatologists. 'Hardly any branch of the speciality was not altered or improved by his work.' Established therapy on a rational basis.

'Hebra nose' rhinoscleroma affecting the nasal lobule and upper lip giving rise to a tapir- or rhinoceros-like appearance.

Hebra's prurigo obs. Form of prurigo seen in malnourished subjects in Vienna. Possibly papular urticaria in atopics.

Hecht AF US paediatrician and geneticist *fl*. 20th cent. BEALS–HECHT SYNDROME.

Heck JW US dental surgeon *fl*. 20th cent.

Heck's disease focal epithelial hyperplasia.

Heerfordt CF Danish ophthalmologist 1871–1953.

Heerfordt's syndrome uveoparotid fever; uveitis, parotitis and facial paralysis. A manifestation of sarcoidosis.

Heller J German dermatologist 1864–1931.

Heller's nail deformity median canaliform dystrophy.

Helweg-Larsen HFR Danish geneticist 1917–69.

Helweg-Larsen–Ludvigsen syndrome hypohidrosis with neurolabyrinthitis.

Henoch EH German paediatrician 1820–1910.

Henoch–Schönlein purpura anaphylactoid purpura.

HEP *H*epato*E*rythropoietic *P*orphyria.

Herlitz CG Swedish paediatrician 1902–82.

Herlitz' syndrome epidermolysis bullosa lethalis. Originally described as 'congenital nonsyphilitic pemphigus'.

Hermann J German-born geneticist *fl*. 20th cent.

Hermann's syndrome (synonyms SC PHOCOMELIA SYNDROME (after initials of two patients), ROBERTS' SYNDROME) hypomelia- hypotrichosis-facial haemangioma syndrome.

Heřmanský F Czechoslovakian haematologist 1916–80.

Heřmansk´y–Pudlák syndrome oculocutaneous albinism, haemorrhagic diathesis and pigmented macrophages in reticuloendothelial system.

herpes originally used to designate a spreading or 'creeping' eruption. Now applied to herpes simplex, herpes zoster and herpes gestationis—all conditions in which a vesicular eruption appears to extend or 'creep' in clusters or in a linear fashion (L from Gk *herpēs* an eruption that runs on and spreads [Hipp], from *herpein* to creep, crawl).

herpetiform herpes-like. Grouped vesicles resembling herpes (L *herpetiformis*, from Gk *herpēs*).

Herxheimer K German dermatologist 1861–1942. JARISCH–HERXHEIMER REACTION; PICK–HERXHEIMER DISEASE.

Hess AF US physician 1875–1933.

Hess (capillary) test a tourniquet test used to determine capillary fragility.

hetero- comb. form meaning other, other of two, different (Gk *heteros* other, one of two).

heterochromia the presence of two or more colours when only one is normal (New L from Gk *hetero*, *chrōma* colour, *ia*).

hibernoma (synonym brown-fat tumour) a benign mesodermal tumour consisting of vacuolated acidophilic cells having the appearance of brown fat (L *hibernus* pertaining to winter, from similarity to fat pads of some hibernating animals).

hidro- comb. form meaning sweat (Gk *hidrōs* sweat, not to be confused with hydro-, comb. form for water).

hiemalis pertaining to winter (L *hiemalis*, from *hiems* winter, *-alis* belonging to).

Higashi O Japanese paediatrician *fl*. 20th cent. CHEDIAK–HIGASHI SYNDROME.

Higashi's syndrome craniostenosis and limb abnormalities.

Hill HR US paediatric pathologist *fl*. 20th cent. QUIE–HILL SYNDROME.

Hippocrates Greek physician born on Cos 460 BC, died in Larissa 377 BC. 'Father of Medicine'. Hippocratic oath, facies; aphorisms of Hippocrates; etc.

Hippocratic nails broad, convex clubbed nails; acropachy.

hirsutism, hirsuties specifically, the growth of hair in women in the male sexual pattern but more commonly any abnormal degree of coarse hairiness (L *hirsutus* shaggy).

histi-, histio-, histo- tissue (Gk *histion* web, warp, dim. of *histos* a loom-beam, the warp woven on it). Thus, histiocyte, a (particular) tissue cell.

histiocytosis any condition in which there is a proliferation of histiocytes; histiocytosis-X is an obs. term now called Langerhans' cell histiocytosis.

HIV *H*uman *I*mmunodeficiency *V*irus.

hives term originally used for various eruptions due to internal causes, now more specifically as popular US term for urticaria; 'nettle-rash'.

HLA antigens *H*uman *L*eucocyte *A*ntigens.

Hodgkin T British physician 1798–1866. Introduced the stethoscope and was noted for his reluctance to accept fees.

Hodgkin's disease (many synonyms) a malignant neoplasm affecting lymph nodes and spleen and characterized by the presence of REED–STERNBERG CELLS in the infiltrate.

Hodgkin WE US paediatrician *fl*. 20th cent. RAPP–HODGKIN SYNDROME.

Hoffmann E German dermatologist 1868–1959.

Hoffmann–Zurhelle naevus superficial lipomatous naevus.

Hogg GR Canadian pathologist *fl*. 20th cent. BIRT–HOGG–DUBÉ SYNDROME.

HOHD *Hair, Onychodysplasia, Hypohidrosis, Deafness* syndrome.

Hoigné R Swiss physician *fl.* 20th cent.

Hoigné reaction acute psychotic symptoms due to procaine in procaine penicillin.

Holmes, Sir Gordon M British neurologist 1876–1965.

Holmes–Adie syndrome pupillary dilatation, usually unilateral, responding poorly to light; of unknown causation.

holocrine shedding completely, as applied to sebaceous glands, the secretion of which is formed by the complete disintegration of the glandular cells (Gk *holos* complete, *krinein* to separate).

Homans J US surgeon 1877–1954.

Homans' sign pain in the calf on forced dorsiflexion of the foot. Suggestive of deep vein thrombosis.

HOOD syndrome *Hereditary Osteo-OnychoDysplasia.*

Horan MB Australian paediatrician *fl.* 20th cent.

hordeolum stye (New L variant of Late L *hordeolus*, dim. of *hordeum* barley corn).

hormiguillo local term for minute painless craters seen in tertiary yaws.

hormone a substance secreted by specialized cells which acts on specific target tissue or which regulates metabolic processes; 'chemical messenger' (Gk *hormōn* pres. part. of *horman* to stir up, urge on).

Horner JF Swiss ophthalmologist 1831–86.

Horner's syndrome miosis, enophthalmos, ptosis and absence of sweating due to lesion of ipsilateral cervical sympathetic chain or ganglia.

Houwer AW Mulock Dutch ophthalmologist early 20th cent. GOUGEROT–HOUWER–SJÖGREN SYNDROME.

Howel Evans AW British physician *fl.* 20th cent.

Howel Evans–Clarke syndrome palmoplantar keratoderma with oesophageal carcinoma, found originally in two Liverpool families.

HPV *Human Papilloma Virus.*

HSAN a group of rare *Hereditary Sensory and Autonomic Neuropathies.* Three main types are recognized.

HTLV *Human T-cell Lymphotropic Virus.* See HIV.

Hughes JP British physician *fl.* 20th cent.

Hughes' syndrome segmental aneurysm of pulmonary artery with peripheral venous thrombosis.

Hünermann C German paediatrician 1900–43. CONRADI–HÜNERMANN SYNDROME.

Hunt J Ramsay see RAMSAY HUNT.

Hunter C Scottish-born Canadian physician 1873–1955.

Hunter syndrome a rare type of disorder of mucopolysaccharide metabolism.

Hunter W British pathologist 1861–1937.

Hunter's glossitis superficial atrophy of tongue associated with macrocytic anaemia.

Hunziker N Swiss dermatologist *fl.* 20th cent. LAUGIER–HUNZIKER SYNDROME.

Huriez C French dermatologist 1907–84.

Huriez' syndrome keratoderma and scleroatrophy of hands and feet.

Hurler G Austrian paediatrician 1889–1965.

Hurler's syndrome mucopolysaccharidosis 1H.

Hurst DI US paediatric neurologist *fl.* 20th cent. VASQUEZ–HURST–SOTOS SYNDROME

Hutchinson, Sir Jonathan British surgeon 1828–1913. Out-standing figure in late 19th-century British medicine. Possessed of an extraordinary visual memory, he made wide-ranging contributions to many aspects of medicine and surgery. His output was prodigious. 'A most careful observer and fascinating teacher.'

Hutchinson's angioma angioma serpiginosum.

Hutchinson's disease summer prurigo.

Hutchinson's melanotic freckle (synonym precancerous melanosis of Dubrueilh) melanomatous lesion of malignant quality, usually seen on the face; lentigo maligna.

Hutchinson's teeth barrel-shaped incisors with a deep concentric notch seen in congenital syphilis. 'Pegged', 'screwdriver' teeth.

Hutchinson's triad keratitis, nerve deafness and tooth deformities in congenital syphilis.

Hutchinson–Boeck disease sarcoidosis.

Hutchinson–Gilford syndrome true PROGERIA.

hydro- comb. form meaning water (Gk *hydōr* water).

hydroa a condition characterized by watery vesicles. Now virtually confined to hydroa aestivale and vacciniforme (Gk but origin uncertain. Perhaps altered form of *hidrōa* heat spots [Hipp, Gal]) or from root *hydr-* water). A neuter pl. noun.

hygroma cystic lymphangioma. Also used for fluid-filled tumours of other types (Gk *hygros* moist, wet, *oma*).

hyper- pref. meaning above, excessive, more than normal (Gk *hyper* above).

hypha unit of fungal structure combining into a complex network. Also called mycelial thread. (Gk *hyphē* or *hyphos* weaving, web.)

hypo- pref. meaning under, less, below normal (Gk *hypo* beneath, under).

hysteresis a biomechanical term denoting a property in which the stress-strain relationships differ between loading or un-loading (Gk *hysteresis*, from *hysterein* to be behind, come later).

hystrix warty or spiny forms of naevi and ichthyosis (Gk *hystrix* porcupine, from *hys* pig, *thrix, trichos* hair, bristle).

-ia suff. denoting condition, state (New L formation and equivalent to Fr *-ie* and English *-y*).

-iasis comb. form meaning, in applied usage, diseased or abnormal condition (Gk *iasis* mode of healing, treatment).

IBIDS *Ichthyosis, Brittle hair, Intellectual impairment, Decreased fertility, Short stature.*

-ic, ical- relating or pertaining to. Interchangeable but modern usage favours *-ic* as shorter (Gk *ikos*, L *icus*, Late L *icalis* relating to).

I-cell disease (synonym Leroy's syndrome) mucolipidosis II, showing coarse cytoplasmic inclusions in cultivated fibroblasts.

ichthammol ammonium ichthyosulphonate, a neutralized distillate of bituminous schists.

ichthyol a natural tar-like substance derived from bituminous deposits rich in fossilized fish (Gk *ichthys* fish).

ichthyosis a group of disorders of keratinization characterized by fine scaling and a feeling of dryness of the skin (Gk *ichthya* rough fish skin [Hipp], from *ichthys* fish, *osis*).

ICS *InterCellular Substance*, the matrix holding epidermal cells together.

icterus jaundice (New L from Gk *ikteros* the jaundice [Hipp]).

-id, -ide suff. deriving from two sources, implying either a taxonomic or a patronymic relationship (L *idus*, akin to Gk *ides*

Chapter 83: *Glossary of Dermatological Terms*

descendent, of; or Gk *eidēs* of the appearance of, similar to, from *eidos* form, shape). In dermatology the term 'ide', 'id', denotes a reaction occurring in a part remote from the primary lesion, usually but not invariably due to an immunological reaction to the agent concerned or to its component parts, e.g. tuberculide, syphilide, trichophytide. (Distinguish 'id', a psychological term derived from L *id*, neuter sing. of *is* he.)

idio- personal, applying to oneself (Gk *idios* personal, one's own. Therefore, peculiar to the individual).

idiopathic having no known cause, originally used to imply that a disease had its own internal or in-built cause, and was not due to external factors (Late L *idiopatheia* [Gall], from Gk *idios* personal, *pathos* suffering, disease).

ILVEN *Inflammatory Linear Verrucous Epidermal Naevus.*

imbricatus overlapping, layered (L *imbricatus*, past part. of *imbricare*, from *imbrex, imbricis* a gutter tile, from the method of layering these).

impetigo contagious eruption of the skin caused by the *Streptococcus/Staphylococcus* (L *impetēre* to attack, assault).

incarnatus becoming flesh. Term used for ingrowing hairs of pseudofolliculitis. (Ecclesiastical L *incarnatus*, past part. passive of *incarnare* to be made flesh; incarnate).

incontinentia (pigmenti) immoderate, intemperate, incontinent; not held in check (L *incontinentia*, from *incontinens*, from *in* not, *continens*, pres. part. of *continere* to hold, keep together, restrain).

infarct an area of coagulation necrosis due to local ischaemia (L *infarcire* to stuff in) [1].

infra- pref. below, beneath (L *infra* for *infera* below).

inter- pref. between, among, shared (L *inter* between, among).

intertrigo inflammation of apposed skin surfaces such as groins, axillae and inframammary areas (L *inter* between, *tri(tus)*, past part. of *terere* to rub, *igo*, a suff. forming nouns from verbs, indicating diseased condition).

ischaemia state of lack of blood supply to a part or organ; arterial insufficiency (Gk *ischaimos* a staunching of blood, from *ischein*, form of *echein* to have, hold, *aemia*, New L suff. from Gk *haima* blood).

iso- pref. same as, equivalent (Gk *isos* equal to).

isomorphic having the same form (Gk *isos* same, *morphē* form).

isomorphic reaction see KOEBNER PHENOMENON.

itch sensation eliciting desire to scratch; skin disorder characterized by an itch. Colloquially, a term used for scabies (ME *icche*, OE *gicce*, from *giccan* to itch).

Ito M Japanese dermatologist 1884–1982. Incontinentia pigmenti achromians (achromic naevus). Streaky and marbled hypermelanosis, often with central nervous system abnormalities.

Ito's naevus naevus fuscoceruleus acromiodeltoideus.

ITP *Idiopathic Thrombocytopenic Purpura.*

ixodes largest genus of Ixodid or hard ticks (Gk *ixōdēs*, from *ixos* mistletoe or birdlime prepared from mistletoe berry, *eidos* like, in form of) because of the surface stickiness of their bodies.

-itis originally Gk adjectival suff. relating to a term specified; later, used as L noun. In New L and modern medical usage it indicates inflammation.

Jaccoud FS French physician 1830–1913.

Jaccoud's syndrome, disease deforming distal arthropathy in young adults with recent rheumatic fever or systemic lupus erythematosus.

Jackson ADM US paediatrician *fl.* 20th cent.

Jackson–Lawler syndrome a variant of pachyonychia congenita with erupted teeth at birth and sebocystomatosis at puberty.

Jacobi E German dermatologist 1862–1915.

Jacobi's poikiloderma poikiloderma atrophicans vasculare.

Jacquet LML French dermatologist 1860–1914.

Jacquet's (napkin) erythema a dermatitis affecting the area covered by diapers; napkin eruption.

Jadassohn J German dermatologist 1863–1936. One of the great figures responsible for the flowering of dermatology in the late 19th and early 20th centuries. A keen observer and prolific writer. Responsible for the delineation of many diseases: granulosis rubra nasi, pachyonychia congenita, macular atrophy, sebaceous naevus, BORST–JADASSOHN PHENOMENON, FRANCESCHETTI–JADASSOHN SYNDROME, etc.

Jadassohn–Lewandowsky syndrome pachyonychia congenita Type I, with later mucosal leukoplakia.

Jadassohn–Pellizzari anetoderma outmoded term for a form of macular atrophy.

Jaffe HL US orthopaedic pathologist 1896–1979.

Jaffe–Lichtenstein syndrome/disease monostotic form of fibrous dysplasia.

Janeway EG US physician 1841–1911.

Janeway lesions faint macular lesions of thenar and hypothenar eminences in bacterial endocarditis.

Jarisch A Austrian dermatologist 1850–1902.

Jarisch–Herxheimer reaction focal exacerbation of lesions when a disease of infective origin is treated with potent antimicrobial agents. Seen in treatment of early syphilis with penicillin.

jaundice yellowish discoloration of the skin, sclerae and mucous membranes resulting from excess of bile pigments in the blood (ME *jaunice*, from OF *jaunice*, *jaunisse*, from *jaune* yellow, with phonetic accretion of 'd'; derived from L *galbus* yellow).

Jeghers H US gastroenterologist 1904–90. PEUTZ–JEGHERS SYNDROME.

Jessner M German, later US dermatologist 1887–1978.

Jessner–Kanof lesion, infiltration benign lymphocytic infiltration.

Job archetypal patriarch of the Old Testament. Was struck down in his prime with a devastating disease of skin and bowels, from which he eventually recovered [8].

Job's syndrome hyperimmunoglobulin E recurrent infection syndrome, commencing in early childhood and therefore oddly named.

Johanson A US paediatrician *fl.* 20th cent.

Johanson–Blizzard syndrome aplasia cutis of scalp, sparse hair, deafness, dental and other defects.

Johnson FC US paediatrician 1894–1934. STEVENS–JOHNSON SYNDROME.

Jorgensen RJ US physician 1841–1911.

Jorgensen's syndrome a form of ectodermal dysplasia, probably identical with BASAN'S SYNDROME.

Jung LKL US paediatrician *fl.* 20th cent.

Jung's disease pyoderma, folliculitis, atrophy and defective leucocyte and lymphocyte function.

Junin disease a form of haemorrhagic fever in S America due to an arenovirus. Named after a town in Argentina from which cases were isolated.

kairo cancer heat-associated carcinoma from contact with hot body-warmers (Japanese *kairo* a pocket-sized metal benzene-heated warmer).

kala-azar visceral form of leishmaniasis (Hindi *kala* black, Assamese *azar* disease, poison). Also known as Dum-Dum fever after a town near Calcutta, India.

Kallin syndrome name (of patient) given to a family with a variant of simple epidermolysis bullosa associated with anodontia, hair and nail disorders.

Kallman FJ German-born US geneticist and psychiatrist 1897–1965.

Kallman's syndrome X-linked trait of hypogonadotrophic hypogonadism and anosmia; perhaps linked with sex-linked ichthyosis (XLI).

Kamino H US pathologist *fl.* 20th cent.

Kamino bodies eosinophilic globules in dermo-epidermal junction in spindle cell and SPITZ NAEVUS.

kampo (kanpo) a form of treatment using Chinese herbal drugs. Properly, kanpo yaku (Chinese *kan* China, *po* method, *yaku* herbal medicine).

kang cancer epithelioma ab igne occurring over greater trochanter from sleeping on heated beds (Chinese term for a stove or a sleeping platform heated by fire beneath).

Kangri cancer epithelioma ab igne from contact with wicker-covered earthenware pots filled with heated charcoal and held close to the belly or thighs. Named after an area in Kashmir.

Kanof NB US dermatologist 1912–88. JESSNER–KANOF INFILTRATE.

Kanzaki T Japanese dermatologist *fl.* 20th cent.

Kanzaki disease angiokeratoderma corporis diffusum with lysosomal α-N-acetylgalactosaminidase deficiency.

Kaposi M Hungarian-born Austrian dermatologist 1837–1902. Student of Hebra (q.v.) and his successor in Vienna, he was an outstanding figure of 19th-century dermatology. He established dermatitis herpetiformis as an entity and described the 'butterfly' erythema of lupus erythematosus.

Kaposi's sarcoma multiple idiopathic haemorrhagic sarcoma.

Kaposi's varicelliform eruption disseminated primary infection with viruses of herpes simplex, vaccinia and perhaps Coxsackie A16, seen especially in atopic subjects. Now termed 'eczema herpeticum' and 'eczema vaccinatum'.

karyorrhexis fragmentation of cell nucleus (Gk *karyon* nut, nucleus, *rhexis* tearing).

Kasabach HH US paediatrician 1898–1943.

Kasabach–Merritt syndrome giant cavernous haemangioma with intravascular coagulation.

Katayama syndrome, disease acute febrile manifestation of schistosomiasis japonica. Urticarial fever. Named after a rice-field area in the western part of Japan.

Kawasaki T Japanese paediatrician *fl.* 20th cent.

Kawasaki's disease mucocutaneous lymph node syndrome.

Kayser B German ophthalmologist 1869–1954.

Kayser–Fleischer rings grey-green or brown rings of copper deposits on the outer border of the cornea, pathognomic of hepatolenticular degeneration.

keds colloq. name either for members of the Hippoboscidae family of arthropods; or sheep ticks (origin uncertain).

keloid alternative term for cheloid and preferred by some in common usage. But probably incorrect in derivation, which is admittedly disputed (Gk *kēlē* tumour, hernia, *kēlis* stain, spot or *chēlē* cloven hoof, claw, forked probe) (see CHELOID).

kerato- comb. form indicating horn or cornea (Gk *keras, keratos* horn). Thus, relating to horny layer, cornification.

kerion an inflammatory granuloma of hair-bearing areas due to superficial fungal infection, particularly of zoophilic species (Gk *kērion* honeycomb).

kibe old term for a chapped or ulcerated chilblain, especially on the heel (origin uncertain, possibly from Welsh *cibi a* sore on a sheep's hoof).

KID Keratitis Ichthyosis Deafness syndrome.

Kikuchi I Japanese dermatologist *fl.* 20th cent.

Kikuchi's disease necrotizing nongranulomatous lymphangitis with fever, leucopenia and cervical lymphadenopathy.

Kimura T Japanese pathologist 1884–1969.

Kimura's disease angiolymphoid hyperplasia with eosinophilia or a condition similar to this.

Kindler T Austrian-born dermatologist 1890–1975.

Kindler's syndrome (synonym Weary–Kindler syndrome) acrokeratotic poikiloderma.

Kirman BH British psychiatrist *fl.* 20th cent.

Kirman's syndrome idiocy and anhidrotic ectodermal dysplasia.

Kitamura K Japanese dermatologist 1899–1989.

Kitamura's disease reticulate acropigmentation.

Klein D Swiss geneticist 1908–93. FRANCESCHETTI–KLEIN SYNDROME.

Klinefelter HF, Jr US physician b. 1912.

Klinefelter's syndrome (synonym XXY syndrome) eunuchoid habitus, gynaecomastia, infertility and other defects seen in males with an extra X chromosome.

Klippel M French neuropsychiatrist 1858–1942.

Klippel–Trenaunay–Parkes Weber syndrome extensive unilateral capillary naevus of limb with hypertrophy.

Kloepfer HW US anatomist *fl.* 20th cent.

Koch AHR German bacteriologist 1843–1910. Koch's bacillus.

Koch's postulates, law the law of specificity of bacteria. Four conditions must be satisfied to establish the causative organism of a specific disease: the organism must be present in every case; it must be isolated and grown in pure culture; when this is inoculated into susceptible animals it must reproduce the disease; and the organism must be grown again in pure culture.

Koebner (Köbner) H German dermatologist 1838–1904.

Koebner phenomenon, reaction the induction of a lesion of certain diseases, typically psoriasis and lichen planus, following nonspecific trauma to the unaffected skin; isomorphic effect, reaction.

Koenen JHOC Dutch psychiatrist 1893–1956.

Koenen's tumours periungual fibromata occurring in tuberous sclerosis.

Kogoj F Yugoslavian dermatologist 1894–1983.

Kogoj's spongiform pustule epidermal pustule containing polymorphonuclear leucocytes seen in active or pustular phases of psoriasis.

Kohlschütter A Swiss paediatrician *fl.* 20th cent.

Kohlschütter's syndrome amelocerebrohypohidrotic syndrome.

koilonychia spoon-shaped nails (Gk *koilos* hollow, *onyx, onychos* nail).

kokarden naevus resembling a rosette worn on hats (German *kokarde* cockade). See COCKADE.

Kokobera virus a flavivirus originally found in Queensland,

Australia and named after the Koko Bera, an Aboriginal tribe of the area.

Kolopp P Alsace-born French dermatologist 1888–1951. WORINGER–KOLOPP DISEASE.

Koplik H US paediatrician 1858–1927.

Koplik spots irregular red spots with greyish centres seen in oral mucosa during the prodromal period of measles.

Koyanagi Y Japanese ophthalmologist 1880–1954. VOGT–KOYANAGI SYNDROME.

Krabbe KH Danish neurologist 1885–1961.

Krabbe's disease hereditary globoid leucodystrophy.

Krause WJF German anatomist 1833–1910.

Krause's end-bulbs encapsulated receptors found in skin and mucous membranes.

kraurosis obs. term used to describe dry condition of mucous membranes, particularly the vagina. Primary atrophy of the vulva (New L from Gk *krauros* dry, brittle, *osis*).

Kunjin virus a flavivirus originally isolated in Queensland, Australia and so-named by contraction of Koko Munjin, an Aboriginal tribal group in the area.

Küstner H German gynaecologist 1897–1963. PRAUSNITZ–KÜSTNER REACTION.

Kveim MA Norwegian physician 1882–1966.

Kveim (Kveim–Siltzbach) test diagnostic test for sarcoidosis using intradermal injection of sarcoid tissue.

kwashiorkor a disease of malnutrition in which the (African) hair becomes a lighter, reddish colour (Ghanaian term for 'rejected one').

Kyanasur Forest fever a tick-borne haemorrhagic fever due to a togavirus, named after an area of Mysore State, India.

Kyrle J Austrian dermatologist 1880–1926.

Kyrle's disease hyperkeratosis follicularis et parafollicularis in cutem penetrans; hypertrophic keratotic lesions penetrating the dermis.

Laband PF Trinidadian dental and oral surgeon *fl.* 20th cent.

Laband syndrome hereditary gingival fibromatosis with defects of ear, nose, nail and bone, and hepatosplenomegaly.

LADD syndrome *Lacrimo-Auriculo-Dento-Digital* syndrome.

Lafora GR Spanish neuropathologist 1886–1971.

Lafora's disease a neuro-metabolic disease with progressive myoclonus epilepsy, showing PAS-positive intracycloplasmic (Lafora) bodies in many organs.

lagophthalmos inability to close eyelids completely, as in facial nerve paralysis; 'hare-eye' (Gk *lagōs* hare, *ophthalmos* eye).

LAMB *Lentigines, Atrial myxomas, Mucocutaneous myxomas, Blue naevi*.

lamella a layer, leaf or plate; used to describe scaling (L *lamella*, dim. of *lamina* a thin plate).

Langer C, Ritter von Edenberg Austrian anatomist 1819–87.

Langer's lines cleavage lines in skin determined by the disposition of connective tissue in reticular layer.

Langer LO US radiologist *fl.* 20th cent.

Langer–Giedion syndrome trichorhinophalangeal syndrome, Type II.

Langerhans P German pathologist 1847–88.

Langerhans' cells important specialized dopa-negative dendritic mesodermal cells.

Langerhans, islets of clusters of endocrine cells in the pancreas.

Langerhans' layer granular layer of epidermis.

Langhans T German anatomist 1839–1915.

Langhans' cells multinucleated giant cells, as found typically in tuberculous granulomas.

lanuginosa excess or undue persistence of fine downy hair covering mid-term fetus (L *lanugo* soft hair, down). Often misused for vellus hair.

Larssen T Swedish medical statistician *fl.* 20th cent. SJÖGREN–LARSSEN SYNDROME.

LASER (laser) *Light Amplification by the Stimulated Emission of Radiation*.

Lassa fever arenavirus infection, first recognized in Lassa, a 'lonely herdsman's village' in Nigeria.

Lassar O German dermatologist 1849–1907.

Lassar's paste zinc oxide paste with salicylic acid.

Lassueur A Swiss dermatologist 1874–1949. PICCARDI–LASSUEUR–GRAHAM-LITTLE SYNDROME.

Laugier P French dermatologist *fl.* 20th cent.

Laugier–Hunziker syndrome acquired macular hyperpigmentation of buccal mucosa and lips. Banded nail pigmentation may also occur.

LAV *Lymphadenopathy Associated Virus* (later HTLV III). Name originally given to AIDS agent, isolated by Montagnier in France in 1983.

Lawler SD US geneticist *fl.* 20th cent. JACKSON–LAWLER SYNDROME.

Lawrence RD British physician 1892–1968.

Lawrence–Seip syndrome (synonyms Seip–Lawrence syndrome, Berardinelli syndrome, lipoatrophic diabetes) total lipoatrophy. Inherited absence of adipose tissue with hyperinsulinism and other features.

Ledderhose G German surgeon 1855–1925.

Ledderhose's disease plantar fibromatosis. Akin to DUPUYTREN'S CONTRACTURE.

Lefèvre P French dermatologist *fl.* 20th cent. PAPILLON–LEFÈVRE SYNDROME.

Legionaire's disease acute respiratory infection caused by various species of genus LEGIONELLA sp.

Legionella a genus of air-borne bacteria first discovered during outbreak of pneumonia at convention of American Legion in 1976.

Leiner C Austrian paediatrician 1871–1930. One of the first paediatric dermatologists.

Leiner's disease, syndrome a desquamative erythroderma of uncertain aetiology affecting young infants and accompanied by diarrhoea, weight loss and increased susceptibility to infections.

Leishman, Sir William B British army surgeon and pathologist 1865–1926.

Leishman–Donovan bodies intracellular phase of flagellate protozoa such as *Leishmania*; amastigotes (Gk *-a-priv, mastix, mastigos* whip, flagellum).

Leishmania a genus of flagellate protozoa of family Trypanosomatidae. Various species are responsible for different forms of leishmaniasis.

Leishmanin test intradermal test for cutaneous Leishmaniasis.

LEND AN EGG extended acronym to describe painful cutaneous nodules comprising *Leiomyoma, Eccrine tumour, Neuroma, Dermatofibroma, Angiolipoma, Neurilemmoma, Endometrioma, Glomus tumour* and *Granular cell tumour*.

Lennert K German histopathologist *fl.* 20th cent.

Lennert's lymphoma a Hodgkin-like lymphoma with massive epithelioid-cell infiltrate; 'epithelioid-cell lymphogranulomatosis'.

lenticularis double-convex, shaped like a lentil (Late L, from dim. of *lens* lentil).

lentigo a pigmented macule having an increased number of melanocytes at the dermo-epidermal junction (L *lentigo*, from *lens*, *lentis* lentil, from an approximation of its shape).

LEOPARD syndrome (widespread) *L*entigos, *E*EG abnormalities, *O*cular hyperteleorism, *P*ulmonary stenosis, *A*bnormal genitals, *R*etarded growth, *D*eafness.

lepidopterism a term used for the ill-effects caused in humans by a structure or product of butterflies and moths (Gk *lepis*, *lepidos* scaly, *pteron* wing).

leprechaunism a rare lethal syndrome of infancy showing wide-set eyes, low-set ears and multiple metabolic and endocrine abnormalities (Irish Gaelic *lupracán leipreachán* and other spellings, from Old Irish *luchorpān*, from *lu* small, *corp* body). A little fellow and a mischievous elf.

leprosy (synonym Hansen's disease) a chronic mycobacterial disease affecting the skin and peripheral nervous system (Gk *lepros* scaly, scabby [Hipp], from *lepra* scale. But the term was originally applied differently or at least more widely and is confused in translation) [9].

Léri A French physician 1875–1930.

Léri syndrome dyschondrosteosis; hereditary dyschondroplasia with short stature, epiphysial ossification and broad diaphyses of long bones.

Leroy E French public health physician *fl.* early 20th cent. FIESSINGER–LEROY SYNDROME, REITER'S SYNDROME.

Leroy JG Belgian geneticist and paediatrician *fl.* 20th cent.

Leroy's syndrome mucolipidosis II; I-cell disease.

Lesch M US paediatrician *fl.* 20th cent.

Lesch–Nyhan syndrome choreoathetosis, retarded mental and physical development and self-mutilation associated with hyperuricaemia due to genetic enzyme deficiency.

Leser E German surgeon 1853–1916.

Leser–Trélat sign rapid development of pruritic seborrhoeic keratoses associated with internal malignancy.

Lester AM British physician 1909–93.

Lester iris, lines areas of pale pigment in the papillary margin of the iris, having a dark clover leaf-like centre. A feature of hereditary osteo-onychodysplasia (nail-patella syndrome).

Letterer E German pathologist 1895–1982.

Letterer–Siwe disease an acute form of generalized histiocytosis of infancy, with seborrhoeic eczema-like eruption and purpura.

leucoderma lack of normal pigmentation of the skin, of various causes; a generic term with limited application (Gk *leukos* white, *derma* skin).

leucoplakia persistent white patches on mucous membranes not attributable to a known disease process (Gk *leuko(s)* white, *plax*, *plakos* flat, plate-like, *-ia*).

leucoplasia lit. white development. Synonymous with LEUCOPLAKIA but indicating continuing process (New L from Gk *leuko(s)* white, *plasis* moulding).

Leventhal ML US obstetrician and gynaecologist 1901–71. STEIN–LEVENTHAL SYNDROME.

Lewandowsky F German dermatologist 1879–1921. JADASSOHN–LEWANDOWSKY SYNDROME.

Lewandowsky's rosacea–like tuberculide a false tuberculide of the face, probably related to rosacea.

Lewandowsky–Lutz syndrome epidermodysplasia verruciformis.

Lewars PD British oral surgeon *fl.* 20th cent.

Lewars' disease pulse granuloma. Chronic mandibular periostitis caused by embedded vegetable matter.

LI *L*amellar *I*chthyosis.

Libman E US physician 1872–1946.

Libman–Sacks endocarditis a verrucous endocarditis that may be associated with systemic lupus erythematosus.

lichen an old term originally applied by Willan to various papular diseases, its usage was modified by Unna (q.v.) and is now restricted to a relatively small number of papular eruptions, of which lichen (rubra) planus is the most common (Gk *leichēn* a tree-moss, lichen or liverwort; a lichen-like eruption on the skin of animals or man [Hipp]. But the association is obscure).

Lichtenstein L US orthopaedic pathologist 1906–77. JAFFE–LICHTENSTEIN SYNDROME.

Lindau A Swedish pathologist 1892–1958. VON HIPPEL–LINDAU DISEASE.

lipometre instrument for photometric assessment of sebum production (Gk *lipos* fat).

Lipschütz B Austrian dermatologist and virologist 1878–1931.

Lipschütz ulcer ulcus vulvae acutum. Single or sparse self-resolving vulval ulcer.

Lisch K Austrian ophthalmologist b. 1907.

Lisch nodules pigmented iris hamartomas occurring in neurofibromatosis.

Lister JM, lst Baron British surgeon 1827–1912. Pioneer of antiseptic surgery (listerism).

Listeria a bacterial genus e.g. *L. monocytogenes*, a microaerophilic Gram-positive bacillus found in soil and as a parasite in vertebrates and invertebrates. Hence listeriosis. After LISTER.

LISUP *L*ow *I*ntensity *S*elective *U*VB *P*hototherapy.

livedo a cyanotic discoloration of the skin of reticulate, patchy or mottled pattern due to venous congestion or arterial disease (L *livere* to be black and blue).

loa loa a filarial worm of genus of filarial nematodes, family Onchocercidae. Cause of loiasis (Congolese, eye-worm).

Lobo J Brazilian physician 1900–79.

Lobo's disease lobomycosis, cheloidiform blastomycosis caused by *Paracoccioides loboi*.

LOD *L*ichenified *O*ncho*D*ermatitis.

Loewenstein (Lowenstein) LW German-born US dermatologist 1885–1959. BUSCHKE–LOEWENSTEIN TUMOUR.

Löffler W Swiss physician 1887–1972.

Löffler's eosinophilic syndrome a transient pulmonary infiltration (febrile pneumonitis) with blood eosinophilia.

Löfgren S Swedish chest physician 1910–78.

Löfgren's syndrome bilateral hilar lymphadenopathy syndrome.

Louis-Bar, Mme D Belgian neurologist *fl.* 20th cent.

Louis-Bar syndrome ataxia telangiectasia.

louse an ectoparasitic insect belonging to the order Anoplura or Mallophaga; dermatologically, head or body louse (*Pediculus*) or pubic louse (*Phthirus*) (OE *lus* louse).

Lowry B Canadian paediatrician and geneticist *fl.* 20th cent. COFFIN–LOWRY SYNDROME.

loxoscelism form of arachnidism caused by spider of family

Loxoscelidae (Gk *loxos* slanting, oblique, *skelos* leg).

Lubarsh O German pathologist 1860–1933.

Lubarsh–Pick disease systemic amyloidosis.

Lucio R Mexican physician 1819–66.

Lucio's phenomenon a distinctive reactional state in the course of diffuse lepromatous LEPROSY.

Ludvigsen K Danish dermatologist *fl.* 20th cent. HELWEG-LARSEN–LUDVIGSEN SYNDROME.

lues a disguised designation for syphilis but originally a term for plague (L *lues* a plague, contagious disease).

lupus a term applied to lesions having an eroded or gnawed quality. Now confined to form of cutaneous tuberculosis, especially lupus vulgaris, and lupus erythematosus, where it is better fitted to describe the discoid form. Used adjectivally as *lupoid*, to describe a gnawed appearance, as in *lupoid sycosis* (L *lupus* wolf, from supposed resemblance to bites of wolf; 'summen clepen cancrum and summen lypum', Lanfranc *c*. 1400; 'a malignant ulcer … very hungry, like vnto a woolfe', Barrough 1590; *OED*).

Lutz W Swiss dermatologist 1888–1958. LEWANDOWSKY–LUTZ SYNDROME.

Lyell A British dermatologist *fl.* 20th cent.

Lyell's syndrome toxic epidermal necrolysis. Originally also included staphylococcal scalded skin syndrome.

Lyme small coastal town in Connecticut, USA, where Lyme disease (borreliosis) was first delineated.

Lyon MF British geneticist *fl.* 20th cent.

Lyon hypothesis inactivation of one of the two X chromosomes in female embryos.

-lysis comb. form meaning loosening, separation or rupture (Gk *lysis*, from *lyein* to loosen, dissolve).

-ma see -OMA.

Macacaceae (Macaca) a large genus of Old World monkeys involving the macaque and rhesus (Portuguese *macaco*, from W African *makaku* monkey).

Machupo an arenavirus causing haemorrhagic fever. Named after a town in Bolivia.

McKusick VA US geneticist *fl.* 20th cent.

McKusick's syndrome metaphyseal chondrodysplasia.

macro- comb. form meaning large, long (Gk *makros* large).

macrocheilia abnormal enlargement of lips (Gk *makro(s)* large, *cheilos* lip).

madarosis loss of eyelashes (Gk *madaros* pulpy, bald; *madarosis* [Gal] loss of eyelashes).

Madelung OW German surgeon 1846–1926.

Madelung's neck a diffuse lipomatosis affecting neck and shoulders, usually of males.

Madura foot parochial name for *mycetoma*, a tumid granulomatous fungal infection of the foot. Named after Madura, now Madurai, a town in S India.

Maffuci A Italian physician 1847–1903.

Maffucci's syndrome dyschondroplasia with haemangiomata.

MAGIC syndrome *M*outh *A*nd *G*enital ulcers with *I*nflamed *C*artilage. A combination of relapsing polychondritis and BEHÇET'S SYNDROME.

main succulente swollen and oedematous hand seen in syringomyelia (Fr *succulente*, from L *suculentus* juice).

Majocchi D renowned Italian dermatologist 1849–1929.

Majocchi's granuloma trichophytic granuloma.

Majocchi's purpura purpura annularis telangiectoides.

Makai E Hungarian surgeon *fl.* 20th cent. ROTHMAN–MAKAI SYNDROME.

mal- comb. form; bad, badly (OF *mal*, from L *malus* bad).

-malacia, -malako comb. form indicating softening of a tissue (Gk *malakia* softness).

malakoplakia an immunodeficiency disease affecting mainly the urinary or gastrointestinal tracts but also, rarely, the skin. So-named after the soft nature of the lesion (Gk *malakos* soft, *plax* flat, plate, plaque, but more directly from Middle Dutch *placken* to beat (metal) flat, thence from Middle Fr *plaque*)

malaria a febrile disease due to infection by protozoa of genus *Plasmodium* transmitted by female *Anopheles* mosquitoes (Italian *mala*, from L *malus* bad, *aria* air).

Malassez LC French physiologist 1842–1909.

Malassezia name previously given to the dimorphic form of the lipophilic yeast *Pityrosporum orbiculare.*

mal de Meleda a characteristic recessive form of genetic palmoplantar keratoderma seen on the island of Meleda (Melita) on the Dalmatian coast.

Malherbe M French surgeon 1845–1915.

Malherbe's benign calcifying epithelioma pilomatricoma.

Malpighi M Italian anatomist and physiologist 1628–94. One of the first microscopists and founders of histology. Malpighi's tubules, vesicles, etc.

Malpighian layer the basal and prickle-cell layers of the epidermis; stratum malpighii.

MALT *M*ucosa-*A*ssociated *L*ymphoid *T*issue (as, for example, Peyer's patches).

mamillaria miliaria profunda (L *mamilla*, dim. of *mamma* breast, teat, nipple).

mange contagious skin disease of domestic and other fur-covered animals, caused by various types of mite (q.v.); earlier, also of humans but now only pejoratively (ME *manjewe*, OF *mangeue* itching, lit. eating, from *manjuer*, *mangier*, from L *manducare* to chew).

Mantoux C French physician 1877–1947.

Mantoux, porokeratosis of a form of dyskeratosis affecting the palms and soles of young adults.

Mantoux test intracutaneous tuberculin test for tuberculosis.

maple syrup urine disease (synonym branched-chain ketonuria) an inborn error of metabolism with increased urinary leucine, isoleucine and valine. Named after syrup made from the sap of the maple tree (OE *mapul* maple).

MaRAS *Ma*jor *R*ecurrent *A*phthous *S*tomatitis. Periadenitis mucosa necrotica recurrens (SUTTON'S ULCER).

Marburg disease a rhabdoviral infection. Named after town in Germany where the disease was first discovered in a consignment of imported monkeys; 'green monkey disease'.

Marek J Hungarian veterinarian and pathologist 1867–1952.

Marek's disease a DNA-virus-induced B-cell lymphoma in poultry.

Marfan AB-J French paediatrician 1858–1942.

Marfan's syndrome a heritable disorder of connective tissue characterized by abnormally long extremities, arachnodactyly and ocular and cardiovascular anomalies.

Margolis E Israeli medicolegal geneticist *fl.* 20th cent. ZIPRKOWSKI–MARGOLIS SYNDROME.

Marie Unna see UNNA, MARIE.

Marie Unna syndrome a genetic form of progressive hypotrichosis with scarring and abnormal hair shafts.

Marinesco G Romanian pathologist and neurologist 1864–1938.

Marinesco–Sjögren syndrome cerebellar ataxia, retarded development, cataracts and skeletal defects.

Marjolin JN French physician 1780–1850.

Marjolin's ulcer squamous cell carcinoma arising in irritated scar tissue.

Marshall D US ophthalmologist b. 1905.

Marshall's syndrome a form of ectodermal dysplasia with congenital myopia and impaired hearing.

Martorell F Spanish vascular surgeon 1906–84. Founded 'Angiologia'.

Martorell's ulcer hypertensive ulcer of the leg.

Martorell's syndrome see TAKAYASU'S ARTERITIS.

Masson CLP French-born Canadian pathologist 1880–1959.

Masson's naevic corpuscles neuroid elements, similar to Meissner's corpuscles (q.v.), found in the deep parts of intradermal naevi.

Masson's pseudosarcoma intravascular papillary endothelial hypoplasia.

mast cell, mastocyte widely dispersed mesenchymal cells found in the bone marrow, dermis and other tissues, the cytoplasm of which contains numerous metachromatically staining granules.

mast cell (German *Mastzelle*, from *mästen* to feed gluttinously, to fatten).

Mauriac C French venereologist 1832–1905.

Mauriac's syndrome neuralgic pain preceding recurrences of herpes simplex.

Mauriac LP French physician 1882–1963.

Mauriac's syndrome juvenile diabetes, dwarfism and hepatomegaly.

Mazzini LY US serologist b. 1894.

Mazzini's test a flocculation test for syphilis.

Mazzoni V Italian physiologist 1880–1940. GOLGI–MAZZONI CORPUSCLE.

Mazzotti L Mexican parasitologist 1900–71.

Mazzotti's test exacerbation of onchocerciasis after diethyl carbamazine. An immunological reaction caused by dying microfilariae.

Meara RH British dermatologist *fl.* 20th cent. DOWLING–MEARA SYNDROME.

measles (synonym morbilli) highly infectious disease caused by a paramyxovirus (pl. construed as sing. From ME *maseles* spots; modern Dutch *mazelen*; origin obscure).

Medina worm *Dranunculus medinensis*, the guinea worm, named after a town in Saudi Arabia.

Mees RA Dutch physician *fl.* 20th cent.

Mees' lines horizontal whitish striations observed on nails in acute arsenical poisoning but also seen with other systemic disease.

Meibom H German anatomist 1638–1700.

Meibomian glands tarsal glands. Modified sebaceous glands lying in a groove in the tarsus of the eyelid.

Meijere see DE MEIJERE.

Meijere's trio group of three hairs growing together as a synchronous group in the same phase of activity.

Meirowsky E US dermatologist 1876–1960.

Meirowsky's phenomenon transient immediate pigment darkening induced particularly by UVA.

Meissner G German histologist 1829–1905.

Meissner's corpuscles sensory nerve endings of the glabrous skin of primates.

melanin a brown-black pigment of human and other vertebrate tissues. Originally coined by Bizio in 1825 for the pigment of cephalopods (Gk *melas* black).

melano- comb. form meaning black, dark (Gk *melano-*, comb. form of *melas, melanos* black)

melasma hypermelanosis of the face, seen chiefly in women; *chloasma* (obs.) (New L from Gk *melasma* [Hipp.] dark spot, from *melas* black).

Meleda see MAL DE MELEDA.

Meleney FL US surgeon 1889–1963.

Meleny's ulcer bacterial synergistic gangrene.

melioidosis a glanders (q.v.)-like infection of rodents and other mammals caused by *Pseudomonas pseudomallei* (Gk *mēlis, mēlidis* a distemper of asses).

Melkersson EG Swedish physician 1898–1932.

Melkersson–Rosenthal syndrome recurrent facial paralysis, facial oedema, granulomatous cheilitis and other associated features.

Melnick M US orofacial geneticist *fl.* 20th cent.

Melnick–Fraser syndrome (synonym BOR syndrome) branchial fistulae, ear pits, hearing loss and renal anomalies.

melorrheostosis thickening of cortex of long bones giving an appearance of a candle down which melted wax has flowed (Gk *melo(s)* limb, *rheo* flow, *osteon* bone, *osis*).

Mendes da Costa S Dutch dermatologist 1862–1941.

Mendes da Costa's syndrome erythrokeratoderma variabilis.

Menkes JH Austrian-born US paediatric neurologist *fl.* 20th cent.

Menkes disease kinky hair. Rare metabolic disorder due to defective copper metabolism.

MEN syndromes *Multiple Endocrine Neoplasia* syndromes of various types according to organs involved.

Merkel FS German anatomist and physiologist 1845–1919.

Merkel cells, touch spots ('tastzellen') nonencapsulated corpuscular epidermal sensory receptors.

Merritt KK US paediatrician b. 1886. KASABACH–MERRITT SYNDROME.

meta- versatile pref. with several shades of meaning: among, after, beyond, between, changed, etc. (Gk *meta*, meanings dependent on the case taken). Also used, *m-*, for 1,3-position of benzene ring.

metophyma inflamed rosaceous nodule of forehead (Gk *metopon* forehead, *phyma* tumour).

Meyerson LB US dermatologist *fl.* 20th cent.

Meyerson's phenomenon a nonspecific papulosquamous reaction around pigmented naevi; sometimes, controversially, to include eczematous reaction and lesions other than pigmented naevi.

Mibelli V Italian dermatologist 1860–1910.

Mibelli, angiokeratoma of familial form of peripheral angiokeratosis.

Mibelli, porokeratosis of single or multiple areas of atrophy surrounded by a raised dyskeratotic edge.

Michaelis LM German-born US biochemist 1875–1949.

Michaelis–Gutmann bodies round basophilic inclusions containing calcium and iron in histiocytes, considered pathognomic for malakoplakia.

'Michelin tyre' baby rare condition in which generalized folding of redundant fat occurs, fancifully resembling logo of Michelin tyres.

micro- pref. meaning small (Gk *mikros* small).

Miescher G Swiss dermatologist 1887–1961. Granulomatosis disciformis chronica progressiva (nondiabetic necrobiosis lipoidica); granulomatous cheilitis.

Mikulicz J (von Mikulicz-Radecki) Polish surgeon, active in Germany 1850–1905.

Mikulicz's syndrome bilateral lacrimal salivary gland swelling, sometimes occurring in sarcoidosis.

Mikulicz's ulcers (synonym MIRAS) minor aphthous ulcers.

Milian GA French dermatologist 1871–1945.

Milian's erythema morbilliform erythema occurring on the ninth day of arsphenamine treatment (obs.).

Milian's white atrophy (synonym atrophie blanche) areas of atrophy with stippled telangiectasia occurring on lower legs and feet, associated with venous incompetence.

miliary similar in size to a millet seed (0.5–1.5 mm) (New L *miliaris* millet-like, from *milium* millet, ia).

milium a tiny white cyst containing laminated keratin (L *milium* millet seed) [1].

Milroy WF US physician 1855–1942.

Milroy's disease, oedema congenital and hereditary lympho-edema of leg Type I.

Mims LC US paediatrician *fl.* 20th cent. FEUERSTEIN–MIMS–SCHIMMELPENNING SYNDROME.

MIRAS MInor Recurrent Aphthous Stomatitis; MIKULICZ'S ULCERS.

Mishima Y Japanese dermatologist *fl.* 20th cent.

Mishima's dual pathway theory a concept of dual origin of malignant melanoma to explain difference in growth rate of various types.

mite colloq. term for any small insect. Properly, a very small arachnid of the subclass Acarina (OE *mite* a small insect; also used for a coin of very small value; 'half-farthing').

Mitsuda K Japanese leprologist 1876–1964.

Mitsuda's antigen, reaction a suspension of heat-killed leprosy bacilli used in an intradermal test for LEPROSY.

Moeller JOL German physician 1819–87.

Moeller's glossitis chronic superficial glossitis; exfoliative glossitis.

Mohr OL Norwegian geneticist 1886–1967.

Mohr's syndrome OFD II.

Mohs FE US surgeon *fl.* 20th cent.

Mohs' micrographic surgical technique method of controlling excision margins of infiltrative skin tumours by microscopy of horizontal sections previously fixed *in vivo*.

mole strictly, a circumscribed pigmented lesion of the skin but often applied to any raised accumulation of melanocytic naevus cells irrespective of pigmentation (OE *māl*, *māel* mole).

Moll JA Dutch anatomist and ophthalmologist 1832–1914.

Moll's glands ciliary glands of the eyelids. Modified sweat glands near free margin of the eyelids.

molluscum properly, a soft cutaneous nodule (L *molluscum*, neuter of *molluscus* rather soft, from *mollis* soft; a fungus growing on a maple tree).

Mondor HJJ French surgeon 1885–1962.

Mondor's disease orig. applied to phlebitis of thoracoepigastric vein; now thought to be lymphangitis (as is the similar condition of penile shaft).

moniliform resembling a string of beads (L *monile* necklace, collar).

Monsel L French army pharmacist *fl.* 19th cent.

Monsel's solution ferric sulphate, now termed basic ferric sulphate. A styptic which acts by denaturing the surface protein of wounds.

Montgomery WF Irish obstetrician 1797–1859.

Montgomery's tubercles apocrine glands in the areola of the breast enlarged during pregnancy.

Montreal type of SECKEL'S SYNDROME a form of bird-headed dwarfism.

Moon H British dental surgeon 1845–92.

Moon's molars (synonyms MULBERRY MOLAR, FOURNIER'S TEETH) malformed molar teeth due to congenital syphilis. A contracted tooth with dome-shaped crown and rough, pitted or irregular surface.

morbilli MEASLES (Med L *morbillis, -i* pustules, dim. of *morbus* disease).

Morgan, Campbell de see DE MORGAN.

Morgan DB US dermatologist *fl.* 20th cent.

Morgan's folds (synonym Dennie–Morgan folds) single or double infraorbital folds in children thought to be indicative of the atopic state.

Morison JR British surgeon 1853–1939.

Morison's paste bismuth-iodoform paste.

morphoea a circumscribed form of scleroderma (Med L *morphea*, L *morphoea* a leprous or scurfy eruption; ultimate origin obscure. ME *morphew, morphu* was probably a different condition).

Morquio L Uruguayan paediatrician 1867–1935.

Morquio's syndrome mucopolysaccharidosis IV.

morsicatio buccarum habit of biting or chewing the buccal mucosa (L *morsus* bite, *bucca* cheek).

Morton TG US surgeon 1835–1903.

Morton's neuroma fibrosis following damage to a plantar digital nerve.

Morvan AM French physician 1819–97.

Morvan's syndrome progressive pain loss, ulceration, loss of soft tissue and resorption of phalanges with muscular atrophy.

mosaic patterned arrangement of small pieces, closely set appearance resembling a mosaic (OF *mosaique*, from Med L *mosaicus*, from Late Gk *mouseion*, from *mouseios* pertaining to the Muses, hence artistic application *fl*). Also used genetically in the same sense as a CHIMAERA.

mosaicism term applied to skin changes resulting from two or more cell lines of different genotypes, genetic or chromosomal.

Moss ML US anatomist and oral biologist *fl.* 20th cent. GORLIN–CHAUDHRY–MOSS SYNDROME.

Moynahan EJ British paediatric dermatologist *fl.* 20th cent.

Moynahan's syndrome 1 xeroderma, talipes and enamel tooth defects; **2** absent hair at birth, sparse hair later, epilepsy, mental retardation.

MSH Melanocyte Stimulating Hormone.

Mucha V Austrian dermatologist 1877–1933.

Mucha–Habermann disease pityriasis lichenoides acuta.

Muckle TJ Canadian pathologist *fl.* 20th cent.

Muckle–Wells syndrome familial urticaria, deafness and amyloidosis.

mudi-chood a peculiar inflammatory dermatosis affecting the nape and shoulders of women in the Kerala state of S India who use oils to dress their long hair (Malayalam *mudi* hair, *chood* heat, from a belief that it is due to the heat of the hair).

Muehrke RC US physician *fl*. 20th cent.

Muehrke's nails whitish bands across whole of nail plate, characteristic but not pathognomic of severe hypoalbuminaemia.

Muir, Sir Edward G British surgeon 1906–73.

Muir–Torre syndrome various combinations of sebaceous neoplasms with or without keratoacanthomas and with low-grade visceral malignancies.

mulberry molar a molar tooth, usually the first, with a flat surface and poorly formed cusps. From resemblance to fruit of the mulberry tree of the Moraceae family (OHG *mulberi*, German *maulbeere*).

mumps an acute infection caused by a paramyxovirus (pl. construed as sing., Engl. dialect *mump* a grimace of the mouth; obs.) 'Swelling of the necke called the mumps' 1598 [*OED*].

Münchhausen, Karl FH, Baron von German soldier and sportsman 1720–97. A teller of wild and improbable stories.

Münchhausen's (Munchausen's) syndrome a chronic factitious disorder seen in those of a psychopathic nature who intentionally and recurrently fabricate lesions, often leading to unnecessary surgery.

Murray J British physician 1843–73.

Murray–Puretić–Drescher syndrome gingival fibromatosis with hyaline fibromas.

Murray Valley fever (synonym Australian X disease) a flaviviral infection, causing encephalitis, named after a river valley area in southern Australia.

Murray Williams G Canadian dermatologist 1921–77.

Murray Williams warts keratotic lesions arising on the site of inflammatory skin conditions.

mycetoma term given to tumid and inflammatory fungal infections of deep tissues usually of the foot, due to various species of fungus (New L from Gk *mykēs*, *mykētos* a fungus, mushroom, *oma*).

myco- comb. form denoting fungus, fungal (New L from Gk *mykēs* fungus).

mycosis fungoides a lymphoma which may present as fungating masses (Gk *mykēs* mushroom, New L *osis* diseased state; L *fungus* mushroom; Gk *eidēs* form, shape). First described by Alibert (q.v.) as 'pian fungoides', later as 'mycosis' from resemblance to mushroom; fully described by Bazin (q.v.) (1862).

Myhre SA US paediatrician *fl*. 20th cent. RUVALCABA–MYHRE SMITH SYNDROME; RUVALCABA–MYHRE–SOTOS SYNDROME.

myiasis disease caused by dipterous larvae (New L from Gk *myia* fly).

myo- comb. form meaning muscle (Gk *mys* muscle).

myoma benign tumour of muscle (Gk *mys*, *oma*).

myrmecia a form of plantar wart due to HPV 1 (Gk *myrmēcia* ant hill or nest).

myx-, myxo- comb. form meaning mucus, nasal discharge, slime (Gk *myxa* mucus, slime).

Naegeli O Swiss dermatologist 1885–1959.

Naegeli–Franceschetti–Jadassohn syndrome reticulate pigmentation, palmoplantar keratoderma and other variable associated defects.

naevus an imprecise term for a circumscribed developmental lesion of skin or mucous membrane involving excess or deficiency of any one of the normal structures; cutaneous hamartoma (L *naevus* birthmark, probably for *gnaevus*, from

Sanskrit root -*gna* relating to birth; something one is born with; LL blemish, fault).

Nager CT Swiss otorhinolaryngologist 1877–1959.

Nager's syndrome acrofacial dysostosis.

NAME *N*aevi, *A*trial myxoma, *M*yxoid neurofibroma and *E*phelides.

Nance WE US geneticist *fl*. 20th cent.

Nance–Horan syndrome X-linked congenital cataracts with supernumerary teeth.

nanism dwarfism (Gk *nanos* dwarf).

Nasu T Japanese pathologist 1915–96.

Nasu disease membranous lipodystrophy, a distinctive form of fat necrosis.

Nazzaro P Italian dermatologist 1921–75.

Nazzaro's syndrome a paraneoplastic syndrome with features of KYRLE'S DISEASE, BAZEX SYNDROME, keratosis pilaris and pityriasis rubra pilaris.

NBIE *N*on-*B*ullous *I*chthyosiform *E*rythroderma.

NCF *N*eutrophil *C*hemotactic *F*actor.

necrobiosis physiological or normal cell death in the midst of living tissue (Gk *nekros* dead, dead body, *bios* life).

necrolysis separation of tissue as the result of its death (Gk *nekros* dead, dead body, *lysis* loosening, from *lyein* to loosen, free).

Neisser ALS Silesian (then Prussian) dermatologist and bacteriologist 1855–1916. Confirmed the LEPROSY bacillus.

Neisseria a genus of Gram-negative diplococci, e.g. *N. gonorrhoeae*.

Nékám L A Hungarian dermatologist 1868–1957.

Nékám's disease (synonyms porokeratosis striata lichenoides, lichen ruber moniliformis) keratosis lichenoides chronica.

Nelson DH US physician *fl*. 20th cent.

Nelson's syndrome progression of an ACTH-secreting pituitary adenoma following bilateral adrenalectomy, showing hyperpigmentation and local pressure effects; ACTH-producing pituitary tumour developing after adrenalectomy.

neo- comb. form meaning new (Gk *neos* new).

neoplasm lit. 'new growth', tumour. A benign or malignant lesion consisting of proliferating cells (New L from Gk *neo*(s) new, *plasma* a moulding, forming).

Nesbit RM US urological surgeon *fl*. 20th cent.

Nesbit's operation a treatment for penile fibromatosis involving excision of ellipses of normal tunica albuginea.

Netherton EW US dermatologist b. 1893.

Netherton's syndrome ichthyosis linearis circumflexa.

Neumann IN Austro-Hungarian dermatologist 1832–1906. Pemphigus vegetans.

Neuman's bipolar aphthosis recurrent orogenital aphthosis of genitals, possibly a forme fruste of BEHÇET'S SYNDROME.

Nézelof C French pathologist *fl*. 20th cent.

Nézelof's immunodeficiency syndrome thymic aplasia, lymphopenia and recurrent pulmonary and viral infections; deficient T-cell responses.

Nicholas J French dermatologist 1868–1960.

Nicholas–Favre disease lymphogranuloma venereum.

Niemann A German paediatrician and pathologist 1880–1921.

Niemann–Pick cells large, pale foamy mononuclear cells seen in NIEMANN–PICK DISEASE.

Niemann–Pick disease form of congenital lipidosis, usually fatal.

nigricans blackish; properly, becoming dark (L pres. part. of *nigricare* to become black, from *niger* black).

Nikolsky (Nikolski) PV Russian dermatologist 1858–1940.

Nikolsky sign epidermal cell separation induced by firm sliding pressure of the finger on apparently normal or perilesional skin of patients with PEMPHIGUS, especially pemphigus foliaceus, and, on the erythematous skin of patients with toxic epidermal necrolysis or SSSS. Not to be confused with lateral extension of a pre-existing bulla by pressure on it, common to many bullous diseases.

nipple the conical projection at the apex of the breast containing the openings of the milk ducts; hence, any projecting apex (prob. ME dim. of *neb* beak or bill (but uncertain)).

nit the egg of the louse; or the encased embryo (ME *nit, nitte,* from OE *hnitu*).

nitidus glistening, shiny (L *nitidus* shining, gleaming).

njovera endemic syphilis colloq. term in Zimbabwe (Shona *njovera*) for sexually transmitted disease.

noma a spreading gangrene, usually around mouth or female pudenda (Gk *nomē* feeding pl. *nomai* eating or corroding sore).

Noonan JA US paediatric cardiologist *fl.* 20th cent.

Noonan's syndrome multisystem disorder with features of Turner's syndrome (q.v.) but with normal chromosome karyotype and equal sex prevalence; familial Turner's syndrome; female pseudo-Turner's syndrome.

Norwegian scabies a form of extensive crusted scabies described by Boeck and seen in elderly, immunocompromised or mentally defective patients.

nummular assuming shape of coin, discoid (L *nummulus* dim. of *nummus* coin).

Nyhan WL US paediatrician *fl.* 20th cent. LESCH–NYHAN SYNDROME.

oast-house disease very light-coloured hair and recurrent oedema occurring with raised methionine (oast-house, a building of particular design used to house kilns for drying hops or malt (OE *āst* burn, prob. from L *aestus* burning, heat).

obliterans destroying, obliterating (L pres. part. of *oblitterare, oblit-* to wipe out, erase).

O'Brien JP Australian dermatopathologist *fl.* 20th cent.

O'Brien's granuloma actinic granuloma.

obturans any structure occluding an opening (L pres. part. of *obturare* to close up, obstruct).

ochre a pigment of clay and iron oxide, of great antiquity; hence, yellow-red in colour (Fr *ocre*, from L *ochra*; Gk *ōchra* yellow-coloured earth).

ochronosis greyish or bluish discoloration of connective tissue and cartilage due to deposition of a pigment derived from oxidized homogentisic acid. Occurs in alkaptonuria (q.v.) and in chronic exposure to phenol and phenolic compounds (Gk *ōchro(s)* yellow, sallow, *osis*).

Ockelbo town in Sweden where cases of an alphavirus infection (Pogosta infection) were first noted.

-ode(s), -oid(es) suff. meaning like, in form of (derivation disputed but probably from Gk *eidos* form, shape).

odontotrichomelic syndrome involving teeth and hair with limb deformities (Gk *odous, odontos* tooth, *thrix, trichos* hair, *melos* limb).

oedema excessive collection of watery fluid in cells, tissues or serous cavities (Gk *oidēma* swelling).

OFD I (synonym PAPILLON–LÉAGE SYNDROME) Oral-Facial-Digital syndrome.

OFD II (synonym MOHR'S SYNDROME) Oral-Facial-Digital syndrome.

Ofuji S Japanese dermatologist *fl.* 20th cent.

Ofuji's disease 1 eosinophilic pustular folliculitis; **2** papuloerythroderma.

Ogna village in Norway from which first cases of epidermolysis bullosa simplex (see GEDDE–DAHL) were recorded.

ointment semisolid preparation in suitable base for application to the skin. Colloq. term used for greasy preparations, as opposed to creams (OF *oignement* irreg., from L *unguentum*, akin to *unctus* past part. of *unguere* to wet, anoint, smear).

oligo- comb. form meaning few, small, scanty (Gk *oligos* few, little).

Oliver CP US paediatrician *fl.* 20th cent. ADAMS–OLIVER SYNDROME.

Ollendorf (Ollendorf-Curth) H German-born US dermatologist *fl.* 20th cent. BUSCHKE–OLLENDORF SYNDROME.

Ollier LXE French surgeon 1830–1900.

Ollier's syndrome enchondromatosis; dyschondroplasia without the cutaneous vascular malformations of Mafucci's syndrome.

Olmsted HC US paediatrician *fl.* 20th cent.

Olmsted's syndrome congenital palmoplantar keratoderma with periorificial plaques and other anomalies.

-oma, -ma suff. now taken to refer to tumour formation but not thus in Gk where -*(o)ma* refers to result of action specified by the preceding element, e.g. diploma, result of folding a paper in two.

Omenn GS US geneticist *fl.* 20th cent.

Omenn's syndrome familial reticuloendotheliosis. A form of severe combined immunodeficiency.

ommochrome a derivative of tryptophan via cynurenine and hydroxykinins that serves as a masking of pigment in the accessory cells of the insect eye; a green, red and brown colouring (GK *omma* eye, *chrōma* colour).

omphalos umbilicus, navel (Gk *omphalos* navel or anything resembling it; central point. Hence the stone in the temple at Delphi, the 'centre of the world').

Omsk city in Russia after which a form of haemorrhagic fever due to *Flavivirus* is named.

onychia inflammation of nail matrix (Gk *onyx, onychos* nail, claw).

onychogryphosis thickening and overcurvature of the nail resembling a ram's horn (New L from Gk *onyx, onychos* nail, Gk *grypōsis*, from *grypos* curved, hooked).

onychoschizia splitting of nail plate into layers (Gk *onyx, onychos* nail, *schizein* to split or cleave).

onychotillomania habit of fiddling with or pulling pieces off the nail, an obsessional or psychopathic trait (Gk *onyx, onychos* nail, *tillein* to pluck, *mania* frenzy).

O'nyong-nyong infection due to mosquito-borne alphavirus (African 'general weakening of the joints').

oo- comb. form meaning egg (Gk *ōion* egg).

Oorthuys JWE Dutch geneticist 1943–92. DELLEMAN–OORTHUYS SYNDROME.

OPD syndrome OtoPalatoDigital syndrome.

ophiasis snake-like, curling; applied to a form of alopecia areata [Cels] (Gk *ophis* serpent, snake).

Opitz JM US geneticist and paediatrician *fl.* 20th cent.

Opitz syndrome (C syndrome, trigonocephaly syndrome)

unusual facies, polydactyly and cardiac abnormalities.

Opitz–Frias syndrome (G syndrome, BBBG syndrome) hyperteleorism with oesophageal abnormalities and hypospadias.

Oppenheim M US dermatologist 1876–1949. Dermatitis striata bullosa pratensis. URBACH–OPPENHEIM DISEASE.

orf ecthyma infectiosum. Highly contagious disease of sheep and goats caused by a parapoxvirus. May infect man by contact (prob. from Old Norse *hrufa* crust, or possibly from *yrfe* cattle).

Oroya fever a febrile illness due to Bartonellosis (from La Oroya, town in central Peru).

ortho- comb. form meaning straight, correct, true (Gk *orthos* straight, upright). Also chemical symbol for substitution in 1,2-position of benzene ring (*o*-).

-osis suff. meaning **1** state or process; or **2** diseased or abnormal condition, production or increase (Gk suff. *-osis* condition).

Osler, Sir William, Bt Canadian physician also active in the USA and Gt Britain 1849–1919. The outstanding clinician, lecturer and medical philosopher of his day. Author of *Aequanimitas* and numerous other publications.

Osler's nodes tender erythematous lesions occurring on pads of fingers and toes, or palms and soles of patients with subacute bacterial endocarditis.

Osler–Vaquez disease polycythaemia vera.

Osler–Rendu–Weber disease, syndrome hereditary haemorrhagic telangiectasia.

osmidrosis bromidrosis; offensive sweat (Gk *osmē* smell, *hidrein* to sweat).

osteopoikilosis condition of mottled or stippled bones (Gk *osteo(n)* bone, *poikilos* mottled).

ostracea resembling an oyster shell (Gk *ostrakon* potsherd or the hard shell of snail, oyster, etc.).

Ota MT Japanese dermatologist 1885–1945.

Ota's naevus oculodermal melanocytosis.

otophyma term given to aberrant rosaceous nodule of ear (Gk *ous, ōtos* ear, *phyma* inflamed swelling).

Oudtshoorn disease erythrokeratolysis hiemalis, named after the town in S Africa where it was first described.

oxyuriasis infestation by worm of genus *Enterobius*; enterobiasis (Gk *oxys* sharp, *oura* tail).

pach-, pachy- comb. forms meaning thick (Gk *pachys* thick).

pachydermoperiostosis hypertrophic osteoarthropathy with thickened skin (Gk *pachys* thick, *derma* skin, *peri* about, around, *osteon* bone). TOURAINE–SOLENTE–GOLÉ SYNDROME.

pachyonychia abnormally thick nails (New L from Gk *pachys* thick, *onyx, onychos* nail, *ia*).

PACK Primary biliary cirrhosis, Anticentromere antibody, CREST syndrome and Keratoconjunctivitis sicca. An extension of primary biliary cirrhosis with limited scleroderma.

Paederus species of rove (blister) beetles which secrete the vesicant pederin.

Paget, Sir James, Bt noted British anatomist, surgeon and pathologist 1814–99. Foremost lecturer of his age, who described many eponymous diseases. First to use the term 'clinical science'.

Paget's disease, extramammary a malignant plaque occurring in anogenital area or axillae and containing characteristic Paget cells.

Paget's disease of the nipple; mammary Paget's disease a marginated scaly or crusted lesion of the nipple containing

intraepidermal Paget cells and associated with intraduct carcinoma of the breast.

Pagetoid reticulosis WORINGER–KOLOPP DISEASE.

Palade GE US pathologist *fl.* 20th cent. WEIBEL–PALADE BODIES.

pangeria generalized form of premature ageing (Gk *pan* all, *gērōn* old man, old, *ia*).

panniculus a layer, covering sheet or garment (L dim. of *pannus* cloth).

papilloma a nipple-like mass projecting from the surface of the skin [1] (L *papilla* nipple, teat, *oma*).

Papillon MM French dermatologist *fl.* 20th cent.

Papillon–Lefèvre syndrome palmoplantar keratoderma with periodontosis.

Papillon-Léage, Mme French stomatologist *fl.* 20th cent.

Papillon-Léage syndrome OFD I.

PAPOVAVIRUS *Papilloma Polyoma Vacuolating Agent VIRUS.*

papyraceus having the consistency of paper; paper-thin, of scars and 'fetus papyraceus' (L *papyrus*, Gk *papyros* the paper reed—a plant of the sedge family, or paper made from it).

PAR Pseudo-Allergic Reactions.

para- pref. a number of meanings dependent on the case taken; basically, beside; but also, beyond, apart from, resembling, diverging from normal (Gk *para*). Also chemical symbol for the 1,4 position of benzene ring (*p*-).

paragonimiasis infection by the lung fluke *Paragonimus westermani*.

Parinaud H French ophthalmologist 1844–1905.

Parinaud's syndrome oculoglandular syndrome.

Parkes Weber F see WEBER, F PARKES.

parvimaculata dappled with small spots (L *parvus* small, *maculata*, past part. of *maculare* to make spotted).

Pasini A Italian dermatologist 1875–1944.

Pasini's albopapuloid form of epidermolysis bullosa.

Pasini and Pierini, idiopathic atrophoderma of a distinctive pattern of sharply defined areas of dermal atrophy, probably an atrophic variant of morphoea.

Passarge E German geneticist *fl.* 20th cent. SCHÖPF–SCHULZ–PASSARGE SYNDROME.

Pasteur L Famous French chemist and microbiologist 1822–95. A dominant figure in 19th-century science. Pasteur's reaction, vaccine, etc.

Pasteurella genus of bacterium named after Pasteur, now called *Yersinia*.

Patau K US geneticist *fl.* 20th cent.

Patau's syndrome trisomy 13.

patch a large macule, more than 2 cm in diameter [1] (ME *pacche, patche*, origin unknown. 'No man seweth a pacche' 1382; 'with twitchis and patches' 1573 [*OED*]).

Paterson DR British otorhinolaryngologist 1863–1939.

Paterson–Brown Kelly syndrome PLUMMER–VINSON SYNDROME.

pathergy a contrived and curious term of imprecise definition; wrong-doing or abnormal reactivity (Gk *pathos* suffering, disease, *ergon* work).

-pathy disease or treatment of disease (Gk *pathos* suffering, disease).

Paul JR US physician 1893–1971.

Paul–Bunnell test for heterophil antibody characteristic of infectious mononucleosis.

Pautrier LMA French dermatologist 1876–1959. Giant lichen; angiolupoid.

Pautrier's abscess, microabscess focal collections of lymphocytes in the epidermis of patients with mycosis fungoides.

PD/AR syndrome Photosensitivity Dermatitis and Actinic Reticuloid syndrome.

peau d'orange a dimpling and induration of the skin, such as may overlie a mammary carcinoma (Fr orange-skin).

PECL Postinflammatory Elastolysis and Cutis Laxa; a variant of anetoderma.

pediculosis a genus of parasitic lice infecting man and other primates, family Pediculidae (L dim. of *pedis* louse).

PEEPO Papular Eruption with Elimination of Papillary Oedema. A term used for papular or dermal eczema.

Pel PK Dutch physician 1852–1919.

Pel–Ebstein fever recurrent febrile episodes of a characteristic nature seen in HODGKIN'S DISEASE.

pelade French term for alopecia areata (Fr from *peler* to peel, pare).

peliosis obs. term for *purpura* (Gk *peliōsis* extravasation of blood [Hipp.], from *peli(os)* livid, dark-coloured, *osis*).

pellagra disease due to dietary deficiency of niacin and tryptophan (either from L *pellis* skin, Gk *agra* seizure, or from Italian *pelle agra* rough skin).

Pellizzari C Italian dermatologist 1851–1925. JADASSOHN–PELLIZZARI ANETODERMA.

pemphigus a group of blistering diseases showing intra-epidermal bullae and acantholysis (New L from Gk *pemphix, pemphigos* a blister).

pemphigoid ('bullous pemphigoid') a blistering disease of the elderly with subepidermal bullae (false L from Gk *pemphix, pemphigoid* pemphigus-like).

penis male organ of copulation (L *penis* tail, penis; akin to Gk *peos* penis).

PEP Polyneuropathy, Endocrinopathy, Pigmentation (see POEMS).

peri- pref. meaning around, about, nearly (Gk *peri*).

perléche (obs.) angular cheilitis (Limousin patois variant of Fr *pourléche*, from *pourlécher* to lick all over).

pernio chilblain (L *pernio* chilblain, frostbite).

perstans persistent (L pres. part. of *perstare* to stand firm, endure).

petechia a punctate haemorrhagic spot 1–2mm in diameter [1] (New L from Italian *petecchia*, ultimate origin obscure).

Peutz JLA Dutch physician 1886–1957.

Peutz–Jeghers syndrome orificial and periorificial lentigines with hamartomatous intestinal polyps.

Peyronie, Fr. de la renowned French surgeon 1678–1747. Surgeon to Louis XV and founder of Royal Academy of Surgery in France.

Peyronie's disease penile fibromatosis.

Pfeiffer RA German geneticist *fl.* 20th cent.

Pfeiffer syndrome acrocephalosyndactyly type V.

phaeochromocytoma (synonym chromaffinoma) benign para-ganglionoma of adrenal medulla or urinary bladder (Gk *phaios* grey, blackish, *chrōma* colour, *kytos* cell, *oma*; thus tumour of cells of dusky colour from their ability to show a strong chromaffin reaction).

phagedaena rarely used term for a rapidly spreading or deepening ulcer (Gk *phagedaina* a cancerous sore [Hipp], from *phagein* to eat).

phakomatosis a term now used for genetic conditions involving neuro-ectodermal, and often ocular structures and consisting of glial overgrowth and vascular malformation (Gk *phakos* lentil,

freckle (mole or birthmark [Gal]), *oma, osis,* applied to lentil-like retinal deposits).

pheromone an odourous secretion that regulates the behaviour of other individuals in a population; in animals, important in sexual attraction, trail marking and as a warning signal (Gk *pherein* to bear, carry, *hormōn,* pres. part. of *horman* to set in motion).

phlebectasia abnormal distension or dilatation of veins (Gk *phleps, phlebos* vein, *ectasia*).

phlegmasia obs. term for severe inflammation (Gk *phlegmasia* inflammation, a fiery heat [Hipp], from *phlegma* heat, fire).

phlycten obs. term for a burn blister; persisting as a small blister or vesicle especially of the eye, e.g. phlyctenular conjunctivitis (Gk *phlyctaina* blister [Hipp]).

phocomelia, phocomely a limb reduction defect in which long bone segments are absent in one or more limbs (New L from Gk *phōkē* seal, *mel(os)* limb, *ia*).

photo- comb. form implying role of light (Gk *phōs, phōtos* light).

phrynoderma dry skin with horny follicular papules, especially as seen in severe vitamin A or essential fatty acid deficiency (Gk *phrynos* toad, *derma* skin, from resemblance to toad skin).

phthiriasis properly, infestation with any type of louse but usually confined to infestation with pubic lice (Gk *phtheir* louse).

***Phthirus* (*Pthirus*)** a genus of louse primarily affecting the pubic hair and occasionally other hairy areas (Gk *phtheir* louse).

phyto- comb. form indicating plant, e.g. phytodermatitis (Gk *phyton* plant, tree).

PIBIDS Photosensitivity, Ichthyosis, Brittle nails, Intellectual impairment, Decreased fertility, Short stature.

Piccardi G Italian physician *fl.* early 20th cent.

Piccardi–Lassueur–Graham-Little syndrome cicatricial alopecia, keratosis pilaris; possibly variant of lichen planopilaris.

PICK Post-Irradiation Conical Keratoses.

Pick F(P)J Austrohungarian dermatologist 1834–1910.

Pick–Herxheimer disease acrodermatitis chronica atrophicans.

Pick L German pathologist 1868–1944. LUBARSH–PICK DISEASE, NIEMANN–PICK DISEASE.

pico- comb. form denoting 10^{-12} SI units. Also used for Picornaviridae, a family of small animal viruses (Italian *piccolo* small).

piebaldism properly, a condition of two or more different colours as shown by patchy absence of normal pigment of skin or hair; the term 'partial albinism' is sometimes wrongly applied to it. (ME from OF *pie* magpie, from L *pica* magpie; ME *balded, bald* smooth, rounded but possibly also white; obscure.) 'Pied' is similar.

piedra a fungal infection of the hair forming superficial nodules on the shaft (Spanish *piedra* stone, from Gk *petra* rock).

Pierini LE Argentinian dermatologist 1899–1987. PASINI AND PIERINI, IDIOPATHIC ATROPHODERMA OF.

piezogenic name given to pedal papules formed of herniated fat, the result of weight-bearing (Gk *piesis, piexis* a pressing, from *piezein* to squeeze, press; *genikos* producing).

pil-, pilo- relating to hair (L *pilus* hair).

pili incarnati an apt term for ingrowing hairs; pseudofolliculitis (L *pilus* hair, Ecclesiastical L *incarnatus,* becoming or be made flesh, past part. passive of *incarnare*).

ping pong patch annular purpura caused by the skin being repeatedly bruised by table-tennis balls (originally Ping-Pong, trademark for table tennis).

pinguecula degenerative nodule of elastic tissue in the inter-palpebral conjunctiva (L dim. noun from *pinguis* fat).

Pinkus F German dermatologist 1868–1947. Emigrated to the US in 1941. Described lichen nitidus. A gifted artist and naturalist.

Pinkus HKB German-born US dermatologist (son of Felix Pinkus) 1905–85. Founder member of American Society of Dermatopathology.

Pinkus tumour premalignant fibroepithelial tumour.

pinta a nonvenereal treponematosis; Mal dal pinto (American Spanish *pinta* coloured spot, from Late L *pincta*, past part. of *pingere* to paint).

Pirquet see VON PIRQUET.

pityriasis a branny scaling of the skin; term applied for conditions showing this (L *pityriasis* scurf [Gal], from Gk *pityron* bran, husks of corn).

PK test see PRAUSNITZ–KÜSTNER TEST (REACTION).

PKU (synonym Folling's disease) *PhenylKetonUria*.

placebo an inactive substance used as a control during tests of drugs or given to patients to induce psychological response by suggestion (L *placebo* 'I shall please', from *placēre* to please; from first words of first antiphon of Vesper Office for the Dead, 'Placebo domino').

plague infectious disease caused by *Yersinia pestis*. Colloq. term for any widespread epidemic disease or infestation (L *plaga* blow, akin to Gk *plēgē* blow, wound, from *plēssein to* strike, smite).

plaque an elevated area of skin 2 cm or more in diameter [1] (Fr *plaque*, prob. from Flemish *placke* a flat disc, a small coin).

-plasia comb. form meaning process of moulding or forming (Gk *plas(is)* a shaping, moulding, *ia*).

plica a fold or twist (New L from L *plicare* to fold, akin to Gk *plekein* to twine).

plica polonica name given to a condition of matted, crusted, verminous hair. Mentioned by Boyle as early as 1684 [*OED*].

Plummer HS US physician 1874–1937.

Plummer–Vinson syndrome (synonym Paterson–Brown Kelly syndrome) dysphagia, postcricoid oesophageal webs, spoon-shaped fingernails and atrophic glossitis.

PMA-NBT test *Phorbol-Myristate Acetate-stimulated NitroBlue Tetrazolium* dye test used to detect chronic granulomatous disease.

pock originally a pustule; later, for pock-mark, pock-hole, the scar or pit left by the 'small' or 'great' pox (OE *poc, pocc*, ME *pokke* a pustule).

POEMS *Polyneuropathy, Organomegaly, Endocrinopathy, M* protein, *Skin* changes.

Pogosta disease (synonym Ockelbo disease) alphavirus infection first noted in Finland. Literally, Pogosta in Finnish refers to a small village around a church.

Pohl–Pincus S German dermatologist *fl.* 19th to early 20th cent.

Pohl–Pincus constriction narrowing of the diameter of the hair shaft following operation, illness or certain mitosis-inhibiting drugs.

poikiloderma dappled or variegated pattern of pigmentation. Usually applied to condition combining this with telangiectasia and atrophy (Gk *poikilos* spotted, mottled, dappled, *derma* skin).

poliosis localized patches of white hair, as in piebaldism, Waardenburg and other syndromes (Gk *poliōsis* becoming grey, from *polios* grey (haired), whitish, as of surf, milk, etc.).

poly- pref. many (Gk *polys* many).

polythelia supernumerary nipples (Gk *polys* many, *thēlē* nipple).

poly X syndrome comprises several anomalies of the sex chromosomes.

pomade a scented ointment, especially for the scalp (1562) in which apples were said to have been an ingredient (Fr *pommade*, from Italian *pomata*, from *pomo* apple, from L *pomum* fruit of a tree).

pompholyx general term for cheiro- (and podo-) pompholyx, term used by Hutchinson in 1876 for an acute, often recurrent deeply seated vesicular or bullous eruption of palms and fingers of unknown cause ('dysidrosis' of Tilbury Fox (q.v.)). Now more loosely but somewhat incorrectly used for any vesicular eruption of palms, fingers or soles (Gk *pompholyx* a bubble).

Pontiac fever a variety of legionellosis presenting as a flu-like illness without pneumonia (after a town in Michigan where cases were first identified).

pore small opening or orifice; applied to opening of sebaceous or sweat ducts onto skin surface (Gk *poros*, L *porus* passage, channel).

poro- comb. form meaning pore, usually the opening of the eccrine sweat duct (Gk *poros* passage, opening).

porphyria name given to a group of inborn errors of metabolism. When unqualified, usually refers to acute intermittent porphyria (Gk *porphyr(os)* purple, *ia*).

port-wine stain capillary angiomatous naevus. But for an accident of history might have been 'claret stain' [10].

Potter EL US pathologist *fl.* 20th cent.

Potter's syndrome a combination of congenital abnormalities resulting from oligohydramnios.

PPD *Purified Protein Derivative* of tuberculin.

PPK *PalmoPlantar Keratoses*.

Prader A Swiss paediatrician *fl.* 20th cent.

Prader–Willi syndrome small stature, obesity, emotional lability, hypotonia, hypogonadism and a characteristic facies.

Prausnitz OCW German bacteriologist 1876–1963.

Prausnitz–Küstner test (reaction) passive transfer test by intradermal injection of serum from sensitized to nonsensitized person and subsequent challenge by sensitizing agent.

prickle cell an epidermal cell, so-named because of its spiny intercellular bridges (OE *pricel*, from stem of *prician* to prick).

primrose, evening a flower of genus *Oenothera* (*prima rosa* first rose).

Pringle JJ British dermatologist 1855–1922. BOURNEVILLE–PRINGLE SYNDROME.

(P)RIST (*Paper disc*) *RadioImmunoSorbent Technique*.

Pritzker MS US dermatologist *fl.* 20th cent. HASHIMOTO–PRITZKER SYNDROME.

pro- pref. indicating before, in front of, anterior to (Gk and L *pro* before, in front of).

proctalgia pain localized to anal region (Gk *prōctos* anus, *algia*).

progeria (synonym HUTCHINSON–GILFORD SYNDROME) a syndrome of premature senility, with dry wrinkled skin, hair loss and a bird-like facies (Gk *pro, gēras* old age).

progrediens advancing, progressing (L pres. part. of *progredior* to advance).

pros- pref. meaning towards, besides, in addition (Gk *pros*).

prosthesis any artificial replacement for a body part (Gk *prosthesis, from pros, thesis* a placing in addition [Hipp]).

Proteus syndrome term aptly coined to denote a disorder of skeletal, hamartomatous and other mesodermal malformations occurring in various combinations; multisystem gigantism. After the Greek sea-god Proteus who changed his shape at will to avoid capture. Hence 'protean', varying in form or shape [11].

prototothecosis infection with species of alga, *Prototheca* (Gk *prōtos* before, first *thēke* a box, sheath, *osis*).

prurigo a term of imprecise definition but in general denoting a number of conditions characterized by intensely irritable papules with no obvious local cause. But retained in usage for other irritable conditions such as Besnier's prurigo (q.v.) (atopic dermatitis), prurigo hiemalis (itching and xerosis), etc. (L *prurigo* itching [Cels], from *prurire* to itch).

pruritus a sensation of itching or a condition in which itching is the predominant symptom (L *pruritus* past part. of *prurire* to itch).

psammoma bodies sand tumour, acervuloma. Concentric laminated bodies found in meningeal tumours (Gk *psammos* sand).

Psaume J French orofacial surgeon *fl*. 20th cent.

Psaume's syndrome orofaciodigital dysostosis.

pseudo- comb. form meaning false, mimicking, taking the place of something else (Gk *pseudēs* false).

pseudopelade a morphological term for a pattern of follicular response to a variety of insults, often unknown, resulting in patches of complete loss of scalp hair (Gk *pseudēs* false, Fr *pelade* hairfall, alopecia).

'pseudothalidomide' syndrome (synonyms, hypomelia-hypotrichosis-facial haemangioma syndrome, ROBERTS' SYNDROME, HERMANN'S SYNDROME (variants)) facial vascular naevus, sparse blond hair, limb malformations and growth retardation.

psittacosis infectious disease due to *Chlamydia* species and transmitted by psittacine birds and other fowls (L *psittacus*, from Gk *psittakos* parrot).

psoriasis a chronic, inflammatory skin disease consisting essentially of well-demarcated dull-red plaques, though with many variants (Gk *psōriasis* being itchy or mangy from *psōra* itch, mange, scab, also of trees overgrown with moss. Earlier names of *lepra*, *alphos* and *psōra* confused in translation and meaning) [9, 12].

pterygium vascular lesions encroaching on the cornea; fusion of eponychium with proximal portion of nail (*pterygium unguis*); web of skin extending from mastoid to achromial process as in Turner's syndrome (q.v.) (*pterygium colli*) (Gk *pterygion* a little wing, from *pteryx* wing).

ptyalism sialorrhoea, excessive salivation (Gk *ptyalon* spittle [Hipp]; *ptyalizein* to have mouth full of spittle [Hipp]).

ptychotropism affinity for the body folds. Originally described as feature of ichthyosiform naevi in the CHILD syndrome but also applicable to other noninflammatory conditions (Gk *ptychē* fold, *tropē* turning) [13].

pubarche first appearance of pubic hair (L *pubes* the soft pubic hair of a person approaching puberty; Gk *archē* beginning).

puberty the period of development of secondary sexual characteristics and of a reproductive capacity (L *pubertas* the age of maturity, from *puber* or *pubes* one who has attained puberty).

Pudlák, P Czechoslovakian physician 1927–93. HEŘMANSKY–PUDLÁK SYNDROME.

Pumphrey RE US otolaryngologist *fl*. 20th cent. BART–PUMPHREY SYNDROME.

PUPPP Pruritic Urticarial Papules and Plaques of Pregnancy.

Puretić B Croatian paediatrician 1922–71.

Puretić S Croatian paediatric dermatologist *fl*. 20th cent.

Puretić syndrome juvenile hyaline fibromatosis (mesenchymal dysplasia). MURRAY–PURETIĆ–DRESCHER SYNDROME.

purpura focal haemorrhage into the skin (L *purpura, from* Gk *porphyra* the purple fish, a gastropod secreting a purple dye).

pyknosis shrinkage and hyperchromatism of a cell or its nucleus following cell death (Gk *pyknos* thick, dense).

pyoderma generic word for any purulent skin condition but often specified as in pyoderma faciale, gangrenosum, vegetans, etc. (Gk *puon* pus, *derma* skin).

Q fever (synonym Query fever) infection caused by *Coxiellia burnettii*. Thus designated in 1937 'until further knowledge should allow a better name'.

Queyrat L French dermatologist 1856–1933. Made syphilis a special study and collected poetry.

Queyrat, erythroplasia of intraepidermal carcinoma of genital mucosa.

Quie PG US immunologist *fl*. 20th cent.

Quie–Hill syndrome a hyperimmunoglobulin E syndrome with defective neutrophil chemotaxis, cutaneous infection and allergic rhinitis.

Quinke HI German physician 1842–1922. Introduced lumbar puncture.

Quinke's oedema angio-oedema.

Quinquaud Ch-E French dermatologist 1842–94. Described folliculitis decalvans.

Rabenhorst syndrome cardio-acro-facial syndrome. Named after family described by Grosse (1974).

racemose grouped, clustered (L *racemus* bunch, cluster, akin to Gk *rax* grape).

Racouchot J French dermatologist b. 1908. FAVRE–RACOUCHOT SYNDROME.

Radcliffe Crocker H British dermatologist 1845–1909. A notable figure of late 19th-century dermatology. Described DERMATITIS REPENS.

Raeder JG Norwegian ophthalmologist 1889–1956.

Raeder's trigeminal syndrome HORNER'S SYNDROME with loss of sweating on the affected side of the face.

Ramírez CO Salvadorean dermatologist 1924–85. Erythema dyschromicum perstans.

Ramsay Hunt J US neurologist 1874–1937.

Ramsay Hunt syndrome auricular herpes zoster with associated facial paralysis.

ranula mucous (sublingual) cyst of the mouth (L *ranula*, dim. of *rana* a frog; LL a swelling in tongue of frog).

Rapp RS US paediatrician *fl*. 20th cent.

Rapp–Hodgkin syndrome form of hypohidrotic ectodermal dysplasia.

Rappaport H US pathologist *fl*. 20th cent.

RAS Recurrent Aphthous Stomatitis.

rash colloq. term for any inflammatory skin eruption (perhaps from OF *rasche* eruptive sores, possibly from L *rasus*, past part. of *radere* to scrape, scratch).

RAST RadioAllergoSorbent Test.

Raynaud M French physician 1834–81.

Raynaud's disease primary idiopathic form of Raynaud's phenomenon.

Raynaud's phenomenon paroxysmal pallor, numbness and coldness of the extremities, often followed by cyanosis, due to digital vasospasm. It occurs in a number of diseases, notably the collagen diseases.

Recklinghausen see VON RECKLINGHAUSEN.

Reed D US pathologist 1874–1964.

Reed–Sternberg cells large cells with characteristic nuclei seen in HODGKIN'S DISEASE.

Refsum SA Norwegian neurologist 1907–91.

Refsum's syndrome heredopathia atactica polyneuritiformis; phytanic acid oxidase deficiency.

Reiter HCJ German bacteriologist 1881–1969.

Reiter's syndrome (synonym Fiessinger–Leroy–Reiter syndrome) nonspecific urethritis, arthritis and iridocyclitis. Patients may develop a rupioid psoriasiform dermatosis.

REM *R*eticular *E*rythematous *M*ucinosis.

Rendu HJLM French physician 1844–1902. Fiessinger–Rendu syndrome (STEVENS–JOHNSON SYNDROME).

Rendu–Osler–Weber syndrome see OSLER–RENDU–WEBER DISEASE.

reticulate lacy, webbed, net-like (L *reticulatus* net-shaped).

retiform in shape of net (L *rete* a net, *-form* shape of).

Reye RDK Australian paediatric pathologist 1912–77.

Reye's tumour infantile digital fibromatosis.

Reynolds TB US physician *fl.* 20th cent.

Reynolds' syndrome primary biliary cirrhosis with scleroderma, Raynaud's phenomenon and telangiectasia.

rhabdomyoma tumour of striated muscle (Gk *rhabdos* rod, *my(s)* muscle, *oma*).

rhagades cracks; fissures (Gk *rhagas*, *rhagados* rent, chink, crack; of the lips [Gal]).

rheo- comb. form denoting flow (Gk *rheein* to flow).

Rheydt type of ichthyosis hystrix gravior, named after a town in Germany from which the first case originated.

rhinophyma term given to rosaceous nodular distortion of nose (Gk *rhis, rhinos* nose, *phyma* inflamed swelling).

rhinoscleroma an indolent progressive infection involving the nose and nasal fossae, with subsequent extension (Gk *rhis, rhinos* nose, *sclēr(os)* hand, *oma*).

rhinosporidiosis a granulomatous nasal mycosis common in Sri Lanka and S India (Gk *rhis, rhinos* nose; New L *sporidium*, dim. from Gk *spora* or *sporos* sowing).

Richner H Swiss ophthalmologist *fl.* 20th cent.

Richner–Hanhart syndrome Type II oculocutaneous tyrosinaemia.

Ricketts HT US pathologist 1871–1910.

rickettsia small coccobacillary organisms transmitted among animals by arthropods. Include agents of typhus, spotted and boutonneuse fevers and tick typhus. After RICKETTS.

Riehl G Austrian dermatologist 1855–1943. Successor to KAPOSI.

Riehl's melanosis distinctive pigmentation of face and neck, perhaps due to cosmetic impurities. Prevalent in Vienna in World War I and also seen during and after World War II.

Rift Valley fever a bunyaviral infection named after the Rift Valley, a geological fault reaching from the Middle East to East Africa.

Riley CM US paediatrician b. 1913.

Riley–Day syndrome familial dysautonomia.

Riley HD, Jr US paediatrician *fl.* 20th cent.

Riley–Smith syndrome macrocephaly, pseudopapilloedema and haemangiomata.

ringworm very old colloq. term for any ring-shaped eruption; more recently used for superficial fungal infections but gradually obsolescent (OE *hring* ring; preTeutonic stem *krengho* is akin to L *cingulum* ring, band. A great variety of uses, all related to a ring or circlet, an object of this shape or a metaphor arising from it).

Ritter G von Rittershain Austrian paediatrician 1820–83. Properly, von Rittershain, as 'Ritter' is a title.

Ritter's disease (so-named; properly, **von Rittershain's disease**). Staphylococcal scalded skin syndrome.

ROAT *R*epeated *O*pen *A*pplication *T*est for eliciting cause of allergic contact dermatitis.

Roberts JB US surgeon 1852–1924.

Roberts' syndrome a variant form of pseudothalidomide syndrome and the hypomelia-hypertrichosis-facial haemangioma syndrome.

Robin P noted French stomatologist 1867–1950.

Robin (Pierre Robin) syndrome cleft palate, micrognathism, glossoptosis and displacement of larynx.

Robinson GC Canadian paediatrician 1878–1960.

Robinson's syndrome familial ectodermal dysplasia with sensorineural deafness and other anomalies.

Rocky mountain (spotted) fever a rickettsial infection occurring in the Rocky Mountain states of N America and elsewhere in N and S America.

Romaña C Argentinian physician *fl.* 20th cent.

Romaña's sign, syndrome unilateral eyelid oedema and lacrimal gland inflammation seen early in American trypanosomiasis (CHAGAS' DISEASE).

Romberg MH von German neurologist 1795–1873.

Romberg's syndrome progressive facial hemiatrophy.

rosacea erythema, telangiectasia and acneiform pustules commonly affecting the central panel of the face, occasionally scalp or elsewhere. Also termed acne rosacea (New L *rosaceus* rose-coloured).

Rosai J US pathologist *fl.* 20th cent.

Rosai-Dorfman disease sinus histiocytosis with massive lymphadenopathy.

Roselli D Italian plastic surgeon *fl.* 20th cent.

Roselli–Gulienetti syndrome a form of ectrodactyly-ectodermal dysplasia-clefting syndrome.

Rosenbach AJF German surgeon 1842–1923.

Rosenbach's erysipeloid infection with *Erysipelothrix insidiosa*, the cause of swine erysipelas.

Rosenthal C German neuropsychiatrist 1892–1937. MELKERSSON-ROSENTHAL SYNDROME.

Rosenthal JW US ophthalmologist *fl.* 20th cent.

Rosenthal–Kloepfer syndrome acromegaloid-cutis verticis gyrata-corneal leukoma syndrome.

roseola a pinkish-red rash 'rose rash', as in roseola infantum, syphilitic roseola, etc. (New L from L *roseus* rosy).

Ross AT US neurologist *fl.* 20th cent.

Ross' syndrome tonic pupils, loss of reflexes, hypohidrosis and compensatory hyperhidrosis.

Ross River virus a togaviral infection, named after a river in N Queensland, Australia.

Rothman M German pathologist 1868–1915.

Rothman–Makai syndrome a form of circumscribed panniculitis.

Rothmund A von, Jr German ophthalmologist 1830–1906.

Rothmund–Thomson syndrome hyperpigmentation, telangiectasia and atrophy, with cataracts and other associated defects.

rotunda rounded (L *rotundus* round, circular).

Roussy G French pathologist 1874–1948. DARIER–ROUSSY SARCOID.

Rowell NR British dermatologist *fl.* 20th cent.

Rowell's syndrome lupus erythematosus with erythema multiforme-like lesions.

Royal malady porphyria variegata. Not to be confused with the 'King's Evil' (see SCROFULA) [14].

RPCFT *Reiter Protein Complement Fixation Test* for syphilis.

RPR *Rapid Plasma Reagin* test. A rapid card test for screening for syphilis.

-rrhagia comb. form meaning a violent flow or discharge (Gk *rhĕgnynai* root, *rhag-* to burst forth).

-rrhexis comb. form meaning breaking, rupture (Gk *rhĕxis*, noun from *rhĕgnynai* a bursting, breaking).

-rrhoea comb. form meaning flow, discharge (Gk *-rrhoia, from rheein* to flow).

rubella German measles (L fem. of *rubellus*, dim. of *ruber* red).

Rubinstein JH US paediatrician *fl.* 20th cent.

Rubinstein-Taybi syndrome broad thumb-hallux syndrome.

Rud E Danish physician 1892–1988.

Rud's syndrome SJÖGREN–LARSSEN SYNDROME with dwarfism, hypogonadism, mental retardation and anaemia.

Ruffini A Italian histologist 1874–1929.

Ruffini's endings, organ of branching nerve endings with expanded tips.

Ruiter M Dutch dermatologist 1900–74. GOUGEROT–RUITER SYNDROME.

Ruiz–Maldonado R Mexican paediatric dermatologist *fl.* 20th cent.

Ruiz–Maldonado syndrome phakomatosis pigmentovascularis; STURGE–WEBER SYNDROME with oculocutaneous melanosis.

rupioid resembling rupia, thick crusted sores (Gk irreg. from *rhypo*(s) filth, *ia*).

Russell A British paediatrician *fl.* 20th cent.

Russell–Silver syndrome growth retardation with somatic asymmetry.

Rutherfurd ME British Public Health physician *fl.* 20th cent.

Rutherfurd's syndrome familial gingival fibromatosis and corneal dystrophy.

rutilism having red hair (L *rutilus* red, yellow-red; as of Germano–Celts ('rutilae comae'); in fact, probably fair or auburn rather than red.

Ruvalcaba RHA Mexican-born US paediatrician and paediatric endocrinologist *fl.* 20th cent.

Ruvalcaba–Myhre–Smith syndrome pigmented genital macules, macrocephaly, intestinal polyps and lipid storage myopathy.

Ruvalcaba–Myhre–Sotos syndrome bony dysplasia and mental deficiency.

Sabouraud RJA French dermatologist 1864–1938. Made outstanding contributions in field of mycology. Elucidated *Trichophyton* sp. and was a leading authority on diseases of the scalp.

Sabouraud's medium (agar) a culture medium for fungi, containing peptone and dextrose.

sabra a species of cactus, *Opuntia ficus-indica.*

sabra dermatitis irritable eruption caused by contact with the glochidia of the Sabra cactus.

Sacks B US physician 1873–1939. LIBMAN–SACKS DISEASE.

SADBE *Squaric Acid DiButyl Ester.*

SADBE *Squaric Acid DiButyl Ester.*

Saethre H Norwegian neuropsychiatrist 1891–1945.

Saethre–Chotzen syndrome a variant of acrocephalosyndactyly Type III.

sairei-to Japanese herbal mixture forming part of Kampo medicine.

Sakati N Saudi Arabian paediatrician *fl.* 20th cent.

Sakati's syndrome form of acrocephalopolysyndactyly with congenital heart disease and skin abnormalities; acrocephalopolysyndactyly Type II.

Sakati–Nyhan syndrome acrocephalopolysyndactyly Type III.

Šalamon T Yugoslavian dermatologist 1914–95.

Šalamon's syndrome sparse brittle hair with anomalies of teeth, nails and eyes.

Salem sarcoidosis beryllium sarcoidal reaction, named after a town in Massachusetts, USA where fluorescent tubes were manufactured.

SALT *Skin-Associated Lymphoid Tissue.*

Samman PD British dermatologist 1914–92.

Samman's syndrome (synonym yellow nail syndrome) thick, curved, slow-growing yellowish nails associated with lymphoedema.

Sanarelli G Italian serologist 1864–1940.

Sanarelli–Shwartzman phenomenon see SHWARTZMAN PHENOMENON.

Sandmann H German paediatrician *fl.* 20th cent.

Sandmann–Åndrä syndrome type of ectodermal dysplasia with hypohidrosis and hypodontia.

Sanfilippo S US paediatrician *fl.* 20th cent.

Sanfilippo's syndrome mucopolysaccharidosis III.

San Joachin valley fever coccidiomycosis. Named after a river valley in California, USA.

SAPHO syndrome *Synovitis-Acne-Pustulosis-Hyperostosis-Osteomyelitis;* a seronegative spondylo-arthropathy.

sarcoidosis a multisystem disease of unknown cause characterized by noncaseating granulomas. First described by Besnier (q.v.) (1889). Many eponyms. (Gk *sarx* flesh, *oid* resembling.)

sarcoma a malignant tumour of mesenchymal origin (Gk *sarx, sarcos* flesh, *-oma*).

Sarcoptes a genus of mite (q.v.), the Sarcoptidae, ectoparasites of warm-blooded animals (Gk *sarx, sarkos* flesh, *koptein* to cut).

SC (phocomelia) syndrome hypomelia-hypotrichosis-facial haemangioma syndrome; pseudothalidomide syndrome. See HERMANN SYNDROME, ROBERTS' SYNDROME.

scabies infestation with *Sarcoptes scabiei.* Colloq. term for itch, mange, 'seven-year itch' (L *scabere* to scratch).

scale a flat plate or flake of stratum corneum [1] (of Teutonic origin; via OF *escale* shell, husk). Variously qualified as collarette, furfuraceous, ichthysiform or psoriasiform.

scalp hair-bearing skin and soft-tissue covering of the head (ME orig. Scandinavian, akin to Old Norse *skál-p,* sheath, Dutch *schelp* shell).

scar fibrous tissue replacing normal tissues destroyed by injury or disease [1] (OF *escare,* from LL *eschara* scab or *eschar* left after a burn or wound, from GK *eschara* hearth, fire [Hipp]).

Schäfer E German dermatologist b. 1897.

Schäfer's syndrome pachyonychia congenita with ophthalmic abnormalities.

Schamberg JF US dermatologist 1870–1934.

Schamberg's disease progressive pigmented purpuric dermatosis.

Schaumann J Swedish dermatologist 1879–1953. BESNIER–BOECK–SCHAUMANN DISEASE.

Schimmelpenning GW German neurologist *fl.* 20th cent. FEUERSTEIN–MIMS–SCHIMMELPENNING SYNDROME.

Schinzel A Swiss geneticist *fl.* 20th cent.

Schinzel–Giedion syndrome complex syndrome with anomalies of teeth and nails, hypertrichosis, telangiectases, simian creases and other features.

Schirmer O German ophthalmologist 1864–1916.

Schirmer's test a method of estimating reduction of lacrimal secretion.

schist- comb. form, meaning divided, split (Gk *schisis*, from *schizein* to cleave, divide).

Schistosoma a genus of trematodes, parasitic blood flukes (Gk *schisis* split, *sōma* body).

schizo- comb. form meaning split, divided (Gk *schizein* to divide).

Schnitzler L French dermatologist *fl.* 20th cent.

Schnitzler's syndrome chronic urticaria with monoclonal IgM paraproteinaemia.

Schönlein JL German physician 1793–1864. HENOCH–SCHÖNLEIN PURPURA.

Schöpf E German dermatologist *fl.* 20th cent.

Schöpf–Schulz–Passarge syndrome cystic eyelids, keratoderma, hypotrichosis, abnormal teeth and nails.

Schüller A Austrian neurologist and radiologist 1874–1958. HAND–SCHÜLLER–CHRISTIAN SYNDROME.

Schultz W German dermatologist 1878–1947.

Schultz–Charlton test (reaction) blanching of the erythema in scarlet fever on intradermal injection of a specific streptococcal antitoxin.

Schwachmann H US paediatrician *fl.* 20th cent.

Schwachmann's syndrome pancreatic insufficiency, growth retardation and bone marrow hypoplasia causing neutropenia.

Schwartz S US physician *fl.* 20th cent. WATSON–SCHWARTZ TEST.

Schweninger E German dermatologist 1850–1924. Personal physician to Bismark.

Schweninger–Buzzi anetoderma outmoded term for a form of macular atrophy.

scler(o)- comb. form meaning hard (Gk *sclēr(os)* hard).

sclerema (neonatorum) a rare disease of infants presenting as a rapidly spreading woody induration of the skin and subcutaneous tissues (New L from Gk *sclēr(os)*, *ma*).

scleroatrophic syndrome see HURIEZ' SYNDROME.

scleroderma a local or generalized hardening of the skin, usually referring to systemic sclerosis (New L from Gk *sclēr(os)*, *derma* skin).

scleroedema, scleredema induration of face, neck and upper trunk (Gk *sclēr(os)*, *oedema* [Hipp], from *oidein* to swell).

sclerosis localized or diffuse induration. A generic term, qualified as in systemic sclerosis (New L from Gk *sclēr(os)*, *osis*).

scorbutic relating to scurvy (New L *scorbuticus*, adjective of *scorbutus* scurvy; OF *scorbute* (1597) and Fr *scorbutique*).

scratch a linear incised superficial wound of the skin, as with the fingernails, thorn, etc.; the act of doing this (origin obscure; possibly from ME *scratte* or *cracchen*, via *scrat* to scratch).

scrofula primary tuberculosis of cervical glands, with or without ulceration of overlying skin (Med L from LL *scrofulae* swelling of neck glands, dim. of *scrofa* a breeding sow (connection obs.), OE *scrofeles*). The 'King's Evil', supposedly curable by the royal touch.

'scrotal shawl' a scrotal fold that envelops the base of the penis. A characteristic of the faciodigitogenital syndrome (Aarskog (q.v.)).

scrotum a fibromuscular sac containing the testes (L prob. variant of *scortum* skin, hide, or of *scrautum* leather bag for holding arrows).

scurf now used to designate pityriasis capitis; previously more generally for scaly or scabby skin (ME from Old Norse akin to OE *sceorf* flakes or scales of dead skin).

scurvy a deficiency disease resulting from lack of vitamin C (origin obscure, a folk word related to Middle Fr *scorbut*, from LL *scorbutus* or from OE *sceorf* scurfy; or perhaps from *sceorfan* to gnaw).

scutular(is) of lesions showing a plate- or saucer-shaped depression as in 'favus cap' (L *scutula*, dim. of *scruta* (*scuta*) a small plate or platter, rhomboid or lozenge-shaped).

seal finger, spaek finger an erysipeloid-like infection of the finger due to an unidentified organism from bites or handling of seals or other marine mammals (Norwegian *spaek*, *spekk* blubber).

Searle's ulcer local Australian term for *Mycobacterium ulcerans* (Buruli ulcer).

sebaceous of or relating to sebum, or glands secreting this (L *sebaceus*, from *sebum* suet, fat, tallow).

sebo-, sebi- comb. form indicating sebum.

seborrhoea abnormally copious secretion of sebum (L *sebum* fat, wax, Gk *rrhoia* stream, flux).

Seckel HPG Swiss paediatrician 1900–60.

Seckel's syndrome bird-headed dwarfism, mental retardation, skeletal defects, etc.

Secrétan H Swiss accident and insurance surgeon 1856–1916.

Secrétan's disease factitious oedema or lymphoedema of a limb by self-application of a tight band. Secrétan commented on the chronicity of the condition but did not invoke a factitious cause [15].

Seip MF Norwegian paediatrician *fl.* 20th cent. LAWRENCE–SEIP SYNDROME.

Seip–Lawrence syndrome see LAWRENCE–SEIP SYNDROME.

Senear FE US dermatologist 1889–1958.

Senear–Usher syndrome pemphigus erythematosus.

Sensenbrenner JA US geneticist *fl.* 20th cent.

Sensenbrenner's syndrome distinctive facies, thin hair, small grey teeth.

serpiginosum creeping, extending, especially in an arciform fashion (Med L *serpigo*, from L *serpere* to creep).

Setleis H US paediatrician *fl.* 20th cent.

Setleis' syndrome bitemporal scars with abnormal eyelashes.

Sézary A French dermatologist 1880–1956.

Sézary's syndrome pruritic erythroderma, lymphadenopathy and the presence in the peripheral blood of more than 10% of atypical mononuclear cells (Sézary cells).

Shabbir G Pakistani dermatologist *fl.* 20th cent.

Shabbir's syndrome laryngo-onycho-cutaneous syndrome.

shagreen with a rough surface, granular. Originally a type of rough granular leather made from horses' or asses' skin, or from shark, ray, etc. (Fr *chagrin*, Turkish *saghri* horse's rump).

shagreen patches collagenous naevi characteristic of tuberous sclerosis.

SHBG *Sex-Hormone-Binding Globulin.*

Sheehan HL British pathologist 1900–88.

Sheehan's syndrome hypopituitarism due to postpartum pituitary necrosis.

Shimpo S Japanese physician *fl*. 20th cent. Shimpo's syndrome (synonyms CROW−FUKASE SYNDROME, TAKATSUKI SYNDROME, PEP, POEMS.

shingles colloq. term for herpes zoster (ME *schingles*, Med L *cingulus* belt, girdle, from L *cingulum* belt, from *cingere to* gird about, equivalent to Gk *zōnē* belt).

Shprintzen RJ US craniofacial scientist *fl*. 20th cent.

Shprintzen's syndrome (synonym velocardiofacial (VCF) syndrome) cleft palate, cardiac abnormalities, typical facies and learning difficulties.

Shulman LE US rheumatologist *fl*. 20th cent.

Shulman's syndrome eosinophilic fasciitis.

Shwartzman G Russian-born US bacteriologist 1896–1965.

Shwartzman phenomenon the development of a haemorrhagic and necrotic lesion at the site of an intradermal injection of an endotoxin 18–36 h after intravenous injection of the same toxin.

sialosis, sialorrhoea ptyalism, excessive salivation (Gk *sialon* saliva, *osis* state of, *rrhoea* flowing).

sicca syndrome (L *sicca* dry, tearless) see SJÖGREN'S SYNDROME.

Siccardi AG Italian geneticist *fl*. 20th cent.

Siccardi's syndrome frequent infection, silver hair, slate-grey pigmentation, lymphadenopathy and hepatosplenomegaly.

Siemens HW German dermatologist 1891–1969, practising in Holland. BLOCH−SIEMENS SYNDROME; CHRIST−SIEMENS− TOURAINE SYNDROME; HALLOPEAU−SIEMENS SYNDROME.

Siemens' syndrome keratosis palmoplantaris areata/striata.

Simonart PJC Belgian obstetrician 1817–47.

Simonart's band, thread a band formed by stretching of adhesions between amnion and fetus.

Simons A German neurologist b. 1879. BARRAQUER−SIMONS DISEASE.

Sindbis fever alphavirus infection. Named after a small village in the Nile Delta.

Sipple JH US physician *fl*. 20th cent.

Sipple's syndrome multiple endocrine neoplasia (familial form Type II).

Siris E US paediatrician *fl*. 20th cent. COFFIN−SIRIS SYNDROME.

SIS *Skin Immune System.*

Sister Joseph superintendent at St Mary's Hospital, Rochester, USA, credited with recognition of umbilical nodule when surgical assistant to Dr WJ Mayo 1856–1939.

Sister Joseph's nodule umbilical metastasis from intra-abdominal neoplasm.

siti endemic syphilis, colloq. term in Botswana (Wolof *siti*).

sixth disease exanthema subitum; roseola infantum.

Siwe SA Swedish paediatrician 1897–1966. LETTERER−SIWE DISEASE.

Sjögren HSC Swedish ophthalmologist 1899–1986.

Sjögren's syndrome keratoconjunctivitis sicca and xerostoma often associated with rheumatoid arthritis, systemic lupus erythematosus or systemic sclerosis. When occurring without these associated diseases, known as SICCA SYNDROME.

Sjögren KGT Swedish psychiatrist and geneticist 1896–1974. MARINESCO−SJÖGREN SYNDROME.

Sjögren–Larssen syndrome a form of congenital ichthyosiform erythroderma with other defects.

skerljero (skorljero, skrljero) local term for endemic syphilis (bejel) from name of village near Rijeka, Slovenia.

Smith DW US paediatrician 1926–81. RUVALCABA−MYHRE− SMITH SYNDROME.

Smith J Ferguson Scottish dermatologist 1888–1978. Described multiple self-healing epitheliomata.

Smith WR US paediatrician *fl*. 20th cent. RILEY−SMITH SYNDROME.

Sneddon IB British dermatologist 1915–87.

Sneddon's syndrome livedo reticularis, cardiovascular lesions and negative antiphospholipid antibodies.

Sneddon–Wilkinson disease subcorneal pustular dermatosis.

sodoku rat-bite fever (Japanese *su* rat, *doku* poison).

solatics term suggested for delusional belief that lesions are due to sunlight.

solehorn a part of the nail formation arising from the proximal hyponychium (German *solen* to soil, become dirty, *horn* horn, keratin). From the muddy colour of the horny debris here.

Solente G French dermatologist *fl*. 20th cent. TOURAINE− SOLENTE−GOLÉ SYNDROME.

Sotos JF US paediatric endocrinologist *fl*. 20th cent. RUVALCABA− MYHRE−SOTOS SYNDROME; VASQUEZ−HURST−SOTOS SYNDROME.

Sotos' syndrome cerebral gigantism.

spaek finger see SEAL FINGER.

SPF *Sun Protection Factor.*

Spiegler E Austrian dermatologist 1860–1908.

Spiegler's tumour eccrine dermal cylindroma.

Spiegler–Fendt sarcoid lymphocytoma cutis.

spirochaete any member of the family Spirochaetaceae, which includes the pathogens *Treponema*, *Borrelia* and *Leptospira* (New L from L *spira*, Gk *speira* something wrapped round or twisted, *chaitē* long flowing hair or mane).

Spitz S US pathologist 1910–56.

Spitz naevus juvenile melanoma.

sporotrichosis a fungal infection of man and animals, caused by *Sporothrix schenckii* (Gk *sporos* sowing, *thrix*, *trichos* hair).

squame a scale or lamina (L *squama* scale, as of fish or serpent).

SSSS *Staphylococcal Scalded Skin Syndrome.*

St Anthony's fire ergotism. Named after a monk of the 3rd–4th cent.

steatocystoma sebaceous cyst (Gk *stear*, *steatos* hard fat, tallow; *kystos* cyst, *oma*).

steatorrhoea excess fat in the stools (Gk *stear*, *steatos* fat, *rrhoia* flow, flux).

Stein IF US gynaecologist 1887–1976.

Stein–Leventhal syndrome polycystic ovary syndrome. Obesity, amenorrhoea, hirsutism and infertility with polycystic ovaries.

Sternberg GM US bacteriologist 1838–1915. REED−STERNBERG CELLS.

Stevens AM US paediatrician 1884–1945.

Stevens–Johnson syndrome (synonym Fiessinger–Rendu syndrome) a severe form of erythema multiforme with mucosal involvement; ectodermosis erosiva pluriorificialis.

Stewart FW US pathologist b. 1894.

Stewart–Treves syndrome lymphangiosarcoma occurring on a lymphoedematous arm after radical mastectomy.

St Helena cellulitis a form of epidemic cellulitis from which no organisms could be isolated, named after the island of St Helena.

Sticker G German dermatologist 1860–1960.

Sticker's syndrome erythema infectiosum.

Still, Sir James British paediatrician 1868–1941.

Still's disease juvenile rheumatoid arthritis.

Strandberg JV Swedish ophthalmologist 1883–1942. GRÖNBLAD–STRANDBERG SYNDROME.

Strauss L US pathologist 1913–85. CHURG–STRAUSS GRANULOMATOSIS.

Streiff EB Italian-born Swiss ophthalmologist 1908–88. HALLERMANN–STREIFF SYNDROME.

strophulus an outmoded term previously used either for papular urticaria (strophulus infantum) or for miliaria (possibly New L from Gk *strophos* a twisting or turn, L *-ulus* dim; or corruption of Med L *scrophulus*, from *scrophulae* misapplied; in either case, the connection is obscure).

STS *Serological Tests for Syphilis.*

Sturge WA British physician 1850–1919.

Sturge–Weber syndrome unilateral facial port-wine naevus with ipsilateral encephalomeningeal angiomatosis. (Many other eponymous titles.)

Sudeck PHM (often misspelt) German surgeon 1866–1938.

Sudeck's atrophy post-traumatic osteoporosis and skin and muscle atrophy.

suffodiens (et abscedens) term applied to burrowing lesion of perifolliculitis capitis (L *suffodire* to tunnel, undermine).

Sulzberger MB US dermatologist 1895–1983. He was a leader of his profession and had 'an immense influence on N American dermatology'. BLOCH–SULZBERGER SYNDROME; SULZBERGER–CHASE PHENOMENON.

Sulzberger–Chase phenomenon induction of immunological nonresponsiveness to a specific antigen by prior oral or systemic administration of the same antigen.

Sulzberger–Garbe syndrome exudative discoid and lichenoid dermatitis.

Summitt RL US paediatrican and geneticist *fl.* 20th cent.

Summitt syndrome an autosomal recessive variant of APERT'S SYNDROME; acrocephalosyndactyly.

SUP *Selective UVB Phototherapy.*

SURT *Sarcoidosis of Upper Respiratory Tract.*

Sutton RL, Sr US dermatologist 1878–1952. Teacher, writer and ardent explorer.

Sutton's naevus (halo naevus) leucoderma acquisitum centrifugum.

Sutton RL, Jr US dermatologist 1908–90. Noted hunter, collector and palaeontologist. Translated Mercurialis' *De Morbis Cutaneis* 1572 from the Latin.

Sutton's ulcer periadenitis mucosa necrotica recurrens.

Sweet RD British dermatologist *fl.* 20th cent.

Sweet's syndrome acute febrile neutrophilic dermatosis.

Sybert VP US paediatrician *fl.* 20th cent.

Sybert-type keratoderma a variant of THOST–UNNA SYNDROME.

sycosis deep inflammation of hair follicles, especially of beard area (Gk *sycōsis* fig-like excrescence, from *sykon* fig, large wart).

Symmers D US pathologist 1879–1957. BRILL–SYMMERS DISEASE.

syndrome a set of symptoms occurring together or the sum of signs in a morbid process (Gk *syndrome* a concurrence).

synophrys profuse growth or midline fusion of eyebrows (Gk *syn* with, together, *ophrys* eyebrow).

syphilis infection with *Treponema pallidum* (after Syphilus, the shepherd in Frascatoro's Latin poem 'Syphilis sive Morbus Gallicus' (1530), portrayed as the first victim of the disease; perhaps from Gk *sys* hog, *philos* loving or from Sipylis, impious son of Niobe who was turned to stone by Apollo on the mountain of that name [16]).

syringocystadenoma tumour of ductal portion of sweat gland (Gk *syrinx* pipe, tube, *kystis* cyst, *adēn, adenos* gland [Hipp]).

syringoma benign tumour of eccrine sweat duct (Gk *syrinx, syringos* tube, pipe, *oma*).

tabes (dorsalis) a form of neurosyphilis; locomotor ataxia. Originally in more general sense of wasting (L *tabes* wasting away, dissolution).

Takatsuki K Japanese physician *fl.* 20th cent.

Takatsuki syndrome (synonyms CROW–FUKASE SYNDROME, PEP, POEMS, Shimpo's syndrome) plasma cell dyscrasia with poly-neuropathy and endocrine disorders.

Takayasu M Japanese surgeon 1860–1938.

Takayasu's arteritis (synonyms Martorell's syndrome, pulseless disease) an obliterative arteritis of unknown aetiology characterized by granulomatous lesions of medium-sized and large arteries.

tanapox a pox virus first seen around the Tana River in Kenya but probably more widely distributed in Tropical Africa.

Tangier disease HDL, *a*-lipoprotein deficiency. After an island in Chesapeake Bay, Virginia, USA.

TAR syndrome *Thrombocytopenia and Absent Radix.*

Tatlock organism a rickettsia (q.v.)-like organism isolated from a patient with Fort Bragg ('pretibial') fever and probably the organism responsible for the Fort Bragg epidemics of 1942–43.

tattoo design marked in skin by pricking in inks or dyes or by the accidental injection of foreign matter into the dermis (Tahitian *ta'tau*; Marquesian *ta'tu* tattoo).

taurodontism molar teeth with enhanced pulp at expense of root. Sometimes a feature of various epidermal dysplasias. A trait common in Neanderthal man (Gk *tauros* bull, *odous, odontos* tooth).

Tay CH Singaporean dermatologist *fl.* 20th cent.

Tay's syndrome atypical ichthyosiform erythroderma with deafness and keratitis.

Taybi H Iranian-born US paediatrician and radiologist *fl.* 20th cent. RUBINSTEIN–TAYBI SYNDROME.

TCR *T-Cell Receptor.*

TDO syndrome *Tricho-Dento-Osseous* syndrome.

TEE *TransEpithelial Elimination.*

telangiectasia, -ectasis condition of dilatation of small blood vessels of skin (New L from Gk *telos* end, *angeion* vessel, *ektasis* dilatation).

tele- pref. meaning far away, far off (Gk *tēle* far away).

tele-, telo- pref. meaning an end, fulfilment (Gk *telos, teleos* an end accomplished).

teleomorph establishment of a perfect state (of fungi) (Gk *telos, teleos* an end accomplished).

TEN *Toxic Epidermal Necrolysis.*

teratogen agent or factor capable of causing developmental abnormality in embryo or fetus (Gk *teras, teratos* monster, *gen* producing).

terebrans   piercing, boring, as in ulcus terebrans (L pres. part. *terebrare* to bore).

tetter   (obs.) term once applied to any of a number of skin diseases of branny, scaly, crusted or eczematous type (OE *teter*, akin to Sanskrit *dadru* skin disease).

thelarche   onset of breast development at puberty; beginning of womanhood (Gk *thēlē* suckling apparatus *archē* onset).

thèque   an aggregation or nest of cells, particularly of naevus cells at the epidermodermal junction (Fr *thèque*, from Gk *thēkē*, L *theca* sheath or small box).

therapy   treatment of disease (New L from Gk *therapeia* fostering, attending on sickness).

thesaurosis   (obs.) storage disease (Gk *thēsauros* a storing-up; treasure, treasury; hence, accumulation of substance by the body).

Thévenard A   French neurologist 1898–1950.

Thévenard's syndrome   hereditary sensory neuropathy; familial ulceromutilating acropathy.

Thibierge G   French dermatologist 1856–1926.

Thibierge–Weissenbach syndrome   calcinosis and telangiectasia with systemic sclerosis.

Thiers J   French neurologist b. 1885. ACHARD–THIERS SYNDROME.

Thomson MS   British dermatologist 1894–1969. ROTHMUND–THOMSON SYNDROME.

Thost A   German physician 1854–1937.

Thost–Unna syndrome   diffuse palmoplantar keratoderma.

thrips   (single) a minute winged insect, genus *Thysanoptera* (L and Gk *thrips* woodworm).

thrush   colloq. term for infection of the oral, pharyngeal and vaginal mucosae with *Candida albicans* (origin obscure; only known from 17th cent. but probably OE or of Scandinavian origin *torsk, trøske*).

tic de lèvres   factitious cheilitis (Fr *lèvres* lips).

tick   ectoparasite of superfamily Ixodoidea comprising hard ticks (Ixodidae) and soft ticks (Argasidae). (ME *tyke, teke*, akin to OE *ticca* a tick.)

tickle   to touch or stroke lightly; to irritate lightly or excite pleasurably, often exciting spasmodic laughter. (Origin uncertain. OE *tinchian, tikelle(n)*; or from *tick* to touch lightly; or transposed from *kittle* ME *kytellen?* echoic.)

Tietz W   US paediatrician *fl.* 20th cent.

Tietz' syndrome   total absence of pigmentation of skin and hair, deaf-mutism, hypoplasia of eyebrows.

Tietze A   German surgeon 1864–1927.

Tietze syndrome   chondritis (usually of the left) manubriosternal and sternoclavicular joints.

Tilbury Fox W   British dermatologist 1836–79. Described impetigo contagiosa.

tinea   a fungal infection of skin, hair or nails caused by one of the dermatophytes *Microsporum, Trichophyton* or *Epidermophyton*, except for its use in terms tinea amiantacea and tinea versicolor (L *tinea* gnawing worm, moth).

TNF   Tumour Necrosis Factor.

TOD   Tricho-Onycho-Dental dysplasia.

Tokelau ringworm   tinea imbricata, caused by *Trichophyton concentricum*. Named after a group of islands in central Pacific Ocean.

tonsurans   shearing, clipping, from appearance of hair in tinea capitis (pres. part. of Late L *tonsurare* to shear, clip, as of a monk's tonsure).

Torre DP   US dermatologist *fl.* 20th cent.

Torre–Muir syndrome   see MUIR–TORRE SYNDROME.

torus   as in torus palatinium, mandibularis, etc. A benign exostosis (L *torus* protuberance, boss, bulge).

Touraine A   French dermatologist 1883–1961. A leading figure in first half of 20th cent. CHRIST–SIEMENS–TOURAINE SYNDROME; COCKAYNE–TOURAINE SYNDROME; DEGOS–TOURAINE SYNDROME.

Touraine–Solente–Golé syndrome   pachydermoperiostosis.

Touton K   German dermatologist 1858–1934.

Touton giant cell   a form of giant cell with a central ring of nuclei typically seen in xanthomas and juvenile xanthogranuloma.

Townes PL   US geneticist *fl.* 20th cent.

Townes' syndrome   imperforate anus with hand, foot and ear anomalies.

TPI   Treponema Pallidum Immobilization test.

trachoma   infection of conjunctiva and cornea by *Chlamydia trachomatis* (Gk *trachōma* roughness).

trachyonychia   excessive ridging or confluent pitting of nails, giving a 'sandpaper' effect. Also loosely used for 20-nail dystrophy (Gk *trachys* rough, *onyx, onychos* nail).

transgrediens   crossing or passing over (L pres. part. of *transgredior* to pass or cross over).

Treacher Collins E   British ophthalmologist 1862–1932.

Treacher Collins–Franceschetti syndrome   (synonym Franceschetti–Klein syndrome) mandibulofacial dysostosis.

Trélat U   French surgeon 1828–90. LESER–TRÉLAT SIGN.

Trenaunay P   French physician b. 1875. KLIPPEL–TRENAUNAY–PARKES WEBER SYNDROME.

Trendelenburg F   German surgeon 1844–1924. BRODIE–TRENDELENBURG TEST.

Treponema   a genus of spirochaetes which includes *Treponema pallidum*, the cause of syphilis (Gk *trepein* to turn, *nēma* a thread).

Treves N   US surgeon 1894–1964. STEWART–TREVES SYNDROME.

TRIC   TRachoma Inclusion Conjunctivitis.

trich-, tricho-   comb. form denoting hair. Numerous combined forms (Gk *thrix, trichos* hair).

trichiasis   aberrant or abnormally directed eyelashes coming into contact with the cornea or conjunctiva (Gk *thrix, trichos* hair, *iasis*).

trichoptilosis   longitudinal splitting of distal hair shaft, which appears feathery (Gk *thrix, trichos* hair, *ptilōsis* plumage, from *ptilon* the downy underfeathers).

trichoschisis   clean transverse fracture of the hair shaft (Gk *thrix, trichos* hair, *schisis* cleavage).

trichotillomania   a compulsion to pluck or twist out hair (Gk *thrix, trichos* hair, *tillein* to pluck, *mania* compulsion).

tripe palms   rugose surface of palmar skin resembling lining of bovine paunch or reticulum (OF *tripe, trippe*, ultimate origin obscure).

trisomy 21   DOWN SYNDROME.

'trisymptome'   a morphological term describing three features of the 'maladie trisymptomatique' of Gougerot: purpura, polymorphic erythema and dermal nodules; a form of leucocytoclastic angiitis.

Tritsch H   German dermatologist *fl.* 20th cent. GREITHER–TRITSCH SYNDROME.

troph-, tropho-, -trophic comb. forms nutrition, nourishment (Gk *trophē* food, sustenance, from *trephein* to nourish).

-tropic suff. meaning a turning towards, affinity for (Gk *tropē*, *tropos* a turn, turning round). The term 'tropism' indicates a turning in a particular direction, bending.

TRPS I *Tricho-Rhino-Phalangeal Syndrome*, Type I, facial, brachyphalangial and hair abnormalities.

TRPS II (synonym LANGER–GIEDION SYNDROME) *Tricho-Rhino-Phalangeal Syndrome*, Type II.

tsetse a dipterous fly of *Glossina* sp. Transmits trypanosomiasis (Tswana, Bantu *tsêtsê* a native word).

tsutsugamushi trombicular mite (q.v.), vectors of scrub typhus or the disease itself (Japanese *tsutsuga* illness, *mushi* insect).

tularaemia a systemic infection due to *Franciscella tularensis* (from Tulare, a county in California, from Spanish *tule* bullrush).

tungiasis infestation with *Tunga penetrans*, a species of genus *Tunga*, class Hexapoda, the chigoe or jigger (Portuguese *tung(a)*, a flea genus).

Turcot J Canadian surgeon 1914–77.

Turcot's syndrome malignant tumours of the central nervous system with polyposis of the colon.

Turner G Grey British surgeon 1877–1951.

Turner's sign, Grey Turner sign ecchymosis in (usually left) flank appearing after onset of acute pancreatitis.

Turner HH US endocrinologist 1892–1970. ULLRICH–TURNER SYNDROME.

Turner's syndrome gonadal dysgenesis due to missing or defective X chromosome.

Turner JG British dental surgeon 1870–1955.

Turner's teeth hypoplastic teeth due to enamel defect following infection or injury to deciduous predecessors.

tylosis the formation of diffuse keratoderma; usually refers to diffuse palmoplantar keratoderma (Gk *tylōsis*, from *tyloun* to become or make callus, *osis*).

Tyson E British anatomist 1649–1708.

Tyson's glands preputial glands, free sebaceous glands of the prepuce.

ulcer a well-defined area of loss of skin and subcutaneous tissue involving the whole thickness of the skin and the underlying tissues, caused by infection, trauma or necrosis (L *ulcus*, from Gk *helkos* a wound: later, a sore, ulcer).

    anaesthetic neurotrophic.

    aphthous aphthae.

    Bazin's ulcerated nodular tuberculosis of calf.

    Buruli caused by *Mycobacterium ulcerans*.

    chiclero (chicle) caused by *Leishmania mexicana*.

    chrome corrosive effect of hexavalent chromium.

    decubitus pressure sore, 'bedsore'.

    eosinophilic form of benign ulcer of tongue.

    factitial form of dermatitis artefacta.

    herpetiform form of painful recurrent mouth ulcer.

    hyperalgesic micro- small painful ulcers of atrophie blanche.

    Jacob's ulcerated basal-cell carcinoma of eyelid.

    Jeddah cutaneous leishmaniasis.

    Lahore cutaneous leishmaniasis.

    Lipschütz ulcus acutum vulvae.

    Malabar tropical ulcer.

    Marjolin's scar epithelioma.

    Martorell's hypertensive ulcer of leg.

    Meleney's progressive infectious gangrene.

    Mikulicz minor aphthous ulcer.

    neurotrophic, neuropathic perforating ulcers in area of sensory nerve loss.

    perforating trophic ulcer of foot, mal perforans.

    phagedaenic rapidly spreading destructive ulcer.

    rodent basal-cell carcinoma.

    snail track mucosal erosion in secondary syphilis.

    soft chancroid.

    steroid unhealing ulcer due to potent topical steroids.

    Sutton's periadenitis mucosa necrotica recurrens.

    tanners CHROME ULCER.

    terebrans widely and deeply extending destructive form of RODENT ULCER.

    tropical chronic infective leg ulcer occurring in hot, humid climates.

    varicose misnomer for venous ulceration of leg.

ulerythema ophryogenes keratosis pilaris atrophicans involving the eyebrows (Gk *oulē* scar, *erythema* redness, *ophrys* eyebrow).

umbilicus navel (L *umbilicus* navel, centre, related to Gk *omphalos*).

Unna, Marie German dermatologist, wife of PG Unna's eldest son Karl, 1881–1977.

Unna, Marie Unna syndrome a form of hereditary hypotrichosis.

Unna PG German dermatologist 1850–1929. Outstanding figure in late 19th- and early 20th-century dermatology. Pioneer in cutaneous histopathology. Indefatigable writer. With Hebra (q.v.), dominated European dermatology of the era.

Unna's naevus 1 erythema nuchae; 'salmon patch'; **2** papillated pigmented naevus with melanocytes confined to papillary dermis.

UNTS *Unilateral Naevoid Telangiectasia Syndrome*.

urachus the urinary canal of the fetus (Gk *ourachos*, from *ouron* urine, *echein* to hold).

Urbach E Czech-born US dermatologist 1893–1946.

Urbach–Oppenheim disease necrobiosis lipoidica.

Urbach–Wiethe syndrome lipoid proteinosis.

urticaria an eruption of itching weals, of physical, systemic or (less commonly) contact origin; nettle-rash, hives (L *urtica* nettle, from *urere* to burn, *aria* condition of, characterized by).

urticata related to wealing (New L adj. from past part. of *urticare* to sting).

Usher BD Canadian dermatologist 1899–1978. SENEAR–USHER SYNDROME.

uveitis inflammation of uveal tract; iridocyclitis (Med L from *uva*, *uvae* grape, *itis*).

vagabond's disease a pejorative term for infestation with pediculosis corporis (Fr *vagabond*, from L *vagabundus* one who strolls around, from *vagare* to wander).

Valley fever coccidiomycosis.

van Creveld S Dutch paediatrician 1894–1971. ELLIS–VAN CREVELD SYNDROME.

van der Woude A US geneticist *fl.* 20th cent.

van der Woude syndrome cleft lip/palate with mucous cysts of lower lip.

Vaquez LH French physician 1860–1936. OSLER–VAQUEZ DISEASE.

variabil-is, -e variable, changeable (L *variabilis*, from *variare* to diversify, variegate).

varians diverse, changing (L pres. part. of *variare* to diversify, change).

varicella disease caused by varicella-zoster virus; chickenpox (Late L irreg. dim. of *variola* spotted).

variola smallpox (Med L dim. of *varius* spotted).

Vasquez SB US paediatrician *fl*. 20th cent.

Vasquez–Hurst–Sotos syndrome hypogonadism, gynaeomastia, mental retardation, short stature and obesity.

vegetans exuberant; vigorous (L pres. part. of *vegetare* to enliven).

vel alternative, or (L conjunction, imperative of *volo*, *velle* will, wish, choose whichever you wish).

veld (veldt) desert sore; Barcoo rot. Parochial term relating to S African pasture lands (Dutch *veld*, *veldt*, *velt* unenclosed country).

vellus the short downy hair that replaces lanugo before or soon after birth on all hair-bearing areas except the scalp (L *vellus* wool, down, fleece).

venenata poisoned, imbued with poison (L past part. *venenare* to poison).

venereal relating to or associated with sexual intercourse (L *venereus*, from *Venus*, *Veneris* goddess of love).

vermiculatus worm-eaten; resembling the tracks of worms (L *vermiculatus*).

vernix caseosa cheesy material on skin surface of near-term fetus and neonate (Med L *vernix* varnish, *caseosa* cheeselike).

verruca a wart, colloquially of the foot (L *verruca* steep place, height, of warts 'like the eminences of little hills' [Sennertus]).

verruga Peruana cutaneous bartonellosis (Spanish *verruga* wart, *Peruana* of Peru).

Vidal EJ-B French dermatologist 1825–93. Early worker in cutaneous pathology. Elucidated the group of lichen diseases.

Vidal's disease lichen simplex.

Vincent JH French bacteriologist 1862–1950.

Vincent's angina pseudomembranous or ulceromembranous angina. Acute fusospirochaetal infection of the tonsils. See VINCENT'S DISEASE, with which it may coexist.

Vincent's disease acute ulcerative gingivitis, necrotizing ulcerative gingivitis; ulceromembranous gingivitis. An acute infection of the gums, associated with *Borrelia vincenti* and *Bacillus fusiformis*.

Vinson PP US surgeon 1890–1959. PLUMMER–VINSON SYNDROME.

VIP *Vasoactive Intestinal Polypeptide*.

Virchow RLK German pathologist 1821–1902. Outstanding figure in 19th-century pathology. In 1847 founded *Virchows Archiv* and edited this for 55 years. His famous proposition 'omnis cellula e cellula' laid the foundations of modern scientific pathology. Physician, anthropologist, ethnologist, social reformer and politician. Was challenged to a duel by Bismarck, inspired Schliemann to excavate Troy and received the Copley Medal of the Royal Society.

Virchow's syndrome a form of bird-headed dwarfism without mental retardation. See SECKEL'S SYNDROME.

vitiligo a primary loss of pigmentation from skin and hair, of unknown cause (L *vitiligo* a skin disease, possibly from *vitium* flaw, blemish).

VLA *Very Late Antigens*.

Vogt A Swiss ophthalmologist 1879–1943.

Vogt–Koyanagi syndrome (synonym Harada's syndrome) uveomeningo-encephalitis, iridocyclitis, choroiditis, deafness followed by vitiligo, poliosis and alopecia. Seen in the Far East.

Vohwinkel KH German dermatologist 1900–49.

Vohwinkel's syndrome hereditary mutilating keratoderma.

Voigt CA Austrian anatomist 1809–90.

Voigt's lines FUTCHER'S LINES.

von Hippel E German ophthalmologist 1867–1939.

von Hippel–Lindau disease, syndrome retinocerebral angiomatosis, with hypernephroma, phaeochromocytoma, etc.

von Mikulicz see MIKULICZ.

von Pirquet CF Austrian paediatrician 1874–1929.

von Pirquet's (Pirquet's) reaction a local skin reaction at the site of the scarified application of Old Tuberculin.

von Recklinghausen FD German pathologist 1833–1910. Osteitis fibrosa cystica; haemochromatosis.

von Recklinghausen's disease neurofibromatosis.

von Rittershain G, Ritter see RITTER G VON RITTERSHAIN.

von Sallmann L Austrian-born US ophthalmologist 1892–1975. WITKOP–VON SALLMANN SYNDROME.

von Willebrand EA Finnish physician 1870–1949.

von Willebrand's disease a bleeding disease due to deficiency or abnormality of plasma coagulation factor VIII.

Vörner H German dermatologist 1869–1938.

Vörner's disease epidermolytic palmoplantar hyperkeratosis.

vulgaris common, ordinary (L *vulgaris* belonging to the masses, common, from *vulgus* the mass of the people as in 'odi profanum vulgus' (Horace); source obscure).

vulva strictly, womb or matrix but now applied to external female genitalia (L *vulva*, *volva* wrapping, seed covering).

Waardenburg PJ Dutch ophthalmologist 1886–1979.

Waardenburg's syndrome piebaldism, lateral displacement of medial canthi, hypertrophy of nasal root and other defects.

Wachters DHJ Dutch pathologist *fl*. 20th cent. Keratoderma palmoplantaris varians.

Waldenström JG Swedish physician 1906–96.

Waldenström's macroglobulinaemia macroglobulinaemia with monoclonal gammopathy.

Waldenström's syndrome idiopathic hyperglobulinaemic purpura.

Waldeyer HWG German anatomist 1836–1921.

Waldeyer's ring oropharyngeal ring of lymphoid tissue surrounding oropharynx; tonsillar ring.

Wallace HJ British dermatologist 1909–84. An outstanding clinician and man of great charisma.

Wallace's lines demarcation lines at the edge of the foot which mark the limit of extension of diseases affecting the legs from those affecting the feet.

wart (synonym verruca) a benign keratotic tumour. Colloquially used for any horny excrescence on the skin but properly so for lesions induced by the papovavirus and variously qualified (ME *werte*, from OE *wearte*, wart).

Waterhouse R British physician 1873–1958. Noted after-dinner speaker and palaeontologist.

Waterhouse–Friderichsen syndrome acute fulminating meningococcal septicaemia with acute adrenal insufficiency from haemorrhage into the adrenal glands.

Watson CJ US physician *fl*. 20th cent.

Watson–Schwartz test a test for urine porphyro- and urobilinogen, giving a red colour with Ehrlich's reagent. The two pigments can be separated by the addition of chloroform.

Watson GH British paediatrician *fl.* 20th cent.

Watson's syndrome pulmonary stenosis, café au lait macules and dull intelligence.

wattle a fleshy lobe or fold of skin pendent from the neck or throat of certain animals and birds. Colloq. term for cervical auricles (origin obscure, possibly from *wartle*, dim. of wart).

weal (misspelt as wheal (q.v.)) a transient circumscribed oedematous swelling as in urticaria or dermographism (modern variant of *wale*, OE *walu*).

Weary PE US dermatologist *fl.* 20th cent.

Weary's poikiloderma 1 hereditary sclerosing poikiloderma; **2** hereditary acrokeratotic poikiloderma (Weary–Kindler syndrome).

Weber, F Parkes British physician and dermatologist 1863–1962. Prodigious recorder of syndromes and rare diseases. Numerous eponymous diseases.

Weber–Christian disease relapsing febrile nonsuppurative panniculitis.

Weber–Cockayne syndrome simple epidermolysis bullosa of hands and feet.

Wegener F German pathologist 1907–90.

Wegener's granulomatosis granulomatous destruction of the respiratory tract, necrotizing arteritis and diffuse or focal glomerulitis.

Weibel ER Swiss anatomist *fl.* 20th cent.

Weibel–Palade bodies endothelium-specific inclusions usually occurring on the venous side of the microvasculature.

Weil A German physician 1848–1916.

Weil's disease haemorrhagic jaundice; icteric leptospirosis.

Weissenbach RJE French physician 1885–1963. THIBIERGE–WEISSENBACH SYNDROME.

Wells GC British dermatologist *fl.* 20th cent.

Wells' syndrome eosinophilic cellulitis.

Wells MV British-born Canadian physician *fl.* 20th cent. MUCKLE–WELLS SYNDROME.

Wells RS British dermatologist *fl.* 20th cent. HAY–WELLS SYNDROME.

wen (obs.) term previously used colloquially to describe any benign lump, particularly sebaceous or epidermoid cysts on the scalp (OE *wenn*).

Werlhof P G German physician 1699–1769. First physician to Court of Hanover.

Werlhof's disease idiopathic thrombocytopenic purpura.

Werner CWO German physician 1879–1936.

Werner's syndrome pangeria, with short stature, cataracts, scleroderma-like skin changes, vascular disease and diabetes mellitus.

Westerhof W Dutch dermatologist *fl.* 20th cent.

Westerhof's syndrome hereditary hypo- and hypermelanotic macules.

wheal common misspelling for weal (q.v.), except for rare use as verb or past part. (originally OE *hwele* a pimple or pustule) but properly used to describe lesions of bites of itch-MITE or harvest-bug (wheal worm).

Whipple GH US pathologist 1878–1976. Shared Nobel Prize 1934. Coined term 'thalassaemia'.

Whipple's disease intestinal lipodystrophy, a rare disease of uncertain aetiology with associated hyperpigmentation, leg nodules and cardiac changes.

Whitfield A British dermatologist 1868–1947.

Whitfield's ointment benzoic acid compound ointment.

whitlow acute paronychia or purulent infection (abscess) of distal finger pulp; felon. Also, specifically, herpetic or melanotic whitlow (ME *whitflawe*, but origin uncertain; possibly Dutch or Low German).

Wickham LF French dermatologist 1861–1913.

Wickham's striae characteristic pattern of white streaking seen on papules of lichen planus.

Wiedemann H-R German paediatrician b. 1915. BECKWITH–WIEDEMANN SYNDROME.

Wiedemann–Rautenstrauch syndrome neonatal progeroid syndrome.

Wiethe C Austrian otorhinolaryngologist 1888–1949. URBACH–WIETHE SYNDROME.

Wilkinson DS British dermatologist *fl.* 20th cent. SNEDDON–WILKINSON DISEASE.

Willan R British dermatologist and physician 1757–1812. Founder of British dermatology. His classification of skin diseases, with that of Alibert (q.v.), dominated European dermatology in first half of the 19th century. *On Cutaneous Diseases*, Vol. 1 (1796), continued by his pupil Bateman (q.v.). Also a general physician and antiquarian.

Willan's lepra psoriasis circinata

Willi H Swiss paediatrician 1900–71. PRADER–WILLI SYNDROME.

Williams see MURRAY WILLIAMS.

Wilson SA Kinnear British neurologist 1878–1937. Eloquent lecturer and left-handed golfer.

Wilson's disease hepatolenticular degeneration.

Wilson, Sir WJ Erasmus British dermatologist 1809–84. A notable 19th-century dermatologist. His enthusiastic views and beliefs on the value of publicizing dermatology were not approved by the Establishment of the day but he was often in advance of his time (*On Healthy Skin* 1845–76; and his support of the value of sea-bathing). A generous benefactor, he brought 'Cleopatra's needle' (and Turkish baths) to London and endowed permanent lectures at the Royal College of Surgeons.

Wilson's disease exfoliative dermatitis (erythroderma).

Winchester P US radiologist *fl.* 20th cent.

Winchester syndrome dwarfism, joint destruction and corneal opacities with hypertrichosis and hyperpigmentation.

Winer WH US dermatologist *fl.* 20th cent.

Winer's pore dilated follicular pore extending to subcutaneous fat.

Winterbottom TM British physician 1766–1859. Active in Sierra Leone.

Winterbottom's syndrome enlargement of posterior cervical lymph nodes in Gambian form of African trypanosomiasis.

Wiskott A German-born US paediatrician 1898–1978.

Wiskott–Aldrich syndrome thrombocytopenic purpura, eczema and recurrent infection.

Wissler H Swiss paediatrician 1906–83.

Wissler's syndrome, Wissler–Fanconi syndrome 'subsepsis allergica' ('hyperergica').

witkop Afrikaans term for favus.

Witkop CJ, Jr US oral surgeon and geneticist *fl.* 20th cent.

Witkop–von Sallmann syndrome hereditary benign intra-epithelial dyskeratosis.

Witkop–Brearley–Gentry syndrome hypoplastic enamel, onycholysis, hypohidrosis.

Wood RW US physicist 1868–1955. Published book of satirical poetry.

Wood's light a source of ultraviolet radiation from which most visible rays have been excluded by the use of a filter. This photo-emission causes fluorescence in certain skin conditions, especially some fungal infections, and porphyrins.

Woolf CM US zoologist *fl.* 20th cent.

Woolf–Dolowitz–Aldous syndrome (Woolf's syndrome) deaf mutism, piebaldism and heterochromia iridis.

Woringer F French dermatologist 1903–64.

Woringer–Kolopp disease pagetoid reticulosis; epidermotrophic lymphoblastoma.

wrinkle a furrow or skin crease, normally present as fine lines which becomes deeper and thicker with age and light exposure (origin obscure).

Wyburn–Mason R British neurologist 1911–83.

Wyburn–Mason syndrome cerebroretinal arteriovenous malformation with ipsilateral vascular or pigmented naevus.

xanth-, xantho- comb. form meaning yellow, usually applied in dermatology to lesions occurring as a result of disordered lipid metabolism (Gk *xanthos* yellow, golden).

xanthelasma symmetrical yellow plaques of eyelids due to lipid deposition (Gk *xanthos* yellow, *elasma* a beaten metal plate).

xero- comb. form meaning dry (Gk *xeros* dry).

xerotica dried out (New L adj. *xeroticus*, from Gk *xeros* dry).

XLI se*X*-Linked *I*chthyosis.

XTE *X*eroderma, *T*alipes, *E*namel defects.

yaws a nonvenereal infectious and contagious spirochaetal disease seen in tropical regions (Carib Indian *yaws*, akin to Caribbean of Lesser Antilles *yáya*).

yeast term used generically for any of a group of saprophytic unicellular fungi. Colloquially, used as term for infection by *Candida albicans* (OE *gist*, ME *yest*, akin to Gk *zestos*, past part. of *zeein* to boil, seethe).

Yersin AEJ Swiss bacteriologist 1863–1943. Discovered cause of plague.

Yersinia renamed genus of several members of *Pasteurella*; after YERSIN.

Zeis E German ophthalmologist 1807–68.

Zeis glands sebaceous glands opening into follicles of eyelashes.

Zellweger H Swiss paediatrician working later in USA *fl.* 20th cent.

Zellweger's syndrome neonatal adrenoleukodystrophy; infantile REFSUM'S SYNDROME; cerebrohepatorenal syndrome.

Zinsser F US-born German dermatologist 1865–1952. COLE-ENGMAN–ZINSSER SYNDROME.

Zinsser H US bacteriologist and immunologist 1878–1940. BRILL-ZINSSER DISEASE.

Ziprkowski L US dermatologist *fl.* 20th cent.

Ziprkowski–Margolis syndrome deaf-mutism with heterochromic irides and hypomelanosis.

Zollinger RM US surgeon *fl.* 20th cent.

Zollinger–Ellison syndrome hypersecretion of gastric hydrochloric acid and intractable peptic ulcer.

zona an area with specific boundaries or distinctive characteristics.

Zonana J US paediatrician and geneticist *fl.* 20th cent. BANNAYAN–ZONANA SYNDROME.

Zoon JJ Dutch dermatologist 1902–58. Plasma cell balanitis.

zoster a shortened term for herpes zoster, often preferred (Gk *zōstēr* belt).

Zumbusch L, Ritter von Austrian dermatologist working in Germany 1874–1940. Generalized form of pustular psoriasis.

Zurhelle E German dermatologist 1899–1965. HOFFMANN–ZURHELLE NAEVUS.

Acknowledgements

The author wishes first to acknowledge the debt he owes to Arthur Rook, the progenitor of this textbook, who had always intended that it should be of particular value to dermatologists who might not have ready access to reference libraries. In its small way, this glossary may help to sustain this ideal.

Invaluable assistance has been provided by many contributors and by other colleagues, here and abroad, who have gone to particular trouble to provide information. Further contributions from these sources will be welcome and will enhance any further editions of this chapter.

The author also wishes to acknowledge the debt he owes to many librarians and their research staff, whose diligent searches cast light on many obscure places. He is also grateful to Dr R. K. Winkelmann and to the International Committee of Dermatology for permission to make use of material in their invaluable *Glossary of Basic Dermatologic Lesions*.

He is particularly indebted to Colin Badcock, M.A. for his expert guidance and illuminating comments on classical derivations.

His thanks are due, finally, to Mrs Joan MacNab and to Mrs Eve Daintith for their unfailing patience and expertise in setting out and proof-reading the manuscript.

REFERENCES

1 (Main reference) Winkelmann RK, ed. *Glossary of Basic Dermatology Lesions*. Uppsala: International League of Dermatological Societies, Committee on Nomenclature and *Acta Derm Venereol* 1987; (Suppl. 130).

2 Goolamali SK, Andison AC. The origin and the use of the word 'acne'. *Br J Dermatol* 1977; **96**: 291–4.

3 Atherton DJ. Allergy and atopic eczema, I. *Clin Exp Dermatol* 1981; **6**: 191–203.

4 Jackson R. The lines of Blashko: a review and reconsideration. *Br J Dermatol* 1976; **95**: 349–60.

5 Brewin TB. Empirical: one word, two meanings. *J Roy Coll Phys Lond* 1994; **28**: 78–9.

6 Smith LA, Allen FV. Erythermalgia (erythromelalgia) of the extremities: a syndrome characterized by redness, heat and pain. *Am Heart J* 1938; **16**: 136–41.

7 Hunter D. *The Diseases of Occupations*. London: Hodder & Stoughton, 1978: 714–17.

8 Kahn J. *Job's Illness: Loss, Grief and Integration. A Psychological Interpretation*. Oxford: Pergamon, 1975: 8–12.

9 Verbov JL. Skin diseases in the Old Testament. *Practitioner* 1976; **216**: 229–36.

10 Mulliken JB. Capillary (port-wine) and other Telangiectatic stains. In Mulliken JB, Young AE, eds. *Vascular Birthmarks*. Philadelphia: Saunders, 1988: 170.

11 Tibbles JAR, Cohen MM. The Proteus syndrome: the Elephant Man diagnosed. *Br Med J* 1986; **293**: 683–5.

12 Glickman FS. Lepra, psora, psoriasis. *J Am Acad Dermatol* 1986; **14**: 863–6.

13 Happle R. Psychotropism as a cutaneous feature of the CHILD syndrome. *J Am Acad Dermatol* 1990; **23**: 763–6.

14 Macalpine I, Hunter R. *Porphyria: A Royal Malady*. London: British Medical Association, 1968.

15 Reading G. Secrétan's syndrome: hard oedema of dorsum of the hand. *Plast Reconstr Surg* 1980; **65**: 182–7.

16 Glickman FS. Syphilus. *J Am Acad Dermatol* 1985; **12**: 593–6.

BIBLIOGRAPHY

Main references are indicated by asterisks (*).

Baxter JH, Johnson C. *Medieval Latin Word-list*. Oxford: Oxford University Press, 1934.

Beerman H. *Contributors to Dermatology*. New York: Medical Lay Press, 1953.

Beighton P, Beighton G. *The Person behind the Syndrome*. Berlin: Springer-Verlag, 1997.

Bergsma D, ed. *Birth Defects Compendium*, 2nd edn. London: Macmillan, 1979.

Buyse ML, ed. *Birth Defects Encyclopedia*. Boston: Blackwell Scientific Publications, 1990.

Blakiston's Gould Medical Dictionary. New York: McGraw-Hill, 1979.

Butterworths Medical Dictionary, 2nd edn. (Critchley M, ed.) London: Butterworth, 1978.

Butterworth T. *Manual of Dermatologic Syndromes*, 2nd edn. Philadelphia: Lippincott, 1972.

Chambers Twentieth Century Dictionary (Macdonald AM, ed.) Edinburgh: Chambers, 1979.

Churchill's Illustrated Medical Dictionary. New York: Churchill Livingstone, 1989.

Dictionary of Word Origins (O'Kill B, ed.). Harlow: Longman, 1983.

Dorland's Illustrated Medical Dictionary, 27th edn. Philadelphia: Saunders, 1988.

Ellis H, Bailey HH, Bishop WJ. *Notable Names in Medicine and Surgery*, 4th edn. London: Lewis, 1983.

Firkin BG, Whitworth JA. *Dictionary of Medical Eponyms*, 2nd edn. New York: Parthenon, 1995/6.

Gold S. *A Biographical History of British Dermatology*. London: British Association of Dermatologists, 1995/6.

International Dictionary of Medicine and Biology. New York: Churchill Livingstone, 1986.

Jablonski S. *Illustrated Dictionary of Eponymic Syndromes and Diseases and their Synonyms*. Philadelphia: Saunders, 1979.

Larousse Dictionnaire Encyclopédique. Paris: Larousse, 1970.

*Leider M, Rosenblum M. *A Dictionary of Dermatological Words, Terms and Phrases*. West Haven, Conn.: Dome Laboratories, 1976.

*Lewis CT, Short C. *A Latin Dictionary*. Oxford: Clarendon Press, 1900.

*Liddell HG, Scott R. *Greek-English Lexicon*. Oxford: Clarendon Press, 1940.

Lin AM, Imaeda S. A dermatologic gazetter. *Int J Dermatol* 1990; **29**: 468–70.

Lourie JA. *Medical Eponyms: Who was Coudé?* London: Pitman, 1982.

Magalini SI, Scrascia E, eds. *Dictionary of Medical Syndromes*, 2nd edn. Philadelphia: Lippincott, 1981.

Manson's Tropical Diseases, 16th edn. (Manson-Bahr PH, Sir, ed.) London: Ballière Tindall, Cassell, 1965.

Norman JM, ed. *Morton's Medical Bibliography*, 5th edn. Aldershot: Scolar, 1991.

Oxford English Dictionary, compact edn. Oxford: Oxford University Press, 1979.

Partridge E. *Origins: A Short Etymological Dictionary of Modern English*, 4th edn. London: Routledge & Kegan Paul, 1966.

Radcliffe-Crocker H. *Diseases of the Skin*, 3rd edn. London: Lewis, 1903.

Rattner H. A consideration of dermatologic nomenclature. *Arch Dermatol* 1958; **77**: 1–7.

Rook A, Dawber R. *Diseases of the Hair and Scalp*. Oxford: Blackwell Scientific Publications, 1982.

Salmon MA, Lindenbaum RH. *Developmental Defects and Syndromes*. Aylesbury: HM & M, 1978.

Stedman's Medical Dictionary (Hensyl WR, ed.) Baltimore: Williams & Wilkins, 1989.

*Winkelmann RK, ed. *Glossary of Basic Dermatology Lesions*. Uppsala: International League of Dermatological Societies Committee on Nomenclature and *Acta Derm Venereol* 1987 (Suppl. 130).

Index

definition, 127, 667–8
due to rubbing, 130
genitocrural, 3168–9
giant, of Pautrier, 669
linear lesions, 128
see also lichen simplex
lichenoid drug eruptions, 1916–17, 3366, 3368, 3380, *3380*
lichenoid melanodermatitis, 1910
lichenoid tissue reaction, 197, 1814, 1899, 1916–19
lichens, *790, 796*
lidocaine, 840, 2774, 3601
lightning burns, 952
lightning pains, 2777
lignans, 3555
lignocaine, 840, 2774, 3601
Liliaceae, *790*
limewater, 3522, 3532
limonene, 828, 858
lincomycin, 3335, 3409
lincosamides, 3335
lindane, 844, 1441, 1462, 3505
linea alba, 453, 3269
linea nigra, 1780
linear focal elastosis, 2027
linear furrows, 2004–5
linear IgA disease, **1880–3**
 clinical features, *1851,* 1882
 differential diagnosis, 652
 drug-induced, 3390
 electron microscopy, 185
 immunology, *176, 177, 1853*
 immunostaining, *3084*
 ocular involvement, 3001
 oral involvement, 3086
 paraneoplastic, 2716
 and ulcerative colitis, 2722
linear lichenoid dermatosis, 128, 525, 529, **670**
linear subcutaneous bands, 2567
lingual erythema migrans, 1605, 3057, **3102–3,** 3557
lingual thyroid, 3067
lingual tonsils 3048, 3067
liniment, 3523
link proteins, *66, 68*
linoleic acid, 56, 692–3, 1944, 3321
linolenic acid, 692–3, 3321
Linuche unguiculata, 1476
lion fish, 1479
lip
 acquired lesions, 3129–47
 allergic contact dermatitis, 757
 anatomy, 3125
 angio-oedema, 3146
 burning sensation, 3146
 carcinoma, 3144–5
 chapping, 3131
 cleft, 3125–6
 congenital anomalies, 3125–30
 dermatoses, 3142–4
 double, 3127
 fibrous lumps, 3131
 fissure, 3143–4
 haemangioma, 3129
 haemorrhagic crusting, 3133
 hypopigmentation, 3146
 inflammation *see* cheilitis
 injuries, 3144
 leukokeratosis, 1341, 1676

leukoplakia, 3130
lichen planus, 3143
loss of sensation, 3146
lupus erythematosus, 3142
melanotic macules, 1721
mucous cyst, 3057, 3144
oedema, 2290
piercing, 3146
pits and sinuses, **603–4,** 3126–7
proliferative vascular lesions, 3131
racial variations in, 3125
in reactive perforating collagenosis, 3146
in sarcoidosis, 3142
senile haemangioma, 2092, 3021, *3022,* 3130
solar keratosis, 1341, 1676, **3137–8,** 3248
squamous cell carcinoma, 1692
surgery on, 3597
tattoos, 3146
telangiectasia, 3129, 3130
ulcers, 3146
vasculitis, 3146
venous lake, 3130
vermilion zone, 3125
lip-lick cheilitis, 698
lip salves, 3523
 contact cheilitis due to, 3131
lip shave, 3138, 3627
lip–tip syndrome, 3146
lipaemia retinalis, 2612
lipectomy, 3630
lipid disorders, 2600–15
lipid storage diseases, 2613–15, 2642
lipidosis, 2287
lipids
 in acne vulgaris, 1943, 1944
 epidermal, 55–6
 metabolism, 1485–6, 2602–4
lipoarabinomannan, 1184
lipoatrophy, 2064–5, 2407, 2426
 insulin, 2426, 2676–7
 localized, 2426–7
 semicircular, 433, 2427
 see also lipodystrophy
lipoblast, 2403
lipocortin, 3311–12, 3548
lipocyte, 2403–4
lipodermatosclerosis, 347, 2159, 2255, 2256, 2284, 2424
lipodystrophy, 2287, **2426–31**
 acquired generalized, 2429
 centrifugal, 2427
 congenital generalized, 2428
 insulin, 2426, 2676–7
 partial, **2429–30,** 2729
 partial face-sparing, 2431
lipoedema, 2287
lipoglycoproteinosis, **2640–1,** *2812,* 2986, *2987*
lipogranuloma
 sclerosing, 920, 2422, 2423, 2984, 3195
 scrotum, 3199
lipoid dermatoarthritis *see* multicentric reticulohistiocytosis
lipoid proteinosis, **2640–1,** *2812,* 2986, *2987*
lipoidal antigen tests, 1257–8
lipoma, **2431**
 benign, *367*
 congenital, 549–50
 frontalis-associated, 2432

in Gardner's syndrome, 389
 granular cell, 2432–3
 oral, 3115
 removal, 3625–6
 subcutaneous, 2778
lipomatosis, 2433–5
 congenital, 550
 encephalocraniocutaneous, 549
 multiple, *367*
lipomyelomeningocoele, 607
Liponyssoides sanguineus, 1470–1
lipophagic panniculitis, 2411
lipoprotein (a), 2603–4
lipoprotein lipase, 2602
 deficiency, 2612
lipoproteins
 high-density, 2603
 in hyperlipidaemias, 2600, *2601,* 2602
 intermediate density, 2602
 low-density, 2602–3
 metabolism, 2602–4
 very low-density, 2602–3
liposarcoma, *2348,* **2369**
liposomes, flattened, 115
liposuction, 3630
lipotechoic acid, 1101
β-lipotrophin, 1762
lipoxygenase, 3318, *3319*
lipstick
 contact cheilitis due to, 3131
 dermatitis, 757
liquid nitrogen, 3573, 3574
liquid paraffin, 3522
liquids as vehicles, 3522
Liriodendron tulipifera, 849
Lisch nodules, 378, *379,* 380, 1778, *1779,* 3007
lisinopril, 3442
Listeria monocytogenes, 491, 1131, 1137
listeriosis, 491, **1137**
Listrophoridae, 1457, 1466
lithium
 adverse effects, 3359, 3428–9
  acne, 1975
  alopecia, 2916
  erythroderma, 675
  keratoderma, 1587
  lichen stomatitis, 1917
  psoriasis, 1592
  teratogenicity, 520, 3358
  xerostomia, *3119*
lithium succinate, 643
livedo, 2736
 with nodules, *2207,* **2209–10**
 with ulceration, 659, 2210, **2248–50,** 2286
livedo annularis *see* livedo reticularis
livedo racemosa *see* livedo reticularis
livedo reticularis, **963–6,** 1777, 2212
 congenital, 452, **583–4,** 964, *965*
 definition, 963
 in DLE, 2452
 idiopathic with systemic involvement, 965–6
 physiological, 452, 584, 964, 2173–4
 persistent, 609
 secondary, 966
 in SLE, 2475
 with summer ulceration, 659, 2210, **2248–50,** 2286
livedo vasculitis *see* livedo with ulceration

trifluridine, 1066
trigeminal nerve lesions in leprosy, 1229
trigeminal neuralgia, *3123*
trigeminal trophic syndrome, 2775–6
triglycerides, 2404, 2602–3
triglycidyl isocynaurate, 852
triiodothyronine, 2705
trimeprazine, 705
trimethadione, 2916, 3358, 3435
trimethoprim, 3331–2, 3358, 3405, 3408
trimethylamine, 2001
trimethylpsoralen, 1621
trinitrotoluene, 838, 1793, 2965
triparanol, 1529, 2916, 2965, 3498
triphalangeal thumbs with
    onychodystrophy, 405
triphenylmethane dyes, 3531, 3534
tripotassium dicitratobismuthate, 3498
trisomy 13, 374, 399, 612, *2812*
trisomy 18, 374, 581, 2020, *2812*, 2893
trisomy 21 *see* Down's syndrome
tristimulus colorimetry, 725
trisymptome, 2179
    see also vasculitis, cutaneous
triton tumour, 2364
tromantadine, 840
Trombiculidae, 1457, 1470
trombidiosis, 1470
tropical phagedena, **1157–8**, 2267
tropical spastic paraparesis, 1055
tropisetron, 3428
tropoelastin, 2060
Trousseau's sign, 2716
true fats and oils, 3522
TRUE test, 804
trunk
    allergic contact dermatitis, 758
    folliculitis, 1123
    seborrhoeic dermatitis, 640–1
    skin biopsy, 188
Trypanosoma, 1378, 1404, 1406–7, 1409
trypanosomiasis, 1406–7
    African, **1407–8**
    American (South American), **1408–10**,
        1446, 2984
trypanosomiasis cruzi, **1408–10**, 1446, 2984
tryptase
    in mast cells, 239–40, 2337
    in mastocytosis, 2340
    in urticaria, 2115
tryptophan, 2054, 2102, *2103*, 2659, 3292,
    3393
TSC *see* tuberous sclerosis complex
tsetse flies, 1407, 1429
TSLS, 1130–1
TSP, 1055
TSST-1, 1104
tsutsugamushi disease, 1170–1, 1470
TTP, 2145, 3117
Tubegauze, 3298
tubercle, 1188–9
    naked, 2681
tubercles of Montgomery, 3149
tuberculide, 637, 2104, 2108
    aetiology, 1199
    definition, 1199
    lichenoid, 1201
    nodular, 1201–2
    papular, 1199–201
    papulonecrotic, 1199–200, 2180, 3193
tuberculin, 859

tuberculin test, 136, 1185–6
tuberculoid infiltrate, 1189
tuberculosis, **1187–206**
    agalactosyl IgG in, 1185
    BCG vaccination, 1205–6
    congenital, 491, 1198
    cutaneous, 1189–99
    diagnosis, 1202–3
    differential diagnosis, *2683*
    ear involvement, 3028
    epidemiology, 1182–3
    and erythema nodosum, 1191, 2197
    following tattooing, 1814
    genitocrural involvement, 3167, 3186,
        3193, 3210, 3222
    heat-shock proteins in, 1185
    histopathology, 1188–9
    history, 1181, 1182
    and HIV infection, 1076, 1182, 1184–5,
        1187, 1204
    immunology, 1183–5
    immunopathology, 1184
    in immunosuppressive therapy, 2752
    leg ulcers in, 2266–7
    miliary, 1188, 1194
    multidrug resistant, 1204
    natural history, 1187–8
    oral involvement, 3092, *3122*
    orificial, 1188, 1193–4, 3193
    penile involvement, 3188
    perianal involvement, 3174
    polymerase chain reaction in diagnosis,
        1203
    preceding vasculitis, 2169
    primary, 1188
    prognosis, 1202
    pulmonary, 2734
    secondary, 1188
    tests, 1185–6
    treatment, 1203–4, 3336–8
    warty, 1188, *1189*, 1191–2, 1204
tuberculosis cutis orificialis, 1188, 1193–4,
    3193
tuberculosis verrucosa cutis, 1188, *1189*,
    1191–2, 1204
tuberculous chancre, 1188, 1190–1
tuberin, 385
tuberous sclerosis complex (TSC), **384–8**,
    2710, 2739
    in adolescence, 3265
    genetics, *365*, *367*
    hypomelanotic macules, 1800–1
    investigation, 132
    ocular involvement, 3008
    oral lesions, 3068, *3122*
    poliosis in, 2964
    premature puberty in, 3266
    renal involvement, 2729
d-tubocurarine, 3359
tubulin, 51
tuftsin deficiency, 513, 2748
tularaemia, **1150**
tulipalins, 736, 756
tuliposides, 736
tulips, 789, *790*, 846
Tumbu fly, 1430
tumoral calcinosis, 2665
tumour angiogenic factor, 1652
tumour necrosis factor, 3490
    in inflammation, 268
    receptors, 268

TNF-α, 268
    in delayed hypersensitivity, 330
    effect on keratinocytes, 49
    in granulomas, 248
    in irritant contact dermatitis, 720
    keratinocyte-derived, 296
    synthesis by mast cells, 2338
TNF-β, 268
    in tuberculosis, 1184, 1185
tumour-suppressor genes, 219–20, 1654–5
tumours
    amputation stump, 906, 2364
    apocrine gland, 1703–5
    definition, 127
    eccrine gland, 1705–12
    in the elderly, 3286
    epidermal, **1651–93**
        and apoptosis, 1656
        benign, 1651
        history, 1651–2
        malignant, 1651, 1677–94
        mechanisms of carcinogenesis, 1652–5
        premalignant, 1670–7
    external ear, 3039–44
    follicular infundibulum, 1697
    hair follicle, 1378–83
    lips, 3144–5
    lymphatic system, 2295–6
    metastatic malignant, 179, **2371–2**
    muscle, 2366–9
    nail apparatus and adjacent structures,
        2844–53
    ovarian, 2898
    and pregnancy, 3271–2
    radiation-induced, 3570–1
    sebaceous gland, 1701–3
    shave biopsy, 3604–5
    in situ, 1651
    skin appendages, **1695–715**
    trichogenic adnexal, 1700–1
    umbilical, 3165
    in xeroderma pigmentosum, 409
    see also malignant disease
tungiasis, 1435
Tungidae, 1433, 1435
Tupaia, 29
Tupaioidea, 29
turban tumour, *367*, 1708, **1713–14**
Turcot syndrome, 389
turf cancer, 938
turf toe, 908
Turner's syndrome, **375–6**
    angiokeratoma corporis diffusum in,
        2640
    differential diagnosis, 2037
    ears in, 3016
    lymphoedema in, 2283
Turolopsis glabrata, 3212
turpentine, 822, 850, 858
twenty-nail dystrophy, 1908, 2828, 2843–4
twin spotting, 362
twin studies in psoriasis, 1591
twistometry, 121
two-hit hypothesis, 219, *220*
tylosis, 1566, 2710, 3061, *3120*
tympanic membrane, 3013
tympanic sulcus, 3014
typhoid, 1143
typhus
    epidemic, 1168–9
    murins/endemic, 1169